CLINICAL DISORDERS OF FLUID AND ELECTROLYTE METABOLISM

THIRD EDITION

Edited by

MORTON H. MAXWELL, M.D.

Department of Medicine
Cedars-Sinai Medical Center, Los Angeles

Department of Medicine
Center for Health Sciences
University of California, Los Angeles

CHARLES R. KLEEMAN, M.D.

Department of Medicine
Center for Health Sciences
University of California, Los Angeles

McGRAW-HILL BOOK COMPANY
New York St. Louis San Francisco Auckland Bogotá Düsseldorf
Johannesburg London Madrid Mexico Montreal New Delhi
Panama Paris São Paulo Singapore Sydney Tokyo Toronto

CLINICAL DISORDERS OF FLUID
AND ELECTROLYTE METABOLISM

Copyright © 1980, 1972, 1962 by McGraw-Hill, Inc. All rights reserved.
Printed in the United States of America. No part of this publication may be
reproduced, stored in a retrieval system, or transmitted, in any form or by any
means, electronic, mechanical, photocopying, recording, or otherwise, without
the prior written permission of the publisher.

1 2 3 4 5 6 7 8 9 0 H D H D 7 8 3 2 1 0 9

This book was set in Plantin by Precision Typographers Inc. The editors were
J. Dereck Jeffers and Henry C. De Leo; the designer was Hermann Strohbach;
the production supervisor was Milton J. Heiberg. New drawings were done by
Allyn-Mason, Inc.
Halliday Lithograph Corporation was printer and binder.

Library of Congress Cataloging in Publication Data

Maxwell, Morton H   ed.
    Clinical disorders of fluid and electrolyte
metabolism.

        Includes bibliographies and index.
        1.   Body fluid disorders.   2.   Water-electrolyte
imbalances.   I.   Kleeman, Charles R., joint author.
II.   Title.
RC630.M39 1979   616.3'99   78-31989
ISBN 0-07-040994-3

£46.80

CLINICAL DISORDERS
OF FLUID AND
ELECTROLYTE
METABOLISM

Editing a book is a long and arduous task,
most often performed at night and during weekends.
This task was greatly facilitated by our patient and sympathetic wives.
It is, therefore, reasonable and pleasurable
to dedicate this book to our wives.
We also wish to dedicate it to all of our contributors;
for this is really their book.

Contents

List of Contributors

ALLEN I. ARIEFF, M.D.
Chief, Nephrology Service
Fort Miley VA Medical Center;
Associate Professor of Medicine
University of California, San Francisco
San Francisco, California

WILLIAM H. BLAHD, M.D.
Chief, Nuclear Medicine Service
VA Wadsworth Medical Center;
Professor of Medicine
University of California, Los Angeles
Los Angeles, California

MICHAEL J. BLUMENKRANTZ, M.D.
Coordinator, VA Cooperative Dialysis Study
VA Wadsworth Medical Center;
Assistant Professor of Medicine
School of Medicine
University of California, Los Angeles
Los Angeles, California

NEAL S. BRICKER, M.D.
Professor of Medicine
Director, Institute of Kidney Diseases
School of Medicine
University of California, Los Angeles
Los Angeles, California

JACK W. COBURN, M.D.
Chief, Nephrology Section
VA Wadsworth Medical Center;
Professor of Medicine
School of Medicine
University of California, Los Angeles
Los Angeles, California

JORDAN J. COHEN, M.D.
Professor of Medicine
Tufts University School of Medicine;
Chief, Nephrology Division
New England Medical Center Hospital
Boston, Massachusetts

ROBERT G. DLUHY, M.D.
Associate Professor of Medicine
Harvard Medical School;
Senior in Medicine
Associate Director
Endocrinology-Hypertension Unit
and Clinical Research Center
Peter Bent Brigham Hospital
Boston, Massachusetts

ERNST J. DRENICK, M.D.
Professor of Medicine
School of Medicine
University of California, Los Angeles;
Chief, General Medicine Section
VA Wadsworth Medical Center
Los Angeles, California

FRANKLIN H. EPSTEIN, M.D.
Professor of Medicine
Harvard Medical School
Physician-in-Chief
Beth Israel Hospital
Boston, Massachusetts

THOMAS F. FERRIS, M.D.
Professor and Chairman
Department of Medicine
University of Minnesota, Twin Cities
Minneapolis, Minnesota

LAURENCE FINBERG, M.D.
Professor and Chairman
Department of Pediatrics
Montefiore Hospital and Medical Center of Albert
 Einstein College of Medicine
Bronx, New York

LEON G. FINE, M.D.
Associate Professor of Medicine
Chief, Division of Nephrology
School of Medicine
University of California, Los Angeles
Los Angeles, California

STANLEY S. FRANKLIN, M.D.
Clinical Professor of Medicine
School of Medicine
University of California, Los Angeles;
Chief of Nephrology
Cedars-Sinai Medical Center
Los Angeles, California

ARTHUR GORDON, M.D.
Director, Nephrology Service
Cedars-Sinai Medical Center, Los Angeles;
Associate Clinical Professor of Medicine
School of Medicine
University of California, Los Angeles
Los Angeles, California

RICHARD M. HAYS, M.D.
Professor of Medicine
Director, Division of Nephrology
Albert Einstein College of Medicine
Bronx, New York

JAMES T. HIGGINS, JR., M.D.
Professor of Medicine
Chief, Division of Nephrology
Department of Medicine
Medical College of Ohio
Toledo, Ohio

GEORGE J. KALOYANIDES, M.D.
Professor of Medicine and Hypertension
Head, Division of Nephrology and Hypertension
Department of Medicine
Health Sciences Center
State University of New York
Stony Brook, New York

JEROME P. KASSIRER, M.D.
Professor and Associate Chairman
Department of Medicine
Associate Physician-in-Chief
Tufts University School of Medicine
New England Medical Center Hospital
Boston, Massachusetts

CHARLES R. KLEEMAN, M.D.
Professor of Medicine
Emeritus Chief, Division of Nephrology
School of Medicine
Director, Center for Health Enhancement Education
 and Research
University of California, Los Angeles
Los Angeles, California

KAREN KLEEMAN, M.D.
Resident in Medicine
Beth Israel Hospital and Harvard School of Medicine
Boston, Massachusetts

M. KLEEREKOPER, M.D.
Clinical Assistant Professor of Medicine
University of Michigan Medical School;
Deputy Director, Bone and Mineral Research
 Laboratory
Fifth Medical Division
Henry Ford Hospital
Detroit, Michigan

JAMES P. KNOCHEL, M.D.
Professor of Internal Medicine
University of Texas
Southwestern Medical School
Dallas, Texas;
Associate Chief of Staff for Research
Chief, Renal Section
VA Medical Center
Dallas, Texas

JOEL D. KOPPLE, M.D.
Professor of Medicine
School of Medicine
University of California, Los Angeles;
Medical Investigator
VA Wadsworth Medical Center
Los Angeles, California

KIYOSHI KUROKAWA, M.D.
Assistant Chief, Nephrology Section
VA Wadsworth Medical Center;
Associate Professor of Medicine
School of Medicine
University of California, Los Angeles
Los Angeles, California

FRANCISCO LLACH, M.D., F.A.C.P.
Chief, Nephrology Section
Associate Professor of Medicine
University of Oklahoma
College of Medicine
VA Medical Center
Oklahoma City, Oklahoma

AMNON LICHT, M.D.
Assistant Professor of Medicine
Program in Kidney Diseases
School of Medicine
University of California, Los Angeles
Los Angeles, California

W. C. MACKAY, Ph.D.
Associate Professor
Department of Zoology
University of Alberta
Edmonton, Alberta
Canada

MORTON H. MAXWELL, M.D.
Director, Hypertensive Division
Department of Medicine
Cedars-Sinai Medical Center
Los Angeles, California;
Clinical Professor of Medicine
School of Medicine
University of California, Los Angeles
Los Angeles, California

R. CURTIS MORRIS, JR., M.D.
Professor of Medicine and Pediatrics
General Clinical Research Center
University of California, San Francisco
San Francisco, California

PATRICK J. MULROW, M.D.
Professor and Chairman
Department of Medicine
Medical College of Ohio
Toledo, Ohio

ROBERT G. NARINS, M.D.
Associate Professor of Medicine
Director of Clinical Services, Nephrology
Peter Bent Brigham Hospital
Boston, Massachusetts

ALLEN R. NISSENSON, M.D.
Assistant Professor of Medicine
School of Medicine
University of California, Los Angeles;
Director, Dialysis Program
Center for the Health Sciences
University of California, Los Angeles
Los Angeles, California

A. MICHAEL PARFITT, M.B. Chir.
Clinical Associate Professor of Medicine
University of Michigan Medical School;
Director, Bone and Mineral Research Laboratory
Fifth Medical Division
Henry Ford Hospital
Detroit, Michigan

SIDNEY F. PHILLIPS, M.D.
Professor of Medicine
Mayo Medical School
Consultant in Gastroenterology
Mayo Clinic
Rochester, Minnesota

H. JOHN REINECK, M.D.
Assistant Professor of Medicine
The University of Texas
Health Science Center at San Antonio
San Antonio, Texas

TELFER B. REYNOLDS, M.D.
Professor of Medicine
University of Southern California
School of Medicine
Los Angeles, California

R. WILLIAM SCHMIDT, M.D.
Chief, Hemodialysis Unit
Fort Miley VA Medical Center;
Assistant Professor of Medicine
University of California, San Francisco
San Francisco, California

BODIL M. SCHMIDT-NIELSEN, M.D.
Research Scientist
Mt. Desert Island Biological Laboratory
Salsbury Cove, Maine

RAYMOND G. SCHULTZE, M.D.
Professor and Executive Vice Chairman
Department of Medicine
School of Medicine
University of California, Los Angeles
Los Angeles, California

ANTHONY SEBASTIAN, M.D.
Associate Professor of Medicine
General Clinical Research Center
University of California, San Francisco
San Francisco, California

BRAMAH N. SINGH, M.D. (New Zealand) Ph.D. (Oxford) M.R.C.P. (London)
Director of Inpatient Cardiology
Cedars-Sinai Medical Center, Los Angeles;
Associate Professor of Medicine
School of Medicine
University of California, Los Angeles
Los Angeles, California

JAY H. STEIN, M.D.
Chairman and Professor
Department of Medicine
Director, Division of Renal Diseases
The University of Texas
Health Science Center at San Antonio
San Antonio, Texas

RICHARD WEITZMAN, M.D.
Assistant Professor of Medicine
School of Medicine
University of California, Los Angeles;
Head, Hypertension Section
Division of Nephrology and Hypertension
Harbor General Hospital
Torrance, California

GORDON H. WILLIAMS, M.D.
Associate Professor of Medicine
Harvard Medical School;
Physician, Director, Endocrinology-Hypertension Unit
and Clinical Research Center
Peter Bent Brigham Hospital
Boston, Massachusetts

Preface

The widespread acceptance of *Clinical Disorders of Fluid and Electrolyte Metabolism* as the standard and most authoritative textbook in the field has been gratifying.

When the first edition was published in 1962, nephrology was not yet a recognized subspecialty, and research in fluid and electrolyte metabolism was limited to a relatively small group of investigators, most of whom had backgrounds in physiology or biochemistry. Over the ensuing years it became apparent that aberrations of mineral and acid-base homeostasis are critically important in clinical situations as diverse as cardiac surgery and diarrhea. In fact, since the composition of the extracellular fluid—the *milieu intérieur* of Claude Bernard—vitally influences the function of every organ in the body, a basic understanding of fluid and electrolyte metabolism is required for all medical subspecialties. This widespread applicability is reflected in the massive proliferation of published articles in this field.

The primary reason for this new edition is to update the book, i.e., to keep up with recent advances. A secondary reason is to continually try to improve and clarify the presentation. We hope we have achieved both of these goals.

Clinical Disorders of Fluid and Electrolyte Metabolism, third edition, presents a comprehensive review of all aspects of fluid and electrolyte metabolism, both basic and clinical. The book should prove useful at every level of medicine, from the medical student to the academic and practicing specialist. In every area the editors have attempted to present, first, the basic underlying physiological and biochemical mechanisms and then, in the same or separate accompanying chapters, detailed discussions of various disease entities and clinical syndromes, emphasizing the rational application of the underlying pathophysiology in diagnosis and treatment. This format permits a student of this subject to find in-depth discussions of underlying physiology, while the clinician faced with an immediate problem can easily find the necessary practical solution, frequently in diagrammatic or tabular form. Extensive references provide documentation of the material within each chapter and serve as a guide for further study.

Obviously, complete uniformity of style and concept cannot be achieved with multiple contributors. However, to our knowledge there are no major contradictions, and the overlapping and repetition which do occur were intended to emphasize certain important principles or clinical entities.

ACKNOWLEDGMENTS

Allen I. Arieff and R. William Schmidt, the authors of Chapter 26, gratefully acknowledge editorial work by Ms. J. Witte, artwork by Bob Surface (Medical Research Graphics, San Francisco) and secretarial work by Ms. M. Marcy and Ms. D. Michel. The work was supported by contract #AM-5-2204 and grant #AM-18350, both from the

NIAMDD of the National Institutes of Health, and by Veterans Administration Research Funds MR1S-0508.

A. M. Parfitt and M. Kleerekoper, the authors of Chapter 8, wish to thank the staff of the Department of Medical Art and Photography, Henry Ford Hospital, for preparing the figures, and Ms. Jessie Miller and Cath Messana for typing the manuscript.

R. Curtis Morris, Jr., and Anthony Sebastian, the authors of Chapter 18, wish to thank Ms. Kathleen Imberg for her expert typing and sustained high spirit. We are greatly indebted to Ms. Jane Wiley and the nursing staff of the General Clinical Research Center.

Morton H. Maxwell
Charles R. Kleeman

CLINICAL DISORDERS OF FLUID AND ELECTROLYTE METABOLISM

1

Dynamics of body water and electrolytes

RICHARD M. HAYS

THE PROPERTIES OF WATER IN LIVING SYSTEMS

In 1913, L. J. Henderson wrote, in his monograph *The Fitness of the Environment*, that life as we know it would not be conceivable without the unique properties of water:

The physiologist has found that water is invariably the principal constituent of active living organisms. Water is ingested in greater amounts than all other substances combined, and it is no less the chief excretion. It is the vehicle of the principal foods and excretory products, for most of these are dissolved as they enter or leave the body. Indeed, as clearer ideas of the physico-chemical organization of protoplasm have developed it has become evident that the organism itself is essentially an aqueous solution in which are spread out colloidal substances of vast complexity. As a result of these conditions there is hardly a physiological process in which water is not of fundamental importance.

The following properties appear to be extraordinarily, often uniquely, suited to a mechanism which must be complex, durable, and dependent on a constant metabolism: heat capacity, heat conductivity, expansion on cooling near the freezing point, density of ice, heat of fusion, heat of vaporization, vapor tension, freezing point, solvent power, dielectric constant and ionizing power, and surface tension (1).

Henderson's observation was based on the known physical properties of water; it was not until 1933, when Bernal and Fowler published their pioneer theory of water and ionic solutions (2), that the biologic role of water could be understood in terms of its structure. Years of intensive work since then have served only to confirm Henderson's conclusion.

THE WATER MOLECULE

The unique properties of liquid water are based largely on the structure of the water molecule (Fig. 1-1). The molecule is V-shaped, with the

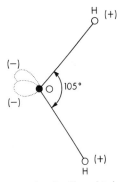

Figure 1-1. The water molecule. The orbitals of the "lone pair" of electrons are indicated at the oxygen atom, and the weakly positive charges at the hydrogen atoms. Hydrogen bonding to neighboring water molecules is thereby made possible.

oxygen at the apex of the V. The angle between the hydrogen-oxygen bonds is 105°, close to the tetrahedral angle (109°28′). The distribution of electrons in the water molecule is such that the hydrogen atoms are slightly positively charged and the oxygen negatively charged, with two "lone pairs" of electrons oriented approximately tetrahedrally, as shown in the figure.

This distribution of charge gives the water molecule two important properties: First, it has a relatively high dipole moment, so that it is readily oriented in an electric field; second, by virtue of electrostatic attraction between negative and positive sites in neighboring molecules (hydrogen bonding), water can achieve an extensive lattice-like structure even in its liquid state. While this structure is not as complete and rigid as ice (Fig. 1-2), liquid water does retain, over short ranges and for short periods, the tetrahedrally coordinated structure of ice.

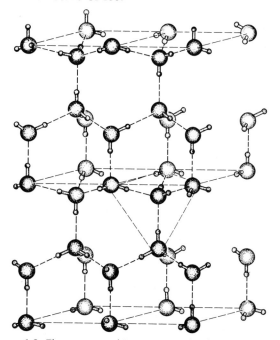

Figure 1-2. The structure of ice. Water molecules, with oxygen shown as large spheres and hydrogen as small spheres, are linked to adjoining water molecules by hydrogen bonds (dashed lines). The extensive hydrogen bonding is responsible for the crystalline structure of ice. (*From L. Pauling*, The Nature of the Chemical Bond, *3d ed., Cornell University Press, Ithaca, N.Y., 1960.*)

CONSEQUENCES FOR LIVING SYSTEMS

Dielectric constant

A number of biologically important properties result directly from the structure of water. Because of their high dipole moment, water molecules orient themselves readily in an external electric field. The field created by the oriented molecules opposes, and thereby reduces, the external field. The ease with which water molecules can engage in this type of "electrical buffering" gives water a high dielectric constant and permits water to act as an effective solvent for electrolytes. When sodium chloride, for example, dissolves in water, the electrostatic attraction between sodium and chloride is markedly reduced by the intervening water molecules, which tend to orient themselves in hydration shells around the individual ions. This is important not only in terms of ion solubility but permits the independent movement of ions in solution.

Icelike structure

Water is a highly associated liquid, as a result of hydrogen bonding between neighboring water molecules. Its high boiling point and the comparative ease with which it freezes reflect this quasi-crystalline structure. The high specific heat of water (the energy required to raise its temperature 1°C) is another consequence of its extensive hydrogen bonding and is of considerable importance in stabilizing body temperature in mammals. The large amount of heat lost upon evaporation of water as perspiration reflects the breaking of hydrogen bonds as water passes from the liquid to the vapor phase, providing the major avenue of heat loss from the body.

A question of current interest is the degree to which water assumes a true icelike structure in the vicinity of proteins and other solutes in living cells. Frank and Evans, in an important series of experiments in 1945 (3), showed that water does indeed become more highly organized in the presence of simple nonpolar gas molecules. A number of workers have suggested that cell membranes, proteins, and other substances may in a similar fashion induce microscopic "icebergs" in the water immediately associated with them and that this highly structured water may be important in such phenomena as the permeability and stabilization of cell membranes (4–6), the masking of active groups in proteins (7), and the anesthetic action of nonpolar gases such as chloroform and nitrous oxide (8).

This brief consideration of the properties of water, as related to its structure, serves to emphasize the unique role of water in the living system. We turn now to a consideration of body water and electrolytes in man. The discussion will begin with a brief summary of the units of measurement used in describing fluid and electrolyte composition.

UNITS OF SOLUTE MEASUREMENT

Forty-five to sixty percent of the human body consists of a dilute aqueous solution in which water is the solvent and in which the solutes are organic and inorganic substances. It is essential in discussing the physiology of the body fluids to express solute concentration in a consistent fashion. Different units serve different purposes. In the case of sodium, for example, we may be interested in knowing that the total body sodium of a 70-kg man is about 5000 milliequivalents (meq), or 115 grams (g), or 71 milliequivalents per kilogram (meq/kg) of body weight. The usual plasma sodium concentration is 142 milliequivalents per liter (meq/L). In discussing the integrity of the extracellular fluid volume, however, we must know that sodium contributes 142 milliosmoles per liter (mosm/L).

Any discussion of fluid and electrolytes must therefore be based on a complete understanding of the units of measurement.

ATOMIC WEIGHT

Atomic weight is an arbitrary number. The weight of 1 atom of oxygen was chosen as 16 to be the relative standard of reference. Relative to this standard, sodium has an atomic weight of 23, and chlorine has an atomic weight of 35.5. The proportion by weight[1] of the various elements in

---

[1] Although the term *mass* is technically correct, by convention the word *weight* will be used in its place in this text. Atomic weights will also be rounded off to the nearest 0.5.

a compound can be calculated with the use of atomic weights. For example, in 58.5 g sodium chloride (NaCl), there are 23 g sodium (Na) and 35.5 g chlorine (Cl). Table 1-1 lists the atomic weights of those elements which occur in the body fluids or are frequently used in biochemical reagents.

MOLECULAR WEIGHT, MOLE, AND MILLIMOLE

The molecular weight of a substance is the sum of the atomic weights of all the elements specified in the formula of that substance. A mole (mol) of a substance is its molecular weight expressed in grams, and a millimole (mmol) is $\frac{1}{1000}$ of a mole, or its weight in milligrams. Because of the small concentrations of most substances in the body fluids, the term *millimole* is the one most frequently employed. The terms *mole* and *millimole* may be used for all substances, regardless of whether they are organic or inorganic, ionized or nonionized. A mole, when applied to an element, is equal to the gram atomic

Table 1-1. Atomic weights of biologically important elements

ELEMENT	SYMBOL	ATOMIC WEIGHT
Aluminum	Al	26.98
Bromine	Br	79.92
Calcium	Ca	40.08
Carbon	C	12.01
Chlorine	Cl	35.46
Chromium	Cr	52.01
Copper	Cu	63.54
Hydrogen	H	1.01
Iodine	I	126.91
Iron	Fe	55.85
Magnesium	Mg	24.32
Manganese	Mn	54.94
Mercury	Hg	200.61
Nitrogen	N	14.01
Oxygen	O	16.00
Phosphorus	P	30.98
Potassium	K	39.10
Silver	Ag	107.88
Sodium	Na	22.99
Sulfur	S	32.07
Tungsten	W	183.86
Zinc	Zn	65.38

weight of that element. Examples are shown in Table 1-2. Although the concentrations of most of the electrolytes in the body fluids are properly expressed as milliequivalents per liter, in theory calcium and phosphorus should be recorded as millimoles per liter.

The concentrations of gases are also expressed in terms of molecular equivalents. One mole of any gas (e.g., oxygen, carbon dioxide, nitrous oxide) under standard conditions of temperature and pressure occupies a constant volume of 22.4 liters, or 1 mmol occupies 22.4 mL. Carbon dioxide (CO_2), the gas which is most important in electrolyte balance, is expressed as millimoles per liter. This is often used interchangeably with milliequivalents per liter, because presumably 1 mmol CO_2 will form 1 meq HCO_3^- .

$$CO_2 + H_2O \rightleftharpoons H^+ + HCO_3^- \qquad (1\text{-}1)$$

This assumption is not completely true, however, since in some situations bicarbonate conceivably could partially dissociate to hydrogen and a carbonate ion. However, this reaction is minimal below a pH of 8 and therefore is of little physiologic consequence.

$$H^+ + HCO_3^- \rightleftharpoons H^+ + H^+ + CO_3^{2-} \qquad (1\text{-}2)$$

Carbon dioxide content (or combining power) is therefore preferably expressed as millimoles per liter. Carbon dioxide is still occasionally expressed as volumes percent (vol percent),[2] i.e., milliliters of CO_2 gas per 100 milliliters of blood. To convert volumes percent of carbon dioxide to

millimoles per liter, the following formula may be used:

$$\frac{mm\ CO_2}{L} = \frac{vol\ percent\ CO_2 \times 10}{22.4} \qquad (1\text{-}3)$$

ELECTROCHEMICAL EQUIVALENCE— MILLIEQUIVALENTS

Electrolytes combine with each other in proportion to their ionic valence, rather than in proportion to their weights. Chemically, the standard of reference is the electric charge (+) of 1 atomic weight (1 g) of hydrogen. One equivalent (eq) of an ion is that amount which can replace or combine with one gram of hydrogen; this amount of the ion is therefore chemically "equivalent" to one gram of hydrogen. Expressed differently, one equivalent of a substance is the atomic, or formula, weight divided by the ionic valence and provides a quantitative index of the combining proportions of all ionic species. The electrolyte concentrations in the dilute body fluids are more easily expressed as milliequivalents (1 meq equals $\frac{1}{1000}$ eq).

The principle of electrochemical equivalence may be illustrated as follows: 1 mmol sodium is 23 mg, and 1 mmol chlorine is 35.5 mg. If we were to add 23 mg sodium and 35.5 mg chlorine to 1 L water, we would have a millimolar solution of sodium chloride:

$$\underset{(1\ mmol)}{23\ mg\ Na^+} + \underset{(1\ mmol)}{35.5\ mg\ Cl^-} \rightarrow \underset{(1\ mmol)}{58.5\ mg\ NaCl} \qquad (1\text{-}4)$$

If we were to add equal weights of sodium and chlorine, however, there would be an excess of sodium ion in solution:

$$35.5\ mg\ Na^+ + 35.5\ mg\ Cl^- \rightarrow$$
$$58.5\ mg\ NaCl + 12.5\ mg\ Na^+ \qquad (1\text{-}5)$$

Electrolytes do not combine gram for gram or milligram for milligram; they combine equivalent for equivalent or milliequivalent for milliequivalent. In the case of univalent ions, 1 eq equals 1 mol, and 1 meq equals 1 mmol. In Eq. (1-4), therefore, 1 meq sodium reacted with 1 meq chlorine.

---

[2] *Percent* means "per hundred." Therefore, any concentration expressed as percent refers to units per deciliter solution. By usage, most of the therapeutic solutions of electrolytes are expressed gravimetrically per deciliter water. Thus *0.9 percent saline solution* refers to 0.9 g of sodium chloride per deciliter water, and *5 percent glucose solution* means 5 g of dextrose per deciliter water, i.e., 50 g/L. To make it more confusing, however, some solutions are also equated in terms of *normal*, or *isotonic*, and still others in terms of moles per liter; i.e., a $\frac{1}{6}$ molar lactate solution contains $\frac{1}{6}$ mL of sodium lactate per liter of water. Also by convention, most of the nonelectrolytes of the body fluids (e.g., glucose, urea, creatinine, uric acid, cholesterol) are expressed as milligrams per deciliter, or mg/dL, of blood or plasma. A blood glucose concentration of 80 mg/dL means 80 mg of glucose per 100 mL of blood.

Table 1-2. Ionized and nonionized substances expressed as moles and millimoles

SUBSTANCE	FORMULA	MOLECULAR WEIGHT	MOLE, mol		MILLIMOLE, mmol	
Glucose	$C_6H_{12}O_6$	$6(12) + 12(1) + 6(16) = 180$	180	g	180	mg
Potassium chloride	KCl	$39 + 35.5 = 74.5$	74.5	g	74.5	mg
Sodium bicarbonate	$NaHCO_3$	$23 + 1 + 12 + 3(16) = 84$	84	g	84	mg
Calcium chloride	$CaCl_2$	$40 + 2(35.5) = 111$	111	g	111	mg
Ammonium chloride	NH_4Cl	$14 + 4(1) + 35.5 = 53.5$	53.5	g	53.5	mg
Bicarbonate	HCO_3^-	$1 + 12 + 3(16) = 61$	61	g	61	mg
Sulfate	SO_4^{2-}	$32 + 4(16) = 96$	96	g	96	mg
Sodium ion	Na^+		23	g	23	mg
Calcium ion	Ca^{2+}		40	g	40	mg

Multivalent ions have a greater chemical combining power than univalent ions. Since electrochemical neutrality must be preserved in all reactions, a divalent ion, which has two electric charges, will react with two univalent ions. Therefore 1 mmol divalent ion supplies 2 meq; i.e., 1 mmol calcium (2 meq) reacts with 2 mmol chloride (2 meq) in the reaction

$$Ca^{2+} + 2\ Cl^- \rightleftharpoons CaCl_2 \qquad (1\text{-}6)$$

It is apparent that 1 mmol of a substance will contain 3 meq if the valence is 3.

Dividing the number of milligrams of a univalent electrolyte by its molecular (or atomic) weight yields the number of milliequivalents. For example, 23 mg sodium divided by the atomic weight of sodium, 23, yields a value of 1; i.e., 23 mg sodium is 1 meq. With multivalent substances, the numerator must be multiplied by the valence; i.e., 40 mg calcium multiplied by its valence ($40 \times 2 = 80$) and divided by its atomic weight ($80 \div 40$) yields 2 meq. Since in the interpretation of laboratory results we are largely concerned with converting milligrams per deciliter to milliequivalents per liter, the numerator must be multiplied by 10. The final equation then becomes

$$\frac{mg/dL}{\text{Atomic weight}} \times valence \times 10 = \frac{meq}{L} \qquad (1\text{-}7)$$

The utility of expressing most of the electrolyte concentrations in milliequivalents per liter is apparent from Table 1-3. The total concentration of cations is equal to that of the anions, and electroneutrality exists. When concentrations are expressed as milligrams per deciliter, however, gross inequality exists, and nothing useful is learned about chemical interrelationships. The largest component, by weight, in the anion column is protein, which in terms of acid-base balance is seldom of importance.

Having emphasized the greater utility of electrochemical as opposed to gravimetric concentrations, it must be pointed out that even the term *milliequivalents per liter* is not ideally applicable to all the electrolytes in all circumstances. For example, as already mentioned, in problems of calcium and phosphorus metabolism, these ions are properly measured as millimoles per liter. The ionized (diffusible) calcium fraction depends on the proportion of calcium not bound to plasma proteins; the usual laboratory determination includes all the serum calcium and is not properly

Table 1-3. Normal plasma electrolyte concentrations

ELECTROLYTE	mg/dL	meq/L
Cations		
Sodium	326	142
Potassium	16	4
Calcium	10	5
Magnesium	2.5	2
Total cations	354.5	153
Anions		
Chloride	362	104
Bicarbonate	60	27
Phosphate	3.5	2
Sulfate	1.5	1
Organic acids	15	6
Protein	7000	13
Total anions	7442	153

expressed as milliequivalents per liter.[3] Serum "phosphorus" consists of variable proportions of phosphate and monohydrogen and dihydrogen phosphate (PO_4^{3-}, HPO_4^{2-}, $H_2PO_4^-$), so that no valence can be assigned to this substance. Plasma proteins are usually expressed as grams percent (g percent), or grams per deciliter (g/dL) plasma (see fn. 2). Although they are included in the anion column (Table 1-3), their electrochemical equivalence is affected by pH and other factors; at times they may even act as weak cations.

OSMOLES AND MILLIOSMOLES

The concepts of osmosis, osmotic pressure, effective osmotic pressure, and oncotic pressure will be described in a succeeding section. The osmotic effect of a substance in solution depends only on the number of particles dissolved and is independent of their weight, electric charge, valence, or chemical formula. This is based upon the fact that 1 mol of any element, regardless of weight, contains the same number of molecules (Avogadro's number: 6.061×10^{23} particles per mole). If a molecule in solution dissociates into two or three particles, the osmotic pressure is doubled or tripled, respectively. Units of osmotic force are conveniently expressed as osmoles (osm) and milliosmoles (mosm).

For substances which do not dissociate into smaller parts (e.g., glucose, urea), 1 mol equals 1 osm, and 1 mmol equals 1 mosm. This also applies to substances which carry electric charges; i.e., 1 mmol of sodium (23 mg) equals 1 mosm. It is obvious in the case of sodium that 1 mosm also equals 1 meq. Divalent and trivalent ions exert no more osmotic pressure than univalent ions, despite their higher chemical equivalences. Thus, for magnesium (Mg^{2+}): 1 mmol (24.5 mg) = 1 mosm = 2 meq; for phosphate (PO_4^{3-}): 1 mmol (95 mg) = 1 mosm = 3 meq. One millimole of sodium chloride (58.5 mg), which dissociates into

---

[3] Serum calcium can be accurately recorded as milliequivalents per liter if the total number of milliequivalents is partitioned into ionized and nonionized fractions; the nonionized fraction may then be classified into calcium proteinates and other nonionized components of calcium salts, such as citrates and phosphates.

sodium and chloride in solution, contributes twice as many osmotically active particles as a nonionized substance, so that 1 mmol = 2 meq = 2 mosm.

SUMMARY

The essential points to remember about the units of measurement discussed above are

1. A millimole equals $\frac{1}{1000}$ of the gram atomic, or molecular, weight of a substance and is independent of valence.
2. A milliequivalent equals $\frac{1}{1000}$ of an equivalent, which is the gram atomic, or formula, weight divided by the ionic valence, or the electrochemical combining power of 1 g atom of hydrogen. If the valence is 2 or 3, 1 mmol contains 2 or 3 meq.
3. A milliosmole equals $\frac{1}{1000}$ of an osmole. It is independent of valence, electric charge, or mass and is a measure of the number of discrete particles in solution.

These relationships may be clarified by referring to Table 1-4.

CONCENTRATIONS

By usage, most of the concentrations in therapeutic solutions of electrolytes are expressed as percent, i.e., weight per deciliter water (see fn. 2). This method of expressing compositions is inaccurate unless the temperature is specified; it is also semantically incorrect, as *1 percent* means "1 part in 100" of the same units.

The more appropriate unit is the molal concentration, or the molality (m), in which the concentration of solute is expressed as moles per 1000 grams solvent. A molal solution of sodium chloride contains 58.5 grams sodium chloride dissolved in 1000 grams water. A given solution has the same molality at all temperatures. The molar concentration, or molarity (M), is the number of moles of solute per liter of solution at some specified temperature, usually dissolved in one liter of water. (see fn. 2). Because of the expansion and contraction of liquids with changes in temperature, the molarity of any given solution varies with the temperature. At low concentrations, as

Table 1-4. Relationship between various units of measurement

SUBSTANCE	FORMULA	ATOMIC OR MOLECULAR WEIGHT	MOLES,* mol	EQUIVALENTS,* eq	OSMOLES,*† osm
Sodium	Na	23	1	1	1
Chloride	Cl	35.5	1	1	1
Sodium chloride	NaCl	58.5	1	2 ($1Na^+, 1Cl^-$)	2 (Na, Cl)
Calcium	Ca	40	1	2 (Ca^{2+})	1 (Ca)
Calcium chloride	$CaCl_2$	111	1	4 ($Ca^{2+}, 2Cl^-$)	3 (Ca, Cl, Cl)
Sodium sulfate	Na_2SO_4	142	1	4 ($2 Na^+, SO_4^-$)	3 (Na, Na, SO_4)
Glucose	$C_6H_{12}O_6$	180	1		1
Urea	NH_2CONH_2	60	1		1

* Multiply by 1000 to obtain millimoles, milliequivalents, or milliosmoles.
† Calculation of osmoles assumes 100 percent dissociation and the properties of an ideal solution.

occur in the body fluids, the solutes may be expressed as millimoles per kilogram (millimolal, mm) or millimoles per liter (millimolar, mM). The difference between molal and molar concentrations is negligible in the range of concentrations and temperature of the body fluids.

The definitions of osmolality and osmolarity and of osmolal and osmolar are similar, the unit of concentration being the osmole instead of the mole.

Since about 90 percent of the serum electrolytes are univalent, total ionic concentration in terms of milliequivalents closely approximates osmolal concentration. By adding the osmolal concentrations of the serum electrolytes (cations and anions), a theoretical value of about 310 mosm/kg serum water, or 310 mosm/L, is derived. By actual measurement, serum osmolality in health is about 285 mosm/L. This is because osmolality is expressed chemically in terms of ideal solutions of sodium chloride, ignoring interionic and other effects that are seen in real solutions and in the serum.

Isotonic, hypertonic, and hypotonic solutions

In clinical usage the term *tonicity* is interchangeable with *osmolality*. A solution is said to be isotonic when it is isosmotic with (has the same osmotic pressure as) the body fluids in health. An isotonic solution when given intravenously will neither decrease nor increase the size of the red blood cells. Since the osmolality of a solution is determined by the number rather than the kind of particles, an isotonic solution need not contain substances identical with those in the plasma. Thus, solutions of 5% glucose in water and 0.9% sodium chloride[4] are isotonic.

A hypertonic solution (e.g., 5% NaCl) has a higher osmolality (greater solute concentration) than the body fluids. A hypotonic solution (e.g., 0.45% NaCl) has a lower osmolality (smaller solute concentration) than the body fluids.

VOLUMES OF THE FLUID COMPARTMENTS OF THE BODY

TOTAL BODY WATER

Early estimates of body water content in man were obtained by the desiccation of cadavers.

[4] Unfortunately, isotonic sodium chloride solution (0.9 percent of NaCl), is usually "normal saline solution," presumably because this concentration of sodium chloride is isotonic with normal body fluids. This is semantically incorrect. A truly normal solution should contain all the important solutes of the plasma in ideal concentrations. W. M. Clark (1952) aptly comments, "The normal solution is one designed to meet the convenience of the analyst and its constitution is dependent upon the use that the analyst makes of it."

There was considerable variation in the values reported, caused largely by the variety of illnesses leading to death (9).

The modern approach to the determination of total body water (the *dilution technique*) was successfully applied by Hevesy and Hofer (10) in 1934, and subsequently, between 1940 and 1960, by a number of workers in studies of normal living subjects (11–14). The oxides of deuterium (D_2O) and tritium (THO), isotopic forms of water, as well as antipyrine were used in these determinations. It will be profitable to describe the dilution technique briefly, since the principles involved apply to all dilution studies of body composition. A known amount of labeled water is given by mouth or intravenously, and blood samples are taken until equilibrium is reached. In the case of water, the concentration of isotope in serum reaches equilibrium within two hours. At this point mixing and distribution of labeled water are regarded as complete, and the *apparent volume of distribution* of the labeled water can then be determined from the relationship

$$V_F = \frac{C_1 V_1 - C_E V_E}{C_F} \qquad (1\text{-}8)$$

where C_1 = concentration of test substance administered

V_1 = volume of test substance administered

C_E = concentration of test substance lost in urine during equilibration time

V_E = volume of urine excreted before equilibration has been achieved

C_F = concentration of test substance after equilibrium has been achieved

V_F = amount of final volume of body water into which test substance has diffused at equilibrium

The labeled water lost in urine is small, approximating 0.4 percent of the administered dose (15), and, in practice, the term for urinary loss of labeled water is omitted, giving the simplified equation

$$V_F = \frac{C_1 V_1}{C_F} \qquad (1\text{-}9)$$

Measured by this method, the *total body water for adults was found to vary from 45 to 60 percent of body weight*. The large range of variation is due mainly to the reciprocal relationship between body water and body fat content, since there is virtually no water in neutral fat. An obese individual, therefore, has less body water in relation to weight than a lean individual. If one takes a value for water of 58 percent of body weight for an adult male, for example, and assumes 16 percent of his body weight as fat, his body water would be 70 percent of his fat-free body weight. Estimates of body water based on fat-free body weight are more constant than those based on body weight not corrected for fat.

Table 1-5. Mean values for total body water in normal human beings in percent of body weight

AGE, YEARS	MEN	WOMEN
10–16	58.9	57.3
17–39	60.6	50.2
40–59	54.7	46.7
60+	51.5	45.5

Table 1-5 summarizes a number of studies of body water in normal subjects in which D_2O, THO, and antipyrine were used. A significant difference between males and females is apparent, largely related to differences in body fat content. The sex difference is a constant finding throughout most of early life as well (Fig. 1-3).

The mean values for total body water, therefore, have been well established for both males and females of all age groups. A number of circumstances have made this measurement a relatively reliable one: D_2O and THO are small molecules and penetrate all phases of body water rapidly, with good mixing; water is not extensively metabolized over the period required for equilibration, nor is there appreciable binding of the labeled molecules. There is a small amount of exchange of isotopic hydrogen with body proteins and carbohydrates, but this is of the order of 2 percent of body weight (12) and does not represent a significant error. Finally, it is possible to compare results of the dilution technique with those obtained from desiccation and specific gravity determinations, with fair agreement.

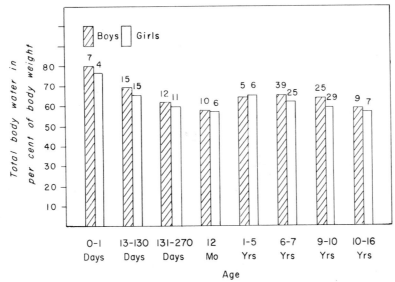

Figure 1-3. Sex differences in relative amounts of total body water at various age levels in infants, children, and adolescents. (*From L. P. Novak,* Compartments, Pools and Spaces in Medical Physiology, *eds. P. E. Bergher and C. C. Lushbaugh, U.S. Atomic Energy Commission Symposium 11, 1967.*)

However, when we turn to a consideration of the major subdivisions of total body water, namely, the extracellular and intracellular fluid volumes, more serious problems of measurement and interpretation are encountered.

THE MAJOR COMPARTMENTS OF BODY WATER

Total body water exists in two major compartments: intracellular and extracellular fluid. By definition, the extracellular fluid includes all body water which is external to the cells. The extracellular fluid, in turn, may be divided into a number of compartments as follows:

1. Plasma
2. Interstitial fluid and lymph
   a. In rapid exchange with plasma
   b. Slowly exchanging with plasma (including dense connective tissue and cartilage)
3. Inaccessible bone water
4. Transcellular fluids

In addition, the pleural, pericardial, peritoneal, and the synovial and joint fluids should be listed. The above division is arbitrary and is based somewhat more on functional than anatomic considerations. This applies particularly to the interstitial fluid, which is functionally and structurally in close relationship with plasma and contains phases that are in rapid exchange with plasma, and phases such as the fluid of connective tissue, in which tracers equilibrate much more slowly (16). Not only is the extracellular fluid of connective tissue and cartilage slow to equilibrate with plasma but a portion of the general interstitial space is now believed to consist of a gel matrix, which may retard the passage of solutes (17) and therefore equilibrate slowly. The sarcolemma of muscle fibers, composed of filamentous and gel-like layers (18), also represents a structure which may be slow to equilibrate.

The so-called transcellular fluids have been described by Edelman and Leibman (19) as "a variety of fluid collections which are not simple transudates and which have the common property of being formed by the transport activity of cells." These include the fluids of salivary glands, the pancreas, the liver and biliary tree, the thyroid gland, the gonads, the skin, the mucous membranes of the respiratory and gastrointestinal tracts, and the kidneys, in addition to the cavitary fluids of the eye, the cerebrospinal fluid, and the intraluminal fluid of the gastrointestinal tract. The electrolyte composition of these fluids differs from that of an ultrafiltrate of plasma, and many of the tracers used to measure extracellular fluid volume may be either excluded from, or unduly concentrated in, these compartments.

MEASUREMENTS OF THE EXTRACELLULAR FLUID VOLUME

In view of the complexities of the extracellular fluid, it will not surprise the reader to learn that precise determination of its volume is difficult or even impossible. With current methods for using the dilution technique, it is essential to employ a tracer that is excluded from cells. However, if large saccharides such as inulin and sucrose are chosen in an effort to avoid penetration into cells, one encounters an equally serious problem: the failure of these tracers to penetrate the entire extracellular space within a reasonable length of time.[5] On the other hand, small ions such as chloride or bromide do penetrate the cell membranes of some tissues (19) and give correspondingly high values for extracellular volume. The range of values for extracellular volume obtained by a number of investigators using a variety of indicators is shown in Table 1-6. The range is large, from approximately 16 percent of body weight (inulin) to 28 percent (bromine). The problem remains, therefore, of finding a tracer which is small enough to equilibrate throughout the entire extracellular space within a reasonable time and which remains extracellular. Edelman and Leibman (19) have approached the problem by proposing that plasma, interstitial fluid and

[5] Studies by Goodford and Leach [*J. Physiol.* (*London*), **186**:1, 1961], for example, have shown that hyaluronidase treatment increases the estimated inulin space of guinea pig smooth muscle, suggesting that extracellular mucopolysaccharides may restrict diffusion of large tracers such as inulin.

Table 1-6. Mean values for extracellular fluid in men and women in percent of body weight

METHOD	MEN	WOMEN
Inulin	15.6	
Mannitol	16.6	
Thiosulfate	16.3	16.0
$^{35}SO_4$	18.0	
Br	28.4	25.1
^{36}Cl	26.8	
^{24}Na	26.2	

Source: Data (with the exception of $^{35}SO_4$) are from C. L. Comar and F. Bronner (eds.), *Mineral Metabolism, an Advanced Treatise*, Academic Press, Inc., New York, 1964, p. 14.

lymph, and connective tissue may be viewed as being in functional equilibrium (capable of being labeled rapidly or slowly by large saccharides), and that this "functional" extracellular space represents 21 percent of the total body weight of a healthy young adult male. To this they have added two compartments which they regard as inaccessible to saccharides, the transcellular volume and inaccessible bone water, giving a total extracellular volume of 27 percent of body weight (45 percent of body water) (Table 1-7).

While the values obtained appear reasonable, they must be regarded as approximations. The question of how completely large saccharides can label the interstitial fluid has already been discussed; in addition, there is some experimental evidence that even saccharides can eventually penetrate cells over long equilibration periods (20).

Studies of the distribution of inorganic radiosulfate ($^{35}SO_4$) by Barratt and Walser (21) and other workers have shown that the distribution of this substance, when extrapolated back to "zero time," may provide a useful estimate of extracellular volume. Studies carried out in man with radiosulfate (22, 23) yield values of 17 to 19 percent of body weight. The pattern of distribution of the saccharides and of sulfate appears to differ significantly, with sulfate overestimating extracellular volume in some tissues and entering some transcellular spaces in experimental animals (21).

Estimates of the extracellular volume must therefore be tentative, depending critically on the technique used. It is nevertheless possible to employ a given technique to measure *changes* in ex-

Table 1-7. Body water distribution in a healthy young adult male*

COMPARTMENT	PERCENT OF BODY WEIGHT	PERCENT OF TOTAL BODY WATER	LITERS
Plasma	4.5	7.5	3
Interstitial lymph	12	20	8.5
Dense connective tissue and cartilage	4.5	7.5	3
Inaccessible bone water	4.5	7.5	3
Transcellular	1.5	2.5	1
Total extracellular	27	45	19
"Functional" extracellular[+]	21	35	14.5
Total body water	60	100	42
Total intracellular	33	55	23

* All figures rounded to nearest 0.5.

+ Minus bone water and transcellular water.

Source: After I. S. Edelman and J. Leibman, *Am. J. Med.,* **27:**256, 1959.

tracellular volume in altered physiologic states, and such measurements have provided useful information. We may now consider briefly one subdivision of the extracellular fluid, the plasma (and whole blood) volume.

PLASMA VOLUME AND TOTAL BLOOD VOLUME

The plasma volume has been measured by determining the volume of distribution of labeled albumin. T-1824, a dye which combines with albumin, or albumin tagged with radioactive iodine (^{131}I) has been used (24, 25). Since albumin is not confined to the vascular compartment and readily escapes into interstitial fluid and lymph (26), it is necessary to determine the volume of distribution of albumin after a relatively short period of equilibrium or to extrapolate back to "zero time." Measured plasma volume is especially suspect in traumatic injury, burns, and other circumstances where plasma protein may leak from the vascular system.

The *red cell mass* is measured by labeling red cells with radioactive chromium (^{51}Cr), phosphorus (^{32}P), or iron (^{59}Fe), or with carbon monoxide. Total blood volume (plasma volume plus red cell mass) may then be estimated by (1) adding the independently determined plasma volume and red cell mass (27) and (2) determining either the plasma volume (PV) or the red cell mass (RCM) and solving for the total blood volume (TBV) using one of the following relationships:

$$TBV = \frac{RCM}{VH} \times 100 \qquad (1\text{-}10)$$

or

$$TBV = \frac{PV}{100 - VH} \times 100 \qquad (1\text{-}11)$$

where VH is the venous hematocrit (Hct). One important source of error in the second type of estimate is the fact that the "large vessel" hematocrit, as determined from sampling a given vein, is not necessarily representative of "whole body hematocrit," which would include the hematocrit of smaller vessels in various organs of the body. The whole body hematocrit is believed to be between 85 and 92 percent of the large vein hematocrit.

Table 1-8 summarizes values from a number of studies of plasma volume (T-1824 method) and of total blood volume. Total blood volume was determined by both the "summation method," in which plasma and red cell volumes were determined simultaneously by appropriate tracers and the values combined, and by the indirect method, in which plasma volume was determined and was divided by 100 − Hct; the latter values are somewhat higher.

INTRACELLULAR FLUID VOLUME

The volume of the intracellular space cannot be determined directly but must be estimated by sub-

Table 1-8. Plasma and blood volume in healthy subjects (in percent of body weight)

	MEN	WOMEN
Plasma volume	4.5 (4.1–4.8)	4.5 (4.1–4.8)
Total blood volume (summation method)	7.3 (6.8–7.8)	6.2 (6.1–6.3)
Total blood volume $\left(\dfrac{PV}{100 - VH} \times 100 \right)$	8.2	7.7 (7.4–8.0)

Source: Data are from P. L. Altman and D. S. Dittmer (eds.), *Biology Data Book,* Federation of American Societies for Experimental Biology, Washington, 1964, p. 263. Data for total blood volume (summation method) include the values of F. D. Moore, K. H. Olesen, J. D. McMurrey, H. V. Parker, M. R. Ball, and C. M. Boyden, *The Body Cell Mass and Its Supporting Environment,* W. B. Saunders Company, Philadelphia, 1963.

tracting the extracellular fluid volume from that of total body water. The volume obtained depends critically on the value for extracellular fluid volume one chooses (see Table 1-6). Assigning a value of 27 percent for total extracellular fluid (Table 1-7), the total intracellular fluid volume becomes 33 percent of body weight, or 55 percent of total body water. The intracellular space, then, is the largest of the fluid spaces of the body.

SUMMARY

The distribution of body water is summarized in Fig. 1-4. The values, as discussed in this section, represent approximations and are subject to the uncertainties mentioned.

The fluid compartments of the body do not, of course, exist as fixed spaces of water with identical composition. They are in constant interchange with each other, and, as the result of several features of cell structure and function, they differ strikingly in their composition. The remainder of this chapter will deal with the ion and protein composition of the body and the major fluid compartments, and the forces regulating interchange between compartments.

THE MAJOR ELECTROLYTES AND THEIR DISTRIBUTION

TOTAL BODY COMPOSITION

The total body content of sodium, potassium, and chloride (determined by the technique of neutron activation) is shown in Table 1-9, as well as the

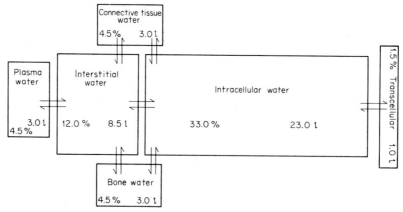

Figure 1-4. Body water compartments in a normal 70-kg man shown as percentage of body weight and in liters. (*After Edelman and Leibman.*)

Table 1-9. Total and exchangeable sodium, potassium, and chloride in healthy subjects

	TOTAL CONTENT,	EXCHANGEABLE, meq	
ION	meq	MEN	WOMEN
Sodium	3710±7% S.D.	2835	2597
Potassium	3640±8% S.D.	3367 (16–30 yr)	2681 (16–30 yr)
		2611 (61–90 yr)	2079 (61–90 yr)
Chloride	2147±6%	2058	1869

Source: Data for total body content are from S. H. Cohn, C. Abesamis, J. Zanzi, J. F. Aloia, S. Yasumura, and K. J. Ellis, *Am. J. Physiol.*, **232**:419, 1977. The data are means of the values for six white males, ages 40–49. Data for exchangeable fraction are from F. D. Moore, K. H. Olesen, J. D. McMurrey, H. V. Parker, M. R. Ball, and C. M. Boyden, *The Body Cell Mass and Its Supporting Environment*, W. B. Saunders Company, Philadelphia, 1963.

amount of these electrolytes that are in dynamic exchange (determined by isotope dilution).

Of the approximately 3600 meq of potassium in the body, close to 90 percent is exchangeable, and virtually all of this 90 percent is within cells. A very different situation exists in the case of sodium, of which a significant fraction (24 percent) is nonexchangeable. Much of the nonexchangeable sodium is locked within the crystalline phase of bone. Of the exchangeable sodium, approximately 85 percent is in extracellular water; 15 percent may be within body cells and in other nonextracellular sites. Of interest also is the observation that age appears to influence the size of the exchangeable potassium pool, but not that of the sodium pool.

ELECTROLYTE COMPOSITION OF THE FLUID COMPARTMENTS: SERUM

The electrolyte composition of the serum, interstitial fluid, and intracellular fluid is shown in Table 1-10. The values for serum are shown in two ways: as milliequivalents per liter of serum and as milliequivalents per liter of serum water. The first is the method of reporting used by all clinical chemistry laboratories, and simply gives the ionic concentration in a given volume of serum. Since the concentration of solids (notably proteins and lipids) in serum is approximately 7 percent, the values per liter of serum water can be found by dividing milliequivalents per liter of serum by 0.93 (Table 1-10). While the concentrations in terms of serum water are more accurate, the first method is nevertheless accurate enough to be generally accepted. If the lipid content of the serum is markedly increased, however, there will be a corresponding decrease in the reported concentrations of ions per liter of serum, while their concentrations per liter of serum *water* will be unaffected.

Several features of the ionic composition of the serum deserve comment. First, sodium and chloride are the major cations and anions, with potas-

Table 1-10. Electrolyte composition of the body fluids

ELECTROLYTES	SERUM, meq/L	SERUM WATER, meq/L	INTERSTITIAL FLUID, meq/L	INTRACELLULAR FLUID (MUSCLE), meq/kg H_2O
Cations				
Sodium (Na^+)	142	152.7	145	±10
Potassium (K^+)	4	4.3	4	156
Calcium (Ca^{2+})	5	5.4		3.3
Magnesium (Mg^{2+})	2	2.2		26
Total cations	153	165	149	195
Anions				
Chloride (Cl^-)	102	109.7	114	±2
Bicarbonate (HCO_3^-)	26	28	31	±8
Phosphate (HPO_4^{2-})	2	2.2		95
Sulfate (SO_4^{2-})	1	1.1		20
Organic acids	6	6.5		
Protein	16	17.2		55
Total anions	153	165	145	180+

sium maintained at the relatively low concentration of 4 meq/L. Sodium and chloride are free in solution; in contrast, appreciable fractions of calcium and magnesium are protein-bound. Approximately 35 to 45 percent of the total serum calcium is bound to protein (27), and an additional 5 to 15 percent is complexed to anions such as phosphate and citrate. Of the serum magnesium, approximately 30 percent is protein-bound, an additional 15 percent is in the form of complexes, and approximately 55 percent is in the free ionic form (28).

INTERSTITIAL FLUID AND THE GIBBS-DONNAN DISTRIBUTION

Since water and electrolytes can diffuse freely across the capillary endothelium and the diffusion of serum proteins is restricted, it has been customary to consider the interstitial fluid as an ultrafiltrate of serum, relatively free of protein and with a somewhat different electrolyte composition. The difference in composition is partly the result of the fact that the serum proteins, which have a net negative charge at pH7.4 and therefore behave as anions, are at a relatively higher concentration on the vascular side of the capillary endothelium. This gives rise to an important asymmetry of ion distribution between serum and interstitial fluid, an example of the *Gibbs-Donnan distribution*. A brief description of the Gibbs-Donnan distribution follows, based on the discussion in West and associates (29).

Imagine a membrane separating two fluid compartments. Sodium chloride is placed in one compartment and the sodium salt of a large protein anion (NaR) in the other. NaCl can pass across the membrane, but the large anion cannot. Initially, the NaR is at concentration a and the NaCl at concentration b:

$$
\begin{array}{cc|cc}
\textbf{(1)} & & \textbf{(2)} & \\
a & \text{Na}^+ & \text{Na}^+ & b \\
a & \text{R}^- & \text{Cl}^- & b \\
\end{array}
$$

The NaCl in compartment (2) diffuses into compartment (1), until equilibrium is reached. Let x represent the net concentration of NaCl that has

passed from (2) to (1) at equilibrium. Then, since the Na$^+$ and Cl$^-$ concentrations in (2) must remain equal to preserve electroneutrality:

$$
\begin{array}{cc|cc}
\textbf{(1)} & & \textbf{(2)} & \\
a + x & \text{Na}^+ & \text{Na}^+ & b - x \\
a & \text{R}^- & & \\
x & \text{Cl}^- & \text{Cl}^- & b - x \\
\end{array}
$$

The term *equilibrium* indicates that the rate of diffusion of NaCl from (2) to (1) equals the rate from (1) to (2). The rate of diffusion of NaCl from (2) to (1) is proportional to the product of the concentrations of Na$^+$ and Cl$^-$ in (2), namely, $(b - x)^2$; the rate of diffusion from (1) to (2) is proportional to the product of the Na$^+$ and Cl$^-$ concentrations in (1), namely, $(a + x)x$. At equilibrium

$$(a + x)x = (b - x)^2 \qquad (1\text{-}12)$$
$$\textbf{(1)} \qquad\qquad \textbf{(2)}$$

or

$$[\text{Na}_1^+][\text{Cl}_1^-] = [\text{Na}_2^+][\text{Cl}_2^-] \qquad (1\text{-}13)$$

where the brackets denote concentrations. This is the fundamental Gibbs-Donnan equation. At equilibrium, $[\text{Na}_2^+]$ and $[\text{Cl}_2^-]$ are equal, and their product is a square, while $[\text{Na}_1^+]$ and $[\text{Cl}_1^-]$ are unequal, and their product is not a square. Since the sum of the factors in a square is less than the sum of the factors in a nonsquare giving the same product, the total of $[\text{Na}^+]$ and $[\text{Cl}^-]$ in (1) will exceed the total in (2).

To summarize:

1. When an impermeant anion is present on one side of a membrane, the concentration of a diffusible positive ion will be *greater* on the side containing the anion than on the *opposite* side, and the concentration of a diffusible anion *less*.
2. The total number of diffusible ions will be greater on the side containing the anion. There will therefore be a difference in osmotic pressure under these conditions, a fact of importance which will be taken up in a later section of this chapter.

Returning to the problem of the distribution of ions across the capillary bed, the concentration of anions other than protein will be lower, and the concentration of cations will be higher in serum water in comparison to interstitial fluid, as the result of the presence of protein in the serum. A factor of 0.95 has been used to estimate electrolyte concentration in interstitial fluid; using sodium and chloride as examples, the Gibbs-Donnan relationship would be expressed as follows:

$$[Cl^-]_{IF} = \frac{Cl_S^-}{0.95 \times H_2O_S} \qquad (1\text{-}14)$$

$$[Na^+]_{IF} = \frac{0.95 \times Na_S^+}{H_2O_S} \qquad (1\text{-}15)$$

where H_2O_S is serum water expressed as the volume fraction.

The estimates for sodium, potassium, bicarbonate, and chloride concentrations in interstitial fluid appear in Table 1-10. Because of uncertainty regarding the correct factor for divalent ions, values for calcium, magnesium, phosphate, and sulfate are omitted. It should be emphasized as well that the correction factor for univalent ions may not be entirely correct, since the interstitial fluid is not really a simple aqueous solution of electrolytes. In addition to having a protein concentration which has been estimated to be as high as 2 percent (30) the interstitial fluid contains a variety of polysaccharides, including hyaluronic acid and chondroitin sulfate, which may contribute to the total anionic charge, the binding of multivalent ions, and other physical properties of the interstitial fluid (31). Under the circumstances, it is not yet possible to give a completely accurate description of the concentration and physical state of ions in the interstitial fluid.

INTRACELLULAR ELECTROLYTES

As one proceeds from serum through interstitial fluid to the intracellular fluid, the problem of determining the precise ionic composition becomes progressively more difficult. The composition varies from tissue to tissue and is easily altered as the result of manipulating the tissue under study. In addition, the problem of accurately defining intracellular and extracellular fluid volumes is as troublesome in the case of an individual tissue as in the body as a whole.

Skeletal muscle

Since skeletal muscle composes a large fraction of body weight and is a major depot of body electrolytes, its composition has been studied extensively. A brief discussion of one such study of human skeletal muscle by Bergstrom (32) will serve to illustrate the problems involved in the determination. Bergstrom employed a biopsy needle to obtain 2- to 30-mg samples of quadriceps femoris from human volunteers. Visible fat was removed and the muscle blotted free of blood and quickly weighed. The samples were then dried to constant weight and their water content determined by difference. The electrolyte content of the dried samples was then determined by the technique of activation analysis, in which radioactive isotopes of the ions are formed by irradiation with neutrons. From their characteristic spectra, the total amounts of sodium, chloride, potassium, and phosphorus could be determined. It was assumed that chloride was confined to the extracellular phase of muscle water. Since the chloride concentration in plasma water was known, the total extracellular water could be estimated from the total chloride present (correcting for the Gibbs-Donnan equilibrium); extracellular water was then subtracted from total water to give the volume of intracellular water, and the potassium, sodium, and phosphorus concentrations per liter of intracellular water estimated. Bergstrom obtained values of 4 meq/kg water for sodium, 167 meq/kg water for potassium, and 110 mmol/kg water for phosphorus.

Aside from the inevitable errors of weighing and counting, an additional source of error is encountered in this study: the difficulty of estimating extracellular fluid volume. Chloride penetrates cells; therefore the assumption that it is entirely extracellular will lead to a value for extracellular volume which is too high and a value for intracellular volume which is too low. The use of high-molecular-weight substances such as inulin to measure extracellular space may, on the other hand, yield values which are too low, as has already been discussed. Therefore we must again regard the values reported by investigations in this area as approximations. In Table 1-10 are summarized a number of studies of human muscle electrolytes in which a variety of techniques were used for the determination of extracellular volume and ion concentration. Mean values with ranges are shown. The reader is referred to the discussions of Bergstrom (32), Kernan (33), Bittar (34), and Walser (35) for further treatment of this subject.

It is clear that the concentrations of intracellular ions differ dramatically from those of the extracellular fluid. Potassium is the predominant cation, with magnesium in high concentration as well. Phosphate, sulfate, and protein are the major anions. Sodium, chloride, and bicarbonate, the predominant ions of the extracellular fluid, are present in much lower concentration within cells. There is abundant evidence that this state of affairs is brought about by the metabolic activity of living cells in the form of active transport mechanisms for specific ions; this will be reviewed in the concluding section of the chapter. However, the extent to which intracellular binding of ions contributes to this disequilibrium deserves consideration as well.

Ion binding

The sum of the total intracellular anions and cations in Table 1-10 exceeds that of the serum. Since cells and extracellular fluid have been found to have equal osmolalities (36), it is probable that a portion of the intracellular ions is osmotically inactive, i.e., bound to proteins and other constituents of the cell. Magnesium, for example, binds readily to a variety of cell lipoproteins and nucleoproteins, ribonucleic acids, and free adenosine-triphosphate (see Ref. 27), and it has been estimated that as much as 30 percent of intracellular magnesium may be bound (37). There has been considerable controversy regarding the extent to which potassium is bound to the cytoplasm. Ling (38), for example, has argued that cell proteins bind potassium selectively and that this accounts for the intracellular accumulation of potassium in preference to sodium. However, there is no evidence that proteins and other anionic molecules isolated from cells bind potassium *preferentially* (39, 40), and while it is entirely possible that some potassium is bound, it is

probable that the cell accumulates most of its potassium as the result of metabolically determined exchanges at the cell membrane.

Cellular organelles

The data for intracellular electrolyte concentrations describe, of course, mean concentrations for total intracellular water. Since cells are not uniform in their internal structure but contain a variety of organelles (mitochondria, nuclei, endoplasmic reticulum, etc.), it is probable that important differences in electrolyte concentration exist in these various compartments. Isolated mitochondria, for example, appear to have a composition similar to that of intracellular fluid when they are suspended in a simple sucrose medium (41). However, in more complex media and when allowed to respire, mitochondria display a dramatic ability to accumulate calcium, inorganic phosphate, and magnesium to levels far in excess of their initial values (Fig. 1-5) (42, 43). Little is known about the ionic composition of other cell organelles; there is some evidence that sodium

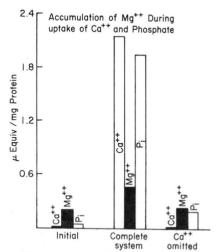

Figure 1-5. The uptake of calcium, magnesium, and inorganic phosphorus by mitochondria from a simple incubation medium (initial), a complete medium (containing succinate Mg^{2+}, Ca^{2+}, phosphate, adenosine triphosphate, and NaCl), and the complete medium with Ca^{2+} omitted. Calcium and phosphate accumulation are strikingly increased in the complete system. (*From Carafoli, Rossi, and Lehninger.*)

may be accumulated in the cell nucleus and play a role in facilitating the inward movement of amino acids for nucleoprotein synthesis (44).

SUMMARY

The extracellular and intracellular compartments differ greatly in their ionic composition, especially with respect to sodium, chloride, potassium, and magnesium. While the composition and extent of ion binding in serum is well understood, there remain a number of questions regarding ionic composition, binding, and distribution in the interstitial and intracellular fluids. It is clear, nevertheless, that ions within and outside the cell are at far different concentrations and that these concentration differences can be maintained only by the expenditure of energy. The remaining sections of this chapter will be concerned with the forces responsible for fluid and electrolyte movement and their relationship, as far as it is understood, to the distribution of ions between the fluid compartments.

FORCES RESPONSIBLE FOR WATER AND SOLUTE MOVEMENT

The major forces responsible for water movement between body compartments are hydrostatic and osmotic pressure. This is not to say that other modes of water transfer can be ignored; the process of pinocytosis (the ability of the cell membrane to engulf and transfer droplets of fluid outside the cell to the cell interior), for example, has been described in cells such as *Amoeba proteus* (45) and in some mammalian tissues (46). However, until the importance of pinocytosis (and other processes such as electroosmosis) is better established, hydrostatic and osmotic forces remain the principal ones to be considered.

HYDROSTATIC PRESSURE

Hydrostatic pressure in human beings is provided by the mechanical pressure of the heart. The mean pressure in the larger arteries is approxi-

mately 95 mmHg (millimeters of mercury). By the time the blood reaches the capillary bed (the site of fluid exchange), its hydrostatic pressure has been reduced to 32 mmHg (approximately 0.04 atm), and the *net* pressure (hydrostatic minus colloid osmotic pressure) is even less (see Fig. 1-8). This small net hydrostatic pressure is sufficient to transfer a small amount of plasma water and solutes from the arterial end of the capillary bed to the interstitial space. The process is reversed at the venous end of the bed, where water filtered at the arterial end returns to the vascular space.

A somewhat different state of affairs exists at the specialized capillary bed of the renal glomerulus. Here, because the vessels connecting the aorta and afferent arterioles are short and direct, the glomerular capillary pressure approaches the arterial pressure. Ultrafiltration of plasma takes place at a net pressure of approximately 45 mmHg (47). Most of the glomerular filtrate returns to the peritubular capillaries after first being resorbed across the tubular epithelium. Recovery of the filtrate is not complete, however, since 1 to 2 L of water per day leave the body as urine.

In both types of capillary bed, then, a relatively low hydrostatic pressure provides a force for water transfer. The amount of fluid transferred across the capillary bed by hydrostatic pressure is relatively small, the major mode of exchange of solutes and water being by diffusion across the capillary endothelium. Ultrafiltration across the glomerulus, however, is a process of great magnitude.

OSMOTIC PRESSURE

Osmotic pressure is a familiar concept to students of biology. It can be illustrated by a simple experiment in which a membrane is tied over an inverted thistle tube (Fig. 1-6). The membrane may be assumed to be semipermeable (i.e., permeable to water but not to a solute such as sucrose). If the thistle tube is partly filled with a solution of sucrose in water and placed in a beaker of pure water, it will be seen that water enters the tube, causing the fluid in the stem to rise. The fluid will continue to rise until its hydrostatic pressure (causing the water to flow outward) just balances the inflow of water caused by

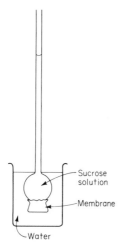

Figure 1-6. Osmosis through a membrane. (*From S. Glasstone, Textbook of Physical Chemistry, 2d ed., Van Nostrand, Princeton, N.J., 1946.*)

osmosis. This experiment illustrates the flow of water from a more dilute to a more concentrated solution when the two solutions are separated by a semipermeable membrane (osmosis); it also demonstrates the reality of "osmotic pressure," in that it can be opposed by a hydrostatic pressure within the tube.

Our understanding of osmotic pressure in quantitative terms was aided greatly by the observation of Pfeffer in 1877 (48) that osmotic pressure was proportional to the concentration of sucrose on the solution side of the membrane and to the absolute temperature (*T*). van't Hoff (49) showed the formal analogy between the laws governing osmotic pressure and Boyle's law for gases. Since, as Pfeffer had shown, π (osmotic pressure) was proportional to solute concentration (*C*), and the concentration *C* in moles per liter is the reciprocal of the volume in liters containing 1 mole (*V*), it followed that for a solution

$$\frac{\pi}{C} = \text{constant} \qquad (1\text{-}16)$$

and

$$\pi V = \text{constant} \qquad (1\text{-}17)$$

Further,

$$\frac{\pi}{T} = \text{constant} \qquad (1\text{-}18)$$

and, combining the two laws for solutions,

$$\pi V = RT \qquad (1\text{-}19)$$

where *R* is a constant. The more familiar expression for van't Hoff's law is

$$\Delta \pi = \Delta CRT \qquad (1\text{-}20)$$

van't Hoff was able to show that *R* for 1 mole of solute had approximately the same value as the gas constant per mole, and it became customary to view osmotic pressure as being derived from the "impacts of the molecules of dissolved substance on the semipermeable membrane" (49), analogous to the pressure produced by gas molecules striking the walls of the container. This view of osmotic pressure was not entirely satisfactory, however; one of its difficulties was the emphasis on the pressure generated by the solutes, whereas flow proceeded in the opposite direction, from pure water to solution. A more satisfactory picture of osmotic pressure can be developed by considering the chemical potential of *water* on either side of the membrane. The addition of solute to the water on one side of the membrane reduces its chemical potential; this can be demonstrated thermodynamically by considering the change in entropy (degree of order) of a pure solvent when solutes are mixed with the solvent. It can be shown that there is an increase in the randomness, or thermodynamic probability, of the resulting solution and hence a decrease in its chemical potential. With this approach, it is possible to view osmosis as the movement of water from a region of higher to a region of lower chemical potential, across an intervening semipermeable membrane. Readers interested in the derivation of the relevant equations are referred to the excellent discussion by Dick (50).

OSMOTIC VERSUS HYDROSTATIC PRESSURE

The relatively great power of osmotic pressure can be seen if one realizes that an 0.1 *M* sucrose solution produces an osmotic pressure of approximately 2.5 atm (1900 mmHg) at 30° C. This greatly exceeds the hydrostatic pressure which the body can achieve; indeed, a difference in osmotic pressure of only 6 mosm across a semipermeable membrane can move as much water as the entire hydrostatic pressure generated by the heart. It must be kept in mind, however, that the entire discussion of osmotic pressure thus far has rested on the assumption that the membranes involved are truly semipermeable. Biologic as well as most synthetic membranes are far from semipermeable, and the meaning of osmotic pressure in relation to "leaky membranes" must now be considered.

LEAKY MEMBRANES

If one places distilled water on one side of a semipermeable membrane and an 0.1 M solution on the other, an osmotic pressure will be generated which will be directly proportional to the solute concentration (or, more properly, the activity of the solute), without regard to the solute used. An 0.1 M solution of sucrose, for example, will exert the same osmotic pressure across a *semipermeable* membrane as an 0.1 M solution of urea (after correction for their activity coefficients).

Where the membrane is permeable to molecules of the solute as well as to solvent molecules, however, this proportionality (based on the van't Hoff relation) no longer holds. Solute molecules will move more or less rapidly from the more concentrated to the less concentrated solution, in a direction opposite to that of the solvent, and osmotic flow of water will be significantly less than predicted. This can be seen in experiments carried out by Grim (51) in which a leaky collodion membrane separated two compartments: one filled with a solution of a given solute, the other filled with distilled water. It can be seen from Fig. 1-7 that the rate of movement of water into the solution compartment (dV/dt) varied greatly with the solute employed. The relatively large molecule, sucrose, produced the highest flow; the smaller molecule, ethylene glycol, a far smaller flow. Urea, the smallest molecule employed, actually produced a "negative osmotic flow," in which the net movement of water proceeded from solution to distilled water. The experiment clearly shows that the osmotic force generated across a leaky membrane depends critically on the interaction between the membrane and the solutes. While solute size may be the critical fac-

tor, other properties of the solute (e.g., its solubility in the membrane) may play an important role as well.

A completely comparable situation exists in biologic membranes, which are far from semipermeable. A number of studies on a variety of tissues, including red cells, renal tubular epithelium, nerve, gastrointestinal epithelium, and amphibian skin and bladder have shown that smaller hydrophilic solutes such as urea, formamide, ethylene glycol, and glycerol, which penetrate cell membranes with relative ease, exert far less than their expected osmotic pressure. Solutes may traverse these epithelia via relatively large channels in the cell membrane (52–55). A more appropriate expression of van't Hoff's law as it applies to such epithelia (and to many synthetic membranes) would be

$$\Delta\pi = \sigma\Delta CRT \qquad (1\text{-}21)$$

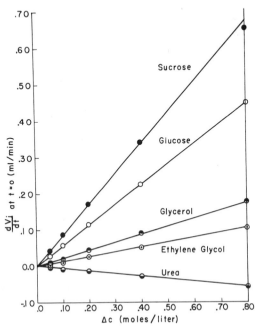

Figure 1-7. The influence of concentration difference (ΔC) and the nature of the solute on osmotic transport rates (dVi/dt) across leaky membranes. (*From E. Grim*, Proc. Soc. Exp. Biol. Med., *83:195, 1953.*)

ONCOTIC PRESSURE

Because of the leakiness of cell membranes, the effective osmotic pressure of small solutes may be considerably reduced, as seen above. This is true, for example, in the case of the capillary bed, where the ions of the plasma can pass freely between the vascular and interstitial compartments, except in so far as they are restrained by Donnan forces. This restraint renders them relatively ineffective in maintaining an osmotic pressure difference between the two compartments. The plasma proteins, although they constitute only a small fraction of the total number of dissolved particles in the plasma, are large enough to remain confined to the plasma compartment, and therefore contribute the major effective osmotic force, preventing excessive fluid loss from the capillaries. This effect of the plasma proteins (particularly albumin) is referred to as the oncotic pressure. The capillary circulation will now be considered as the first example of the relationship between hydrostatic and osmotic forces in the transfer of solutes and water.

THE CAPILLARY CIRCULATION

Movement of water, metabolites, ions, and proteins between the plasma and interstitial fluid is made possible by the existence of the capillary circulation. The total filtering surface of the capillary bed is enormous, of the order of 6300 m² in the adult.

There are two basic conditions that the capillary bed must meet: First, it must be highly permeable, permitting the rapid exchange of material from plasma to cells via the interstitial fluid (and in the reverse direction, from cells back to plasma). Second, it must maintain fluid balance: fluid delivered to the interstitial space at the arterial end must be recovered at the venous end of the capillary. If balance were not maintained, the body would be perpetually edematous, with the interstitial fluid chronically expanded by fluid incompletely recovered by the capillaries. Alternatively, if recovery exceeded delivery, a state of chronic cellular dehydration would exist. How capillaries can maintain their high permeability and yet achieve precise fluid balance has interested biologists for many years.

CAPILLARY PERMEABILITY

The capillaries are highly permeable, and the hydrostatic pressure at the arterial end of the capillary has been shown by Landis (56) to average 32 mmHg. Outward movement of water is therefore favored at the arterial end. To achieve fluid balance, forces must exist at the venous end of the capillary that will result in a net return of water to the circulation. Starling (57) originally proposed that a balance of hydrostatic pressure and colloid osmotic pressures was responsible for fluid balance. At the arterial end, hydrostatic pressure exceeds the colloid osmotic pressure of plasma proteins (25 mmHg), and there is a net outward movement of fluid. At the venous end, hydrostatic pressure drops to 15 mmHg, and the colloid osmotic pressure now exceeds hydrostatic pressure, with a resulting net resorption of fluid. This balance of osmotic and hydrostatic forces is shown in Fig. 1-8.

The basic validity of Starling's proposal has been shown by many studies of the capillary circulation. Some modifications of the traditional model have been proposed, however (30). There appear to be clear-cut differences in the permeability and surface area of the arterial and venous capillaries; both area and permeability are greater at the venous end of the bed. The protein concentration in the interstitial fluid is not negligible but

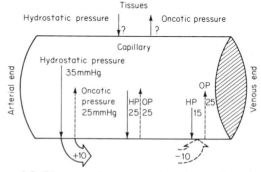

Figure 1-8. Diagrammatic representation of a capillary showing the forces involved in the Starling equilibrium. At the arterial end, hydrostatic pressure exceeds oncotic pressure, and there is a net outflow of fluid. At the venous end, hydrostatic pressure is reduced, and oncotic pressure now results in a net reabsorption of fluid. Modifications of this scheme are discussed in the text; of particular importance is the finding that tissue oncotic pressure may be substantial. (*From Maxwell*, Postgrad. Med., *23:427, 1958.*)

is now believed to be of the order of 2 percent. Hydrostatic tissue pressure has been difficult to measure directly but may be in the range of 0 to +5 mmHg (30). While these findings have added additional variables to the calculation of fluid balance along the capillary bed, the results are still consistent with Starling's proposal, and we may continue to view the partition of body fluids between the circulation and interstitial fluids as the result of a balance between hydrostatic and colloid osmotic pressures.

WATER MOVEMENT ACROSS THE CELL

Early studies of water movement across amphibian skin (58, 59) and capillary wall (60) provided evidence that water flow occurred by Poiseuille flow across channels or "pores" in the cell membrane. The advantage of Poiseuille, or bulk, flow for the osmotic transfer of water can be seen if one compares the expressions for diffusion (the movement of individual water molecules across a membrane, driven by the difference in concentration or osmotic pressure across the membrane) with the expression for Poiseuille flow.

For diffusion:

$$\omega_T = \frac{n\pi r^2 D \, \Delta P}{RT \, \Delta X} \qquad (1\text{-}22)$$

For Poiseuille flow:

$$L_p = \frac{n\pi r^4 D \, \Delta P}{8\eta \overline{V} \, \Delta X} \qquad (1\text{-}23)$$

where ω_T = net flow predicted from diffusion
L_p = total osmotic flow
n = number of channels
r = radius of aqueous channel open to diffusion or flow
D = free diffusion coefficient of water
$\overline{V}$ = partial molar volume of water
R = gas constant
T = absolute temperature
η = bulk viscosity coefficient of water
$\Delta P/\Delta X$ = osmotic pressure gradient across the membrane

The important difference between the two expressions is in the role of the r term. Diffusion is proportional to πr^2, the total area open to the water molecules; Poiseuille flow is proportional to πr^4. This means that for pore radii significantly greater than the radius of a water molecule (approximately 1.5 Å), flow will be the dominant mechanism for water movement, and there will be an increasingly large discrepancy between flow and diffusion as r increases.

Discrepancies of this sort between total osmotic flow and the flow predicted from diffusion alone have been noted in a variety of tissues (61), with Poiseuille flow appearing to account for 100 times more water movement than does diffusion in the vasopressin-treated toad bladder. However, work in a number of laboratories (62–64) has shown that the rate of diffusion of water across the cell membrane can be greatly underestimated if one does not take into account the retarding effects of unstirred layers and tissue components in series with the cell membrane on the measured diffusion rates. In addition, it is possible to block the movement of small solutes such as urea with agents such as phloretin without interfering with osmotic water flow, and also to reduce osmotic water flow without reducing urea transport (65–67). Thus, there appear to be independent pathways for the movement of water and of small solutes across the cell membrane. This does not mean that aqueous channels are absent from the membrane; indeed, there is evidence that water flow does take place in such channels (68). However, such channels appear to have very small radii, since they exclude solutes which are not much larger than a water molecule. We are left with a tentative description of the cell membrane as a membrane penetrated by protein channels of narrow radius, involved largely or exclusively with water flow, and by a smaller number of wider channels involved in selective solute transport.

SOLUTE TRANSPORT IN THE LIVING CELL

THE CELL MEMBRANE

Early studies (69, 70) established the predominantly lipid nature of the plasma membrane and the arrangement of lipid molecules in a bilayer with the hydrophilic portions of the molecules facing in an outward direction. The exact confor-

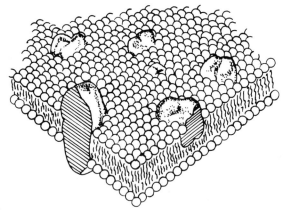

Figure 1-9. Lipid-globular protein mosaic model of the cell membrane, in which globular proteins are imbedded in one leaflet of the lipid bilayer, or traverse the entire bilayer. (*From S. J. Singer, Ann. N.Y. Acad. Sci., 195:16, 1972.*)

mation of membrane proteins and the way in which they were arranged in the bilayer were a subject of debate. It now appears that the proteins are largely globular and are inserted into the bilayer as shown in Fig. 1-9. This is the lipid-globular protein mosaic model for membrane structure, proposed independently by Lenard and Singer (71) and by Wallach and Zahler (72). The proteins may occupy a surface position or may traverse the bilayer. The latter type of protein is probably the most important in relation to transport, since it is a logical pathway for the movement of electrolytes and other hydrophilic solutes, which can penetrate the lipid phase of the membrane only at very low rates. Some of these proteins may be aggregates of two or more identical or similar polypeptide chains which form a water-filled channel through the membrane. Lipophilic solutes, on the other hand, can cross the lipid bilayer directly, and the water molecule may cross both the protein and lipid components of the membrane. The relative rates at which water, glycerol (a hydrophilic molecule), and diacetin (a lipid-soluble ester of glycerol) cross the red cell membrane are shown in Table 1-11.

TRANSPORT MECHANISMS

Solutes may cross the cell membrane by simple diffusion, facilitated diffusion, or by an energy-

Table 1-11. Permeability coefficients of representative molecules across ox red cell membrane

MOLECULE	PERMEABILITY COEFFICIENT, cm/s
Water	47×10^{-4}
Glycerol	2×10^{-4}
Diacetin	1000×10^{-4}

Source: From R. Whittam, *Transport and Diffusion in Red Blood Cells,* Monographs of the Physiological Society, no. 13, The Williams & Wilkins Company, Baltimore, 1964.

linked process of active transport. Their movement may be coupled to the movement of other solutes or to water flow. While it is not possible to deal with this complex topic in any detail, some basic features of transport can be described.

Permeability coefficient

Imagine a membrane separating two large aqueous compartments (Fig. 1–10). Compartment

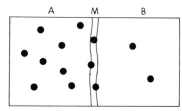

Figure 1-10. Diffusion of a solute from compartment A across a membrane (M) to compartment B.

A contains a solute to which the membrane is permeable. Individual solute molecules enter the membrane phase, and move, on the average, toward solution B, finally entering B. The amount of solute reaching B (solute flux Φ) will depend directly on the area of the membrane available for diffusion (A), the difference in concentration of solute in compartments A and B (ΔC), the time allowed for the process to take place (t), and the ease with which the molecules of the particular solute penetrate the membrane (expressed as the permeability coefficient K). Since the compartments are large, the buildup of solute concentration in compartment B, and its movement in the opposite direction into compartment A, can be considered to be negligible. The flux will vary inversely with the thickness of the membrane (ΔX).

These terms can be combined in the following expression:

$$\Phi = \frac{KA \; \Delta Ct}{\Delta X} \qquad (1\text{-}24)$$

In biologic studies, the thickness of the membrane is not accurately known, and the ΔX term is omitted, giving the expression

$$\Phi = KA \; \Delta Ct \qquad (1\text{-}25)$$

It is customary to refer to the *permeability coefficient* of a given membrane for a given solute or solvent and rearrange the expression:

$$K = \frac{\Phi}{A \; \Delta Ct} \qquad (1\text{-}26)$$

The usual dimensions of the permeability coefficient are centimeters per second, and the term expresses the movement of solute or solvent across a unit area of a particular membrane per unit of concentration difference per unit time.

Simple diffusion

Imagine an experiment in which solute flux (Φ) is determined over a wide range of solute concentration in compartment A. For every tenfold increase in concentration, there is a tenfold increase in Φ. In other words, the rate of movement of solute from A to B is a linear function of its concentration. (Fig. 1–11).

In a second experiment, diffusion is allowed to take place until the concentration of solute in A and B are equal. At this point, it is observed that there is no further change in solute concentration, i.e., solute cannot move "uphill" against a concentration gradient to accumulate in compartment B. Of course, *bidirectional* movement from A to B, and B to A, continues to take place, but at equal rates.

The two properties that have been described, linearity with concentration and inability to move against a concentration gradient, are characteristic of simple diffusion.

Facilitated diffusion

Facilitated diffusion is also a passive process, unable to move against a concentration gradient.

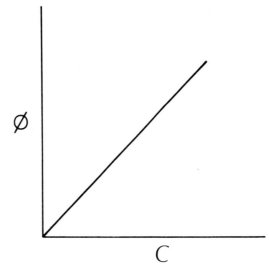

Figure 1-11. Simple diffusion, in which unidirectional flux of a solute (Φ) is a linear function of the solute concentration (C).

However, unlike simple diffusion, facilitated diffusion shows saturation (Fig. 1–12). In addition, a specific solute moving across a cell membrane by facilitated diffusion moves more rapidly than other solutes of comparable size and solubility. Both of these features can be understood if we

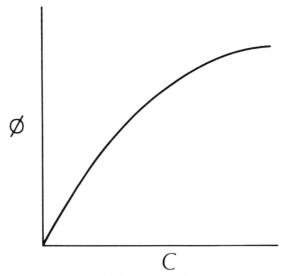

Figure 1–12. Facilitated diffusion, in which Φ shows saturation as C increases.

assume that specific components of the membrane (membrane proteins, as a rule) have a structure that "recognizes" and binds certain solutes. Since there is preferential binding of certain solutes, these solutes will move across the membrane at a relatively high rate. Since the number of binding sites is limited, transport will show saturation at high solute concentrations. Furthermore, there will be competition between solutes of similar structure for binding sites.

The reality of facilitated diffusion has been illustrated in a recent experiment by Kasahara and Hinkle (73). These workers extracted and isolated a membrane protein from human erythrocytes, which, when incorporated into liposomes (small lipid vesicles), proved to be a specific carrier for D-glucose. D-Glucose was transported into the liposome at a considerably faster rate than L-glucose, as in the intact human red cell (Fig. 1-13). Since there was no energy source available, accumulation of D-glucose above its concentration in the outside medium did not take place.

Active transport

The process of active transport is distinguished by its ability to move solutes against an electrochemical concentration gradient (74). Inherent in this definition is the requirement of an energy source, since work must be done to move solutes in an "uphill" direction (75). The simplest ex-

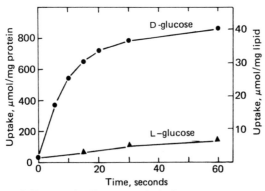

Figure 1-13. D- and L-Glucose uptake by liposomes containing D-glucose transporting protein extracted from human erythrocytes. Acceleration of D-glucose uptake is shown. (*From Kasahara and Hinkle.*)

ample of active transport would be one in which equal concentrations of a nonelectrolyte (e.g., glucose) are present on either side of a membrane and, with time, a net accumulation of glucose in one compartment is observed. The role of metabolic energy in the process is shown when net accumulation ceases upon the addition of a metabolic inhibitor.

When a charged species is being transported, it is more difficult to determine whether the process is active or passive, since both chemical and electric gradients influence its movement. For example, the movement of potassium from an extracellular to an intracellular position may proceed against a steep concentration gradient, but down an electric gradient, since the cell interior is generally negative in relation to the outside medium. Potassium movement would be characterized as active if the favorable potential gradient were not large enough to offset the unfavorable concentration gradient.

More complex problems arise when the movement of several ions across epithelia is considered. Consider an epithelial tissue such as the frog skin or certain segments of the renal tubule, which transport sodium and chloride from the outside, or urinary surface, to the inside, or nutrient surface. An electric potential difference can be measured across such membranes, in which the inside surface is positive in relation to the outside surface. In considering the system, we would say that ionic movement proceeds against a concentration gradient, but additional questions arise. Are both sodium and chloride being "actively transported"? Are one or both ions responsible for the potential generated across the membrane?

Ussing and Zerahn, in their classic experiments on the isolated frog skin (76) were able to provide clear-cut answers to these questions. They employed the apparatus shown in Fig. 1–14, in which the frog skin (S) was mounted between two identical salt solutions and the potential measured by two bridges (A and A') located close to the membrane and connected to a potentiometer (p). A second circuit entered the chambers via electrodes B and B'. Current could be passed through this second circuit by batteries at D; the current passed was read on a microammeter

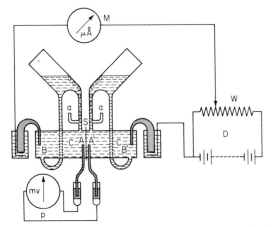

Figure 1-14. The short-circuiting apparatus of Ussing and Zerahn.

(M). In an experiment, the spontaneous potential generated by active transport could be brought to zero ("short-circuited") by means of the battery circuit; under these conditions, a current was observed on the ammeter. Ussing and Zerahn then determined, in short-circuited skins, the net movement of isotopically labeled sodium ions; this net movement proved, when expressed as current, to be identical to the current required to bring the spontaneous potential to zero. Several important conclusions emerged from these experiments: First, sodium was the only actively transported ion, since it was the only ion showing net transport when the potential difference across the skin was abolished; second, sodium moving in the non-short-circuited skin toward the region of positive potential could be properly described as moving against an electrochemical gradient; and, third, the chloride ion moved passively across the skin, its asymmetric movement being the response of a negatively charged ion to the positive potential established by active sodium transport. The total potential across the cell was attributed to the sum of an inward diffusion potential created by sodium entry across the outward-facing surface, and a more complex set of events across the inward-facing surface in which potassium moved into the cell in exchange for sodium across the pump and then diffused out of the cell to generate the second component of the total potential (see Fig. 1-16A). This scheme has been modified, as will be discussed shortly.

It should be noted that while chloride movement is passive in the frog skin, it has an important influence on the magnitude of the sodium potential. If, for example, the skin is made virtually impermeable to chloride by treating it with copper sulfate or by substituting a nonpenetrating anion like sulfate for the chloride, the sodium potential becomes very large, since it is not effectively dissipated by the "shunting" effect of the accompanying anion.[6] Skins which are highly permeable to chloride, on the other hand, would have a lower potential at any given rate of sodium transport. It has recently been proposed that the resistance to accompanying anions may depend partly on the ease with which the anion can traverse the tight junctions between epithelial cells (77). Coupled or "neutral" anion and cation transport also reduces potential.

While chloride is not responsible for the direction of the potential in frog skin, there are tissues in which chloride transport does establish the direction of the potential. These include the thick ascending limb of the loop of Henle (78), the cornea (79), the dogfish rectal gland (80, 81), and the gill (82). Bidirectional transport also influences potential.

THE ROLE OF ACTIVE TRANSPORT

A number of functions are served by the process of active transport, and it is useful to consider first the functions that apply to all cells and finally those that apply to the more specialized group of transporting epithelia.

TRANSPORT AND CELL METABOLISM

All cells require substrates to support their metabolism and often must gather these substrates from the surrounding extracellular fluid. Muscle cells, for example, may require glucose during ac-

---

[6] The potential generated by the active transport of a cation may be dissipated in another way; the movement of a second cation in the opposite direction. An example is Na^+/K^+ exchange, where potassium moves passively down the potential gradient established by active sodium transport.

tivity at a considerably higher rate than can be produced by simple diffusion. A complex transport system for the accumulation of glucose is present in the outer membrane of muscle cells and is capable of meeting this metabolic requirement (83). Similiar systems exist for the accumulation of amino acids. An example of this type of transport is discussed at the conclusion of the chapter.

THE MAINTENANCE OF CELL VOLUME.

In the discussion of the Gibbs-Donnan equilibrium, it was pointed out that if an impermeant anion (or cation) were present on one side of a membrane, the total concentration of diffusible ions at equilibrium would be greater on the side of the impermeant ion. This relatively larger ionic concentration (plus, of course, the presence of the impermeant anion) produces a difference in osmotic pressure across the membrane. In a system in which living cells, containing a high concentration of protein anions, are surrounded by extracellular fluid, a considerable osmotic pressure difference would be expected. This would be compensated for by a movement of water (and then of ions) into the cell, cell swelling, and the generation of an intracellular hydrostatic pressure sufficient to balance the difference in osmotic pressure. This solution to the problem would be unphysiologic, to say the least, and could result in the rupture of the cell membrane. The problem is solved instead by the outward active transport of sodium. Transport in this direction generates a potential difference across the cell membrane, with the inside negative in relation to the outside. The negative inside potential has two effects: it enhances the inward movement of potassium, and it inhibits, by repulsion, the inward movement of chloride. Net ionic movement is outward, and this balances the osmotic pressure difference across the cell membrane, maintaining cell volume. As pointed out by Leaf (84), the importance of active transport in maintaining cell volume can be demonstrated by cooling the cell to 0°; outward transport of sodium is greatly re-

duced, the potential difference decreases, sodium and chloride enter the cell, potassium leaks out, and the cell swells. The relationship of ion transport to cell volume is shown schematically in Fig. 1-15.

The result of the outward transport of sodium is, of course, the marked difference in intracellular and extracellular ion distribution summarized earlier in Table 1-10. Potassium is the major intracellular cation, and sodium the major extracellular cation.

RADIAL AND DIRECTIONAL TRANSPORT

The accumulation of substrates and the active extrusion of sodium are, therefore, general require-

REGULATION OF CELL VOLUME

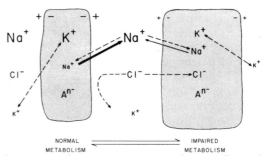

Figure 1-15. Schematic representation of a normally metabolizing cell and a cell whose metabolism has been reversibly inhibited. In the normally metabolizing cell (left), Na^+ diffuses into the cell and K^+ out (dashed lines). However, active ion transport extrudes Na^+ (solid arrow) and causes K^+ uptake sufficient to maintain high intracellular K^+ content and low intracellular Na^+ content, respectively, in the steady state. The cell membrane potential is shown (+) outside and (−) inside. The membrane potential is depicted as preventing entry of chloride into the cell, A^{n-} represents nondiffusible polyvalent intracellular anions (such as proteins and nucleic acids). The situation in a swollen cell is depicted at right. Inhibition of metabolism slows or stops the ion pump so that Na^+ entering the cell by diffusion cannot be extruded and the K^+ lost from the cell cannot be replaced. The cell membrane potential diminishes, and chloride now enters the cell. This requires further entry of Na^+ into the cell to preserve electric neutrality. The increased solute content of the cell results in secondary entry of water, and the cell becomes swollen. (*From Leaf.*)

ments of living cells. Muscle cells, red blood cells, bacteria, and many other nonpolar cells engage in this type of transport, which proceeds in a *radial* fashion over the entire cell membrane. A second, and distinctive, type of transport takes place across polar cells (cells whose opposite surfaces differ in structure and function); this can be described as directional transport and is typical of a wide variety of epithelial cells. These cells border fluid-filled compartments such as the renal tubule or gastrointestinal tract and are involved in the secretion of material into, and resorption of material from these compartments. These epithelial cells are capable, then, of net transfers of solute and water and perform a critical role in maintaining body homeostasis. The renal tubular epithelial cells, for example, are responsible for the resorption of 99 percent of the salt and water and virtually all of the glucose and amino acids filtered at the glomerulus; they regulate acid-base balance by secretion of hydrogen ions into the tubular fluid and potassium balance by secretion of potassium. Movement of ions across these cells is characterized by a series of steps in which the ions are transported across specific sites in the membrane (often accompanied by exchanges with other ions), bound to specific carriers, and eventually secreted or resorbed. One step or more may be under endocrine control.

THE MOLECULAR BASIS OF ACTIVE TRANSPORT

There has been considerable progress in our understanding of the molecular basis of active transport since the previous edition of this text was written. Sodium-potassium-activated ATPase remains the most completely characterized transport system, but there is increasing awareness of the role of other systems in both mammalian and nonmammalian cells.

SODIUM-POTASSIUM-ACTIVATED ATPASE

In 1957, Skou (85) described the properties of an enzyme found in the leg nerve of the shore crab which appeared to have an important relationship to active sodium transport. The important characteristics of this enzyme, sodium-potassium-activated ATPase, were that it was involved in the hydrolysis of ATP (the principal source of energy for active transport), that it was maximally activated only in the presence of sodium and potassium (magnesium was required as well), and that it was present in the outer membrane of the nerve cell. All these features suggested strongly that the enzyme was involved in the sodium-transporting system. Since Skou's report, considerable evidence has accumulated confirming the importance of this enzyme. It is present in an enormous number of cell membranes, its activity is inhibited by cardiac glycosides which also inhibit active sodium transport in vivo, and its activity in a given tissue can be shown to vary in relationship to the level of sodium transport taking place in the tissue. A number of examples of the last point can be given. Tosteson and his associates (86) have found that the red cell Na^+–K^+–ATPase in a strain of sheep with a genetically determined low concentration of potassium in their red blood cells is lower than in normal sheep, who are able to maintain a high Na^+–K^+ gradient. The activity of Na^+–K^+–ATPase in the kidney increases under circumstances in which sodium transport is increased (87), such as removal of the opposite kidney or administration of adrenal steroids; activity is reduced following adrenalectomy. Activity increases in the presence of increased renal potassium excretion (88). The activity of the enzyme in the gills of euryhaline fish rises strikingly when the fish goes from fresh water to salt water, an adapatation which allows the increased excretion of sodium in salt water (89, 90).

A major advance has been the isolation of Na^+–K^+–ATPase from the dogfish rectal gland by Hokin and coworkers (91) who have been able to incorporate the enzyme into artificial liposomes and, using ATP as a source of energy, demonstrate the coupled transport of sodium and potassium. The ratio of sodium to potassium transport in their preparation was approximately 3:2, and transport was inhibited by ouabain.

OTHER TRANSPORT SYSTEMS

$Na^+–K^+–ATPase$ does not appear to be the only transport system for sodium. Whittenbury and Proverbio (92), in their studies of sodium extrusion from guinea pig kidney cortex slices, described at least two sodium pumps, one inhibited by ouabain and presumably dependent on $Na^+–K^+–ATPase$, the second inhibited by ethacrynic acid. Studies on the isolated perfused rat kidney (93) have suggested the presence of three distinct transport mechanisms: one dependent on $Na^+–K^+–ATPase$ and responsible for approximately one-half of total sodium reabsorption; a second associated with bicarbonate reabsorption, inhibited by acetazolamide and responsible for 15 to 20 percent of sodium reabsorption; and a residual system, uncharacterized, but inhibited by cooling. The problem of multiple sodium pumps has been reviewed by Whittenbury and Grantham (94).

Sodium and potassium are not the only ions that are transported by the ATPase system. For example, a magnesium-calcium ATPase which is capable of actively transporting calcium has been isolated from the sarcoplasmic reticulum of rabbit muscle (95).

COUPLED TRANSPORT

Until now we have considered directional transport across epithelia largely in terms of the movement of single solutes across the cell. There is increasing evidence, however, that the movement of anions and cations, as well as ions and inorganic solutes, may proceed in a coupled fashion, as well as singly, across certain epithelial membranes. An early suggestion that sodium and chloride may move as an ion pair was made by Shanes (96) in his studies of ion transport across nerve. Nellans and coworkers (97) estimated that approximately 20 percent of the total sodium and chloride influxes across the brush border of rabbit ileum are mediated by a coupled NaCl influx. Coupled NaCl movement has recently been proposed for the gill of seawater fish (98) and for the dogfish rectal gland (81).

The observation that sodium influences the movement of organic solutes such as glucose and amino acids across cell membranes was first made in studies of the small intestine (99) and has now been reported in a variety of cells (100–102). Studies of the renal proximal tubule have shown that D-glucose and sodium appear to cross the brush border together in a charged sodium-glucose carrier complex (103, 104); a similar relationship between sodium and amino acid transport in proximal tubule has been described (105, 106). There is a mutual enhancement of sodium and organic solute reabsorption by the proximal tubule when both components of the coupled transport system are present. For example, when glucose or amino acids are present in the luminal fluid perfusing the isolated rabbit proximal tubule, fluid absorption and transepithelial potential difference are enchanced (106, 107). On the other hand, the presence of sodium enhances the reabsorption of α-methyl-D-glycoside (108) and amino acids (109). One may visualize a carrier in the luminal membrane whose affinity to sodium is enhanced by organic solutes, and vice versa. The process of cotransport appears to be dependent on the ability of the cell to maintain a low intracellular concentration of sodium by active extrusion of sodium across the basolateral membrane. Sodium in the luminal solution can then move across the luminal membrane down its electrochemical gradient, with cotransport of the organic solute. Thus, while cotransport itself may not be an active process, it depends on and is responsive to the active transport of sodium across the opposite border of the cell. Figure 1-16 depicts a number of the transport mechanisms considered in this section.

SOLVENT DRAG

Another type of coupling which is of importance is solvent drag, the coupling of water and solute transport. This was first described by Andersen and Ussing (59), who noted that the movement of solutes across the toad skin was accelerated in the presence of an osmotic water flow, to produce a net movement of solute in the "downstream" direction. While the discovery of solvent drag first appeared to support the view that solutes and water traversed common channels in the cell

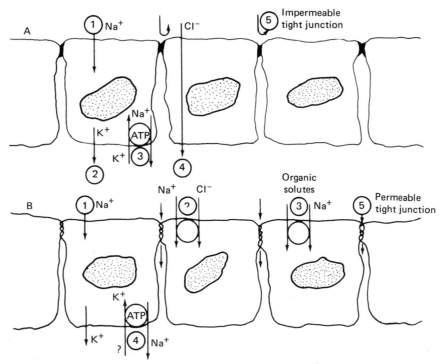

Figure 1-16. A. Representation of Ussing's hypothesis for transepithelial transport. Sodium enters the cells passively (1). Potassium leaves the cells following its electrochemical gradient (2). Ion concentrations are maintained by the action of a tightly coupled Na–K–ATPase (3). Chloride moves passively, following the potential differences generated by the transport of sodium (4). The junctions are impermeable to ion movements (5). B. New concepts of epithelial organization. In addition to the electrogenic sodium path (1), at least two other systems for Na entry into the cells have been described: a neutral system in which Na and Cl movements are coupled (2) and a system in which the movements of Na and organic solutes are coupled (3). The pumped movements at the basal surface very likely are electrogenic (4). The permeability of the tight junctions varies considerably among different epithelia (5). More than one individual process for sodium entry can be found in the same epithelium. Chloride can move either following the electrochemical gradient created by the cation pump as in Ussing's model or possibly through an independent anion active transport system. (*From Erlij.*)

membrane, it is more likely that the coupling of water and solute movement takes place in the intercellular spaces (110).

TRANSPORT AND EPITHELIAL STRUCTURE

Transport across epithelia depends on events at the two cell surfaces and on the overall organization of the epithelium itself. Of importance here are the orientation of the epithelial cells, the mutual interaction of cells via gap junctions, and the roles of the tight junction and lateral intercellular space.

THE ORIENTATION OF EPITHELIAL CELLS

Reabsorptive epithelial cells are polar in nature, with their luminal surface (often microvillar in structure) facing a solution such as tubular urine, gastrointestinal fluid, or bile. The opposite (serosal) surface faces interstitial fluid and nutrient capillaries. In an epithelium such as that of the renal tubule, the luminal surface is the site of the coupled transport systems described earlier. Active transport may also take place across the surface. The serosal or basolateral surface is the site of active sodium extrusion. It is also the site of hormone attachment and of the membrane-bound adenyl cyclase. Although the two cell surfaces are spatially separated, there is a high degree of interaction between them, mediated by changes in intracellular potential, changes in intracellular ion concentration, intracellular "messengers" such as cyclic AMP, and other feedback mechanisms.

MUTUAL INTERACTION OF CELLS

In 1965, Loewenstein and coworkers (111) demonstrated free electric communication between adjoining epithelial cells. Subsequent studies (112) showed that solutes can be transferred laterally from cell to cell, apparently through specialized "gap junctions." The permeability of the transfer pathway depends critically on the level of intracellular calcium (113). The finding of lateral communication between epithelial cells raises the possibility that specialized cells within an epithelium may contribute to overall epithelial function.

THE ROLE OF THE TIGHT JUNCTION.

In 1963, Farquhar and Palade (114) published their important study of junctional complexes between epithelial cells. These complexes are present as bands encircling the apical end of epithelial cells and are responsible for the tight cell-to-cell adherence typical of epithelia. The structure of a representative junctional complex is shown in Fig. 1-17. Functionally, the junctional complexes act as seals, separating the solutions on opposite sides of the epithelium. However, it has become clear that there are great differences in the degree of "tightness" of junctional complexes, especially with respect to their permeability to ions. This was suggested in a number of studies employing cable analysis (115, 116). In a study of the *Necturus* gallbladder, a tissue characterized by a low transepithelial resistance and potential, Fromter (117) showed that the separate ohmic resistances across the mucosal and serosal cell membranes were in fact quite high (4470 and 2880 ohms/cm^2, respectively), and concluded that the very low resistance measured across the en-

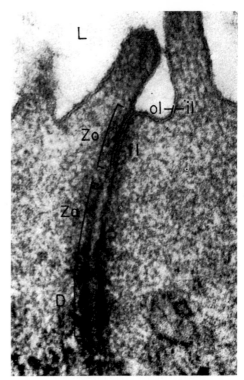

Figure 1-17. Junctional complex between two epithelian cells of the mucosa of the gallbladder (guinea pig), showing the occluding zonule (Zo) followed by adhering zonule (Za), followed by the desmosome (D). The trilaminar structure of the apical cell membrane can be clearly distinguished and traced into the occluding zonule. The fusion line (fl) is also visible within the junction. ×155,000. (*From Farquhar and Palade.*)

tire epithelium (324 ohms/cm^2) was the result of a low-resistance shunt pathway between the cells through the junctional complex. As a consequence of these and other studies, epithelia have been classified as high-resistance, high-potential epithelia, with truly tight junctional complexes (renal collecting duct, frog skin, urinary bladder, gastric mucosa) and low-resistance, low-potential epithelia, with relatively ion-permeable tight junctions (proximal tubule, small intestine choroid plexus). The renal distal tubule occupies a somewhat intermediate position. Support for the key role of the tight junction has been provided by the morphologic studies of Erlij and his associates (77), who showed a correlation between the

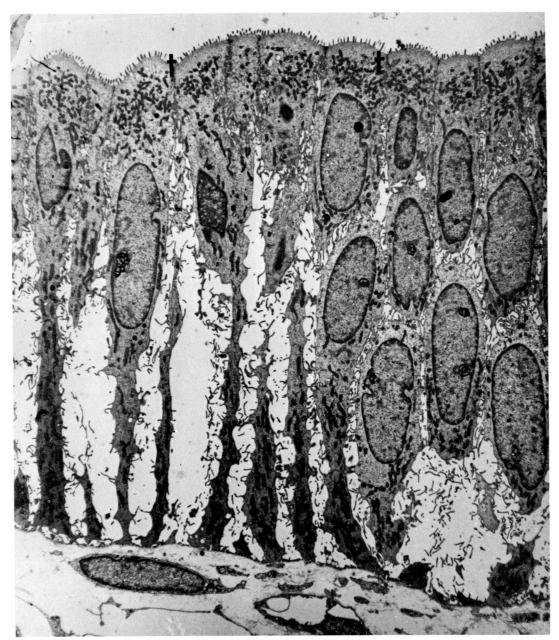

Figure 1-18. Rabbit gallbladder epithelium transporting sodium chloride and water from its luminal (upper) surface to its serosal surface, showing the extreme degree to which the intercellular spaces can expand. The epithelial cells are closely joined near their luminal surface by a tight junction: the intercellular channels below this junction may change their dimensions greatly, as suggested by comparing the left and right portions of the figure. (Approximately ×2100.) (*From O. H. Wheeler, G. I. Kaye, R. T. Whitlock, and N. Lane, J. Cell. Biol., 30:237, 1966.*)

electric properties of a variety of epithelia and the extent to which the electron-dense metal lanthanum penetrated the junctional complex.

The physiologic importance of this diversity among epithelia is not entirely clear. However, it is advantageous for structures such as the proximal tubule, which are engaged in high rates of solute and water reabsorption, to be able to transport sodium without building up high transmembrane potentials, since such adverse potentials would increase the energy required for transport.

THE LATERAL INTERCELLULAR SPACE

In series with the tight junction there is a relatively long and open intercellular channel, termed the *lateral intercellular space* (Fig. 1-18). In reabsorptive epithelia, it is a site into which sodium is actively transported across the basolateral cell membrane. In their studies of the role of the lateral intercellular space, Diamond and Bossert (118) pointed out that its permeability properties and dimensions exerted an important effect on the osmolality of the fluid emerging from both reabsorptive and secretory epithelia. While the original proposals of Diamond and Bossert will probably require modification (see 119, 120) there is little doubt that the intercellular space is of major importance in regulating water and solute transport. As discussed earlier, solvent drag probably takes place in these long channels. In addition, and also of major importance, is the observation that sodium transport into the lateral intercellular space of the proximal tubule appears to be responsive to changes in the oncotic pressure of the peritubular capillaries, a subject that will be discussed in Chap. 3.

REFERENCES

1. Henderson, L. J.: *The Fitness of the Environment*, The Macmillan Company, New York, 1913.
2. Bernal, J. D., and R. H. Fowler: A theory of water and ionic solution, with particular reference to hydrogen and hydroxyl ions, *J. Chem. Phys.*, **1**:515, 1933.
3. Frank, H. S., and M. W. Evans: Free volume and entropy in condensed systems. III. Entropy in binary liquid mixtures; partial molal entropy in dilute solutions; structure and thermodynamics in aqueous electrolytes, *J. Chem. Phys.*, **13**:507, 1945.
4. Hempling, H. G.: Permeability of the Ehrlich ascites tumor cell to water, *J. Gen. Physiol.*, **44**:365, 1960.
5. Hays, R. M., and A. Leaf: The state of water in the isolated toad bladder in the presence and absence of vasopressin, *J. Gen. Physiol.*, **45**:933, 1962.
6. Hechter, O.: Role of water in the molecular organization of cell membranes, *Fed. Proc.*, **24**(suppl. 15):91, 1965.
7. Klotz, I. M.: Protein hydration and behavior, *Science*, **128**:815, 1958.
8. Pauling, L.: A molecular theory of general anesthesia, *Science*, **134**:15, 1961.
9. Forbes, R. M., H. H. Mitchell, and A. R. Cooper: Further studies on the gross composition and mineral elements of the adult human body, *J. Biol. Chem.*, **223**:969, 1956.
10. Hevesy, G., and E. Hofer: Die Verweilzeit des Wassers im Menschilchen Korper, Untersucht mit Hilfe von "Schwerem" Wasser als Indicator, *Klin. Wochenschr.*, **13**:1524, 1934.
11. Moore, F. D.: Determination of total body water and solids with isotopes, *Science*, **104**:157, 1946.
12. Pace, N., L. Kline, H. K. Schachman, and M. Harfenist: Studies on body composition. IV. Use of radioactive hydrogen for measurement in vivo of total body water, *J. Biol. Chem.*, **168**:459, 1947.
13. Edelman, F. S., J. M. Olney, A. H. James, L. Brooks, and F. D. Moore: Body composition: Studies in the human being by the dilution principle, *Science*, **115**:447, 1952.
14. Steele, J. M., E. Y. Berger, M. F. Dunning, and B. B. Brodie: Total body water in man, *Am. J. Physiol.*, **162**:313, 1950.
15. Schloerb, P. R., B. J. Friis-Hansen, I. S. Edelman, A. K. Solomon, and F. D. Moore: The measurement of total body water in the human subject by deuterium oxide dilution: With considerations of the dynamics of deuterium distribution, *J. Clin. Invest.*, **29**:1296, 1950.
16. Kruhøffer, P.: Inulin as an indicator for the extracellular space, *Acta Physiol. Scand.*, **11**:16, 1946.

17. Ogston, A. G., and C. F. Phelps: The partition of solutes between buffer solutions and solutions containing hyaluronic acid, *Biochem. J.*, **78**:827, 1961.

18. Mauro, A., and W. R. Adams: The structure of the sarcolemma of the frog skeletal muscle fiber, *J. Biophys. Biochem. Cytol.*, **10**(suppl.): 177, 1961.

19. Edelman, I. S., and J. Leibman: Anatomy of body water and electrolytes, *Am. J. Med.*, **27**:256, 1959.

20. White, H. L., and D. Rolfe: Whole body inulin and sucrose spaces in the rats, *Am. J. Physiol.*, **188**:151, 1957.

21. Barratt, T. M., and M. Walser: Extracellular fluid in individual tissues and in whole animals: The distribution of radiosulfate and radiobromide, *J. Clin. Invest.*, **48**:56, 1969.

22. Ryan, R. J., L. R. Pascal, T. Inoye, and L. Bernstein: Experiences with radiosulfate in the estimation of physiologic extracellular water in healthy and abnormal men, *J. Clin. Invest.*, **35**:1119, 1956.

23. Pluth., J. R., J. Cleland, C. K. Meador, W. N. Tauxe, J. W. Kirklin, and F. D. Moore: Effect of surgery on the volume distribution of extracellular fluid determined by the sulfate and bromide methods, in P. E. Bergner and C. C. Lushbaugh (eds.), *Compartments, Pools and Spaces in Medical Physiology*, U.S. Atomic Energy Commission Symposium 11, 1967, p. 217.

24. Moore, F. D., J. D. McMurrey, H. V. Parker, and I. C. Magnus: Body composition: Total body water and electrolytes: Intravascular and extravascular phase volumes, *Metabolism*, **5**:447, 1956.

25. Crispell, K. R., B. Porter, and R. T. Nieset: Studies of plasma volume using human serum albumin tagged with radioactive iodine[131], *J. Clin. Invest.*, **29**:513, 1950.

26. Rothschild, M. A., A. Bauman, R. S. Yalow, and S. A. Berson: Tissue distribution of I[131] labelled human serum albumin following intravenous administration, *J. Clin. Invest.*, **34**:1354, 1955.

27. Bassett, S. H.: Disorders of calcium and phosphorus metabolism, in M. H. Maxwell and C. R. Kleeman (eds.), *Clinical Disorders of Fluid and Electrolyte Metabolism*, 1st ed., McGraw-Hill Book Company, New York, 1962, chap. 5.

28. Walser, M.: Magnesium metabolism, *Rev. Physiol Biochem. Pharmacol.*, **59**:185, 1967.

29. West, E. S., W. R. Todd, H. S. Mason, and J. T. van Bruggen: *Textbook of Biochemistry*, 4th ed., The Macmillan Company, New York, 1966, chap. 5.

30. Wiederhielm, C. A.: Dynamics of transcapillary fluid exchange, *J. Gen. Physiol.*, **52**(pt. 2):29s, 1968.

31. Laurent, T. C.: The exchange of macromolecules from polysaccharide Media, in G. Quintarelli (ed.), *The Chemical Physiology of Mucopolysaccharides*, Little, Brown and Company, Boston, 1968.

32. Bergstrom, J.: Muscle electrolytes in man, *Scand. J. Clin. Lab. Invest.*, **14**(suppl. 68), 1962.

33. Kernan, R. P.: *Cell K*, Butterworth, Inc., Washington, 1965.

34. Bittar, E. E.: *Cell pH*, Butterworth, Inc., Washington, 1964.

35. Walser, M.: Extracellular fluid in individual tissues in relation to extracellular fluid in the body as a whole, in P. E. Bergner and C. C. Lushbaugh (eds.), *Compartments, Pools and Spaces in Medical Physiology*, U.S. Atomic Energy Commission Symposium 11, 1967, p. 241.

36. Maffly, L. H., and A. Leaf: Intracellular osmolarity of mammalian tissues, *J. Clin. Invest.*, **37**:916, 1958.

37. Nanninga, L. B.: Calculation of free magnesium, calcium and potassium in muscle, *Biochim. Biophys. Acta*, **54**:338, 1961.

38. Ling, G. N.: *A Physical Theory of the Living State: The Association-Induction Hypothesis*, Blaisdell Publishing Company, New York, 1962.

39. Fenichel, I. R., and S. B. Horowitz: Intracellular transport, in R. M. Dowben (ed.), *Biological Membranes*, Little, Brown and Company, Boston, 1969, chap. 6.

40. Lev, A. A.: Determination of activity and activity coefficients of potassium and sodium ions in frog muscle fibres, *Nature*, **201**:1132, 1964.

41. Gamble, J. L., Jr., and R. C. Hess: Mitochondrial electrolytes, *Am. J. Physiol.*, **210**:765, 1966.

42. Vasington, F. D., and J. V. Murphy: Ca^{++} uptake by rat kidney mitochondria and its dependence on respiration and phosphorylation, *J. Biol. Chem.*, **237**:2670, 1962.

43. Carafoli, E., C. S. Rossi, and A. L. Lehninger: Cation and anion balance during active accumulation of Ca^{++} and Mg^{++} by isolated mitochondria, *J. Biol. Chem.*, **239**:3055, 1964.

44. Allfrey, V. G., R. Meudt, J. W. Hopkins, and A. E. Mirsky: Sodium dependent "transport" reactions in the cell nucleus and their role in protein and nucleic acid synthesis, *Proc. Natl. Acad. Sci. USA*, **47**:907, 1961.

45. Mast, S. O., and W. L. Doyle: Ingestion of fluid by *Amoeba*, *Protoplasma*, **20**:555, 1934.

46. Palade, G. E.: The endoplasmic reticulum, *J. Biophys. Biochem. Cytol.*, **2**(suppl.):85, 1956.

47. Pitts, R. F.: *Physiology of the Kidney and Body Fluids*, 2d ed., Year Book Medical Publishers, Inc., Chicago, 1968.

48. Pfeffer, W.: *Osmotische Uentersuchungen*, W. Engelmann, Leipzig, 1877.

49. van't Hoff, J. H.: Die Rolle des osmotischen Druckes in der Analogie zwischen Loesungen und Gasen, *Z. F. Physikal. Chem.*, **1**:481, 1887.

50. Dick, D. A. T.: *Cell Water*, Butterworth, Inc., Washington, 1966.

51. Grim, E.: Relation between pressure and concentration difference across membranes permeable to solute and solvent, *Proc. Soc. Exp. Biol. Med.*, **93**:195, 1953.

52. Hays, R. M., S. H. Harkness, and N. Franki: The movement of urea and other small molecules across the toad bladder, in B. Schmidt-Nielsen (ed.), *Proceedings of the International Colloquia on Urea and the Kidney*, Exerpta Med., Amsterdam, 1970, p. 149.

53. Lief, P. D., and A. Essig: Urea transport in the toad bladder; coupling of urea flows, *J. Memb. Biol.*, **12**:159, 1973.

54. Eggena, P.: Inhibition of vasopressin-stimulated urea transport across the toad bladder by thiourea, *J. Clin. Invest.*, **52**:2963, 1973.

55. Levine, S. D., and R. E. Worthington: Amide transport channels across toad urinary bladder, *J. Memb. Biol.*, **26**:91, 1976.

56. Landis, E. M.: Microinjection studies of capillary blood pressure in human skin, *Heart*, **15**:209, 1930.

57. Starling, E. H.: On the absorption of fluids from the connective tissue spaces, *J. Physiol. (London)*, **19**:312, 1896.

58. Koefoed-Johnsen, V., and H. H. Ussing: The contributions of diffusion and flow to the passage of D_2O through living membranes, *Acta Physiol. Scand.*, **28**:60, 1953.

59. Andersen, B., and H. H. Ussing: Solvent drag on non-electrolytes during osmotic flow through isolated toad skin and its response to antidiuretic hormone, *Acta Physiol. Scand.*, **39**:228, 1957.

60. Pappenheimer, J. R.: Passage of molecules through capillary walls, *Physiol. Rev.*, **33**:387, 1953.

61. Hays, R. M.: The movement of water across vasopressin-sensitive epithelia, in F. Bronner and A. Kleinzeller (eds.), *Current Topics in Membranes and Transport*, vol. 3, Academic Press, New York, 1972, p. 341.

62. Hays, R. M., and N. Franki: The role of water diffusion in the action of vasopressin, *J. Memb. Biol.*, **2**:263, 1970.

63. Schafer, J. A., and T. Andreoli: Cellular constraints to diffusion: The effect of antidiuretic hormone on water flows in isolated membrane collecting tubules, *J. Clin. Invest.*, **51**:1264, 1972.

64. Parisi, M., and Z. F. Piccini: The penetration of water into the epithelium of toad urinary bladder and its modification by oxytocin, *J. Memb. Biol.*, **12**:227, 1973.

65. Levine, S., N. Franki, and R. M. Hays: Effect of phloretin on water and solute movement on the toad bladder, *J. Clin. Invest.*, **52**:1435, 1973.

66. Levine, S. D., R. D. Levine, R. E. Worthington, and R. M. Hays: Selective inhibition of osmotic water flow by general anesthetics on toad urinary bladder, *J. Clin. Invest.*, **58**:980, 1976.

67. Hays, R. M.: Antidiuretic hormone, *N. Engl. J. Med.*, **295**:659, 1976.

68. Finkelstein, A.: Nature of the water permeability increase induced by antidiuretic hormone (ADH) in toad urinary bladder and related tissues, *J. Gen. Physiol.*, **68**:137, 1976.

69. Gorter, E., and F. Grendel: On bimolecular layers of lipoids on the chromocytes of the blood, *J. Exp. Med.*, **41**:439, 1925.

70. Danielli, J. F., and H. A. Davson: A contribution to the theory of permeability of thin films, *J. Cell. Physiol.*, **5**:495, 1935.

71. Lenard, J., and S. J. Singer: Protein conformation in cell membrane preparations as studied by optical rotatory dispersion and circular dichroism, *Proc. Natl. Acad. Sci. USA*, **56**:1828, 1966.

72. Wallach, D. F. H., and P. H. Zahler: Protein conformations in cellular membranes, *Proc. Natl. Acad. Sci. USA*, **56**:1552, 1966.

73. Kasahara, M., and P. C. Hinkle: Reconstitution of

D-glucose transport catalyzed by a protein fraction from human erythrocytes in sonicated liposomes, *Proc. Natl. Acad. Sci. USA,* **73**:396, 1976.

74. Rosenberg, T.: On accumulation and active transport in biological systems. I. Thermodynamic considerations, *Acta Chem. Scand.,* **2**:14, 1948.

75. Kedem, O.: Criteria of active transport, in A. Kleinzeller and A. Kotyk (eds.), *Membrane Transport and Metabolism,* Czechoslovak Academy of Science, Prague, 1961, p. 87.

76. Ussing H. H., and K. Zerahn: Active transport of sodium as the source of electrical current in the short circuited isolated frog skin, *Acta Physiol. Scand.,* **23**:110, 1951.

77. Erlij, D.: Solute transport across isolated epithelia, *Kidney Int.,* **9**:76, 1976.

78. Burg, M., and N. Green: Function of the thick ascending limb of Henle's loop, *Am. J. Physiol.,* **224**:659, 1973.

79. Zadunaisky, J. A.: Active transport of chloride in frog cornea, *Am. J. Physiol.,* **211**:506, 1966.

80. Hayslett, J. P., D. A. Schon, M. Epstein, and C. A. M. Hogben: In vitro perfusion of the dog-fish rectal gland, *Am. J. Physiol.,* **226**:1188, 1974.

81. Stoff, J. S., P. Silva, M. Field, J. Forrest, A. Stevens, and F. H. Epstein: Cyclic AMP regulation of active chloride transport in the rectal gland of marine elasmobranchs, *J. Exp. Zool.,* **199**:443, 1977.

82. Garcia-Romen, F., and J. Maetz: The mechanism of sodium and chloride uptake by the gills of a fresh water fish *Carassius auratus.* I. Evidence for an independent uptake of sodium and chloride ions, *J. Gen. Physiol.,* **47**:1195, 1964.

83. Park, C. R., H. E. Morgen, M. J. Henderson, D. M. Nejen, E. Cadenas, and R. L. Post: The regulation of glucose uptake in muscle as studied in the perfused rat heart, *Recent Prog. Horm. Res.,* **17**:493, 1961.

84. Leaf, A.: Regulation of intracellular fluid volume and disease, *Am. J. Med.,* **49**:291, 1970.

85. Skou, J. C.: Influence of some cations on adenosine triphosphatase from peripheral nerves, *Biochim. Biophys. Acta,* **23**:394, 1957.

86. Tosteson, D. C., R. H. Moulton, and M. Blaustein: Enzymatic basis for difference in active cation transport in two genetic types of sheep red cells, *Fed. Proc.,* **19**:128, 1960.

87. Katz, A. I., and F. H. Epstein: Role of sodium potassium-activated adenosine triphosphatase in reabsorption of sodium by kidney, *J. Clin. Invest.,* **46**:1999, 1967.

88. Epstein, F. H., and P. Silva: Role of Na, K-ATPase in renal function, *Ann. N.Y. Acad. Sci.,* **242**:519, 1974.

89. Kamiya, M., and S. Utida: Sodium-potassium-activated adenosine triphosphatase activity in gills of fresh water, marine and euryhaline teleosts, *Comp. Biochem. Physiol.,* **31**:671, 1969.

90. Epstein, F. H., A. I. Katz, and G. E. Pickford: Sodium- and potassium-activated adenosine triphosphatase of gills: Role in adaptation of teleosts to salt water, *Science,* **156**:1245, 1967.

91. Hilden, S., and L. E. Hokin: Active potassium transport coupled to active sodium transport in vesicles reconstituted from purified sodium and potassium ion-activated adenosine triphosphatase from the rectal gland of *Squalus acanthias, J. Biol. Chem.,* **250**:6296, 1975.

92. Whittembury, G., and F. Proverbio: Two modes of Na extrusion in cells from guinea pig kidney cortex slices, *Arch. Gen. Physiol.,* **316**:1, 1970.

93. Besarab, A., P. Silva, and F. H. Epstein: Multiple pumps for sodium reabsorption by the perfused kidney, *Kidney Int.,* **10**:147, 1976.

94. Whittembury, G., and J. J. Grantham: Cellular aspects of renal sodium transport and cell volume regulation, *Kidney Int.,* **9**:103, 1976.

95. Warren, G. B., P. A. Toon, N. J. M. Birdsall, A. G. Lee, and J. C. Metcalfe: Reconstruction of a calcium pump using defined membrane components, *Proc. Natl. Acad. Sci. USA,* **71**:622, 1974.

96. Shanes, A.: Electrochemical aspects of physiological and pharmacological action in excitable cells. Part I. The resting cell and its alteration by extrinsic factors, *Pharmacol. Rev.,* **10**:59, 1958.

97. Nellans, H. N., R. A. Frizell, and S. G. Schultz: Coupled sodium-chloride influx across the brush border of rabbit ileum, *Am. J. Physiol.,* **225**:467, 1973.

98. Silva, P., R. Solomon, K. Spokes, and F. H. Epstein: Ouabain inhibition of gill Na-K-ATPase: Relationship to active chloride transport, *J. Exp. Zool.,* **199**:419, 1977.

99. Reid, E. W.: Intestinal absorption of solutions, *J. Physiol. (London),* **28**:241, 1902.

100. Christensen, H. N., T. R. Riggs, and N. E. Ray: Concentrative uptake of amino acids by erythrocytes in vitro, *J. Biol. Chem.*, **194:**41, 1952.

101. Christensen, H. N., and T. R. Riggs: Concentrative uptake of amino acids by the Ehrlich mouse ascites carcinoma cell, *J. Biol. Chem.*, **194:**57, 1952.

102. Schultz, S. G., and P. F. Curran: Coupled transport of sodium and organic solutes, *Physiol. Rev.*, **50:**637, 1970.

103. Frömter, E., and K. Luer: Electrical studies on sugar transport kinetics of rat proximal tubule, *Pfluegers Arch.*, 343:R47, 1973.

104. Ullrich, K.: Renal tubular mechanisms of organic solute transport, *Kidney Int.*, **9:**134, 1976.

105. Evers, J., H. Murer, and R. Kinne: Phenylalanine transport by isolated renal plasma membrane vesicles, *Biochim. Biophys. Acta*, **426:**598, 1976.

106. Kokko, J. P.: Proximal tubular potential difference: Dependence on glucose, HCO_3 and amino acids, *J. Clin. Invest.*, **52:**1362, 1973.

107. Burg, M. B.: Mechanism of fluid absorption by proximal convoluted tubules, *Proc. Sixth Int. Cong. Nephrol.*, S. Karger AG, Florence, Italy, 1975.

108. Ullrich, K. J., G. Rumrich, and S. Kloss: Specificity and sodium dependence of the active sugar transport in the proximal tubule of the rat kidney, *Pfluegers Arch.*, **351:**35, 1974.

109. Ullrich, K. J., G. Rumrich, and S. Kloss: Sodium dependence of the amino acid transport in the proximal convolution of the rat kidney, *Pfluegers Arch.*, **351:**49, 1974.

110. Ussing, H. H.: Effects of ADH in transport paths in toad skin, in H. H. Ussing and N. A. Thorn (eds.), *Alfred Benzon Symposium V: Transport Mechanisms in Epithelia,* p. 11, Munksgaard, Copenhagen, 1973.

111. Loewenstein, W. R., S. J. Socolar, S. Higashino, Y. Kanno, and N. Davidson: Intercellular communication: Renal, urinary bladder, sensory, and salivary gland cells, *Science*, **149:**295, 1965.

112. Loewenstein, W. R.: Membrane junctions in growth and differentiation, *Fed. Proc.*, **32:**60, 1973.

113. Loewenstein, W. R.: Cell surface membranes in close contact. Role of calcium and magnesium ions, *J. Colloid Interface Sci.*, **25:**34, 1967.

114. Farquhar, M. G., and G. E. Palade: Junctional complexes in various epithelia, *J. Cell. Biol.*, **17:**375, 1963.

115. Boulpaep, E. L.: Electrophysiological properties of the proximal tubule: Importance of cellular and intracellular transport pathways, in G. Giebisch (ed.), *Electrophysiology of Epithelial Cells,* Schatteur, Stuttgart, 1971, p. 258.

116. Shiba, H.: Heaviside's "Bessel cable" as an electric model for flat simple epithelial cells with low resistive junctional membranes, *J. Theor. Biol.*, **30:**59, 1971.

117. Fromter, E.: The route of passive ion movement through the epithelium of *Necturus* gallbladder, *J. Memb. Biol.*, **8:**259, 1972.

118. Diamond, J. M., and W. H. Bossert: Functional consequences of ultrastructural geometry in "backwards" fluid transporting epithelia, *J. Cell. Biol.*, **37:**694, 1968.

119. Sackin, H., and E. L. Boulpaep: Models for coupling of salt and water transport. Proximal tubular reabsorption in Necturus kidney, *J. Gen. Physiol.*, **66:**671, 1975.

120. Diamond, J. M.: Twenty-first Bowditch lecture: The epithelial junction: Bridge, gate and fence, *Physiologist*, **20:**10, 1977.

2

Comparative physiology of electrolyte and water regulation, with emphasis on sodium, potassium, chloride, urea, and osmotic pressure*

B. M. SCHMIDT-NIELSEN / W. C. MACKAY

In order to reach a deeper understanding of how the mammalian organism regulates and maintains its internal environment we must view the mammal in its proper place among other vertebrates. The mechanisms by which mammals maintain homeostasis have evolved from the ancestral lower vertebrates. Therefore, a study of osmoregulatory and excretory functions in the various taxonomic groups can help elucidate general and common mechanisms. In this context, then, information gained about animals which represent branching points on the phylogenetic tree may be of particular importance, even though the group may no longer be important in terms of numbers or distribution.

The extracellular fluid composition is quite similar in most vertebrates. With some notable exceptions among the fishes, the total osmotic concentration ranges around 250 to 350 mosm with sodium and chloride ions constituting 80 to 90 percent of the total osmolality.

Vertebrates inhabit three major types of environments: freshwater, marine, and terrestrial. Some are strictly adapted to only one type of en-

vironment; others can tolerate slow or abrupt changes from one type of environment to another. In the majority of vertebrates, the composition of the body fluids is kept reasonably constant even in the face of large variations in the environment.

Each environment places particular stresses or demands on the animal, because the osmotic concentration and ionic composition of the environment may differ notably from those of the body fluids. Thus, freshwater forms will tend to gain water and lose salts by diffusion, while marine forms with body fluids hypoosmotic to the environment will lose water by osmosis and gain salt by diffusion and drinking. For terrestrial animals the problem is most often evaporative water loss to the environment and a limited access to freshwater.

The degree to which the environment taxes the osmoregulatory systems of an animal depends not only upon the ionic and osmotic concentration difference between the animal and its surroundings but also upon the permeability of the integument. Thus, aquatic forms which obtain their oxygen through gills or across the skin have large surfaces permeable to oxygen and carbon dioxide in close contact with the water. These surfaces are quite permeable to water and some-

* This work was supported by Grant AM 09975-05 and 15972-07 from the National Institutes of Health, Bethesda, Maryland.

what less so to salts. Aquatic vertebrates such as aquatic mammals and reptiles are much less exposed to their environment, since they utilize aerial gas exchange and the skin has an exceedingly low permeability.

The end product of nitrogen excretion is also a determining factor in osmoregulation. Urea excretion in animals unable to produce an osmotically concentrated urine requires a higher rate of urine flow than does uric acid excretion.

The osmoregulatory mechanisms involve a number of organs. In freshwater fishes, the gills and kidneys play the most important role. In marine fishes, the gills carry out a much greater proportion of the osmoregulatory work than do the kidneys. In addition, the gut is involved in osmoregulation. In amphibians, the skin, kidneys,

and bladder perform all the osmoregulatory functions. In most reptiles, the skin is unimportant, while the kidneys, and in some the salt gland, carry out the function. In birds, as in reptiles, salt glands and kidneys are both important. In mammals, the kidney alone has taken over all osmoregulation.

EXTRACELLULAR FLUID COMPOSITION

The internal environment of any particular group of vertebrates is determined by two factors: (1) the genetic pool from which the animal has evolved and (2) the environment to which it is adapted.

In the present chapter we shall deal exclusively with the regulation of the extracellular fluid com-

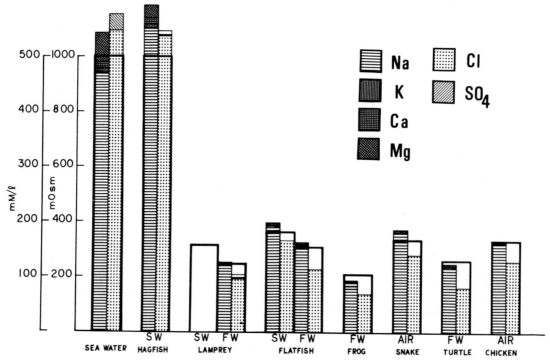

Figure 2-1. Extracellular fluid composition of vertebrates which do not utilize urea in osmoregulation. The dark line surrounding each bar gives the osmotic concentration. Concentrations of some of the constituents of the extracellular fluid are given within each bar. The osmolality can be read directly from the osmolar scale. The concentration of all the ionic constituents can be read directly from the left-hand scale. The composition of seawater is given for comparison. Abbreviations below each bar indicate the environment to which the animal is adapted: seawater, SW; freshwater, FW; terrestrial conditions, AIR.

partment. In recent years considerable attention has been given to the volume and solute regulation of the intracellular compartment. The literature has been reviewed in several recent publications (17, 104, 242).

MARINE ADAPTATION

The body fluid composition of marine vertebrates shows that genetic adaptation to the environment has been achieved in three different ways:

1. No osmoregulation. The body fluids are isosmotic to the sea, and the extracellular fluid has substantially the same ionic composition as seawater. Little energy is spent for osmoregulation and ion regulation.
2. Slight hyperosmoregulation. The body fluids are slightly hyperosmotic to the seawater due to a high urea concentration. This prevents osmotic water loss and thereby reduces the energy requirement, but permits the animal to maintain a lower plasma sodium concentration than that of the seawater.
3. Hypoosmoregulation. The body fluids have about one-third the osmolality of the seawater. This requires a highly developed, energy-requiring, osmoregulatory system but permits the animal to maintain plasma sodium and chloride concentrations almost as low as those found in freshwater or terrestrial animals. The lower plasma sodium concentration may be very important for muscle and nerve function.

The hagfish, belonging to the most primitive class of vertebrates, Cyclostomata, are in osmotic equilibrium with the seawater (Fig. 2-1). The ionic composition of the plasma is also quite similar to that of seawater with the exception that the plasma concentrations of Mg^{2+}, Ca^{2+}, and SO_4^{2-} are lower (205) (Table 2-1). Thus, the hagfish shows no osmoregulation and only a minimum of ion regulation. In this respect, it is much like many marine invertebrates. The lampreys, also belonging to the class Cyclostomata, are, in many respects, more advanced than the hagfish. Lampreys breed in freshwater but migrate to the sea as adults or remain in freshwater or brackish water for their whole life cycle. The marine lampreys have been poorly investigated, but it is clear that their body fluids are considerably hypoosmotic (315 mosm) to the seawater.

The sharks and rays (Elasmobranchii), belonging to the class Chondrichthyes, are slightly hyperosmotic to seawater due to the retention and accumulation of urea, which accounts for more than one-third of the plasma osmolality (Table 2-1, Fig. 2-2) (279). Another subclass of Chondrichtyes, the Holocephali, also has high plasma urea and is slightly hyperosmotic to the seawater (90).

Apparently the bony fishes (Osteichthyes) represent a branching point. One subclass, Actinopterygii, gave rise to several orders of fishes, including the teleosts, which do not maintain a high plasma urea and which are hypoosmotic to the seawater. The other subclass, Sarcopterygii, is ancestral to the amphibians, reptiles, and mammals. The living marine fish belonging to this subclass, the coelacanth, has been found (116, 221) to have high plasma urea much like the sharks and rays.

In all the marine forms which have a high plasma urea, the plasma sodium and chloride concentrations are considerably lower than those of seawater (Table 2-1, Fig. 2-2). In shark plasma, the sodium concentration is about 270 meq/L. The chloride concentration is about 260 meq/L (38).

The marine teleosts are distinctly hypoosmotic to their environment. Plasma osmolality is around 380 mosm compared to seawater with an osmolality of 1000 mosm. Sodium and chloride ions are the major osmotically active components in the plasma (171, 264).

Among the amphibians, only a few are able to survive in water of high salinity. The crab-eating frog, *Rana cancrivora*, has been found to survive in 80 percent seawater (112). It regulates much like the sharks, rays, and coelacanths by accumulating urea in the blood in concentrations up to 350 meq/L. The sodium and chloride concen-

Table 2-1. Extracellular fluid composition of vertebrates (concentrations in mmol)

ANIMAL	HABITAT*	mosm	[Na+]	[K+]	[Ca2+]	[Mg2+]	[Cl-]	[SO42-]	[HPO42-]	UREA	OTHER	REF.
Seawater	....	1000	459	9.8	10.1	52.5	538	26.6				
Cyclostoma												
Epatretus (hagfish)	SW	1002	554	6.8	8.8	23.4	532	1.7	2.1	3	....	205, 233
Lampetra (lamprey)	FW	248	120	3.2	1.9	2.1	96	2.7	...	0.4	(HCO3-) 6.4	233, 300
Elasmobranchii												
Squalus (dogfish shark)	SW	1075	269	4.3	3.2	1.1	258	1	1.1	376	(TMAO) 75	38
Carcharhinus (freshwater shark)	SW	....	288	6	5.7	3.8	288	...	...	356	(TMAO) 47	289
	FW	....	245	6	4.5	1.4	219	0.5	4.0	169	....	289
Potamotrygon (freshwater stingray)	FW	308	150	6	7	4	149	...	7	1	(TMAO) 0	290
Teleostei												
Platichthys (flounder)	SW	335	166	3.6	4.2	1.2	146	...	...	...	....	171
	FW	276	134	3.3	3.9	0.7	114	...	...	...	....	171
Anguilla (eel)	SW	371	178	3	...	...	155	...	...	...	....	264
	FW	323	155	3	...	...	106	...	...	...	....	264
Carassius (goldfish)	FW	293	142	2	6	3	107	...	...	...	....	114
Crossopterygii												
Latimeria (coelacanth)	SW	932	197	5.8	4.8	5.3	187	4.8	...	377	(HCO3-) 9.6	117
Dipnoi (lungfish) Protopterus	FW	470	....	8.2	2.1	...	44.1	...	...	...	(CO2) 35	237
Amphibia												
Rana esculenta (frog)	FW	210	92	3	2.3	1.6	70	...	...	2	....	1a, 188
Scaphiopus (toad)	FW	279	144	4.7	...	...	98	...	...	23	(NH3) 2.5	171
	Ter.	691	247	6.7			184			263	(NH3) 12	171
Rana cancrivora (frog)	FW	290	125	9	...	...	98	...	...	40	....	112
	80% SW	830	252	14	...	...	227	...	...	350	....	112
Amphiuma (congo snake)	FW	....	109	4.3	3.1	1.1	85	...	...	...	....	1a
Reptilia												
Pelamis (sea snake)	Marine	....	264	11			198	...	...	...	....	73
Alligator	FW	278	140	3.6	5.1	3.0	111	...	...	...	(HCO3-) 18	48
Ctenosaura (false iguana)	Ter.	....	159	2.9	2.9	1.0	133	...	2.3		(HCO3-) 15	1a
											...	
Aves												
Anas (duck)	SW	313	147	3.0	2.5		112	...	1.7		....	134
Anas (duck)	FW	294	138	3.1	2.4		103	...	1.6		....	134
	Dehyd.	411	190	...	...		142	...	...		....	134
Zenaidura (mourning dove)	FW	372	176	...	...		136	...	...		....	280
											...	

* SW = seawater; FW = freshwater; Ter. = terrestrial.

trations are up to 250 meq/L in the saltwater-adapted frog (Table 2-1). Other amphibians, such as *Xenopus* and *Scaphiopus,* have also been found to accumulate urea when under osmotic stress (191–193).

Among the reptiles, turtles, snakes, and crocodiles can successfully adapt to seawater. Most of them do not retain urea and are distinctly hypoosmotic to their environment. The marine turtle maintains a blood osmolality of around 375 mosm

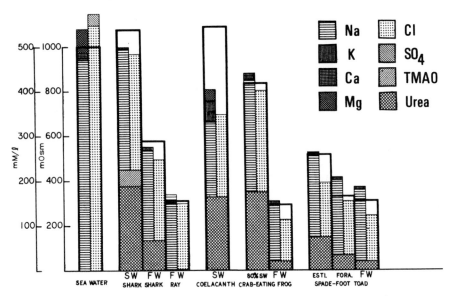

Figure 2-2. Extracellular fluid composition of vertebrates which utilize urea in osmoregulation. Symbols are the same as in Fig. 2-1. Osmolality and urea and trimethylamine oxide (TMAO) concentrations can be read directly from the osmolar scale. Abbreviations below each bar indicate the environment to which the animal is adapted: seawater, SW; freshwater, FW; estivating in soil, ESTI; foraging in terrestrial habitat, FORA.

and the saltwater crocodile an osmolality of 350 mosm. The reptiles have minimal diffusional exchange with their environment, because they are air-breathers and their integument has a low permeability to water and electrolytes.

FRESHWATER ADAPTATION

All freshwater vertebrates are hyperosmotic to their environment. The osmotic concentration of the plasma ranges between 220 and 300 mosm in most freshwater vertebrates. The freshwater forms have a reduced plasma osmolality compared to their marine relatives. This reduction is well illustrated in forms migrating between seawater and freshwater, and in estuarine forms exposed to changes in salinity in their environment. The osmolality change is primarily due to a change in plasma sodium and chloride concentration (Fig. 2-1). In Table 2-2, the plasma sodium level is given for euryhaline forms of fish, amphibians, and reptiles. In all these vertebrates, it appears that the animals regulate actively at the two levels of plasma Na$^+$ concentration.

Energetically, it is to the advantage of a freshwater animal to reduce the osmotic gradient be-

Table 2-2. Plasma sodium and plasma chloride in euryhaline fishes, amphibians, and reptiles (concentrations in mmol)

ANIMAL	FRESHWATER		SEAWATER		
	[NA$^+$]	[Cl$^-$]	[Na$^+$]	[Cl$^-$]	REF.
Anguilla anguilla (eel)	155	106	178	155	264
Rana cancrivora (crab-eating frog)	125	98	252	227	112
Malaclemys (diamondback terrapin)	101		164		77

tween itself and its environment. All the water which enters the animal by diffusion must be excreted as a dilute urine via the kidney. Energy-requiring active transport is involved in producing a dilute urine by the renal tubules. Accumulation of urea in the body fluids is uncommon among freshwater forms. The freshwater elasmobranchs, which have invaded freshwater recently, are the only forms in which urea is found in more than minimal concentrations (Fig. 2-2). The plasma urea concentration is greatly reduced compared with that of its marine relatives but is still more than 100 mmol/L (289, 291). The truly landlocked stingray, *Potamotrygon*, found 4000 miles from the coast in the Orinoco and Amazon drainage system, have negligible plasma urea concentrations and show the same low plasma osmolality as other freshwater fishes (291).

TERRESTRIAL ADAPTATION

The ability to maintain a constant internal environment is most highly developed in the mammals. Reptiles and amphibians show large varia-

tions in blood osmolality with changing water intake, and particularly during estivation (Table 2-3). The spadefoot toad, *Scaphiopus*, for example, lives in very dry desert regions and makes use of temporary desert ponds for the short period the larvae must spend in water. This animal spends much of its time underground and obtains water from the soil by osmosis, its body fluids being kept slightly hypertonic to the soil water by the accumulation of urea in its blood (236) (Table 2-3). The blood osmolality rises during estivation. After 44 days in dry soil, the plasma osmolality reached 691 mosm/L, the result of a 240 mmol/L increase in urea and 85 to 100 mmol/L increases in Na^+ and Cl^- concentrations (192, 193). In turtles and tortoises, the blood osmolality increases 60 to 80 mosm with dehydration. In the desert tortoise, *Goptherus agassizii*, the increase could be accounted for by the increase in blood urea concentration (54, 105). The plasma sodium concentration of the freshwater turtle decreases from a normal value of 144 meq/L to 80 meq/L in hibernating animals (80). Most birds maintain rather constant plasma osmolalities. However, the Savannah sparrow, *Passerculus sandwichensis bel-*

Table 2-3. Plasma composition of reptiles and amphibians in various habitats (concentrations in mmol)

ANIMAL	HABITAT*	mosm	[Na⁺]	[K⁺]	[Cl⁻]	UREA	REF.
Amphibia							
Scaphiopus couchi (spadefoot toad)	Ter. emerging from estivation	456	184	4	122	148	
	Ter. foraging	326	165	6	118	69	192, 193
	FW	305	159	5	102	39	
Rana cancrivora (crab-eating frog)	FW	290	125	9	98	40	112
	80% SW	830	252	14	227	350	
R. esculenta (green frog)	FW	210	92	3	. . .	2	188
Reptilia							
Natrix cyclopion (water snake)	FW	262	134	6	96	. . .	82
Alligator mississippiensis	FW	278	140	4	111	. . .	48
Pituophis melanoleucus (gopher snake)	Ter.	335	180	6	141	. . .	66
Phrynosoma cornutum (horned toad)	Ter.	315	121	. . .	120	. . .	232
Pelamis platurus (sea snake)	Marine	. . .	264	11.4	198	. . .	73

* Ter. = terrestrial; FW = freshwater; SW = seawater.

dingi, which lives in salt marshes, is able to tolerate an increase in osmotic concentration of its body fluids from a normal level of 370 mosm to 490 to 610 mosm due to increased plasma electrolytes (225). The freshwater-dwelling subspecies of the Savannah sparrow, *P. sandwichensis brooksi,* cannot tolerate a plasma osmolality greater than 400 mosm (225).

NITROGEN METABOLISM

The metabolic end products of nitrogen metabolism in vertebrates are determined by evolution as well as by habitat. The three major nitrogenous waste products excreted by all vertebrates are ammonia, urea, and uric acid. A number of other compounds such as allantoin, trimethylamine oxide (TMAO), creatine, and creatinine are also excreted, but since they do not make up a large fraction of the nitrogenous waste products, their synthesis or accumulation will not be considered in detail.

Vertebrates can be divided roughly into three groups: ammonotelic, ureotelic, and uricotelic, according to the predominance of the excretory product, ammonia, urea, or uric acid. There is considerable overlap between these groups (Fig. 2-3).

SUMMARY OF BIOLOGIC ROLE OF NITROGENOUS WASTE PRODUCTS

Ammonia is the predominant excretory product in the majority of aquatic lower vertebrates, freshwater or marine. It is a highly soluble, easily diffusible substance and can, consequently, diffuse out into the surrounding water through the skin or gills. Ammonium ions can also be exchanged for sodium ions in the gills of freshwater fishes which actively take up sodium from the medium (101, 161, 176). The kidneys play a very minor role in ammonia excretion in freshwater or marine fishes.

Ammonia, in concentrations higher than a few milligrams per 100 mL, is toxic to the organism. Consequently, vertebrates which may, in any way, be exposed to dehydration and resulting retention of ammonia do not depend upon ammonia production exclusively. Thus, fishes and adult amphibians which leave the water for periods of time detoxify ammonia formed by catabolism by converting it into urea.

The *urea* molecule is highly soluble in water and is distributed in the total water space of the animal. Vertebrates can acquire a pronounced tolerance to urea. It is found in concentrations up to 350 mmol/L in the body fluids of several fishes and amphibians. In the African lungfish, after protracted estivation, the concentration may be as high as 1000 mmol/L (276). Another important function of urea is its role in osmoregulation. As mentioned earlier, several marine fishes and amphibians maintain a high plasma urea concentration and thereby avoid osmotic outflux of water from the body. The same is the case in burrowing estivating fishes and amphibians, where urea not only serves as a nontoxic storage product but also raises the osmotic concentration of the animal above that of the soil and prevents water loss (236). Finally, in mammals, urea plays a rather unique role. It is not stored in the body fluids but is accumulated in the inner medulla of the kidney in concentrations up to 1000 mmol/L. It serves an osmotic function in the renal concentrating mechanism by raising the osmotic concentration in the medullary tissue and thereby raising the osmotic concentration of the urine in the collecting duct.

Uric acid synthesis and excretion became important to the first truly terrestrial vertebrates, the reptiles. The very low solubility of uric acid or urates permits their excretion as a crystalline paste, which does not, like urea, tie up water osmotically. The terrestrial animal, faced with a scarcity of water, can thus conserve water. An amphibian excreting urea must return to water periodically in order to be able to take up enough water to excrete the stored urea. A reptile can excrete the uric acid continuously on a minimal water intake.

SUMMARY OF BIOSYNTHESIS OF NITROGENOUS WASTE PRODUCTS

Ammonia is formed by deamination of amino acids and by the degradation of purines via uric

PHYLOGENY AND NITROGEN EXCRETION
IN THE VERTEBRATES

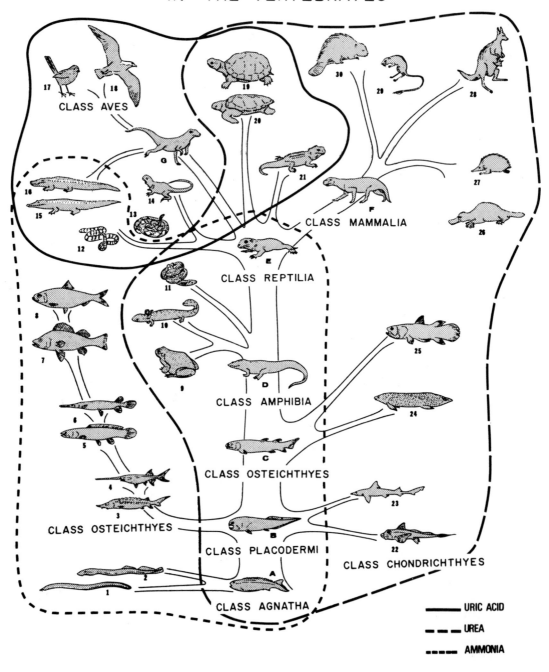

acid, allantoin, etc., to urea and ammonia (Fig. 2-4). *Urea* is synthesized from ammonia through the ornithine cycle (Fig. 2-5), and it is also formed through the degradation of purines to urea (Fig. 2-4). *Uric acid* is formed from the degradation of purines to uric acid (Fig. 2-4); it is also formed through synthesis of NH_3, CO_2, ATP, glycine, and formate via ribose 1-phosphate and hypoxanthine to uric acid. Thus, an animal can form all these three waste products or any combination thereof, depending upon enzyme activities. An animal can excrete virtually all its nitrogenous waste as ammonia if it deaminates amino acids and breaks down its purine all the way to ammonia (Fig. 2-3). If an animals possesses no urease, it can excrete the amino nitrogen in the form of ammonia and the purine nitrogen in the form of urea. This is the case in most teleosts. An animal possessing all the enzymes of the ornithine cycle can convert a certain amount of its amino nitrogen into urea. The relative amounts of urea and ammonia excreted depend upon the amounts of the rate-limiting enzymes of the ornithine cycle and the rate at which ammonia is removed from the body. Animals which do not possess a complete ornithine cycle are unable to produce urea from ammonia but can still form urea from the breakdown of purine and arginine.

In the following account, the distribution of these enzymes among vertebrates and the changes that can take place during development and adaptation to the environment will be discussed. We have preferred to deal with the vertebrates phylogenetically because of the profound effect evolution has had upon nitrogen excretion.

NITROGEN METABOLISM OF CYCLOSTOMES (SUPERCLASS AGNATHA)

The most primitive living vertebrates, the jawless lampreys and hagfish, are ammonotelic. The hagfish is exclusively marine and is in osmotic equilibrium with the seawater in which it lives, while the lamprey, which spawns in freshwater but can invade the sea, has a lower plasma osmolality than the seawater (about 300 mosm). In neither of these does urea constitute a significant fraction of the plasma osmolality. Read (229) found the freshwater-adapted Pacific lamprey to excrete 91.7 percent of its waste nitrogen as ammonia, 87.3 percent via the gills, and 4.4 percent via the kidneys. Urea is excreted only through the kidneys and constitutes 0.5 percent of the total nitrogen excreted.

The ornithine urea cycle was found to be incomplete in the lamprey. Only carbamoyl phosphate synthetase and arginase were found in the liver; the remaining ornithine cycle enzymes could not be detected. Read (229), assuming that the ancestors possessed a functioning ornithine cycle, concluded that deletion or repression of the genes controlling the production of the remaining enzymes has occurred during evolution.

NITROGEN METABOLISM OF CARTILAGINOUS FISHES (CLASS CHONDRICHTHYES)

The living forms include the sharks, rays, skates (subclass Elasmobranchii), and the ratfish (subclass Holocephali). In both these subclasses, urea serves an osmoregulatory function. In marine

Figure 2-3. Phylogeny and nitrogen excretion in the vertebrates. The solid and dashed lines enclose groups which utilize that form of nitrogen as a major excretory product. Extinct ancestral forms of the major groups are indicated by a letter: A, ostracoderm Anaspida (*Pterolepis*); B, arthrodire (*Dinichthys*); C, crossopterygian (*Osteolepis*); D, labyrinthodont (*Diplovertebron*); E, cotylosaur (*Semoria*); F, therapsid (*Lycaenops*); G, thecodont. Existing forms are indicated by a number: 1, hagfish Myxine (*Epatretus*); 2, lamprey (*Lampetra*); 3, sturgeon (*Scaphyrhynchus*); 4, paddlefish (*Polyodon*); 5, bowfin (*Amia*) 6, gar pike (*Lepidosteus*); 7, yellow perch (*Perca*); 8, herring (*Clupea*); 9, bullfrog (*Rana*); 10, mud puppy (*Necturus*); 11, apod (*Ichthyophis*); 12, sea snake (*Pelamis*); 13, rattle snake (*Crotalus*); 14, false iguana (*Ctenosaura*); 15, crocodile (*Crocodylus*); 16, alligator (*Alligator*); 17, Savannah sparrow (*Passerculus*); 18, sea gull (*Larus*); 19, desert tortoise (*Gopherus*); 20, green turtle (*Chelonia*); 21, Tuatara (*Sphenodon*); 22, ratfish (*Hydrolagus*); 23, dogfish shark (*Squalus*); 24, lungfish (*Protopterus*); 25, coelacanth (*Latimeria*); 26, duckbill platypus (*Ornithorhynchus*); 27, spiny ant-eater (*Echidna*); 28, great gray kangaroo (*Macropus*); 29, kangaroo rat (*Dipodomys*); 30, beaver (*Castor*).

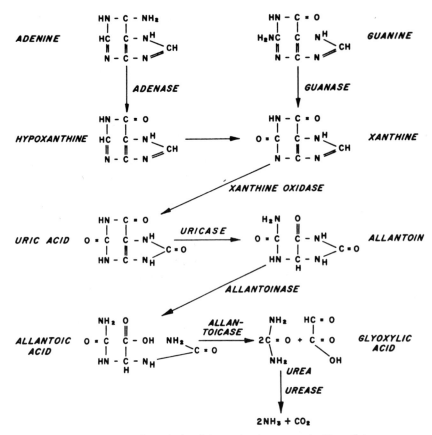

Figure 2-4. Pathway for breakdown of purine ammonia. (*From C. L. Prosser and F. A. Brown.*)

sharks and rays, the plasma urea concentration is about 350 mmol; in the ratfish, about 200 to 300 mmol. In the sharks and rays, it has been shown that the high plasma urea concentration is maintained through (1) a high production of urea, (2) low permeability to urea of gills and other integuments, and (3) urea conservation by the excretory organs. The urine has a much lower urea concentration than plasma; i.e., urea is actively resorbed from the glomerular filtrate along the nephron. Similarly, the rectal gland fluid (see later) also has a very low urea concentration (36, 37,39). By measuring ^{14}C-labeled bicarbonate incorporation, urea was found to be formed via the ornithine pathway and via the purine pathway (261).

The ornithine urea cycle has been found to be complete in the elasmobranchs (298). Earlier workers failed to demonstrate the presence of carbamoyl phosphate synthetase in elasmobranch liver. However, by devising a procedure whereby homogenates could be prepared preserving the integrity of the mitochondria, the enzyme was demonstrated in significant amounts. The results also indicated that glutamine rather than ammonia is the true substrate for carbamoyl phosphate synthetase (136, 298).

In the ratfish, *Hydrolagus colliei*, the complete ornithine urea cycle was demonstrated by Read (228). Comparison of the enzyme concentrations indicated arginine succinate synthetase to be the rate-limiting enzyme.

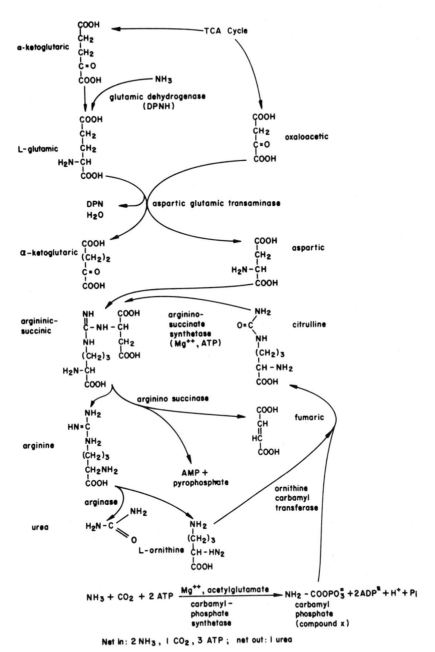

Figure 2-5. Modified ornithine cycle for urea production. (*From
C. L. Prosser and F. A. Brown.*)

Many elasmobranchs are able to invade freshwater. Under these conditions, the blood urea concentration decreases to values around 100 mmol/L. A decrease in blood urea concentration can be caused by a decreased synthesis or an increased loss. An increased loss is brought about automatically by the increase in glomerular filtration rate (GFR) which accompanies adaptation to freshwater. Since a high blood urea concentration in a freshwater animal increases the osmotic gradient across the integuments and thereby causes an increased water influx, Watts and Watts (298) expected to find an adaptive decrease in ornithine cycle enzymes. To the contrary, they observed that acclimation to freshwater of *Raja circulares* caused an increase in ornithine cycle enzyme activity. It was concluded that the maintenance of a minimum urea level is more important as a long-term homeostatic control mechanism than as a simple osmoregulatory device. It has been postulated that the proteins and enzymes of marine elasmobranch tissue are especially adapted to the high plasma and tissue urea concentration (145) and for the maintenance of normal cardiac function (291). Later investigators suggested no specific biochemical effect of urea upon elasmobranch enzymes (182, 183). Urea production changes with the need for maintaining a high plasma osmolality. Thus, in *Raja erinacea* urea production decreased following transfer to 50 percent seawater (107). On the other hand, to an elasmobranch fully adapted to freshwater, such as the stingray *Potamotrygon*, urea is no longer of importance. *Potamotrygon* is found 4000 miles from the ocean in the Amazon River. Thorson et al. (290) found its plasma urea to be less than 1 mmol/L. The urea production is decreased, and the renal tubules do not resorb urea actively.

NITROGEN METABOLISM OF BONY FISHES (CLASS OSTEICHTHYES)

These fishes represent a branching point. The ray-finned fishes, which include all our most common fishes (orders Chondrostei and Holostei and subclass Teleostei), are ammonotelic. The fleshy-finned fishes (superorder Crossopterygii and order Dipnoi) are known to be predominantly ureotelic.

Ray-finned fishes. The teleosts are adapted to marine, brackish, and freshwater habitats. All of them, regardless of habitat, excrete 80 to 90 percent of their nitrogenous waste as ammonia. The major portion is excreted through the gills. The rest of the nitrogenous waste is excreted through the kidneys in the form of trimethylamine oxide, creatinine, creatine, and urea. Urea constitutes less than 4 percent of the total nitrogen excreted. The ammonia excreted through the gills of the sculpin is derived partly (40 percent) from plasma amino acids (not glutamine) deaminated in the gills, and partly (60 percent) from blood ammonia (108). The ornithine cycle was previously believed to be incomplete in the ray-finned fishes. Recently, low but significant levels of all the ornithine cycle enzymes have been detected in liver homogenates from a number of freshwater and marine teleostean fishes (136). It has not been shown, so far, if measurable amounts of urea are formed via the ornithine cycle in these fishes. Urea production from purines has been demonstrated (109). The detection of the enzymes indicates that the difference between the ammonotelic and ureotelic fishes might lie in the manner of expression rather than in possession of structural genes for the ornithine cycle.

One marine teleost, the mudskipper, can live completely out of water for 12 to 24 h. In seawater, it excretes urea and ammonia, the ratio of urea nitrogen to ammonia nitrogen being 0.60. After a period out of water, this ratio was raised to 0.67, possibly indicating an increased synthesis of urea (recalculated from Gordon et al. [113]). There have not been any assays of the ornithine cycle in the mudskipper published so far.

Fleshy-finned fishes. The living fleshy-finned fishes include three orders of lungfish and the famous living fossil, the coelacanth, *Latimeria chalamnae*. The lungfishes are all freshwater forms. The African lungfish *Protopterus* survives protracted periods of drought by remaining motionless in a mud cocoon. During this estivation, which may last up to 7 to 11 years, it does not excrete nitrogenous waste, and urea accumulates in its body fluids in concentrations up to 1000 mmol/L (4 percent of body weight) (276). The Australian lungfish *Neoceratodus* never estivates and is fully aquatic. *Protopterus*, when in water, eliminates 50 percent of its nitrogenous end products as urea (110). *Neoceratodus* eliminates a large fraction as ammonia and only 2 to 3 percent as urea (110). The rate of incorporation of ^{14}C-labeled bicarbonate into urea by liver slices was 100 times greater in *Protopterus* than in *Neoceratodus*. The level of the ornithine cycle enzymes in liver slices was 10 to 100 times greater in *Protopterus* than in *Neoceratodus*. The activity of carbamoyl phosphate synthetase in *Neoceratodus* liver was low and of the same order of magnitude (0.45 mmol/g tissue per h) as in the teleosts.

The coelacanth is a marine fish. In its plasma, urea has been demonstrated in concentrations around 355 mmol/L (221). Enzyme assays demonstrated the presence of the ornithine cycle enzymes arginase and carbamoyltransferase synthetase in concentrations comparable to those of frogs and other ureotelic animals (32, 111).

NITROGEN METABOLISM OF AMPHIBIANS (CLASS AMPHIBIA)

The living amphibians belong to three orders: frogs and toads (Anura), salamanders and newts (Urodela), and wormlike burrowing types (Apoda). With the adaptation to spending some time out of water, ureotelism became more predominant, just as it is predominant in the lungfish when it estivates in its mud cocoon. Urea is formed via the ornithine cycle and from purine breakdown. There are, however, wide variations among the amphibians in the relative amounts of ammonia and urea being excreted.

Anurans. Anurans have been studied quite intensively. The eggs of most frogs or toads are laid in water where they hatch to fully aquatic tadpoles. After metamorphosis, the young frog spends part of its time on land and part of its time in the pond. Some anurans are almost completely aquatic (i.e., *Xenopus*); others are more terrestrial, such as various species of toads. Many anurans estivate in burrows in the ground during the winter or during periods of drought. Some anurans can tolerate brackish water or seawater, the most noteworthy being the crab-eating frog, *Rana cancrivora*, which can tolerate 80 percent seawater (112).

The tadpoles of various frogs excrete most of their nitrogen as ammonia (204). In *R. catesbeiana*, the ratio (urea N_2)/(urea N_2 + ammonia N_2) in the urine is 10 percent in the tadpole but rises sharply to 60 percent during the period of metamorphosis. During the same period, the activity of the enzymes of the ornithine cycle in the liver increases fivefold or more, and carbamoyl phosphate synthetase increases more than 20-fold (30). The ability of the kidney to excrete urea by active secretion into the renal tubule develops at the same time (97) during metamorphosis, and the arginase activity in the kidney increases (234). In contrast, in the aquatic frog, *Xenopus*, the ratio (urea N_2)/(urea N_2 + ammonia N_2) rises insignificantly during metamorphosis, from 14 percent in the early states to 24 percent in the fully grown adult (7).

Frogs *R. cancrivora* (112), *Xenopus laevis* (7, 142), and *R. pipiens* (240), exposed to various salinities, react initially by decreasing the urea excretion and accumulating urea in the body fluids. In *Xenopus* and in *R. cancrivora* an increase in ornithine cycle enzyme activity has been demonstrated during acclimation in saline solutions (8, 142, 191). When acclimated for several months to a 420-mosm saline solution, the urea concentration in the tissue water had increased to about 100 mmol/L. The rate of urea production had increased 26-fold (147, 281).

During estivation, *Xenopus* and the spadefoot toad, *Scaphiopus*, accumulate urea in the blood in high concentrations (6, 192, 193). The ratio (urea N_2)/(urea N_2 + ammonia N_2) in the urine is increased from 22 percent before estivation to 75 percent immediately after estivation. The carbamoyl phosphate synthetase is increased sixfold in the estivating animal, indicating an increase in urea production (6). Many of the frogs secrete urea actively into the renal tubules. The mechanism serves to maintain a lower plasma urea concentration than would be found if urea were excreted by filtration alone. This may serve an osmoregulatory function, since it helps to maintain a lower plasma osmolality than would otherwise be found and thus reduces water influx through the skin (169). The fact that the more aquatic species have higher rates of urea secretion and higher renal arginase activity (18, 44) supports this hypothesis.

Urodeles. Urodeles have been studied much less than the anurans. The fully aquatic *Necturus* excretes only 11 percent of the total nitrogen as urea and 89 percent as ammonia. The skin (not the gills) serves as the major route of ammonia excretion (86). Another urodele, the red eft, which spends part of its life cycle on land, changes from ammonia to urea excretion during its terrestrial period but reverts to ammonia when it returns to the water (208). There is no information on the ornithine cycle enzymes in these animals.

NITROGEN METABOLISM OF REPTILES (CLASS REPTILIA)

The living reptiles belong to four orders: the turtles and tortoises (Chelonia), the sphenodon (Rynchocephalia), the lizards and snakes (Squamata), and the crocodiles (Crocodilia).

The adult reptiles, as the first fully terrestrial vertebrates, synthesize uric acid from amino nitrogen and purines and lack the enzymes which break down uric acid to urea and ammonia (226). Presumably, the early reptiles, from which the mammals developed, were still semiaquatic in their habitat, like the present-day turtles. Members of Chelonia and Rhynchocephalia are ammonoureouricotelic. Most members of Squamata are only ammonouricotelic, but a few exceptions are also ureotelic. The relative amounts of ammonia urea and uric acid excreted vary among the species and with habitat.

Uric acid is always excreted by active tubular secretion in addition to being filtered. Urea is also secreted in the sphenodon and quite likely in the freshwater turtle. Ammonia appears to be formed in the renal tubules of the crocodilians.

Chelonia. Chelonians are found in all types of habitats: freshwater, marine, semiaquatic, and fully terrestrial. However, in all cases, the eggs

are laid on land in a moist place. All chelonians excrete ammonia, urea, and uric acid. Urea may be excreted by tubular secretion. Chelonians have the ornithine cycle enzymes in addition to the enzymes for synthesis of uric acid (156, 157). The proportion of these excretory products varies greatly with the habitat of the species. Thus, the freshwater turtle excretes 4 to 44 percent ammonia, 45 to 95 percent urea, and 1 to 24 percent uric acid. The desert tortoise, on the other hand, excretes 6 to 8 percent ammonia, 15 to 50 percent urea, and 20 to 50 percent uric acid (54). There is, however, no reliable evidence for a shift between urea and uric acid production with a change in water intake within a species. Rogers (235) found a decrease in urea concentration/uric acid concentration in bladder urine of turtles after 20 days' dehydration compared with hydrated turtles. This decrease can easily be explained as a diffusion of urea out of the bladder, since the urine remained in the bladder during the 20 days of dehydration.

When tortoises or turtles are dehydrated or are hibernating, urea accumulates in the blood (up to 100 mmol/L has been measured) (54, 105). In the tortoise, large amounts of uric acid are stored in the bladder during dehydration.

The euryhaline diamondback terrapin accumulates urea up to about 115 mmol/L in the plasma when it is maintained in seawater. Its total plasma osmolality, however, only rises to 460 mosm (106). The marine turtle (*Caretta caretta*), although partly ureotelic, does not accumulate urea in the plasma in high concentrations as do the ureotelic fishes and amphibians. It maintains a plasma osmolality of around 340 to 400 mosm (260).

The renal excretion pattern shows that uric acid is actively secreted into the tubules in turtles and tortoises. Urea appears to be excreted mostly by glomerular filtration, but a weak tubular secretion cannot be excluded (54).

Rhynchocephalia. The sphenodon, a primitive reptile which lives in moist caves, has been found to be ammonoureouricotelic (127). It maintains a plasma urea concentration around 5 to 10 mmol/L. In the animals maintained on high-protein intake, the percentage of total nitrogen excretion was distributed as 4 percent ammonia N_2, 27 percent urea N_2, and 65 percent uric acid N_2 (127). In the animals on low-protein diets, relatively less urea and more uric acid were excreted: 3.7 percent ammonia N_2, 11 percent urea N_2, and 81 percent uric acid N_2.

The sphenodon was found to excrete urea by active tubular secretion. The urea clearance exceeded the GFR by 24 percent (245).

Squamata. The lizards and snakes have mostly adopted uricotelism as the adult pattern of nitrogen excretion. However, several of the lizards belonging to the skink family have been found to be partly ureotelic (245 and unpublished observations). During embryonic development all lizards and snakes go through the stages of ammonotelism and ureotelism. Embryos of snakes produce ammonia for the first few days but rapidly convert to urea production via the ornithine cycle (91). During embryonic development, urea is the primary excretory product of the oviparous snake *Coluber*. In the terminal stages of development, there is a shift from urea to uric acid. This occurs the last 6 to 10 days of a 68-day incubation period (91). Packard (215) suggests that the urea production is an adaptation to the environment. The water-permeable eggs are deposited in moist soil, from which they absorb water, and double their weight during the incubation period (45, 91). The absorption of water appears to be due to the accumulation of urea. In the viviparous placental snake *Thamnophis*, almost half of the nitrogenous waste produced by the embryo is absorbed by the mother. The embryo produces predominantly urea during the greater part of the gestation period. The shift to uric acid production occurs during the last 2 days of the 72-day gestation period (215). Packard (215) suggests that the shift to uric acid represents a biochemical metamorphosis associated with the transition from embryonic to free-living existence.

The ornithine cycle appears to be completely repressed after uric acid production has begun (31). Khalil (155) found no arginase in the liver of adult lizards and snakes, which excrete about 95 percent of their nitrogenous waste as uric acid. The enzyme xanthine oxidase, which catalyzes the reaction of hypoxanthine or xanthine to uric

acid, was found in the liver of snakes but not in lizards. It is present in the kidneys of both snakes and lizards (155).

Adaptation to an aquatic environment involves, in some reptiles, a shift toward ammonotelism. This apparently is not true of the freshwater snake. Dantzler (unpublished observations) found the ammonia concentration in the urine of *Natrix* to be 1 to 2 mmol/L and the rate of excretion to be 6 to 15 μmol/g per h. (Ammonia N_2)/(ammonia N_2 + uric acid N_2) was only about 2.5 to 5 percent (calculated from Dantzler's data).

In the sea snake, on the other hand, the ammonia concentration in the urine was around 60 mmol/L (B. Schmidt-Nielsen, unpublished). In the terrestrial, blue-tongued lizard, the ammonia concentration in the urine was around 2 to 5 mmol/L, and the rate of excretion was around 5 to 10 μmol/kg per h.

Crocodilia. The crocodilians are descendants of the terrestrial ruling reptiles and are secondarily adapted to an amphibious mode of life. They, like aquatic squamatans, reflect their terrestrial ancestry in that, in spite of their habitat, the urea cycle does not function in the adult.

The crocodilians, however, have adapted to their environment by ammonia excretion. Ammonia nitrogen normally constitutes 30 percent of total nitrogen excreted and uric acid about 46 percent. Fasting reduces the amount excreted as uric acid, while dehydration reduces the amount excreted as ammonia (47, 48). It is suggested that ammonia is formed by deamination of amino acids directly in the renal tubules. (122).

NITROGEN METABOLISM OF BIRDS (CLASS AVES)

The adult birds are predominantly uricotelic. During the first day of embryonic development, the embryo produces about 25 percent of its nitrogen in the form of ammonia and 25 percent as urea, but the pattern quickly changes to the adult pattern. Packard (215) relates this to the fact that bird eggs, in contrast to snake eggs, are laid in a dry site. Uric acid is deposited as insoluble waste in the egg, and does not increase the osmolality of the egg. Arginase activity can be measured in the embryo up to the eighteenth day and has even been demonstrated in the liver of adult birds (29).

The adult terrestrial bird excretes 87 percent of its waste nitrogen as uric acid and only 3 to 4 percent as ammonia, while the more aquatic duck excretes only 52 percent as uric acid and 32 percent as ammonia. Thus, birds, like reptiles, appear to adapt to an aquatic habitat by increasing the ammonia excretion (282). The mechanism has not been investigated.

RENAL EXCRETION

SUMMARY OF KIDNEY STRUCTURE

The renal excretory organs of vertebrates consist of two compact kidneys, the kidney ducts or ureters, the cloaca, and, in some cases, a bladder. The cloaca and bladder are, in many lower vertebrates, important functional parts of the excretory system, since considerable transport of water and solutes takes place across their epithelium.

The kidneys are located between the dorsal body wall and the peritoneum. The relative size and extent of the kidneys vary greatly in different animals. In some fishes, the kidneys stretch as two narrow bands almost as far as the head. In other forms, the kidneys are rounded organs close to the cloaca.

In adult vertebrates, the kidneys may be of three types: pronephric, with no true glomeruli but a nephrostome in the tubule; mesonephric, which has a glomerulus in the tubule and, in many cases, also has a nephrostome; metanephric, with only glomeruli, no nephrostomes.

The basic unit of the kidney, the nephron in adult vertebrates, consists of (1) renal corpuscle with a glomerulus, (2) neck segment, (3) proximal segment parts I and II, (4) intermediate segment, (5) distal segment, (6) collecting tubules. (The vertebrate nephron is quite distinct from the nephridia of the chordate *Amphioxus*, just below the vertebrate level.) Many collecting tubules join a collecting duct. Several collecting ducts join the ureter—usually one from each kidney. The two ureters open into the cloaca or into a urinary sinus. The bladder, when present in lower vertebrates, is a diverticulum to the cloaca. The tubules in lower vertebrates are highly convoluted,

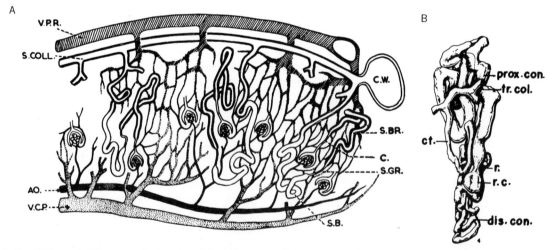

Figure 2-6. Frog kidney. *A.* Diagrammatic drawing of the kidney of a frog. V.P.R., renal portal vein; S. Coll., collecting duct; C.W., ureter; S.BR., proximal tubule; C., neck segment; S.GR., intermediary segment; S.B., distal tubule; AO., renal artery; V.C.P., renal efferent vein. *B.* Reconstruction of a single renal nephron. r.c., Renal corpuscle; prox. con., proximal tubule; dis. con., distal tubule; ct., initial collecting tubule; tr. col., collecting duct. (*From W. von Möllendorff.*)

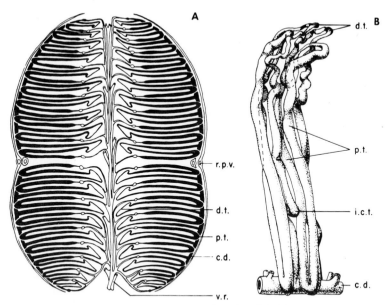

Figure 2-7. Reptile kidney *A.* Crocodile kidney lobule. v.r., Vena revehns; c.d., collecting duct; p.t., proximal tubule; d.t., distal tubule *(Adapted from W. von Möllendorff.) B.* Two crocodile renal nephrons. c.d., Collecting duct; p.t., proximal tubule; d.t., distal tubule; i.c.t., initial collecting tubule.

and there is no loop of Henle in fishes, amphibians, or reptiles. The tubules are arranged parallel to one another, and the collecting ducts run at right angles to the tubules (Figs. 2-6,2-7). In bird kidneys, the majority of the tubules are arranged as in lower vertebrates; however, some of the tubules have a loop of Henle, and these loops, as in the mammalian kidney, are arranged parallel to the collecting ducts (Fig. 2-8).

The vertebrate nephron shows many variations as adaptations to the habitat of the animal and the particular functional requirements. The number and size of the glomeruli are related to habitat. Freshwater teleosts generally have more and larger glomeruli than do marine teleosts. The length and development of the different parts of the nephron vary greatly among vertebrates, and one or several parts of the nephron may be entirely missing.

For example, the *Myxines*, with no osmoregu-lation and little ion regulation, have atubular kidneys with large glomeruli draining directly into the collecting duct. Some marine teleosts, which, as hypoosmoregulators, have no excess water to excrete and no ability to produce a concentrated urine, have aglomerular nephrons, and only the second segment of the proximal tubule is present (Fig. 2-9).

The blood supply to the kidney of most of the lower vertebrates differs from that of mammals in that a renal portal system is present in addition to the arterial blood supply. The caudal vein splits up into a second capillary net which joins the postglomerular capillary net surrounding the nephrons.

The renal portal circulation is not found in Cyclostomata. It is found in Elasmobranchii, Holostei, marine Teleostei, Dipnoi, Amphibia, Reptilia, and Aves. It is missing in some freshwater teleosts (126, 197).

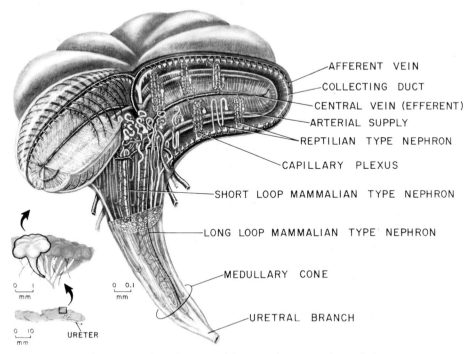

AFFERENT VEIN
COLLECTING DUCT
CENTRAL VEIN (EFFERENT)
ARTERIAL SUPPLY
REPTILIAN TYPE NEPHRON
CAPILLARY PLEXUS
SHORT LOOP MAMMALIAN TYPE NEPHRON
LONG LOOP MAMMALIAN TYPE NEPHRON
MEDULLARY CONE
URETRAL BRANCH
URETER

Figure 2-8. A three-dimensional drawing of a section of avian kidney showing types of nephrons present, their relative positions in kidney, and their relationship to other renal structures. [*Reprinted with the permission of E. J. Braun and W. H. Dantzler (27).*]

SUMMARY OF KIDNEY FUNCTION

The main function of the kidney in all freshwater animals is to excrete water which enters the body by diffusion. The GFR is high in freshwater forms compared with that in most marine forms (Table 2-4). GFR is regulated according to habitat. It decreases in fishes migrating from freshwater to saltwater, in amphibians going from water to land (247), and in terrestrial reptiles becoming dehydrated (54, 232). Reduction in filtration rate is mostly caused by a reduction in number of functioning glomeruli rather than in the amount filtered by each nephron. The hormonal control is obviously different in fishes versus amphibians and reptiles. In fishes (131, 175, 238) the

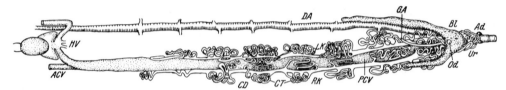

Figure 2-9. Aglomerular teleost kidney. Schematic drawing of the two kidneys from the pipefish, viewed ventrally. DA, Dorsal aorta; GA, gastrointestinalis; Bl, bladder; Ad, adrenal gland; Ur, ureter; Od, oviduct; PCV, vena card. posterior; RK, right kidney; CT, renal tubules; CD, collecting duct; LK, left kidney; ACV, vena card. ant.; HV, vena hepatica. (*From W. von Möllendorff.*)

Table 2-4. Urine flow and glomerular filtration rate in freshwater, marine, and terrestrial vertebrates

ANIMAL	HABITAT*	BODY WEIGHT, kg	URINE FLOW, mL/kg/DAY	GFR, mL/kg/DAY	GFB,† mL/m²/DAY	REF.
Cyclostomata						
Eptatretus stouti	SW	0.1	4–10	4–10	33	205
Petromyzon marinus	FW	0.1	302	671	1,438	
Elasmobranchii						
Mustelus canis	SW	7.8	15	45	875	38
Squalus acanthus	SW	20	33.5	102.9	1,290	
Pristis microdon	FW	10	150–450	450	9,570	
Teleostei						
Lophius piscatorius	SW	4.1–7.2	26.6	0	(504 urine flow)	164
Ameiurus nebulosus	FW	1.0	154	225	2,250	
Platichthys flesus	SW	0.20	14.4	57.6	724	
	FW	0.20	42.8	99.8	1,260	
Amphibia						
Rana clamitans	FW	0.15	317	822	4,400	
R. catesbeiana	FW	0.48	256	619	4,800	
R. cancrivora	FW	0.010–0.055	575	1,400	4,200	
	80% SW	0.010–0.055	36	600	1,800	
Reptilia						
Pseudemys scripta	FW	1.5	31.7	114	1,300	54
Hemidactylus species	Ter.	0.005	61.3	250	446	232
Phrynosoma cornutum	Ter.	0.030	47.3	85	266	232
Natrix cyclopion	FW	0.8	109	236	2,170	167
Pituophis melanoleucus	Ter.	. . . .	. . . .	. . . .	. . . .	160
Sphenodon	Ter.	0.8	5.9	15.6	143	
Crocodylus actutus	FW	2.5	29.6	230	3,140	
Aves						
Gallus domesticus	(FW loaded)	1.5	417	3,050	35,000	252
	(SW loaded)		261	2,980	34,000	25
Anas platyrynchos	FW	2.25	. . . .	3,140	41,000	252
	SW	2.23	. . . .	3,060	40,200	
Mammalia						
Seal						
Fasting	SW	20	12.0	3,600	93,500	
Fed	SW	20	24.0	7,200	187,000	
Dog	Ter.	10	15–600	6,190	131,500	
Man	Ter.	70	7–300	2,840	113,500	

* SW = seawater; FW = freshwater; Ter. = terrestrial.

† GFR is calculated in milliliters per square meter of body surface (BS) per day. BS is calculated from body weight (BW) by the equation BS (m²) = (BW$^{0.67}$/10) (kg). Since physiologic functions are proportional to body surface area rather than to weight, it is more meaningful to compare GFRs per square meter of body surface than per kilogram of body weight, particularly when animals with greatly different body weights are compared.

‡ B. Schmidt-Nielsen (in preparation).

SOURCE: Except where noted, the data in this table are taken from table 4 in Ref. 224.

Table 2-5. Urine flow (V) and urine composition in lower vertebrates (concentrations in mmol)

ANIMAL	HABITAT*	V, mL/kg PER DAY	INULIN OR CREATININE U/P	mosm	[Na$^+$]	[K$^+$]	[Mg^{2+}]	[Cl$^-$]	[SO$_4^{2-}$]	[UREA]	REF.
Eptatretus (hagfish)	SW	4–8	1.05	. . .	533	11	29	548	14.6	8.8	87 205, 227
Lampetra (lamprey)	FW	496	1.76	29	12	2	. . .	1	. . .	. . . .	192, 300
Squalus (shark)	SW	15	2.93	800	240	2	40	240	70	100	38, 152
Pristis (sawfish)	FW	250	. . . .	54	. . .	. . .	. . .	. . .	. . .	. . .	277
Platichthys (flounder)	FW	28.1	. . . .	86	37	1.4	2.2	24	. . .	. . . .	171
	SW	3.8	. . . .	328	112	3.2	11.5	133			
Opsanus (toadfish)	SW	4.3	. . . .	331	72	8	. . .	104	. . .	. . . .	165
	FW	20.9	. . . .	213	87	7	. . .	39			175
Carassius (goldfish)	FW	330	1.45	36	. . .	. . .	. . .	. . .	. . .	. . . .	175
Rana cancrivora (crab-eating frog)	FW	576	2.50	185	. . .	. . .	. . .	5			
	80% SW	33	17.45	430	20	21	. . .	12	. . .	230	111, 257
R. esculenta (green frog)	FW	610	2.27	26	5	2					
Pseudemys (turtle)	FW	32	3.59	. . .	. . .	. . .	. . .	. . .	. . .	39.6	54
Gopherus (desert tortoise)	Ter.	48	2.37	. . .	. . .	. . .	. . .	. . .	. . .	13.8	
Malaclemys (diamondback terrapin)	FW	24	. . . .	57	1	5					
	SW	4.4	. . . .	207	28	31	. . .	. . .	. . .	. . . .	13
Anas (duck)	Ter., FW	57.7	. . . .	241	9	37	. . .	12			
	SW	52.5	. . . .	441	76	46	. . .	124	. . .	. . . .	133

* SW = seawater; FW = freshwater; Ter. = terrestrial.

neurohypophyseal hormone arginine vasotocin (AVT) increases GFR, but in amphibians (238) and reptiles (52, 54) it decreases GFR by constricting the afferent arteriole. The renal plasma flow (RPF) in animals with a renal portal circulation is about 10 to 20 times greater than the GFR. It can be measured as the paraaminohippurate (PAH) clearance. In freshwater teleosts which do not have the portal circulation, RPF is only two to three times the GFR. The urine in most freshwater forms is extremely dilute (20 to 40 mosm), and the urine flow is high (Table 2-5). Nitrogenous waste is not excreted by the kidneys but is excreted by the gills of most freshwater fishes. It is excreted primarily by the kidneys of

higher aquatic animals, such as amphibians, and exclusively by the kidneys of reptiles, birds, and mammals.

In marine fishes, the kidneys serve in excreting the divalent ions, SO$_4^{2-}$ and Mg^{2+} primarily, while Na$^+$ and Cl$^-$ are excreted via the gills. The urinary sinus plays an important role in resorption of Na$^+$, Cl$^-$, and water, and in concentrating the divalent ions in the urine. A small fraction of the nitrogenous waste is excreted by the kidneys of marine teleosts in the form of trimethylamine, trimethylamine oxide, and creatinine (Table 2-5).

In terrestrial forms, the kidneys serve as the major organs for excretion of nitrogenous waste, regardless of the form in which it is excreted.

Water is conserved by the kidneys of most terrestrial forms, and the major sites for water resorption appear to be the cloaca, bladder, or intestine. Na^+ and K^+ ions may be excreted as urate or as soluble salts with water. However, the capacity of the kidneys for excretion of soluble salts is greatly limited in most vertebrates, since kidneys without a countercurrent mechanism cannot concentrate the urine osmotically above the plasma concentration. Only the kidneys of birds and mammals have the ability to produce a urine with a higher osmolality than that of the blood. This is achieved through the countercurrent arrangement of nephrons, capillaries, and collecting ducts. The countercurrent system in the bird kidney, however, operates rather differently from that in mammals. More detailed descriptions for the various classes of vertebrates follow. For fishes, an excellent and detailed description has been given by Hickman and Trump (126). For amphibians, the literature has been reviewed by Deyrup (64); for birds, by Sperber (281).

KIDNEYS OF CYCLOSTOMES

Structure of kidney. The primitive fishes hagfish and lamprey have very different kidney morphologic features and functions. The hagfish kidneys consist of paired anterior pronephroi and paired mesonephroi. The function of the pronephros in the mature hagfish is not well understood, but it does not appear to function as a kidney. The mesonephric kidneys, located caudad to the pronephros, consist of 15 to 20 very large renal corpuscles, measuring 0.5 to 1.5 mm, attached to two straight archinephric ducts (ureters) (162). The ureters have a short, blind end, then a glomerular segment about 10 cm long. The glomeruli are arranged segmentally along the ureters and are attached to the ureters by extremely short ducts. Thus, true nephrons are lacking. The caudal segment of the ureter is 5 to 6 cm long. Two thin urinary ducts connect the ureter with the cloaca. The cells of the ureter resemble proximal tubular cells; they are tall and columnar, and have apical brush borders. The bases of the cells are invaginated. There are many

small mitochondria. The glomeruli are supplied by branches of segmental arteries from the dorsal aorta. A dense capillary network surrounds the ureter. This is supplied by postglomerular arterioles and by arteries directly from the aorta. There is no renal portal circulation (197).

The functioning lamprey kidneys are elongated organs with a triangular cross section. In the river lamprey, *Petromyzon fluviatilis* (197, 306, 307), each kidney has one very long glomus (9 cm long and 0.25 mm wide) surrounded by a continuous urinary space (304). No difference in size of the glomus between seawater- and freshwater-acclimated fish has been noted (305). The glomus has been formed by the fusion of many originally separate glomeruli. The neck segments of the nephrons radiate from the glomus. The nephrons consist of a ciliated neck segment or proximal segment (70 μm) with brush border and a narrow segment (45 μm) connecting it with the archinephric duct. The latter tubular segment has not been well described, and whether it is a typical distal segment is not clear.

Function of kidney. The hagfish, which is an osmoconformer, has a very ineffective kidney function (see Table 2-5). The filtration rate is low [7.2 mL/kg/day; single-nephron glomerular filtration rate (SNGFR) is 20 nL/min] (285). The urine is isosmotic with the blood, and there is little or no Na^+ resorption from the filtrate and no water resorption (194, 205). The lack of a tubule is also evident, as there is little or no secretion of divalent ions. The urine concentrations of Mg^{2+}, Ca^{2+}, SO_4^{2-}, and $H_2PO_4^-$ are slightly higher than in the plasma. Secretion, if it occurs, is very slight (194, 199, 205, 227). Furthermore, the kidney does not secrete phenol red, which is secreted by all tubular kidneys. In the archinephric ducts, however, some urea secretion takes place, K^+ is secreted, and 50 percent of the filtered glucose is resorbed (87, 286).

The river lamprey, which has been the best studied, spawns in freshwater. The young migrate to freshwater lakes or brackish water in estuaries. They return to rivers in the fall or spring before they spawn. They are able to hypoosmoregulate in seawater and hyperosmoregulate in freshwater. During anadromous migration, a breakdown in the osmoregulatory mechanism occurs (220). Bentley and Follett (12) found that the GFR was 496 mL/kg/day in freshwater, and decreased to 160 mL/kg/day in 100 mmol/L NaCl. The urine flow rate ranges from 0 to 6.2 mL/kg/day in 50 percent seawater (220) and to 160 mL/kg/day in freshwater. In lampreys in 50 percent seawater, the urine was never hyperosmotic to the blood, but Ca^{2+}, Mg^{2+}, and SO_4^{2-} are excreted in high concentrations (220).

Fractional Na^+ and Cl^- resorption were 91 and 33 percent, respectively, in freshwater. When the animal was injected with salt or transferred to salt water, the fractional resorption decreased. Urine osmolality in freshwater is comparable to that of freshwater teleosts (181).

KIDNEYS OF CARTILAGENOUS FISHES

Structure of kidney. The mature shark kidneys consist of a caudal thick part and a long, ribbonlike anterior part located against the dorsal body wall on each side of the midline.

In the cranial end of the kidney, hematopoietic tissue is found. The ribbonlike part has segmentally arranged nephrons, four to six nephrons per segment. The last four segments have 50 to 60 nephrons each. Each nephron has a long, ciliated neck segment. The proximal segment (up to 1 cm long), consisting of two distinct parts (126), is followed by a distal segment and a collecting tubule. The spatial arrangement of each tubule shows great complexity (60, 284). There are at least two highly coiled proximal tubular segments and several distal tubular segments. Each tubule bends back on itself to form a countercurrent loop system consisting of five tubule segments surrounded by connective tissue. The terminal distal tubule segment is one of these five tubules. It joins the collecting tubule. Juxtaglomerular cells are apparently absent in elasmobranchs (49). The ureters lead to the urogenital sinus in the female or the cloaca in the male. In the mature female skate a bilobed urinary bladder is attached caudally and dorsally to the urogenital sinus. Several ureters empty directly into the urinary bladder (163).

The kidneys of the ratfish (Holocephali) are similar in many ways to those of the shark. They differ, however, in the following respects: the glomeruli are less open, much of the volume is occupied by mesangial cells, the first segment of the proximal tubule is less complex with fewer mitochondria than that of the shark (126).

Function of kidney. The body fluids of sharks, skates, and rays are slightly hyperosmotic to the seawater in which they live, due to the accumulation of urea and trimethylamine oxide. The body fluids of the ratfish are probably isosmotic with the seawater, and its plasma urea concentration is slightly lower than that of the shark. The hyperosmolality in the elasmobranchs causes an osmotic influx of water which must be excreted through the kidneys.

The GFR in the marine elasmobranch (40 to 100 mL/kg/day) (250) is similar to that of marine teleosts. When placed in 75 percent seawater, the GFR increases threefold and the fractional resorption of water decreases (98, 250). The urine is always slightly hypoosmotic to the plasma. In skates or sharks acclimated to dilute seawater urine osmolality is about 50 to 75 percent of the plasma (284). The dilution of the urine takes place in the distal segment of the tubule as well as along the collecting duct (284). Na^+ is resorbed in the tubules. The Na^+ concentration in the urine is on the average slightly lower than in the plasma, but frequently exceeds the plasma concentration (126, 250, 284). Sodium-potassium-activated ATPase (Na^+–K^+–ATPase) does not participate in the bulk resorption of Na^+ (121). Micropuncture studies indicate that divalent ions (Mg^{2+}, SO_4^{2-}, and HPO_3^{2-}) are secreted into the second proximal tubule of the nephron (284).

The tubules effectively resorb urea, leaving less than 10 percent of filtered urea in the urine and a urine urea concentration of one-third or less of that in the plasma (152, 278). Urealike molecules with an amide group, such as acetamide and methylurea, are also resorbed, while thiourea is not resorbed (249). Trimethylamine oxide is also actively resorbed in   e distal segment or initial collecting tubule (46). Urea resorption appears to be linked to Na^+ resorption. In *Squalus acanthius* the ratio of urea to Na^+ resorption was fixed at a value of 1.6 over a wide range of filtered Na^+ concentrations (250). The urea transport seems to involve a special carrier which can be poisoned by chromate administration (119).

The urine urea concentration becomes lower than that of the plasma in a late distal segment. It has been suggested that the countercurrent arrangement of the five tubular segments is important for the urea resorption mechanisms (20). When elasmobranchs are acclimated to lower salinities, the fraction of filtered urea resorbed decreases sharply (98, 107).

In the true freshwater stingray, investigated by Thorson and coworkers (290), blood urea is low (0.75 mmol/L), and urea is not resorbed by the tubules (Goldstein and Forster, personal communication).

KIDNEYS OF BONY FISHES

Structure of kidney. The kidneys of the ray-finned fishes Chondrostei and Holostei are incompletely described. In Holostei (freshwater), the tubules are mesonephric, with some open nephrostomes (197). The tubules are segmentally arranged. The nephron consists of a relatively large glomerulus with a short neck region and a proximal segment with two parts, the second part with less developed brush border than the first. Collecting tubule and collecting duct connect the tubules to the ureter. A renal portal circulation is present (197).

The Teleostei show considerable variation in the kidneys. Ogawa (212) divides them into five types according to the shape and fusion of the two kidneys. Generally, they consist of a head kidney and a trunk kidney. The head kidney consists primarily of lymphoid, hematopoietic, and chromaffin tissue. The trunk kidney consists of nephrons and hemapoietic tissue. The renal tubules show great variation (126).

On the basis of glomerular development and nephron segments present, Homer Smith reached the conclusion that teleosts originated in freshwater. In true freshwater teleosts, where the excretion of a large volume of dilute urine is required, the glomeruli are relatively large, and the

nephron consists of the following segments: neck segment; proximal segment, parts I and II; distal segment; collecting tubule. An intermediate segment may or may not be present. All these segments are also found in the euryhaline teleosts, which spend part of their life cycle in freshwater. The only exception is the killifish, which lacks the distal segment (4, 197).

In many marine teleosts, several segments are missing, and the glomeruli, if present, are modified or reduced in size. In recent invaders of the sea, such as the ocean catfish and the marine eel, all the nephron segments are present. A large number of marine teleosts, however, do not have the distal segment. Finally, a number of marine teleosts, such as the sea horse, the goosefish, and the toadfish, and also Antarctic teleosts, have aglomerular tubules (Fig. 2-9). The only segments left are the second part of the proximal tubule and the collecting tubule (68, 126, 186, 207). Thus, the tubules clearly reflect their function.

The arterial blood supply to the kidney comes from one or several branches of the dorsal aorta. These branches break up into finer branches which supply the glomeruli. The renal portal blood circulation comes from the vena caudalis. In some of the freshwater teleosts, which have a very rich renal arterial blood supply, the renal portal circulation is missing.

The kidneys of the fleshy-finned fishes, the lungfishes (Dipnoi), have been well described by several investigators. The kidney of *Neoceratodus* has been described by Gunther (quoted from 197). A description of kidney structure of *Lepidosiren* and *Protopterus* is summarized by Hickman and Trump (126) from several sources. The kidneys have 8 to 10 lobes. The nephron consists of a renal corpuscle with a glomerulus and an inconspicuous mesangial region, a ciliated neck segment, a proximal tubule containing first and second segments with cell structure resembling that of teleost nephrons, a ciliated intermediate segment lined by low, cuboidal, ciliated cells, a distal segment with a striated cytoplasm formed by elongated perpendicular mitochondria, and a collecting duct system.

The glomeruli are supplied from the arteria

coeliaca. The tubular capillary net is, in addition, supplied from the renal portal system (vena caudalis).

Function of kidney. Among the ray-finned fishes, only the teleosts have been studied extensively. The GFR is considerably higher in freshwater than in marine teleosts (Table 2-4). Furthermore, the GFR changes in euryhaline fishes when they move from a freshwater to a saltwater habitat. The aglomerular fishes form the primary urine, not by filtration, but by secretion. Presumably, the secretion of water is secondary to the secretion of solute into the tubule; the nature of the solute has not yet been determined (246). It seems that the ability to form urine by tubular secretion is not confined to the aglomerular teleost. Marshall and Grafflin (185) found that they could render the sculpin functionally aglomerular with a dose of phlorhizin. It then continued to form urine by tubular secretion. Hickman (123) has shown that the southern flounder *Paralichthys lethostigma* shows seasonal variations in filtration rate. In the winter months, the filtration rate decreases virtually to zero, but the urine flow remains constant and higher than the filtration rate. In the summer months, however, the filtration rate is higher and exceeds the urine flow two- to threefold. In the eel tubular fluid secretion was dominant when the eel was acclimated to freshwater, but not to seawater (246). Recent observations (68) on Antarctic fish suggest that the aglomerular condition in fishes may be an adaptation to prevent urinary loss of glucoproteins with biological antifreeze properties. Antarctic teleosts were all aglomerular.

The regulation of the glomerular filtration in euryhaline fishes may be hormonal. The GFR in fishes increases with injections of the neurohypophyseal hormone, AVT (131, 175, 216). Angiotensin produces diuretic and natriuretic effects in the American eel (211). This could be due to AVT release, since angiotensin causes release of vasopressin in mammals (202, 262). In the aglomerular toadfish, however, the rate of urine production is not affected by AVT, although it is regulated. Thus, it is five times higher in freshwater than in seawater.

The tubular resorption of water is around one-third to one-half of the filtered water. This fraction is about the same in freshwater and in marine teleosts. In freshwater fishes, the urine osmolality is low, indicating an efficient ion resorption and low tubular permeability to water. In marine teleosts, glomerular or aglomerular, the urine is, under normal conditions, slightly hypoosmotic to the plasma (U/P osmolar 0.85) (95). In the Antarctic teleosts the urine was essentially isosmotic to the plasma (67).

The euryhaline glomerular teleosts are able to regulate the urine osmolality. In the sole *Platichthys flesus* and in the eel *Anguilla rostrata* the urine osmolality is 45 to 50 mosm when the fish is in freshwater. When the fish is transferred to seawater, the urine osmolality rises, over 48 h, to 200 to 280 mosm (246). The rise in urine osmolality is due to a slight increase in tubular water resorption (inulin U/P rises from 2.8 to 4.0) but must be due primarily to increased divalent ion secretion, since monovalent ion concentrations rise only slightly (123, 125, 246). In *Fundulus kansae*, it was observed (92) that the urine osmolality rises about 200 mosm above the plasma concentration on the second day following transfer to seawater, then gradually falls to the plasma level within the next 10 days. This transient hyperosmolality of the urine could possibly be due to Na^+ influx via the tail into the renal portal vein.

Low urine osmolality is found only in fishes with a distal tubular segment. Na^+ concentrations are very low in the urine of freshwater as well as of marine teleosts (Table 2-5). High urine Na^+ and Cl^- concentrations are found only when the fish is disturbed by handling or is under unnatural restraint. This is true in glomerular as well as aglomerular fish (95).

From present evidence, it cannot be ascertained if the water permeability of any part of the renal tubule increases when the fish is transferred to seawater, since the changes in urine osmolality could be due to changes in divalent ion secretion.

In the aglomerular teleost *Opsanus tau* (165), adaptation to freshwater does not involve the production of a dilute urine, presumably because a distal tubule is lacking. The osmolar U/P was 0.85 in freshwater and 0.90 in seawater. The urine Cl⁻ concentration was very low in both media. The urine Na⁺ concentration was higher in the urine in freshwater (107 mmol/L) than in seawater (about 15 mmol/L), presumably because divalent ion secretion was more prevalent during seawater adaptation. With a fivefold increase in the urine flow, the renal Na⁺ loss is increased more than 30-fold in freshwater. This places a greater burden on the Na⁺ uptake mechanisms in the gills.

Diuretics, furosemide, and ethacrynic acid produce marked natriuresis and chloruresis in the freshwater catfish (128). Similar observations were made in seawater eels (246) and in marine teleost (Lasix, Edecrin, Brinaldrix) (123).

The amount of Mg^{2+} secreted rises 30-fold when a euryhaline fish is transferred from freshwater to seawater (246). The secretory mechanism for Mg^{2+} is independent of the Na⁺ resorption mechanism (16). In aglomerular Antarctic teleost, divalent ion secretion is very strong with the Mg^{2+} urine/plasma ratio ranging between 50 and 250 (67).

Teleosts secrete phenol red, PAH, and Diodrast actively into the renal tubules (95), and these substances compete for the same transport system. The uphill transport takes place both at the peritubular and the luminal membranes of proximal tubular cells (158). The maximal rate of PAH secretion was the same in the glomerular sculpin (138 mg/kg per day) and the aglomerular goosefish (137 mg/kg per day).

In glomerular as well as in aglomerular teleosts, the urinary sinus modifies the urine composition through a coupled Na⁺, Cl⁻ and water resorption. Divalent ions are concentrated in the bladder urine as a result of this fluid resorption (16, 230, 231).

In the fleshy-finned lungfish *Protopterus,* the GFR was found by Sawyer (237) to be around 14 to 30 mL/kg per h. The filtration rate ceases completely during estivation, when all nongaseous exchange with the environment comes to a halt. Sawyer (237), investigating the effect of AVT on the renal function of *Protopterus,* found that the GFR is more than tripled by doses of AVT as low as 0.5 μg/kg. The Na⁺ excretion is increased 60- to 100-fold.

Under normal conditions, one-half to two-thirds of the filtered water is resorbed. The urine osmolality is extremely low, about 16 to 20 mosm. Na⁺ concentrations are about 5 mmol/L; NH_4^+, 3 to 4 mmol/L; and urea, 0.1 to 0.6 mmol/L. Thus, the kidney function of a nonestivating lungish is quite similar to that of a freshwater teleost.

In the coelecanth *Latimeria chalumnae* bladder urine and plasma taken from living animals have been analyzed. From this information some deductions can be made as to renal function. Osmolality is identical in urine and plasma. Na⁺ concentration is essentially the same in both fluids. Cl⁻ is lower in urine. Mg^{2+} and total P are more than 5 times higher and SO_4^{2-} is more than 20 times higher than in plasma, suggesting tubular secretion of these ions. In contrast to elasmobranchs, urea concentration was identical in plasma and urine, indicating no active resorption of urea (116).

KIDNEYS OF AMPHIBIANS

Structure of kidney. The mesonephric kidneys of adult amphibians consist of two flattened oblong organs. The number of nephrons varies greatly in different species. In the salamander *Salamandra maculosa,* it is only 800; in the bullfrog *Rana catesbeiana,* it is 6400 to 8150 (cited in Deyrup [64]).

The nephron has all the typical segments. The cell structure of the tubular segments is much like those in teleosts. The largest renal corpuscles are found in salamanders (127 × 165 μm). In frogs and toads, they are smaller (85 μm) (197). The glomeruli are supplied with blood from several arteriae renalis, 50 in salamanders, 5 to 6 in frogs. All amphibians have a functioning renal portal system, but there are considerable variations in the final circulation pattern (197). The portal vein, the vena portarum iliaca, is a continuation of the vena iliaca.

The arrangement of the highly convoluted tubules within the kidney is shown in Fig. 2-6. The collecting ducts, running at right angles to the tubules, join the ureter. The two ureters open into the dorsal side of the cloaca. The urine collects in the bladder, which opens into the ventral side of the cloaca. The bladder, a bilobed diverticulum to the cloaca, is well developed in adult frogs and toads. It is absent in the tadpole, but develops gradually during metamorphosis.

Function of kidney. The function of the amphibian kidney is primarily, as in freshwater fishes, that of excreting excess water. In addition, however, the kidney function must adapt to the change in osmoregulatory demands placed on the animal when it leaves the pond and becomes dehydrated, when it hibernates or estivates, or when it is exposed to saline water.

In the freshwater frog *R. clamitans,* GFR is about 30 mL/kg/h (247); in *R. esculenta,* about 60 mL/kg/h; and in tadpoles of *R. clamitans*, about 44 mL/kg/h (97). Dehydration causes a gradual decrease in GFR (247). Thus, in *R. clamitans,* it decreases to 15 percent of the control value after the frog has lost water corresponding to 14 percent of its body weight. A greater degree of dehydration results in complete cessation of glomerular filtration. The frog or toad burrowing in the ground is also exposed to dehydration, and GFR goes to zero.

Exposure to saline water also affects the GFR. In *R. esculenta* transferred from freshwater to an 0.8% NaCl solution, the GFR decreased abruptly but then in the course of 5 to 8 h rose to values equal to or higher than the control value (188). In *R. cancrivora,* which can adapt to 80 percent seawater, the GFR is inversely proportional to the osmolality of the medium. It is 55 mL/kg per h in freshwater and is reduced to one-half at 300 mosm and one-third at 600 mosm (275).

An amphibian hibernating during the winter at the bottom of a pond will be exposed to a steady influx of water, but because the temperature is lower and also because of changes in the skin, the rate of water influx is decreased. In frogs exposed to temperatures of 5°C in the laboratory, the GFR was reduced to about one-fourth the rate at 20 to 25°C (247). The GFR is regulated by the antidiuretic hormone AVT. The hormone presumably causes constriction of the afferent arteriole to the glomerulus (239). The nephrons function intermittently. In *Necturus* (103) following a single injection of AVT (20 mg/kg body weight), many glomeruli could be seen to have reduced blood flow and in many cases there was a total shutdown of flow. In the frog kidney, the tubular maximum for glucose resorption (Tm glucose) and tubular maximum for PAH secretion (Tm PAH) are both proportional to GFR (94, 247), indicating that GFR is proportional to the number of functioning glomeruli.

The overall tubular resorption of water is, under normal experimental conditions, about two-thirds to four-fifths of filtered water (247, 248). The proximal resorption of water is about 30 percent of the filtrate in *Necturus* (103) and *R. catesbeiana* (169). Proximal fluid and sodium transport are partially inhibited by Diamox, ouabain, and ethacrynic acid. Significant transepithelial Na^+ and Cl^- concentration difference is maintained when the lumen contains a poorly permeant nonelectrolyte solute (299).

Expansion of extracellular fluid volume reduces proximal resorption (14) and morphologically changes the tight junctions (141). When an amphibian is exposed to dehydration or saline solution, or treated with AVT, the tubular water resorption increases, and the free-water clearance decreases (56, 188, 238, 239, 247). This is caused primarily by an increased permeability of the distal tubule to water (103). In *R. cancrivora,* tubular resorption of water increased with increasing medium osmolality. The creatinine U/P ratio rose from 2 to 3 in freshwater to values as high as 40 at medium concentration of 600 mosm. The tubular resorption of water is under the control of AVT (238). The tubular as well as the glomerular effect of AVT can be blocked by probenecid (56). AVT also enhances tubular resorption of Na^+ (143). The diluting segment consists of two distinct parts of the distal tubule. In the first part there is active Cl^- transport (lumen positive); in the second part Na^+ is actively transported (287).

The osmolality of the urine is normally very low in frogs, 20 to 40 mosm. In the dehydrated frog, the urine osmolality is increased, but even severe dehydration does not cause the osmolality of the urine (that has not been exposed to the bladder) to increase to that of the blood. Mayer (188) found that the urine of frogs placed in 0.8% saline solution had urine osmolality of 168 mosm when the plasma osmolality was 260 mosm. In *R. cancrivora* exposed to medium con-

centrations from 300 to 800 mosm the urine osmolality was usually 100 to 200 mosm below that
of the plasma (112).

In amphibians adapted to freshwater, the primary solutes in the urine are Na$^+$, Cl$^-$ and K$^+$,
and urea. Na$^+$ and Cl$^-$ are very effectively resorbed by the tubules (15, 187), and urea is actively secreted into the tubules by the adult frog.
The active secretion of urea was first demonstrated by Marshall (184) and later confirmed by
others (96, 247). The secretion is limited by a tubular maximum and is subject to competition
(96). The urea derivative thiourea is also secreted
by the same mechanism, but not methylurea and
acetamide (248). Micropuncture studies have
shown (169, 170, 296) that the secretion takes
place along the proximal and distal tubular segments.

The tubular urea secretion is found in many
amphibians to varying degrees, but not in all (Ref.
43 and B. Schmidt-Nielsen, unpublished). *R.
cancrivora* does not secrete urea when it is acclimated to higher salinities. However, it does not
resorb urea actively either, as do the elasmobranchs. The urine urea concentration is about
the same as that of the blood (257), indicating that
urea diffuses back passively across the tubule or
collecting duct epithelium. *R. cancrivora* thus
conserves urea mainly by having a high tubular
permeability to urea and a low GFR.

The bladder plays an important role in amphibians. When the frog is in water and the level of
AVT in the blood is low, the bladder has a low
permeability to water and urea. Dehydration,
which causes release of AVT, increases the bladder permeability to water and to urea and also enhances active transport of Na$^+$ from mucosal to
serosal sides. The effect of AVT on the bladder
is greatest in the more terrestrial frogs and toads
and is missing or minimal in fully aquatic forms
(175). Amphibian bladders have been used extensively for the study of water and solute movement
across epithelial membranes.

KIDNEYS OF REPTILES

Structure of kidney. The kidneys of reptiles
are well described by von Möllendorff (197). In

chelonians, the kidneys are compact organs located deep in the pelvis. In lizards, the two kidneys, located close to the cloaca, often join caudad. In snakes, the kidneys are elongated organs.
In most reptiles, the tubules are arranged in lobules which follow one another in the craniocau-
dal direction. Each lobule has a ventrally located
collecting duct which joins the ureter; a branch
of the arteria renalis supplies the glomeruli
within the lobule with arterial blood; and a
branch from the vena renalis afferens supplies the
tubules with renal portal blood. The highly convoluted tubules, arranged parallel to each other,
run at a right angle to the collecting ducts.

The number of tubules per kidney varies from
1600 to 2000 in some lizards to 15,000 in some
snakes. The size of the renal corpuscles is about
the same as in amphibians. The largest (216 ×
140 μm) are found in the turtle (*Testudo*). The
smallest (54 × 77 μm) are found in the lizard
(*Lacerta*).

The tubules have all the typical segments. The
total length of the tubule varies from 4 to 16 mm.
The structure of the tubular cells differs from
those of lower vertebrates in that proximal and,
particularly, distal tubular cells have narrow lateral fingerlike interdigitations; the basal cell
membranes, however, are smooth and have no interdigitations or basal infoldings (57, 253) such as
one finds in fishes, amphibians, and mammals
(58).

The initial collecting tubule, which is much
wider than the distal tubule, is, in some lizards,
lined with mucus-secreting cells. The collecting
ducts join the ureters, which, as in amphibians,
open into the dorsal side of the cloaca. A bladder
is present in all chelonians and in some lizards
and snakes.

Function of kidney. For recent reviews, see
Dantzler (50b) and Dantzler and Holmes (55).
Reptiles have adapted to all types of habitats:
freshwater, marine, and terrestrial. In all reptiles,
regardless of habitat, the kidney is the only organ
for excretion of waste nitrogen. In freshwater-
adapted reptiles, a primary function is also that of
excreting excess water. In marine and in some
terrestrial reptiles, excess salt is excreted via the
salt gland.

GFR is highly variable in the ureotelic freshwater-adapted turtle *Pseudemys scripta.* It increases following a water load and decreases when the animal is dehydrated. When water corresponding to 10 percent of body weight has been lost, the glomerular filtration ceases. In the more terrestrial chelonian, the desert tortoise *Gopherus agassizii,* and in all the squamatans and crocodilians investigated, the GFR appears to be less variable. Water load in most of these animals causes an increase in GFR, but dehydration or salt load has less effect. The comparison, however, is not valid in all cases, since the degree of dehydration varies as shown in Table 2-6.

Salt loading has a variable effect on GFR. Salt loading increases plasma osmotic pressure but causes, at the same time, an increase in extracellular space. Reptiles, in which GFR decreases more readily with dehydration, respond to salt loading by a decreased GFR. Thus, in the freshwater turtle, even a modest salt loading (a 20-mosm increase in plasma osmolality) causes complete glomerular shutdown. In the desert tortoise, however, the filtration rate ceased only after a 100-mosm increase in plasma osmolality (54).

In freshwater snakes, moderate infusion of salt (3.6 mmol/kg/h) reduced the filtration rate to half (52). A comparison between the effect of salt loading on the freshwater snake *Natrix sipedon* and the desert snake *Pituophis melanoleucus* (160) showed that, with identical loading in the two species, GFR decreased slightly in the freshwater snake and increased about 60 percent in the desert snake.

The antidiuretic hormone AVT has been found to regulate the filtration rate in freshwater turtles and in freshwater snakes (52, 54).

The question of whether or not the variations in filtration rate are caused by intermittent tubular function has been investigated in reptiles by measuring Tm PAH (52, 54). Dantzler (52) concludes, on the basis of his findings of exaltation of PAH clearance during rising GFR in the water snake, that there is true intermittency of glomerular function. SNGFR was estimated in *Sceloporus cyanogenus* to be 4.6 nL/min (285).

The tubular resorption of water is about one-half to three-fourths of the filtered water in chelonians (54), in the squamatans (166, 232), and in

Table 2-6. Reptiles: Glomerular filtration rate in normal, water-loaded, and dehydrated animals (in mL/kg per h)

	HABITAT*	NORMAL	WATER-LOADED, 10–15% OF BODY WT	DEHYDRATED, 5–18% OF BODY WT	REF.
Chelonians					
Pseudemys scripta	FW	4.7	10.3	0 (10%)	54
Gopherus agassizii	T(D)	4.7	15.1	. . . .	54
Chelonia mydas mydas	SW	(14.3)	. . . .	. . . .	132
Squamatans					
Hemidactylus spp.	T(W)	10.4	24.3	3.33 (18%)	232
Tiliguas scincoides	T(W)	15.9	24.5	0.68 (10%)	253
Phrynosoma cornutum	T(D)	3.54	5.52	2.14 (5%)	232
Tropidurus spp.	T(D)	3.62	1.23	4.53 (5%)	232
Natrix sipedon	FW	28.1	. . . .	. . . .	167
Pituophis melanoleucus	T(D)	10.8	. . . .	. . . .	160
Laticauda columbrina	SW	(0.5)†	. . . .	. . . .	253
Rhynchocephalians					
Sphenodon	T(W)	0.36	0.65	. . . .	‡
Crocodilians					
Crocodylus acutus	FW	9.6	15.2	6.1 (10%)	252
C. johnstoni	FW	6.0	3.3	1.9 (10%)	253
C. porosus	SW	1.5	18.8	0.68 (10%)	252

* FW = freshwater; SW = seawater; T(W) = terrestrial wet habitat; T(D) = terrestrial dry habitat.

† One animal only.

‡ B. Schmidt-Nielsen (in preparation).

Table 2-7. Reptiles: Osmolal U/P of ureteral urine

ANIMAL	HABITAT*	NORMAL	WATER LOAD	DEHYDRATION	REF.
Chelonians					
Pseudemys scripta	FW	0.62	0.60	0.84	54
Gopherus agassizii	T(D)	0.36	0.57	. . .	
Squamatans					
Hemidactylus spp.	T(W)	0.64	0.74	0.74	232
Tiliguas scincoides	T(W)	0.50	0.43	0.66	253
Phrynosoma cornutum	T(D)	0.93	0.90	0.97	232
Tropidurus spp.	T(D)	0.96	0.99	0.97	232
Natrix cyclopion	T(W)	0.43	0.37	. . .	167
Rhynchocephalians					
Sphenodon	T(W)	0.89	0.65	. . .	†
Crocodilians					
Crocodylus acutus	FW	0.80	0.82	0.84	252
C. johnstoni	FW	0.71	0.83	0.94	253
C. porosus	SW	0.95	0.45	. . .	253

* FW = freshwater; SW = seawater; T(W) = terrestrial wet habitat; T(D) = terrestrial dry habitat.
† B. Schmidt-Nielsen (in preparation).

the sphenodon (245). In the crocodile *Crocodylus acutus* (252), the tubular water resorption is about seven-eighths of filtered water. Water loading, which increases GFR, does not decrease fractional tubular water resorption appreciably in any of the reptiles. Dehydration, on the other hand, increases fractional tubular water resorption in freshwater turtles and snakes but has less effect in other reptiles (54, 166, 285). AVT administration likewise increases fractional tubular water resorption in the freshwater turtles (54) and snakes, and decreases free-water clearance (C_{H_2O}/C_{in}) (52). In the water snake, Dantzler (52) clearly demonstrated that the tubular effect of AVT is more pronounced than the glomerular effect.

The osmolality of the urine collected at the ureteral openings of various reptiles is shown in Table 2-7. Compared to fishes and amphibians, it is remarkable how poorly these reptiles are able to dilute the urine and how little the urine osmolality varies with the state of hydration of the animal. Micropuncture studies on the lizard *Sceloporus cyanogenys* (285) showed that the osmolality of the fluid in the distal tubule or collecting duct is unaffected by the state of hydration of the animal or by the injection of AVT. It appears from these and other findings (115) that the water permeability of the distal tubule or collecting duct system in many reptiles is insensitive to AVT. In this respect, then, they function like the thick as-

cending limb of the mammalian loop of Henle.

Na^+ is resorbed isosmotically in the proximal tubule of reptiles, as in mammals, as shown by micropuncture studies. About 35 percent of filtered Na^+ and water was resorbed in the proximal tubule of the lizard *Sceloporus cyanogenys* (285). In the water snake, the total tubular Na^+ resorption was found to be 91 percent of the filtered Na^+, while distal tubular Na^+ resorption was estimated to be 32 percent of filtered Na^+ (167). Saline loading reduced total Na^+ resorption to 70.5 percent. Similar observations were made on the lizard *Sceloporus* (285). In the lizards *Phrynosoma* and *Tropidurus*, total tubular Na^+ resorption was only around 50 percent of filtered Na^+. In the sea turtle *Chelonia mydas mydas*, urinary Na^+ and K^+ excretion increased when saline solution was injected (intramuscularly). The major part of injected salt was, however, excreted extrarenally (132). The Na^+ concentration in the urine of the seawater-adapted turtle was only 11 mmol/L and the K^+ concentration 8.1 mmol/L (130). It is quite possible that divalent ions are excreted in the urine, but measurements are lacking.

The Na^+ resorption is under the control of adrenal cortical hormones (22). Thus, adrenalectomy reduced tubular Na^+ resorption (82). Aldosterone increased Na^+ resorption in saline-solution-loaded animals (167). Dehydration decreased tubular Na^+ resorption in *Sphenodon*

(245) and in *Sceloporus* (B. Schmidt-Nielsen, in preparation). In the snake the response was the opposite (52). It is quite likely that the decreased Na^+ resorption is a response to AVT (243, 297).

In crocodilians, Na^+ and Cl^- ions are resorbed, presumably, in the distal tubule, and NH_4^+ and HCO_3^- are secreted. This mechanism may be an exchange mechanism of Na^+ for H^+ and Cl^- for HCO_3^-, similar to that observed across fish gills. The mechanism results in an extremely low loss of electrolytes in the urine of the crocodile, and may be an electrolyte-conserving mechanism for this freshwater reptile, which cannot produce a dilute urine. Under normal conditions, the Na^+ concentration of ureteral urine is 61 mmol/L and the Cl^- concentration 45 mmol/L, while cloacal urine collected from the undisturbed crocodile has Na^+ and Cl^- concentrations as low as 1 to 6 mmol/L (48, 252).

Urea is a nitrogenous waste product in chelonians and in *Sphenodon* and in lizards of the skink family (245 and unpublished observations). It is excreted mostly by glomerular filtration, but active secretion contributes to its excretion. Urea clearance exceeds the filtration rate at high urine flow in *Pseudemys scripta* (54), and in *Sphenodon* the urea clearance exceeds the filtration rate by 20 percent (245).

Uric acid is excreted by active tubular secretion in all reptiles, the uric acid clearance being 4 to 10 times the GFR. Acute metabolic alkalosis increases C_{urate}/GFR (53). Urate is not secreted by the same transport mechanism as PAH (50a).

The osmolality of the final urine can, to some degree, be modified in the cloaca, where Na^+ and Cl^- resorption takes place (258). In the crocodile (252) and in the sphenodon (245), the urine osmolality is decreased, while the urine is stored in the cloaca. In the lizard *Amphibolurus* from dry salt lakes in Australia the urine becomes hyperosmotic to the plasma in the cloaca. The mechanism is unknown (28). Cloacal regulation does not appear to be under AVT control (269).

KIDNEYS OF BIRDS

Structure of kidney. The kidneys of birds (27, 197, 281) are compact organs situated dorsad,

deep in the pelvis. Like the reptilian kidneys, they are divided into numerous lobules, but, unlike the reptilian kidney, the renal tissue consists of two parts—a cortical and a medullary part. The medullary part is also called the *cone*, or *papilla*. At the tip of each cone, several collecting ducts open into a branch of the ureter. There are several cortical lobules for each cone. (See Fig. 2-8.)

Within each lobule, two types of nephrons are found:

1. Reptilian-type (RT) metanephric tubules consisting of the usual sequence of segments. These tubules, found entirely in the cortical part of each lobule, are convoluted and run at right angles to the collecting ducts.
2. Metanephric mammalian-type (MT) tubules with a loop of Henle which reaches down into the medullary part. In these tubules, the proximal segment is followed by a thin loop segment which runs parallel to the collecting duct in the renal cone.

Each cone is surrounded by a connective tissue sheath. It consists of a ring of collecting ducts which surround straight capillaries, and thin descending segments of the loop of Henle. Concentric layers of thick ascending segments of the loop of Henle surround the collecting ducts (223).

The capacity to produce a concentrated urine is associated with the total number of loops of Henle or with the relative abundance of medullary cone tissue (144, 223).

Function of kidney. All birds are essentially terrestrial, although some may spend most of their time on the ocean or on freshwater. Birds generally have a greater evaporative water loss than reptiles, due to evaporation from respiratory passages during flight and evaporative cooling during heat stress (9). Water conservation is, therefore, essential to most birds.

Water conservation is achieved through (1) the excretion of precipitated urate in concentrations up to 3000 times that of the blood (the urates aid in the excretion of Na^+ and K^+ ions in an osmotically inactive form) (23, 195, 269), (2) the ability to produce a concentrated urine, and (3) extrarenal hyperosmotic salt excretion. All birds excrete most of their nitrogenous waste as uric acid, but the proportion of NH_4^+ to uric acid in the urine varies with habitats. All birds can produce a urine more concentrated than the blood.

It is interesting that in birds physiologic adaptation to drinking water of a high salinity has been achieved in two different ways: In oceanic birds, such as sea gulls, terns, pelicans, petrels, and cormorants, the kidneys apparently do not concentrate the urine to a high degree, and a major portion of ingested salt is excreted extrarenally via the salt gland (139, 254). In the birds belonging to the order Passeriformes which have adapted to salt marshes, extrarenal salt excretion has not developed, and the kidneys have developed a high capacity for concentrating the urine.

Birds have a much higher GFR than lower vertebrates, mainly because their kidneys have more nephrons. SNGFR was 13 to 16 nL/min in MT nephrons and 6.3 nL/min in RT nephrons (27). The SNGFR in RT tubules in birds is thus not much higher than that in reptiles (see page 00). GFR appears to be more stable in birds than in reptiles. The duck *Anas platytrynchos* can adapt to drinking saline solutions, but there is little effect on GFR. GFR in ducks maintained on saline solution (284 mmol NaCl and 6 mmol KCl) was 128 mL/kg/h, and in the freshwater-maintained bird 131 mL/kg/h. In the rooster *Gallus domesticus* the GFR varied from 105 mL/kg/h in the dehydrated bird (6 percent loss of body weight) to 127 mL/kg/h during water loading (9 percent of body weight). Salt loading (10 to 15 mmol NaCl/kg body weight) did not result in a significant decrease in GFR (274). Increasing salt loads do, however, decrease the GFR, as observed by Dantzler (51). Thus, a salt load of 30 mmol/kg body weight caused a 25 percent decrease in GFR, and a load of 45 mmol/kg body weight caused a 60 percent decrease in GFR. A decrease in the number of functioning glomeruli, with a decreasing GFR, was suggested by the linear relationship between Tm PAH and GFR. It has been shown (27) that a significant shift in glomerular filtration between RT and MT nephrons occurs following a salt load. In the desert quail SNGFR remained relatively constant in MT nephrons following a salt load (40 mmol/kg body weight) but filtration ceased in all RT nephrons. The glomerular intermittency was caused by vasoconstriction at the level of the afferent arterioles (24). At more moderate salt loads, only a portion of RT nephrons ceased to function. This regulation is probably under the control of AVT, but this has not been proven (3, 27).

In birds, the tubular resorption of water varies over a much greater range than in reptiles. In the rooster, inulin U/P varied from a minimum of 3 in water-loaded birds to a maximum of 100 to 120 in dehydrated birds. On the average, 90 and 98.8 percent filtered water was resorbed during hydration and dehydration, respectively. The tubular water resorption is clearly regulated by AVT (3, 271).

Regulation of the osmotic concentration of the urine is well developed in birds. The domestic fowl chicken and turkey are able to regulate the osmotic concentration of the urine from a minimum of 50 mosm to a maximum of around 500 mosm. Average osmolar U/P ratio in water-loaded roosters was 0.37, the same as in water-loaded freshwater snakes. Maximum osmolar U/P ratio in dehydrated roosters was about 1.58.

Many desert-dwelling birds are able to concentrate the urine 2 to 2.8 times the plasma osmolality (270). Birds living in salt marshes, all of the order Passeriformes, are able to concentrate the urine to the same or higher degrees. The Savannah sparrow *Passerculus sandwichensis* (family *Fringilidae*) can apparently drink saline water from the salt marshes which they inhabit. *P. sandwichensis beldingi* inhabits salt marshes year round. *P. sandwichensis brooksi* breeds in freshwater marshes but winters in southern California, where it often occurs in salt marshes. *P. sandwichensis beldingi* can concentrate the urine up to 2100 mosm and reach an osmolar U/P of 5. *P. sandwichensis brooksi* can concentrate the urine up to 1000 mosm (osmolar U/P 2.2). Both species can tolerate serum osmotic concentrations exceeding 400 mosm (225).

Other birds, such as the swamp sparrow (*Melospiza*), the seaside sparrow (*Ammospiza*), and the crossbill *Loxia curviostra sitkensis,* can also tolerate saline water drinking and concentrate chloride in the urine, but information on osmotic concentrating ability is lacking (59, 224).

Oceanic birds do not seem to concentrate the urine very highly. In the gull *Larus glaucescens,* acclimated to saltwater, Na^+ and Cl^- concentrations in cloacal urine are around 50 to 150 mmol/L and K^+ around 20 to 50 mmol/L. In birds acclimated to increasing salt concentrations up to full-strength seawater (139), the ratio of Na^+ to K^+ in spontaneously voided urine was approximately 1, even when the birds were acclimated to full-strength seawater and a large fraction of ingested Na^+ and Cl^- was excreted via the salt gland. Gulls acclimated to freshwater still excrete a major portion of injected Na^+ and K^+ extrarenally (137).

AVT, in addition to increasing tubular water resorption, also increases Na^+ but not K^+ resorption in the renal tubules of the domestic fowl (271). This increase in electrolyte resorption is only observed following a large injection of antidiuretic hormone (21). During dehydration, a larger amount of Na^+ is resorbed than during water loading (274). Thus, birds, some reptiles, and amphibians all have a renal natriferic effect of AVT.

Uric acid is secreted by the renal tubules of birds, as first shown by Mayrs in 1924 (189). Uric acid clearance is identical to PAH clearance (282). The ratio C_{urate}/C_{in} was found in the chicken to vary from 7.5 to 15.8 (263) and in the duck to be about 10. In the duck, about 30 percent of total nitrogen is excreted as NH_4, 62 percent as uric acid, and 2.7 percent as urea. Divalent cations are incorporated into avian urate precipitates in high concentrations (196). The urea clearance exceeded the inulin clearance by as much as 80 percent at high urine flows but decreased to less than 10 percent of the GFR at the lowest urine flows (282). A similar decrease in urea clearance with increasing tubular water resorption was observed in the chicken (275). The results indicate either active tubular urea secretion or tubular synthesis of urea and a high tubular back-diffusion of urea.

The countercurrent system in bird kidneys, which is somewhat similar to that found in the mammalian kidneys, is responsible for the ability of bird kidneys to produce a hyperosmotic urine. Na^+ and Cl^- accumulate in the tissue of the renal cones during the production of a concentrated urine (275). Urea, which comprises 50 percent of total solutes in the mammalian renal papilla, con-

stitutes only 0.4 percent of total solutes in the cone of the bird kidney.

The cloaca of birds plays an important role in modification of the urine. Skadhauge (272) showed that urine, after it enters the cloaca, is regurgitated as far as to the caeca and that fluid is resorbed, particularly during dehydration. In the gull, spontaneously voided urine samples had a much lower Na^+/K^+ ratio than cloacal samples that were withdrawn artificially (138). These data indicate that Na^+ resorption is predominant in the cloaca. In the chicken, the hyperosmotic urine which enters the cloaca from the ureters remains hyperosmotic to the plasma during the stay in the cloaca due to hyperosmotic resorption (via intercellular spaces) across the intestinal epithelium (272).

Even in the Australian xerophilic parrot, whose kidneys can produce a urine with a urine-to-plasma osmotic ratio of 2.6, the stay in the cloaca does not change the osmolality of the urine. Forty percent of the Na^+ is resorbed by a mechanism which shows saturation kinetics. K^+ is secreted (270).

EXTRARENAL SALT EXCRETION MECHANISMS

Fishes, reptiles, and birds, which in their habitats are exposed to a high salt intake, excrete salt via extrarenal routes. Extrarenal salt excretion is also found in some terrestrial reptiles with a moderate salt but limited water intake.

Since the kidneys of fishes and reptiles cannot produce a urine with a higher osmotic concentratin than that of blood, they cannot excrete excess salt through the kidneys without a considerable water expenditure. Even certain birds, with some capacity for concentrating the urine, excrete salt extrarenally whenever they must depend upon seawater for drinking. The organs for salt excretion are gills in most fishes, rectal glands in elasmobranchs, and nasal or supraorbital glands in reptiles and birds.

SALT EXCRETION THROUGH GILLS

Fishes that are hypoosmotic to the seawater in which they live lose water and gain salt by diffusion. To make up for the water loss, the fishes drink seawater, which further increases the salt load. Since the salt concentration in seawater is about three times that of the extracellular fluid of the fish, the excess salt must be excreted in a concentration greater than three times that of the blood in order for the fish to gain free water.

Chloride cells in gills. The chloride cells, to which the function of salt excretion has been assigned (149, 154, 198, 219), are formed near the base of the secondary lamellae of the gill arches and also in other branchial epithelia both inside and outside the oral cavity. In seawater-adapted fish the chloride cells are characterized by an apical cavity filled with mucopolysaccharide. The cavity makes contact with the external environment through a relatively small opening in the surrounding respiratory epithelial cells (61, 149). Chloride cells are generally columnar and contain an extensive network of branching tubules which are continuous with the basal and lateral cell surface. In addition, they contain many mitochondria which are associated with the tubular network. The Na^+–K^+–ATPase which has been implicated in salt secretion by fish gills is associated with this tubular system (151). When the salinity of the external medium is raised, the number and size of the chloride cells increase. The opercular skin of some fishes contain typical gill chloride cells at much higher density than the gills (148). The marine elasmobranchs also have chloride cells in their gills (71).

Function of gills. The excretion of salt through the gills was first best demonstrated in the eel using an in vivo perfused heart-gill preparation. Keys (161), using a very sensitive chloride method, showed that the active excretion of salt takes place across the gill epithelium, since chloride is moved from the lower concentration in the perfusion solution (196 mmol/L) to the higher concentration in the medium (534 mmol/L).

The rate of chloride secretion appears to depend upon the internal chloride concentration. Secretion does not take place unless the plasma Cl^- concentration is increased above that found in the freshwater-acclimated eel (161).

The potential difference across the gill meas-

ured in seawater-acclimated fish is approximately $+20$ mV (inside positive) (135) and hence Cl^- is secreted across a large electrochemical gradient (135). The active chloride transport has been studied with opercular skin mounted in an Ussing-type flux chamber (150). Transport ceases in chloride-free medium and is inhibited by ouabain, furosemide, and anoxia. The potential across the isolated membrane is about the same as that measured in vivo across the gills. This potential is primarily due to differential permeability of the gill to Na^+ and K^+ and hence it changes in response to changes in the ionic composition of the external environment. The gill of seawater-acclimated eels is approximately 34 times more permeable to K^+ than to Na^+; therefore changes in external K^+ concentration have a much more marked effect on potential than do changes in external Na^+ concentration (135). External Cl^- has essentially no effect on gill potential (180).

In addition to the net Cl^- transport a considerable exchange-diffusion takes place across the gills. The fluxes of Na^+ and Cl^- of euryhaline fish are much greater in seawater than in freshwater (201). Thus, Na^+ in the blood exchanges with Na^+ in the medium at a rate many times faster than the net excretion rate. In the flounder, *Platichthys*, Na^+ influx and efflux were 2.25 and 2.60 mmol/100 g per hour, while net efflux was 0.35 mmol/100 g per hour (201). The same is true for Cl^-. When saltwater-acclimated flounder are transferred to freshwater, the Na^+ influx is immediately reduced from 2.25 to 0.42 mmol/100 g per hour (201) and the gill potential reverses to -70 mV (222). In both the flounder and trout the decrease in Na^+ flux on transfer to freshwater can be accounted for by the change in potential across the gill (159, 222). However, in the mullet and sea perch, the changes in fluxes cannot be accounted for entirely by the observed changes in potential (180). The large chloride fluxes observed in seawater (200) occur against an electrochemical gradient and hence the immediate reduction in Cl^- flux which occurs when fish are placed in Cl^--free seawater must be due to an exchange-diffusion mechanism. Extrusion of both Na^+ and Cl^- is stimulated by addition of K^+ to the external medium. This stimulatory effect of K^+ on both Na^+ and Cl^- efflux is blocked by thiocyanate ion even though the potential is unaffected (83, 180). The exact mechanism of action of thiocyanate is not known, but it selectively inhibits anion transport in many epithelia (83). In the opercular skin studies, thiocyanate partially inhibited net Cl^- transport (148).

THE ELASMOBRANCH RECTAL GLAND

The blood of the marine elasmobranchs has lower Na^+ and Cl^- concentrations than that of the seawater (Fig. 2-1). Consequently, these ions can enter the body by diffusion. Since the body fluids are slightly hyperosmotic to the seawater, the elasmobranch, unlike the marine teleost, does not suffer an osmotic loss of water and thus has no need for drinking seawater. Experimental evidence confirms that it does not drink (278). The discovery by Burger and Hess (39) that a constant excretion of an almost pure NaCl solution (6300 μmol/kg per day, recalculated from Burger—see Ref. 36) takes place via the rectal gland even in the starving fish showed that a constant influx of NaCl must take place, presumably via the gills (36, 39). This influx takes place even though the gills of marine elasmobranchs are much less permeable to sodium and chloride than are the gills of marine teleosts (40, 177).

Structure of rectal gland. The rectal gland, a finger-shaped organ, is located in the caudal portion of the body cavity. It is drained by a single duct into the intestine, posterior to the spiral valve. In the dogfish *Squalus,* it is composed of branching, tightly packed, blind-ending tubules which drain into a central collecting duct (34). In the stingray *Urolophus,* the gland is somewhat S-shaped (70) and lobulated, the central duct branches, and there are a number of lobular ducts.

There is a peripheral arterial supply to a capillary network which courses centrally to a venous drainage via sinusoidal vessels. It should be noted that in the elasmobranch the capillary blood flow is concurrent in direction with the flow of secretion in the tubules (34, 35, 70). This vascular arrangement is different from that of the salt gland in birds and reptiles, in which the capillary blood flow is countercurrent to the tubular flow (89, 254).

Electon microscopy of the tubular cells shows that the lateral borders have numerous deep interdigitations. Basal infoldings are not extensive in the stingray rectal glands, according to Doyle (70), but are well developed in the dogfish *Squalus* (34).

Function of rectal gland. The rectal gland of *Squalus acanthias* excretes continuously at a fairly constant rate of about 12 mL/kg per day (36). This is approximately equal to the simultaneously measured urine flow of 11 mL/kg per day. Secreted fluid is isosmotic with the blood (this is in contrast to the highly hyperosmotic fluid secreted by birds and reptiles). The solutes secreted are primarily Na^+ and Cl^-. The urea concentration in the secreted fluid is only about 40 mmol/L, i.e., about one-tenth the concentration in the plasma. The rate of Na^+ excretion is 10.5 μmol/kg per day. In the shark *Hemiscyllium plagiosum,* 75 percent of the total NaCl excretion is via the rectal gland (301). Dogfish in which the rectal gland is surgically removed survive for periods of at least 21 days without a change in plasma or urinary osmolality. The urine flow and urine Cl^- concentrations are increased; hence increased salt loss via the kidney (37) makes up for the lack of rectal gland function.

The rectal gland does not appear to be under nervous control (36), and no hormone has yet been found which controls its secretion, although many have been tried (36). Receptors which control secretion appear to be sensitive to three types of stimuli: osmotic concentration, salt concentration, volume changes (36, 37). Secretion can most easily be stimulated by injection of 2 mL/kg body weight of a 4% NaCl solution. The increased secretion is initiated after a delay of approximately 1 h (36). This suggests hormonal involvement. When the rectal gland is perfused in vitro, it continues to secrete a fluid at similar rates and of similar composition to that observed in vivo (120, 267). Both Na^+ and Cl^- are secreted against an electrochemical gradient, but since the blood side is 4 to 10 mV positive, Cl^- is transported against a larger gradient than is Na^+ (120, 267). When the secretory rate is stimulated by theophylline, the electric potential across the tubule increases from 7 to 20 mV (blood side positive) indicating increased electrogenic Cl^- transport.

These experiments have also provided some evidence concerning the control of secretory rate. Both increased perfusion rate (120) and the presence of theophylline (283) elevate secretory rate. Hence secretion in vivo could be regulated by changes in blood flow to the gland or at the cellular level by some agent which elevates cAMP levels in the tubules.

THE REPTILIAN AND AVIAN SALT GLANDS

Many marine birds, such as gulls, cormorants, and petrels, spend considerable time out at sea with no access to freshwater. They feed on fishes and marine invertebrates and must replace the water lost by evaporation from their lungs by drinking seawater. For a long time, it was an open question how they manage to excrete excess salt obtained through their food and the seawater ingested. K. Schmidt-Nielsen and collaborators (254–256) found that when cormorants or gulls were given seawater by stomach tube or intravenously, a nasal secretion started which lasted for several hours. The fluid dripping off the tip of the beak had an osmotic cencentration two to three times that of the blood (Table 2-8). It was found that the secretion came from a supraorbital gland which was given the name *salt gland*. Extrarenal salt excretion has subsequently been demonstrated in many species of birds and reptiles. Marine birds all possess well-developed salt glands. Most terrestrial birds lack salt glands; however, some desert birds, such as the ostrich and a few others, have salt glands (41, 95). Salt glands may be particularly important to young terrestrial birds which experience high evoporative water loss in the nest (213, 218). In reptiles, the salt gland is found in the marine iguana, the sea snake, sea turtle, and many terrestrial forms.

Structure of salt glands. The salt glands of birds and reptiles are located in the nasal or orbital region (254) except in snakes, which have oral salt glands (79) (Fig. 2-10). They are not homologous structures but glands of different embryonic origins which have acquired similar functions in birds and reptiles (75, 254). The glands in birds and reptiles are composed of several lobules. Each lobule has a central canal from which densely packed blind tubules radiate. Each tubule is about 700 μm long and 1.0 to 1.5 μm in cross section (1, 69). The cells are cuboidal. The vascular system differs from that of the elasmobranch rectal gland in that an arteriole runs between the tubules to the central duct. Here it splits up into capillaries which turn back and run close to the tubules. The flow in the capillaries is thus countercurrent to the flow in the tubules (Fig. 2-11). This arrangement may play a significant role in the production of a hyperosmotic secretion.

The ultrastructure of the cells of reptilian salt glands differs from that of avian salt glands. In reptiles (1), the cells have elaborate lateral borders with numerous interdigitations much like those of the elasmobranch rectal gland. In the gull, the cells have deep basal and lateral infoldings which may be connected with one another and which may form continuous channels through the cells (69). The basal lateral membranes are rich in Na^+–K^+–ATPase (84).

Table 2-8. Composition of salt gland fluid

ANIMAL	Mosm	CONCENTRATION, mmol			
		[NA$^+$]	[K$^+$]	[Cl$^-$]	REF.
Dogfish shark	1018	540	7	533	39
Marine iguana	. . . .	1434	235	1256	
Green sea turtle	. . . .	713	29	782	76
Land iguana	. . . .	692	214	486	
Sea snake	. . . .	620	28	635	73
Chuckwalla	. . . .	150	1102	827	206
False iguana	Normal	77	320	. . . .	288
	hyperkalemic	67	537	. . . .	
Herring gull	. . . .	718	24	720	254
Duck	. . . .	482	14	494	140

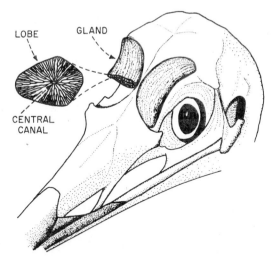

Figure 2-10. The salt glands of birds are located above the orbit. Each gland consists of many lobes about 1 mm in diameter, arranged longitudinally in the gland. Every lobe has a central canal with branching secretory tubules arranged around it. The gland drains via a duct into the nasal region. (*From K. Schmidt-Nielsen.*)

Function of salt glands. In birds and reptiles, the salt gland does not secrete continuously. In birds, the secretion starts following seawater ingestion. It can be artificially induced by injection of hypertonic saline solutions, or even hyper-

tonic sucrose solutions. The maximum rate of fluid secretion from avian salt glands is considerably greater than that in reptiles (Table 2-9). The maximum ion concentrations are not much different (Table 2-8). Hence, the rate of ion excretion via the salt gland is much greater in birds than in reptiles (Table 2-10).

The salt gland secretion of reptiles and birds living in a marine habitat is high in Na^+, while terrestrial reptiles secrete a fluid which is rich in K^+ (Table 2-8). The composition of the salt gland fluid changes in response to the salt intake (Table 2-8). In terrestrial lizards, as much as 40 percent of the anion is bicarbonate (258).

The mechanism of function and control of the avian and reptilian salt gland has been extensively studied and is reviewed by Peaker and Linzell (218). Reptilian salt glands appear to be controlled, at least partly, by osmoreceptors (73, 81), as a sucrose load will elicit a response comparable to that elicited by a similar osmotic load of NaCl (73). The avian salt glands are under the control of osmoreceptors located near the heart (118), which cause the gland to secrete via parasympathetic nerve pathways. Secretion can be stimulated by acetylcholine and blocked by atropine, epinephrine, and acetazolamide (88).

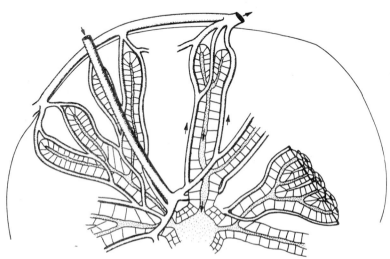

Figure 2-11. Cross section of a single lobe of avian salt gland. The blood vessels and capillaries of each lobe are arranged so that the flow of blood in the capillaries is countercurrent to the flow of fluid in the secretory tubules. (*From K. Schmidt-Nielsen.*)

Table 2-9. Maximum flow rate of salt gland secretion

SPECIES	FLOW RATE, mL/kg BODY WT/h	REF.
Herring gull	30	254
White duck	12	93
Sea snake	1.54	78
Chuckwalla	0.54	81
False iguana	0.17	288
Dogfish shark	3.00	37

SALT UPTAKE MECHANISMS

Animals that are hyperosmotic to their environment lose salt by diffusion through the integuments and in the urine. Probably the greatest loss is in the urine, since most freshwater forms have a high urine flow and the urine can never become sodium- and chloride-free. To compensate for this loss, salt is actively taken up from the medium by the gill epithelium of fishes, the skin of amphibians, and the epithelium of the pharynx of cloaca of turtles.

SALT UPTAKE THROUGH GILLS

The mechanism for salt uptake by fish gills has been most thoroughly investigated in teleost fishes. Freshwater fishes, when depleted of salt, are able to take up salt from solutions of 1 mM and will reduce the salt concentration of the solution to 0.2 mM (161) by active uptake of salt across their gills. This uptake appears to involve two separate and independent mechanisms, one in which Cl$^-$ is taken up in exchange for HCO$_3^-$, produced by carbonic anhydrase in the gills, and a second in which Na$^+$ is taken up in exchange for NH$_4^+$ or H$^+$ (62, 101, 161, 173, 176). The Cl$^-$ mechanism will also accumulate Br$^-$, but no other anion. The Na$^+$ mechanism is, however, specific for Na$^+$ (161). It is not clear whether all freshwater fishes use this coupled mechanism all the time. Ammonia excretion does not appear to be so tightly linked to Na$^+$ uptake as HCO$_3^-$ excretion is to Cl$^-$ uptake, but good correlations have been observed between NH$_4^+$ plus H$^+$ excretion and Na$^+$ uptake (63, 172). In fish the gills are the acid-base regulatory organs. The coupling of Na$^+$ uptake to NH$_4^+$ or H$^+$ excretion and Cl$^-$ uptake to HCO$_3^-$ excretion provides a mechanism for acid-base regulation. Recent evidence indicates that internal ion balance is closely linked to the pH regulatory function (19, 42). The importance of these exchange mechanisms for acid-base regulation is further supported by the demonstration of a Na$^+$ for H$^+$ or NH$_4^+$ exchange system in a seawater teleost and a marine elasmobranch (85, 217).

SALT UPTAKE THROUGH SKIN

The skin is the most important organ of ion regulation in freshwater amphibians, because it actively takes up Na$^+$ and Cl$^-$ from the medium to

Table 2-10. Maximum rate of salt gland electrolyte secretion

SPECIES	HABITAT	SECRETION RATE, μmol/100 g BODY WT/h			REF.
		NA$^+$	K$^+$	Cl$^-$	
Black-backed gull	Marine	1760	. .	. . . .	73
Herring gull	Marine	1500	. .	. . . .	73
Ringbill gull	Marine	1160	67	1120	73
White duck	Marine	692	17	692	93
Cormorant	Marine	383	8	333	73
Marine iguana	Marine (coastal)	255	51	237	76
Sea snake	Marine (pelagic)	218	9	169	73
Green sea turtle	Marine (pelagic)	134	5	. . . .	132
Banded sea snake	Marine	73	3	74	81
Land iguana	Terrestrial	26	5	18	76
Chuckwalla	Terrestrial	3	31	. . . .	81
False iguana	Terrestrial	1	9	. . . .	288

replace salt which is lost by diffusion across the skin and in the urine (161).

More aquatic species are able to maintain Na^+ and Cl^- balance at the lowest external concentrations, while more terrestrial forms show the highest uptake rates for Na^+ (203). Frogs are able to control the Na^+ permeability of the skin. Thus, frogs placed in running distilled water are able to survive for 2 to 3 months (190). An electric potential of approximately 50 to 100 mV (inside positive) exists across the skin of frogs both in vivo and in vitro as a result of the active transport of Na^+. Because frog skin readily lends itself to in vitro studies, it has been used extensively as a model for active transport studies, and the literature has been reviewed elsewhere (153, 292–294). Cl^- movements across the frog skin in vitro were thought to be passive down the electrochemical gradient created by the sodium transport (292). However, Cl^- has been found to be actively transported in vivo when the frog is in its normal freshwater medium (102, 161). Cl^- transport was later shown also in vitro when the external salt concentration was low (2, 99).

Cl^- is also actively transported in vivo by larval frogs and salamanders (65, 102, 146). In fact, in vivo salt uptake by amphibians shows exchange of Na^+ for NH_4^+ or H^+, and exchange of Cl^- for HCO_3^-. Thus, the mechanism is similar to that found in teleosts (65, 101, 161). The Cl^- uptake mechanism will also transport Br^-, but the Na^+ transport system is specific for Na^+ as in the fish gill. Ammonia may diffuse across the gill and be trapped outside by combination with an H^+ ion to form NH_4^+ outside the epithelial cell.

Na^+ uptake by the skin is under hormonal control. AVT and other neurohypophyseal hormones increase Na^+ transport as they increase the water permeability of the skin. Long-term depletion of body Na^+ (161) activates the Na^+ transport mechanism. This is presumably the effect of aldosterone.

Amphibians do not drink water but rather maintain water balance by taking up water across the skin. They cope with water loss incurred while spending time on land by increasing the rate of water uptake by the skin when they return to the pond. This increase is due to an increased permeability of the skin mediated by posterior pituitary hormone (10, 33, 239). As the animal becomes dehydrated, the neurohypophyseal hormone AVT is released, causing increased skin and bladder permeability. The net effect of dehydration or the injection of neurohypophyseal hormone on water balance is to cause a net water uptake, and hence an increase in the weight of the animal when it is placed in water. This was first noted by Brunn (33) and is sometimes referred to as the *Brunn effect*.

The magnitude of water uptake following dehydration generally is higher in preferentially terrestrial species than in more aquatic forms (175). This is due to a greater response of the skin to posterior pituitary hormone (11, 175). The pelvic region of the skin is most sensitive to AVT (302); it is better vascularized than other areas and in some terrestrial forms, it has grooves on the surface which carry water by capillary action over the whole skin when only the pelvic surface is in contact with water (44, 168). The increased water permeability of the skin caused by AVT is apparently due to an increase in the size of water-filled pores. Thus, AVT greatly increases the osmotic bulk flow of water through the skin but has only a small effect on diffusional permeability (175). This mode of action of AVT is very significant under conditions of dehydration. Thus, the release of AVT does not result in increased water loss by diffusion, but it preadjusts the skin for rapid water uptake when the animal returns to water.

SALT UPTAKE THROUGH THE CLOACA

Freshwater turtles, which utilize aquatic gas exchange across oral and cloacal membranes, lose salt and gain water in a manner similar to that of the freshwater amphibians and fishes. The magnitudes of these fluxes are smaller in the turtles than in the fishes and amphibians (74). The freshwater, soft-shelled turtle can take up salt from dilute solutions, and is able to maintain salt balance in solutions as dilute as 0.005 mM (80). Salt loss is compensated for by active salt uptake across the walls of both the pharynx and the

Table 2-11. Composition of fluids (mmol) involved in salt and water regulation in a marine teleost (*Paralichthys lethostigma*)

FLUID	mosm	[Na$^+$]	[K$^+$]	[Ca^{2+}]	[Mg^{2+}]	[Cl$^-$]	[SO$_4^{2-}$]
Seawater	912	432	9	9	49	504	
Plasma	337	180	4	3	1	160	0.2
Urine	333	15	2	19	140	127	60
Rectal	337	21	1	12	180	126	106

SOURCE: Ref. 125.

cloaca; however, the cloaca seems to be the major site of salt uptake (72). In vitro studies indicate that the major ion taken up by the cloaca, cloacal bursa, and pharynx is Na$^+$, since the observed short-circuit current could be accounted for by the net Na$^+$ transport (80). Cl$^-$ fails to follow Na$^+$ uptake in equivalent quantities; hence other anions must be involved (72). No significant K$^+$ uptake has been demonstrated in freshwater turtles. The ability of turtles actively to take up salts from dilute solutions is correlated with habitat (74). The most highly aquatic turtles are able to take up salt most readily. Cloacal Na$^+$ absorption may be a common feature of all reptiles and birds (258, 269). Turtles use this ability to achieve salt uptake from their environment. Other reptiles utilize cloacal salt uptake to reduce loss via the kidneys.

SALT UPTAKE THROUGH THE GUT

Marine teleosts maintain water balance by drinking seawater, actively absorbing salt (NaCl) and water from the gut, and excreting the excess salt across the gills (Table 2-11). Hence, in these animals, the gut is an important organ of osmotic regulation. The seawater drunk by marine fishes rapidly becomes isosmotic with the blood due to passive diffusion of Na$^+$ and Cl$^-$ into the blood across the esophagus and to a lesser extent by the osmotic entry of water (129). The seawater in the gut is isosmotic with the blood by the time it reaches the small intestine, where absorption of salt and water takes place (265). Salt is actively absorbed from the fish gut, and water follows passively. In vivo studies have demonstrated that the major ions absorbed are Na$^+$ and Cl$^-$ (125, 265) (Tables 2-11 and 2-12). Measurements of electric potentials and unidirectional fluxes in vitro demonstrated that both Na$^+$ and Cl$^-$ are transported, but active chloride transport is the dominant feature (5). Freshwater fishes do not drink; however, fishes adapted to saline water drink increasing quantities with increasing external salinity from media which are approximately isosmotic with the blood (one-third seawater) to double-strength seawater (179, 265). The salt transport mechanism by the gut is activated further by acclimation to increasing external salinity (273). This increase in gut salt transport appears to be mediated by the pituitary-interrenal axis (128). In the teleosts, cortisol (hydrocortisone) rather than aldosterone is the hormone responsible for stimulating sodium transport (128). The increase in salt and water transport by the teleost gut on acclimation to seawater is due to increases in the osmotic permeability of the gut to water as well as in-

Table 2-12. Rate of salt and water uptake and excretion by a marine fish (*Paralichthys lethostigma*)

	μmol/kg/h						H$_2$O
	Na$^+$	K$^+$	Ca^{2+}	Mg^{2+}	Cl$^-$	SO$_4^{2-}$	(mL/kg/DAY)
Seawater drunk	1956	41	43	226	2282	128	109.5
Rectal excretion	23	1	13	200	140	117	26.7
Renal excretion	3	0.3	3	26	23	11	4.3
Extrarenal excretion (calculated)	1930	40	26	0	2119	0	78.8

SOURCE: Ref. 125.

creases in Na^+ and Cl^- transport (273). The acclimation process of gut transport on transfer to seawater has been studied in the eel. Gut salt transport increases slowly, reaching a maximum on the fifth day of transfer to seawater and then decreasing to a new steady-state level by the fourteenth day (214).

COMPARISON OF OSMOREGULATION BETWEEN MAMMALS AND LOWER VERTEBRATES

Mammals are the only fully terrestrial vertebrates which are ureotelic. Thus, they do not have the advantage of the reptiles that nitrogenous waste can be excreted in an isosmotic urine with a minimum of water. Mammals must, in order to excrete urea and conserve water, form an osmotically concentrated urine. With the ability to concentrate the urine, the need for extrarenal salt excretion disappeared, because the mammalian countercurrent kidney is almost as efficient in concentrating salt as urea. Thus, in mammals, the kidney has taken over all the osmoregulatory functions which are normally shared by skin, gills, salt glands, and kidney in lower vertebrates.

REFERENCES

1a. Abel, J. H., and R. A. Ellis: Histochemical and electron microscopic observations on the salt secreting lacrymal glands of marine turtles, *Am. J. Anat.*, **118**:337, 1966.

1b. Altman, P. L., and D. S. Dittmer: *Blood and Other Body Fluids*, Federation of American Societies for Experimental Biology, Washington, 1961.

2. Alvarado, R. H., A. M. Poule, and T. L. Mullen: Chloride balance in *Rana pipiens*, *Am. J. Physiol.*, **229**:861–868, 1975.

3. Ames, E., K. Steven, and E. Skadhauge: Effects of arginine vasotocin on renal excretion of Na^+, K^+, Cl^-, and urea in the hydrated chicken, *Am. J. Physiol.*, **221**:1223–1228, 1971.

4. Anderson, Bettina G., and Richard D. Loewen: Renal morphology of freshwater trout, *Am. J. Anat.*, **143**:93–114, 1975.

5. Ando, M., S. Utida, and H. Nagahama: Active transport of chloride in eel intestine with special reference to sea water adaptation, *Comp. Biochem. Physiol.*, **51A**:27–32, 1975.

6. Balinsky, J. B., M. M. Cragg, and C. Baldwin: The adaptation of amphibian waste nitrogen excretion to dehydration, *Comp. Biochem. Physiol.*, **3**:236, 1961.

7. Balinsky, J. B., E. L. Choritz, C. G. L. Coe, and G. S. van der Schans: Urea cycle enzymes and urea excretion during the development and metamorphosis of *Xenopus laevis*, *Comp. Biochem. Physiol.*, **22**:53, 1967.

8. Balinsky, J. B., S. E. Dicker, and A. B. Elliott: The effects of long-term adaptation to different levels of salinity on urea synthesis and tissue amino acid concentrations in *Rana cancrivora*, *Comp. Biochem. Physiol.*, **43B**:71–82, 1972.

9. Bartholomew, G. A., and T. J. Cade: The water economy of land birds, *The Auk*, **80**:504, 1963.

10. Bentley, P. J.: Neurohypophyseal hormones in amphibia: A comparison of their actions and storage, *Gen. Comp. Endocrinol.*, **13**:39, 1969.

11. Bentley, P. J., A. K. Lee, and A. R. Main: Comparison of dehydration and hydration of two genera of frogs (*Heleioporus* and *Neobatrachus*) that live in areas of varying aridity, *J. Exp. Biol.*, **35**:677, 1958.

12. Bentley, P. J., and B. K. Follett: Kidney function in a primitive vertebrate, the cyclostome *Lampetra fluviatilis*, *J. Physiol. (London)*, **169**:902, 1963.

13. Bentley, P. J., W. L. Bretz, and K. Schmidt-Nielsen: Osmoregulation in the diamondback terrapin, *Malaclemys terrapin centrata*, *J. Exp. Biol.*, **46**:161, 1967.

14. Bentzel, Carl J.: Proximal tubule structure-function relationships during volume expansion in *Necturus*, *Kidney Int.*, **2**:324–335, 1972.

15. Bentzel, C. J., B. Parsa, and D. K. Hare: Osmotic flow across proximal tubule of Necturus: Correlation of physiologic and anatomic studies, *Am. J. Physiol.*, **217**:570, 1969.

16. Beyenbach, Klaus W., and Leonard B. Kirschner: Kidney and urinary bladder functions of the rainbow trout in Mg and Na excretion, *Am. J. Physiol.*, **229**:389–393, 1975.

17. Bishop, Stephen H.: Nitrogen metabolism and excretion: Regulation of intracellular amino acid

concentrations, in *Estuarine Processes,* vol. 1, *Uses, Stresses and Adaptation to the Estuary,* Academic Press, Inc., New York, 1976, pp. 414–431.

18. Boernke, William E.: Natural variations in hepatic and kidney arginase activities in Minnesota anuran amphibians, *Comp. Biochem. Physiol.,* **47B:**201–207, 1974.

19. Bornanein, M., B. De Renzis, and J. Maetz: Branchial Cl transport, anion stimulated ATPase and acid base balance in *Anguilla anguilla* adapted to freshwater: Effects of hyperonia, *J. Comp. Physiol.,* **117:**313–322, 1977.

20. Boylan, John W.: A model for passive urea reabsorption in the elasmobranch kidney, *Comp. Biochem. Physiol.,* **42A:**27–30, 1972.

21. Bradley, E. L., W. N. Holmes, and A. Wright: The effects of neurohypophysectomy on the pattern of renal excretion in the duck (*Anas platyrhynchos*), *J. Endocrinol.,* **51:**57–65, 1971.

22. Bradshaw, S. D., V. H. Shoemaker, and K. A. Nagy: The role of adrenal corticosteroids in the regulation of kidney function in the desert lizard *Dipsosaurus dorsalis, Comp. Biochem. Physiol.,* **43A:**621–635, 1972.

23. Braun, Eldon J.: *Effect of Uric Acid on Ion Excretion in Birds,* XXVIIth International Congress of Physiological Sciences, Paris, 1977.

24. Braun, Eldon J.: Intrarenal blood flow distribution in the desert quail following salt loading, *Am. J. Physiol.,* **231:**1111–1118, 1976.

25. Braun, Eldon J.: Renal response of the starling (*Sturnus vulgaris*) to an intravenous salt load, *Am. J. Physiol.* In press.

26. Braun, Eldon J., and William H. Dantzler: Effects of water load on renal glomerular and tubular function in desert quail, *Am. J. Physiol.,* **229:**222–228, 1975.

27. Braun, Eldon J., and William H. Dantzler: Function of mammalian-type and reptilian-type nephrons in kidney of desert quail, *Am. J. Physiol.,* **222:**617–629, 1972.

28. Braysher, M. L.: The excretion of hyperosmotic urine and other aspects of the electrolyte balance of the lizard *Amphibolurus maculosus, Comp. Biochem. Physiol.,* **54A:**341–345, 1976.

29. Brown, G. W.: Studies in comparative biochemistry and evolution. I. Avian liver arginase, *Arch. Biochem. Biophys.,* **114:**184, 1966.

30. Brown, G. W., and P. P. Cohen: Biosynthesis of urea in metamorphosing tadpoles, in W. D. McElroy and B. Glass (eds.), *A Symposium on the Chemical Basis of Development,* The Johns Hopkins Press, Baltimore, 1958.

31. Brown, G. W., and P. P. Cohen: Comparative biochemistry of urea synthesis. III. Activities of urea-cycle enzymes in various higher and lower vertebrates, *Biochem. J.,* **75:**82, 1960.

32. Brown, G. W., and S. G. Brown: Urea and its formation in coelacanth liver, *Science,* **155:**570, 1967.

33. Brunn, F.: Beitrag zum Kentniss der Wirkung von Hypophysenextrakten auf den Wasserhaushalt des Frosches, *Z. Ges. Exp. Med.,* **25:**170, 1921. From J. Maetz, *Proc. Zool. Soc. London,* **9:**107, 1963.

34. Bulger, R. E.: Fine structure of the rectal (salt-secreting) gland of the spiny dogfish, *Squalus acanthias, Anat. Rec.,* **147:**95, 1963.

35. Bulger, R. E.: Electron microscopy of the stratified epithelium lining of the excretory canal of the dogfish rectal gland, *Anat. Rec.,* **151:**589, 1965.

36. Burger, J. W.: Further studies on the function of the rectal gland in the spiny dogfish, *Physiol. Zool.,* **35:**205, 1962.

37. Burger, J. W.: Roles of the rectal gland and the kidneys in salt and water excretion in the spiny dogfish, *Physiol. Zool.,* **38:**191, 1965.

38. Burger, J. W.: Some aspects of liver function in the spiny dogfish (*Squalus acanthias*), in P. W. Gilbert, R. F. Mathewson, and D. P. Rall (eds.), *Sharks, Skates, and Rays,* The Johns Hopkins Press, Baltimore, 1967.

39. Burger, J. W., and W. N. Hess: Function of the rectal gland in the spiny dogfish, *Science,* **131:**670, 1960.

40. Burger, J. W., and D. C. Tosteson: Sodium influx and efflux in the spiny dogfish, *Squalus acanthias, Comp. Biochem. Physiol.,* **19:**649, 1966.

41. Cade, T. J., and L. Greenwald: Nasal salt secretion in falconiform birds, *Condor,* **68:**338, 1966.

42. Cameron, J. N.: Branchial ion uptake in Arctic gragling: Resting values and effects of acid-base disturbance, *J. Exp. Biol.,* **64:**711–725, 1976.

43. Carlisky, N. S.: Urea excretion and arginase in anuran kidney, in B. Schmidt-Nielson (ed.), *Urea*

and the Kidney, Excerpta Medica Foundation, Amsterdam, 1970.

44. Christensen, C. U.: Adaptations in the water economy of some anuran amphibia, *Comp. Biochem. Physiol.,* **47A:**1035–1049, 1974.

45. Clark, H.: Eggs, egg-laying and incubation of the snake, *Elaphe emorgi* (Baird and Girard), *Copeia,* **30:**90, 1953.

46. Cohen, J. J., M. A. Krupp, and C. A. Chidsey: Renal conservation of trimethylamine oxide by the spiny dogfish, *Squalus acanthias, Am. J. Physiol.,* **194:**229, 1958.

47. Coulson, R. A., and T. Hernandez: Source and function of urinary ammonia in the alligator, *Am. J. Physiol.,* **194:**873, 1959.

48. Coulson, R. A., and T. Hernandez: *Biochemistry of the Alligator,* Louisiana State University Press, Baton Rouge, 1964.

49. Crockett, David R., Jeffery W. Gerst, and Shaw Blankenship: Absence of juxtaglomerular cells in the kidneys of elasmobranch fishes, *Comp. Biochem. Physiol.,* **44A:**673–675, 1973.

50a. Dantzler, W. H.: Comparison of renal tubular transport of urate and PAH in water snakes: Evidence for differences in mechanisms and sites of transport, *Comp. Biochem. Physiol.,* **34:**609–623, 1970.

50b. Dantzler, W. H.: Renal function (with special emphasis on nitrogen excretion), in C. Gans and W. R. Dawson (eds.), *Biology of the Reptilia,* Academic Press, Inc., New York, 1976, pp. 447–503.

51. Dantzler, W. H.: Renal response of chickens to infusion of hyperosmotic sodium chloride solution, *Am. J. Physiol.,* **210:**640, 1966.

52. Dantzler, W. H.: Glomerular and tubular effects of arginine vasotocin in water snakes (*Natrix sipedon*), *Am. J. Physiol.,* **212:**83, 1967.

53. Dantzler, W. H.: Effect of metabolic alkalosis and acidosis on tubular urate secretion in water snakes, *Am. J. Physiol.,* **215:**747, 1968.

54. Dantzler, W. H., and B. Schmidt-Nielsen: Excretion in fresh-water turtle *Pseudemys scripta* and desert tortoise *Gopherus agassizii, Am. J. Physiol.,* **210:**198, 1966.

55. Dantzler, William H., and W. N. Holmes: Water and mineral metabolism in reptilia, *Chem. Zool.,* **9:**277–336, 1974.

56. Dantzler, W. H., D. P. Shaffner, P. J. S. Chiu, and

57. Davis, L. E., and B. Schmidt-Nielsen: Ultrastructure of the crocodile kidney (*Crocodylus acutus*) with special reference to electrolyte and fluid transport, *J. Morphol.,* **121:**255, 1967.

58. Davis, Lowell E., Bodil Schmidt-Nielsen, and Hilmar Stolte: Anatomy and ultrastructure of the excretory system of the lizard, *Sceloporus cyanogenys, J. Morphol.,* **149:**279–326, 1976.

59. Dawson, W. R., V. H. Shoemaker, H. B. Tordoff, and A. Borut: Observations on metabolism of sodium chloride in the red crossbill, *The Auk,* **82:**606, 1965.

60. Deetjen, Peter, and Dorothy Antkowiak: The nephron of the skate, *Raja erinacea, Mt. Desert Island Biol. Lab.,* **10:**5–7, 1970.

61. Degnam, K. J., K. J. Karnaky, and J. A. Zadunaisky: Active chloride transport in the *in vitro* opercular skin of a teleost (*Fundulus heteroclitus*), a gill-like epithelium rich in chloride cells, *J. Physiol.,* **271:**155–191, 1977.

62. De Renzis, G.: The branchial chloride pump in the goldfish, *Carassius auratus*: Relationship between Cl^-/HCO_3^- and Cl^-/Cl^- exchanges and the effects of thiocyanate, *J. Exp. Biol.,* **63:**587–602, 1975.

63. De Renzis, G., and J. Maetz: Studies on the mechanism of chloride absorption by the goldfish gill: Relation with acid-base regulation, *J. Exp. Biol.,* **59:**339–358, 1973.

64. Deyrup, I. J.: Water balance and kidney, in J. A. Moore (ed.), *Physiology of the Amphibia,* Academic Press, Inc., New York, 1964, pp. 251–328.

65. Dietz, T. H., L. B. Kirschner, and D. Porter: The roles of sodium transport and anion permeability in generating transepithelial potential differences in larval salamanders, *J. Exp. Biol.,* **46:**85, 1967.

66. Dietz, T. H., and E. D. Brodie: Blood ion concentrations as a function of developmental stage in the gopher snake, *Pituophis melanoleucus catenifer, Comp. Biochem. Physiol.,* **30:**673, 1969.

67. Dobbs, G. H. III, and A. L. DeVries: Renal function in Antarctic teleost fishes: Serum and urine composition, *Marine Biol.,* **29:**59–70, 1975.

68. Dobbs, Gary H. III, Yuan Lin, and Arthur L.

DeVries: Aglomerularism in Antarctic fish, *Science*, **185**:793–794, 1974.

69. Doyle, W. L.: The principal cells of the salt-gland of marine birds, *Exp. Cell Res.*, **21**:386, 1960.

70. Doyle, W. L.: Tubule cells of the rectal salt-gland of *Urolophus*, *Am. J. Anat.*, **111**:223, 1962.

71. Doyle, W. L., and D. Gorecki: The so-called chloride cell of the fish gill, *Physiol. Zool.*, **34**:81, 1961.

72. Dunson, W. A.: Sodium fluxes in fresh-water turtles, *J. Exp. Zool.*, **165**:171, 1967.

73. Dunson, W. A.: Salt gland secretion in the pelagic sea snake *Pelamis*, *Am. J. Physiol.*, **215**:1512, 1968.

74. Dunson, W. A.: Concentration of sodium by freshwater turtles, in D. S. Nelson and F. C. Evans (eds.), *Proceedings of the Second National Symposium on Radioecology*, 1969.

75. Dunson, W. A.: Reptilian salt glands, in *Exocrine Glands*, University of Pennsylvania Press, Philadelphia, 1969.

76. Dunson, W. A.: Electrolyte excretion by the salt gland of the Galápagos marine iguana, *Am. J. Physiol.*, **216**:995, 1969.

77. Dunson, W. A., and M. K. Dunson: Interspecific differences in fluid concentration and secretion rate of sea snake salt glands, *Am. J. Physiol.*, **227**:430–438, 1974.

78. Dunson, W. A., R. K. Packer, and M. K. Dunson: Sea snake: An unusual salt gland under the tongue, *Science*, **173**:437–441, 1971.

79. Dunson, W. A.: Some aspects of electrolyte and water balance in three estuarine reptiles, the diamondback terrapin, American and "salt water" crocodiles, *Comp. Biochem. Physiol.*, **32**:161, 1970.

80. Dunson, W. A., and R. D. Weymouth: Active uptake of sodium by soft-shell turtles (*Trionyx spinifer*), *Science*, **149**:67, 1965.

81. Dunson, W. A., and A. M. Taub: Extrarenal salt excretion in sea snakes (*Laticauda*), *Am. J. Physiol.*, **213**:975, 1967.

82. Elizondo, R. S., and S. J. LeBrie: Adrenal-renal function in water snakes, *Natrix cyclopion*, *Am. J. Physiol.*, **217**:419, 1969.

83. Epstein, F. H., J. Maetz, and G. De Renzis: Active transport of chloride by the teleost gill: Inhibition by thiocyanate, *Am. J. Physiol.*, **224**:1295–1299, 1973.

84. Ernst, S. A., C. C. Goertemiller, Jr., and R. A. Ellis: The effect of salt regimens on the development of (Na$^+$-K$^+$)-dependent ATPase activity during the growth of salt glands of ducklings, *Biochim. Biophys. Acta.*, **135**:682–692, 1967.

85. Evans, D. H.: The effects of various external cations and sodium transport inhibitors on sodium uptake by the sailfin molly *Poecilia latipinna*, acclimated to seawater, *J. Comp. Physiol.*, **96**:111–115, 1975.

86. Fanelli, G. M., and L. Goldstein: Ammonia excretion in the neotenous newt *Necturus maculosus* (Rafinesque), *Comp. Biochem. Physiol.*, **13**:193, 1964.

87. Fänge, R.: Structure and function of the excretory organs of myxinoids, in A. Biodal and R. Fänge (eds.), *The Biology of Myxine*, Universitets Forlaget, Oslo, 1963.

88. Fänge, R., K. Schmidt-Nielsen, and M. Robinson: Control of secretion from the avian salt gland, *Am. J. Physiol.*, **195**:321, 1958.

89. Fänge, R., K. Schmidt-Nielsen, and H. Osaki: The salt gland of the herring gull, *Biol. Bull.*, **115**:162, 1958.

90. Fänge, R., and K. Fugelli: Osmoregulation in chimaeroid fishes, *Nature (London)*, **196**:689, 1962.

91. Fitch, H. S.: Natural history of the racer *Coluber constrictor*, *Univ. Kans. Publ. Mus. Natur. Hist.*, **15**:351, 1963.

92. Fleming, W. R., and J. G. Stanley: Effects of rapid changes in salinity on the renal function of a euryhaline teleost, *Am. J. Physiol.*, **209**:1025, 1965.

93. Fletcher, G. L., I. M. Stainer, and W. N. Holmes: Sequential changes in the adenosinetriphosphatase activity and the electrolyte excretory capacity of the nasal glands of the duck (*Anas platyrhynchos*) during the period of adaptation to hypertonic saline, *J. Exp. Biol.*, **47**:375, 1967.

94. Forster, R. P.: The nature of the glucose reabsorptive process in the frog renal tubule: Evidence for intermittency of glomerular function in the intact animal, *J. Cell. Comp. Physiol.*, **20**:55, 1942.

95. Forster, R. P.: A comparative study of renal func-

tion in marine teleosts, *J. Cell. Comp. Physiol.*, **42**:487, 1953.

96. Forster, R. P.: Active cellular transport of urea by frog renal tubules, *Am. J. Physiol.*, **179**:372, 1954.

97. Forster, R. P., B. Schmidt-Nielsen, and L. Goldstein: Relation of renal tubular transport of urea to its biosynthesis in metamorphosing tadpoles, *J. Cell. Comp. Physiol.*, **61**:239, 1963.

98. Forster, Roy P., Leon Goldstein, and Jeffrey K. Rosen: Intrarenal control of urea reabsorption by renal tubules of the marine elasmobranch, *Squalus acanthias*, *Comp. Biochem. Physiol.*, **42A**:3–12, 1972.

99. Garcia-Romeau, F., and J. Ehrenfeld: Chloride transport through the nonshort-circuited isolated skin of *Rana esculenta*, *Am. J. Physiol.*, **228**:845–849, 1975b.

100. Garcia-Romeau, F., and J. Ehrenfeld: *In vivo* Na$^+$ and Cl$^-$ independent transport across the skin of *Rana esculenta*, *Am. J. Physiol.*, **228**:839–844, 1975a.

101. Garcia Romeau, F., and J. Maetz: The mechanism of sodium and chloride uptake by the gills of a fresh-water fish *Carassius auratus*. I. Evidence for an independent uptake of sodium and chloride ions, *J. Gen. Physiol.*, **47**:1195, 1964.

102. Garcia Romeau, F., A. Salibián, and S. Pezzani-Hernández: The nature of the *in vivo* sodium and chloride uptake mechanism through the epithelium of the Chilean frog, *J. Gen. Physiol.*, **53**:816, 1969.

103. Garland, H. O., I. W. Henderson, and J. Anne Brown: Micropuncture study of the renal responses of the urodele amphibian *Necturus maculosus* to injections of arginine vasotocin and an anti-aldosterone compound, *J. Exp. Biol.*, **63**:249–264, 1975.

104. Gilles, R.: Mechanisms of ion and osmoregulation, in O. Kinne (ed.), *Marine Ecology, a Comprehensive Integrated Treatise on Life in Oceans and Coastal Water*, vol. II, *Physiological Mechanisms*, part 1, John Wiley & Sons, Inc., London, 1975, pp. 259–347.

105. Gilles-Baillien, M.: Seasonal variations in blood and urine constituents of the tortoise *Testudo hermanni hermanni* Gmelin, *Arch. Int. Physiol. Biochim.*, **77**:427, 1969.

106. Gilles-Baillien, M.: Urea and osmoregulation in the diamondback terrapin *Malaclemys centrata centrata* (Latreille), *J. Exp. Biol.*, **52**:691–697, 1970.

107. Goldstein, Leon, and Roy P. Forster: Osmoregulation and urea metabolism in the little skate *Raja erinacea*, *Am. J. Physiol.*, **220**:742–746, 1971.

108. Goldstein, L., R. P. Foster, and G. M. Fanelli, Jr.: Gill blood flow and ammonia excretion in the marine teleosts, *Myoxocephalus scorpius*, *Comp. Biochem. Physiol.*, **12**:489, 1964.

109. Goldstein, L., and R. P. Forster: The role of uricolysis in the production of urea by fishes and other aquatic vertebrates, *Comp. Biochem. Physiol.*, **14**:567, 1965.

110. Goldstein, L., P. A. Janssens, and R. P. Forster: Lungfish *Neoceratodus forsteri*: Activities of ornithine-urea cycle and enzymes, *Science*, **157**:316, 1967.

111. Gordon, M. S., K. Schmidt-Nielsen, and H. M. Kelly: Osmotic regulation in the crab-eating frog (*Rana cancrivora*), *J. Exp. Biol.*, **38**:659, 1961.

112. Goldstein, Leon, Susan Harley-DeWitt, and Roy P. Forster: Activities of ornithine-urea cycle enzymes and of trimethylamine oxidase in the coelacanth, *Latimeria chalumnae*, *Comp. Biochem. Physiol.*, **44B**:357–362, 1973.

113. Gordon, M. S., I. Boëtius, D. H. Evans, R. McCarthy, and L. C. Oglesby: Aspects of the physiology of terrestrial life in amphibious fishes, *J. Exp. Biol.*, **50**:141, 1969.

114. Grant, F. B., P. K. T. Pang, and R. W. Griffith: The 24-hour seminal hydration response in goldfish (*Carassius auratus*). I. Sodium, potassium, calcium, magnesium, chloride and osmolality of serum and seminal fluid, *Comp. Biochem. Physiol.*, **30**:273, 1969.

115. Green, Brian: Aspects of renal function in the lizard *Varanus gouldii*, *Comp. Biochem. Physiol.*, **43A**:747–756, 1972.

116. Griffith, R. W., B. L. Umminger, B. F. Grant, P. K. T. Pang, L. Goldstein, and G. E. Pickford: Composition of bladder urine of the coelacanth, *Latimeria chalumnae*, *J. Exp. Biol.*, **196**:371–380, 1976.

117. Griffith, R. W., P. K. T. Pang, A. K. Sriuastava, and G. E. Picford: Serum composition of freshwater stingrays (Potamotrygonidae) adapted to

fresh and dilute seawater, *Biol. Bull.*, **144**:304–320, 1973.

118. Hanwell, A., J. L. Linzell, and M. Peakes: Nature and location of the receptors for salt-gland secretion in the goose, *J. Physiol.*, **226**:453–472, 1972.

119. Hays, Richard M., Sherman D. Levine, Jack D. Myers, Henry O. Heinemann, Michael A. Kaplan, Nicholas Franki, and Henry Berliner: Urea transport in the dogfish kidney, *J. Exp. Zool.*, **199**:309–315, 1977.

120. Hayslett, J. P., D. A. Schan, M. Epstein, and C. A. M. Hogben: *In vitro* perfusion of the dogfish rectal gland, *Am. J. Physiol.*, **226**:1188–1192, 1974.

121. Hayslett, John P., Lee M. Jampol, John N. Forrest, Mark Epstein, H. Victor Murdaugh, and Jack D. Myers: Role of Na-K-ATPase in the renal reabsorption of sodium in the elasmobranch, *Squalus acanthias, Comp. Biochem. Physiol.*, **44A**:417–422, 1973.

122. Hernandez, T., R. A. Coulson, and J. D. Herbert: Synthesis of renal ammonium bicarbonate from ^{14}C labeled amino acids in crocodilia, *Comp. Biochem. Physiol.*, **46B**:417–425, 1973.

123. Hickman, C. P.: Glomerular filtration and urine flow in the euryhaline southern flounder, *Paralichthys lethostigma*, in seawater, *Can. J. Zool.*, **46**:427, 1968.

124. Hickman, C. P.: Urine composition and kidney tubular function in the southern flounder, *Paralichtys lethostigma*, in seawater, *Can. J. Zool.*, **46**:439, 1968.

125. Hickman, C. P.: Ingestion, intestinal absorption, and elimination of seawater and salts in the southern flounder, *Paralichthys lethostigma, Can. J. Zool.*, **46**:457, 1968.

126. Hickman, C. P., and B. Trump: The kidney, in W. S. Hoar and D. J. Randall (eds.), *Fish Physiology*, vol. 1, Academic Press, Inc., New York, 1969.

127. Hill, L., and W. H. Dawbin: Nitrogen excretion in the tuatara, *Sphenodon punctatus, Comp. Biochem. Physiol.*, **31**:453, 1969.

128. Hirano, T., and S. Utida: Effects of ACTH and cortisol on water movement in isolated intestine of the eel, *Anguilla japonica, Gen. Comp. Endocrinol.*, **11**:373, 1968.

129. Hirano, T., and W. Mayer-Gostan: Eel esophagus

as an osmoregulatory organ, *Proc. Natl. Acad. Sci. USA.*, **73**:1348–1350, 1976.

130. Holmes, W. N.: Some aspects of osmoregulation in reptiles and birds, *Arch. Anat. Microsc. Morphol. Exp.*, **54**:491, 1965.

131. Holmes, W. N., and R. L. McBean: Studies on the glomerular filtration rate of rainbow trout, *Salmo gairdneri, J. Exp. Biol.*, **40**:335, 1963.

132. Holmes, W. N., and R. L. McBean: Some aspects of electrolyte excretion in the green turtle, *Chelonia mydas mydas, J. Exp. Biol.*, **41**:81, 1964.

133. Holmes, W. N., G. L. Fletcher, and D. J. Stewart: The patterns of renal electrolyte excretion in the duck (*Anas platyrhynchos*) maintained on freshwater and on hypertonic saline, *J. Exp. Biol.*, **48**:487, 1968.

134. House, C. R.: Osmotic regulation in the brackish water teleost *Blennius pholis, J. Exp. Biol.*, **40**:87, 1963.

135. House, C. R., and J. Maetz: On the electrical gradient across the gill of the seawater-adapted eel, *Comp. Biochem. Physiol.*, **47A**:917–924, 1974.

136. Huggins, A. K., G. Skutsch, and E. Baldwin: Ornithine-urea cycle enzyme in teleostean fish, *Comp. Biochem. Physiol.*, **28**:587, 1969.

137. Hughes, M. R.: Cloacal and salt-gland ion excretion in the seagull, *Larus glaucescens*, acclimated to increasing concentrations of sea water, *Comp. Biochem. Physiol.*, **32**:315–325, 1970.

138. Hughes, M. R.: Renal and extrarenal sodium excretion in the common tern *Sterna hirundo, Physiol. Zool.*, **41**:210, 1968.

139. Hughes, M. R.: Cloacal and salt-gland ion excretion in the sea gull *Larus claucescen* acclimated to increasing concentrations of sea water, *Comp. Biochem. Physiol.*, **32**:315, 1970.

140. Hughes, M. R., and F. E. Ruch, Jr.: Sodium and potassium in spontaneously produced salt gland secretion and tears of ducks, *Anas platyrhynchos*, acclimated to fresh and saline waters, *Can. J. Zool.*, **47**:1133, 1969.

141. Humbert, Fabienne, Alain Grandchamp, Claude Pricam, Alain Perrelet, and Lelio Orci: Morphological changes in tight junctions of *Necturus maculosus* proximal tubules undergoing saline diuresis, *J. Cell. Biol.*, **69**:90–96, 1976.

142. Janssens, P. A.: Urea production and transami-

nase activity in *Xenopus laevis* Daudin, *Comp. Biochem. Physiol.*, **13**:217, 1964.

143. Jard, S., and F. Morel: Action of vasotocin and some of its analogues on salt and water excretion by the frog, *Am. J. Physiol.*, **204**:222, 1963.

144. Johnson, Oscar W., and Robert D. Ohmart: The renal medulla and water economy in vesper sparrows (*Pooecetes gramineus*), *Comp. Biochem. Physiol.*, **44A**:655–661, 1973.

145. Jones, M. E.: Vertebrate carbamoyl phosphate synthetase I and II separation of arginine-urea and pyrimidine pathways, in B. Schmidt-Nielsen (ed.), *Urea and the Kidney*, Excerpta Medica Foundation, Amsterdam, 1970.

146. Jørgensen, C. B., H. Levi, and K. Zerahn: On active uptake of sodium and chloride ions in anurans, *Acta. Physiol. Scand.*, **30**:178, 1954.

147. Jurss, Von Karl, and Wolfram Schlisio: Osmotic and ionic regulation in *Xenopus laevis* Daud during adaptation to different osmotic environments. IV. Changes in the nitrogen excretion, urea and glycogen levels of the liver, and blood sugar (in German, with English abstract), *Zool, Jb. Physiol. Bd.*, **79**:1–8, 1975.

148. Karnaky, Karl J. Jr., and William B. Kinter: Killifish opercular skin: A flat epithelium with a high density of chloride cells, *J. Exp. Zool.*, **199**:355–364, 1977.

149. Karnaky, K. J., S. A. Ernst, and C. W. Philpott: Teleost chloride cell. 1. Response of pupfish *Cyprinodon variegatus* gill Na-K-ATPase and chloride cell fine structure to various high salinity environments, *J. Cell. Biol.*, **20**:144–156, 1976a.

150. Karnaky, Karl J. Jr., Kevin J. Degnan, and Jose A. Zadunaisky: Chloride transport across isolated opercular epithelium of killifish: A membrane rich in chloride cells, *Science*, **195**:203–205, 1977.

151. Karnaky, K. J., L. B. Kinter, W. B. Kinter, and C. E. Stirling: Teleost chloride cell II. Autoradiographic localization of gill Na-K-ATPase in killifish *Fundulus heteroclitus*, adapted to low and high salinity environments, *J. Cell. Biol.*, **70**:157–177, 1976b.

152. Kempton, R.: Studies on the elasmobranch kidney. II. Reabsorption of urea by the smooth dogfish *Mustelus canis*, *Biol. Bull.* (*Woods Hole*), **104**:45, 1953.

153. Keynes, R. D.: From frog skin to sheep rumen: A survey of transport of salts and water across multicellular structures, *Q. Rev. Biophys.*, **2**:177, 1969.

154. Keys, A. B., and E. N. Willmer: Chloride secreting cells, cited in the gills of fishes, with special reference to the common eel, *J. Physiol.* (*London*), **76**:368, 1932.

155. Khalil, F.: Excretion in reptiles, IV. Nitrogenous constituents of the excretion of lizards, *J. Biol. Chem.*, **189**:443, 1951.

156. Khalil, F., and G. Haggag: Ureotelism and uricotelism in tortoises, *J. Exp. Zool.*, **130**:423, 1955.

157. Khalil, F., and G. Haggag: Xanthine oxidase and arginase in the liver and kidney of reptiles, *Z. Vergl. Physiol.*, **43**:269, 1960.

158. Kinter, William B.: Structure and function of renal tubules isolated from fish kidneys, *Fortschr. Zool.*, **23**:223–231, 1975.

159. Kirschner, L. B., L. Greenwald, and M. Saunders: On the mechanism of sodium extrusion across the irrigated gill of seawater-adapted rainbow trout (*Salmo gairdneri*), *J. Gen. Physiol.*, **64**:148–165, 1974.

160. Komadina, S., and S. Solomon: Comparison of renal function of bull and water snakes (*Pituophis melanoleucus* and *Natrix spiedon*), *Comp. Biochem. Physiol.*, **32**:333, 1970.

161. Krogh, A.: *Osmotic Regulation in Aquatic Animals*, Dover Publications, Inc., New York, 1939.

162. Kuhn, K., H. Stolte, and E. Reale: The fine structure of the kidney of the hagfish (*Myxine glutinosa* L.): A thin section and freeze-fracture study, *Cell. Tissue Res.*, **164**:201–213, 1975.

163. Lacy, Eric R., Bodil Schmidt-Nielsen, Erik Swenson, and Thomas Maren: The urinary bladder in the little skate, *Raja erinacea*, *Mt. Desert Island Biol. Lab.*, **15**:56–57, 1975.

164. Lalou, B.: Excretion renale chez un poisson euryhalin, le flet (*Platichthys-flesus* L.): Caracteristiques de l'urine normale en eau douce et en eau de mer et effets des changements de milieu, *Comp. Biochem. Physiol.*, **20**:925, 1967.

165. Lalou, B., I. W. Henderson, and W. H. Sawyer: Renal adaptations by *Opsanus tau*, a euryhaline aglomerular teleost, to dilute media, *Am. J. Physiol.*, **216**:1266, 1969.

166. LeBrie, S. J., and I. D. W. Sutherland: Renal

function in water snakes, *Am. J. Physiol.*, **203**:995, 1962.

167. LeBrie, S. J., and R. S. Elizondo: Saline loading and aldosterone in water snakes *Natrix cyclopion*, *Am. J. Physiol.*, **217**:426, 1969.

168. Lillywhite, H. B., and P. Licht: Movement of water over toad skin: Functional role of epidermal sculpturing, *Copeia*, **1974** (1):165–171, 1974.

169. Long, William Scott: Renal handling of urea in *Rana catesbeiana*, *Am. J. Physiol.*, **224**:482–490, 1973.

170. Long, W. S.: Renal secretion of urea in *Rana catesbeiana*, in B. Schmidt-Nielsen (ed.), *Urea and the Kidney*, Excerpta Medica Foundation, Amsterdam, 1970.

171. Macfarlane, N. A. A.: Effects of hypothysectomy on osmoregulation in the euryhaline flounder, *Platichthys flesus* (L), in sea water and in fresh water, *Comp. Biochem. Physiol.*, **47A**:201–217, 1974.

172. Maetz, J.: Branchial sodium exchange and ammonia excretion in the goldfish *Carassius auratus*. Effects of ammonia-loading and temperature changes, *J. Exp. Biol.*, **56**:601–620, 1972.

173. Maetz, J.: Na^+/NH_4, Na^+/H^+ exchanges and NH_3 movement across the gill of *Carassius auratus*, *J. Exp. Biol.*, **58**:255–275, 1973.

174. Maetz, J.: Transport of ions and water across the epithelium of fish gills, in *Lung Liquids*, Excerpta Medica, Amsterdam, 1976. Also in *Ciba Found. Symp.*, **35**:138–159.

175. Maetz, J.: Physiological aspects of neurohypophyseal function in fishes with some reference to the amphibia, *Symp. Zool. Soc. London*, **9**:107, 1963.

176. Maetz, J., and F. Garcia Romeau: The mechanism of sodium and chloride uptake by the gills of a freshwater fish, *Carassius auratus*. II. Evidence for NH_4^+ and HCO_3^-/Cl^- exchanges, *J. Gen. Physiol.*, **47**:1209, 1964.

177. Maetz, J., and B. Lalou: Les Échanges de sdoium et de chlore chez un elasmobranche, *Scyliorhinus*, mesurés a l'aide des isotopes ^{24}Na et ^{36}Cl, *J. Physiol.* (*Paris*), **58**:249, 1966.

178. Maetz, J., and G. Campanini: Potentials transépithéliaux de la branchie d'anguille *in vivo* en eau douce et en eau de mer, *J. Physiol.* (*Paris*), **58**:248, 1966.

179. Maetz, J., and E. Skadhauge: Drinking rates and gill ionic turnover in relation to external salinities in the eel, *Nature* (*London*), **217**:371, 1968.

180. Maetz, J., and M. Bornanein: Biochemical and biophysical aspects of salt excretion by chloride cells in teleosts, *Forschr. Zool.*, **23**:321–362. Gustav Fisher Verlag, Stuttgart, 1975.

181. Malvin, R. L., E. Carlson, S. Legan, and P. Churchill: Creatinine reabsorption and renal function in freshwater lamprey, *Am. J. Physiol.*, **218**:1506, 1970.

182. Malyusz, M.: O_2 consumption and K^+/Na^+ balance of elasmobranch kidney slices after replacement of urea by thiourea or acetamide, *Comp. Biochem. Physiol.*, **47A**:271–275, 1974.

183. Malyusz, M., and V. Thiemann: The effect of urea, thiourea and acetamide on the renal and branchial enzyme-pattern of the dogfish *Scyliorhinus canicula*, *Comp. Biochem. Physiol.*, **54B**:177–179, 1976.

184. Marshall, E. K., Jr.: The secretion of urea in the frog, *J. Cell. Comp. Physiol.*, **2**:349, 1932.

185. Marshall, E. K., Jr., and A. L. Grafflin: The function of the proximal convoluted segment of the renal tubule, *J. Cell. Comp. Physiol.*, **1**:161, 1932.

186. Marshall, E. K., and H. W. Smith: The glomerular development of the vertebrate kidney in relation to habitat, *Biol. Bull.* (*Woods Hole*), **49**:135, 1930.

187. Maude, D. L., I. Shehadeh, and A. K. Solomon: Sodium and water transport in single perfused distal tubules of *Necturus* kidney, *Am. J. Physiol.*, **211**:1043, 1966.

188. Mayer, N.: Adaptation de *Rana esculenta*: á des milieux variés: Etude spéciale de excretion renale de l'eau et des electrolytes au cours des changements de milieux, *Comp. Biochem. Physiol.*, **29**:27, 1969.

189. Mayrs, E. B.: Secretion as a factor in elimination by the bird's kidney, *J. Physiol.* (*London*), **58**:276, 1924.

190. McAfee, R. D.: Survival of *Rana pipiens* in deionized water, *Science*, **178**:183–185, 1972.

191. McBean, R. L., and L. Goldstein: Ornithine-urea activity in *Xenopus laevis*: Adaptation in saline, *Science*, **157**:931, 1967.

192. McClanahan, L., Jr.: Adaptations of the spadefoot

toad, *Scaphiopus couchi,* to desert environments, *Comp. Biochem. Physiol.,* **20:**73, 1967.

193. McClanahan, L. L., V. H. Shoemaker, and R. Ruibal: Structure and function of the cocoon of a ceratophryd frog, *Copeia,* **1976** (1):179–185, 1976.

194. McFarland, W. N., and F. W. Munz: A re-examination of the osmotic properties of the pacific hagfish, *Polistotrema stouti, Biol. Bull.,* **114:**348, 1958.

195. McNabb, Roger A.: Urate and cation interactions in the liquid and precipitated fractions of avian urine and speculations on their physico-chemical state, *Comp. Biochem. Physiol.,* **48A:**45–54, 1974.

196. McNabb, Roger, and F. M. Anne McNabb: Avian urinary precipitates: Their physical analysis, and their differential inclusion of cations (Ca, Mg) and anions (Cl), *Comp. Biochem. Physiol.,* **56A:**621–625, 1977.

197. Möllendorff, W. von: *Handbuch der Mikroskopischen Anatomie des Menschen,* Verlag von Julius Springer, Berlin, 1930.

198. Morris, R.: The mechanism of marine osmoregulation in the lamprey (*Lampertra flaviatilis L.*) and the causes of its breakdown during the spawning migration, *J. Exp. Biol.,* **35:**649, 1958.

199. Morris, R.: Studies on salt and water balance in *Myxine glutinosa* (L.), *J. Exp. Biol.,* **42:**359–371, 1965.

200. Motais, R.: Les Mecanismes d'échanges ioniques branchiaux chez les téléostéens, *Ann. Inst. Océanogr. (Monaco),* **45:**1, 1967.

201. Motais, R., F. Garcia Romeau, and J. Maetz: Exchange diffusion effect and euryhalinity in teleosts, *J. Gen. Physiol.,* **50:**391, 1966.

202. Mouw, David, Jean-Philippe Bonjour, Richard L. Malvin, and Arthur Vander: Central action of angiotensin in stimulating ADH release, *Am. J. Physiol.,* **220:**239–242, 1971.

203. Mullen, T. L., and R. H. Alvarado: Osmotic and ionic regulation in amphibians, *Physiol. Zool.,* **49:**11–23, 1976.

204. Munro, A. F.: The ammonia and urea excretion of different species of amphibia during their development and metamorphosis, *Biochem. J.,* **54:**29, 1953.

205. Munz, F. W., and W. N. McFarland: Regulatory function of a primitive vertebrate kidney, *Comp. Biochem. Physiol.,* **13:**381, 1964.

206. Nagy, K. A.: Water and electrolyte budgets of a free-living desert lizard, *Sauromalus obesus, J. Comp. Physiol.,* **79:**39–62, 1972.

207. Nash, J.: The number and size of glomeruli in the kidneys of fishes with observations on the morphology of the renal tubules of fishes, *Am. J. Anat.,* **47:**425, 1931.

208. Nash, G., and G. Fankhauser: Nitrogen excretion in developing newts, *Science,* **130:**714, 1959.

209. Natochin, Yu V., G. P. Gisev, O. A. Goncharevskaya, E. A. Lavrova, and E. I. Shakhmatova: Effect of diuretics on the secretion and reabsorption of ions in the kidney of marine teleosts, *Comp. Biochem. Physiol.,* **43A:**253–258, 1972.

210. Nishimura, Hiroko: Renal responses to diuretic drugs in freshwater catfish *Ictalurus punctatus, Am. J. Physiol.,* **232**(3):F278–F285, 1977.

211. Nishimura, Hiroko, and Wilbur H. Sawyer: Vasopressor, diuretic and natriuretic responses to angiotensins by the American eel, *Anguilla rostrata, Gen. Comp. Endocrinol.,* **29:**337–348, 1976.

212. Ogawa, M.: Comparative study of the external shape of the teleostean kidney with relation to phylogeny, *Sci. Rept. Tokyo Kyoidu Daigaku,* **B10:**61, 1961.

213. Ohmart, R. D.: Physiological and ecological observations concerning the salt-secreting nasal glands of the roadrunner, *Comp. Biochem. Physiol.,* **43A** 311–316, 1972.

214. Oide, M., and S. Utida: Changes in water and ion transport in isolated intestines of the eel during salt adaptation and migration, *Mar. Biol.,* **1:**102, 1967.

215. Packard, G. C.: The influence of ambient temperature and aridity on modes of reproduction and excretion of amniote vertebrates, *Am. Natur.,* **100:**667, 1966.

216. Pang, Peter K. T.: Osmoregulatory functions of neurohypophysial hormones in fishes and amphibians, *Am. Zool.,* **17:**739–749, 1977.

217. Payan, P., and J. Maetz: Branchial sodium transport mechanisms in *Scyliothinus canicula:* Evidence for Na^+/NH_4^+ exchanges and for a role of carbonic anhydrase, *J. Exp. Biol.,* **58:**487–502, 1973.

218. Peaker, M., and J. L. Linzell: *Salt Glands in*

Birds and Reptiles, Monogr. Physiol. Soc., no. 32, Cambridge University Press, New York, 1975.

219. Philpott, C. W., and D. E. Copeland: Fine structure of chloride cells from three species of fundulus, *J. Cell. Biol.,* **18:**389, 1963.

220. Pickering, Alan D., and R. Morris: Osmoregulation of *Lampetra fluviatilis* L. and *Petromyzon marinus* (Cyclostomata) in hyperosmotic solutions, *J. Exp. Biol.,* **53:**231–243, 1970.

221. Pickford, G. E., and F. B. Grant: Serum osmolality in the coelacanth, *Latimeria chalumnae:* Urea retention and ion regulation, *Science,* **155:**568, 1967.

222. Potts, W. T. W., and F. B. Eddy: Gill potentials and sodium fluxes in the flounder *Platichthys flesus, J. Comp. Physiol.,* **87:**29–48, 1973.

223. Poulson, T. L.: Countercurrent multipliers in avian kidneys, *Science,* **148:**389, 1965.

224. Poulson, T. L.: Salt and water balance in seaside and sharp-tailed sparrows, *The Auk,* **86:**473, 1969.

225. Poulson, T. L., and G. A. Bartholomew: Salt balance in the Savannah sparrow, *Physiol. Zool.,* **35:**109, 1962.

226. Prosser, C. L., and F. A. Brown: *Comparative Animal Physiology,* W. B. Saunders Company, Philadelphia, 1961.

227. Rall, D. P., and J. W. Burger: Some aspects of hepatic and renal excretion in *Myxine, Am. J. Physiol.,* **212:**354, 1967.

228. Read, L. J.: Enzymes of the ornithine-urea cycle in the Chimaera *Hydrolagus colliei, Nature (London),* **215:**1412, 1967.

229. Read, L. J.: A study of ammonia and urea production and excretion in the freshwater adapted form of the Pacific lamprey, *Entosphenus tridentatus, Comp. Biochem. Physiol.,* **26:**455, 1968.

230. Renfro, J. Larry: Interdependence of active Na^+ and Cl^- transport by the isolated urinary bladder of the teleost, *Pseudopleuronectes americanus, J. Exp. Zool.,* **199:**383–390, 1977.

231. Renfro, J. L.: Water and ion transport by the urinary bladder of the teleost *Pseudopleuronectes americanus, Am. J. Physiol.,* **228:**52–61, 1975.

232. Roberts, J. S., and B. Schmidt-Nielsen: Renal ultrastructure and excretion of salt and water by three terrestrial lizards, *Am. J. Physiol.,* **211:**476, 1966.

233. Robertson, J. D.: The chemical composition of the blood of some aquatic chordates, including members of the *Tunicata, Cyclostomata* and *Osteichthyes, J. Exp. Biol.,* **31:**424, 1954.

234. Robinson, R. R., and B. Schmidt-Nielsen: Distribution of arginase within the kidneys of several vertebrate species, *J. Cell. Comp. Physiol.,* **62:**147, 1963.

235. Rogers, L. J.: The nitrogen excretion of *Chelodina longicollis* under conditions of hydration and dehydration, *Comp. Biochem. Physiol.,* **18:**249, 1966.

236. Ruibal, R., L. Tevis, and V. Roig: The terrestrial ecology of the spadefoot toad *Scaphiopus hammondii, Copeia,* **3:**571, 1969.

237. Sawyer, W. H.: Diuretic and natriuretic responses of lungfish (*Protopterus aethiopicus*) to arginine vasotocin, *Am. J. Physiol.,* **210:**191, 1966.

238. Sawyer, W. H.: Evolution of antidiuretic hormones and their functions, *Am. J. Med.,* **42:**678, 1967.

239. Sawyer, W. H., and M. K. Sawyer: Adaptive responses to neurohypophyseal fractions in vertebrates, *Physiol. Zool.,* **25:**84, 1952.

240. Scheer, B. T., and R. P. Markel: The effect of osmotic stress and hypophysectomy on blood and urine urea levels in frogs, *Comp. Biochem. Physiol.,* **7:**289, 1962.

241. Schmidt-Nielsen, Bodil: Renal transport of urea in elasmobranchs, *Alfred Benzon Symposium V, Copenhagen, 1972.* in H. H. Ussing and N. A. Thorn (eds.), *Transport Mechanisms in Epithelia,* Academic Press Inc., New York, 1973, pp. 608–621.

242. Schmidt-Nielsen, Bodil: Comparative physiology of cellular ion and volume regulation, *J. Expt. Zool.,* **194:**207–219, 1975.

243. Schmidt-Nielsen, Bodil: Regulation of volume and osmolality of the urine in the lower vertebrates, *Alfred Benzon Symposium XI, Osmotic and Volume Regulation,* 1977. In press.

244. Schmidt-Nielsen, B.: The excretory system, in D. B. Dill and E. F. Adolph (eds.), *Handbook of Physiology,* sec. 4. *Adaptation to the Environment,* American Physiological Society, Washington, 1964.

245. Schmidt-Nielsen, Bodil, and Deanne Schmidt: Renal function of *Sphenodon punctatum, Comp. Biochem. Physiol.,* **44A:**121–129, 1973.

246. Schmidt-Nielsen, Bodil, and J. Larry Renfro: Kidney function of the American eel, *Am. J. Physiol.*, **228**:420–431, 1975.

247. Schmidt-Nielsen, B., and R. P. Forster: The effects of dehydration and low temperature on renal function in the bull frog, *J. Cell. Comp. Physiol.*, **44**:233, 1954.

248. Schmidt-Nielsen, B., and C. R. Shrauger: Handling of urea and related compounds by the renal tubules of the frog, *Am. J. Physiol.*, **205**:483, 1963.

249. Schmidt-Nielsen, B., and L. Rabinowitz: Methylurea and acetamide: Active reabsorption by elasmobranch renal tubules, *Science*, **146**:1587, 1964.

250. Schmidt-Nielsen, Bodil, Bruno Truniger, and Lawrence Rabinowitz: Sodium linked urea transport by the renal tubule of the spiny dogfish, *Comp. Biochem. Physiol.*, **42A**:13–25, 1972.

251. Schmidt-Nielsen, B., K. J. Ullrich, G. Rumrich, and W. S. Long: Micropuncture study of urea movements across the renal tubules of *Squalus acanthias*, *Bull. Mt. Desert Island Biol. Lab.*, **6**:35, 1966.

252. Schmidt-Nielsen, B., and E. Skadhauge: Function of the excretory system of the crocodile (*Crocodylus acutus*), *Am. F. Physiol.*, **212**:973, 1967.

253. Schmidt-Nielsen, B., and L. E. Davis: Fluid transport and tubular intercellular spaces in reptilian kidneys, *Science*, **159**:1105, 1968.

254. Schmidt-Nielsen, K.: The salt-secreting gland of marine birds, *Circulation*, **21**:955, 1960.

255. Schmidt-Nielsen, K., C. B. Jørgensen, and H. Osaki: Extrarenal salt excretion in birds, *Am. J. Physiol.*, **193**:101, 1958.

256. Schmidt-Nielsen, K., and W. J. L. Sladen: Nasal salt secretion in the Humboldt penguin, *Nature (London)*, **181**:1217, 1958.

257. Schmidt-Nielsen, K., and P. Lee: Kidney function in the crab-eating frog (*Rana cancrivora*), *J. Exp. Biol.*, **39**:167, 1962.

258. Schmidt-Nielsen, K., A. Borut, P. Lee, and E. Crawford: Nasal salt excretion and the possible function of the cloaca in water conservation, *Science*, **142**:1300, 1963.

259. Schmidt-Nielsen, Bodil, and Yogendra Patel: Renal urea and water reabsorption in the little skate, *Raja erinacea*, *Bull. Mt. Desert Island Biol. Lab.*, **12**:94–98, 1972.

260. Schoffeniels, E., and R. R. Tercafs: L'osmorégulation chez les Batraciens, *Ann. Soc. R. Zool. Belg.*, **96**:23–39, 1965-6b.

261. Schooler, J. M., L. Goldstein, S. C. Hartman, and R. P. Forster: Pathways of urea synthesis in the elasmobranch, *Squalus acanthias*, *Comp. Biochem. Physiol.*, **18**:271, 1966.

262. Shade, Robert E., and Leonard Share: Vasopressin release during nonhypotensive hemorrhage and angiotensin II infusion, *Am. J. Physiol.*, **228**:149–154, 1975.

263. Shannon, J. A.: The excretion of uric acid by the chicken, *J. Cell. Comp. Physiol.*, **11**:135, 1938.

264. Sharratt, B. M., I. C. Jones, and D. Bellamy: Water and electrolyte composition of the body and renal function of the eel (*Anguilla anguilla* L.), *Comp. Biochem. Physiol.*, **11**:9, 1964.

265. Shehadeh, Z. H., and M. S. Gordon: The role of the intestine in salinity adaptation of the rainbow trout *Salmo gairdneri*, *Comp. Biochem. Physiol.*, **30**:397, 1969.

266. Siegel, N. J., D. A. Schon, and J. P. Hayslett: Evidence for active chloride transport in dogfish rectal gland, *Am. J. Physiol.*, **230**:1250–1254, 1976.

267. Siegel, N. J., P. Silva, F. H. Epstein, T. H. Maren, and J. P. Hayslett: Functional correlates of the dogfish rectal gland during *in vitro* perfusion, *Comp. Biochem. Physiol.*, **51A**:593–597, 1975.

268. Skadhauge, Erik: Cloacal resorption of salt and water in the galah (*Cacatua roseicapilla*), *J. Physiol.*, **240**:763–773, 1974.

269. Skadhauge, Erik: Excretion in lower vertebrates: Function of gut, cloaca, and bladder in modifying the composition of urine, *Fed. Proc.*, **36**:2487–2492, 1977.

270. Skadhauge, Erik: Renal concentrating ability in selected West Australian birds, *J. Exp. Biol.*, **61**:269–276, 1974.

271. Skadhauge, E.: The effect of unilateral infusion of arginine vasotocin into the portal circulation of the avian kidney, *Acta Endocrinol.*, **47**:321, 1964.

272. Skadhauge, E.: The cloacal storage of urine in the rooster, *Comp. Biochem. Physiol.*, **24**:7, 1968.

273. Skadhauge, E.: The mechanism of salt and water absorption in the intestine of the eel (*Anguilla anguilla*) adapted to waters of various salinities, *J. Physiol. (London)*, **204**:135, 1969.

274. Skadhauge, E., and B. Schmidt-Nielsen: Renal function in domestic fowl, *Am. J. Physiol.*, **212**:793, 1967.

275. Skadhauge, E., and B. Schmidt-Nielsen: Renal medullary electrolyte and urea gradient in chickens and turkeys, *Am. J. Physiol.*, **212**:1313, 1967.

276. Smith, H. W.: Metabolism of the lung-fish, *Protopterus aethiopicus, J. Biol. Chem.*, **88**:97, 1930.

277. Smith, H. W.: The absorption and excretion of water and salts by the elasmobranch fishes. I. Fresh water elasmobranchs, *Am. J. Physiol.*, **98**:279, 1931.

278. Smith, H. W.: The absorption and excretion of water and salts by the elasmobranch fishes. II. Marine elasmobranchs, *Am. J. Physiol.*, **98**:296, 1931.

279. Smith, H. W.: The retention and physiological role of urea in the elasmobranchii, *Biol. Rev.*, **11**:49, 1936.

280. Smyth, M., and G. A. Bartholomew: Effects of water deprivation and sodium chloride on the blood and urine of the mourning dove, *The Auk*, **83**:517, 1966.

281. Sperber, I.: Excretion, in A. J. Marshall (ed.), *Biology and Comparative Physiology of Birds*, Academic Press, Inc., New York, 1960, pp. 469–492.

282. Stewart, D. J., W. W. Holmes, and G. Fletcher: The renal excretion of nitrogenous compounds by the duck (*Anas platyrhynchos*) maintained on freshwater and on hypertonic saline, *J. Exp. Biol.*, **50**:527, 1969.

283. Stoff, J. S., P. Silva, M. Field, J. Forrest, A. Stevens, and F. H. Epstein: Cyclic AMP regulation of active chloride transport in the rectal gland of marine elasmobranchs, *J. Exp. Zool.*, **199**:443–448, 1977.

284. Stolte, H., and B. Schmidt-Nielsen: Comparative aspects of fluid and electrolyte regulation by the cyclostome, elasmobranch and lizard kidney, *Alfred Benzon Symposium XI, Osmotic and Volume Regulation*, 1977. In press.

285. Stolte, Hilmar, Bodil Schmidt-Nielsen, and Lowell Davis: Single nephron function in the kidney of the lizard, *Sceloporus cyanogenys, Zool. Jb. Physiol. Bd.*, **81**:219–244, 1977.

286. Stolte, H., R. G. Galaske, G. M. Eisenback, C. Lechene, B. Schmidt-Nielsen, and J. W. Boylan: Renal tubule ion transport and collecting duct function in the elasmobranch little skate, *Raja erinacea, J. Exp. Zool.*, **199**:403–410, 1977.

287. Stoner, Larry C.: Isolated, perfused amphibian renal tubules: The diluting segment, *Am. J. Physiol.*, **233**(5):F438–F444, 1977.

288. Templeton, J. R.: Nasal salt excretion in terrestrial lizards, *Comp. Biochem. Physiol.*, **11**:223, 1964.

289. Thorson, T. B., C. M. Cowan, and D. E. Watson: Body fluid solutes of juveniles and adults of the euryhaline bull shark *Carcharhinus leucas* from freshwater and saline environments, *Physiol. Zool.*, **46**:29–42, 1973.

290. Thorson, T. B., C. M. Cowan, and D. E. Watson: *Potamotrygon* spp: Elasmobranchs with low urea content, *Science*, **158**:375, 1967.

291. Urist, M. R.: Calcium and other ions in blood and skeleton of Nicaraguan fresh-water shark, *Science*, **137**:984, 1962.

292. Ussing, H. H.: The use of tracers in the study of active ion transport across animal membranes, *Symp. Quant. Biol.*, **13**:193, 1948.

293. Ussing, H. H.: The alkali metal ions in isolated systems and tissues, in H. H. Ussing, P. Kruhøffer, J. H. Thaysen, and N. A. Thorn, *The Alkali Metal Ions in Biology*, Springer-Verlag OHG, Berlin, 1960.

294. Ussing, H. H.: The frog skin potential, *J. Gen. Physiol.*, **43** (suppl.):135, 1960.

295. van Liew, J. B., P. Deetjen, and J. W. Boylan: Glucose reabsorption in the rat kidney: Dependence on glomerular filtration, *Pflueger Arch.*, **295**:232, 1967.

296. Walker, A. M., and C. L. Hudson: The role of the tubule in the excretion of urea by the amphibian kidney, *Am. J. Physiol.*, **118**:153, 1937.

297. Walter, Roderich, Clark W. Smith, P. K. Mehta, S. Boonjarern, Jose A. L. Arruda, and Neil A. Kurtzman: Conformational considerations of vasopressin as a guide to the development of biological probes and therapeutic agents, in Thomas E. Andreoli, Jared J. Grantham, and Floyd C. Rector, Jr., (eds.), *Disturbances in Body Fluid Osmolality*, American Physiological Society, Washington, 1977, pp. 1–36.

298. Watts, D. C., and R. L. Watts: Carbamoyl phosphate synthetase in the Elasmobranchii: Osmo-

regulatory function and evolutionary implications, *Comp. Biochem. Physiol.,* **17**:785, 1966.

299. Whittembury, Guillermo, F. Diezi, J. Diezi, K. Spring, and G. Giebisch: Some aspects of proximal tubular sodium chloride reabsorption in *Necturus* kidney, *Kidney Int.,* **7**:293–303, 1975.

300. Wikgren, B.: Osmotic regulation in some aquatic animals with special reference to the influence of temperature, *Acta Zool. Fenn.,* **71**:1, 1953.

301. Wong, T. M., and D. K. O. Chan: Physiological adjustments to dilution of the external medium in the lip-shark *Hemiscyllium plagiosum* (Bennett) II. Branchial renal and rectal gland function, *J. Exp. Zool.,* **200**:85–96, 1977.

302. Yorio, T., and P. J. Bentley: Asymmetrical permeability of the integument of tree frogs (Hylidae), *J. Exp. Biol.,* **67**:197–204, 1977.

303. Youson, John: Absorption and transport of ferritin and exogenous horseradish peroxidase in the opisthonephric kidney of the sea lamprey. II. The tubular nephron, *Cell Tissue Res.,* **157**:503–516, 1975.

304. Youson, J. H., S. J. Hansen, and I. M. Campbell: A quantitative comparison of the kidneys of the landlocked sea lamprey of the Great Lakes and the anadromous sea lamprey of the Atlantic, *Petromyzon marinus* L., *Can. J. Zool.,* **52**(12);1447–1455, 1974.

305. Youson, J. H., and D. B. McMillan: The opisthonephric kidney of the sea lamprey of the Great Lakes, *Petromyzon marinus* L. I. The renal corpuscle, *Am. J. Anat.,* **127**:207, 1970.

306. Youson, J. H., and D. B. McMillan: The opisthonephric kidney of the sea lamprey of the Great Lakes, *Petromyzon marinus* L. II. Neck and proximal segments of the tubular nephron, *Am. J. Anat.,* **127**:233, 1970.

3

Regulation of sodium balance

H. JOHN REINECK / JAY H. STEIN

INTRODUCTION

Sodium salts constitute more than 90 percent of the total solute contained in the extracellular fluid (ECF). Since sodium is actively extruded from the intracellular to the extracellular fluid, its salts are largely confined to the latter compartment (1), where the concentration of sodium is maintained relatively constant by alterations in antidiuretic hormone (ADH) release (2) and water intake (3). Therefore, the control of the extracellular fluid volume is dependent upon the regulation of sodium balance. Since sodium salts are excreted primarily by the kidney, it follows that the regulation of sodium balance will be determined by the relationship between sodium intake and the renal handling of sodium.

This relationship is demonstrated in Fig. 3-1, which schematically portrays a sodium balance study in a normal individual (4). In the initial period, the individual is on a 10 meq sodium diet and in the steady state, as denoted by a constant weight and a urinary sodium excretion equal to the intake. As sodium intake is increased to 150 meq per day, a period of positive sodium balance ensues that lasts 3 to 5 days (see hatched area in Fig. 3-1). With the increase in total body solute, ADH and the thirst mechanism are activated so that water retention occurs until the serum osmolality stabilizes at approximately the same level as was present on the 10 meq sodium intake. By the fifth day, sodium intake and urinary sodium excretion are again equivalent, body weight is constant, and the subject is in a new steady state at an increased level of extracellular fluid volume. If the individual is then placed back on the 10 meq sodium intake, reversal of the previous sequence of events occurs. This simplified example clearly illustrates the relationship between sodium balance and the regulation of extracellular fluid volume. The rise in sodium excretion that occurs as sodium intake increases is presumably a consequence of an increase in extracellular fluid volume, denoted by the period of positive sodium balance and the increase in body weight. Yet, as straightforward as the relationship may seem, the factors that regulate the crucial homeostatic machinery are very complex. We will attempt to describe in detail the various components of the afferent limb of this regulatory system, which perceives changes in ECF volume, and the efferent mechanisms, which determine the renal handling of sodium.

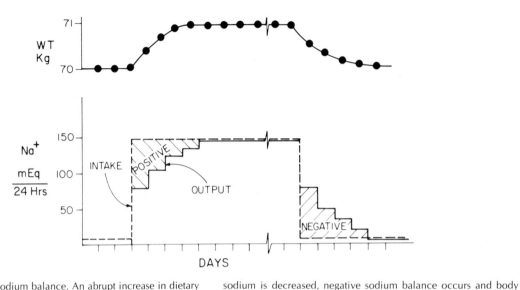

Figure 3-1. Normal sodium balance. An abrupt increase in dietary sodium intake results in a period of positive sodium balance and concomitant weight gain lasting 3 to 5 days. Thereafter urinary sodium equals sodium intake and weight stabilizes. When dietary sodium is decreased, negative sodium balance occurs and body weight decreases. After 3 to 5 days, a steady state is again achieved.

PERCEPTION OF CHANGES IN EXTRACELLULAR FLUID VOLUME

The status of the extracellular fluid volume should be viewed in terms of the relationship between the volume of fluid contained in that compartment and the holding capacity of the compartment. The latter is determined by the capacity of the vascular tree and the compliance of the interstitial space. Peters noted in 1935 that the capacity of the vascular bed is variable and that expansion must therefore be viewed as a "fullness" of these fluid compartments (5). The vasodilation that accompanies normal pregnancy results in sodium retention not because of an absolute deficit of extracellular fluid volume, but because of an expanded capacity of the ECF (6). Cirrhosis (7), arteriovenous fistula (8), and even assumption of the upright posture (9) are other examples of relative volume depletion that result in sodium retention. On the other hand, exposure to cold (10) and immersion in water (11) are examples of relative increases in extracellular fluid volume, enhancing sodium excretion.

If the kidney is to respond appropriately to either absolute or relative changes in extracellular fluid volume, there must be some mechanism for perceiving these changes. Whether this afferent limb of volume control is of extrarenal or renal origin is not known. Furthermore, the role of known volume receptors in the control of sodium excretion is also unclear. The possible components of the afferent limb are summarized in Table 3-1.

The extracellular fluid space comprises venous, arterial, capillary and interstitial components. The search for the afferent receptor of volume has involved manipulations and measurements of pressure and volumes in these various compartments.

Thoracic inferior vena cava ligation causes a profound antinatriuresis resulting in edema and ascites formation (12). This observation suggests

Table 3-1. Possible afferent components of ECF volume control

1. Intravascular receptors
    Cardiac atria
    Arterial baroreceptors
2. Interstitial volume or pressure
3. Intrarenal hemodynamic and compositional receptors
4. Juxtaglomerular apparatus

that thoracic venous pressure may be important in sensing extracellular volume. Verney demonstrated in 1947 that venous baroreceptors were important in the release of ADH (2). Gauer, Henry, and Sieker placed these volume receptors in the atria (13). While there is little doubt that these baroreceptors have an important effect on ADH release and therefore on water excretion, there is no evidence that they play any role in determining urinary sodium excretion. Cardiac denervation has no effect on the natriuretic response to saline loading (14). Furthermore, the acute closure of an arteriovenous fistula, which is associated with a marked increment in urinary sodium excretion, decreases pressure on the venous side of the circulation. It therefore seems unlikely that a venous baroreceptor signals the retention or excretion of sodium.

Stimulation of arterial baroreceptors is also known to effect ADH release (15). Sodium retention, however, may occur with high, normal, or low mean arterial pressures, so that these receptors cannot be the sole sensor for the maintenance of sodium balance. That changes in cardiac output may be a primary determinant of alterations in sodium excretion has also been suggested (16). As noted above, however, arteriovenous fistula closure results in enhanced sodium excretion despite a fall in cardiac output (8). Additionally, other sodium-retaining states, including cirrhosis (7) and fever (17), are associated with a high cardiac output.

All these observations must, however, be interpreted with caution. It is possible that in nonpathologic states, venous and arterial pressure as well as cardiac output may be involved in the determination of sodium excretion and that some unknown factors override these determinants in sodium-retaining states.

The possibility that interstitial volume or pressure is an important determinant of sodium excretion is suggested by several observations. The infusion of hyperoncotic albumin, which increases the vascular volume and depletes the interstitial compartment, results in no change or only a modest increase in urinary sodium excretion (18–22). The administration of plasma or isooncotic solutions expands the vascular space

without altering interstitial volume or pressure (23) and results in a significantly greater natriuretic response. The magnitude of the increment in sodium excretion accompanying saline infusion exceeds that seen with either hyperoncotic or isooncotic expansion (22, 24). Since saline infusion expands both vascular and interstitial volume, these observations suggest that expansion of the latter compartment may be involved in the perception of changes in extracellular fluid volume. As will be discussed below, however, compositional changes in the blood in response to different modalities of expansion vary, and these changes may directly affect the renal handling of sodium.

Volume changes may also be recognized within the kidney. The renin-angiotensin-aldosterone system is a potential control mechanism for sodium excretion. Tobian et al. have demonstrated the baroreceptor activity of the juxtaglomerular apparatus and the reciprocal relationship between perfusion pressure and renin release (25). Increased aldosterone release would then be the efferent limb of the mechanism for enhanced sodium reabsorption in volume-depleted states. As is discussed in the following section, however, this mechanism cannot fully account for the maintenance of sodium balance. The possibility that angiotensin may effect sodium excretion by altering renal hemodynamics will also be discussed.

Fitzgibbons et al. (26) and Osgood and associates (27) have demonstrated that constriction of the aorta before acute saline loading markedly blunts the natriuretic response to expansion when compared with the findings when the aorta is constricted after saline is administered. In other words, by preventing any hemodynamic perception of expansion at the level of the kidney, the natriuretic response to saline adminstration is decreased. While these findings may in some way be due to an effect on the efferent limb of volume regulation, they are also consistent with an intrarenal afferent receptor of extracellular fluid volume which requires exposure of the kidney to the hemodynamic effects of volume expansion.

In summary, the location and indeed the existence of a single extrarenal afferent receptor of extracellular fluid volume is without certain proof. It is, in fact, likely that more than a single afferent receptor exists and that the kidney itself may be intimately involved in perceiving the "fullness" of the extracellular fluid space.

RENAL REGULATION OF SODIUM EXCRETION

GENERAL CONCEPTS

The urinary excretion of sodium is determined by the difference between the rate of filtration and tubular reabsorption. Plasma is composed of 93 percent water and 7 percent solids (protein, lipids, etc.), the latter components containing virtually no sodium. Since only the fluid component of plasma is filtered, this would tend to increase the concentration of sodium in glomerular filtrate over that of plasma. On the other hand, the Donnan effect (see Chap. 1) tends to cancel this

change. Thus, the sodium concentration of the glomerular filtrate is essentially equal to that of plasma, and the filtered load of sodium is the product of the glomerular filtration rate (GFR) and the plasma sodium concentration.

GLOMERULAR FILTRATION RATE AND GLOMERULAR-TUBULAR BALANCE

In normal human beings the filtered load of sodium is approximately 14 meq per minute. The urinary excretion rate is about 1 percent of this amount, or 0.14 meq per minute, indicating that 99 percent is reabsorbed. If the GFR were increased by only 1 percent and reabsorption did not change in parallel, urinary sodium excretion would double. Conversely, small decreases in the GFR would produce a relatively large fall in sodium excretion. One might even suggest that the entire efferent limb of sodium regulation was determined by changes in the GFR not balanced by

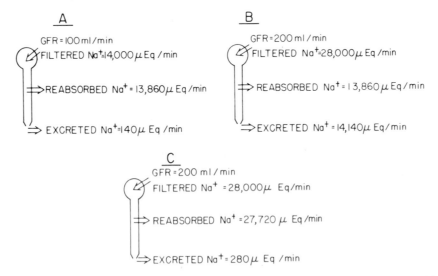

Figure 3-2. Schematic illustration of the relationship between filtered sodium load and tubular reabsorption of sodium. A. Filtered sodium equals 14,000 μeq/min and 99 percent is reabsorbed, leaving 1 percent, or 140 μeq/min excreted. B. If the GFR is doubled and the rate of tubular reabsorption is unaltered, this twofold rise in the GFR would result in a greater than tenfold increase in urinary sodium excretion. C. The GFR is again doubled. However, the rate of tubular reabsorption also doubles, resulting in only a twofold increase in sodium excretion.

appropriate alterations in sodium transport. This type of mechanism would be extremely precarious, however, because frequent major alterations in the GFR can occur with changes in posture, protein feedings, and other maneuvers.

There is, however, abundant evidence that a relationship does exist between filtration and reabsorption; it is schematically represented in Fig. 3-2. In the first panel is the control situation. The GFR is 100 ml/min, the filtered load is 14,000 μeq/min, and sodium excretion is 140 μeq/min, or 1 percent of the filtered load. If the GFR is doubled, the filtered sodium load increases to 28,000 μeq/min. If sodium reabsorption remained constant, sodium excretion would be massive, 14,140 μeq/min (panel B). This is not what normally occurs. As shown in panel C, sodium reabsorption tends to increase parallel with the filtered load, and sodium excretion is only modestly elevated. This coupling between changes in filtered sodium load and renal-tubular sodium reabsorption has been termed glomerular-tubular balance. It occurs when the filtered load changes in either direction.

The coupling between filtration and sodium reabsorption has been extensively studied, primarily in the proximal convoluted tubule. The mechanism does not appear to be intrinsic to the tubule; Burg and Orloff found that in the isolated perfused rabbit proximal convoluted tubule, absolute reabsorption was independent of perfusion rate (28). Imai et al. found similar results at physiologic flow rates (29); at lower perfusion rates, however, these authors found a direct relationship between reabsorption and flow and suggested that substrate delivery (glucose, alanine, and bicarbonate) could be rate-limiting for sodium reabsorption under these circumstances, thus contributing to glomerular-tubular balance.

The bulk of evidence, however, indicates that factors extrinsic to the proximal convoluted tubule are responsible for the phenomenon and suggests that hemodynamics and compositional changes in the postglomerular circulation are intimately involved. According to this view, Starling forces along the peritubular capillary are important determinants of proximal reabsorption. Brenner (30–36) and Windhager (37, 38) and their

colleagues have demonstrated quite conclusively that peritubular capillary oncotic pressure and proximal tubular reabsorption vary directly. Alterations in postglomerular resistance will cause directionally similar changes in the GFR, filtration fraction,[1] and peritubular capillary oncotic pressure, while peritubular capillary hydrostatic pressure will change in the opposite direction. Thus, at any given RPF, an increase in GFR will be accompanied by an increase in peritubular oncotic pressure and a decrease in peritubular hydrostatic pressure, resulting in enhanced proximal tubular reabsorption. Contrariwise, in a situation in which the GFR falls while renal plasma flow remains constant, the opposite sequence occurs. Even in circumstances in which the GFR and renal plasma flow are altered concomitantly, the peritubular oncotic force (the product of the capillary oncotic pressure and plasma flow) may be a major determinant of glomerular-tubular balance. For example, if the GFR and plasma flow are increased proportionately and the protein concentration in the efferent arteriole remains unchanged, more reabsorbate would have to enter the peritubular capillary in order to reduce the protein concentration in this vessel to the level seen prior to increasing the GFR, even at a constant oncotic and hydrostatic pressure. A more detailed discussion of these so-called physical factors is presented below.

Although changes in proximal tubular sodium reabsorption may be of paramount importance in the maintenance of glomerular-tubular balance, the distal nephron may also participate if incomplete compensation occurs proximally. Thus, under normal circumstances there is a direct relationship between filtration rate and tubular sodium reabsorption that would tend to minimize changes in sodium excretion as the filtered load is varied.

ALDOSTERONE

The need for aldosterone in the maintenance of normal sodium balance is illustrated by the renal

---

[1] Filtration fraction $= \dfrac{\text{GFR}}{\text{renal plasma flow (RPF)}}$

salt wasting which occurs in adrenal insufficiency. Since volume depletion stimulates and expansion suppresses aldosterone secretion (39), it has been attractive to credit this hormone with an important role in regulating urinary sodium excretion and ECF volume. Clearance and micropuncture studies have demonstrated the importance of aldosterone in the tubular reabsorption of sodium, especially along the distal nephron, where it affects potassium secretion as well (40).

The specific site of action of aldosterone has recently been questioned. Hierholzer et al. showed an effect of aldosterone on sodium reabsorption along the distal convoluted tubule in the rat (41). However, recent in vitro studies (42, 43) performed on isolated rabbit tubules failed to show any effect of this hormone along the distal convoluted tubule, at least as reflected by changes in the transtubular potential difference. Rather, aldosterone had a major electrogenic effect in the cortical collecting tubule, implying that miner-

alocorticoid-dependent electrogenic sodium transport is located along this segment. Uhlich and colleagues have further demonstrated that the hormone increases net sodium reabsorption along the papillary collecting duct by increasing sodium transport (44) and diminishing sodium back leak (45).

The mechanism by which aldosterone affects sodium transport is still not clear. Schmidt et al. have presented interesting data indicating that mineralocorticoid stimulates sodium-potassium–activated ATPase (Na^+–K^+–ATPase) on the peritubular border of distal tubular cells and therefore exerts its effect by decreasing the intracellular concentration of sodium and increasing that of potassium (46).

All of these studies indicate that aldosterone may affect net sodium reabsorption; however, several observations indicate that aldosterone is not solely responsible for regulating sodium excretion. First, the hormone appears to require about 30 to 60 minutes to exert its effect on sodium transport, presumably because its action requires the synthesis of an intracellular or membrane-bound protein (43). Yet, changes in sodium excretion occur immediately after assuming the erect position or during hemorrhagic hypotension. Second, patients with adrenal insufficiency on a fixed dosage of both mineralocorticoid and cortisone can still maintain sodium balance (47). Third, the chronic administration of mineralocorticoid causes only a transient period of salt retention, after which sodium balance is restored (48–50).

The latter so-called DOCA escape phenomenon is illustrated in Fig. 3-3. Once again we have our 70-kg subject, who is now ingesting 100 meq of sodium per day and is in the steady state. After mineralocorticoid is administered, a period of sodium and water retention ensues that lasts for 3 to 5 days. Then, in spite of continued mineralocorticoid administration, a natriuresis occurs and the subject goes back into balance, albeit at a higher level of extracellular volume. These studies have been interpreted to indicate that the sodium-retaining action of mineralocorticoid is overcome by a factor or factors which become operative as extracellular fluid volume is expanded. Thus, although the presence of mineralocorti-

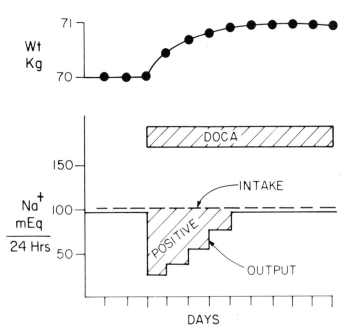

Figure 3-3. "DOCA escape" phenomenon. When an individual on a constant sodium intake receives mineralocorticoid, a period of positive sodium balance and weight gain occurs. After 3 to 5 days, however, a new steady state ensues, with sodium excretion again equal to sodium intake, and no further weight gain occurs.

coids may be necessary for normal sodium transport, it seems doubtful that alterations in secretion of the hormone play a major role in the regulation of extracellular fluid volume, at least in the uncomplicated physiologic setting.

It would therefore seem clear that factors other than filtration rate and aldosterone secretion must play a role in the regulation of urinary sodium excretion. Unequivocal proof of this postulate was obtained by de Wardener and his colleagues in a group of classic experiments published in 1961 (50).

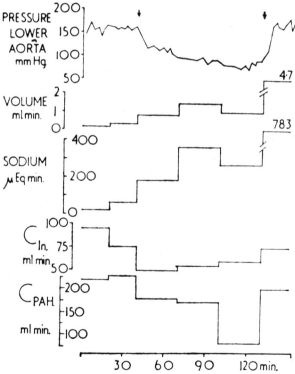

Figure 3-4. The de Wardener experiment. A dog receiving mineralocorticoid was volume expanded with isotonic saline. Despite a fall in renal perfusion pressure, the GFR (C_I) and RPF (C_{PAH}), that was achieved by inflating an aortic balloon proximal to the renal arteries, a large increase in urinary sodium excretion occurred. This group of studies provided unequivocal evidence that factors other than the GFR and mineralocorticoid were involved in determining urinary sodium excretion. (*From de Wardner, Mills, Clapham, and Hayter.*)

THE DE WARDENER EXPERIMENT

At the time this study was performed, there was still to be disproved a prevalent view that an unmeasurable increase in the GFR might determine the natriuresis which occurs with expansion of the extracellular fluid volume. Therefore, de Wardener decreased the GFR and the filtered load of sodium by reducing the perfusion pressure to the kidney of the dog with an inflatable balloon placed cephalad to the renal artery. In addition, supraphysiologic doses of mineralocorticoid were given before and during the experiment. Yet, in spite of these maneuvers and a resultant marked fall in the GFR, a natriuresis occurred when a large infusion of isotonic saline was given to the animal (Fig. 3-4). Although the natriuresis was certainly greater when the balloon was deflated and the filtered load increased, these studies provided unequivocal evidence that a natriuresis could occur after expansion of the extracellular fluid volume which was independent of changes in the GFR and aldosterone secretion. Since that time, a number of laboratories have examined other possible factors involved in the efferent limb of volume regulation. The main possibilities are summarized in Table 3-2 and will be discussed individually.

PERITUBULAR CAPILLARY FORCES

Ludwig initially proposed that tubular reabsorption was a totally passive phenomenon caused by a fall in hydrostatic pressure in the postglomerular capillaries coupled with the concentration of nonfilterable solutes in the capillary circulation

Table 3-2. Possible efferent components of ECF volume other than GFR and aldosterone

1. Peritubular capillary forces
   Hydrostatic pressures
   Colloid osmotic pressures
2. Medullary blood flow
3. Redistribution of renal blood flow or glomerular filtrate
4. Humoral substances
   "Natriuretic hormone"
   Antidiuretic hormone
5. Sympathetic nerve activity

(51, 52). This view was quite intuitive, since Starling's classic description of the forces affecting solute and water movement across the capillary was not published until 67 years later (53). Yet, tubular transport cannot be explained on the basis of the Ludwig hypothesis alone. First, active transport of sodium has been demonstrated in virtually every portion of the nephron (54). Second, pure passive reabsorption is not compatible with the ability of the mammalian kidney to both concentrate and dilute the final urine. These two points in particular dissuaded a number of investigators from considering seriously the role of the capillary circulation in the regulation of salt and water balance. However, although there is clearly active transport of sodium or chloride or both, along the nephron, changes in hydrostatic and oncotic pressure in the peritubular capillary circulation may modify the net reabsorption of electrolytes. Interestingly, Green, Windhager, and Giebisch found that an effect of oncotic pressure

on proximal tubular sodium reabsorption could be demonstrated only in the presence of an intact active transport system (55). Thus, the active transport of sodium and other electrolytes in no way obviates a role for passive forces in altering the composition of the final urine.

In order to understand more clearly the role of these so-called physical factors, a few basic comments are warranted. Fig. 3-5 is a schematic representation of the hydrostatic forces along the capillary circulation of the rat kidney. These values were obtained in the Munich-Wistar rat, which is endowed with surface glomeruli accessible for micropressure measurements (56, 57). Along the glomerular capillary, net ultrafiltration is favored at least in a portion of the glomerulus, because of the greater transcapillary hydrostatic pressure gradient (ΔP). As filtration occurs, the transcapillary colloid osmotic pressure difference ($\Delta \pi$) rises until it equals ΔP, when filtration occurs. The reverse forces are operative in the peritubular capillary (58, 59). Because of the marked pressure drop from the glomerulus to the peritubular capillary, $\Delta \pi$ exceeds ΔP and reabsorption of filtrate into the capillary occurs.

$$\Delta P = P_c - P_I$$
$$\Delta \pi = \pi_c - \pi_I$$

where P_c and P_I = the capillary and interstitial hydrostatic pressure
π_c and π_I = the capillary and interstitial colloid osmotic pressures, respectively

Thus the fluid exchange across the capillary wall at any point can be expressed by

$$\mathcal{J}_v = K[(\pi_c - \pi_I) - (P_c - P_I)] \qquad (3\text{-}1)$$

where $\mathcal{J}_v$ = the net transcapillary fluid flux
K = the effective hydraulic permeability of the capillary wall

Although it has recently become popular to consider these passive forces totally as a function of the mass balances shown in Eq. (3-1), it must be remembered that the events which alter either ΔP or Δp are primarily hemodynamic. For exam-

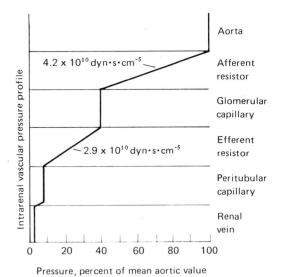

Figure 3-5. Intrarenal vascular pressures. Despite a large drop in pressure along the afferent arteriole, the difference between glomerular capillary pressure and intratubular pressure ($\Delta \pi$ exceeds the transcapillary oncotic pressure difference ($\Delta \pi$) and net filtration occurs. Because of a resistor at the level of the efferent arteriole, however, peritubular capillary pressure falls and $\Delta \pi$ now exceeds $\Delta \pi$ favoring the capillary uptake of reabsorbate. (*From Brenner, Deen, and Robertson.*)

ple, increases in renal blood flow caused by various stimuli (e.g., vasocilator agents, extracellular volume expansion, etc.) are usually associated with a fall in filtration fraction (FF). As originally derived by Bresler (60)

$$C_E = C_A \frac{1}{1 - FF} \qquad (3\text{-}2)$$

where C_E = efferent arteriolar protein concentration
where C_A = afferent arteriolar protein concentration

Rearranging:

$$FF = 1 - \frac{C_A}{C_E} \qquad (3\text{-}3)$$

From Eq. (3-3), it is clear that at any given c_A, a fall in filtration fraction will decrease c_E. In addition, vasodilatation will increase P_c because of the fall in resistance at the efferent arteriole. Thus, renal vasodilatation will decrease oncotic and increase hydrostatic pressure in the efferent arteriole, both alterations which would tend to decrease capillary uptake.

Although the relationship between capillary uptake and the Starling forces acting across the peritubular capillary seems straightforward, a rather complex mechanism is required to explain how alterations in these parameters may modify urinary sodium excretion. The initial Ludwig hypothesis suggesting a direct osmotic gradient between peritubular capillary and tubular lumen does not seem plausible. Recent observations have led to the development of a pump-leak model schematically shown in Fig. 3-6. This model is clearly applicable only to the proximal tubule. Electrophysiologic studies by Boulpaep and others have demonstrated that the proximal convoluted tubule possesses typical characteristics of a leaky epithelium (61): when an electric current is passed along the proximal convoluted tubule, there is significant shunting across some high conductance pathway. Virtually all evidence points to the tight junction or lateral intercellular space or both as the site of this shunt pathway. In this model, sodium moves into the cell down a concentration gradient and then is actively trans-

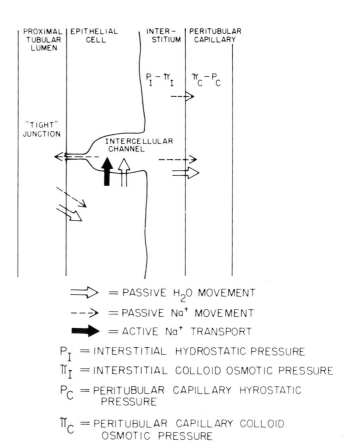

= PASSIVE H₂O MOVEMENT

= PASSIVE Na⁺ MOVEMENT

= ACTIVE Na⁺ TRANSPORT

P_I = INTERSTITIAL HYDROSTATIC PRESSURE

π_I = INTERSTITIAL COLLOID OSMOTIC PRESSURE

P_C = PERITUBULAR CAPILLARY HYROSTATIC PRESSURE

π_C = PERITUBULAR CAPILLARY COLLOID OSMOTIC PRESSURE

Figure 3-6. Schematic representation of the "pump-leak" model of proximal tubular sodium reabsorption. Filtered sodium is passively reabsorbed from the tubular lumen into the epithelial cell down a concentration gradient. It is then actively transported into the lateral intercellular channel, which communicates directly with the interstitial space. The uptake of reabsorbate from the interstitium into the peritubular capillary is determined by the Starling forces across the capillary wall. If the net force for uptake of reabsorbate into the capillary is decreased, conductive and geometric changes in the tight junction interspace complex may occur that favor increased "backleak" of reabsorbate into the tubular lumen, diminishing net absorption.

ported into the interspace, with water following because of the osmotic gradient created by the sodium transport. In the original formulation of this model, a markedly hypertonic interstitium was predicted, but recent work has suggested that only a small osmotic gradient need be generated to have the system function efficiently. Fluid moves from the intercellular channel into the interstitium down a hydrostatic pressure gradient generated in the channel. The reabsorbate entering the interstitium is then removed at a rate determined by the Starling forces acting across the peritubular capillary. If the rate of reabsorption exceeds the rate of capillary uptake, interstitial volume will increase. For example, a decrease in capillary oncotic pressure or a rise in capillary hydrostatic pressure or both would decrease the rate of uptake from the renal interstitium. The alteration in interstitial volume may then lead to a change in the conductance or the geometry of the tight junction–intercellular channel complex, with a resultant increase in the flux of sodium back into the lumen of the proximal tubule (backleak). The net effect of this alteration would be a decrease in net sodium transport in the proximal tubule, even though active transport was unchanged. Although a number of aspects of this model are still controversial, the general description seems to be a reasonable working hypothesis. In any case, from this model, one can see how alterations in the Starling forces in the peritubular capillary circulation may modify net sodium transport in the proximal convoluted tubule.

Both clearance and micropuncture studies have been utilized to confirm this general relationship between capillary forces and urinary sodium excretion. Earley and his coworkers have presented a series of ingenious clearance studies which clearly demonstrate that changes in renal blood flow, perfusion pressure, or plasma oncotic pressure may alter tubular sodium transport (62–64). Micropuncture studies by Brenner and his associates (30–36) and Windhager et al. (37, 38) have shown a direct relationship between peritubular capillary oncotic pressure and proximal tubular sodium reabsorption. Spitzer and Windhager developed a technique which allowed them to perfuse the peritubular capillary circulation with solutions of varying protein concentrations. In these studies, they noted a direct relationship between the oncotic pressure of the perfusate and proximal tubular sodium reabsorption (Fig. 3-7). Similarly, Brenner and associates found that both fractional and absolute sodium reabsorption in the proximal tubule varied directly with the peritubular capillary colloid osmotic pressure.

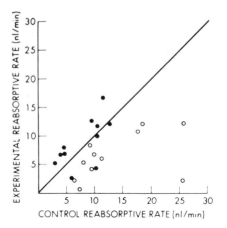

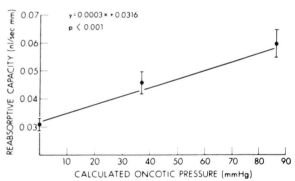

Figure 3-7. Effect of peritubular capillary oncotic pressure on proximal tubular sodium reabsorption. In the top panel free-flow micropuncture studies were performed during a control period and an experimental period during which peritubular capillaries were perfused with either saline (o) or 8% dextran solution (●). Proximal reabsorption fell with the saline perfusion, which decreased oncotic pressure, and rose with the dextran perfusion, which increased oncotic pressure. The bottom panel illustrates the direct relationship between peritubular oncotic pressure and proximal reabsorption obtained by the split droplet technique. (*From Spitzer and Windhager.*)

Alterations in perfusion pressure may also modify proximal tubular transport. In several models, proximal tubular transport decreases in association with an increase in renal perfusion pressure (65–67). This may be a primary mechanism for the so-called pressure diuresis and natriuresis, although other investigators have suggested that sodium transport may also be decreased in Henle's loop, the collecting duct, and/or juxtamedullary nephrons when perfusion pressure is increased (68–70).

Recent studies by Fitzgibbons and associates (26) and Osgood et al. (27) have demonstrated that renal perfusion pressure per se, or some consequence of its alteration, may be of even greater importance than was previously thought. In the de Wardener experiment (50) (Fig. 3-4), renal perfusion pressure was decreased after an acute saline load had been administered for a finite period. In the studies mentioned above, however, perfusion pressure was reduced just before administering the volume load: surprisingly, no natriuresis occurred in the rat after a 10 percent body weight Ringer load, despite a constant GFR and a markedly reduced plasma protein concentration. In addition, no change in proximal reabsorption was observed in this group of studies. These studies do not contradict the findings of de Wardener but rather indicate that intrarenal events may be of primary importance in determining the natriuretic response to volume expansion. It would seem that a reduction in perfusion pressure before volume expansion markedly attenuates these intrarenal adjustments.

MEDULLARY BLOOD FLOW

A theory has been formulated to explain how hemodynamic alterations may change sodium transport in the distal, as well as the proximal, nephron. Earley proposed that an increase in medullary blood flow, as may occur during extracellular volume expansion, may depress sodium reabsorption in the ascending limb of Henle's loop as a consequence of a dissipation of the usual hypertonicity of the medullary interstitium (71). The theory is as follows: States associated with an increase in medullary blood flow will "wash out" the hypertonic medullary interstitium. This will decrease the abstraction of water from the descending limb of Henle's loop that normally occurs because of the high medullary osmolality. Thus, an increased volume of fluid with the same total content of sodium will be delivered to the water-impermeable ascending limb. If there is a lower limit to the sodium concentration which can be generated along the ascending limb, then more sodium will be delivered to the distal portions of the nephron. Although this hypothesis has not been adequately tested, it does seem to be a reasonable model to explain at least a portion of the natriuresis seen in settings such as extracellular volume expansion.

REDISTRIBUTION OF BLOOD FLOW AND/OR FILTRATE

Alterations in the distribution of renal blood flow might affect urinary sodium excretion (72–74). According to this original theory, juxtamedullary nephrons may have a greater sodium reabsorption capacity than more superficial nephrons, and thus redistribution of flow to deep nephrons would result in sodium retention. Utilizing an inert gas washout technique, Thornburn et al. produced data to support this hypothesis (74). In a recent review, however, Lameire, Lifschitz, and Stein (75) compiled data from a large number of studies employing the radio-labeled microsphere method; there was no correlation between the changes in distribution and urinary sodium excretion. They concluded that there was no clear-cut evidence that redistribution of blood flow is a major determinant of urinary sodium excretion.

Glomerular filtration could conceivably be redistributed without a redistribution of renal blood flow. Multiple laboratories have utilized micropuncture methods as well as a technique which determines the nephron uptake of ^{14}C-ferrocyanide (Hanssen technique) to determine the distribution of the nephron GFR. The results are somewhat conflicting (75), yet it would seem fair to say that there is generally no evidence to suggest that a redistribution of glomerular filtrate has not been consistently noted in a given experimental setting. Therefore, it is unlikely that distributional changes in either renal blood flow or glomerular filtration are important determinants of urinary sodium excretion.

It should also be noted that the original hypothesis (that larger juxtamedullary nephrons could reabsorb more sodium) was based strictly on anatomic data. Recently, Kokko and his associates have begun a systematic evaluation of the transport characteristics of isolated rabbit proximal tubules from superficial and juxtamedullary nephrons (76, 77). Although fascinating electrophysiologic differences have been noted, the physiologic significance of the findings is unclear. It is also worth noting that recent studies by Stein and associates have indicated that sodium transport may even be inhibited to a greater extent in juxtamedullary nephrons during Ringer loading (78). This phenomenon is discussed in greater detail below.

"NATRIURETIC HORMONE"

Since the classic studies of de Wardener demonstrated that factors other than the GFR and aldosterone are involved in the control of urinary sodium excretion, a great deal of interest has centered on the identification and isolation of a humoral substance affecting sodium transport. de Wardener himself hypothesized the existence of such a "natriuretic hormone" (50). Later studies by de Wardener and various associates described a substance, found in extracts of plasma and urine in both human beings and animals, which inhibited sodium reabsorption in vivo and in vitro (79–82). Buckalew has also proposed the existence of a natriuretic hormone based on the finding of an inhibitor of toad bladder sodium transport in dialysates of plasma from volume-expanded animals (83–86). Numerous other investigators have reported humoral inhibitors of sodium reabsorption (87–97).

A series of studies by Bricker and associates have examined the possible role of such a humoral factor in the control of sodium excretion in uremic man and animals (98–103). These authors suggest that during a period of nephron loss, transient sodium retention occurs that leads to the release of a humoral inhibitor of sodium transport. Interpreting data obtained by in vitro microperfusion techniques, they suggest a distal site of action of this substance (104). Recently, this group has also reported that the renal tubule of uremic animals is more sensitive to the "hormone" (105) and that a similar substance can be found in the urine of volume-expanded normal dogs (106).

These studies suggest the existence of some as yet unidentified hormonal factor which is an important regulator of urinary sodium excretion. It should be emphasized, however, that the search for the chemical nature of such a substance has been unsuccessful (107). The aforementioned studies of Fitzgibbons et al. (26) and Osgood and colleagues (27) on renal perfusion pressure also argue strongly against the existence of a hormone of extrarenal origin. Indeed, these studies cast grave doubt on the physiologic importance of such a hormone, at least in the natriuretic response to acute ECF volume expansion. Thus, while the search for a humoral regulator of sodium balance other than aldosterone continues, its existence is still uncertain.

SYMPATHETIC ACTIVITY

Altered adrenergic nervous activity can modify urinary sodium excretion by influencing Starling forces in the peripheral capillary bed, by changing the central blood volume and thus the distribution of the ECF, or by changing renal hemodynamics. A more direct effect of the autonomic nerve activity on renal sodium handling has also been demonstrated. A large number of studies in anesthetized animals have shown that either anatomic or pharmacologic unilateral renal denervation leads to a significant ipsilateral increase in sodium excretion (108–110). Conversely, renal nerve stimulation decreases sodium excretion (111, 112).

The mechanism by which renal nerve activity alters sodium excretion remains controversial. Several authors have demonstrated that an increase in GFR or renal blood flow occurs with renal denervation (113, 114). Recent studies in the rat and dog, however, describe diminished proximal reabsorption of sodium even in the absence of measureable changes in GFR or renal blood flow (115–117). Bello-Reusse et al. have examined the possible role of hemodynamic factors more closely (118). These investigators found a marked fall in proximal tubular sodium transport in association with only small changes in peritubular capillary hydrostatic pressure after renal denervation. Furthermore, glomerular capillary pressure and nephron GFR were unchanged by this maneuver. These findings suggest that alterations in renal hemodynamics are not involved in the diminished sodium reabsorption seen in this model and that a direct effect on tubular transport may be operative. Anatomic and histochemical studies have indicated innervation of renal tubules in the rat (119, 120). Additionally, several in vitro studies have demonstrated that catecholamines directly affect active sodium transport (121, 122).

It should be noted, however, that several investigators have studied the effect of chronic unilateral denervation in the conscious animals and have found no effect on sodium excretion (123–124). Furthermore, Lifschitz found that renal denervation failed to blunt either the antinatriuretic response to hemorrhage or the natriuretic response to volume expansion in awake dogs (125). Therefore, further studies are needed to define better the role of the renal nerves in the physiologic control of urinary sodium excretion.

ANTIDIURETIC HORMONE (ADH)

The importance of ADH in the control of water excretion is well known and accepted. Because ECF volume, as well as tonicity, affects the release of the hormone (126), various investigators have sought to define a role for this hormone in the control of sodium excretion.

Kurtzman et al. have demonstrated that the infusion of pharmacologic doses of ADH causes a significant increase in urinary sodium excretion without changing GFR or RBF. When increases in renal perfusion pressure were prevented by nitroprusside administration, the natriuretic response persisted (127). Chan and Sawyer administered ADH to animals undergoing a water diuresis and also observed a natriuretic response (128). It is possible that in the latter studies, transient volume expansion occurred secondary to water retention and caused the increased sodium excretion. Humphreys and coworkers found, however, that either exogenous or endogenous ADH released during a water diuresis increased urinary sodium excretion. The authors suggested that the natriuretic response was due to diminished loop reabsorption resulting from medullary washout (129).

The effect of ADH on sodium transport has been studied more directly. Numerous investigators have shown that the hormone increases rather than decreases sodium transport across anuran membranes (130–132). Burg and associates, studying the isolated cortical collecting duct, found that ADH caused a transient rise in the electric potential (133) and an increased lumento-bath transport, without altering movement of sodium in the opposite direction (134). Thus, in the cortical collecting tubule, ADH appears to increase sodium reabsorption.

The effect of ADH on papillary collecting duct sodium transport has also been examined. Ullrich and associates, studying the rat papilla in vivo (135), and Tadokoro et al., using an in vitro preparation (136), described an increased backleak of sodium in response to ADH. If these studies are correct, the effect of ADH on net sodium transport along the cortical and papillary segments of the collecting duct differs not only in mechanism but also in direction. With all these various complicated results, there is currently no definite evidence to suggest that ADH plays a role in the regulation of sodium balance.

SEGMENTAL ANALYSIS OF SODIUM TRANSPORT

In this final section we will describe the qualitative and quantitative aspects of sodium transport in the various nephron segments.

PROXIMAL TUBULE

The proximal tubule normally reabsorbs from 50 to 75 percent of the filtered load of sodium. Reabsorption along this segment is isotonic, as evidenced by tubular fluid to plasma osmolar and sodium concentration ratios of unity (137). That the reabsorption of sodium is at least in part due to active transport has been shown by several well-supported observations. First, inhibitors of Na^+-

K^+–ATPase decrease proximal sodium reabsorption by approximately 35 percent (138). Second, while the exact quantitative value of the early proximal tubular transepithelial potential differential (PD) is controversial, most investigators agree that it is oriented lumen-negative (139). Finally, if a poorly reabsorbable substance such as raffinose or mannitol is placed within the proximal tubular lumen in vivo (140, 141) or in vitro (142), the steady-state ratio of tubular fluid to plasma sodium in the steady state is less than unity. All of these findings can be explained only by an active transport process. We reemphasize, however, that passive forces also appear to be involved in the proximal reabsorption of sodium.

Several investigators have demonstrated by both in vivo and in vitro methods that sodium transport along the proximal convoluted tubule is linked to the active reabsorption of bicarbonate, glucose, and amino acids (29, 143–146). According to the theory first proposed by Rector and colleagues, a significant portion of proximal tubular sodium reabsorption is passive, following bulk fluid reabsorption which is dependent on active bicarbonate and glucose reabsorption (147). Subsequently, amino acid transport was shown to influence net sodium reabsorption (146). Recent studies in vivo in the rat and in vitro in the isolated rabbit tubule have described a small but consistent negative PD in the early proximal convoluted tubule which is produced by glucose and amino acid transport (143–145). In the latter portion of the proximal tubule, the tubular fluid to plasma chloride ratio exceeds 1, presumably because of the preferential reabsorption of bicarbonate (148, 149) more proximally. This gives rise to the development of a positive PD caused by diffusion of chloride down its concentration gradient.

In the straight portion of the proximal tubule (pars recta) sodium reabsorption also occurs. Because this tubular segment is inaccessible to micropuncture, information regarding it is derived solely from in vitro microperfusion studies of isolated rabbit tubules. When straight proximal tubules from superficial nephrons are perfused with a solution identical to that found at the end of the convoluted tubule, this segment similarly develops a lumen-positive PD, and a significant portion of net sodium transport is dependent on this passive chloride gradient (76, 150). Nonetheless, active sodium reabsorption also occurs, since either cooling the bath or adding ouabain to it inhibits sodium reabsorption (150). Recent studies demonstrated intrinsic differences between straight proximal tubules of superficial and deep nephrons, the former being more permeable to chloride and the latter more permeable to sodium (76). The significance of this finding is not clear, however, since net fluid reabsorption did not differ in the pars recta of the two nephron populations.

In addition to reabsorbing sodium, the straight tubule actively secretes organic solutes (151, 152). In fact, when the segment is exposed to high concentrations of para-aminohippurate, net fluid secretion is observed. Such secretory activity could alter net sodium and fluid transport in this segment.

In summary, proximal reabsorption is due, at least in part, to active transport of sodium. In addition, a portion of sodium reabsorption may be linked to the development of a positive potential difference across the late proximal tubule as well as to bulk flow of reabsorbate. Finally, net sodium reabsorption is further modulated by the Starling forces across the proximal tubule. The relative importance of each of these phenomena is unclear.

Dirks, Cirksena, and Berliner were the first to directly demonstrate by micropuncture that saline loading diminished fractional sodium reabsorption along the proximal convoluted tubule (153). Fig. 3-8 summarizes the results of these important studies in the dog. The horizontal axis is the tubular fluid to plasma inulin ratio in a segment of proximal tubule during hydropenia, while the vertical axis represents the inulin ratio obtained from the same tubule during isotonic saline loading. Since reabsorption in the proximal tubule is isotonic, a fall in the tubular fluid to plasma inulin ratio is indicative of a decrease in both fractional water and sodium transport. As can be noted from the figure, the tubular fluid to plasma inulin ratio fell markedly during saline loading. This alteration persisted even when the total kidney GFR was markedly decreased. Subsequent studies in many laboratories have confirmed this finding and, in addition, described decreased absolute reabsorption along this segment during volume expansion. Conversely, sodium-retaining states have been shown to enhance proximal reabsorption. Weiner et al. demonstrated that marked ECF volume depletion increased sodium reabsorption along this segment (154), while Bank and Anyedjian described salt retention and enhanced proximal reabsorption in animals with ascites and edema secondary to bile duct obstruction (155). Cirksena and associates also found that saline loading failed to decrease proximal reabsorption in the setting of acute inferior thoracic vena cava obstruction (156). Thus, proximal tubular sodium reabsorption appears to respond appropriately to changes in extracellular fluid volume.

LOOP OF HENLE

Current concepts of sodium transport along the loop of Henle are largely derived from in vitro microperfusion studies performed on isolated rabbit tubules. The descending limb of Henle's loop has been studied by Kokko, who found this segment to be virtually impermeable to sodium (157).

The thin ascending limb of Henle's loop effects net sodium reabsorption. In vitro studies by Imai and Kokko provide a model for passive sodium transport from lumen to interstitium (158). Recent observations by Johnston et al. in the rat demonstrate a sodium concentration gradient from lumen to vasa recta in hydropenic rats, suggesting that passive flux of sodium may indeed occur (159). The thick ascending segment of Henle's loop has been extensively studied by Burg and his colleagues (160–162) and Rocha and Kokko (163). These investigators found a lumen-positive *PD* generated by active chloride transport. Their findings suggest that sodium reabsorption in this segment occurs passively down an electrochemical gradient.

Absolute sodium reabsorption along the loop of Henle of superficial nephrons varies directly with changes in delivery to that segment (22, 164–

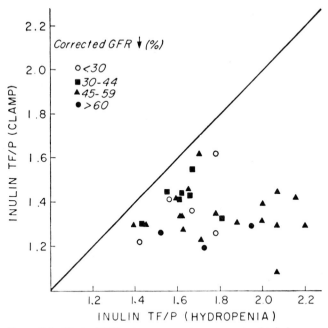

Figure 3-8. Effect of ECF volume expansion on proximal tubular sodium reabsorption. The inulin TF/P values are an index of fractional sodium and water reabsorption. The horizontal axis represents hydropenic values and the vertical axis those obtained during saline loading while clamping the renal artery. Despite falls in the GFR to less than 30 percent of control, proximal reabsorption is significantly decreased by saline loading. (*From Dirks, Cirksena, and Berliner.*)

168). The change in fractional reabsorption (i.e., the percentage of delivered sodium reabsorbed) along Henle's loop as a function of delivery is less certain. Landwehr and coworkers (165) found an increase in this parameter in response to volume expansion, while Kunau et al. (167), studying varying degrees of expansion, described decreased fractional reabsorption. Yet in both studies absolute sodium reabsorption was markedly increased. Thus there is no evidence that sodium transport in the loop of Henle, at least of superficial nephrons, is inhibited by extracellular volume expansion. We caution, however, that sodium reabsorption along the loop of Henle of deep nephrons may be affected by changes in ECF volume. Recent studies by Stein and associates have demonstrated a greater delivery of so-

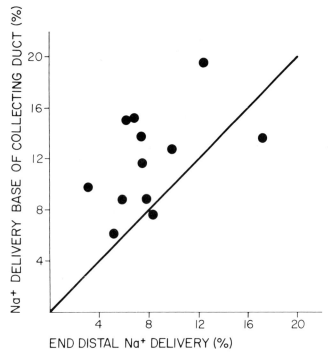

Figure 3-9. In ten of twelve studies sodium delivery to the base of the papillary collecting duct exceeded delivery to the end of distal tubule of superficial nephrons. This finding suggests a greater inhibition of sodium reabsorption in juxtamedullary nephrons in response to ECF volume expansion. (*From Stein, Osgood, and Kunau.*)

dium to the base of the papillary collecting duct than to the late distal tubule of superficial nephrons (Fig. 3-9) (169). These studies were interpreted to indicate a greater inhibition of sodium transport in inner than in outer cortical nephrons during expansion of the extracellular fluid volume. Further studies localized this greater inhibition of sodium transport to the loop of Henle of these nephrons (78). Juxtamedullary nephrons have a thin ascending limb in which sodium transport occurs because of a concentration gradient developed by the accumulation of urea in the medullary interstitium. (See Chap. 12.) Saline loading markedly decreases the hypertonicity of the medullary interstitium and may, therefore, abolish this concentration gradient and markedly decrease sodium transport in the thin ascending limb of these nephrons. In contrast, the loop of

Henle of superficial nephrons of the rat is made up only of a thick ascending limb, which presumably transports sodium chloride only by an active process that is seemingly not impaired by volume expansion.

DISTAL CONVOLUTED TUBULE

Net sodium reabsorption occurs along the distal convoluted tubule. Electric measurements indicate a lumen-negative *PD*, the magnitude increasing progressively along the length of the segment (170). While the sodium concentration of the tubular fluid varies depending on the model studied, the tubular fluid to plasma sodium concentration gradient is normally less than unity and progressively decreases along the length of the segment. Thus sodium reabsorption occurs against an electrochemical gradient, indicating an active transport process. Unlike the proximal convoluted tubule, which, as discussed above, has a low electric resistance and high sodium chloride permeability, the electric resistance is high along the distal convoluted tubule (171). This property allows the establishment and maintenance of a high transepithelial sodium concentration gradient.

Micropuncture studies of sodium transport along the distal convoluted tubule during ECF volume expansion demonstrate increased absolute and decreased fractional reabsorption (166, 167). Furthermore, the in vivo microperfusion studies of Morgan and Berliner describe a direct correlation between perfusion rate and sodium reabsorption along this segment. Saline loading did not qualitatively or quantitatively alter this relationship (168).

COLLECTING DUCT

Important physiologic differences appear to distinguish the cortical collecting tubule and papillary collecting duct. While some of these observed differences may be caused by the methods utilized and the species under study, it seems appropriate to discuss these two portions of the terminal nephron separately.

Cortical collecting tubule

A large number of in vitro microperfusion studies have demonstrated net sodium reabsorption along this nephron segment. The nature of this sodium transport is not entirely clear, however. A lumen-negative *PD* has been reported (133, 134, 172–174) and Grantham et al. (172) found this segment capable of generating and maintaining a sizable sodium concentration gradient. The removal of sodium from the perfusate abolishes this electric potential, and ouabain inhibits sodium transport and causes transepithelial depolarization (133, 172). These results suggest that active electrogenic sodium transport occurs along the cortical collecting duct. Further studies by Kokko's group have shown that the negative *PD* is maintained only in the presence of mineralocorticoids (42, 43). These authors suggest that mineralocorticoids are necessary for active sodium transport in this nephron segment.

Electric resistance is high in the cortical collecting tubule when compared with the proximal convoluted tubule (133, 173), and measurements of undirectional sodium flux indicate that little backleak of sodium occurs. These findings are supported by the observations of Tischer and Yarger, who found that lanthanum permeability across the tight junction of the cortical collecting tubule was quite low (175).

In summary, the cortical collecting tubule is capable of effecting net sodium reabsorption and maintaining a large concentration gradient for sodium. Recent in vitro studies suggest that this phenomenon is mineralocorticoid-dependent.

Medullary collecting duct

The ability of this terminal portion of the nephron to reabsorb sodium is now well established. Studies utilizing micropuncture and microcatheterization techniques have demonstrated that the lowest tubular fluid sodium concentrations are achieved and the steepest transepithelial concentration gradients can be maintained along this segment (40). Recent studies in the hamster by Rau and Fromter describe a significant negative electric potential that is abolished by the substitution of choline for sodium in the tubular lu-

men. The magnitude of this *PD* varies directly with the sodium concentration of the fluid perfusing the segment (176). These findings indicate that active electrogenic sodium transport occurs along the terminal collecting duct.

Micropuncture studies comparing end distal delivery and urinary excretion of sodium suggest that fractional reabsorption in the collecting duct is depressed by ECF volume expansion. Stein and colleagues found no difference in end distal sodium delivery in animals volume-expanded with Ringer's solution or hyperoncotic albumin; yet urinary sodium excretion was significantly greater in the former group (22). Sonnenberg (166) and Malnic et al. (137) also found an inverse relationship between ECF volume and fractional collecting duct sodium reabsorption. It must be stressed, however, that these studies compared late distal delivery in superficial nephrons and urinary excretion of sodium as an index of sodium reabsorption. Such an extrapolation may be invalid if nephron heterogeneity of sodium reabsorption exists. Indeed, as previously mentioned, there does seem to be a much greater inhibition of sodium transport in more inner cortical nephrons during extracellular expansion. Thus, this type of comparison is not a valid marker of net collecting duct transport.

In fact, Diezi et al. (177) and Stein, Osgood, and Kunau (169) have found a marked increase in absolute sodium reabsorption along the papillary collecting duct in ECF volume expansion when this parameter was measured by direct micropuncture studies. Therefore it does not seem that collecting duct sodium transport is impaired during acute expansion of the extracellular volume, but it would seem that the collecting duct must participate in the regulation of sodium balance in the steady state.

REFERENCES

1. Pitts, R. F.: *Physiology of the Kidney and Body Fluids: Volume and Composition of the Body Fluids*, Year Book Medical Publishers, Inc., Chicago, 1968.
2. Verney, E. B.: Croonan Lecture: The antidiuretic

hormone and the factors which determine its release, *Proc. R. Soc. London Biol.,* **135:**25, 1947.

3. Woolf, A. V.: Osmometric analysis of thirst in man and dog, *Am. J. Physiol.,* **161:**75, 1950.

4. Strauss, M. B., E. Lamdin, W. P. Smith, and D. J. Bleifer: Surfeit and deficit of sodium: A kinetic concept of sodium excretion, *Arch. Intern. Med.,* **102:**527, 1958.

5. Peters, J. P.: *Body Water: The Exchange of Fluids in Man,* Charles C Thomas, Publisher, Springfield, Ill., 1935.

6. Ferris, T. F.: Medical complications during pregnancy, in *Renal Disease,* chap. 1, W. B. Saunders Company, Philadelphia, 1975.

7. Papper, S., and J. D. Rosenbaum: Abnormalities in the excretion of water and sodium in "compensated" cirrhosis of the liver, *J. Lab. Clin. Med.,* **60:**967, 1962.

8. Epstein, F. H., R. S. Post, and M. McDowell: The effect of an arterial venous fistula on renal hemodynamics and electroyte excretion, *J. Clin. Invest.,* **32:**233, 1953.

9. Epstein, F. H., A. V. N. Goodyer, F. D. Lawrason, and A. S. Relman: Studies of the antidiuresis of quiet standing: The importance of changes in plasma volume in glomerular filtration rate, *J. Clin. Invest.,* **30:**63, 1951.

10. Wesson, L. G.: *Physiology of the Human Kidney: Sodium Chloride Monovalent Anions,* Grune & Stratton, Inc., New York, 1969.

11. Arborelius, M., U. I. Baldwin, and B. Lilja: Hemodynamic changes in man during emersion with the head above water, *Aerospace Med.,* **43:**592, 1972.

12. Davis, J. O., and D. S. Howell: Mechanisms of fluid and electrolyte retention in experimental preparation in dogs. II. Thoracic inferior vena cava obstruction, *Circ. Res.,* **1:**171, 1953.

13. Gauer, O. H., J. P. Henry, and H. O. Sieker: Cardiac receptors in fluid volume control, *Prog. Cardiovasc. Dis.,* **4:**1, 1961.

14. Gilmore, J. P., and J. M. Daggetti: Response of the chronic cardiac denervated dog to acute volume expansion, *Am. J. Physiol.,* **210:**509, 1966.

15. Share, L.: Vasopressin: Its bioassay and the physiologic control of its release, *Am. J. Med.,* **42:**701, 1967.

16. Borst, J. G. G.: The characteristic renal excretion patterns associated with excessive or inadequate circulation, *Ciba Foundation Symposium on the Kidney,* J. and A. Churchill, Ltd., London, 1954.

17. Latham, W.: The urinary excretion of sodium and potassium during the pyrogenic reaction in man, *J. Clin. Invest.,* **35:**947, 1956.

18. Goodyer, A. V. N., E. R. Peterson, and A. S. Relman: Some effects of albumin infusions on renal function and electrolyte excretion in normal man, *J. Appl. Physiol.,* **1:**671, 1949.

19. Welt, L. G., and J. Orloff: The effects of increase in plasma volume on the metabolism and excretion of water in electrolytes by normal subjects, *J. Clin. Invest.,* **30:**751, 1951.

20. Orloff, J., and W. D. Blake: Effects of concentrated salt-poor albumin on metabolism and excretion of water and electrolyte in dogs, *Am. J. Physiol.,* **164:**167, 1951.

21. Howards, S. S., B. B. Davis, F. G. Knox, F. S. Wright, and R. W. Berliner: Depression of fractional sodium reabsorption by the proximal tubule of the dog without sodium diuresis, *J. Clin. Invest.,* **47:**1561, 1968.

22. Stein, J. H., R. W. Osgood, S. Boonjarern, and T. F. Ferris: A comparison of the segmental analysis of sodium reabsorption during ringer's and hyperoncotic albumin infusion in the rat, *J. Clin. Invest.,* **52:**2313, 1973.

23. Earley, L. E., and T. M. Daugharty: Sodium metabolism, *N. Engl. J. Med.,* **281:**72, 1969.

24. Martino, J. A., and L. E. Earley: Demonstration of the role of physical factors as determinants of natriuretic response to volume expansion, *J. Clin. Invest.,* **46:**1963, 1967.

25. Tobian, L., A. Tomboulian, and J. Janecek: Effect of high perfusion pressure on the granulation of juxtaglomerular cells in an isolated kidney, *J. Clin. Invest.,* **38:**605, 1959.

26. Fitzgibbons, J. P., F. J. Gennari, H. B. Garfinkel, and S. Cortell: Dependents of saline-induced natriuresis upon exposure of the kidney to the physical effects of extracellular fluid volume expansion, *J. Clin. Invest.,* **54:**1428, 1974.

27. Osgood, R. W., N. H. Lameire, M. I. Sorkin, and J. H. Stein: Effect of aortic clamping on proximal reabsorption and sodium excretion in the rat, *Am. J. Physiol.,* **1:**F92, 1977.

28. Burg, M. B., and J. Orloff: Control of fluid absorption in renal proximal tubules, *J. Clin. Invest.,* **47:**2016, 1968.

29. Imai, M., D. W. Seldin, and J. P. Kokko: Effect of perfusion rate on the fluxes of water, sodium, chloride and urea across the proximal convoluted tubule, *Kidney Int.*, **11**:18, 1977.

30. Brenner, B. M., K. H. Falchuk, R. I. Keimowitz, and J. L. Troy: The relationship between peritubular capillary protein concentration and fluid reabsorption by the renal proximal tubule, *J. Clin. Invest.*, **48**:1519, 1969.

31. Falchuk, K. H., B. M. Brenner, and M. Tadokoro: Oncotic and hydrostatic pressure in peritubular capillaries and fluid reabsorption by proximal tubule, *Am J. Physiol.*, **220**:1427, 1971.

32. Brenner, B. M., and J. H. Galla: Influence of postglomerular hematocrit and protein concentration on rat nephron fluid transfer. *Am. J. Physiol.*, **220**:148, 1971.

33. Brenner, B. M., and J. L. Troy: Postglomerular vascular protein concentration: Evidence for causal role in governing fluid reabsorption in glomerular tubular balance by the renal proximal tubule, *J. Clin. Invest.*, **50**:336, 1971.

34. Brenner, B. M., J. L. Troy, and T. M. Daugharty: On the mechanism of inhibition of fluid reabsorption by the renal proximal tubule of the volume expanded rat, *J. Clin. Invest.*, **50**:1596, 1971.

35. Daugharty, T. M., I. F. Ueki, and D. P. Nicholas: Comparative renal effects of isotonic and colloid-free volume expansion in the rat, *Am. J. Physiol.*, **222**:225, 1972.

36. Brenner, B. M., J. L. Troy, and T. M. Daugharty: Quantitative importance of changes in postglomerular colloid osmotic pressure in mediating glomerular tubular balance in the rat, *J. Clin. Invest.*, **52**:190, 1973.

37. Lewy, J. E., and E. E., Windhager: Peritubular control of proximal tubular fluid reabsorption in the rat kidney, *Am. J. Physiol.*, **214**:943, 1968.

38. Spitzer, A., and E. E. Windhager: Effect of peritubular oncotic pressure changes on proximal fluid reabsorption, *Am. J. Physiol.*, **218**:1188, 1970.

39. Davis, J. O.: A critical evaluation of the role of receptors in the control of aldosterone secretion and sodium excretion, *Prog. Cardiovasc. Dis.*, **4**:27, 1961.

40. Hierholzer, K., and M. Wiederholt: Some aspects of distal tubular solute and water transport, *Kidney Int.*, **9**:198, 1976.

41. Hierholzer, K., M. Wiederholt, H. Holzgreve, G. Giebisch, R. M. Klose, and E. E. Windhager: Micropuncture study of renal transtubular concentration gradients of sodium and potassium in adrenalectomized rats, *Pfluegers Arch.*, **285**:193, 1965.

42. Gross, J. B., M. Imai, and J. P. Kokko: A functional comparison of the cortical collecting tubule and the distal convoluted tubule, *J. Clin. Invest.*, **55**:1284, 1975.

43. Gross, J. B., and J. P. Kokko: Effects of aldosterone and potassium sparing diuretics on electrical potenial differences across the distal nephron, *J. Clin. Invest.*, **59**:82, 1977.

44. Uhlich, E., C. Baldamus, and K. Ullrich: Einfluss von Aldostern auf den Natrium Transport in den Sammelrohren der Saugetiernier, *Pfluegers Arch.*, **308**:111, 1969.

45. Uhlich, E., R. Halbach, and K. J. Ullrich: Einfluss von Aldosteron auf den Ausstrom Markierten Natriums auf den Sammelrohren der Ratte *Pfluegers Arch.*, **320**:261, 1970.

46. Schmidt, U., J. Schmid, H. Schmid, and U. C. Dubach: Sodium- and potassium-activated ATPase: A possible target of aldosterone, *J. Clin. Invest.*, **55**:655, 1975.

47. Rosenbaum, J. D., S. Papper, and M. M. Aschley: Variations in renal excretion of sodium independent of change in adrenal cortical hormone dosage in patients with Addison's disease, *J. Clin. Endocrinol. Metab.*, **15**:1459, 1959.

48. August, J. T., D. H. Nelson, and J. W. Thorn: Response of normal subjects to large amounts of aldosterone, *J. Clin. Invest.*, **37**:1549, 1958.

49. Strauss, M. B., and L. E. Earley: An inquiry into the role of sodium retaining steroids in the homeostasis of body fluids in man, *Trans. Assoc. Am. Physicians*, **72**:200, 1959.

50. De Wardener, H. E., I. H. Mills, W. F. Clapham, and C. J. Hayter: Studies on the efferent mechanism of the sodium diuresis which follows the administration of intravenous saline in the dog, *Clin. Sci.*, **21**:249, 1961.

51. Ludwig, C., E. Nieren, and W. Harbereitung: Handworterbuch der Physiologie, Rudolph, Wagner, Braunschweig, Friedr. Vieweg & Sohn, Brunswick, Germany, **2**:628, 1844.

52. Ludwig, C.: *Lehrbuch der Physiologie des Menschen*, C. F. Winker, Heidelberg, 1861.

53. Starling, E. H.: *The Fluids of the Body*, Keener, Chicago, 1908.

54. Schultz, S. G.: Transport across epithelia: Some basic principles: Symposium on membrane transport in the kidney, *Kidney Int.*, **9**:65, 1976.

55. Green, R., E. E. Windhager, and G. Giebisch: On protein oncotic pressure effects on proximal tubular movement in the rat, *Am. J. Physiol.*, **226**:265, 1974.

56. Brenner, B. M., J. L. Troy, and T. M. Daugharty: Dynamics of glomerular ultrafiltration in the rat, *J. Clin. Invest.*, **50**:1776, 1971.

57. Brenner, B. M., W. M. Deen, and C. R. Robertson: *The Physiologic Basis of Glomerular Ultrafiltration: Kidney and Urinary Tract Physiology*, University Park Press, Baltimore, 1973.

58. Deen, W. M., C. R. Robertson, and B. M. Brenner: Model of peritubular capillary control of isotonic fluid reabsorption by the renal proximal tubule, *Biophys. J.*, **13**:340, 1973.

59. Blantz, R. C., and B. G. Tucher: Determinants of peritubular capillary fluid uptake in hydropenia and saline in plasma expansion, *Am. J. Physiol.*, **228**:1927, 1975.

60. Bresler, E. H.: Problem of volume component of body fluid homeostasis, *Am. J. Med. Sci.*, **232**:93, 1956.

61. Boulpaep, E. L.: Electrical phenomena in the nephron: Symposium on membrane transport in the kidney, *Kidney Int.*, **9**:88, 1976.

62. Earley, L. E., and R. M. Friedler: The effects of combined renal vasodilatation and pressor agents on renal hemodynamics in the tubular reabsorption of sodium, *J. Clin. Invest.*, **45**:542, 1965.

63. Martino, J. A., and L. E. Earley: Demonstration of role of physical factors as determinants of natriuretic response to volume expansion, *J. Clin. Invest.*, **46**:1963, 1967.

64. Martino, J. A., and L. E. Earley: Relationship between intrarenal hydrostatic pressure and hemodynamically induced changes in sodium excretion, *Circ. Res.*, **23**:371, 1968.

65. Earley, L. E., J. A. Martino, and R. M. Friedler: Factors affecting sodium reabsorption by proximal tubule as determined during blockade of distal sodium reabsorption, *J. Clin. Invest.*, **45**:1668, 1966.

66. Dirks, J. H., and J. F. Seely: Micropuncture studies on effect of vasodilators on proximal tubular sodium reabsorption in the dog, *Clin. Res.*, **15**:478, 1967.

67. Koch, K. M., H. F. Aynedijian, and N. Bank: Effect of acute hypertension on sodium reabsorption by the proximal tubule, *J. Clin. Invest.*, **47**:1696, 1968.

68. Stumpe, K., H. Lowitz, and B. Ochwadt: Fluid reabsorption in Henle's loop and urinary excretion of sodium and water in normal rats and rats with chronic hypertension, *J. Clin. Invest.*, **49**:1200, 1970.

69. Bank, N., H. Aynedjian, V. Bansal, and D. Goldman: Affect of acute hypertension on sodium transport by the distal nephron, *Am. J. Physiol.*, **219**:275, 1970.

70. Kunau, R. T. and N. H. Lameire: The effect of an acute increase in renal perfusion pressure on sodium transport in the rat kidney, *Cir. Res.*, **39**:689, 1976.

71. Earley, L. E., and R. M. Friedler: Observations on the mechanism of decreased tubular reabsorption of sodium and water during saline loading, *J. Clin. Invest.*, **43**:1928, 1964.

72. Goodyer, A. V. N., and C. A. Jaeger: Renal response to non-shocking hemorrhage: Role of the autonomic nervous system and of the renal circulation, *Am. J. Physiol.*, **180**:69, 1955.

73. Barger, A. C.: Renal hemodynamic factors in congestive heart failure, *Ann. N.Y. Acad. Sci.*, **139**:276, 1966.

74. Thornburn, G. D., H. H. Kopald, J. A. Herd, M. Hollenberg, C. C. C. O'Morchoe, and A. C. Barger: Intrarenal distribution of nutrient blood flow determined with krypton-85 in the unanesthetized dog, *Circ. Res.*, **13**:290, 1963.

75. Lameire, N. H., M. D. Lifschitz, and J. H. Stein: Heterogeneity of nephron function, *Ann. Rev. Physiol.*, **39**:159, 1977.

76. Kawamura, S., M. Imai, D. W. Seldin, and J. P. Kokko: Characteristics of salt and water transport in superficial and juxtamedullary straight segments of proximal tubules, *J. Clin. Invest.*, **55**:1269, 1975.

77. Jacobson, H. R. and J. P. Kokko: Intrinsic differences in various segments of the proximal convoluted tubule, *J. Clin. Invest.*, **57**:818, 1976.

78. Osgood, R. W., H. J. Reineck, and J. H. Stein: Ef-

fect of volume expansion on sodium transport in the proximal tubule of juxtamedullary nephrons, *Clin. Res.*, **25**:444A, 1977.

79. Clarkson, E. M., L. B. Talner, and H. E. de Wardener: The effects of plasma from blood volume expanded dogs on sodium potassium and PAH transport of renal tubule fragments, *Clin. Sci.*, **38**:1617, 1970.

80. Clarkson, E. M. and H. E. de Wardener: Inhibition of sodium in potassium transport in separated renal tubule fragments incubated in extracts of urine obtained from salt-loaded individuals, *Clin. Sci.*, **42**:607, 1972.

81. Nutbourne, D. M., J. D. Howse, R. W. Schrier, L. B. Talner, M. G. Ventom, P. J. Verroust, and H. E. de Wardener: The effect of expanding the blood volume of a dog on the short circuit current across an isolated frog skin incorporated in the dog's circulation, *Clin. Sci.*, **38**:629, 1970.

82. Brown, P. R., K. G. Koutsaimanis, and H. E. de Wardener: Effect of urinary extracts from salt-loaded man on urinary sodium excretion by the rat, *Kidney Int.*, **2**:1, 1972.

83. Buckalew, V. M., F. J. Martinez, and W. E. Green: The effect of dialysates and ultrafiltrates of plasma of saline loaded dogs on toad bladder sodium transport, *J. Clin. Invest.*, **49**:926, 1970.

84. Buckalew, V. M.: Variable factors affecting ultrafiltration of a humoral sodium transport inhibitor, *Nephron*, **9**:66, 1972.

85. Buckalew, V. M., and D. B. Nelson: Natriuretic and sodium transport inhibitory activity in plasma of volume expanded dogs, *Kidney Int.*, **5**:12, 1974.

86. Buckalew, V. M., and K. A. Diamond: Effect of vasopressin on sodium excretion and plasma antinatriferic activity in the dog, *Am. J. Physiol.*, **231**:28, 1976.

87. Sealey, J. E., J. D. Kirshman, and J. H. Laragh: Natriuretic activity in plasma and urine of salt loaded man and sheep, *J. Clin. Invest.*, **48**:2210, 1969.

88. Blythe, W. B., D. D'avila, H. J. Gitelman, and L. G. Welt: Further evidence for humoral natriuretic factor, *Cir. Res.*, **8**(suppl. 2):21, 1971.

89. Cort, J. H., and B. Lichardus: Natriuretic hormone, *Nephron*, **5**:401, 1968.

90. Kramer, H. G., H. C. Gonick, and F. Kruck: Natriuretisches Hormon, *Klin. Wochenschr.*, **50**:893, 1972.

91. Kramer, H. G., B. Gospodinov, and F. Kruck: Humorale Hemmung des Epithelialen Natrium Transports nach Akutr Expansion des Extracellular Volumens, *Klin. Wochenschr.*, **52**:801, 1974.

92. Gonick, H. C., and L. F. Saldanha: A natriuretic principle derived from kidney tissue of volume expanded rats, *J. Clin. Invest.*, **56**:247, 1975.

93. Viskoper, J. R., J. W. Czaczkes, N. Schwartz, and T. D. Ullmann: Natriuretic activity of a substance isolated from human urine during excretion of the salt load, *Nephron*, **8**:540, 1971.

94. Viskoper, J. R., H. Wald, N. Schwartz, and J. W. Czaczkes: Natriuretic material obtained from urine, *Nephron*, **9**:220, 1972.

95. Kaloyanides, G. J., and M. Azer: Evidence for a humoral mechanism in volume expansion natriuresis, *J. Clin. Invest.*, **50**:1603, 1971.

96. Sonnenberg, H., A. T. Veress, and J. W. Pearce: A humoral component of the natriuretic mechanism in sustained blood volume expansion, *J. Clin. Invest.*, **51**:2631, 1972.

97. Johnston, C. I., and J. O. Davis: Evidence from cross circulation studies for a humoral mechanism in the natriuresis of saline loading, *Proc. Soc. Exp. Biol. Med.*, **121**:1058, 1966.

98. Slatopolsky, E., I. O. Elkan, C. Weerts, and N. S. Bricker: Studies on the characteristics of the control system governing sodium excretion in uremic man, *J. Clin. Invest.*, **47**:521, 1968.

99. Schultze, R. G., H. F. Shapiro, and N. S. Bricker: Sudies on the control of sodium excretion in experimental uremia, *J. Clin. Invest.*, **48**:869, 1969.

100. Bourgoignie, J. J., K. H. Hwang, C. S. Espinel, S. Klahr, and N. S. Bricker: A natriuretic factor in the serum of patients with chronic uremia, *J. Clin. Invest.*, **51**:1514, 1972.

101. Bourgoignie, J. J., K. H. Hwang, E. Ipakchi, and N. S. Bricker: The presence of a natriuretic factor in urine of patients with chronic uremia: The absence of the factor in nephrotic uremic patients, *J. Clin. Invest.*, **53**:1559, 1974.

102. Schmidt, R. W., J. J. Bourgoignie, and N. S. Bricker: On the adaptation in sodium excretion in chronic uremia: The effects of "proportional reduction" of sodium intake, *J. Clin. Invest.*, **53**:1736, 1974.

103. Webber, H., K. Y. Lin, and N. S. Bricker: Effect of sodium intake on single nephron glomerular

filtration rate and sodium reabsorption in experimental uremia, *Kidney, Int.*, 8:14, 1975.

104. Fine, L. G., J. J. Bourgoignie, K. H. Hwang, and N. S. Bricker: On the influence of the natriuretic factor from the urine of patients with chronic uremia on bioelectric properties and sodium transport of the isolated mammalian collecting duct, *J. Clin. Invest.*, 58:590, 1976.

105. Fine, L. G., J. J. Bourgoignie, H. Webber, and N. S. Bricker: Enhanced end organ responsiveness of the uremic kidney to the natriuretic factor, *Kidney, Int.*, 10:364, 1976.

106. Favre, H., K. H. Hwang, R. W. Schmidt, N. S. Bricker, and J. J. Bourgoignie: An inhibitor of sodium transport in the urine of dogs with normal renal function, *J. Clin. Invest.*, 56:1302, 1975.

107. Levinsky, N. G.: Non-aldosterone influences on renal sodium transport, *Ann. N.Y. Acad. Sci.*, 139:295, 1966.

108. Bricker, N. S., R. A. Straffon, E. P. Mahoney, and J. P. Merrill: The functional capacity of the kidney denervated by autotransplantation in the dog, *J. Clin. Invest.*, 37:185, 1958.

109. Blake, W. D. and A. N. Jurf: Renal sodium reabsorption after acute renal denervation in the rabbit, *J. Physiol. (London)*, 196:65, 1968.

110. Bonjour, J. P., P. C. Churchill, and R. L. Malvin: Change in tubular reabsorption of sodium and water after renal denervation in the dog, *J. Physiol. (London)*, 204:571, 1969.

111. Blendis, L. M., R. B. Auld, E. A. Alexander, and N. G. Levinsky: Effect of renal beta and alpha adrenergic stimulation on proximal sodium reabsorption in dogs, *Clin. Sci.*, 43:569, 1972.

112. Gill, J. R. and A. G. T. Kasper: Effect of renal alpha adrenergic stimulation on renal proximal tubular sodium reabsorption, *Am. J. Physiol.*, 223:1201, 1972.

113. Sartorius, O. W., and H. Burlington: Acute effects of denervation on kidney function in the dog, *Am. J. Physiol.*, 185:407, 1956.

114. Blake, W. D.: Relative roles of glomerular filtration and tubular reabsorption in denervation diuresis, *Am. J. Physiol.*, 202:777, 1962.

115. Bello-Reusse, E., R. E. Colindres, E. Pastoriza-Munoz, R. A. Mueller, and C. W. Gottschalk: Effects of acute unilateral renal denervation in the rat, *J. Clin. Invest.*, 56:208, 1975.

116. Bello-Reusse, E., D. L. Trivino, and C. W. Gottschalk: Effect of sympathetic renal nerve stimulation on proximal water and sodium reabsorption, *J. Clin. Invest.*, 57:1104, 1976.

117. Nomura, G., T. Takabatake, S. Aria, D. Uno, M. Shimao, and N. Hattori: Effect of acute unilateral renal denervation on tubular sodium reabsorption in the dog, *Am. J. Physiol.*, 232:F16, 1977.

118. Bello-Reusse, E., E. Pastoriza-Munoz, and R. E. Colindres: Acute unilateral renal denervation in rats with extracellular volume expansion, *Am. J. Physiol.*, 232:F26, 1977.

119. Muller, J., and L. Barajas: Electron microscopic and histochemical evidence for a tubular innervation in the renal cortex of the monkey, *J. Ultrastruct. Res.*, 41:533, 1972.

120. Barajas, L., and J. Muller: The innervation of the juxtamedullary apparatus and surrounding tubules. A quantitative analysis by serial section electron microscopy, *J. Ultrastruct. Res.*, 43:107, 1973.

121. Handler, J. S., R. Bensinger, and J. Orloff: Effect of adrenergic agents on toad bladder response to ADH, 3' 5' AMP, and theophylline, *Am. J. Physiol.*, 215:1024, 1968.

122. Field, M., and I. McColl: Ion transport in rabbit ileomucosa. III. Effects of catecholamines, *Am. J. Physiol.*, 225:852, 1973.

123. Grabfield, G. P., and D. Swanson: Studies on denervated kidney: Effects of unilateral denervation in acute experiments on sodium chloride excretion, *Arch. Int. Pharmacodyn. Ther.*, 61:92, f1939.

124. Berne, R. M.: Hemodynamics and sodium excretion of denervated kidney in anesthetized and unanesthetized dog, *Am. J. Physiol.*, 171:148, 1952.

125. Lifschitz, M. D.: Lack of a role for renal nerves in renal sodium reabsorption in conscious dogs, *Clin. Sci. Mol. Med.*, 54:567, 1978.

126. Leaf, A., and A. R. Mamby: An antidiuretic mechanism not regulated by extracellular fluid tonicity, *J. Clin. Invest.*, 31:60, 1952.

127. Kurtzman, N. A., P. W. Rogers, S. Boonjarern, and J. A. L. Arruda: Effect of infusion of pharmacologic amounts of vasopressin on renal electrolyte excretion, *Am. J. Physiol*, 228:890, 1975.

128. Chan W. Y., and W. H. Sawyer: Saluretic actions of neurohypophysial peptides in conscious dogs, *Am. J. Physiol.*, 201:799, 1961.

129. Humpreys, M. H., R. M. Friedler, and L. E. Earley: Natriuresis produced by vasopressin or hemorrhage during water diuresis in the dog, *Am. J. Physiol.*, **219**:658, 1970.

130. Ussing, H., and K. Zerahn: Active transport of sodium as the source of electric current in the short circuited isolated frog skin, *Acta Physiol. Scand.*, **23**:110, 1951.

131. Koefoed-Johnson, V., and H. Ussing: The contributions of diffusion and flow to the passage of D_2O through living membranes, *Acta Physiol. Scand.*, **28**:16, 1953.

132. Leaf, A.: Membrane effects of antidiuretic hormone, *Am. J. Physiol.*, **42**:745, 1967.

133. Burg, M., L. Isaccson, J. Grantham, and J. Orloff: Electrical properties of isolated perfused rabbit renal tubules, *Am. J. Physiol.*, **215**:788, 1968.

134. Frindt, G., and M. Burg: Effect of vasopressin on sodium transport and cortical collecting tubules, *Kidney Int.*, **1**:224, 1972.

135. Ullrich, K. J., C. Baldamus, E. Uhlich, and G. Rumrich: Einfluss von Calciumionen und Antidiuretischem Hormon auf den Transtubularen Natrium Transport en der Rattennier, *Pfluegers Arch.*, **310**:369, 1969.

136. Tadokoro, M., I. Hauraguchi, M. Teruoka, and F. Sakai: Microperfusion experiments in collecting duct of the isolated rat renal medulla in-vitro, *Jpn. J. Pharmacol.*, **18**:272, 1968.

137. Malnic, G., R. Klose, and G. Giebisch: Micropuncture study of distal tubular potassium in sodium transport in the rat nephron, *Am. J. Physiol.*, **211**:529, 1966.

138. Gyory, A. Z., V. Brendel, and R. Kinne: Effect of cardiac glycosides and sodium ethacrynate on transepithelial sodium transport in in-vivo micropuncture experiments and on isolated plasma membranes sodium-potassium-ATPase in-vitro of the rat, *Pfluegers. Arch.*, **335**:287, 1972.

139. Burg, M. B., and J. J. Grantham: Ion movement in renal tubules, *Membranes in ion transport*, John Wiley & Sons, Inc., Interscience Publishers, New York, **3**:49, 1970.

140. Windhager, E. E., and G. Giebisch: Micropuncture study of renal tubular transfer of sodium chloride in the rat, *Am. J. Physiol.*, **200**:581, 1961.

141. Kashgarian, M. H., H. Soteckle, C. W. Gottschalk, and K. J. Ullrich: Transtubular electrochemical potentials of sodium and chloride in proximal and distal renal tubules of rats during antidiuresis and water diuresis, *Pfluegers Arch.*, **277**:89, 1963.

142. Kokko, J. P., M. B. Burg, and J. Orloff: Characteristics of sodium chloride and water transport in the renal proximal tubule, *J. Clin. Invest.*, **50**:69, 1971.

143. Kokko, J. P.: Proximal tubule potential difference. Dependence on glucose, HCO_3 and amino acids, *J. Clin. Invest.*, **52**:1362, 1973.

144. Barratt, L., F. Rector, J. Kokko, and D. W. Seldin: Factors governing the transepithelial potential differences across the proximal tubule of the rat kidney, *J. Clin. Invest.*, **53**:454, 1974.

145. Fromter, E., and K. Gebner: Free flow potential profile along rat kidney proximal tubule, *Pfluegers Arch.*, **351**:69, 1974.

146. Burg, M., C. Patlak, N. Green, and D. Villey: Organic solutes in fluid absorption by renal proximal convoluted tubules, *Am. J. Physiol.*, **231**:627, 1976.

147. Rector, F. C., M. Martinez-Maldonado, F. P. Brunner, and D. W. Seldin: Evidence for passive reabsorption of sodium chloride in proximal tubule of rat kidney, *J. Clin. Invest.*, **45**:1060, 1966.

148. Fromter, E., G. Rumrich, and K. Ullrich: Phenomenologic description of Na, Cl, and HCO_3 absorption from proximal tubules of the rat kidney, *Pfluegers Arch.*, **340**:3, 1973.

149. Weinstein, S. W., and J. Szyjewicz: Early postglomerular plasma concentrations of chloride, sodium and inulin in the rat kidney, *Am. J. Physiol.*, **231**:822, 1976.

150. Schaffer, J. A., C. S. Patlak, and T. E. Andreoli: A component of fluid absorption linked to passive ion flow in the superficial pars recta, *J. Gen. Physiol.*, **66**:445, 1975.

151. Grantham, J., R. Irwin, P. Qualizza, D. Tucker, and F. Whittier: Fluid secretion in isolated proximal straight renal tubules. Effect of human uremic serum, *J Clin. Invest.*, **52**:2441, 1973.

152. Grantham, J., P. Qualizza, and R. Irwin: Net fluid secretion in proximal straight tubules in-vitro: Role of PAH, *Am. J. Physiol.*, **226**:191, 1974.

153. Dirks, J. H., W. J. Cirksena, and R. W. Berliner: The effect of saline infusion on sodium reabsorp-

tion by the proximal tubule of the dog, *J. Clin. Invest.*, **44**:1160, 1965.

154. Weiner, M., E. Weinman, M. Kashgarian, and J. Hayslett: Accelerated reabsorption in the proximal tubule produced by volume depletion, *J. Clin. Invest.*, **50**:1379, 1971.

155. Bank, N., and H. Anyedjian: Micropuncture of renal salt and water retention in bile duct obstruction, *J. Clin. Invest.*, **55**:994, 1975.

156. Cirksena, W. J., J. A. Dirks, and R. W. Berliner: Effect of thoracic cava obstruction on response of proximal tubule sodium reabsorption to saline infusion, *J. Clin. Invest.*, **45**:179, 1966.

157. Kokko, J. P.: Sodium chloride and water transport in the descending limb of Henle, *J. Clin. Invest.*, **49**:1838, 1970.

158. Imai, M., and J. Kokko: Sodium, urea and water transport in the thin ascending limb of Henle. Generation of osmotic gradients by passive diffusion of solutes, *J. Clin. Invest.*, **53**:393, 1974.

159. Johnston, P. A., C. A. Battilana, F. B. Lacy, and R. L. Jamison: Evidence for a concentration gradient favoring outward movement of sodium from the thin loop of Henle, *J. Clin. Invest.*, **59**:234, 1977.

160. Burg, M. D., and N. Green: Function of the thick ascending limb of Henle's loop, *Am. J. Physiol.*, **224**:659, 1973.

161. Burg, M., L. Stoner, J. Cardinal, and N. Green: Furosemide effect on isolated perfused tubules, *Am. J. Physiol.*, **225**:119, 1973.

162. Burg, M., and N. Green: Effect of ethacrynic acid on the thick ascending limb of Henle's loop, *Kidney Int.*, **4**:301, 1973.

163. Rocha, A. S., and J. P. Kokko: Sodium chloride and water transport in the medullary thick ascending limb of Henle: Evidence for active chloride transport, *J. Clin. Invest.*, **52**:612, 1973.

164. Dirks, J., and J. Seely: Effect of saline infusion and furosemide on the dog distal nephron, *Am. J. Physiol.*, **219**:114, 1970.

165. Landwehr, D., R. Klose, and G. Giebisch: Renal tubular sodium and water reabsorption in the isotonic sodium chloride loaded rat, *Am. J. Physiol.*, **212**:1327, 1967.

166. Sonnenberg, H.: Proximal and distal tubular function in salt-deprived and salt-loaded deoxycorticosterone acetate escaped rats, *J. Clin. Invest.*, **52**:263, 1973.

167. Kunau, R. T., H. L. Webb, and S. C. Borman: Characteristics of sodium reabsorption in the loop of Henle and distal tubule, *Am. J. Physiol.*, **227**:1181, 1974.

168. Morgan, T., and R. W. Berliner: A study by continuous microperfusion of water and electrolyte movements in the loop of Henle and distal tubule of the rat, *Nephron*, **6**:388, 1969.

169. Stein, J. H., R. W. Osgood, and R. T. Kunau: Direct measurement of papillary collecting duct sodium transport in the rat: Evidence for heterogeneity of nephron function during Ringer's loading, *J. Clin. Invest.*, **58**:767, 1976.

170. Wright, F.: Increasing magnitude of electrical potential along the renal distal tubule, *Am. J. Physiol.*, **220**:624, 1971.

171. Boulpaep, E., and J. Seely: Electrophysiology of proximal and distal tubules in the autoperfused dog kidney, *Am. J. Physiol.*, **221**:1084, 1971.

172. Grantham, J. J., M. Burg, and J. Orloff: The nature of transtubular Na and K transport in isolated rabbit renal collecting tubules, *J. Clin. Invest.*, **49**:1815, 1970.

173. Helman, S. I., J. Grantham, and M. Burg: Effect of vasopressin on electrical resistance of renal cortical collecting tubules, *Am. J. Physiol.*, **220**:1825, 1971.

174. Stoner, L. C., M. Burg, and J. Orloff: Ion transport in cortical collecting tubules: Effect of amiloride, *Am. J. Physiol.*, **227**:453, 1974.

175. Tischer, C. C., and W. E. Yarger: Lanthanum permeability of tight junctions along the collecting duct of the rat, *Kidney Int.*, **7**:35, 1975.

176. Rau, W., and E. Fromter: Electrical properties of the medullary collecting duct of the golden hamster kidney. I. The transepithelial potential difference, *Pfluegers Arch.*, **351**:113, 1974.

177. Diezi, J., P. Michoud, J. Aceves, and G. Giebisch: Micropuncture study of electrolyte transport across papillary collecting duct of the rat, *Am. J. Physiol.*, **224**:623, 1973.

4

Potassium: physiology and pathophysiology

RAYMOND G. SCHULTZE / ALLEN R. NISSENSON

INTRODUCTION

Potassium is the major intracellular cation of most animal and plant tissues and therefore plays a primary role in the maintenance of the intracellular fluid (ICF) volume. Omnivores and carnivores ingest moderate amounts of this ion, but herbivores ingest very large quantities. Only diets rich in carbohydrates in the form of processed sugars contain little potassium. As a result of the large dietary intake of potassium, mammals have evolved a highly efficient mechanism of potassium excretion. Potassium conservation, when required by a low potassium intake, is less efficient.

Spontaneous diseases of potassium metabolism are rare. The hyperkalemic and hypokalemic forms of periodic paralysis and an inherited form of chronic hypokalemia are the primary examples of these disorders. Serious problems with potassium balance may arise as part of other disease processes, however. For example, hyperkalemia occurs when the ability of the kidney to excrete this ion is lost while intake continues. Hypokalemia results when renal excretion is uncontrolled due to the presence in the plasma of ex-

cessive mineralocorticoids or because of loss of the body fluids containing large amounts of this ion, e.g., diarrheal fluid.

Perhaps the most clinically important abnormalities of potassium metabolism are those which are iatrogenic. For instance, the ingestion of some drugs may result in inappropriate potassium retention, whereas the administration of others may cause the loss of potassium in excess of intake.

In this chapter, the anatomy of body potassium, the mechanisms controlling potassium excretion, and the disorders of potassium balance will be reviewed.

ANATOMY OF BODY POTASSIUM

Chemical measurements of the potassium content of adult human cadavers have revealed a mean value of approximately 55 meq/kg body weight (1). More recently, estimates of total body potassium have been made by measuring the gamma emissions of ^{40}K (2). Naturally distributed potassium is primarily ^{39}K, but a constant proportion is ^{40}K, a gamma emitter. By utilizing a whole body counter and correcting for errors introduced by the geometry of the body, it is possible to measure the total body content of ^{40}K and then calculate the total body potassium (3). The average value of 53 meq/kg body weight obtained by this method is in excellent agreement with the value obtained by the chemical analysis of cadavers (4, 5).

A third method measures body potassium by a dilution technique (6). A known amount of the radioactive isotope ^{42}K is infused intravenously, and measurements of the specific activity of the isotope in a sample of plasma are done repetitively over a 48-h period. An estimate of total body potassium, usually referred to as "exchangeable potassium," can then be calculated from the "dilution" of the known original dose in the sample. The major problem of this method is that it takes more than 48 h for the injected isotope to be distributed equally in the total body potassium. Potassium excretion during this time complicates the calculation. In general, the calculated values for exchangeable potassium are about 15 percent less than measurements of total body potassium utilizing ^{40}K (4, 6).

Of the 3700 meq of potassium found in the body, more than 95 percent is located in intracellular water. Since skeletal muscle holds most of the intracellular water, it also contains the majority of the body's potassium. Fat contains little water and little potassium. As the body ages, total body potassium as a function of body weight decreases because the muscle mass declines and fat increases (7). In middle age, total body potassium for each kilogram of body weight is about 10 percent less than that of a young adult, and in the elderly, 20 percent less (5). Women have a higher percentage of fat per unit of body weight; their values for potassium per kilogram of body weight are about 75 percent of those of men.

The average concentration of potassium in human ICF is thought to be about 150 meq/kg H_2O. It should be emphasized that this is an *average* value and that tissues may vary in their potassium content. Furthermore, potassium may be compartmentalized within cells, as has been demonstrated in the heart muscle (8). In any event, cells behave osmotically as though nearly all of the intracellular potassium were osmotically active.

The reason for the high intracellular potassium

concentrations cannot be easily deduced. Indeed, there are mammalian cells such as sheep erythrocytes in which the predominant intracellular cation is sodium, not potassium. It is of interest that many enzymes are stimulated by potassium and inhibited or unaffected by sodium (9). Perhaps, as has been suggested by some biologists, life began in the ocean when the predominant cation was potassium rather than sodium.

POTASSIUM PHYSIOLOGY

POTASSIUM INTAKE

As noted in the introduction, potassium is found in foods of both animal and vegetable origin. Without resorting to synthetic foods, it is almost impossible to devise a diet that contains no potassium. The dietary intake of potassium averages 1 to 1.5 meq/kg body weight per day in humans. Some herbivores ingest 10 times this amount.

POTASSIUM OUTPUT

Under normal conditions, ingested potassium may be lost from the body by one of three routes. In temperate climates, a small amount of potassium, less than 5 meq/day, is lost in sweat. Larger amounts may be lost by this route in the tropics, where 4 to 6 L of sweat containing a total of 25 to 50 meq of potassium may be formed each day (10).

Ordinarily less than 10 percent of ingested potassium (7 to 15 meq) is found in the stool. The amount to be found depends on both the water and the bacterial content. "Dry" stools may contain 130 meq/L of water, but since the water content is low, losses are small. Liquid stools may contain up to 20 meq potassium per liter of water (11).

More than 90 percent of ingested potassium is excreted in the urine. If potassium intake is gradually increased, the excretion rate in the urine follows pari passu without a detectable increase in total body potassium. The excretory process is so efficient that under appropriate conditions, potassium excretion may exceed the amount filtered through the glomerulus. Potassium conservation, however, is less efficient. The minimum potassium excretion rate is related to the total body potassium deficit. As a rough approximation, when the total body deficit is 50 to 150 meq, potassium excretion is usually reduced to 15 to 25 meq/day. When the deficit reaches 150 to 350 meq, urinary potassium excretion may be reduced to 5 to 15 meq/day. When the deficit is in excess of 350 meq, the kidneys are capable of removing nearly all potassium from the urine, and excretion may be reduced to 1 to 5 meq/day (14). Unfortunately, deficits in total body potassium of this degree may be associated with significant morbidity.

THE EXCRETION OF POTASSIUM BY THE KIDNEY

Potassium excretion by the kidney has been studied closely for more than four decades, and although the mechanisms involved are not completely understood, the major features are clear. Early studies utilizing clearance methodology established that both the experimental animal (12, 15) and the human (14, 16) were capable of secreting potassium, since under some conditions the amount found in the urine exceeds the amount filtered. A careful analysis of the data revealed that potassium excreted remained relatively constant despite wide variation in glomerular filtration rate (GFR) (17). On the basis of this observation, Berliner and Kennedy (18) suggested that it was likely that most of the filtered potassium was absorbed in the first portion of the nephron and that secretion at a distal site accounted for the potassium found in the urine. Malvin, Wilde, and Sullivan (19) added support for this concept when they examined nephron transport of potassium with a technique that stops the flow of urine within the tubule for a time so that the action of the tubular epithelium on the filtrate becomes exaggerated. These investigators found that samples of urine that had been exposed for a time to the epithelium of the distal convoluted tubule and collecting duct contained much more potassium than samples which had been exposed to the epithelium of the thick ascending limb. Thus, the potassium in the urine appeared to be secreted by

the distal nephron or collecting duct and was not derived from filtered potassium.

For the past decade, potassium transport by parts of single nephrons has been studied by micropuncture techniques in vivo and microperfusion techniques in vitro. Although most micropuncture studies have been performed on rats, there are data available from dogs and monkeys (20, 21). To a large degree, the micropuncture studies support the broad conclusions about the sites of potassium transport derived from clearance studies.

The concentration of potassium in glomerular filtrate has been determined directly by measuring the potassium in fluid obtained from Bowman's space (22). This feat is possible in the Wistar strain of rats developed in Munich. The concentration of potassium in this fluid is very close to that of plasma, and, therefore, it appears that potassium is freely filtered through the glomerular capillary wall.

The fate of filtered potassium along the nephron can be determined in the experimental animal infused with inulin by collecting tubular fluid and measuring the potassium and inulin concentrations of the collected fluid and of simultaneously collected plasma. The ratio of tubular fluid to plasma potassium concentrations divided by the ratio of the tubular fluid to plasma inulin concentrations $(TF/P_K)(TF/P_{in})^{-1}$ gives the fraction of filtered potassium remaining in the fluid at the site of puncture. The ratio falls as potassium is absorbed and increases when potassium is added.

The initial 60 percent of the proximal tubule is accessible to micropuncture. Fluid collected from this segment of the nephron has been reported to have potassium concentrations from 0.8 to 1.2 times the simultaneous concentration in plasma (23). This wide variation in values may be due to methodological problems. Most of the recently reported values are grouped between 0.9 and 1.0 times that of plasma. It seems reasonable to assume, then, that the fractional reabsorption of potassium proceeds at a rate comparable to that of sodium and water (24, 25, 26). These values also suggest that proximal reabsorption of potassium may be passive, especially if the middle portion of the proximal convoluted tubule is electrically positive compared to the extracellular fluid (ECF) space. On the other hand, Beck et al. (27) have suggested that potassium transport in the proximal tubule is active. They administered acetazolamide to dogs after obtaining control measurements of potassium and water absorption in the proximal tubule of dog nephrons. As expected, the drug inhibited sodium, bicarbonate, and water absorption but did not interfere with potassium absorption. Thus, TF/P_K ratios in proximal tubular filtrate fell from a control value of 1.00 to 0.85 after acetazolamide, and fractional potassium reabsorption was unchanged. Additional studies will be required to establish firmly the presence of an active potassium transport mechanism inferred from this experiment.

The pars recta of the proximal tubule is capable of secreting potassium. The process is related to the secretion of organic anions, as has been demonstrated in vitro by Grantham et al. (28). Recently, Jamison et al. (29) have confirmed in vivo that potassium is added to tubular filtrate by the pars recta *or* descending limb of Henle's loop of juxtamedullary nephrons. These investigators have found that the amount of potassium in the tubular filtrate collected at the tip of Henle's loop of juxtamedullary nephrons exceeds the amount filtered by at least 10 to 15 percent. Thus, an amount equal to 60 to 80 percent of the original filtered load is added between the last accessible portion of the proximal tubule and the inner medulla. It seems likely that both the pars recta and the thin limb of Henle's loop contribute to the added potassium in the tubular filtrate. While the pars recta contributes via the active secretion of organic anion, the contribution along the thin limb is probably passive. As this segment of the nephron descends into the medulla, the potassium concentration in the medullary interstitium increases progressively (29). The fluid leaving the straight portion of the proximal tubule has a relatively low potassium concentration. Thus, potassium may enter the filtrate from the interstitial fluid down a concentration gradient.

In the thick portion of the ascending limb of Henle's loop, where chloride is the actively transported ion species, potassium is passively absorbed along with sodium. Absorption is avid.

Less than 10 percent of the filtered potassium reaches the earliest segment of surface distal tubules (24, 30, 31). Thus, the ascending limb may reabsorb an amount of potassium equal to the original filtered load because it reabsorbs almost all of the potassium added in the proximal portion of the loop. Absorption of potassium by this nephron segment is independent of the amount which must be excreted (32).

Even when potassium is infused intravenously during a micropuncture study, reabsorption of potassium by the nephron from the glomerulus to the first segment of the distal tubule is about 90 percent complete. In fact, the same amount of potassium reaches this point along the nephron no matter what the dietary intake: high, low, or in-between (24, 25).

As predicted by Berliner and Kennedy (12) and confirmed by Malvin, Wilde, and Sullivan (19), micropuncture studies have demonstrated that the distal convoluted tubule plays the major role in potassium excretion. When the diet is deficient in potassium, reabsorption of this ion continues in both the distal convoluted tubule and the collecting duct. When dietary intake of potassium is sufficient, secretion of this ion into the tubular fluid occurs primarily in the last half of the distal convoluted tubule, and/or the cortical collecting tubule. Grantham, Burg, and Orloff (33) have found that perfused isolated rabbit cortical collecting tubules are quite capable of secreting potassium when the sodium content of the urine is relatively high. The secretion of potassium appears to be directly coupled to sodium reabsorption in this segment.

The medullary collecting tubule has been found to reabsorb potassium under many conditions, including that of a high potassium intake. In states of sodium depletion, however, this segment secretes potassium when potassium intake is large (30, 34). Secretion of potassium has also been observed during potassium infusions (35) and in chronic metabolic alkalosis (36).

In summary, under all dietary conditions studied thus far, potassium is freely filtered and reabsorbed with sodium and water in the proximal convoluted tubule. No variation in reabsorption occurs in this segment when dietary intake is varied. Potassium is added to the filtrate in both the pars recta of the proximal tubule and the descending limb of Henle's loop. The amount secreted along the latter segment may vary with the potassium dietary load (29). However, under all dietary conditions, potassium is avidly reabsorbed in the thick ascending limb so that only 5 to 10 percent of the original amount filtered remains at the beginning of the distal convoluted tubule. In states of total body potassium deficiency, reabsorption continues in the distal convoluted tubule and collecting duct. In physiologic circumstances requiring potassium excretion, potassium is secreted by the distal convoluted tubule with the bulk of the ion being added in the last half of this segment. The collecting tubule reabsorbs a part of the secreted potassium except when secretion rates are very high when, under several conditions, potassium may be secreted by the collecting tubule.

TUBULAR MECHANISMS OF POTASSIUM EXCRETION

The mechanism of distal tubular potassium secretion has been under intensive study for some time. It has been found that the electrical potential difference (*PD*) between the filtrate and peritubular fluid is small in the early distal tubule, approximately 10 mV, but large in the late distal tubule, approximately 50 mV (37). The *PD* is oriented lumen-negative. For a time, data from micropuncture studies, in which potassium secretion was measured at the same time as the *PD* across the tubule, seemed to show that secretion and the degree of electronegativity of the lumen were correlated. Subsequently, the degree of electronegativity and the rate of potassium secretion have been dissociated (38).

Giebisch and his coworkers (24, 25) have measured the TF/P_K ratios and simultaneously the *PD* between tubular fluid and interstitial fluid. Under most conditions studied thus far, potassium concentration in the luminal fluid of the distal tubule has been less than predicted from the known electrochemical gradients. This observation has lead to the suggestion that while the predominant movement of potassium in the distal tubule is

down a favorable electrochemical gradient from cell to lumen, there is an active pump at the luminal border which returns potassium to the cell. Thus, the net amount of potassium secreted is the result of these two processes: outward diffusion and back reabsorption. When reabsorption exceeds passive secretion, as in states of potassium depletion, potassium is conserved. When the reverse is true, potassium is secreted.

The rate of entry into the filtrate from the distal tubular cell water appears to be a function of the chemical activity of potassium in the cell. The accumulation of potassium in the distal tubule cell is the result of a sodium-potassium coupled pump located in the cell membrane separating cellular and peritubular fluid. In potassium-depleted states, the rate of entry of potassium into the cell across the peritubular membrane is slow, and cellular potassium is low. Secretion is reduced. In states of potassium loading and metabolic alkalosis, which are associated with a high rate of potassium excretion, entry of potassium into distal tubular cells is enhanced, cell potassium content is high, and the rate of secretion into the tubular fluid is high (32). Thus, physiologic control of potassium excretion could be achieved by controlling intracellular potassium. The rate of entry into filtrate is also a function of the rate of flow past the secreting site (39, 40, 41). Thus, physiologic control of potassium excretion could also be achieved by controlling distal tubular flow rate.

PHYSIOLOGIC CONTROL OF POTASSIUM EXCRETION
(See also Chaps. 7 and 14)

As noted above, potassium secretion by the distal tubule is dependent on the distal tubular intracellular potassium concentration, and therefore on the uptake of potassium by the peritubular cell membrane. It is known that mineralocorticoids may stimulate potassium excretion, and an early study demonstrated that this effect could occur without a change in sodium excretion (42). Furthermore, in the absence of mineralocorticoids, the rate of potassium excretion at any given plasma level of the ion is diminished. Normal potassium excretion is restored by the administration of a mineralocorticoid hormone. Early micropuncture studies demonstrated that in the absence of aldosterone, the rate of potassium secretion by the distal convoluted tubule was markedly impaired. In fact, TF/P_K ratios, which normally reach 2 to 5 in this segment of the nephron, were always found to be under 1 (43, 44). More recent micropuncture evidence suggests that aldosterone stimulates peritubular potassium uptake and thereby increases the intracellular potassium content (45, 46). These data support the view that aldosterone may regulate potassium excretion by varying distal tubular intracellular potassium concentration.

The second most important factor in the regulation of potassium excretion is the rate of flow of filtrate past the site of secretion (39, 40, 41, 47). The steady-state luminal potassium concentration is reached with great rapidity, and a tenfold increase in tubular flow rate does not substantially change this relationship. Thus, at a given level of intracellular potassium concentration and intraluminal electronegativity, the rate of potassium secretion will be directly related to the rate of filtrate flow through the distal tubule. Based on these observations, it is believed that diuretics which act on the thick ascending limb to reduce filtrate absorption augment potassium excretion by increasing the flow of filtrate past the potassium secretory site (38).

The dependence of potassium excretion on the distal tubular flow rate may explain the changes in excretion observed when sodium intake is altered. Large loads of potassium are easily excreted when dietary intake of sodium is high but are excreted with difficulty when salt is severely restricted or the organism is volume-depleted (25). Thus, a high-sodium diet will enhance the *potential* for potassium excretion whereas a sodium-deficient diet will make excretion of a potassium load more difficult. Clearly, however, a control system for potassium excretion by the kidney must be capable of varying potassium excretion widely at all levels of sodium intake.

It has been well documented that potassium excretion can be altered by changes in acid-base equilibrium (see also Chap. 6). Thus, the immediate response to an increase in blood pH due to

hypocapnia or increased plasma sodium bicarbonate is an increase in potassium excretion (48, 49, 50). Since both of these maneuvers tend to increase the potassium content of body cells, including the cells of the distal tubule, the increase in potassium excretion is easily understood. On the other hand, decreases in pH due to hypercapnia or increased hydrogen ion entry into the ECF reduce intracellular potassium, and a transient reduction in potassium excretion follows (48, 51).

The immediate effect of the pH change does not persist (52). In respiratory alkalosis, the rate of potassium excretion rapidly returns to normal and the total body potassium content remains unaltered. In respiratory and metabolic acidosis, the initial decrease in potassium excretion is reversed, and potassium excretion exceeds control values. In the steady-state phase, a respiratory or metabolic acidosis is associated with mild or moderate total body potassium deficit (53, 54, 55, 56, 57). Diabetic ketoacidosis is associated with a marked potassium deficiency which is due to continued urinary potassium losses. The high urinary loss of potassium is due to the excretion of large amounts of keto acids. In metabolic alkalosis, the initial increase in potassium excretion becomes greater and the steady-state phase of this disorder is associated with a large total body potassium deficit (50).

The increased potassium excretion in respiratory and metabolic acidosis and in metabolic alkalosis are associated with increased sodium excretion, and thus it seems likely that an increased rate of filtrate flow past the distal tubular secretory site may contribute to an inappropriately high rate of potassium excretion (52). In metabolic alkalosis, a high intracellular potassium concentration has been found in the cells of the distal convoluted tubule, and this factor must also contribute greatly to the persistently high rate of potassium excretion found in this disorder (38, 58).

Of the factors just enumerated, only aldosterone and distal tubular flow rate appear to have a role in the *physiologic regulation* of potassium excretion. The action of aldosterone on distal tubular cells described above represents the efferent side of a regulatory loop. The afferent side appears to be a direct effect of potassium on aldosterone secretion by the adrenal gland. Two sites of action of potassium have been described: (1) the synthesis of pregnenolone (an aldosterone precursor) from cholesterol is stimulated by acute elevations in plasma potassium, and (2) the conversion of corticosterone to aldosterone is enhanced by chronic elevations in potassium intake (59, 60). On the other hand, decreased potassium intake leading to potassium deficiency is associated with decreased aldosterone secretion.

Potassium intake may also affect filtrate flow through the distal tubule. It has been clearly demonstrated that acute increases in plasma potassium inhibit proximal reabsorption of filtrate (61). The resulting increase in flow through the distal tubule would favor increased potassium excretion. Studies of proximal filtrate reabsorption in states of potassium depletion have not addressed the question of total filtrate absorption, although it is known that bicarbonate absorption is enhanced in this setting and it is conceivable that total filtrate absorption may also be enhanced. If the latter is true, the resulting fall in filtrate flow through the distal tubule would reduce potassium secretion.

The major control of day-to-day potassium excretion appears to be the hormone aldosterone. Since this hormone is also known to be a major determinant of sodium excretion, it is reasonable to ask how the hormone can control the excretion of both ions at once.

An analysis of the possible interrelated mechanisms for the control of both ions is presented in Table 4-1. The successful control of potassium excretion by a single hormone may well depend on the interrelationship between distal tubular flow rate and aldosterone. For example, when sodium intake is elevated and sodium and filtrate load to the distal nephron is enhanced, it is possible that distal intracellular potassium concentration falls because of the reduction in plasma aldosterone which follows the increased sodium intake. The reduction in intracellular potassium concentration prevents excessive potassium losses due to an increased distal tubular fluid flow rate. Conversely, a low sodium intake may lead to a somewhat decreased distal tubular flow rate, but stimulates aldosterone secretion. As a result of higher aldosterone levels, potassium uptake by distal tubular cells is stimulated. As distal tubular intracellular potassium concentrations increase, potassium secretion increases, thus offsetting the reduced tubular fluid flow rate. Large potassium loads not only increase aldosterone secretion at any level of sodium intake but also decrease proximal sodium absorption. These two factors increase potassium excretion by increasing distal tubular potassium secretion and distal tubular fluid flow rate. Further analysis of how potassium excretion could be controlled during ingestion of other combinations of sodium and potassium intake is presented in Table 4-1. It should be noted that experimental data are not available to verify all of the suggestions in the table. However, none of the available evidence con-

Table 4-1. Changes in determinants of K excretion with variations in dietary Na and K

DIET		ALDOSTERONE SECRETION	DISTAL TUBULAR FLOW RATE	DISTAL TUBULAR INTRACELLULAR K	Na EXCRETION	K EXCRETION
Na	K					
N	N	+ +	+ +	+ +	N	N
↑	N	+	+ + +	+	↑	N
↓	N	+ + +	+	+ + +	↓	N
N	↑	+ + +	+ +	+ + +	N	↑
N	↓	+	+ +	+	N	↓
↑	↑	+ +	+ + +	+ +	↑	↑
↓	↓	+ +	+	+ +	↓	N or ↓
↑	↓	+	+ + +	+	↑	↓
↓	↑	+ + +	+ +	+ + +	↓	↑

tradicts the scheme. The possible role of the pars recta of the proximal tubule and the thin descending limb of Henle's loop have not been included in this analysis of the control of potassium excretion because of the limited information currently available on this subject. It is also possible that a hormone other than aldosterone may be operative in controlling potassium excretion (62).

THE CONTROL OF THE PLASMA POTASSIUM CONCENTRATION

Simple observation of normal individuals leads to the conclusion that plasma potassium concentration is carefully controlled. Values for plasma potassium are consistently between 3.5 and 4.5 meq/ L despite large variations in dietary potassium intake. The mechanism which keeps plasma potassium concentrations within such narrow limits is not completely understood. However, recent experiments have suggested a major role for the glucoregulatory hormones in this process (63).

For many years it has been known that insulin profoundly affects the movement of potassium across cell membranes (64). It has been commonly accepted that insulin lowers the plasma potassium concentration. Indeed, insulin is frequently used to treat hyperkalemia. The explanation for this effect has been that insulin lowers plasma potassium through its effect on entry of glucose into cells. This explanation is not correct. Rather, insulin stimulates the efflux of sodium by an energy-dependent process associated with the stimulation of Mg^{2+}-dependent Na^+-K^+-ATPase. The efflux of sodium is associated with an increase in intracellular potassium (65, 66).

In response to the intravenous infusion of potassium, insulin secretion is stimulated and plasma insulin levels may reach four to five times control values (67, 68) (see also Chap. 24). Plasma glucagon levels also increase as a direct result of potassium infusion (67). It is likely that the role of glucagon is to protect the animal from hypoglycemia. It should be noted that the effect of potassium on glucagon is direct; hypoglycemia need not be present before glucagon levels increase.

In the absence of insulin, little infused potas-sium is able to enter cells (68). Thus, it takes considerably less potassium to raise the plasma potassium level of animals made diabetic with alloxan than it does in normal animals. On the other hand, in states of potassium depletion, insulin secretion is impaired in response to a given glucose load (69).

The clinical implications of these observations are important. Patients with diabetes mellitus may not be able to tolerate well either large potassium loads or impairment of renal potassium excretion. Indeed, there is abundant evidence that the insulin-deficient patient taking the potassium-sparing diuretic triamterene is particularly prone to develop hyperkalemia, especially when renal function is even mildly impaired (70). It has also been shown that when the ECF of a diabetic patient becomes acutely hypertonic, plasma potassium levels may increase quickly (71, 72, 73). This effect is thought to be due to the rapid shift of water from the intracellular to the extracellular space, and as the water moves through the pores of the cell membrane, potassium follows due to a solvent drag effect.

There is experimental evidence that indicates that the sympathetic nervous system is also involved in the control of plasma potassium levels (63). The infusion of alpha-adrenergic agents such as epinephrine and norepinephrine produces an acute hyperkalemic response due to the release of potassium from liver cells. The action of epinephrine on muscle differs from its action on the liver. Potassium uptake by skeletal muscle is stimulated by epinephrine and isoproternol, a beta-adrenergic effect. This effect is blocked by propranolol.

These observations imply that agents which have beta-adrenergic–stimulating properties may be useful in treating hyperkalemia. Indeed, salbutamol has been used in the treatment of hyperkalemic periodic paralysis (74). Beta-adrenergic blockers, on the other hand, may be useful in treating hypokalemia (75). More importantly, beta blockade may prevent adequate control of plasma potassium in patients with a tendency to develop hyperkalemia. Patients at risk are those with insulin insufficiency, severe renal failure, those patients who exercise vigorously, and those who ingest large amounts of potassium. Although there are no reports of patients experiencing hyperkalemia while taking propranolol, such patients may exist and simply may not have been detected (63).

ADAPTATION TO A HIGH POTASSIUM INTAKE

When a large dose of potassium is administered to animals not previously ingesting a high-potassium diet, hyperkalemia may occur, and the sudden potassium load may be fatal. However, if dietary potassium is gradually increased, the administration of a previously lethal potassium load is well tolerated (76). Careful studies show that plasma potassium levels do not become as elevated, and potassium excretion is enhanced so that the load is more rapidly excreted. The adaptation appears to be chronic in cattle and sheep (77, 78). These animals continuously ingest large amounts of potassium. Uremic humans and animals also demonstrate an adaptive response to the administration of large potassium loads (62).

The renal response to chronic high potassium loads appears to be intrinsic to the kidney (79). Isolated perfused kidneys from normal animals are able to increase fractional potassium excretion twofold as the concentration of potassium in the perfusion fluid is increased from 4 to 10 meq/L. Kidneys from potassium-adapted animals have a fractional potassium excretion five times greater than kidneys from nonadapted animals. Fractional excretion remains constant as the potassium concentration in the perfusion fluid increases.

A complete understanding of the mechanism by which renal potassium excretion is increased in response to chronic high potassium loads remains elusive. Na^+–K^+–ATPase has been given a primary role since chronic potassium loading increases the renal activity of this enzyme (80). Initial increases are found in the outer medulla, but more prolonged administration of high potassium loads stimulates an increase in cortical and papillary activities of the enzyme as well. The outer medulla appears to be most sensitive to increased potassium loads since changes in this region occur earlier and at lower levels of potassium administration. When the activity of the enzyme is blocked by the administration of ouabain, renal potassium excretion is markedly impaired.

The effect of potassium on the kidney Na^+–K^+–ATPase appears to require mineralocorticoids but is not due solely to the effects of these hormones (80). Thus, potassium-increased Na^+–K^+–ATPase activity occurs in response to a high-potassium diet in adrenalectomized animals given only small amounts of mineralocorticoid to prevent death. The action of a substance not synthesized in the adrenal gland may be responsible for the renal potassium adaptation.

The site of potassium adaptation remains uncertain and may involve different segments of the nephron in different animals. The earliest and most pronounced area of increased Na^+–K^+–ATPase activity is the outer medulla. Yet, structures in this area are now known to secrete potassium. However, the thick ascending limbs of Henle's loops, which are prominent in this area, avidly absorb this cation. Jamison et al. (29) have demonstrated that large amounts of potassium are added to the tubular filtrate in the pars rectae or descending thin limb and removed by the thick ascending limb. In potassium-loaded animals, the amount of potassium added to and removed from the filtrate is 50 to 100 percent greater. It is possible that the increased Na^+–K^+–ATPase found by several investigators relates to this phenomenon and not to increased secretion. In the rabbit, the cortical collecting tubule is capable of secreting large amounts of potassium (81), and some investigators have observed secretion by the collecting tubule in the rat (30, 34, 35, 36). More studies will be required to explain some of the ambiguities in the current data.

The colon also plays a role in potassium adaptation. Potassium excretion by this organ is enhanced by potassium loading and in conditions in which the renal excretion of the cation is impaired. Thus, when the glomerular filtration rate declines to less than 5 mL/min, potassium excretion by the colon increases markedly. The increased excretion appears to be correlated with a rise in colon Na^+–K^+–ATPase and can be blocked with ouabain. While mineralocorticoids appear necessary for the increase in $Na^+–K^+–ATPase$ to occur, these hormones may play only a permissive and not a regulatory role (82).

POTASSIUM PATHOPHYSIOLOGY (See also Chaps. 5 and 14)

THE CONSEQUENCES OF HYPERKALEMIA

Plasma potassium concentrations are normally 3.5 to 4.5 meq/L. Levels of plasma potassium greater than 7.0 meq/L are dangerous, and plasma levels greater than 8.5 meq/L are frequently fatal. The cause of death is usually cardiac arrest, but occasionally, respiratory paralysis occurs before the heart stops.

Marked elevations in plasma potassium cause abnormalities of both heart and skeletal muscle function by lowering the resting electrical potential of muscle cells and thereby preventing repolarization. Thus, in the presence of hyperkalemia, skeletal muscle fibers may contract and then relax, paralyzed. The first symptom the patient may observe is weakness in the lower extremities which gradually proceeds to paralysis as more and more fibers become involved (83). The paralysis begins in the lower extremities, gradually ascends, and may eventually involve the muscles of respiration and cause death from pulmonary insufficiency.

Heart muscle is in a manner analogous to skeletal muscle, and the abnormalities can be followed on the electrocardiogram (84). The T waves in the precordial leads change first. Initially, they become tented and taller, but later they become broad. The second change observed is the lengthening of the P-R interval, and then the P wave gradually disappears. Finally the R wave decreases in amplitude and the QRS complex widens. Shortly before the heart stops, the QRS complex and T wave merge to form a sine wave. Ventricular fibrillation soon follows. Throughout the process, the contractile force of the heart is progressively impaired. In some patients, the pathophysiologic effects of hyperkalemia involve the heart first before the skeletal muscle, and in these instances, death may occur without any noticeable premonitory signs and symptoms. Therefore, the physician must be aware of the conditions in which hyperkalemia may occur and anticipate the problem.

THE CONSEQUENCES OF POTASSIUM DEPLETION

Most forms of potassium depletion are associated with hypokalemia. The most important exception to this statement is the potassium depletion which may be present in some forms of metabolic acidosis, but in the absence of hypokalemia. In diabetic ketoacidosis, for example, plasma potassium levels may be elevated despite potassium losses of 5 meq/kg body weight. The clinical consequences of potassium depletion, however, are associated with hypokalemia. The adverse consequences of potassium deficiency may be divided into four categories: metabolic, cardiovascular, neuromuscular, and renal.

The most notable adverse metabolic effect of potassium deficiency is impaired glucose tolerance. Potassium is required for normal insulin release, and it can be shown that insulin secretion in response to increases in plasma glucose is impaired when total body potassium is deficient (85). Potassium-depleted young animals also have impaired protein anabolism, perhaps because of the lack of insulin stimulation.

The cardiovascular consequences of potassium depletion are multiple. Changes in electric activity may be seen on the electrocardiogram. T waves are decreased in amplitude and U waves develop. The combined T-U wave may make it appear that there is a prolonged Q-T interval. In chronic severe hypokalemia, the myocardium may undergo lysis, and muscle cells are replaced by fibrous tissue (86). A prominent round-cell infiltration may be found.

Premature atrial and ventricular contractions have been associated with hypokalmia, but these arrhythmias are most common in those patients who are taking digitalis (87). Serious ventricular arrhythmias, secondary to hypokalemia, have rarely been reported in patients not taking one of the cardiac glycosides. However, in a few patients with a severe preexisting heart disease, hypokalemia may produce arrhythmias (88). Severe chronic hypokalemia may be associated with salt and water retention, congestive heart failure, and marked impairment of cardiac function.

In addition to the adverse affects potassium depletion has on cardiac muscle, it also has serious effects on smooth and striated muscle, and these effects may occasionally result in a fatality. Cross-striations of skeletal muscle are lost in moderately severe potassium depletion and rhabdomyolysis, and permanent loss of muscle mass may occur in severe potassium depletion. Striated and smooth muscle may also become paralyzed in hypokalemia. As the plasma potassium falls and the intracellular to extracellular potassium concentration ratio increases, the resting potential becomes so great that depolarization and the subsequent stimulation of contraction cannot occur. Weakness and eventually paralysis are the end results. The lower extremities are usually the first to be involved, but the respiratory muscles soon follow. Weakness of the diaphragm usually precedes involvement of the accessory muscles of respiration. Thus, patients with severe hypokalemia may present with a picture of ascending paralysis and respiratory insufficiency of rapid onset (89).

Involvement of the smooth muscle leads to decreased bowel motility and may result in an ileus or severe gastric atony by mechanisms entirely analogous to the effect of hypokalemia on striated muscle. Urinary retention due to bladder paralysis may be a manifestation of the same process.

Many potassium-depleted patients complain of alterations of sensorium. Memory impairment, disorientation, and confusion may occur. How many of these symptoms are the result of the hypokalemia itself and how many are due to secondary complications of the effects of hypokalemia such as anoxia and metabolic alkalosis is unclear (90).

The kidney in potassium depletion has been well studied. In man, microscopic examination of cells of the proximal convoluted tubule reveals vacuolization (86). The vacuoles disappear rapidly when the potassium deficit is repaired. There have been reports of more severe changes in potassium with prolonged potassium depletion. An interstitial nephritis characterized by round-cell infiltration has been noted (91). The reversibility of this lesion is unclear.

Renal function is impaired in potassium depletion. Best known of the impairments is the inability to concentrate the urine. Impairment of concentrating ability is usually insignificant until the total body potassium losses exceed 200 meq. Then the maximum urinary osmolality falls rapidly from about 1200 mosm/kg to 300 to 400 mosm/kg. The major cause of the defect appears to be a reduction in the ability of the medullary thick ascending limb to pump sodium chloride into the medullary interstitium (91).

The potassium-depleted kidney also secretes more ammonia than a normal kidney under similar systemic conditions (92). As a result, the minimal urinary pH is greater than normal. Potassium depletion also enhances bicarbonate and sodium absorption in the proximal tubule (93). The mechanism for this effect is probably related to the fact that in potassium-depleted states, the intracellular hydrogen ion concentration of proximal tubular cells is increased. Thus, hydrogen ion secretion and subsequent bicarbonate reabsorption are enhanced.

Renin secretion by the kidney in states of potassium depletion is increased, but the mechanism responsible is not understood (94, 95). The high renin secretion rate may be one of the factors responsible for the polydipsia that is characteristic of potassium-depleted patients. Increased renin secretion stimulates thirst by increasing the circulating angiotensin II level, and angiotensin II directly stimulates the thirst center (96). Direct stimulation of the thirst center by potassium depletion has also been suggested.

HYPOKALEMIA AND POTASSIUM DEFICIENCY

The measurement of the concentration of potassium in serum or plasma has become readily accessible since the invention of the flame photometer. On the other hand, measurement of total body potassium remains technically difficult. Therefore, the clinical assessment of total body potassium is usually done by measurement of the serum or plasma potassium concentrations.

Potassium concentrations in normal people range from 3.6 to 4.5 meq/L. Although many authors give 5.5 meq/L as the upper limit of normal, values in normal individuals above 4.5 meq/L are unusual and may be due to the release of the ion from platelets or red cells. Serum concentrations are 0.2 to 0.4 meq/L higher than plasma because potassium is released from platelets as the clot forms (113).

Hypokalemia in the majority of clinical settings denotes a total body potassium deficiency. However, a deficit of 200 meq is usually present before hypokalemia is observed. It has been suggested that once the plasma potassium has fallen to 3 meq/L, an additional decrease of 1 meq/L will occur for each additional 100 to 400 meq decrement in total body potassium (97).

Hypokalemia may also occur without a deficit in total body potassium. A shift of potassium from extracellular to intracellular fluid will occur when plasma pH increases, when plasma bicarbonate concentration rises (93), or when plasma insulin levels increase (63). In these instances, hypokalemia is not associated with potassium deficiency. On the other hand, normokalemia may be present in spite of a large deficit in total body potassium. Chronic respiratory acidosis, cirrhosis of the liver, uremia, and congestive heart failure are examples of disease states in which this may occur (49). The deficit of potassium in these patients is probably due to metabolic abnormalities related to the primary disease, since even with massive potassium supplementation, potassium stores do not change. Of course, correctable potassium deficits may also occur in these patients due to some of the mechanisms listed in Table 4-2. However, in general, the administration of potassium to this group of patients only results in higher rates of potassium excretion rather than net positive potassium balance.

There are several reports in the literature which suggest that commonly used diuretics (chlorthalidone, furosemide) in some manner shift potassium from ECF to ICF (98, 99). Indeed, measurements of total body potassium have failed to detect potassium deficiencies in patients receiving these drugs despite the presence of hypokalemia.

Under some circumstances, plasma potassium concentrations are normal or high despite severe total body potassium deficits. The primary example is diabetic ketoacidosis, in which plasma potassium concentrations may be normal or high, but a deficit of 10 meq/kg of body weight may be present.

Clearly, the value of the plasma potassium concentration for any patient must be integrated with the clinical history and physical examination in order to assess appropriately its relationship to total body potassium stores.

CAUSES OF POTASSIUM DEPLETION AND HYPOKALEMIA

REDUCED INTAKE OF POTASSIUM

On occasion, a reduced intake of potassium may contribute to potassium deficiency, but this factor alone is probably only rarely a cause of potassium depletion since most diets contain large amounts of potassium. Diets high in carbohydrate food made from refined sugars are an exception to the general rule. These diets may contain only small amounts of potassium. Patients with alcoholism may ingest only small amounts of potassium since most of their calories come from low-potassium alcoholic beverages. However, other factors may play an important role in producing potassium deficits in alcoholic patients. For instance, magnesium deficiency, which is associated with renal potassium wasting, is relatively common in alcoholics. Patients with anorexia nervosa frequently are potassium deficient, but these patients commonly abuse cathartics and lose large quantities of potassium in the stool.

POTASSIUM DEPLETION DUE TO GASTROINTESTINAL LOSSES (See also Chap. 22)

Salivary, pancreatic, or bile fistulas have been associated with potassium depletion. In part, this may be due to the relatively high potassium content of the fluid which is lost, but other factors such as starvation or a high rate of catabolism may contribute to the deficiency.

Vomiting and nasogastric suction are also as-

Table 4-2. Causes of potassium depletion and/or hypokalemia

I. EXTRACELLULAR TO INTRACELLULAR POTASSIUM SHIFTS

A. Decreased blood hydrogen ion concentration (increased pH)
B. Increased plasma bicarbonate concentration
C. Increased plasma insulin
D. Familial hypokalemic paralysis
E. Administration of diuretics

II. DECREASED POTASSIUM INTAKE

A. Carbohydrate diet
B. Alcoholism
C. Anorexia nervosa
D. Geophagia

III. GASTROINTESTINAL LOSSES

A. Salivary, pancreatic, or bile fistula
B. Protracted, voluminous vomiting or gastric suction
C. Diarrhea, especially that associated with excessive secretion of vasoactive intestinal peptide
D. Laxative or enema abuse
E. Ureterosigmoidostomy
F. Villous adenoma of colon or rectum
G. Malabsorption

IV. INCREASED URINARY LOSSES

A. Excessive mineralocorticoid effect
  1. Primary hyperaldosteronism
    a. Adrenal adenoma
    b. Idiopathic hyperaldosteronism
    c. Indeterminate hyperaldosteronism
    d. Glucocorticoid-remediable hyperaldosteronism
  2. Adrenal hyperplasia
  3. Adrenal cortical adenoma
  4. Excessive secretion of ACTH from pituitary or an ectopic site
  5. Some forms of secondary hyperaldosteronism
    a. Renal vascular hypertension
    b. Hemangiopericytomas of the kidney
    c. Bartter's syndrome
    d. Birth-control pills
  6. Congenital adrenal hyperplasia due to 17-hydroxylase deficiency
  7. Licorice or carbenoxolone ingestion
B. Intrinsic renal disease
  1. Renal tubular acidosis
  2. Fanconi syndrome
  3. Rarely in chronic pyelonephritis, polycystic disease, and interstitial nephritis
  4. After prolonged amphotericin administration
  5. During a postobstructive or post-ATN diuresis
  6. Posttransplantation
C. Diuretic induced
  1. Thiazides
  2. Loop diuretics
  3. Carbonic anhydrase inhibitor
  4. Organomercurials, large loads of nonreabsorbable anion
  5. Carbenicillin or penicillin
D. Idiopathic or familial
  1. Bartter's syndrome
  2. Liddle's syndrome
  3. Familial hypokalemia associated with hypomagnesemia
E. Hypomagnesemia

V. LEUKEMIA WITH LYSOZYMURIA

sociated with the development of hypokalemia. The major loss of potassium is not due to the loss of gastric fluid but rather to a profound kaliuresis. As a result of the loss of hydrochloric acid and the subsequent development of metabolic alkalosis, large amounts of bicarbonate are excreted in the urine. The flow of bicarbonate past the potassium secretory site increases the rate at which this cation is secreted into the tubular fluid and causes substantial losses. An increase in aldosterone secretion, as a result of volume depletion, further stimulates potassium losses in this condition (100).

Diarrheal fluid may contain as much as 30 meq/L of potassium. Thus, potassium losses in viral, bacterial, or endotoxic diarrheas may be quite large. Perhaps the most spectacular disorder of this type is the diarrhea associated with non-beta cell islet tumors of the pancreas (101). This tumor releases a substance called vasoactive intestinal polypeptide which increases the secretion of fluids from the small bowel. The volume of diarrheal fluid passed per day may exceed 10 L and daily potassium losses by this route may be as great as 200 to 300 meq. The diarrhea can be completely cured by the removal of the tumor.

Villous adenoma is a peculiar tumor of the colon and rectum that is associated with large potassium losses. Most of these patients have a continuous, bothersome rectal discharge, but occasionally the secretions from the tumor are small and unnoticed. Removal of the tumor, when that is possible, eliminates the problem (102). Increased losses of potassium in the stool have also been associated with ganglioneuroblastomas (103) and the Mediterranean type of abdominal lymphoma (104).

One of the more common causes of hypokalemia in patients presenting without an obvious etiology is the chronic ingestion of cathartics (105, 106, 107). Usually patients abusing these agents have a serious emotional disorder and do not readily admit to their habit. Frequent use of enemas will produce a similar picture. This cause of potassium depletion must be suspected in every patient in whom a diagnosis of potassium depletion is not readily apparent.

The diagnosis of hypokalemia due to gastrointestinal losses can frequently be made from the history and physical examination. During the development of hypokalemia due to vomiting, the urine contains large amounts of both sodium and potassium and is relatively alkaline, but when vomiting stops and the patient's condition stabilizes, the urine contains little sodium or potassium and the urine is acid. The change is due to the volume depletion which accompanies this disorder. When potassium losses occur through the colon, the urine contains very small amounts of potassium, usually less than 20 meq/day and often less than 10 meq/day. The presence of more than 20 meq of potassium per day in the urine in patients who are not losing gastric or duodenal fluid strongly suggests that the hypokalemia and potassium deficiency are due to renal losses.

HYPOKALEMIA ASSOCIATED WITH INCREASED URINARY LOSSES

MINERALOCORTICOIDS (See also Chaps. 14 and 23)

As noted earlier, mineralocorticoids play a key role in the regulation of potassium excretion. Thus, as might be surmised, many of those conditions which give rise to excessive mineralocorticoid secretion are associated with hypokalemia. Primary hyperaldosteronism is the classic disorder associated with potassium deficiency. Four forms of this

disorder are known to exist (108). A single adrenal adenoma may produce the characteristic clinical picture of hypertension, hypokalemia, hypernatremia, metabolic alkalosis, and renal potassium wasting. In other patients with what is called idiopathic hyperaldosteronism, there is no adenoma, but one finds small, often microscopic, nodules throughout the zona glomerulosa of both adrenals. The presenting clinical picture of this form of adrenal hyperplasia is quite similar to that of an adenoma except that hypokalemia is less severe and renin levels are not as suppressed. Unfortunately, the response to bilateral adrenalectomy in this form of the disease is not as salutary.

A small percentage of patients with hyperaldosteronism will have the indeterminate form of the disease in which the adrenal glands are normal grossly and microscopically. Two forms of hyperaldosteronism which respond to the administration of adrenal hormones have been described. Glucocorticoid-responsive hyperaldosteronism is a form of the disorder which is ameliorated by replacement doses of glucocorticoids. The second form, which is clinically a mild disorder, is responsive to desoxycorticosterone. The diagnosis of primary hyperaldosteronism is made by demonstrating elevated plasma aldosterone levels without a diurinal variation. Quadratic analysis of several variables as described by Biglieri will separate those patients with an adenoma from the 20 to 50 percent with hyperplasia (idiopathic type) (108).

Hyperaldosteronism, secondary to a disease associated with edema formation, is not usually characterized by hypokalemia unless the patient has been treated with diuretics. Other forms of secondary hyperaldosteronism, however, are frequently associated with renal potassium losses. Renal vascular hypertension with excessive renin production from one kidney may be associated with hypokalemia, but this is not a constant feature of the disease (109). Patients with small renal tumors called hemangiopericytomas have secondary hyperaldosteronism due to the secretion of renin from these neoplasms. Hypokalemia may be severe in these patients. These tumors often cannot be diagnosed with angiography and are suspected only when a unilateral elevation of renin is seen in the absence of vascular disease (110, 111). On occasion, hypernephromas and Wilm's tumors will secrete renin (112, 114). These tumors are large and may be diagnosed with a combination of an IVP, angiography, and ultrasound.

Congenital adrenal hyperplasia is associated with a deficiency of either adrenal 11-hydroxylase or 17-hydroxylase (115, 116). As a result of those enzyme abnormalities, these patients have a cortisol deficiency and high ACTH levels which stimulate the adrenals to produce large quantities of steroid hormones, many of which have mineralocorticoid effects. Sodium retention, hypertension, and hypokalemia result from their action. The administration of a glucocorticoid suppresses ACTH, and the production of adrenal steroids subsides.

The ingestion of European licorice, which contains glycyrrhizic acid, or carbenoxolone, a drug used in Europe to treat gastric ulcers, may produce a picture of Cushing's syndrome and an associated hypokalemia (117, 118). These agents have both a glucocorticoid and mineralocorticoid effect. Stopping either agent reverses the disorder.

INTRINSIC RENAL DISEASE

Renal tubular acidosis (RTA) is one of the few diseases which causes hypokalemic acidosis. Patients with either type 1 or type 2 of this disorder may have profound loss of potassium in the urine. The cause of the loss is thought to be an increased flow of filtrate past the potassium-secreting site because of the inability of the tubular epithelium to reabsorb filtered bicarbonate (119). More recently, work with the isolated collecting tubule suggests that the increased potassium loss may also be due to the higher pH of filtrate passing through the collecting duct (120). The potassium loss is observed in both types of RTA and may also be seen in the Fanconi syndrome.

On rare occasions, patients with chronic pyelonephritis, polycystic disease, and interstitial nephritis have also been reported to have potassium wasting. The mechanism involved is unclear (121, 122, 123).

Hypokalemia may be seen in three diuretic states: postobstruction, after acute renal failure, and immediately after successful renal transplants. These processes are usually self-limiting.

DRUG INDUCED RENAL POTASSIUM WASTING

The most common cause of renal potassium wasting is generally thought to be the administration of diuretics. The thiazides, loop diuretics, and the organomercurials inhibit the absorption of filtrate in the thick ascending limb and early distal tubule. The increased flow of filtrate past the potassium secretory site increases secretion, especially when severe secondary hyperaldosteronism is present. Thus, the immediate response to the administration of these diuretics is not only an increase in sodium excretion but also an increase in the rate of potassium excretion. Acetazolamide inhibits the proximal absorption of bicarbonate and produces what is essentially a proximal renal tubular acidosis. Potassium losses occur during the short period of time this drug is effective in eliciting a natriuresis.

Over the long term (3 to 6 months), administration of diuretics does not appear to be associated with large deficits in total body potassium. Repeated measurements of total body potassium in patients receiving long-term diuretic therapy generally fail to show values significantly less than control. Even when potassium supplements are given, total body potassium content remains constant (98, 99).

The administration of several antibiotics is associated with an increased loss of potassium in the urine. The administration of amphotericin B is associated with reduced renal function in almost all patients receiving the drug, and hypokalemia from a mild kaliuresis is frequently present. In most patients, renal function returns to normal and potassium losses cease when the drug is stopped (124). Gentamicin has also been reported to increase the renal loss of potassium, but the mechanism is unknown (125). The intravenous administration of carbenicillin has been associated with hypokalemia. This drug is usually given in large doses (20 to 40 g/day) and is rapidly excreted. The high rate of distal tubular flow produced by the osmotic effect of the drug and the fact that in the urine, carbenicillin is a nonresorbable anion combine to cause large potassium losses (126).

Excessive renal potassium losses have been observed in magnesium deficiency, but the locus of potassium loss by the kidney is unknown (127, 128, 129). Frequently, the hypokalemia characteristic of this condition is associated with hypocalcemia. Thus, the combined presence of hypokalemia and hypocalcemia should alert the physician to measure the serum magnesium.

Acute leukemias have been associated with hypokalemia and inappropriate losses of potassium in the urine. The excretion of lysozymes has been implicated as the cause, but avid potassium uptake by leukemic cells or a relative magnesium deficiency due to rapid growth of the leukemic cell mass have not been ruled out as contributing factors.

Finally, there are several reports of a familial form of hypokalemia in which chronic renal potassium wasting is the major feature (130).

OTHER DISORDERS ASSOCIATED WITH HYPOKALEMIA

In 1962, Bartter described a disorder in two black children which was characterized by severe hypokalemia, hyperreninemia, hyperaldosteronism, and profound losses of potassium in the urine (131). Both children had growth retardation and were normotensive. On microscopic examination of the kidneys, marked hypertrophy and hyperplasia of the juxtaglomerular apparatus and hyperplasia of the medullary interstitial cells were found. Subsequently, the disorder has been recognized in patients without growth retardation.

Many explanations of the pathophysiology of Bartter's syndrome have been offered, but none are completely satisfactory. The original suggestion that vascular insensitivity to angiotensin II or renal salt wasting with secondary hyperreninemia and hyperaldosteronism might be causal have not held up. Recent clinical evidence has raised the possibility that excessive prostaglandin synthesis

and release may play a key role. The overproduction of prostaglandin E has been found in patients with the syndrome, and the administration of indomethacin, which inhibits prostaglandin synthesis, reverses completely most manifestations of the disorder. Significant kaliuresis and hypokalemia persist, however, and potassium supplements are required. Stein has made the suggestion that the fundamental disorder is renal potassium wasting which leads to potassium deficiency. In the potassium-depleted state, prostaglandin synthesis is increased and high levels of PGE cause peripheral vasodilation, inadequate circulation, hyperreninemia, and secondary hyperaldosteronism (132).

Liddle and his associates have described a patient with all the clinical characteristics of primary hyperaldosteronism, hypertension, hypokalemia, and metabolic alkalosis (133). However, measurements of plasma aldosterone were normal. Triamterene, but not spironolactone, corrected the abnormalities. This finding suggests that there is a defect in the cell membranes of these patients. Indeed, abnormal membrane sodium transport by the red cells of the patients with this syndrome has been reported (134).

HYPERKALEMIC DISORDERS

The clinical states associated with an elevated serum potassium are outlined in Table 4-3. The distinction between pseudo- and true hyperkalemia is important. Pseudohyperkalemia is an in vitro phenomenon caused by the release, upon standing, of intracellular potassium by red blood cells, or by white blood cells and platelets, in patients with marked leukocytosis or thrombocytosis (135, 136, 137). Potassium is released from platelets in the process of clot formation (113, 138). Thus, *serum* potassium levels may be up to 0.5 meq/L greater than the simultaneously determined *plasma* potassium levels. Both vigorous arm exercise before blood drawing and tight application of tourniquet before venipuncture may result in cellular potassium release and spuriously elevated potassium levels (139).

Table 4-3. Causes of hyperkalemia

I. PSEUDOHYPERKALEMIA

  A. Thrombocytosis
  B. Hemolysis
  C. Leukocytosis

II. TRUE HYPERKALEMIA

  A. As a result of decreased renal excretion
    1. Oliguric renal failure
      a. Acute
      b. Chronic
    2. Pharmacologic blockade of potassium secretion
      a. Triamterene
      b. Spironolactone
      c. Amiloride
    3. Relative or absolute hypoaldosteronism
      a. Hyporeninemic aldosteronism
      b. Adrenal cortical insufficiency
    4. Isolated defect in renal excretion of potassium
      a. Congenital
      b. Acquired
  B. As a result of cell leak/transcellular K shifts
    1. Acidosis
      a. Metabolic
      b. Respiratory
    2. Rapid release of cell K
      a. Crush injury
      b. From malignant cells after chemotherapy
        i. Lymphomas
        ii. Leukemia
        iii. Myeloma
      c. Succinylcholine depolarization of cell membrane
      d. Acute digitalis poisoning
      e. Following arginine infusion
      f. Idiopathic or familial hyperkalemic episodic paralysis
  C. As a result of high K intake
    1. Oral K supplementation
    2. Intravenous K administration
      a. Rapid administration of K solutions
      b. K penicillin in high doses
      c. Rapid transfusion of aged blood
  D. Increased extracellular osmolality
    1. Glucose
    2. Mannitol
    3. Saline

TRUE HYPERKALEMIA

True hyperkalemia may be the result of decreased potassium excretion by the kidneys in patients with severe renal failure, transcellular shifts of potassium, or excessive potassium intake in the presence of limited excretory capacity. In some patients with severe chronic renal failure, hyperkalemia occurs when there is a decrease in potassium excretion by the colon.

DECREASED RENAL POTASSIUM EXCRETION

Significant, often fatal, hyperkalemia is commonly seen in untreated patients with oliguric acute renal failure. There are multiple factors which contribute to the elevated potassium levels. Potassium may be released from damaged cells in patients with burns, trauma, or extensive infections. A considerable amount of potassium may be administered in the transfusion of old blood. Ordinarily the kidneys could excrete the additional load of potassium, however, in this disorder, the GFR is less than 1 mL/min and the urine formed is less than 250 mL/day. The flow of filtrate past the potassium secretory sites is simply too low to allow for significant excretion. Thus, as a result of the markedly reduced excretory capacity, the liberation of potassium from cells secondary to cell injury or the development of metabolic acidosis, hyperkalemia is a common finding in oliguric acute renal failure. Hyperkalemia is less severe but not absent in patients with nonoliguric renal failure (24-h urine volume greater than 800 mL).

Most patients with chronic renal failure have normal plasma potassium levels (140). This finding reflects the ability of the remaining nephrons in the diseased kidneys and the gastrointestinal tract to adapt to the patient's renal disease. As long as the 24-h urine volume is greater than 1 L, and severe constipation does not occur, external potassium balance remains normal even when the glomerular filtration rate is less than 5 mL/min.

The mechanisms by which external potassium balance is maintained when renal mass is markedly decreased have been studied in both experimental animals and humans. In dogs, adaptation to an 80 percent reduction in nephron mass occurs within 24 h after subtotal nephrectomy (62). By that time, a fourfold increase in potassium excretion per nephron occurs, and within a week potassium excretion by the residual nephron population exceeds 90 percent of the dietary intake. The adaptation occurs as rapidly and as completely in adrenalectomized animals maintained on minimal doses of mineralocorticoid hormones. The rate of potassium excretion was also shown to be independent of the rate of sodium excretion. This study suggests that in experimental renal insufficiency in dogs, the adaptive increase in potassium excretion is not mineralocorticoid dependent, and the existence of a kaliuretic hormone is possible. Evidence from studies in uremic rats suggests that an increase in the activity of $Na^+-K^+-ATPase$ in the distal nephron or collecting duct may play a role in increasing potassium excretion per nephron in renal failure (141).

In patients with chronic renal disease, markedly increased rates of potassium excretion per nephron have been demonstrated, and the amount of potassium excreted may exceed the amount filtered. The mechanism(s) inducing the increased rate of potassium excretion are as unclear in the human as in experimental animals. Although there is no evidence that increased aldosterone secretion rates play a role in increasing nephron potassium excretion in humans, it is clear that normal levels are required. Uremic patients with even mild mineralocorticoid deficiency cannot increase potassium excretion per nephron appropriately. It is also evident that fecal potassium excretion contributes significantly to potassium loss when creatinine clearance is less than 5 mL/min (142, 143). As much as 25 to 30 meq of potassium per day may be excreted in the stool. The mechanism of the increased stool potassium in chronic renal failure has not been completely elucidated. Decreased intestinal water reabsorption and increases in colonic $Na^+-K^+-ATPase$ have been implicated as possible mechanisms responsible for intestinal potassium excretion. The importance of the intestinal excretory route in patients with chronic renal failure is well illustrated by the occasional dialysis patient who develops severe hyperkalemia following an increase in intake of constipating aluminum hydroxide phosphate binders.

Pharmacologic blockade by the aldosterone antagonist spironolactone or the non-aldosterone-dependent diuretics amiloride and triamterene decreases potassium secretion by distal portions of the nephron (144). The administration of these agents to patients ingesting or receiving large amounts of potassium may lead to severe hyperkalemia. Patients with even mild degrees of renal failure may also develop hyperkalemia, and these agents should never be used in patients with renal failure or uremia.

Either a relative or an absolute deficiency of aldosterone may result in hyperkalemia. Isolated hypoaldosteronism has been observed in a number of elderly patients with adult-onset diabetes, mild renal insufficiency, mild metabolic acidosis, inability to conserve sodium on a very low-salt diet, hyperkalemia, and low plasma renin activity (144–150). Glucocorticoid secretion appears normal. An acquired abnormality of the juxtaglomerular apparatus with decreased renin production and decreased angiotensin II–stimulated aldosterone secretion has been suggested as the mechanism. Why the hyperkalemia per se does not stimulate aldosterone release in these patients as normally occurs is unclear, but that it does not suggests that in addition to a defect in renin release, there may be an independent abnormality in aldosterone production.

Hypoaldosteronism may also result from administration of heparin and related compounds (151). Heparin may produce its effect either by inhibiting renin secretion or by a direct effect on the adrenal cortex.

Enzymatic defects which result in decreased mineralocorticoid production have been described and may be associated with hyperkalemia. Certain forms of the adrenogenital syndrome, as well as a 21-hydroxylase and an 18-hydroxydehydrogenase deficiency have been associated with hyperkalemia (152–156).

Patients in Addisonian crisis often develop hyperkalemia, though this is not invariably present in uncomplicated Addison's disease (157, 158). Normally, a patient with Addison's disease who ingests sufficient sodium can excrete enough potassium in the urine to maintain external potassium balance. When a crisis occurs, however, sodium depletion and oliguria are present, hypotension and tissue hypoxia develop, and cellular potassium release increases. The inability of the adrenals to increase aldosterone production results in decreased renal potassium excretion and hyperkalemia.

A small group of patients with an inability to excrete potassium normally but with normal adrenal and renal function have been described (159). These patients have a number of other abnormalities, including hypertension, short stature, and a mild renal tubular acidosis. The etiology of the hyperkalemia is unclear but seems to be related to decreased distal nephron potassium secretion. Thiazide diuretics seem effective in normalizing serum potassium levels.

TRANSCELLULAR POTASSIUM SHIFTS

Both metabolic and respiratory acidosis may be associated with hyperkalemia as a result of intracellular buffering of excess hydrogen ions. When hydrogen ions enter cells, potassium leaks out. The precise interrelationships between transmembrane hydrogen and potassium fluxes remain to be defined (58).

Tissue damage from a multitude of causes, including crush injuries, burns, and rhabdomyolysis, may result in rapid cell breakdown and release of potassium and result in hyperkalemia. Muscle injury in particular may cause a rapid rise in potassium load to the kidneys which exceeds their potassium excretory ability. A protein released from damaged muscle is nephrotoxic and, thus, the increased potassium load may not be rapidly excreted by the damaged kidney.

Rapid malignant cell lysis after chemotherapy, particularly in lymphomas, leukemia, and myeloma, have been reported to cause hyperkalemia (160, 161). Hyperkalemia is rare after treatment of nonhematologic or mesenchymal tumors.

During normal cellular depolarization, potassium leaks from cells. This leakage can be exaggerated and lead to hyperkalemia after the administration of depolarizing muscle relaxants such as succinylcholine (162, 163). Patients with excessive cellular breakdown, e.g., those with trauma or burns, as well as patients with renal failure, seem particularly susceptible to this effect of depolarizing agents. Tubocurare and magnesium sulfate may alleviate the potassium leak (164).

Digitalis glycosides act to inhibit cell membrane ATP. When these agents are given in excess or taken in a suicide attempt, the marked inhibition of $Na^+-K^+-ATPase$ leads to reduction of cellular potassium uptake. Net cellular potassium loss results in hyperkalemia (165, 166).

Arginine hydrochloride, an amino acid used intravenously to treat severe metabolic alkalosis, may lead to hyperkalemia, probably as a result of its displacement of intracellular potassium, independent of cellular or blood pH changes (167).

INCREASED POTASSIUM INTAKE

The administration of large amounts of potassium to normal individuals usually does not result in hyperkalemia. However, in patients with impaired ability to excrete potassium (e.g., chronic renal failure, Addison's disease, sodium-retaining states with oliguria) excessive oral or intravenous administration of potassium may lead to hyperkalemia (168). It is a widespread practice to give patients starting on diuretics a potassium supplement in anticipation of an increased urinary loss of potassium. If the diuretic does not produce a diuresis and kaliuresis, however, hyperkalemia may ensue. Furthermore, these patients frequently use salt substitutes which contain large amounts of potassium. Many of these preparations contain 10 to 13 meq/g. The additional potassium load may contribute to the danger (169, 170, 171).

Intravenous potassium administration may also cause hyperkalemia, particularly if potassium has been added to a solution without sufficient mixing. Mixing has been noted to be particularly difficult when solutions are added to plastic bags (172, 173). The rapid infusion of high-dose potassium penicillin salts (1.7 meq of potassium per 1 million units potassium penicillin G) and the rapid transfusion of aged blood after potassium has been released from metabolically inactive red cells also produce hyperkalemia (174, 175).

A sudden increase in ECF osmolality by the intravenous administration of hypertonic solutions of mannitol, glucose, and saline has been associated with hyperkalemia in a small group of patients (176, 177). The increased ECF osmolality causes a rapid shift of fluid from the ICF to the ECF space and intracellular potassium enters the ECF by a solvent drag effect. Most patients who demonstrate this abnormality have insulin insufficiency or mild mineralocorticoid depletion (178).

A step-by-step diagnostic approach to patients with elevated serum potassium is outlined in Fig. 4-1. It is not designed to be all-encompassing but to provide a logical sequence of clinical and laboratory tests to be performed to determine the cause of a given patient's hyperkalemia.

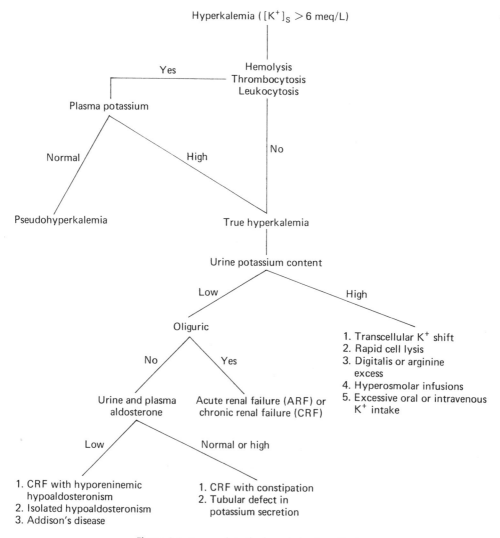

Figure 4-1. Approach to the hyperkalemic patient.

FAMILIAL KALEMIC EPISODIC PARALYSES (FKEP)

Three syndromes of episodic muscle weakness, known as hypo-, normo-, or hyperkalemic periodic paralyses have been described. Though rare, these syndromes may lead to permanent muscle atrophy, and thus early diagnosis and treatment are desirable.

Familial hypokalemic episodic paralysis is the most common of the three disorders (180). It is inherited as an autosomal dominant with variable penetrance. The syndrome usually becomes clinically evident in the first and second decades of life, but attacks may decrease in frequency by the fourth or fifth decade or may even cease altogether. Males are more frequently affected than females. Individual episodes of weakness and paralysis often begin during sleep or after a high carbohydrate meal. Rest after vigorous exercise, cold temperatures, trauma, tension, and infections have also been noted to induce an attack (180). Each episode may last up to 24 h and usually involves trunk and proximal limb muscles with sparing of the muscles of respiration. Neither mechanical nor electrical stimuli evoke a muscle response during an episode (185).

A number of biochemical abnormalities have been noted during these episodes, but the precise etiology of each of these remains unknown. Plasma potassium levels fall to less than 3 meq/L because of a shift of extracellular potassium to the intracellular space. The shift is associated with a decline in urinary potassium excretion and an increase in urinary 17-hydroxycorticosteroids, 17-ketosteroids, and aldosterone. This observation has lead to the thought that a nonaldosterone mineralocorticoid might be stimulating potassium entry into body cells (181). No documentation for this hypothesis exists. Two additional findings are of interest. Blood levels of lactate and pyruvate increase, and vacuolization of the muscle cells characterizes the biopsy of muscle cells (182).

For many years, treatment consisted of a low-carbohydrate diet with potassium supplementation which appeared to be beneficial in ameliorating or preventing attacks. More recently, acetazolamide, a carbonic anhydrase inhibitor, has been shown to be beneficial, perhaps by causing a mild metabolic acidosis and decreasing cellular uptake of potassium (183, 184).

Familial hyperkalemic episodic paralysis (adynamia episodica hereditaria) has also been described and is inherited as an autosomal dominant (179, 186). In contradistinction to patients with hypokalemic periodic paralysis, patients with this disorder have an *increase* in serum potassium during episodes of muscle weakness. Affected individuals suffer attacks more frequently, and at an earlier age than those with the hypokalemic variety. Vigorous exercise, cold temperature, emotional stress, and general anesthesia may precipitate an attack. The attacks are usually of rapid onset and short duration. Head and neck muscles, along with the muscles of the extremities, may be affected. The episodes have been associated with an increase in urinary potassium and a decrease in urinary sodium excretion. Serum sodium, chloride, phosphate, and glucose fall while serum bicarbonate rises (187).

Again, the etiology of this condition is unknown, but therapy with thiazide diuretics, acetazolamide, and mineralocorticoids has been effective in preventing attacks (187). Of interest is a report that acetazolamide prevents the attacks as well as the fall in blood glucose, even when the serum potassium was elevated, suggesting that the effect of this agent is to correct a primary abnormality of glucose transport or metabolism that might be causing the syndrome. The frequency and severity of attacks seem to decrease dramatically after adolesence.

Familial normokalemic episodic paralysis has also been described but is not clearly a distinct entity and has many of the features of both the hypokalemic and hyperkalemic forms.

THERAPY OF DISORDERS OF POTASSIUM METABOLISM

HYPERKALEMIA

Severe hyperkalemia associated with paralysis of skeletal muscle or marked changes on the electrocardiogram represents a medical emergency and must be treated immediately and aggressively. Treatment may be divided into two stages. During the first stage of treatment, the objective is to restore toward normal the ratio of intracellular to extracellular potassium concentrations. This prevents the muscle membranes from remaining depolarized and alleviates paralysis of skeletal muscle and the abnormal conduction of electrical impulses in the heart. The second stage of therapy is designed to remove the excess potassium from the body.

Three measures are commonly used to counteract the immediate effects of hyperkalemia. Bicarbonate ions induce the cellular uptake of potassium by a poorly understood direct effect and by raising the pH of the blood. Two or three ampuls of sodium bicarbonate (each ampul contains 44 meq $NaHCO_3$) can be rapidly infused over a period of several minutes. The effect of the infusion may be followed on the electrocardiogram and is usually evident within a minute or two. The movement of potassium into the cells returns the ratio of intracellular to extracellular potassium chemical activity toward normal and ameliorates the effect of the potassium overload. The treatment is usually effective over a period of several hours, but the patient should be monitored with electrocardiograms and measurements of plasma potassium until measures to reduce the total body potassium content can be taken.

In less drastic situations or as a follow-up to initial treatment with sodium bicarbonate, an intravenous insulin infusion can be used to stimulate the uptake of potassium by cells. A loading dose of 1 unit of insulin per 10 kg body weight followed by 1 unit/kg/h is a reasonable approach. A minimum of 2 or 3 g of glucose should be administered with each unit of insulin to prevent hypoglycemia. The hypokalemic effects of insulin may be noted within 30 min and in most circumstances will last as long as insulin is infused. When the administration of insulin is stopped, plasma potassium levels may rise rapidly. If there is a high rate of entry of potassium into the ECF from damaged cells, as in a crush injury, insulin may not be successful in controlling the plasma potassium level.

The effects of hyperkalemia on the heart can also be temporarily ameliorated by the rapid infusion of a solution of ionized calcium. Three ampuls of 10% calcium gluconate may be infused intravenously over 3 to 5 min while the electrocardiogram is monitored. The onset of action may be noted within 1 to 5 min, but the action is relatively transient.

After one of these immediate steps to lower plasma potassium has been taken, the second stage of therapy directed at reducing total body potassium must be instituted. The resin, sodium polystyrene sulfonate (Kayexalate), is an effective cation exchanger: 1 g of resin will bind approximately 1 meq of potassium in the gastrointestinal tract. The resin may be given orally in doses of 15 to 30 g two to four times per day. To prevent constipation, 50 mL of 20 or 25% sorbitol for each 15 g of resin should be used as a vehicle. Sorbitol may also induce a mild diarrhea, thus aiding the bowel excretion of both potassium and sodium liberated in the exchange. The resin may also be administered in a retention enema. The usual dose with this method is 50 g of resin in 200 mL of 25% sorbitol. The desired retention time of 30 to 60 min may be achieved with the use of an inflated rectal catheter.

In some patients with renal failure peritoneal or hemodialysis may be used to remove potassium from the body. Access to the intravascular compartment can be obtained through a femoral vein catheter obviating the need for a Scribner shunt.

HYPOKALEMIA

The treatment of hypokalemia is usually not urgent. However, when plasma potassium levels are below 2 meq/L and the presence of paralysis or arrhythmias are noted, intravenous administration of potassium chloride is justified. As much as 40 meq of potassium per hour may be given via solutions which contain no more than 60 meq/L. Up to 400 meq KCl can be administered intravenously per day. When the plasma potassium concentration reaches 2.5 meq/L, the rate of administration should be slowed to 10 meq/h, and solutions should contain no more than 30 meq/L.

Pain at the site of infusion may limit the rate at which the solutions of potassium are given. Administration into a central venous catheter is dangerous since there is a limited time for mixing with blood returning to the heart.

Postoperatively it may be necessary to administer potassium intravenously to avoid potassium depletion. In most instances, the daily administration of 30 to 50 meq is sufficient to make up for potassium lost in urine and other body fluids. Each bottle of replacement intravenous fluid should contain a fraction of the desired daily dose. Once oral feedings have been resumed, intravenous potassium administration should be stopped.

Hypokalemia is the most commonly treated electrolyte abnormality in the practice of ambulatory medicine. Potassium supplements are usually prescribed along with diuretics or glucocorticoid hormones. As indicated above, however, symptoms from mild hypokalemia (3.0 to 3.5 meq/L) are unusual, and since many patients receiving diuretics do not have potassium levels below 3.0 meq/L, the administration of potassium to this group has been challenged (188). The long-term effects of even moderate hypokalemia do not appear to be associated with an increased morbidity or mortality.

There are reasons for not treating patients with potassium. The Boston Collaborative Drug Surveillance Program recently reported a review of 16,000 hospitalized medical patients who had received KCl during their hospitalization (189). Of these patients, 87 percent did not have an identified potassium deficiency and were given KCl "prophylactically." Of the patients receiving supplemental potassium, 5.8 percent developed complications of the therapy. In over half, hyperkalemia was noted. KCl was implicated in the death of 0.15 percent of the patients. The deaths associated with the administration of KCl exceeded the deaths caused by drugs commonly recognized for their potentially lethal reactions.

Over the past several years, considerable evidence has accumulated that hypertensive patients treated with diuretics will not suffer severe potassium deficits despite the absence of potassium supplements (98, 190, 191). Total body potassium measured by the ^{40}K technique has been found to be unchanged from normal values. When patients are given potassium supplements of approximately 40 meq/day, no change in total body potassium or plasma potassium can be detected. Thus, it has been suggested by several authors that potassium supplementation may be unwarranted in hypertensive patients treated with diuretics because of the lack of evidence for the existence of significant potassium deficits.

Lawson and his associates have reported studies of potassium balance in 21 patients receiving thiazides or loop diuretics for edema (99). They found that the administration of up to 50 meq of potassium per day had no effect on plasma potassium or total body potassium. A number of these patients were on long-term digoxin therapy and showed no evidence of arrhythmias or cardiac glycoside toxicity even though potassium supplements were stopped.

What guidelines might be used to aid the physician in the use of potassium supplementation? There is general agreement that potassium should be administered to any patient with a plasma potassium of less than 2.5 meq/L on repeated examination even if the patient is asymptomatic. If a patient has symptoms *suggestive* of hypokalemia (fatigue or lethargy) and plasma potassium levels between 2.5 and 3.0 meq/L, potassium supplements are also indicated. If there are *clear-cut* symptoms of potassium depletion or hypokalemia and the serum potassium is between 3.0 and 3.5 meq/L, supplementation is also warranted. Usually 30 to 50 meq/KCl per day is enough to reverse the symptoms.

Patients taking digitalis have always been considered an especially vulnerable group. Potassium antagonizes the action of cardiac glycosides, and most physicians feel very uncomfortable treating patients with a combination of diuretics and cardiac glycosides without giving supplemental potassium. However, the relationship between digitalis toxicity and hypokalemia in patients is confusing. Two studies have shown no difference between potassium levels in patients with and those without digitalis toxicity (192, 193), whereas another study has shown that digitalis toxicity occurs at lower plasma digitalis levels in the presence of hypokalemia (194). Until a definitive, well-controlled examination of the importance of potassium supplements in this group is carried out, potassium should be given to digitalized patients receiving diuretics in an effort to keep potassium levels above 3.5 meq/L.

Two products can be recommended: 10% KCl may be given orally; a dose of 15 mL twice daily (40 meq) is well tolerated, especially when given in fruit juice. When given as a single dose, gastric irritation may result. In situations where the total body deficit is large, this dose may be given every 4 h.

KCl also comes impregnated in a wax tablet in a dose of 8 meq per tablet which dissolves slowly as it moves through the gastrointestinal tract. There have been very few reports of intestinal ulcerations from this preparation, and it is probably tolerated more readily than 10% KCl. The slight extra cost is probably returned in the form of better compliance.

REFERENCES

1. Shohl, A. T.: *Mineral Metabolism*, Reinhold Publishing Corp., New York, 1939.
2. Burch, R. R. J., and F. W. Spiers: Measurement of the g-radiation from the human body, *Nature*, **172**:519, 1953.
3. Miller, C. E., and A. P. Remenchik: Problems involved in accurately measuring the K content of the human body, *Ann. N.Y. Acad. Sci.*, **110**:175, 1963.
4. Bartter, J., and G. B. Forbes: Correlation of potassium-40 data with anthropometric measurements, *Ann. N.Y. Acad. Sci.*, **110**:264, 1963.
5. Edelman, I. S., and J. Liebman: Anatomy of body water and electrolytes, *Am. J. Med.*, **27**:56, 1959.
6. Corsa, L., J. M. Olney, R. W. Steenberg, M. R. Ball, and F. D. Moore: Measurment of exchangeable potassium in man by isotope dilution, *J. Clin. Invest.*, **29**:1280, 1950.
7. Pierson, R. N., D. H. Lin, and R. A. Phillips: Total body potassium in health: Effects of age, sex, height and fat, *Am. J. Physiol.*, **226**:206, 1974.
8. Weatherall, M.: Location of fractions of potassium in rabbit auricles, *Proc. R. Soc. London Biol.*, **156**:83, 1962.
9. Ussing, H. H.: The alkali metal ions in isolated systems and tissues, in *Handbuch der Experimentellen Pharmakologic*, vol. 13, Springer-Verlag OHG, Berlin, 1960.
10. Tinckler, L. F.: Fluid and electrolyte observations in tropical surgical practice, *Br. Med. J.*, **1**:1263, 1966.
11. Fordtran, J. S.: Speculations on the pathogenesis of diarrhea, *Fed. Proc.*, **26**:1405, 1967.
12. Berliner, R. W., and T. J. Kennedy, Jr.: Renal tubular secretion of potassium in the normal dog, *Proc. Soc. Exp. Biol. Med.*, **67**:542, 1948.
13. Keith, N. M., A. E. Osterberg, and H. E. King: The excretion of potassium by the normal and diseased kidney, *Trans. Assoc. Am. Physicians*, **55**:219, 1940.
14. Squires, R. D., and E. J. Huth: Experimental potassium depletion in normal human subjects: I. Relationship of ionic intakes to renal conservation of potassium, *J. Clin. Invest.*, **38**:1134, 1959.
15. Mudge, G. H., J. Foulkes, and A. Gilman: The renal secretion of potassium, *Proc. Soc., Exp. Biol. Med.*, **67**:545, 1948.
16. McCance, R. A., and E. M. Widdowson: Alkalosis with disordered kidney function, *Lancet*, **2**:247, 1937.
17. Davidson, D. G., N. G. Levinsky, and R. W. Berliner: Maintenance of potassium excretion despite reduction of glomerular filtration during sodium diuresis, *J. Clin. Invest.*, **37**:58, 1958.
18. Berliner, R. W., T. J. Kennedy, Jr., and G. Hilton: Renal mechanisms for secretion of potassium, *Am. J. Physiol.*, **162**:348, 1950.
19. Malvin, R. L., W. S. Wilde, and L. P. Sullivan: Localization of nephron transport by stop-flow analysis, *Am. J. Physiol.*, **194**:135, 1958.
20. Bennett, C. M., J. R. Clapp, and R. W. Berliner: Micropuncture study of the proximal and distal tubule in the dog, *Am. J. Physiol.*, **213**:1254, 1967.
21. Bennett, C. M., B. M. Brenner, and R. W. Berliner: Micropuncture study of nephron function in the rhesus monkey, *J. Clin. Invest.*, **47**:203, 1968.
22. Le Grimellec, C. T., P. Poujeol, and C. de Rouffignac: H^3-inulin and electrolyte concentrations

in Bowman's capsule in rat kidney, *Pflügers Arch.*, **354**:117, 1975.

23. Schultze, R. G.: Recent advances in the physiology and pathophysiology of potassium excretion, *Arch. Intern. Med.*, **131**:885, 1973.

24. Malnic, G., R. N. Klose, and G. Giebisch: Micropuncture study of renal potassium excretion in the rat, *Am. J. Physiol.*, **206**:764, 1964.

25. Malnic, G., R. M. Klose, and G. Giebisch: Micropuncture study of distal tubular potassium and sodium transport in rat nephron, *Am. J. Physiol.*, **211**: 529, 1966.

26. Marsh, D. J., K. J. Ullrich, and G. Rumrich: Micropuncture analysis of the behavior of potassium ions in the rat cortical tubules, *Pflügers Arch.*, **277**:107, 1963.

27. Beck, L. H., D. Senesky, and M. Goldberg: Sodium-independent active potassium reabsorption in the proximal tubule of the dog, *J. Clin. Invest.*, **52**:2641, 1973.

28. Grantham, J., P. B. Qualizza, and R. L. Erwin: Fluid secretion in proximal straight tubules *in vitro*: Role of PAH, *Am. J. Physiol.*, **226**:191, 1974.

29. Jamison, R. L., F. B. Lacy, J. P. Pennell, and V. M. Sanjana: Potassium secretion by the descending limb or pars rects of the juxtamedullary nephron in *vitro*, *Kidney Int.*, **9**:323, 1976.

30. Wright, F. F., N. Strieder, N. B. Fowler, and G. Giebisch: Potassium secretion by distal tubule after potassium adaptation, *Am. J. Physiol.*, **221**:437, 1971.

31. Duarte, C. G., F. Chomety, and G. Giebisch: Effective amiloride ouabain and furosemide on distal tubular function in the rat, *Am. J. Physiol.*, **221**:632, 1971.

32. Giebisch, G.: Some reflections on the mechanism of renal tubular potassium and transport, *Yale J. Biol. Med.*, **48**:315, 1975.

33. Grantham, J. J., M. B. Burg, and J. Orloff: The nature of transtubular Na and K transport in isolated rabbit renal collecting tubules, *J. Clin. Invest.*, **49**:1815, 1970.

34. Peterson, L., and F. S. Wright: Effect of sodium intake on renal potassium excretion, *Physiologist*, **17**:305, 1974.

35. Bank, N., and H. S. Aynadjian: A micropuncture study of potassium excretion by reminant kidney, *J. Clin. Invest.*, **52**:1480, 1973.

36. Mello-Aires, M., and G. Malnic: Renal handling of sodium and potassium during hypochloremic alkalosis in the rat, *Pflügers Arch.*, **331**:215, 1972.

37. Wright, F. S.: Increasing magnitude of electrical potential along the renal distal tubule, *Am. J. Physiol.*, **220**:624, 1971.

38. Wright, F. S.: Sites and mechanisms of potassium transport along the renal tubule, *Kidney Int.*, **11**:415, 1977.

39. Kunau, R. P., H. L. Webb, and S. C. Borman: Characteristics of the relationship in the flow rate of tubular fluid and potassium transport in the distal tubule of the rat, *J. Clin. Invest.*, **54**:1488, 1974.

40. Khuri, R. N., M. Wiederholt, N. Strieder, and G. Giebisch: Effects of flow rate and potassium intake on distal tubular potassium transfer, *Am. J. Physiol.*, **228**:1249, 1975.

41. Reineck, H., J. Stein, and T. Ferris: Studies on distal tubular potassium transport in Sprague-Dawley rats, *Am. J. Physiol.*, **229**:1403, 1975.

42. Barger, A. C., R. E. Berlin, and J. T. Tulenko: Infusion of aldosterone, 9-alpha fluorohydrocortisone and antidiuretic hormone in the renal artery of normal and adrenalectomized unanesthetized dogs: Effect on electrolyte and water excretion, *Endocrinology*, **62**:304, 1958.

43. Heirholzer, K.: Micropuncture study of renal transtubular concentration gradients of sodium and potassium in adrenalectomized rats, *Pflügers Arch.*, **285**:193, 1965.

44. Courtney, M. A.: Renal tubular transfer of water and electrolytes in adrenalectomized rats, *Am. J. Physiol.*, **216**:589, 1969.

45. Wiederholt, M., W. Scnoormans, F. Fisher, and C. Berlin: Mechanism of action of aldosterone on potassium transfer in the rat kidney, *Pflügers Arch.*, **345**:159, 1973.

46. Wiederholt, M., S. K. Agulian, and R. N. Khuri: Intracellular potassium in the distal tubule of the adrenalectomized and aldosterone treated rat, *Pflügers Arch.*, **347**:117, 1974.

47. Reinek, H. J., R. W. Osgood, T. F. Ferris, and J. H. Stein: Potassium transport in the distal tubular collecting duct of the rat, *Am. J. Physiol.*, **229**:1403, 1975.

48. Malnic, G., M. Mello-Aires, and G. Giebisch: Potassium transport across the renal distal tubular epithelium during acid-base disturbances, *Am. J. Physiol.*, **221**:1192, 1971.

49. Gennari, F. J., M. B. Goldstein, and W. B. Schwartz: The nature of renal adaptation to chronic hypocapnia, *J. Clin. Invest.*, **51**:1722, 1972.

50. Kassirer, J. P., and W. B. Schwartz: The response of normal man to selective depletion of hydrochloric acid, *Am. J. Med.*, **40**:10, 1966.

51. Barker, E. S., R. B. Singer, J. R. Elkinton, and J. K. Clark: The renal response of man to acute experimental respiratory alkalosis and acidosis, *J. Clin. Invest.*, **36**:515, 1957.

52. Gennari, F. J., and J. J. Cohen: Role of the kidney in potassium homeostasis: Lessons from acid base disturbances (editorial), *Kidney Int.*, **8**:1, 1975.

53. DeSousa, R. C., J. T. Harrington, E. S. Ricanati, J. W. Shelkrot, and W. B. Schwartz: Renal regulation of acid-base equilibrium during chronic administration of mineral acid, *J. Clin. Invest.*, **53**:465, 1974.

54. Satorius, O. W., J. C. Roemmelt, and R. F. Pitts: The renal regulation of acid-base balance in man: IV. The nature of the renal compensations in ammonium chloride acidosis, *J. Clin. Invest.*, **28**:423, 1949.

55. Polak, A., G. F. Haynie, R. M. Hays, and W. B. Schwartz: Effects of chronic hypercapnia on electrolyte acid-base equilibrium: I. Adaptation, *J. Clin. Invest.*, **40**:1223, 1961.

56. Schwartz, W. B., N. C. Brackett, Jr., and J. J. Cohen: The response of extracellular hydrogen ion concentration to graded degrees of chronic hypercapnia: Physiologic limits of the defense of pH, *J. Clin. Invest.*, **44**:291, 1965.

57. Carter, N. W., D. W. Seldin, and H. C. Teng: Tissue and renal response to chronic respiratory acidosis, *J. Clin. Invest.*, **38**:949, 1959.

58. Adler, S., and D. S. Fraley: Potassium and intracellular pH, *Kidney Int.*, **11**:433, 1977.

59. Boyd, J. E., W. P. Palmore, and P. J. Mulrow: Role of potassium in the control of aldosterone secretion in the rat, *Endocrinology*, **88**:556, 1971.

60. Boyd, J. E., and T. J. Mulrow: Further studies of the influence of potassium on aldosterone production in the rat, *Endocrinology*, **90**:299, 1972.

61. Brandis, M., J. Keyes, and E. E. Windhager: Potassium-induced inhibition of proximal tubular fluid reabsorption in rats, *Am. J. Physiol.*, **222**:421, 1972.

62. Schultze, R. G., D. D. Taggart, H. Shapiro, J. P. Pennell, S. Caglar, and N. S. Bricker: The adaptation in potassium secretion associated with nephron reduction in the dog, *J. Clin. Invest.*, **50**:1061, 1971.

63. Knochel, J. P.: Role of glucoregulatory hormones in potassium homeostasis, *Kidney Int.*, **11**:443, 1977.

64. Zierler, K. L.: Hyperpolarization of muscle by insulin in a glucose-free environment, *Am. J. Physiol.*, **197**:524, 1959.

65. Gavryck, W. A., R. D. Moore, and R. C. Thompson: Effect of insulin on membrane-bound Na^+–K^+–ATPase extracted from frog skeletal muscle, *J. Physiol.*, **252**:43, 1975.

66. Moore, R. D.: Effect of insulin on sodium pump in frog skeletal muscle, *J. Physiol.*, **232**:23, 1973.

67. Santeusanio, F., G. R. Falooma, J. P. Knochel, and R. H. Unger: Evidence for a role of endogenous insulin and glucagon in the regulation of potassium homeostasis, *J. Lab. Clin. Med.*, **81**:809, 1973.

68. Hiatt, N., L. Morgenstern, M. B. Davidson, G. Bonorris, and A. Miller: Role of insulin in the transfer of infused potassium tissue, *Horm. Metab. Res.*, **5**:84, 1973.

69. Conn, J. W.: Hypertension, the potassium ion and impaired carbohydrate tolerance, *N. Engl. J. Med.*, **273**:1135, 1965.

70. Walker, B. R., D. M. Capuzzi, F. A. Alexander, R. G. Familiar, and R. C. Hoppe: Hyperkalemia after triamterene in diabetic patients, *Clin. Pharmacol. Ther.*, **13**:643, 1972.

71. Noreno, M., C. Murphy, and C. Goldsmith: Increase in serum potassium resulting from the administration of hypertonic mannitol and other solutions, *J. Lab. Clin. Med.*, **73**:291, 1969.

72. Goldfarb, S., B. Strunk, I. Singer, and M. Goldberg: Paradoxical glucose-induced hyperkalemia: Combined aldosterone-insulin deficiency, *Am. J. Med.*, **59**:744, 1975.

73. Goldfarb, S., M. Cos, I. Singer, and M. Goldberg: Acute hyperkalemia induced by hyperglycemia:

Hormonal mechanisms, *Ann. Intern. Med.*, **84**:426, 1976.

74. Wang, P., and T. Chausen: Treatment of attacks in hyperkalemic familial periodic paralysis by inhalation of salbutamol, *Lancet*, **1**:221, 1976.

75. Conway, M. J., J. A. Seibel, and R. P. Eaton; Thyrotoxicosis and periodic paralysis: Improvement with beta blockade, *Ann. Intern. Med.*, **81**:332, 1974.

76. Thatcher, J. S., and A. W. Radike: Tolerance to potassium intoxication in the albino rat, *Am. J. Physiol.*, **151**:138, 1974.

77. Anderson, R. S., and E. C. Pickering: Effects of intravenous infusion of potassium chloride on potassium and sodium excretion and the rate of urine formation in the cow, *J. Physiol.*, **164**:180, 1962.

78. Scott, D.: The effects of intravenous infusion of KCl or NaCl on the renal excretion of potassium in sheep, *Q. J. Exp. Physiol.*, **54**:25, 1969.

79. Silva, P., B. D. Ross, A. N. Charney, A. Besarab, and F. H. Epstein: Potassium transport by the isolated perfused kidney, *J. Clin. Invest.*, **56**:862, 1975.

80. Silva, P., J. P. Hayslett, and F. H. Epstein: The role of Na-K-activated adenosine triphosphatase and potassium adaptation: Stimulation of enzymatic activity by potassium loading, *J. Clin. Invest.*, **52**:2665, 1973.

81. Grantham, J., J. M. B. Burg, and J. Orloff: The nature of transtubular Na and K transport in isolated rabbit renal collecting tubules, *J. Clin. Invest.*, **49**:1815, 1970.

82. Silva, P., A. N. Charney, and F. H. Epstein: Potassium adaptation and Na-K-ATPase activity in the mucosa of colon, *Am. J. Physiol.*, **229**:1576, 1975.

83. Emanuel, M., and R. G. Metcalf: Quadriplegia in hyperkalemia, *J. Maine Med. Assoc.*, **157**:134, 1966.

84. Fisch, C.: Relation of electrolyte disturbances to cardiac arrhythmias, *Circulation*, **47**:408, 1973.

85. Sagild, U., V. Andersen, and P. B. Andreasen: Glucose tolerance and insulin responsiveness in experimental potassium depletion, *Acta Med. Scand.*, **169**:243, 1961.

86. Welt, L. G., W. Hollander, Jr., and W. B. Blythe: The consequences of potassium depletion, *J. Chron. Dis.*, **11**:213, 1960.

87. Mason, D. T., R. Zelis, G. Lee, J. L. Hughes, J. F. Span, Jr., and E. A. Amsterdam: Current concepts and treatment of digitalis toxicity, *Am. J. Cardiol.*, **27**:546, 1971.

88. Steiness, E., and K. H. Olsen: Cardiac arrhythmias produced by hypokalemia and potassium loss during maintenance digoxin therapy, *Br. Heart J.*, **38**:167, 1976.

89. Weiner, M., and F. H. Epstein: Signs and symptoms of electrolyte disorders, *Yale J. Biol. Med.*, **43**:76, 1970.

90. Mitchell, W., and F. Feldman: Neuropsychiatric aspects of hypokalemia, *Can. Med. Assoc. J.*, **98**:49, 1968.

91. Schwartz, W. B., and A. S. Relman: Effects of electrolyte disorders on renal structure and function, *N. Engl. J. Med.*, **276**:383, 1967.

92. Tannen, R. L.: Relationship of ammonia production and potassium homeostasis, *Kidney Int.*, **11**:453, 1977.

93. Kunau, R. T., Jr., A. Frick, F. C. Rector, Jr., and D. W. Seldin: Micropuncture study of the proximal tubular factors responsible for maintenance of alkalosis during potassium deficiency in the rat, *Clin. Sci.*, **34**:223, 1968.

94. Abbrecht, P. H., and A. J. Vander: Effect of chronic potassium deficiency on plasma renin activity, *J. Clin. Invest.*, **49**:1510, 1970.

95. Sealey, J. E., I. Clark, M. B. Bull, and J. H. Laragh: Potassium balance in the control of renin secretion, *J. Clin. Invest.*, **49**:2119, 1970.

96. Fitzsimmons, J. T.: The role of a renal thirst factor in drinking induced by extracellular stimuli, *J. Physiol.*, **201**:349, 1969.

97. Scribner, B. H., and J. M. Burnell: Interpretation of the serum potassium concentration, *Symposium: Water and Electrolytes, Metabolism*, **5**:468, 1956.

98. Leemhuis, M. P., K. J. van Damme, and A. Struyvenberg: Effects of chlorthalidone on serum and total body potassium in hypertensive patients, *Acta Med. Scand.*, **200**:37, 1976.

99. Lawson, D. H., K. Boddy, J. M. B. Gray, M. Mahaffey, and E. Mills: Potassium supplements in patients receiving long-term diuretics for oedema, *Q. J. Med.*, **179**:469, 1976.

100. Seldin, D. W., and F. C. Rector, Jr.: The genera-

tion and maintenance of metabolic alkalosis, *Kidney Int.*, **1**:306, 1972.

101. Verner, J. V., and A. B. Morrison: Endocrine pancreatic islet disease with diarrhea, *Arch. Intern. Med.*, **133**:492, 1974.

102. Roy, A. D., and J. Ellis: Potassium-secreting tumors of the large intestine, *Lancet*, **1**:795, 1959.

103. Cameron, D. G., H. A. Warner, and A. J. Szabo: Chronic diarrhea in an adult with hypokalemic nephropathy and osteomalacia due to a functioning ganglioneuroblastoma, *Am. J. Med. Sci.*, **253**:417, 1967.

104. Scizffers, M. J., M. Levey, and G. Hermann: Intractable watery diarrhea, hypokalemia and malabsorption in a patient with mediterranean type of abdominal lymphoma, *Gastroenterology*, **55**:111, 1968.

105. Schwartz, W. B., and A. S. Relman: Metabolic and renal studies in chronic potassium depletion resulting from over use of laxatives, *J. Clin. Invest.*, **32**:258, 1953.

106. Fleischer, N., H. Brown, D. Y. Graham, and S. Delenna: Chronic laxative-induced hyperaldosteronism and hypokalemia simulating Bartter's syndrome, *Ann. Intern. Med.*, **70**:791, 1969.

107. Wolff, H. T., F. Kruck, and P. Vecsei: Psychiatric disturbance leading to potassium depletion, sodium depletion, raised plasma renin concentration and secondary hyperaldosteronism, *Lancet*, **1**:257, 1968.

108. Biglieri, E. G., J. Stockigt, and M. Schambelan: Adrenalmineralocorticoids causing hypertension, *Am. J. Med.*, **52**:623, 1972.

109. Simon, N., S. S. Franklin, K. H. Bleifer, and M. H. Maxwell: Clinical characteristics of renal vascular hypertension, *JAMA*, **220**:1209, 1972.

110. Robertson, T. W., A. Klidjian, L. J. Harding, G. Walters, M. R. Lee, and A. H. T. Robb-Smith: Hypertension due to a renin secreting tumor, *Am. J. Med.*, **43**:963, 1967.

111. Kihara, I., S. Kitamura, T. Hoshino, S. Hitoshi, and T. A. Watanabe: Hitherto unreported vascular tumor of the kidney: A proposal of juxtaglomerular cell tumor, *Acta Pathol. Jap.*, **18**:197, 1968.

112. Voute, P. A., Jr., J. Vander Meer, N. Stougaard, and W. Kloosteziel: Plasma renin activity in Wilm's tumor, *Acta Endocrinol.*, **67**:197, 1971.

113. Hartmann, R. C., and S. M. Mellinkoff: The relationship of platelets to the serum potassium concentration, *J. Clin. Invest.*, **34**:938, 1955.

114. Conn, J. W., E. L. Cohen, C. T. Lucas, W. J. McDonald, G. H. Mayer, W. Blugh, Jr., W. C. Eveland, J. J. Bookstein, and J. Lapides: Primary reninism, *Arch. Intern. Med.*, **130**:682, 1972.

115. Bongiovanni, A. M.: Disorders of adrenalcorticol steroid biogenesis, in J. B. Stanbury, J. J. Wyngaarden, and D. S. Fredrickson (eds.), *The Metabolic Basis of Inherited Disease*, McGraw-Hill Book Company, New York, 1972, p. 857.

116. Biglieri, E. G., M. A. Herron, and N. Brust: 17-Hydroxylation deficiency in man, *J. Clin. Invest.*, **45**:1946, 1966.

117. Conn, J. W., D. R. Rovner, and E. L. Cohen: Licorice-induced pseudo-aldosteronism, *JAMA*, **205**:492, 1968.

118. Horwich, L., and R. Galloway: Treatment of gastric ulceration with carbenoxolone sodium: Clinical and radiologic evaluation, *Br. Med. J.*, **2**:550, 1968.

119. Sebastian, A., E. McSherry, and R. C. Morris, Jr.: Renal potassium wasting in renal tubular acidosis, *J. Clin. Invest.*, **50**:667, 1971.

120. Boudry, J. F., L. C. Stoner, and M. B. Berg: Effect of acid lumen pH on potassium transport in renal cortical collecting tubules, *Am. J. Physiol.*, **230**:239, 1976.

121. Eastham, R. D., and M. McElligott: Potassium-losing pyelonephritis, *Br. Med. J.*, **1**:898, 1956.

122. Mahler, R. F., and S. W. Stanbury: Potassium-losing renal disease, *Q. J. Med.*, **97**:21, 1956.

123. Jones, N. R., and I. H. Mills: Reversible renal potassium loss with urinary tract infection, *Am. J. Med.*, **37**:305, 1964.

124. McGurdy, D. K., M. Frederic, and J. R. Elkinton: Renal tubular acidosis due to amphotericin B, *N. Engl. J. Med.*, **278**:124, 1968.

125. Holmes, A. M., C. M. Hesling, and T. M. Wilson: Drug-induced secondary hyperaldosteronism in patients with pulmonary tuberculosis, *Q. J. Med.*, **39**:299, 1970.

126. Lipner, H. I., F. Ruzany, M. Dasgupta, P. D. Lief, and N. Bank: The behavior of carbenicillin as a non-reabsorbable anion, *J. Lab. Clin. Med.*, **86**:183, 1975.

127. Shils, M. E.: Experimental human magnesium depletion, *Medicine*, **48:**61, 1969.

128. Medalle, R., and C. Waterhouse: A magnesium-deficient patient presenting with hypocalcemia and hyperphosphatemia, *Ann. Intern. Med.*, **79:**76, 1973.

129. Whang, R., H. J. Morosi, and D. Rogers: The influence of sustained magnesium deficiency on muscle potassium repletion, *J. Lab. Clin. Med.*, **70:**895, 1976.

130. Gitelman, H. J., J. B. Graham, and L. G. Welt: A new familial disorder characterized by hypokalemia, hypomagnesemia, *Trans. Assoc. Am. Physicians*, **79:**221, 1966.

131. Bartter, F. C., P. Pronove, J. R. Gill, and R. C. MacCartle: Hyperplasia of the juxtaglomerular complex with hyperaldosteronism and hypokalemic alkalosis, *Am. J. Med.*, **33:**11, 1962.

132. Kunau, R. T., and J. H. Stein: Disorders of hypo- and hyperkalemia, *Clin. Nephrol.*, **7:**173, 1977.

133. Liddle, G. W., T. Bledsoe, and W. S. Coppage, Jr.: A familial renal disorder simulating primary aldosteronism, but with negligible aldosterone secretion, *Trans. Assoc. Am. Physicians*, **76:**199, 1963.

134. Gardner, J. D., A. Lapey, A. P. Simopoulos, and E. L. Bravo: Abnormal membrane sodium transport in Liddle's syndrome, *J. Clin. Invest.*, **50:**2253, 1971.

135. Salomon, J.: Spurious hypoglycemia and hyperkalemia in myelomonocytic leukemia, *Am. J. Med. Sci.*, **267:**359, 1974.

136. Bronson, W. R., T. V. De Vita, P. P. Carbone, and E. Cotlove: Pseudohyperkalemia due to release of potassium from white blood cells during clotting, *N. Engl. J. Med.*, **274:**369, 1966.

137. Bellevue, R., H. Dosik, G. Speigel, and B. D. Gussoff: Pseudo-hyperkalemia and extreme leukocytosis, *J. Lab. Clin. Med.*, **85:**660, 1975.

138. Hartman, R. C., J. V. Auditore, and D. P. Jackson: Studies on thrombocytosis. I. Hyperkalemia due to release of potassium from platelets during clotting, *J. Clin. Invest.*, **37:**699, 1958.

139. Skinner, S. L.: A cause of erroneous potassium levels, *Lancet*, **1:**478, 1961.

140. Van Yperscle de Strihou, C.: Potassium homeostasis in renal failure, *Kidney Int.*, **11:**491, 1977.

141. Schon, D. A., P. Silva, and J. P. Hayslett: Mechanism of potassium excretion in renal insufficiency, *Am. J. Physiol.*, **227:**1323, 1974.

142. Hayes, C. P., M. E. McLeod, and R. R. Robinson: An extrarenal mechanism for the maintenance of potassium balance in severe chronic renal failure, *Trans. Assoc. Am. Physicians*, **80:**207, 1967.

143. Wilson, D. R., T. S. Ing, A. Metcalfe-Gibson, and O. M. Wrong: The chemical composition of faeces in uremia, as revealed by *in vivo* faecal dialysis, *Clin. Sci.*, **35:**197, 1968.

144. Goldberg, M.: The renal physiology of diuretics, in J. Orloff and R. W. Berliner (eds.), *Handbook of Physiology*, sec. 8, *Renal Physiology*, American Physiologic Society, Washington, D.C., 1973, p. 1003.

145. McNay, J. L., and E. Oran: Possible predisposition of diabetic patients to hyperkalemia following administration of the potassium-retaining diuretic amiloride (MK 870), *Metabolism*, **19:**58, 1970.

146. Hudson, J. B., A. V. Chobanian, and A. S. Relman: Hypoaldosteronism. A clinical study of a patient with an isolated adrenal mineralocorticoid deficiency resulting in hyperkalemia and Stokes-Adams attacks, *N. Engl. J. Med.*, **257:**529, 1957.

147. Perez, G., L. Siegel, and G. E. Schreiner: Selective hypoaldosteronism with hyperkalemia, *Ann. Intern. Med.*, **76:**757, 1972.

148. Weidmann, P., R. Reinhart, P. Rowe, J. W. Coburn, M. H. Maxwell, and S. G. Massry: Syndrome of hyporeninemic hypoaldosteronism and hypokalemia in renal disease, *J. Clin. Endocrinol. Metab.*, **36:**965, 1973.

149. Schambelan, M., J. R. Stockigt, and G. G. Biglieri: Isolated hypoaldosteronism in adults, *N. Engl. J. Med.*, **287:**573, 1973.

150. Michelis, M. F., and H. V. Murdaugh: Selective hypoaldosteronism, *Am. J. Med.*, **59:**1, 1975.

151. Schlatmann, R. J. A. F. M., A. P. Jansen, H. Prenen, J. K. Vanderkorst, and C. L. H. Majoor: The natriuretic and aldosterone-suppressive action of heparin and some related polysulfated polysaccharides, *J. Clin. Endocrinol. Metab.*, **24:**25, 1960.

152. David, R., S. Golan, and W. Drucker: Familial aldosterone deficiency enzyme defect, diagnosis and clinical course, *Pediatrics*, **41:**403, 1968.

153. Jacobs, D. R., and J. B. Posner: Isolated analdosteronism II. The nature of the adrenal cortical

enzymatic defect and the influence of diet and various agents on the electrolyte balance, *Metabolism*, **13**:225, 1964.

154. Ulick, S., E. Gautier, K. K. Vetter, J. R. Markello, S. Yaffe, and C. U. Lowe: An aldosterone biosynthetic defect in a salt losing disorder, *J. Clin. Endocrinol. Metab.*, **24**:669, 1964.

155. Paver, W. K. A., and G. J. Pauline: Hypertension and hyperpotassemia without renal disease in a young male, *Med. J. Aust.*, **2**:305, 1964.

156. Weinstein, S. F., D. M. Allan, and S. A. Mendoza: Hyperkalemia, acidosis and short stature associated with a defect in renal potassium excretion, *J. Pediatr.*, **85**:355, 1974.

157. Pollen, R. H., and R. H. Williams: Hyperkalemic neuromyopathy in Addison's disease, *N. Engl. J. Med.*, **263**:273, 1960.

158. Van Dellen, R. G., and D. C. Parnell: Hyperkalemic paralysis in Addison's disease, *Mayo Clin. Proc.*, **44**:904, 1969.

159. Spitzer, A., C. M. Edelman, Jr., L. D. Goldberg, and P. H. Hanneman: Short stature, hyperkalemia and acidosis. A defect in renal transport of potassium, *Kidney Int.*, **3**:251, 1973.

160. Morse, B. M., and S. J. Shattil: Metabolic complications of aggressive therapy of chronic lymphocytic leukemia, *Am. J. Med. Sci.*, **267**:311, 1974.

161. Muggia, F. M.: Hyperkalemia and chemotherapy, *Lancet*, **1**:602, 1973.

162. Weintraub, H. D., D. V. Heisterkamp, and L. H. Cooperman: Changes in plasma potassium concentration after depolarizing blockers in anesthetized man, *Br. J. Anesth.*, **41**:1048, 1969.

163. Cooperman, L. H.: Succinylcholine-induced hyperkalemia in neuromuscular disease, *JAMA*, **213**:1867, 1970.

164. Aldrete, J. A., A. Zabler, and J. K. Aikawa: Prevention of succinylcholine-induced hyperkalemia by magnesium sulfate, *Can. Anaesth. Soc. J.*, **17**:477, 1970.

165. Smith, T. W., and J. T. Willerson: Suicidal and accidental digoxin ingestion. Report of five cases with serum digoxin level correlations, *Circulation*, **44**:29, 1971.

166. Bismuth, C., M. Gaultier, F. Conso, and H. L. Efthymiou: Hyperkalemia in acute digitalis poisoning. Prognostic significance and therapeutic implications, *Clin. Toxicol.*, **6**:153, 1973.

167. Hertz, P., and J. A. Richardson: Arginine-induced hyperkalemia in renal failure patients, *Arch. Intern. Med.*, **130**:778, 1972.

168. Hultgren, H. N., R. Swenson, and G. Wettach: Cardiac arrest due to oral potassium administration, *Am. J. Med.*, **58**:139, 1975.

169. Sopko, J. A., and R. M. Freeman: Salt substitutes as a source of potassium, *JAMA*, **238**:608, 1977.

170. Snyder, E. L., T. Dixon, and E. Bresnitz: Abuse of salt "substitute," *N. Engl. J. Med.*, **292**:320, 1975.

171. Haddad, A., and E. Strong: Potassium in salt substitutes, *N. Engl. J. Med.*, **292**:1082, 1975.

172. Lankton, J. W., J. N. Siler, and J. L. Neigh: Hyperkalemia after administration of potassium from non-rigid parenteral fluid containers, *Anaesthesia*, **39**:660, 1973.

173. Williams, R. H. P.: Potassium overdosage: A potential hazard of non-rigid parenteral fluid containers, *Br. Med. J.*, **1**:714, 1973.

174. Simon, G. E., and J. R. Bove: The potassium load from blood transfusion, *Postgrad. Med.*, **49**:61, 1971.

175. Bostic, O., and W. F. C. Duvernoy: Hyperkalemic cardiac arrest during transfusion of stored blood, *J. Electrocardiol.*, **5**:407, 1972.

176. Makoff, D. L., J. A. De Silva, and B. J. Rosenbaum: On the mechanism of hyperkalemia due to hyperosmotic expansion with saline or mannitol, *Clin. Sci.*, **41**:383, 1971.

177. Moreno, M., C. Murphy, and C. Goldsmith: Increase in serum potassium resulting from the administration of hypertonic mannitol and other solutions, *J. Lab. Clin. Med.*, **73**:291, 1969.

178. Goldfarb, S., M. Cox, I. Singer, and M. Goldberg: Acute hyperkalemia induced by hyperglycemia: Hormonal mechanisms, *Ann. Intern. Med.*, **84**:426, 1976.

179. Gamstorp, I.: *Adynamia episodia heretaria*, *Acta Paediatr. Scand.*, **45**(Suppl.):1, 1956.

180. Pearson, C. M., and K. Kalyanararnon: Periodic paralysis, in J. B. Stanbury, J. B. Wyngaarden, and D. S. Fredrickson (eds.), *The Metabolic Basis of Inherited Diseases*, McGraw-Hill Book Company, New York, 1972.

181. Streeten, D. H. P., and P. J. Speller: The role of mineralocorticoids in the pathogenesis of hypo-

kalemic periodic paralysis, *J. Clin. Endocrinol. Metab.*, **39**:326, 1974.

182. McArdle, B.: Familial periodic paralysis, *Br. Med. J.*, **12**:226, 1956.

183. Griggs, R. C., W. K. Engel, and J. S. Resnick: Acetazolamide treatment of hypokalemic periodic paralysis, *Ann. Intern. Med.*, **73**:39, 1970.

184. Resnick, J. S., W. K. Engel, R. C. Griggs, and A. C. Stam: Acetazolamide prophylaxis in hypokalemic periodic paralysis, *N. Engl. J. Med.*, **278**:582, 1968.

185. Hoffman, W. W., and R. A. Smith: Hypokalemic periodic paralysis studied *in vitro*, *Brain*, **93**:445, 1970.

186. Meyers, K. R.: A summary review of the diagnosis and pathology of the primary familial periodic paralyses, *Ann. Clin. Lab. Sci.*, **5**:216, 1975.

187. Hoskins, B., F. Q. Vroom, and M. A. Jarrell: Hyperkalemic periodic paralysis. Effects of potassium, exercise, glucose, and acetazolamide on blood chemistry, *Arch. Neurol.*, **32**:579, 1975.

188. Kassirer, J. T., and J. P. Harrington: Diuretics and potassium metabolism: A reassessment of the need, effectiveness and safety of potassium therapy, *Kidney Int.*, **11**:505, 1977.

189. Lawson, D. H.: Adverse reactions to potassium chloride, *Q. J. Med.*, **NS XLIII**: 433, 1974.

190. Edmonds, C. J., and B. Jasani: Total body potassium in hypertensive patients during prolonged diuretic therapy, *Lancet*, **1**:8, 1972.

191. Croxon, N. S., J. M. Neutze, and M. B. John: Exchangeable potassium in heart disease: Long-term effects of potassium supplements and amiloride, *Am. Heart J.*, **84**:53, 1972.

192. Smith, P. W., and E. Haber: Digoxin intoxication: The relationship of clinical presentation to serum digoxin concentration, *J. Clin. Invest.*, **49**:2377, 1970.

193. Beller, G. A., T. W. Smith, W. H. Abelmann, E. Haber, and W. B. Wood, Jr.: Digitalis intoxication: A prospective clinical study with serum level correlations, *N. Engl. J. Med.*, **284**:989, 1971.

194. Shapiro, W., and K. Taubert: Hypokalemia and digoxin-induced arrhythmias, *Lancet*, **2**:604, 1975.

5

Serum electrolytes and the heart

KAREN KLEEMAN / BRAMAH N. SINGH

INTRODUCTION

The basic functions of the heart—rhythmic excitation, conduction, and contraction—depend essentially on the translocation of a number of electrolytes across the membranes of myocardial cells. It is therefore not surprising that electrolyte disturbances may produce major disorders of cardiac rhythm and conduction as well as myocardial function. The deleterious changes induced by serum and myocardial tissue electrolyte imbalances are commonly but not invariably reflected in the electrocardiogram (ECG), which records at the body surface the transmitted mass movement of ionic currents generated within the heart muscle during each cardiac cycle. Although many of the characteristic ECG patterns of electrolyte disturbances have been appreciated for decades, advances in the knowledge of cardiac electrophysiology have been particularly striking in the past 10 years (1–3), related in part to the application of the voltage clamp technique to the study of various types of cardiac fibers (4). The knowledge, albeit incomplete, that has accrued from such studies is beginning to define the ionic basis for the genesis of different forms of cardiac ar-

rhythmias and conduction disturbances with greater precision. Enough is now known to place our recognition and treatment of many such disorders in the clinic on an increasingly rational physiologic basis.

MYOCARDIAL ELECTROPHYSIOLOGY

Like all cells, those in the heart have membranes which permit the passage of certain ions and block that of others. This selective permeability produces an electric potential difference across the cell membrane of the unstimulated or "resting" cell: the voltage is determined by the ionic permeabilities characteristic of the membrane and the ionic concentrations inside and outside the cell, in accordance with the Hodgkin-Katz-Goldman constant field equation:

$$E_M = \frac{g_K E_K + g_{Na} E_{Na} + g_{Cl} E_{Cl} + g_{Ca} E_{Ca}}{g_K + g_{Na} + g_{Cl} + g_{Ca}} \quad (5\text{-}1)$$

This equation describes not only the resting potential but also the transmembrane voltage (E_M) at any given instant. $E_{(ion)}$ is the equilibrium potential for that ion, determined by its concentration gradient across the cell according to the Nernst equation; $g_{(ion)}$ is the membrane conductance for that ion. Conductance, a concept similar to permeability, measures the ease with which an ionic species flows across a membrane in response to an electrochemical driving force. Its value ranges from 0 (no conductance) to 1 (the ion species flows freely across the membrane without any impediment).

Resting myocardial cells and Purkinje fibers have a very high potassium conductance and near-zero conductance for other ionic species, so their resting potential—about −85 mV, inside negative—approaches the potassium equilibrium potential (E_K). However, the conductance of cardiac cells for different ionic species is not constant, but undergoes sequential alterations with each heart beat. These changes permit the flow of specific membrane currents in an orderly temporal sequence, which is the basis for the transmembrane voltage changes evident during the transcription of the action potential, the "anatomy" of which may vary somewhat in different cardiac fibers (Fig. 5-1).

Each ionic current of a cardiac cell has its own unique character, being specific with respect to its voltage dependence and (in some cases) time dependence. It has been shown experimentally that each current has a limited voltage range over which it flows across the membrane, i.e., the conductance of that ion is voltage-dependent. Some currents also have various time dependencies: they cease to flow after a given interval, even if the transmembrane voltage remains within their active range. Furthermore, they may require a fi-

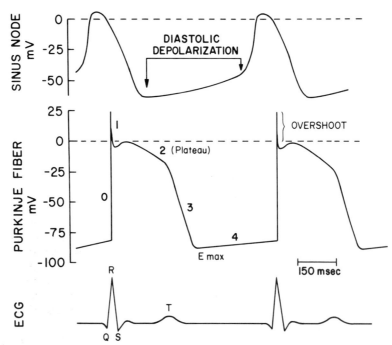

Figure 5-1. Transmembrane potentials from the sinus node and a Purkinje fiber. Note the spontaneous diastolic depolarization in the upper panel, characteristic of pacemaker fibers. The lower panel shows the correlation of time sequence of changes in the action potential and that of the surface electrogram. Alterations in depolarization will be reflected in changes in the QRS duration of the surface record; those in repolarization will be associated with alterations in the Q-T$_c$ interval.

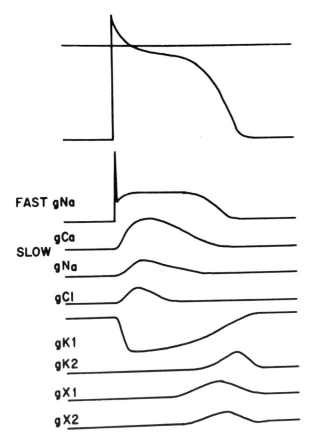

Figure 5-2. Diagrammatic representation of various ionic channels involved in the generation of cardiac action potential; g_{Na}, g_K, etc., represent membrane conductance to sodium, potassium, etc. (see text). (*From Y. Watanabe and L. S. Dreifus,* Cardiac Arrhythmias, *Grune & Stratton, Inc., New York, 1977.*)

voltage clamp. The channels are thought to be conformations of charged molecules, such as proteins or phospholipids. Because of their charge, such molecules assume an open or close configuration in response to changes in the potential difference between the membrane surfaces. Thus, they determine membrane conductance for the ion species for which they are specific.

In the discussion that follows, we will describe the voltage dependence of each current in terms of the transmembrane potential, which is how these currents have been described experimentally. However, it is emphasized that the potential *between* the membrane surfaces, which is what actually controls the currents, is not in fact the same as the *transmembrane* potential difference. It has an additional determinant, which cannot be measured simply because it affects only this "intramembrane" potential. The cell membrane has a layer of fixed negative charges on its outer and inner surfaces which influences the electric field within the membrane. Certain cations, notably calcium and hydrogen ions, appear to bind to these negative charges. In so doing they may alter the intramembrane potential, thereby altering the character of the various ionic currents.

The study of intramembrane potential is a relatively new and complex area of biophysics that is still of only potential interest to clinicians, but it may eventually enable us to explain the complicated effects of calcium and hydrogen ions on the electrophysiologic properties of cardiac cells.

THE ACTION POTENTIAL

Figure 5-1 shows the configuration and voltage scale of action potentials recorded from a spontaneously active sinus node cell and a Purkinje fiber which is stimulated to fire. The surface ECG correlate of the Purkinje fiber potential is also included in the figure for comparison.

The numbered phases of the Purkinje fiber action potential have been clearly delineated in different animal species, but less is known about the nature of the ionic currents flowing during these phases. Phase 0, the upstroke which depolarizes

nite period for activation or reactivation after they have shut off. More complex relationships between voltage and time dependencies have been described for some currents.

Ionic currents flow through plasma membrane "channels" which can discriminate between ionic species, probably on the basis of molecular size. It is the properties of these channels that determine current voltage and time dependence. Figure 5-2 represents the activation patterns of the various ionic channels involved in the generation of the cardiac action potential, as demonstrated by the cell, is carried largely by an inward sodium current (i_{Na}). The channels which carry this current normally open over a transmembrane potential range of about −65 mV (the "threshold" for sodium current) to −40 mV and rapidly close as the inward flow of sodium ions further depolarizes the cell. These channels take only a few milliseconds to close but much longer to "recover," i.e., become responsive to a second stimulus. In ventricular muscle, recovery may require 400 ms (2).

Clinically, the most significant property of the sodium channels is the way in which their activation depends upon the transmembrane resting potential. These channels carry their maximum current at the fastest rate when the cell is depolarized to threshold from a resting potential which is greater (more negative) than −90 mV (5). At smaller resting membrane potentials, the sodium channels are not fully activated and they carry less current, so the upstroke becomes slower and briefer. As may be seen in Fig. 5-3, as the resting

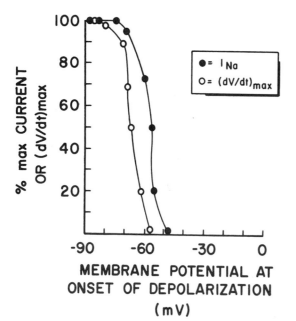

Figure 5-3. Relation of magnitude of Na^+ current and of $(dV/dt)_{max}$ of the action potential upstroke to membrane potential at the onset of depolarization. (*From L. S. Gettes, Pharmacol. Ther. [B.], 2:787, 1976.*)

potential becomes more positive than −70 mV the maximum sodium current falls off rapidly, until at potentials beyond −50 mV the channels do not open at all. As discussed below, conduction velocity is directly related to the rapidity and amplitude of the action potential upstroke, so that the cell that is depolarized at rest (resting membrane potential smaller, i.e., less negative than normal) conducts slowly.

Phase 1 (*rapid repolarization*) is attributed in part to a chloride current (i_{Cl}) activated at about −10 mV and in part to the result of the inactivation of g_{Na} occurring at voltages near 0 mV. The chloride current has no known significance; it has a very long recovery time (about 1 s), so it probably flows little, if at all, at usual heart rates (6).

Phase 2 is the plateau of the action potential. It is longest in Purkinje fibers, slightly shorter in ventricular muscle, and quite short in atrial muscle. Very little current flows in the plateau voltage range.

The current which has aroused much interest among cardiac electrophysiologists recently encompasses both phase 0 and the plateau. This is the slow inward current (*slow response*), so-called because the channels that carry it differ substantially from the sodium channels that open rapidly to permit the passage of a large, fast current (*fast response*). The slow current is essentially a calcium current (i_{Ca}). Its threshold is about −35 mV (7), so it is activated as the fast sodium current depolarizes the cell; its magnitude, like that of the sodium current, is affected by the membrane resting potential (7), but not as dramatically. The slow channels begin to inactivate at about −20 mV, but their inactivation is time-dependent, with a long time constant of about 500 ms in ventricular muscle (8), so that the slow current starts to fall off significantly only near the end of the plateau. The properties of the fast (i_{Na}) and slow (i_{Ca}) channels are compared and contrasted in Table 5-1.

Repolarization (phase 3) is primarily the function of an outward current, i_x, carried largely by potassium (9). This current has important time- as well as voltage-dependent properties; it is activated very slowly in the plateau range, but its

Table 5-1. Comparison of properties of rapid and slow inward currents in cardiac muscle

ELECTROPHYSIOLOGIC PROPERTY OR OTHER ASSOCIATED FEATURES	RAPID CURRENT (FAST RESPONSE)	SLOW CURRENT (SLOW RESPONSE)
Activation or inactivation of kinetics	Rapid	Slow
Dependent on extracellular ion concentration of	Sodium	Calcium
Abolished by	Tetrodotoxin	Verapamil
Threshold of activation	−60 to −70 mV	−30 to −40 mV
Resting membrane potential	−80 to −90 mV	−40 to −70 mV
Conduction velocity	0.5 to 3.0 ms	0.01 to 0.1 ms
Overshoot	+20 to +35 mV	0 to +15 mV
Maximal rate depolarization of phase 0 (V_{max})	100 to 1000 V·s	1 to 10 V·s
Action potential amplitude	100 to 130 mV	35 to 75 mV
Response to stimulus	All or none	Affected by characteristics of stimulus
Safety factor for conduction	High	Low
Recovery of excitability	Prompt, ends with repolarization	Delayed, outlasts full repolarization
Relationship to nodal tissues	Probably nil	Probably mediates pacemaker potentials
Pathologic conditions (ischemia, ouabain toxicity)	Significance unknown	Appears significant
Catecholamines	Produce little effect	Cause significant enhancement

magnitude increases as the inactivation of i_{Ca} begins to repolarize the membrane. As membrane potential becomes more negative, i_x continues to increase, and repolarization speeds up. This curious behavior of i_x may be due to the transient accumulation of potassium at the outer surface of the membrane during repolarization. Such an accumulation might be expected to decrease the potassium concentration gradient and so retard the outward current, but paradoxically it appears to increase membrane potassium conductance, and so it increases the outward current i_x. This inverse relationship between potassium conductance and the driving force for potassium appears to be shared by the channels for other potassium currents and may account for many of the observed effects of hyper- and hypokalemia, discussed below.

Another current which contributes to repolarization is a "background" potassium current, i_{K1} (1); it is voltage-dependent only. It flows very little at plateau voltages, but it increases as repolarization begins and continues until resting potential is reached.

Phase 4 of the action potential corresponds to diastole. In atrial and ventricular muscle, phase 4 is flat, as no net current flows. In Purkinje fibers and other potential pacemaking cardiac tissues, however, a net inward current flows, depolarizing the cell. Normally, the Purkinje fiber is fully depolarized by a stimulus conducted from above before the slow phase 4 depolarization reaches threshold. However, if no stimulus reaches the Purkinje fiber, or if its depolarization is sufficiently accelerated, it will reach threshold itself and produce a spontaneous action potential capable of propagating throughout the heart; thus it is a "latent" pacemaker. Pacemaker current in the Purkinje fiber has a potassium and a sodium component. The potassium current, i_{K2}, flows outward during the end of repolarization, from about −60 to −90 mV, but then undergoes time-dependent *inactivation* during diastole. As i_{K2} decreases, the cell begins to depolarize; as the threshold for i_{Na} is approached, a small inward sodium current is activated and depolarization continues (1, 10).

An action potential from a pacemaker cell in the sinoatrial node is shown in Fig. 5-1. This cell is characterized by a small resting (or maximum diastolic) potential of about −60 mV, a marked spontaneous diastolic depolarization to a firing threshold of about −40 mV, and a slow upstroke of low amplitude. The ionic basis for the maximum diastolic potential of the sinus node is not certain. The value may depend on both calcium and potassium, calcium conductance being greater and potassium conductance a good deal less than the conductances for these ions in resting Purkinje fibers; the maximum diastolic potential would then be further from the potassium equilibrium potential of −110 mV and closer to the calcium equilibrium potential of +65 mV.

Spontaneous depolarization in the sinoatrial node is apparently produced, as in the Purkinje fiber, by the decay of an outward current plus the gradual activation of an inward current. The outward current in this case decays over a range of −60 to −40 mV and appears to be primarily a potassium current (11), which may be equivalent to i_x in the cardiac muscle cell (12). The inward current appears to be a calcium current, the same current which produces the plateau in Purkinje fibers and muscle cells, activated near −40 mV. This current continues on to produce the upstroke of the sinoatrial node action potential. Drugs such as verapamil (13) which inhibit calcium entry decrease the slope of diastolic depolarization and the slope and amplitude of the upstroke (14); these drugs can slow the sinus rate to the point of sinus arrest (15). Catecholamines appear to accelerate the sinus rate by shifting the calcium threshold to more negative potentials, thus increasing the calcium current (16). Acetylcholine slows the individual pacemaker cell by increasing potassium conductance so that decay of the outward potassium current is slower (1), but it may also decrease calcium conductance, reducing the inward calcium current (17).

The action potential of the upper atrioventricular (AV) node is very similar to that of the sinoatrial node. Spontaneous diastolic depolarization occurs, but more slowly, so that under normal circumstances these cells are depolarized by a stimulus from above and do not reach threshold spontaneously. Calcium antagonists depress or suppress the upstroke of the slow-channel, i_{Ca}-dependent AV action potential just as they do that of the sinus node (15).

Of particular significance in the context of electrolyte disturbances is the recent description by Lederer and Tsien (18) of a new current system they designate *transient inward current* (TI). The TI was found to be induced by cardiac glycosides or high external calcium concentrations; it is manifested as a small, rapid depolarization which follows full repolarization. The TI is sensitive to external calcium and is inhibited by manganese ions, which block calcium entry. These observations suggest that TI represents a transient calcium influx (19); sodium, potassium, chloride and hydrogen ions appear to have been excluded as potential charge carriers for the TI (4). Transient depolarizations of this type (also called *oscillatory afterpotentials*, see above) may constitute a significant mechanism for the arrhythmogenicity associated with digitalis intoxication (20).

CONDUCTION

The path followed by the cardiac impulse from the sinus node pacemaker cell to the farthest subepicardial ventricular muscle cell is well known. Conduction of the spontaneously initiated action potential along this path occurs by successive depolarization of contiguous areas of cell membrane by the upstroke of an action potential occurring upstream. A larger and faster upstroke will depolarize contiguous areas of membrane to threshold faster, and so the impulse will be conducted more rapidly along its path. It follows, therefore, that conduction velocity in the heart is directly related to the rate and magnitude of the action potential upstroke, which is itself determined by the resting potential of the cell. Thus, any influence—such as hyperkalemia or severe hypokalemia—which decreases the resting potential of cardiac cells will result in slower conduction.

The resting potential of the cells in the sinus and AV nodes is so small that the sodium current, which produces the large, fast upstroke in cardiac muscle and Purkinje fibers, is completely inactivated and does not flow at all. The small, slow, calcium-dependent upstroke might be expected to result in slow conduction, and it does; nodal conduction has a rate of 0.02 to 0.06 m/s versus 1 m/s in muscle (21). Slow AV conduction ensures that the atria will contract before the ventricles.

The action potential will propagate with no loss of magnitude and thus no drop in conduction velocity as long as each area activated responds with a sodium spike (6). However, where conduction is dependent upon the calcium current it becomes *decremental*: that is, the size of the upstroke progressively decreases and conduction slows. If the upstroke is further decreased by hypoxia, electrolyte imbalance, or drugs, depolarization may fail to reach threshold at some point, and conduction will fail (22).

THE "UNIVERSAL" ACTION POTENTIAL

It is likely that in early embryonic life, all cardiac cell membranes have the same electric properties (23). As differentiation proceeds, this uniformity is lost, and each type of cardiac cell develops its own distinctive pattern of cyclic current changes. However, more similarities than differences remain between Purkinje fibers and ventricular muscle, ventricular and atrial muscle, and sinus and AV nodal cells. Moreover, the embryonic commonality of all cardiac cells is not blotted out by differentiation, merely suppressed. If a resting sinoatrial node cell is hyperpolarized by externally applied current to the activation range of the sodium channels, a small sodium current will develop upon stimulation (24). And if normal atrial (12) or ventricular muscle cells (25) or Purkinje fibers (26, 27) are depolarized to a resting potential in the sinoatrial range, they will develop spontaneous depolarizations apparently dependent on inward calcium current.

If a muscle cell or Purkinje fiber is first depo-larized by hyperkalemia or hypoxia to a resting potential at which the sodium channels are fully inactivated and is then exposed to catecholamines, which increase the inward calcium current, it will develop a slow, small, calcium-dependent action potential that will conduct but is very prone to block (28, 29). "Sick" fibers of this sort have recently been implicated as a potential source of troublesome reentrant arrhythmias (29).

THE ELECTROCARDIOGRAM AS A REFLECTION OF THE ACTION POTENTIAL

The deflections of the surface ECG reflect the summated action potentials of the cardiac muscle masses, the mass of the sinus node and specialized conducting system being too small for their perturbations to be recorded at the body surface.

The P wave of the ECG reflects depolarization (phase 0) of atrial muscle. Atrial repolarization occurs during the P-R interval but is not normally seen because it is slower than depolarization and more spread out over time; the net current flowing at any instant is not great enough to record itself on the ECG. The P-R interval reflects slow conduction of the slow-response action potential through the AV node. The QRS deflection is the summated phase 0 depolarization of the ventricular muscle mass; its width reflects the speed of conduction throughout the ventricle. The ST segment corresponds to the plateau (phase 2) of the action potential; it terminates as soon as some part of the ventricular muscle begins to repolarize.

The T wave corresponds to the repolarization (phase 3) of ventricular muscle. It is not as tall as the QRS deflection because repolarization is slower and more dispersed in time than depolarization. Its height will be increased if the speed of repolarization is accelerated, so that more total current flows at any instant.

Repolarization is a very sensitive process subject to alteration by a multitude of influences which may affect the T wave. Some of the electrolyte derangements which do affect the T wave have been studied in individual cells and can be explained specifically in terms of changes in the repolarization currents i_x and i_{K1}. The U wave, markedly accentuated in hypokalemia, is frequently present in certain surface leads of the human ECG. Its precise origin is still debated. Hoffman and Cranefield (30) believe that the U wave is the surface record of repolarization of the ventricular Purkinje system, i.e., it is the Purkinje fiber T wave.

CONTRACTION

A detailed discussion of the mechanism of cardiac contraction is beyond the scope of this chapter. However, the role of calcium in excitation-contraction coupling merits emphasis. The entry of calcium during the action potential is essential for contraction. Figure 5-4 shows tension development as a function of membrane potential in a strip of ventricular muscle (31). It can be seen that tension is not generated until the threshold for the inward calcium current is reached. All inotropic agents act by increasing the amount of calcium entering the cytoplasm during the action po-

tential. Catecholamines increase the inward calcium current, while cardiac glycosides transport calcium intracellularly by another mechanism (32).

The well-known sliding filament model of contraction is described in detail by Wikman-Coffelt et al. (33). The interaction of actin and myosin, with hydrolysis of adenosine triphosphate (ATP) and shortening of cardiac muscle, cannot take place without calcium. In vivo, actin is kept apart from myosin by a complex of the proteins tropomyosin and troponin; calcium binding to troponin relieves this inhibition and permits actin-myosin interaction and contraction. If more calcium is made available, more actin-myosin interaction occurs and a stronger contraction develops. Contraction continues until the calcium is removed from troponin and actin reinhibited. Calcium removal is accomplished by a pump located in the sarcoplasmic reticulum, the energy for which is provided by ATP hydrolyzed by a calcium-activated ATPase. The sarcoplasmic reticulum gathers up cytoplasmic calcium and so permits relaxation. Mitochondria also take up free cytoplasmic calcium but are not thought to play a dominant role in relaxation (34).

CARDIAC REFRACTORINESS AND THE ORIGIN OF ARRHYTHMIAS

Normal cardiac rhythm is maintained by (1) the dominance of a single pacemaker discharging with the highest frequency; (2) fast and generally uniform conduction in predetermined pathways of impulse transmission; and (3) long and uniform duration of the action potential and of the refractory period of the myocardial fiber. The duration of the Purkinje fiber action potential normally outlasts that of the ventricular action potential, thus providing the safety factor for the orderly conduction of the depolarizing impulse. Myocardial cells differ from the excitable cells in nerve and skeletal muscle in having an unusually long refractory period; that is, following the passage of an action potential they require not one or two but several hundred milliseconds of recovery time before they can generate another propagating action

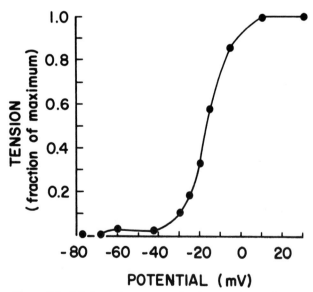

Figure 5-4. Relation between strength of contraction and membrane potential in ventricular muscle under voltage clamp conditions. [*From G. W. Beeler and H. Reuter, J. Physiol. (London), 207:191, 1970.*]

potential in response to a stimulus. The prolonged refractory period limits the number of times the heart can contract per minute, obviating the hemodynamic catastrophe that would occur if tetanic myocardial contraction resulted from an excessively rapid train of impulses.

The long refractory period in cardiac muscle reflects the time-dependent properties of three membrane ionic currents: slow inactivation of i_{Ca} and slow activation of i_x, which lengthen the plateau, and the long recovery time of i_{Na}. AV nodal cells have a shorter action potential but a refractory period which far outlasts full repolarization; its length could result from slow inactivation of i_x, slow recovery of i_{Ca}, or both, at the low resting membrane voltage of nodal fibers.

There is still a paucity of knowledge regarding changes in ionic currents and relevant membrane conductances involved in the recognized categories of arrhythmogenesis: altered impulse generation (arrhythmias caused by enhanced automaticity), impulse propagation (reentrant arrhythmias), and excitability (4, 20, 35). The relationship of these final pathways of arrhythmogenesis to alterations in the action potential duration has not been established, but it is recognized that conditions such as anoxia and ischemia and the use of halothane, all of which markedly accelerate repolarization, are proarrhythmic (36). Conversely, interventions which produce "pure" and homogenous prolongation of the action potential duration with a corresponding lengthening of the absolute refractory period are antiarrhythmic (37), but again, the membrane currents mediating this salutary effect have not been clearly identified.

It is reasonably clear, however, that depression of conduction velocity or unidirectional block may occur as a consequence of attenuated fast response or following its replacement by the slow response, as can occur in cells depolarized by hypoxia or hyperkalemia (22, 28, 29); these are conducive to reentry (29). Reentry which may also result from inhomogeneity in repolarization in subjacent myocardial fibers.

The ionic mechanism underlying enhanced automaticity under pathologic conditions is not clearly understood, but it may be mediated by slow-response–dependent potentials. Of particular interest are the low-voltage oscillations which may be induced in myocardial fibers in sodium-free calcium-rich solutions, hypokalemia, or ischemia; the precise mechanisms for the oscillations of the membrane potential under these conditions possibly are different, but they may all give rise to potentially lethal regenerative depolarizations (29).

CARDIOVASCULAR EFFECTS OF SERUM ELECTROLYTE DISORDERS

Most electrolyte-induced cardiac abnormalities encountered clinically are due to changes in serum potassium, since the imbalance of this ion not only affects nearly all aspects of cardiac function but can also be produced readily by numerous disease states and drug therapies. Fluctuations in serum potassium levels also have clinically significant repercussions on the pharmacologic actions of different therapeutic agents—in particular, cardiac glycosides and local anesthetic antiarrhythmic agents (38). Potassium will therefore receive major emphasis in this chapter, with less extensive discussion of disorders of calcium and magnesium and a passing reference to sodium and the interactions between digitalis and serum electrolyte concentrations. Several signs and symptoms and the etiology of electrolyte disorders have been presented elsewhere in this volume (39; see also Chap. 11).

HYPERKALEMIA

In cardiac muscle hyperkalemia produces two dominant electrophysiologic effects which largely account for the associated electrocardiographic alterations. The first is the depression of conduction velocity, the second an increase in potassium conductance (g_K). Since the resting potential of muscle and Purkinje fibers is essentially the potassium equilibrium potential, increasing extracellular potassium, which decreases the potassium equilibrium potential according to the Nernst equation, will decrease the resting potential. As discussed above, the magnitude of the sodium current—the primary determinant of conduction velocity in muscle and Purkinje fibers—diminishes steadily as the transmembrane resting potential becomes smaller. The consequent sluggish conduction, resulting from reduced upstroke velocity of phase 0, accounts for the disappearing P wave, widening QRS, and the eventual sine wave pattern of the hyperkalemic ECG (see below).

The maximum diastolic potential of the sinoatrial node is independent of changes in extracellular potassium within the range compatible with life (40). This phenomenon, and possibly the early acceleration of AV conduction within a certain range of extracellular potassium concentration, may be ascribed to the second prominent electrophysiologic effect of hyperkalemia, an increase in K conductance. It is intriguing that there appears to be an inverse relationship between g_K and the transmembrane driving force for potassium flow (6). It seems that in hyperkalemia, where the concentration gradient for outward potassium flow is diminished, g_K increases; while in hypokalemia, with an increased gradient, g_K falls (1). Since g_K is already near maximum in resting Purkinje fibers and muscle cells, a small further increase is of little consequence; but it may be that in nodal cells, which normally have a comparatively low g_K, g_K can increase enough to compensate for the depolarizing effect of high extracellular potassium. The resting potential of sinoatrial and AV node cells would not therefore change, or might even increase slightly if g_K rose enough to hyperpolarize the cells.

Although hyperkalemia cannot significantly increase Purkinje and muscle cell g_K at rest, it does increase g_K during repolarization; thus it exaggerates the normal tendency of the repolarizing potassium currents i_x and i_{K1} to speed up as repolarization proceeds.

ELECTROCARDIOGRAPHIC PATTERNS OF
HYPERKALEMIA

Myocardial fibers from various parts of the heart may react somewhat differently to alterations in external potassium concentration, although the effects on atrial, ventricular, and Purkinje fibers are qualitatively similar (41). Atrial fibers are more sensitive to hyperkalemia than those in the ventricular myocardium, while fibers in the nodal and conducting tissues are rather resistant; these properties are reflected in the sequence of evolution of the electrophysiologic and ECG alterations in hyperkalemia (Fig. 5-5). The first change is an increase in the rate of repolarization (phase 3 of the action potential), responsible for the early peaked "tent-shaped" T waves and shortening Q-T_C interval of the ECG. The T-wave amplitude may remain unaltered or may increase somewhat. T-wave

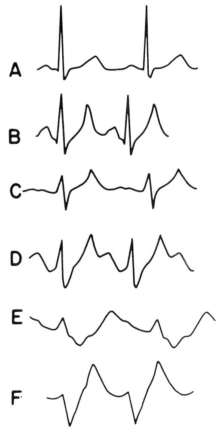

Figure 5-5. Electrocardiographic changes of hyperkalemia. It is a normal record. B through F are arranged to illustrate serial changes of elevated potassium levels. (*From C. R. VanderArk, F. Ballantyne, and E. W. Reynolds,* Complex Electrocardiography I, *1973.*)

changes usually become apparent with serum K_o^+ levels between 5.5 and 6 meq/L (42). AV conduction may be accelerated at this level, and conduction may improve in patients with AV block (43). Ventricular rate may increase in patients with atrial fibrillation (44). As K_o^+ rises further, slowed conduction through ventricular muscle and the His-Purkinje system is reflected in a widening QRS and lengthening P-R interval. At a potassium level of 7 to 7.5 meq/L, slow conduction through atrial muscle is evident as a shrinking, flattened P wave; the QRS continues to widen, and AV nodal conduction is slowed. Eventually, at potassium levels of 8 to 9 meq/L or higher, conduction through atrial muscle fails and the P wave disappears; however, the sinus node, which is relatively resistant to hyperkalemia, may continue to fire. The impulse still travels down through atrial specialized internodal conducting fibers and through the AV node to stimulate the ventricles, producing a "sinoventricular" rhythm (40). The sine wave pattern, with a wide QRS merging with an opposing T wave (Fig. 5-6), presages the development of ventribular fibrillation or asystole if appropriate emergency treatment is not instituted promptly. The wide QRS complexes in the advanced stages of hyperkalemia may also blend with T waves of opposite polarity and simulate complexes of ventricular origin; if the rate is rapid, the mistaken diagnosis of ventricular tachycardia may be made and the correct one of hyperkalemia missed.

Hyperkalemia can also produce ST-segment depression, rarely ST-segment elevation, perhaps as a result of the early onset of repolarization (as in the "early repolarization" normal ECG variant). If such an ST-segment elevation accompanies a simultaneously produced intraventricular conduction defect resulting in QS complexes, the ECG pattern may mimic that of acute transmural myocardial infarction (45). T waves simulating those of hyperkalemia have also been reported in patients with tachycardia, subendocardial infarction, and massive cerebrovascular accident (45).

It is generally believed (46) that K_o^+ concentration, rather than changes in total body K^+ or K_i^+, accounts for the ECG patterns, since changes in K_o^+ affect the K_i^+/K_o^+ ratio more significantly. However, the correlation of serum K_o^+ with ECG

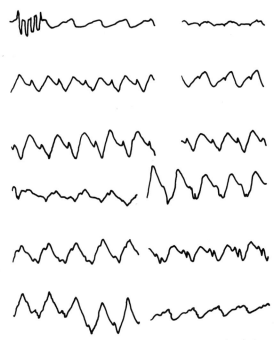

Figure 5-6. Hyperkalemia with a sine wave pattern simulating ventricular tachycardia. (*From C. R. VanderArk, F. Ballantyne, and E. W. Reynolds,* Complex Electrocardiography I, *1973.*)

changes may vary over a wide range, and, occasionally, relatively minor alterations in K_o^+ may be accompanied by striking changes in surface ECG (47). It should also be recognized that the known ECG features of hyperkalemia have been produced experimentally as a result of a virtually "pure" change in serum K_o^+. In the clinical context, the basic patterns may be altered substantially by the associated electrolyte and acid-base abnormalities, concomitant drug therapy, or underlying heart disease. For example, the inverted T waves of left ventricular hypertrophy may become upright, and digitalis may "normalize" the early T-wave changes of hyperkalemia (45). Since most patients with hyperkalemia have varying degrees of acidosis or hyponatremia, it is of particular significance that both acidosis and hyponatremia augment the ECG features and the dangerous electrophysiologic effects of high serum K_o^+. Hyponatremia and acidosis of a significant degree may make a K_o^+ of 6 meq/L a life-threatening emergency; conversely, a K_o^+ of 8 to 8.5 meq/L has been reported with no ECG changes when Na^+ and pH were normal (47). The cardiotoxicity of hyperkalemia may also be potentiated by associated hypocalcemia.

It is important to recognize that although ECG changes correlate poorly with absolute serum K^+ levels, they accurately reflect the electrophysiologic condition of the heart and the patient's risk of dangerous arrhythmias.

ARRHYTHMIAS AND CONDUCTION DISTURBANCES IN HYPERKALEMIA

The overall effects of hyperkalemia on cardiac rhythm and conduction are complex. A gradual stepwise increase in K_o^+ produces a biphasic and usually reproducible sequence: an initial increase followed by a profound decrease in impulse generation and conduction in all cardiac tissues. Clinically, virtually any arrhythmia or conduction disturbance may arise in the setting of hyperkalemia, depending on the rate of increase in K_o^+, associated abnormalities of Na_o^+, Ca_o^{2+}, or pH, underlying disease of the heart and of the conducting system, the status of the autonomic nervous system, and concomitant drug therapy. As in the case of ECG alterations, the observed changes in rhythm and conduction caused by hyperkalemia may be accounted for by diminished conduction velocity or increased potassium conductance or both.

A mild to moderate elevation in K_o^+ (to 6 meq/L) may accelerate AV conduction and shorten the P-R interval, but it is not practical to use IV potassium to improve AV transmission in patients with unstable AV block. Progressive increases in K_o^+ (to levels beyond 6 meq/L) retard AV conduction, but true AV nodal block greater than first degree is rarely seen (48) in cases of uncomplicated hyperkalemia, presumably because of the relative insensitivity to K_o^+ of the cells in the N region of the AV node (46). As already discussed, progressively higher levels of K_o^+ produce a symmetrical generalized slowing of intraventricular conduction, and in patients with latent disease of the conducting system, gross abnormalities may become electrocardiographically

manifest with hyperkalemia. Various forms and combinations of reversible fascicular blocks may be encountered in patients with hyperkalemia, and the QRS morphology may come to resemble the pattern of right or left bundle branch block (49–51). Changes in serum potassium are also clinically significant in patients with artificial pacemakers. Very high levels of K_o^+ increase the threshold of excitability, such that pacemakers may fail because of conduction block out of the pacing site (52). Retardation of conduction in the conducting tissue may be inhomogenous and be associated with unidirectional block. It may thus predispose to reentrant ectopic beats (48). Ventricular fibrillation may occur when ventricular conduction slows to the point where some fibers have recovered excitability before depolarization of others is complete (53). Ventricular tachycardia is not a particularly common arrhythmia in hyperkalemia, but it has been reported in a patient with hyperkalemic periodic paralysis (54).

Although hyperkalemia has little effect on the firing frequency of the normal sinoatrial nodal pacemaker over a wide range of K_o^+, elevated K_o^+ tends to suppress ectopic pacemaker activity in working muscle and Purkinje fibers, probably by increasing potassium conductance so that the inward potassium pacemaker currents decay very slowly. When serum potassium is increased very rapidly, progressive sinus bradycardia (55) or even cardiac arrest following suppression of all pacemakers (48) may occur. These findings are attributable to a sudden marked increase in potassium conductance, which increases outward potassium current to a level where no pacemaker, even the sinus node, is able to depolarize to threshold potential.

TREATMENT OF HYPERKALEMIA

The cardiotoxicity of hyperkalemia is often a medical emergency. The immediate treatment is directed toward the reversal of the deleterious consequences of high external potassium, toward the lowering of serum potassium by driving potassium into the cells, and toward the reduction in the amount of total body potassium. The long-term management is aimed at the control of the underlying disorder and the correction of the precipitating cause. Serum potassium levels between 5 and 7 meq/L associated with narrow QRS complexes may respond to the rectal or oral administration of sodium polystyrene sulfonate resin (Kayexalate), 12 to 16mg tid or qid. The presence of widened QRS or arrhythmias, however, requires urgent treatment. Temporary transvenous ventricular pacing is the preferred modality for asystole, bradycardia, or AV block; tachyarrhythmias caused by hyperkalemia are best treated by the prompt intravenous infusion of sodium or calcium ions under electrocardiographic control.

The infusion of 10 to 20 mL of a 10% solution of calcium gluconate usually produces a beneficial response within 2 min, the effect persisting for 15 to 120 min. Calcium presumably acts by binding to the plasma membrane and altering intramembrane potential. The observed effect is an apparent shift in the activation range of a number of currents—i_{Na}, i_{K1}, and i_{K2}—to more positive transmembrane potentials (56). Hyperkalemia reduces the sodium current by shifting the resting potential to a level where some sodium channels are inactivated; calcium treatment shifts the voltage dependence of i_{Na} correspondingly, reactivating these channels. More available channels means that a larger sodium current flows, resulting in a greater upstroke velocity and faster conduction.

High or low serum sodium (within the range compatible with life) does not have recognizable effects on the heart when other electrolytes are in balance. Hyperkalemia changes this situation, however. When hyperkalemia has reduced the number of available sodium channels, hyponatremia further decreases the sodium current, action potential upstroke, and conduction velocity. Hypertonic saline enhances the i_{Na} and so increases conduction velocity (57). Although hypertonic sodium chloride has been reported to be effective in the treatment of hyperkalemia, sodium bicarbonate ($NaHCO_3$) is now generally used because of the associated acidosis. $NaHCO_3$ may be given as an IV bolus of 45 meq or as an infusion of 90 meq in 500 mL of 10% dextrose in water. A salutary effect is apparent in about 5 min, and lasts several hours. A rapid control of hyperkalemic toxicity may also be achieved by the administration of 50 mL of 50% dextrose with 10 to 25 units of regular insulin, which induces a shift of extracellular potassium into the cell. The onset of action of this regimen occurs within 15 to 60 min, and the effects last several hours. Once the clinical emergency of hyperkalemic cardiotoxicity has been contained, as indicated by the reversal of QRS widening, conduction defects, and arrhythmias, excess potassium ion may be removed from the body by the continued administration of cation exchange resin or by a program of hemo- or peritoneal dialysis.

HYPOKALEMIA

In contrast to hyperkalemia, the major electrophysiologic effects of low extracellular potassium concentration are on cardiac repolarization. These electrophysiologic changes can be ascribed largely to decreased potassium conductance, which appears to result in some way from the increased concentration gradient of potassium across the cell membrane. The decrease in g_K impedes the flow of the repolarization currents i_x and i_{K1}, so that repolarization is prolonged, producing the flat, broad T wave of hypokalemia.

Since the resting potential of working ventricular myocardial cell and Purkinje fiber essentially follows the potassium equilibrium potential, hypokalemia, according to the Nernst equation, should hyperpolarize these cells, with resultant fast conduction and decreased ectopic automaticity. However, the hypokalemic fall in g_K oversets these predictions, causing the resting potential to deviate from the potassium equilibrium potential. In the Purkinje fiber, a decrease in extracellular potassium from 5.4 to 2.7 does not change the resting potential, because g_K is approximately halved (6). At a potassium level of less than 2.7, the Purkinje fiber is actually *depolarized* at rest because of the marked decrease in g_K (6). The slight QRS widening that occurs in severe hypokalemia reflects slow conduction, which may be due to both the decrease in resting potential and the slowing of repolarization to the point where the cell is still partly depolarized when the next conducted impulse impinges on it. Prolonged AV conduction and block have been

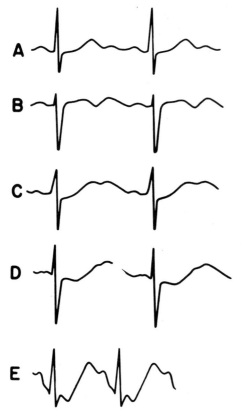

Figure 5-7. Electrocardiographic changes of hyperkalemia. A is a normal record with a typical U wave. B through E are arranged to illustrate serial changes of hypokalemia. (*From C. R. VanderArk, F. Ballantyne, and E. W. Reynolds,* Complex Electrocardiography I, 1973.)

ascribed to the latter effect—that is, it is suggested that AV node cells are still partly refractory when each new conducted impulse arrives, so that their upstroke is diminished correspondingly (45). Both QRS and PR will usually remain within the normal range, their widening detectable only in serial ECGs (45).

ELECTROCARDIOGRAPHIC PATTERNS OF HYPOKALEMIA

From the above electrophysiologic considerations, the ECG patterns of hypokalemia may be inferred. They correlate reasonably well with levels of serum potassium. Progressively severe hypokalemia shows itself in an enlarging U wave, a broad and progressively flattening T wave, ST depression, and, when potassium is very low, in prolonged QRS and P-R intervals (Fig. 5-7). Characteristic ECG changes have been reported in 10 percent of patients with potassium levels between 3 and 3.5, 35 percent with levels between 2.7 and 3, and 78 percent with a level lower than 2.7 meg/L (58). Although not specific, the U wave is particularly helpful in the electrocardiographic recognition of hypokalemia. The normal U wave has the same polarity as the T wave, while having 5 to 50 percent of its amplitude; however, when the U wave voltage exceeds that of the T wave, hypokalemia should be suspected. Moreover, as the severity of hypokalemia increases, the T waves become diminutive and the U waves become prominent, with accompanying ST-segment depression (Fig. 5-8a). It is known, however, that prominent U waves may occur in left ventricular hypertrophy (42) and following the use of drugs that delay cardiac repolarization: quinidine, procainamide, and certain phenothiazine compounds (59, 60). Hypernatremia and alkalosis are also likely to aggravate the electrophysiologic and electrocardiographic manifestations of hypokalemic cardiotoxicity.

ARRHYTHMIAS AND CONDUCTION DISTURBANCES IN HYPOKALEMIA

Unless the degree of hypokalemia is extreme, conduction disturbances are usually minor, and severe hypokalemia may be present without cardiac arrhythmias. Significant AV conduction problems, including complete AV block, have nevertheless been encountered. Ectopic, reentrant, and potentially lethal ventricular and atrial arrhythmias may be induced by hypokalemia. Since hypokalemia decreases potassium conductance, the decay of the pacemaker current (i_{k2}) in the Purkinje fibers is accelerated, producing unifocal or multifocal ectopic beats (Fig. 5-8a). It is noteworthy that hypokalemia provides the ideal setting for reentry to multiply a single ectopic beat into ventricular tachycardia or ventricular fibrilla-

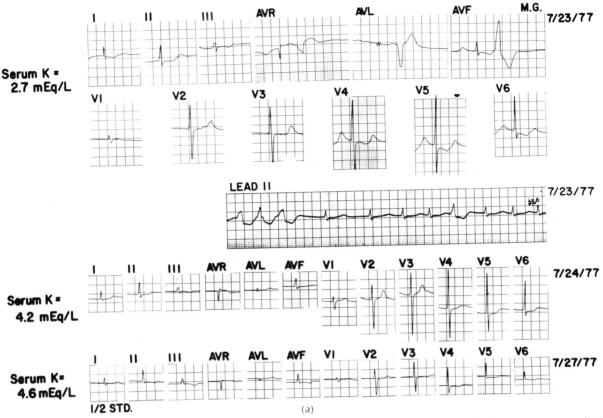

Figure 5-8. (a) Electrocardiographic features and ventricular arrhythmias in a patient with diuretic-induced hypokalemia. Note the prominence of U waves and diminutive T waves, particularly apparent in V2 in the top panel; effect of hypokalemia on intraventricular conduction, apparent at 2.7 meq/L, resolves when serum potassium is restored to 4.6 meq/L. (*From B. N. Singh, unpublished observations, 1977.*) (b) Simultaneous recording of leads I, II, III from a patient with Conn's syndrome showing *torsade de pointes*. Sinus rhythm is shown in the first beat and in the last three beats in which the Q-T appears prolonged; precise measurement is impossible because the succeeding P waves are merged with the preceding T waves. The first four beats of the arrhythmia show tachycardia, bidirectional in leads II and III, succeeded by a run of tachycardia with wide QRS complexes in which the QRS axis rotates, in an undulating fashion, the differences being well shown by comparison of the three leads. The last run of *torsade de pointes* is prolonged, and the QRS complex is more uniform, with a closer resemblance to classic ventricular tachycardia, the arrhythmia terminating with another change in axis for the last four beats. (*From D. M. Krikler and P. V. L. Curry, Br. Heart J., 38:118, 1976.*)

tion. First, slow repolarization exaggerates the normal differences in the timing of repolarization throughout the heart, so that ectopic beats are more likely to fall in the "vulnerable period" of the T-U complex. Second, because Purkinje fibers are rapidly depolarizing during diastole, they are at a lower than normal membrane potential when they are fully depolarized by conducted stimulus. Thus they have a lower upstroke velocity, conduct more sluggishly, and are prone to block (61).

A complex interplay of ectopy and reentry has been suggested as the mechanism of the unusual

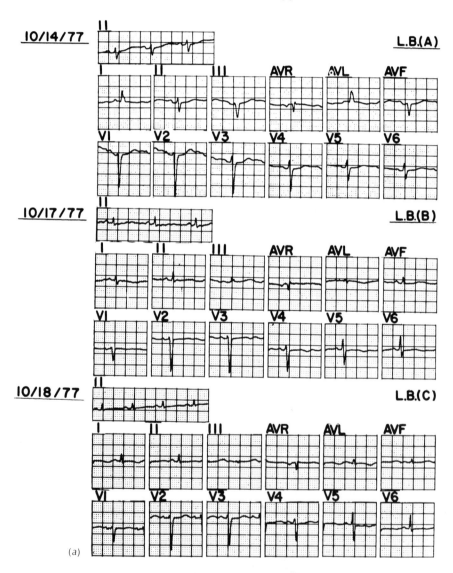

(a)

Figure 5-9. (a) ECG patterns in a patient on liquid protein diet for 5 months with a 90-lb weight loss. The initial tracing (10/14/77) is compatible with hypokalemia, but the serum level was 3.9 meq/ L, serum magnesium, 1.8 meq/L and calcium, 8.8 mg/100 dl. (*From B. N. Singh, et al, JAMA, in press, 1978.*) (*b*) Ventricular arrhythmias (*torsade*) in the same patient (see Fig. 5-9(*a*) associated with

bidirectional ventricular tachycardia called *torsade de pointes* (Fig. 5-8*b*), frequently reported in the context of hypokalemia, rarely in that of hypomagnesemia (62). *Torsade* has occurred following ordinary gastrointestinal and diuretic-induced potassium loss, in Conn's syndrome, and in hypokalemic familial periodic paralysis (62). If the arrhythmia is due to hypokalemia, it may respond to potassium replacement. It is of interest that the arrhythmia is usually initiated by an extrasystole occurring late rather than early in diastole and may often be self-terminating, presenting with recurrent syncope. However, *torsade* does have a dangerous propensity to degenerate into ventricular fibrillation, especially if treated with agents which further delay the repolarization phase of the cardiac action potential. ECG features virtually identical to those of hypokalemia associated with sudden death from *torsade* have recently been described in young female patients on liquid protein (300 calories daily with and without potassium supplements) weight-reducing diets (63). In such patients serum potassium is not always low, and other electrolytes may be normal. *Torsade* has been treated successfully in one patient (Fig. 5-9) by diphenylhydantoin, an antiarrhythmic compound which accelerates rather than delays cardiac repolarization.

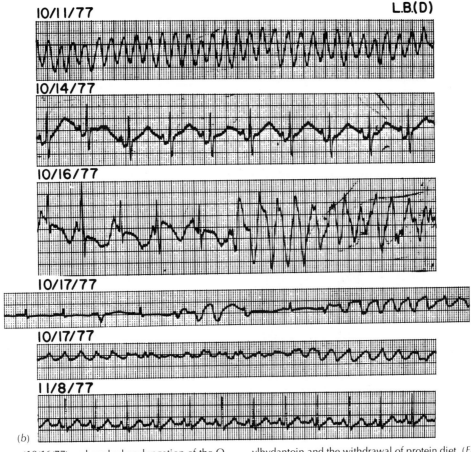

(b)

prominent U waves (10/16/77) and marked prolongation of the Q-U interval. Complete resolution of the changes occur on diphenylhydantoin and the withdrawal of protein diet. (*From B. N. Singh, et al.,* JAMA, *in press, 1978.*)

TREATMENT OF HYPOKALEMIA

Patients with hypokalemia who have a deficit of total body potassium require replacement therapy, usually 5 to 10 g of potassium chloride daily in divided doses, given orally. Parenteral administration may be necessary in cases of hypokalemia associated with arrhythmias and conduction disturbances. However, intravenous administration of potassium should be undertaken in conjunction with a careful monitoring of the ECG and frequent determinations of serum potassium even in cases of severe electrolyte deficits. Rapidly rising serum potassium is dangerous not only to the normokalemic patient becoming hyperkalemic but also to the hypokalemic patient receiving potassium replacement. Since the effects of excess potassium depend on the extracellular to intracellular *gradient* of potassium rather than on absolute potassium levels, untoward reactions may be precipitated even in the hypokalemic patient during rapid infusion of potassium ion.

POTASSIUM BALANCE AND CARDIAC CONTRACTILITY

There is a remarkable paucity of data, clinical as well as experimental, in regard to alterations in cardiac inotropy with varying levels of serum potassium. Acutely induced hypokalemia in the experimental animal has been associated with a positive inotropic effect (64), the mechanism of which is poorly understood; in contrast, chronic severe potassium deficiency may lead to cardiac enlargement and, presumably, diminished contractility (65). Experimentally it has been shown that calcium uptake by the sarcoplasmic reticulum requires potassium ions (66) and that uptake is reduced in the sarcoplasmic reticulum of chronically potassium-depleted hearts (67). In chronically potassium-depleted cats, cardiac contractility was found to be depressed to a degree corresponding to the reduction in the sarcoplasmic reticulum calcium binding (68). The clinical significance of the experimental observations is, however, uncertain. It is also known that a rapid increase in serum potassium tends to depress contractility and may exacerbate congestive heart failure, but again

the mechanism of this negative inotropic effect is not understood. It is conceivable that the acceleration of repolarization with the shortening of the action potential may decrease the amount of calcium that can enter the myocardial cell before each heartbeat (1). No clinical studies of ventricular function in hyperkalemia have been reported, but in dogs, systemic arterial pressure and left ventricular dp/dt (index of contractility) remained unchanged until serum potassium levels exceeded 10 meg/L. The left ventricular filling pressure rose progressively thereafter, with parallel reductions in contraction and conduction velocity that suggest the reduction in cardiac performance may have resulted from asynchronous activation of the ventricular myocardium (55).

POTASSIUM AND MYOCARDIAL INFARCTION

Potassium ion may play a particularly significant role in the genesis of arrhythmias following coronary occlusion (69). Rapid egress of potassium from the ischemic myocardium into the venous effluent may precede ventricular ectopy, and both potassium loss and ectopy can be reduced by procainamide (70). Myocardial ischemia leads to an increase in the K_o^+/K_i^+ ratio, and regional hyperkalemia may induce focal inhomogeneity of refractoriness and conduction, changes which favor ventricular fibrillation. Of interest is the observation that during myocardial ischemia a striking epicardial conduction delay may precede the onset of ventricular arrhythmias (71). Similarly, it has been demonstrated in vitro that high concentrations of K_o^+ in conjunction with epinephrine may retard conduction in strands of Purkinje fibers and papillary muscle to the extent that reentry could develop (29). It is conceivable that the local release of potassium and catecholamines may induce reentrant arrhythmias by a similar mechanism in ischemic muscle in patients with acute myocardial infarction. Of much interest are the observations of Dyckner et al. (72), who found a significant degree of hypokalemia in 15 percent of 444 patients with acute myocardial infarction. The cause of hypokalemia was not clear, but the hypokalemic patients had a significant higher incidence of sinus bradycardia, atrial flutter and fibrillation, ventricular premature beats, and ventricular tachycardia. These findings are of practical significance insofar as the actions of most antiarrhythmic drugs used in the control of dysrhythmias complicating infarction may be potassium-dependent (73).

CARDIAC ELECTROPHYSIOLOGICAL EFFECTS OF ALTERED SERUM CALCIUM

Serum calcium levels outside the physiologic range primarily affect repolarization with relatively trivial influence on depolarization or AV conduction. However, only extremely high or low serum calcium levels produce electrophysiologic abnormalities of clinical significance.

Repolarization

In ventricular muscle (74) and Purkinje fibers (75), hypercalcemia virtually abolishes the plateau phase of the action potential (Fig. 5-10) without affecting the resting membrane potential.

As the plateau abbreviates, so does the ST segment of the ECG. In Purkinje fibers, all phases of repolarization are accelerated (75, 76), but only initial repolarization is accelerated in ventricular muscle (74). Since the total time required for repolarization in the ventricular muscle mass does not decrease, and perhaps because repolarization throughout the ventricle does not become better synchronized, the T wave does not narrow or increase in amplitude, as it does in hyperkalemia. In Fig. 5-10, from Hoffman and Suckling (74), it may be seen that the overall rate of repolarization (slope of phase 3) is actually decreased at the very high calcium concentration used in that experiment; this slowing may account for the widening T wave at calcium levels above 16 mg/dL.

Hypercalcemia increases the inward calcium current and thus exerts a positive inotropic effect in heart muscle. Logically, therefore, it would seem that the plateau should be lengthened, not shortened. However, the increase in i_{Ca} is more than countered by enhancement of the repolarization currents i_x and i_{K1}. In Purkinje fibers, i_x

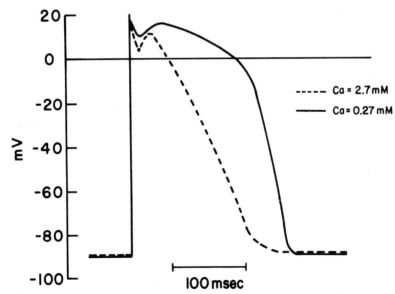

Figure 5-10. A tracing of transmembrane action potentials recorded from a papillary muscle in varying external calcium levels. Note the abbreviation of the plateau phase in high calcium concentration. (*From Hoffman and Suckling*, Am. J. Physiol., *186:317, 1956.*)

appears to be activated early by the higher (more positive) plateau produced by the surge of calcium current (76); Isenberg (77) produced a high plateau and rapid repolarization by injecting calcium into Purkinje fibers with a microelectrode (Fig. 5-11). i_{K1} is also activated early, but apparently by increased extracellular rather than intracellular calcium (76). It may be that increased membrane calcium binding raises the activation range of i_{K1}, like that of i_{Na}, to more positive transmembrane potential (76). The response of the repolarization currents in ventricular muscle cells is assumed to be similar, though not identical (76), but it has not been studied specifically.

Low extracellular calcium lengthens the plateau, presumably because activation of the repolarization currents (and so *onset* of repolarization)

is delayed, but does not affect the *rate* of repolarization in ventricular muscle (74). Thus the ST segment lengthens, but the T wave does not.

Depolarization

In shifting the activation range of i_{Na} to more positive transmembrane potentials, hypercalcemia increases the amplitude of i_{Na} in a cell depolarized by hyperkalemia. Paradoxically, in a normal cell the shift actually *decreases* the amplitude of i_{Na} by accentuating the difference between the resting potential and threshold potential, which is known to decrease the action potential upstroke. Since high extracellular calcium diminishes upstroke velocity in ventricular muscle cells (75), it will diminish conduction velocity and widen the QRS.

Atrioventricular conduction

The basis for hypercalcemic depression of AV conduction has not been demonstrated experimentally. However, it is known that high calcium perfusion increases the sinus rate (78), enhancing the slope of diastolic depolarization presumably by increasing the inward calcium current. If it is assumed that a similar process occurs in the closely related AV node cells, then it might be expected that these cells will depolarize to a greater than usual degree by the time of arrival of an oncoming conducted action potential. Since the amplitude of i_{Ca} falls with a decrease in the potential from which the cell is depolarized to threshold (7), the upstroke of the AV node cell would be diminished and conduction would slow. Thus the P-R interval would be prolonged, and block might occur in susceptible hearts.

The electrocardiographic effects of altered serum calcium are predictable from the known effects on transmembrane potentials and currents. A typical tracing from a patient with severe hypocalcemia is shown in Fig. 5-12. The major change is a lengthening of the ST segment with a resultant increase in te Q-T_C interval. The duration of the T wave is not usually affected by hypocalcemia, but it may develop a more peaked

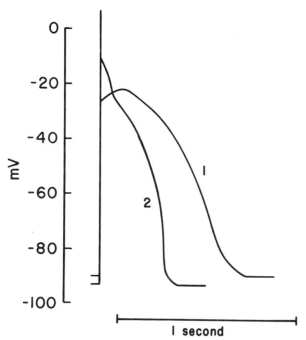

Figure 5-11. Transmembrane action potential changes illustrating the effect of iontophoretically injected Ca²⁺ in cardiac Purkinje fibers. In the superimposed tracings, *1* represents the control action potential and *2* after iontophoresis. Note the hyperpolarization and considerable shortening of the action potential duration, consistent with the possibility that the level of intracellular Ca²⁺ can affect the potassium permeability in cardiac muscle. (*From G. Isenberg,* Nature, *253:273, 1975.*)

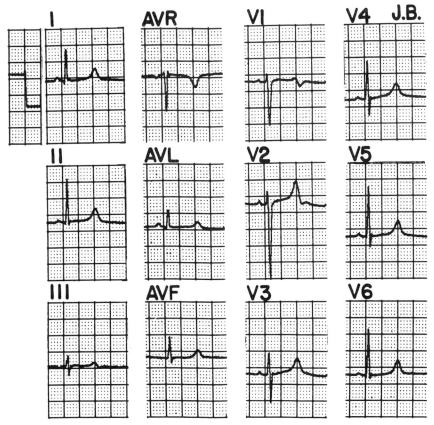

Figure 5-12. Effect of hypocalcemia (4.6 mg/100 dL) on the ECG in a patient with idiopathic hypoparathyroidism. Note the prolonged Q-T$_c$ interval caused by the lengthening of the ST segment without change in the width of T wave or QRS. There is no change in AV conduction. (*Courtesy of V. Kamdar and G. Braunstein, unpublished observations, 1977.*)

appearance; a decrease in the duration of the QRS complex is trivial, not recognizable clinically. Similarly, changes in P wave and P-R intervals are not usually seen in clinical hypocalcemia. As might be expected, a marked decrease in the length of the ST segment is the major electrocardiographic manifestation of hypercalcemia, reflected in a decrease in the Q-T$_c$ interval. When serum calcium is below 16 mg/dL, the T wave is not usually altered in duration, but it may be somewhat less peaked in appearance. At serum calcium levels above 16 mg/dL, the T wave may broaden, with the Q-T$_c$ interval tending to return

toward a more normal duration. Hypercalcemia may slightly prolong the QRS and the PR interval, though not dramatically.

CARDIAC ARRHYTHMIAS IN HYPOCALCEMIA AND HYPERCALCEMIA

Arrhythmias and disturbances of conduction in the clinic are rare in hypocalcemia as well as hypercalcemia, an observation which is consistent with the finding that, in the presence of normal levels of K_o^+ and Mg_o^{2+}, extremely large fluctuations in Ca_o^{2+} are needed to affect the shape or amplitude of the cardiac action potential (34). Sporadic cases of cardiac dysrhythmias and conduction defects in hypocalcemic and hypercalcemic syndromes have been reported (45). However, for a given level of serum calcium outside the physiologic range, only a few patients will develop abnormalities of rhythm and conduction.

The prolongation of the Q-T$_C$ interval produced by hypocalcemia may or may not contribute to arrhythmogenesis. It is not known whether prolongation reflects homogenous or heterogenous lengthening of repolarization throughout the heart. If this reflected a homogenous lengthening of repolarization, the absolute refractory period would be prolonged, with a consequent reduction in excitability and in the probability of an arrhythmia. Indeed, isolated or "pure" prolongation of the action potential duration as in hypothyroidism (79) or by the chronic administration of the drug amiodarone (80) has been shown to constitute an antiarrhythmic mechanism. Thus, at least under certain circumstances, hypocalcemia may also be antiarrhythmic, and it is conceivable that calcium-chelating agents in digitalis intoxication may exert their salutary effect, at least in part, through this mechanism. Prolongation of the Q-T$_C$ interval as an isolated phenomenon also occurs as a hereditary syndrome (81) in which recurrent episodes of ventricular tachycardia or ventricular fibrillation form the basis for syncope or sudden death. In such cases it is likely that delayed repolarization is not homogenous; the temporal dispersion in the recovery of excitability may lead to reentrant arrhythmias. A similar mechanism may be postulated to be responsible for certain arrhythmias noted in hypocalcemia. Ectopy is uncommon in hypocalcemia, but supraventricular tachycardia with sinoatrial block (82), 2:1 AV block (83), as well as complete heart block responding to intravenous calcium infusion (84) have all been reported, especially in children. Although ventricular fibrillation may be produced with relative ease in experimental hypocalcemia in animals (42), hypocalcemia as a cause of ventricular tachycardia or fibrillation is rare in clinical practice. A patient with recalcitrant ventricular fibrillation was, however, reported recently; successful defibrillation could be achieved only after serum calcium was restored toward normal levels (85). As might be predicted, hypocalcemia facilitates the development of intraventricular and atrioventricular block and ventricular fibrillation in patients with hyperkalemia (86). Patients with renal failure are particularly prone to develop both these electrolyte disturbances.

Hypercalcemia rarely produces arrhythmias except in the digitalized patient. In primary hyperparathyroidism, first-degree and second-degree AV block of the Wenckebach type, sinus arrest, and paroxysmal atrial fibrillation have been reported (87, 88). The arrhythmias were abolished by removal of the parathyroid adenoma. It is recognized that acute rises in serum calcium can produce sinus bradycardia or even sinus arrest (86).

Severe hypercalcemia will produce extrasystoles, ventricular tachycardia, and ventricular fibrillation in intact experimental animals (75). Hypercalcemia accelerates pacemaker activity in Purkinje fibers by shifting the activation range of the pacemaker current i_{K2} to more positive potentials (10), so that the outward potassium current starts to decay even before full repolarization is reached. As discussed above, hypercalcemia may slow conduction by decreasing i_{Na}. It also shortens the refractory period in Purkinje fibers, since repolarization is accelerated, thus providing the necessary background to reentrant arrhythmias. Thus it seems reasonable that high calcium should be considered as a possible pathogenetic factor if arrhythmias develop in a hypercalcemic patient.

CARDIAC FAILURE AND ALTERED SERUM CALCIUM

Despite the dependence of contraction on calcium, chronic hypocalcemia does not appear to be associated with heart failure, but marked reduction in ventricular function may follow acutely induced depression of serum calcium levels. Heart failure caused by hypocalcemia has been reported in neonatal hypocalcemia (89), in the "hungry bone syndrome" immediately following surgery for severe hyperparathyroidism (90), and intraoperatively after rapid transfusion of calcium-binding citrated whole blood (91). Failure may be marked, with acute hypotension or pulmonary edema. Hypocalcemia should be suspected when failure develops following parathyroid surgery or therapy with effective calcium-lowering agents such as mithramycin or intravenous phosphate.

CALCIUM AND CARDIOMYOPATHY

Calcium overload is toxic to cells, all of which maintain a low cytoplasmic free calcium by energetically gathering up that ion into mitochondria and sarcoplasmic reticulum and by extruding it to the extracellular fluid. It is now felt that calcium may be the final mediator of cellular destruction for a variety of agents which produce experimental cardiac necrosis. The toxic agents—catecholamines, cardiac glycosides, vitamin D—all increase cytoplasmic calcium and in massive doses appear to overwhelm the cell with it. Cell death is ascribed to exhaustion of ATP supply caused by activation of calcium-stimulated ATPases and to poisoning of mitochondria by calcium overload (92–95).

It has been suggested that myopathic and some failing hearts may share a common defect: poor calcium uptake by the sarcoplasmic reticulum. This deficiency has been observed in human hearts removed from transplant patients with severe atherosclerotic coronary disease (96), and experimentally in potassium-depletion cardiomyopathy (67), bacterial infective cardiomyopathy (97), failure consequent on hypertrophy (98) and on pulmonary hypertension (99), the hereditary cardiomyopathy of the Syrian hamster (100) (an animal that dies young with a necrotic heart), and in fragmented sarcoplasmic reticulum exposed to ethanol (101). It is possible that when the sarcoplasmic reticulum loses its usual capacity, mitochondria, which bear in most cell types the primary responsibility for clearing excess calcium from the cytoplasm, start to take up more and more calcium in an attempt to maintain homeostasis (47, 69, 102). As mitochondria become more and more burdened with calcium, phosphorylation rate and metabolic efficiency progressively fall (69). This possibility awaits experimental verification, but it permits the hope that drugs such as verapamil (13) that inhibit calcium entry into cardiac cells might slow the relentless course of some progressive cardiomyopathies or protect the myocardium of the patient with acute coronary occlusion (103). Verapamil can completely prevent myocardial necrosis in the cardiomyopathic Syrian hamster (104).

MAGNESIUM

There is still a paucity of data dealing with the cardiac effects of alterations in the tissue and serum levels of magnesium ions. It is recognized, however, that magnesium is essential for basic metabolic processes, including oxidative phosphorylation, and for the maintenance of cell volume [as a cofactor for membrane sodium-potassium-activated ATPase ($Na^+–K^+–ATPase$)] and mitochondrial integrity (105). Cardiac muscle has high concentrations of magnesium (106), but translocations of this cation, as far as is known, are not involved in the normal action potential, in conduction or in contraction; nor does magnesium deficiency or excess, except at the point of near-paralysis, have specific, readily recognizable cardiac effects.

Magnesium deficiency and cardiac arrhythmias

Magnesium deficiency has been most clearly associated with arrhythmias caused by digitalis toxicity (vide infra), but there have been a few case reports of arrhythmias caused by magnesium deficiency per se in nondigitalized patients: supraventricular tachycardia refractory to all measures but magnesium replacement (107), paroxysmal ventricular fibrillation (108), asystole, and ventricular tachycardia (109). The latter two occurred in a 13-year-old girl successfully treated for diabetic ketoacidosis, a condition in which large quantities of magnesium are commonly lost and in which concomitant acidosis and hypokalemia may obscure magnesium depletion as the source of arrhythmias.

The arrhythmias of magnesium deficiency are

probably due to the loss of intracellular potassium, since without adequate magnesium, cells are unable to maintain normal concentrations of intracellular potassium. The potassium released by cells is subsequently lost from the body, and this manifests as hypokalemia (110). It will be difficult or impossible to replace the lost potassium until magnesium deficiency is corrected, since the administered potassium is not retained by the cells.

Experimentally, it has been shown that perfusion with low magnesium shortens the effective or absolute refractory period of cardiac muscle cells and lengthens their relative refractory period (111). Within each cardiac cycle there is therefore a somewhat longer period during which a premature impulse will find a partially refractory myocardium and will induce the low-amplitude, slowly conducting action potentials which may produce ventricular ectopy or fibrillation. Perfusion with high magnesium concentration has the opposite effect, lengthening the effective refractory period and shortening the relative refractory period. Ghani and Rabah (112) showed that intravenous magnesium increased the threshold for ventricular premature contractions and ventricular fibrillation in normal as well as in digitalized dogs.

ECG changes in magnesium depletion

Reproducible changes in the electrocardiogram can be demonstrated in animals by moderate to severe magnesium depletion; similar changes have been noted in some but not all severely magnesium-depleted human subjects (113, 114). The changes are, however, best seen in the experimental situation, where the picture is not distorted by other primary electrolyte deficiencies, cardiomyopathy, congestive heart failure, or associated drug therapy.

Animals with early magnesium depletion, before the onset of hypokalemia, develop tall, peaked T waves, slight widening of the QRS, and sometimes mild ST depression. These changes may reflect a relative hyperkalemia caused by the loss of intracellular potassium (115). Animals and human subjects with severe magnesium deficiency (0.2 to 0.6 meq/L [110]) and secondary hypokalemia and hypocalcemia show prolonged P-R interval, wide QRS, slight ST depression, and broad and flat or inverted T waves (110, 115). Shils (110) found T-wave abnormalities most clear-cut in his magnesium-depleted subjects and also observed prolonged Q-T intervals compatible with hypocalcemia. The observed changes did not, however, regress with magnesium repletion alone, but required correction of the coexistent hypocalcemia and hypokalemia. Clear ECG changes occurred in only three of the six subjects, and all those subjects who showed ECG changes were also markedly symptomatic from their electrolyte deficiencies (tetany, weakness, etc.).

The ECG changes seen in alcoholic cardiomyopathy can resemble those of magnesium deficiency, but the effect of magnesium depletion and repletion on the ECG in this disorder has not been studied.

Magnesium and ischemic heart disease

In Europe and Canada, much more than in the United States, epidemiologists have noted that ischemic heart disease is less prevalent in regions with hard drinking water (116–118). Hard water is high in magnesium, and the suggestion has been made that it is the higher cardiac muscle magnesium content that protects against the development of coronary artery disease in hard-water areas (119). Two lines of evidence support this hypothesis. In some studies of accidental death victims from hard- and soft-water areas, the hard-water drinkers were found to have higher cardiac muscle or coronary artery magnesium levels (120, 121). These findings, however, have not gone unchallenged (122). There are more convincing data suggesting that patients dying of cardiac conditions tend to have lower myocardial magnesium than do those dying of other causes (119, 123). Clearly, further work is needed in determining the precise significance of altered magnesium metabolism in different cardiac disorders and of the role of magnesium in the genesis and control of cardiac arrhythmias.

EFFECTS OF ELECTROLYTES ON THE ACTION OF ANTIARRHYTHMIC DRUGS AND DIGITALIS

Although alterations in the serum levels of K^+, Ca^{2+}, Na^+, and Mg^{2+} all may change the cardiac actions of many antiarrhythmic drugs and digitalis, in the clinical setting the effects of altered potassium concentration are the most striking and of the greatest therapeutic significance.

ANTIARRHYTHMIC DRUGS

It is known that those antiarrhythmic drugs which have potent local anesthetic effects on nerve (e.g., quinidine, lidocaine, procainamide), exert their principal electrophysiologic effects by depressing the upstroke velocity of phase 0 and that of phase 4. Both these parameters, at least in the Purkinje fibers, are also affected importantly by alterations in K_o^+. Since the resting membrane potential in cardiac muscle is a function of the ratio K_i^+/K_o^+, a small decrease in K_o^+ will hyperpolarize the cells, and this itself would increase the maximal rate of depolarization (MRD). Consequently, drugs such as quinidine and lidocaine, which act by depressing the MRD, would be much less effective in low-potassium solution (38). Clinical relevance of this fact to the treatment of dysrhythmias is illustrated by the case of a patient with a ventricular tachycardia and a serum potassium of 3.1 meq/L. The patient failed to respond to 2 mg propranolol IV plus 500 mg lidocaine IV plus 2 mg/min lidocaine infusion, but after serum potassium had been raised to 4.4 meq/L by an infusion of 60 meq of potassium chloride, sinus rhythm was restored by lidocaine, 2 mg/min (124). Resistance to the effects of antiarrhythmic agents may be particularly relevant in patients with acute myocardial infarction and in those after open-heart surgery, in whom varying levels of hypokalemia may be encountered (72, 125).

As might be expected, mild increases in serum potassium may function as an antiarrhythmic mechanism by depressing phase 4 depolarization in Purkinje fibers, and by reducing the resting membrane potential, which will reduce the MRD.

Thus, the effects of hyperkalemia and local anesthetic antiarrhythmic drugs on the MRD and conduction velocity will be additive; in low dose ranges, the therapeutic effects of these drugs will be potentiated, whereas with high doses, toxicity will be augmented by hyperkalemia. As with hyperkalemic cardiotoxicity, the toxic effects on atrioventricular and intraventricular conduction of the drugs that act by depression of the MRD can be reversed by the administration of sodium chloride or sodium lactate (126).

DIGITALIS

The cellular mechanisms whereby digitalis glycosides exert their inotropic, antiarrhythmic, and arrhythmogenic actions in cardiac muscle are still not completely understood, although there have been rapid advances recently in our knowledge of their action on the heart. The interaction of digoxin and serum electrolytes in the clinical context has long been appreciated and is particularly noteworthy in relation to AV conduction and to the genesis of arrhythmias in glycoside cardiotoxicity. Normal cardiac contraction depends upon the calcium which enters the cytoplasm before each heartbeat. The slow calcium current probably provides about 10 percent of the total amount of calcium required for maximum force development (127), the source of the remainder still being uncertain. It is possible that the slow current triggers the release of the remaining calcium from the sarcoplasmic reticulum, as in skeletal muscle (128), but the evidence for this is not entirely convincing. On the other hand, Langer (129, 130) has proposed that the source of the calcium is a glycoprotein coat, external to the sarcolemma, the sialic acid residues of which bind calcium. This calcium can be displaced from its binding sites, and its presence thereby demonstrated, by the heavy metal lanthanum (131). The calcium is thought to enter the cell via a carrier which exchanges intracellular sodium for extracellular calcium and which is stimulated by increases in the ratio Na_i^+/Na_o^+.

All positive inotropic agents, including digitalis, increase the amount of intracellular calcium for excitation-contraction coupling, but they accomplish this in different ways. Adrenergic stimulants increase the slow inward calcium current, but digitalis does not (132). Digitalis has two effects, both of which probably contribute to increased inotropy (133). Glycoside binding to sarcolemmal Na^+–K^+–ATPase, its probable receptor (134), appears to alter membrane structure in such a way that the amount of externally bound calcium increases (135, 136). More calcium is then available to be transported inward for contraction. In Langer's still controversial formulation (137, 138), the sodium/calcium exchange system is coupled to the sodium-potassium pump. Digitalis inhibits Na^+–K^+–ATPase, which provides energy to the sodium-potassium pump; consequently, Na_i^+ increases, which in turn stimulates sodium-calcium exchange and increases intracellular calcium. The loss of intracellular potassium produced by pump inhibition does not increase inotropy (139, 140), but may be related to digitalis toxicity (140–142).

ELECTROPHYSIOLOGY OF DIGITALIS-TOXIC ARRHYTHMIAS

Although digitalis-toxic arrhythmias have been well described, the precise mechanisms of their causation have not. In in vitro preparations, the appearance of arrhythmias is temporally related to Na^+–K^+–ATPase inhibition (143), and evidence of an indirect nature links digitalis-toxic arrhythmias to myocardial potassium loss (140, 141). However, the precise sequence of events from Na^+–K^+–ATPase inhibition to the appearance of arrhythmias has not yet been established.

Digitalis is said to enhance automaticity, an effect thought to be the basis for the ventricular and supraventricular premature contractions as well as the ectopic ventricular and junctional tachycardias produced by toxic concentrations of glycosides. In fact, digitalis may *suppress* the pre-existing pacemaker mechanism of ventricular cells (144), and it is likely that it increases automaticity, like contractility, by mechanisms unique to itself (18, 19). Electrophysiologic studies over a

decade ago demonstrated differences between digitalis-induced "repetitive ventricular response" and "normal" idioventricular rhythm. Idioventricular rhythms in the absence of digitalis usually do not develop in the face of a faster supraventricular rate; in contrast, digitalis-toxic ventricular rhythms may be *induced* by rapid supraventricular rates. Such arrhythmias generally do not appear unless the underlying rate is rapid. It is common knowledge that the usual forms of idioventricular rhythms are susceptible to overdrive suppression, whereas digitalis-toxic rhythms demonstrate the phenomenon of postpacing acceleration; that is, the faster a digitalis-toxic preparation is paced, the earlier the ectopic tachycardia will appear and the more rapid will be its rate (144, 145).

This anomalous behavior has been explained by the electrophysiologic demonstration of the phenomenon of the "transient depolarization" or "oscillatory afterpotential" (OAP). Recordings of action potentials from atrial or ventricular specialized conducting fibers exposed to digitalis (146) show that repolarization is followed by a small secondary depolarization, the OAP (18, 19). The OAP appears to have the same electrophysiologic characteristics as the repetitive ventricular response of digitalis toxicity. Its amplitude is generally small (though higher glycoside concentrations increase it), but both its amplitude and its coupling interval depend on the preceding cycle length; in a cell paced at a faster rate, a more closely coupled, higher-amplitude OAP is produced. A premature beat similarly evokes a high-amplitude OAP. If the OAP has sufficient amplitude to attain threshold, it will produce a premature contraction resembling a reentrant beat (147). This beat in turn will be followed by an OAP, which may then reach threshold; thus a self-sustaining tachycardia, like the accelerated junctional and ventricular rhythms seen clinically, can develop in digitalis toxicity.

Even OAPs which are not of sufficient amplitude to reach threshold can be manipulated experimentally to produce complex rhythm disturbances, and all of the characteristic digitalis-toxic arrhythmias can be so reproduced (147). The ionic mechanism underlying OAP is still not entirely understood (20). However, it is known that OAPs cannot be induced in the absence of calcium, and very high concentrations of calcium can evoke trains of OAPs in the absence of digitalis (148). OAPs can be abolished by manganese ion (147) or the drug verapamil (149), both of which block calcium entry into myocardial cells.

DIGITALIS AND CALCIUM

Hypercalcemia may aggravate all forms of cardiac toxicity produced by digitalis. Since digitalis increases cellular calcium uptake, and OAPs are calcium-dependent, the synergism between calcium and digitalis with respect to the generation of ectopic beats, bigeminy, and accelerated rhythms appears to be reasonably clear. Why calcium should enhance digitalis-induced sinus bradycardia and atrioventricular block is less clear, since the ionic bases of these disturbances of rhythm are not known.

Hypercalcemia increases the amount of calcium bound to the sarcolemma (136), but it has not been experimentally verified that calcium entry into cardiac cells increases likewise, though this seems a logical assumption. Calcium also inhibits Na^+–K^+–ATPase, but it takes only a rather low concentration of calcium to do this (134), and the effect is probably not increased by hypercalcemia.

At least one of the calcium antagonists (verapamil, nifedipine, D_{600}) has been shown to inhibit the development of digitalis-toxic tachycardia and AV block (150). Though none of these drugs is currently available for clinical use in the United States, they may prove effective in the immediate treatment of digitalis-toxic arrhythmias. In this context, it is of interest that insensitivity to digoxin in the presence of hypocalcemia has recently been reported (151). The significance of the observation that ectopic beats produced by excess digitalis are suppressed by lowering calcium concentration by Na_2 edetic acid (EDTA) (152, 153), needs to be evaluated in light of the finding that Na_2 EDTA is equally effective in suppressing ectopic tachyarrhythmias in digitalized and nondigitalized patients (153).

DIGITALIS AND POTASSIUM

It is generally known that hypokalemia predisposes to digitalis toxicity, and potassium replacement can avert and reverse digitalis-induced arrhythmias. For example, of 12 stable patients taking digitalis and diuretics placed on low-potassium diets by Steiners and Olesen (154), six developed ventricular extrasystole, bigeminy, or first-degree AV block within one week, although their mean serum potassium level was still near normal (3.4 meq/L). Experimentally, hypokalemic dogs given digitalis infusions develop ventricular tachycardia much faster than normokalemic animals similarly treated (155). Both potassium depletion and acute hypokalemia without depletion, as may be produced by carbohydrate infusion with or without insulin, are capable of provoking digitalis-toxic arrhythmias (156).

The effect of potassium on the electrophysiologic perturbations produced by digitalis has not been extensively studied. Ferrier and Moe (19) found that the amplitude of digitalis-induced oscillatory afterpotentials could be altered by changing the extracellular potassium concentration. Subthreshold OAPs seen at 4 mmol K^+ reached threshold and produced self-sustaining tachycardias at 2 mmol K^+. OAPs are suppressed by increased potassium in both atrium and ventricle (146).

It is unlikely that all possible mechanisms for the interaction of digitalis and potassium have been fully elucidated. It is reasonably certain, however, that potassium inhibits the binding of digitalis to its membrane receptor. When myocardial cells are first exposed to digitalis and then to increased extracellular potassium, some of the bound digitalis is released (157); when myocardial cells are bathed in potassium during digitalis infusion, digitalis uptake is less in higher extracellular potassium concentrations (158). The implication, therefore, is that higher potassium, while suppressing arrhythmias, will also decrease inotropy, as has been documented experimentally (159, 160). Of interest is the observation that hypokalemia may predispose to digitalis toxicity independently of increased glycoside binding or a change in inotropy (155, 156), so that arrhythmias and contractility may not necessarily be suppressed equally by increases in potassium concentration.

Although their findings have not as yet been verified in human beings, Gelbart et al. (155) showed that *chronically* potassium-depleted dogs have markedly impaired inotropic responses to digitalis and to isoprenaline. From their findings Gelbart et al. infer that potassium repletion in patients not only averts arrhythmias, but restores the normal inotropic response.

The increased sensitivity to digitalis in the presence of hypokalemia may prove troublesome in renal dialysis and excessive diuresis and during both gastrointestinal loss of K^+ ions and the administration of dextrose or steroids. The loss of intracellular K^+ caused by chronic heart failure may also predispose to digitalis toxicity, accounting for the increased sensitivity of the severely diseased heart to digitalis. These observations provide the basis for the widespread use of potassium therapy in digitalis toxicity complicated by atrial or ventricular arrhythmias. However, the effects of IV infusion may prove hazardous in digoxin toxicity if administration is at an inappropriately rapid rate; this may occasionally produce a striking depression of conduction, be it sinoatrial, intra-atrial, atrioventricular, or intraventricular (48). Of particular interest is the interaction of potassium and digitalis on AV conduction, since both extremes, high and low serum K^+, may depress AV conduction. It is known that moderate hyperkalemia may improve AV conduction in patients with AV block induced by digitalis, with higher levels of potassium acting synergistically with the glycoside in slowing conduction velocity through the AV node. Since the effect of varying K_o^+ levels on the AV node in this setting may not be predictable, it is prudent to avoid intravenous potassium administration in unstable AV block complicating digitalis toxicity.

It should be mentioned that *hyperkalemia* is a manifestation of acute massive digitalis overdose, since digitalis, by inhibiting $Na^+-K^+-ATPase$, hinders movement of potassium into the cell. In a study of 91 patients with digitalis overdose, the initial serum potassium was found to provide the best guide to prognosis (161).

DIGITALIS AND MAGNESIUM

Magnesium has been used sporadically to treat digitalis-toxic arrhythmias since 1935 (162), and magnesium deficiency is known to enhance digitalis toxicity in animals and humans (163). Digitalis-toxic arrhythmias develop at a lower glycoside dose and persist longer in hypomagnesemic animals (164). Consistently in animal studies, and individually in several human case reports and small series, magnesium infusion has been found to reverse or abort digitalis-toxic arrhythmias (165–170). Spector et al. (166) found that IV magnesium sulfate immediately restored sinus rhythm in dogs infused with cardiac glycosides to the point of ventricular tachycardia. Ghani and Smith (165) obtained identical results in digitalis-toxic, normomagnesemic animals, which were made mildly hypermagnesemic to arrest ventricular tachycardia; these authors also showed that pretreatment of normomagnesemic animals with magnesium increased the glycoside level at which ventricular tachycardia occurred. In case reports of digitalis-toxic patients, paroxysmal atrial tachycardia, atrial flutter, premature ventricular contractions, ventricular tachycardia resistant to lidocaine, and ventricular fibrillation recurring after numerous cardioversions were all found to respond immediately to magnesium infusion.

It should be emphasized that a number of digitalis-toxic patients are likely to be magnesium-depleted, even though their serum magnesium levels may be normal (171, 172). Congestive heart failure by itself may accelerate urinary magnesium loss (173) as do furosemide and ethacrynic acid (169, 174). It is noteworthy that hypomagnesemia was found in 21 percent of digitalis-toxic and 10 percent of nontoxic patients in one small series (175).

The mechanism through which magnesium counteracts digitalis toxicity is still unknown. At the cellular level, increases in extracellular magnesium appear to increase the resting potential, action potential amplitude, and maximum rate of depolarization and conduction velocity (176), all of which are decreased by digitalis. Magnesium depletion has been found to increase myocardial digoxin uptake in one study (177) but not in another (166). Although magnesium is needed for the activation of Na^+–K^+–ATPase, the amount required is probably minimal, and increases in the available magnesium do not appear to reverse the enzyme inhibition produced by digitalis (166).

The best available evidence suggests that magnesium opposes digitalis toxicity by inhibiting the loss of intracellular potassium produced by digitalis. In the isolated myocardium, perfusion with high Mg^{2+} concentrations can completely reverse glycoside-induced potassium loss without decreasing contractility (140). The reversal is effected by blocking potassium egress rather than by increasing uptake, indicating that it is not brought about by reactivation of the sodium-potassium pump (140).

Although potassium loss is only a suspected, not a proven mechanism of digitalis toxicity, Seller et al. (178) found that the toxic dose of digitalis was increased by administration of potassium-sparing diuretics such as triamterene. These drugs decrease potassium loss from the heart as well as from the kidney (141). As with magnesium, the diuretics did not decrease contractility, so their protective effect cannot be ascribed to the displacement of digitalis from its receptors (178).

Digitalis-toxic patients, even with near normal serum magnesium levels, may require, and usually tolerate easily, very large quantities of IV magnesium. The recommendations for treatment of patients with and without magnesium depletion vary. Iseri et al. (170), from their experience and a review of the literature, recommend 10 to 15 mL of 20% magnesium sulfate IV over 1 min, followed by 500 mL of 2% magnesium sulfate over 6 h by IV infusion, the latter to be repeated if deficiency is documented.

Hypermagnesemia has its own toxic effects, though in general these become significant only at levels not readily attained, even by a program such as that described above. Atrioventricular and intraventricular conduction slow, with prolonged PR and QRS, at 6 to 10 meq/L; sinoatrial and atrioventricular block occur at about 15 meq/L and cardiac arrest at levels above 25 meq/L (179), though neuromuscular blockade with respiratory paralysis ensues much earlier, at about 12 meq/L. Patients with renal insufficiency need the most careful surveillance, since they become hypermagnesemic readily, and digitalis-toxic patients in renal failure are likely to be hypermagnesemic when first seen (179).

REFERENCES

1. Noble, D.: *The Initiation of the Heartbeat*, Clarendon Press, Oxford, 1977.
2. Fozzard, H. A.: Cardiac muscle: Excitability and passive electrical properties, *Prog. Cardiovasc. Dis.*, **19**:343, 1977.
3. Strauss, H. C., E. N. Prystowsky, and M. M. Scheinman: Sino-atrial and atrial electrogenesis, *Prog. Cardiovasc. Dis.*, **19**:385, 1977.
4. Hauswirth, O., and B. N. Singh: Voltage clamp in heart muscle in relation to the genesis and the pharmacological control of cardiac arrhythmias, *Pharmacol. Rev.* In press, 1978.
5. Weidmann, S.: The effect of the cardiac membrane potential on the rapid availability of the sodium carrier system, *J. Physiol. (London)*, **27**:213, 1955.
6. Vassalle, M.: Generation and conduction of impulses in the heart under physiological and pathological conditions, *Pharmacol. Ther. [B]*, **3**:1 1977.
7. New, W., and W. Trautwein: Inward membrane currents in mammalian myocardium, *Pflügers Arch.*, **334**:1, 1972.
8. Beeler, G. W., and H. Reuter: Membrane calcium currents in ventricular myocardial fibers, *J. Physiol. (London)*, **207**:191, 1970.
9. Noble, D., and R. W. Tsien: Outward membrane currents activated in the plateau range of potentials in cardiac Purkinje fibers, *J. Physiol. (London)*, **200**:205, 1969.
10. McAllister, R. E., D. Noble, and R. W. Tsien: Reconstruction of the electrical activity of cardiac Purkinje fibers, *J. Physiol. (London)*, **251**:1, 1975.
11. Irisawa, H.: Electrical activity of rabbit sinoatrial node as studied by a double sucrose gap method, in P. Rulunt (ed.), *Symposium and Colloquium on the Electrical Field of the Heart*, Presses Académiques Européenes, Brussels, 1972.

12. Brown, H. F., A. Clark, and S. J. Noble: The pacemaker current in frog atrium, *Nature New Biol.*, **235**:30, 1972.

13. Qingh, B. N., and E. M. Vaughan Williams: A fourth class of antidysrhythmic action? Effect of verapamil on ouabain toxicity, on atrial and ventricular intracellular potentials and on other features of cardiac function, *Cardiovasc. Res.*, **6**:109, 1972.

14. Wit, A. L., and P. F. Cranefield: Effect of verapamil on the sinoatrial and atrioventricular nodes of the rabbit and the mechanism by which it arrests re-entrant atrioventricular nodal tachycardia, *Circ. Res.*, **35**:413, 1974.

15. Zipes, D. P., and J. C. Fischer: Effects of agents which inhibit the slow channel on sinus node automaticity and atrioventricular conduction in the dog, *Circ. Res.*, **34**:184, 1974.

16. Vassort, G., O. Rougier, D. Garneir, M. P. Sauviat, E. Coraboeuf, and Y, M. Gargouil: Effects of adrenaline on membrane inward currents during the cardiac action potential, *Pflügers Arch.*, **309**:70, 1969.

17. Ikemoto, Y., and M. Goto: Nature of the negative inotropic effect of acetylcholine on the myocardium. An elucidation in the bullfrog atrium, *Proc. Jpn. Acad.*, **51**:501, 1975.

18. Lederer, W. J., and R. W. Tsien: Transient inward current underlying arrhythmogenic effects of cardiotonic steroids in Purkinje fibers, *J. Physiol. (London)*, **263**:73, 1976.

19. Ferrier, G. R., and G. K. Moe: Effect of calcium on acetylstrophanthidin-induced transient depolarizations in canine Purkinje tissue, *Circ. Res.*, **33**:508, 1973.

20. Arnsdorf, M. F.: Membrane factors in arrhythmogenesis: Concepts and definitions, *Prog. Cardiovasc. Dis.*, **19**:413, 1977.

21. Sano, T., and S. Yamagishi: Spread of excitation from the sinus node, *Circ. Res.*, **16**:423, 1965.

22. Cranefield, P. F., H. O. Klein, and B. F. Hoffman: Conduction of the cardiac impulse. I. Delay, block, and one-way block in depressed Purkinje fibers, *Circ. Res.*, **28**:199, 1971.

23. Hagiwara, S.: The Ca-dependent action potential, *Membranes*, **3**:359, 1975.

24. Kreitner, D.: Evidence for the existence of a rapid sodium channel in the membrane of rabbit sinoatrial cells, *J. Mol. Cell. Cardiol.*, **7**:655, 1975.

25. Katzung, B. G., and J. A. Morgenstern: Effects of extracellular potassium on ventricular automaticity and evidence for a pacemaker current in mammalian ventricular myocardium, *Circ. Res.*, **40**:105, 1977.

26. Hauswirth, O., D. Noble, and R. W. Tsien: The mechanism of oscillatory activity at low membrane potentials in cardiac Purkinje fibers, *J. Physiol. (London)*, **200**:255, 1969.

27. Imanishi, S.: Calcium sensitive discharges in canine Purkinje fibers, *Jpn. J. Physiol.*, **21**:443, 1971.

28. Pappano, A. J.: Calcium-dependent action potentials produced by catecholamines in guinea pig atrial muscle fibers depolarized by potassium, *Circ. Res.*, **27**:379, 1970.

29. Cranefield, P. F.: *The Conduction of the Cardiac Impulse*, Futura Publishing Company, New York, 1975.

30. Hoffman, B. F., and P. F. Cranefield: *Electrophysiology of the Heart*, McGraw-Hill Book Company, New York, 1960.

31. Beeler, G. W., and H. Reuter: The relation between membrane potential, membrane currents and activation of contraction in ventricular myocardial fibers, *J. Physiol. (London)*, **207**:211, 1970.

32. Schwartz, A.: Is the cell membrane Na^+–K^+–ATPase enzyme system the pharmacological receptor for digitalis? *Circ. Res.*, **39**:2, 1976.

33. Wikman-Coffelt, J., C. Fenner, A. F. Salel, T. Kamiyama, and D. T. Mason: Myofibrillar proteins and the contractile mechanism in the normal and failing heart, in D. T. Mason (ed.), *Congestive Heart Failure: Mechanisms, Evaluation and Treatment*, Dun-Donnelley Publishing Corporation, New York, 1976, p. 53.

34. Solaro, R. J., and F. N. Briggs: Calcium conservation and the regulation of myocardial contraction, *Recent Adv. Stud. Cardiac Struct. Metab.*, **4**:359, 1974.

35. Gettes, L. S.: Possible role of ionic changes in the appearance of arrhythmias, *Pharmacol. Ther. [B]*, **2**:787, 1976.

36. Singh, B. N., and O. Hauswirth: Comparative mechanisms of action of antiarrhythmic drugs, *Am. Heart J.*, **87**:367, 1974.

37. Singh, B. N., and E. M. Vaughan Williams: A third class of antiarrhythmic action. Effects on

atrial and ventricular intracellular potentials, and other pharmacological actions on cardiac muscle of MJ1999 and AH3474, *Br. J. Pharmacol.,* **39:**675, 1970.

38. Singh, B. N., and E. M. Vaughan Williams: Effect of altering potassium concentration on the action of lidocaine and diphenylhydantoin on rabbit and ventricular muscle, *Circ. Res.,* **29:**286, 1971.

39. Weiner, M. W., and F. H. Epstein: Signs and symptoms of electrolyte disorders, in M. H. Maxwell and C. R. Kleeman (eds.), *Clinical Disorders of Fluid and Electrolyte Metabolism,* McGraw-Hill Book Company, New York, 1979, chap. 16.

40. DeMello, W. C., and B. F. Hoffman: Potassium ions and electrical activity of specialized cardiac fibers, *Am. J. Physiol.,* **199:**1125, 1960.

41. Paes de Carvalho, A.: Role of potassium ions in the electrophysiological behavior of mammalian cardiac muscle, in E. Bajusz (ed.), *Electrolytes and Cardiovascular Diseases,* S. Karger, Basel and New York, 1965, p. 55.

42. Surawicz, B.: Arrhythmias and electrolyte disturbances, *Bull. N.Y. Acad. Sci.,* **43:**1160, 1967.

43. Bettinger, J. C., B. Surawicz, J. W. Bryfagle, B. N. Anderson, and S. Bellet: The effect of intravenous administration of potassium chloride on ectopic rhythms, ectopic beats, and disturbances of AV conduction, *Am, J. Med.,* **21:**521, 1956.

44. Fisch, C., E. F. Steinmetz, and R. B. Chevalier: Transient effect of intravenous potassium on AV conduction and ventricular ectopic beats, *Am. Heart J.,* **60:**220, 1959.

45. VanderArk, C. R., F. Ballantyne, III, and E. W. Reynolds, Jr.: Electrolytes and the electrocardiogram, in A. N. Brest (ed.), *Complex Electrocardiography I,* F. A. Davis Company, Philadelphia, 1973, p. 269.

46. Zipes, D.: Electrolyte derangements in the genesis of arrhythmias, in L. S. Dreifus and W. Likoff (eds.), *Cardiac Arrhythmias,* Grune & Stratton, Inc., New York, 1973, p. 55.

47. Merrill, J. P., H. D. Levine, W. Somerville, and S. Smith: Clinical recognition and treatment of acute potassium intoxication, *Ann. Intern. Med.,* **37:**797, 1950.

48. Fisch, C.: Relation of electrolyte disturbances to cardiac arrhythmias, *Circulation,* **47:**408, 1973.

49. Bashour, T., I. Hsu, H. J. Garfinkel, R. Wickra-

mesakaran, and J. C. Rios: Atrioventricular and intraventricular conduction in hyperkalemia, *Am. J. Cardiol.,* **35:**199, 1975.

50. Nair, M. R. S., and W. F. C. Duvernoy: Reversible fascicular block due to hyperkalemia, *Cardiovasc. Med.,* **2:**985, 1977.

51. O'Neil, J. P., and E. K. Chung: Unusual electrocardiographic finding: Bifascicular block due to hyperkalemia, *Am. J. Med.,* **61:**573, 1976.

52. O'Reilly, M. V., D. P. Murnaghan, and M. B. Williams: Transvenous pacemaker failure induced by hyperkalemia, *JAMA,* **228:**336, 1974.

53. Surawicz, B.: Ventricular fibrillation, *Am. J. Cardiol.,* **28:**268, 1971.

54. Lisak, R. P., J. Lebeau, S. H. Tucker, and L. P. Rowland: Hyperkalemic periodic paralysis and cardiac arrhythmia, *Neurology,* **22:**810, 1972.

55. Ettinger, P. O., T. J. Regan, and H. A. Oldewurtel: Hyperkalemia, cardiac conduction, and the electrocardiogram: A review, *Am. Heart J.,* **88:**360, 1974.

56. Kass, R. S., and R. W. Tsien: Multiple effects of calcium antagonists on plateau currents in cardiac Purkinje fibers, *J. Gen. Physiol.,* **66:**169, 1975.

57. Ballantyne, F., III, L. D. Davis, and E. W. Reynolds, Jr.: Cellular basis for reversal of hyperkalemic electrocardiographic changes by sodium, *Am. J. Physiol.,* **229:**935, 1975.

58. Surawicz, B., H. Brown, B. Crum, R. Kemp, S. Wagner, and A. J. Bellet: Quantitative analysis of the electrocardiographic pattern of hypopotassemia, *Circulation,* **16:**750, 1957.

59. Kelley, H. G., J. E. Foy, and S. G. Laverty: Thioridazine hydrochloride (mellaril): Its effect on the electrocardiogram and a report of two fatalities with electrocardiographic abnormalities, *Can. Med. Assoc. J.,* **89:**546, 1963.

60. Ban, T. A., and A. St. Jean: The effect of phenothiazines on the electrocardiogram, *Can Med. Assoc. J.,* **91:**537, 1964.

61. Singer, D. H., R. Lazzarra, and B. F. Hoffman: Interrelationships between automaticity and conduction in Purkinje fibers, *Circ. Res.,* **21:**537, 1967.

62. Krikler, D. M., and P. V. L. Curry: Torsade de pointes, an atypical ventricular tachycardia, *Br. Heart J.,* **38:**117, 1976.

63. Singh, B. N., T. D. Gaarder, T. Kanegae, M.

Goldstein, J. Z. Montgomerie, and H. Mills: Liquid protein diets and *torsade de pointes*, *JAMA*, **240:**115, 1978.

64. Brace, R. A., D. K. Anderson, W.-T. Chen, J. B. Scott, and F. J. Haddy: Local effects of hypokalemia on coronary resistance and myocardial contractile force, *Am. J. Physiol.*, **227:**590, 1974.

65. Surawicz, B., H. A. Brawun, W. B. Crum, R. L. Kemp, S. Wagner, and J. Bellet: Clinical manifestations of hypopotassemia, *Am. J. Med. Sci.*, **233:**603, 1957.

66. Duggan, P. F.: Calcium uptake and associated adenosine triphosphatase activity in fragmented sarcoplasmic reticulum: Requirement for potassium ions, *J. Biol. Chem.*, **252:**1620, 1977.

67. Kim, N. D., and C. E. Harrison, Jr.: $^{45}Ca^{2+}$ accumulation by mitochondria and sarcoplasmic reticulum in chronic potassium depletion cardiomyopathy, *Recent Adv. Stud. Cardiac Struct. Metab.*, **4:**551, 1974.

68. Sack, D. W., N. D. Kim, and C. E. Harrison, Jr.: Myocardial function and subcellular calcium metabolism in chronic potassium deficiency, *Recent Adv. Stud. Cardiac Struct. Metab.*, **5:**203, 1975.

69. Harris, A. S., A. Bisteni, R. A. Russell, J. C. Bringham, and J. E. Firestone: Excitative factors in ventricular tachycardia resulting from myocardial ischemia. Potassium a major excitant, *Science*, **119:**200, 1954.

70. Regan, T. J., M. A. Harman, Q H. Lehan, W. M. Burke, and H. A. Oldewurtel: Ventricular arrhythmias and K^+ transfer during myocardial ischemia and intervention with procaineamide, insulin or glucose solution, *J. Clin. Invest.*, **46:**1657, 1967.

71. Waldo, A. L., G. A. Kaiser, R. J. Castany, and B. F. Hoffman: A study of arrhythmias associated with acute myocardial infarction, *Circulation*, **38:**200, 1968.

72. Dyckner, T., C. Helmers, T. Lundman, and P. O. Wester: Initial serum potassium level in relation to early complications and prognosis in patients with acute myocardial infarction, *Acta Med. Scand.*, **197:**207, 1975.

73. Singh, B. N.: The rational basis of antiarrhythmic therapy: The clinical pharmacology of commonly used antiarrhythmic drugs, *Angiology*, in press, 1978.

74. Hoffman, B. F., and E. E. Suckling: Effect of several cations on transmembrane potentials of cardiac muscle, *Am. J. Physiol.*, **186:**317, 1956.

75. Temte, J. V., and L. D. Davis: Effect of calcium concentration on the transmembrane potentials of Purkinje fibers, *Circ. Res.*, **20:**32, 1967.

76. Kass, R. S., and R. W. Tsien: Control of action potential duration by calcium ions in cardiac Purkinje fibers, *J. Gen. Physiol.*, **67:**599, 1976.

77. Isenberg, G.: Is potassium conductance of cardiac Purkinje fibers controlled by $(Ca^{2+})_i$? *Nature*, **253:**273, 1975.

78. Seifen, E., H. Schaer, and J. M. Marshall: Effects of calcium on the membrane potentials of single pacemaker fibres and atrial fibres in isolated rabbit atria, *Nature*, **202:**1223, 1964.

79. Freedberg, A. S., J. G. Papp, and E. M. Vaughan Williams: The effect of altered thyroid state on atrial intracellular potentials, *J. Physiol. (London)*, **207:**357, 1970.

80. Singh, B. N., and E. M. Vaughan Williams: The effect of amiodarone, a new anti-anginal drug on cardiac muscle, *Br. J. Pharmacol.*, **39:**657, 1970.

81. Jervell, A., and F. Lange-Nielsen: Congenital deaf mutism, functional heart disease with prolongation of the Q-T interval and sudden death, *Am. Heart J.*, **54:**59, 1957.

82. Johnson, J. D.: Hypocalcemia and cardiac arrhythmias, *Am. J. Dis. Child.*, **115:**373, 1968.

83. Castellanos, A.: Unusual forms of heart block in infancy, *Br. Heart J.*, **22:**713, 1960.

84. Griffin, J. H.: Neonatal hypocalcemia and complete heart block, *Am. J. Dis. Child.*, **110:**672, 1965.

85. Kambara, H., B. J. Held, and J. Phillips: Hypocalcemia and intractable ventricular fibrillation, *Ann. Intern. Med.*, **86:**583, 1977.

86. Johnson, J. D., and R. Jennings: Hypocalcemia and cardiac arrhythmias, *Am, J. Dis. Child.*, **115:**373, 1968.

87. Crum, W. D., and H. J. Till: Hyperparathyroidism with Wenckebach's phenomenon, *Am. J. Cardiol.*, **6:**838, 1960.

88. Voss, D. M., and E. H. Drake: Cardiac manifestations of hyperthyroidism with presentation of a previously unreported arrhythmia, *Am. Heart J.*, **72:**235, 1967.

89. Troughton, D., and S. P. Singh: Heart failure and

neonatal hypocalcemia, *Br. Med. J.*, **4**:76, 1972.

90. Falko, J. M., C. A. Bush, M. Tzagaurnis, and F. B. Thomas: Congestive heart failure complicating the hungry bone syndrome, *Am. J. Med. Sci.*, **271**:85, 1976.

91. Denlinger, J. K., and M. L. Nahrwald: Cardiac failure associated with hypocalcemia, *Anesth. Anal. (Cleve.)*, **55**:34, 1976.

92. Dleckenstein, A., J. Janke, H. J. Döring, and O. Leder: Myocardial fiber necrosis due to intracellular calcium overload—a new principle in cardiac pathophysiology, *Recent Adv. Stud. Cardiac Struct. Metab.*, **4**:563, 1974.

93. Dleckenstein, A., J. Janke, H. J. Döring, and O. Leder: Key role of calcium in the production of noncoronarogenic myocardial necrosis, *Recent Adv. Stud. Cardiac Struct. Metab.*, **6**:21, 1975.

94. Bloom, S., and D. L. Davis: Calcium as mediator of isoproterenol-induced myocardial necrosis, *Am. J. Pathol.*, **69**:459, 1972.

95. Nirdlinger, E. L., and P. O. Bramante: Subcellular myocardial ionic shifts and metabolic alterations in the course of isoproterenol-induced cardiomyopathy of the rat, *J. Mol. Cell. Cardiol.*, **6**:49, 1974.

96. Harigaya, S., and A. Schwartz: Rate of calcium binding and uptake in normal animal and failing human cardiac muscle. Membrane vesicles (relaxing system) and mitochondria, *Circ. Res.*, **25**:781, 1969.

97. Tomlinson, C. W., S. L. Lee, and N. S. Dhalla: Abnormalities in heart membranes and myofibrils during bacterial infective cardiomyopathy, *Circ. Res.*, **39**:82, 1976.

98. Sordahl, L. A., W. B. McCallum, W. G. Wood, and A. Schwartz: Mitochondria and sarcoplasmic reticulum function in cardiac hypertrophy and failure, *Am. J. Physiol.*, **224**:497, 1973.

99. Suko, J., J. H. K. Vogel, and C. A. Chidsey: Intracellular calcium and myocardial contractility. III. Reduced calcium uptake and ATPase of the sarcoplasmic reticular fraction prepared from chronically failing hearts, *Circ. Res.*, **27**:235, 1970.

100. Owens, K., R. C. Ruth, W. B. Weglicki, A. C. Stam, and E. H. Sonnenblick: Fragmented sarcoplasmic reticulum of the cardiomyopathic Syrian hamster: Lipid composition, Ca^{++} transport,

and Ca^{++} stimulated ATPase, *Recent Adv. Stud. Cardiac Struct. Metab.*, **4**:541, 1974.

101. Swartz, M. H., D. I. Repke, A. M. Katz, and E. Rubin: Effects of ethanol on calcium binding and calcium uptake by cardiac microsomes, *Biochem. Pharmacol.*, **23**:2369, 1974.

102. Wrogemann, K., M. C. Blanchaer, J. H. Thakar, and B. J. Mezon: On the role of mitochondria in the hereditary cardiomyopathy of the Syrian hamster, *Recent Adv. Stud. Cardiac Struct. Metab.*, **6**:231, 1975.

103. Singh, B. N., H. J. Smith, and R. M. Norris: Reduction in infarct size following experimental coronary occlusion by administration of verapamil, *Recent Adv. Stud. Cardiac Struct. Metab.*, **10**:435, 1975.

104. Hasmin, G., and E. Bajusz: Prevention of myocardial degeneration in hamsters with hereditary cardiomyopathy, *Recent Adv. Stud. Cardiac Struct. Metab.*, **6**:219, 1975.

105. Seelig, M. S.: Myocardial loss of functional magnesium. I. Effect on mitochondrial integrity and potassium retention, *Recent. Adv. Cardiac Struct. Metab.*, **1**:615, 1972.

106. Lazzara, R., K. Hyatt, W. D. Love, J. Cronvich, and G. E. Burch: Tissue distribution, kinetics and biologic half-life of Mg^{28} in the dog, *Am. J. Physiol.*, **204**:1086, 1963.

107. Chadda, K. D., E. Lichstein, and P. Gupta: Hypomagnesemia and refractory cardiac arrhythmia in a nondigitalized patient, *Am. J. Cardiol.*, **31**:98, 1973.

108. Loeb, H. S., R. J. Pietras, R. M. Gunnar, and J. R. Tobin: Paroxysmal ventricular fibrillation in two patients with hypomagnesemia, *Circulation*, **37**:210, 1968.

109. McMullen, J. K.: Asystole and hypomagnesemia during recovery from diabetic ketoacidosis, *Br. Med. J.*, **1**:690, 1977.

110. Shils, M. E.: Experimental human magnesium depletion, *Medicine (Baltimore)*, **48**:61, 1969.

111. Watanabe, Y., and L. S. Dreifus: Electrophysiological effects of magnesium and its interactions with potassium, *Cardiovasc. Res.*, **6**:79, 1972.

112. Ghani, M. F., and M. Rabah: Effect of magnesium chloride on electrical stability of the heart, *Am. Heart J.*, **94**:600, 1977.

113. Miller, J. R., and T. R. VanDellen: Electrocardi-

ographic changes following intravenous administration of magnesium sulfate, combined effect with digitalis, *J. Lab. Clin. Med.*, **26**:1116, 1941.

114. Seelig, M. S.: Electrocardiographic patterns of magnesium depletion appearing in alcoholic heart disease, *Ann. N.Y. Acad. Sci.*, **162**:902, 1969.

115. Seta, K., R. Kleiger, E. E. Hellerstein, B. Lown, and J. J. Vitale: Effect of potassium and magnesium deficiency on the electrocardiogram and plasma electrolytes of pure-bred beagles, *Amer. J. Cardiol.*, **17**:516, 1966.

116. Schroeder, H. A.: Relation between mortality from cardiovascular disease and treated water supplies, *JAMA*, **172**:1902, 1960.

117. Morris, J. N., M. Crawford, and J. A. Heady: Hardness of local water supplies and mortality from cardiovascular disease, *Lancet*, **1**:860, 1961.

118. Stitt, F. W., D. G. Clayton, M. D. Crawford, and J. N. Morris: Clinical and biochemical indicators of cardiovascular disease among men living in hard and soft water areas, *Lancet*, **1**:122, 1973.

119. Chipperfield, B., and J. R. Chipperfield: Heart muscle magnesium, potassium, and zinc ion concentrations after sudden death from heart disease, *Lancet*, **1**:293, 1973.

120. Crawford, T., and M. D. Crawford: Prevalence and pathological changes of ischemic heart disease in a hard-water and in a soft-water area, *Lancet*, **1**:229, 1967.

121. Anderson, T. W., D. Hewitt, L. C. Neri, G. Schreiber, and F. Talbot: Water hardness and magnesium in heart muscle, *Lancet* **2**:1390, 1973.

122. Chipperfield, M. R., G. Behr, and P. Burton: Magnesium and potassium content of normal heart muscle in areas of hard and soft water, *Lancet*, **1**:121, 1976.

123. Behr, G., and P. Burton: Heart muscle magnesium, *Lancet*, **2**:450, 1973.

124. Parmintuan, J. C., L. S. Dreifus, and Y. Watanabe: Comparative mechanisms of antiarrhythmic drugs, *Am. J. Cardiol.*, **26**:512, 1970.

125. Singh, B. N., P. J. Hurley, and J. D. K. North: The use of amiloride in potassium depletion before cardiac surgery, *Am. Heart J.*, **78**:22, 1969.

126. Bellet, S., G. Hamdan, A. Somlyo, and R. Lara: The reversal of cardiotoxic effects of quinidine by molar lactate. An experimental study, *Am. J. Med. Sci.*, **237**:165, 1959.

127. Solaro, R. J., R. M. Wise, J. S. Shiner, and F. N.

Briggs: Calcium requirements for cardiac myofibrillar activation, *Circ. Res.*, **34**:525, 1974.

128. Fabiato, A., and F. Fabiato: Calcium release from the sarcoplasmic reticulum, *Circ. Res.*, **40**:119, 1977.

129. Langer, G. A., J. S. Frank, and A. J. Brady: The myocardium, in Guyton and Cowley (eds.), *Cardiovascular Physiology II*, vol. 9 of *International Review of Physiology*, University Park Press, Baltimore, 1976.

130. Wendt, J. R., and G. A. Langer: The sodium-calcium relationship in mammalian myocardium: Effect of sodium deficient perfusion on calcium fluxes, *J. Mol. Cell. Cardiol.*, **9**:551, 1977.

131. Langer, G. A., and J. S. Frank: Lanthanum in heart cell culture. Effect on calcium exchange correlated with its localization, *J. Cell. Biol.*, **54**:441, 1972.

132. McDonald, T. F., H. Nawrath, and W. Trautwein: Membrane currents and tension in cat ventricular muscle treated with cardiac glycosides, *Circ. Res.*, **37**:674, 1975.

133. Blaad, B. E., and D. Noble: Glycoside-induced inotropism of the heart—more than one mechanism? *J. Physiol. (London)*, **266**:76P, 1977.

134. Schwartz, A.: Is the cell membrane Na^+–K^+-ATPase enzyme system the pharmacological receptor for digitalis? *Circ. Res.*, **39**:2, 1976.

135. Gervais, A., L. K. Lane, B. M. Annex, G. E. Lindenmayer, and A. Schwartz: A possible mechanism of the action of digitalis, *Circ. Res.*, **40**:8, 1977.

136. Nayler, W. G.: Some factors which influence the amount of calcium stored at the superficially located sites in cardiac muscle cells, *Recent Adv. Stud. Cardiac Struct. Metab.*, **5**:73, 1975.

137. Okita, G. F., F. Richardson, and B. F. Roth-Schechter: Dissociation of the positive inotropic action of digitalis from inhibition of sodium- and potassium-activated adenosine triphosphatase, *J. Pharm. Exp. Ther.*, **185**:1, 1973.

138. Langer, G. A.: The relationship between myocardial contractility and the effects of digitalis on ionic exchange, *Fed. Proc.*, **36**:2231, 1977.

139. Langer, G. A., and P. A. Poole-Wilson: Dissociation of the inotropic effect of acetylstrophanthidin in myocardium and the increase of K^+ efflux, *J. Physiol.*, **248**:13P, 1975.

140. Shine, K. I., and A. M. Douglas: Magnesium ef-

fects in rabbit ventricle, *Am. J. Physiol.*, **228:**1545, 1975.

141. Seller, R. H., S. Banath, T. Namey, M. Neff, and C. Swartz: Cardiac effect of diuretic drugs, *Am. Heart J.*, **89:**493, 1975.

142. Noack, E., and K. Greeff: Calcium uptake and storage in isolated heart mitochondria influenced by sodium and potassium ions, *Recent Adv. Stud. Cardiac Struct. Metab.*, **5:**165, 1975.

143. Okita, G. T., R. E. Ten Eick, and F. Richardson: Inhibition of Na^+-K^+-ATPase and digitalis action: Dissociation from inotropic effects and its role in digitalis cardiotoxicity, *Ann. N.Y. Acad. Sci.*, **242:**658, 1974.

144. Vassalle, M., K. Greenspan, and B. F. Hoffmann: Analysis of arrhythmias induced by ouabain in intact dogs, *Circ. Res.*, **13:**132, 1963.

145. Hagemeijer, F., and B. Lown: Effect of heart rate on electrically induced repetitive ventricular responses in the digitalized dog, *Circ. Res.*, **27:**333, 1970.

146. Hashimoto, K., and G. K. Moe: Transient depolarizations induced by acetylstrophanthidin in specialized tissue of dog atrium and ventricle, *Circ. Res.*, **32:**618, 1973.

147. Ferrier, G. R.: Digitalis arrhythmias: Role of oscillatory afterpotentials, *Prog. Cardiovasc. Dis.*, **19:**459, 1977.

148. Foster, P. R., V. Elharrar, and D. P. Zipes: Accelerated ventricular escapes induced in the intact dog by barium, strontium and calcium, *J. Pharm. Exp. Ther.*, **200:**373, 1977.

149. Rosen, M. R., J. P. Ilvento, H. Gelband, and C. Merker: Effects of verapamil on electrophysiologic properties of canine cardiac Purkinje fibers, *J. Pharm. Exp. Ther.*, **189:**414, 1974.

150. Chiou, C. Y., M. H. Malagodi, B. V. R. Sastry, and P. Posner: Effects of a calcium antagonist, 6-(N,N-diethylamino) hexyl-3,4,5-trimethoxybenzoate, on digitalis-induced arrhythmias and cardiac contractions, *J. Pharm. Exp. Ther.*, **198:**444, 1976.

151. Chopra, D., P. Janson, and C. T. Sawin: Insensitivity to digoxin associated with hypocalcemia, *N. Engl. J. Med.*, **296:**917, 1977.

152. Surawicz, B.: Use of the chelating agent, EDTA, in digitalis toxicity and cardiac arrhythmias, *Prog. Cardiovasc. Dis.*, **2:**432, 1959.

153. Surawicz, B., M. G. McDonald, V. Kaljot, and

J. C. Bettinger: Treatment of cardiac arrhythmias with salts of EDTA, *Am. Heart J.*, **58:**493, 1959.

154. Steiness, E., and K. H. Olesen: Cardiac arrhythmias induced by hypokalemia and potassium loss during maintenance digoxin therapy, *Br. Heart J.*, **38:**167, 1976.

155. Gelbart, A., R. J. C. Hall, and R. H. Goldman: Digoxin-induced arrhythmias in hypokalemia, *Lancet*, **2:**850, 1976.

156. Hall, R. J., A. Gelbart, M. Silverman, and R. H. Goldman: Studies on digitalis-induced arrhythmias in glucose- and insulin-induced hypokalemia, *J. Pharm. Exp. Ther.*, **201:**711, 1977.

157. Anderson, G. J., J. C. Bailey, J. Reiser, and A. Freeman: Electrophysiological observations on the digitalis-potassium interaction in canine Purkinje fibers, *Circ. Res.*, **39:**717, 1976.

158. Prindle, H. K., C. L. Skelton, S. E. Epstein, and F. I. Marcus: Influence of extracellular potassium concentration on myocardial uptake and inotropic effect of tritiated digoxin, *Circ. Res.*, **28:**337, 1971.

159. Goldman, R. H., J. Coltart, E. Schweizer, G. Snidow, and D. C. Harrison: Dose response *in vivo* to digoxin in normo- and hyperkalemia: Associated biochemical changes, *Cardiovasc. Res.*, **9:**515, 1975.

160. Lee, G., R. Zelis, and D. T. Mason: Linear dose response and quantitative attenuation by potassium of the inotropic action of acetylstrophanthidin, *Clin. Pharm. Ther.*, **22:**34, 1977.

161. Bismuth, C., M. Gaultier, M. Gonnet, and J. Pallet: L'hyperkaliémie dans l'intoxication digitalique massive, *Biomed. (Express)*, **19:**152, 1973.

162. Zwillinger, L.: Magnesium and the heart, *Klin. Wochenschr.*, **14:**1429, 1935.

163. Sellers, R. H., J. Cangiano, K. E. Kim, S. Mendelssohn, A. N. Brest, and C. Swartz: Digitalis toxicity and hypomagnesemia, *Am. Heart J.*, **79:**57, 1970.

164. Kleiger, R. E., and S. Katsutaka: Effects of chronic depletion of potassium and magnesium upon the action of acetylstrophanthidin, *Am. J. Cardiol.*, **17:**520, 1966.

165. Ghani, M. F., and J. R. Smith: The effectiveness of magnesium chloride in the treatment of ventricular tachyarrhythmias due to digitalis intoxication, *Am. Heart J.*, **88:**621, 1974.

166. Specter, M. J., E. Schweizer, and R. H. Goldman:

Studies on magnesium's mechanism of action in digitalis-induced arrhythmias, *Circulation*, **52**:1001, 1975.

167. Enselberg, C. D., H. G. Simmons, and A. A. Mintz: The effects of magnesium upon cardiac arrhythmias, *Am. Heart J.*, **39**:703, 1950.

168. Szekely, P., and N. A. Wynne: Cardiac arrhythmias caused by digitalis, *Clin. Sci.*, **10**:241, 1951.

169. Lim, P., and E. Jacob: Magnesium deficiency in patients on long-term diuretic therapy for heart failure, *Br. Med. J.*, **3**:620, 1972.

170. Iseri, L. T., J. Freed, and A. R. Bures: Magnesium deficiency and cardiac disorders, *Am. J. Med.*, **58**:837, 1975.

171. Martin, H. E.: Clinical magnesium deficiency, *Ann. N.Y. Acad. Sci.*, **162**:891, 1969.

172. Mendelson, J. H., M. Ogata, and N. K. Mello: Effects of alcohol ingestion and withdrawal on magnesium states of alcoholics: Clinical and experimental findings, *Ann. N.Y. Acad. Sci.*, **162**:918, 1969.

173. Lazarra, R. K., T. K. Yun, W. C. Black, J. J. Walsh, and G. E. Burch: Magnesium and potassium metabolism in patients with idiopathic cardiomyopathy and chronic congestive heart failure, *Proc. Soc. Exp. Biol. Med.*, **120**:110, 1965.

174. Duarte, C. G.: Effects of ethacrynic acid and furosemide on urinary calcium, phosphate, and magnesium, *Metabolism*, **17**:867, 1968.

175. Beller, G. A., W. B. Hood, Jr., T. W. Smith, W. H. Abelmann, and W. E. C. Wacker: Correlation of serum magnesium levels and cardiac digitalis intoxication, *Am. J. Cardiol.*, **33**:225, 1974.

176. Watanabe, Y., and L. S. Dreifus: Electrophysiological effects of magnesium and its interactions with potassium, *Cardiovasc. Res.*, **6**:79, 1972.

177. Goldman, R. H., R. E. Kleiger, E. Schweizer, and D. C. Harrison: The effect on myocardial ³H-digoxin of magnesium deficiency, *Proc. Soc. Exp. Biol. Med.*, **136**:747, 1971.

178. Seller, R. H., J. Greco, S. Banach, and R. Seth: Increasing the intropic effect and toxic dose of digitalis by the administration of antikaliuretic drugs: Further evidence for a cardiac effect of diuretic drugs, *Am. Heart J.*, **90**:56, 1975.

179. Smith, P. K., A. W. Winkler, and H. E. Hoff: Electrocardiographic changes and concentration of magnesium in serum following intravenous injection of magnesium salts, *Am. J. Physiol.*, **126**:720, 1939.

6

Acid-base metabolism

JORDAN J. COHEN / JEROME P. KASSIRER

INTRODUCTION

The chemical principles that define the nature of acids and bases and that govern the level of acidity apply not only to simple chemical systems but to complex biologic systems as well. In applying these principles to normal and disordered hydrogen ion metabolism in man, however, it is crucial to have clearly in mind the prevailing physiologic context within which the pertinent chemical reactions take place. As is the case with other aspects of fluid and electrolyte metabolism, the metabolism of hydrogen ion can be understood fully only in relation to the physiologic processes that influence input to and output from the organism (external balance) and that maintain body fluid concentrations within viable limits. When viewed from this physiologic perspective, it is clear that the acidity of body fluids is a dynamic variable, impinged upon continuously by a wide variety of competing forces.

The following discussion will review the chemical principles that define the nature of acids and bases and their interactions, describe the physiologic mechanisms that normally constrain and perturb body fluid acidity, and examine the clinical disturbances of acid-base equilibrium.

SECTION I

Chemical considerations

Hydrogen ions are protons freed of their associated electrons. In aqueous solutions, individual protons are bound to one or more water molecules, but, in accordance with standard practice, hydrogen ions will be designated here by the symbol H^+.

A large array of molecules, both inorganic and organic, contain linkages with hydrogen that may rupture, yielding hydrogen ions. A consequence of this dissociation process is the simultaneous generation of an equal number of sites for potential recombination with hydrogen ion. This principle of hydrogen ion chemistry provides the foundation for the definition of acids and bases: an acid is any molecular species that functions as a proton donor, and a base, any molecular species that functions as a proton receptor. Thus, the relationship between an undissociated acid and its conjugate, dissociated base can be described as follows:

$$\text{Acid} \rightleftharpoons \text{base} + H^+ \qquad (6\text{-}1)$$

Both inorganic and organic acid-base pairs are commonly encountered in biologic systems; carbonic acid–bicarbonate (H_2CO_3/HCO_3^-), monobasic-dibasic phosphate ($H_2PO_4^-/HPO_4^{2-}$), ammonium-ammonia (NH_4^+/NH_3), and lactic acid–lactate are some examples. In addition, many protein molecules (e.g., hemoglobin) contain acidic groups that may dissociate, yielding a series of corresponding conjugate bases.

For an individual acid molecule, the cycle of dissociation and subsequent recombination is a never-ending process. For a given acid species, however, the process of dissociation progressively reduces the number of molecules at risk of dissociation and thereby reduces the absolute rate of dissociation. Conversely, this process increases the number of molecules available for recombination and thereby increases the absolute rate of recombination. When the rates of these opposing reactions exactly counterbalance each other, a state of chemical equilibrium is said to exist, and no further net change occurs.

A useful concept derived from a rigorous analysis of the physical chemistry of equilibrium states (22) is embodied in the so-called mass action expression. This expression states that, at equilibrium, the ratio of the concentration products of opposing reaction sets is a constant. Applying this formulation to the reaction shown in Eq. (6-1) yields

$$\frac{[H^+] \times [\text{base}]}{[\text{Acid}]} = K \qquad (6\text{-}2)$$

$$\frac{[H^+] \times [\text{base}]}{[\text{acid}]} = K \qquad (6\text{-}2)$$

This equation may be rearranged to highlight the property of acidity as follows:

$$[H^+] = K \times \frac{[\text{acid}]}{[\text{base}]} \qquad (6\text{-}3)$$

The factor K in Eq. (6-3) is termed the *dissociation constant* and is a measure of the strength of a given acid.[1] The strength of an acid can be appreciated best in terms of the tenacity by which the hydrogen ion clings to its locus on individual acid-base molecules. The tenacity of hydrogen ion bonding varies greatly among acid-base pairs and, hence, the point at which equilibrium is established differs widely. At one end of the spectrum are acids that dissociate freely since their corresponding bases have a very low affinity for hydrogen ions; these acids have high dissociation constants and are considered strong acids. At the other end of the spectrum are acids that dissociate sparingly, since their corresponding strong bases have a very high affinity for hydrogen ions; these acids have low dissociation constants and are considered weak acids.

The process of dissociation-recombination occurs whenever an acid-base substance is placed in solution. In aqueous solutions, water is a crucial participant in this process because water itself possesses a locus for hydrogen ion dissociation. Hence, chemical equilibrium involves not only the acid-base solutes in the solution but water and its conjugate base, the hydroxyl ion. Thus,

$$\text{HOH} \rightleftharpoons H^+ + OH^- \qquad (6\text{-}4)$$

and, at equilibrium,

$$\frac{[H^+] \times [OH^-]}{[\text{HOH}]} = K_{\text{HOH}} \qquad (6\text{-}5)$$

---

[1]Since the dissociation constant is influenced by temperature and by other physicochemical properties of the solution in question, it is truly constant only in reference to a particular set of conditions.

Since the molar concentration of undissociated water varies negligibly in dilute solutions, it follows from Eq. (6-5) that the concentrations of hydrogen and hydroxyl ions at equilibrium are complementary to each other (i.e., they exhibit a constant ion product). By convention, however, the concentration of the hydrogen ion in pure water (which is, of course, equivalent to that of hydroxyl ions) serves as a neutral reference point (7).

The hydrogen ion concentration (or, more precisely, activity[2]) of water is increased by the addition of any acid and decreased by the addition of any base. Adding a strong acid increases H^+ concentration more than adding an equimolar amount of a weaker acid does, because a greater number of the strong acid molecules relinquish their hydrogen ions (and a greater number of hydroxyl ions recombine with protons) before equilibrium is reestablished. Similarly, adding a strong base decreases hydrogen ion concentration more than adding an equimolar amount of a weaker base does, because more protons will migrate from water to the stronger base (and more hydroxyl ions will be generated) before equilibrium is reestablished.

In complex solutions containing multiple acid-base solutes, the concentration of hydrogen ions at equilibrium is determined by the composite influence of the hydrogen ion affinities of each of the individual molecular species present, in conjunction with their relative concentrations. As a general statement,

$$[H^+] = K_1 \frac{[acid_1]}{[base_1]} = K_2 \frac{[acid_2]}{[base_2]}$$
$$= \cdots = K_n \frac{[acid_n]}{[base_n]} \quad (6\text{-}6)$$

[2] The activity coefficient of hydrogen ions is assumed to vary only slightly in response to the small variations in temperature and ionic strength that occur in biologic systems such as those under consideration here. For this reason, the distinction between hydrogen ion concentration and hydrogen ion activity will be ignored and the terms used interchangeably.

It is clear from Eq. (6-6) that any change in the acidity of such a complex solution must involve a redistribution of hydrogen ions among all of the acid-base pairs present. If one adds an acid or a base to such a solution, the *change* in hydrogen ion concentration that results will be smaller than if one added the same acid or base to pure water. The ability of solutions containing acid-base pairs to resist changes in acidity is termed *buffering* and the acid-base pairs themselves are termed *buffers*.

The extent to which such buffering occurs in a given solution is a function of the initial hydrogen ion concentration and the dissociation constants and respective concentrations of the individual buffer pairs present. A well-mixed, homogenous solution can have only one hydrogen ion concentration (the isohydric principle). Therefore, one need know the dissociation constant and the component concentrations of but a single buffer pair in order to monitor the acid-base behavior of any homogenous system, no matter

Table 6-1. Equivalent values for pH and hydrogen ion concentration

pH	$[H^+]$, neq/L
7.70	20
7.65	22
7.60	25
7.55	28
7.50	32
7.45	35
7.40	40
7.35	45
7.30	50
7.25	56
7.20	63
7.15	71
7.10	79
7.05	89
7.00	100
6.95	112
6.90	126
6.85	141
6.80	158

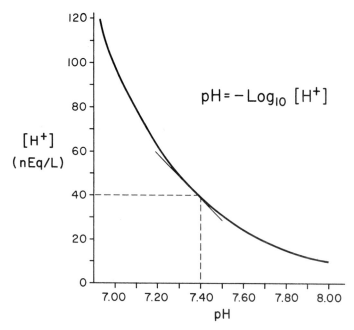

Figure 6-1. Relationship between pH and hydrogen ion concentration (in nanoequivalents per liter), the two most commonly employed units for specifying the level of acidity. A tabular form of this relationship is presented in Table 6-1. Note that the normal arterial blood pH of 7.40 corresponds to a hydrogen ion concentration of 40 neq/L. Furthermore, over the pH range 7.20 to 7.50, each 0.01 unit change in pH is approximately equivalent to a 1.0 neq/L change (in opposite direction) in hydrogen ion concentration; this approximation is illustrated by the solid straight line. These easily remembered relationships facilitate conversion of the most frequently encountered blood pH measurements to their corresponding hydrogen ion concentrations.

how complex. As will become evident, this principle simplifies the analysis of acid-base changes in living organisms because it permits us to focus attention virtually exclusively on the physiologically preeminent buffer pair, carbonic acid–bicarbonate.

Acidity is often measured in terms of the pH unit, which is defined as the negative logarithm of the hydrogen ion concentration:

$$pH = -\log [H^+] \qquad (6\text{-}7)$$

Use of the pH unit has become well established among chemists because it allows the very wide range of hydrogen ion concentrations encountered in chemical systems to be designated by a manageable numerical scale. Because the range of hydrogen ion concentrations encountered in living systems is small and so does not pose this problem, the acidity of body fluids is frequently designated directly in equivalent, linear units of hydrogen ion concentration (Table 6-1). The unit usually selected for numerical convenience is nanoequivalents per liter (i.e., millimicroequivalents per liter or 10^{-9} equivalent per liter).

Figure 6-1 depicts the relationship between the nanoequivalent per liter scale and the pH scale over the range of plasma acidity encountered in man. Conversion from pH units to nanoequivalents per liter is facilitated by certain fortunate numerical relationships noted in the legend of this figure.

SECTION II

Physiologic considerations

DETERMINANTS OF BODY FLUID ACIDITY

In discussing the acidity of living organisms, attention is usually centered on the acid-base equilibrium of plasma. In so doing, it is assumed that the acidity of this readily accessible body fluid correlates reasonably well with the acidity of other major fluid compartments. This assumption is bolstered by the rapid diffusion-equilibrium achieved between plasma and interstitial fluid and by the relative ease with which hydrogen ions traverse cell membranes.

It must be kept in mind, however, that the acid-base composition of plasma may fail to reflect all of the important physiologic events that may affect local acidity and, hence, certain vital functions (52). For example, acid-base composition within cells, within the cerebrospinal fluid, and on the surface of bone all appear to be influenced in part by factors that do not invariably produce corresponding changes in plasma acidity. Nevertheless, the acidity of the plasma compartment is of undoubted importance to the body as a whole, and an understanding of acid-base equilibrium in plasma does provide a reliable framework for the diagnosis and treatment of clinical disturbances of hydrogen ion metabolism.

CARBONIC ACID–BICARBONATE BUFFER SYSTEM

Among the many buffer pairs that equilibrate with extracellular hydrogen ion concentration, the carbonic acid–bicarbonate pair is of overwhelming physiologic importance in the regulation of acidity. This pair is not only the dominant buffer in the extracellular fluid but, even more important, it is the only buffer whose component concentrations can be varied independently by physiologic regulatory systems.

Fig. 6-2 depicts the relevant chemical reactions involving carbonic acid and bicarbonate and lists various forms of the mass action relationship derived from them. Two equivalent sets of mass action expressions are shown, one utilizing hydrogen ion concentration units and the other utilizing pH units as the measure of acidity.

As can be seen, carbon dioxide normally produced by the tissues is dissolved in plasma and achieves a concentration proportional to its partial pressure (Pa_{CO_2}). Carbonic acid is formed from the hydration of dissolved carbon dioxide; this reaction is reversible and reaches equilibrium virtually instantaneously, owing to the ubiquity and abundance of the enzyme carbonic anhydrase. Consequently, a fixed concentration ratio is established between dissolved carbon dioxide and carbonic acid.[3] As a corollary, the concentration of carbonic acid, like the concentration of dis-

solved carbon dioxide, is directly proportional to the Pa_{CO_2}.

Although carbonic acid molecules have two hydrogen atoms, only one has a sufficiently weak bond to permit appreciable dissociation within the range of hydrogen ion concentrations found in the extracellular fluid. This dissociation yields equivalent numbers of hydrogen and bicarbonate ions. Equilibrium is established quickly in this reversible reaction as the rate of recombination of hydrogen and bicarbonate ions counterbalances the ongoing rate of dissociation.

It is important to note the physiologic context within which this dissociation-recombination process occurs. As will be discussed shortly, bicarbonate serves as a major anionic constituent of the extracellular compartment and is maintained at relatively high concentration by the kidneys. As a consequence, the dissociation of carbonic acid must proceed in the face of a large quantity of its conjugate base. For this reason, the statistical likelihood of recombination is greatly enhanced and equilibrium is reached at a concentration of hydrogen ions that is correspondingly very low.

The mass action expression governing equilibrium for the dissociation of carbonic acid is shown as Eq. (1) of Fig. 6-2. Algebraic rearrangement yields Eqs. (2) and (3), which focus attention on hydrogen ion concentration; substituting Pa_{CO_2} for carbonic acid concentration yields Eqs. (4) and (5), which contain variables readily measurable by most clinical laboratories. Incorporating the appropriate constants for blood plasma at normal body temperature and selecting convenient units of measure yield Eqs. (6) and (7) of Fig. 6-2.

These mass action expressions *always* govern

---

[3] This concentration ratio favors dissolved carbon dioxide over carbonic acid by approximately 800:1. However, since no practical purpose is served by treating these substances separately, both are regarded, by convention, as being carbonic acid. As a consequence, the *apparent* concentration of carbonic acid is some 800-fold greater than its actual concentration. The interpretation of acid-base data is unaffected by this convention, however, since the *apparent* dissociation constant for carbonic acid (793.4 neq/L, pK = 6.1) is correspondingly lower than its true value.

$$P_a CO_2$$

$$\downarrow$$

$$\text{DISSOLVED} \quad CO_2 + H_2O \underset{\text{CARBONIC ANHYDRASE}}{\rightleftharpoons} H_2CO_3 \rightleftharpoons H^+ + HCO_3^-$$

$$\frac{[H^+] \times [HCO_3^-]}{[H_2CO_3]} = K \qquad (1)$$

$$[H^+] = K \times \frac{[H_2CO_3]}{[HCO_3^-]} \qquad (2) \qquad\qquad pH = pK + \log \frac{[HCO_3^-]}{[H_2CO_3]} \qquad (3)$$

$$[H^+] = K \times \frac{\alpha\, Pa\, CO_2}{[HCO_3^-]} \qquad (4) \qquad\qquad pH = pK + \log \frac{[HCO_3^-]}{\alpha\, Pa\, CO_2} \qquad (5)$$

$$[H^+] = 24 \times \frac{Pa\, CO_2}{[HCO_3^-]} \qquad (6) \qquad\qquad pH = 6.1 + \log \frac{[HCO_3^-]}{.0301\, Pa\, CO_2} \qquad (7)$$

Figure 6-2. Equilibrium expressions for the carbonic acid-bicarbonate buffer system. The pertinent chemical reactions are shown at the top of the figure. Equation (1) defines the interrelationships among hydrogen ion, bicarbonate ion, and carbonic acid concentrations at chemical equilibrium. Arithmetic refinements of this expression, using hydrogen ion concentration as the measure of acidity, are shown on the left-hand side as Eqs. (2), (4), and (6) ("Henderson" equations). The equivalent, inverse logarithmic expressions, using pH units as the measure of acidity, are shown on the right-hand side as Eqs. (3), (5), and (7) (*Henderson-Hasselbalch* equations). The numerical values of the constants used in Eqs. (6) and (7) are those appropriate for blood plasma at normal body temperature when bicarbonate ion concentration is measured in milliequivalents per liter, Pa_{CO_2} in millimeters of mercury, and hydrogen ion concentration in nanoequivalents per liter (10^{-9} equivalent per liter), or pH units, respectively.

the interrelationships among Pa_{CO_2} (in mmHg), bicarbonate concentration (in meq/L), and hydrogen ion concentration (in neq/L or pH units, respectively) because of the rapidity with which chemical equilibrium is established within the organism, during both the hydration of carbon dioxide and the dissociation of carbonic acid. As a result, no matter how rapidly physiologic or pathophysiologic events may be altering acid-base equilibrium, the acid-base values observed at any instant in blood plasma always conform to these equations.

From a physiologic perspective then, plasma acidity can be considered to be a dependent variable, its value being a passive reflection of the prevailing levels of Pa_{CO_2} and bicarbonate concentration. Changes in plasma acidity, whether they be physiologic adjustments or pathophysiologic disturbances, can be mediated only through changes in Pa_{CO_2} and/or bicarbonate concentration. Because these two variables can change independently, this buffer pair functions as the crucial link between the chemical process of buffering on the one hand and the physiologic process of acidity regulation on the other. Accordingly, intelligent appraisal of body fluid acidity depends upon an understanding of the physiologic factors that impinge upon the levels of Pa_{CO_2} and plasma bicarbonate.

DETERMINANTS OF PLASMA BICARBONATE CONCENTRATION

The physiologic regulatory system responsible for the negative feedback control of plasma bicarbonate concentration is depicted in Fig. 6-3. As is apparent from this figure, the regulation of bicarbonate concentration is a byproduct of the maintenance of external hydrogen ion balance. The basic features of this system are analogous to those of the physiologic control systems main-

taining the external balance of most other noncatabolized substances in the body; variations (largely random) in the rate of input produce some alteration in body composition that is counterbalanced by an appropriate adjustment in the rate of output (usually renal). The control system regulating hydrogen ion balance differs from that regulating the balance of most other substances, however, because of the enormous disparity between the large amount of hydrogen ion that passes through the body and the vanishingly low concentration of free hydrogen ions that is tolerated by the living organism.

HYDROGEN ION INPUT

Unlike sodium and other electrolytes, all of which gain access to body fluids directly as a result of

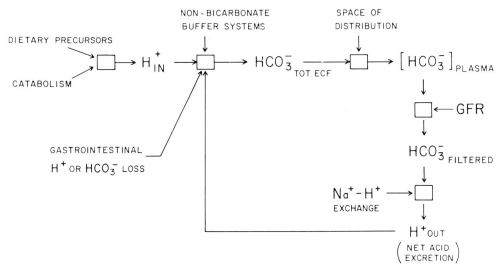

Figure 6-3. Block diagram of the physiologic control system that maintains external hydrogen ion balance and stabilizes plasma bicarbonate concentration. Each block represents the physiologic transfer function that converts the respective inputs into the indicated output. When bicarbonate is titrated by the addition of acid or by the loss of base, restoration of bicarbonate (alkali) stores depends upon the kidney's ability to augment net acid excretion. When bicarbonate stores are increased by the addition of base or by the loss of acid, removal of the bicarbonate excess depends upon the kidney's ability to lower net acid excretion, even to neg-

ative values. Within this context, plasma bicarbonate concentration is seen to be a complex physiologic variable, the value of which is refashioned at every instant by a continuous interplay among the following five factors (Table 6-2): (1) hydrogen ion input (positive or negative), which is normally a consequence of endogenous acid production; (2) hydrogen ion or bicarbonate ion loss from the gastrointestinal tract, which is negligible under *normal* circumstances; (3) the availability of nonbicarbonate buffers; (4) the space of distribution of bicarbonate; and (5) the rate of net acid excretion by the kidney (positive or negative).

ingestion, acids (and bases) are only rarely present as such in the diet. Rather, hydrogen ions are normally introduced into body fluids by endogenous acid production (49). By this process, certain neutral precursor substances are broken down by normal metabolic processes, yielding a variety of strong acids. These endogenous acids are derived either from the breakdown of common constituents of the diet or from the catabolism of body tissues. Consequently, factors that alter the rate of cellular metabolism may lead to variation in hydrogen ion input even in the face of a constant dietary intake of acid precursors.

As shown in Fig. 6-4, three metabolic processes contribute to the endogenous acid load: oxidation of the sulfhydryl groups of cystine and methionine to form sulfuric acid; hydrolysis of phosphoesters to form phosphoric acid; and the incomplete breakdown of neutral carbohydrates, fats, and proteins to form organic acids (36, 38, 50). Some endogenously generated organic acids are true end products of metabolism (e.g., uric acid, creatinine) and contribute, albeit only minimally, to the normal acid load. Other organic acids are metabolic intermediates (e.g., acetoacetic acid, β-OH butyric acid, lactic acid) and contribute to the acid load only when generated faster than they can be converted to carbon dioxide and water.

The overall rate of hydrogen ion input cannot be determined with the same accuracy as is possible for sodium and other electrolytes, both because the contribution of the diet cannot be assessed precisely and because the contribution of catabolic processes cannot be measured directly. Under normal dietary conditions, however, endogenous acid production appears to average approximately 1 meq/kg per day in adults (49) and 2 to 3 meq/kg per day in infants and young children (2). The presence of acids as such in the diet

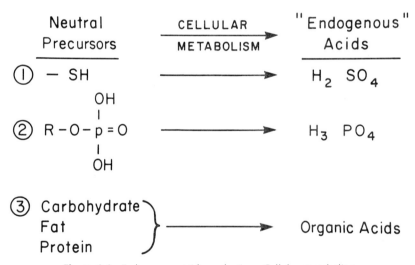

Figure 6-4. Endogenous acid production. Cellular metabolism serves to convert a variety of neutral precursor substances into strong acids. Three major classes of such endogenous acids are recognized: sulfuric acid derived from the oxidation of sulfhydryl groups; phosphoric acid derived from the hydrolysis of phosphoesters; and organic acids derived from the breakdown of carbohydrates, fats, and proteins.

will, of course, augment the hydrogen load derived from endogenous acid production. Conversely, the ingestion of bicarbonate or other strong base, or of organic acid anions that may be converted to bicarbonate by cellular metabolism (e.g., citrate, acetate), will tend to offset the endogenous hydrogen ion load.

BODY BUFFERING

The addition of a large quantity of strong acid, such as that produced each day by cellular metabolism, to a solution lacking in buffers would result in a large increment in hydrogen ion concentration. When acid is added to body fluids, however, titration of body buffers permits this large acid influx to occur without a significant change in acidity.

Among the immediately available buffer solutes, bicarbonate is the most prevalent and plays the pivotal role in the buffering of strong acids. During the titration of body buffers by hydrogen ions, bicarbonate is converted to carbonic acid and thence to carbon dioxide and water (Fig. 6-5). The small amount of carbon dioxide generated by this titration is excreted by the lungs together with the very much larger amount of carbon dioxide derived from cellular metabolism (see below). Approximately 50 percent of the daily endogenous hydrogen ion load is buffered in this reaction with bicarbonate (59, 62, 63). The remainder is accounted for by other hydrogen ion acceptors, including dibasic phosphate and hemoglobin and other proteins (Fig. 6-5). The net effect on body fluid composition of the daily endogenous acid load is thus a depletion of bicarbonate stores and a conversion of some nonbicarbonate buffer bases to their respective acid forms.

Only very small alterations in body composition are, of course, produced over a single day by the normal rate of endogenous acid production. Nevertheless, this process cannot continue unopposed, since each of the available base components would eventually be converted completely to its corresponding acid form, and the acidity of body fluid would rise progressively. It should be apparent that body buffering, despite its critical role in blunting the immediate impact of acid loads, makes no direct contribution to *external* hydrogen ion balance. Body buffering merely substitutes one change in body composition, namely, the conversion of certain bases to their acid forms, for another, much less desirable change, namely a marked increase in hydrogen ion concentration. Until body composition is restored by replacing the deficit of available base, positive hydrogen ion balance and a tendency for acidification of body fluids will persist.

The central role played by bicarbonate ion in the maintenance of hydrogen ion balance is illustrated in Fig. 6-6. The importance of this ion stems from the fact that it is the only base consumed during buffering that can be regenerated by the kidney and returned to body fluids. The amount of bicarbonate required to backtitrate nonbicarbonate buffers and to replenish bicarbonate content fully following the influx of acid is termed the *bicarbonate debt* and is precisely equivalent to the amount of hydrogen ion originally buffered.

RENAL CONTRIBUTION TO HYDROGEN ION BALANCE

The kidneys make an indispensable contribution to external hydrogen ion balance by regulating the bicarbonate content of the body. When the buffering of ingested or endogenous acid reduces the baseline content of bicarbonate and creates a bicarbonate debt, the kidney generates new bicarbonate ions and replenishes body stores (Fig.6-6). Conversely, when a bicarbonate surplus arises during the buffering of ingested or endogenous base, the kidney excretes the excess bicarbonate ions into the urine. In order to understand fully the role of the kidney in effecting these adjustments, attention will first be focused on the mechanisms by which the renal tubule recaptures the bicarbonate that is normally filtered.

Bicarbonate reabsorption

Although bicarbonate ions are freely filtered at the glomerulus, they are not able to traverse the

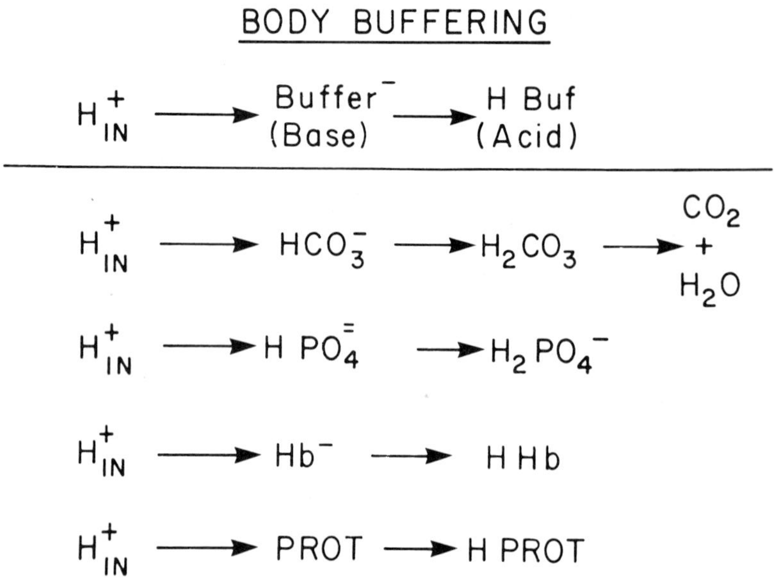

BODY BUFFERING

$$H^+_{IN} \longrightarrow \begin{matrix} Buffer^- \\ (Base) \end{matrix} \longrightarrow \begin{matrix} H\ Buf \\ (Acid) \end{matrix}$$

$$H^+_{IN} \longrightarrow HCO_3^- \longrightarrow H_2CO_3 \longrightarrow \begin{matrix} CO_2 \\ + \\ H_2O \end{matrix}$$

$$H^+_{IN} \longrightarrow H\ PO_4^= \longrightarrow H_2PO_4^-$$

$$H^+_{IN} \longrightarrow Hb^- \longrightarrow H\ Hb$$

$$H^+_{IN} \longrightarrow PROT \longrightarrow H\ PROT$$

Figure 6-5. Body buffering. Body fluids contain numerous substances that can function as hydrogen ion acceptors (bases) or donors (acids) in the range of normal acidity. These substances, called "buffers," account for the resistance to change in acidity displayed by body fluids when challenged with the addition of a strong acid or base. When endogenous (or exogenous) hydrogen ions are added to body fluids, as depicted here, most react with the base components of the common buffer substances, bicarbonate, dibasic phosphate, hemoglobin (Hb), and other proteins.

tubule epithelium with similar ease and must be conserved by an indirect mechanism. This mechanism, outlined in Fig. 6-7, is initiated by a process referred to as sodium-hydrogen exchange.[4] When those sodium ions that electrically balance bicarbonate in the glomerular filtrate are reabsorbed by the tubule cell, electroneutrality is maintained by the secretion of an equivalent number of hydrogen ions. These secreted hydrogen ions, in turn, prevent filtered bicarbonate from reaching the final urine by converting the bicarbonate into carbonic acid and thence to carbon dioxide and water; these latter substances are highly diffusable and readily conserved.

The cycle is completed within the renal tubule cell, where these reactions proceed in the reverse direction, the combination of carbon dioxide and water producing the carbonic acid from which secreted hydrogen ions are derived. As can be seen in Fig. 6-7, this cellular process makes available not only hydrogen ions for secretion but an equivalent number of bicarbonate ions for conservation; these are the bicarbonate ions, rather than those originally filtered, that are returned to body fluids.

Thus, bicarbonate ions have an evanescent existence in the kidney, being filtered from the plasma, converted by secreted hydrogen ion into carbon dioxide and water, and regenerated anew by the tubule epithelium. The essence of the kidney's contribution to hydrogen ion balance may be said to reside in its ability to direct hydrogen ions derived from a virtually limitless intracellular source (i.e., carbon dioxide and water) into the tubule lumen, while directing the associated bicarbonate ions back into the extracellular fluid. Note that under *all* circumstances, the rate at which the kidney returns bicarbonate to the body

[4]The term *sodium-hydrogen exchange* is not meant to imply the presence of a carrier-mediated transport process but is used merely as a shorthand description of that portion of sodium reabsorption that is balanced electrically by the secretory movement of hydrogen.

is equivalent to the rate at which filtered sodium ions are exchanged for hydrogen.

This indirect mechanism of bicarbonate reabsorption is utilized by all of the nephron segments that are concerned with bicarbonate conservation, but the various segments differ markedly in their quantitative contribution to the overall process. The proximal convoluted tubule is the most important site of bicarbonate reclamation. Both clearance studies and micropuncture experiments indicate that approximately 90 percent of filtered bicarbonate is normally conserved by the proximal tubule. This observation correlates well with the abundant carbonic anhydrase activity present at the luminal surface of proximal epithelial cells, a location that facilitates the rapid interconversion of carbon dioxide and carbonic acid essential for efficient bicarbonate reabsorption. The loop of Henle appears to play a minor, if any, role in bicarbonate conservation. When bicarbonate excretion is to be prevented, therefore, the distal convoluted tubule and collecting duct must remove whatever bicarbonate escapes proximal reabsorption.

Acid excretion

Mere conservation of body bicarbonate by the process shown in Fig. 6-7 requires only that the rate of hydrogen secretion be equivalent to the rate of bicarbonate filtration. When body bicarbonate is to be augmented, however, the rate of hydrogen secretion must *exceed* the rate of bicarbonate filtration, and the excess hydrogen ions must gain access to the final urine. A tiny but physiologically critical fraction of these excess hydrogen ions remains in solution in urine as free protons and serves to increase urinary hydrogen ion concentration. In human beings, the maximum urinary hydrogen ion concentration that can be achieved is approximately $10^{-4.0}$ mol/L or 0.1 mmol/L (pH ~ 4.0). Even though this concentration represents a level more than 1000-fold higher than that in plasma, the amount of hydrogen ion that it actually represents is trivial. Nevertheless, the ability of the kidney to generate an acid urine contributes importantly to the formation of titratable acid and ammonium, the two principal carriers of bulk urinary hydrogen ion excretion.

TITRATION OF ALKALI STORES

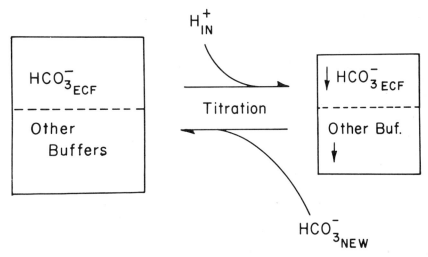

Figure 6-6. Reversible titration of alkali stores. The addition of hydrogen ions to the extracellular fluid, as depicted in Fig. 6-5, titrates bicarbonate and nonbicarbonate buffers to their acid forms, reducing the store of available alkali. The addition of new bicarbonate ions, derived from the kidney, serves to reverse this process. Note that the quantity of new bicarbonate required to replenish alkali stores fully is precisely equivalent to the original load of hydrogen ion.

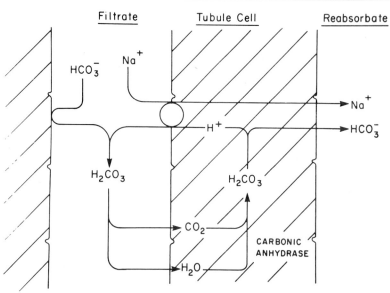

Figure 6-7. Bicarbonate "reabsorption." This schematic diagram represents the indirect mechanism employed by the kidney to prevent excretion of filtered bicarbonate. The fraction of filtered sodium that is reabsorbed in exchange for hydrogen ions derived from cellular carbonic acid is returned to the plasma in association with the bicarbonate ions generated in equivalent numbers. When secreted hydrogen ions encounter filtered bicarbonate in the lumen, bicarbonate is converted to carbonic acid and then to carbon dioxide and water, which are readily reabsorbed.

Titratable acid is the amount of hydrogen ion present in the urine in combination with the base components of all filtered buffer substances that are excreted (Fig. 6-8). The degree to which urinary buffers convey secreted hydrogen ions depends on the *amount* and *nature* of the various buffers present and on the degree of urinary acidification. Normally, approximately half the total urinary hydrogen ion is excreted in the form of titratable acid. Phosphate is the urinary buffer substance that normally accounts for the majority of titratable acid. At normal plasma hydrogen ion concentrations, 80 percent of this buffer solute is in the dibasic form; at the hydrogen ion concentration of maximally acid urine, however, virtually all of the phosphate excreted is in the monobasic form.

Ammonium, the other major repository of urinary hydrogen ion, is much more responsive to alterations in hydrogen ion input than is titratable acid. As indicated in Fig. 6-9, the enzymatic release of ammonia (NH_3) from glutamine within the renal tubule cell is the principal source of urinary ammonium (44, 45, 46). Two important properties of ammonia account for its central role in hydrogen ion excretion. First, being a nonionized substance, it diffuses freely across cell membranes. Second, being a very strong base, it removes secreted hydrogen ions from solution with great efficiency. In so doing, freely diffusible ammonia is converted into poorly diffusible ammonium ions, which are thereby trapped in the urine. As tubular fluid hydrogen ion concentration rises as a result of hydrogen ion secretion, the concentration of free ammonia base in the urine falls, enhancing the net rate of ammonia secretion. Therefore, both the rate at which the renal epithelial cells generate ammonia and the extent to which the urine is acidified are critical determinants of the rate of urinary ammonium excretion.

REGULATION OF RENAL ACID EXCRETION

When the organism is confronted with an acid load, the kidney must return more bicarbonate to body fluids than it receives in the glomerular filtrate; it accomplishes this by maintaining a rate of sodium-hydrogen exchange in excess of the rate of bicarbonate filtration, thus generating titratable acid and ammonium for excretion. When confronted with an alkali load, on the other hand, the kidney must return less bicarbonate to the body than it receives in the glomerular filtrate; it does this by allowing the rate of sodium–hydrogen ion exchange to fall short of the rate of bicar-

bonate filtration, thus permitting some of the filtered bicarbonate to escape into the urine.

The quantitative contribution of the kidney to external hydrogen ion balance in all circumstances can be calculated as the sum of urinary ammonium and titratable acidity minus urinary bicarbonate. Note that this quantity, which is termed *net acid excretion,* has a positive value when hydrogen ion output is preponderant and a negative value when bicarbonate output is preponderant.

In the average adult, the rate of net acid excretion (and new bicarbonate generation) normally required to balance endogenous acid production is only some 50 to 100 meq/day. This quantity, however, represents less than 2 percent of the hydrogen ions actually secreted by the kidney; at a normal filtration rate of 180 L/day and a normal

TITRATABLE ACIDITY

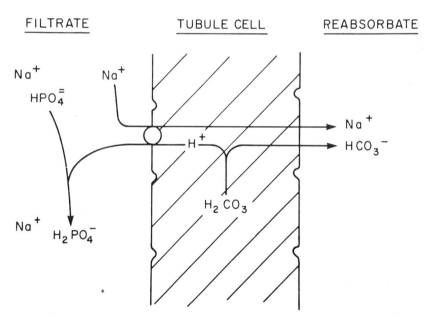

Figure 6-8. Titratable acidity. During the process of urinary acidification, when some hydrogen ions secreted by the tubule cell combine with filtered buffers that are destined for excretion, titratable acidity is formed; phosphate is the major filtered buffer that functions in this capacity. The amount of hydrogen ion excreted as titratable acid can be measured by back-titrating the urine to the hydrogen ion concentration of the original filtrate (i.e., that of plasma). Note that, for each hydrogen ion excreted in this form, a new bicarbonate ion is generated by the kidney and returned to the body.

URINARY AMMONIUM

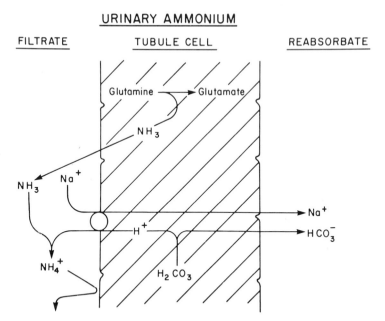

Figure 6-9. Urinary ammonium. When cellular ammonia (NH_3), derived largely from glutamine, diffuses into the tubule lumen and combines with secreted hydrogen ion, urinary ammonium (NH_4^+) is formed. Because the positively charged ammonium ion does not readily penetrate the tubule epithelium, it is "trapped" in the luminal fluid and excreted in the final urine. Note that, for each hydrogen ion excreted as ammonium, a new bicarbonate is generated by the kidney and returned to the body.

plasma bicarbonate concentration of 25 meq/L, the daily rate of hydrogen ion secretion required simply to prevent the excretion of filtered bicarbonate is of the order of 4500 meq.

The mechanisms responsible for the exceedingly fine adjustments in the rate of sodium-hydrogen exchange apparently required to control acid excretion are not clear. It seems highly improbable that these adjustments stem simply from the imperceptibly small changes in body fluid acidity induced by ordinary variations in endogenous acid production. Moreover, recent studies have demonstrated a clear dissociation between systemic hydrogen ion concentration and the augmented renal acid excretion elicited by prolonged acid feeding (19).

An alternative explanation to account for the day-to-day regulation of acid excretion hinges on the recognition that endogenous acids burden the extracellular fluid not only with hydrogen ions but with an equivalent number of relatively nonreabsorbable anions (i.e., sulfate, phosphate, and the various organic acid anions). Let us assume that the fraction of filtered sodium reabsorbed in association with chloride remains constant as long as dietary salt intake, extracellular volume, and renal sodium avidity are stable. As a corollary, the fraction of filtered sodium reabsorbed by the exchange process would also remain constant. Under these circumstances, merely replacing a nonreabsorbable bicarbonate ion (which has a relatively high affinity for hydrogen) with an equally nonreabsorbable endogenous acid anion (which has a very low affinity for hydrogen) would relinquish secreted hydrogen ions, formerly engaged in bicarbonate conservation, for excretion into the urine as net acid. According to this view, regulation of renal acid excretion in the face of a variable rate of endogenous acid production would be a byproduct of sodium homeostasis and of the inherent, relatively static, permeability characteristics of the renal epithelium. This hypothesis is supported by abundant experimental data indicating that renal acid excretion can be influenced importantly simply by altering the anion composition of the filtrate (5, 12, 19, 27, 58).

Several factors other than endogenous acid production are also known to influence bicarbonate reabsorption and acid excretion by the kidney. Perhaps chief among these is the carbon dioxide tension of body fluids. Prolonged changes in carbon dioxide tension have profound effects on tubular hydrogen ion secretion and thereby alter the level of plasma bicarbonate concentration that the kidney functions to maintain. Whether hydrogen transport is affected directly or indirectly through changes in chloride and/or sodium transport is not clear. Regardless of the mechanism, however, chronic hypercapnia accelerates hydrogen ion secretion, producing a sustained elevation in plasma bicarbonate concentration, whereas chronic hypocapnia leads to a dampening of hydrogen ion secretion and a sustained reduction in plasma bicarbonate concentration. A more detailed discussion of the influence of carbon dioxide tension in the kidney is found in subsequent sections of this chapter that deal with acid-base disturbances of respiratory origin.

Changes in extracellular fluid volume also influence the rate of tubular hydrogen ion secretion but do not alter the steady-state level of plasma bicarbonate concentration unless coupled with other factors. Effective extracellular volume is, of course, a major determinant of the rate of tubular sodium reabsorption. Expansion of the extracellular volume dampens reabsorption and promotes sodium excretion, whereas contraction of volume stimulates sodium conservation. In view of the dependence of overall hydrogen ion secretion on the magnitude of sodium transport, it is not surprising that alterations in extracellular volume have an influence on the rate of bicarbonate reabsorption. For example, the fall in proximal tubule sodium reabsorption induced by acute volume expansion is accompanied by a roughly proportionate fall in proximal bicarbonate reabsorption. It is important to recognize, however, that significant excretion of bicarbonate into the urine occurs in such acute experiments only when volume expansion is totally or partially the result of the provision of alkaline salts. When volume expansion is produced without the provision of alkali (e.g.,

by the administration of normal saline), virtually all of the bicarbonate that escapes proximal reabsorption is conserved at distal sites. When "isometric" expansion is produced in normal animals by infusing solutions containing sodium, chloride, and bicarbonate in concentrations identical to those in normal plasma, a reduction in the transport of all of these electrolytes occurs; as a result, very little change in plasma electrolyte composition is observed. Consequently, despite the reduction in bicarbonate reabsorption which accompanies volume expansion, expansion per se does not lead to a significant alteration in acid-base equilibrium. By similar reasoning, it can be concluded that volume contraction per se does not influence acid-base equilibrium either; when the process responsible for contracting extracellular volume does not alter the concentration of plasma electrolytes, no change in the fraction of filtered sodium conserved in exchange for hydrogen ion need occur and, hence, no alteration in the steady-state level of plasma bicarbonate concentration would be anticipated.[5]

Changes in body potassium stores have also been thought to influence renal bicarbonate reabsorption and acid excretion, presumably by altering intracellular acidity. Whether the reduction in hydrogen ion secretion thought to accompany potassium surfeits or the accelerated hydrogen ion secretion thought to accompany potassium deficits has a significant influence on the physiologic regulation of hydrogen ion balance is not well established. The role of potassium in abnormalities of acid-base equilibrium is discussed later.

GASTROINTESTINAL CONTRIBUTION TO HYDROGEN ION BALANCE

As indicated in Fig. 6-3, the secretion of hydrogen ion by the stomach and of bicarbonate by the pancreas, biliary tree, and small intestine carries

---

[5]As discussed in the section on metabolic alkalosis, volume contraction is often the consequence of processes that do alter bicarbonate and chloride concentrations. Under these circumstances, the concentration-induced stimulus to renal sodium conservation may play an important role in perpetuating the abnormal electrolyte composition of the plasma.

the potential for serious disruptions of external hydrogen ion balance. Under normal circumstances, these enteric secretions are virtually completely reabsorbed and, hence, have no *net* impact on bicarbonate stores; but when acid gastric juice or alkaline small intestinal fluids are lost from the body, the level of bicarbonate may be markedly affected. Further discussion of the role of the gastrointestinal tract is deferred to subsequent sections in which derangements of hydrogen ion metabolism are considered.

DETERMINANTS OF PLASMA CARBON DIOXIDE TENSION

Although the physiologic control system regulating carbon dioxide balance and, hence, Pa_{CO_2} is much less complicated than that regulating hydrogen ion balance, the two systems exhibit the same basic features: endogenous production of the substance by metabolic processes; its conversion to an altered form during transport from point of origin to site of elimination; and a regulated mode of excretion.

CARBON DIOXIDE INPUT

Under basal conditions, cellular processes in normal adults generate approximately 20,000 mmol of carbon dioxide daily. The rate of production is altered when energy requirements change but is remarkably constant from day to day in normal individuals if the level of exercise is reasonably stable.

This large carbon dioxide input into body fluids does not contribute to the daily hydrogen ion load or to the corresponding bicarbonate debt discussed in the preceding section. Carbon dioxide homeostasis affects hydrogen ion metabolism only through its influence on carbonic acid concentration and, correspondingly, through its impact on the equilibrium concentration of free hydrogen ions (Fig. 6-2).

CARBON DIOXIDE TRANSPORT

The carbon dioxide produced in tissues is transported by the blood to the pulmonary capillaries for excretion. Although the amount of carbon dioxide that can be transported is greatly enhanced by certain properties of hemoglobin, which binds carbon dioxide, the process of diffusion is the fundamental driving force responsible for the steady flow of carbon dioxide from the tissue to the blood and from the blood to the alveolar spaces of the lungs. Accordingly, a progressive gradient of carbon dioxide tension is found between body tissues and alveoli.

As carbon dioxide is generated by cellular metabolism, it diffuses into red blood cells, where a portion is hydrated under the catalytic influence of carbonic anhydrase to form carbonic acid. Hydrogen ions relinquished by the dissociation of this carbonic acid combine with certain basic groups of hemoglobin that are made even more avid for hydrogen by the low oxygen tension in venous blood. Bicarbonate ions, generated in equivalent numbers during this process, diffuse back into the plasma in exchange for chloride. A lesser but significant portion of the carbon dioxide entering the bloodstream reacts directly with certain amino acid residues on hemoglobin (and other proteins) to form carbamino compounds. When blood reaches the pulmonary capillaries, this entire sequence is reversed, as carbon dioxide diffuses out of blood into the alveolar spaces and as the affinity of hemoglobin for hydrogen is lessened by the high oxygen tension in the pulmonary capillaries.

The physiologic importance of this cycle centers on the removal of carbon dioxide from solution and its temporary conversion to bicarbonate and carbamino compounds. This process permits much larger quantities of carbon dioxide to be transported from the tissues to the lungs than could otherwise be accommodated by the carbon dioxide gradient. The analogy between this cycle and the process of body buffering during endogenous acid production is apparent. Just as body buffering permits large quantities of hydrogen ion to flow through body fluids without large changes in hydrogen ion concentration, so these mechanisms for transporting carbon dioxide permit large quantities of this substance to pass through the system with minimal changes in carbon dioxide tension. Moreover, just as body buffering makes no direct contribution to external hydrogen ion balance, so the buffering of carbonic acid by hemoglobin makes no direct contribution to external carbon dioxide balance. External balance is determined by the rates of carbon dioxide production and elminination and not by the intermediate mode of transport.

CARBON DIOXIDE EXCRETION

The rate at which carbon dioxide is excreted from the body is the product of alveolar ventilation and alveolar carbon dioxide concentration. Since the concentration of carbon dioxide in alveolar gas is proportional to its partial pressure, the following proportionality may be written:

$$CO_2 \text{ excretion} \sim P_{A_{CO_2}} \times \text{alveolar ventilation}$$

Since diffusion equilibrium for carbon dioxide is achieved with ease across the alveolar capillary wall, *alveolar* carbon dioxide tension ($P_{A_{CO_2}}$) and *arterial* plasma carbon dioxide tension ($P_{a_{CO_2}}$) are virtually identical. Furthermore, in the steady state, the rate of carbon dioxide excretion is equivalent to the rate of carbon dioxide production. Under steady-state circumstances, therefore, the following relationship governs $P_{a_{CO_2}}$:

$$P_{a_{CO_2}} \sim \frac{CO_2 \text{ production}}{\text{alveolar ventilation}}$$

Table 6-2. Physiologic factors impinging on plasma acidity

I. THROUGH PLASMA BICARBONATE CONCENTRATION
1. Rate of hydrogen ion input (positive or negative)
2. Rate of hydrogen ion or bicarbonate ion loss via the gastrointestinal tract
3. Availability of nonbicarbonate buffers
4. Space of distribution for bicarbonate
5. Rate of net acid excretion by the kidney (positive or negative)

II. THROUGH PLASMA CARBON DIOXIDE TENSION (CARBONIC ACID CONCENTRATION)
1. Rate of carbon dioxide production
2. Rate of alveolar ventilation

Thus, plasma carbon dioxide tension can be regarded as a complex physiologic variable, the value of which is determined at every instant by a continuous byplay between the rate of carbon dioxide production and the rate of alveolar ventilation (Table 6-2).

The regulation of carbon dioxide excretion is extremely efficient under normal circumstances, owing to the exquisite sensitivity of the medullary respiratory centers to changes in $P_{a_{CO_2}}$. Thus, moment-to-moment changes in the rate of carbon dioxide production in a healthy subject are responded to swiftly by appropriate changes in the rate of alveolar ventilation, the level of $P_{a_{CO_2}}$ being only transiently and minimally affected.

SECTION III

Clinical disturbances of acid-base equilibrium

DEFINITION OF TERMS

The simple mass action expression formulated by Henderson (30),

$$[H^+] \text{ (neq/L)} = 24 \frac{P_{a_{CO_2}} \text{ (mmHg)}}{[HCO_3] \text{ (meq/L)}} \quad (6\text{-}8)$$

will be used as a point of departure for examining the limited variety of ways in which plasma acid-

ity may be disturbed. The interrelationships expressed by the Henderson equation are depicted graphically in Fig. 6-10. Nomograms of this general type are useful in visualizing the impact on acidity of the various disturbances to be considered and in following the pathways traversed by acid-base equilibrium in response to physiologic and pathologic processes (13). Arterial carbon dioxide tension and plasma bicarbonate concen-

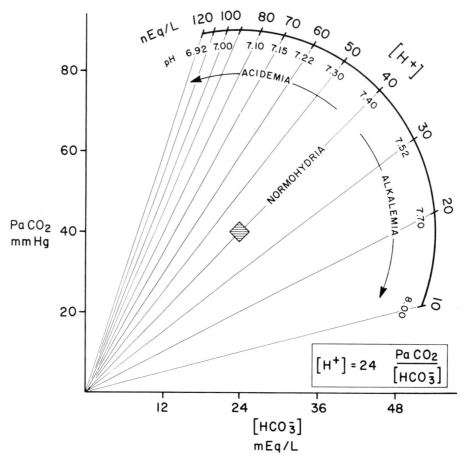

Figure 6-10. A graphic representation of the relationships in plasma among carbonic dioxide tension (Pa_{CO_2}), bicarbonate concentration, and hydrogen ion concentration at chemical equilibrium. The algebraic form of these relationships is shown in the lower right. Carbon dioxide tension is depicted in mmHg on the vertical axis and bicarbonate concentration is depicted in milliequivalents per liter on the horizontal axis. Hydrogen ion concentration (depicted in both nanoequivalents per liter and pH units) is displayed by a series of isobars radiating from the origin. The normal ranges for these parameters in arterial blood are indicated by the shaded zone near the center of the figure. As can be seen, normal levels of hydrogen ion concentration (normohydria) can result from certain abnormal combinations of Pa_{CO_2} and bicarbonate concentration. The terms acidemia and alkalemia are used to denote increases and decreases in hydrogen ion concentration, respectively.

tration average approximately 40 mmHg and 24 meq/L, respectively, in normal individuals. Consequently, normal arterial hydrogen ion concentration is approximately 40 neq/L (pH 7.40).

Abnormalities of acid-base equilibrium can be initiated either by changes in Pa_{CO_2} or by changes in plasma bicarbonate concentration (Fig. 6-11). Increases and decreases in Pa_{CO_2}, denoted by the terms *hyper-* and *hypocapnia*, initiate acid-base disturbances referred to as respiratory acidosis and respiratory alkalosis, respectively. Changes in bicarbonate concentration, termed *hyper-* and *hypobicarbonatemia* initiate acid-base disturbances called metabolic acidosis and metabolic alkalosis.

In each of the four cardinal acid-base disturbances so defined, the initiating process not only alters acid-base equilibrium directly but sets in motion certain secondary physiologic responses that serve to change the value of the countervailing variable. Thus, as shown in Fig. 6-12, the metabolic disturbances induce a ventilatory response that secondarily alters the level of Pa_{CO_2}, whereas the respiratory disturbances induce buffer and renal responses that secondarily alter the level of bicarbonate concentration. As a general rule, these adaptive responses tend to lessen the impact on acidity but fall short of returning hydrogen ion concentration to normal levels.

In the absence of other limiting disease processes, each of these secondary physiologic responses pursues a characteristic time-course and produces readjustments in acid-base equilibrium that are highly dependent, quantitatively, on the

magnitude of the initiating change. It is reasonable, therefore, to regard the secondary physiologic adaptations as part and parcel of the acid-base disturbances to which they are wedded and not as independent abnormalities in their own right.

In accordance with these principles, a *simple* acid-base disturbance refers to the presence of a single initiating abnormality coupled with its anticipated secondary physiologic response. By contrast, a *mixed* acid-base disturbance refers to the coexistence of two or more independent abnormalities. In order to recognize and unravel such mixed disturbances of acidity, the limits of the secondary physiologic adjustments to each of the primary disorders, and the relevant response times, must be known; these considerations are discussed in greater detail below.

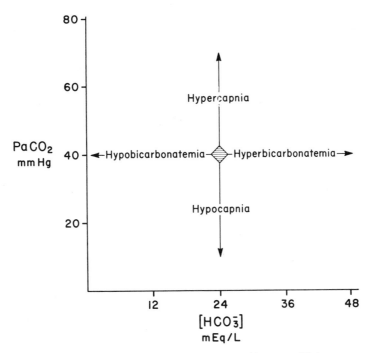

Figure 6-11. Disturbing influences on acid-base equilibrium. "Metabolic" acid-base disturbances are initiated by changes in plasma bicarbonate concentration (hypo- or hyperbicarbonatemia), whereas "respiratory" acid-base disturbances are initiated by changes in Pa_{CO_2} (hypo- or hypercapnia).

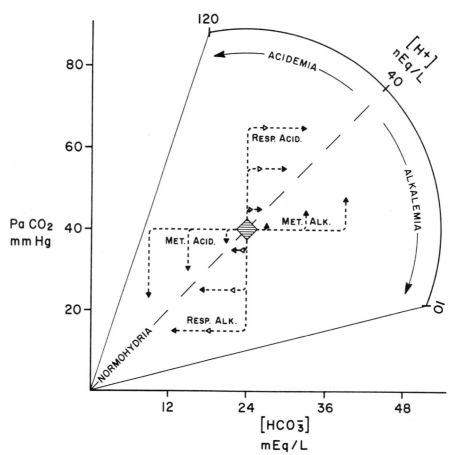

Figure 6-12. Pathways of clinical acid-base disturbances. Each of the four cardinal acid-base disturbances is composed of an initiating abnormality (in either Pa_{CO_2} or bicarbonate concentration) and a physiologic adaptive response in the countervailing variable. Metabolic acidosis and alkalosis are initiated, respectively, by some degree of hypo- or hyperbicarbonatemia, which elicits an adaptive, secondary change in Pa_{CO_2}. Respiratory acidosis and alkalosis are initiated, respectively, by some degree of hyper- or hypocapnia, which elicits adaptive changes in bicarbonate con-

centration. As indicated by the two arrowheads on the pathways denoting respiratory disturbances, the adaptive changes in bicarbonate elicited by these disorders are of dual origin, body buffers (open arrowheads) and the kidney (closed arrowheads). Note that in each of the four classes of acid-base disorders, the secondary, physiologic responses are roughly proportional to the magnitude of the initiating changes but fail to return hydrogen ion concentration completely to normohydric levels.

PRACTICAL CONSIDERATIONS

Attention to the practical aspects of blood sampling, specimen handling, and analytic methodology are of critical importance for an accurate appraisal of acid-base equilibrium in the clinical setting; failure to adhere to proper procedures can

introduce serious artifacts and thwart meaningful interpretation of the acid-base data.

Arterial blood provides the most reliable data for assessing the acid-base status of the extracellular compartment as a whole, because it is relatively uninfluenced by local factors. The most accessible sites for direct arterial puncture are the brachial, radial, and femoral vessels. The risks associated with direct needle puncture of such large vessels are well known and include trauma to adjacent structures, hematoma formation, and arterial spasm. In addition, the discomfort and anxiety associated with direct arterial puncture may lead to hyperventilation and a transient reduction in Pa_{CO_2}; this "artifactual" influence on acid-base equilibrium can be minimized by allowing patients to relax for a few moments between puncturing the vessel and removing the blood sample. When frequent assessment of acid-base equilibrium is required, it is often desirable to place an inlying arterial catheter rather than risk multiple arteriotomies.

Freely flowing capillary blood obtained by finger stick, especially if "arterialized" by prior warming of the hand, provides a close approximation of arterial blood and is especially useful for acid-base assessment in infants and young children. Venous blood drawn without stasis can be used for acid-base measurements, but cognizance must be taken of the greater variability of the data obtained and of the necessary discrepancies between venous and arterial values; the P_{CO_2} of venous blood is approximately 5 to 7 mmHg higher, the bicarbonate concentration approximately 1 to 3 meq/L higher, and the hydrogen ion concentration approximately 3 to 5 neq/L higher (pH 0.03 to 0.05 units lower) than are the respective values for arterial blood.

Samples for Pa_{CO_2} and pH measurements must be prevented from clotting. Heparin is by far the most suitable anticoagulant for this purpose, because the small quantity required (less than 100 units/mL of blood) does not alter the acid-base composition of the blood or interfere with subsequent analyses. Other anticoagulants [e.g., edetic acid (EDTA), citrate, oxalate] should not be used.

Carbon dioxide diffuses so readily that even brief exposure of the blood sample to room air may lead to a significant distortion of the acid-base values; consequently, syringes must be filled carefully to avoid aspiration of air, capped immediately, and delivered promptly to the laboratory. If vacuum containers are used for collecting specimens, care must be taken to fill the container completely.

Even when anaerobic conditions are strictly maintained during sampling, changes in the acid-base status of the specimen occur continuously in vitro because of continuing cellular metabolism. If possible, therefore, measurements should be made immediately. If a delay of greater than 5 to 10 minutes is unavoidable, the specimen should be cooled (e.g., by immersing the syringe in crushed ice) in order to retard the rate of cellular metabolism; even with this precaution, measurements should be completed within one hour after sampling.

Both hydrogen ion concentration (pH) and carbon dioxide tension can be measured directly by standard electrochemical techniques. Bicarbonate concentration is generally estimated from the total carbon dioxide (tCO_2) released from an acidified serum sample; since approximately 95 percent of the CO_2 released is derived from bicarbonate ions under virtually all circumstances,[6] the value obtained for tCO_2 (in mmol/L) may be substituted for true bicarbonate concentration in the Henderson equation (Fig. 6-10) without invalidating subsequent clinical interpretations. Measurements in the same blood sample of any two of the three variables in this equation are, of course, sufficient to permit calculation of the third.

METABOLIC ACIDOSIS

Metabolic acidosis refers to those acid-base disturbances initiated by a reduction in plasma bicarbonate concentration.

PATHOPHYSIOLOGY

Plasma bicarbonate concentration may be reduced either by a disproportionate loss of bicar-

---

[6]The remainder of the total CO_2 is derived from carbonic acid and dissolved carbon dioxide. If a measurement of Pa_{CO_2} is available, the combined concentration of dissolved carbon dioxide and carbonic acid (in mmol/L) may be obtained by multiplying Pa_{CO_2} (in mmHg) by the factor 0.03. The actual bicarbonate concentration may then be calculated by subtracting this value from the total CO_2.

bonate ions as such or by the addition of a strong acid that consumes bicarbonate during the process of buffering. The degree to which plasma bicarbonate falls during metabolic acidosis is a function not only of the magnitude of the bicarbonate loss or of the acid load but of the rate of the offending process and of the speed with which the kidney is able to replenish bicarbonate stores. If the kidneys themselves are not responsible for the acidosis, and if renal function is normal, acid excretion may, with sufficient time, increase to a level of 200 to 400 meq/day or greater (54).

SECONDARY PHYSIOLOGIC ADJUSTMENTS IN RESPIRATION

As illustrated in Fig. 6-10, the effect on acid-base equilibrium of a reduction in bicarbonate concentration is an increase in plasma acidity. The physiologic response to this primary alteration in acid-base equilibrium is an increase in alveolar ventilation and a corresponding decrease in Pa_{CO_2}. This ventilatory response appears to result from a direct effect on the medullary respiratory centers of the small but definite changes in cerebral interstitial fluid bicarbonate and hydrogen ion concentrations that occur during metabolic acidosis (42). The time-course of the adjustments in ventilation during metabolic acidosis is influenced importantly, however, by the delay imposed by the blood-brain barrier on the equilibration of bicarbonate between plasma and cerebral interstitial fluid. As shown in Fig. 6-13, during the rapid onset of severe metabolic acidosis, the abrupt fall in plasma bicarbonate concentration characteristically outstrips the secondary decrements in Pa_{CO_2}, giving rise to extreme elevations in plasma hydrogen ion concentration. Several hours may elapse before full ventilatory adjustments occur and maximal blunting of the acidemia is accomplished. Similarly, during the rapid repair of a severe metabolic acidosis, the restoration of a normal or near normal level of plasma bicarbonate is frequently associated with persisted hyperventilation and a consequent marked reduction in plasma hydrogen ion concentration; frankly alka-

lemic levels of plasma hydrogen ion concentration may even be encountered.

Studies of the quantitative relationships between plasma bicarbonate concentration and Pa_{CO_2} in patients with various degrees of stable, uncomplicated metabolic acidosis indicate that the level to which Pa_{CO_2} falls when a steady state is achieved is roughly proportional to the prevailing decrement in plasma bicarbonate; on the average, a reduction in plasma bicarbonate concentration of 1.0 meq/L is associated with a 1.0 to 1.3 mmHg reduction in Pa_{CO_2}[7] (1, 37, 43, 68). This relationship is illustrated in Fig. 6-14.

These observations find application in clinical medicine when used as adjuncts to historical and other laboratory data in distinguishing patients with uncomplicated metabolic acidosis from those in whom an independent respiratory acid-base abnormality is also present. If respiratory readjustments fall short of the anticipated level (i.e., if Pa_{CO_2} is higher than expected for a given decrement in plasma bicarbonate), an element of respiratory acidosis is probably present; conversely, if respiratory adjustments appear excessive (i.e., if Pa_{CO_2} is lower than expected), an independent element of primary respiratory alkalosis is probably present (see the section on mixed acid-base disturbances). When making such inferences, allowances must be made for the lag in ventilatory adjustments anticipated during intervals of rapid change in plasma bicarbonate concentration (Fig. 6-13).

DIAGNOSIS AND CLINICAL MANIFESTATIONS

When metabolic acidosis is the only pathologic process affecting acid-base equilibrium, laboratory data reveal a reduced plasma bicarbonate concentration in association with some degree of acidemia (Fig. 6-14). If bicarbonate concentration

---

[7]The minimal value for plasma carbon dioxide tension that can be achieved is approximately 10 mmHg. Such extreme reductions in Pa_{CO_2} typically occur in uncomplicated metabolic acidosis only when plasma bicarbonate concentration is reduced to extremely low levels (i.e., less than 5 meq/L).

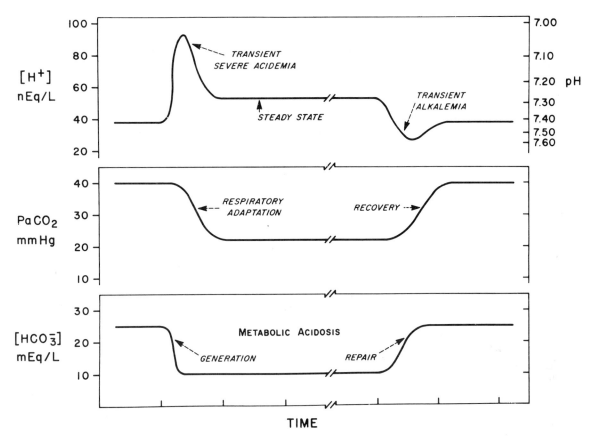

Figure 6-13. Schematic time-course of the changes in plasma acid-base equilibrium during the generation and repair of metabolic acidosis. Metabolic acidosis is initiated by a reduction in plasma bicarbonate concentration that elicits a secondary, adaptive response in Pa_{CO_2}. When a large decrement in bicarbonate concentration occurs abruptly, as in the illustration presented here, there is typically a delay in the development of secondary hypocapnia and in the expected attenuation of the degree of acidity (see Fig. 6-14). This delay probably reflects the obstacle posed by the blood-brain barrier in achieving equilibration between plasma and cerebral interstitial fluid. Similarly, when severe metabolic acidosis is rapidly repaired, hypocapnia often persists for several hours; as a result, transient reductions in hydrogen ion concentration, even to frankly alkalemic levels, are often seen before completely normal acid-base equilibrium is restored.

is less than 10 meq/L, an element of metabolic acidosis can be diagnosed with confidence even if a measurement of hydrogen ion concentration or Pa_{CO_2} is not available; bicarbonate concentration is rarely, if ever, reduced to levels this low solely by the secondary physiologic responses to respiratory alkalosis (see below).

Obvious hyperventilation is frequently the initial clue to the presence of metabolic acidosis. Manifestations of central nervous system dys-function, including stupor and coma, may dominate the clinical picture. Cardiovascular manifestations of metabolic acidosis are also common and include depressed cardiac contractility and peripheral vasodilation, changes that may result in congestive heart failure, hypotension, or marked alteration in tissue perfusion. In addition, the threshold for the induction of ventricular fibrillation appears to be significantly reduced in metabolic acidosis. Gastrointestinal dysfunction may

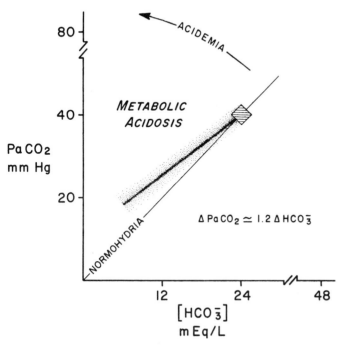

Figure 6-14. Effect of metabolic acidosis on acid-base equilibrium. The initiating event is a reduction in plasma bicarbonate concentration that produces an increase in hydrogen ion concentration (see Fig. 6-10). In response to this change, the respiratory system produces a secondary reduction in carbon dioxide tension that has an ameliorating effect on the level of acidity. The extent of this physiologic response of the respiratory system is roughly proportional to the fall in plasma bicarbonate concentration, each meq/L decrement in [HCO_3^-] being associated, on the average, with an approximately 1.2 mmHg reduction in Pa_{CO_2}. The biologic variation typical of such physiologic responses is indicated by the shaded area.

be manifested by anorexia, nausea, and vomiting. It has been speculated that the morbidity and mortality rates associated with metabolic acidosis may, in part, reflect the effects of increased intracellular acidity on crucial enzyme systems.

Critical alterations in the distribution of body potassium also occur frequently during metabolic acidosis. The elevated extracellular hydrogen ion concentration produced by this acid-base disturbance appears to favor movement of hydrogen ions into cells in exchange for potassium. As a result,

hyperkalemia is a common finding in severe metabolic acidosis and may necessitate rapid correction of the acidemia in order to avoid or reverse life-threatening cardiac arrhythmias. Similarly, the shift of potassium out of cells during acidosis may mask the presence of a severe degree of potassium depletion; for example, significant potassium deficits often accompany the metabolic acidosis produced by prolonged diarrhea or uncontrolled diabetes (see below), but serum potassium may be normal or even elevated when such patients are first encountered. In these circumstances, serum potassium concentration usually falls markedly during or after correction of the acidosis.

THERAPEUTIC PRINCIPLES

Repair of the altered body composition produced by metabolic acidosis centers on the provision of adequate amounts of bicarbonate. If plasma bicarbonate concentration is only moderately depressed, and if the cause of the acidosis can be treated or is self-limited, bicarbonate replacement therapy may not be necessary, because the normal kidney can replete body bicarbonate stores over a period of several days. If, however, the cause of the acidosis cannot be eliminated (e.g., chronic renal failure), long-term alkali therapy may be necessary. Bicarbonate, or an organic anion that can be converted to bicarbonate (e.g., citrate), may be administered orally for this purpose in a dose adjusted empirically to maintain the desired plasma bicarbonate concentration.

If bicarbonate concentration is markedly depressed, rapid therapeutic intervention may be required even if the underlying cause can be removed quickly (e.g., diabetic acidosis). Rapid correction of metabolic acidosis is accomplished most reliably by the intravenous administration of sodium bicarbonate. As a general rule, therapy should be designed to replace only about one-half of the total bicarbonate deficit over the initial 12 hours of treatment in order to avoid the consequences of abrupt changes in extracellular acid-base equilibrium. When this precaution is observed, tetany, altered mental status, and convulsions rarely occur.

In estimating the amount of bicarbonate required to produce a desired increment in plasma bicarbonate concentration, the effect of nonbicarbonate buffers on the fate of administered bicarbonate must be considered. For the same reason that 50 percent of an infused hydrogen ion load is buffered by extracellular bicarbonate (the remainder being accommodated by other buffers), no less than 50 percent of an administered bicarbonate load is dissipated immediately by hydrogen ions relinquished from other buffers. Thus, in selecting an appropriate dose of bicarbonate, the desired increment in plasma concentration must be multiplied by an *apparent* space of distribution at least twice as large as the normal extracellular fluid volume (i.e., approximately 40 percent of body weight). The apparent space of bicarbonate distribution may be even larger in patients with severe metabolic acidosis (i.e., plasma bicarbonate less than 5 meq/L) (25). Estimates of bicarbonate requirements serve only as rough guidelines and must be adjusted to suit individual circumstances; this is particularly true when increased acid production or bicarbonate losses continue during the period of therapy.

Other alkalinizing agents (e.g., lactate, citrate) offer no advantage over bicarbonate in the urgent treatment of metabolic acidosis, since their net effect on acid-base equilibrium is achieved only through their capacity to increase bicarbonate concentration. If cardiac or renal failure precludes administration of adequate amounts of bicarbonate (with sodium), it may be necessary to institute peritoneal dialysis or hemodialysis.

CAUSES OF METABOLIC ACIDOSIS

As indicated in Fig. 6-15 and Table 6-3, two groups of metabolic acidoses can be identified according to the presence or absence of an elevated concentration of undetermined anions. The undetermined anion concentration, often referred to as the anion gap, consists of the net negative charges on plasma proteins and the negative charges contributed by the numerous inorganic and organic anions normally present in the plasma. The contribution made by these plasma constituents to the electroneutrality of this compartment is conventionally estimated by subtracting the sum of the measured chloride and bicarbonate concentrations from the measured concentration of sodium. Defined in this way, the undetermined anion concentration normally ranges between 8 and 12 meq/L.

Table 6-3. Causes of metabolic acidosis

NORMAL UNDETERMINED ANION CONCENTRATION	ELEVATED UNDETERMINED ANION CONCENTRATION
Loss of bicarbonate	Overproduction of organic acids
Diarrhea	Diabetic ketoacidosis
Small-bowel losses	Prolonged starvation
Ureterosigmoidostomy	Alcoholic ketoacidosis
Ileal-loop bladder	Methyl alcohol ingestion
Carbonic anhydrase inhibitors	Ethylene glycol ingestion
Dilutional acidosis	Paraldehyde ingestion
Disproportionate failure of renal tubular function	Salicylate intoxication
Renal tubular acidosis	Lactic acidosis
Tubulointerstitial renal disease	Renal insufficiency
Urinary tract obstruction	Uremic acidosis
Addition of hydrochloric acid	Acute renal failure
Ammonium chloride	
Lysine − HCl	
Arginine − HCl	

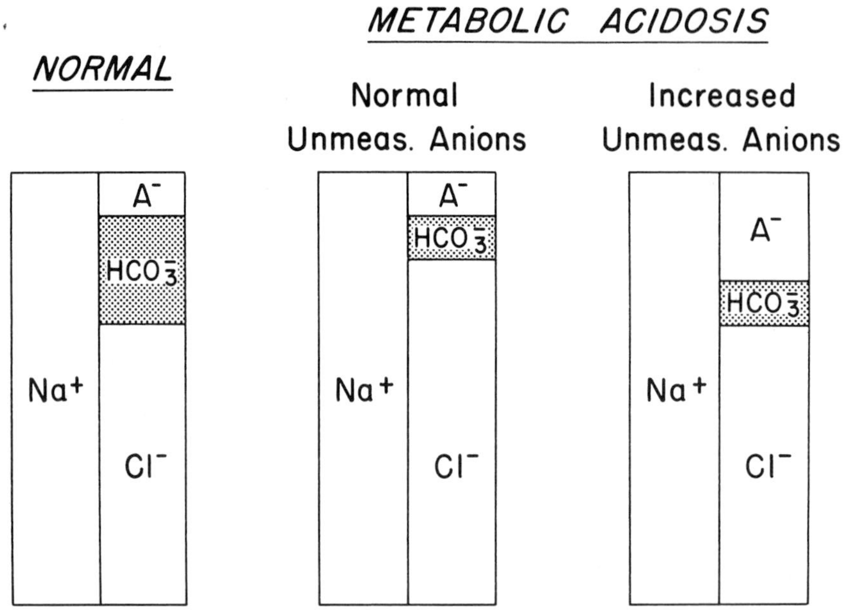

METABOLIC ACIDOSIS

NORMAL

Normal
Unmeas. Anions

Increased
Unmeas. Anions

Figure 6-15. Patterns of extracellular electrolyte composition under normal conditions and during metabolic acidosis. Under all circumstances, sodium ions account for the bulk of cation equivalents, whereas chloride and bicarbonate ions account for most of the anion equivalents. The normal discrepancy between sodium concentration and the sum of chloride and bicarbonate concentrations is defined as the "unmeasured anion" concentration and is composed of the anionic groups of proteins as well as numerous other organic and inorganic anions. Defined in this way, the concentration of undetermined anions normally ranges between 8 and 12 meq/L. Reductions in bicarbonate concentration can be offset either by an increase in chloride concentration or by an increase in the concentration of unmeasured anions. The latter pattern is characteristic of those forms of metabolic acidosis that result from the overproduction of organic acids (see Table 6-3).

Normal undetermined anion concentration

The causes of metabolic acidosis associated with a normal undetermined anion concentration are listed in the left-hand column of Table 6-3. These conditions can be subclassified as follows: a loss of bicarbonate as such from the body; a disproportionate failure of renal tubular function; and the addition of hydrochloric acid to body fluids.

Loss of bicarbonate. Bicarbonate can be lost from the body through either the gastrointestinal tract or the kidney. The most common cause of gastrointestinal bicarbonate loss is diarrhea, during which bicarbonate derived from pancreatic and intestinal secretions is incompletely absorbed. The bicarbonate concentration of diarrheic stool is almost always higher (and the chloride concentration lower) than that of plasma and may reach levels as high as 70 to 80 meq/L under some circumstances. Infants and children are particularly prone to develop acidosis as a result of diarrhea, because of the relatively large bicarbonate losses that occur over a short time (65). Small-bowel losses of bicarbonate may also occur via nasogastric suction or by direct drainage following abdominal surgery.

Significant metabolic acidosis, caused in part by the loss of bicarbonate, is a frequent complication in patients with ureterosigmoidostomy. The temporary retention of chloride-rich urine in the sigmoid colon results in the reabsorption of chloride in exchange for extracellular bicarbonate, which is subsequently evacuated with the stool. Reabsorption of urinary ammonium as well as renal damage from infection and other causes may also contribute importantly to the development of acidosis in these patients. Although the loss of bicarbonate and absorption of ammonium can be retarded by frequent enemas or the use of rectal tubes to reduce contact time between urine and colonic mucosa, the frequent occurrence of chronic metabolic acidosis is one of the many factors that limits the usefulness of this method of urinary diversion. Fortunately, urinary diversion using the ileal-loop bladder technique is associated with a much lower incidence of metabolic complications. Unless stomal obstruction develops, producing marked distention of the ileal conduit, external drainage of the urine is usually sufficiently prompt to avoid significant bicarbonate losses.

Carbonic anhydrase inhibitors (e.g., acetazolamide) induce a loss of bicarbonate from the kidney because carbonic anhydrase activity plays a crucial role in renal bicarbonate reabsorption. Prolonged administration results in a sustained reduction in plasma bicarbonate and a reciprocal increase in plasma chloride; in response to the usual therapeutic doses, plasma bicarbonate is rarely reduced to levels lower than 17 to 18 meq/L.

Mild metabolic acidosis can result from a marked and sudden increase in the space of bicarbonate distribution, which causes existing bicarbonate to be diluted or "lost" in a larger volume, thereby reducing its plasma concentration. Such dilutional acidosis is occasionally seen during rapid reexpansion of a severely volume-contracted patient when such reexpansion is accomplished with saline or other fluids lacking in bicarbonate or equivalent base (23).

Disproportionate failure of renal tubular function. Several varieties of congenital and acquired renal tubular diseases result in some limitation of bicarbonate reabsorption or urinary acidification or both in the absence of significant glomerular dysfunction. Patients with such defects may develop severe metabolic acidosis, often accompanied by extreme potassium depletion. This group of disorders is referred to as renal tubular acidosis and is discussed in Chap. 18.

Tubulointerstitial renal diseases and urinary tract obstruction, disorders in which selective damage to tubular cells occurs, are also charac-

terized by the development of moderately severe metabolic acidosis. The undetermined anion concentration in these conditions remains normal or near normal as long as glomerular function is not severely impaired (see below). Patients with this form of hyperchloremic metabolic acidosis differ from those with renal tubular acidosis in two important respects: first, they have no measurable defect in urinary acidification, and second, they do not excrete administered bicarbonate abnormally.

Addition of hydrochloric acid. The reduction in extracellular bicarbonate concentration caused by titration of body fluids with hydrochloric acid is, of course, associated with an increase in the concentration of chloride and not of undetermined anion. This form of metabolic acidosis also occurs after the administration of ammonium chloride (51) or of certain synthetic amino acid preparations containing the cationic amino acids lysine, arginine, and/or histamine (29). Each of these substances yields hydrochloric acid during the course of cellular metabolism.

Elevated undetermined anion concentration

The causes of metabolic acidosis characterized by an elevation of undetermined anion concentration are listed in the right-hand column of Table 6-3. With the exception of renal insufficiency, each of the conditions listed involves the overproduction of organic acids. Hence, the challenge presented to the organism in each instance is qualitatively similar to the challenge presented during the normal physiologic process of endogenous acid production; as these acids are delivered to the extracellular fluid, hydrogen ions are relinquished and body buffers are titrated. The decrement in plasma bicarbonate concentration is associated with a reciprocal increment in undetermined anion concentration, which is attributable to an accumulation of the corresponding organic acid anions.

The physiologic response of the kidney to the overproduction of endogenous acid involves conservation of existing bicarbonate stores and augmentation of net acid excretion to replace bicarbonate deficits. Difficulty frequently arises, however, because the kidney's ability to regenerate bicarbonate is easily outstripped by the very high rate to which acid production can increase in some pathologic settings. Under such circumstances, bicarbonate concentration often falls precipitously, symptoms develop suddenly, and emergency treatment is mandatory. If acid production increases gradually, however, plasma bicarbonate concentration may show only a slight reduction because renal acid excretion may keep pace with the increased acid load.

Diabetic ketoacidosis. Diabetic ketoacidosis is a prototype for metabolic acidosis caused by increased organic acid production (21). In uncontrolled diabetes mellitus, the metabolism of fat stores causes an overproduction of acetyl-CoA and, in most instances, a consequent release of acetoacetic acid into the circulation. The nitroprusside test provides a semiquantitative assay for acetoacetic acid, and a positive reaction in the serum serves to confirm the diagnosis of diabetic ketoacidosis. On occasion, however, β-OH butyric acid, which does not react with nitroprusside, contributes to the increased acid load in uncontrolled diabetes. In such cases, there may be a discrepancy between the increment in undetermined anion concentration and the degree of positivity in the serum nitroprusside reaction. A similar discrepancy occurs when an element of lactic acidosis is superimposed on diabetic acidosis (see below).

The ability of the patient with diabetes to respond to developing ketoacidosis may be compromised by coexistent renal insufficiency secondary either to diabetic nephropathy or to the volume deficits induced by osmotic (glucose) diuresis. In rare instances, osmotic diuresis is so intense, and volume depletion so severe, that vascular collapse and acute tubular necrosis supervene.

Severe potassium deficits commonly develop during diabetic acidosis as a result of potassium losses from the kidney, the gastrointestinal tract, or both; such deficits often are not reflected in a proportionate degree of hypokalemia until the acidemia is at least partially corrected. Patients receiving digitalis must be monitored with particular caution during the correction of diabetic acidosis because of the high risk of serious cardiac arrhythmias in the face of potassium deficiency.

Proper treatment of diabetic acidosis requires provision of adequate amounts of insulin and replacement of fluid and electrolyte losses. The need for exogenous bicarbonate is highly variable and should be determined largely by the clinical state. Since the organic acids produced in diabetic acidosis are not end products of metabolism, the circulating organic anions derived from them can reenter cells to be metabolized if the ability to utilize glucose is restored. In the metabolism of these anions, hydrogen ions are reclaimed from the acid forms of body buffers, and bicarbonate is regenerated stoichiometrically. In theory, therefore, additional bicarbonate from exogenous or renal sources is required only to replace organic acid anions that are lost in the urine and hence no longer available for reutilization. Although these losses may be large, the kidney can ordinarily repair the deficits without assistance within a few days if renal function is normal.

These theoretical considerations notwithstanding, when ketoacidosis is severe, sufficient bicarbonate should be given promptly to reduce the risks associated with acidemia per se and to provide a margin of safety until the underlying metabolic derangement is reversed by insulin therapy.

Prolonged starvation. Prolonged starvation may result in metabolic acidosis by a process qualitatively similar to that seen in diabetes mellitus. Even under extreme circumstances, however, plasma bicarbonate concentration rarely falls to levels lower than 17 to 18 meq/L and administration of bicarbonate is rarely necessary. In such patients, the serum nitroprusside test is usually weakly positive.

Alcoholic ketoacidosis. Alcholic ketoacidosis, an occasional sequela of heavy alcohol abuse, occurs most often in premenopausal women (17). The major source of hydrogen ion in most instances is β-OH butyric acid; consequently, the serum nitroprusside reaction, as in the occasional diabetic patient with predominant β-OH butyric acidosis, is typically negative or only weakly positive even in the face of severe metabolic acidosis. It is difficult to establish a firm diagnosis of β-OH butyric acidosis, because assay techniques for this substance are not readily available; the diagnosis should be suspected, however, in any patient with unexplained metabolic acidosis (and an increased unmeasured anion concentration) in whom the plasma nitroprusside reaction is negative and the plasma lactate is normal.

Methyl alcohol. Methyl alcohol ingestion may produce rapid and profound metabolic acidosis (9) but the mechanisms responsible for the acidosis are not entirely clear. Although methyl alcohol is converted to formaldehyde and thence to formic acid by the same metabolic pathways traversed by ethyl alcohol, quantitative considerations exclude formic acid as the major cause of the acidosis. Since formaldehyde functions to uncouple oxidative phosphorylation in tissue preparations, it has been postulated that the acidosis results from the release of large quantities of Krebs cycle organic acids. Furthermore, because hypotension is common in patients with severe methyl alcohol intoxication, it is reasonable to speculate that lactic acid overproduction may often be a contributing factor (see below).

Even though, methyl alcohol–induced acidosis is self-limited once ingestion ceases, the rapidity with which it develops frequently results in an alarming clinical picture requiring prompt therapy. Moreover, there is some evidence that the retinal damage that often complicates methyl alcohol ingestion is lessened by prompt correction of the acid-base disturbance. Large amounts of bicarbonate are usually required to replenish deficits and to neutralize the large acid load. Attempts have been made to retard the rate of formaldehyde and formic acid production, including hemodialysis to remove unmetabolized methyl alcohol (34) and intravenous administration of ethyl alcohol to inhibit metabolic conversion to the toxic products (6). Since both methyl and ethyl alcohol are central nervous system depressants, however, the administration of ethyl alcohol must be undertaken with great caution.

Ethylene glycol. The metabolic acidosis seen in association with ethylene glycol ingestion is usually overshadowed by the central nervous system and renal toxicity which characteristically dominate the clinical picture produced by this poison (18). Although ethylene glycol is partially converted to oxalic acid, the amount of oxalic acid produced is insufficient to account for the severe acidosis which is occasionally seen. The mecha-

nisms have not been clarified. Abundant oxalate crystals are usually present in the urine sediment, however, and their identification may aid in establishing the correct diagnosis.

Paraldehyde. Paraldehyde ingestion, especially if prolonged, may also result in severe metabolic acidosis (8). As in methyl alcohol and ethylene glycol ingestion, however, the precise mechanisms responsible for the acidosis are unclear. It is known that paraldehyde gradually decomposes to acetic acid during storage, especially when exposed to sunlight, and it had been thought that the acidosis might result from the ingestion of this degradation product. However, the amount of acetic acid that could be ingested, even under extreme circumstances, is insufficient to account for the severity of the acid-base disturbance often observed. Moreover, ingestion of either fresh or decomposed paraldehyde produces similar abnormalities in experimental animals. Production of acetic acid in vivo has been postulated as a mechanism, but elevated plasma acetate concentrations have not been found in intoxicated patients. A firm diagnosis of this condition depends upon the availability of adequate historical data.

Salicylate intoxication. Salicylate intoxication results in a complex acid-base disturbance caused by direct effects of the salicylate molecule on both respiration and metabolism (64, 71). The features of the acid-base disturbance observed in a particular individual depend upon the specific interaction between these independent drug effects. An early response to salicylate overdosage is primary hyperventilation (respiratory alkalosis), which is thought to result from a heightened sensitivity of the medullary respiratory center to carbon dioxide. The resulting reduction in Pa_{CO_2} would be expected to cause plasma bicarbonate to fall slightly in keeping with the physiologic adaptive responses evoked by respiratory alkalosis (see below). However, greater reduction in plasma bicarbonate concentration, sufficient to elevate hydrogen ion concentration to frankly acidemic levels, occurs when the independent metabolic effects of the salicylate molecule cause a large outpouring of organic acids from cells.

Salicylates affect intermediary metabolism by several mechanisms, including the uncoupling of oxidative phosphorylation and the inhibition of dehydrogenase and aminotransferase enzyme systems; the increased production of organic acids is thought to be related to these biochemical derangements. The nature and relative importance of the specific organic acids generated under the direct influence of salicylates remain unclear; the Krebs cycle intermediaries, citric and succinic acids, and the fatty acid metabolites, acetoacetic and β-OH butyric acids, have been incriminated.

The magnitude of both the respiratory and the metabolic effects of salicylates appears, in general, to be dose-dependent. An even more important factor, however, is a marked age-related difference in susceptibility to the metabolic derangements; infants and young children appear to be very sensitive to the metabolic effects, whereas adults typically exhibit some resistance to them. Consequently, metabolic acidosis appears relatively early in the course of intoxication and usually dominates the clinical picture in the pediatric age group, whereas respiratory alkalosis frequently dominates in adults.

The diagnosis of salicylate intoxication may be suggested by history and by a positive ferric chloride test of the urine but should be confirmed by measuring the serum salicylate level; values above 30 mg/dL are generally regarded as being within the toxic range.

The key to therapy of this intoxication is removal of the offending salicylate molecule. Removal of salicylate can usually be accomplished by forced diuresis, but peritoneal or hemodialysis may be necessary in severely intoxicated patients or in the presence of renal insufficiency. When renal function is unimpaired, excretion of salicylates can be enhanced by alkalinizing the renal tubular fluid, because an alkaline medium favors the dissociation (ionization) of salicylic acid and thereby retards nonionic back-diffusion of the acid form into the plasma. Some caution must be exercised, however, whenever bicarbonate is administered to a patient with salicylate intoxication. Even a relatively small increase in bicarbonate concentration in the presence of overriding respiratory alkalosis could depress hydrogen ion concentration to dangerously low levels. Conversely, failure to administer sufficient

bicarbonate in the presence of metabolic acidosis may permit a fatal elevation of hydrogen ion concentration to occur. Clearly, acid-base parameters must be monitored frequently in order to provide appropriate guidelines for bicarbonate administration.

Lactic acidosis. Lactic acidosis is now recognized as one of the leading causes of serious metabolic acidosis (40). In normal individuals, a small amount of lactic acid, derived from the reduction of pyruvic acid, enters the circulation but is promptly removed by the liver; the liver reoxidizes the lactic acid to pyruvic acid, which is then metabolized to carbon dioxide and water. Consequently, lactic acid production normally makes no *net* contribution to the endogenous acid load. Steady-state plasma lactate concentration in healthy subjects is approximately 1.0 meq/L and hence contributes only slightly to the normal undetermined anion concentration.

The accelerated cycle of lactic acid production and utilization in strenuous exercise provides a useful physiologic model for understanding the derangements seen in pathologic states of lactic acidosis (Table 6-4). During strenuous exercise,

Table 6-4. Causes of lactic acidosis

OVERPRODUCTION OF LACTIC ACID
Excessive oxygen (energy) demands
Severe voluntary exercise
Prolonged generalized convulsions
Decreased oxygen delivery
Shock
Cardiac arrest
Cardiopulmonary bypass
Severe hypoxia ($Pa_{O_2} < 30-35$ mmHg)
Very severe anemia
Interference with oxygen utilization
Phenformin
Isoniazid overdosage
Idiopathic ("spontaneous")
Diabetic mellitus
Leukemia
Other chronic diseases
UNDERUTILIZATION OF LACTIC ACID
Hepatic failure
Ethanol intoxication

the marked outpouring of lactic acid may temporarily outstrip the ability of the liver and other organs to remove it. As a result, transient reductions in bicarbonate concentration and corresponding elevations in plasma lactate occur. The eventual utilization of this lactate accounts, in part, for the "oxygen debt" acquired during voluntary exercise. A clinical reflection of this physiologic process is seen in the transient lactic acidosis that often accompanies prolonged, generalized convulsions.

The common denominator between strenuous exercise and most of the pathologic conditions associated with lactic acidosis is anaerobic glycolysis. Under anaerobic conditions, the ratio of reduced to oxidized nicotinamide-adenine dinucleotide (NADH:NAD) is increased, and lactic acid formation is prompted (Fig. 6-16). The degree of acidosis produced by the increased lactic acid release may be magnified by the presence of hepatic dysfunction, which could limit the rate of lactate reutilization.

The delivery of insufficient oxygen to sustain optimum aerobic conditions appears to be directly responsible for the lactic acidosis that occurs during shock, cardiac arrest, cardiopulmonary bypass, severe hypoxia, and very severe anemia. The magnitude of the acidosis seen under these circumstances is highly variable, and the success of therapy is dependent upon the ease with which the underlying condition can be reversed.

Even when the delivery of oxygen is adequate, lactic acidosis could, in theory, occur if oxygen utilization by the tissues were impeded. Such a mechanism is thought to produce the lactic acidosis seen in association with phenformin therapy and that reported with isoniazid overdosage.

"Spontaneous" lactic acidosis, i.e., that occurring in the absence of a detectable cause for lactic acid overproduction, is seen occasionally in seriously ill patients and is usually a preterminal event (70). Patients with diabetes mellitus and leukemia seem especially prone to develop this form of metabolic acidosis.

The diagnosis of lactic acidosis can be established with certainty only by the finding of an elevated serum lactate concentration. If the concentration of undetermined anions is elevated, however, and if other causes for this finding appear unlikely from history and routine laboratory tests (e.g., serum ketones, creatinine, salicylate), a presumptive diagnosis of lactic acidosis may be made with reasonable confidence even when a lactate determination is not available.

The onset of lactic acidosis is often abrupt, because the rate of lactic acid production is often extremely high. As a result, therapy must be instituted quickly. The rate of bicarbonate administration required to keep pace with the continuing rate of acid production varies considerably and can be determined for individual patients only by monitoring acid-base parameters frequently. It is often necessary to administer such large quantities of bicarbonate (e.g., 100 to 300 meq per hour) that the risk of marked hyperosmolality and serious vascular congestion is great; if concomitant diuretic therapy fails to produce adequate sodium and water losses, dialysis may be required to prevent or treat these complications.

Unfortunately, even prompt and vigorous alkali therapy often fails to avert death. For this reason, other therapeutic approaches have been attempted, including the administration of oxidizing agents (e.g., methylene blue), in an effort to improve the oxidative state of cells, and the administration of vasodilating agents (e.g., nitroprusside), in an effort to improve tissue perfusion. The efficacy of such approaches remains uncertain.

Uremic acidosis. Uremic acidosis refers to the acid-base disturbance that stems from chronic renal insufficiency per se; the resulting decrement in plasma bicarbonate is a consequence not of increased acid production but of a failure of tubular function (i.e., Na^+/H^+ exchange) to keep pace with the normal demands for bicarbonate reabsorption and net acid excretion (28, 56).

In contrast to patients with predominant tubulointerstitial renal disease, in whom acidosis often appears before the development of marked glomerular insufficiency, patients with more generalized forms of renal damage typically do

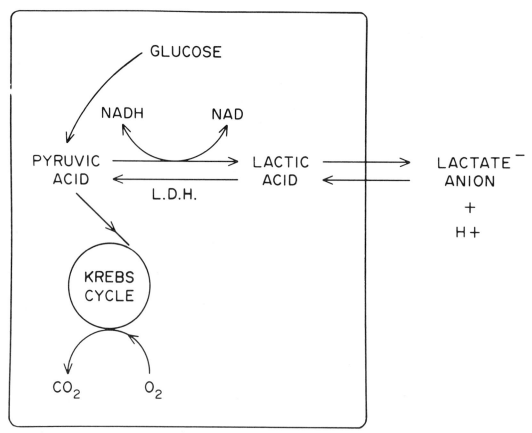

Figure 6-16. Schematic representation of the cellular production of lactic acid. Glycolytic pathways convert glucose to pyruvic acid, which normally enters the Krebs cycle for further oxidation. The equilibrium relationships between pyruvic acid and its reduced counterpart, lactic acid, is governed by the ratio of NADH:NAD. When this ratio is increased (e.g., under anaerobic conditions), enzymatic conversion via lactic dehydrogenase to lactic acid is fostered. When lactic acid is released from cells into the circulation, its relatively high dissociation factor guarantees the immediate release of its hydrogen ions for extracellular buffering. The utilization of lactate (largely by the liver) proceeds by the reverse reactions, body buffers releasing hydrogen ions to reconstitute lactic acid for further metabolism.

not manifest clinically significant reductions in plasma bicarbonate until much later in the course of their disease; as a rule, by the time acidosis is recognized, the coexisting degree of glomerular dysfunction has resulted in retention of numerous anions (e.g., sulfate, phosphate) and elevation of plasma undetermined anion concentration. Hence, uremic acidosis is an exception to the rule that an elevated undetermined anion concentration signifies an increase in endogenous acid production.

The impairment in net acid excretion in patients with chronic renal insufficiency can usually be ascribed to an inability of the remaining renal parenchyma to generate sufficient quantities of ammonia. Surprisingly, the ability of the diseased kidney to acidify the urine maximally and to excrete titratable acid is generally well preserved. Occasionally, uremic acidosis can be traced to an incomplete conservation of filtered bicarbonate that results in frank renal bicarbonate wasting.

When renal function is only moderately impaired (serum creatinine less than approximately 4 mg/dL), the associated acidosis is typically quite mild and often goes undetected; the undetermined anion concentration may not be noticeably elevated under these circumstances. It is when chronic renal insufficiency is of greater severity that more striking degrees of metabolic acidosis are encountered and the undetermined anion concentration is typically elevated. It is important to emphasize, however, that chronic renal failure per se, even when quite severe, does not often cause plasma bicarbonate concentration to fall to levels lower than 12 to 15 meq/L. This is not to say that more severe metabolic acidosis is unusual in patients with advanced renal insufficiency, but rather that when it occurs, it is usually the consequence of an inadequate response of the diseased kidney to an increased acid load or to an extrarenal loss of bicarbonate.

Certain special features of persistent metabolic acidosis deserve comment.[8] As a general rule, patients with long-standing metabolic acidosis exhibit fewer outward signs of their deranged acid-base equilibrium than do patients with comparable acute reductions in bicarbonate concentration. Mental status may be particularly well preserved despite striking biochemical abnormalities. Similarly, the increase in rate and depth of respirations resulting from chronic metabolic acidosis may escape the notice of both the patient and the physician.

Another striking feature of chronic metabolic acidosis is the tendency for bone to be demineralized. Although there are many other explanations for disordered bone metabolism in patients with chronic renal failure, it is likely that acidosis plays at least a contributory role in many cases (48). It has been suggested, in fact, that dissolution of alkaline bone salts may be an important adaptive mechanism for averting more severe degrees of acidosis in chronic renal failure (28, 35). Evidence suggests that as long as kidney function remains markedly impaired, a portion of the daily endogenous acid load is retained. Nevertheless, bicarbonate concentration does not usually fall progressively, as might be expected if acid balance were continuously positive. In order to reconcile the apparently relentless retention of hydrogen ion with the observed tendency for bicarbonate concentration to stabilize (albeit at a reduced level), it has been postulated that the large alkali reserve normally sequestered in bone is mobilized under the influence of chronic acidosis and utilized for buffering (49).

Chronic uremic acidosis may be treated by the provision of sufficient exogenous base to offset the positive balance of hydrogen ion. Ordinarily, only modest doses of bicarbonate are required. Adequate treatment is difficult in a small fraction of patients, however, because of an inability to tolerate the accompanying sodium loads.

Acute renal failure. Although acute renal failure invariably causes some degree of metabolic acidosis because of the retention of endogenous acid, plasma bicarbonate concentration typically falls by only 1 to 2 meq/L per day if the rate of cellular acid production is normal (approximately 1 meq/kg per day). Consequently, severe acidosis is not a common feature of the early stages of uncomplicated acute renal failure and rarely becomes a problem if periodic peritoneal dialysis or hemodialysis is employed to control the uremic state. Acid production is occasionally augmented greatly during acute renal failure, however, because of coexisting fever, soft-tissue trauma, steroid administration, or other factors; under these circumstances, acidosis may develop more rapidly and may require treatment.

METABOLIC ALKALOSIS

Metabolic alkalosis refers to those acid-base disturbances initiated by an elevation in plasma bicarbonate concentration.

PATHOPHYSIOLOGY

Because of the constraints imposed by electroneutrality, elevations in bicarbonate concentra-

---

[8]Persistent metabolic acidosis is seen most commonly in patients with chronic renal failure but is also encountered in patients with chronic diarrhea, ureterosigmoidostomy, and renal tubular acidosis.

tion can occur only if accompanied by a reduction in chloride concentration of at least equivalent magnitude. Consequently, the pattern of plasma anion composition is similar in all forms of metabolic alkalosis and, by contrast to metabolic acidosis, does not help to distinguish among the various mechanisms that can produce this acid-base disturbance.

In considering the pathophysiology of metabolic alkalosis, it is imperative that a sharp distinction be drawn between the production of the elevated bicarbonate level on the one hand and the maintenance of that elevated level on the other.

Production of alkalosis

Elevations in plasma bicarbonate can be produced in three ways: administration of alkali; loss of hydrogen ion; and disproportionate loss of chloride.

Administration of alkali. The administration of bicarbonate, or of bicarbonate precursors (e.g., citrate, lactate, acetate), at rates greater than the rate of endogenous acid production leads to a direct increase in plasma bicarbonate concentration. However, alkali surfeits acquired in this way are normally excreted very promptly, and hence are not often responsible for significant increments in plasma bicarbonate concentration.

Loss of hydrogen ion. Negative hydrogen ion balance (output greater than input) also leads to an increment in body alkali stores. Common examples are the loss of hydrochloric acid from the stomach and the excretion of more acid by the kidney than that produced by cellular metabolism. Excess bicarbonate is derived from the latter source (1) during the action of those diuretics that can promote hydrogen as well as sodium and potassium losses in the urine (e.g., thiazides, furosemide, ethacrynic acid), (2) during the renal response to respiratory acidosis (see below), and (3) in association with various forms of hyperadrenocorticism.

In some animals, depletion of cellular potassium stores appears to cause hydrogen ions to shift into cells, generating a bicarbonate surplus for the extracellular compartment. There is little evidence, however, that this mechanism is of importance in humans. (The relationship between potassium deficits and metabolic alkalosis is discussed in greater detail below.)

Disproportionate loss of chloride. Whenever fluid lost from the body differs in anion composition from that of the extracellular fluid, plasma anion composition is altered. Accordingly, when chloride losses are disproportionately large with respect to simultaneous bicarbonate losses, the plasma concentration of bicarbonate rises as the remaining bicarbonate is restricted to a smaller space of distribution. Such disproportionate chloride losses occur commonly via the kidney in response to potent diuretic agents, most of which promote the excretion of sodium and potassium in association, almost exclusively, with chloride. The element of metabolic alkalosis attributable to this mechanism would, of course, compound that attributable to the renal loss of hydrogen ion, which can also occur as a consequence of diuretic administration. In rare instances, disproportionate loss of chloride may occur via the colon.

Maintenance of metabolic alkalosis

Unlike metabolic acidosis, metabolic alkalosis is frequently perpetuated by the normal kidney. The reason for this becomes clear when one contrasts the renal response to alkali administration with the renal response to a loss of hydrogen ion or chloride or both.

When metabolic alkalosis is produced by a surfeit of administered alkali, it is accompanied by an equivalent surfeit of administered cation, usually sodium. Hence, the metabolic alkalosis produced by alkali administration is associated with an expansion of extracellular volume, the accompanying hypochloremia resulting simply from an enlarged space of chloride distribution. If renal function is normal, the metabolic alkalosis, the volume expansion, and the hypochloremia are all rapidly repaired as the bicarbonate surfeit escapes reabsorption and is excreted with the unneeded cation. Owing to the efficiency with which excess bicarbonate can be excreted by the normal kidney in the presence of volume expansion, *sus-*

tained metabolic alkalosis can result from the administration of alkali only if renal function is markedly reduced, if the rate of alkali administration remains extremely high, or if a volume-independent stimulus for sodium retention is present (66).

Conversely, when metabolic alkalosis and hypochloremia are produced by a loss of hydrogen ion or a disproportionate loss of chloride, no additional sodium (or other cation) is made available to the organism. Consequently, for the kidney to excrete the surplus bicarbonate, a loss of body sodium must occur. This tendency toward sodium depletion is quickly forestalled, of course, by the heightened sodium avidity engendered by the resulting deficit in effective extracellular volume. However, in order to prevent further excretion of sodium in the presence of hypochloremia and a reduced filtered chloride load, the kidney must maintain an accelerated rate of sodium-hydrogen exchange and thus perpetuate the metabolic alkalosis (31). If frank cation (sodium and/or potassium) deficits also occur during the development of metabolic alkalosis, as they often do, the kidney will attempt not only to conserve remaining body cation but to retain administrated cation as well. If these deficient cations are made available with nonreabsorbable anions, rather than with chloride, the enhanced cation avidity may augment sodium-hydrogen exchange further and produce additional surplus bicarbonate (69).

This discrepancy between the availability of reabsorbable anion (chloride) in the glomerular filtrate and the heightened stimulus to conserve filtered sodium accounts for the maintenance of metabolic alkalosis in most forms of this acid-base disturbance. As a corollary, the administration of sodium chloride is sufficient in these instances to repair the chloride deficit and return sodium-hydrogen exchange to normal (31).[9] In some less common forms of metabolic alkalosis (e.g., hyperadrenalism), however, the administration of sodium chloride does not result in a dampening of sodium-hydrogen exchange; chloride deficits and metabolic alkalosis persist, and administered chloride escapes into the urine. The failure of the kidney to retain administered chloride in these instances implies that sodium-hydrogen exchange is being stimulated by factors other than the discrepancy between sodium avidity and the availability of reabsorbable anion.

Even though the mechanisms responsible for these differences require further clarification, the recognition that chloride-responsive and chloride-resistant forms of metabolic alkalosis occur provides a useful means for classifying the various causes of this acid-base disturbance, as will be discussed below.

POTASSIUM AND METABOLIC ALKALOSIS

The complex relationship between metabolic alkalosis and potassium metabolism deserves special comment. For many years, potassium depletion was considered to be the initial event responsible for the induction and subsequent maintenance of the elevated bicarbonate concentration seen in the common forms of metabolic alkalosis. Studies in animals had suggested that loss of cellular potassium caused a shift of extracellular hydrogen ions (derived from carbonic acid) into cells and, thereby, produced an increase in extracellular bicarbonate concentration (16, 41). The failure of the kidneys to excrete this surplus bicarbonate was also attributed to potassium depletion, on the assumption that the resulting increase in hydrogen ion concentration within the renal tubule cell directly enhanced the rate of sodium-hydrogen exchange.

Such a causal role for potassium depletion in metabolic alkalosis appeared to be supported by the virtually invariable association between metabolic alkalosis and potassium depletion. More recent evidence indicates, however, that the potassium deficit commonly encountered in metabolic alkalosis (as high as 300 to 500 meq) is, in fact, a consequence of the alkalosis and not its cause. Most convincing is the observation that

[9]This physiologic fact does not lessen the importance of including potassium in the replacement therapy for patients with metabolic alkalosis; as a rule, considerable quantities of potassium chloride must be administered to correct coexisting potassium deficits.

plasma anion composition can be returned to normal in most instances by the administration of chloride salts even when associated potassium deficits are not repaired (33).

Several mechanisms operate during the induction and maintenance of metabolic alkalosis that promote the development of potassium deficiency. First, the process responsible for the loss of hydrogen, chloride, or both may cause some potassium to be lost from the body as well (e.g., vomiting, diuretic administration). Second, renal potassium wasting is characteristic of metabolic alkalosis and is explained by the same process that fosters the high rate of bicarbonate reabsorption: the disparity between the availability of reabsorbable anion (chloride) in the glomerular filtrate and the simultaneous need to conserve body sodium accelerates not only sodium-hydrogen exchange but also sodium-potassium exchange (60). Third, urinary potassium losses may be augmented even further if sufficient volume depletion has occurred to stimulate aldosterone secretion. It should be noted, parenthetically, that the degree of hypokalemia encountered in metabolic alkalosis may be out of proportion to the size of the potassium deficit to the extent that alkalemia causes hydrogen ions to shift out of cells in exchange for potassium.

It has been suggested that degrees of potassium depletion more severe than those commonly seen as a consequence of metabolic alkalosis can themselves produce and sustain an elevated plasma bicarbonate concentration. This possibility is considered in more detail below.

SECONDARY PHYSIOLOGIC ADJUSTMENTS IN RESPIRATION

As illustrated in Fig. 6-10, the effect on acid-base equilibrium of an elevation in plasma bicarbonate concentration is a reduction in hydrogen ion concentration. The physiologic response to this primary alteration in acid-base equilibrium is a reduction in alveolar ventilation and a corresponding increase in Pa_{CO_2}. Although an incre- ment in bicarbonate concentration alters hydrogen ion concentration less than does the same absolute decrement in bicarbonate concentration, the adaptive elevation in Pa_{CO_2} induced by metabolic alkalosis has less leverage on returning hydrogen ion concentration toward normal than does the secondary reduction in Pa_{CO_2} induced by metabolic acidosis (see Fig. 6-10). In addition to these mathematical considerations, the magnitude of the ventilatory response in metabolic alkalosis is typically much smaller than it is in metabolic acidosis of comparable severity; in uncomplicated metabolic alkalosis, each meq/L increment in bicarbonate concentration appears, on the average, to evoke only a 0.4- to 0.7-mmHg increment in Pa_{CO_2}. This relationship is depicted in Fig. 6-17. Hence, metabolic alkalosis rarely evokes a rise in Pa_{CO_2} of more than 10 to 15 mmHg, unless the alkalosis is very severe (61). The probable explanation for this seemingly restrained respiratory response is that the degree of hypoventilation necessary to produce greater elevations in Pa_{CO_2} would also result in significant reduction in Pa_{O_2}.

DIAGNOSIS AND CLINICAL MANIFESTATIONS

When metabolic alkalosis is the only abnormality affecting acid-base equilibrium, laboratory studies reveal an elevated plasma bicarbonate concentration in association with some degree of alkalemia, despite the respiratory readjustments (Fig. 6-17). If bicarbonate concentration is greater than 40 meq/L, some element of metabolic alkalosis is virtually assured, even if a measurement of Pa_{CO_2} or hydrogen ion concentration is not available; bicarbonate is rarely increased to such high levels solely by the secondary physiologic responses initiated by respiratory acidosis (see below). Metabolic alkalosis may coexist with other acid-base disturbances of acidity. In such cases, the acid-base parameters alone may not be diagnostic but the presence of metabolic alkalosis may be suggested by the clinical history or by the existence of unexplained potassium or chloride deficits.

The clinical findings associated with metabolic

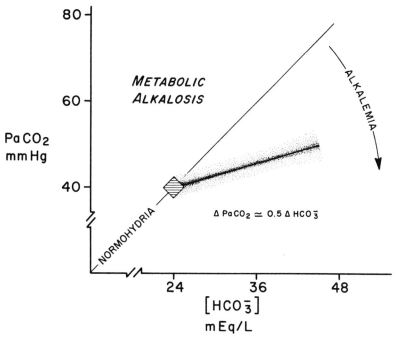

Figure 6-17. Effect of metabolic alkalosis on acid-base equilibrium. The initiating event is an elevation of plasma bicarbonate concentration, which produces a reduction in hydrogen ion concentration (see Fig. 6-10). In response to this primary alteration in acid-base equilibrium, secondary hypoventilation occurs and carbon dioxide tension is somewhat increased. Although the extent of this response is, as indicated, roughly proportional to the increase in plasma bicarbonate concentration, the change in Pa_{CO_2} is of more limited magnitude than the analogous response seen during metabolic acidosis (see Fig. 6-14). The biologic variation typical of such physiologic responses is indicated by the shaded area.

alkalosis are nonspecific and rarely aid in the diagnostic process. Heightened neuromuscular excitability may result in tetany or generalized convulsions, especially if alkalosis is extremely severe. Since potassium deficits regularly accompany metabolic alkalosis, the manifestations of this electrolyte disorder (e.g., muscle weakness, cardiac arrhythmias) often dominate the clinical picture.

CAUSES OF METABOLIC ALKALOSIS

Table 6-5 divides the causes of metabolic alkalosis into two large groups according to their responsiveness to administered chloride. As can be seen, the common causes fall into the chloride-responsive group.

Chloride-responsive alkalosis

Loss of acid gastric fluid, whether by vomiting or gastric suction, leads commonly to significant metabolic alkalosis. Experimental studies of selective hydrochloric acid depletion suggest that the kidney responds initially to this form of metabolic alkalosis by increasing the excretion of bicarbonate in association with that of sodium and potassium (39). As sodium is lost, however, extracellular volume contracts, and the kidney very shortly beings to conserve sodium avidly. Thereafter, augmented sodium-cation exchange, enhanced by the disproportion between the requirement for quantitative sodium reabsorption and the reduced availability of filtered chloride, sustains the alkalosis and enhances the excretion of administered potassium.

Table 6-5. Causes of metabolic alkalosis

CHLORIDE-RESPONSIVE	CHLORIDE-RESISTANT	MISCELLANEOUS
Vomiting	Hyperaldosteronism	Administration of alkali
Gastric suction	Bartter's syndrome	"Milk-alkali" syndrome
Use of certain diuretics	Cushing's syndrome	
Abrupt relief of chronic hypercapnia	Licorice ingestion	
Villous adenoma of the colon	Severe K$^+$ depletion	
Congenital chloride diarrhea		

The magnitude of the alkalosis depends, of course, on the degree of gastric acidity and on the amount of gastric fluid lost. In extreme situations (e.g., continuous gastric suction in Zollinger-Ellison syndrome) loss of HCl from the stomach may result in plasma bicarbonate concentrations in excess of 60 to 70 meq/L.

The potent diuretics in common use (e.g., thiazides, furosemide, ethacrynic acid) promote the excretion of sodium (and potassium) almost exclusively in association with chloride (i.e., without a proportionate increase in bicarbonate excretion). Net acid excretion is also frequently augmented during the diuresis. As a consequence both of the disproportionate chloride loss and of the direct loss of acid, extracellular bicarbonate concentration rises. Because patients receiving diuretics are frequently advised to adhere to a diet low in salt and, hence, low in chloride, it is common for diuretic-induced metabolic alkalosis to persist for long periods. For the same reason, supplemental potassium administered without chloride to patients receiving diuretics and a low-salt diet may not be retained in amounts adequate to repair accumulated deficits (60).

Abrupt relief of chronic hypercapnia results in metabolic alkalosis by a rather circuitous route. As discussed below, bicarbonate concentration is elevated significantly (by as much as 12 to 15 meq/L) as a normal physiologic response to chronic hypercapnia (respiratory acidosis). If sudden improvement in alveolar ventilation (e.g., tracheostomy, assisted ventilation) then reduces Pa_{CO_2} abruptly, acid-base equilibrium may be displaced to a point indistinguishable from that resulting from any form of primary metabolic alkalosis and will remain there until plasma bicarbonate can be reduced appropriately. Correction of the alkalosis requires excretion of the excess bicarbonate by the kidney and, as in the other forms of metabolic alkalosis discussed above, can be accomplished fully only if exogenous chloride is made available (57).

Villous adenoma of the colon may be associated with large losses of fluid and electrolyte into the stool. Metabolic alkalosis is occasionally seen under such curcumstances and is presumed to result from disproportionately large chloride losses. Sizable potassium deficits are frequently incurred as well (4). Congenital chloride diarrhea is a rare disorder of infancy that appears to result from malabsorption of chloride and typically induces alkalosis responsive to chloride administration (20).

In each of the above forms of metabolic alkalosis, the urine is virtually chloride-free (urine chloride concentration less than 10 meq/L), and alkalosis is readily corrected by chloride administration. In treating patients with chloride-responsive metabolic alkalosis, the most suitable form and rate of chloride administration is determined by the clinical situation. Since large potassium deficits are almost always present, potassium chloride is generally the most reasonable choice. Precautions concerning the rate and avenue of potassium chloride administration are discussed elsewhere. If the chloride deficit is too severe to permit safe repletion solely with potassium chloride, additional chloride may be provided as the sodium salt. Indeed, sodium chloride administration is often warranted in patients with metabolic alkalosis because of concomitant volume contraction. If sodium intake must be curtailed, on the other hand, chloride may be administered with ammonium or as the monohydrochloride of lysine or arginine. The latter agents are also particularly useful in the management of extreme alkalosis.

When evaluating the effect of therapy for metabolic alkalosis, it should be recalled that both sodium chloride and potassium chloride correct alkalosis by suppressing renal acid excretion and increasing renal alkali excretion. Accordingly, the first sign that alkalosis is responding to therapy is a rise in urine pH as excessive alkali stores are excreted. Simultaneously, plasma bicarbonate concentration begins to fall. After sufficient chloride has been administered, appreciable amounts of chloride appear in the urine.

Chloride-resistant alkalosis

The chloride-resistant nature of an unexplained metabolic alkalosis (and hypochloremia) can be easily determined by measuring urinary chloride; a value greater than 10 to 15 meq/L (if recent diuretic administration is excluded) is prima facie evidence that the kidney is unable to retain administered chloride normally.

Resistance to chloride therapy characterizes some of the less common causes of metabolic alkalosis, as listed in Table 6-5. With the exception of severe potassium depletion, each of these conditions is characterized by hyperadrenocorticism. Consequently, it has been presumed that a direct stimulating effect of adrenal steroids on renal sodium-cation exchange sustains the increased plasma bicarbonate concentration despite normal dietary chloride intake. Attempts to produce experimental metabolic alkalosis in man by long-term administration of mineralocorticoids have, however, been largely unsuccessful. As a result, the possibility has been raised that potassium deficits, which are usually sizable in the presence of hyperadrenocorticism, may play an important role in perpetuating the alkalosis in these instances (32).

In primary hyperaldosteronism, the degree of metabolic alkalosis is quite variable, but its presence frequently provides the clue to the diagnosis. In Bartter's syndrome, a disorder in which hyperplasia of the juxtaglomerular complex and excess renin production appear to be responsible for a high rate of aldosterone secretion, metabolic alkalosis and potassium depletion are characteristic features. Metabolic alkalosis is also seen in association with Cushing's syndrome, particularly that form of the syndrome resulting from the ectopic production of ACTH-like material by certain neoplasms. In such instances, alkalosis may appear quite abruptly and may be unusually severe. Excessive licorice ingestion may result in a mild metabolic alkalosis and significant potassium depletion because of the steroid-like action of a major component of licorice, glycyrrhizic acid.

Chloride-resistant metabolic alkalosis may also occur in patients who have no evidence of hyperadrenocorticism. In these patients, very striking potassium deficits have been noted, serum potassium concentrations usually falling to levels of 2 meq/L or less. As a consequence, it has been postulated that severe potassium depletion, per se, produces a change in renal tubular function that prevents normal chloride conservation until some portion of the potassium deficit is repaired (24). As mentioned above, more moderate degrees of potassium depletion, such as those ordinarily accompanying the common forms of metabolic alkalosis, do not produce chloride resistance since they do not prevent retention of administered chloride and correction of the alkalosis. It is conceivable, however, that the development of more extensive potassium deficits might, in some cases, convert a chloride-responsive alkalosis into a chloride-resistant one.

Miscellaneous causes of metabolic alkalosis

As noted above, sustained metabolic alkalosis results from the administration of bicarbonate or other base when the rate of administration is extremely high or when altered renal function imposes a limitation on alkali excretion. In either case, correction usually follows interruption of the alkali load. An interesting example of this etiology of metabolic alkalosis is the milk-alkali syndrome (47). If the ingestion of moderately large amounts of absorbable alkali and calcium salts eventually results in nephrocalcinosis and subsequent renal insufficiency, continued alkali ingestion may give rise to sustained metabolic alkalosis.

RESPIRATORY ACIDOSIS

Respiratory acidosis refers to those acid-base disturbances initiated by an elevation in carbon dioxide tension.

PATHOPHYSIOLOGY

An elevation in carbon dioxide tension (hypercapnia) occurs whenever CO_2 excretion lags behind CO_2 production (positive CO_2 balance). Overproduction of CO_2 by itself, however, is never responsible for significant hypercapnia; in the presence of a normal respiratory system, increased CO_2 production stimulates alveolar ventilation sufficiently to maintain Pa_{CO_2} at nearly normal levels. Therefore, with the exception of the adaptive increase in Pa_{CO_2} elicited by metabolic alkalosis, the presence of hypercapnia can be interpreted as signifying some impediment to alveolar ventilation.

SECONDARY PHYSIOLOGIC RESPONSES

The changes in acid-base equilibrium that occur during respiratory acidosis are indicated in Figs. 6-18 and 6-19. From a consideration of the Henderson relationship (Fig. 6-10), it is clear that the isolated effect of an increment in Pa_{CO_2} on acid-base equilibrium is a proportionate increment in hydrogen ion concentration; the resulting acidemia can be ameliorated only by a secondary elevation in bicarbonate concentration. This elevation in bicarbonate occurs in two distinct steps (Fig. 6-18), the first related to the titration of nonbicarbonate tissue buffers and the second to renal adaptive mechanisms.

A small increase in bicarbonate concentration is observed within moments of the onset of hy-

percapnia, as hydrogen ions derived from carbonic acid are removed from solution by nonbicarbonate buffers (e.g., hemoglobin). This immediate change is quite small, however, increasing the level of plasma bicarbonate concentration only 3 to 4 meq/L above normal even when hypercapnia is extreme (Pa_{CO_2} 80 to 90 mmHg) (10). This modest increase in plasma bicarbonate in vivo contrasts sharply with the large increase observed during in vitro titration of whole blood with carbon dioxide over the same range of carbon dioxide tensions. The seemingly lower in vivo buffer capacity is attributable, at least in part, to the fact that some bicarbonate generated by blood buffers must diffuse into the poorly buffered interstitial space in the intact organism.

The net effect of the tissue buffer response to acute hypercapnia is that plasma hydrogen ion concentration is elevated by approximately 0.75 neq/L for each mmHg increase in Pa_{CO_2} (Fig. 6-19). Since the contribution of body buffering during the acute phase of hypercapnia is so clearly limited, it is relatively easy under these circumstances to recognize the coincidental presence of a complicating metabolic acid-base disturbance. Thus, if hypercapnia is known to be of recent onset, and bicarbonate concentration is found to be greater than 28 to 30 meq/L, a metabolic alkalosis must also be present. Similarly, if plasma bicarbonate concentration is lower than 25 to 26 meq/L in a patient with acute hypercapnia, a cause for a coexistent metabolic acidosis should be sought (see the section on mixed acid-base disturbances, below).

Several hours after the acute titration of tissue buffers, the renal response to persistent hypercapnia begins to be manifested by a further, gradual rise in plasma bicarbonate (Fig. 6-18). Under the influence of persistent hypercapnia, the rate of sodium-hydrogen exchange by the renal tubule is accelerated; as a consequence, the rate of net acid excretion (largely in the form of augmented ammonium excretion) transiently exceeds the rate of endogenous acid production, negative hydrogen ion balance develops, and new bicarbonate is generated. The persistent acceleration of sodium-

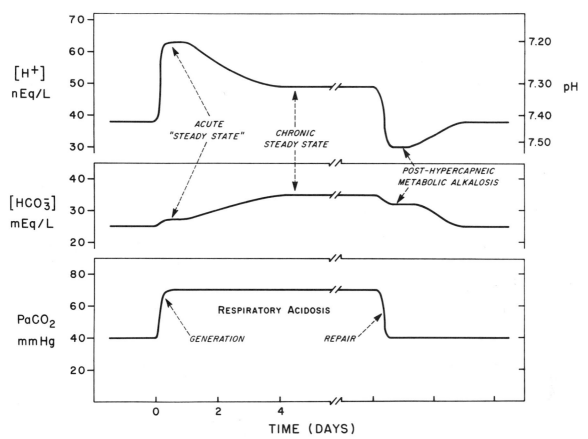

Figure 6-18. Schematic time-course of the changes in plasma acid-base equilibrium during the generation and repair of respiratory acidosis. Respiratory acidosis is initiated by an elevation in Pa_{CO_2}. In the illustration presented here, Pa_{CO_2} is assumed to rise abruptly from 40 to 70 mmHg and to remain at this level for at least several days. The small elevation in plasma bicarbonate concentration that occurs immediately results from the titration of tissue buffers and serves to attenuate to a slight degree the rise in hydrogen ion concentration (see Fig. 6-19). For the next several hours no additional changes can be detected; hence, this interval is termed an acute "steady state." Thereafter, renal adaptive responses cause a further increase in bicarbonate concentration and a further dampening of the acidemia; a new, chronic steady state is generally achieved within a few days. When chronic respiratory acidosis is rapidly repaired, as in this example, a transient state of posthypercapneic metabolic alkalosis supervenes until the adaptive surplus in alkali stores is excreted (see text).

hydrogen exchange during hypercapnia insures the conservation of these new bicarbonate ions as they are recycled through the kidney by glomerular filtration. As bicarbonate stores are being augmented by this process, chloride stores are correspondingly depleted as a result of the enhanced urinary chloride excretion which oc-

curs in association with the increased excretion of ammonium (55).

Studies in animals indicate that a highly predictable relationship exists between the degree of chronic hypercapnia and the level at which plasma bicarbonate concentration stabilizes after full physiologic adaptation (55). Observations in

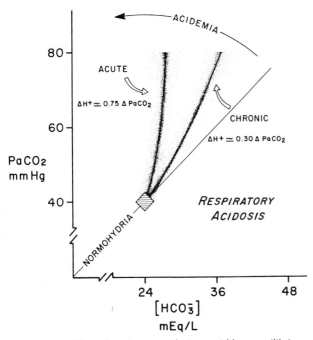

Figure 6-19. Effect of respiratory acidosis on acid-base equilibrium. The initiating event is an increase in carbon dioxide tension that elevates plasma hydrogen ion concentration (see Fig. 6-10). The acidifying effect of hypercapnia is ameliorated by secondary elevations in bicarbonate concentration that result, acutely, from a titration of nonbicarbonate buffers and, chronically, from an adaptation in the renal handling of bicarbonate. The impact of these secondary adjustments in bicarbonate concentration on the steady-state level of plasma acidity is indicated; note that the changes in plasma hydrogen ion concentration typically seen during both acute and chronic respiratory acidosis are roughly proportional to the increment in Pa_{CO_2}. The shaded areas connote the biologic variation characteristic of such responses. The time-course over which acid-base adjustments to hypercapnia occur is shown in Fig. 6-18.

patients with chronic, stable respiratory acidosis appear to confirm the presence of a predictable pattern of response when no complicating acid-base disturbances are present (11, 67). These findings in experimental animals and in man indicate that chronic hypercapnia is associated with an increment in hydrogen ion concentration of approximately 0.3 neq/L for each mmHg increment in Pa_{CO_2} (Fig. 6-19).

This empiric relationship between the change in Pa_{CO_2} and the anticipated alteration in hydrogen ion concentration may be used as an aid in detecting the presence of other acid-base disorders in patients known to have chronic respiratory acidosis (15). In this regard, it is noteworthy that certain complicating acid-base disturbances occur with considerable frequency in patients with long-standing respiratory failure. An element of metabolic alkalosis often results from the loss of gastric acid or from the use of diuretics, for example. Similarly, sudden reductions in Pa_{CO_2} often occur as a consequence of tracheostomy, mechanical ventilation, or both. In each of these circumstances, plasma bicarbonate concentration may remain elevated and thus hydrogen ion concentration may fall to levels lower than anticipated for the level of Pa_{CO_2} observed; frank alkalemia may even result (see Fig. 6-18).

Failure to recognize and correct superimposed metabolic alkalosis in patients with underlying pulmonary dysfunction can have important clinical consequences, since relative or absolute alkalemia may abrogate an important stimulus to respiration in such patients. If plasma acid-base values are diagnostically inconclusive, a measurement of urine chloride concentration may help to exclude the presence of the most common forms of superimposed alkalosis (see Table 6-5). In the absence of recent diuretic administration, the finding of abundant urinary chloride provides reasonable assurance that a superimposed, chloride-responsive alkalosis is not present.

An element of metabolic acidosis or of acute respiratory acidosis would, of course, cause hydrogen ion concentration to rise to levels *higher* than anticipated for the level of Pa_{CO_2} observed. If a superimposed element of metabolic acidosis is very severe, plasma bicarbonate concentration may fall to levels frankly lower than normal and be easily recognized. However, if the superimposed metabolic acidosis is of only moderate severity, bicarbonate concentration may be suppressed only partially, toward normal. Under these circumstances, the acid-base parameters can be indistinguishable from those encountered during partial physiologic adaptation to hypercapnia alone, and a valid judgment about the complex origin of the acid-base disturbance will depend upon clinical and other laboratory data (15) (see the section on mixed acid-base disturbances).

DIAGNOSIS AND CLINICAL MANIFESTATIONS

Clinical manifestations of respiratory acidosis vary markedly according to the rapidity with which hypercapnia develops. Acute hypercapnia is often associated with marked anxiety, severe breathlessness, reduced mental capacity, and stupor or coma in unusually severe instances. Chronic hypercapnia appears to be tolerated better but may also be responsible for confusion, loss of memory, and somnolence. Asterixis often accompanies both acute and chronic hypercapnia. Signs and symptoms of increased intracranial pressure are not uncommon and appear to be related to the well-established vasodilating effects of carbon dioxide on cerebral (and other) blood vessels; frank papilledema may be found when hypercapnia is severe. A reduction in alveolar ventilation is always associated with some degree of hypoxia as well as with hypercapnia in individuals breathing room air. Consequently, inadequate oxygenation may be an important factor contributing to the symptoms of respiratory acidosis. In patients with long-standing hypercapnia, attempts to alleviate hypoxia by administering high inspired-oxygen concentrations should be made with considerable caution, because if such therapy raises Pa_{O_2} above the patient's normal level, it will remove the hypoxic drive to respiration and result in even further reduction in alveolar ventilation.

CAUSES OF RESPIRATORY ACIDOSIS

Alveolar hypoventilation may result from disease or malfunction within any element in the regulatory system controlling respiration, including the respiratory center, the respiratory muscles, the thoracic cage, pleural space, lung parenchyma, and the airways. Table 6-6 separates the common

causes of respiratory acidosis into two groups in accordance with their usual mode of onset and duration. This classification also underscores the biphasic time-course of the secondary, biologic responses to hypercapnia.

Acute hypercapnia is seen in association with sudden suppression of the respiratory center, as may occur during general anesthesia or sedative overdosage. Acute respiratory failure frequently accompanies cardiac arrest, and the resulting hypercapnia may contribute more importantly than associated metabolic factors (e.g., lactic acid overproduction) to the severe acidemia commonly observed in this situation. An abrupt reduction in alveolar gas exchange, resulting in carbon dioxide retention, may occur during pneumothorax or severe pulmonary edema. Alveolar ventilation may also be limited by acute obstruction of the airways, during bronchospasm, laryngospasm or aspiration of foreign bodies. Similarly, acute hypercapnia results from improperly adjusted mechanical ventilators.

Treatment of acute respiratory acidosis, regardless of etiology, must be directed at prompt removal of the underlying cause. It is imperative to restore adequate ventilation swiftly in order to prevent extreme elevations in hydrogen ion concentration (and severe hypoxia). Although circumstances may require the administration of bicarbonate to blunt the developing acidemia, such therapy is a temporizing maneuver at best and should not divert attention away from correcting the hypercapnia.

Table 6-6. Causes of respiratory acidosis

ACUTE	CHRONIC
General anesthesia	Obstructive pulmonary disease
Sedative overdosage	Primary alveolar hypoventilation
Cardiac arrest	Brain tumor
Pneumothorax	Respiratory nerve damage (e.g.,
Pulmonary edema	poliomyelitis)
Severe pneumonia	Primary myopathy involving respiratory muscles
Bronchospasm	
Laryngospasm	Restrictive disease of the thorax
Aspiration of foreign body	(e.g., scleroderma)
Mechanical ventilators	Prolonged pneumonia

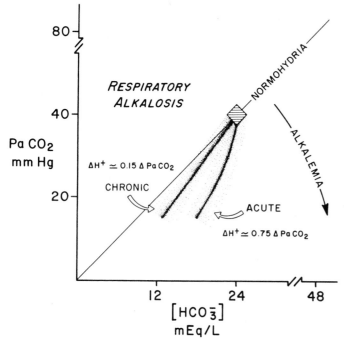

Figure 6-20. Effect of respiratory alkalosis on acid-base equilibrium. The initiating event is a decrease in carbon dioxide tension that reduces plasma hydrogen ion concentration (Fig. 6-10). This alkalinizing effect of hypocapnia is ameliorated by secondary reductions in bicarbonate concentration that result, acutely, from a titration of tissue buffers and, chronically, from an adaptation in the renal handling of bicarbonate. The impact of these secondary adjustments in bicarbonate concentration on the steady-state level of plasma acidity is indicated; note that the changes in plasma hydrogen ion concentration typically seen during both acute and chronic respiratory alkalosis appear to be roughly proportional to the decrement in Pa_{CO_2}. The shaded areas connote the biologic variation characteristic of such responses.

The great majority of patients with long-standing respiratory acidosis have underlying chronic obstructive pulmonary disease. Some of the other, less common causes of sustained hypercapnia are listed in Table 6-6.

RESPIRATORY ALKALOSIS

Respiratory alkalosis refers to those acid-base disturbances initiated by a reduction in carbon dioxide tension.

PATHOPHYSIOLOGY

Increased alveolar ventilation is the only process that can result in a period of negative carbon dioxide balance and, hence, in a reduction in carbon dioxide tension (hypocapnia). Primary hyperventilation and respiratory alkalosis, therefore, are synonymous. Hyperventilation may occur because of increased neural or chemical stimulation (or dis-inhibition) of the respiratory center or may be produced by mechanical ventilation.

SECONDARY PHYSIOLOGIC RESPONSES

The changes in acid-base equilibrium associated with primary hyperventilation are shown in Fig. 6-20 and are, for the most part, the obverse of those seen during respiratory acidosis. As Pa_{CO_2} falls, the tendency for hydrogen ion concentration to be reduced is opposed by a secondary reduction in plasma bicarbonate concentration. The decrements in bicarbonate induced by hypocapnia, like the analogous increments induced by hypercapnia, are the consequence of the immediate response of tissue buffering and of a more protracted response of renal adaptive mechanisms.

The biologic importance of these secondary responses is underscored by noting how extreme an effect even modest hyperventilation would have on hydrogen ion concentration if no change in bicarbonate were to occur. As can be seen from Fig. 6-10, an increase in alveolar ventilation sufficient to reduce Pa_{CO_2} from 40 to 20 mmHg would, in the face of a normal bicarbonate level, cause hydrogen ion concentration to fall to the dangerously low level of 20 neq/L (pH 7.70). It is interesting to contrast this situation with that prevailing in metabolic alkalosis, in which such alarming reductions in hydrogen ion concentration could be produced only by extreme elevations in bicarbonate concentration, even if secondary hypercapnia failed to occur.

During acute hypocapnia, tissue buffering produces a change in plasma bicarbonate concentration somewhat greater in magnitude than that observed during acute hypercapnia of comparable degree, a decrement in bicarbonate of some 3 to

4 meq/L occurring within minutes after Pa_{CO_2} is lowered to 20 to 25 mmHg (3). The resulting change in plasma hydrogen ion concentration, however, is strikingly similar to that observed during acute elevations in CO_2 tension. On the average, each mmHg reduction in Pa_{CO_2} results in an immediate fall in plasma hydrogen ion concentration of approximately 0.75 neq/L (Fig. 6-20).

If hypocapnia persists, plasma bicarbonate concentration falls further as a consequence of renal adaptation; a dampening of renal sodium-hydrogen exchange occurs, causing a transient suppression of net acid excretion and a reduction in the rate of bicarbonate reabsorption. Studies in animals indicate that these physiologic responses are complete within 2 to 4 days and result in a highly predictable relationship between the degree of chronic hypocapnia and the level at which plasma bicarbonate stabilizes; each mmHg reduction in Pa_{CO_2} is associated with a fall in plasma bicarbonate concentration averaging 0.4 to 0.5 meq/L (14, 26), a decrement sufficient to limit the fall in hydrogen ion concentration dramatically (Fig. 6-20). Though not yet well studied, changes of this magnitude probably occur in man as well. If so, it would appear that plasma hydrogen ion concentration is maintained at more nearly normal levels during uncomplicated chronic hypocapnia than is the case during uncomplicated chronic hypercapnia.

DIAGNOSIS AND CLINICAL MANIFESTATIONS

The acid-base parameters themselves are diagnostic of some element of respiratory alkalosis only when hypocapnia is associated with alkalemia. When hypocapnia is associated with acidemia, a separate element of respiratory alkalosis may be diagnosed only if the degree of hypocapnia is clearly beyond the range anticipated in response to the coexisting metabolic acidosis (see the section on mixed acid-base disturbances).

Acute respiratory alkalosis is frequently accompanied by numbness and paresthesias of the lips and extremities and may be associated with carpopedal spasm and light-headedness (53). Chronic respiratory alkalosis is typically accom-

panied by few symptoms other than those associated with the underlying disease process (see below). It is particularly noteworthy that marked hypocapnia can be sustained without a clinically evident increase in respiratory effort. For this reason, the physical examination should not be relied on in the diagnosis of respiratory alkalosis.

CAUSES OF RESPIRATORY ALKALOSIS

Table 6-7 lists some of the common causes of respiratory alkalosis. Most are associated with the abrupt appearance of hypocapnia, but in many instances the process may be sufficiently prolonged to permit full, chronic adaptation to occur. Consequently, no attempt has been made to separate these conditions into acute and chronic subgroups.

The mechanisms by which these conditions lead to hyperventilation differ markedly. Anxiety and hysteria appear to act through cortical pathways, which accounts for the improvement that often follows reassurance or sedation. Rebreathing into a closed system (e.g., a paper bag) may also be helpful, as it interrupts the positive feedback that may result from the symptoms of hypocapnia.

Table 6-7. Causes of respiratory alkalosis

Anxiety, hysteria
Fever
Salicylate intoxication
Central nervous system diseases
   Cerebrovascular accident
   Trauma
   Infection
   Tumor
Congestive heart failure
Pneumonia
Pulmonary emboli
Hypoxia
   Lowered barometric pressure
   Ventilation-perfusion imbalance
Hepatic insufficiency
Gram-negative septicemia
Mechanical ventilators

Fever and salicylate intoxication appear to stimulate the respiratory center more directly. Various central nervous system lesions of vascular, traumatic, infectious, and neoplastic origin, if located in the vicinity of the medullary respiratory centers, may also enhance stimulatory inputs or interrupt normal inhibitory pathways.

Numerous intrathoracic processes such as congestive heart failure, pneumonia, and pulmonary emboli may induce hyperventilation by stimulating the afferent limbs of certain neural reflex mechanisms. Hypoxia stimulates ventilation through chemoreceptor mechanisms and may result in hypocapnia if carbon dioxide excretion is unimpeded (e.g., high altitude, marked perfusion-ventilation imbalance).

The mechanisms responsible for the primary hyperventilation common in severe hepatic insufficiency and in gram-negative septicemia are not yet known. Since respiratory alkalosis may be an early manifestation of each of these disorders, however, unexplained hyperventilation may be an important clue to their presence.

Finally, mechanical ventilators may produce respiratory alkalosis if they are improperly adjusted. This complication can be avoided only by assessing acid-base equilibrium frequently in patients on assisted or controlled ventilation.

Treatment of respiratory alkalosis must be directed to removing the underlying cause. Attempts to return Pa_{CO_2} toward normal by increasing the carbon dioxide content of inspired air have not been rewarding.

MIXED ACID-BASE DISTURBANCES

Figure 6-21 depicts the range of Pa_{CO_2}-bicarbonate relationships characteristic of the graded degrees of each of the simple acid-base disorders. Given the wide variety of pathophysiologic processes that can alter plasma bicarbonate and Pa_{CO_2}, as discussed in the preceding sections, it is evident that the presence of one acid-base abnormality does not preclude the development of additional disturbances that may have independent effects on acid-base equilibrium. Coexistence of

two or more simple acid-base disorders is referred to as a mixed acid-base disturbance.

If the coexistence of independent acid-base abnormalities shifts the relationship between Pa_{CO_2} and bicarbonate concentration to a point clearly outside the range of responses characteristic of any single disorder, the presence of the mixed disturbance will be evident from an analysis of the acid-base parameters themselves. The acid-base values will fall outside all of the stippled areas in Fig. 6-21. It is important to recognize, however, that a mixed disturbance may be present even when acid-base parameters fall within the range of responses for a single disorder. This may occur if one of the disorders is of relatively small magnitude, if the two disorders have opposing effects on the same parameter (e.g., metabolic acidosis superimposed on metabolic alkalosis), or if three (or more) disturbances combine to masquerade as a single disorder. Consequently, acid-base values that fall within the range for a given simple disturbance can be said to be consistent with, but not necessarily diagnostic of, that disturbance.

It is clear from an examination of Fig. 6-21 that certain mixed disturbances are characterized by a normal or near normal hydrogen ion concentration. Thus, the presence of both chronic respiratory acidosis and metabolic alkalosis, or of both metabolic acidosis and respiratory alkalosis, may be overlooked if one focuses only on the level of acidity and fails to appreciate the abnormalities in plasma bicarbonate concentration and Pa_{CO_2}. It is also clear that other combinations of simple disturbances tend to cause extreme shifts in hydrogen ion concentration because bicarbonate concentration and Pa_{CO_2} are diverted in opposite directions. Thus, in patients with both metabolic acidosis and respiratory acidosis and in those with both metabolic alkalosis and respiratory alkalosis, relatively small abnormalities in Pa_{CO_2} and bicarbonate concentration can produce alarmingly high or alarmingly low concentrations of hydrogen ion, respectively.

Mixed acid-base disturbances are encountered with surprising frequency in hospitalized patients. Moreover, virtually every conceivable combination of simple disturbances can occur. The

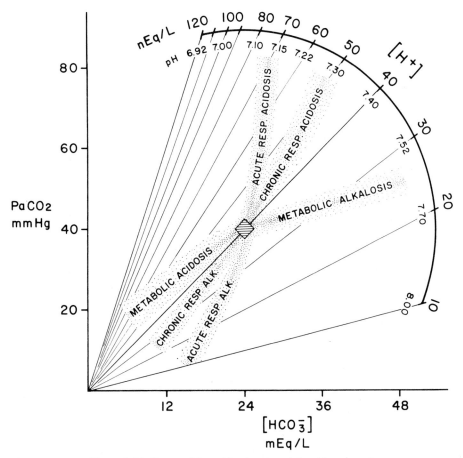

Figure 6-21. Range of Pa_{CO_2}-bicarbonate relationships characteristic of graded degrees of simple acid-base disorders. Acid-base values falling outside the stippled areas denote the presence of a mixed acid-base disturbance. Values falling within the stippled areas are consistent with, but not necessarily diagnostic of, the corresponding simple disorder.

more common mixed disorders will be discussed in the following sections.

RESPIRATORY ACIDOSIS AND METABOLIC ACIDOSIS

This combination of disturbances is characterized by acid-base values falling between the zones for acute respiratory acidosis and simple metabolic acidosis (Fig. 6-21). Elements of respiratory and metabolic acidosis frequently coexist in patients with cardiopulmonary arrest; such patients often develop lactic acidosis because of poor tissue perfusion and hypercapnia because of inadequate ventilation. Patients with severe pulmonary edema may develop a similar picture. As noted above, this combination of disturbances may produce extreme degrees of acidemia, plasma hydrogen ion concentration occasionally reaching levels well in excess of 100 neq/L (pH < 7.0).

The existence of this mixed disturbance is readily apparent when plasma bicarbonate is low and Pa_{CO_2} is high. It should be clear from the examination of Fig. 6-21, however, that this mixed disturbance can also be recognized in patients with moderately severe respiratory acidosis even when bicarbonate concentration is "normal," rather than elevated, as well as in patients with moderately severe metabolic acidosis even when Pa_{CO_2} is "normal."

METABOLIC ACIDOSIS AND RESPIRATORY ALKALOSIS

This combination is commonly encountered during the rapid correction of severe metabolic acidosis, as indicated schematically in Fig. 6-13. During treatment, plasma bicarbonate concentration often returns toward normal more swiftly than the secondary hypocapnia (originally induced by the acidosis) can abate. As a consequence, the degree of hypocapnia often remains inappropriately great with respect to the then-current decrement in plasma bicarbonate concentration for a period of several hours or more; hydrogen ion concentration during such intervals may be normal or even frankly low.

Patients with salicylate intoxication commonly manifest elements of both metabolic acidosis and respiratory alkalosis, reflecting the independent effects of the salicylate molecule on both cellular metabolism and ventilation. Patients with gram-negative sepsis may also develop this mixed disturbance, reflecting the frequent occurrence of primary hyperventilation on the one hand and of lactic acidosis and/or renal failure on the other.

The diagnosis of this mixed disturbance is straightforward if acid-base equilibrium falls between the zone for simple metabolic acidosis and that for chronic respiratory alkalosis (Fig. 6-21). If acid-base equilibrium falls between the zones for acute and chronic respiratory alkalosis, however, consideration must also be given to the possibility that only respiratory alkalosis is present but that insufficient time has elapsed for full renal adaptation to have occurred.

RESPIRATORY ALKALOSIS AND METABOLIC ALKALOSIS

Although these two disturbances do not coexist often, when they do, hydrogen ion concentration may, of course, be driven to extremely low levels. Patients with hepatic insufficiency, who frequently have persistent hyperventilation, may develop this combination of acid-base disturbances if they are treated with potent diuretics or if they lose gastric fluid. Similarly, patients with an underlying metabolic alkalosis may develop respiratory alkalosis if ventilation is stimulated (e.g., pulmonary embolus, sepsis) or if mechanical ventilation is utilized.

This mixed disturbance can be diagnosed readily if the level of Pa_{CO_2} is subnormal and if plasma bicarbonate concentration is frankly elevated. As can be seen from Fig. 6-21, acid-base values falling anywhere between the zone for acute respiratory alkalosis and that for metabolic alkalosis would be consistent with this combination of disturbances.

METABOLIC ALKALOSIS AND RESPIRATORY ACIDOSIS

This combination of disturbances is seen relatively frequently, because patients with carbon dioxide retention secondary to severe pulmonary disease often develop metabolic alkalosis as a result of vomiting or diuretic administration. In addition, patients with long-standing hypercapnia and secondary hyperbicarbonatemia caused by renal adaptation are primed to develop "post-hypercapneic" metabolic alkalosis if a sudden improvement in ventilation (e.g., tracheal suction, mechanical ventilation) returns Pa_{CO_2} toward normal; this alkalosis persists until the adaptive increase in bicarbonate stores is removed by renal excretion (Fig. 6-18).

This mixed disturbance is readily identified when the plasma bicarbonate concentration is elevated beyond the range appropriate for full adaptation to the observed level of Pa_{CO_2}, i.e., when acid-base equilibrium falls between the zone for simple metabolic alkalosis and chronic respiratory acidosis in Fig. 6-21.

ACUTE RESPIRATORY ACIDOSIS AND CHRONIC RESPIRATORY ACIDOSIS

Patients fully adapted to an elevated level of Pa_{CO_2} may experience a sudden deterioration of pulmonary function that causes Pa_{CO_2} to rise even further. Under these circumstances, acid-base equilibrium falls in the area intermediate between the zone for acute and chronic respiratory acidosis. It should be noted, however, that a similar acid-base picture (i.e., an elevated Pa_{CO_2} coupled with a level of plasma bicarbonate concentration intermediate between the ranges appropriate for acute and chronic hypercapnia) can also be seen in patients with a stable degree of hypercapnia in whom full adaptation has not yet occurred, in patients with chronic respiratory acidosis in whom mild to moderate metabolic acidosis has supervened, and in patients with acute respiratory acidosis complicated by metabolic alkalosis.

The fact that more than one combination of simple disturbances can give rise to the same acid-base picture underscores the need to consider not only the acid-base values themselves but also historical and other laboratory information in reaching definitive conclusions regarding diagnosis and therapy.

REFERENCES

1. Albert, M. S., R. B. Dell, and R. W. Winters: Quantitative displacement of acid-base equilibrium in metabolic acidosis, *Ann. Intern. Med.*, **66**:312, 1967.

2. Albert, M. S., and R. W. Winters: Acid-base equilibrium of blood in normal infants, *Pediatrics*, **37**:728, 1966.

3. Arbus, G. S., L. A. Hebert, P. R. Levesque, B. E. Etsten, and W. B. Schwartz: Characterization and clinical application of the "significance band" for acute respiratory alkalosis, *N. Engl. J. Med.*, **280**:117, 1969.

4. Babior, B. M.: Villous adenoma of the colon, *Am. J. Med.*, **41**:615, 1966.

5. Bank, N., and W. Schwartz: Influence of anion penetrating ability on urinary acidification and excretion of titratable acid, *J. Clin. Invest.*, **39**:1516, 1960.

6. Bartlett, G. R.: Inhibition of methanol oxidation by ethanol in the rat, *Am. J. Physiol.*, **163**:619, 1950.

7. Bates, R. G.: *Determination of pH; Theory and Practice*, John Wiley & Sons, Inc., New York, 1964.

8. Beier, L. S., W. H. Pitts, and H. C. Gonick: Metabolic acidosis occurring during paraldehyde intoxication, *Ann. Intern. Med.*, **58**:155, 1963.

9. Bennett, I. L., Jr., F. H. Cary, G. L. Mitchell, Jr., and M. N. Cooper: Acute methyl alcohol poisoning: Review based on experience in outbreak of 323 cases, *Medicine (Baltimore)*, **32**:431, 1953.

10. Brackett, N. C., Jr., J. J. Cohen, and W. B. Schwartz: Carbon dioxide titration curve of normal man, *N. Engl. J. Med.*, **272**:6, 1965.

11. Brackett, N. C., Jr., C. F. Wingo, O. Muren, and J. T. Solano: Acid-base response to chronic hypercapnia in man, *N. Engl. J. Med.*, **280**:124, 1969.

12. Clapp, J. R., F. Rector, Jr., and D. Seldin: Effects of unreabsorbed anions on proximal and distal transtubular potentials in rats, *Am. J. Physiol.*, **202**:781, 1962.

13. Cohen, J. J.: A new acid-base nomogram featuring hydrogen ion concentration. Henderson revisited, *Ann. Intern. Med.*, **66**:159, 1967.

14. Cohen, J. J., N. E. Madias, C. J. Wolf, and W. B. Schwartz: Regulation of acid-base equilibrium in chronic hypocapnia: Evidence that the response of the kidney is not geared to the defense of extracellular $[H^+]$, *J. Clin. Invest.*, **57**:1483, 1976.

15. Cohen, J. J., and W. B. Schwartz: Evaluation of acid-base equilibrium in pulmonary insufficiency: An approach to a diagnostic dilemma (editorial), *Am. J. Med.*, **41**:163, 1966.

16. Cooke, R. E., W. E. Segar, D. B. Cheek, F. E. Coville, and D. C. Darrow: The extrarenal correction of alkalosis associated with potassium deficiency, *J. Clin. Invest.*, **31**:798, 1952.

17. Cooperman, M. T., F. Davidoff, R. Spark, and J. Pallotta: Clinical studies of alcoholic ketoacidosis, *Diabetes*, **23**:433, 1974.

18. Dammin, G. J.: Consequences of ethylene glycol poisoning, *Am. J. Med.*, **32**:891, 1962.

19. DeSousa, R. C., J. T. Harrington, E. S. Ricanati, J. W. Shelkrot, and W. B. Schwartz: Renal regu-

lation of acid-base equilibrium during chronic administration of mineral acid, *J. Clin. Invest.*, **53**:465, 1974.

20. Evanson, J. M., and S. W. Stanbury: Congenital chloridorrhaea or so-called congenital alkalosis with diarrhea, *Gut*, **6**:29, 1965.

21. Felig, P.: Diabetic ketoacidosis, *N. Engl. J. Med.*, **290**:1360, 1974.

22. Gardiner, W. C., Jr.: *Rates and Mechanisms of Chemical Reactions*, W. A. Benjamin, Inc., New York, 1969.

23. Garella, S., B. S. Chang, and S. I. Kahn: Dilution acidosis and contraction alkalosis: Review of a concept (editorial), *Kidney Int.*, **8**:279, 1975.

24. Garella, S., J. A. Chazan, and J. J. Cohen: Saline-resistant metabolic alkalosis or "chloride-wasting nephropathy." Report of four cases with severe potassium depletion, *Ann. Intern. Med.*, **73**:31, 1970.

25. Garella, S., C. L. Dana, and J. A. Chazan: Severity of metabolic acidosis as a determinant of bicarbonate requirements, *N. Engl. J. Med.*, **289**:121, 1973.

26. Gennari, F. J., M. B. Goldstein, and W. B. Schwartz: The nature of the renal adaptation to chronic hypocapnia, *J. Clin. Invest.*, **51**:1722, 1972.

27. Giebisch, G., G. Malnic, R. Klose, and E. Windhager: Effect of ionic substitutions on distal potential differences in rat kidney, *Am. J. Physiol.*, **211**:560, 1966.

28. Goodman, A. D., J. Lemann, Jr., E. J. Lennon, and A. S. Relman: Production, excretion, and net balance of fixed acid in patients with renal disease, *J. Clin. Invest.*, **44**:495, 1965.

29. Heird, W. C., R. B. Dell, J. M. Driscoll, Jr., B. Grebin, and R. W. Winters: Metabolic acidosis resulting from intravenous alimentation mixtures containing synthetic amino acids, *N. Engl. J. Med.*, **287**:943, 1972.

30. Henderson, L. J.: The theory of neutrality regulation in the animal organism, *Am. J. Physiol.*, **21**:427, 1908.

31. Kassirer, J. P., P. M. Berkman, D. R. Lawrenz, and W. B. Schwartz: The critical role of chloride in the correction of hypokalemic alkalosis in man, *Am. J. Med.*, **38**:172, 1965.

32. Kassirer, J. P., A. M. London, D. M. Goldman, and W. B. Schwartz: On the pathogenesis of metabolic alkalosis in hyperaldosteronism, *Am. J. Med.*, **49**:306, 1970.

33. Kassirer, J. P., and W. B. Schwartz: Correction of metabolic alkalosis in man without repair of potassium deficiency. A re-evaluation of the role of potassium, *Am. J. Med.*, **40**:19, 1966.

34. Keyvan-Larijarni, H., and A. M. Tannenberg: Methanol intoxication: Comparison of peritoneal dialysis and hemodialysis treatment, *Arch. Intern. Med.*, **134**:293, 1974.

35. Lemann, J., Jr., J. R. Litzow, and E. J. Lennon: The effects of chronic acid loads in normal man: Further evidence for the participation of bone mineral in the defense against chronic metabolic acidosis, *J. Clin. Invest.*, **45**:1608, 1966.

36. Lemann, J., Jr., and A. S. Relman: The relation of sulphur metabolism to acid-base balance and electrolyte excretion. The effects of DL-methionine in normal man, *J. Clin. Invest.*, **38**:2215, 1959.

37. Lennon, E. J., and J. Lemann, Jr.: Defense of hydrogen ion concentration in chronic metabolic acidosis, *Ann. Intern. Med.*, **65**:265, 1966.

38. Lennon, E. J., J. Lemann, Jr., and A. S. Relman: The effects of phosphoproteins on acid balance in normal subjects, *J. Clin. Invest.*, **41**:637, 1962.

39. Needle, M., G. Kaloyanides, and W. B. Schwartz: Effects of selective depletion of hydrochloric acid on acid-base and electrolyte equilibrium, *J. Clin. Invest.*, **43**:1836, 1964.

40. Oliva, P. B.: Lactic acidosis, *Am. J. Med.*, **48**:209, 1970.

41. Orloff, J., T. J. Kennedy, Jr., and R. W. Berliner: The effect of potassium in nephrectomized rats with hypokalemic alkalosis, *J. Clin. Invest.*, **32**:538, 1953.

42. Pappenheimer, J. R.: The ionic composition of cerebral extracellular fluid and its relation to control of breathing, *Harvey Lect.*, **61**:71, 1965–1966.

43. Pierce, N. F., D. S. Fedson, R. C. Brigham, R. C. Mitra, R. B. Sack, and A. Mondal: The ventilatory response to acute base deficit in humans, *Ann. Intern. Med.*, **72**:633, 1970.

44. Pitts, R. F.: Renal production and excretion of ammonia, *Am. J. Med.*, **36**:720, 1964.

45. Pitts, R. F., J. deHaas, and J. Klein: Relation of renal amino and amide nitrogen extraction to ammonia production, *Am. J. Physiol.*, **204**:187, 1963.

46. Pitts, R. F., L. A. Pilkington, and J. C. M. deHaas: N[15] Tracer studies on the origin of urinary ammonia in the acidotic dog, with notes on the enzymatic synthesis of labelled glutamic acid and glutamines, *J. Clin. Invest.*, **44**:731, 1965.

47. Punsar, S., and T. Somer: The milk-alkali syndrome: A report of three illustrative cases and a review of the literature, *Acta Med. Scand.*, **173**:435, 1963.

48. Reidenberg, M. M., B. L. Hoog, B. J. Channick, C. R. Shuman, and T. G. Wilson: The response of bone to metabolic acidosis in man, *Metabolism*, **15**:236, 1966.

49. Relman, A. S.: Renal acidosis and renal excretion of acid in health and disease, in W. Dock and I. Snapper (eds.): *Advances of Internal Medicine*, vol. 12, Year Book Medical Publishers, Inc., Chicago, 1964.

50. Relman, A. S., E. J. Lennon, and J. Lemann, Jr.: Endogenous production of fixed acid and the measurement of the net balance of acid in normal subjects, *J. Clin. Invest.*, **40**:1621, 1961.

51. Relman, A. S., P. F. Shelborne, and A. Talman: Profound acidosis resulting from excessive ammonium chloride in previously healthy subjects: A study of two cases, *N. Engl. J. Med.*, **264**:848, 1961.

52. Robin, E. D.: Of man and mitochondria—intracellular and subcellular acid-base relations, *N. Engl. J. Med.*, **265**:780, 1961.

53. Saltzman, H., A. Heyman, and H. Sieker: Correlation of clinical and physiological manifestations of sustained hyperventilation, *N. Engl. J. Med.*, **268**:1431, 1963.

54. Satorius, O. W., J. C. Roemmelt, and R. F. Pitts: The renal regulation of acid-base balance in man. IV. The nature of the renal compensation in ammonium chloride acidosis, *J. Clin. Invest.*, **28**:423, 1949.

55. Schwartz, W. B., N. C. Brackett, Jr., and J. J. Cohen: The response of extracellular hydrogen ion concentration to graded degrees of chronic hypercapnia, *J. Clin. Invest.*, **44**:291, 1965.

56. Schwartz, W. B., P. W. Hall, III, R. M. Hays, and A. S. Relman: On the mechanisms of acidosis in chronic renal disease, *J. Clin. Invest.*, **38**:39, 1959.

57. Schwartz, W. B., R. M. Hays, A. Polak, and G. D. Haynie: Effects of chronic hypercapnia on electrolyte and acid-base equilibrium. II. Recovery, with special reference to the influence of chloride intake, *J. Clin. Invest.*, **40**:1238, 1961.

58. Schwartz, W. B., R. Jenson, and A. S. Relman: Acidification of urine and increased ammonium excretion without change in acid-base equilibrium: Sodium reabsorption as stimulus to acidifying process, *J. Clin. Invest.*, **34**:673, 1955.

59. Schwartz, W. B., K. J. Orning, and R. Porter: The internal distribution of hydrogen ions with varying degrees of metabolic acidosis, *J. Clin. Invest.*, **36**:373, 1957.

60. Schwartz, W. B., C. van Ypersele de Strihou, and J. P. Kassirer: Role of anions in metabolic alkalosis and potassium deficiency, *N. Engl. J. Med.*, **279**:630, 1968.

61. Shear, L., and I. S. Brandman: Hypoxia and hypercapnia caused by respiratory compensation for metabolic alkalosis, *Am. Rev. Respir. Dis.*, **107**:836, 1973.

62. Singer, R. B., J. K. Clark, E. S. Barker, A. P. Crosley, Jr., and R. Elkinton: The acute effects in man of rapid intravenous infusion of hypertonic bicarbonate solution. I. Changes in acid-base balance and distribution of the excess buffer base, *Medicine (Baltimore)*, **34**:51, 1955.

63. Swan, R. C., and R. F. Pitts: Neutralization of infused acid by nephrectomized dogs, *J. Clin. Invest.*, **34**:205, 1955.

64. Tenney, S. M., and R. M. Miller: The respiratory and circulatory actions of salicylate, *Am. J. Med.*, **19**:498, 1955.

65. Teree, T. M., E. Mirabel-Font, A. Ortiz, and W. B. Wallace: Stool losses and acidosis in diarrheal disease of infancy, *Pediatrics*, **36**:704, 1965.

66. Van Goidsenhoven, G. M-T., O. V. Gray, A. V. Price, and P. H. Sanderson: The effect of prolonged administration of large doses of sodium bicarbonate in man, *Clin. Sci.*, **13**:383, 1954.

67. van Ypersele de Strihou, C., L. Brasseur, and J. de Coninck: The "carbon dioxide response curve" for chronic hypercapnia in man, *N. Engl. J. Med.*, **275**:117, 1966.

68. van Ypersele de Strihou, C., and A. Frans: The pattern of respiratory compensation in chronic uraemic acidosis, *Nephron*, **7**:37, 1970.

69. van Ypersele de Strihou, C., and J. Morales-Barria: The influence of dietary sodium and potassium intake in the genesis of furosemide induced alkalosis, *Clin. Sci.*, **37**:859, 1969.

70. Waters, W. C., III, J. D. Hall, and W. B. Schwartz: Spontaneous lactic acidosis: The nature of the acid-base disturbance and considerations in diagnosis and management, *Am. J. Med.*, **35**:781, 1963.

71. Winters, R. W., J. S. White, M. C. Hughes, and N. K. Ordway: Disturbances of acid-base equilibrium in salicylate intoxication, *Pediatrics*, **23**:260, 1959.

7

Renal function: General concepts

NEAL S. BRICKER / RAYMOND G. SCHULTZE / AMNON LICHT

INTRODUCTION

To write a chapter on normal renal function in a multiauthored text as comprehensive and wide ranging as this one necessarily involves a selective approach, for many specific renal functions are considered in detail in other chapters. We have therefore limited the scope of our presentation, dealing almost exclusively with the kidney as an organ of excretion. We have made an effort to deal conceptually with the major role that the kidney, as an excretory organ, plays in the maintenance of life and well-being. In so doing, we have addressed the biologic phenomena that underlie renal functions, ranging from the physical events that influence glomerular filtration and proximal tubular fluid reabsorption to certain of the intricate biologic control systems responsible for regulating the tubular transport of several of the most important constituents of body fluids.

The selectivity of the approach is perhaps most evident in the limited number of individual functions and control systems treated in depth. These include the formation of glomerular filtrate and the regulation of the filtration process; volume control and the regulation of sodium excretion; urinary concentrating and diluting mechanisms; the regulation of acid-base homeostasis; and the renal excretion of potassium. The list is not entirely an arbitrary one, for these same functional systems are not only among the most vital but also among the most thoroughly investigated. Moreover, the knowledge of the characteristics of these systems in health provides the key to the understanding and interpretation of the alterations and adaptations in the same systems that occur in chronic progressive renal disease.

There has been great progress in the understanding of normal mechanisms of renal function. In part, this relates to the rapid expansion of basic information about how living cells and their subcellular component parts function, for these data have provided increasing insight into how whole organs function. In part, the progress relates to the fact that an ever-increasing number of investigators, using an ever-expanding armamentarium of experimental methods and techniques, have directed their efforts to the search for information about the kidneys. But there is a significant element in our advancing knowledge of normal physiology that stems paradoxically from the distortion of normal physiologic mechanisms produced by disease. The diverse consequences of disease can lead to many and varied perturbations of a normal physiologic system, thereby revealing the component parts of the system in a manner that the investigator may not be able to reproduce de novo in the laboratory.

However, while the study of disease processes can lead to clarification of normal physiologic mechanisms, the reverse relationship is, if anything, more impressive. For the interpretation of renal function in pathologic states must necessarily proceed from knowledge in depth of the manner in which the kidneys function in health. Indeed, within a relatively short period of time, the clinical approach to a growing number of diseases of the kidneys and disorders of body fluids has been stripped of empiricism and transformed into an increasingly rational, objective, and quantitative exercise. Knowledge of normal physiology has contributed enormously to this transformation.

FUNCTIONAL COMMITMENTS OF THE NORMAL KIDNEY

The kidney functions primarily as an excretory organ. But it is a highly specialized organ of excretion, for it excretes a host of different substances simultaneously and yet is capable of discriminating between individual solutes, regulating the excretion rates of many key substances independently of a variety of others. In a descriptive sense, the role of the kidney in the excretion of many solutes and of water is to preserve their constancy in the extracellular fluid and thus to assure the preservation of *balance*.

BALANCE AND ITS MAINTENANCE

The term *balance* connotes the maintenance of a constant amount of a substance within the body. In essence, what goes in must come out. The maintenance of balance requires that the combined rates of elimination of the substance by all routes, metabolic as well as excretory, remain equal to the combined rates of acquisition by all routes. For many solutes, the rates of acquisition vary over a wide range (because of dietary variations), while the rates of nonrenal elimination do not vary proportionately. Operationally, therefore, what the organism must do is add up these various rates, establish the difference between total accession and total nonrenal elimination, and then effect the excretion of just that quantity of the substance which will establish balance. Often this is accomplished with the aid of extrarenal control systems which detect displacements from the steady state.

The nature and quantitative contribution of the kidneys to the maintenance of balance varies with different substances. For some solutes, of which urea and creatinine are the prime examples (1), the kidney exercises no discriminatory role, and the rate of excretion is determined exclusively by the plasma level, so that the higher the concentration of the solute in the plasma, the greater is the amount filtered into the functioning nephrons, and the greater is the rate of excretion per nephron. Balance is maintained for these solutes, but not because of any finely tuned regulatory function of the kidneys (active transport by the tubular epithelial cells appears to play a minor role at most in regulating the excretion rates of both urea and creatinine). Excretion rates therefore will continue to approximate accession rates simply because any increase in production will lead to a rise in plasma levels; the amount of the substance filtered, thus, will increase, and excretion rates will rise until a new steady state (i.e., balance) is achieved. A decrease in production rates will initiate the opposite sequence. When the nephron population diminishes in chronic renal disease, excretion rates will fall below production rates with each decrement in renal function, and urea and creatinine will accumulate in the body fluids. But as the plasma levels rise, the filtered load per remaining nephron will rise, and the total excretion rates will return to their previous level. Thus balance for urea and creatinine will be reestablished, but at a higher plasma concentration.

There is a second category of solutes for which the kidneys make a quantitatively limited, but regulated, contribution to total excretion. In contrast to their passive role in urea and creatinine excretion, the kidneys play an important role in regulating body fluid concentrations for these substances. Phosphate and urate are prime examples of such solutes. Renal excretion appears to be closely regulated by tubular transport systems which remain responsive to the homeostatic requirements of the body.

Finally, for many solutes, including sodium, potassium, chloride, glucose, amino acids, and hydrogen, the maintenance of external balance is primarily if not exclusively a renal phenomenon. For most of these solutes, only a small fraction of the filtered load is excreted, and the precise rate of excretion is determined by closely regulated tubular transport systems.

THE CONCEPT OF CONTROL SYSTEMS

A substantial part of the understanding of normal renal function involves a consideration of how excretion rates for multiple solutes can be regulated simultaneously. This understanding must begin with the definition of the general manner in which the kidney handles each substance (i.e., by filtration alone, by filtration and resorption, by filtration and secretion, or by filtration, reabsorption, and secretion). Then the search for information must be directed toward defining the events which can modulate the component parts of a given excretory system (i.e., glomerular versus tubular) and thereby regulate the excretion rate.

The total picture requires an understanding of the events which control the modulators. In other words, is there a control system operative within the organism which assesses the excretory requirement and directs the activity of a factor or factors that will initiate the required changes at the level of the nephron? A control system must have a detector element that will recognize even very small dislocations from the steady state of the solute in question. The control system will also need an integrating element (or elements) capable of collecting and interpreting heterogenous messages from different parts of the body. In addition, there must be a means of transmitting the collated information to the kidney in order to

effect the necessary changes in function. Presumably the detector element for most control systems resides in an extrarenal location. A case in point is the phosphorus control system, in which the entrance of phosphate into the extracellular fluid (ECF) leads to a reciprocal fall in ionized calcium that is then detected by the parathyroid glands in the neck. Some detectors, however, may reside within the kidney [e.g., the macula densa lying in the distal tubular wall (2)]. The integrating elements, if they exist, will reside in the central nervous system.

Finally, with regard to the effector limb, for at least some control systems, information is transferred to the kidney via a hormone. Two such effector hormones that are well characterized are the antidiuretic hormone (ADH), which modulates the renal excretion of water, and the parathyroid hormone (PTH), which modulates the renal excretion of phosphate and may contribute to the modulation of calcium excretion. Aldosterone plays some part in the regulation of sodium excretion and perhaps a larger part in the regulation of potassium excretion, and it is also possible that there may be a natriuretic hormone which contributes to the fine regulation of sodium excretion.

In all probability there are control systems governing the renal excretion of many different solutes. Unfortunately, however, knowledge of most of these is either limited or nonexistent; thus this category of information must occupy a relatively small part of this chapter. Whatever the nature of the effector element of a control system, it must retain solute specificity despite any coupled steps in the tubular transport of the regulated solute with any other solute. For example, PTH, which modulates tubular reabsorption of phosphate, also inhibits proximal tubular reabsorption of sodium (3). Yet the biologic control system for sodium must be capable of overriding any interfering effects of PTH on sodium transport.

ENDOCRINE AND METABOLIC FUNCTIONS

The contribution of the kidneys to well-being is by no means limited to the excretion of solutes and water. The kidney plays a crucial role in the production of the active metabolite of vitamin D, 1,25-dihydroxycholecalciferol (4, 5). The juxtaglomerular apparatus, which resides in the wall of the afferent arteriole is thought to be involved in the synthesis of renin and in the production of an erythropoietic hormone (6) from a plasma substrate. It has also been shown recently that cells from the renal medulla synthesize prostaglandins in tissue culture (7), and, with the aid of histochemical techniques, collecting tubules have been shown to be possible sites of prostaglandin synthesis (8).

The normal physiologic functions of these biologically active compounds and the control systems regulating their synthesis and release are coming under close scrutiny. From a metabolic point of view, the kidney may under certain conditions serve as an important organ for glucose production. It may also contribute to the breakdown of some peptide and protein molecules.

GENERAL CHARACTERISTICS OF URINE FORMATION

The formation of urine begins with the flow of blood through the glomerular capillaries in large volume and at a high rate. Within the capillary lumina, approximately 25 percent of the water and solutes are diverted from the moving stream of plasma and rerouted through the triple-layered glomerular membrane into Bowman's space and the tubular lumen. The three layers of the glomerular filter are the capillary endothelial cells, the basement membrane, and the epithelial cells. These are presented schematically in Fig. 7-1. This transposed fluid is the *glomerular filtrate*. Because the filtering membranes are freely permeable to water and low-molecular-weight solutes, the glomerular filtrate closely resembles the plasma from which it was formed.[1] Glomerular filtrate, therefore, contains the majority of sol-

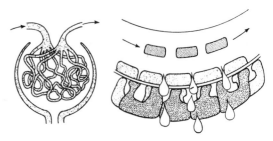

Figure 7-1. The diagram at the left is a schematic drawing of a normal glomerulus, showing the afferent arteriole breaking up into capillary loops and the capillary loops in turn reuniting to form the efferent arteriole. The diagram at the right is a schematic representation of a single capillary loop in a normal glomerulus. The three stippled rectangles are red blood cells in transit. The upper portion of the glomerular membrane is deleted, and only a single line is shown. Each of the three layers of the glomerular membrane is shown for the lower boundary. From capillary lumen downward, these layers include the endothelial cells, the basement membrane, and the epithelial cells with their discrete foot processes. (*From Disease-a-Month, Oct., 1955.*)

utes and water that must be excreted, but the amounts of most substances filtered greatly exceed those that ultimately appear in the urine. The extra quantity of these solutes and of water must be retrieved from the tubular fluid as it flows down the length of the nephron. The reclamation of these particles requires their transfer across the tubular epithelial cells and their subsequent entry into the peritubular capillary plasma. There are some solutes, on the other hand, that are filtered in quantities smaller than those found in the urine. These substances must be transferred into the tubular fluid by the tubular epithelial cells by a process referred to as secretion. The majority of the secreted solutes are transported from the per-

---

[1] The only major difference resides in the virtual absence of plasma proteins from the filtrate (9). This in turn will introduce small compositional changes caused by two phenomena: First, 100 ml of whole plasma contains only about 93 ml of water, the remainder of the volume being occupied by protein molecules. Consequently, the low-molecular-weight solutes that existed in the plasma in 100 ml of fluid (93 ml of water and 7 ml of protein) will be delivered into the glomerular fil-

trate in 93 ml of water. This means that all completely filtrable solutes will be approximately 7% more concentrated in the glomerular filtrate than in the plasma because of the "plasma water" effect. The second difference between golmerular filtrate and plasma relates to the charge on the protein molecules, which at the pH of body fluids is predominantly negative. By virtue of the Gibbs-Donnan equilibrium, the distribution of charged particles will be altered such that the concentration of cations in the glomerular filtrate will be somewhat lower than in the plasma and the concentration of anions will be somewhat higher. The plasma water and Gibbs-Donnan effects are additive for anions; they tend to be offsetting for cations.

itubular capillary surface of the epithelial lumen into the tubular lumen. However, ammonia and, in a special sense, hydrogen ions are produced de novo within the epithelial cells and are secreted only across the luminal border of the epithelial cells. Finally, for some solutes, most notably potassium and uric acid, transtubular movements are bidirectional. The removal from the tubular fluid occurs via resorption; reentry into the tubular fluid occurs via secretion.

Fine regulation of the amount of any substance excreted in the urine theoretically could be mediated by controlled changes in either the glomerular filtration rate (GFR) or the rate of tubular transport. However, it is more difficult to conceive of changes in the GFR affecting fine regulation; for when the GFR changes, the delivery of all filtered solutes changes *pari passu*. Consequently, if an increase in the GFR were utilized to increase the excretion of one specific solute, the rate of tubular transport of all resorbed solutes would have to increase to avoid a change in their excretion rates. There is evidence that for certain solutes which are excreted in precisely modulated quantities, final control is accomplished by modifications of tubular transport. Thus, logically, increasing attention has been focused on the nature of the tubular transport systems and on the events that alter their activity. Nevertheless, the formation of glomerular filtrate is an extremely critical step in the formation of urine and warrants separate consideration.

FORMATION OF GLOMERULAR FILTRATE

In a normal adult man the volume of glomerular filtrate equals approximately 120 ml/min, or 170 L/day. This process of glomerular filtration is an entirely passive one that depends exclusively upon physical forces.

In the normal adult, from 500 to 600 ml of plasma traverse the renal circulation each minute. Because the weight of the two kidneys combined is far less than 1 percent of total body weight, it is evident that the kidneys are preferentially perfused and thus must have a very low-resistance vascular bed. There are relatively few subdivisions between the aorta and the glomerular capillaries, and the individual arterial branches are short and have relatively large cross-sectional diameters. Thus there is limited dissipation of hydrostatic pressure by frictional resistance proximal to the glomerular capillaries.

The major force promoting filtration is the blood pressure within the glomerular capillaries. The two main forces opposing ultrafiltration across the glomerular capillaries are the colloid oncotic pressure, which arises from the nonfiltered protein molecules in the glomerular capillary plasma, and the hydrostatic pressure in Bowman's space. There are several differences between the Starling forces in glomerular capillaries and those in systemic capillaries (10): hydrostatic pressure remains relatively constant in glomerular capillaries, whereas it declines markedly along the length of extrarenal capillaries; glomerular capillaries are less permeable to protein than are systemic capillaries; in contrast to systemic capillaries, plasma oncotic pressure rises along the course of glomerular capillaries; and the hydrostatic pressure in Bowman's space is considerably higher than in the systemic analogue (11). These relationships are presented schematically in Fig. 7-2.

The rate of formation of glomerular filtrate is also influenced heavily by the ultrafiltration coefficient (K_f) of the glomerular capillaries (10, 11). The relationship between the relevant physical forces and K_f is described in the following equation:

$$\text{GFR} = k_f \, (P_{GC} - P_T - \Pi_{GC} + \Pi_F) \qquad (7\text{-}1)$$

where K_f = the ultrafiltration coefficient (hydraulic conductivity per unit area times glomerular surface area)

P_{GC} = the mean glomerular capillary hydrostatic pressure

P_T = the hydrostatic pressure in Bowman's space

Π_{GC} = the mean effective colloid osmotic pressure of the glomerular capillary plasma

Π_F = the colloid osmotic pressure of the glomerular filtrate

(A more detailed treatment of this formulation may be found in Ref. 11.)

In the final analysis, the number of perfused

Glomerular capillary hydraulic and
oncotic pressures,
mmHg

	Afferent end	Efferent end
P_{GC}	45	45
P_T	10	10
Π_{GC}	20	35
$P_{UF} = P_{GC} - P_T - \Pi_{GC}$	15	0

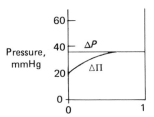

Dimensionless distance along idealized
glomerular capillary

Figure 7-2. Hydraulic and colloid osmotic pressure profiles along an idealized glomerular capillary in the rat. $\Delta P = P_{GC} - P_T$ and $\Delta\Pi = \Pi_{GC} - \Pi_G$ where P_{GC} and P_T are the hydraulic pressures in the glomerular capillary and Bowman's space, respectively, and Π_{GC} and Π_T are the corresponding colloid osmotic pressures. (P_{GC} net ultrafiltration pressure.) (*From W. M. Deen, C. R. Robertson et al., Fed. Proc., 33:14, 1974.*)

glomeruli and the number of potent capillary loops per glomerulus will serve as prepotent determinants of the total GFR. In health, the latter factors are thought to remain constant; in certain intrinsic renal diseases any or all of the factors may be altered markedly.

REGULATION OF THE GLOMERULAR FILTRATION RATE

Generally, the amount of salt and water filtered exceeds the amount excreted into the urine by over a hundredfold. Consequently, uncontrolled changes in the GFR could prove extremely disruptive to the regulation of salt and water balance. Indeed, the precise regulation of the excre-

tion rates of many different solutes could be perturbed seriously by wide fluctuations in the GFR. Thus, on a priori grounds, a regulatory mechanism should exist. It must function to keep pressure differences constant across a filtering bed in the face of substantial changes in cardiac output, blood pressure, and peripheral resistance. It has been demonstrated that renal blood flow tends to remain quite constant in nervated, denervated, and isolated kidneys (12), in the face of marked changes in mean arterial blood pressure. This phenomenon is known as *autoregulation.* Moreover, the GFR is autoregulated in a manner comparable with that of renal plasma flow (13), and the GFR will often remain stable even when renal blood flow changes. The regulatory mechanisms undoubtedly require controlled modulation of the key intrarenal resistances, and it seems very likely that a control system exists which is capable of exercising a discriminant influence over the tone of the afferent and the efferent arterioles. Despite a great deal of work and the proposal of many theories, however, the mechanism of autoregulation has not been fully identified. One contemporary theory (14), for example, suggests that when a spontaneous change in the GFR does occur, the sodium concentration of the tubular fluid reaching the macula densa will change, the macula densa will sense this change and transmit the information to the juxtaglomerular cells in the wall of the contiguous afferent arteriole, and the rate of renin release from the juxtaglomerular granules will be altered. The change in renin activity will, in turn, change the activity of angiotensin, and angiotensin may then lead to vasoconstriction of the afferent, the efferent, or both types of arterioles. Further details of this feedback loop will be considered in a later section of this chapter. Other theories of autoregulation have been reviewed (15) and may be consulted for reference.

TUBULAR MODIFICATIONS OF THE GLOMERULAR FILTRATE

As the glomerular filtrate begins its descent through the nephron, it rapidly loses its original identity. Of the original volume, in excess of 170

L per 24 h in a normal adult, less than 1.5 L of urine will ordinarily remain at the end of the collecting ducts. Of 1100 g of sodium chloride that is filtered, less than 10 g will generally remain in the final urine, and of the approximately 400 g of sodium bicarbonate filtered, only trace amounts will be excreted. Similarly, virtually all the filtered glucose and amino acids will be resorbed, 85 to 95 percent of the filtered phosphate will be resorbed, and varying (but substantial) fractions of many other filtered solutes will be removed from the tubular fluid. On the other hand, certain substances such as ammonia, hydrogen ions, potassium ions, and urate will be added to the tubular fluid as it moves from glomerulus to renal papilla.

The fact that filtration is a nonselective process and that the volume of glomerular filtrate is so large in relation to the volume of the final urine demands that the single layer of epithelial cells lining the tubules perform a large number of highly complex functions simultaneously. Not only must there be a high degree of discrimination in regulating the individual rates of excretion of a number of different substances but the various transport processes must allow for changes in the movement of one substance without disturbing the regulated patterns of excretion of all other substances. Before considering the manner in which tubular transport of specific solutes is regulated, the general types of transport mechanisms available to the epithelial cells, as well as the nature of the epithelial cell per se, will be discussed briefly.

TUBULAR EPITHELIAL CELLS

Two contiguous renal tubular epithelial cells are depicted schematically in Fig. 7-3. In each cell a large body of cytoplasm is shown surrounded by a very thin external plasma membrane. Within the cytoplasm, only the intracellular fluid and mitochondria are shown. The nucleus and the other subcellular units have been omitted. The cytoplasm of the epithelial cell, in common with that of other living cells, has a low concentration of sodium and a high concentration of potassium. It must maintain these relationships despite the fact

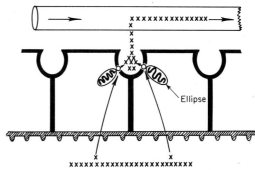

Figure 7-3. Schematic drawing of two contiguous epithelial cells from the proximal tubule. The x's represent sodium ions in the tubular fluid which enter the tubular epithelial cells across the luminal plasma membrane. The circles with the attached arrows depict the sodium pumps in the intercellular region of the plasma membrane. The ellipse on either side of the intercellular space represents a mitochondrion. The cylinder at the top of the diagram depicts a peritubular capillary. The plasma membrane is depicted differently at the luminal than at the intercellular and peritubular capillary surfaces for reasons which are discussed in the text.

that the surrounding extracellular fluid is sodium-rich and potassium-poor and that there is constant traffic of substantial quantities of both sodium and potassium through the cell water. The plasma membrane, though anatomically a continuous structure, is depicted differently at the surface of the cell facing the tubular lumen (from which microvilli project) than at the lateral and peritubular capillary surfaces. This is to indicate that the functional properties of the different segments of the membrane may differ. At the junction of the two cells, there is a lateral intercellular space (16). There is a good possibility that a significant part of the sodium transported by the epithelial cells may be deposited within this space before it enters the peritubular capillaries.

The mitochondrion is the cell's energy transducer. Substrates of the Krebs cycle are oxidized, and their electrons are transferred through the electron transport chain of the mitochondria to molecular oxygen. The energy derived from this electron transport system is diverted into the structure of adenosine triphosphate (ATP). The ATP, in turn, yields its energy to the various cellular processes that are energy-requiring, and the most important of these from a quantitative point of view in the renal tubule is the transport of sodium ions across the lateral and peritubular capillary plasma membranes. Thus, the location of the mitochondria in juxtaposition to the transporting segment of the plasma membrane should simplify the transfer of energy to the membrane for the active transport of sodium ions in a manner which will be discussed subsequently.

THE PLASMA MEMBRANE

The plasma membrane is an extremely thin structure, less than 100 Å in thickness, which is rich in lipids but also contains protein. Although a number of new and more sophisticated models of the plasma membrane have been proposed, the classic Davson-Danielli model still provides a conceptual framework for describing transmembrane movements of solutes and water. The membrane is depicted as consisting of two layers of lipid molecules covered on each side with a layer of protein (see Fig. 7-4) (17). Within the structure of the lipoprotein membrane are a series of hypothetical pores which are believed by many observers to constitute water-filled channels through which certain solutes and water may cross the membrane. Within the matrix of the membrane there must also exist a group of constituent molecules, probably low-molecular-weight proteins, which serve as the "carriers" or "receptors" in the transport systems for various solutes. The ATPase system (an enzyme or a group of enzymes that hydrolyze ATP and effect the transfer of the energy from ATP to the carrier molecules) also resides either within or very close to the plasma membrane. Indeed there is a substantial body of opinion which holds that the ATPase enzyme system and the carrier, at least for sodium, are one and the same.

The plasma membrane serves as a barrier to the movement of all particles, both charged and uncharged, between the cell interior and the fluid surrounding the cell. The degree of resistance to movement varies considerably for different particles, but because of its lipid matrix the plasma membrane tends to be quite permeable to lipid-soluble substances, which dissolve in the membrane as they pass through it. There is also a high

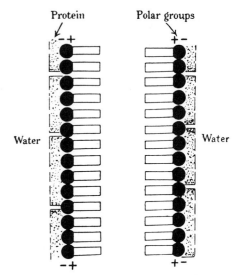

Figure 7-4. The Davson-Danielli model of the plasma membrane. The clear rectangles with black globular ends are lipid molecules. The hydrophilic ends (globules) of the lipid molecules face a layer of protein molecules (the shaded rectangles oriented in a longitudinal direction are the protein molecules); and the hydrophobic tails (clear rectangles) of the lipid molecules face each other. The protein molecules face the ICF at one border of the plasma membrane and the ECF at the other border. The entire structure is approximately 90 to 100 Å in thickness.

degree of permeability to water and to urea molecules, because they are presumed to move through the water-filled pores. It is generally believed that the *passive* movement of other low-molecular-weight lipid-insoluble substances across the membrane also occurs through these pores. The freedom with which these movements take place within the membrane must be influenced by the diameter of the pores; by the dimensions, electric charge, and other physical properties of the transported species; and, for ions, by any charge along the length of the pore channels. The actual rate at which a substance passes through a membrane depends upon the balance between the factors responsible for the movement (such as the chemical and electrochemical concentration gradients) and the factors impeding the movement (such as the permeability or conductance of the membrane for the species involved) (18).

A final mechanism of transmembrane movement of solutes is through pinocytosis (18).

THE MECHANISMS OF TRANSPORT

Although a detailed discussion of transport mechanisms may be found in Chap. 1, a brief description of these processes is indicated. Transport across the plasma membrane traditionally is classified as active or passive depending upon whether energy from cellular metabolism is involved.

Passive transport

The transport of a substance across a plasma membrane is termed *passive* if it can be accounted for entirely on the basis of physical forces and does not involve the direct utilization of metabolic energy from the cell in which the transport occurs. The two principal forces involved in passive transport are the chemical concentration gradient and the electric potential gradient. The latter is involved only in the movement of charged particles. In addition, the movement of water through a pore will influence the associated movement of solutes within the same pore through the mechanisms of solvent drag and bulk flow.

Chemical concentration gradient. When a solute exists in the fluid compartments in contact with both sides of a permeable membrane, the solute will move across the membrane in both directions. However, if there is a greater concentration of the solute on one side of the membrane than on the other, the rate of collision of particles with the membrane will be greater on that side; thus the movement of particles from the side of high concentration to that of low concentration will exceed the simultaneous movement in the opposite direction.

Electric potential gradient. When there is an electric potential gradient across a membrane, such that one surface is electrically positive to the other, the electric field will influence the movement of all charged particles. Anions will tend to move toward the side where positive charges pre-

dominate, and cations will move preferentially in the opposite direction. For all ions in solution, therefore, the direction of passive movement will depend upon the combined effect of the chemical concentration gradient and the electric potential gradient. For uncharged solutes only the chemical concentration gradient is involved.

Solvent drag effect and bulk flow. Solvent drag ordinarily plays a limited role in the movement of solutes across biologic membranes. The drag effect may be described as follows: As water molecules move through a pore in a lipid membrane, they will exert a frictional force on all solute particles simultaneously in transit in the same pore. The effect will be to accelerate the movement of particles migrating in the same direction as the water and to impede the movement of particles migrating in the opposite direction.

If the pores are sufficiently large to allow for groups of water molecules to exist simultaneously, any force (e.g., osmotic or hydrostatic) which favors the flow of water across the membrane will result in movement of "solution" such that the water molecules in transit will carry with them the solutes dissolved in the water in the parent solution. Bulk flow could represent an important mechanism in the transfer of solutes and water out of the proximal tubule.

Active transport

Active transport of a solute particle across a membrane implies that the movement cannot be accounted for by physical forces alone. Thus, the transport cannot be explained on the basis of the combined effects of the chemical concentration gradient, the electric potential gradient, solvent drag, and bulk flow. Active transport, therefore, usually takes place "uphill" in a thermodynamic sense, and a source of energy must be made available to make the system go. The energy is derived from metabolism of the epithelial cells which are engaged in the active transport. According to one prevailing concept, a solute species which is actively transported enters into chemical combination with a constituent of the cell membrane termed the *carrier*. Carrier molecules, as previously suggested, may be low-molecular-weight proteins. The solute-carrier complex moves across the finite distance of the membrane and then dissociates, releasing the transported species. The energy from metabolism is delivered to the carrier-solute complex either from the high-energy phosphate bond of ATP or from a phosphorylated high-energy intermediate compound which is in equilibrium with ATP. When a high-energy phosphate bond is utilized in transport, its replenishment is necessary and occurs primarily via the oxidation of metabolic substrates. A substantial portion of the total oxygen consumed by the kidney and of the total substrate utilized is directed to the transport of a single ion, sodium.

Because the resorption of sodium is the principal energy-consuming process in the renal tubular epithelial cells and because sodium transport per se may influence the movements of water, urea, hydrogen, potassium, etc., the mechanisms of sodium excretion, which are also discussed in detail in Chap. 3, will be considered here.

RENAL EXCRETION OF SODIUM

THE BIOLOGY OF SODIUM EXCRETION

When a normal person subsists on a salt-free diet, the urine is excreted essentially free of sodium ions. Even when the salt intake is as much as 25 g/day, external sodium balance may be maintained by the excretion of less than 2 percent of the filtered sodium. Thus, with a normal number of functioning nephrons under all but the most unusual circumstances, in excess of 98 out of every 100 filtered sodium ions must be resorbed by the tubular epithelial cells. The process of transporting a sodium ion across the epithelial cell of the proximal tubule involves several interrelated steps. These are depicted schematically in Fig. 7-5. Sodium ions are thought to enter the cell across the luminal plasma membrane, either by moving passively down an electrochemical gradient through water-filled pores in the membrane or by combining with carriers. Once within the cytoplasm, sodium diffuses across the cell through the cell water, and this process is thought

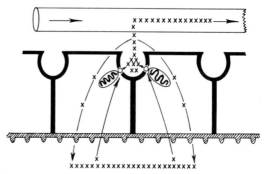

Figure 7-5. Schematic representation of two contiguous epithelial cells transporting sodium ions. The general details of the drawing are the same as those shown in Fig. 7-3. The x's again represent sodium ions which enter the cell across the luminal border, diffuse across the cells, and are transported via a carrier-mediated active transport system across the intercellular border into an intercellular space. Sodium ions then either diffuse into the peritubular capillary, where they are returned to the systemic circulation, or they leak back across the plasma membrane, into the cell interior, and back into the tubular fluid from which they originated.

to be passive in nature. It is not clear whether a sodium ion in transit enters a large pool of intracellular sodium or whether the "transportable pool" of sodium is small and compartmentalized in narrow intracellular channels. The movement across the lateral or peritubular capillary membranes is uphill thermodynamically and thus requires the input of energy from cellular metabolism.

Once a sodium ion has crossed the lateral (or contraluminal) membrane, it still must be transferred into the peritubular capillary plasma before resorption is complete. There is a growing belief that the great majority of sodium ions which are moved across the tubular epithelial cells may be deposited, not in the interstitial fluid between the contraluminal membrane and the peritubular capillary, but rather in intercellular spaces such as are depicted in Fig. 7-5. If this does in fact occur, sodium ions might accumulate in high concentration in the intercellular spaces. Two fates would then be open to any individual sodium ion: first, it could move from the microcosm of high sodium activity into the peritubular capillary plasma with the resorbed water. Thus its reclamation will have been completed. Second, it might leak back across the lateral plasma membrane, through the cytoplasm, through the luminal membrane, and back into the tubular fluid from which it originated.

A backleak of sodium does occur, and the magnitude of the leak would determine the net efficiency of the sodium resorptive process; for the greater the magnitude of the backleak, the greater would be the total number of sodium ions which must be actively pumped to achieve a given rate of *net* resorption. The major factor determining the direction in which a sodium ion will move after it is transported into the intercellular space may well be physical in nature, for the movement into the peritubular capillaries presumably involves no carrier mechanism and is governed by the same forces that influence distribution of fluid across other capillaries. An increase in hydrostatic pressure within the capillary would serve to retard the entry of water and sodium ions into the capillary lumen, and the plasma protein concentration in the peritubular capillary plasma would represent a second force influencing the direction and rate of passive sodium movements. Because of the unique arrangement of the circulation in the kidney, a change in the fraction of the renal plasma flow which is filtered across the glomeruli will produce a corresponding change in peritubular plasma protein concentration and thus in oncotic pressure. If filtration fraction (the ratio of the GFR to renal plasma flow) diminishes so that a smaller percentage of renal plasma flow is filtered, the protein molecules (which are virtually all nonfilterable) will enter the postglomerular capillaries in a larger volume of plasma. Thus oncotic pressure will decrease, and the forces favoring sodium and water entry into the capillaries will diminish. Conversely, an increase in filtration fraction would tend to promote the movement of sodium ions into the peritubular capillaries and thereby facilitate sodium resorption. Another factor, one of lesser importance, which might theoretically influence the movement of sodium ions from intercellular spaces to capillaries, would be the volume of interstitial fluid through which the ions must diffuse. An increase in this volume would create an increase in path length and thus might serve to facilitate reentry

of the sodium ions into the epithelial cells and to increase the backleak. A decrease in interstitial fluid volume such as might obtain with either a reduction in capillary hydrostatic pressure or an increase in peritubular capillary oncotic pressure should facilitate entry of the sodium ions into the capillary lumen.

It has been suggested that in addition to the mechanism responsible for the transcellular transport of sodium, there is a second "neutral" sodium pump located in the peritubular plasma membrane (19). The latter is believed to be a sodium-potassium exchange pump that serves to maintain the constancy of intracellular sodium and potassium concentrations and of cell volume (19). Figure 7-6 is a schematic depiction of both theoretical sodium pumps.

The resorption of positively charged sodium ions requires that an equivalent number of negatively charged ions accompany the sodium or that the difference between sodium ions and anions be compensated for by the movement into the tubular fluid of cations. Electric neutrality is satisfied by both mechanisms. Sodium resorption is accompanied by the concomitant resorption of anions (principally chloride), and a portion of the

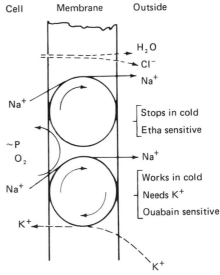

Figure 7-6. Schematic characterization of the two modes of Na extrusion. (*From G. Whittenbury, Pflügers Arch., 316:1, 1970.*)

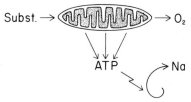

Figure 7-7. Schematic drawing of a mitochondrion (shown in the ellipse). A substrate of the Krebs cycle is oxidized, and the electrons are transported through the electron transport chain and ultimately are received by oxygen. At three points in the electron transport process energy is conserved. The energy from the electrons is transmitted through a series of high-energy intermediate compounds to adenosine triphosphate (ATP). ATP, or an intermediate in equilibrium with the ATP, serves as the definitive source of energy for the sodium pump.

resorbed sodium is attended by the secretion of both hydrogen (throughout the nephron) and potassium (primarily in the distal nephron).

THE ENERGETICS OF SODIUM TRANSPORT

In Fig. 7-7 a mitochondrion is shown synthesizing ATP. As electrons are transferred from a substrate through the electron transport chain of the mitochondrion to molecular oxygen, energy is conserved at three points. At each of these energy conservation sites, finite quantities of energy are trapped and transferred through a series of intermediate compounds. The last step in this sequence involves the addition of a high-energy phosphate bond to adenosine diphosphate (ADP), forming ATP. Either ATP per se or some high-energy intermediate molecule derived from ATP serves as the source of free energy for sodium transport. It is both of interest and of considerable importance that a stoichiometric relationship exists between net sodium transport and oxygen consumption of the kidney. (With a normal rate of sodium resorption of approximately 14.5 meq/min, the minimal energy expenditure is 14 cal/min, or about 1 cal/meq of Na^+.) This stoichiometry reveals that the more sodium that is transported, the more ATP is utilized. The replenishment of the ATP stores requires an increase in metabolism and thus in oxygen consumption (see Fig. 7-7). Therefore, not only is sodium transport

one of the key energy-consuming processes of the renal tubular epithelial cells but it serves as a major determinant of the overall rate of epithelial cell metabolism.

CONTRIBUTIONS OF VARIOUS SEGMENTS OF THE NEPHRON TO SALT AND WATER RESORPTION

The total amount of sodium which enters the nephrons in a 24-h period in a normal adult approximates 24,000 meq. About 75 percent of this amount (roughly 18,000 meq) is resorbed in the proximal tubules. The majority of the sodium ions that are resorbed proximally are accompanied by chloride ions; however, somewhat over 4000 resorbed sodium ions are attended by the inward movement (i.e., secretion) of hydrogen ions.[2] The secreted hydrogen ions combine with the filtered bicarbonate which is present in the tubular fluid, converting it to carbonic acid, which in turn is dehydrated to carbon dioxide and water. Thus the hydrogen ion entry operationally results in the resorption of bicarbonate[3] (see Chap. 6).

The proximal tubule is highly permeable to water, and as solute is resorbed, water moves across passively in isosmotic quantities. Thus approximately 75 percent of the filtered water also is resorbed by the end of the proximal tubule. At the last accessible portion of the proximal tubule (i.e., the last segment of the proximal tubule that is accessible to micropuncture), not only is the tubular fluid greatly reduced in volume but it remains isosmotic.

Structurally, the proximal tubule seems ideally designed for the resorption of large quantities of

[2] This calculation assumes that 80 percent of the filtered bicarbonate is reabsorbed in the proximal tubule and that all bicarbonate resorption takes place by hydrogen ion secretion; if bicarbonate is resorbed as an ion, the calculations are in excess of the true number.

[3] The actual bicarbonate that returns to the peritubular capillary fluid is not the filtered bicarbonate which, as indicated, is decomposed to carbon dioxide and water. Rather the bicarbonate ion left behind in the renal tubular epithelial cell when the hydrogen ion was secreted (both having arisen from intracellular carbonic acid) moves across the contraluminal or lateral membrane and constitutes the resorbed ion. This will be discussed in greater detail later in the chapter.

salt and water. The luminal border of the tubular epithelial cells is characterized by innumerable microvilli which protrude into the tubular lumen. The existence of these invaginations provide an extremely large surface area with which sodium ions may collide and begin their traffic across the cell.

Evidence would indicate that net sodium resorption does not occur in the descending limb of the loop of Henle; indeed, as will be indicated in the discussion of the concentrating mechanism, sodium ions may actually reenter the tubular fluid in the thin descending limb from the medullary interstitial fluid. As the tubular fluid passes the hairpin turn of the loop and enters the ascending limb of the loop of Henle, net resorption of sodium chloride resumes. It has become evident in recent years that it is the chloride ion rather than sodium that is actively transported by the thick ascending limb (20). The resorption of sodium appears to be largely if not completely passive. The NaCl that is resorbed by the ascending limb is transported into the medullary interstitial fluid and serves as the principal osmotic force allowing for the subsequent removal of water from the collecting ducts in the concentrating process (see Chap. 12). The ascending limb apparently is relatively watertight, so that the removal of solute occurs without the simultaneous diffusion of water molecules. Consequently, the urine entering the early distal tubule is hypoosmotic.

The patterns of distal tubular behavior in the human kidney are unknown. It was previously believed, on the basis of micropuncture studies in the rat, that, in addition to sodium resorption in the distal tubule under the influence of ADH, water moved out of the distal tubular fluid into the cortical interstitium until the fluid became isosmotic. However, recent micropuncture studies in the dog (21) and monkey (22) failed to confirm this pattern. Rather, the distal tubule appeared to behave more as an inert conduit than as an equilibrating segment for water. The fluid leaving the distal tubule, which we will presume hereafter to be hypoosmotic in man, enters the collecting duct where additional sodium is resorbed and where variable quantities of water are resorbed. Water movements across the collecting duct epithelia take place from the tubular fluid into the medullary interstitial fluid. The driving force for this movement is the osmotic gradient created by the previous resorption of sodium by the ascending limb of the loop of Henle. The permeability of the collecting duct to water is influenced greatly by the ADH; when ADH activity is maximal, water will be resorbed in the collecting ducts until the urine approaches osmotic equilibrium with the hyperosmotic medullary interstitium. On the other hand, in the absence of ADH a small proportion of the water reaching the collecting duct will be resorbed, and the urine will be excreted as a very dilute solution. With intermediate concentrations of ADH the osmolality of the final urine will vary between markedly dilute and maximally concentrated.

GLOMERULAR-TUBULAR BALANCE

We have already emphasized that the amount of sodium filtered greatly exceeds the amount excreted under normal conditions of living. We also have noted that small changes in the GFR could prove very disruptive to the maintenance of sodium balance if tubular resorption remained fixed. (For example, if the GFR increased by 2 ml/min and none of the extra filtered sodium were resorbed, NaCl excretion would increase by almost 24 g/day.) The term *glomerular-tubular balance* (see Chap. 3) describes a phenomenon that is very important biologically and is of considerable interest scientifically. The term implies that proximal tubular resorption of sodium (and water) changes in parallel with changes in the GFR so as to maintain the percentage of the filtrate resorbed relatively constant. A constant *fraction* of the filtered sodium (and water) thus continues to be resorbed in the proximal tubule despite increases or decreases in the GFR. This property of the proximal tubule prevents large changes in sodium delivery out of the proximal tubule from occurring with spontaneous changes in the GFR. Hence, glomerular-tubular balance may be viewed as a buffering device that protects against potentially harmful and undesirable changes in sodium excretion. But it does not seem to affect the fine adjustments in sodium excretion necessary for the maintenance of sodium balance.

The characteristics and mechanism of glomerular-tubular balance have come under intense scrutiny in recent years, and a summary of the pertinent data follows.

The evidence for glomerular-tubular balance

The existence of glomerular-tubular balance was suggested a number of years ago by Wesson, Anslow, and Smith on the basis of clearance data in dogs undergoing massive osmotic diuresis (24). These investigators postulated that when a change in the GFR occurred, proximal tubular resorption adjusted so as to accommodate approximately two-thirds of the change in the filtered load of sodium. This assessment has now been confirmed and amplified by micropuncture studies. Micropuncture experiments have shown that approximately the same percentage of filtrate is resorbed at a given point in the nephron before and after experimental reduction of the GFR by means of constricting the aorta between the renal arteries or constricting a renal artery per se. Fractional resorption, moreover, tends to remain the same when the GFR rises to its previous level after release of the constriction.

The basis of glomerular-tubular balance

The manner in which proximal tubular sodium resorption changes with changes in the GFR so as to keep the proportion of filtered sodium resorbed relatively constant is unknown. The theories that have been proposed, however, are almost as ingenious as the phenomenon itself and merit brief consideration.

Geometry theory. The geometry theory suggests that the changes in sodium resorption that accompany changes in the GFR relate to the altered geometry of the tubular lumen initiated by an increase in tubular volume (or tubular radius) (25). In essence, an increase in the GFR would increase the volume of fluid in the proximal tubule; this would stretch the luminal surface of the tubular wall, increasing the surface area available for penetration by sodium ions and thereby allowing an increase in the rate of resorption of sodium. On a priori grounds, this theory must be held suspect, since the luminal border in reality consists of myriads of microvilli projecting into the tubular lumen rather than a smoothly lined cylinder. Increasing the volume of the tubule, therefore, would not necessarily increase the surface area available for sodium resorption; it might simply change the direction of projection of the microvilli.

The evidence for the geometry theory stems from the fact that the so-called intrinsic resorption capacity of the tubule, designated C, was initially found by Gertz et al. (26, 27) to vary directly with the volume of the tubular fluid or with r^2, the square of the radius.[4] This relationship was also observed by Rector, Brunner, and Seldin (28) and Landwehr, Klose, and Giebisch (29). However, there are now several sets of data that open the geometry theory to serious question. One fundamental requisite for the geometry theory is that the volume of the proximal tubule must vary with the GFR, for resorption varies with the GFR. There are conflicting data regarding this matter. Rector et al. found the required relationship when the GFR was diminished by constricting the aorta of rats (28). On the other hand, Baines, Leyssac, and Gottschalk were unable to confirm this relationship (32). More difficult for the geometry theory is the fact that the ratio $C/\pi\tau^2$ has been found not to remain constant under at least three different experimental conditions. The first of these involves raising ureteral pressure and thereby increasing proximal tubular volume (31). The ratio $C/\pi\tau^2$ has also been found to change when τ^2 (i.e., tubular volume) is changed by renal venous constriction (33). Finally, a dissociation between C and τ^2 has been demonstrated when blood pressure is increased by bilateral carotid artery constriction (34). Thus the case against "geometry" seems strong, and at the very least the theory cannot be accepted as fact at this time.

A hormonal feedback loop. The second generic explanation for the maintenance of glomerular-tubular balance involves a humoral mediator which would be released with spontaneous changes in either the GFR or proximal tubular sodium resorption and which would tend to restore the status of glomerular-tubular balance to-

---

[4] The intrinsic resorptive capacity represents the rate of tubular fluid resorbed per unit length of tubule.

ward its initial level. Thurau and Schnermann (14) proposed the following mechanism: With a spontaneous change in the GFR, the composition of the tubular fluid reaching the macula densa in the wall of the distal tubule would change. The cells of the macula densa would serve as sensor elements. These cells are always exposed to hypotonic fluid delivered from the ascending limb of the loop of Henle. With a change in the GFR, the amount and/or the concentration of sodium reaching the early distal tubule would change, and this would lead to an alteration in the rate of renin release by the juxtamedullary cells which reside in the wall of the afferent arteriole contiguous with the macula densa. The renin would increase the local concentration of angiotensin, and this in turn would influence the GFR through its vasoactive effect on the afferent arteriole. According to this hypothesis, an increase in tubular fluid sodium (concentration or mass) would lead to an increased rate of renin release, an increase in angiotensin activity, and a decrease in the GFR in that nephron. A decrease in delivery of sodium to the macula densa would result in a reduction in renin release and a subsequent rise in the GFR.

The second type of feedback loop was proposed by Leyssac (30). Leyssac suggested that if proximal intratubular pressure decreases (as might occur with a primary increase in sodium resorption), a change would occur at the level of the macula densa, renin would be released, and angiotensin would be liberated and would reach the proximal tubular epithelial cells. According to Leyssac, the angiotensin would inhibit proximal tubular sodium resorption, thereby restoring intratubular volume and pressure toward its original level. If primary changes in proximal tubular pressure lead to corresponding changes in the GFR, this mechanism might serve not only to control the constancy of proximal tubular sodium resorption but to prevent changes in the GFR. Thus it could explain the phenomenon of glomerular-tubular balance.

Any theory that involves a sensing role by the macula densa and the subsequent release of renin and modulation of local concentrations of angiotensin must satisfy one important condition: If the GFR changes, there must be a finite period of time during which resorption of sodium will proceed at its original rate, and thus glomerular-tubular balance will be disturbed. The restoration would occur only after the change had been detected and sufficient time had elapsed for a hormone to be released and to effect an end-organ alteration. In order to determine whether there is a period of time during which glomerular-tubular balance is disturbed, Brenner, Bennett, and Berliner (31) measured fractional water resorption in individual rat tubules using micropuncture techniques before, immediately after, and from 5 to 30 min after constricting the aorta and thus reducing the GFR. In collections obtained as soon as 15 to 45 s after initiating a decrease in the GFR, no disruption of glomerular-tubular balance was observed. These data, thus, do not support the view that a humoral feedback mechanism is primarily responsible for the maintenance of glomerular-tubular balance.

The phenomenon of glomerular-tubular balance is seen in whole kidneys and in single nephrons studied in situ. The balance, however, does not exist in single isolated perfused proximal tubules studied in vitro (35). It thus seems most likely that glomerular-tubular balance is explained by the same "physical factors" that were described in the discussion of proximal tubular sodium resorption. A decrease in filtration rate will reduce the degree to which colloid osmotic pressure rises in the glomerular capillaries. Peritubular capillary oncotic pressure will therefore diminish, and this decrease will result in a reduction in salt and water resorption in the proximal tubule (36). An increase in the glomerular filtration rate should have the opposite effect.

The control system governing sodium excretion. A control system for the regulation of sodium balance, as indicated in the introductory section, must be concerned with the regulation of the extracellular fluid volume. Sodium is the principal cation of ECF and with its two major anions, chloride and bicarbonate, contributes well over 90 percent of the total pool of solute particles. On the other hand, ICF sodium concentration is very low in most cell types. Therefore, when sodium is added to body fluids, it will remain almost entirely within the extracellular compartment. The addition of sodium ions will serve transiently to increase the osmotic pressure of ECF, and water will move out of the cells into the extracellular space. The rise in osmolality of the ECF produced by the added sodium chloride will initiate an increase in the rate of release of ADH, and more water will be resorbed from the collecting ducts. In some instances, the thirst mechanism may be activated, and water intake will increase. A primary increase in sodium mass, therefore, will promote an expansion of ECF volume. Conversely, a decrease in sodium mass will initiate a corresponding decrease in ECF volume.

The complexities of regulating the excretion rate of sodium make it extremely unlikely that the mechanisms of control reside entirely within the nephron. Rather, it seems essential that a biologic control system exists that has the general design shown in Fig. 7-8. The component parts of the system are three:

1. *The detector element.* Detector elements presumably monitor some function of volume rather than the mass of sodium or the concentration of sodium. But the location and the precise nature of the detector elements remain unknown. Most of the existing data would be explained if the detector element sensed "effective" arterial blood volume (37, 38). The receptors might detect the degree of stretch or some properties of the transmural pressure gradient neither in arterial walls nor in the chambers of the heart.
2. *The integrating element.* Judging from other regulatory systems, there may be numerous volume stimuli arising simultaneously from different parts of the body. Some could be of an excitatory nature, others of an inhibitory nature. All presumably would be channeled

into the central nervous system, and the summation of the stimuli would be transmitted to the effector system.
3. *The effector element.* The effector element includes the nephron, which is the end organ, a transmission system through which information is conveyed to the nephron, and one or more mechanisms for modifying sodium resorption.

MODULATORS OF SODIUM EXCRETION

If one were to design a mechanism for modulating a function as important as the regulation of sodium excretion, it is unlikely that the control apparatus would include only a single effector device. Rather, there would be several regulators, each of which could, if the situation dictated, take over as the definitive mechanism but would, under normal operating conditions, serve in a supportive role, One of the regulators, however, would be designed as the "fine dial," which could modify sodium excretion by effecting small changes in the percentage of filtered sodium ions resorbed. Evidence now emerging suggests that the actual control system for sodium does include multiple effector components, but information about the hierarchy of these components (in terms of their relative roles) under normal conditions is controversial. Several of the proposed regulatory mechanisms will be described. These include changes in the GFR and a subset of this mechanism, which involves redistribution of glomerular filtrate between cortical and juxtamedullary nephrons; changes in aldosterone activity; changes in intrarenal "physical factors" (e.g., peritubular capillary hydrostatic pressure and oncotic pressure); changes in nerve stimulation; and changes in the activity of a natriuretic hormone. The information is evolving so rapidly and from so many different laboratories that the true role of, and interplay between, these various factors may well be revealed within the near future.

Changes in glomerular filtration rate

Because normally only a small percentage of the filtered sodium is excreted (and because changes

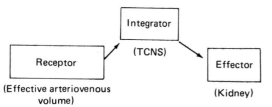

Figure 7-8. Biologic control system for the regulation of external sodium balance. (*From N. S. Bricker, et al., Yale J. Biol. Med.,* **48:**293, 1975.)

in the GFR are attended by proportional changes in proximal tubular resorption that minimize "downstream" sodium delivery and thus changes in sodium excretion) controlled changes in the GFR could in theory initiate changes in sodium excretion with sufficient precision to satisfy the requirements for balance imposed by the normal daily variation in salt intake (39, 40, 41). Two considerations, however, make it unlikely that changes in the GFR could effect very small and highly precise alterations in sodium excretion. The first of these is that the GFR, as described above, is determined to a substantial degree by pressure differences across a filtering membrane. To change sodium excretion by 1 sodium ion out of 400 or 500 filtered sodium ions thus would require extraordinarily small but extraordinarily precise modifications in one of the physical determinants of glomerular filtration. That this might occur in response to small changes in dietary salt intake cannot be ruled out, but there exists no precedent for it. The second a priori consideration that weighs against the GFR as the fine modulator has already been discussed. If GFR changes are used to alter sodium excretion, all other filtered solutes would be delivered in greater or lesser amounts as the filtered load of sodium changed; hence the resorption of many other solutes, the excretion rates of which are carefully regulated, would have to change every time the dictates of sodium balance required an alteration in the filtered load of sodium.

A third consideration that would seem to weigh against the GFR as the fine modulator of sodium excretion is the fact that sodium modulation can continue in the absence of regulation of the GFR. Thus, when changes in the GFR are prevented by putting a band around the aorta, sodium excretion may increase appropriately as the intake of sodium increases either acutely or chronically (42).

Redistribution of glomerular filtrate

Recent studies by Barger and colleagues (43, 44) have raised the possibility that an increase or decrease in sodium excretion may be accompanied by redistribution of glomerular filtrate between the cortical and juxtamedullary nephrons. In the-

ory, the cortical nephrons should be oriented functionally more toward the excretion of sodium than are the juxtamedullary units because the latter have longer proximal tubules and longer ascending limbs of the loops of Henle. Thus overall glomerular-tubular balance for the cortical glomeruli should be weighted in the direction of glomerular preponderance, whereas the opposite relationship would obtain for the deep units. Thorburn et al. (45) have demonstrated changes in regional blood flow using radioactive krypton washout curves; they have also shown redistribution of blood flow between cortex and outer medulla using radioautography of "snap frozen" kidneys and perfusion of the renal vasculature with plastic materials (43). There is also some direct evidence for a disproportionate increase in filtration in superficial nephrons during both acute (46, 47) and chronic (48) volume expansion. However, there is opposing evidence about redistribution both of plasma flow and of filtrate using radioactive microspheres (49) or antiglomerular basement membrane (50). Thus with these techniques, it has been shown that deep rather than superficial flow increases disproportionately during volume expansion. Further, recent micropuncture studies in rats and dogs have shown that filtration in superficial nephrons does not increase out of proportion to the total GFR during acute saline loading (51, 52, 53). We feel that very precise control of sodium excretion rates would be as difficult to obtain with "redistribution" of glomerular filtrate (or renal plasma flow) between two groups of nephrons as with changes in the total GFR; thus we would favor the view that this mechanism may play a supportive role in the regulatory system but does not serve as the fine regulatory device.

Changes in aldosterone activity

Aldosterone changes the capacity of epithelial cells to transport sodium. It does so by increasing the rate of entry of sodium ions across the luminal plasma membrane into the "transportable pool of sodium ions" (54) and/or by inducing the synthesis of new protein involved in the energy-producing reactions which provide ATP for the active transport of sodium ions (55). Aldosterone is present in body fluids normally, and the rate of secretion increases in many salt-retaining states. Conversely, in the absence of mineralocorticoid hormone, salt losing occurs. Thus, aldosterone is closely linked to the regulation of sodium excretion, and until recently it was widely held that aldosterone is the principal regulator of sodium balance. This view requires reappraisal.

The evidence challenging the role of aldosterone as the fine regulator of sodium excretion is substantial. Two of the major categories of information will be cited. Continued high dosage of aldosterone will lead to sodium retention for only a short period of time, after which the so-called escape phenomenon occurs. Escape is characterized by a spontaneous restoration of the capacity to maintain salt and water balance albeit with a somewhat expanded ECF volume. Clinically, salt and water balance are maintained in patients with aldosterone-secreting tumors. At the other extreme is the well-known clinical observation that patients with Addison's disease given a fixed dose of mineralocorticoid hormone are capable of maintaining salt balance despite normal variations in dietary salt intake. Thus sodium regulation can occur in the absence of changes in aldosterone activity. While this does not necessarily mean that the regulatory system *normally* utilizes a mechanism other than aldosterone for effecting fine modulation, it would tend to favor such a conclusion. At this point, therefore, we would suggest that aldosterone activity conditions the capacity of the epithelial cells to transport sodium but that some other factor serves as the fine regulator.

The "third factor"

That some factor or factors other than changes in the GFR and in aldosterone activity influence sodium excretion was demonstrated convincingly by De Wardener et al. in 1961 (56, 57). In dogs maintained on high levels of mineralocorticoid hormones (thereby excluding mineralocorticoid insufficiency, or changes in mineralocorticoid hormone activity), IV salt loading resulted in a marked increase in sodium excretion. It was possible to elicit this natriuretic effect of saline in-

fusion even though the GFR did not increase. Thus some factor other than a reduction in mineralocorticoid hormone activity and an increase in the GFR was instrumental in promoting an increase in sodium excretion. The mediator has been referred to descriptively as "third factor." A number of observers favor the view that third factor is a natriuretic hormone, but there is also evidence that physical factors within the renal parenchyma may influence sodium excretion. It is possible that third factor may actually consist of more than one regulatory factor.

Intrarenal "physical factors." The possible role of hydrostatic pressure and plasma oncotic pressure in the peritubular capillaries on transepithelial movement of sodium has already been described. A decrease in intratubular hydrostatic pressure or an increase in peritubular capillary oncotic pressure would facilitate the movement of sodium ions from the interstitial fluid into the capillary plasma. This in turn could lead to a decrease in the backleak of sodium and hence to an increase in net sodium resorption. It also is theoretically possible that, by accelerating the removal of sodium ions sequestered in intracellular spaces, the active transport of sodium might be influenced directly by mechanisms that are now obscure. (58). A series of studies reported by Earley and colleagues (59–61) have demonstrated that during salt loading changes do occur in physical factors within the kidneys. Moreover, Spitzer and Windhager (62) and Brenner and associates (63) have shown that changes in peritubular capillary oncotic pressure induced by infusing varying concentrations of dextran into an efferent arteriole or albumin intra-aortically alter sodium transport in individual nephrons. It has also been shown recently that proximal tubular reabsorption of sodium, chloride, and water is partially flow-dependent (64). Thus a role of intrarenal factors in regulation of sodium excretion seems to have been established. What remains to be determined is whether these factors are capable of exercising the type of fine regulation required for the ongoing maintenance of sodium balance. Several situations have been described in which the physical forces seem to go in a direction opposite to that predicted for regulation, but the methods for measuring various physical parameters within the kidney are still too limited to permit final judgment. Our own opinion is that the physical forces may play the prepotent role in regulating sodium excretion under certain adverse or threatening physiologic circumstances, such as massive loading of IV saline solution or severe volume depletion (65), but that under normal conditions changes in physical factors play only a supportive role in regulation.

Renal nerves. It has been known for many years that denervation of the kidney causes sodium excretion to increase (66). Recent anatomic studies have clearly demonstrated adrenergic innervation of rat proximal and distal tubules (67). Subsequent experiments have shown that direct renal stimulation increases tubular sodium reabsorption in the absence of changes in the GFR, renal blood flow (RBF) or intrarenal redistribution of blood flow (68). DiBona et al. have also presented evidence that neither angiotensin II nor prostaglandins play a role in mediating the effects of low-level direct renal nerve stimulation (69). Thus it seems clear that nerve stimulation can change sodium reabsorption. However, it has not been established that renal nerves represent a key element in the efferent limb of the sodium control system.

A natriuretic hormone. The precision with which sodium excretion is regulated has acted as a major stimulus to the continuing search for a rapidly acting regulatory hormone that serves as the definitive modulator of sodium excretion. The evidence for the existence of a natriuretic hormone has grown progressively, yet this evidence remains largely phenomenologic. Since the original paper by de Wardener et al. (56) pointing to the existence of third factors, many scientists throughout the world have attempted to isolate the natriuretic hormone. A few of the pertinent observations follow. Sedlakova and his associates (70) and Buckalew and his associates (71) presented evidence supporting the existence of a dialyzable inhibitor of sodium transport in salt-loaded animals, and Sedlakova and associates (70) developed additional information suggesting that the substance may be a peptide synthesized in the anterior hypothalamus. A low-molecular-weight substance was also found in the plasma of salt-loaded animals which inhibits the uptake of para-aminohippurate (PAH) by rabbit kidney cortical slices (72). Laragh et al. described a nondialyzable factor with a molecular weight as great as 50,000 in blood and urine of sheep and human beings subjected to salt loading. This factor, when injected into rats, produced a striking natriuretic response (73). More recently, a factor with similar biologic characteristics was found in normal dogs in which values for fractional sodium excretion were increased following 4 days of high salt ingestion and administration of a potent mineralocorticoid hormone (74). Using the technique of reinfusing urine, investigators also found evidence for the existence of a potent natriuretic factor whose action is largely independent of change of mineralocorticoid hormones, prostaglandins, urea, or vasopressin (75). The natriuretic factor that has been obtained from normal dogs after "escape" and from uremic dogs and patients has a molecular weight of less than 1000, is inactivated by two different peptidases, is acidic, nonvolatile, and lipid-insoluble. After acid hydrolysis, several acidic amino acids are detectable in the chromatographic fraction or urine that possesses natriuretic activity (76).

There is a long list of well-organized physiologic agents which increase sodium excretion. Among the more possible candidates for a role as natriuretic hormones are the vasodilators, including those made in the kidney (bradykinin and prostaglandins) and other hormones such as vasopressin, oxytocin, PTH, and calcitonin, all of which can increase sodium excretion, at least some by inhibiting tubular sodium reabsorption. It is thus essential to demonstrate that the effects of any incompletely purified new natriuretic hormone extracted from blood or urine were not due to these recognized hormones. Micropuncture studies in salt-loaded rats (77) and dogs (78) have shown that inhibition of sodium resorption occurs in proximal tubules. However, it is not inconceivable that the proximal tubular effect of salt loading relates primarily to physical factors and that the natriuretic hormone which might serve as the final modulator of sodium excretion acts at a more distal site in the nephrons (79).

It is attractive to invoke the existence of a natriuretic hormone which serves as the precise regulator of sodium excretion. The rate of release of the hormone would be tuned to the need for maintaining the constancy of ECF volume, and thus there would normally be a given level of hormone activity under the usual conditions of life and an increased level of hormone activity with increased levels of salt intake. An increase in natriuretic hormone activity could help to explain the escape phenomenon and the continued sodium excretion in the syndrome of inappropriate antidiuretic hormone (ADH) secretion; and inappropriately low levels of natriuretic hormone activity could play a major role in the pathogenesis of some edema-forming states. However, available evidence is too preliminary to permit a definitive assessment of the existence of such a hormone. If there is a natriuretic hormone, its site of synthesis remains unknown, its molecular nature is unknown, and its mechanism of action at the level of the tubular epithelial cells is incompletely understood.

SUMMARY

The regulation of sodium balance and the maintenance of the constancy of ECF volume are intimately related functions. Changes in sodium balance in general lead to corresponding changes in ECF volume, and, conversely, changes in ECF volume exercise a feedback control over the rate of renal excretion of sodium. The rate of acquisition of sodium may vary widely under conditions of normal day-to-day living, and the rate of extrarenal losses of sodium may also vary. Thus the constancy of ECF volume, which is so essential to the maintenance of a normal physiologic state, is continually being threatened. The kidney, which operates as the end organ of the homeostatic control system, must therefore excrete into the urine a precisely regulated amount of sodium. This amount represents the difference between total accession rates and total extrarenal excretion rates. Both the overall control system and the specific determinants of sodium excretion by the kidney represent fascinating and rapidly evolving areas of normal and pathologic physiology.

The control of sodium excretion appears to be too important a process for the well-being of the organism to have only a single regulator, and the efferent limb of the sodium control system presumably involves several factors, including intrarenal physical factors and perhaps a natriuretic hormone. However, one of the control factors must be dominant under the usual conditions of day-to-day living, and, despite the inadequate evidence, we would lean in the direction of a natriuretic hormone serving as the key regulator.

CONCENTRATING AND DILUTING MECHANISMS

THE CONCENTRATING MECHANISM

The ability to excrete a concentrated urine represents a major evolutionary advance which is enjoyed only by mammals and some birds. Mature human beings may concentrate their urine to approximately four times the osmolality of plasma, and thus when water must be conserved, solute may be excreted in a quarter of the volume of water in which it is contained in the plasma. From a physiologic point of view, the elaboration of a concentrated urine means that, in addition to resorbing water together with solute in isosmotic quantities, the nephron is able to abstract pure water without any solutes.

The concentration of urine takes place in the medulla of the kidney. It owes its existence to three anatomic structures and their unique interrelationships. These three medullary structures are the long loops of Henle, the vasa recta capillary loops, and the collecting ducts. The structures lie in close proximity to each other and are surrounded by interstitial fluid, which permits the traffic of solute and water between the component parts.

The fact that loops of Henle are found only in mammals and birds, both of which are able to elaborate concentrated urine, was viewed as early as 1909 by Peter (80) as evidence that this unusual anatomic unit contributes to the concentration of urine. In 1942 Kuhn and Ryffel (81) originated the concept of the countercurrent multiplier system for urine concentration. In 1951 Hargitay and Kuhn (82) reproposed the theory with preliminary experimental evidence for supporting the view that the loops of Henle represent the site of countercurrent multiplication, serving to create a hypertonic interstitial fluid in the inner medulla that in turn serves as the osmotic force for the outward diffusion of water from the collecting ducts.

General properties

In the discussion of salt and water excretion, it was noted that the tubular fluid remains isosmotic throughout the accessible portion of the proximal tubule but becomes dilute by the time it reaches the first portion of the distal tubule accessible to micropuncture. At the bend of the loop of Henle, the tubular fluid is markedly hypertonic. The solutes which account for the rise in osmolality are sodium chloride and urea. Within the ascending limb of the loop of Henle, chloride is actively transported, sodium is passively transported, and both are transferred out of the tubular fluid, without water, into the medullary interstitium. (The movement of urea will be considered separately.)

As the urine courses through the distal tubule, further solutes are removed with or without proportional amounts of water, under the influence of ADH, into the surrounding isosmotic cortical interstitial fluid, so that urine entering the cortical collecting tubule is isosmotic or hypoosmotic to the plasma. The urine then moves through the cortical and into the medullary collecting ducts. Under the influence of the ADH the collecting ducts become freely permeable to water, which moves along the osmotic gradient into the hypertonic medullary interstitium. As water diffuses out of the collecting duct, the urea concentration of the tubular fluid rises, and urea then diffuses into the medullary interstitic fluid, where it ultimately constitutes a substantial part of the total medullary solute content. More will be said of the special role of urea in the concentrating process below. By the end of the papillary collecting duct, osmotic equilibrium is achieved, and the urine attains the same hypertonicity as the surrounding medulla.

When ADH activity is diminished or absent, the collecting duct is relatively impermeable to water, and osmotic equilibrium will not be attained. The tubular fluid, consequently, will remain hypoosmotic to the plasma. Any solute resorption that occurs as the urine traverses the collecting ducts will result in a further lowering of the osmolality of the final urine.

Specific properties

The countercurrent multiplier system. It has been known for many years that the concentration of chloride in homogenates of kidney slices increases progressively from the corticomedullary junction through the inner medulla (83, 84). In 1955 (85, 86) it was also shown that the concentration of sodium is higher in the inner medulla than in the renal cortex. In dehydrated dogs, sodium concentration of slices from the renal papilla may exceed 300 meq/L (87). A similar gradient exists for urea. In 1951, Hargitay and Kuhn (88) demonstrated that the osmolality of slices of rat kidney also increases from the cortex through the inner medulla.

Thus the chloride concentration, the sodium concentration, the urea concentration, and the total solute concentration increase progressively in the dehydrated animal as the papillary tip is approached. An explanation for this resides in the operation of a countercurrent multiplier system between the descending and ascending limbs of the loop of Henle. The system must work so as to allow a solution flowing through a hairpin-shaped tube to undergo a progressive increase in osmolality as it descends toward the tip of the tube and then a progressive decrease in osmolality as it ascends from the tip.

The process may be described by beginning at the top of the two limbs of the loop and progressing toward the bend. The thick ascending limb is thought to initiate the procedure by actively transporting chloride from the tubular urine into the medullary interstitial fluid that lies between the two limbs (20, 89).[5] The addition of the chlo-

---

[5] According to current theory (90, 91) there is no biologic need for active transport of sodium chloride in the thin ascending limb of Henle; but there is controversy about this issue (92, 93).

ride (plus sodium) to the interstitium increases its osmolality; it thus becomes hypertonic to the fluid in the descending limb. In consequence of this gradient, water will diffuse out of the descending limb, and sodium chloride may diffuse into the descending limb. As a result both the sodium concentration in the descending limb and the osmolality increase. The urine coursing down the thin descending limb becomes increasingly hypertonic as it approaches the bend of the loop; the urine rising in the ascending limb becomes increasingly hypotonic. The maximum osmolality must occur at the tip of the loop, and thereafter the continuing resorption as the fluid rises up the ascending limb will decrease the osmolality. To make the system work it is necessary to theorize that the ascending limb is relatively impermeable to water, for if water were to diffuse out of this segment with the resorption of solute, no concentration gradient would be engendered between the interstitial fluid and the urine in the descending limb.

Contribution of the vasa recta and the concept of a countercurrent exchange mechanism. The elaboration of a hypertonic medullary interstitium creates an effective osmotic force for the movement of water out of the tubular fluid coursing down the collecting duct. However, to make this system theoretically sound, some disposition must be made of the vasa recta capillary blood which flows through the medulla in close proximity to the loops and the collecting duct. The general properties of capillary walls are such that salt and water will move freely across in the direction of their respective concentration gradients. Consequently it might be expected that water would diffuse out of the capillary plasma and into the interstitial fluid, whereas sodium would escape from the interstitial fluid and enter the capillary plasma. Both of these events would diminish considerably the osmotic pressure of the medullary interstitium and thereby decrease the volume of water that would diffuse out of the collecting duct. Moreover, the flow of plasma perfusing the capillary loops under most conditions is several times more rapid than the flow of tubular fluid passing through the collecting ducts. Thus the plasma could serve to dissipate the hyperton-

icity of the medulla and in theory could render the concentrating mechanism impotent.

The theoretical explanation for the continued and efficient concentration of the urine in the presence of vasa recta flow rates which exceed urine flow rates invokes a countercurrent exchange mechanism between the descending and ascending limb of the vasa recta (87). The vasa recta have an anatomic configuration somewhat similar to the loops of Henle, although the descending and ascending limbs communicate via cross bars which allow for short-circuiting of some solutes traversing the capillary loop. The operation of the countercurrent exchanger is thought to be as follows:

As the plasma flows down the descending limb of the capillary in the direction of the increasing medullary concentration gradient, water will move out of the capillary plasma, and solute (sodium, chloride, and urea) will enter the plasma. Thus the osmolality of the plasma will increase progressively at the expense of the hypertonicity of the medullary interstitium. However, as the plasma flows up the ascending segment of the capillary, the diffusion gradients will be reversed, water will move back into the plasma, and solute will return to the interstitium. The net removal of solute from the interstitium and the net addition of water to the interstitium will be very much diminished by the countercurrent flow of the plasma through the inner medulla. The exchange of solutes and water between the two limbs of the capillary, occurs entirely by passive mechanisms; thus the system does not involve active transport and is incapable of multiplying the gradient in the manner accomplished in the loops of Henle. Any event which serves to increase the rate of blood flow through the vasa recta may wash out the medullary concentrate gradient and decrease the effectiveness of the concentrating mechanism by lowering the maximum obtainable medullary osmolality (94). Conversely, a reduction in medullary blood flow might in theory increase the maximum attainable osmolality.

The role of urea in the concentrating process. Urea, the major end product of protein metabolism excreted in the urine, appears to enjoy a unique relationship in the operation of the concentrating mechanism and water conservation. Under normal circumstances about half the total concentration in the medulla is made up of sodium salts. Much of the remainder is urea, which reaches high concentrations in the medullary interstitium. This is a consequence of a cyclic trapping process involving medullary interstitium loops of Henle and cortical and medullary portions of the collecting ducts (90, 91, 95, 96). As noted above, under the influence of ADH, the cortical and medullary collecting ducts become highly permeable to water; water diffuses down its chemical gradient from tubular fluid to interstitial fluid. In consequence of this, the concentration of urea in the tubular fluid increases in the papillary region of the collecting duct. The permeability to urea (perhaps under the influence of ADH) increases (97, 98), and there is accelerated diffusion of urea from the collecting duct fluid to the interstitial fluid. During antidiuresis, urea enters the pars recta (99) and the ascending limb of Henle's loop, and, as a result, more urea may enter the distal tubule in the normal kidney than is initially filtered (100). As long as the plasma flow through the ascending vasa recta is normal, this recycling of urea serves to maintain a corticopapillary concentration gradient for urea in the immediate regions of the kidney. Because of the selective permeabilities to sodium, urea, and water of the different tubular segments in the inner medulla and renal papilla, the high chemical concentration of urea in these regions may serve as a force for the entry of additional sodium from the loop of Henle, and thereafter of water from the collecting duct into the interstitial fluid. Urea thus plays an important and unique part in the urinary concentrating process.

Influence of high rates of solute excretion on the concentrating mechanism. It has long been known that, during osmotic diuresis induced, for example, by the infusion of mannitol, the osmolality of urine will fall progressively toward that of the plasma as solute excretion increases (101, 102). Alternatively, the highest achievable osmolality of the urine (and the highest osmolal urine/plasma ratios) are achieved when rates of solute excretion are low (103, 104, 105). The relationship between solute excretion and urine concentration is of considerable importance in understanding concentrating defects in certain pathologic states, and the explanation for this relationship emerges readily within the framework of the present model of urine concentration.

In discussing the mechanism of changes in osmolality with osmotic diuresis, it will be assumed for the sake of simplicity that the resorption of sodium chloride by the ascending limb of the loops of Henle remains constant despite an increase in load caused by inhibition of proximal tubular sodium resorption. Thus the number of nonurea osmotically active particles transferred to the medullary interstitium would remain constant. When the rate of solute excretion is low, the volume of tubular fluid entering and traversing the collecting ducts will be small, and as the urine courses through the inner medulla water will diffuse out of the tubule into the interstitium until osmotic equilibrium is achieved. Because of the small volume of tubular fluid and the relatively large quantity of medullary solute, the achievement of osmotic equilibrium will occur after the diffusion of a limited quantity of water. But the final osmolality of the urine will be very high, because at osmotic equilibrium, the total number of solute particles in tubular fluid plus medullary interstitium will be high in relationship to the total pool of water molecules.

As the rate of distal solute delivery increases, larger volumes of tubular fluid will enter the collecting ducts. Water will again diffuse out of the collecting ducts until the tubular fluid and medulla approach osmotic equilibrium. However, larger volumes of water must enter the medullary interstitium before this equilibrium is achieved, and the final osmolality of the interstitium will be diminished. Consequently, at osmotic equilibrium, the final osmolality of the urine will be lower. At extremely high rates of solute excretion, large quantities of free water will diffuse out of the urine (as much as 5 to 6 ml/100 ml of glomerular filtrate), yet the final osmolality of the urine and presumably of the medullary interstitium may be little higher than the plasma osmolality. It is even possible with extreme osmotic diuresis to effect the excretion of a dilute urine despite the presence of maximum ADH activity. The explanation for this phenomenon is that the urine emanating from the distal tubule in human beings is probably hypotonic, and when very large volumes of hypotonic urine enter the collecting ducts, osmotic equilibrium with the medullary interstitium will fail to be achieved. Even if it is, both urine and medulla may be more dilute than the plasma.

In summary, it is generally agreed that urine is concentrated by a combination of countercurrent multiplication and countercurrent exchange. There is, however, continued debate on several points. These include (1) the means whereby the osmolality of fluid within the descending limb of Henle rises (i.e., whether this is due primarily to solute entry, to water abstraction, or to both); (2) whether the reabsorption of Na^+ (Cl^-) from the thin ascending limb is active or passive; and (3) whether vasopressin increases the permeability of the medullary portion of the collection duct to urea.

THE DILUTING MECHANISM

In comparison with the complexities of the concentrating process, the process of dilution seems relatively simple (106, 107). Conceptually, there are only two major considerations: solute must be removed from the urine by active transport, and water must be prevented from leaving the tubular fluid in isosmotic amounts.

The process of dilution begins in the ascending limb of the loop of Henle, where solute is removed from the urine without the simultaneous removal of water. As already indicated, the tubular fluid entering the distal tubule is hypotonic. It has also been indicated that as the fluid traverses the distal tubule and the collecting ducts, the rate of movement of water into the interstitium depends upon the presence or absence of ADH. When this hormone is absent or is present in low activity, water diffusion out of the collecting ducts will be restricted and the hypoosmolality of the tubular fluid will not be dissipated. Moreover, any continuing transport of solute out of the urine in the distal segments of the nephron will further serve to dilute the urine further as it courses toward the papillary orifice.

The ability to decrease the osmolality of the urine is also influenced by the rate of solute excretion. The greater the volume of isosmotic fluid leaving the proximal tubule, the less will the osmolality of the solution be reduced by the net resorption of any given amount of solute. Consequently, with increasing rates of solute excretion in the absence of any ADH, the urine osmolality will approach the plasma osmolality asymptotically. However, although the osmolality of the final urine rises, the amount of free water excreted may stay the same or even increase. Thus the primary function of the diluting mechanism, the excretion of free water, will not be impaired, despite the fact that the urinary osmolality is substantially above the minimum values attainable (40 to 50 mosm/kg) at normal rates of solute excretion.

RENAL REGULATION OF ACID-BASE HOMEOSTASIS

The processes of metabolism normally result in the addition of acid to body fluids. Each day, in a normal person, at least 40 to 60 meq of hydrogen ions is added to the ECF. The regulatory system thus has as its first charge the protection of the organism against this incursion. By defining the mechanism of regulation that occurs under normal conditions, it becomes possible to explain the more drastic threats to the economy of acid-base homeostasis that occur in many disease states. The present discussion will focus upon the component parts of the regulatory system and especially upon the contribution of the definitive organ of regulation in the maintenance of acid-base homeostasis, the kidney (see also Chap. 6). In Fig. 7-9, the major steps in the acid-base regulatory system are depicted schematically. Hydrogen ions are shown entering the ECF after their release from the metabolism of protein. The hydrogen ions combine with bicarbonate ions in the circulation, forming carbonic acid. Each hydrogen ion incorporated into the structure of a bicarbonate ion thus is removed from the ECF. Only a small portion of the newly formed carbonic acid molecules will dissociate, rereleasing their hydrogen ions into circulation. Carbonic acid is actually a rather strong acid, and in aqueous solution it should release a large majority of the

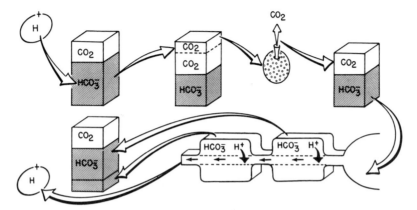

Figure 7-9. Schematic representation of the acid-base regulatory system tracing the fate of a typical hydrogen ion that enters body fluids in the course of normal metabolic processes. The details of this system are described in the text. *From N. S. Bricker and S. Klarh, Modern Treatment, 5:635, 1968.)*

protons accepted from the solution. However, in body fluids carbonic acid is rapidly converted to carbon dioxide (CO_2) and water (H_2O), so that relatively few molecules of carbonic acid (H_2CO_3) actually exist in solution.

The buffering of the hydrogen ions by bicarbonate results in two changes in the composition of the ECF. First, the concentration of bicarbonate diminishes. Second, the concentration of carbonic acid, or more correctly the partial pressure of carbon dioxide (P_{CO_2}), increases (see Fig. 7-9). Thus the protection of the ECF against the incursion of hydrogen ions, although largely successful, nevertheless leads to an alteration in the ratio of proton donor (carbonic acid) to proton acceptor (bicarbonate) in the major conjugate acid-base pair of the extracellular fluid. The result must be a decrease in the pH of the ECF. Were this to continue, acidosis would be progressive and ultimately lethal.

The compensatory mechanisms which prevent progressive acidosis are accomplished by two organs of regulation, the lungs and the kidneys. The role of the lungs is to excrete the excess carbon dioxide engendered by the buffering of the hydrogen ions by bicarbonate.[6] The decrease in pH and the increase in the P_{CO_2} in body fluids re-

sult in a stimulation of the respiratory center; this in turn leads to an increase in both the rate and depth of respiration, and the P_{CO_2} is restored to its normal level of 40 mmHg. The role of the kidneys is to restore the bicarbonate concentration in plasma to its original level. This involves two functional contributions: first, via a process referred to as bicarbonate reclamation, all the bicarbonate entering the glomerular filtrate (approximately 4500 meq per 24 h) must be conserved, for were even a small fraction of the filtered bicarbonate to be lost in the urine, the ability to maintain acid-base homeostasis would be compromised. Second, via a process referred to as bicarbonate regeneration, the bicarbonate consumed in the original buffering of metabolic hydrogen ions must be regenerated and restored to the body fluids.

A singular mechanism accomplishes both processes. Within the tubular epithelial cells, carbon dioxide and water combine to form carbonic acid. This reaction is catalyzed by carbonic anhydrase. A portion of the carbonic acid molecules dissociate, liberating free hydrogen ions capable of crossing the luminal border of the cell membrane and entering the tubular fluid, presumably in exchange for resorbed sodium ions (see Fig. 7-9). As long as bicarbonate ions are present in the tubular fluid, those hydrogen ions that combine with the bicarbonate will result in the formation of

---

[6] The lungs also excrete the very large quantities of carbon dioxide produced from oxidative metabolism.

carbonic acid, which in turn will be dehydrated into water and carbon dioxide (in the proximal tubule, luminal carbonic anhydrase catalyzes this dehydration reaction). Thus hydrogen entry will result in the dissipation of tubular fluid bicarbonate. However, the filtered bicarbonate has been converted into carbon dioxide and water rather than returned to the ECF. The bicarbonate ions that do return to the ECF are those that were left behind in the cells after the hydrogen ions were secreted. Under steady-state conditions, one bicarbonate ion is dissipated from the tubular fluid, and another enters the ECF. Thus from an operational point of view, filtered bicarbonate is resorbed from the tubular fluid and restored to the ECF quantitatively.

In addition to bicarbonate, two other buffers exist in the tubular fluid, phosphate and ammonia. When a hydrogen ion combines with either a phosphate ion or an ammonia molecule, it is effectively removed from the tubular fluid, allowing entry of additional hydrogen ions. Once again, the bicarbonate left behind in the epithelial cells will be restored to the peritubular capillaries, but in this instance it will represent the de novo addition of new bicarbonate rather than the "resorption" of a filtered bicarbonate. Thus each hydrogen ion that enters the tubular fluid and is buffered by phosphate or ammonia will allow the return of a new bicarbonate to the ECF. Under steady-state conditions, the number of new bicarbonate ions regenerated will equal the number consumed in the ECF in the original buffering of the metabolic hydrogen ions, and the number of hydrogen ions excreted into the urine (buffered by phosphate and ammonia) will equal the number entering the ECF hydrogen ion concentration and bicarbonate concentration will remain constant despite the continued entrance of hydrogen ions.

How the control system operates to maintain acid-base homeostasis with such precision is unknown. One component of the control system relates to the quantitative aspects of bicarbonate resorption. In health, as indicated, virtually no bicarbonate is lost in the urine. However, if an exogenous load of bicarbonate is given to a normal person, the extra bicarbonate is excreted promptly and the normal concentration of bicarbonate in the serum reestablished. On the other hand, in a variety of acid-base abnormalities, the kinetics of bicarbonate resorption are altered, often in a compensatory and thus appropriate direction. A number of events are known to influence bicarbonate resorption. ECF volume expansion or contraction will reduce or increase, respectively, both the blood level of bicarbonate at which bicarbonaturia begins (i.e., the threshold) and the maximum rate of bicarbonate resorption (the Tm) (108–110). Parathyroid hormone is known to inhibit bicarbonate resorption (111, 112), and potassium depletion may be associated with an increased capacity for bicarbonate resorption (113). There are other factors that influence bicarbonate resorption (114–117), key among them being the P_{CO_2} of arterial blood.

A key element in the control system relates to the influence of the role of hydrogen ion accession in body fluids on the renal tubular production of hydrogen ions and de novo synthesis of bicarbonate. When hydrogen ion production increases markedly, as in ketoacidosis or lactic acidosis, the increased load of hydrogen ions entering the extracellular fluid will result in a decrease in plasma bicarbonate. The bicarbonate which buffers the added hydrogen ions will be converted to carbonic acid: the largest part of the carbonic acid will be dehydrated to carbon dioxide and water, and the increase in P_{CO_2} will be followed by an increased rate of pulmonary excretion of carbon dioxide. The kidneys must then regenerate a substantially increased quantity of bicarbonate. This requires that the rate of hydrogen ion excretion in combination with phosphate and ammonia increase markedly, for an increase in hydrogen ions bound to nonvolatile buffers (rather than an increase in free hydrogen ions in solution) is the only effective way to increase net excretion of hydrogen. (Even at the lowest urinary pH attainable, approximately 4.5, the number of hydrogen ions in solution is trivial in relation to the number excreted in combination with buffers.) Moreover, by virtue of their physicochemical properties, both phosphate and ammonia will have combined with a near maximum number of hydrogen ions at a urine pH below 5. Lowering the urinary pH from 5 to 4.5, for example, will increase the number of bound hydrogen ions by an insignificant amount. Hence, in an acid urine, the only way to increase net hydrogen ion excretion is to increase the excretion rate of buffer. With the development of metabolic acidosis, some increase in phosphate excretion may occur, but phosphate excretion normally is attuned to the rate of phosphate entry into the ECF, and the control system for phosphate seems to be designed primarily to effect external phosphate balance rather than to control acid-base homeostasis. Thus titratable acid excretion (i.e., phosphate-bound protons) will increase only modestly, making a limited contribution to the increased hydrogen ion excretion.[7] The primary mechanism of protection relates to ammonia excretion, and it seems likely that modulation of the rate of ammonia production in the tubular epithelial cells represents the key effector element in the acid-base control system both in health and in conditions of increased hydrogen ion production.

THE CONTROL OF AMMONIA PRODUCTION AND SECRETION

Ammonia (NH_3) is synthesized in the tubular epithelial cells from amino acid precursors, the principal one of which is glutamine. As NH_3 is generated in the renal tubular cell, it will diffuse freely across the cell membranes and will enter the tubular fluid. Within the tubular fluid, NH_3, which is a strong base, will combine with freely dissociated hydrogen ions and will be converted to a new species, NH_4^+. This buffering process thus will increase the opportunity for further entry into the tubular fluid of both additional NH_3 and H^+ species. When metabolic acidosis is induced experimentally, by feeding ammonium chloride, ammonia excretion increases progressively over at least a several-day period (118), and in human beings with severe metabolic acidosis ammonia excretion rates in excess of 400 meq/day may occur.

The events which limit the rate of synthesis of

---

[7] If the underlying cause of the acidosis results in liberation of phosphate from the cells (as may occur in diabetic ketoacidosis), the extra phosphate excreted in the urine will contribute to the enhancement of hydrogen ion excretion and thus to enhancement of bicarbonate ion regeneration.

ammonia from glutamine in the face of metabolic acidosis have been investigated intensively for a number of years. The extraction of glutamine from renal arterial blood increases within 60 min of the administration of an increased acid load (119). An increase in ammonia-producing enzymes (i.e., in glutaminase I, glutamic dehydrogenase, and glutaminase II enzymes) occurs in experimental metabolic acidosis in some species, but the requirement of this enzyme adaptation of an increase in the rate of ammonia excretion is challenged by two observations: first, in the dog, glutaminase adaptation does not occur after an acid load has been given, although ammonium excretion rates increase appropriately (120). Second, Goldstein (121) found that in rats rendered acidotic the inhibition of synthesis of deoxyribonucleic acid-dependent ribonucleic acid (DNA-dependent RNA) in the kidney by Dactinomycin prevented the increase in glutaminase I activity but did not block the increased rate of ammonia excretion.

Interest has been focused on whether ammonia production and renal gluconeogenesis are coupled events. Goodman and associates found that renal cortical slices from rats in which metabolic acidosis is produced in vivo have an increased capacity for glucose production from amino acid precursors of ammonia as well as an increased capacity for ammonia production (122). Cortical slices from rats with metabolic alkalosis exhibit decreased gluconeogenesis. Similar findings were observed by Goorno (123) in the dog. Kamm and associates (124) also found that changing the pH of the media used to incubate kidney slices influences renal gluconeogenesis in vitro. They postulated that enhanced renal gluconeogenesis in acidosis is due to a direct stimulation of one of the enzymatic steps between oxalacetate and glucose. Kamm subsequently suggested that increased conversion of glutamic acid to glucose may enhance glutaminase activity and thereby increase ammonia production from glutamine (125).

Recently several arguments have been raised against the hypothesis that gluconeogenesis is the primary mechanism controlling ammonia production. Preuss (126) found that the acute administration of ammonium chloride to rats resulted in an adaptive increase in ammonia production within 4 h, but gluconeogenesis did not increase until after 12 h. Further evidence against a central regulatory role of gluconeogenesis comes from the studies of Pitts (127, 128) using ^{14}C-glutamine in acidotic and alkalotic dogs. Pitts suggested that gluconeogenesis is not the primary process controlling ammonia production and proposed that access of glutamine to glutaminase I and other oxidative enzymes within mitochondria is augmented. In states characterized by increased ammoniagenesis, Adam and Simpson (129) have adduced support for this thesis in studies on mitochondria from acidotic rats. It would appear, therefore, that chronic metabolic acidosis specifically enhances the transport of glutamine into the mitochondria.

In summary, ammoniagenesis appears to be a critical and decisive event in the overall operation of the acid-base control system. The present evidence, we believe, supports the view that the role of production of ammonia by the kidney is linked closely to the continuing need for acid-base homeostasis. In Chap. 8 there is a more detailed discussion of all aspects of acid-base physiology and pathophysiology.

POTASSIUM

The total amount of potassium in a normal adult human being approximates 3500 meq. Of this, the greatest part by far is intracellular. However, a small but very important fraction of total body potassium resides in the ECF. Potassium is acquired in the diet principally from protein, and normally from 30 to 100 meq of potassium is ingested daily. Very small quantities of potassium are ordinarily lost in stool and sweat, and the predominant route of excretion is through the kidney. Hence the kidney is the primary end organ in the potassium regulatory system. The control system is complex and appears to have multiple component parts only some of which are understood. The primary charge of the control system is to maintain excretion rates of potassium equal to accession rates. A more immediate goal is to control the concentration of potassium in the ECF within rather narrow limits, for if values fall outside these limits, abnormalities of life-threatening proportions can evolve. Because potassium is predominantly an intracellular cation, the control system, in the final analysis, must be oriented to protect the intracellular content of potassium, as well as the ECF concentration of potassium.

In addition to the plasma and the intracellular potassium concentrations, potassium excretion can be influenced by the pH of the ECF, the pH of the ICF, and the rate of delivery of sodium to the distal portions of the nephron. Finally, mineralocorticoid hormone activity contributes to the modulation of potassium excretion by the kidney.

It has been known for a number of years that potassium may be excreted into the urine in quantities greater than are filtered at the glomeruli (130). From this observation it became evident that a mechanism must exist in the nephron for secreting potassium ions into the tubular fluid. Berliner and associates in one of several key pioneering observations demonstrated that the rate of potassium excretion into the urine is not influenced decisively by experimental reduction of the GFR (131); hence the filtered load of potassium is not the principal determinant of the rate of potassium excretion. Rather, the interplay between tubular resorption and tubular secretion of potassium must determine the ultimate rate of excretion.

Within recent years, a very concerted effort has been made to gain a deeper understanding of the manner in which the kidney excretes potassium, and the new knowledge is extensive. The key observations are summarized below. Micropuncture studies of the accessible portion (about two-thirds) of the proximal tubule of mammals have shown that the ratio of the potassium concentration in tubular fluid to that in plasma ranges from 0.8 to 1.2 (132–137).

The fact that the tubular fluid/plasma (TF/P) ratios for potassium remain close to unity indicates that the fraction of filtered potassium resorbed proximally is the same as the fraction of filtered water resorbed. Although these data could reflect a passive mode of potassium resorption in the proximal tubule, it seems more likely, on the basis of several different observations (136, 138, 139) that the resorption of potassium is an active process. In the rat, only about 5 to 10 percent of the filtered potassium reaches the first accessible portion of the distal tubule (133), suggesting that net potassium resorption continues along the short loops of Henle. On the other hand, in micropuncture studies of long loops of Henle by de Rouffignac and Morel in *Psammomys* (140) and Jamison in the rat (141) potassium appeared to reenter the long loops of Henle, and indeed in the studies of Jamison more potassium was found in tubular fluid of long loops of Henle (close to the bend) than was filtered at the glomerulus. It is very unlikely that any active transport of potassium takes place in the thin descending portion of the loop of Henle (142); however, potassium could diffuse into the tubular fluid in this segment of the nephron. In the thick ascending limb, it is possible that potassium, along with sodium, is resorbed passively; however, active resorption of potassium has not been excluded. In the distal tubules of cortical glomeruli of the rat, the direction of net movement of potassium depends upon the diet of the animal. In animals on a low-potassium diet, further removal occurs in both the distal tubule and the collecting duct such that as little as 1 percent of the filtered potassium may be excreted (133). However, in rats receiving a moderate intake of potassium, potassium ions are added to the tubular fluid in the distal tubule in amounts that may approximate 75 percent of the total excreted. In rats on a high-potassium diet, considerably more potassium may be added to the tubular fluid, and the final excretion rate may be more than twice as great as the filtered load of potassium.

The presence of a negative potential difference (*PD*) in the lumen of cortical distal tubular segments favors the passive entry of potassium into the tubular fluid (143). However, in studies to determine the relation between *PD* and potassium transport, the steady-state luminal ion concentration in the early distal segment was well below that expected with a purely passive mechanism (135). Moreover, ouabain caused the luminal potassium concentration to rise, a finding which also supports the concept of active potassium reabsorption (144). Recent evidence suggests that potassium secretion may be intimately tied to the transport of potassium from blood to cytoplasm across the peritubular cell membrane, while the resorptive mechanism may be located at the lu-

minal surface of the cell (145). If this interpretation is correct, net potassium secretion into the tubular fluid would represent the interplay between active resorption across the luminal membrane and passive diffusion down an electrochemical gradient across the same membrane. Which of these two mechanisms (i.e., active resorption and passive secretion) would serve as the fine regulator of the amount of potassium delivered into the urine remains to be established; nor is it clear how such an interplay would affect the excretion of two or more times the amount of potassium entered, as occurs in reduced chronic renal failure.

Under many experimental and clinical conditions, there is an inverse relationship between potassium and hydrogen ion excretion. For example, when ECF alkalosis is induced by infusion of bicarbonate-containing solutions or by hyperventilation, the urinary excretion of potassium increases and the urinary excretion of hydrogen ion decreases. Induction of respiratory acidosis increases hydrogen ion excretion and decreases potassium excretion. Infusion of potassium in large quantities results in an increase in potassium excretion and a decrease in hydrogen ion excretion. In many forms of potassium depletion, potassium excretion into the urine is diminished; the urine remains acid, however, despite the development of extracellular alkalosis. Finally, administration of carbonic anhydrase inhibitors typically results in a decrease in hydrogen ion excretion and an increase in potassium excretion. Berliner and associates (148) suggested some years ago that there was an exchange in the distal part of the nephron between sodium ions resorbed and either potassium or hydrogen ions secreted. They suggested, furthermore, that some form of competition exists between potassium and hydrogen secretion. However, on the basis of recent micropuncture studies it is no longer reasonable to consider that hydrogen and potassium ions compete for secretion in the strict sense of carrier-mediated transport (147).

That potassium secretion is in some manner dependent upon sodium delivery to the distal nephron is supported by a variety of data. Experimentally it is difficult to achieve maximum potassium secretory rates in the absence of appreciable rates of sodium excretion. Moreover, Seldin et al. (150) have shown that the induction of potassium depletion by desoxycorticosterone is inhibited when sodium is restricted. In patients with congestive heart failure, in whom distal sodium delivery is diminished in consequence of an increase in fractional sodium resorption in the proximal tubule, potassium excretion may increase briskly when distal sodium delivery is increased by diuretic administration. Thus the entry of potassium into the distal tubular lumen apparently depends upon the availability of sodium in the tubular fluid. However, Giebisch et al. have studied the quantitative aspects of this relationship and were able to demonstrate that, even in animals maintained on a very low salt diet, the amount of sodium resorbed in the distal tubule exceeded by far the amount of potassium secreted. Many sodium ions were resorbed for every potassium ion secreted. Thus although the load of sodium reaching the exchange site influences the capacity of the nephron to deliver potassium into the tubular fluid, there does not seem to be a 1:1 exchange of sodium for potassium in the distal tubule. In vitro studies of isolated perfused cortical collecting tubules (149, 150) have also shown that while there is an interrelationship between active sodium resorption and potassium secretion, there is no rigid linkage suggestive of an exchange pump. On a continuing basis a successful control system must be capable of regulating potassium excretion independently of changes in sodium excretion, for potassium balance must be maintained without regard for any changes in sodium intake if potassium homeostasis is to be protected.

Aldosterone is known to influence potassium excretion. This hormone acts at a distal site in the nephron, but the precise mechanism of action remains unknown. In light of the foregoing comments it appears that aldosterone (and other mineralocorticoid hormones) could act either by increasing the permeability of the apical plasma membrane to potassium or by increasing the rate of sodium resorption and thereby increasing the role of potassium secretion. Clinically, potassium concentrations of the ECF influence the rate of production of aldosterone, and, conversely, such excess levels of aldosterone as those observed in primary aldosteronism lead to potassium depletion. In adrenal insufficiency, on the other hand, potassium retention and hyperkalemia typically occur.

In summary, although the majority of total body potassium resides within the cell water, a small but critical fraction is found in the ECF. The careful control of both total body potassium and ECF potassium concentration is essential for continued well-being and is the charge of the potassium control system. This system is intricate and not entirely understood. It responds to the potassium which enters body fluids from the diet and serves to effect the excretion of the same amount of potassium from the body. The excretion takes place almost entirely via the kidneys in health. (In uremia, the amount of potassium excreted in the feces may increase appreciably.) In the presence of sudden large loads of potassium, the cells sequester much of the added cation, thereby protecting the organism from potentially dangerous increases in the plasma potassium concentration. Ultimately, however, the kidneys must excrete the added potassium. Present information suggests that potassium is completely filtered at the glomerulus and largely resorbed in the proximal tubule. In the distal tubule a relatively small percentage of the filtered potassium occurs (this has been observed in the rat) while potassium simultaneously leaks downhill into the tubular fluid.

The balance between active resorption and passive secretion determines net entry of potassium into the distal tubular fluid and thus net excretion into the urine. Aldosterone influences this balance in a manner yet to be clarified. Whether there is another hormone or extrahormonal mechanisms that play a key role in modulating potassium excretion also remains to be determined. However, there are other factors known to influence potassium excretion. These include the pH of the ECF; the pH of the ICF, especially in the renal tubular epithelial cells; the potassium concentration of the ECF; the potassium content of the renal tubular cells; and finally the delivery of sodium to the distal tubule where sodium and potassium exchange occurs.

REFERENCES

1. Smith, H. W.: *The Kidney Structure and Function in Health and Disease,* Oxford University Press, New York, 1951.
2. Reiss, E., J. M. Canterbury, M. A. Bergovitz, and E. L. Kaplan: The role of phosphate in the secretion of parathyroid hormone in man, *J. Clin. Invest.,* **49:**2146, 1970.
3. Wen, S.: Micropuncture studies of phosphate transport in proximal tubule of the dog. The relationship to sodium reabsorption, *J. Clin. Invest.,* **53:**143, 1974.
4. Deluca, H. F.: The kidney as an endocrine organ involved in function of vitamin D, *Am. J. Med.,* **58:**39, 1975.
5. Kolata, G. B.: Vitamin D: Investigation of a new steroid hormone, *Science,* **188:**635, 1975.
6. Erslev, A.: Renal biogenesis of erythropoietin, *Am. J. Med.,* **58:**25, 1975.
7. Muirhead, E. E., G. Germain, B. E. Leach, J. A. Pitcock, P. Stephenson, B. Brooks, W. L. Brosius, E. G. Daniels, and J. W. Himman: Production of renomedullary prostaglandins by renomedullary interstitial cells grown in tissue culture, *Circ. Res.,* **31**(suppl.):161, 1972.
8. Janszen, F. H. A., and D. H. Nugteren: Histochemical localization of prostaglandin synthetase, *Histochemie,* **23:**159, 1971.
9. Leber, P. D., and D. J. Marsh: Micropuncture study of concentration and fate of albumin in rat nephron, *Am. J. Physiol.,* **219:**358, 1970.
10. Pappenheimer, J. R., E. M. Renkin, and L. M. Borrero: Filtration, diffusion and molecular sieving through peripheral capillary membranes: A contribution to the pore theory of capillary permeability, *Am. J. Physiol.,* **167:**13, 1951.
11. Brenner, B. M., J. L. Troy, and T. M. Daugharty: The dynamics of glomerular ultrafiltration in rat, *J. Clin. Invest.,* **50:**1776, 1971.
12. Foster, R. P., and J. P. Maes: Effect of experimental neurogenic hypertension on renal blood flow and glomerular filtration rate in intact denervated kidney of unanesthetized rabbits with adrenal glands demedullated, *Am. J. Physiol.,* **150:**534, 1947.
13. Brenner, B. M., J. L. Troy, T. M. Daugharty, and W. M. Deen: Dynamics of glomerular ultrafiltration in rat. II Plasma flow dependence of GFR, *Am. J. Physiol.,* **223:**1184, 1972.
14. Thurau, K., and J. Schnermann: Die Natriumkozentration an den Macula densa-Zellen als regulierender Faktor für das Glomerulumfiltrat (Micropunktransnerache), *Klin. Wochenschr.,* **43:**410, 1965.
15. Pitts, R. F.: *Physiology of the Kidney and Body Fluids,* 2d ed., Year Book Medical Publishers, Inc., Chicago, 1968.
16. Tisher, C. C., R. E. Bulger, and H. Valtin: Morphology of renal medulla in water diuresis and vasopressin-induced antidiuresis, *Am. J. Physiol.,* **220:**87, 1971.
17. Davson, H., and J. F. Danielli: *The Permeability of Natural Membranes,* Cambridge University Press, London, 1952.
18. Harris, E. J.: *Transport and Accumulation in Biological Systems,* 3d ed., University Park Press, Baltimore, 1972.
19. Maude, D. L.: Mechanism of salt transport and some permeability properties of rat proximal tubule, *Am. J. Physiol.,* **218:**1590, 1970.
20. Burg, M., and N. Green: Function of the thick ascending limb of Henle's loop, *Am. J. Physiol.,* **224:**659, 1973.
21. Bennett, C. M., J. R. Clapp, and R. W. Berliner: Micropuncture study of the proximal and distal tubule in the dog, *Am. J. Physiol.,* **213:**1254, 1967.
22. Bennett, C. M., B. M. Brenner, and R. W. Berliner: Micropuncture study of nephron function in the Rhesus monkey, *J. Clin. Invest.,* **47:**203, 1968.
23. Stoner, L., M. Burg, and J. Orloff: Ion transport in cortical collecting tubule: Effect of amiloride, *Am. J. Physiol.,* **227:**453, 1974.
24. Wesson, L. G., Jr., W. P. Anslow, Jr., and H. W. Smith: The excretion of strong electrolytes, *Bull. N.Y. Acad. Med.,* **24:**586, 1948.
25. Brunner, F. P., F. C. Rector, Jr., and D. W. Seldin: Mechanism of glomerulotubular balance. II. Regulation of proximal tubular reabsorption by tubule volume, as studied by stopped-flow microperfusion, *J. Clin. Invest.,* **45:**603, 1966.
26. Gertz, K. H.: Transtubulare Natrienchloridflusse und Permeabilitat für Nichtelektrolyte im proxi-

malen und distalen Konvolut der Rattenniere, *Pfluegers Arch. Ges. Physiol.*, **276**:336, 1963.

27. Gertz, K. H., J. A. Mangos, G. Braun, and H. D. Pagel: On the glomerular tubular balance in the rat kidney, *Pfluegers Arch. Ges. Physiol.*, **285**:360, 1967.

28. Rector, F. C., Jr., F. P. Brunner, and D. W. Seldin: Mechanism of glomerulotubular balance. I. Effect of aortic constriction and elevated uretero-pelvic pressure on glomerular filtration rate, fractional reabsorption, transit time, and tubular size in the proximal tubule of the rat, *J. Clin. Invest.*, **45**:590, 1966.

29. Landwehr, D. M., R. M. Klose, and G. Giebisch: Micropuncture study of sodium reabsorption in saline-loaded rats, *Fed. Proc.*, **25**:460, 1966.

30. Leyssac, P. P.: Intrarenal function of angiotensin, *Fed. Proc.*, **26**:59, 1967.

31. Brenner, B. M., C. M. Bennett, and R. W. Berliner: The relationship between glomerular filtration rate and sodium reabsorption by the proximal tubule of the rat nephron, *J. Clin. Invest.*, **47**:1358, 1968.

32. Baines, A. D., P. P. Leyssac, and C. W. Gottschalk: Proximal tubular volume and inulin clearance in non-diuretic rats, *Int. Congr. Nephrol. Free Commun.*, **2**:152, 1966.

33. Lewy, J. E., and E. E. Windhager: Peritubular control of proximal tubular fluid reabsorption in the rat kidney, *Am. J. Physiol.*, **214**:943, 1968.

34. Koch, K. M., H. S. Aynedhian, and N. Bank: Effect of acute hypertension on sodium reabsorption by the proximal tubule, *J. Clin. Invest.*, **47**:1696, 1968.

35. Burg, M. B., and J. Orloff: Control of fluid absorption in the renal proximal tubule, *J. Clin. Invest.*, **47**:2016, 1968.

36. Brenner, B. M., J. L. Troy, T. M. Daugharty, and R. M. MacInnes: Quantitative importance of changes in postglomerular colloid osmotic pressure in mediating glomerulotubular balance in the rat, *J. Clin. Invest.*, **52**:190, 1973.

37. Epstein, F. H., R. S. Post, and M. McDowell: The effect of an arteriovenous fistula on renal hemodynamics and electrolyte excretion, *J. Clin. Invest.*, **32**:233, 1953.

38. Peters, J. P.: *Body Water in the Exchange of Fluids in Man*, Charles C Thomas, Publisher, Springfield, Ill., 1935.

39. Wesson, L. G., Jr.: Glomerular and tubular factors in the renal excretion of sodium chloride, *Medicine*, **36**:281, 1957.

40. Ploth, D. W., and J. Schnermann. Dependency of autoregulation of nephron-filtration (N-GFR) on maintenance of distal fluid delivery (abstract), *Proc. Intern. Congr. Nephrol.*, 6th, Florence, 1975.

41. Marshand, G. R., T. J. Burke, J. A. Haas, J. C. Romero, and F. G. Knox: Regulation of filtration rate in sodium-depleted and -expanded dogs, *Am. J. Physiol.*, **232**:F325, 1977.

42. Levinsky, N. G.: Non-aldosterone influences on renal transport, *Ann. N.Y. Acad. Sco.*, **139**:295, 1966.

43. Barger, A. C.: Renal hemodynamic factors in congestive heart failure, *Ann. N.Y. Acad. Sci.*, **139**:276, 1966.

44. Barger, A. C., and J. A. Herd, The renal circulation, *N. Engl. J. Med.*, **284**:482, 1971.

45. Thorburn, G. D., H. H. Kopald, J. A. Herd, H. Hollenberg, C. C. C. O'Morchoe, and A. C. Barger: Intrarenal distribution of nutrient blood flow determined with 85 Kr in the unanesthetized dog, *Circ. Res.*, **13**:290, 1963.

46. deRouffignac, C., and J. P. Bunvalet: Variations in glomerular filtration rate of single superficial and deep nephrons under various conditions of sodium intake in the rat, *Pfluegers Arch.*, **319**:141, 1970.

47. Jamison, R. L., and F. R. Lacy: Effect of saline infusion on superficial and juxtamedullary nephrons in rat, *Am. J. Physiol.*, **221**:690, 1971.

48. Horster, M., and K. Thurau: Micropuncture studies on the filtration rate of single superficial and juxtamedullary glomeruli in the rat, *Pfluegers Arch. Ges. Physiol.*, **301**:162, 1968.

49. Stein, J. H., S. Boonjarern, C. B. Wilson, and T. F. Ferris: Alterations in intrarenal blood flow distribution: Methods of measurement and relationship to sodium balance, *Circ. Res.*, **32**(suppl. I):61, 1972.

50. Wallin, J. D., F. C. Rector, Jr., and D. W. Seldin: Effect of volume expansion on intrarenal distribution of plasma flow in the dog, *Am. J. Physiol.*, **223**:125, 1972.

51. Mandin, H., A. H. Israelit, F. C. Rector, Jr., and D. W. Seldin: Effect of saline infusions on intrarenal distribution of glomerular filtrate and prox-

imal reabsorption in the dog, *J. Clin. Invest.*, **50**:514, 1971.

52. Davidman, M., E. A. Alexander, R. C. Lalone, and N. G. Levinsky: *Nephron*, function during volume expansion in the rat, *Am. J. Physiol.*, **223**:188, 1972.

53. Daugharty, T. M., I. F. Uck, D. P. Nicholas, and B. M. Brenner: Comparative renal effects of iso-oncotic and colloid-free volume expansion in the rat, *Am. J. Physiol.*, **222**:225, 1972.

54. Sharp, G. W. G., and A. Leaf: Mechanism of action of aldosterone, *Physiol. Rev.*, **49**:593, 1966.

55. Edelman, I. S.: Aldosterone and sodium transport, in K. W. McKerns (ed.), *Functions of the Adrenal Cortex*, Appleton-Century-Crofts, Inc., New York, 1968.

56. deWardener, H. E., I. H. Mills, W. F. Clapham, and C. J. Hayter: Studies on the efferent mechanism of the sodium diuresis which follows the administration of intravenous saline in the dog, *Clin. Sci.*, **21**:249, 1961.

57. Mills, I. W., H. E. deWardener, and C. J. Hayter: Studies on the afferent mechanism of the sodium chloride diuresis which follows intravenous saline in the dog, *Clin. Sci.*, **21**:259, 1961.

58. Giebisch, G.: Coupled ion and fluid transport in the kidney, *N. Engl. J. Med.*, **287**:913, 1972.

59. Earley, L. E., and R. M. Friedler: Observations of the mechanism of decreased tubular reabsorption of sodium and water during saline loading, *J. Clin. Invest.*, **43**:1928, 1964.

60. Earley, L. E., and R. M. Friedler: The effects of combined vasodilation and pressor agents on renal hemodynamics and the tubular reabsorption of sodium, *J. Clin. Invest.*, **45**:542, 1966.

61. Daugharty, T. M., L. J. Belleau, J. A. Martino, and L. E. Earley: Interrelationship of physical factors affecting sodium reabsorption in the dog, *Am. J. Physiol.*, **215**:1442, 1968.

62. Spitzer, A., and E. E. Windhager: Proximal tubular fluid reabsorption during microperfusion of single efferent arterioles in rat kidneys, *Proc. Intern. Union Physiol. Sci.*, **7**:413, 1968.

63. Brenner, B. M., K. H. Flachuk, R. I. Keimowitz, and R. W. Berliner: Relation between peritubular capillary protein concentration and fluid reabsorption by the rat proximal tubule, *J. Clin. Invest.*, June 1969, (Abstr.).

64. Imai, M., D. W. Seldin, and J. P. Kokko: Effect of perfusion rate on the fluxes of water, sodium, chloride and urea across the proximal convoluted tubule, *Kidney Int.*, **11**:18, 1977.

65. Stein, J. H., R. W. Osgood, S. Boonjarern, J. W. Cox, and T. F. Ferris: Segmental sodium reabsorption in rats with mild and severe volume depletion, *Am. J. Physiol.*, **227**:351, 1974.

66. Blake, W. D.: Relative rules of glomerular filtration and tubular reabsorption in denervation diuresis, *Am. J. Physiol.*, **202**:777, 1962.

67. Barajas, L., and J. Muller: The innervation of juxtaglomerular apparatus and surrounding tubules; a quantitative analysis by serial section electron microscopy, *J. Ultrastruct. Res.*, **43**:107, 1973.

68. Slick, G. L., A. J. Aguilera, E. J. Zambraski, G. F. DiBona, and G. J. Kaloyanides: Renal neuroadrenergic transmission, *Am. J. Physiol.*, **229**:60, 1975.

69. DiBona, G. F., E. J. Zambraski, A. J. Aguilera, and G. J. Kaloyanides: Neurogenic control of renal tubular sodium reabsorption in the dog, *Circ. Res.*, **40**(suppl. I)I:127, 1977.

70. Sedlakova, E., B. Lichardus, and J. H. Cort: Plasma saluretic activity: Its nature and relation to oxytocin analogs, *Science*, **164**:580, 1969.

71. Buckalew, V. M., Jr., F. J. Martinez, and W. E. Green: Dialyzable inhibitor of toad bladder sodium transport in plasma of volume expanded dogs, *Clin. Res.*, **17**:236, 1969.

72. Bricker, N. S., S. Klahr, M. L. Purkerson, and R. G. Schultze: On an in vitro assay system for a humoral substance present in plasma and serum during extracellular fluid volume expansion and uremia, *Nature*, **219**:1058, 1968.

73. Laragh, J. H., J. E. Sealey, and J. D. Kirschman: Natriuretic activity in plasma and urine of salt-loaded man and sheep, *J. Clin. Invest.*, In press., Abstr.

74. Favre, H., J. H. Hwang, R. W. Schmidt, N. S. Bricker, and J. J. Bourgoignie: An inhibitor of sodium transport in the urine of dogs with normal renal function, *J. Clin. Invest.*, **56**:1302, 1975.

75. Harris, R. H., and W. E. Yarger: Urine-reinfusion natriuresis: Evidence for potent natriuretic factors in rat urine, *Kidney Int.*, **11**:93, 1977.

76. Bourgoignie, J. J., H. Favre, M. A. Kaplan, Ch. Eun, K. H. Hwang, and N. S. Bricker: On the natriuretic factor of serum and urine from patients

with chronic uremia. Central nervous control of Na⁺ balance, *International Workshop at Cologne 1975*, Georg. Thieme, Stuttgart, 1976.

77. Cortney, M. A., M. Mylle, W. E. Lassiter, and C. W. Gottschal: Renal tubular transport of water solute and PAH in rats with isotonic saline, *Am. J. Physiol.*, **209:**1199, 1965.

78. Dirks, J. H., W. J. Cirksena, and R. W. Berliner: The effect of saline infusion on sodium reabsorption by the proximal tubule of the dog, *J. Clin. Invest.*, **44:**1160, 1965.

79. Fine, L. G., J. J. Bourgoignie, K. H. Hwang, and N. S. Bricker: On the influence of the natriuretic factor from patients with chronic uremia on the bioelectric properties and sodium transport of the isolated mammalian collecting tubule, *J. Clin. Invest.*, **58:**590, 1976.

80. Peter, K.: Untersuchungen über Bau und Entwicklung der Niere, *Jena*, 1909.

81. Kuhn, W., and K. Ryffel: Herstellung Konzentrierter losungen aus verdunnten durch blosse membranwirkung. Ein modellversuch zur funktion der niere, *Z. Physiol. Chem.*, **276:**145, 1942.

82. Hargitay, B., and W. Kuhn: Das Multiplikationsprinzip als Grundlage er Harnkonzentrierung in der Niere, *Z. Electrochem.*, **55:**539, 1951.

83. Glimstedt, G.: Quantitative histotopochemische Untersuchungen über die Nieren. 1. Die Verteiling der Chloride, *Z. Mikr. Anat. Forsch.*, **52:**335, 1942.

84. Ljungberg, E.: On the reabsorption of chloride in the kidney of rabbit, *Acta Med. Scand.*, **1**(suppl. 186):189, 1947.

85. Krakusin, J. S., and R. B. Jennings: Radioautographic localization of Na²² in the rat kidney, *Arch. Pathol. (Chicago)*, **59:**471, 1955.

86. Ullrich, K. J., F. O. Drenskhahn, and K. H. Jarusch: Untersuchungen zum Problem der Harnkonzentrierung und-verdunnung, *Pfluegers Arch. Ges. Physiol.*, **261:**62, 1955.

87. Berliner, R. W., N. G. Levinsky, D. G. Davidson, and M. Eden: Dilution and concentration of the urine and the action of antidiuretic hormone, *Am. J. Med.*, **24:**730, 1958.

88. Hargitay, B., and W. Kuhn: Likalisation des Konzentrierungsprozesses in der Niere durch directe Kryoskipie, *Helv. Physiol. Pharmacol. Acta*, **9:**196, 1951.

89. Rocha, A. S., and J. P. Kokko: Sodium chloride and water transport in the medullary thick ascending limb of Henle. Evidence for active chloride transport, *J. Clin. Invest.*, **52:**613, 1973.

90. Kokko, J. P., and F. C. Rector, Jr.: Countercurrent multiplication system without active transport in inner medulla, *Kidney Int.*, **2:**214, 1972.

91. Stephenson, J. L.: Concentration of urine in a central core model of the renal counterflow system, *Kidney Int.*, **2:**85, 1972.

92. Marsh, D. J.: Solute and water flows in thin limbs of Henle's loop in the hamster kidney, *Am. J. Physiol.*, **218:**824, 1970.

93. Marsh, D. J., and S. P. Azen: Mechanism of NaCl reabsorption by hamster thin ascending limbs of Henle's loop, *Am. J. Physiol.*, **228:**71, 1975.

94. Valtin, H.: *Renal Functions: Mechanisms Preserving Fluid and Solute Balance in Health*, Little, Brown and Company, Boston, 1973.

95. Pennell, J. P., F. B. Lacy, and R. L. Jamison: An in vivo study of the concentration process in the descending limb of Henle's loop, *Kidney Int.*, **5:**335, 1974.

96. Pennell, J. P., V. Sanjana, N. R. Frey, and R. L. Jamison: The effect of urea infusion on the urinary concentration mechanism in protein-depleted rats, *J. Clin. Invest.*, **55:**399, 1975.

97. Morgan, T., and R. W. Berliner: Permeability of loop of Henle, vasa recta, and collecting duct to water, urea and sodium, *Am. J. Physiol.*, **215:**108, 1968.

98. Rocha, A. S., and J. P. Kokko: Permeability of medullary nephron segments to urea and water, effect of vasopressin, *Kidney Int.*, **6:**379, 1974.

99. Kawamura, S., and J. P. Kokko: Urea secretion by the straight segment of the proximal tubule, *J. Clin. Invest.*, **58:**604, 1976.

100. Armen, T., and H. W. Reinhardt: Transtubular movement of urea at a different degree of water diuresis, *Pfluegers Arch. Eur. J. Physiol.*, **326:**270, 1971.

101. Mudge, G. H., J. Foulks, and A. Gilman: Effect of urea diuresis on renal excretion of electrolytes, *Am. J. Physiol.*, **158:**218, 1949.

102. Wesson, L. G., Jr., and W. P. Anslow, Jr.: Excretion of sodium and water during osmotic diuresis in the dog, *Am. J. Physiol.*, **153:**465, 1948.

103. DeWardener, H. F., and F. del Greco: Influence

of solute excretion rate on production of hypotonic urine in man, *Clin. Sci.*, **14**:715, 1955.

104. Strauss, M. B., and L. G. Welt (eds.): *Diseases of the Kidney*, 2d ed., Little Brown and Company, Boston, 1971, vol. 2.

105. Tisher, C. C., R. W. Schrier, and J. S. McNeil: Nature of the urine concentration mechanism in the macaque monkey, *Am. J. Physiol.*, **223**:1128, 1972.

106. Jamison, R. L., and F. B. Lacy: Evidence for urinary dilution by the collecting tubule, *Am. J. Physiol.*, **223**:898, 1972.

107. Jamison, R. L., J. Buerkert, and F. B. Lacy: A micropuncture study of collecting tubule function in rats with hereditary diabetes insipidus, *J. Clin. Invest.*, **50**:2444, 1971.

108. Purkerson, M. L., H. Lubowitz, R. W. White, and N. S. Bricker: On the influence of extracellular fluid volume expansion on bicarbonate reabsorption in the rat, *J. Clin. Invest.*, **48**:1754, 1968.

109. Kurtzman, N., M. White, and P. Rogers: Effect of potassium and extracellular volume on renal bicarbonate reabsorption, *Metabolism*, **22**:481, 1973.

110. Crumb, C. K., M. Martinez-Maldonado, G. Eknoyan, and W. Suki: Effects of volume expansion, purified parathyroid extract and calcium on renal bicarbonate absorption in the dog, *J. Clin. Invest.*, **54**:1289, 1974.

111. Karlinsky, M., D. Sager, N. Kurtzman, and V. Pillay: Effect of parathormone and cyclic adenosine monophosphate on renal bicarbonate reabsorption, *Am. J. Physiol.*, **227**:1226, 1974.

112. Beck, N., K. Kim, M. Walak, and B. Davis: Inhibition of carbonic anhydrase by parathormone and cyclic AMP in rat renal cortex in vitro, *J. Clin. Invest.*, **55**:149, 1975.

113. Kumau, R. T., A. Frick, F. C. Rector, Jr., and D. W. Seldin: Micropuncture study of the proximal tubular factors responsible for the maintenance of alkalosis during potassium deficiency in the rat, *Clin. Sci.*, **34**:223, 1968.

114. Pitts, R. F., and R. S. Alexander: The nature of the renal tubular mechanisms for acidifying the urine, *Am. J. Physiol.*, **144**:239, 1945.

115. Rector, F. C., Jr., N. W. Carter, and D. W. Seldin: The mechanism of bicarbonate reabsorption in the proximal and distal tubules of the kidney, *J. Clin. Invest.*, **44**:278, 1965.

116. Vieira, F. L., and G. Malnic: Hydrogen ion secretion by rat renal cortical tubules as studies by antimony microelectrodes, *Am. J. Physiol.*, **214**:710, 1968.

117. Deetjen, P., and T. Maren: The dissociation between renal HCO_3^- reabsorption and H^+ secretion in the skate, *Raja crimacea*, *Pfluegers Arch.*, **346**:25, 1974.

118. Pitts, R. F.: Renal excretion of acid, *Fed. Proc.*, **7**:418, 1948.

119. Lotspeich, W. D.: Metabolic aspects of acid-base change, *Science*, **155**:1066, 1967.

120. Rector, F. C., Jr., and J. Orloff: The effect of the administration of sodium bicarbonate and ammonium chloride on the excretion and production of ammonia. The absence of alterations in the activity of renal ammonia-producing enzymes in the dog, *J. Clin. Invest.*, **38**:366, 1959.

121. Goldstein, L.: Actinomycin D inhibition of adaptation in the rat, *Nature*, **205**:1330, 1965.

122. Goodman, A. D., R. E. Fuisz, and G. F. Cahill, Jr.: Renal gluconeogenesis, in acidosis, alkalosis and potassium deficiency: Its possible role in regulation of renal ammonia production, *J. Clin. Invest.*, **45**:612, 1966.

123. Goorno, W. E., F. C. Rector, Jr., and D. W. Seldin: Relation of gluconeogenesis to ammonia production in the dog and rat, *Am. J. Physiol.*, **213**:969, 1967.

124. Kamm, D. E., R. E. Fuisz, A. D. Goodman, and G. F. Cahill: Acid-base alterations and renal gluconeogenesis: Effect of pH, bicarbonate concentration and P_{CO_2}, *J. Clin. Invest.*, **46**:1172, 1967.

125. Kamm, D. E.: Effect of acidosis and alkalosis on renal cortical glutamate metabolism, *Clin. Res.*, **17**:434, 1969, (Abstr.).

126. Preuss, H. G.: Pyridine nucleotides in renal ammonia metabolism, *J. Lab. Clin. Med.*, **72**:370, 1968.

127. Pitts, R. F., L. A. Pilkington, M. B. MacLeod, and E. Leal-Pinto: Metabolism of glutamine by the intact functioning kidney of the dog, Studies in metabolic acidosis and alkalosis, *J. Clin. Invest.*, **51**:557, 1972.

128. Pitts, R. F.: Control of renal production of ammonia, *Kidney Int.*, **1**:297, 1972.

129. Adam, W., and D. P. Simpson: Glutamine transport in rat kidney mitochondria in metabolic acidoses, *J. Clin. Invest.*, **54**:165, 1974.

130. McCance, R. A., and E. M. Widdowson: Alka-

losis with disordered kidney functions, *Lancet,* **233:**247, 1937.

131. Davidson, D. G., N. G. Levinsky, and R. W. Berliner: Maintenance of potassium excretion despite reduction of glomerular filtration during sodium diuresis, *J. Clin. Invest.,* **37:**548, 1958.

132. Bloomer, H. A., F. C. Rector, Jr., and D. W. Seldin: The mechanism of potassium reabsorption in the proximal tubule of the rat, *J. Clin. Invest.,* **42:**277, 1963.

133. Giebisch, G., G. Malnic, R. M. Klose, and E. E. Windhager: Effect of ionic substitutions on distal potential differences in the rat kidney, *Am. J. Physiol.,* **211:**560, 1966.

134. Litchfield, J. B., and P. A. Bott: Micropuncture study of the renal excretion of water, K, Na and Cl in the rat, *Am. J. Physiol.,* **203:**667, 1962.

135. Malnic, G., R. M. Klose, and G. Giebisch: Micropuncture study of distal tubular potassium and sodium transport in the rat nephron, *Am. J. Physiol.,* **211:**529, 1966.

136. Malnic, G., R. M. Klose, and G. Giebisch: Microperfusion study of distal tubular potassium and sodium-transfer in the rat kidney, *Am. J. Physiol.,* **211:**548, 1966.

137. Brenner, B. M., and R. W. Berliner: The transport of potassium, in J. Orloff and R. W. Berliner (eds.): *Handbook of Physiology,* sec. 8, *Renal Physiology,* American Physiology Society, Washington, D.C. 1973.

138. Barratt, L. J., F. C. Rector, J. P. Kokko, and D. W. Seldin: Factors governing the transepithelial potential difference across the proximal tubule of the rat kidney, *J. Clin. Invest.,* **53:**454, 1974.

139. Beck, L. H., D. Senesky, and M. L. Goldberg: Sodium independent active potassium reabsorption in proximal tubule of the dog, *J. Clin. Invest.,* **52:**2641, 1974.

140. deRouffignac, C., and F. Morel: Micropuncture study of water, electrolytes and urea movements along the loops of Henle in *Psammomys, J. Clin. Invest.,* **48:**474, 1969.

141. Jamison, R. L.: Micropuncture study of superficial and juxtamedullary nephrons in the rat, *Am. J. Physiol.,* **218:**46, 1970.

142. Rocha, A. S., and J. P. Kokko: Membrane characteristics regulating potassium transport out of the isolated perfused descending limb of Henle, *Kidney Int.,* **4:**326, 1973.

143. Wright, F. S.: Increasing magnitude of electrical potential along the renal distal tubule, *Am. J. Physiol.,* **220:**624, 1971.

144. Duarte, C. G., F. Chamety, and G. Giebisch: Effect of amiloide, ouabain and furosemide on distal tubular function in the rat, *Am. J. Physiol.,* **221:**632, 1971.

145. Mello-Aires, M. de., G. Giebisch, and G. Malnic: Kinetics of potassium transport across a single distal tubule of rat kidney, *J. Physiol. (London),* **232:**47, 1973.

146. Burg, M., L. Stoner, J. Cardinal, and N. Green: Furosemide effect on isolated perfused tubules, *Am. J. Physiol.,* **225:**119, 1973.

147. Stoner, L. C., M. B. Burg, and J. Orloff: Ion transport in cortical collecting tubule: Effect of amiloide, *Am. J. Physiol.,* **227:**453, 1974.

148. Berliner, R. W., T. J. Kennedy, and J. Orloff: Relationship between acidification of the urine and potassium metabolism, *Am. J. Med.,* **11:**274, 1951.

149. Malnic, G., M. de Mello-Aires, and G. Giebisch: Potassium transport across renal distal tubules during acid-base disturbances, *Am. J. Physiol.,* **221:**1192, 1971.

150. Seldin, D. W., L. G. Welt, and J. H. Kort: The role of sodium salt and adrenal steroids in the production of hypokalemic alkalosis, *Yale J. Med.,* **29:**229, 1956.

8

The divalent ion homeostatic system—physiology and metabolism of calcium, phosphorus, magnesium, and bone

A. M. PARFITT / M. KLEEREKOPER

INTRODUCTION AND SCOPE

There are several reasons for considering calcium, phosphorus, and magnesium together. In contrast to most other electrolytes, their major ionic species in body fluids are divalent. They all are important constituents of bone mineral, and they both affect and are affected by the metabolism and turnover of bone. They influence one another, are acted upon by the same agents, and are often disturbed in the same diseases.

This chapter presents the physiology of the divalent ions as a basis for understanding the clinical syndromes described in Chap. 19. The discussion will include the body content, distribution, and function, the relationships to the composition, structure, and turnover of bone, the normal pathways of absorption, transport, and excretion, the hormonal and nonhormonal control of ion movements, and how these elements fit together into a homeostatic system.

The physical chemistry of divalent ions is more complex than of univalent ions, and a brief account of the thermodynamic concept of ion activity must be given. Because of its charge, each ion in solution has an electrostatic field around it

which restricts the mobility of other ions and so reduces their potential for chemical reaction, referred to as activity or effective concentration (1). The ratio of effective to actual concentration is defined as the activity coefficient. This varies with pH and with temperature but is mainly a function of the total ionic strength of the solution. These factors are all fairly constant for blood, so that the usual practice of ignoring activity coefficient corrections to plasma concentrations leads to negligible error. Activity coefficients are both lower and more variable for divalent than for univalent ions (Table 8-1) and are important for the physicochemical state of the divalent ions in interstitial and intracellular fluids, for the equilibrium between interstitial fluid and bone mineral (and so for both mineralization and calcium homeostasis), and for the pathogenesis of both soft-tissue calcification and calcium-containing renal calculi.

As well as the nonspecific effects of ionic charge there are also specific effects due to ion-pair formation. For most strong electrolytes the constituent ions are either aggregated into crystals, linked by covalent bonds as amorphous solids, or fully dissociated in aqueous solution.

Table 8-1. Activity coefficients for major ions at ionic strength of plasma, 0.16

Na^+	0.74	Ca^{2+}	0.36
K^+	0.72	Mg^{2+}	0.40
Cl^-	0.72	HPO_4^{2-}	0.23
HCO_3^-	0.74	$H_2PO_4^-$	0.62

Source: From Neuman and Neuman (1).

Table 8-2. Comparison of different units for concentrations of divalent ions

	AW*	mmol/L	meq/L	mg/dL
Ca	40	1	2	4.0
Mg	24	1	2	2.4
P	31	1	1.8†	3.1

* AW = atomic weight.
† At pH 7.4 only (see text).

Weak electrolytes in solution remain partly undissociated and can also exist in another state, in which specific ions of opposite charge are held together by an electrostatic force but remain in solution (2). It is convenient to refer to such ion pairs as complexes even though the association is electrostatic rather than covalent. The ability to form ion pairs is much greater for multivalent than for monovalent ions (3). The reversible equilibrium between free ions and ion pairs can be described in terms of the law of mass action and hence by an association constant, just as with other chemical equilibria.

Throughout both this chapter and Chap. 19, SI units will be used where possible, and concentrations of substances in body fluids will usually be expressed in mmol/L; these are compared with more traditional units in Table 8-2. Because of its dependence on pH, the meq is an inconvenient unit for phosphate; the reasons for this dependence will be explained later. For convenience, concentrations of inorganic phosphate are normally expressed in terms of elemental phosphorus, and the qualifying term *inorganic* is omitted unless the context permits confusion with organic phosphate. The term *plasma phosphate* therefore refers to the plasma inorganic orthophosphate phosphorus.

BODY CONTENT AND DISTRIBUTION OF DIVALENT IONS

A major theme of this chapter will be the distinction between total body content of ions and their concentration in plasma and other body fluids. Some pertinent data are summarized in Table 8-3. They are based mainly on chemical analysis of cadavers (4); in vivo measurement of total body calcium and phosphorus by neutron activation and whole body counting gives results about 10 to 20 percent less than those based on chemical analysis (5). The values obviously will vary with age, sex, and the proportion of lean body mass to total body weight. Almost all the calcium in the body is in bone, so that the total body content of calcium depends almost entirely on the amount of bone, and changes in external balance depend almost entirely on the net movement of calcium in and out of bone. About 85 percent of total body phosphorus and 60 percent of total body magnesium is in bone, so that the total body content of phosphorus and magnesium is more dependent on changes in the soft tissues. The different body components listed in Table 8-3 will be discussed

Table 8-3. Representative values for normal body content and distribution of divalent ions

TISSUE	% BW	kg	Ca mmol/kg	Ca mmol	Ca % T	P mmol/kg	P mmol	P % T	Mg mmol/kg	Mg mmol	Mg % T
Bone	10	7	4500	31,350	99.5	2,700	19,000	85	120	840	65
Muscle	45	32	1.5	48		60	1,900	9	9	280	22
ECF*	20	14	2.5	35		1.2	17		0.9	13	
RBC†	3	2	0.02	0.04	0.05	20	40	6	4.0	8	13
Other	22	15	4.0	60		80	1,200		10	150	
Total (T)	100	70	450	31,500	100	320	22,200	100	20	1300	100

* ECF = extracellular fluid.
† RBC = red blood cells.

in more detail, beginning with the extracellular fluid (ECF).

TRANSPORT AND PHYSICAL STATE OF THE DIVALENT IONS IN THE ECF

The main difference between plasma and interstitial fluid is the protein content, which affects ion concentrations in three ways. The first is the distinction between plasma and plasma water. The proteins and other macromolecules in blood occupy about 6 percent of the total volume, so that the water content of plasma is normally about 94 mL/dL. A precise value can be calculated from the formula $99.5 - 0.8$ TP (6), where TP = total protein, but this formula takes no account of the possibility of protein binding of water. Ideally, all solute concentrations should be referred to plasma water rather than to plasma; this is usually disregarded but is important if the concentration of macromolecules is increased. Second, at the normal pH of blood the proteins behave as anions because many of the COOH groups are dissociated. Consequently, in a protein-free solution in equilibrium with plasma, preservation of electric neutrality requires that the concentration of cations be reduced and the concentration of other anions increased (Chap. 1). Such protein-free solutions may be generated either by dialysis, which involves net movement of ions but not of water, or by ultrafiltration, which involves net movement of water also. According to the Gibbs-Donnan theory of semipermeable membranes, charged macromolecules are treated as independent ions. Their restricted mobility across the membrane results in concentration differences for other ions which should be the same for all ions with the same charge (6, 7). An alternative theory, more in keeping with current concepts of the physical chemistry of macromolecules, is that the plasma proteins bind both water and a sufficient number of all cations in plasma to balance the anions exactly, thus forming nondiffusible complexes which carry no net charge (7). These different approaches have an important bearing on the interpretation of in vivo ultrafiltration experiments. According to the traditional concept, a Gibbs-Donnan correction must be applied to convert concentrations in an ultrafiltrate into concentrations in plasma water (6, 7), but according to the newer concept, ionic concentrations, or more accurately activities, are the same in an ultrafiltrate as in plasma water without the need to apply a Gibbs-Donnan correction (7). The Gibbs-Donnan correction factors for the divalent ions are given in Table 8-4. They are calculated from experimentally determined plasma: ultrafiltrate ratios for monovalent ions (6). Third, proteins have specific binding affinity for many ions, but the magnitude of this depends on how the nonspecific anion effect is calculated. Calculations of protein binding according to both the Gibbs-Donnan and the charge-neutralization concepts are shown in Table 8-4. The newer concept gives a lower value for protein-bound phosphate and higher values for protein-bound calcium and magnesium, which will be used in subsequent discussions.

Plasma calcium

Of the total calcium in plasma, about half is associated with various anions and about half is ionized. Strictly speaking, all calcium in the body is ionized, but the term usually refers to the free ionic fraction in blood which is physiologically active. This can be measured by spectrophotometry after ultrafiltration (8, 9), by potentiometry with a specific calcium ion electrode (10), or by gel filtration (11). Calcium that forms ion pairs with anions such as bicarbonate, or is bound to low-molecular-weight organic anions such as citrate, is collectively known as complexed calcium.

Table 8-4. Effect of plasma protein (7.2 g/dL) on divalent ion concentrations in plasma and plasma ultrafiltrates

	Ca	P	Mg
1. Plasma water correction factor	1.07	1.07	1.07
2. Gibbs-Donnan (G-D) correction factor	0.95	1.06	0.95
3. Predicted ultrafiltrable factor using G-D [(1) × (2)]	1.02	1.13	1.02
4. Measured ultrafiltrable factor	0.56	0.96	0.76
5. Degree of protein binding using G-D concept {100[1−(4)(3)]}	45%	15%	25%
6. Degree of protein binding using charge neutralization {100[1−(4)(1)]}	48%	10%	29%

Table 8-5. Representative values for plasma calcium fractions

	mmol/L	%
Free ions	1.10	44
Protein-bound	1.15	46
Complexed		
$\quad$ CaHCO$_3^-$	0.10	
$\quad$ CaHPO$_4$	0.04	
$\quad$ Ca citrate	0.04	
$\quad$ Unidentified	0.07	
$\quad$ Total complexed	0.25	10
Total diffusible	1.35	54
Total	2.50	100

Total diffusible = free ions + complexed.

Both ionized and complexed calcium will cross biologic or synthetic membranes, and so together they constitute the diffusible or ultrafiltrable calcium (Table 8-5), which has been determined in a variety of ways. Protein-bound calcium is non-diffusible or nonultrafiltrable. About nine-tenths of this fraction is bound to albumin and about one-tenth to various globulins (12). The binding of calcium to albumin occurs by chelation to a pair of adjacent carboxyl groups on glutamyl or aspartyl residues (13, 14). There are about 12 independent binding sites per albumin molecule, each having a critical three-dimensional relationship to the imidazole group of an adjacent histidine residue, which acts as an electron donor (13, 14). The apparent association constant varies with both ionic strength and pH but is unaffected by temperature. The normal plasma albumin concentration is about 0.7 mmol/L, so that with a free ionized calcium of 1.1 mmol/L only about 10 to 15 percent of the binding sites are occupied. Consequently, when excess calcium is added to blood, either in vitro or in vivo, all the fractions increase in the same proportion, and the ultrafiltrable fraction as a percentage of the total does not change (15). This could be predicted from the equilibrium defined by McLean and Hastings (16), who first analyzed the relationship of calcium to protein in detail. According to their formulation, Ca^{2+} + protein^{2-} = Ca protein, so that:

$$\frac{[Ca^{2+}] \times [\text{protein}^{2-}]}{[\text{Ca protein}]} = k \qquad (8\text{-}1)$$

where Ca protein + protein^{2-} = total protein, and k is the dissociation constant. A graphic representation of this equation is shown in Fig. 8-1. From the same equilibrium it also follows that the percent of ultrafiltrable calcium varies with the concentration of protein; all such values given in the text or in the tables assume a normal plasma protein level of 7.2 g/dL. The protein binding of calcium therefore acts as a buffer which reduces by about half the change in ionized calcium resulting from acute gains or losses of calcium by the blood. This does not seem to apply in the rat, in which calcium infusion produces almost as much increase in diffusible calcium as in total calcium (17). Another consequence of the large excess of unfilled binding sites is that competition for binding by magnesium has no significant effect on ionized calcium (15). Adding phosphate to blood in vitro has no effect on ultrafiltrable calcium until the total inorganic phosphate concentration is about 6 mmol/L (15), so that any effect seen in vivo is due to factors other than simple saturation of blood. The most important factor modifying the binding is pH, an increase in pH causing an increase in binding and a fall in ionized calcium concentration and vice versa. This is due partly to competition between H^+ ions and Ca^{2+} ions for the binding sites (13) but also involves changes in conformation of the albumin molecule (14). Changes in P_{CO_2} do not affect calcium binding other than via changes in pH (6, 18).

The concentration of the complexed fraction is less certain, because it is usually estimated as the difference between free ionized calcium and ultrafiltrable calcium, but direct measurement of the major complexes has recently been accomplished by gel filtration (11). Complexed calcium includes calcium bound to organic ions such as citrate, isocitrate, and lactate (1, 8) and forming ion pairs with inorganic ions such as HPO_4^{2-} and HCO_3^- (1, 12). According to the most recent estimates, the $CaHCO_3^+$ ion pair is the most abundant single form of complexed calcium (11, 18). This provides another mechanism whereby changes in pH lead to changes in free ionized calcium, since a rise in pH will lead to a rise in HCO_3^-, increased formation of the $CaHCO_3^+$ complex, and a fall in ionized calcium. However, the combined effect of both mechanisms is to produce a change in ionized calcium of only 0.04 mmol/L for each 0.1-unit change in pH (10, 18). The metabolic alka-

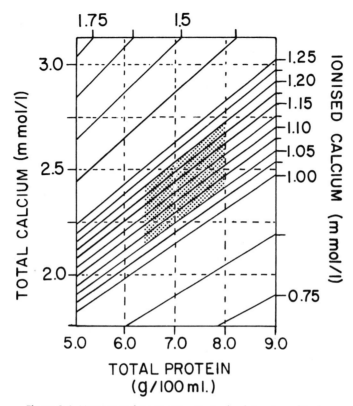

Figure 8-1. Nomogram for estimating ionized calcium (mmol/L of plasma water) from total calcium (mmol/L of plasma) and total protein (g/dL of plasma). (*From McLean and Hastings.*)

losis associated with gastric acid secretion produces a relatively greater change, possibly also caused by increased calcitonin secretion (19). The possible importance of calcium complexes with citrate and isocitrate in regulating the urinary excretion of calcium is discussed later. Representative values for concentrations of plasma calcium fractions are given in Table 8-5.

Plasma phosphate

Using 10% trichloracetic acid, the total phosphorus in plasma can be divided into an acid-insoluble fraction comprising mainly phospholipids and an acid-soluble fraction comprising a small amount of organic ester phosphate and all of the inorganic phosphate (Table 8-6) (20). Inorganic orthophosphate is distributed among four ionic

species resulting from the successive dissociation of orthophosphoric acid (Fig. 8-2):

$$H_3PO_4 \rightleftharpoons H^+ + H_2PO_4^-$$
$$\rightleftharpoons H^+ + HPO_4^{2-} \rightleftharpoons H^+ + PO_4^{3-} \quad (8\text{-}2)$$

This equilibrium is governed by pH, and over the pH range of body fluids the concentrations of undissociated phosphoric acid and fully dissociated trivalent phosphate are extremely small and for most purposes can be disregarded (12). At pH 7.4

Table 8-6. Partition of total plasma phosphorus into different fractions, with concentrations in mmol/L

Acid-soluble	1.30
Organic ester	0.10
Inorganic*	1.20
Acid-insoluble (phospholipids)	2.60
Total	3.90

* Inorganic includes orthophosphate and pyrophosphate.

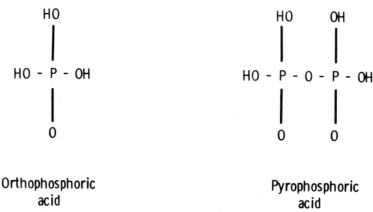

Orthophosphoric
acid

Pyrophosphoric
acid

Figure 8-2. Structures of phosphoric acids of biologic importance.

the concentration ratio $HPO_4^{2-}:H_2PO_4^-$ is 4:1, so that the apparent valence is 1.8, but the activity ratio (Table 8-1) is only 1.5:1. The ionic radius of $H_2PO_4^-$ is smaller than of HPO_4^{2-}, and partly for this reason the monovalent and divalent ions may be transported differently across cells and their membranes. Consequently, changes in their proportion brought about by changes in pH may be of physiologic importance. Inorganic phosphate also includes pyrophosphate, which comprises the anions produced by the dissociation of pyrophosphoric acid, $H_4P_2O_7$ (Fig. 8-2). The concentration of pyrophosphate in body fluids is very small—about 3 μmol/L in plasma (21)—but it has important functions in bone which are quite distinct from those of orthophosphate.

Based on comparison of the measured ultrafiltrable phosphate concentration (9, 15) with that predicted from the charge neutralization concept (Table 8-4), about 10 percent of the inorganic phosphate is nondiffusible and presumably protein-bound, but nothing is known of the protein concerned or the nature of the binding. Using in vivo ultrafiltration by prolonged venous occlusion, less than 5 percent of plasma phosphate was nondiffusible (6). Calculations using previously published stability constants suggested that sodium phosphate was the most abundant complex (9), but a more recent analysis indicated that at concentrations found in biological fluids complexing of phosphate to sodium does not occur

(22). The values for free phosphate ions shown in Table 8-7 are derived by subtracting the value for protein-bound phosphate and the calculated values for the calcium and magnesium complexes (9, 12) and dividing the remainder in the ratio of 4:1. No direct measurements of free phosphate ion concentrations in biologic fluids are available. When calcium is added to serum in vitro, above a concentration of about 4.5 to 5.0 mmol/L there is a fall in the ultrafiltrable phosphate, usually ascribed to the formation of a nondiffusible colloidal complex of calcium phosphate with protein (23), but this does not occur in normal conditions. In the presence of a normal total calcium, raising the phosphate concentration as high as 8 mmol/L does not affect the diffusibility of phosphate or calcium (15).

Table 8-7. Representative values for plasma inorganic orthophosphate fractions

	mmol/L	%
Free HPO_4^{2-}	0.81	68
Free $H_2PO_4^-$	0.20	17
Protein-bound	0.12	10
Complexed		
$CaHPO_4$	0.04	
$MgHPO_4$	0.03	
Total complexed	0.07	5
Total diffusible*	1.08	
Total	1.20	100

* Total diffusible = free ions + complexed ions.

Plasma magnesium

Like calcium, magnesium is also bound to plasma proteins, mainly albumin, and the mechanism and sites of binding are the same as for calcium (13, 24). Measurements of ultrafiltrable magnesium are less consistent than for calcium, results varying from 60 to 80 percent (12, 25). Since the binding sites appear not to discriminate between Ca and Mg, and since the proportion of complexes to free ions is about the same for both, the reason for the lesser protein binding of magnesium is not clear. If the protein-bound magnesium is taken as 0.21 mmol/L (Table 8-8), less than 5 percent of the binding sites on albumin are normally occupied by magnesium, and calcium and magnesium together occupy less than 20 percent of the total binding sites. A normal level of calcium reduces magnesium binding by about 12 percent and a normal level of magnesium reduces calcium binding by about 5 percent (13). The effect of pH on binding is qualitatively the same as for calcium, but no data on the magnitude of this effect in human beings are available.

There is not yet a specific ion electrode for magnesium, and the available data for ionized magnesium are based on spectrophotometry (9) or ion-exchange adsorption (26). By analogy with calcium it is likely that $MgHCO_3^+$ is the most abundant complex, but no data are available. The values for the other complexes shown in Table 8-8 were calculated from published association constants (9, 12).

Table 8-8. Representative values for plasma magnesium fractions

	mmol/L	%
Free ions	0.50	60
Protein bound	0.21	25
Complexed		
$MgHCO_3$	?	
$MgHPO_4$	0.03	
Mg citrate	0.04	
Unidentified	?	
Total complexed	0.13	15
Total diffusible*	0.63	
Total	0.84	100

* Total diffusible = free ions + complexed ions.

Interstitial fluid and connective tissue

The concept that all extravascular and extracellular fluid has the same composition, the *milieu intérieur* of Claude Bernard, must be modified in the light of increasing evidence that each organ regulates the composition of its own interstitial fluid for its own special needs (27). Nevertheless, the water of connective tissue throughout the body must normally be in osmotic equilibrium with the plasma, from which it is separated only by capillary endothelium. It is widely assumed that this endothelium behaves as a semipermeable membrane and that interstitial fluid is an ultrafiltrate or dialysate of plasma, with a very low protein content and a composition determined by the principles already outlined. This simple model may be adequate for monovalent ions, but for the divalent ions the position is more complex. In many organs the capillary endothelium is more permeable to protein than is supposed by the model (28, 29). Studies with labeled albumin indicate that about 40 percent of the protein in plasma enters tissue fluid each day and that as much as 50 percent of the total exchangeable pool of plasma proteins is outside the blood (30). If this is distributed throughout the remainder of the ECF, the interstitial fluid protein concentration would be about 1.4 g/dL, assuming a plasma protein level of 7.2 g/dL, a plasma volume of 3 L, and a total ECF volume of 18 L (31). Direct measurements of interstitial fluid protein concentration in human beings are not available, but in lymph, values from 1.1 to 2.4 g/dL have been found (29). In rat subcutaneous tissue fluid, obtained by implanting a Millipore filter diffusion chamber for 4 weeks, the protein content was about 60 percent of the plasma level (32). Capillary permeability may have been increased by a chronic inflammatory response to the foreign body, but this would not apply to fluid obtained by micropuncture from guinea pig muscle, which had a protein content of 40 percent of the plasma level (33). Even the smallest of these various estimates of interstitial fluid protein content would significantly modify the total calcium and magnesium concentrations.

A more important defect in the simple model is

that it fails to confront the central paradox that the bulk of the so-called extracellular fluid is not fluid at all (34). To explain why this is so, a brief digression must be made into the structure and chemistry of connective tissue (35), a topic which is also important for the understanding of bone. As well as joining all the cells of the body together, connective tissue mediates all transport between the capillaries and the cells in a manner which reflects the space-filling, water-adsorbing, and cation-binding properties of the ground substance. The main chemical constituents of ground substance are a family of macromolecules called glycosaminoglycans (GAG) or acid mucopolysaccharides. These are long-chain polymers, each repeating unit comprising a uronic acid and a glycosamine. All the COOH groups of the uronic acids of the GAG molecules are fully dissociated at physiologic pH, and so are negatively charged. The most abundant GAG is hyaluronic acid (HA), in which the repeating unit consists of glucuronic acid and acetyl glucosamine. This is a single-chain unbranched molecule of enormous length (2 to 3 μm) containing several thousand repeating units (molecular weight $> 10^6$) arranged in a random coil; it has a small peptide at one end. In chondroitins 4-sulfate and 6-sulfate, the repeating unit has sulfated galactosamine instead of glucosamine. The SO_3H groups are also fully dissociated and negatively charged. The chains are much shorter, but a large number of them are attached to a central polypeptide core to form a proteoglycan (PG) or protein polysaccharide, so that the total molecule may be even larger than HA. Both HA and PG are diffuse molecules that are dispersed over a large volume of water in much the same way that the branches of a tree are dispersed in space (35). The total volume thus occupied by a diffuse macromolecule is known as its domain, which may be 10^3 to 10^4 times as large as the volume of its constituent atoms and as much as 0.4 μm in diameter. Within a domain, movement of water, ions, and other solutes is restricted, and some larger molecules may be excluded completely. Solutions of HA and PG molecules either form viscous liquids or, at the temperature of the body, they may adsorb and immobilize a large volume of water to form gels,

which are elastic and deformable but not fluid. These are given greater rigidity by the formation of three-dimensional networks with the collagen and reticulin fibrils, which are either wrapped around by the coiled HA molecules (35) or covalently bound to PG molecules (36). Further strength is given by the entanglement of adjacent diffuse molecules at the periphery of their domains. There is thus formed a structure which prevents the macroscopic flow of water (37) and resists the extrusion of water by compression (38), even though it contains a large quantity of water and permits the slow diffusion of water and ions, both through and between the domains. A unified concept of the ground substance, consistent with both electrochemical measurements and with electron microscopic appearances, views it as a two-phase gel (39). One phase has a low-water, high-colloid content, with a high density of negative charge, and the other phase consists of submicroscopic vacuoles of high-water, low-colloid content, which permits greater diffusion of water and ions. All interstitial water is a component of one or the other phase, and the proportion between the two phases varies between different tissues and in the same tissue at different times, probably because of variation in the degree of GAG aggregation.

The density of negative charge varies from 25 to 170 meq/kg tissue water in different connective tissues (40) and is even higher than this within the domains. The charges are fixed, not only because the COO^- and SO_3^- groups cannot escape from the domains but because movement of the entire domain through tissue space is restricted. This has complex effects on the concentration and flow of ions within the ground substance. Each domain tends to accumulate cations and to exclude anions, to form a macromolecule-water-cation complex which carries no net charge (41), analogous to the uncharged protein-water-cation complexes present in blood. For most GAGs the order of affinity for cations is Ca > Mg > Na > K (35, 41). As well as nonspecific electrostatic attraction of all cations, these affinities reflect more specific binding of divalent ions. The calcium-binding capacity per gram of chondroitin SO_4 (CS) is 20 times greater than of albumin (42) and can be as high as one atom of calcium for each glucuronic acid unit (43). At physiologic pH, the affinity of CS for calcium is fairly low (44); nevertheless, the presence of CS in solution increases the total calcium concentration by 25 percent and reduces the phosphate concentration by 10 percent (43). Calcium binding is greater to PGs than to nonaggregated GAGs, probably because of chelate formation with pairs of SO_3^- or COO^- groups on adjacent GAG chains on the PG molecule (45). Hyaluronic acid binds calcium more avidly than nonaggregated CS. Assuming that ionic activities are the same throughout the water phase in equilibrium with blood, indirect estimates based on potential difference measurements between different tissues indicate that the ionized calcium and magnesium levels in tissue water are about 1½ to 2 times those in plasma in loose connective and subcutaneous tissue, and even higher in dense connective tissue (40), although in the absence of a separate fluid phase the concept of concentration is somewhat ill-defined.

Unfortunately, confirmation of these estimates by direct analysis is not possible, and there are no data for the divalent ion composition of normal human interstitial fluid. Edema fluid obtained by drainage through Southey's tube has a very low protein content (46, 47) and the same calcium content as an ultrafiltrate of plasma (47, 48); however, a large increase in volume and consequent dilution of macromolecules abolishes the special character of interstitial fluid, so that measurements made on edema fluid give no useful information on normal tissue fluid (34). Calculated concentrations of ionized calcium and magnesium are about 5 to 15 percent higher than in plasma in fluids accumulating in the pleural and peritoneal spaces (which should be in equilibrium with interstitial fluid) (28, 49), and about 50

percent higher than plasma in lymph (28). Phosphate levels are usually close to the plasma level in both edema and pleural fluid (49) but are only about half the plasma level in lymph (28). The values for calcium and phosphate in rat subcutaneous fluid (32) are given in Table 8-9; the calcium level is probably consistent with the protein level, but the phosphate level is lower than expected.

It is evident from the foregoing that the total quantity of divalent ions in interstitial fluid is very uncertain and probably quite variable. Calculations based on total plasma concentrations are probably closer to the truth than the more usual calculations based on plasma ultrafiltrable concentrations, but small changes in the physicochemical state of connective tissue macromolecules could significantly modify the amount of mineral sequestered within their domains.

Apart from plasma, the only other readily accessible component of the ECF is the cerebrospinal fluid (CSF), but this is not, as was once hoped, a simple ultrafiltrate of plasma (28). The CSF calcium is lower and the CSF magnesium higher than the corresponding values in plasma ultrafiltrates (50). Furthermore, both levels are probably regulated in some manner, since the CSF calcium responds only minimally to clinical or experimental variation in plasma calcium (51).

INTRACELLULAR AND SOFT-TISSUE CONTENT OF DIVALENT IONS

The composition of any organ is determined by the composition and relative amounts of its cells, connective tissue, and interstitial fluid, but most analyses of tissue have not attempted to separate these three components.

Table 8-9. Divalent ion content of rat subcutaneous interstitial fluid

	INTERSTITIAL FLUID (IF)		ULTRAFILTRATE OF IF	
	CONCENTRATION	% PLASMA	CONCENTRATION	% IF
Ca (mmol/L)	2.20	88	1.56	71
P (mmol/L)	1.77	84	1.63	92
Protein (g/dL)	5.09	62	0.04	0.5

Source: From Rasmussen (32).

Calcium

The calcium content of organs other than bone varies from 1 to 10 mmol/kg of tissue (4). This wide variation reflects mainly differences in the kind and amount of connective tissue, since much of the tissue calcium is bound to the GAGs or PGs of the ground substance, or to acidic phospholipids in the cell membrane. The calcium content of red cells (Table 8-3) is only about 0.02 mmol/L (52). An additional compartment, located outside the cell membrane but separated from interstitial fluid by a barrier of high-molecular-weight proteins, has been found in skeletal and cardiac muscle (53). The calcium concentration within this compartment is higher than in ECF, providing a local reservoir of calcium to sustain the contractile properties of these cells. The calcium content of the interstitial fluid of muscle is about 1.6 mmol/kg water, similar to the estimated value for other tissues (54). The calcium content of many tissues increases progressively with age because of dystrophic mineralization of connective tissue.

The calcium inside cells may be complexed with other ions, such as orthophosphate or pyrophosphate, or bound to organic molecules, such as ATP, but much the largest part is sequestered within organelles such as mitochondria or the sarcoplasmic reticulum (55). The free cytosol calcium concentration is usually estimated to be 10^{-3} mmol/L or less, corresponding to an ECF/ICF gradient of more than 1000:1 (56–58), but may be up to 10 times greater at normal body temperature (59).

Phosphate

Most of the soft-tissue and intracellular (IC) phosphorus is in the form of organic phosphate compounds such as phosphorylated intermediates of glycolysis, creatine phosphate, and adenosine mono-, di-, and triphosphates, an account of which would encompass the whole field of biochemistry and so is outside the scope of this chapter. In the red cell, the major phosphate-containing component is 2,3-diphosphoglycerate. The total IC inorganic phosphate in the liver is about twice the ECF level (60), but the free inorganic phosphate concentration in cell cytosol is only about half of the ECF concentration (61, 62); in the red cell this relationship holds when the plasma level varies between 0.6 and 1.8 mmol/L (63). Phosphate is frequently referred to as a major intracellular anion, but its contribution to the ionic structure of IC water is quite small. Organic phosphate compounds, particularly adenosine phosphate, behave as anions at the pH inside cells; for example, ATP has an effective valence of 3.5 and provides about 10 to 30 meq/L of anion (64). Like calcium, much of the IC inorganic phosphate is bound to other ions (including calcium and magnesium) or is sequestered within mitochondria or other organelles. The IC inorganic phosphate is normally in equilibrium with both EC phosphate and IC glyceraldehyde-3-phosphate. This is the point at which inorganic phosphate enters the glycolytic pathway to form 1,3-diphosphoglycerate and so to participate in the regeneration of ATP. Because of the relatively constant composition of cells, gains or losses of nitrogen by the body are usually accompanied by corresponding gains or losses of extraosseous phosphorus. For muscle, the molar ratio of phosphorus to nitrogen is 0.03 (65, 66), and with muscle-wasting, phosphorus and nitrogen are lost from the cells in this proportion (66). The relationship between potassium, the major IC cation, and phosphate is more variable. Glycogen deposition in the liver is accompanied by influx of potassium but not of phosphate (67), but loss of potassium from muscle as a result of hypokalemia is accompanied by loss of phosphorus in a molar ratio (P/K) of about 0.6 (66).

Magnesium

Like calcium, some tissue magnesium is bound to connective tissue macromolecules, but the proportion of the total is smaller. Magnesium is frequently listed as a major IC cation, but indirect estimates of the free cytosol concentration give values which vary between 0.2 mmol/L for red cells (68) and 1.0 mmol/kg in liver (69), or from about 0.25 to 1.2 times the ECF concentration, so that its contribution to the ionic structure of IC water is negligible. Total IC magnesium content is about 10 times higher; for example, total red cell magnesium is 2.0 mmol/L (70). About 80 percent of muscle magnesium is nonelutable (71) and cannot readily be mobilized (72). Some IC magnesium is in the form of magnesium-containing metalloenzymes, but much is bound to other ions, such as orthophosphate and pyrophosphate (64), or to such organic compounds as ATP (73) or protein (69), or is sequestered within mitochondria. The total IC binding sites are normally about one-half saturated and so serve to stabilize the IC free magnesium concentration (69). The total IC magnesium in many tissues is about one-tenth of total IC phosphate; there is an approximate relationship between the metabolic activity of a cell and its ionic composition, active cells tending to have higher total concentrations of K, Mg, and P and lower concentrations of Na and Ca (74). The magnesium content of muscle is closely correlated with the potassium content (25, 66), and in potassium depletion, magnesium is lost with potassium in a molar ratio (Mg/K) of 0.05, but the reason for this is not known. Possibly both potassium and magnesium are linked in some way with glycogen stores or with structural cytoplasmic proteins.

CELLULAR AND SUBCELLULAR ASPECTS OF DIVALENT ION METABOLISM

Transcellular movements of divalent ions

The magnitude of the concentration gradient between EC and IC fluids is much greater for calcium than for phosphate or magnesium. As with sodium, the lowest ECF concentration of calcium compatible with life would still be far above the IC concentration, so that passive loss of IC ion cannot occur. By contrast, with depletion of either inorganic phosphate or magnesium, the ECF concentration may fall below the normal IC level so that substantial loss of IC ion can occur by passive diffusion.

For both sodium and calcium, the large electrochemical gradient between the ECF and ICF is presumed to be maintained by active transport across the cell membrane (56–58). In cardiac muscle and nerve, calcium extrusion is directly coupled to sodium transport, but in red cell and liver, calcium and sodium transport are independent (75). Ion transport is easily depressed by cell injury leading to a rise in intracellular sodium or calcium or both. The cell membrane is much less permeable to calcium than to sodium, so that much less energy is consumed by the calcium pump than by the sodium pump (57). The low cytosol calcium ion concentration is also maintained by active transport into and release from mitochondria and microsomes (55–58, 76), which may be more important than the cell membrane pump in the minute-to-minute regulation of cytosol calcium concentration (56, 76). Mitochondria accumulate calcium and phosphate ions together to form insoluble amorphous tricalcium phosphate (76), a reaction which releases H^+ ions into the cytosol. Consequently, deficiency of intracellular phosphate reduces mitochondrial calcium uptake; uptake of phosphate may be the primary event most directly coupled to electron transport (77). Mitochondria also accumulate calcium in a form which can be rapidly released. A substantial influx of calcium may exceed the limited capacity of the organelles to store calcium phosphate so that calcium overload may lead to mitochondrial disruption and cell injury (78).

Much less is known about the transmembrane movements of phosphate and magnesium. For a membrane potential of -60 mV, the intracellular phosphate concentration should be much lower than the indirectly estimated value determined by passive diffusion of about half the EC concentration, suggesting active inward transport. The movement of inorganic phosphate into cells which follows the administration of glucose, insulin, or epinephrine (79) is consistent with this, but obviously other explanations are possible. In the red cell HPO_4^{2-} enters and leaves by either passive or facilitated diffusion (63), but $H_2PO_4^-$ is transported by a saturable mobile carrier (80). Conversely, in the isolated kidney cell, $H_2PO_4^-$ moves by passive diffusion, and the cell membrane is much less permeable to HPO_4^{2-} (81). A similar difference is found in mitochondria, which are impermeable to HPO_4^{2-} but accumulate

$H_2PO_4^-$ against a concentration gradient by means of a phosphate carrier (64). In several systems, including nerve fibers and cultured tumor cells, both influx and efflux of phosphate are dependent largely on simultaneous transport of sodium (82, 83). The relationship of transepithelial phosphate transport to sodium will be considered in a later section.

For magnesium, if the indirect estimate of cytosol concentration is correct, both active extrusion from the cell and active uptake by mitochondria would be necessary, but little is known of the details except that both cell membrane and mitochondrial pumps are probably less active than for calcium, since the gradients are much smaller (61).

Exchangeable pools of divalent ions

When an ion labeled with a radioactive tracer is injected into the blood in vivo, the rate of disappearance of the radioactivity can be extrapolated back to the time of injection to estimate the amount in which the tracer appears to be distributed. This is referred to as the exchangeable or miscible pool. Although many of the assumptions underlying such analysis are open to serious question, the concept of the exchangeable pool is useful if not overinterpreted. If the size of the pool were fixed, it would determine the extent of change in plasma concentration which would result from short-term gains or losses of the ion in question, but, as will be demonstrated, the complexity of the exchanges between ECF and bone precludes such a simple relationship. For calcium, the exchangeable pool is about 1 percent of the total body calcium or about 250 mmol (84). This includes all of the calcium in the ECF, most of the connective tissue and cell membrane calcium, and about 0.5 percent of the calcium in bone.

In man, ^{32}P given IV is distributed over most of the ECF within a few minutes. The rapidly exchangeable pool is about 0.6 mmol/kg body weight, and the pool turns over about 10 times daily (85). The pool size is about double the total ECF phosphate, and the rest of the pool is presumably all intracellular. How much of this is available to buffer short-term changes in the plasma in man is not known. Exchangeable phosphate in bone will be considered in a later section. Radioactive phosphate is incorporated so quickly into organic compounds that conclusions concerning the kinetics of inorganic phosphate transport cannot be drawn from such experiments with any confidence (86). The tissue turnover of phosphate determined by the rapidity of ^{32}P exchange is primarily a function of the rate of glycolysis and so is high in red cells, intermediate in liver and heart, and low in resting muscle and nervous tissue (87).

For magnesium, the exchangeable pool in man is about 2 mmol/kg body weight (88–90), which is about 10 percent of the total body magnesium. This presumably includes all of the ECF magnesium, but the location of the remainder is unclear. In vitro, about 20 to 30 percent of the magnesium in bone (91) and muscle (71, 72) is both exchangeable and readily elutable, but if the same applied in vivo, the exchangeable pool would be about 25 percent of the total body magnesium. Both in the dog and in the sheep, magnesium in muscle is much less readily exchangeable than in other soft tissues, especially the heart (92, 93). The value of 2 mmol/kg probably includes about 1 percent of magnesium in bone and about 20 percent of magnesium in muscle and other soft tissues. Bone magnesium will be further considered in a later section.

Metabolic functions of divalent ions

Many functions can be assigned to the divalent ions on the basis of in vitro experiments. At the cellular and subcellular level, the need for ionic calcium is ubiquitous. It plays an essential role in cell aggregation and communication, membrane integrity and permeability, microtubular function, ion transfer, cell division and growth, blood coagulation, skeletal and cardiac muscle contraction, and in coupling a wide variety of electric, chemical, and hormonal stimuli to their responses (61, 94–97). Apart from its role in the regulation of bone mineralization and turnover, which will be considered later, inorganic phosphate is important mainly in regulating the intracellular distribution of calcium and magnesium, and as a substrate for the regeneration of ATP from ADP. This occurs directly in the mitochondria via oxidative phosphorylation and indirectly in the cytosol via anaerobic glycolysis. Inorganic phosphate also participates directly in the phosphorylation of glycogen to glucose-1-phosphate, an action catalyzed by phosphorylase-a (64). Magnesium functions as a chelating agent in many biologic systems (98) and is essential for the activation of a variety of enzymes, including adenylate cyclase, ATPase, and enzymes involved in many aspects of intermediary metabolism, protein synthesis, and the transfer of genetic information (64, 98, 99). However, for most of the many vital functions dependent on the divalent ions, a significant impairment occurs only at concentrations lower than could ever exist in vivo. The physiologic functions of the divalent ions, which are important to an understanding of the clinical effects of excess or deficiency, will be examined in Chap. 19.

BONE AND BONE MINERAL IN RELATION TO DIVALENT ION METABOLISM

THE COMPOSITION AND STRUCTURE OF BONE IN RELATION TO MINERAL HOMEOSTASIS (100–103)

Bone is a specialized connective tissue that consists of a mineralized organic matrix in which cells are dispersed. The matrix comprises fibers of collagen within a ground substance containing abundant PG and glycoprotein complexes. Bone mineral contains mainly calcium, phosphate, and carbonate in an approximate molar ratio of 10:6:1 with variable amounts of magnesium, sodium, potassium, chloride, citrate, fluoride, and pyrophosphate (Table 8-10) (104). Young bone contains about 30 percent organic material by volume, about 40 percent mineral, and about 30 percent water, of which 20 percent is in the tissues and 10 percent bound to the crystals of mineral; in old bone the water content is only about 3 percent (1).

Table 8-10. Major ions in bone mineral*

CATION		ANION	
Ca^{2+}	6.66	PO_4^{3-}	4.02
Mg^{2+}	0.18	CO_3^{2-}	0.79
Na^+	0.32	Citrate^{3-}	0.05
K^+	0.02	Cl^-	0.02

* Expressed in mmol/g of dry, fat-free bone.
Source: From Armstrong and Singer (104).

Bone matrix (102, 103)

The fibrous protein collagen accounts for about 90 percent by weight of bone matrix. Of total body collagen, which represents about one-third of total body protein, about 60 percent is in bone and about 30 percent is in skin. The tropocollagen macromolecule is a semirigid rod about 300 nm long and 1.5 nm wide, composed of three polypeptide α chains, each containing about 1000 amino acid residues. Each α chain forms a helix around its own long axis, and the three α chains are coiled around each other like a piece of rope. Glycine (32 percent), alanine (13 percent), proline (11 percent), and hydroxyproline (11 percent) are the most abundant amino acids in the α chain, and tryptophane and cystine are absent. Hydroxyproline and hydroxylysine (0.6 percent) are found only in connective tissue proteins. The tropocollagen molecules are arranged end to end in a parallel and overlapping manner to form fibrils, but the precise three-dimensional organization which gives rise to the typical cross-banding at 70-nm intervals is uncertain (105, 106). The fibrils each have a central core of ground substance similar to that in which they are embedded (107).

The ground substance of bone is organized in a way similar to that of other connective tissues, but glycoproteins are more abundant. Like PGs, these are protein-carbohydrate complexes, but the side chains are mostly 1- to 3-unit oligosaccharides of many different kinds, so that a higher proportion of the molecule is protein (103). Some glycoproteins containing sialic acid are specific for bone; they are bound to chondroitin sulfate, the commonest GAG in bone, and, like PGs, have a high binding capacity for divalent ions.

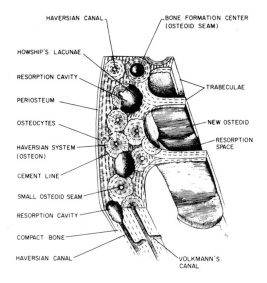

CROSS AND LONGITUDINAL SECTION OF BONE SHOWING THE REMODELING UNITS
IN CORTICAL BONE AND ON ENDOSTEAL SURFACES

Figure 8-3. Diagram of bone structure to show anatomic relationship between the periosteal, haversian, cortical endosteal, and trabecular endosteal surfaces. (*Courtesy of Z. F. G. Jaworski.*)

Bone structure (100, 101)

A typical bone (an organ) has solid cortical bone (tissue) on the outside and a network of plates and bars about 200 μm thick known as trabeculae on the inside, between which is the hematopoietic marrow. This arrangement gives rise to four surfaces—periosteal, intracortical or haversian, inner cortical or cortical endosteal, and trabecular endosteal, the latter three being in continuity (Fig. 8-3). Each of these surfaces is always in one of three functional states (Fig. 8-4): forming surfaces are covered by osteoblasts, resorbing surfaces by osteoclasts, and quiescent surfaces by flat lining cells. These cells, sometimes referred to as resting osteoblasts or surface osteocytes, separate the bone from the bone marrow or from the contents of haversian canals (Fig. 8-5). Although they appear to be in contact, the electron microscope reveals gaps between them through which large molecules can readily pass. Trabecular bone provides only 20 percent of the total volume of bone but nearly 70 percent of the total surface. The structural unit of cortical bone is the haversian

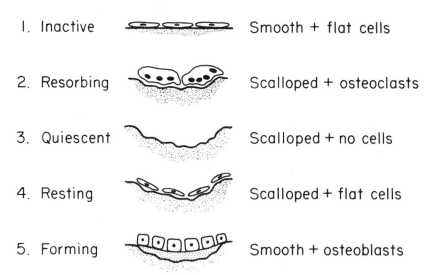

Figure 8-4. Diagrammatic representation of different states of the bone surface during normal remodeling, classified on the basis of surface configuration and endosteal cell morphology.

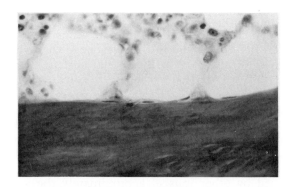

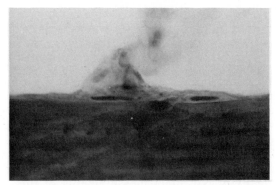

Figure 8-5. Flat endosteal lining cells of human trabecular bone separating bone marrow above from bone below. Upper panel ×400; lower panel ×1000. (*Courtesy of A. R. Villanueva.*)

system, or osteon. This is a cylinder of concentric lamellae about 200 μm in diameter, with its long axis roughly parallel to that of the bone. It has a central canal about 60 μm in diameter containing blood vessels which are continuous at the endosteal surface with those of the bone marrow (100). Bone contains lacunae and canaliculi within which are osteocytes and their cell processes, maintaining contact with each other and with the cells on the surface. In the young adult no part of the bone is farther than 20 μm from a living cell or farther than 5 μm from a canaliculus.

The circulation of bone, macro and micro

Bone has an abundant blood supply, with estimates ranging from 2.5 to 20 mL per 100 g/min, or from 5 to 25 percent of the cardiac output (108, 109). Even the lowest figure is far higher than is needed to support the metabolic demands of the

tissue. The passage of mineral ions and water from blood to bone can be traced from the arterioles and capillaries, through the ground substance of the connective tissue in the bone marrow or within haversian canals, between the cells lining the bone surfaces to enter the extracellular fluid (ECF) compartment adjacent to the bone (110, 111), and thence via surface pores to reach the canalicular-lacunar system (Fig. 8-6). This is largely filled by osteocytes and their processes, which are separated from the bone by extensions of the fluid compartment on the surface. From the canaliculi (diameter, 200 nm) radiate microcanaliculi (diameter, 50 nm) that form channels between adjacent bundles of collagen fibrils (111). The surface area for exchange between the crystals of bone mineral and the bone ECF is more than 30 times greater at the canalicular-lacunar level than at the gross surface, and more than 3000 times greater at the microcanalicular level

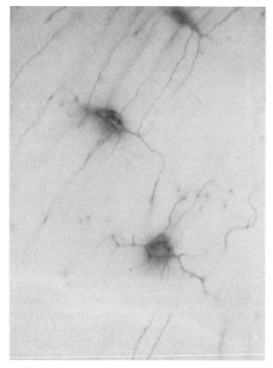

Figure 8-6. Osteocytes in human cortical bone lying in lacunae connected by canaliculae. Magnified ×1000. (*Courtesy of A. R. Villanueva.*)

(111). Little is known of the microcirculation through bone except that it is rapid; in the rat, all osteocyte lacunae can be reached by tetracycline within 30 minutes (111). Bone water is completely exchangeable (112), but because of its intimate relationship to the crystals and the small size of the microcanaliculi, much of the water cannot be penetrated by medium-sized molecules such as polyethylene glycol (MW, 4000 daltons) (113). Nevertheless, even large molecules such as horseradish peroxidase freely enter the bone ECF (101), and proteins such as albumin can be found in some osteocyte lacunae within 15 min (114). Water probably percolates from the surface through the microcanaliculi and possibly even smaller channels (115) and is somehow pumped by the osteocytes along the canaliculi, either within or around the cell processes (111).

Bone mineral (102, 103)

Bone mineral exists in two physical forms, amorphous and crystalline. The amorphous form consists mainly of brushite ($CaHPO_4 \cdot 2H_2O$) and tricalcium phosphate [$Ca_3(PO_4)_2$]. It is most abundant when the mineral is first formed and becomes progressively transformed into the crystalline form with time. The crystals are needles or plates of dimensions between 5 and 10 nm; about one-fifth of the calcium and phosphate ions are in surface positions (111). Bound to the surface of each crystal is a thin film of water, the hydration shell, containing ions in solution and ions adsorbed to the crystal surface (1). The lattice structure of the crystals, which is the arrangement of the constituent ions in space, conforms to that of naturally occurring minerals called apatites, the general formula of which is $3(Ca_3(PO_4)_2)Ca \cdot X_2$. This is not a molecular formula but specifies the relative proportions of the smallest number of ions needed for one unit cell, the imaginary parallelopiped which represents the repeating unit of the crystal structure. According to the majority view (102), bone mineral is mainly hydroxyapatite ($X_2 = OH_2^-$) with traces of fluoroapatite ($X_2 = F_2^-$), but there is considerable uncertainty concerning the location of the substantial amount of carbonate in bone. One possibility

is that carbonate is substituted for phosphate in the crystal lattice with appropriate adjustment for electroneutrality and is also present in the hydration shell adsorbed to the crystal surface. Other possibilities are that carbonate is substituted for hydroxyl groups ($X_2 = CO_3^{2-}$) to form carbonate-apatite, or exists as a separate crystalline phase of calcium carbonate (116). Quite apart from this uncertainty about crystal structure, the exact composition of bone mineral is indeterminate, because some of its constituent ions can be replaced by other ions of approximately the same radius, producing minor defects in the shape of the crystals which do not affect the overall structure (1, 117). Such substitution can occur at the time the crystal is formed or by exchange with existing crystals. In vitro, interactions between bone mineral and solution involve diffusion into the hydration shell, exchange within the layer of ions bound to the crystal surface, exchange at the crystal surface, and exchange within the crystal; the same four processes probably occur in vivo (1). The composition of the hydration shell is variable, most likely reflecting the composition of the bone ECF. No direct measurements of this are available, but there is much more potassium in bone than can be accounted for by the mineral or by the cells (118). In vitro equilibration experiments with powdered bovine bone (27) suggested that the concentrations of calcium and magnesium in bone ECF were about one-third of those in plasma and the concentration of potassium much higher (Table 8-11). The concentration of albumin in bone fluid is also about one-third that in plasma, so that the proportion of free to protein-bound calcium would be the same in both fluids (114). But bone fluid calcium and magnesium could be maintained at a higher level in vivo by cellular activity (for example, by H^+ ion pro-

Table 8-11. Electrolyte concentrations, in mmol/L, of bovine bone ECF* compared with bovine plasma

	Ca	Mg	Na	K	P	Cl	UA†	TOTAL
Plasma	1.5	0.7	140	4	1.8	100	44	292
Bone ECF	0.5	0.4	125	25	1.8	130	19	302

* Estimated by in vitro equilibration.

† UA = unmeasured anion.

Source: From Neuman (27).

duction) as will be discussed later. If there are gradients in vivo between plasma and bone fluid, they must be maintained by the activity of the flat lining cells on the surface (Fig. 8-5) (111).

The osteocyte and perilacunar bone

The 1- to 2-μm-thick layer of bone lining the walls of osteocyte lacunae differs from bone elsewhere in several respects (111, 119). In perilacunar bone the collagenous fibers are more loosely packed and less densely mineralized, the mineral is more amorphous, more soluble, and more easily removed by acid or edetic acid (EDTA), and the bone is more permeable than is found elsewhere and so is more accessible to mineral exchange. These differences are maintained by the osteocyte and do not persist if the cell dies. This metabolically reactive bone is of particular importance in calcium homeostasis and its identity may be maintained by cyclical removal and replacement, a specialized form of bone turnover termed osteocytic mini-remodeling (61). When studied by electron microscopy, both resorptive and formative phases can be identified (111). By light microscopy, using thick ground sections, the proportion of activated osteocytes (including both resorptive and formative phases) is normally about 40 percent (120), and in thin, toluidine blue–stained sections the proportion of resorptive osteocytes is about 4 percent (61).

BONE TURNOVER AND THE REMODELING SYSTEM (100, 111, 117)

Bone turnover is the removal of old bone tissue and its replacement by new. During growth, removal and replacement often occur on different surfaces to produce changes in size and shape, a process known as modeling. After maturity the new bone occupies the same anatomic location as the old, a process known as remodeling. The remodeling system is not concerned in the long-term regulation of normal plasma concentrations of any of the divalent ions, but disturbances in remodeling can produce short-term changes in these concentrations.

Bone resorption (117, 121)

Bone is removed as a whole, both mineral and matrix, by osteoclastic resorption, which accomplishes the nearly simultaneous digestion of collagen, depolymerization of mucopolysaccharides, and dissolution of mineral. Mineral is probably removed first, but matrix follows soon after, the proportion remaining the same (122). Mononuclear cells resembling monocytes and macrophages may also participate in resorption both directly and as precursors to osteoclasts. The chemistry of resorption is complex and involves the production by the osteoclasts of many different compounds. These include lactic, citric, and carbonic acids, which help to dissolve the mineral, lysosomal enzymes, and collagenase which digest matrix both intra- and extracellularly, and glycoproteins and hyaluronic acid, the functions of which are obscure (117, 121). In vitro, some product of bone matrix digestion provides a chemotactic stimulus for the migration of mononuclear cells to the site of resorption, a mechanism which enables resorption to continue after the initial stimulus is withdrawn (123).

Osteoclasts are multinucleated giant cells lying in irregular indentations of the bone surface known as Howship's lacunae. They make contact with the bone at a central ruffled border where resorption is occurring, surrounded by a peripheral clear zone which is inactive and which forms a seal between the cell and the bone surface (111, 124). The *extent* of bone surface undergoing resorption is determined by the number of osteoclasts, and the *speed* of advance of the resorption front through tissue space is determined by the volume of bone resorbed per osteoclast nucleus in unit time, an expression of cell activity. The *rate* of resorption expressed as volume of bone resorbed in unit time either per unit volume of existing bone or per whole skeleton is determined by the product of cell activity and cell number. These distinctions between extent, speed, and rate must be kept in mind during any discussion of bone resorption.

Normally, there are two populations of osteoclasts, active cells with predominant ruffled borders and a membrane potential of about −9 mV, and inactive cells with predominant clear zones and a membrane potential of about -24 mV (117, 124). The relative prevalence of these cells represents the relative durations of active and resting stages. Changes in the mean activity of the entire population of osteoclasts may be accomplished by varying the proportion which are turned on by parathyroid hormone or by other stimuli. It is not known how long the cell can remain in the active state, or whether intermediate degrees of activity are possible. Sustained changes in bone resorption are accomplished mainly by changing the rate of recruitment of new osteoclasts from local or blood bone precursors; this is the main determinant of the number of cells. In bone adjacent to osteoclasts, the osteocytes may enlarge their lacunae a few days before the bone is resorbed from the surface, but these cells do not participate in bone resorption independently (111, 119). Osteoclasts which begin a new focus of resorption on a bone surface tend to avoid bone which has never been mineralized, but once resorption is initiated, bone of all kinds is removed. Normally, about 0.5 percent of the endosteal surface is covered by osteoclasts and about 5 percent by Howship's lacunae, most of which therefore are without osteoclasts. The fraction of the bone surface at which resorption is occurring at one time is unknown, but it must lie between these limits.

Bone formation

Bone is made by osteoblasts in two stages—matrix synthesis and mineralization—which are separated in both time and space. Matrix formation involves the biosynthesis of collagen and of the proteoglycans, glycoproteins, and other components of the ground substance (102, 103). The biosynthesis of collagen involves assembly of the pro-α chain of protocollagen followed by hydroxylation of some of the proline and lysine residues. Three pro-α chains are assembled in the Golgi apparatus into the three-stranded molecule of procollagen, which is transferred to secretory granules. After extrusion from the cell, the amino terminal region of each procollagen strand is cleaved to form nascent α chains. Most of these develop cross-links between them to form tropo-collagen, which polymerizes to the collagenous fibril, but some α chains are degraded to smaller peptides (100). An indication of the speed of collagen synthesis is that tritiated proline can be demonstrated in osteoid by autoradiography within 6 hours of its administration (125). Once the fibrils are incorporated into osteoid there is a gradual increase in collagen cross-linking and a reduction in both the amount and degree of polymerization of the proteoglycans (102). These and other less well-understood changes, collectively known as matrix maturation, must be completed before mineralization can begin, and this normally takes about 10 days. With the normal rate of matrix apposition of 1 μm/day, a layer of as yet unmineralized matrix (the osteoid seam) of about 10 μm thickness lies beneath the osteoblasts (100, 111). This is separated from the mineralized bone by the zone of demarcation where tetracycline and other bone-seeking substances are deposited (Fig. 8-7). Normally, about 15 percent of the endosteal surface is covered by osteoid seams. As new bone is formed, some of the osteoblasts on the surface become buried within the bone as osteocytes.

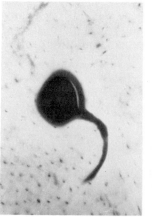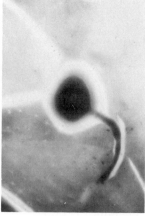

Figure 8-7. Osteoid seam in dog cortical bone. Left: Bright field illumination; right: ultraviolet illumination. Two separate pairs of fluorescent labels can be seen; the most recent label is close to the zone of demarcation. An earlier pair of labels has been truncated by the resorption space in which the seam formed. Note Volkmann's canal entering the haversian canal at four o'clock. Magnified ×250. (*Courtesy of A. R. Villanueva.*)

Most bone formation in the adult occurs in apposition to an existing surface, the finished product consisting of lamellar bone in which alternating layers are distinguishable by the different orientations of the collagen fibers. When bone is laid down in locations where there was no bone before, although the biosynthesis of collagen and formation of fibers is the same, the fibers are dispersed at random, with no preferred orientation, and mineralization occurs diffusely, without recognizable osteoid seams. Such bone is referred to as woven or fibrous bone.

Mineralization

The chemical basis of this is uncertain. Studies by electron microprobe in vivo demonstrated rapid initial deposition of mineral with a Ca/P ratio of 1.35, which increased slowly to 1.60 over a few days, consistent with an initial amorphous phase with gradual transition to crystalline hydroxyapatite (126). It is possible that brushite, tricalcium phosphate, octocalcium phosphate, and hydroxyapatite are formed in succession (Table 8-12) (127). Alternatively, a trimer of amorphous tricalcium phosphate or three dimers of amorphous brushite (128) could be the immediate precursors of apatite. Either scheme involves only the sequential addition of the calcium and phosphate ions present in extracellular fluid, but these steps

are phase transformations, not true chemical reactions. Modification of step 4 by substituting carbonic acid for water would permit the formation of carbonate apatite. The H^+ ions generated at steps 2 and 4 must be neutralized or removed for the process to continue. The relationship of mineralization to the composition of plasma is unclear. Most experimental work has been conducted on the mineralization of cartilage during endochondral ossification, which differs in several respects from the mineralization of bone. With respect to a defined solid phase, the ion activity product of a solution may be below the minimum level required for precipitation (the formation product), above the level of spontaneous precipitation (the solubility product), or between these two points in the so-called metastable range where precipitation can be induced by seeding. The activity product of plasma is most likely above the solubility product of hydroxyapatite but below the formation product of either brushite or tricalcium phosphate (1), since crystals of the former will grow in plasma but crystals of the latter will dissolve. The initiation of mineralization therefore requires the active participation of cells; from a broad biologic viewpoint, this is the rule over a wide range of species, types of calcifiable matrix, and chemical varieties of mineral (129). In bone, these cells are the osteoblasts and the most recent generation of osteocytes within the osteoid

Table 8-12. Chemical reactions involved in possible scheme of mineralization*

OVERALL
$10Ca^{2+} + 6HPO_4^{2+} + 2H_2O \rightleftharpoons Ca_{10}(PO_4)_6(OH)_2 + 8H^+$
Hydroxyapatite

POSSIBLE STEPS:

1.	$4Ca^{2+} + 4HPO_4^{2-} \rightleftharpoons$	$4CaHPO_4$
		Secondary calcium phosphate
2.	$4CaHPO_4 + 2Ca^{2+} \rightleftharpoons$	$2Ca_3(PO_4)_2 + 4H^+$
		Tertiary calcium phosphate
3.	$2Ca_3(PO_4)_2 + Ca^{2+} + 2HPO_4^{2-} \rightleftharpoons$	$Ca_8(PO_4)_4(HPO_4)_2$
		Octocalcium phosphate
4.	$Ca_8(PO_4)_4(HPO_4)_2 + 2Ca^{2+} + 2H_2O \rightleftharpoons$	$Ca_{10}(PO_4)_6(OH)_2 + 4H^+$
		Hydroxyapatite

* Note especially the generation of H^+ ions at steps 2 and 4; the reactions will be halted if these are not neutralized or removed.

seam. The mineral ions destined to reach the zone of demarcation probably travel through or around the cell processes joining these cells. Apart from facilitating ion transport, the cell sequesters mineral in mitochondrial granules (130) and in extracellular membrane-bound matrix vesicles (131), and maintains concentration gradients between the plasma and the fluid phase at sites of mineralization (132). Analysis of this fluid, which can be aspirated directly by micropuncture of epiphyseal cartilage, suggests several conclusions about cartilage mineralization (100, 132, 133). First, the levels of calcium and phosphate are too low to initiate mineralization unaided. Second, the inorganic phosphate level is normally equal to that of ECF, but when the extracellular phosphate level falls as a result of vitamin D depletion, a fluid:ECF gradient can be established which is abolished by local application of dinitrophenol. Third, the fluid contains two PG fractions, one capable of promoting crystallization and the other of inhibiting mineralization, possibly by binding calcium. Fourth, the bicarbonate concentration is higher than that of ECF, and the pH of the fluid is around 7.6. These differences are maintained by a mechanism dependent on carbonic anhydrase and are abolished by carbonic anhydrase inhibition and by systemic ammonium chloride administation (133). The role of PG complexes in mineralization is incompletely understood (42). The PG content is high in newly formed osteoid but low in the zone of demarcation (102). Since ^{35}S-labeled chondroitin sulfate is incorporated into new bone, the fall in PG content is probably due to removal of the protein core with liberation of unattached GAG molecules (42). This would reduce the calcium-binding capacity and increase the availability of free calcium for mineralization, but the amount released is probably too small to be important (134). PGs also form a macromolecular net within which a rise in pH could markedly increase the concentration of PO_4^{3-} (135). Mineral may also be sequestered and made available at a critical location by binding to acidic phospholipids such as phosphatidyl serine (128), which could be broken down by a specific lipase at the mineralization front (136).

Bone cells and cartilage cells contain an enor-

mous amount of calcium, mostly sequestered in electron-dense granules so that the cytosol calcium concentration is maintained at the low level characteristic of all cells (137). These mitochondrial granules contain calcium, phosphate, magnesium, phospholipid, RNA, and protein. They increase in number in chondrocytes during endochondral ossification and in osteoblasts engaged in bone formation. Calcium ions destined for mineral deposition are actively taken up by cells, sequestered within these granules, and subsequently extruded. The granules may be stabilized in colloidal form by some mineralization inhibitor and probably represent the smallest transportable form of solid calcium phosphate (76). Alternatively, calcium and phosphate may be sequestered and extruded independently (138). A variety of complex particles containing mineral within a membrane have been isolated from calcifying cartilage and bone. These particles, known as matrix vesicles (131), originate from cells from which they are budded off by reversed pinocytosis. They have an outer trilaminar membrane rich in lipids and phospholipids, and they contain alkaline phosphatase, adenosine triphosphatase, and pyrophosphatase (probably all the same enzyme) but no acid phosphatase, and so are not lysosomal in origin. The phosphatase activity is probably needed to destroy a variety of inhibitors of mineralization (139). As well as possibly containing mineral as preformed mitochondrial granules, they may be extruded from the cells unmineralized and then actively accumulate calcium and phosphate ions (131). In cartilage they remain in situ, and when the cells from which they originate have matured and begun to degenerate, the vesicle membrane disrupts, depositing its lipids at the zone of demarcation or mineralization front and making the mineral ions available to the solid phase. A similar mechanism operates in woven bone mineralization, but matrix vesicles have not been isolated from lamellar bone.

An alternative view concerning the solubility of the initial solid phase is that plasma is in the metastable region (106). The minimum ion product at which amorphous calcium phosphate will form in vitro from a protein-free electrolyte solution of the same ionic strength and pH as plasma is 2.0 mmol/L^2, which was thought to be within the physiologic range (140). However, this is still well above the maximum ion product ($Ca^{2+} \times HPO_4^{2-}$) of 0.9 derived from the data in Tables 8-5 and 8-7, which would support spontaneous formation of amorphous calcium phosphate only at pH 7.6 (140). If no local increase in ion product was necessary, mineralization could be initiated by epitactic seeding or heterogenous nucleation by collagen. Epitaxy is the induction of crystal deposition from a metastable solution by the provision of crystals which are physically similar to, but chemically different from those desired. Collagen has a crystalline structure with a period similar to that of hydroxyapatite and can undoubtedly function in this manner (102). One theory is that the three-dimensional stacking of the collagen molecules creates spaces at regular intervals within the fibrils known as hole zones. Inside these zones phosphorylation of serine residues (both in collagen and in associated glycopeptides) is followed by binding of inorganic phosphate ions which gain access by diffusion; this in turn permits nucleation of bone mineral inside the fibrils. Although widely accepted, this mechanism has met with many arguments (106). An alternative theory is that mineralization is initiated by the binding of calcium ions to noncollagenous matrix proteins which then undergo a conformational change that favors the subsequent addition of phosphate ions and the formation of the solid phase (106). These possibilities are not mutually exclusive and neither excludes the participation of cells.

The distribution of the physical density of bone determined by microradiography suggests that mineralization is about 50 to 70 percent complete within a few days (111, 141). This abrupt change (referred to as primary mineralization) depends mainly on the formation of new crystals and is probably under the direct control of the osteoblast. The mineral density then increases slowly to about 90 percent of maximum over the next 3 to 6 months and to about 95 percent of maximum over many years (Fig. 8-8). This gradual change, referred to as secondary mineralization, involves displacement of crystal-bound water, depends mainly on the growth of existing crystals, and is only indirectly under cellular control via changes in the composition of the bone ECF. This distinction between primary and secondary mineralization must not be confused with the transition from amorphous to crystalline mineral (126).

Restraint on crystal growth—the role of pyrophosphate

Since an ion product of only 0.2 mmol/L^2 is needed to maintain the continued growth of bone mineral crystals (104), there must normally be some way of preventing such growth from occurring. Within the depths of mature bone, mineralization probably continues to increase until inward diffusion of further ions is prevented by the reduction in water content (1). At quiescent bone surfaces the estimated ion product in human bone ECF is 0.3 mmol/L^2, assuming that the concentration of Ca^{2+} is one-third that of plasma (Table 8-11), and the concentration of HPO_4^{2+} is the same. This is still above the level needed for continued crystal growth, but the difference is probably within the margin of error of the estimation. The pH in bone fluid may be sufficiently low to increase the apparent solubility of bone mineral and thus permit equilibrium at the bone-fluid interface (142), as will be discussed later in relation to calcium homeostasis. Another possibility is that the bone surface is covered by pyrophosphate, a naturally occurring inhibitor of mineralization. Pyrophosphate is a byproduct of many biosynthetic reactions (143) and can be derived from nucleoside triphosphates such as adenosine triphosphate (ATP) by removal of the two terminal phosphate groups instead of the single orthophosphate needed to produce adenosine diphosphate (ADP). Activation of adenyl cyclase produces pyrophosphate as well as cyclic adenosine monophosphate (AMP) from ATP. The turnover of pyrophosphate is very high and is mainly intracellular, but the concentration in body fluids is small—2 to 6 μmol/L (21). Pyrophosphate is rapidly hydrolyzed to orthophosphate under the influence of the enzyme pyrophosphatase, which may be identical with alkaline phosphatase. Pyrophosphate inhibits the transformation of amor-

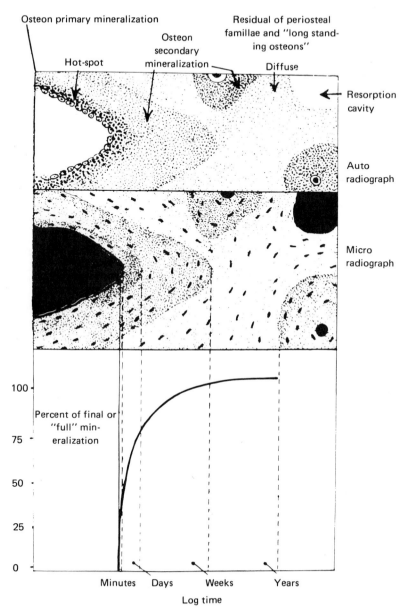

Figure 8-8. Comparison of autoradiograph and microradiograph of same area to illustrate distinction between primary and secondary mineralization and to demonstrate completeness of mineralization as a function of time. (*Courtesy of J. Jowsey.*)

BONE REMODELLING UNIT

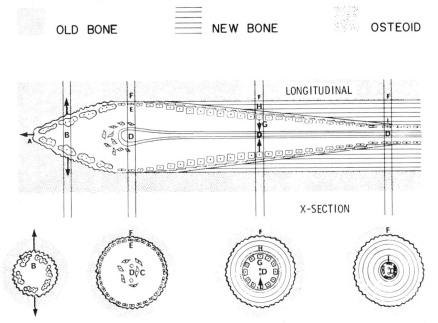

Figure 8-9. Diagram showing a longitudinal section through a cortical remodeling unit (above). Corresponding transverse sections at different levels (below) showing cortical remodeling cycles at different stages of development. (A) Apex of advancing osteoclastic front moving from right to left; (B) multinucleated osteoclasts advancing centrifugally to enlarge a small resorption space; (C) spindle-shaped mitotically active mesenchymal cells; (D) capillary loop; (E) mononuclear cells (? postosteoclasts) lining quiescent zone between resorption and formation; (F) cement line separating new bone from old; (G) osteoblasts advancing centripetally during radial closure; (H) osteoid seam separating osteoblasts from recently formed bone; (I) flattened cells lining canal of completed haversian system. [*From A. M. Parfitt (111).*]

phous to crystalline bone material and blocks heterogenous nucleation and aggregation (21). Crystals coated with pyrophosphate neither grow nor dissolve, despite large changes in the calcium phosphate ion product in the ambient solution. It has been postulated that all quiescent bone surfaces are normally covered with pyrophosphate bound to apatite crystals and that the pyrophosphate must be hydrolyzed before either resorption or formation can occur (144).

The supracellular organization of bone remodeling and turnover (100, 111)

Cortical bone turns over by the creation of new osteons. A hole is excavated by a cutting cone of osteoclasts (Fig. 8-9) which advances longitudinally through the cortex. Immediately behind, the hole is refilled by a closing cone of osteoblasts. On the trabecular surface the cells are arranged as if a cutting cone and closing cone had been cut open longitudinally and unfolded over the surface. There are thus created anatomically discrete structures, the cortical or trabecular remodeling units, which travel through the cortex or across the trabecular surface to carry out the functions of bone turnover in an ordered and predictable manner, each lasting for about the same period of time and replacing about the same volume of old bone by new. Precursor cell proliferation, osteoclastic resorption, and osteoblastic formation follow one another in unvarying succession, but the nature of the close spatial and temporal coupling between these processes is still unknown. One theory is that osteoclasts modulate directly into osteoblasts (61) and that osteoprogenitor cells, osteoclasts, osteoblasts, and osteocytes form a continuous series. It is more likely that osteoclasts are derived both from local preosteoclasts in bone and from blood-borne precursors resembling monocytes which originate in the spleen or in the bone marrow, and that osteoblasts are derived from local preosteoblasts in bone (111). The interrelations between the different bone cells may be important in relation to the presence or absence of hormone receptors in different cell types; mononuclear macrophages, which are putative precursors of osteoclasts, have both parathyroid hormone (PTH)- and calcitonin (CT)-sensitive adenylate cyclase receptors (145). Conceivably the extent of the coupling between resorption and formation could differ according to the origin of the osteoclasts.

Nevertheless, the usual existence of this coupling has important implications concerning the effect of a change in the remodeling system on the composition of the ECF, since changes in bone resorption, however produced, are usually followed by changes in bone formation of similar magnitude (111, 146).

The major determinant of the rate of bone turnover is the rate of recruitment of new osteoclasts from precursor cells, referred to as activation; in a steady state bone turnover is independent of the rate at which individual osteoclasts and osteoblasts work (111). The magnitude of normal bone turnover is uncertain, kinetic methods tending to give higher estimates than histomorphometric methods. On the assumption that turnover in trabecular bone is the same per unit area of surface as in cortical bone, various histologic methods led to an estimate of whole body bone turnover of 4 percent per annum (111). This is much less than the 12 to 15 percent usually derived from kinetic analysis, the difference being attributed to the inclusion of long-term exchange (111). However, trabecular bone turnover may be considerably higher than predicted from the surface/volume ratio. If the ilium is representative, trabecular bone turnover may be as high as 40

percent per annum, and the histomorphometric estimate of whole body bone turnover closer to 10 percent per annum, in reasonable agreement with the best kinetic data. This corresponds to daily exchanges of about 6.0 to 7.5 mmol for calcium, 3.6 to 4.5 mmol for phosphate, and 0.12 to 0.15 mmol for magnesium.

The change in bone or mineral balance produced by sustained changes in the remodeling system depends on the rate of activation of new remodeling units and on the net balance between resorption and formation in each unit. This depends, in turn, on both the *duration* and on the *speed* of cellular action. Changes in the rate of bone turnover alter the *magnitude* but not the *direction* of any change in balance already occurring on a particular surface. Normally, the bone balance within each remodeling unit is slightly positive on the periosteal surface, zero or slightly negative on the haversian surface, and increasingly negative on the endosteal surface after the age of about 35. Even in the elderly, the degree of negative balance is only a small part of the bone turned over.

The total time taken for the complete cycle of remodeling to unfold in a particular location (σ) is usually about 3 to 4 months, 20 days (σ_R) for resorption and 80 days for formation (σ_F). These time relationships determine the occurrence of transient changes in bone and mineral balance after a change in bone turnover rate during the 8 months or longer it takes to attain a new steady state (147). These changes are reversible, in contrast to the irreversible changes caused by amplification of an existing trend. The sequential changes in balance produced by five stages in the life history of a single remodeling unit are shown in Fig. 8-10, on the assumption that all of the bone removed is eventually replaced. For the first 20 days resorption occurs alone. For the next 80 days resorption continues at the same rate, and formation gradually increases until a complete structure, as shown in Fig. 8-9, is formed. Resorption and formation then remain equal as the remodeling unit continues to advance longitudinally for an unknown time (σ_{LA}). When the unit stops advancing, resorption gradually diminishes over about 20 days, but formation continues at the

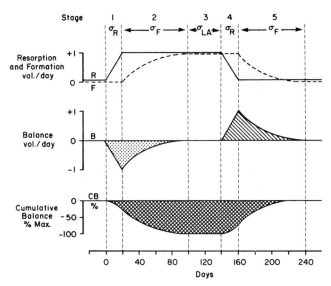

Figure 8-10. Changes in resorption and formation rates (upper panel) and in bone balance (middle panel) in arbitrary units of bone volume per day and in cumulative balance (lower panel) as percent of maximum deviation in balance, during five stages in the evolution of a single remodeling unit. Curvilinear segments are due to more rapid bone formation at beginning of osteon closure. σ_R = duration of resorption in cross section (20 days), σ_F = duration of formation in cross section (80 days), and σ_{LA} = duration of longitudinal advance during which resorption and formation continue at the same rate; this duration is unknown but is arbitrarily taken as $\frac{1}{2}\sigma_F$. Note that entire life span of remodeling unit = $3\sigma_F$.

same rate. Finally, after cessation of resorption, formation continues alone at a diminishing rate for a further 80 days until a new osteon is completed. These five stages are less clearly defined in trabecular remodeling units. The extent to which mineral homeostasis is disturbed by the remodeling unit is determined by the balance at any one time, but the extent to which bone mass is disturbed is determined by the cumulative balance (Fig. 8-10). This is the size of the hole created by the remodeling unit, which is about 0.02 mm³. Note that when the daily balance is maximally negative the cumulative negative balance is small, and when the cumulative balance is maximally negative (0.02 mm³) the daily balance is zero.

At any one time bone and mineral balance re-

flects the sum total of a large number of such systems at all stages of development. The sequential changes in whole body bone and mineral balance produced by seven stages in the response to an abrupt but temporary increase in activation and initiation of new remodeling units are shown in Fig. 8-11. As before, it is assumed that no net gain or loss of bone occurs by the end of the se-

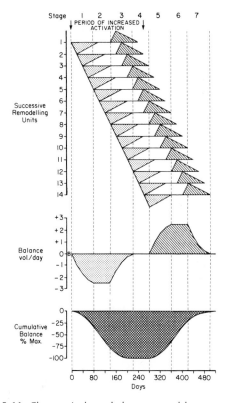

Figure 8-11. Changes in bone balance caused by succession of new remodeling units initiated after an increase in activation at time zero (upper panel). Each of units 1 to 14 is similar to the middle panel of Fig. 8-10, except that curvilinear segments are shown as linear for simplicity. No further new units are initiated after t = 250 days, when activation returns to the previous level. Summation of bone balances of individual units at different phases at the same time (shown in middle panel) leads to seven stages in total response. For example, at 220 days the different stages of negative balance in units 8 to 11 offset exactly the different stages of positive balance in units 1 to 4, units 5 to 7 being in zero balance. The cumulative balance is shown in lower panel; scales as in Fig. 8-10.

quence. For the first 80 days (σ_F) the balance gets progressively more negative. For the next 60 days ($\sigma_R + \sigma_{LA}$) the negative balance remains at the same level, as the continued addition of new units offsets the progressive changes in existing units. The negative balance then gradually diminishes over the next 80 days as the oldest systems enter their replacement phase. The balance then returns to zero, and a new steady state is achieved in which the magnitude of the bone and mineral deficit remains unchanged for as long as the increase in turnover persists. When activation returns to the previous level, after 20 days (σ_R) the balance becomes increasingly positive, and the next three stages are mirror images of the first three (Fig. 8-11). The relationship between daily and cumulative balance is similar for the aggregate of all units as for a single unit. An increase in bone turnover will therefore cause a negative bone and mineral balance for approximately 8 months, and a decrease in bone turnover will cause a positive balance for approximately 8 months. In both cases reverse changes of equal magnitude and equal duration occur when turnover returns to normal.

Noncoupled bone turnover during growth and repair (111)

Although bone formation normally does not occur except in apposition to a surface where resorption has recently been completed, there are important physiologic and pathologic exceptions to this rule. During growth, resorption and formation occur mostly on separate surfaces and can be regulated independently. Bone laid down on the outer surface may be removed from the inner surface by the advancing resorption front within a few weeks or months. In animals that never stop growing, such as the rat, bone turnover is of this kind throughout life. Pathologic bone resorption induced by osseous metastases, myeloma, or a variety of abnormal humoral agents may be initiated by osteoclasts but is often continued by mononuclear cells of various kinds (148, 149) and is not directly coupled to subsequent formation. The link between resorption and formation may also be broken in severe hyperparathyroidism,

primary or secondary, with osteitis fibrosa (150). Nevertheless, bone formation may increase to a variable extent either as a compensatory repair mechanism or as a separate response to the same pathologic process. When this occurs, formation may outstrip resorption, leading to osteosclerosis. Such noncoupled bone formation may be in apposition to an existing surface or may occur directly in fibrous connective tissue without the need for an adjacent bone surface. In either case the bone is fibrous or woven in texture. Woven bone occurs physiologically during early embryologic development and pathologically in Paget's disease, fracture repair, osteitis fibrosa, osteogenic tumors, myelofibrosis, in relation to osseous metastases, and in ectopic ossification.

MINERAL TURNOVER AND THE HOMEOSTATIC SYSTEM (111, 117)

Exchange of calcium between blood and bone, short-term, long-term, and intermediate

Examination of bone by autoradiography shows that uptake of radioactive calcium and of other bone-seeking isotopes occurs rapidly over all free bone surfaces regardless of the age or degree of mineralization of the bone, so that rapid exchangeability is a function of proximity to the circulation, not of the physical properties of the bone mineral. The previous belief that the exchangeability or availability of bone was determined solely by its age was a consequence of studying only young, small animals. When almost all bone surfaces are engaged in resorption or formation there is inevitably a close correlation between the age of bone and its distance from the surface. Only in the adults of larger animals are extensive quiescent surfaces found. Uptake of labeled calcium ions at bone surfaces which are not growing can occur only in exchange for unlabeled calcium ions which are released. These opposite processes can be described by a single rate constant so that the surface calcium behaves as a single compartment (151). This includes calcium ions within the surface lining cells, calcium ions dissolved in the bone ECF and in the hydration shell, and calcium ions bound to the cyrstal surface or in surface positions in the crystal lattice (1). The surface compartment is in reversible equilibrium with the systemic ECF, so that after a single dose of radiocalcium the surface activity gradually fades because of return to the blood. The equilibration between bone and ECF can also be studied by incubating bone in vitro. In such a system calcium and phosphate ions can either be released or taken up by bone according to whether the ion product in the ambient fluid is below or above the level of equilibration (117). The magnitude of rapid surface exchange depends on the kinetic model used. Estimates have varied from 50 to 150 mmol/day (111, 152), but even the smallest estimate is at least six times larger than the amount of calcium turned over by resorption and formation, sufficient to replace the entire ECF calcium at least once every day.

Some radioactivity is trapped as "hot spots" at sites of new bone formation but there is also a gradual buildup of diffuse radioactivity via the microcirculation to become evenly distributed throughout the bone. Some labeled ions penetrate the bone crystals and so remain for a very long time but are gradually returned to the circulation by a process of long-term exchange. The distinction between rapid surface exchange and long-term diffuse exchange is useful, but in reality there is a continuous spectrum of residence time of calcium ion in bone from a few minutes to many decades.

Intermediate residence times measured in days or weeks reflect superficial exchange in surface bone below the 1- to 4-μm depth of the rapidly exchangeable pool and in the walls of canaliculi and lacunae. Exchange in these locations will be modified by the physical properties of bone which alter its diffusion impedance (115, 153). The most important of these is water content, which declines as the bone ages because of the progression of secondary mineralization, reaching a minimum of about 3 percent in fully mature cortical bone. The main determinant of the overall reactivity of bone with ions in the ECF is therefore the mean age of the skeleton, which varies directly with chronologic age and inversely with mean bone turnover since skeletal maturity (154).

Aging also increases the perfection and size of the crystals, thus further reducing exchangeability (1). Increase in bone turnover increases the proportion of young, incompletely mineralized bone and so increases the fraction of bone mineral accessible to diffusion. The diffusion impedance of perilacunar bone is also kept low by the activity of osteocytes and is further reduced by exposing the bone to a low pH or a high citrate concentration (111, 119).

The calcium homeostatic system in bone

Regulation of plasma calcium displays three main features. First, there is a steady-state level with oscillation between fairly narrow limits, which varies directly with the prevailing level of PTH secretion. Second, there are mechanisms for the correction of errors in the steady-state level which are partly, but not wholly, dependent on acute changes in PTH secretion. Third, regulation is neither very rapid nor very precise, the apparent stability of plasma calcium reflecting the small magnitude of the disturbing signals rather than unusual efficiency of the homeostatic system (155). There is an important conceptual distinction between the determination of particular steady-state level of plasma calcium and the correction of deviations from that level (117). This distinction also applies to the control of plasma sodium; resetting of the osmostat causes hyponatremia even though the components of the feedback loop are functioning normally, the system defending a low level of sodium as if it were normal (156).

It is evident from the normal coupling between resorption and formation that the remodeling system which regulates bone turnover and bone mass cannot be concerned in the normal steady-state control of plasma calcium. Bone turnover may be very low in hypothyroidism and very high in hyperthyroidism, but the difference in mean plasma calcium between these two conditions is less than 0.25 mmol/L despite a difference in turnover of more than twentyfold (117). In Paget's disease associated with hypoparathyroidism a large increase in bone turnover is accompanied by hypocalcemia (117). In a cortical remodeling unit some of the mineral ions removed by osteoclasts will almost immediately be redeposited at the closely adjacent sites of new bone formation which are supplied by the same blood vessels (Fig. 8-9). In trabecular bone there is a greater possibility of the products of resorption escaping into the general circulation, but the statistical coupling of resorption and formation over a wide range still holds. Even the transient changes in net bone balance consequent on changes in turnover (Figs. 8-10 and 8-11), and the more sustained changes which alter bone mass in disease, produce only minimal changes in plasma calcium for reasons which will become clearer when the renal handling of calcium is described.

The nature of the equilibrium between blood and bone. Because plasma calcium homeostasis is not regulated by bone resorption and bone turnover, some have concluded that it is regulated entirely by extraskeletal mechanisms (157, 158). A more reasonable conclusion is that the participation of bone in calcium homeostasis depends on a completely different cell system. Whatever the nature of the fluxes of calcium between plasma and the rapidly exchangeable bone surface compartment, the plasma calcium level must normally be such that the inward and outward fluxes are equal. The mechanisms giving rise to these fluxes could therefore regulate the plasma calcium by altering the level at which equilibration between ECF and bone occurred. This equilibrium can be considered at two levels. The first concerns movements of ions between the solution and the solid phase, which do not involve changes in the amount of mineral. The second concerns the solubility factors that determine the growth or dissolution of the solid phase.

In vitro the exchange of labeled for unlabeled calcium ions is isoionic, an ion entering the crystal only to take up a position just vacated by another ion (117). Such one-for-one exchange cannot affect the amount of calcium either in the solution or in the solid phase and so cannot participate in calcium homeostasis. But calcium can also undergo heteroionic exchange with sodium, hydronium (H_3O^+) or magnesium, and phosphate likewise with carbonate or citrate. Calcium ions

can also accumulate in the hydration shell at the expense of the solution in response to the electrostatic effect of binding of pyrophosphate ions (159), so that at this level calcium and phosphate can move independently.

Early studies on the plasma composition in rickets suggested that the solubility of bone mineral determined its equilibrium with the ECF and accounted for the frequently observed reciprocal relationship between calcium and phosphate levels in blood. However, because of the complexity and varying composition of its crystal structure, bone mineral does not have a fixed solubility. Possible mechanisms of reconciling the ion activity product in plasma with the solubility product of HA were discussed previously. Bone mineral cannot be in direct equilibrium with plasma but must be in equilibrium with the bone fluid with which it is in contact. Consequently, the ionic composition of bone fluid and plasma must differ.

Chemical disequilibrium and biologic equilibrium. The chemical disequilibrium between blood and bone must somehow be reconciled with the biologic equilibrium deduced from autoradiography. Two theories have been proposed. According to Neuman, the apparent solubility of bone mineral is higher in vivo than in vitro because the pH at the solid solution interface is maintained at 7.1, thus stabilizing amorphous brushite ($CaHPO_4 \cdot 2H_2O$) as the mineral phase at the bone surface. This ensures a constant ion activity product in the bone fluid and reversible deposition or dissolution of the mineral which reproduces in bone ECF the ionized calcium and phosphate levels normally found in plasma (142). This is thought to be achieved by the continuous production of lactic acid by osteocytes under the influence of parathyroid hormone, with outward gradients for both H^+ ions and lactate between bone fluid and blood. At least 80 percent of glucose utilization by bone is accounted for by aerobic glycolysis; if lactate production by rat bone is extrapolated to human beings on the basis of body weight, the amount is about 10,000 mmol/day (160). According to Talmage, the concentrations of calcium and phosphate in the bone ECF are the same in vivo as in vitro (Table 8-11). The

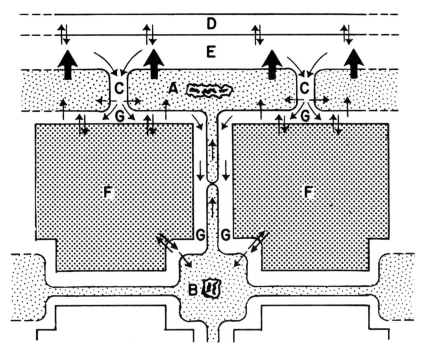

Figure 8-12. Model of calcium homeostasis based on outwardly directed calcium pump in surface osteocytes (modified after Talmage). (A) Surface osteocyte; (B) deep osteocyte (nature of junction and/or communication between these cells is unclear); (C) pore between adjacent surface osteocyte; (D) blood vessel; (E) connective tissue between blood vessel and bone surface; (F) bone; (G) extracellular fluid between osteocytes (surface and deep) and bone. Large unidirectional arrows indicate active pumping of calcium out of surface osteocytes into connective tissue fluid. Other unidirectional arrows indicate passive flow of calcium along a concentration gradient. Bidirectional arrows indicate reversible movements of calcium between compartments of same concentration. Ionic calcium concentration is believed to be about 1.2 mM/L in (D) and (E) and about 0.4 mM/L in (G). [*From A. M. Parfitt (117).*]

concentration gradient for calcium between plasma and bone ECF across the layer of surface lining cells is balanced by an outward flux maintained by cellular activity (110, 111, 161). Under the influence of parathyroid hormone, calcium ions are pumped out of the surface lining cells away from bone toward the connective tissue ECF in equilibrium with the plasma (Fig. 8-12). These calcium ions flow into the surface cells through their inner walls, facing the bone, or are derived from the osteocytes in deeper regions of bone traveling toward the surface along the canaliculi, either within or outside the cell processes. Chick calvaria appear to maintain exactly such an outward flux (117), but subsequent experiments suggested that this was the result of inadequate buffering of lactate. Active inward transport of potassium could still be demonstrated, but inward and outward fluxes of calcium and phosphate were believed to be passive (162, 163). The issue is obviously far from settled, but the agreement between these investigators concerning the existence of the blood-bone equilibrium must not be obscured by their disagreement concerning its mechanism. Both sides agree that the plasma calcium is somehow regulated by events at quiescent bone surfaces and that concentration differences must exist between plasma and the bone fluid. The application of this concept to clinical medicine need not await resolution of the controversy concerning its mechanism. A hydraulic analogy for both suggested mechanisms and for a possible combination of them is depicted in Fig. 8-13, and a physical model embodying this analogy for the Talmage concept has been built and successfully tested (161). Either or both of these mechanisms would permit the control of plasma calcium in a manner which did not require indefinitely sustained changes in the net gain or loss of calcium by the skeleton. An increase in bone mineral solubility caused by increased H^+ ion production or an increase in the activity of the outwardly directed calcium pump will raise the plasma calcium to a new level at which influx and efflux of calcium at the bone surface again come into equilibrium, the net loss of calcium by bone amounting only to a few hundred milligrams. Conversely, with a decrease in bone mineral solubility or a decrease in

the activity of the pump, equilibration at the bone surface is attained at a lower calcium level than normal, with a net gain of calcium by bone of a few hundred milligrams.

The existence of two separate systems in bone, one concerned with bone turnover and bone mass and the other with plasma calcium homeostasis, is an example of the separate control of content and of concentration mentioned earlier. It is of cardinal importance and will be referred to repeatedly, both in the remainder of this chapter and in Chap. 19.

The role of bone in the metabolism of phosphate, magnesium, and other ions.

All ions in solution in body fluids are able to enter the hydration shell of bone mineral, but the depth of further penetration is variable and is the main determinant of the rapidity of exchange. Three groups of ions can be recognized (164). Potassium and chloride (and urea) are confined to the hydration shell and are most rapidly and completely exchangeable. Magnesium, sodium, and carbonate can penetrate the surface positions in the crystal lattice and are less exchangeable. Finally, calcium and phosphate can penetrate the crystal interior and are most slowly exchangeable. The composition of the hydration shell, of the surface-bound ion layer, and of the crystal surface reflect, in varying degrees the composition of the bone ECF and thus indirectly the systemic ECF. Bone behaves like a gigantic ion exchange column but is subject to the limitations previously mentioned concerning age, water content, and diffusion impedance and to additional constraints arising from differences in ionic or molecular radius (153, 165). Within these limitations, bone therefore tends to resist changes in ion composition but cannot exert homeostatic regulation for any ion other than calcium. The unique position of calcium is due to the cell-mediated transport system located on quiescent surfaces, as previously described. This buffering action of bone may reduce the impact of acute changes, but once a change in composition is established, the same action of bone may delay the return to normality (1).

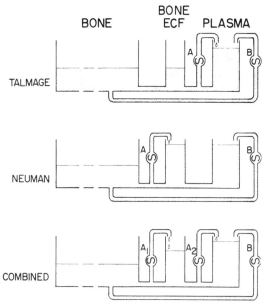

Figure 8-13. Hydraulic analogies for various models of calcium homeostasis discussed in the text. Heights of water in the various tanks represent the concentrations of calcium in designated compartments. Pump A operates continuously to maintain gradient between bone ECF and plasma (Talmage) or to increase apparent solubility of bone mineral (Neuman). Pump B operates intermittently to replace sudden losses of calcium from perilacunar bone. [*After A. M. Parfitt (117).*]

Phosphate. Most of what was said concerning exchange of calcium between blood and bone applies also to phosphate. Rapid uptake of ^{32}P occurs over all free bone surfaces, which in young, small animals are all recently formed and of low mineral density (166), but there is considerable variability between different bones and between different surfaces (167). More prolonged fixation depends on growth and new bone formation. ^{32}P forms hot spots in cortical bone in forming osteons, just like labeled calcium (168). Both in vitro (104) and in vivo (169) the fraction of the total mineral which is exchangeable is the same for phosphate as for calcium, although the kinetics may differ slightly (1). If the same applies in man, the exchangeable bone phosphorus would total about 100 mmol, but the turnover of this is much slower than the extraosseous pool. Although phosphate ions can leave bone without calcium ions by heteroionic exchange for citrate of carbonate, this selective loss can occur only on a very small scale, and there is essentially no independent skeletal reserve of phosphate. If the skeleton is a storehouse for phosphate, it is one whose contents are available only if the walls are pulled down; mobilization of a substantial amount of skeletal phosphate can occur only as a consequence of loss of whole bone mineral. In growing animals severe phosphate depletion leads to profound demineralization of bone, which enables soft-tissue phosphate to be preserved (170). There may be a greater net loss of mineral than of matrix (122), but whether this occurs because of impaired mineral deposition or increased mineral dissolution is unclear. In some circumstances phosphate depletion may also impair bone formation and increase bone resorption, as discussed later. For the most part bone can contribute to the prevention of hypophosphatemia only at the expense of providing calcium to the ECF, whether it is needed or not.

Magnesium. The state of magnesium in bone and its availability to body fluids is still uncertain. Crystallographic data (1) and the elution of 70 percent of the magnesium from ground bovine bone with dilute acid (171) suggested that it was confined to the hydration shell and the crystal surface. Synthetic apatite crystals exclude magnesium from the lattice interior and about 90 percent of magnesium in such crystals is surface-limited and readily exchangeable (172). By contrast, in powdered human bone only 30 percent of the magnesium was elutable and the same fraction exchangeable with ^{28}Mg (25). In the rat a similar fraction of 25 percent was found (173). If bone mineral behaves like synthetic apatite, the remainder could be located only in the noncrystalline amorphous fraction of bone mineral. In the young rat, the in vivo exchangeable bone magnesium is only slightly less than the in vitro elutable magnesium (173). Both elutable (in vitro) and exchangeable (in vivo) bone magnesium fall with age (173, 174), probably because of enlargement of crystals and consequent reduction in surface area. In the dog there is a sevenfold variation between bones and a fourfold variation between animals in the uptake of ^{28}Mg. Autoradiography showed localization of ^{28}Mg in the metaphyses adjacent to the growth plate (175); whether magnesium hot spots occur in mature animals is not known.

The size of the in vivo rapidly exchangeable bone magnesium pool in man is uncertain. If, like calcium and phosphate, this was confined to the 2 to 3 percent of bone close to a surface, it would be less than 1 percent of the total bone magnesium, or about 8 mmol. The total exchangeable pool of about 140 mmol would then make up about 20 percent of soft-tissue magnesium as well as all the ECF magnesium. However, although the existence of a skeletal reserve of magnesium has been denied (88), the amount available to offset depletion is probably much more than 1 percent of the total. The response of bone magnesium pools to dietary deficiency in the rat (173) and to the hypermagnesemia of renal failure in human beings (91) indicated that the elutable pool correlates with the plasma magnesium at the time of study, and the nonelutable pool correlates with the plasma magnesium at the time the bone was formed. Withdrawal of magnesium from the elutable pool can occur within a few days in response to hypomagnesemia, and bone magnesium can be restored by intravenous magnesium too quickly to be explained by bone turnover (176). Surface-limited magnesium ions in crystals located far from a free bone surface must therefore be accessible to the circulation of bone water and are therefore slowly exchangeable. This may reflect the smaller size of the magnesium ion relative to the calcium or phosphate ion. Continued bone formation during hypomagnesemia will reduce the nonelutable magnesium pool at a rate dependent on growth and bone turnover, and so will be much more rapid in young animals than in old (177). Availability of magnesium via this mechanism depends on the normal process of bone resorption. Despite the variation in the proportional changes in elutable and nonelutable fractions, total bone magnesium concentration is highly correlated with plasma magnesium according to the relationship (25): Bone magnesium (as percent ash) = 0.6 plasma magnesium (mmol/L) + 0.2.

Sodium and potassium. The skeleton contains about 320 mmol of sodium and about 16 mmol of potassium per kilogram of fat-free bone (Table 8-10), for a total amount of 1400 mmol of sodium (112) and 75 mmol of potassium (178) in a 70-kg body. The rapidly exchangeable fraction for sodium in vivo is about 45 percent in young animals and about 25 percent in the adult human (112), so that total bone sodium is only 30 percent less than total ECF sodium and about 15 percent of total exchangeable sodium is in bone. The rapidly exchangeable bone sodium is in the bone-tissue fluid and in the hydration shell (179). The remainder is located deep in the crystal lattice and is only very slowly exchangeable (180). Potassium ions cannot enter the crystal (118), so that apart from a small amount in bone cells, potassium must be either in the bone-tissue fluid or in the hydration shell. Potassium is almost completely exchangeable in vitro but only about 60 percent exchangeable in vivo (178). Why bone-tissue fluid actively accumulates potassium is unknown. Bone sodium and potassium are mobilized more easily by metabolic acidosis than by depletion of the ion (181), but up to 10 percent of bone sodium can be withdrawn even in adult animals (182). This ability of bone to release sodium is impaired by parathyroidectomy (183). In the growing rat, sodium depletion depresses bone formation and leads to osteopenia (184), and in

human subjects receiving nourishment only by the intravenous route, retention of calcium and phosphate in bone does not occur unless sodium is also provided (185). Normal bone turnover exchanges less than 1 mmol of sodium and less than 0.1 mmol of potassium daily.

Hydrogen ion and bicarbonate. The importance of the skeleton as a buffer source and the effect of chronic acidosis on bone have been debated for many years; this reflects in part continued uncertainty about the state of bone carbonate. As with magnesium, both changes in surface ion content and changes in bone composition and mass brought about by remodeling may interact with the ECF. Acute metabolic acidosis induced by ammonium chloride reduces bone carbonate (or bicarbonate) with a parallel loss of sodium and potassium (182, 186), probably by withdrawal from the hydration shell. Like the soft-tissue buffers, this component of bone buffering is readily available, accessible by simple diffusion but of small capacity. Acute respiratory changes in P_{CO_2} also lead to corresponding changes in CO_2 in bone (187). Chronic metabolic acidosis as in renal failure leads to progressive reduction of carbonate within the crystal lattice with a corresponding increase in phosphate (188). This probably reflects changes in the composition of the ECF at the time new crystals of bone mineral were formed (189), but balance studies in normal subjects given ammonium chloride suggested that selective dissolution of calcium carbonate could occur from mature bone within a few weeks (190). Chronic accumulation of H^+ ions may also be buffered by net loss of whole bone. Although conveniently measured by the amount of calcium liberated, it is the phosphate, hydroxyl, and carbonate ions in bone which are actually responsible for the buffering. This component is made available only slowly, and requires the active intervention of cells but is of considerable magnitude. At normal body pH and phosphate ion distribution, dissolution of bone mineral neutralizes 0.92 meq of H^+ ion for each mmol of calcium liberated, according to the equation:

$$46H^+ + 5[Ca_{10}(PO_4)_6(OH)_2]$$
$$\rightarrow 50Ca^{2+} + 24HPO_4^{2-} + 6H_2PO_4^- + 10H_2O$$
$$(8\text{-}3)$$

If the phosphate liberated is used to increase urinary titratable acidity maximally, an additional 0.48 for a total of 1.40 meq of H^+ ions is neutralized. Replacement of carbonate by phosphate would neutralize 1.20 meq of H^+ ions per mmol, and selective loss of calcium carbonate would neutralize 2 meq of H^+ ions for each mmol of calcium released (191). The converse changes take place during growth. Net formation of new bone releases 0.92 meq of H^+ ions for each mmol of calcium incorporated, which may contribute to metabolic acidosis in rapidly growing infants (191, 192), Conversely, experimental chronic metabolic acidosis leads to increased net bone resorption and to loss of bone (193, 194), but it is not known how bone resorbing cells are stimulated by H^+ ion accumulation. The possible role of parathyroid hormone in this process will be discussed later.

Interactions between calcium, phosphate, and magnesium in blood and bone

Although the calcium and phosphate levels in plasma do not conform to a fixed solubility product, a rise in plasma phosphate is often followed by a fall in plasma calcium. Direct precipitation of mineral in the blood or soft tissues could not occur until the plasma phosphate rose to at least 2 mmol/L (195) or even higher (12), depending on the initial solid phase, but a much smaller increase than this produced by phosphate administration will lower ionized calcium (196). Part of this fall is due to increased formation of $CaHPO_4$ ion-pair complexes in plasma (3), but any increase in plasma phosphate will also be transmitted to the bone fluid. Whichever theory of the composition of this fluid is correct, there will be immediate deposition of amorphous mineral at the bone surface and a fall in ionized calcium in the bone fluid which will be transmitted back to the plasma. Similarly, hypophosphatemia leads by a converse series of events to a rise in both bone fluid and plasma ionized calcium. If parathyroid function is normal, appropriate changes in PTH secretion will restore a normal ionized calcium, as explained later.

The lowering of plasma calcium by phosphate infusion is accompanied by a fall in the level of intravenously administered strontium, and both calcium and strontium are returned to the circulation 24 to 48 h later (197). This can be explained in part by increased deposition of amorphous calcium phosphate at the bone surface with coprecipitation of strontium, but it may also result from sequestration and subsequent release of colloidal calcium phosphate by macrophages in the soft tissues, especially the liver (198, 199). The fall in plasma calcium induced by phosphate infusion is greater in patients with bone disease or hypercalcemia than in normal subjects (200) and the fall is markedly reduced by the administration of ethane hydroxy diphosphonate (EHDP), a synthetic analogue of pyrophosphate which isolates the bone from the bone fluid (201). Hyperphosphatemia also leads to a fall in plasma magnesium (195), but the mechanism of this is unclear.

In embryonic or fetal bone in tissue culture, raising the phosphate level in the ambient fluid decreases both spontaneous resorption and that induced by parathyroid hormone and increases collagen synthesis. Conversely, lowering the phosphate level inhibits collagen synthesis and bone formation (202, 203). But phosphate administration in vivo has no effect on PTH-induced bone resorption even though net release of calcium from bone is depressed (204, 205). This was interpreted as an effect on bone formation but more likely reflected the ion fluxes at the bone surface as already described. Phosphate depletion increases the release of calcium from bone (206); the cellular mechanism of this is not clear, but in the parathyroidectomized rat, both osteoclastic and osteocytic resorption are increased (207). This may be due in part to increased synthesis of 1,25-dihydroxycholecalciferol, the active metabolite of vitamin D. In larger animals and human beings phosphate administration increases both bone resorption and formation, probably by inducing secondary hyperparathyroidism (203). Although there is some evidence that phosphate supplements increase the accumulation of osteoblasts in man (208) no role for plasma phosphate in the normal regulation of bone resorption and formation has been established.

Increasing the magnesium concentration has

no effect on bone resorption in tissue culture (209) but does increase calcium release by heteroionic exchange (210). Conversely, a low magnesium level reduces both calcium release from bone and bone resorption in vitro (210). In vivo, bone resorption is depressed by magnesium depletion and increased by magnesium repletion in both the rat (211) and the dog (212). However, variations in plasma magnesium within the normal range have not been shown to affect calcium, phosphorus, or bone metabolism in any species.

BONE AS A SINK AND AS A RESERVOIR

The preceding discussion has identified two entirely different ways in which ions can move between bone and body fluids, shown diagrammatically in Fig. 8-14. The remodeling system

removes and replaces whole volumes of bone by means of osteoclastic resorption and osteoblastic formation, whereas the homeostatic system regulates the exchange and transfer of ions between the bone fluid and the surface mineral by means of the surface lining cells and the osteocytes. The former process is slow, irreversible, microscopic in scale, and entirely dependent on cell function. It is of relatively small magnitude (5 to 10 mmol of calcium daily) but of large capacity since it has potential access to the entire skeleton. The latter process is rapid, reversible, ultramicroscopic in scale, and, while requiring cell function to be set at a certain level, operates primarily by physicochemical mechanisms. It is of relatively large magnitude (50 to 100 mmol of calcium daily) but of small capacity, having access only to the mineral close to the bone surface. These characteristics are summarized in Table 8-13. In a normal

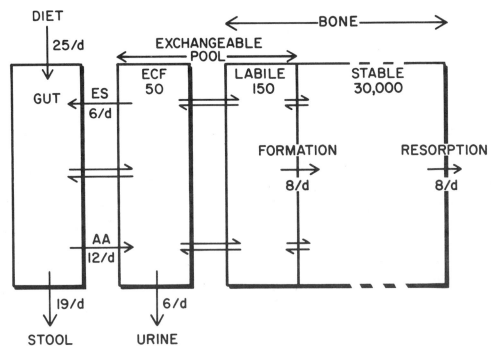

Figure 8-14. Schematic representation of calcium balance and turnover. Numerical values are expressed in mmol. Single arrows identify irreversible processes; double arrows identify reversible processes. ES = endogenous secretion and AA = absolute absorption.

Table 8-13 Contrasting characteristics of two types of exchange of ions between bone and body fluids*

CHARACTERISTIC	REMODELING	HOMEOSTASIS
Rate	Slow	Rapid
Kinetics	Irreversible	Reversible
Scale	Microscopic	Ultramicroscopic
Mechanism	Cellular	Physicochemical†
Magnitude	Small	Large
Capacity	Large	Small

* One is based on resorption and formation (remodeling), the other on the biologic equilibrium at the bone surface (homeostasis).
† The level of equilibrium is determined by cellular activity, but ionic exchanges at a particular level are physicochemical.

young adult both systems are in equilibrium, in the sense that for each system the number of ions entering and leaving bone is the same in the long term. Sustained gains or losses are usually mediated only by the remodeling system, and it is often assumed that a change in external balance reflects the net difference between bone resorption and bone formation. However, short-term transient gains or losses can occur in either system, and the different mechanisms underlying both sustained and transient changes in the mineral content of bone will now be summarized and some estimates formed of their possible magnitude.

The discussion will focus mainly on gains or losses of calcium and phosphorus which require changes in the total amount of mineral, in contrast to gains or losses of magnesium which may involve only the exchangeable magnesium pool. Calcium is almost all in bone, whereas there are significant amounts of magnesium and phosphorus in the soft tissues, so that storage and release from bone can be more easily demonstrated for calcium than for magnesium or phosphorus. It is convenient to describe these changes in terms of the amount of calcium stored each day, but if the bone mineral changes in amount and not in composition each mmol of calcium will be accompanied by about 0.6 mmol of phosphorus and 0.03 mmol of magnesium.

Storage of mineral in bone may be either a homeostatic response which prevents excessive accumulation of mineral in the ECF or a primary process tending to cause excessive depletion from

the ECF. Conversely, release of mineral from bone may be either a homeostatic response which prevents excessive depletion of mineral from the ECF or a primary process tending to cause excessive accumulation in the ECF. In both cases the homeostatic system in bone may respond at least temporarily to a homeostatic burden imposed by the remodeling system. Although the main emphasis is on physiologic defense mechanisms, the consequences of some pathologic processes will be described briefly for comparison.

Storage of mineral in bone

When calcium gluconate or chloride is infused at a rate of 0.4 mmol/kg body weight over 4 h to normal human subjects, about 40 to 60 percent of the infused calcium is still present in the body after 24 h (213), for an average retention of about 15 mmol. In the dog, short-term storage of mineral in bone is proportional to the increase in blood level (117). When repeated daily infusions of 13.75 mmol were given for 5 to 16 days, continued retention of 4 to 8 mmol of calcium and to 3 to 6 mmol of phosphorus daily was found, the highest cumulative retention of calcium amounting to about 130 mmol in 16 days (214). Similarly, single intravenous infusions of sodium phosphate produce short-term retention of both phosphate and calcium (195, 200), and continued oral administration to 40 to 60 mmol of sodium phosphate for 6 to 18 days produced continued retention of 3.5 mmol of calcium and 9.5 mmol of phosphate daily (215). The mechanism of these short-term and presumably transient effects has not been clearly established, and several possibilities must be examined.

Completion of primary mineralization. With a normal bone turnover of 10 percent per annum, the total amount of unmineralized osteoid is about 0.5 percent of the total bone volume. With an increase from zero to 70 percent of maximum mineral content this could accept about 100 mmol of calcium, but it is most unlikely that an abrupt acceleration of primary mineralization contributes significantly to short-term mineral storage, numerous statements to this effect notwithstanding. Mineralization requires both normal maturation of the matrix and the transport of mineral across the layer of osteoblasts, both of which limit the extent to which the prevailing rate of mineralization can be augmented. Normal osteoid is virtually free of mineral, but in osteomalacia the osteoid may paradoxically contain scattered foci of mineral detectable by electron microscopy (100). If the osteoid volume was increased twentyfold to 10 percent, enlargement of these foci with an increase of osteoid mineralization from 1 to 1.5 percent of maximum could store 120 mmol of calcium. Continued intravenous phosphate administration for 10 days may produce radiographic healing of rickets (216), but in adults with osteomalacia, although the foci of mineral within the osteoid may enlarge, normal mineralization is not resumed (217). Except when hypophosphatemia is a rate-limiting factor, there is no evidence that phosphate administration will augment primary mineralization to a significant extent.

Completion of secondary mineralization. Normally, mineralization in cortical bone increases from about 70 to nearly 95 percent of maximum in about three months at an exponentially decreasing rate. In trabecular bone, with its higher surface/volume ratio, secondary mineralization is largely complete in about one month. With a normal bone turnover of 10 percent per year, an abrupt completion of secondary mineralization throughout the skeleton could store about 100 mmol of calcium. The rate of secondary mineralization is limited primarily by the rate of diffusion of ions into bone of progressively decreasing water content and permeability, but a modest acceleration could probably be induced by raising the calcium-phosphate ion activity product. Possibly about 10 percent of the theoretical maximum, or about 10 mmol of calcium, could be stored by this mechanism.

Temporary expansion of the bone surface–perilacunar compartment. The amorphous mineral immediately adjacent to free bone surfaces, which is in equilibrium with the bone fluid and with the ECF, contains about 150 mmol of calcium. The bone fluid is also in equilibrium with the perilacunar bone, and from the rapidity

with which plasma constituents gain access to the lacunae it is likely that equilibration is only 30 to 60 minutes slower than with the surface compartment. From the number of osteocytes per mm^3 of bone it can be estimated that the low-density permeable zone around the lacunae contains about 0.5 percent of total bone mineral or an additional 150 mmol of calcium. A 10 percent increase in the size of this combined surface and perilacunar compartment could therefore store about 30 mmol of calcium. If the pericanalicular surface was included to a depth of 1 μm, almost 20 percent of the total bone mineral would be involved, but there is no evidence that bone of low density and high permeability is present around the canaliculae as well as the lacunae, and it is likely that the total amount of pericanalicular bone mineral can vary only between much narrower limits and that exchange with the bone fluid is much slower.

As well as changes in the total amount of mineral, minute-to-minute changes occur by heteroionic exchange both in the ionic concentrations within the hydration shell and in the composition of the crystals. This also involves the bone surface and perilacunar compartments, but similar changes probably also occur over progressively longer time scales at the canalicular and microcanalicular levels. A 1 percent increase in the calcium content of the bone surface–perilacunar compartment by means of heteroionic exchange for sodium or magensium could store 3 mmol of calcium.

It is likely that most short-term storage of mineral occurs in the surface and perilacunar compartment by one or the other of these mechanisms. For example, the presence of increased amounts of low-density, incompletely mineralized bone in osteomalacia may account for the increased temporary storage of calcium in response to a standard calcium infusion (218).

Growth. During normal growth the calcium content of the skeleton increases from about 700 to about 20,000 mmol in 20 years, an average increase of about 4 mmol of calcium, 2.5 mmol of phosphorus, and 0.1 mmol of magnesium per day. During the period of most rapid growth in adolescence the rates of storage would be two to three times as high.

Reduction in bone turnover. An evolving osteon in cortical bone represents a hole with a volume of 0.02 mm^3 which exists for 4 to 12 months. Similar deficits exist on the trabecular surface as incompletely refilled Howship's lacunae. With a normal bone turnover of 10 percent per year, remodeling units of 2000 μm total length advancing by 20 μm/day represent about 1 percent of the total bone volume. Consequently, about 300 mmol of calcium is temporarily missing from bone at one time because of remodeling. A reduction of bone turnover to 5 percent per annum will reduce the amount of temporarily missing bone to about 0.5 percent of the total and so store about 150 mmol of calcium over about 100 days, or about 1.5 mmol of calcium, 1 mmol of phosphorus, and 0.04 mmol of magnesium daily. Much larger amounts would be stored when a pathologically increased turnover is returned to normal. For example, with an abrupt fall from 40 to 10 percent, the net deposition will be six times larger or 9 mmol of calcium, 6 mmol of phosphorus, and 0.25 mmol of magnesium daily. In practice, bone turnover falls gradually rather than abruptly, so that lesser rates of storage over a longer period of time are seen.

Woven bone formation. Pathologic osteosclerosis consists in the deposition of woven bone within the marrow space leading to an increase in total trabecular bone mass. A threefold increase in trabecular volume throughout 25 percent of the skeleton over 1 year would represent a total increase of 3000 mmol of calcium or about 8 mmol/day, but except in rare instances the total amount and rate of accumulation of pathologic woven bone would be considerably smaller than this.

Healing of metabolic bone disease. Severe osteomalacia responding maximally to vitamin D, calcium and phosphate supplements may store as much as 25 mmol of calcium, 16 mmol of phosphate, and 0.7 mmol of magnesium per day. Such a rate could not be sustained for more than a few weeks, and most balance studies have shown storage of about 5 to 10 mmol of calcium per day

(219). Resorption of incompletely mineralized bone and its replacement by bone of normal composition also occurs in osteomalacia and provides for slower storage of mineral over a longer time period. In osteitis fibrosa cystica, surgical cure of primary hyperparathyroidism is followed by an abrupt cessation of osteoclastic resorption and the rapid appearance of osteoblasts at all previously resorbing surfaces. Because the switchover from resorption to formation is accomplished within a few days rather than being spread over several months, as when caused simply by a reduction in bone turnover, the magnitude of storage can be as high as 40 mmol of calcium, 25 mmol of phosphorus, and 1 mmol of magnesium daily (220), but the amounts are usually much smaller.

Circadian and seasonal variation in mineral balance

A normal young adult is in mineral equilibrium in the long-term, but there are temporary gains and losses of mineral at different times of the day. In most persons there will be a calcium retention of about 2 mmol during the day and a calcium loss of about 2 mmol to provide continued urinary excretion during the night (221). Much of this fluctuation in balance could be borne by the interstitial and connective tissue pools of calcium, since small changes in net charge or alterations in sodium or potassium content could significantly modify the calcium-binding capacity of the macromolecular network (40). Nevertheless, it is likely that bone also participates, and the amounts are well within the capacity for short-term gain and loss by the bone surface–perilacunar compartment. These shifts could also be accomplished by cyclical fluctuation in the activity of existing osteoclasts and osteoblasts without a change in their number. For the anatomic reasons explained earlier, such a transient uncoupling of the remodeling cycle either from augmentation of osteoclastic resorption or suppression of osteoblastic formation is more likely to occur on the trabecular surface than within the cortex.

There may also be periodic changes in balance over longer time intervals of weeks or months, such as the menstrual cycle, and a seasonal fluctuation with net calcium retention in the summer and net loss in the winter (222). This may be related to seasonal changes in vitamin D metabolism, but nothing is known of its anatomic basis.

Withdrawal of mineral from bone

Under most conditions hypocalcemia is a more frequent threat than hypercalcemia, and several mechanisms exist for the acute removal of calcium from bone. The experimental counterpart to infusion of calcium is removal of calcium either by dialysis or, more usually, by the infusion of a chelating agent such as edetic acid (EDTA). When the plasma calcium is reduced by 25 to 30 percent by EDTA infusion over a 2-h period, the preinfusion level is restored in about 4 h in the dog and about 12 h in human beings (223). In the dog, the magnitude of calcium mobilized is proportional to the ECF deficit, analogous to the effects of a calcium infusion (117). There is no evidence that augmentation of intestinal absorption or renal tubular reabsorption contributes significantly to this repair, so that the deficit in ECF calcium, amounting to about 10 mmol in human beings, must be replenished from bone. More prolonged demands on bone mineral content are made by a low-calcium diet, which may lead to a negative calcium balance for many weeks and cumulative losses of 100 mmol or more (222, 224).

Mobilization of calcium from the bone surface–perilacunar compartment. Temporary withdrawal of mineral is probably mediated by the same compartment as temporary storage. Removal of calcium without phosphate can occur by alteration in hydration-shell composition or by heteroionic exchange, but the extent of this is probably small. Redistribution of the total rapidly exchangeable mineral could repair about one-half to two-thirds of the deficit in ECF calcium produced by EDTA infusion, but complete repair requires mobilization of additional mineral under the influence of increased parathyroid hormone secretion. Dissolution of 10 percent of the amorphous mineral in the bone surface–perilacunar compartment could provide 15 mmol of calcium, 9 mmol of phosphorus, and 0.4 mmol of magne-

sium. Other mechanisms are extension of the low-density perilacunar zone to a greater distance from the osteocytes and augmentation of the activity of osteoclasts. It is unlikely that the calcium-phosphate ion activity product in bone ECF could ever fall low enough to permit dissolution of apatite.

Increased normal bone resorption without increased bone turnover. Although an increase in the proportion of active osteoclasts occurs as part of the response to acute hypocalcemia and could also be concerned in the normal mobilization of calcium at night, it is not known how long the cells can remain in the activated state in response to a longer lasting stimulus such as dietary calcium deprivation (224). An increase in bone resorption caused by increased osteoclast activity could lead to a deficit of bone which never gets repaired, in contrast to increased resorption in the normal remodeling sequence which initiates its own repair.

Increase in bone turnover. A fourfold increase in bone turnover from 10 to 40 percent per annum will increase the amount of temporarily missing bone from 1 to 4 percent of the total. If this increase were spread over 60 days, an additional 15 mmol of calcium, 9 mmol of phosphorus, and 0.4 mmol of magnesium would be added to the ECF each day. If each remodeling cycle is normal, this amount will all be replenished when the bone turnover rate returns to the previous level, but if the distance traveled by the resorption front also increases, more bone may be removed by each cycle than is replaced. There is an additional nonreversible component to the mobilization of bone mineral because the amplitude of any existing negative balance will be proportionately increased, and an existing net loss of 1 to 2 mmol/day caused by involutional bone loss will increase to 4 to 8 mmol/day, so that the total extra burden from a fourfold increase in turnover, including both reversible and irreversible components, could be as high as 21 mmol of calcium each day. However, as explained earlier, after the completion of two full sigmas the reversible loss would cease but the irreversible loss would continue at the same rate.

Aging and involutional bone loss. After the age of 50 the total bone mass declines by about 2 percent per annum in women and somewhat more slowly in men. This represents a loss of about 2 mmol/day of calcium, 1.25 mmol/day of phosphorus, and 0.05 mmol/day of magnesium. This is so whether the skeleton is thought to be responding in an appropriate manner to increased demand for calcium, or delivering a slow calcium infusion into the circulation for reasons unrelated to calcium homeostasis.

Pathologic bone resorption. Primary or secondary tumors in bone cause a local increase in bone resorption which is not coupled to subsequent formation; they may remove up to 15 to 20 mmol of calcium each day. The same may occur in severe hyperparathyroid bone disease with osteitis fibrosa when the normal coupling between resorption and formation is broken (150).

Development of metabolic bone disease. An increase in the amount of osteoid from 0.5 to 10 percent of the total bone mass over a 5-year period will be associated with a negative calcium balance of approximately 2 mmol/day. If bone turnover continues at its normal value of 10 percent per annum and no mineralization occurred at all in the newly formed bone, this amount of osteoid could accumulate in 1 year with a negative balance of approximately 8 mmol/day. During the development of osteitis fibrosa cystica there may be, as well as an increase in turnover, a replacement of normal lamellar bone by incompletely mineralized woven bone, which can produce an additional loss of calcium amounting to 5 mmol/day, assuming that the woven bone was mineralized to the extent of 75 percent of the lamellar bone.

EXTERNAL BALANCE AND TURNOVER OF THE DIVALENT IONS

The net difference between all routes of gain and loss of substances by the body is the external balance. After birth, all constituents of the body are ultimately derived from the diet, so that the gains by the body are determined by net absorption (NA), which is the difference between dietary intake (I) and fecal excretion (F) (Fig. 8-15); in this context, the contents of the gastrointestinal (GI) tract are considered to be outside the body. Loss from the body normally occurs in the urine and to a smaller extent from the skin. Mineral losses in sweat may be significant in a very hot and humid climate, but under most conditions this can be disregarded. Consequently, the difference between net absorption and urinary excretion, the two components of external turnover, determines the external balance which in turn determines the body content. Turnover can take place only via the blood, so that the components of external turnover are also major determinants of the plasma and ECF composition. Interchange between the body and the contents of the GI tract is also a form of external turnover; this may be disturbed in disease but normally has little homeostatic impact for the divalent ions.

In Table 8-14 average values for daily external turnover for the divalent ions are compared with similar values for sodium and potassium and expressed as a percentage of the amounts of each ion in the ECF, in the soft tissues, in bone, and in the whole body. For the major intracellular ions—potassium, magnesium, and phosphate—

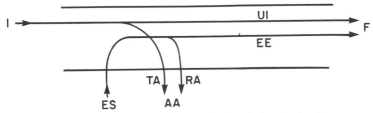

Figure 8-15. Intestinal exchanges of mineral. I = intake, ES = endogenous secretion, TA = true absorption, RA = reabsorption (of ES), AA = absolute (total) absorption (TA + RA), UI = unabsorbed intake (I − TA), EE = endogenous excretion (ES − RA), and F = fecal excretion (UI + EE).

Table 8-14. External turnover of divalent and monovalent ions in relation to magnitudes of different body compartments

	Ca	P	Mg	Na	K
External turnover, mmol/day	5	30	4	150	60
ECF content, mmol	35	17	13	2,000	70
External turnover, %ECF/day	14	175	30	7.5	86
Renal clearance, mL/min	3	16	4	0.7	10
Soft-tissue content, mmol	120	3,200	530	1,400	4,000
External turnover, %ST/day	4	0.9	0.7	11	1.5
Bone content, mmol	31,350	19,000	840	1,400	75
External turnover, %bone/day	0.016	0.15	0.5	11	80
Total body content, mmol	31,500	22,200	1,400	4,800	4,200
External turnover, %total/day	0.016	0.13	0.3	3.1	1.4

the ECF turnover and renal plasma clearance are high, and soft-tissue turnover is low. For the major extracellular ion—sodium—the opposite is true. Calcium occupies an intermediate position for both ECF and soft tissue. For the major constituents of bone, external turnover is a very small fraction of the total osseous and total body content.

The external balance for the divalent ions should be zero in healthy adults, provided it is averaged over an appropriate time. As already mentioned, there are short-term circadian variations and long-term seasonal and other fluctuations in balance, but the magnitude of these does not usually exceed 5 mmol of calcium daily. During growth, the external balance is normally continuously positive. The mineral content of the body of a neonate is about 700 mmol of calcium, 550 mmol of phosphorus, and 35 mmol of magnesium, so that attainment of an adult skeleton requires an average retention of about 4 mmol of calcium, 2.5 mmol of phosphorus, and 0.1 mmol of magnesium daily during the first 20 years of life. The rates for calcium vary from about 1.5 to 2 mmol between 3 and 6 years to about 10 mmol daily at the peak of the adolescent growth spurt; phosphate and magnesium are stored in the same proportions as in bone, with additional amounts for soft-tissue growth (225). After the age of about 45, because of involutional bone loss, the "normal" balance becomes negative to the extent of about 1.5 mmol of calcium and 1 mmol of phosphorus daily.

NUTRITIONAL ASPECTS

The question of the dietary calcium requirement is still debated among nutritionists and others interested in the pathogenesis of involutional bone loss (226, 227). Normal persons are able to conserve calcium in time of need by increasing the efficiency of absorption and decreasing the rate of loss in the urine (228) by mechanisms which will be described later. When calcium balance is studied in normal individuals at different levels of intake, the minimum level at which calcium equilibrium is attained (which is the classic way of defining the nutritional requirement) reflects primarily the intake prevailing before the experiment began. Some, but not all, normal persons can eventually adapt to substantially lower intakes (228). Whatever the efficiency of adaptation, the calcium intake needed to maintain bone mass is much higher than that needed to maintain plasma calcium, which is probably close to zero.

In the United States and other wealthy countries most dietary calcium comes from milk and milk products, whereas in poorer countries vegetable sources are relatively more important. Most of the difference in mean calcium intake between countries is due to differences in milk consumption. The absolute amount provided by cereals and other nondairy sources is fairly constant, so that total calcium intake is approximated by the total dairy product calcium plus 6 mmol daily (229). Individual intakes are much more variable than community intakes and less easily predicted from this formula. High-protein foods such as meats, fish and eggs, provide only 5 to 10 percent of the total calcium intake in almost all countries. Some nondairy foods, such as chocolate, nuts, parsley, dried fruits, string beans, canned fish, tea, and caviar have a very high calcium content but are normally eaten in insufficient quantities to be nutritionally significant. The calcium in drinking water (mainly as bicarbonate) varies considerably, and hard water may contain 1.5 to 3 mmol/L of calcium, but this is unlikely to be important unless other sources are defective or consumption of water unusually high. In the United Kingdom and probably also in the United States, the majority of the population have intakes between 10 and 40 mmol daily, with a mean of about 25 mmol.

The availability or utilization of calcium varies with different foods. In spinach the calcium is present mainly as insoluble oxalate, while the lactose in milk enhances absorption. Other components of the diet have relatively little effect on calcium. The calcium/phosphorus ratio is important in rats, both very high and very low ratios interfering with calcium absorption. In human beings, wide variations in phosphate intake have very little effect (230, 231), although they alter calcium metabolism in other ways. Fatty acids can form insoluble soaps with calcium which are not absorbed, but fat absorption is normally so efficient that wide variations in fat intake have no effect on calcium absorption unless fat absorption is impaired, either from disease or from functional immaturity in infants. Many cereal foods, especially those made from unrefined flour, contain phytic acid (inositolhexaphosphoric acid), which forms an insoluble and unabsorbably complex with calcium and magnesium (232). In the United Kingdom during World War II the extraction of flour was increased, and to offset the increase in phytate content it was fortified with extra calcium by government decree. Interest in phytate has recently been renewed by the suggestion that the high incidence of nutritional rickets in Indian migrants to the United Kingdom is related to the high phytate content of *chapatis* made from unleavened flour, but other factors are probably of greater importance. For most clinical purposes nutritional assessment with respect to calcium can be based on the total daily intake or, more simply, on the total consumption of dairy foods.

In wealthy countries dairy products and meat each provide about half the total daily intake of phosphorus of about 40 to 50 mmol, other sources such as grains and vegetables being much less important. These priorities are reversed in poorer countries. The molar Ca/P ratio of milk is about 1, much higher than in most other foods, so that the Ca/P ratio of whole diets depends mainly on the milk intake. The phosphorus intake varies over a narrower range between different countries than does the calcium intake. Most organic phosphate esters in meat, phosphoproteins in milk, and phospholipids in eggs are hydrolyzed in the gut and so are utilized as readily as dietary inorganic orthophosphate. Vegetable sources of phosphorus are readily available in human beings but not in the chick (230). Much of the phosphorus in grains is in the form of phytate. When the intake of this is habitually small, about half a phytate load is hydrolyzed by intestinal phytase (probably an alkaline phosphatase) and the phosphorus made available for absorption (230), but when the intake is habitually large, the activity of intestinal phytase is enhanced. Dietary phytate normally has as little significance for the nutrition of phosphate as it does for calcium, although it may be important for trace elements such as zinc.

Magnesium is a major constituent of all cells and so is present in all foods except fats; consequently, no single class of food is dominant in providing the normal dietary intake of 8 to 16 mmol. In green vegetables it is chelated to the porphyrin group of chlorophyll. Virtually any diet providing enough nutrients to support life would also contain enough magnesium (227).

GASTROINTESTINAL ABSORPTION AND FECAL EXCRETION OF THE DIVALENT IONS (231–234)

The function of the intestinal tract as a whole determined by combined balance and isotope studies will be described first, before considering the cellular mechanisms underlying the gross changes.

Data from balance and isotope studies

In considering the completeness of absorption, it is important to distinguish between *net* absorption, *absolute* absorption, and *true* absorption (Fig. 8-15). Net absorption (NA) is defined as the difference between intake (I) and fecal excretion (F), determined by the metabolic balance method.

$$NA = I - F \qquad (8\text{-}4)$$

Net absorption can be expressed as a fraction of intake (β), where $\beta = (I - F)/I$, or as a percentage of intake, where NA% = $\beta \times 100$. NA is also the difference between absolute absorption (AA) and endogenous gastrointestinal secretion (ES), sometimes called digestive juice secretion:

$$NA = AA - ES \text{ or } AA = I - (F - ES) \qquad (8\text{-}5)$$

Absolute absorption includes absorption of dietary intake (true absorption, or TA) and absorption of endogenous secretion (reabsorption, or RA). That part of endogenous secretion which escapes absorption is called endogenous fecal excretion (EE), which can be estimated by measurement of fecal radioactivity after intravenous administration of labeled material. Therefore:

$$AA = TA + (ES - EE) \qquad (8\text{-}6)$$

Combining Eqs. (8-5) and (8-6),

$$TA = I - (F - EE) \qquad (8\text{-}7)$$

True absorption can be expressed as a fraction of intake (α), where $\alpha = [I - (F - EE)]/I$ or as a percentage of intake where TA% = $\alpha \times 100$. The same relationships can be derived by considering that total fecal excretion consists of endogenous excretion and unabsorbed dietary intake (UI) so that F = EE + (I − TA). True absorption can also be estimated by measuring cumulative fecal radioactivity or whole body retention of radioactivity (corrected for urinary excretion) after oral administration of labeled material. Both these methods are subject to a small error because of secretion of some absorbed radioactivity. Endogenous secretion and absolute absorption can be measured from the same combined balance and isotope studies needed to measure net absorption and true absorption, by making an assumption about the relationship between absorption of dietary intake and the absorption of endogenous secretion. If these are equal, then

$$ES = \frac{EE}{1 - \alpha} \text{ and } AA = TA + EE\frac{\alpha}{1 - \alpha} \qquad (8\text{-}8)$$

This assumption is probably not correct for any of the divalent ions. Endogenous secretion can also be estimated from average values for the volume and composition of the known intestinal secretions—saliva, gastric juice, bile, pancreatic juice and succus entericus (Table 8-15) (231, 235–238). But ions may be extruded by the intestinal mucosa directly and not just as part of a fluid secretion, so that total endogenous secretion could be greater than total digestive juice secretion.

Completeness of absorption must be distinguished from rapidity of absorption. The normal

Table 8-15. Volume and divalent ion concentrations of intestinal secretions

	VOL,	Ca		P		Mg	
	L/day	mmol/L	mmol/day	mmol/L	mmol/day	mmol/L	mmol/day
Saliva	1.0	1.3	1.3	4.0	4.0	0.3	0.3
Gastric secretion	1.5	1.0	1.5	1.0	1.5	0.7	1.0
Bile	1.0	1.5	1.5	5.0	5.0	0.7	0.7
Pancreatic secretion	1.5	1.0	1.5	1.0	1.5	0.4	0.6
Intestinal secretion	1.0	1.2	1.2	1.0	1.0	0.4	0.4
Total	6.0		7.0		13.0		3.0

Source: From Sunderman and Bremer; Davenport; Code; Altman and Dittmer (235–238).

intestine has considerable functional reserve; if absorption in proximal segments is reduced, absorption in distal segments may increase so that the same total amount is absorbed over a longer portion of intestine and over a longer time period. The rapidity of absorption can be studied by measuring the time course of plasma or forearm radioactivity after an oral dose of labeled material. This is also affected by the rapidity of uptake in bone and soft tissues and the rate of urinary excretion. From the time course of plasma radioactivity after separate oral and IV administration, both rapidity and completeness can be calculated; this technique has been used for calcium (239) but not for phosphorus or magnesium. Rapidity of absorption can also be determined by perfusion of short segments using a triple lumen tube and measurement of the rate of disappearance of labeled ions in relation to an inert marker (240). Results of both isotope administration and intestinal perfusion depend on the absorption of inorganic salts which require no digestion; the results do not necessarily indicate how the same elements will be absorbed from food.

Calcium. Representative values for calcium of the various quantities discussed in the previous section are shown in Table 8-16. Two values are given for endogenous secretion and absolute absorption. The lower values assume that only 85 percent of ES_{Ca} is available for absorption at the same efficiency as dietary calcium (241) because it enters the gut distal to the sites of most active absorption, so that $ES_{Ca} /(1 - 0.85\alpha_{Ca})$. The higher values are estimated from the volume and composition of the digestive juices (Table 8-15) and imply that, like the calcium in bile (242), most digestive juice calcium is absorbed with *greater* efficiency than dietary calcium. This apparent paradox is discussed further in the next section. Endogenous secretion is unaffected by raising the plasma calcium, and very little of a parenteral load of calcium appears in the stool (231).

The values in Table 8-16 apply only to the stated intake. Based on available balance data, net calcium absorption has a curvilinear relationship to intake, with a steep initial rise (Fig. 8-16). At intakes below 80 μmol/kg body weight per day, net absorption is negative because fecal excretion exceeds intake. Above this level fractional net absorption rises to a peak and then declines slowly, whereas absolute net absorption increases progressively (231). Fractional true absorption is highest at the lowest intake and falls with increasing intake (Fig. 8-16). The same applies to individual calcium loads; frequent small doses of

Table 8-16. Representative values for various components of absorption, secretion, and excretion of divalent ions by intestinal tract*

QUANTITY, μm/kg BW/day		Ca	P	Mg
Intake	(I)	350	700	150
Endogenous secretion	(ES)	80/100	150/190	20/40
True absorption	(TA)	150	500	70
Reabsorption	(RA)	35/50	100/140	10/30
Absolute absorption	(AA)	180/200	600/640	80/100
Endogenous excretion, ES - RA	(EE)	50	50	10
Unabsorbed intake, I - TA	(UI)	200	200	80
Total fecal excretion	(F)	250	250	90
Net absorption, I - F	(NA)	100	450	60
Urinary excretion	(U)	100	450	60
Fractional total absorption	(α)	0.43	0.71	0.47
Fractional net absorption	(β)	0.29	0.64	0.40

* Higher values for endogenous secretion and absolute absorption and reabsorption are based on volume and composition of intestinal secretions, lower values on parenteral administration of radioactive material.

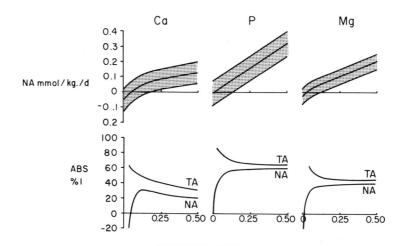

Figure 8-16. Absorption of divalent ions as functions of intake. NA = net absorption, TA = true absorption, and %I = percent of intake. (*After R. Wilkinson.*)

a calcium supplement are better absorbed than fewer large doses, even when the total daily intake is the same (243). These changes reflect the properties of the calcium transport system and are not indicative of adaptation, which is a change in α at the same intake after prolonged use of an intake higher or lower than is customary (231). More calcium is absorbed whenever the demand for calcium is increased, as normally happens during growth, pregnancy, and lactation. The high calcium absorption of infancy is a consequence of rapid growth rather than of age as such, but both basal calcium absorption and the ability to increase absorption in response to a low calcium intake decline progressively after the age of about 50 (231, 244). The mechanism of all these changes will be discussed in the section on vitamin D.

After a single dose of labeled calcium given with an inert carrier but no food, the plasma radioactivity usually peaks at 1 h, and absorption is usually complete within 2½ to 4 h (239). When the dose is given during a meal the peak plasma increment may be delayed for 4 h, and significant absorption occurs beyond 8 h (245). The peak increase in stable plasma calcium after an oral load occurs at about 1½ to 2 h (246). A detailed kinetic analysis (239) led to a model characterized

by a delay of 20 min before the onset of calcium absorption caused by transit out of the stomach, attainment of a peak absorption rate at 40 to 60 min after ingestion, and completion of absorption within 2½ h. Absorption from the proximal component (duodenum and upper jejunum) was nine times higher per unit length than from the distal component. The rate of absorption from the duodenum and jejunum, whether determined indirectly from plasma or forearm radioactivity curves or directly by intubation and perfusion (247), correlates well with net calcium absorption determined by balance studies.

Phosphorus. Representative values for phosphorus of the various quantities discussed in the previous section are shown in Table 8-16. Endogenous secretion and excretion and absolute absorption cannot be measured accurately; as for calcium two values are given, but they are only approximate (231). Based on available balance studies, net phosphate absorption is a linear function of intake such that $NA_P = I_P - 10\ \mu mol/kg$ body weight per day (Fig. 8-16). The form of the relationships between fractional true and fractional net absorption and intake is similar to those for calcium, except that mean net absorption according to the model is always positive (Fig. 8-16); this extrapolation may not be valid at very low intakes. Over the customary range of intakes, net fractional absorption is about twice as high for phosphorus as for calcium.

After administration of ^{32}P, the peak plasma radioactivity is attained after 1 h (248), and the peak increment in stable plasma phosphate after an oral load occurs after 1½ h (249). These intervals are about the same as for calcium, even though phosphorus appears to be absorbed more rapidly than calcium in the rat, as judged by the earliest appearance of radioactivity in the systemic circulation.

Magnesium. Representative values for magnesium of the various quantities discussed in the previous section are shown in Table 8-16. As for phosphorus, the two values given for endogenous secretion and excretion and absolute absorption are only approximate. Based on available balance studies, net absorption of magnesium is a linear function of intake over the customary range of intakes, such that $NA_{Mg} = 0.40I_{Mg} - 3$ mmol/kg body weight per day (Fig. 8-16). At very low intakes NA_{Mg} can be negative because fecal magnesium excretion is greater than intake, but this is much less apparent than for calcium. At very high intakes the linear relationship no longer holds, and NA_{Mg} is less than is predicted from the above equation. The form of the relationships between fractional true and fractional net absorption and intake are similar to those for phosphorus (Fig. 8-16). Over the customary range both are intermediate between corresponding values for calcium and for phosphorus (Table 8-16). The peak increase in plasma radioactivity after an oral dose of labeled magnesium is at 6 h, and the level is still raised after 24 h (250).

The mechanisms of divalent ion absorption

Morphologic aspects (251, 252). The intestinal mucosa is thrown into folds and corrugations so that even on a macroscopic scale the surface is large in relation to the volume of the luminal contents. On a smaller scale the mucosa consists of villi about 1 mm long and 0.1 mm in diameter, which further increase the surface area. Each villus consists mainly of columnar cells that absorb

nutrients and goblet cells that secrete mucus. There is a very rapid turnover of cells, new cells arising by mitosis in the crypts between the villi and migrating to the tips of the villi in about 5 days (in human beings) to replace the approximate loss of 250 g of cellular debris shed into the lumen daily. The luminal pole of each columnar cell is folded into microvilli about 1 μm long and 0.1 μm in diameter, which increase the surface area another fortyfold. The surface of the microvilli contains pores of about 0.4 nm radius. The spaces between the microvilli are filled with a filamentous material which projects into the lumen and forms a continuous layer called the glycocalyx or fuzzy coat. This is composed of GAG and PG molecules which differ from those of mucus but which, as in connective tissue, have binding capacity for divalent ions because of their fixed negative charge. Within the microvilli are microfilaments or microtubules, which presumably facilitate the transfer of absorbed material to the body of the cell. The microvilli and the glycocalyx together constitute the brush border of the cell. Adjacent mucosal cells are joined at their luminal poles by tight and intermediate junctions (Fig. 8-17), but the basal half of the cells are separated by lateral intercellular spaces which become distended during the absorption of sodium and water. Substances which enter the cell through the brush border can leave by crossing the plasma membrane either at the basal surface or at the lateral surface to enter the intercellular spaces. Entry to these spaces is also possible by a shunt or paracellular pathway through the tight junctions. The luminal fluid immediately adjacent to and between the villi forms the so-called unstirred layer which does not mix readily with the remainder of the luminal contents. The unstirred layer forms an additional barrier to be traversed by substances undergoing absorption (253), but its importance for divalent ions is unknown.

Intraluminal concentrations and other digestive aspects. The concentration of substances in the intestinal lumen is obviously of critical importance in understanding the mechanisms of transport across the mucosa, but data of this kind for the divalent ions in human subjects are very sparse. The same distinction between total, ultra-

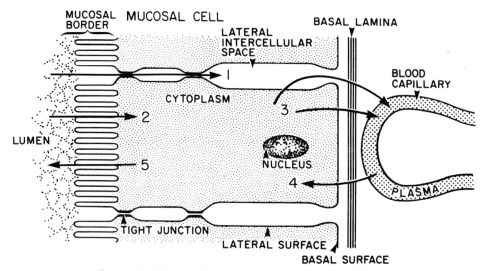

Figure 8-17. Diagram of intestinal mucosal cell to show different sites of movement of ions involved in absorption. 1. Paracellular route across tight junctions. 2. Influx across brush border. 3. Efflux across basolateral surface. 4. Influx across basolateral surface. 5. Efflux across brush border. (*After R. H. Wasserman.*)

filtrable, and free ionized concentrations applies to the contents of the GI tract as well as to the plasma. In addition, much of the divalent ion content, particularly in the distal ileum and colon, is not in solution but is in precipitated solid form.

In milk, the free ionized concentration is less than 1 mmol/L, only about 3 percent of the total calcium concentration. The remainder forms colloidal complexes with casein, lactalbumin, and phosphate. In fruits and vegetables, much of the calcium may be complexed to organic acids such as tartrate. It is usually presumed that all the dietary calcium is converted to the free ionic form by the action of gastric HCl, but there are no data for intraluminal ionized calcium after a meal in human beings. Conversion of the calcium in food to a form suitable for absorption also involves the formation of micelles with bile and lecithin, which facilitate passage into solution and contact with the brush border (231). If some dietary calcium persists in complexed form beyond the site of most active absorption in the duodenum, it could be less efficiently absorbed than calcium in intestinal secretions such as bile.

Most of the phosphorus in milk is inorganic, but most of the phosphorus and magnesium in meat, vegetables, and other nondairy sources is intracellular and so is in complex organic form. Liberation of free ions therefore requires a much longer period of digestion than for calcium. Another factor is intraluminal pH, which gets progressively more alkaline beyond the duodenum (231). If hydrolysis of organic phosphate esters in food is accomplished by intestinal alkaline phosphatase, it presumably takes place mainly in the ileum, the need for an alkaline pH for optimum *digestion* of dietary phosphate contrasting with the need for an acid pH for optimum *solubilization* of phosphate and calcium. On the other hand, the pH optimum of alkaline phosphatase is so high, and its localization so predominantly in the duodenum where the pH is normally low, that it may have nothing to do with ester hydrolysis. Direct evidence concerning the site and mechanisms of this process are lacking.

After ingestion of a high-calcium milk meal, the total dissolved calcium concentration was about 15 mmol/L in the stomach and fell progressively to about 1 to 1.5 mmol/L in the distal ileum. After a low-calcium meat meal, the dissolved calcium concentration was about 1 to 1.5

mmol/L at all levels (254). These values may be too low, because the autoanalyzer method does not detect some strongly bound complexes of calcium; in the fasting state higher values of about 2 mmol/L at all levels were found after ashing (255). In the dog, total dissolved concentration was higher in the ileum (8 mmol/L) than more proximally. There are no data for intraluminal phosphorus or magnesium concentrations after a meal, but fasting phosphorus concentration in human beings was also about 2 mmol/L at all levels (255). In the fowl, intestinal ionized calcium concentrations are much less affected by diet than the total calcium, varying between 2 and 6 mmol/L in the duodenum and jejunum and between 0.8 and 2.5 mmol/L in the ileum (256, 257). Ultrafiltrable phosphorus concentrations

were about 8 to 12 mmol/L in the duodenum, 3 to 4 mmol/L in the jejunum, and 1 to 2 mmol/L in the ileum. Both ionized calcium and ultrafiltrable phosphate concentrations progressively decline with increasing distance beyond the jejunum, even though total calcium and phosphate concentrations progressively increase. These relationships are maintained at all levels of dietary intake. The available data are consistent with the same pattern in human beings.

The concentrations in human fecal fluid determined by in vivo dialysis are about 20 mmol/L for calcium, 5 mmol/L for phosphorus, and 25 mmol/L for magnesium (258, 259). These values fell to about 2, 3, and 1 mmol/L respectively on an electrolyte-free diet, suggesting that most of the calcium and magnesium remaining in solu-

Table 8-17. Estimates of absolute absorption, AA, and net absorption, NA, of water, L/day and divalent ions, mmol/day, at different levels of the intestinal tract*

SECRETION	SALIVARY +GASTRIC	BILIARY +PANCREATIC	INTESTINAL
H_2O	2.5	2.5	1.0
Ca	2.8	3.0	1.2
P	5.5	6.5	1.0
Mg	1.3	1.3	0.4

	Diet→	Stomach		Duodenum + Jejunum		Ileum		Colon		Feces
H_2O	2.0	4.5	4.5	7.0	2.5	3.5	0.7	0.7	0.1	0.1
Ca	25	27.8	27.8	30.8	23.3	24.5	18.5	18.5	18.0	18.0
P†	50	55.5	55.5	62.0	54.5 (39.5)	55.5 (40.5)	22.5	22.5	18.0	18.0
Mg	10	11.3	11.3	12.6	11.1	11.5	7.0	7.0	6.0	6.0

										TOTAL
	H_2O			4.5		2.8		0.6		7.9
AA	Ca			7.5		6.0		0.5		14.0
	P†			7.5 (22.5)		33.0 (18.0)		4.5		45.0
	Mg			1.5		4.5		1.0		7.0

	H_2O			−0.5		1.8		0.6		1.9
NA	Ca			1.7		4.8		0.5		7.0
	P†			−4.5 (10.5)		32.0 (17.0)		4.5		32.0
	Mg			−1.1		4.1		1.0		4.0

* Food is assumed to mix completely with saliva and gastric secretion in the stomach, with bile and pancreatic secretion in the proximal duodenum and with intestinal secretion in the proximal ileum. Values in each box represent sum of digesta received from earlier stage and secretions. Values between boxes represent transfers to next stage.

† Values enclosed in parentheses are for the second of two different assumptions concerning partition of phosphorus absorption between segments (see text).

Table 8-18. Theoretical total concentrations, mmol/L, of divalent ions in luminal contents and absorbate at different levels of the intestinal tract

| | CONTENTS | | | | | | ABSORBATE | | |
	DIET	STOMACH	DUODENUM	ILEUM	COLON	FECES	DUODENUM/JEJUNUM	ILEUM	COLON
Ca	12.5	6.2	4.4	7.0	26.4	180	1.7	2.1	0.8
P*	25.0	12.3	8.9	15.9 (11.6)	32.1	180	1.7 (5.0)	11.8 (6.4)	7.5
Mg	5.0	2.5	1.8	3.3	10.0	60	0.3	1.6	1.7

* Values enclosed in parentheses are for the second of two different assumptions concerning partition of phosphorus absorption between segments (see text).

tion in the feces originates in the diet, whereas most of the phosphorus is endogenous.

A model of absolute and net absorption at different levels can be constructed (Table 8-17) which permits upper limits for intraluminal concentrations to be estimated. Data required for the model are the volume and composition of the dietary intake and of the intestinal secretions (Table 8-15) and the amounts of water absorbed at different levels (235, 236). These values are only approximate because digestive juice concentrations tend to vary inversely with secretion rates, which change after each meal. There are no data for the volume of luminal contents transferred from the duodenum to the jejunum, so these segments are combined. It is assumed that net calcium absorption is divided between the combined duodenum and jejunum, ileum, and colon in the same proportion as in the dog (260). For partition of phosphorus absorption, two alternative assumptions were made. First, that absolute cal-

cium and phosphorus absorption in the duodenum and jejunum are equimolar, because vitamin D has its major action at this site and variations in vitamin D status lead to equimolar changes in calcium and phosphorus absorption (261). Second, that absolute phosphate absorption is distributed along the small intestine in the same proportion as absolute calcium absorption. Absorption of magnesium is assumed to be the same per unit length through the small bowel, as was found by intubation and perfusion in human beings (262). Significant absorption from the colon is inferred from the effects of rectal administration for both phosphorus (263) and magnesium (264). From the amounts of water and divalent ions present at different levels, theoretical total concentrations can be calculated (Table 8-18). These are lowest in the upper small intestine for all three substances and increase progressively thereafter because of preferential absorption of water. From the lengths of the different segments

Table 8-19. Estimated values for peak absorption of water and divalent ions at different levels of the intestinal tract*

	DUODENUM/JEJUNUM	ILEUM	COLON
Length, m	1.2	1.8	1.0
Transit time, h	2	4	24
H_2O, L/m per h	0.63	0.13	0.02
Ca, mmol/m per h	1.04	0.28	0.02
P,† mmol/m per h	1.04 (3.12)	1.53 (0.83)	0.17
Mg, mmol/m per h	0.21	0.21	0.04

* Food and water intake is presumed to occur as three equal meals, the digesta of which remain separated as far as the colon, so that total daily absorption occurs over 6 h in the duodenum and jejunum and 12 h in the ileum.

† Values enclosed in parentheses are for the second of two different assumptions concerning partition of phosphorus absorption between segments (see text).

Table 8-20. Comparison of absorptive fluxes calculated from the model, Table 8-17, with absorptive fluxes measured by intubation and perfusion in human beings

	Ca		P*		Mg	
	DJ	I	DJ	I	DJ	I
Intraluminal concentration, mmol/L	4.4	2.0	8.9	2.0	1.8	?
Flux calculated from model, mmol/m per h	1.04	0.28	1.04	1.53	0.21	0.21
			(3.12)	(0.83)		
Measured flux at specified concentration, mmol/m per h	0.84	0.20	3.50	0.34	0.22	?

* Values enclosed in parentheses are for the second of two different assumptions concerning partition of phosphorus absorption between segments (see text).
Source: Figures for calcium: From Wensel, Rich, Brown, and Volwiler; Ireland and Fordtran; Soergel, Mueller, Gustke, and Geenen (240, 244, 247). Figures for phosphorus:From Juan, Liptak, and Gray; Gray, Walton, Lovell, Williams, Dove, and Shapiro (265, 266); Walton and Gray (personal communication). Figures for magnesium: From Branna, Vergne-Marini, Pak, Hull, and Fordtran (262).
DJ = Duodenum + jejunum

and estimates of transit times (235, 236), peak absolute absorption rates after meals at different levels can be calculated (Table 8-19). The value for calcium is about four times greater in the duodenum and jejunum than in the ileum, even though net absorption occurs predominantly in the ileum. These values can be compared with those determined experimentally by intubation and perfusion in human beings (Table 8-20) (240, 244, 247, 262, 265, 266). In view of the number of steps in the calculations, there is reasonable agreement for calcium and magnesium. For phosphate the data agree much more closely with the second assumption of the model than with the first. However, the first assumption is more consistent with the digestive factors previously discussed, so that the difference between absorption of inorganic salts and absorption from food could be greater for phosphorus than for calcium. Also, net secretion of phosphorus in the upper small intestine and net absorption more distally is consistent with findings in the rat (267) and in the horse (268).

Comparison of the apparent concentrations calculated from the model (Table 8-18) with the various results previously assembled suggests that precipitation of calcium and magnesium as insoluble phosphates, carbonates, and soaps begins in the terminal ileum, progresses further in the colon, and is very extensive in the feces. Total fecal phosphate is correlated closely with the sum of total fecal calcium and magnesium (269). Some

of the precipitated calcium is probably derived from intestinal secretions, but much of the undissolved magnesium is contained in bacteria and cellular debris. Data obtained in the dog and fowl suggest that precipitation occurs more and more proximally as the dietary calcium intake increases (257, 270).

Cellular and subcellular aspects. Transport of divalent ions across the intestinal mucosa involves the same types of mechanisms as ion transport across other epithelial membranes. Passive diffusion, facilitated diffusion, carrier-mediated active transport, and solvent drag all occur under different conditions; these terms will be used according to the definitions given in Chap. 1. As well as any activity gradients which may exist between the luminal contents and the plasma, there is also an electric gradient with the mucosal surface negative to the serosal surface. This will oppose the absorption of calcium and magnesium but facilitate the absorption of phosphorus. In the chick, the magnitude of this potential difference is in the range found in other leaky epithelia with high permeability to water (256). In the rat, the potential difference will balance an intraluminal calcium concentration of about 6.5 mmol/L, so that net absorption at lower concentrations requires active transport (271). Similar calculations have not been performed for phosphorus and magnesium.

Calcium (231–234). Both in vitro studies using the everted gut sac technique and in vivo intubation and perfusion studies have shown that the mucosa is able to establish an ion activity gradient between the luminal and serosal surfaces, indicating net active transport against an electrochemical gradient. The results of one study using the Ussing short-circuit technique suggested that calcium was transported as a counter ion to active phosphate transport (272), but other studies using the same technique have reaffirmed the majority view. The transport mechanism requires metabolic energy, is saturable, is specific for calcium, and (as will be discussed in more detail later) is stimulated by vitamin D. The intraluminal concentration at which saturation occurs varies from 2 to 10 mmol/L in different species. Active transport occurs at all levels, including the colon, but beyond the duodenum it is easier to demonstrate in vivo than in vitro. All studies are in agreement that the lumen-plasma flux is highest in the duodenum and is also high in the jejunum, which fits with the model developed in the previous section.

Both in vitro and in vivo studies indicate an additional passive diffusional component that is nonsaturable and proportional to intraluminal concentration (229, 231, 273). Figure 8-18 illustrates how a measured total net inward (lumen to plasma) flux can be resolved into a saturable and a nonsaturable component, with provision also for a constant outward (plasma to lumen) flux. Also

shown is how the relationship between net absorption and calcium intake (determined from balance studies) can likewise be resolved into an active and a diffusional component (273). The former is more important at low intakes and the latter at high intakes, with estimates of their relative magnitude at a normal intake varying between 1:1 and 3:1 (229, 231).

The mucosal cell is presumed to resemble other cells in having a low intracellular free-calcium concentration. Most of the intracellular calcium is sequestered in electron-dense granules found mainly in the microvilli and in mitochondria; both uptake and release of calcium by these granules are metabolically controlled. The first step in absorption is mucosal uptake: calcium binds to some constituent of the cell membrane by a rapid nonsaturable process which precedes entry into the cell (231). This occurs at the brush border down a concentration gradient, either by simple diffusion without requiring energy or possibly by facilitated diffusion. The total mucosal cell calcium can increase three- to fivefold during absorption (274), but the calcium entering the cell exchanges with only a small fraction of the total cell calcium (274), most of it being stored temporarily in mitochondrial granules (274). The form in which calcium travels through the cytosol and the possible role of microtubules and

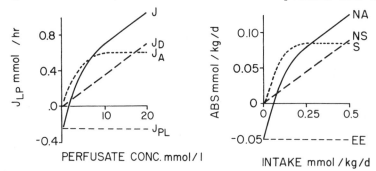

Figure 8-18. Left: Partition of total in vitro flux into saturable and nonsaturable components. J_{LP} = net lumen-to-plasma flux, J_D = flux caused by diffusion, J_A = flux caused by active transport, J_{PL} = plasma-to-lumen flux, and $J_{LP} = J_D + J_A - J_{PL}$. Right: Partition of net in vivo absorption (NA) into saturable (S) and nonsaturable (NS) components. ES = exogenous secretion and NA = NS + S − E. (*After R. Wilkinson.*)

other organelles in calcium transport are unknown (275). Calcium leaves the cell at the basal and lateral walls by an active transport mechanism that requires sodium. Under different experimental conditions either brush border influx or basolateral efflux may be rate-limiting. In addition, there is active efflux at the brush border and passive influx at the basal and lateral walls (276). Values for all four fluxes in the rat duodenum and ileum are shown in Fig. 8-19.

Calcium also travels via the paracellular pathway across the tight junctions to enter the lateral spaces. This is the most likely location of the diffusional component, which is thereby able to increase progressively with increasing luminal concentration even at levels far higher than normally occur, without producing a dangerous increase in intracellular free-calcium concentration.

The molecular basis of active calcium transport is still unclear. A calcium-binding protein occurs in the intestine and its role in absorption has been extensively studied; this will be discussed in the section on vitamin D. There are at least three different kinds of membrane-bound adenosine triphosphatase (ATPase) that may be related to calcium transport. These enzymes may serve the dual function of mobile carrier and energy source. First, in common with all other cells, the mucosal cells contain an ouabain-sensitive, Mg^{2+}-dependent Na^+–K^+–ATPase (sodium-potassium-activated ATPase) which subserves sodium transport (277). This is found in all parts of the cell membrane but is concentrated mainly at the basolateral surface. By maintaining an electric gradient, the sodium pump could facilitate entry of calcium at the brush border, and it has also been postulated that calcium extrusion at the basolateral surface is coupled by exchange-diffusion with passive sodium influx. This could explain the dependence of calcium efflux on sodium, but inhibition of the sodium pump with ouabain has no effect on calcium transport (277). Second, there is an Mg^{2+}-dependent Ca^{2+}–ATPase located only at the brush border, which is probably also a nonspecific alkaline phosphatase (278). This enzyme is related to vitamin D status and may be concerned in facilitated diffusion into the cell, but it can be inhibited by phenylalanine without impairing calcium transport (279). Finally, there is a Ca^{2+}-dependent Na^+–ATPase, which is not inhibited by ouabain, is located only at the basolateral surface, and is specific for calcium (280). This enzyme is the most plausible candidate for the basolateral calcium

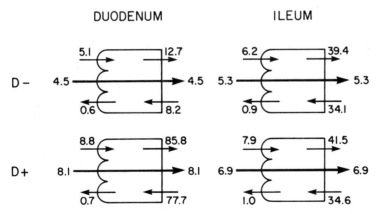

Figure 8-19. Calcium fluxes across intestinal mucosa. For each cell the luminal pole is on the left and the basal pole on the right. Net inward flux is resultant of lumen-to-mucosa flux and mucosa-to-lumen flux at the luminal pole, and resultant of mucosa-to-plasma and plasma-to-mucosa flux at basal pole. D− = vitamin D–deficient rats. D+ = vitamin D–replete rats. Note that vitamin D increases influx at both poles and efflux at the basal pole. Flux is expressed as mmol per 0.5 h per gram of mucosal tissue. *(From M. K. Younoszai, E. Urban, and H. P. Schedl.)*

pump and would also explain the requirement for sodium; as will be discussed in a subsequent section it is stimulated by PTH, either directly or indirectly. Whether the dependence of active basolateral efflux on sodium is related to the depressant effect of sodium depletion (281) or the stimulant effect of sodium loading on calcium absorption (282) is not known.

Phosphorus. Much less is known about phosphorus than about calcium absorption. Intubation and perfusion studies indicate that the relationship between net absorption and luminal concentration is linear above 1.5 mmol/L in human beings and 2 mmol/L in the rat but curvilinear at lower levels (231, 265). Phosphorus can be absorbed against an electrochemical gradient, and as for calcium, the data can be resolved into a saturable active component and a nonsaturable diffusional component, but the latter is relatively more important at normal intakes than for calcium. Phosphorus is enhanced by bulk movement of sodium and water, so the diffusional component may be partly dependent on solvent drag. Active transport of phosphorus occurs throughout the small intestine but is greatest in the jejunum and least in the ileum (283). Phosphorus absorption is enhanced by vitamin D at all levels.

The intracellular free-phosphate concentration in the mucosal cell is not known, so that no model of active and passive fluxes such as that given for calcium can be constructed. Entry into the mucosal cell may require alkaline phosphatase and involves uptake by brush border vesicles, a process which is rapid, saturable, and dependent on sodium transport (284). $H_2PO_4^-$ is taken up in preference to HPO_4^{2-} so that uptake (and absorption) is enhanced by a low pH. Oral ^{32}P labels all regions and organelles of the cell, but absorbed ^{32}P mixes with only a small fraction of the total intracellular inorganic phosphate pool, suggesting passage through restricted channels such as microtubules (285). Extrusion from the cell is dependent on the $Na^+-K^+-ATPase$ which subserves sodium transport and may be rate-limiting (286, 287).

Although many studies indicate that the transport processes of calcium and phosphorus are quite independent, in vivo their absorption is partly related (261). Active transport of calcium requires some phosphorus (231), and active transport of phosphate in the duodenum (but not in the jejunum) requires some calcium (283). There are also digestive factors which affect their relative availability. Provided dietary phosphorus is adequate, the vitamin D–dependent component of calcium absorption is accompanied by an equimolar absorption of phosphorus, but if dietary phosphate is defective, vitamin D can promote the absorption of calcium without phosphorus. In normal circumstances it is evident that most phosphorus is absorbed without calcium. Extreme reduction in dietary phosphorus may impair calcium absorption, and a large excess of either may reduce absorption because of precipitation of insoluble calcium phosphate. There are probably three components to normal phosphorus absorption—calcium-coupled, vitamin D–dependent; noncalcium-coupled, vitamin D–dependent; and noncalcium-coupled, vitamin D–independent (261).

Magnesium. Intubation and perfusion studies in human beings indicate a relationship between luminal concentration and net inward flux of magnesium similar to that of phosphorus (262). Magnesium absorption is only about half as rapid as calcium absorption. The data can be resolved into a saturable active component and a nonsaturable diffusional component, but direct evidence for active transport against an electrochemical gradient was suggestive rather than conclusive (262). Most of the data in other species suggest that the saturable component occurs by facilitated diffusion rather than by active transport (288). Like phosphorus absorption, magnesium absorption is enhanced by bulk flow of sodium and water, so that part of the nonsaturable component may be related to solvent drag rather than passive diffusion. It is likely that the saturable component is dependent partly on vitamin D, which increases magnesium absorption in human beings but to a much lesser extent than it does calcium absorption (289). Apart from this, calcium and magnesium resorption are unrelated. Contrary to findings in the rat, calcium has no depressant effect on magnesium transport in human beings even in eightfold excess (262), and magnesium loading may even enhance calcium absorption (290, 291), probably by increasing fecal phosphate excretion.

THE RENAL EXCRETION OF DIVALENT IONS

All constituents of the urine are ultimately derived from either the diet or the contents of the body. If external balance is zero and losses from the skin are disregarded, the rate of urinary excretion is equal to net absorption, any difference between them representing a gain or loss by the body, so that

$$U_X V = NA_X - B_X \qquad (8\text{-}9)$$

where U_X = Urinary concentration of substance X
V = Rate of urine formation
NA_X = Net absorption of substance X
B_X = External balance of substance X

Consequently, the normal ranges for excretion of urinary constituents and the historical, geographic, cultural, and seasonal variations in these normal ranges are simply a reflection of the dietary habits and the characteristics of intestinal absorption prevailing in a particular community at a particular time. From the point of view of the preservation of body composition, the function of the kidney is to match urinary excretion to net absorption over a wide range. However, the kidney is also concerned with the regulation of plasma concentrations. From this viewpoint one function of the kidney is to supply components of the extracellular fluid by the process of tubular reabsorption. The fundamental expression of renal physiology is that the excretion of a substance is the difference between the filtered load and tubular reabsorption (counting tubular secretion as negative reabsorption), or in symbols:

$$U_X V = P_X \cdot GFR - TR_X \qquad (8\text{-}10)$$

Consequently, the normal ranges for excretion of negative reabsorption), or in symbols:

$$U_X V = P_X \cdot GFR - TR_X \qquad (8\text{-}10)$$

Here U_X and P_X are urinary and plasma concen-

trations, and TR_X is tubular reabsorption of substance X. Consequently, combining Eqs. (8-9) and (8-10):

$$P_X \cdot GFR - TR_X = NA_X - B_X \qquad (8\text{-}11)$$

Data derived from measurements on the urine can be expressed in several ways. The simplest is concentration (V_X). Concentrations of divalent ions at different levels in the nephron are critical to understanding the mechanisms of tubular reabsorption or secretion, but concentrations in the final urine are determined mainly by water excretion and are important primarily in the pathogenesis of urinary tract stones. The most usual method is amount ($U_X V$) per unit of time, either 1 min or 24 h. For some purposes urinary creatinine is a useful referent. The expression (U_X/U_{Cr}) reduces the dependence on accurate urine collection and relates excretion rate to muscle mass, so partly reducing the variation of excretion with age and sex (292). The use of body weight as a referent ($U_X V/kg$) also reduces interindividual variation, because dietary intake tends to vary with body size. Finally, the use of creatinine clearance as a referent [$(U_X V/C_{Cr}) \cdot 100$] provides an index of excretion per unit of functioning renal mass or per nephron and is also the most appropriate expression for considering the role of the kidney in the homeostatic control of plasma concentrations.

The overall function of the kidney in relation to the sometimes conflicting requirements of preserving body content and maintaining plasma concentrations of divalent ions will be examined first and more detailed consideration then given to intrarenal and cellular mechanisms.

A model for the homeostatic function of the kidney

The simplest model of the kidney is the outlet tap of a water tank in which the level represents either concentrations in body fluids or some other function of body content (Fig. 8-20). In a steady state, the level in the tank adjusts itself automatically such that output exactly equals input and the level depends on the relationship between hydrostatic pressure and flow for a particular setting

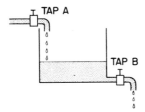

Figure 8-20. Simple hydraulic model of kidney. Height of water in tank represents concentration of substances in ECF. Tap A controls input; tap B (kidney) controls output.

of the tap. For substances such as urea the setting of the tap is relatively fixed, so that the level varies directly with input. For other substances the setting of the tap can be homeostatically controlled so the level can be kept constant in the face of varying inputs. The characteristics of the tap can be studied by examining the changes in flow (dependent variable) as a function of the level in the tank (independent variable). But in the steady state, flow is equal to input, so the level in the tank is the dependent variable which changes as a function of two independent variables—variation in flow (or load) and variation in the setting of the tap.

Much of the information about the renal handling of divalent ions has been gained from short-term acute experiments which do not always give a true picture of chronic steady-state behavior. The distinction between transient and steady-state effects can be illustrated with the model (Fig. 8-21). For example, further opening of tap A (increase in load) will lead to a progressive increase in level until outflow again equals inflow. Restoration of the same level can be achieved by further opening of tap B, which will cause an immediate increase in outflow followed by a gradual fall until outflow and inflow are again equal. Similarly, further closing of tap B (reduced excretory capacity) will cause an immediate fall in outflow and then a progressive rise in level until outflow equals inflow. Restoration of the same level can be accomplished by further closing of tap A, which will cause an immediate fall in inflow and a delayed fall in outflow. Note that in each case the *transient* effect of a change in the setting of tap B is an immediate change in outflow but that the *steady-state* effect is a change in the level in

the tank, with restoration of the same outflow as before. In just the same way, the steady-state effect of a change in the renal handling of a substance is a change either in plasma concentration or in some other function of body content such as ECF volume, not a change in urinary excretion rate. Only if there is a change in load can there be a steady-state change in urinary excretion, but this does not necessarily have to result from a change in NA. For an organic substance such as glucose the change in load may reflect a change in metabolic production rate, and for calcium and phosphate a quasisteady state can be established by the slow dissolution of bone mineral. This causes increased rates of urinary excretion with a change in body composition which is too slow to be detected over a short period.

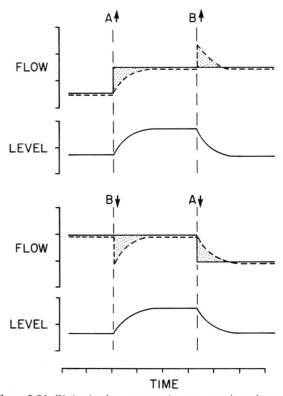

Figure 8-21. Distinction between transient states and steady states produced by partial opening (up arrow) or partial closing (down arrow) of taps A and B in Fig. 8-20. Solid line represents flow through tap A; dashed line, flow through tap B.

Saturable and nonsaturable mechanisms of tubular reabsorption: An analysis of the TM concept. Transport across the renal tubular epithelium, as across other biologic membranes, is either active and potentially saturable or passive and nonsaturable. If the epithelium is permeable to the substance being transported, as it is for sodium in the proximal convoluted tubule, transport is opposed by passive diffusion in the opposite direction and is gradient-limited (293). For such substances, the concentrations needed to demonstrate saturation may be impossible to attain in vivo. If the epithelium is impermeable, transport is capacity-limited, giving rise to a maximum rate of tubular reabsorption, or Tm, a concept first developed for glucose. It is evident that all substances for which there is a plasma threshold below which excretion is close to zero and reabsorption almost complete must be reabsorbed by active transport.

Studies of the renal handling of glucose during glucose infusion indicated that as the filtered load was increased by raising the plasma level, reabsorption increased also; at first to the same extent, then at a progressively decreasing rate, until finally the maximum reabsorption rate, the Tm, was reached, above which further increments in filtered load were completely excreted (294). Sometimes a Tm is illustrated by plotting urinary excretion (U_XV) against filtered load ($P_X \cdot GFR$), but the effects of altering filtered load by a change in P_X and by a change in GFR are usually not the same. When U_XV is plotted against plasma level (P_X) (Fig. 8-22), the relationships between plasma level, GFR, Tm, and threshold can be demonstrated geometrically. In addition, different values for renal clearance (U_XV/P_X) are represented by a family of lines of different slope radiating from the origin. The curvilinear lower segment of the Tm line (or splay region) gives rise to three thresholds: the appearance threshold, which is the plasma concentration at which a substance first

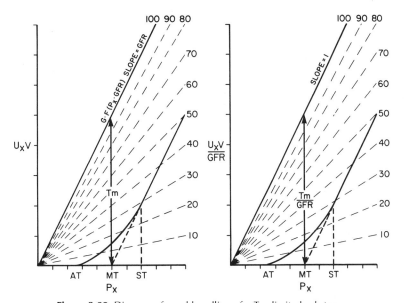

Figure 8-22. Diagram of renal handling of a Tm-limited substance. On left, U_XV plotted against P_X. On right, U_XV GFR plotted against P_X. Vertical distance between lines representing filtration and excretion is Tm on left, Tm/GFR on right. Dashed lines radiating from origin represent different values for fractional reabsorption of X. AT = appearance threshold, MT = mean threshold, and ST = saturation threshold.

appears in the urine; the saturation threshold, which is the plasma level above which no further increase in reabsorption occurs; and the mean threshold (numerically equal to Tm/GFR), which is the point where the extrapolation of the linear upper segment of the line intersects the baseline. Two explanations for splay have been put forward: dispersion in the relationship between glomerular filtration and tubular reabsorptive capacity in individual nephrons; and a relationship between transport rate and intraluminal concentration analogous to the Michaelis-Menten relationship between reaction rate and substrate concentration. An anatomic basis for glomerular-tubular dispersion has been found by microdissection (295) and is further supported by the obvious differences between superficial and deep nephrons, but the importance of transport kinetics in determining splay remains unproved (296). Both theories interpret a change in Tm/GFR as a consequence of a change in the amount of transport carrier per nephron, and hence V_{max}, but a change in splay without a change in Tm/GFR is attributed on the one hand to an alteration in glomerular-tubular dispersion and on the other to a change in the Michaelis constant (K_m). Homer Smith believed that a Tm was a biologic constant like height and was unrelated to GFR. The subsequent demonstration that Tm_g could be altered by a variety of maneuvers threatened at one time to discredit the concept of Tm altogether, but most of the variation can be eliminated if data are expressed as Tm_g/GFR rather than as absolute values (297). Variation of Tm with GFR is partly a consequence of differences in renal size between individuals, those with larger kidneys having higher values for both quantities. There is also a functional relationship demonstrable in an individual. This is obscured in many experiments because GFR and ECF volume usually change in the same direction, so that an increase in Tm consequent on an increase in GFR may be offset by a decrease in Tm caused by a decrease in the proximal reabsorption of sodium (298), as will be discussed later. This change in viewpoint concerning Tm does not require a revival of the concept of glomerular intermittency, so vehemently denied by Homer Smith. Although the recruitment of temporarily inactive nephrons into active use is an obvious explanation for a functional relationship between GFR and Tm, the relationship can be explained equally well by citing the dependence of reabsorption on peritubular blood flow or the degree of tubular dilatation (297). Whatever the explanation, Tm/GFR is a reasonable index of maximum reabsorption per unit of functional renal tissue and is probably related to the mean maximum reabsorptive capacity of single nephrons.

Graphic demonstration of Tm/GFR is simplified if $U_X V$/GFR rather than $U_X V$ is plotted against P_X (Fig. 8-22), where the quantity $U_X V$/GFR is an index of load per nephron. This assumes that an increase in absolute load or a decrease in GFR have the same effect on plasma level, which for the divalent ions is usually the case. A plot of this kind enables results from different subjects or from the same subject at different times to be shown on the same chart. The family of lines of different slope radiating from the origin denote different values for fractional clearance (C_X/GFR) rather than absolute clearance.

The relationship between plasma concentration and load: Fractional versus absolute values for reabsorption and excretion. This method of data presentation has the further advantage of making more explicit the role of the kidney in regulating plasma concentrations. From Eq. (8-10) can be derived two alternative methods of interpreting data concerning simultaneous plasma and urine concentrations of a test substance and of creatinine, using creatinine clearance as a simple method of estimating GFR. If Eq. (8-10) is divided throughout by filtered load ($P_X \cdot C_{Cr}$), then:

$$\frac{U_X V}{P_X \cdot C_{Cr}} = 1 - \frac{TR_X}{P_X \cdot C_{Cr}} \qquad (8\text{-}12)$$

which states that fractional excretion (clearance as a fraction of GFR) = 1 − fractional reabsorption. Alternatively, if Eq. (8-10) is divided throughout only by GFR then:

$$\frac{U_X V}{C_{Cr}} = P_X - \frac{TR_X}{C_{Cr}} \qquad (8\text{-}13)$$

The relationship between these methods is shown in Fig. 8-22; it is evident that unless the line relating excretion to plasma level has no intercept, both absolute and fractional clearances must vary with load. In fact, the clearance of any reabsorbed substance increases with plasma level as a rectangular hyperbole, approaching the GFR as an asymptote. Consequently, clearances of threshold substances, either absolute or fractional, cannot be interpreted except in relation to the plasma level, and so despite their widespread use they are inappropriate for considering the tubular reabsorption of the Tm substances in general and of the divalent ions in particular.

By rearrangement of Eq. (8-13) it follows that

$$P_X = \frac{U_X V}{C_{Cr}} + \frac{TR_X}{C_{Cr}} \qquad (8\text{-}14)$$

Above the splay region $TR_X/GFR = Tm_X/GFR$ where $Tm_X = Tm$ for substance X. This is simply an arithmetic consequence of the definitions. The truth of Eq. (8-14) does not by itself establish a primary role for the kidney in homeostasis; such a conclusion confuses a tautology with a physiologic relationship. Nevertheless, if there are no significant extrarenal mechanisms of plasma homeostasis, the plasma level can be resolved into, and can be considered as determined by, its two components of $U_X V/GFR$ (or load per nephron) and TR_X/GFR (or reabsorption per nephron). One reservation must be made. Since tubular reabsorption cannot be measured directly but only determined as the difference between filtered load and urinary excretion, any attempt to examine experimentally the relationship between plasma level and tubular reabsorption suffers from a methodologic flaw. The two quantities P_X and $P_X - (U_X/GFR)$ both contain the common variable P_X, so that any correlation between them may be artefactual. This difficulty is circumvented if stability of Tm/GFR is established in the conventional manner at several different plasma levels. A self-consistent model of renal handling can then be constructed which has considerable explanatory and predictive power.

In terms of the hydraulic analogy, the relationship of plasma level to its components can be shown by replacing the tap by a sluice gate (Fig. 8-23). The width of the gate represents GFR, the height of the gate represents Tm_X/GFR, and the GFR. Furthermore, different characteristics of the

THE KIDNEY AS A SLUICE GATE

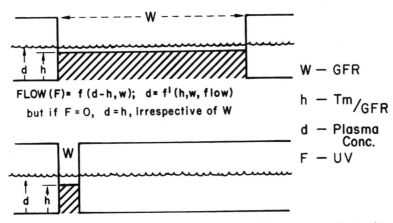

Figure 8-23. Hydraulic analogy for regulation of plasma concentrations by the kidney. W = width of sluice gate permitting escape of water from a reservoir (analogous to GFR), h = height of sluice gate (analogous to Tm/GFR), d = depth of water in reservoir (analogous to plasma concentration), and F = flow of water (analogous to UV). F is a function (f) of height of water above gate (d − h) and width of gate (w); d is a function (f′) of height and width of gate, and flow.

splay region can be represented by different shapes of the gate (158). The partition of the plasma level into its components can also be shown graphically by inverting the axes of Fig. 8-22 to make plasma level the dependent variable (Fig. 8-24). A change in U_xV/GFR (load per nephron) because of a change either in U_xV or in GFR will drive the values along the prevailing Tm line to the left or right. Conversely, a change in Tm_x/GFR (reabsorption per nephron) without a change in U_xV/GFR will drive the values either up or down to a new Tm line. Any shift can be resolved into components of movement in these two directions; for example, movement from point 1 to point 2 in Fig. 8-24 results from an increase in U_xV/GFR and a corresponding fall in Tm_x/GFR with no change in plasma level.

With these general concepts in mind, models based on this method of data analysis will be developed for the renal handling of each of the di-

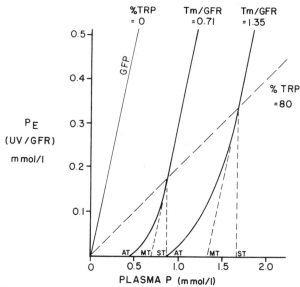

Figure 8-25. Tm/GFR model of renal handling of phosphate. Upper and lower values for Tm_P/GFR were established by Bijvoet (300). Curvilinear segments have same shape, so that proportions between AT, MT, and ST are constant, and saturation occurs at TRP of 80 percent at all values of Tm_F/GFR. [*From A. M. Parfitt and B. Frame (301).*]

valent ions. For convenience of exposition the previous order of presentation will be changed and phosphate taken first.

Models for the renal handling of divalent ions

Phosphate. From data summarized in Table 8-4 the glomerular filtrate/plasma ratio (GF/P) for phosphate should be 0.96. Direct measurement by micropuncture in the rat gave a value of 0.93 (299). Little error is introduced by the common practice of ignoring this correction and assuming that GF/P for phosphate is unity. Numerous studies have demonstrated that phosphate reabsorption in human beings and the dog (but not the cat) conforms to a Tm/GFR model (300, 301) with a normal range of 0.7 to 1.4 mmol/L (Fig. 8-25), but there are three important differences from glucose reabsorption (301). First, provided ECF volume is stable, Tm_g/GFR for glucose is subject to only slight variation at different times in the same person, whereas changes in Tm_P/GFR for

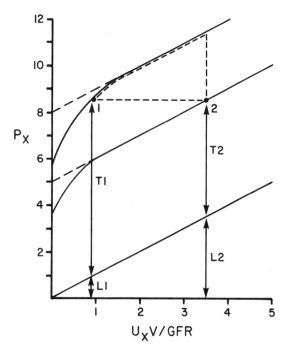

Figure 8-24. Inversion of Fig. 8-22 (right) showing plasma concentration (P_x) as a function of load (U_xV/GFR). Plasma level can be partitioned into tubular reabsorption (TR_x/GFR) and load (U_xV/GFR). If load increases (L1 → L2) and plasma level remains unchanged, tubular reabsorption must increase (T1 → T2).

phosphate are produced by a wide variety of hormonal and other factors, both physiologic and pathologic. Second, for glucose the normal plasma level is well below the appearance threshold, so that normally the urine is virtually free of glucose. For phosphate the normal plasma level is close to the mean threshold (Tm_P/GFR), so that normally the urine always contains phosphate. Finally, the plasma level of glucose is determined entirely by extrarenal mechanisms, including the action of various hormones on the uptake and release of glucose by liver and muscle. In contrast, there is no important extrarenal mechanism except net absorption for the regulation of the plasma level of phosphate, which is therefore determined entirely by load per GFR and Tm_P/GFR. Tubular reabsorption normally supplies about 190 mmol daily to the ECF and accounts for about 90 percent of the plasma phosphate in the fasting state and about 80 percent at other times (Table 8-21); only when GFR is substantially reduced does load per GFR make a significant contribution to the plasma level. This difference from glucose has an important bearing on the effect of a reduction in tubular reabsorption (decrease in Tm/GFR). For glucose, impaired reabsorption is manifested by glucosuria; any tendency to hypoglycemia is prevented by the very efficient extrarenal mechanisms of glucose homeostasis. However, for phosphate, impaired tubular reabsorption produces only a transient increase in phosphate excretion, and the steady-state effect is a fall in plasma level and no change in urinary excretion (Fig. 8-21). This distinction is obscured by the usual practice of describing agents which decrease tubular reabsorption as phosphaturic, a term which emphasizes the ephemeral at the expense of the permanent.

The general acceptance of the Tm_P/GFR concept has been delayed by the existence of a renal counterpart to Heisenberg's uncertainty principle: the process of measurement alters that which is being measured. The classic method of determining Tm_P depends on prolonged IV infusion to permit observation at multiple plasma levels. Apart from being cumbersome and inconvenient to repeat, this procedure may induce changes in phosphate reabsorption for a variety of reasons including (but not necessarily limited to) hypocalcemia, volume expansion, potassium depletion, and pyrogen-induced changes in renal blood flow (301). Although these problems can often be circumvented, the data obtained by phosphate infusion are sometimes too variable to be of clinical use. Fortunately, this obstacle has now been largely overcome by the development of a method for estimating Tm_P/GFR without saturating the transport mechanism. By expressing data obtained in different subjects in units of Tm_P/GFR, their titration curves could be superimposed (300). In each subject the difference between the appearance and saturation thresholds was proportional to Tm_P/GFR. Saturation of the transport mechanism occurred when fractional reabsorption was less than 80 percent, so that the ratio of mean threshold/saturation threshold was a constant value of 0.8 (Fig. 8-25). Furthermore, the form of the curvilinear segment appears to be the same in all normal individuals over a wide range of values for Tm_P/GFR and is also of the same form as the curvilinear segment for glucose titration curves. The ratio of appearance threshold/mean threshold has a constant value of 0.643 for both substances. Consequently, by expressing this form as a mathematically defined function it is possible to estimate the location of the Tm_P/GFR

Table 8-21. Representative normal values for Tm/GFR and components of fasting plasma ultrafiltrable, UF, concentrations of divalent ions

	Ca	P	Mg
Tm/GFR	0.80–1.00*	0.70–1.40	0.60–1.00
Fasting plasma UF concentration	1.20–1.40	0.80–1.45	0.60–0.75
Tubular reabsorption, TR/GFR	1.16–1.38	0.60–1.35	0.58–0.74
Load, UV/GFR	0.01–0.04	0.05–0.20	0.01–0.02

* After two-component model of Mioni, D'Angelo, Ossi, Bertaglia, Marcon, and Maschio (313).

line corresponding to any point on the U_PV/GFR-plasma phosphate plot. These observations suggest that glomerular-tubular dispersion rather than transport kinetics is the major determinant of splay, at least with respect to differences between normal persons in the fasting state. If this is true in other circumstances also it is unlikely that a change in splay could occur in the absence of a change in Tm_P/GFR, since nephron dispersion is much less likely to be subject to homeostatic control than a carrier-substrate K_m; Tm_P/GFR is therefore an appropriate index of phosphate reabsorption even though the kidney is normally operating in the splay region. In the dog, variation in protein intake may lead to substantial changes in phosphate excretion at the same plasma level with no change in Tm_P/GFR (302), so that changes in the form of the curvilinear splay region may modulate the physiologic with circadian variation in phosphate excretion. However, most agents which produce acute changes in phosphate excretion after a single dose produce corresponding changes in Tm_P/GFR after repeated administration (294).

Although the Tm_P/GFR model is based on data derived from acute short-term infusion studies, data from more long-term observation also show excellent conformity to the model. As will be described later, variations in plasma phosphate caused by variations in parathyroid status can be completely explained in terms of the model by differences in Tm_P/GFR. Variations in load per GFR caused by variation in dietary intake produce predictable changes in plasma phosphate with no evidence of a change in Tm_P/GFR, at least during the first few days. The data points are driven to the left or right along a prevailing Tm_P/GFR line in accordance with the model, the plasma level adjusting automatically so that $U_PV = NA_P$. After a few days, adaptive changes in Tm_P/GFR take place which permit the altered load to be excreted with less change in plasma level. This adaptation is partly dependent on changes in PTH secretion but can occur in the absence of PTH both in the rat (303) and in human beings (301). Adaptation may involve changes in the size of some phosphate pool within the renal tubule cells and also in vitamin D metabolism, as discussed later.

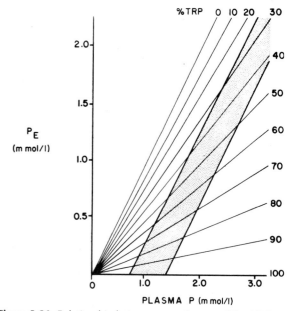

Figure 8-26. Relationship between normal range of Tm_P/GFR and fractional reabsorption. Note that increasing load ($P_E = U_PV$/GFR) at constant Tm_P/GFR automatically reduces %TRP and increases fractional excretion. (*From A. M. Parfitt and B. Frame (301).*)

Changes in phosphate load in either direction produce the changes in fractional excretion and reabsorption predicted by the model, even though Tm_P/GFR remains constant (Fig. 8-26). Even when an adaptive change in Tm_P/GFR occurs, most of the observed change in fractional excretion and reabsorption is caused by the change in load (301), so that these commonly used indices of tubular reabsorption are quite inappropriate, at least in this context.

Most measurements of phosphate excretion are made either over a short period in the fasting state or on pooled 24-h or longer collections, neither of which permit study of the circadian rhythm (294, 304). Phosphate excretion is usually lowest in the early morning, rises through the early afternoon to about three to five times the early morning rate, and falls during the night. These changes are in part the result of parallel changes in plasma phosphate, but there is probably also a change in tubular reabsorption of phosphate possibly caused by changes in PTH and in cortisol secretion. Whether this reflects an alteration in splay or in Tm/GFR is not known. Apart from its physiologic importance, the circadian rhythm complicates the interpretation of short-term experiments.

Magnesium. Based on the data summarized in Table 8-4, GF/P for magnesium should be 0.76, but direct measurements in the rat gave results 4 percent higher than in plasma ultrafiltrate (299), and a value of 0.8 has been assumed in the following discussion. Magnesium has been much less studied than phosphate, but the available data obtained during magnesium infusion indicate that magnesium reabsorption conforms to a Tm/GFR model in human beings, and probably also in the dog, with a lower limit of 0.6 mmol/L and a poorly defined upper limit of 1 to 1.5 mmol/L (Fig. 8-27) (305, 306). For magnesium, as for phosphate, the normal plasma ultrafiltrable level is close to the prevailing Tm_{Mg}/GFR, but there is a much sharper threshold with less splay than for phosphate, saturation occurring when the fractional reabsorption is less than 95 percent.

The shape of the curvilinear segment, how constant this shape is in normal persons, and whether or not changes in splay modulate physiologic changes in excretion are all unknown.

Several other resemblances to phosphate are evident. First, there is no evidence for any important extrarenal mechanism for regulating plasma magnesium, which is therefore determined entirely by load per GFR and tubular reabsorption according to the relationship: $P_{Mg(UF)} = U_{Mg}/GFR + Tm_{Mg}/GFR$. Second, tubular reabsorption accounts for about 90 percent of the plasma magnesium in the fasting state and about 80 percent at other times (Table 8-21), supplying about 110 mmol daily to the ECF. As for phosphate, load per GFR makes a significant contribution only when GFR is reduced. Third, the steady-state effect of impaired tubular reabsorption is a fall in plasma level with no change in urinary excretion. Finally, variations in load per GFR caused by variation in dietary intake are associated with changes in plasma magnesium that are predictable in terms of the model without a change in Tm_{Mg}/GFR, so that the reduction in urinary excretion of magnesium is an automatic consequence of the fall in plasma magnesium, with no active conservation (305, 306). In the long term there is suggestive evidence for adaptive changes in Tm_{Mg}/GFR, but this is less well established than for phosphate. As for phosphate, changes in load produce predictable changes in fractional excretion and reabsorption despite no change in Tm_{Mg}/GFR (Fig. 8-28).

There is an appreciable circadian variation in magnesium excretion, with an approximately twofold difference between the highest rate in the late morning and the lowest rate in the late evening. This is partly due to such factors as posture, activity, and food ingestion, but there is probably also an intrinsic rhythm in tubular reabsorption, the cause of which is unknown (304, 307).

Calcium. Based on the data summarized in Table 8-4, the GF/P for calcium should be 0.56. Direct measurement by micropuncture in the rat gave a value of 0.63 (299); a value of 0.6 will be assumed in the ensuing discussion. The relationship between either $U_{Ca}V$ or $U_{Ca}V/GFR$ and plasma ultrafiltrable calcium ($P_{Ca(UF)}$) can be ex-

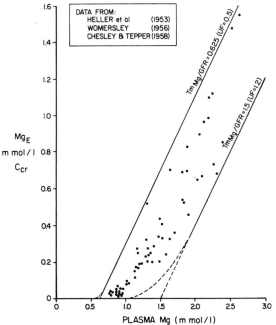

Figure 8-27. Tm/GFR model of renal handling of magnesium. Points have been experimentally determined by cited authors. Tm_{Mg}/GFR line is drawn on assumption that ultrafiltrable factor for *magnesium = 0.8.* [*From A. M. Parfitt (305).*]

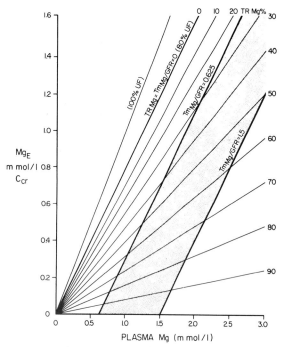

Figure 8-28. Relationship between normal range for Tm_{Mg}/GFR and fractional reabsorption. Note that increasing lod ($Mg_E = U_{Mg}V$/GFR) at constant Tm_{Mg}/GFR automatically decreases the percent TR_{Mg} and increases fractional magnesium clearance.

amined during calcium infusion (Fig. 8-29). The relationship is similar whether the latter is raised continuously or in a step-wise manner (308, 309); however, when calcium is given as a large single injection the peak increase in urinary excretion is delayed for i to 2 h, when the plasma level may have fallen to normal (310). Since hypercalcemia suppresses PTH secretion, it might be supposed that the results would refer to the hypoparathyroid rather than to the normal state, but consistent discrimination is obtained between different levels of parathyroid function, so that tubular reabsorption probably does not change significantly during the course of the infusion. Calcium is usually infused as the gluconate ion, which may reduce reabsorption caused by the formation of a calcium complex within the tubular lumen (311). Although calcium excretion is slightly lower at the same plasma-ionized calcium level when calcium chloride is used, the difference is too small to alter any of the conclusions drawn from cal-

cium gluconate infusion. The titration curves for calcium resemble those for phosphate and magnesium in having a threshold, a curvilinear lower segment, and a linear upper segment. In one study a Tm for calcium was apparently reached (312), but this has never been confirmed. All other studies have shown a progressive increase in the tubular reabsorption of calcium, whether absolute or per unit of GFR, however high the plasma calcium, with no evidence for a Tm. This is paradoxical, since the concentration of calcium may be much lower in urine than in plasma, so that there must be an active and hence saturable component to calcium reabsorption.

Two approaches to this paradox have been proposed. First, Mioni and colleagues (313) have demonstrated that when the line relating load per GFR to plasma level has a slope of less than unity, tubular reabsorption can be resolved into two components—a fractional (gradient-limited) component related to the slope, which increases progressively with plasma level, and an absolute (capacity-limited) component related to the intercept, which reaches a Tm (Fig. 8-30). When applied to

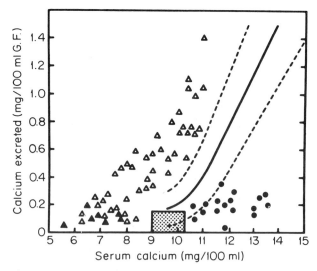

Figure 8-29. Relationship between calcium excretion per deciliter of creatinine clearance (Ca_E) and plasma calcium determined by infusion of calcium gluconate into normal subjects (between dotted lines) and patients with hypoparathyroidism (triangles) and hyperparathyroidism (closed circles). (*From M. Peacock, W. G. Robertson, and B. E. C. Nordin.*)

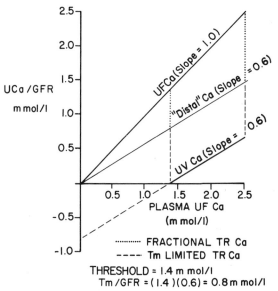

Figure 8-30. Partition of tubular reabsorption calcium into fractional component of 40 percent of filtered load in proximal tubule and absolute (Tm-limited) component in the distal tubule. (*After G. Mioni, A. D'Angelo, E. Ossi, E. Bertaglia, G. Marcon, and G. Maschio.*)

calcium the fractional component of reabsorption is about 40 to 50 percent of the filtered load, and $P_{Ca(UF)}$ can be resolved into its components of load per GFR and reabsorption per GFR:

$$P_{Ca(UF)} = 0.4\, P_{Ca(UF)} + \frac{Tm_{Ca}}{GFR} + \frac{U_{Ca}V}{GFR}$$

so that   (8-16)

$$0.6\, P_{Ca(UF)} = \frac{Tm_{Ca}}{GFR} + \frac{U_{Ca}V}{GFR}$$

The Tm component has a range of about 0.80 to 0.94 mmol/L (Table 8-21). By appropriate transformation of the data the curvilinear splay segment was found to be of the same mathematical form as for glucose and phosphate (313), so that the same anatomically determined glomerular-tubular dispersion might account for splay for all three substances. But this may be fortuitous, since the Tm component of reabsorption is probably located only in the distal nephron for calcium and in the proximal nephron for glucose.

The second approach is the proposal by Marshall and Nordin of a single component Tm/GFR

(capacity-limited) model in which the K_m is so high that the plasma level needed to attain transport saturation is incompatible with life (314). By combining data from normal subjects and patients with osteomalacia, to define the curvilinear splay segment with greater precision, they calculated a Tm/GFR of about 2.05 mmol/L, much higher than on the Mioni model (Fig. 8-31). Further discussion of these models will be postponed until a subsequent section, but fortunately the tubular reabsorption of calcium can be assessed without resolving this conflict. The observed relationship between $U_{Ca}V$/GFR and P_{Ca} can be compared with the relationship determined by calcium infusion (Fig. 8-29), and $P_{Ca(UF)}$ can be resolved into its components of load per GFR and tubular reabsorption, which is of great value in

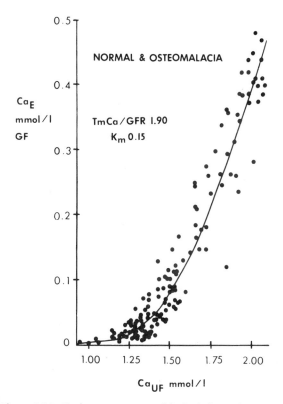

Figure 8-31. Single-component model of tubular reabsorption of calcium obtained by combining calcium infusion data from normal subjects and from patients with osteomalacia. (*From D. H. Marshall.*)

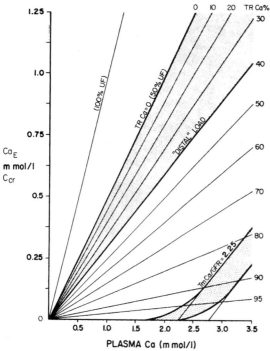

Figure 8-32. Relationship between normal range for Tm_{Ca}/GFR (two-component model) and fractional reabsorption. Note that increasing load ($Ca_E = U_{Ca}V/GFR$) at a constant Tm_{Ca}/GFR automatically decreases $\%TR_{Ca}$ and increases fractional calcium clearance.

clarifying the pathogenesis of hypercalcemia. Tubular reabsorption normally supplies about 260 mmol to the ECF daily (Table 8-21). As for phosphate and magnesium, changes in load produce predictable changes in fractional excretion and reabsorption despite no change in Tm_{Ca}/GFR (Fig. 8-32).

The most important difference between calcium and the other divalent ions is the existence of a major homeostatic system for calcium in

bone, as already discussed. Consequently, the kidney does not play the dominant role in determining the plasma level that it does for phosphate and magnesium. Nevertheless, the tubular reabsorption of calcium is subject to much more prompt and precise homeostatic control than the tubular reabsorption of phosphate or magnesium. The blood-bone equilibrium and the tubular reabsorption of calcium are both controlled by PTH, and both must normally be set at the same level, otherwise one homeostatic system would be systematically undoing the work of the other (117). The difference in the mechanisms of plasma homeostasis between calcium and the other divalent ions is well shown in the different responses to dietary deprivation. With both phosphate and magnesium, as already discussed, renal conservation is a passive consequence of the fall in plasma level, and tubular reabsorption does not change significantly for some time. With calcium, renal conservation occurs with little or no fall in plasma calcium, because of an immediate increase in tubular reabsorption, probably mediated by increased PTH secretion (305, 315). Renal conservation of calcium in response to cellulose phosphate (305) may be more effective than in response to dietary calcium restriction alone (315), possibly because hypomagnesemia acts as an additional stimulus to PTH secretion. Nevertheless, the pattern of prompt reduction in urinary calcium with minimal change in plasma calcium on the first day, with little or no change thereafter, is the same as with dietary calcium deprivation. This is in contrast to the renal conservation of sodium, which takes 3 to 4 days to become maximally effective but is eventually much more complete than for calcium (Table 8-22). This immediate, short-term response must be distinguished from the gradual, further reduction in urinary calcium over many months (228), which

Table 8-22. Urinary conservation on low dietary intake: Comparison of divalent ions with sodium

| | PLASMA CONCENTRATION | CHANGE IN URINARY EXCRETION | | INCREASE IN TUBULAR REABSORPTION |
		TIME TO NADIR, DAYS	% REDUCTION	
Sodium	No change	4–5	95–99	Large
Phosphate	Fall	3–4	80–90	Slight
Magnesium	Fall	1–2	90–95	None
Calcium	No change	1–2	25–50	Moderate

probably takes place by a different mechanism. Long-term adaptation of urinary excretion to calcium intake can be expressed as a power function: $U_{Ca}V = kI^{0.2}$, where the usual value of k is 1.6 with a range of 0.3 to 3.6 (292).

The circadian rhythm of calcium excretion resembles that of magnesium in timing, magnitude, and partial dependence on posture, activity, and food ingestion, but there is somewhat stronger evidence of an intrinsic rhythm unrelated to these factors (307, 316).

Intrarenal mechanisms of divalent ion excretion

Membrane transport of divalent ions has been studied less intensively in the kidney than in the gut. One difficulty with the kidney is that raising the plasma level increases the concentration to the same extent on both sides of the tubular epithelium. There is also significant heterogeneity among nephrons, and only limited access is possible to luminal concentrations at different locations in the nephron. Two main types of nephron can be recognized (317). The majority are cortical or superficial nephrons with relatively small glomeruli, lower single-nephron GFR, and short loops of Henle which penetrate only a short distance into the outer medulla and so do not participate in the concentrating mechanism. The remainder are juxtamedullary nephrons with larger glomeruli and higher single-nephron GFR and long loops of Henle which penetrate almost to the papilla and are entirely responsible for the generation of medullary hypertonicity (Fig. 8-33). The proportions differ in different species. Both types share the same collecting ducts.

Most of the information concerning intrarenal mechanisms has been obtained by the techniques of micropuncture and microperfusion. The tubular fluid/plasma (TF/P) ratio of inulin concentrations is an estimate of fractional water reabsorption, so that absolute and fractional reabsorption of solutes in different nephron segments can be calculated. In small rodents and in the dog, both proximal and distal tubules of superficial nephrons lie close to the surface of the kidney and are accessible to micropuncture, but the loop of Henle is inaccessible. Conversely, in small ro-

dents, but not in the dog, the hairpin turn of the loop of Henle of juxtamedullary nephrons is accessible to micropuncture at the papilla, whereas proximal and distal tubules are very difficult to puncture. In the desert rat (*Psammomys*), as an adaptation to the need for strict water conservation the papillae are hypertrophied and easy to puncture, and all nephrons have long loops of Henle.

Changes in the distribution of blood flow between the two types of nephron may be important to the regulation of sodium excretion (317), but there is no information on the possible importance of this mechanism for the divalent ions. By combining data for the two types of nephron in different species a composite picture can be built

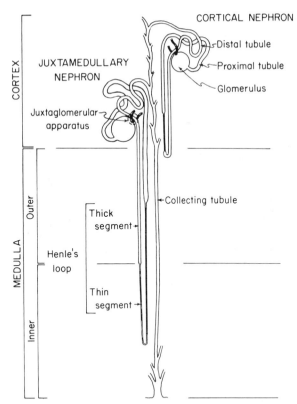

Figure 8-33. Comparison of cortical and juxtamedullary nephrons. Note that micropuncture of proximal and distal convoluted tubules is possible only for cortical nephrons, and micropuncture of hairpin turn of loop of Henle is possible only for juxtamedullary nephrons. (*From L. P. Sullivan.*)

up, but the validity of this for the human kidney must clearly be regarded as provisional.

Functional and structural organization of the nephron. About 80 to 90 percent of the filtered loads of sodium (and its attendant anions) and of water are reabsorbed either in the proximal tubule or in the loop of Henle. This bulk flow out of the nephron imposes constraints on all other solutes, and similar fractions for the divalent ions are also reabsorbed at these sites by mechanisms linked in various ways to the reabsorption of salt and water. For each major ion and for water there are additional reabsorptive mechanisms, located more distally, which permit the excretion of each substance to be regulated independently.

Because of its importance for the divalent ions, reabsorption of salt and water at different sites in the nephron will be described briefly; further details are given in Chaps. 3, 12, and 13 and elsewhere (318). The proximal tubular epithelium shows a general structural resemblance to the intestinal mucosa (Fig. 8-17). The cells have a brush border with microvilli, glycocalyx, and associated unstirred layer at the luminal or apical pole; they are separated by lateral intercellular spaces and are held together by tight junctions (319, 320). These are highly permeable to water, sodium, and chloride. Sodium enters the cell down a concentration gradient at the luminal pole and is actively transported into the lateral intercellular space, which is hypertonic with respect to the lumen (321). The osmotic gradient across the tight junction leads to reabsorption of water and the electric gradient to reabsorption of bicarbonate, chloride, and other anions. The bulk reabsorption of sodium, chloride, and water creates concentration gradients favoring reabsorption of all other constituents of the tubular fluid. Because of the paracellular leak across the tight junctions, which permits passive back-flux, the gradients across the entire epithelium are very small; the potential difference is about -2 mV (lumen-negative) in the early proximal tubule, and about $+2$ mV in the late proximal tubule and pars recta. No significant concentration gradient for sodium can be established, so that its reabsorption is gradient-limited rather than capacity-limited. By the end of the proximal tubule, the glomerular filtrate has been reduced in bulk by about 65 percent but not much changed in composition.

The descending limb of the loop of Henle is permeable to water but not to sodium or chloride, the concentrations of which rise progressively because of the abstraction of water into the hypertonic medullary interstitial fluid. By the hairpin turn the volume has been reduced to about 15 percent of the glomerular filtrate by the reabsorption of a further 20 percent of filtered water, and the sodium concentration has risen to 2 or 2½ times that of plasma. The ascending limb of the loop is permeable to sodium and chloride but not to water, so that the concentrations begin to fall progressively from the hairpin turn. In the thin segment these changes are passive, but in the thick diluting segment there is active reabsorption of chloride. This establishes a potential difference of $+6$ to $+12$ mV, which leads to passive reabsorption of sodium and of other cations (including calcium and magnesium). About 25 percent of the filtered sodium is reabsorbed at this site with a fall in luminal sodium concentration to about half that of plasma.

In the distal convoluted tubule the tight junctions between the cells are relatively impermeable to salt and water. Active reabsorption of sodium establishes a large concentration gradient for sodium and a large negative potential difference that inhibits reabsorption and may enhance secretion of other cations but favors reabsorption of anions. Finally, in the collecting duct the details of sodium reabsorption are similar, but permeability to water can be increased by antidiuretic hormone, thus permitting reabsorption of water without sodium. The characteristics of salt and water reabsorption at different sites in the nephron are summarized in Table 8-23. The collecting duct, once regarded simply as a passive conduit, may be the most important site in the regulation of the excretion of sodium, potassium, and hydrogen ion as well as water under physiologic conditions (322).

For many years it was believed that the fractional reabsorption of sodium in the proximal tubule was constant and that the regulation of sodium excretion was accomplished by variation either in GFR ("first factor") or in the distal tu-

Table 8-23. Characteristics of sodium and water reabsorption at different sites along the nephron

	WATER	SODIUM		PERMEABILITY	
	FR%*	FR%	TF/P†	WATER	SODIUM
Proximal tubule	65	65	1.0	High	High
Descending limb	20	0	2.3	High	Low
Ascending limb	0	25	0.6	Low	High
Distal tubule	2	5.5	0.4	Low	Low
Collecting duct	12.2	4	0.6	Variable	Low
	FE% ‡	FE%	U/P§		
Urine	0.8	0.5	0.6		

* FR = fractional reabsorption.
† TF/P = tubular fluid/plasma concentration ratio.
‡ FE = fractional excretion.
§ U/P = urine/plasma concentration ratio.

bular reabsorption of sodium under the influence of salt-retaining hormones secreted by the adrenal cortex ("second factor"). When it was first established that proximal tubular sodium reabsorption could vary inversely with ECF volume, the "third factor" was introduced. Because of the multiplicity and complexity of the mechanisms involved, including hemodynamic, physical, and humoral factors, this term is now obsolete, but it is still useful to distinguish between aldosterone- and nonaldosterone-dependent changes in sodium reabsorption and excretion, because these have quite different effects on the excretion of the divalent ions. The former occur primarily in the distal convoluted tubule and are unaccompanied by any immediate changes in divalent ion excretion. By contrast, the latter occur in the proximal tubule, ascending limb, and collecting duct and are frequently accompanied by changes in the excretion of phosphate, magnesium, and calcium in the same direction. Sodium and chloride reabsorption in the ascending limb and in the distal tubule and collecting duct varies with load so that if the extent of proximal reabsorption changes, reabsorption at more distal sites changes in the opposite direction because of a corresponding change in load. The nephron thus works as a whole to minimize variation in the amount of sodium chloride and water reaching the urine. For example, infusion of parathyroid hormone reduces proximal reabsorption of sodium substantially but leads to only a modest increase in uri-

nary sodium excretion. By contrast, expansion of ECF volume by the intravenous infusion of sodium chloride inhibits sodium reabsorption in the proximal tubule, ascending limb, and collecting duct, so that urinary sodium excretion increases substantially.

Phosphate. Under normal conditions phosphate is actively reabsorbed more completely than salt and water and against an electrochemical gradient in the first 10 to 20 percent of the length of the proximal tubule; the tubular fluid/plasma ultrafiltrate ratio (TF/UF) falling from 1.0 in the glomerular filtrate to about 0.7, so that this short segment reabsorbs 35 to 40 percent of the filtered phosphate load but only 10 to 20 percent of the filtered water (323, 324). Presumably the active transport mechanism has more capacity per unit length in the early than in the late proximal tubule, as was found also for glucose and amino acids. Along the remainder of the proximal tubule, phosphate is reabsorbed in parallel with salt and water; the TF/UF remains unchanged at about 0.7, so that at the end of the proximal tubule about 25 percent of the filtered load remains (Table 8-24).

At high plasma phosphate levels maintained by phosphate infusion two types of response have been found in the rat. In some experiments TF/UF for phosphate rises progressively along the proximal tubule in parallel with the rise in TF/P for insulin; absolute phosphate reabsorption remains unchanged or actually declines (323,

Table 8-24. Characteristics of divalent ion reabsorption at different sites along the nephron

	P		Mg		Ca	
	FR%	TF/UF*	FR%	TF/UF	FR%	TF/UF
Proximal tubule	75	0.7	45	1.6	61	1.1
Descending limb	5	(1.3)	−3	2.8	9	2.0
Ascending limb	−5	1.7	48	0.6	20	0.6
Distal tubule	5	1.3	4	0.5	5	0.4
Collecting duct	5	19	2	5.0	3	2.5
	FE%	U/P	FE%	U/P	FE%	U/P
Urine	15	19	4	5	2	2.5

* TF/UF = tubular fluid/plasma ultrafiltrable concentration ratio. Other abbreviations as in Table 8-23.

325). This indicates a reduction in fractional reabsorption consistent with a Tm and is analogous to the effect of increased load on whole kidney reabsorption (301). In another study TF/UF for phosphate rose to about 1.0 but did not increase further along the nephron, with an increase in absolute reabsorption (326). This discrepancy could reflect strain or species differences in the rat, or more careful avoidance of volume expansion in the latter experiments.

There is considerable uncertainty concerning the handling of phosphate by the remainder of the nephron. Comparison of fluid aspirated from late proximal and early distal sites of the same nephron indicates that under different conditions either a small net addition of phosphate or net reabsorption of a further 5 to 10 percent filtered load can occur at some site in between (327, 328). No papillary micropuncture data are available, but the results could be explained by a bidirectional flux of phosphate in the loop of Henle (329), with net reabsorption in the pars recta and net secretion in the ascending limb, possibly along the electric gradient established by chloride reabsorption; however, microperfusion in the rat demonstrated slight bidirectional fluxes for phosphate in the proximal tubule but not in the loop of Henle (330). Comparison of distal puncture fluid with urine suggests that an additional 10 percent of the filtered load is reabsorbed either in the late distal tubule or collecting duct (327). In the rat, ^{32}P injected at the distal puncture site can be recovered quantitatively in the urine even after parathyroidectomy (331), which appears to rule out phosphate reabsorption in between. But with smaller doses of ^{32}P some distal reabsorption can be demonstrated after microinjection (332). Urine from juxtamedullary nephrons could have a lower phosphate content than urine from superficial nephrons, but even complete reabsorption in juxtamedullary nephrons fails to account for the difference between distal micropuncture site and urine in some experiments (327). Nevertheless, distal reabsorption is probably greater in juxtamedullary than in superficial nephrons (332). The distal tubule and collecting duct are important in the final regulation of excretion of many other substances, and these segments contain PTH-sensitive adenylate cyclase and show inhibition of phosphate reabsorption in response to PTH. Consequently, a separate distal reabsorption site will be presumed to exist, at least in the dog and in human beings (Table 8-24). By performing micropuncture during phosphate infusion in the dog, the whole kidney Tm_P/GFR could be divided into separate proximal and distal components of approximately equal magnitude (325). Since at normal blood levels much more phosphate is reabsorbed proximally than distally, the proximal Tm/GFR must have little splay, whereas the distal Tm/GFR must have a wide splay.

The constancy of TF/UF for phosphate along most of the proximal tubule indicates that the reabsorption of phosphate is closely linked to the reabsorption of sodium and water. A decrease in sodium reabsorption caused by expansion of ECF volume is accompanied by decreased phosphate reabsorption and increased phosphate excretion even when calcium is added to the infusate to prevent any increase in PTH secretion (333, 334). Conversely, when sodium reabsorption is enhanced by ECF volume contraction, proximal phosphate reabsorption is increased and phosphate excretion is reduced. These changes occur by increases or decreases in the proximal Tm_P/GFR with no change in the distal Tm/GFR (325). However, because of the wide splay in the distal Tm/GFR, distal phosphate reabsorption at normal blood levels varies directly with load so that the change in urinary excretion is usually less than the change in proximal reabsorption. The link with sodium reabsorption is caused partly by the sodium requirement of the active transport mechanism for phosphate, which is discussed below, and partly by a nonspecific consequence of the bulk reabsorption of salt and water.

The relative contribution of the transcellular and paracellular routes to phosphate transport is unknown, but the tight junction appears to be impermeable to phosphate, and active reabsorption in the early (and probably late) proximal tubule must presumably be transcellular. The intracellular free phosphate ion concentration is as uncertain in the renal tubule as in other cells so that whether active influx at the luminal pole or active efflux at the basal pole is the principal driving force is unknown, but net inward fluxes probably represent the balance between fluxes in opposite directions at both poles, as in the intestinal mucosal cell (284, 320). Most data place the active step at the luminal pole, implying that the free phosphate concentration is higher inside the cell than outside. The cyclic AMP–dependent step in phosphate reabsorption is located at the luminal pole, as will be discussed later (335). Furthermore, vesicles composed of brush border membranes isolated from the luminal pole of proximal tubule cells demonstrate transport of phosphate coupled as a counter ion to active sodium transport, whereas in vesicles obtained from basolateral membranes phosphate transport is independent of sodium and occurs passively down an electrochemical gradient (284). If sodium was replaced by potassium, phosphate transport was concentration-dependent. The net flux represented the sum of the active and passive components, as in the intestine (Fig. 8-18). In this in vitro system HPO_4^{2-} coupled to the sodium ion was transported in preference to $H_2PO_4^-$ (284), whereas in the intact nephron $H_2PO_4^-$ appears to be preferentially reabsorbed (336). This accounts for the apparent reciprocal relationship between phosphate and bicarbonate reabsorption (325) and may also explain the accelerated reabsorption of phosphate in the earliest segment of the proximal tubule. The persistent reduction in phosphate reabsorption that occurs in chronic metabolic acidosis despite a subnormal cAMP response to PTH is unexplained.

The effect of calcium on renal phosphate transport, both in experimental animals and in human subjects, is the subject of conflicting reports (325). In patients with hypoparathyroidism, raising a subnormal plasma calcium to normal by giving calcium supplements intravenously (337) or by mouth (338) reduces the high Tm_P/GFR toward normal. However, in some cases of familial hypophosphatemic vitamin D refractory rickets, the low Tm_P/GFR is unaffected by PTH but increased by calcium infusion to a greater extent than can be explained by suppression of PTH (339). In acute experiments calcium at low to moderate levels potentiates the action of PTH and may substitute for it (340), but at high levels calcium opposes the action of PTH, possibly by inhibiting the generation of cAMP (341).

Large increases·or decreases in glucose reab-

sorption induce reciprocal changes in phosphate reabsorption, suggesting competition for a common carrier. There is no evidence that this mechanism operates within the physiologic range, and the effect can be explained as a consequence of the change in the potential difference across the tubular epithelium generated by glucose reabsorption. The same probably applies to the apparent competition between phosphate and amino acid reabsorption (325).

Magnesium. In both the rat and the dog, the TF/UF for magnesium increases to about 1.5 along the proximal tubule, indicating reabsorption of only 45 percent of the filtered load (Table 8-24), significantly less than for sodium and water (342). In the rat, the TF/UF rises to over 3 at the hairpin turn, and even higher values occur in the desert rat because of the medullary recycling between the ascending and descending limbs. At the distal puncture sites, the TF/UF falls to about 0.6 because of reabsorption of a further 50 percent of the filtered load in the ascending limb of the loop, a higher proportion than of sodium and water (Table 8-24). With magnesium infusion, there is some reduction in fractional reabsorption in the proximal tubule but no change in absolute reabsorption.

Magnesium transport in the distal tubule and beyond is less well characterized, but in the dog about 5 percent of the filtered load is reabsorbed beyond the distal puncture site, either in the late distal tubule or in the collecting duct. In the rat about 5 percent of the filtered load is reabsorbed in the early distal tubule with no reabsorption beyond the distal puncture site. With magnesium loading, net secretion of magnesium can be demonstrated in the descending limb of the loop of Henle in the rat (343). In the dog, comparison of distal puncture sites and urine during magnesium loading suggested net secretion in the terminal nephron segments (344), but the discrepancy could be explained by increased magnesium excretion by juxtamedullary nephrons. It is generally believed that the human nephron more closely resembles that of the dog than that of the rat. Results from the former species, therefore, are summarized in Table 8-24.

Decreases or increases in excretion of sodium produced by a wide variety of maneuvers are accompanied by parallel changes in magnesium excretion (307, 325, 345). In most circumstances the change in magnesium clearance is about double the change in sodium clearance, the disparity being somewhat less during mannitol-induced osmotic diuresis. This probably reflects the proportionally greater magnesium than sodium reabsorption in the ascending limb.

Very little is known of the cellular mechanisms of magnesium reabsorption. Reabsorption in the distal tubule and collecting duct occurs against an electrochemical gradient, presumably by an active transport mechanism which is specific for magnesium, but nothing is known of its nature. There may be an additional transport mechanism shared with calcium, since increasing the plasma concentration of either ion decreases the reabsorption and increases the excretion of the other (307, 325, 345). The relationship between whole kidney Tm/GFR for magnesium and reabsorption at specific sites in the nephron is unknown. Like phosphate, the intracellular free magnesium concentration in the renal tubule cell is as uncertain as in other cells, so that active transport for magnesium might be located either at the luminal or basolateral poles. The concentration of magnesium in renal tissue water, like that of potassium, decreases from cortex to inner medulla, in contrast to sodium and calcium, for which the gradient is in the opposite direction (346). The concentration of magnesium is higher than of calcium in the cortex but much less in the papilla; however, these measurements do not discriminate between intra- and extracellular magnesium. Ingestion of rapidly metabolizable nutrients such as glucose or ethanol produces a transient decrease in proximal reabsorption and increase in excretion of magnesium for a few hours despite a fall in sodium excretion. This has been attributed to enhancement of sodium reabsorption and retardation of chloride reabsorption in the proximal tubule (347). The altered magnesium reabsorption is probably not of physiologic significance; sustained ingestion of ethanol has no effect on urinary magnesium or magnesium balance (348).

Calcium. In the dog, the TF/UF for calcium normally remains at about 1.1 along the proximal tubule, leaving 35 to 40 percent of the filtered load remaining at the end (Table 8-24) (349, 350). In the rat, the TF/GF for calcium increases to 1.2 in the immediate postglomerular segment, indicating less rapid reabsorption of calcium than of water; subsequently the TF/UF remains at the same level, indicating reabsorption in parallel with water. During mannitol-induced osmotic diuresis, TF/UF for calcium consistently falls below 1.0, indicating active transport against an electrochemical gradient, a mechanism which appears not to operate under normal circumstances (349). With calcium infusion TF/UF rises to about 1.2 to 1.4 in both dog and rat, indicating decreased fractional but unchanged absolute reabsorption (351, 352). This suggests a limited reabsorptive capacity, but during microperfusion of the nephron, calcium reabsorption increases in direct proportion to intratubular concentration over a wide range (353). The paradoxical effect of hypercalcemia may depend on the formation of filtrable but nonreabsorbable complexes with phosphate; the TF/UF or TF/GF for calcium is also increased by complex formation with sulfate (345) or ferrocyanide (354). Reduced tubular reabsorption of complexed calcium also accounts for the increase in urinary calcium produced by the intravenous infusion of sodium citrate and isocitrate (355) and EDTA (223), the greater effect of calcium gluconate than calcium chloride infusion on calcium excretion (356), the exaggerated calciuretic response to saline infusion in adrenalectomized dogs (357), and the paradoxical increase in calcium excretion produced by sodium phosphate infusion, which is the opposite of the effect produced by long-term oral administration (358). The physiologic importance of differential reabsorption of the various normal components of complexed calcium (Table 8-5) is unknown.

TF/UF for calcium increases along the descending limb in the rat but is less than TF/P for sodium at the hairpin turn, suggesting either net reabsorption of calcium or net addition of sodium (359). Possibly some reabsorption of calcium continues beyond the proximal puncture site in the pars recta, as for phosphate. In the hamster, comparison of proximal and papillary puncture sites suggests that addition of calcium occurs in the descending limb, but these sites sample different types of nephron. However, there is evidence from intranephron injection of radiocalcium for medullary recycling of calcium in the loop of Henle in the rat (360). This process is much more pronounced in the desert rat, in which much higher TF/UF values at the papilla are found for all ions.

In the ascending limb a further 20 to 25 percent of the filtered load of calcium is reabsorbed, the TF/UF falling progressively to about 0.5 in the early distal tubule (Table 8-24). Reabsorption of calcium, as of sodium, varies directly with load at this site and so is gradient-limited. With saline infusion, distal TF/UF values may be as low as 0.3 for both calcium and sodium. Distal TF/UF for calcium is not altered by moderate hypercalcemia in the dog but is increased in the rat; however, the calcium/sodium ratio is increased by calcium infusion in both species. About 8 percent of the filtered load of calcium is reabsorbed in the distal tubule and collecting duct, a somewhat higher fraction than for magnesium and a somewhat lower fraction than for sodium and possibly phosphate. These are the major sites of physiologic control of calcium excretion, calcium reabsorption in the distal nephron being increased by parathyroid hormone and metabolic alkalosis and decreased by chronic metabolic acidosis, phosphate depletion, and calcium infusion (349, 350).

It is evident from the parallel changes in TF/UF along the nephron that calcium reabsorption is linked with sodium and water reabsorption both in the proximal tubule and in the ascending limb. As for phosphate and magnesium, acute changes in sodium excretion are usually accompanied by parallel changes in calcium excretion. The change in calcium clearance is usually about the same as or slightly greater than the change in sodium clearance. This relationship is discussed further below.

Less is known of the cellular mechanisms of calcium transport in the kidney than in the gut. A calcium-binding protein has been extracted from the kidney (361); its concentration varies with the tubular reabsorption of calcium (362) but its function is unknown. The Mioni model of whole kidney calcium handling (Fig. 8-30) can be related to intrarenal mechanisms if the fractional component of reabsorption (represented by the slope) corresponds to sodium-linked reabsorption in the proximal tubule, and the Tm component (represented by the intercept) is located in the ascending limb, distal tubule, and collecting duct. On this interpretation the splay in the whole kidney titration curve would correspond to the load dependence of calcium reabsorption in the ascending limb. However, the fractional component in the model corresponds to only 40 to 50 percent of the filtered load, whereas about 60 to 65 percent of the filtered load is reabsorbed in the proximal tubule. Moreover, the distribution of reabsorption among different nephron segments is similar for calcium and magnesium, although the whole kidney handling of these ions is quite different.

In the dog, metabolic inhibitors such as dinitrophenol and sodium azide increase calcium excretion with no change in sodium excretion, presumably by depression of an active transport mechanism which is specific for calcium (363). As mentioned previously, there may be a shared transport mechanism for calcium and magnesium as well as independent mechanisms for each ion. Because the intracellular free-calcium concentration is very low, transport across the tubular epithelium could be accomplished by passive influx at the luminal pole and active efflux at the basolateral surface. A calcium-activated ATPase has been localized to the plasma membrane (364, 365) but not to a specific pole of the cell. Alternatively, calcium efflux could occur by exchange-diffusion or counter transport against passive sodium influx (350). In this case, independence from sodium could be accomplished by facilitated diffusion at the luminal pole, as in the gut, but in either case calcium is probably pumped into the lateral intercellular space. The calcium concentration in renal tissue water increases progressively from cortex to papilla, the magnitude of change being greater than for sodium (346). Papillary calcium concentration correlates with but is much higher than urinary calcium concentration. Ingestion of rapidly metabolizable nutrients increases calcium as well as magnesium excretion, presumably by the same mechanism (347). Carbohydrate refeeding after total starvation decreases calcium excretion, probably because of reversal of metabolic acidosis.

The relationship between divalent ion excre-

tion and the renal handling of salt and water. A link between sodium and calcium excretion was first found with mannitol diuresis in the dog (358). Later, saline infusion was found to increase the clearance of sodium and ultrafiltrable calcium in parallel, the clearances being approximately equal at high rates of urine flow (345). The correlation was not an artefact due to inclusion of V as a common variable but indicated that the reabsorption of these ions was reduced in proportion to their concentration in glomerular filtrate, with the concentration ratio remaining the same along the nephron. The same relationship was subsequently found when sodium excretion was altered by a variety of other maneuvers. Decreased reabsorption and increased excretion of sodium consequent on ECF volume expansion (307, 325, 345), increased arterial pressure (366), renal vasodilatation (367), and administration of a wide variety of diuretics (368) are accompanied by decreased reabsorption and increased excretion of calcium. Conversely, increased reabsorption and decreased excretion of sodium caused by ECF volume contraction, renal vasoconstriction, or bile duct obstruction (369) are accompanied by decreased calcium excretion. It was postulated and widely accepted that sodium and calcium were actively reabsorbed by a common transport mechanism (345), notwithstanding the steric improbability of a monovalent and a divalent ion having the same affinity for a mobile carrier. Despite an extensive search, no evidence for such a mechanism has been found. Sodium and calcium compete for binding to an ATPase in microsomes of brain and muscle (370), but this observation is unlikely to be relevant to renal physiology. Furthermore, the reabsorption of magnesium, phosphate, and several nonelectrolyte constituents of the glomerular filtrate such as glucose is also influenced by sodium reabsorption. Each of the experimental procedures listed above produces changes in the reabsorption and excretion of magnesium and phosphate in the same direction as for sodium and calcium, but in general the correlation with sodium excretion is less close for phosphate than for magnesium and calcium. Bradykinin and prostaglandin E_2 increase the clearances of sodium, calcium, and magnesium but not phosphate because their effect is exerted beyond the proximal tubule (371). As previously mentioned, the change in calcium clearance is usually about the same or slightly greater than the change in sodium clearance, whereas the change in magnesium clearance is about double the change in sodium clearance. Since the plasma concentrations do not change much, the slope relating urinary calcium to urinary sodium excretion is approximately equal to the Ca/Na ratio of plasma ultrafiltrable concentrations, whereas the equivalent slope for magnesium is about twice as great. A comprehensive and generally accepted explanation for all these observations is not yet possible, but it is likely that the link between sodium and other substances differs at different sites in the nephron (368, 370).

In the proximal tubule, active reabsorption of sodium is the driving force leading to passive reabsorption of chloride and the water. As a result, the concentrations of all other constituents of the glomerular filtrate will tend to increase progressively along the tubule; depending on the permeability of the tubular epithelium, they will be reabsorbed as a passive consequence of the tubular fluid/plasma concentration gradients (372). In addition, the same physical and hemodynamic factors which influence sodium transport across the tubular epithelium probably also influence the reabsorption of other substances. Bulk flow of salt and water will also carry other substances with it by solvent drag. The tight junctions of the proximal tubular epithelium are freely permeable to calcium as well as sodium, with significant passive back-flux for both ions; consequently, this nonspecific mechanism accounts adequately for their parallel reabsorption. Presumably, the permeability to calcium is less in the immediate postglomerular segment, where calcium is reabsorbed more slowly than water. However, the proximal tubular epithelium is relatively impermeable to magnesium, accounting for the lesser reabsorption of magnesium in this segment. In the rat, there is some passive concentration-dependent reabsorption of magnesium when the TF/UF rises above 2. The permeability to phosphate is also low, but the dependence of active phosphate transport on sodium contributes to the coupling between their reabsorption.

In the ascending limb, reabsorption of sodium,

calcium, and magnesium may be linked because all three ions are passively reabsorbed along the electric gradient established by active chloride reabsorption. This theory is consistent with the absence of significant reabsorption of phosphate at this site. If it is true, the driving force predicted by the Nernst equation would be much greater for the divalent ions calcium and magnesium than for the monovalent ion sodium, whereas fractional reabsorption of calcium and sodium is similar at this site and only about twice as high for magnesium. Calcium reabsorption may be less than predicted because it is reabsorbed as the monovalent ion pair $CaCl^-$ (370), and magnesium reabsorption may be less than predicted because the tubular epithelium is much less permeable to this ion (360). An alternative theory is that active reabsorption of calcium and magnesium shares the same source of energy as active reabsorption of sodium.

In the distal tubule and collecting duct, calcium, magnesium, and probably phosphate are reabsorbed by mechanisms which are unrelated to sodium but which subserve the homeostasis of the individual ions. Because of the large transtubular potential difference, any interaction would lead to an inverse rather than a direct relationship between calcium and magnesium reabsorption and sodium reabsorption. Aldosterone-dependent changes in distal sodium reabsorption and sodium excretion have no significant direct effects on the reabsorption of phosphate, magnesium, or calcium. In patients with Addison's disease, glucocorticoid withdrawal leads to increased excretion of magnesium and calcium as well as sodium (373), and the usual postdiuretic retention of sodium and calcium fails to occur (374), but the nephron site of altered reabsorption is unknown. In normal subjects, short-term administration of sodium-retaining steroids has no effect on calcium and magnesium excretion, whether the steroids are given as a single intravenous infusion (375, 376) or for several days by mouth (377). The increase in calcium and magnesium excretion when sodium-retaining steroids are given for a longer period is a consequence of volume expansion (307, 325).

The effect of altered sodium reabsorption on the composition of the urine is profoundly modified by differential reabsorption at more distal sites. The more proximal the site of altered reabsorption, the less likely it is to be reflected in the urine. The load dependence of sodium and calcium reabsorption in the ascending limb and of phosphate reabsorption in the distal tubule has already been mentioned; this will tend to reduce the effect of changes in reabsorption occurring in the proximal tubule alone. The greater effect of decreased sodium reabsorption on magnesium as opposed to calcium excretion probably reflects both the smaller fraction of magnesium normally reabsorbed in the distal nephron and the larger fraction normally reabsorbed in the ascending limb (Table 8-24), which is the major site of sodium-dependent changes.

The effects of infusion of hyperoncotic albumin are an instructive example of this principle. This procedure expands intravascular but not interstitial fluid volume and decreases the proximal reabsorption of sodium, but it has only a modest effect on sodium excretion and no effect on calcium excretion (378, 379). Because of the large rise in plasma albumin concentration, protein-bound calcium increases, ionized calcium falls, and PTH secretion is stimulated. This in turn reduces the proximal reabsorption of sodium and calcium and increases the distal reabsorption of calcium. When the increased PTH secretion is prevented, there is no change in proximal sodium reabsorption but a modest fall in distal reabsorption; suppression of proximal sodium reabsorption presumably requires an increase in interstitial fluid volume rather than in intravascular volume.

The importance of sodium-dependent changes in divalent ion excretion in the long term is unknown, but any effects which persist are smaller in magnitude than are found in acute experiments. This may reflect either a shift in the site of predominant alteration of sodium reabsorption from the proximal tubule and ascending limb to more distal segments, or adaptive changes in individual reabsorptive mechanisms in the distal tubule and collecting duct. Chronic volume expansion caused by aldosterone excess is not accompanied by a sustained increase in urinary phosphate (380); there is only a modest increase in urinary calcium although the calciuretic effect of increased dietary sodium is enhanced. In normal subjects a high salt intake leads to increased urinary calcium for up to a week (381) and possibly longer, but more recent studies have shown no such effect after two weeks (382, 383). The correlation between 24-h excretion rates for sodium and calcium (384) may reflect a correlation between dietary intakes rather than any renal interaction. If there is a sustained increase in urinary calcium following increased salt ingestion, there must be either a negative calcium balance (which can occur only at the expense of bone) or a compensatory increase in calcium absorption, for which there is some evidence both in the rat and in human beings (383).

THE ENDOCRINE AND METABOLIC CONTROL OF BONE AND BONE MINERAL METABOLISM

All hormones probably have effects on bone and its constituent minerals, but for some hormones these effects constitute their main function. These are sometimes referred to collectively as the calciotropic hormones, which include parathyroid hormone (PTH), calcitonin (CT), and the active metabolites of cholecalciferol (CC). Other members of this group await discovery. The effects of pH and acid-base balance will also be described in this section, but other agents which have clinically important action on bone and its mineral will be considered in Chap. 19.

Much of the confusion in this field stems from the widespread failure to relate in vitro dose response curves to the range of hormone concentrations found in vivo (157). Sometimes physiologic and pharmacologic doses have opposite effects because they are acting on different receptors. Each action of a hormone has its own receptor, and each receptor has its own individual dose response curve. The time course of response reflects the plasma concentration, protein binding, membrane penetration, and receptor binding of a hormone, but an unphysiologic spike in concentration may cause a long-lasting unphysiologic response.

PARATHYROID HORMONE

The parathyroid glands, located on either side of the thyroid, are normally four in number, varying from two to six. Each weighs about 30 to 40 mg, somewhat more in women than in men, and increases in weight with age up to about 40 years. About one-third to one-half of the total gland bulk is fat, the proportion increasing parallel with the increase in total weight.

Chemistry and biosynthesis of PTH

The secretory product of the parathyroid gland is an 84-amino-acid-polypeptide of MW 9500 daltons, but biologic activity appears to reside solely in the amino terminal portion of the molecule. The 1-34 fragment is as potent as the parent hormone, and fragments as short as 2-27 retain some biologic activity (385). However, not all of the fragments have been fully tested for all possible actions of the hormone; for example, none has been examined for potency in increasing the tubular reabsorption of calcium. The primary structure has been completely determined for bovine and porcine PTH, which differ in only seven positions, and partly determined for human PTH. The sequences proposed by two laboratories for the first 34 amino acids (counting from the amino terminus) differ in three positions (157), but analysis of biosynthetic human PTH incorporating labeled amino acid precursors favors the Niall rather than the Brewer structure (386). PTH is derived from a larger precursor, pro-PTH, which has an additional hexapeptide at the amino terminus (387). The primary product of messenger RNA translation is an even larger molecule, pre-pro-PTH, which has an additional 25 amino acids at the amino terminus (388). The additional sequence acts as a signal to direct the nascent molecule into the cisternal spaces of the rough endoplasmic reticulum, and the addend is removed within a few seconds to form pro-PTH. This is transported within 10 to 15 min to the Golgi region, where the hexapeptide is cleaved to form PTH, which in turn is degraded intracellularly, secreted directly, or packaged into secretory granules (387). These store only enough hor-

Table 8-25. Turnover of calciotropic hormones

	PTH	1,25-DHCC	CT
Secretion rate, pmol/24 h	5000–10,000	900–1800	600–6000
Plasma concentration, pmol/L	1–10*	60–120	3–30
Metabolic clearance rate,† L/24 h	1,000–5,000	15	200

* Determined from indirectly estimated secretion rate and rate of disappearance.

† MCR = secretion rate/plasma concentration = volume of distribution × 0.693/half-time of disappearance.

mone to maintain a normal secretion rate for a few hours. The intracellular migration of both pro-PTH and PTH occurs along microtubules; if these are disrupted by colchicine or vinblastine, both the conversion of pro-PTH to PTH and the release of PTH from secretory granules are blocked (387, 389–391). The secretion of PTH is enhanced by vitamin A and by cytochalasin B, probably by facilitating the fusion of secretory granules with the cell membrane, but it is unlikely that vitamin A is concerned in the normal control of PTH secretion. In the rat, only about 20 percent of the PTH synthesized is released. The remainder is degraded inside the cell to smaller peptides and amino acids which may be recycled.

Secretion of PTH

Direct measurements of secretion rate have not yet been accomplished in any species, but indirect estimates based on the minimum rate of infusion of bovine PTH needed to restore and maintain normocalcemia in parathyroidectomized animals (expressed as pmol/kg per 24 h) are about 3 to 6 in the dog and 450 to 900 in the rat (Table 8-25) (150, 157).

Regulation by calcium. Secreted PTH is derived from both newly synthesized PTH and the storage granules. The release of preformed hormone is controlled primarily by the ionized calcium level of the blood, and to a lesser extent by magnesium (157, 387), both ions causing changes in the oxygen consumption and ATP content of the glands (392, 393). The reception of these signals by the parathyroid cell probably involves a membrane-bound adenylate cyclase. Studies in which opposite changes were produced in the concentration of both divalent ions indicate that

magnesium is about one-third as potent as calcium on a molar basis in altering PTH secretion (394). Earlier studies of PTH secretion in response to hypocalcemia suggested a proportional control over a wide range of calcium concentrations, but this concept was too simple. PTH secretion is probably also related to the rate of change of ionized calcium (derivative control) and to the duration of the change in ionized calcium (integral control). In the cow, an increase in PTH secretion can be detected within 20 s in response to a fall in ionized calcium of only 0.025 mmol/L (395). When PTH level and plasma calcium are measured simultaneously over a wide range, a sigmoid relationship is seen (Fig. 8-34), the steepest rise in PTH secretion occurring in the region between 2.3 and 1.9 mmol/L of calcium, with smaller increases at lower levels and failure to suppress hormone secretion completely at high levels. The same conclusion is reached if the integrated increment in PTH over a period of time is related to the integrated decrement in plasma calcium. Sustained hypercalcemia pro-

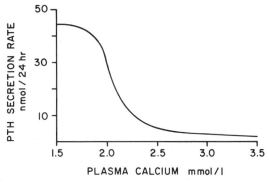

Figure 8-34. Secretory response of the parathyroid glands to acute changes in plasma calcium concentration in the calf. (*After G. P. Mayer.*)

gressively reduces PTH concentration in the venous effluent of the parathyroid, but basal secretion persists for 2 h and in some experiments for as long as 35 h with no further fall, indicating continued hormone synthesis at a low rate despite hypercalcemia (396). The most rapid changes in secretion are probably related mainly to release of preformed hormone; the effects of hypocalcemia on hormone synthesis are more complex. In the rat, incubation of parathyroid tissue in a low-calcium medium for 1 to 2 h had only a slight effect on the rate of synthesis of pro-PTH and the rate of cleavage of pro-PTH to PTH, but it markedly reduced the rate of intracellular degradation and recycling of PTH so that more was available for secretion (387). Conversely, incubation in a high-calcium medium increased the rate of intracellular degradation so that less was available for secretion. More prolonged exposure to a low-calcium concentration increases the uptake of both neutral amino acids and of α-aminoisobutyric acid by the gland, and it increases total hormone synthesis (397). Changes in magnesium level have no effect.

Sustained changes in hormone secretion are accomplished mainly by changing the number of hormone-secreting cells. Normally there is a cycle of alternating activity and quiescence of the parathyroid chief cell (398). Active cells have more intracellular organelles, the endoplasmic reticulum is aggregated into lamellae, the Golgi apparatus is larger and more prominent, and the secretory granules are abundant. Inactive cells have fewer organelles and a high glycogen content, the endoplasmic reticulum is dispersed, and the Golgi apparatus is less prominent. Secretory granules may increase initially because of inhibition of release but eventually become fewer. Several intermediate stages between these two principal cell forms can be demonstrated. The relative numbers of cells in these different stages of the cell cycle reflect the relative periods of time that each cell spends in the different stages, and this is regulated by the level of plasma calcium. A persistently low plasma calcium increases the proportion of active cells because each cell has a shorter period of quiescence between successive bursts of activity (399–401). Conversely, a per-

sistently high plasma calcium decreases the proportion of active cells because the period of quiescence is prolonged. The largest and most sustained increase in hormone secretion involves not just an increase in the proportion of active cells but an increase in the total number of chief cells, or hyperplasia. Increased DNA synthesis and increased mitotic index (401) can be detected in the rat parathyroid within a few hours of low-calcium incubation, but increased cell number may not be demonstrated for several weeks in the intact cow (399).

In summary, the control of parathyroid hormone secretion by calcium is exercised by a hierarchy of five overlapping mechanisms, each with its own time scale (Table 8-26). First, there is increased release of preformed hormone, which operates within seconds and minutes. Second, there is a decrease in intracellular hormone degradation which becomes evident within 1 to 2 h. Third, there is increased total hormone synthesis within 1 to 2 days. Fourth, there is an increase in the proportion of active cells owing to a decrease in the length of the quiescent interval, which becomes evident in about a week. Finally, there is true hyperplasia, which develops gradually over even longer periods. In general, each mechanism does not become operative unless the demand for increased hormone exhausts the capacity or outlasts the time scale of the preceding mechanism in the hierarchy. Only the first, and possibly the second, of these processes is affected by magnesium as well as calcium. It is possible that there are also long-term controls of cell proliferation and functional cell mass which are independent of plasma calcium.

Other influences on PTH secretion. There are a variety of other stimuli to PTH secretion, but none as yet is of established physiologic impor-

Table 8-26. Mechanisms of increasing PTH secretion in response to hypocalcemia

MECHANISM	TIME SCALE
1. Release of preformed hormone ↑	Seconds to minutes
2. Intracellular degradation ↓	Minutes to hours
3. Hormone synthesis ↑	Hours to days
4. Quiescent interval ↓	Days to weeks
5. Hyperplasia	Weeks to months

tance. There is a nocturnal increase in PTH secretion which can be suppressed by calcium infusion but which is not clearly related to a fall in ionized calcium (402, 403). Magnesium and probably other divalent cations such as strontium and barium have an action similar to that of calcium on the rapid secretion of preformed hormone, but it is unlikely that plasma magnesium variation within the physiologic range has any important effect. Severe magnesium depletion leads to suppression of PTH release (404), presumably because one or more of the enzymes required are magnesium-dependent. Several metabolites of vitamin D have recently been implicated in parathyroid control, as will be discussed later. β-Adrenergic stimulation with either epinephrine or norepinephrine increases PTH secretion, and both basal- and agonist-stimulated increments of this mode of secretion are inhibited by propranolol (405). Isolated parathyroid cells contain β-adrenergic receptors, the binding of agonist to which causes cAMP generation and PTH release independent of stimulation by hypocalcemia (406). Finally, cortisol stimulates PTH secretion, both directly as well as by decreasing calcium absorption. Both β-adrenergic stimulation and cortisol may lead to changes in PTH secretion in various disease states, but only the former is likely to be of physiologic significance (407). Changes in plasma phosphate (196) and in acid-base balance (408) probably influence PTH secretion via changes in ionized calcium, but direct effects such as on cell proliferation have not been ruled out. There is no evidence for pituitary control of the parathyroid gland, other than a nonspecific effect of growth hormone on size.

Metabolism of PTH

The fate of secreted PTH is complex and still incompletely understood; it is of importance for the interpretation of PTH radioimmunoassay results (409), as a possible means of regulating hormone concentration (410), and because different metabolites may have different biologic effects. Metabolism occurs mainly in the kidney and in the liver (411). In the dog, the kidney carries out over 60 percent of the total metabolic clearance of in-

fused bovine PTH, but because of technical problems in organ perfusion the products of this metabolism have not been identified (412). Renal uptake of PTH occurs both by glomerular filtration and tubular reabsorption and directly from the peritubular circulation. The renal enzymes that degrade PTH are stimulated by calcium, so that an increase in secretion of PTH indirectly enhances its own disappearance (410). Biologically active PTH-like material is excreted in the urine (413), but whether this is unchanged hormone or a fragment resulting from renal metabolism is unknown; normally it amounts to only 1 percent of the filtered load. The liver carries out about 40 percent of the total metabolic clearance of PTH, and the venous effluent contains the same fragments as can be detected in the systemic circulation (414).

There is general agreement that the largest and most abundant product of PTH metabolism makes up the C-terminal two-thirds or so of the molecule. The half-life of this fragment is at least 20 times that of the native hormone and possibly much longer, and it is biologically inactive (157). According to most estimates, it has a molecular weight on the order of 6000 to 7000 daltons (A2 in Fig. 8-35) so that the other product of hormone

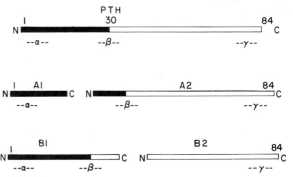

Figure 8-35. Relationship between intact PTH molecule and hypothetical immunoreactive fragments produced by cleavage at different sites. N = amino terminals; C = carboxy terminals. Numbers 1, 30, and 84 refer to amino acid residues. Solid line is the biologically active portion of the molecule. α, β, and γ refer to different antigenic sites. A1 and A2 are fragments which result from cleavage in region of residues 20 to 25. B1 and B2 are fragments which would result from cleavage in region of residues 40 to 45. (*From A. M. Parfitt,* Clin. Endocrinol. Metabol., *3:451, 1974.*)

cleavage (A1) would be too short to have any biologic activity either. However, in the only study attempting to define the cleavage site, it was located no closer to the amino terminus than residue 34 (385). Cleavage at this site would produce a C-terminal fragment of molecular weight only 5000 (B2) and an N-terminal fragment which would be biologically active (B1). A fragment of MW 4500 capable of activating adenylate cyclase has been detected, but the evidence for its presence in vivo was not conclusive (157). Although fragments with the structural requirements for biological activity arise by peripheral metabolism (385), their production is not a prerequisite for hormone action, since the native hormone is able to activate adenylate cyclase receptors (157).

The half-life of infused homologous PTH has not been determined in any species, but the half-life of bovine PTH in the dog is 4 to 8 min (415). The disappearance of endogenous PTH has a half-life of 2 to 4 min in the cow (416) and up to 20 min in human beings (417). The longer values probably reflect mainly the C-terminal metabolite. If a half-life of 4 min is combined with the secretion rate inferred in the dog, the equilibrium concentration of secreted hormone in plasma is only 1 to 2 pmol/L, which is only about 2 percent of the total amount of immunoassayable material. Even the longest half-life of 20 min corresponds to a plasma concentration of only 5 to 10 pmol/L.

The actions of PTH

The most obvious effects of lack of PTH are a fall in plasma calcium and a rise in plasma phosphate; normal levels of PTH secretion prevent these abnormalities by several actions on bone and on kidney. The mechanisms of target cell stimulation by PTH, as by several other peptide hormones, involve both activation of membrane-bound adenylate cyclase and increased cell membrane permeability to calcium; it is not clear whether these are simultaneous or successive mechanisms or whether they are the only signals which link the binding of hormone to receptor with biochemical and physiologic effects.

Bone. PTH has actions on all types of cell in bone and thus influences both the remodeling and the homeostatic systems. These actions subserve three main functions (117). First, in conjunction with its effects on gut and on kidney, PTH determines the steady-state level of plasma calcium. Second, PTH is an important component of the homeostatic feedback mechanism, which detects and corrects deviations in plasma calcium from the steady-state level. Finally, PTH is a major determinant of the prevailing level of bone remodeling and turnover. For all three functions, the effect of PTH is dependent on an adequate supply of 1,25-dihydroxycholecalciferol (1,25-DHCC), the active metabolite of vitamin D (117). These functions are listed in order of importance, but for convenience of exposition they will be described in reverse order.

The Mechanism of Bone Cell Activation by PTH. PTH binds to and activates adenylate cyclase receptors in bone, both binding and activation having similar dose response curves. In isolated but uncharacterized bone cells a response can be obtained with concentrations as low as 10^{-2} pmol/L, but with continued exposure to PTH, generation of cAMP declines markedly after 60 min (117). All types of cell isolated from fetal rat or neonatal mouse calvaria generate cAMP in response both to PTH and to calcitonin, but periosteal cells show a preferential response to CT and true bone cells a preferential response to PTH (418). The former population consists mainly of osteoclastlike cells and their precursors and the latter consists mainly of osteoblasts (419). In the adult rat, osteoblasts, osteocytes, and periosteal cells have both PTH- and CT-sensitive adenylate cyclase receptors, but marrow cells (presumably including some osteoclasts and their precursors) respond only to calcitonin (117).

It is still uncertain whether all of the physiologically important actions of PTH on bone require activation of adenylate cyclase. Modest increases of either exogenous or endogenous PTH can elevate plasma calcium without raising bone cAMP content (420). PTH also increases cell membrane permeability to calcium and the uptake of calcium by bone cells. It is unclear whether calcium uptake is a separate effect of hormone binding to receptor, a consequence of cAMP generation, or the primary response to receptor binding which precedes cAMP generation (117).

PTH and Bone Turnover. Statements concerning bone resorption in both experimental and clinical contexts frequently obscure the important distinctions between extent, speed, and rate of resorption. Nonetheless, PTH undoubtedly increases the rate of bone resorption both in vivo and in vitro. During continued PTH infusion in human beings for 24 h, urinary hydroxyproline excretion increases slowly and stabilizes at about twice the baseline level after 8 h and takes a similar time to decline to normal when the infusion is terminated (421). In tissue and organ culture experiments there are both short-term effects, caused by an increase in osteoclast activity, and longer term effects caused by an increase in osteoclast number, but the lowest effective concentration is about 50 times the normal plasma PTH level in the rat (422). The effects on cell activity are transient and are discussed in the next section, but they may provide a means for perpetuating resorption after the stimulus is withdrawn, and for the local increase in osteoclast number which occurs within a few hours, before there has been time for completion of the proliferative cell cycle.

PTH also increases the recruitment of new osteoclasts in vivo, as shown both by short-term studies in animals and long-term studies in human subjects with increased PTH secretion (117). This increases the activation of bone remodeling cycles, the morphologic basis of increased bone turnover. Short-term increases in osteoclast number may arise by activation of preosteoclasts arrested in the G1 or G2 stages of the proliferating cell cycle, but sustained increases can result only from increased frequency of mitosis in osteoclast progenitor cells. PTH is less able to increase bone turnover if 1,25-DHCC is deficient. The increase in osteoclast activity produced acutely by PTH is not sustained, and continuous exposure to excess PTH may actually depress the speed of advance of the resorption front, although the distance traveled by the front is increased (117). Bone turnover is increased by thyroxine as well as by PTH; these two hormones together are the main determinant of the normal level of bone turnover

in the adult but are not responsible for the increased turnover during growth. Even when both hormones are absent, bone turnover does not stop completely.

Because of the normal coupling between resorption and formation in vivo, a rise in the number of osteoclasts in response to PTH is followed within a few weeks by a rise in the number of osteoblasts as each remodeling cycle progresses to its formative stage. PTH in high doses inhibits lamellar bone formation, but low doses may stimulate woven bone formation in growing animals (150). The synthetic bovine 1–34 peptide stimulates both osteoblasts and chondroblasts in organ culture at doses too low to cause release of calcium (423), but there is no convincing evidence that PTH is concerned in the normal regulation of osteoblast function in adults.

PTH and the Stabilization of Plasma Calcium. A small reduction in ionized calcium leads within a few minutes to an increase in PTH secretion (395). This is the receptor arm of a feedback loop that serves to correct errors in the prevailing steady-state level of plasma calcium. The effector arm of this feedback loop is a rapid release of calcium from bone that is not dependent on an increased number of osteoclasts and is unrelated to bone turnover (117, 157). The rapid hypercalcemic response to PTH requires 1,25-DHCC and varies directly with the prevailing level of plasma calcium and inversely with the level of plasma phosphate. It is augmented by prior administration of calcium and is preceded by a very early fall in plasma calcium, which may be a reflection of sudden movement of calcium into bone cells. This effect of PTH is mediated by increased transport of calcium out of bone ECF, by increased removal of mineral without matrix from the zone of less dense metabolically active bone around the osteocyte lacunae and canaliculae, and by increased resorptive capacity of existing osteoclasts. It thus involves three different cell types whose response probably differs in time course and in sensitivity to PTH. Because of the very large surface area involved, the bone lining cell osteocyte complex is ideally placed to mobilize mineral, even though the total amount available is relatively small. PTH alters the surface morphology of the lining cells (424), increases the number of gap junctions they form with osteocytes (425), and increases pyroantimonate precipitation within the lining cells (426), suggesting increased cell membrane permeability to calcium. When PTH is given at varying time periods after ^{45}Ca, the shorter the time interval the greater is the rise in labeled calcium compared with total calcium (427). This indicates that PTH causes release from bone of those calcium ions which have most recently entered and so are still close to the surface. Concerning the osteocytes, PTH causes an increase in lactate production by these cells within 2 min and an increase in mitochondrial granules inside the cells within 30 min (117). The osteocytes thus show both metabolic and structural changes in response to PTH which occur within the time scale of the early hypercalcemic response. Concerning the osteoclast, previously resting cells become active in response to PTH, as shown by an increase in ruffled border and a decrease in clear zone (124), an increase in RNA and protein synthesis, and depolarization of the cell with an increase in the resting membrane potential (117, 124).

If the demand for calcium is sufficiently prolonged, PTH increases osteoclast proliferation and bone turnover as already described; this will cause a transient net loss of mineral from bone for 4 to 6 weeks, but PTH also causes more sustained effects in and around osteocytes, with more of these cells entering the resorptive phase of the mini-remodeling cycle and with increased mobilization of perilacunar mineral from around all cells (117). These changes are of more pathologic than physiologic significance and merge imperceptibly into the diseased bone of prolonged hyperparathyroidism.

PTH and the Determination of Steady-State Plasma Calcium Level. Neither of the previously described functional systems on which PTH acts is concerned in determining the normal level of plasma calcium. The reasons why the bone remodeling and turnover system cannot subserve this function have been explained, and further discussion is given elsewhere (117, 428). There are also many reasons why the error-correcting mechanism cannot subserve this function either;

the conceptual distinction between error correction and steady-state determination has been explained. Indefinite continuation of the acute hypercalcemic response to PTH cannot account for the sustained hypercalcemia which results from sustained PTH excess. In the dog, this can be produced by PTH infusion at twice the normal secretion rate, much less than the amount needed to release calcium from bone by either of the two established mechanisms (157). In human beings, perilacunar demineralization is not progressive, reflecting the severity of the hyperparathyroid state rather than its duration (117). Even if the observed changes occurred in only 1 year, the net input of calcium into the ECF would be increased by only 1 mmol/day. The effect on plasma calcium of net release from bone by whatever mechanism depends mainly on the kidney. From the normal characteristics of tubular reabsorption of calcium previously described, it can be estimated that to raise the plasma calcium by 0.1 mmol/L would require an increase in the flow of calcium into and out of the ECF of 5 mmol per 24 h. In most patients with primary hyperparathyroidism the net input of calcium from bone estimated either from balance studies or from measurements of bone mass is less than 2 mmol per 24 h (428), sufficient to raise the plasma calcium in the presence of normal renal function by only 0.04 mmol/L.

Because of arguments such as these it is widely held that the determination of normal plasma calcium is the function not of the bone but of the kidney (157, 158). The reasons for believing that the calcium exchanges at quiescent bone surfaces are also concerned in this determination were extensively discussed in a previous section. Despite chemical disequilibrium these surfaces are characterized by biologic equilibrium and are covered by a layer of cells sufficiently extensive to enable concentration gradients between bone ECF and systemic ECF to be maintained. PTH determines the plasma calcium level at which the inward and outward fluxes at the bone surface are equal; as discussed earlier, this is accomplished either by reducing bone fluid pH as a result of lactate production or by increasing the uptake and outward extrusion of calcium by the lining cells, or by both mechanisms. The actions of PTH on this system, as on the remodeling and error-correcting systems, require 1,25-DHCC for their proper expression.

Kidney. PTH decreases the tubular reabsorption of phosphate, sodium, bicarbonate, potassium, and amino acids and increases the tubular reabsorption of calcium, magnesium, and glucose. The effect on phosphate reabsorption was the first of any kind to be established, and for many years the other renal effects were neglected. Phosphate, calcium, and magnesium are regulated directly and independently by PTH, but each is also influenced indirectly by the effect of PTH on sodium reabsorption. Although not the most important, the effects on monovalent ions will therefore be described before the effects on divalent ions; to facilitate cross-reference the order of presentation of the latter will be the same as on pp. 320–331.

Mechanism of Renal Cell Activation by PTH. PTH binds to receptors isolated from the renal cortex in a manner which activates adenylate cyclase and generates cAMP; as in bone, receptor-binding and enzyme activation have similar dose response curves (429, 430). In the rabbit, PTH-sensitive adenylate cyclase is localized to the proximal convoluted tubule, pars recta, the cortical portion of the thick ascending limb, the distal convoluted tubule, and the early branched segment of the collecting duct (431). In the proximal tubule, the receptors are located at the basolateral or contraluminal pole of the cells (Fig. 8-36), although the cAMP generated by hormone-receptor interaction functions at the luminal pole (335, 432). In isolated renal tubules, cAMP release begins within 10 s of exposure to PTH, reaching a peak at 60 s (433). PTH administration in human beings is followed within a few minutes by a brisk but transient rise in plasma cAMP (434). This does not occur in the absence of the kidneys and presumably represents cAMP generated at the basolateral pole which fails to enter the renal tubule cell (Fig. 8-36). Some cAMP does enter the cell, and as in bone this is either preceded or accompanied by entry of calcium (61); cAMP then travels to the luminal pole, and in conjunction with the increase in cytosol calcium activates a protein

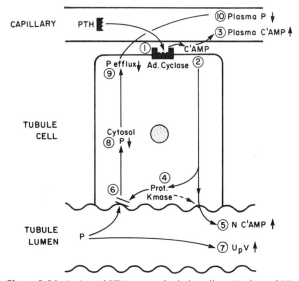

Figure 8-36. Action of PTH on renal tubule cell. 1. Binding of PTH to adenyl cyclase receptor in cell membrane. 2. Entry of some cAMP into cell. 3. Entry of some cAMP into capillary, leading to rise in plasma level of cAMP. 4. Passage of cAMP to luminal pole and activation of protein kinase. 5. Escape of cAMP from cell into tubule lumen leading to rise in NcAMP excretion. 6. Changes in brush border proteins and/or enzymes leading to block in influx of P into tubule cells. 7. P denied entry into cell is excreted. 8. Free cytosol P concentration falls. 9. Efflux out of cell falls. 10. Plasma P falls. (Entry of calcium into cell omitted for simplification.)

kinase which leads to phosphorylation of a variety of different proteins in the brush border (435). Some of the cAMP then escapes from the renal tubule cell into the urine; whether this is cAMP which has initiated metabolic effects without itself being metabolized or whether it is surplus cAMP not required for physiologic function is not known. Urinary cAMP may also originate in muscle or liver, or in the kidney as a result of antidiuretic hormone (ADH) action. Subtraction of the filtered load permits calculation of the nephrogenous cAMP; when measured during a water diuresis this reflects predominantly the action of PTH on the renal tubule (436). After a single dose of PTH in man, there is a large, abrupt, and transient increase in cAMP excretion, the peak occurring about 15 to 30 min after the peak rise in plasma cAMP, but preceding any other measurble effect on urinary excretion (430). During continued infusion of PTH, urinary cAMP remains high throughout the infusion but falls to normal within 30 min after the infusion is terminated (421).

Although PTH, like other polypeptide hormones, does not need to enter the cell to accomplish its physiologic functions, labeled PTH has been demonstrated by autoradiography within renal cell mitochondria, its authenticity confirmed by immunofluorescence (437). A variety of direct effects of PTH on isolated mitochondria have been described (438), but these are probably artifacts, and the presence of PTH within the cell is most likely related to its metabolic degradation. PTH affects mitochondrial function indirectly via the increased intracellular cAMP. This causes release of calcium from mitochondria, and the combination of increased intracellular concentrations of calcium and cAMP and decreased intracellular concentration of phosphate leads to a variety of changes in intermediary metabolism (61, 438), but their physiologic significance is not established.

Sodium, Bicarbonate, Potassium, and Water. After a single injection of PTH in human beings there is an acute increase in the excretion of sodium, potassium, bicarbonate, and water (430, 438). With continued infusion of pharmacologic doses into human subjects for 24 h, sodium, bicarbonate, and potassium excretion reach a peak after 4 to 6 h and then return to the baseline level (421). The plasma bicarbonate falls and remains low but the plasma sodium does not change; the cumulative sodium loss and hydrogen ion retention are sustained with the development of hyperchloremic acidosis. When the infusion is terminated there is a transient period of both sodium retention and hydrogen ion loss. Descriptively, these effects are identical with those which follow carbonic anhydrase inhibition, although PTH probably does not act in this way (439). There is reduction of the threshold for bicarbonate excretion (Tm_{HCO3}/GFR) and establishment of a new steady state in which the components of hydrogen ion excretion are unchanged, the sodium diuresis continuing only for as long as bicarbonate excretion remains elevated. The same changes occur in chronic phosphate depletion (440) but develop too slowly to account for the response to PTH. A low bicarbonate threshold is more common in secondary than in primary hyperparathyroidism partly because of more severe phosphate depletion and partly because calcium has the opposite effect to PTH and increases bicarbonate reabsorption. Consequently, hypercalcemia counteracts and hypocalcemia enhances the effect of PTH excess (441).

Both clearance and micropuncture studies in dogs indicate that the effect of PTH on the reabsorption of sodium, bicarbonate, and water is located in the proximal convoluted tubule (325); altered ion transport occurs at the luminal pole and is reproduced by infusion of cAMP and by the direct application of cAMP to the brush border (335). Like impaired proximal sodium reabsorption from other causes, this is accompanied by impaired reabsorption of phosphate, calcium, and magnesium, although this may be less evident with sodium reabsorption linked to bicarbonate than with sodium reabsorption linked to chloride. Potassium loss may be a further direct consequence of the reduced proximal sodium reabsorption or a nonspecific result of increased distal delivery of sodium.

Phosphate. PTH is the most important single factor controlling Tm_P/GFR, the major determinant of the plasma phosphate level (300). When PTH secretion changes abruptly there is a transient change in urinary phosphate excretion in the same direction, but the steady-state effect of a sustained change in tubular reabsorption caused by altered PTH secretion is a change in plasma phosphate level, not in urinary phosphate excretion. The rapidity of change in phosphate excretion depends on the dose; very large single doses injected directly into the renal artery increase phosphate excretion within a few minutes, but continued infusion in the dog at a rate of two to four times the normal secretion rate may not produce a detectable increase for an hour (442).

In human beings, Tm_P/GFR is inversely re-

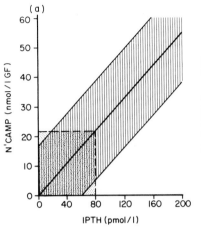

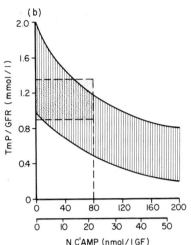

Figure 8-37. (a) Relationship between immunoreactive parathyroid hormone (IPTH) and nephrogenous cyclic adenosine monophosphate (NcAMP). Note that total immunologic activity is 10 to 100 times the indirectly estimated concentration of secreted hormone. Shaded square encloses normal ranges for both variables. Oblique lines enclose 95 percent confidence limits for the regression. (b) Relationship between either IPTH or NcAMP and Tm_P/GFR. Shaded rectangle encloses normal ranges for both variables and curved lines enclose the 95 percent confidence limits for the relationship.

lated both to nephrogenous cAMP (NcAMP) and to plasma PTH over a wide range, but the relationship is curvilinear (Fig. 8-37). Above a certain level of PTH further increments in PTH secretion produce little further decrement of Tm_P/GFR despite further increments in NcAMP, indicating that a significant component of phosphate reabsorption is insensitive to PTH. Conversely, the effect of PTH decrements on Tm_P/GFR increases progressively as PTH declines, but this may be due to hypocalcemia as well as directly to PTH deficiency. The effect of PTH on Tm_P/GFR and cAMP generation is reduced but not abolished by vitamin D deficiency (443). During continued infusion of PTH in normal subjects, Tm_P/GFR reaches its lowest value after about 6 h and then remains stable (421). When the infusion is terminated, Tm_P/GFR shows little change for 6 h and does not return to baseline levels for 24 h. This indicates that although the continued production of cAMP requires the continued secretion of PTH, the metabolic changes induced by cAMP persist for many hours after the cAMP itself has disappeared.

Because of the link between sodium and phosphate reabsorption in the proximal tubule during ECF volume expansion, the phosphaturic effect of PTH has been ascribed in part to its effect on sodium and bicarbonate reabsorption, but it is now clear that the major effect of PTH on phosphate reabsorption is independent of effects on other ions (325, 441). The location of PTH-sensitive phosphate reabsorption along the nephron is subject to the same uncertainties as the location of phosphate reabsorption in general. The bulk of the PTH-sensitive component is located in the proximal convoluted tubule and pars recta (444), but there is probably also a distal component which may be small in magnitude but physiologically important (325).

The PTH-sensitive phosphate transport process is at the luminal pole so that PTH reduces the entry of phosphate from the lumen into the tubule cell and presumably decreases the intracellular phosphate concentration. Paradoxically, PTH also increases both the uptake of labeled phosphate by the renal tubule cell (445) and its incorporation into adenosine triphosphate (ATP)

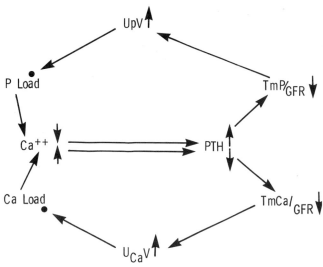

Figure 8-38. Participation of PTH in disposition of excess loads of either calcium or phosphate. In this and subsequent figures the symbol ———● identifies a process which opposes the state to which it is directed, and so closes a feedback loop.

and adenosine diphosphate (ADP), but these changes probably reflect acceleration of intracellular phosphate turnover (442). Under some experimental conditions this may be accompanied by increased efflux of phosphate from the tubule cell into the urine, but net phosphate secretion has not been convincingly demonstrated.

Although PTH determines the basal setting of Tm_P/GFR and participates in the normal circadian rhythm of phosphate excretion, a role for PTH in modulating short-term changes in phosphate excretion under normal conditions has not been established. A large phosphate load sufficient to cause hyperphosphatemia is followed by a transient decline in ionized calcium and an increase in PTH secretion (196) that enables the extra phosphate to be excreted more rapidly (Fig. 8-38). However, a small phosphate load will increase urinary phosphate more quickly than a physiologic increment in PTH secretion, with little elevation in plasma level (446), so that other factors may be more important in fine regulation.

The effect of a PTH-induced fall in Tm_P/GFR on plasma phosphate may be partly offset by increased net loss of phosphate from bone and increased net absorption of phosphate. PTH also increases mobilization of inorganic phosphate from striated muscle (447) and to a lesser extent from liver, but whether this leads to a sustained reduction in intracellular phosphate is not known.

Magnesium. PTH increases the tubular reabsorption of magnesium in human beings, but this is easier to demonstrate in hypoparathyroid than in normal subjects and requires large supraphysiologic doses (305, 306). The effect may be obscured by hypercalcemia, which reduces magnesium reabsorption probably because of competition between calcium and magnesium for the same transport process (307). During continuous infusion of PTH for 24 h there was net retention of magnesium during the infusion despite no significant change in plasma level. When the infusion was terminated, urinary magnesium rose promptly and remained high until the plasma calcium returned to normal 24 h later (421), thus demonstrating both the magnesium-conserving effect of the hormone and the magnesium-wasting effect of hypercalcemia. The lack of effect of small doses of PTH on magnesium reabsorption and the small amount of increase even with large doses in normal persons make it unlikely that changes in PTH secretion are concerned in normal magnesium homeostasis (306). The Tm_{Mg}/GFR was the same in patients with moderate deficiency or excess of PTH as in normal subjects, and in response to magnesium depletion all three groups showed a parallel fall in plasma Mg and in urinary Mg/(mmol/L of C_{Cr}), indicating that renal conservation of magnesium is a passive consequence of the fall in plasma level with no homeostatic increase in tubular reabsorption (305). Since the proximal tubular action of PTH decreases magnesium reabsorption, the magnesium-conserving effect is presumably located in the ascending limb or in more distal sites, although this has not been directly established.

Calcium. PTH is an important factor controlling the tubular reabsorption of calcium, a major determinant of the plasma calcium level in conjunction with the calcium homeostatic system in bone (157, 300). During calcium infusion, calcium excretion/(mmol/L of C_{Cr}) is higher than normal when PTH secretion is deficient and lower than normal when PTH secretion is high (Fig. 8-29) (308); Tm_{Ca}/GFR, whether calculated according to the Nordin or Mioni models, is low in the former case and high in the latter. After parathyroidectomy, urinary calcium excretion may rise for a while even though plasma calcium is falling. In the hamster, the excess calcium which appears in the urine may be enough to account completely for the loss of calcium from the ECF (448), and the same may occur after excision of a parathyroid adenoma in some patients with hyperparathyroidism (449). When normal subjects were given a continuous infusion of PTH for 24 h, neither plasma nor urinary calcium changed significantly for the first 4 h (421). There is thus a temporal dissociation between the effect of PTH on Tm_P/GFR, which fell substantially within 2 h, and on Tm_{Ca}/GFR, which did not begin to increase for 4 h. Thereafter, plasma calcium rose steadily but urinary calcium did not increase for a further 16 h; thus the increase in tubular reabsorption of calcium did not contribute to the rise in plasma calcium but served to prevent the calcium mobilized from bone from being excreted, as observed also many years ago in the rat (450). When the infusion was terminated, urinary calcium continued to rise although the plasma calcium did not fall during the next 8 h, during which either intestinal absorption of calcium or net loss of calcium from bone must have increased to higher rates than during the infusion. Suppression of PTH and consequent decrease in tubular reabsorption enables a calcium load to be more rapidly excreted in the urine (Fig. 8-38).

Micropuncture studies in both the dog (451) and the rat (452) demonstrate that PTH decreases the reabsorption of calcium and sodium in the proximal tubule, and possibly also in the ascending limb of the loop, but strongly stimulates the reabsorption of calcium without sodium beyond the distal puncture site, either in the terminal portion of the distal tubule or in the collecting duct. This is the ideal location for effective calcium conservation (350). For example, the increment in calcium excretion produced by various diuretics is substantially reduced by a low-calcium diet (453, 454), because much of the cal-

cium denied reabsorption in the ascending limb is recaptured more distally when PTH secretion is enhanced. Several lines of evidence suggest that this action of PTH is not mediated directly by increased generation of cAMP. First, there are fewer PTH-sensitive adenylate cyclase receptors in these segments (431). Second, the effects of PTH on calcium reabsorption occur several hours later than its effects on phosphate reabsorption (421). Third, neither cAMP nor dibutyryl (DB) cAMP have been shown to increase tubular reabsorption of calcium (325). Finally, in pseudohypoparathyroidism, calcium reabsorption may respond normally to PTH even though cAMP generation and phosphate reabsorption are deficient (455). Calcium reabsorption in the terminal segment of the distal tubule and in the collecting duct is also increased by thiazide diuretics and by bicarbonate infusion. These agents have in common the delivery of an increased amount of bicarbonate to the site of calcium reabsorption (451), but whether or how this influences calcium transport is not known.

Other Renal Effects. With chronic PTH hypersecretion there is a decreased tubular reabsorption of amino acids that may be associated with amino aciduria (430). As with the low threshold for bicarbonate, this is more common in secondary than in primary hyperparathyroidism because calcium has the opposite effect to PTH on amino acid reabsorption (456). PTH also increases the tubular reabsorption of glucose, so that Tm_g/GFR is increased in hyper- and decreased in hypoparathyroidism (430). This is partly a further instance of the reciprocal relationship between glucose and phosphate reabsorption and is of little clinical significance; renal glycosuria is not found in patients with hypoparathyroidism. The effects of PTH on 1-hydroxylation of 25-HCC is discussed later.

Gut. Chronic PTH excess is associated with an increased gastrointestinal absorption of calcium (157) and magnesium, but this is due principally or perhaps entirely to enhancement of 1,25-DHCC synthesis by the kidney. PTH increases sodium-dependent calcium transport across the basolateral pole of the intestinal mucosal cell (457), but although this occurs very quickly, it is not clear that this is a direct effect of PTH rather than an indirect effect mediated by 1,25-DHCC. PTH in very high concentrations increases passive influx of calcium into isolated intestinal cells (458), but this is a nonspecific effect on membrane permeability. No effect, direct or indirect, of PTH on phosphate absorption has been reported.

VITAMIN D AND ITS METABOLITES (459–464)

Historically, the term *vitamin* D denotes a constituent of the diet that cures rickets (459). This was identified chemically as cholecalciferol (D_3 or CC), a substance also made in the skin from the provitamin 7-dehydrocholesterol in response to sunlight. Although cholecalciferol is a vitamin, its most active metabolite biologically is a steroid hormone, the secretion of which is regulated in accordance with need. The related substance ergocalciferol (D_2 or EC), present in fish liver, is derived from the provitamin ergosterol, which occurs in some plants and fungi. Many an-

alogues of vitamin D have been synthesized, of which the most important are the dihydrotachysterols (DHT_2 and DHT_3), and 1α-hydroxycholecalciferol (1α-HCC).

Chemistry, biosynthesis, and metabolism of vitamin D

In the provitamins the steroid nucleus is intact, but photochemical activation breaks the C9-C10 bond and opens the B ring (Fig. 8-39). CC (D_2) and EC (D_3) have the same nucleus but different side chains; DHT_2 and DHT_3 have a 180° rotation of the A ring, with the same corresponding side chains. CC, whether obtained from the diet or from the skin, is converted in the liver to 25-hydroxycholecalciferol (25–HCC), a transport form readily measured in blood. This in turn is converted in the kidney either to 1α,25-dihydroxycholecalciferol (1,25-DHCC) or to 24,25-dihydroxycholecalciferol (24,25-DHCC) (Fig. 8-40). Other identified metabolites are 25,26-DHCC and 1α,24,25-trihydroxycholecalciferol (1α,24,25-THCC). A series of similar metabolites can be made from EC. DHT is 25-hydroxylated to form 25-HDHT, but because of rotation of the A ring the 3-hydroxy group of DHT is in the same position as the 1-hydroxy group of 1,25-DHCC (Fig. 8-39). It is not known whether 1,25-DHDHT is formed.

Numerical data for vitamin D and its metabolites will be expressed throughout in molar units. For amounts of CC, 1 nanomole (nmol) = 0.384 μg and 1 picomole (pmol) = 0.384 ng; for concentrations of CC, 1 nmol/L = 0.384 ng/mL and 1 pmol/L = 0.384 pg/mL. For 25-HCC and 1,25-DHCC the conversion factors are similar, but with constants of 0.4 and 0.417 respectively. The international unit, defined as the biologic activity of 25 ng of CC, may be used to characterize material which is incompletely purified but is otherwise of only historical interest.

Sunlight and vitamin D synthesis in the skin. Normal skin contains about 1.3 nmol/cm² of 7-dehydrocholesterol and a similar amount of CC (465, 466). The precursor has been variously located in the stratum spinosum of the Malpighian layer and in the sebaceous glands (467). In an

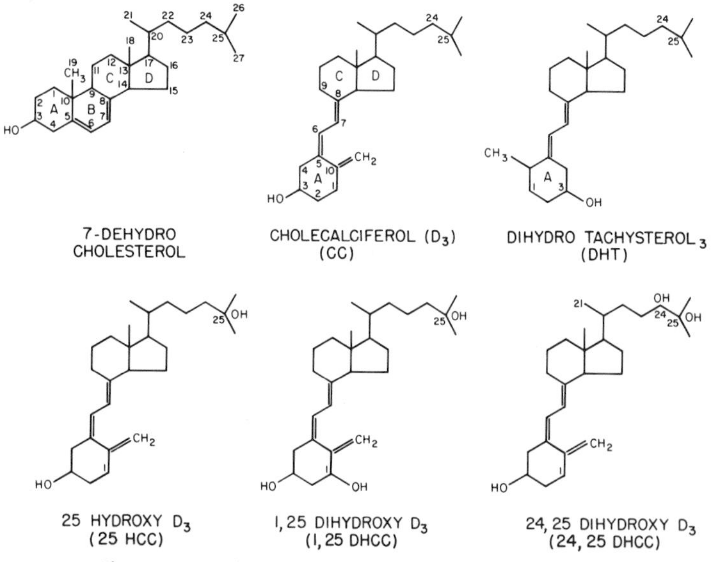

Figure 8-39. Chemical structures of vitamin D and its principal metabolites. Photochemical activation of 7-dehydrocholesterol opens the steroid B ring at the 9 to 10 band. Note 180° rotation of A ring in DHT structure.

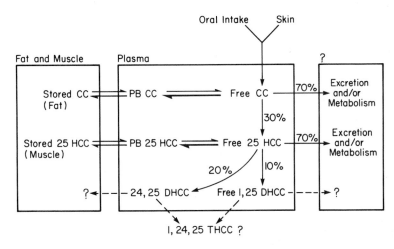

Pathways of vitamin metabolism in normal subject
PB = Protein Bound   CC = Cholecalciferol

Figure 8-40. Schema of normal vitamin D metabolism.

adult these values correspond to a total content of about 18 μmol of CC, and an additional 21 μmol could be made by quantitative conversion of the precursor. The maximum rate of synthesis estimated by irradiation of isolated skin in vitro is 6.5 μmol in 3 h (466), but how long this could be kept up is not known. The provitamin is a by-product of cholesterol biosynthesis, and its availability is not normally a limiting factor in vitamin D production. Photochemical activation of the provitamin requires the absorption of ultraviolet (UV) light of wavelength 285 to 310 nm. Much of the UV energy in sunlight is absorbed by ozone, clouds, and atmospheric pollution. This effect increases with distance from the equator, because of the reduced angle of incidence and the increased path length of the sun's rays. UV light is completely absorbed by glass, and 8 h of exposure to fluorescent lighting has less effect than a 15-min walk in the sun (468). Ranked in order of importance, the factors determining skin synthesis of vitamin D (as determined by plasma 25-HCC levels) are geographic location, indoor or outdoor work, and the season of the year, but there is considerable individual variation (468). Two months' confinement in a submarine reduced plasma 25-HCC by 40 percent (469). Although UV absorption is markedly reduced by

melanin, there is enough provitamin in the stratum corneum for black skin to make about half as much vitamin D as white skin (470), and the rise in plasma 25-HCC is the same in light- and dark-skinned persons for the same degree of UV irradiation (471). Skin pigmentation is unlikely to be a limiting factor in vitamin D synthesis south of the Arctic Circle, but it might protect against vitamin D intoxication in the tropics (472).

Dietary intake and intestinal absorption of vitamin D. Although the normal daily requirement of vitamin D, estimated to be about 25 nmol in children and about 5 nmol in adults, could be met entirely by the skin, many persons in North America and Europe need vitamin D in the diet. Natural sources are few: there are small amounts in eggs, liver, and oily fish, but milk and other dairy products are adequate sources only in the summer. In the United States 25 nmol are added to each quart of milk by federal law, but despite this public health measure as many as 30 percent of children may have intakes below 25 nmol daily and 3 percent below 6.5 nmol daily (473). Until recently, the addition was almost entirely as EC; while this was so, the level of 25-HCC in the blood would represent the contribution of skin synthesis to the total vitamin D status and the level of 25-HEC would represent the contribution of dietary intake, including vitamin supplements. Unfortunately, most of the vitamin D now added to milk is in the form of CC, so that this convenient separation is no longer possible. The widely quoted claim that in the United States only 18 percent of the total vitamin D supply comes from the diet (474) was made without awareness of this change and is a considerable underestimate; it is probably much truer of England. In children, circulating 25-HEC is largely derived from vitamin supplements (475).

Absorption of CC is a two-step process involving rapid uptake by the intestinal mucosa followed by slow transfer to intestinal lymphatics and thence to chylomicra in the blood (460). The first step requires bile salts (especially taurocholate) but is passive and nonsaturable (476); the second step is facilitated by micelle formation with fatty acid and monoglyceride within the intestinal lumen (460). A limited amount of CC is esterified during absorption. It is likely that the entire small intestine has the capacity to absorb vitamin D; the jejunum is normally the major site, but the fractional absorption of labeled vitamin D instilled directly into the intestinal lumen is greatest in the duodenum (477).

With single doses of labeled CC ranging from 100 to 2500 nmol, the peak plasma level occurs after 4 to 8 h. About 80 percent of the dose is normally absorbed, ranging from about 60 to 90 percent in different subjects, but the fraction absorbed during continued administration is not known.

Transport, metabolism, and storage of CC. After dispersion of the chylomicra, CC is carried in the blood bound to an α-globulin which has greater affinity for CC than for EC. In the United States the normal blood level of CC is from 20 to 120 nmol/L, but in England the values are probably about half as much (Table 8-27) (478).

Both CC and EC of whatever origin are taken up rapidly by the liver and hydroxylated in position 25 by an enzyme located in the microsomes of the smooth endoplasmic reticulum (Fig. 8-40). After hepatectomy some formation of 25-HCC is still detectable but the amount is extremely small (479). The conversion of a single dose of labeled CC to 25-HCC is inversely related to body vitamin D stores, an eightfold increase in dose producing only a threefold increase in 25-HCC synthesis (480, 481). This attenuation is less evident with chronic administration, but a tenfold increase in the daily dose is associated with only a fourfold increase in plasma 25-HCC when CC is given but with a tenfold increase when 25-HCC itself is given (482). About 10 to 15 times as much of the parent vitamin as of its metabolite is needed to maintain the same plasma level of 25-HCC. Partial suppression of activity of the calciferol 25-hydroxylase may be accomplished directly through excess vitamin D (481) and indirectly through product inhibition by newly

Table 8-27. Estimated quantitative aspects of vitamin D metabolism at different levels of intake*

INTAKE	CHARACTERISTIC	CC	25-HCC	1,25-DHCC	24,25-DHCC
Minimal	Daily production, nmol/day	5	4	0.9	0.4
	Percent conversion of precursor	—	80	22.5	10
	Plasma concentration, nmol/L	10	15	0.06	4.0
	Plasma pool turnover, %/day	16	9	500	3.3
Average	Daily production, nmol/day	50	15	1.2	3.0
	Percent conversion	—	30	8	20
	Plasma concentration, nmol/L	60	60	0.08	6.0
	Plasma pool turnover, %/day	28	8	500	16
High	Daily production, nmol/day	500	50	1.5	15.0
	Percent conversion	—	10	3	30
	Plasma concentration, nmol/L	250	150	0.10	15.0
	Plasma pool turnover, %/day	67	11	500	33

* Note that a 100-fold increase in intake is associated with a 12-fold increase in production of 25-HCC and with a less than 2-fold increase in production of 1,25-DHCC.

synthesized 25-HCC (483). Exogenous HCC has no effect on enzyme activity. EC is hydroxylated by the same enzyme as CC; this hydroxylase is specific for these substrates and has a low capacity, low K_m, and high V_{max}. By contrast, DHT and the synthetic analogue 1α-HCC are 25-hydroxylated by the same enzyme as cholesterol; this hydroxylase is nonspecific and has a high capacity, high K_m, and low V_{max} and is not inhibited by precursors or products (484). It is probably the second hydroxylase that leads to continued production of some 25-HCC however high the blood level.

Normally, less than 25 percent of the day's supply of CC is 25-hydroxylated (Table 8-27). Some of the remainder is converted to biologically inactive metabolites, many of which form soluble glucuronide conjugates. These are excreted mainly in the bile and ultimately in the stool, and to a smaller extent in the urine. With small single doses only about 5 to 10 percent is excreted in the stool (485), but this fraction increases progressively with the dose. Vitamin D is lipid-soluble, and the bulk of the CC which escapes both 25-hydroxylation and inactivation is stored as such in body fat (Fig. 8-40) (486, 487). Limited amounts are also stored in muscle or as esters in the liver. What determines the balance between inactivation and storage is unknown; after hepatectomy in the rat, labeled CC remains in the circulation for very much longer than normal, suggesting that uptake in fat may somehow be dependent on the presence of the liver (479). When the supply of vitamin D is abundant in the summer, 25-hydroxylation is suppressed and the surplus vitamin is diverted to body stores. When the supply is short in the winter, 25-hydroxylation is enhanced, the plasma level of CC falls, and the stored vitamin D is withdrawn until the same cycle is repeated the following year. With continued administration of pharmacologic doses of CC, the storage pool expands progressively until an equilibrium is reached in which the total loss by excretion and metabolism balances the daily intake (Fig. 8-40) (488, 499). Consequently, the half-life of disappearance from plasma is a function both of the dose and of the duration of treatment. Thus, with a single dose of labeled CC

given to a vitamin D–deficient subject, the half-life may be only a few days, but after prolonged treatment the half-life of biologic activity varies from 2 to as long as 16 months (488).

Transport, metabolism, and storage of 25-HCC. 25-HCC in blood is bound to the same protein as CC—a specific high-capacity, high-affinity α-globulin of MW 55,000 daltons, called D-binding protein (DBP) or transcalciferin (490–492). This is normally only about 2 percent saturated and is unaffected by any mineral or hormone, so that the free 25-HCC concentration is extremely low and is not homeostatically regulated. The normal total plasma level of 25-HCC is about 20 to 100 nmol/L in the United States and about 15 to 50 nmol/L in England, similar to that of CC (Table 8-27) (468, 469). It shows significant seasonal variation, but less than for CC. The combined CC and 25-HCC levels determined by chemical methods agree closely with the total biologic activity in blood determined by the rachitic rat assay, which is about 50 to 200 nmol/L in adults in the United States (493), about half that level in adults in England (488), and about 100 to 250 nmol/L in children in Europe (494). The total plasma pool of 25-HCC is thus about 0.25 μmol, but the total exchangeable pool is higher, estimates varying between 0.5 and 1 μmol (495, 496). Based on plasma disappearance curves which give a half-life of about 20 days, the total daily production of 25-HCC is normally about 10 to 20 nmol in the United States, which represents a turnover of the ECF pool of about 2 to 3 percent per day (Table 8-27) (497, 498). Almost certainly this value would be lower in England.

The most important fate of 25-HCC is conversion either to 1,25-DHCC or to 24,25-DHCC, but only about 20 to 30 percent of the daily supply normally follows this route. Of the remainder, some is excreted unchanged in bile, but at least 85 percent of this is subsequently absorbed; depending on the daily supply of CC, about 20 to 60 nmol of 25-HCC takes part in this enterohepatic circulation daily, with fecal losses of about 2 to 5 nmol per day (499). Oral 25-HCC is absorbed promptly, the peak blood levels occurring 4 h after a single dose (497, 500). The site and mechanism of absorption of 25-HCC, whether secreted in bile or administered by mouth, is presumed to be the same as of dietary CC, but there is no specific information available. Some 25-HCC is converted to more polar, biologically inactive metabolites, a process which may be enhanced by the induction of hepatic microsomal enzymes. The ultimate fate of these metabolites is unknown but probably includes both urinary and fecal excretion. Finally, like CC, some 25-HCC is sequestered in body stores, but because of its lower lipid solubility these are located predominantly in muscle rather than in fat (486). The half-life of disappearance from blood increases with the size of the storage pool, but this effect is less evident than with CC.

The control of 1,25-DHCC and 24,25-DHCC synthesis. 25-HCC is taken up by the kidney where it is hydroxylated, either in position 1 or in position 24 (Fig. 8-40). The 1-hydroxylase is a mitochondrial mixed-function oxidase requiring molecular oxygen and cytochrome P450 and is similar to those involved in the biosynthesis of other steroid hormones. The 24-hydroxylase is also a mitochondrial enzyme but is not dependent on cytochrome P450. It is not located exclusively in the kidney, since some 24,25-DHCC is present in anephric patients. The amount and activity of the renal 1-hydroxylase is regulated much more closely than those of the hepatic 25-hydroxylase, so that the normal plasma 1,25-DHCC level varies over only a twofold range, from about 60 to 120 pmol/L (Tables 8-25 and 8-27), and is unaffected by variation in diet or sun exposure (464). Regulation of 1-hydroxylation has been studied at four levels of organization—in vivo in the intact human subject and whole animals, and in vitro in organ, tissue, and subcellular preparations. The conclusions drawn from these different levels of study are not always in agreement, and many of the results obtained with isolated renal tubules and mitochondria are of dubious physiologic significance (463). Short-term changes in 1-hydroxylation may be mediated by alteration in enzyme activity brought about by changes in mitochondrial uptake of calcium and phosphate, but long-term changes require alteration in the amount of enzyme. Because of its short half-life of 2 h, this is regulated by changes in enzyme synthesis rather than in degradation. (462–464)

In vivo the most important single factor is the overall state of vitamin D nutrition, probably because 1,25-DHCC in some way inhibits 1-hydroxylation. When the plasma 25-HCC is below 25 nmol/L, conversion of a single dose of labeled 25-HCC to 1,25-DHCC is inversely related to body stores (however determined), but at higher levels of 25-HCC there is no detectable formation of 1,25-DHCC (481). Both in the chick and the rat a 50- to 500-fold increase in dietary CC had no effect on plasma 1,25-DHCC (501). Conversely, in severe vitamin D deficiency 1-hydroxylation occurs rapidly and completely and is unresponsive to controls which may operate in vitamin D–replete subjects (462, 481). Between these extremes physiologic regulation occurs by a complex interplay of PTH, plasma phosphate, and plasma calcium and of several other hormones.

The increase in calcium absorption brought about by a low-calcium diet is at least partly mediated by an increase in 1,25-DHCC synthesis, and in the rat this adaptive response can be abolished by parathyroidectomy. PTH is undoubtedly one factor which stimulates 1-hydroxylation, but as yet there is no evidence in human beings for control of 1,25-DHCC synthesis by variation in PTH secretion within the physiologic range. Dietary phosphate depletion also increases both 1-hydroxylase activity in the chick (502) and the plasma 1,25-DHCC level in the rat (503), but only if the plasma phosphate falls more than 50 percent below normal. This effect is probably mediated by some component of the intracellular phosphate pool and is not abolished by parathyroidectomy (503). Since PTH lowers plasma phosphate, its effect on 1-hydroxylation could be indirect; the action of PTH on phosphate reabsorption is located at the luminal pole of the renal tubule cell, so that PTH also lowers intracellular phosphate (Fig. 8-36). Thus calcium depletion, PTH excess, and phosphate depletion all stimulate 1-hydroxylation via a reduction in intracellular phosphate, although PTH most likely has an additional direct effect. Plasma 1,25-DHCC is low in hypoparathyroidism (464), but the relative contributions of PTH deficiency and hyperphosphatemia have not been determined. In primary hyperparathyroidism the increased production of

1,25-DHCC from a single dose of labeled 25-HCC is not correlated with plasma phosphate (504), but in stone-forming patients raised plasma 1,25-DHCC levels are more closely correlated with plasma phosphate than with plasma PTH (505). In women, dietary phosphate depletion lowers plasma phosphate and increases plasma 1,25-DHCC, but in men phosphate depletion leads to no change in plasma phosphate or 1,25-DHCC (505).

Apart from adaptation to a low-calcium diet, increased intestinal absorption of calcium is normally required in three situations—growth, pregnancy, and lactation—in each of which the plasma 1,25-DHCC level is raised (464). Although this could be mediated in part by secondary hyperparathyroidism, there is increasing evidence that each of the main hormones involved—growth hormone, estrogen, and prolactin—are potent stimulators of 1-hydroxylation (464, 506). The general principle seems to be that if a physiologic state increases the demand for calcium, the hormonal cause of the state also ensures that the demand is satisfied, a form of anticipatory regulation that is more efficient than classical negative feedback mechanisms.

In contrast to the precursors CC and 25-HCC, 1,25-DHCC is subject to rapid turnover without storage. The disappearance of 1,25-DHCC from blood occurs in three phases with successive half-lives of 5 min, 1¼ h, and 24 h (507); likewise, after cessation of administration in normal subjects the biologic action of 1,25-DHCC (as shown by urinary calcium) declines, with a half-life of 1 to 2 days (508). The daily production is about 1.2 nmol, a turnover of about 500 percent of the plasma pool daily (Table 8-27). The ultimate fate of 1,25-DHCC is unknown; some unidentified metabolites are excreted both in the urine and in the stools, but there is also side-chain oxidation with formation of carbon dioxide.

In many circumstances there is an inverse relationship between formation of 1,25-DHCC and 24,25-DHCC, possibly because increased activity of the 1-hydroxylase enzyme in some way inhibits 24-hydroxylation. However, the latter process is not controlled, and when 1-hydroxylation is suppressed, 24,25-DHCC is produced in proportion to the body pool of 25-HCC (481). The plasma

24,25-DHCC level is normally about 6 nmol/L and correlates with the plasma level of 25-HCC (509, 510). The plasma pool is about 18 nmol and daily production about 3 nmol, a turnover of 16 percent of the plasma pool per day, much faster than for 25-HCC but much slower than for 1,25-DHCC (Table 8-27). A final metabolite made in the kidney is 1,24,25-THCC. This can arise either by 1-hydroxylation of 24,25-DHCC or by 24-hydroxylation of 1,25-DHCC. It has biologic activity, but its physiologic importance, if any, is unknown. It may be a step in the inactivation and degradation of 1,25-DHCC (463).

The actions of vitamin D and its metabolites

Vitamin D increases the plasma level of calcium by potentiating the action of PTH on the calcium homeostatic system in bone and by increasing intestinal absorption, bone resorption, and renal tubular reabsorption. It increases the plasma level of phosphate directly by the same three mechanisms and also indirectly by inhibiting PTH secretion. It is concerned directly or indirectly in the maintenance of normal osteoblast function and may have a more general effect on protein synthesis in intestine, muscle, and other tissues. Finally, PTH secretion may be inhibited directly as well as indirectly by an increase in plasma calcium. The effects on intestinal calcium absorption and bone resorption are mediated primarily by 1,25-DHCC, but for some of the other effects other metabolites may be more important.

Intestine. Under different experimental conditions, vitamin D appears to enhance either the entry of calcium at the brush border or the exit of calcium at the basolateral pole, or to act on both processes together (460). Increased basolateral efflux may result from increased availability of calcium released from mitochondria, rather than from increased activity of the cell membrane pump (59, 511, 512). Vitamin D also promotes calcium absorption via the paracellular shunt pathway across the tight junctions (513), as well as via the transcellular pathway. The stimulation of intestinal calcium absorption by 1,25-DHCC is a direct effect which does not require the presence of PTH. When 1,25-DHCC is given by mouth, as little as 0.25 nmol/day will significantly increase calcium absorption in normal subjects (508). This occurs even though the plasma level of 1,25-DHCC does not change, suggesting a local action on the intestinal mucosa (514). Like other steroid hormones 1,25-DHCC enters its target cell and associates with a cytoplasmic receptor. The hormone-receptor complex migrates into the nucleus and associates with the nuclear chromatin, leading to an increase in template activity and messenger RNA production (464). The nuclear receptor has much less affinity for 25-HCC or for 1α-HCC. 1,25-DHCC produces its effects by increasing protein synthesis, but what proteins are involved and what functions they serve are still unclear. One of the earliest effects is an increase in cAMP production (515), but whether this is due directly to the hormone or requires prior protein synthesis is not known. The most intensively studied is a calcium-binding protein (CABP) which is present at the absorptive surface but appears to be synthesized by the goblet cells and secreted in the mucus (516). There is an excellent steady-state correlation between intestinal CABP concentration and calcium absorption (513) but no correlation in acute studies, since after a single dose of 1,25-HCC, calcium absorption increases earlier than CABP synthesis (517). This suggests that CABP is not related to the initiation of calcium absorption in response to 1,25-DHCC but may be concerned in the maintenance of calcium absorption on a long-term basis. There is also an intracellular vitamin D–dependent calcium-binding protein which facilitates both the diffusion of calcium into the mucosal cell and the release of calcium from mitochondria (512). In addition, 1,25-DHCC increases the synthesis of the various types of phosphatase which were mentioned earlier. Like CABP, these correlate better with steady-state calcium absorption than with the acute response to 1,25-DHCC. Recently, two new proteins have been detected in the brush borders soon after 1,25-DHCC administration and preceding the increase in calcium absorption (515). These may be concerned in molecular reorganization of the brush border, as has been demonstrated with filipin, a polyene antibiotic which mimics some of the actions of vitamin D (518).

Vitamin D also accelerates the proliferation of intestinal mucosal cells (519) and increases the height of the villi and the surface area of the microvilli (520).

As indicated earlier, vitamin D also promotes the absorption of phosphorus and magnesium. It acts in some way on the saturable rather than the diffusional components, but much less is known about the mechanisms involved. Phosphorus absorption occurs partly as a counter ion to calcium and partly by an unrelated vitamin D–dependent mechanism. No phosphate- or magnesium-binding proteins have been detected.

One of the early clues that vitamin D needed to be further metabolized was the time lag of 10 to 12 h before the onset of increased calcium absorption in the rat (463). With 25-HCC this lag is reduced to 4 to 6 h, and with 1,25-DHCC it is further reduced to about 2 h. Because of its increased potency and speed of action, which are unaffected by nephrectomy, 1,25-DHCC is evidently the principal mediator for vitamin D action on the intestine. 25-HCC binds to intestinal receptors and increases calcium absorption directly, but the amounts required are 100 to 1000 times greater (463, 464). Although this ratio is similar to the ratio of plasma concentrations, the free 25-HCC level is extremely small. Doses of 25-HCC comparable to the normal production rate are ineffective in the absence of the kidneys, but high doses undoubtedly act directly without 1-hydroxylation. This is probably the basis for the traditional distinction between physiologic and pharmacologic doses of vitamin D. A small daily dose (5 to 10 nmol) given to a vitamin D–deficient subject produces a large increase in both calcium absorption and calcium retention, but a much larger dose (50 to 100 nmol) given to a normal subject has no effect. Even larger doses, on the order of 5000 nmol daily or more, will increase calcium absorption and urinary calcium excretion with little change in balance (Fig. 8-41). The apparent difference in sensitivity to vitamin D between a deficient and a replete subject is due to changes in vitamin D metabolism rather than to changes in target cell responsiveness. In the vitamin D–deficient subject conversion of the parent vitamin to 25-HCC and then to 1,25-

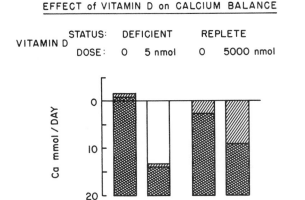

Figure 8-41. Comparison of effect on calcium absorption and calcium balance of a physiologic dose of vitamin D given to a vitamin D–deficient subject, and a pharmacologic dose of vitamin D given to a vitamin D–replete subject.

DHCC is rapid and efficient, whereas in the vitamin D–replete subject both 25 and 1-hydroxylation are suppressed. With a very high dose, the plasma 25-HCC level becomes high enough to act directly, but the 1,25-DHCC level is little changed.

The physiologic importance of 24,25-DHCC in relation to calcium absorption is unclear. In the rat, this compound is inactive unless it is 1-hydroxylated to form 1,24,25-DHCC (463), but in human beings, 24,25-DHCC in doses close to physiologic may increase calcium absorption even in anephric patients (521). 25-HDHT, because of its pseudo-1-hydroxylation, may bind to intestinal receptors and increase calcium absorption without being further metabolized (460).

Bone. The actions of vitamin D on bone are more complex and less well understood than the actions on the gut and include effects on both the remodeling and homeostatic systems. Bone resorption or mineralization induced by vitamin D are accompanied by proportional movements of phosphorus and magnesium, but there is no evidence that vitamin D influences the uptake or release of these substances by mechanisms unrelated to calcium. The healing of rickets and osteomalacia is to a large extent due to increasing the plasma levels of calcium and phosphate. In addition, depressed osteoblast and chondroblast function improve, but whether this is due directly or indirectly to vitamin D is not known.

The best-documented effect is on bone resorption. In the rat, a single dose of either 1,25-DHCC or 25-HCC produces the same sustained increase in calcium absorption, but a sustained increase in plasma phosphate occurs only with 25-HCC, so that this substance is more effective in healing rickets (522). The rise in plasma phosphate evidently requires continued production of 1,25-DHCC and so is not mediated entirely by increased calcium absorption and suppression of PTH. The plasma phosphate rises despite a low-phosphate diet and when urinary phosphate excretion is already very low, so that no significant further enhancement of intestinal absorption or tubular reabsorption can occur. By inference, the increase in plasma phosphate is derived from bone (522). In tissue culture 1,25-DHCC is the only substance which can increase bone resorption at concentrations below the normal plasma level. This occurs whether 1,25-DHCC is given to the animal before death or is added directly to the culture system (523, 524). The effect is potentiated by PTH, but with high doses can occur in its absence and is not mediated by adenylate cyclase activation (525).

In vivo, the release of calcium and phosphate from bone by 1,25-DHCC is more dependent on the presence of PTH than in vitro, but it can occur in the absence of PTH if the animal is phosphate-depleted (464, 522). The effect of 1,25-DHCC-induced bone resorption depends on the level of PTH secretion. If 1,25-DHCC formation is increased because of phosphate depletion, PTH is low and the phosphate released from bone is retained but the calcium is excreted in the urine. The net effect is to raise the plasma phosphate more than the plasma calcium. Conversely, if 1,25-DHCC formation is increased because of calcium deficiency, PTH is also increased and the calcium released from bone is retained but the phosphate is excreted in urine; the net effect is to raise the plasma calcium more than the plasma phosphate. In this way, 1,25-DHCC is able to participate in the regulation of both plasma cal-

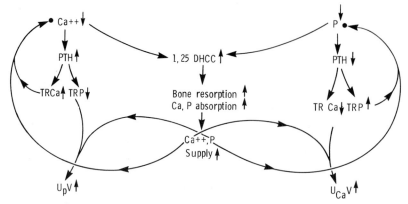

Figure 42. Dual role of 1,25-DHCC in defense against both hypocalcemia and hypophosphatemia, showing how disposal of mobilized calcium and phosphate varies with PTH status. ——→• as in Fig. 8-38.

cium and plasma phosphate (Fig. 8-42) (464, 522). Whether this ingenious system operates in human beings is not known.

1,25-DHCC is also necessary for the release of calcium and phosphate from bone by PTH as well as the converse. The plasma calcium response to PTH in human beings is blunted by acute renal failure, partly because of 1,25-DHCC deficiency (526). In the vitamin D–deficient rat the defective calcemic response to PTH can be restored by giving lactose, which increases intestinal calcium absorption. However, in chicks made vitamin-deficient from birth, the calcemic response to PTH declines progressively to zero within 4 weeks and cannot be restored to normal by raising the plasma calcium level with supplemental calcium (527).

Like PTH, 1,25-DHCC produces short-term effects by increasing the activity of existing osteoclasts and by increasing the dissolution of perilacunar mineral by osteocytes (528); long-term effects are produced by increasing the recruitment of new osteoclasts (523). 25-HCC also stimulates bone resorption directly but the doses required are 100 to 1000 times larger (463, 523). It is probably responsible for the increased osteoclastic bone resorption which occurs in vitamin D intoxication (529), but this has not been directly established. Although transient hypercalcemia will result from vitamin D–stimulated bone

resorption, the long-term steady-state effect of this action of vitamin D is an increase in the activation of remodeling units and in bone turnover, a process which does not significantly influence plasma calcium.

A large body of clinical evidence indicates that 1,25-DHCC also acts synergistically with PTH on the calcium homeostatic system in bone. Normally, only small amounts of each are needed for the functioning of this system, and to a certain extent a large amount of each can compensate for a deficiency of the other. The experimental evidence for participation of vitamin D in the calcium homeostatic system is less extensive than for PTH, but there is no evidence which contradicts this concept. In human beings, vitamin D enhances the rate of exchange between bone and ECF in both normal subjects and patients with hypoparathyroidism (530). When calvaria of mice are incubated in tissue culture, the calcium concentration at equilibrium in the medium is higher with normal bone than with bone from vitamin D–deficient animals; in this system vitamin D increased both lactase production and the passive solubility of bone mineral in the manner required by the Neuman theory (531). Secondly, 1,25-DHCC binds to a cytosol receptor and localizes in the nuclei of bone cells in the same manner as in intestinal cells (532), and it produces changes in endosteal cell morphology similar to those produced by PTH (533). These data are consistent with stimulation of a transcellular calcium pump of the type postulated by Talmage.

There is no unequivocal evidence for a direct role of vitamin D or its metabolites in the process of bone formation. Nevertheless, there is abundant evidence that in vitamin D deficiency the function of bone- and cartilage-forming cells is disturbed in a variety of complex ways which cannot be explained by a reduction in calcium and phosphate levels in the blood (460, 534). DHT has about $1/5$ the potency of 25-HCC in raising the plasma calcium in hypoparathyroidism but has only about $1/50$ the potency of 25-HCC in healing rickets. This tenfold reduction in the relative antirachitic potency of DHT suggests that it lacks some additional action unrelated to raising the plasma calcium which is possessed by 25-HCC (489). Normal rat serum contains a vitamin D–dependent factor which stimulates the uptake of calcium by bone in vitro, an effect which cannot be duplicated by manipulating the calcium and phosphate levels of serum from a vitamin D– deficient rat (535). Although normal calcium uptake could not be restored by human serum, the factor could still be a vitamin D metabolite, since the concentrations of these are much lower in man than in the rat. In the rachitic rat, crystal nuclei appear in cartilage fluid aspirated by micropuncture from the epiphysis within 2 h of vitamin D administration, even though the Ca $\times$ P product is still below 40; the phosphate concentration also rises much sooner in the cartilage fluid than in the plasma after vitamin D administration (132). When labeled vitamin D is given to rats, radioactivity is found in the proliferative chondrocytes (536), and when labeled 25-HCC is given, radioactivity is found in the hypertrophic chondrocytes (537). The substance preferentially accumulated by these cells was not identified in either case, but it would be surprising if it were not carrying out some function. When labeled vitamin D is given with an otherwise vitamin D– free diet for 3 weeks, 25-HCC and 24,25-DHCC are the major metabolites in bone, the level of 1,25-DHCC being rather low (538). There is much indirect evidence that one or the other or both of these metabolites enhances the deposition

of mineral in bone independent of changes in plasma calcium and phosphate levels (539), but their mechanism of action is unknown. For example, the increased calcium absorption produced by 24,25-DHCC in human subjects is accompanied by a slight fall in plasma calcium rather than the rise produced by 1,25-DHCC (521), and when 25-HCC is given to vitamin D– deficient subjects, normal bone mineralization is restored sooner and at lower plasma calcium and phosphate levels than with 1,25-DHCC (540). In the rat, 1,25-DHCC may actually depress bone formation in vivo (539), and in mouse calvaria it causes regression of osteoblasts to flat fibroblast-like cells (523), similar to the effect of PTH.

Kidney. Vitamin D deficiency is characterized by decreased renal tubular reabsorption of phosphate and increased renal tubular reabsorption of calcium (460). These abnormalities cannot both be due entirely to secondary hyperparathyroidism, because they change at different rates with treatment—tubular reabsorption of phosphate increasing within a few days and tubular reabsorption of calcium not falling to normal for many weeks or months. Because of the slow rate at which plasma PTH declines after correction of human vitamin D deficiency (541), the early changes in phosphate reabsorption cannot be due entirely to a fall in PTH. It is likely that vitamin D has a direct phosphate-conserving effect which is mediated principally by 25-HCC. When labeled CC is given there is specific localization of radioactivity in the proximal tubule (542), and there is micropuncture evidence that vitamin D increases phosphate reabsorption at this site (543). 25-HCC consistently increases phosphate reabsorption in acute experiments (325), most likely by inhibiting the activation of adenylate cyclase and the synthesis of cAMP (544). Although changes in sodium reabsorption occurred in the same direction, they were too small to account entirely for the changes in phosphate reabsorption. These responses are most evident when PTH is present but can occur in its absence; 25-HCC opposes the phosphaturic effect of PTH, but some vitamin D is needed for this effect to occur (545), although the amount is less than is needed for the effects on bone. The evidence concerning 1,25-DHCC is conflicting, some studies showing an increase and some a decrease in phosphate reabsorption (546). In human beings, physiologic doses of 1,25-DHCC probably have no significant direct effect on phosphate reabsorption, but high doses may have a PTH-like effect. The fall in Tm_P/GFR with treatment in hypoparathyroidism depends on the restoration of normocalcemia, whether this is accomplished by a large dose of a calcium salt or by a small dose of 1,25-DHCC (338).

Vitamin D probably has a calcium-conserving as well as a phosphate-conserving effect on the kidney, an action in the same direction as that of PTH (547). Both 1,25-DHCC and 25-HCC consistently increase tubular reabsorption of calcium and sodium in clearance experiments, but micropuncture studies show that this effect can be dissociated from sodium; it occurs independent of the presence or absence of PTH and is located in the distal tubule and collecting duct (548). Calcium reabsorption can be enhanced by a physiologic dose of 1,25-DHCC, but a much higher dose of 25-HCC is needed. These data suggest that 25-HCC is the main phosphate-conserving metabolite and 1,25-DHCC the main calcium-conserving metabolite. Since vitamin D increases the plasma levels of both calcium and phosphate

by its actions on gut and bone, the effect on urinary excretion depends on whether the increase in filtered load or in tubular reabsorption is predominant.

Other effects. Muscle contains a specific binding protein for 25-HCC and this compound, but not 1,25-DHCC, increases phosphate accumulation, ATP content, and protein synthesis in muscle (549). Vitamin D stimulates the proliferation and growth of intestinal mucosal cells (519) and possibly of epiphyseal cartilage cells, and so may have a general effect on protein synthesis throughout the body (550). However, the finding of 25-HCC-binding proteins in all nucleated cells probably represents an artifact caused by inadvertent inclusion of the binding protein in plasma (551).

1,25-DHCC, like other steroid hormones, may be part of a feedback loop which regulates the secretion of its own trophic hormone. A calcium-binding protein (possibly vitamin D–dependent) has been found in the parathyroid glands (552), and the chief cells contain cytoplasmic receptors for 1,25-DHCC similar to those found in the gut (464, 553). In the rat, 1,25-DHCC reduces PTH secretion both in vitro and in vivo, but no consistent effect has been obtained in other species. Even in the rat, the structural changes induced by calcium depletion are determined entirely by the plasma calcium level irrespective of vitamin D status (555). There is much clinical evidence which suggests that vitamin D deficiency may stimulate PTH secretion and induce parathyroid hyperplasia directly, as well as via hypocalcemia. However, attempts to demonstrate an effect of 1,25-DHCC on PTH secretion in human beings have so far been unsuccessful. Studies in the dog suggest that this effect of vitamin D–deficiency is mediated by 24,25-DHCC rather than by 1,25-DHCC (556). This makes better physiologic sense, since it would amplify the PTH response to excess or deficiency of calcium or vitamin D (Fig. 8-43).

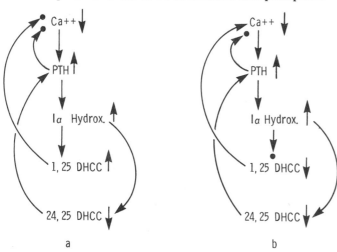

Figure 8-43. Reciprocal changes in 1-hydroxylation and 24-hydroxylation in response to hypocalcemia (a) and vitamin D depletion (b). Note that the reduced plasma 24,25-DHCC level enhances PTH secretion and so facilitates the homeostatic response. ——→● as in Fig. 8-38.

CALCITONIN (557–560)

It is not yet known whether calcitonin (CT) has a physiologic function in human beings, but it has important pharmacologic effects and is customarily included among the calciotropic hormones. It is secreted by the parafollicular cells of the thyroid (better known as C cells). These have a different embryologic origin from the other cells of the thyroid, migrating from the neural crest via the branchial arch. In nonmammalian vertebrates, the C cells retain separate anatomic identity as the ultimobranchial body (UB), but in mammals they are incorporated into the substance of the thyroid. In human beings, C cells are sparse and are concentrated in the midportion of the lateral lobes (561). C cells may also occur in other organs, such as the adrenal and the parathyroid.

Chemistry, biosynthesis, and metabolism of CT

In all species studied CT is a 32 amino acid polypeptide of MW about 3500 daltons. Like PTH there are both resemblances and differences in the amino acid sequence between different species, but only nine amino acid residues are common to all species. Little is known of the details of CT biosynthesis, but preliminary data suggest a prohormone of MW 9000 to 13,000 daltons and a pre-pro-hormone of MW 26,000 to 65,000 daltons which is probably the initial product of messenger RNA translation (562–564). There are multiple immunoreactive forms of CT in the circulation; in contrast to PTH they are all of larger molecular weight and may represent either precursors or dimers and polymers of the basic hormone (565–567). Unlike PTH, the entire molecule is needed for biologic activity, and no shorter fragments have been detected. The synthesis of CT is much less closely coupled to secretion than is the case with PTH, and the capacity for storage of hormone in the form of electron-dense granules is much greater. Consequently, large quantities of CT may accumulate in the thyroid if the secretion rate is reduced.

The plasma concentration of CT in human beings, determined by radioimmunoassay, is in the range of 3 to 30 pmol/L (Table 8-25) (568–570), which is about 50 to 100 times smaller than the concentrations determined by bioassay. Whether this discrepancy reflects artifacts in the bioassay technique or the existence of an additional unidentified hypocalcemic hormone is not clear. In the rat, both human and salmon CT are metabolized by microsomal enzymes in the kidney, although porcine CT is metabolized mainly by the liver. Salmon CT is more resistant than porcine CT to metabolic degradation, which is part of the explanation for its greater biologic activity in human beings. The fate of human CT is unclear. The metabolic clearance rate (MCR) of radioiodinated human hormone determined by disappearance of radioactivity is about 150 mL/min (Table 8-25), about two-thirds of which could be attributed to the kidney (571). If this value is combined with the range of plasma concentrations previously given, the secretion rate (MCR × plasma level) is only about 0.6 to 6 nmol or 0.2 to 2 MCR units per day. On the other hand, the MCR of pharmacologic doses of unlabeled MCR porcine CT in man determined by radioimmunoassay was about 750 mL/min (572), which would correspond to a secretion rate of 3 to 30 nmol or 1 to 10 MCR units daily.

The control of CT secretion (573)

It is still not known whether CT is secreted continuously or intermittently. In the mature rat, thyroidectomy is abruptly followed by transient hypercalcemia caused by the sudden removal of CT (574), but in human beings CT is undetectable in about 30 percent of normal subjects even with the most sensitive assays (569, 570). This may reflect rapid catabolism, since the concentration is always higher in the thyroid vein than in the peripheral circulation (575). The major controlling factor is the calcium concentration in the blood perfusing the thyroid gland, high levels stimulating and low levels inhibiting CT secretion—the opposite relationship to PTH. A response occurs within a few minutes of a rise in plasma calcium and is accompanied by a prompt reduction in the number of storage granules. Less than 30 percent of the hormone released results from increased de novo protein synthesis. In the pig, the acute change in plasma calcitonin is a linear function of plasma calcium in the range 3 to 5 mmol/L (576). In most studies enough calcium has been given to induce hypercalcemia, but a mean rise in plasma calcium of less than 0.1

mmol/L in normal human subjects led to a three-fold increase in plasma CT (568). The response to oral calcium is less consistent, a rise occurring in only two of five subjects (577). Experimental hypocalcemia induced by EDTA infusion lowers high CT levels to normal but does not produce a clear-cut fall in normal subjects because the baseline level is so low. Some early studies suggested that the secretion of a hypocalcemic agent might be controlled indirectly by calcium via a releasing factor from the parathyroid (578). This mechanism does not operate for CT (576) but might do so for some other hypocalcemic hormone. Chronic hypercalcemia leads to sustained degranulation of the C cells and in some species to C cell hyperplasia (557, 559); in patients with chronic hypercalcemia the plasma calcitonin level was found normal with one assay (570) but increased with another (573). Conversely, sustained hypocalcemia leads to cessation of secretion but continued synthesis, leading to a progressive increase in the number of storage granules (557) and an exaggerated increase in plasma CT in response to calcium infusion (579).

Since the most easily demonstrated effect of near physiologic doses of CT in normal subjects is an increase in phosphate excretion, a rise in plasma phosphate concentration would be a logical stimulus to CT secretion. A good correlation was found between fasting plasma phosphate and plasma CT in both normal subjects and those with various diseases (580). Furthermore, the circadian changes in plasma phosphate may be accompanied by parallel changes in plasma CT (569). However, there was no effect of phosphate (or calcium!) on CT release from human thyroid in vitro (581).

Under appropriate experimental conditions CT secretion can also be increased by gastrin, glucagon, β-adrenergic agents, prostaglandin E_2, DB cAMP, and magnesium and decreased by dopamine (557–560). The physiologic importance of these stimuli is not established, but pentagastrin and DB cAMP were the only agents consistently effective in vitro as well as in vivo (581). The rise in plasma magnesium must be two to three times as great as the rise in plasma calcium to achieve the same effect (582). In several species, increased secretion of gastrin and then CT in sequence may mediate the prevention of postprandial hypercalcemia (559), but in the rat, food ingestion is followed by release of CT and gastrin together with no change in plasma calcium (583). These effects have not been shown to occur in human beings.

In normal subjects there is a circadian variation in plasma CT which rises steadily from the early morning through the afternoon and falls toward the evening; the mechanisms and significance of this are unknown.

The actions and effects of CT

Although CT in pharmacologic doses has many actions, it is uncertain whether any of these can be obtained in human beings by doses corresponding to the plasma levels or secretion rates previously mentioned.

Bone. The most obvious effect of CT, and the basis of its discovery, is a fall in plasma calcium usually accompanied by a similar or even greater fall in plasma phosphate. These changes begin within a few minutes and are due to an increase in the net accumulation of calcium and phosphate by bone. This is due partly to decreased bone resorption and partly to increased sequestration of mineral by the osteocyte–bone lining cell system. CT decreases osteoclastic bone resorption in two ways—by blocking the activity of existing osteoclasts and by reducing the number of osteoclasts. Both of these effects are usually easiest to demonstrate when resorption has been increased either experimentally or as a result of disease. The effect on existing cells is shown by a rapid fall, detectable within 30 min, in the release of radioactive calcium from bone in tissue culture (584). This is accompanied by morphologic changes which are demonstrated best by electron microscopy. Within 15 min there begins a progressive flattening and diminution of the ruffled border and a corresponding increase in the extent of clear zone, changes which reach a peak at one hour. Later, the osteoclasts withdraw from the bone surface (585); similar changes may persist in vivo for up to a week (586). There are also changes in cell polarization. The mean membrane potential becomes more negative, with a change from a bimodal to a unimodal distribution, suggesting that previously active cells had become inactive (117, 124). All these changes are the opposite of those produced by PTH. The concentrations of CT in the culture medium used to achieve them are from 1000 to 10,000 times greater than the normal plasma level, but similar effects can be obtained in vivo in the rabbit with doses much closer to the physiologic range (587).

The reduction in the number of osteoclasts can be demonstrated in tissue culture within 48 hours. An effect this swift could be due to a reduction in osteoclast life span, but CT also prevents the increase in number of osteoclasts which occurs in response to the administration of vitamin A or PTH in vitro (584, 588) or of estrogen in vivo (589). In acute experiments the effect of CT on osteoclast proliferation depends on the precise timing of administration. In tissue culture, resorption induced by PTH may escape from the inhibitory effect of CT after a few days, indicating that once precursor cell division has been initiated it cannot be suppressed (590). Similarly, in the intact rat, CT is unable to prevent the osteoclast proliferation set in train by the secondary hyperparathyroidism of nephrectomy (591). Chronic CT excess in the rat is accompanied by a reduction in osteoclast number (588) that can be due only to reduced genesis from precursor cells. Similarly, in patients with chronic endogenous CT hypersecretion caused by medullary carcinoma of the thyroid (MCT), a tumor of the C cells, osteoclasts are absent (592). Bone turnover is markedly reduced because the initial activation of new remodeling cycles is depressed; nevertheless, the plasma calcium is usually normal in these patients.

The acute effect of CT on plasma calcium depends on the prevailing rate of bone turnover. This is not because a reduction in bone turnover (which is a slow process) itself contributes to acute hypocalcemia, but because normally turnover is closely related to the number of osteoclasts present. Thus the hypocalcemic effect diminishes with increasing age and is most evident in conditions such as Paget's disease where bone turnover is very high. The hypocalcemic effect is also directly related to the prevailing level of plasma phosphate and can be enhanced by prior phosphate administration (593).

Although the suppression of osteoclastic resorption undoubtedly contributes to the acute hypocalcemic effect of CT, there is considerable evidence that this is not the only mechanism involved. First, in the rat CT may cause hypocalcemia even though osteoclast proliferation is actually enhanced because of increased PTH secretion (591). Second, the acute hypercalcemia following thyroidectomy in the rat is unaccompanied by any change in urinary hydroxyproline excretion (574). Third, suppression of bone resorption should lead to an equimolar change in plasma calcium and phosphate, but these effects can be dissociated by various maneuvers. For example, when CT is given to rats pretreated with either EHDP (594) or cortisone (595), the plasma phosphate still falls but the plasma calcium rarely changes. Although CT may promote the uptake of phosphate by soft tissues such as the liver (596), there is also increased influx of phosphate into bone. Conversely, in the intact rat CT can temporarily prevent the increased efflux of calcium from the bone surface produced by PTH (597), and in mouse calvaria in tissue culture CT induces net uptake of calcium without phosphate, an effect unrelated to mineral maturation, bone formation, or inhibition of resorption (598). Finally, CT produces striking ultrastructural changes in osteocytes. These cells shrink because of a sudden efflux of water accompanied by extrusion of phosphate, which is soon followed by increased accumulation of mitochondrial granules containing both calcium and phosphate (593). These data together indicate that CT can alter either phosphate or calcium fluxes in a manner which causes storage of mineral in the bone surface–perilacunar compartment (599). There may even be a permanent increase in perilacunar mineralization if this was previously defective (600).

The effect of CT on bone formation is biphasic. Initially, there may be a transient increase, both in the number of osteoblasts and the rate of bone formation, which occurs at sites where bone resorption has recently been terminated (597, 601). In the long term, bone formation is depressed as a result of reduced activation of new bone remodeling cycles and the usual coupling between resorption and formation (592, 602).

Like PTH, CT binds to receptors in bone, stimulates adenylate cyclase and enhances cAMP generation by bone tissue (559, 560), although doses too small to produce these effects may still cause hypocalcemia (603). Cyclic AMP production in response to CT is greatest in cells located close to the periosteum (CT cells), which show a biochemical kinship with osteoclasts (419). CT also blocks the increase in synthesis of acid phosphatase and hyaluronate by these cells in response to PTH but has no effect when given alone (419). Mononuclear phagocytes, which may be circulating precursors of osteoclasts, also have adenylate cyclase receptors for both PTH and CT (145).

The fundamental action of CT on bone cells is not known. One possibility is that CT lowers the intracellular free-calcium ion activity (597), an effect opposite to that of PTH, which could be achieved by increasing the active extrusion of calcium from the cell and by increasing the sequestration of calcium in mitochondria. This may relate to a very early, acute effect of CT in human beings whereby recently administered radioactive calcium increases transiently within a few minutes (604). However, CT does not block the early acute hypocalcemic effects of PTH in the dog (157).

Kidney. The other major target organ for CT is the kidney. It has effects on tubular reabsorption which are in the same direction as those of PTH for sodium and phosphate and in the opposite direction for calcium and magnesium (605).

Sodium. CT causes a prompt increase in urinary sodium excretion that is detectable within 30 min (606). This effect can be obtained by continuous administration of salmon CT in a dose of 0.8 unit per hour (or less than 20 units per day), or with single doses of porcine CT of 8 units (607). As with other natriuretic agents, during continued administration sodium excretion returns to the baseline level, but there is a sustained reduction in ECF volume and body weight and increased secretion of renin and aldosterone (608), indicating that sodium reabsorption at some site in the nephron remains inhibited but that reabsorption at some other site is correspondingly increased. In contrast to PTH, which increases the excretion of sodium paired with bicarbonate, CT causes an equimolar increase in sodium and chloride excretion. These effects persisted unchanged for as long as 39 days on a dose of 63 units daily, and cessation of CT was followed by sodium retention and restoration of body weight and ECF volume to normal. Participation of CT in normal ECF volume regulation would require that CT secretion be stimulated by volume expansion, but no studies along these lines have been published. The renal handling of sodium and chloride has not been examined in patients with MCT.

The site in the nephron at which CT inhibits sodium reabsorption has not been localized, but changes in amino acid excretion and in free-water clearance have suggested an effect in the proximal tubule (430, 605). The natriuretic effect of CT in human beings is inhibited partly by indomethacin (609), suggesting that prostaglandins may somehow be involved. In the thyroparathyroidectomized dog, CT has no effect by itself, but it prevents the reduction in sodium, phosphate, and calcium excretion produced by 25-HCC (610). In patients with hypoparathyroidism, salmon, porcine, and human CT all cause an increase in sodium excretion (611).

Phosphate, Magnesium, and Calcium. CT increases the urinary excretion rate of phosphate, magnesium, and calcium, all of which are correlated in timing, magnitude, dose requirement, and independence from PTH with the increase in sodium excretion. However, in normal subjects, for all three ions the increase in urinary excretion is greater than the increase in urinary sodium relative to their concentrations in ECF, so that their clearances increase more than the clearance of sodium (606, 612). In patients with hypoparathyroidism this is still true for phosphate and magnesium, but the increase in sodium and calcium clearances were similar (611).

The effect on phosphate was initially attributed to increased PTH secretion in response to the hypocalcemia, but it can be demonstrated in hypoparathyroid patients (in whom it may cause a fall in plasma phosphate) and in parathyroidectomized animals. As little as 0.4 unit per hour (or 9.6 units per day) of porcine CT may increase phosphate excretion in normal subjects (613), a dose which has no effect on plasma composition. Micropuncture during increased endogenous CT secretion suggested that the decreased reabsorption of phosphate occurs in the proximal tubule (605). The phosphaturic effect is smaller and less prompt after CT than after PTH administration.

Although increased urinary excretion of phosphate can be obtained with doses which are close to physiologic, there is no evidence that this effect can be sustained. Patients with MCT invariably have normal plasma phosphate levels unless they have primary hyperparathyroidism as well. CT may modulate the splay portion of the titration curve but probably does not change Tm_P/GFR. It is of interest that the circadian increase in plasma CT occurs at about the same time as the circadian increase in urinary phosphate.

Calcitonin also decreases the tubular reabsorption of calcium, but this effect may be obscured by the effect of hypocalcemia. In young animals and in patients with Paget's disease, urinary calcium excretion may fall as a result of the fall in filtered load, but when the plasma calcium does not change urinary calcium excretion invariably increases (606, 612). Continued administration of CT in Paget's disease may lead to a rise in urinary calcium above the control level as the plasma calcium returns to normal. The effect on tubular reabsorption may be more sustained for calcium than for phosphate, although calcium reabsorption has not been studied in patients with MCT. In some circumstances, particularly in the treatment of hypercalcemia, increased urinary calcium excretion may contribute to the hypocalcemic effect of calcitonin.

Mechanism of Renal Actions of CT. Receptors have been isolated from the kidney which bind CT with the same affinity as the receptors in bone (430, 606, 614). The binding initiates adenylate cyclase activation and cAMP generation, but the receptors are anatomically and functionally distinct from those for PTH. They are located in the brush border as well as at the antiluminal pole of the tubule cell. In contrast to the action of PTH, doses of CT that cause phosphaturia may have no effect on plasma or urinary cAMP in human beings, although very high doses cause a modest increase in both (615). In the dog, this is blocked by prior administration of 25-HCC (610). The metabolic degradation of CT by the kidney involves different receptors (430, 605). In contrast to its effect on bone cells, CT inhibits the active extrusion of calcium by renal tubule cells (616), although the effect on mitochondrial calcium accumulation may be in the same direction as the effect of PTH.

Other effects of CT on mineral metabolism. In human beings, CT acutely increases the secretion of water, sodium, calcium, and phosphate by the intestinal mucosa into the lumen and so decreases net absorption (265). Repeated administration paradoxically may increase net absorption of calcium determined by balance studies (617) and increase the absorption of radioactive phosphate (618), but these effects could be mediated by increased synthesis of 1,25-DHCC as a result of increased PTH secretion. In the rat, CT inhibits vitamin D–stimulated intestinal calcium absorption (619); it is not known whether the same occurs in human beings. Contrary to earlier reports, CT has no direct effect on vitamin D metabolism (620).

The physiologic role of CT. From the data given it is evident that no certain physiologic function can yet be assigned to CT. Soon after its discovery it was suggested that PTH and CT were equally important members of a symmetrical double feedback loop for the regulation of plasma calcium, but it is now clear that CT is not concerned in steady-state plasma calcium regulation in human beings and probably not in any species (621). Deficiency or excess of this hormone may not be accompanied by any obvious changes in mineral metabolism. Nevertheless, it has consistently been found that both the magnitude and duration of hypercalcemia in response to a standard calcium infusion are greater in hypothyroid subjects receiving adequate thyroxin replacement than in normal controls (622). Although none of these studies has conclusively ruled out a renal effect, it seems likely that the protection against hypercalcemia by the temporary storage of calcium in bone is defective in such individuals, although it is not clear whether it is the ability to reduce osteoclastic resorption or to augment perilacunar sequestration which is most depressed. In either case the hypercalcemic response to dietary calcium ingestion is minimized, although no harmful effects can yet be attributed to the lack of this mechanism in man. CT may also participate in the normal circadian variation in plasma phosphate and urinary phosphate excretion, but the evidence on this point to date is merely suggestive.

HYDROGEN ION REGULATION AND ACID-BASE BALANCE

This interacts with divalent ion metabolism at several points, some of which have already been mentioned. The most immediate effect of a fall in blood pH is an increase in plasma ionized calcium and a consequent reduction in PTH secretion. However, if metabolic acidosis is continued for more than a few hours, there is decreased tubular reabsorption and increased urinary excretion of calcium, phosphate, and magnesium (623), increased fecal excretion of calcium and phosphate (190, 623), a fall in plasma calcium (total and ionized) and phosphate, stimulation of PTH secretion (624), increased removal of calcium from the bone surface–perilacunar compartment, increased net bone resorption, and loss of intra-cellular phosphate and probably magnesium. PTH may thus participate in a short-term feedback loop that serves to stabilize plasma bicarbonate concentration via its effects on tubular reabsorption of bicarbonate (Fig. 8-44) (625) and in a longer term feedback loop that serves to withdraw buffer from bone in the defense against chronic metabolic acidosis (Fig. 8-44) (626).

In the steady state established after several weeks (498), plasma ionized calcium and PTH return to normal, vitamin D metabolism is normal, fecal calcium and phosphate fall to or below normal, the initial negative phosphate and magnesium balances return to baseline, and there is no persistent change in urinary, fecal, or plasma magnesium. However, decreased tubular reabsorption of calcium and phosphate, slight hypophosphatemia, hypercalciuria and negative calcium balance persist, associated with preferential removal of calcium carbonate from bone. The effects of chronic metabolic acidosis on bone cells and the relationship to lactate production by osteocytes and the abundance of carbonic anhydrase in osteoclasts are not known. The continued withdrawal of calcium carbonate may depend more on the reduced plasma bicarbonate level than on the fall in blood pH.

Metabolic alkalosis has been studied less. When induced acutely by sodium bicarbonate infusion there is a fall in ionized calcium and a brisk increase in PTH secretion (408) and in phosphate excretion (325), but how long this can be sustained is not known. Metabolic alkalosis accompanying calcium carbonate administration increases the size and decreases the exchange-

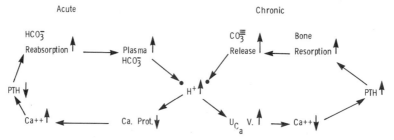

Figure 8-44. Participation of PTH in stabilization of plasma (H$^+$). Note that acute and chronic changes in PTH are in opposite directions.———▸● as in Fig. 8-38.

ability of the rapidly exchangeable calcium pool, and it decreases calcium accretion into bone, in both normal subjects and those with hypoparathyroidism (627). Chronic metabolic alkalosis caused by sodium bicarbonate ingestion is associated with increased tubular reabsorption of calcium and hypocalciuria (215). The long-term effect on bone cell function has not been adequately examined, although decreased bone resorption and positive calcium balance have been reported in response to both sodium and potassium bicarbonate administration (193).

POSSIBLE ADDITIONAL CALCIOTROPIC HORMONES

The interrelationships between three hormones, three minerals, and bone compose a system of formidable complexity, but it is far from certain that all the pieces in this jigsaw have been discovered. The absence of any hormone with a dominant role in the regulation of magnesium metabolism is surprising, and suggestive evidence for an additional hypocalcemic hormone was mentioned earlier. Plasma calcium homeostasis in the rat may show anticipatory regulation, such that appropriate corrective changes occur in advance of, rather than in response to, the disturbing signal, presumably by mechanisms involving the central nervous system (628, 629). This concept has not yet been shown to apply to human beings, although a form of anticipatory regulation probably operates in vitamin D metabolism. Many years ago Nicolaysen postulated an endogenous factor by which calcium absorption is regulated in relation to bodily need. It is widely believed that 1,25-DHCC is Nicolaysen's endogenous factor, but not all investigators are convinced that it is the only one (630). Much indirect evidence suggests that the bone has other means of signaling its needs to the gut and to the kidney than by allowing the plasma levels of calcium and phosphate to fall.

There is good evidence for an unidentified humoral agent which decreases the tubular reabsorption of calcium; blood from a phosphate-depleted rabbit, to which sufficient phosphate has been added to restore a normal concentration, causes hypercalciuria when perfused into an isolated kidney (631). There may also be an agent which inhibits phosphate reabsorption in addition to PTH and CT; in some cases of nonfamilial hypophosphatemic osteomalacia associated with various types of tumor (most notably a hemangiopericytoma), the plasma phosphate returns rapidly to normal after excision of the tumor, an extract of which was found in one case to cause increased phosphate excretion in a puppy (632). The ability of the kidney to adjust phosphate excretion to intake, with little or no change in plasma phosphate or in PTH secretion, has already been mentioned.

There are thus many suggestive pieces of evidence for the existence of undiscovered calciotropic hormones. However, the need to postulate such additional hormones will not be established until levels of PTH and all its biologically active metabolites, of all known metabolites of vitamin D, and of calcitonin have been measured simultaneously in a variety of clinical and experimental situations, a feat which has not yet been accomplished.

REFERENCES

1. Neuman, W. F., M. W. Neuman: *The Chemical Dynamics of Bone Mineral*, The University of Chicago Press, Chicago, 1958.
2. Robinson, R. A., R. H. Stokes: *Electrolyte Solutions*, Butterworth Scientific Publications, London, 1955.
3. Payne, J. W., M. Walser: Ion association. II. The effect of multivalent ions on the concentration of free calcium ions as measured by the frog heart method, *Bull. Johns Hopkins Hosp.*, **105**:298–310, 1959.
4. Widdowson, E. M., J. W. T. Dickerson: Chemical composition of the body, in C. L. Comar, F. Bronner (eds.): *Mineral Metabolism*, Academic Press, Inc., New York, 1964, vol. IIA.
5. Cohn, S. H., A. Vaswani, I. Zanzi, J. F. Aloia, M. S. Roginsky, K. J. Ellis: Changes in body chemical composition with age measured by total-body neutron activation, *Metabolism*, **25**:85–96, 1976.

6. Van Leeuwen, A. M.: Net cation equivalency (base binding power) of the plasma proteins, *Acta Med. Scand.*, **422**(suppl.):1–212, 1964.

7. Terepka, A. R., P. S. Chen, Jr., T. Y. Toribara: Ultrafiltration: A conceptual model and a study of sodium, potassium, chloride and water distribution in normal human sera, *Physiol. Chem. Phys.*, **2**:59–78, 1970.

8. Rose, G. A.: Determination of the ionized and ultrafiltrable calcium of normal human plasma, *Clin. Chim. Acta*, **2**:227, 1957.

9. Walser, M.: Ion association. VI. Interactions between calcium, magnesium, inorganic phosphate, citrate and protein in normal human plasma, *J. Clin. Invest.*, **40**:723–730, 1961.

10. Moore, E. W.: Ionized calcium in normal serum, ultrafiltrates, and whole blood determined by ion exchange electrodes, *J. Clin. Invest.*, **49**:318–334, 1970.

11. Toffaletti, J., H. J. Gitelman, J. Savory: Separation and quantitation of serum constituents associated with calcium by gel filtration, *Clin. Chem.*, **22**:1968–1972, 1976.

12. Marshall, R. W.: Plasma fractions, in B. E. C. Nordin (ed.), *Calcium, Phosphate and Magnesium Metabolism*, Longman, Inc., New York, 1976.

13. Pedersen, K. O.: Protein-bound calcium in human serum. Quantitative examination of binding and its variables by a molecular binding model and clinical chemical implications for measurement of ionized calcium, *Scand. J. Clin. Lab. Invest.*, **30**:321–324, 1972.

14. Eastman, J. W., S. J. Rehfeld, H. Loken: Ultrafiltrable calcium and the conformation of albumin, *Clin. Chim. Acta*, **58**:233–237, 1975.

15. Hopkins, T., J. E. Howard, H. Eisenberg: Ultrafiltration studies on calcium and phosphorus in human serum, *Bull. Johns Hopkins Hosp.*, **91**:1–21, 1952.

16. McLean, F. C., A. B. Hastings: The state of calcium in the fluids of the body. I. The conditions affecting the ionization of calcium, *J. Biol. Chem.*, **108**:285–322, 1935.

17. Rodan, G. A., E. P. Katz: Calcium binding to nondialyzable components of rat blood under in vivo conditions, *Am. J. Physiol.*, **225**:1082–1088, 1973.

18. Pedersen, K. O.: The effect of bicarbonate, P_{CO_2},

and pH on serum calcium fractions, *Scand. J. Clin. Lab. Invest.*, **27**:145–150, 1971.

19. Hughes, W., S. Cohen, D. Arvan, B. Seamonds: The effect of the alkaline tide on serum-ionized calcium concentration in man, *Digestion*, **15**:175–181, 1977.

20. Stearns, G., W. Warweg: Studies of phosphorus of blood. I. The partition of phosphorus in whole blood and serum, the serum calcium and plasma phosphatase from birth to maturity, *J. Biol. Chem.*, **102**:749–765, 1933.

21. Russell, R. G. G., H. Fleisch: Pyrophosphate and diphosphonates, in G. H. Bourne (ed.), *The Biochemistry and Physiology of Bone*, vol. IV, *Calcification and Physiology*, Academic Press, New York, 1976.

22. Smales, F. C.: A computer program for calculating the activities of calcium and orthophosphate ions in biological fluids and related synthetic solutions, *Calcif. Tissue Res.*, **8**:304–319, 1972.

23. McLean, F. C., M. A. Hinrichs: The formation and behavior of colloidal calcium phosphate in the blood, *Am. J. Physiol.*, **121**:580–588, 1938.

24. Frye, R. M., H. Lees, G. A. Rechnitz: Magnesium-albumin binding measurements using ion-selective membrane electrodes, *Clin. Biochem.*, **7**:258–270, 1974.

25. Alfrey, A. C., N. Miller, D. Butkus: Evaluation of body magnesium stores, *J. Lab. Clin. Med.*, **84**:153–162, 1974.

26. Heaton, F. W.: The determination of ionized magnesium in serum and urine, *Clin. Chim. Acta*, **15**:139–144, 1967.

27. Neuman, W. F.: The milieu intérieur of bone: Claude Bernard revisited, *Fed. Proc.*, **28**:1846–1850, 1969.

28. Manery, J. F.: Water and electrolyte metabolism, *Physiol. Rev.*, **34**:334–417, 1952.

29. Courtice, F. C.: Lymph and plasma proteins: Barriers to their movement throughout the extracellular fluid, *Lymphology*, **1**:9–17, 1971.

30. Wiederhielm, C. A.: Dynamics of transcapillary exchange, *J. Gen. Physiol.*, **52**:295–635, 1968.

31. Edelman, I. S., J. Leibman: Anatomy of body water and electrolytes, *Am. J. Med.*, **27**:256–271, 1969.

32. Rasmussen, P.: The concentration of calcium,

inorganic phosphate and protein in the interstitial fluid of rats, *Calcif. Tissue Res.*, **6**:197–293, 1970.

33. Creese, R., J. L. D'Silva, D. M. Shaw: Interfibre fluid from guinea-pig muscle, *J. Physiol. (London)*, **162**:44–52, 1962.

34. Guyton, A. C., A. E. Taylor, R. A. Brace: A synthesis of interstitial fluid regulation and lymph formation, *Fed. Proc.*, **35**:1881–1885, 1976.

35. Schubert, M., D. M. Hamerman: *A Primer of Connective-Tissue Biochemistry*, Lea & Febiger, Philadelphia, 1968.

36. Mathews, M. B.: The interaction of collagen and acid mucopolysaccharides. A model for connective tissue, *Biochem. J.*, **96**:710–716, 1965.

37. McMaster, P. D., R. J. Parsons: The movement of substances and the state of the fluid in the intradermal tissue, *Ann. N.Y. Acad. Sci.*, **52**:992–1003, 1956.

38. Fessler, J. H.: A structural function for mucopolysaccharides in connective tissue, *Biochem. J.*, **76**:125–132, 1960.

39. Gersh, I., H. R. Catchpole: The nature of ground substance of connective tissue, *Perspect. Biol. Med.*, **3**:282–319, 1960.

40. Catchpole, H. R., N. R. Joseph, M. B. Engel: Thermodynamic relations of polyelectrolytes and inorganic ions of connective tissue, *Fed. Proc.*, **25**:1124–1126, 1966.

41. Dunstone, J. R.: Ion-exchange reactions between acid mucopolysaccharides and various cations, *Biochem. J.*, **85**:336–351, 1962.

42. Bowness, J. M.: Present concepts of the role of ground substance in calcification, *Clin. Orthop.*, **59**:233–247, 1968.

43. MacGregor, E. A., J. M. Bowness: Interaction of proteoglycans and chondroitin sulfates with calcium or phosphate ions, *Can. J. Biochem.*, **49**:417–425, 1971.

44. Urist, M. R., D. P. Speer, K. J. Ibsen, B. S. Strates: Calcium binding by chondroitin sulfate, *Calcif. Tissue Res.*, **2**:253–261, 1968.

45. Woodward, C., E. A. Davidson: Structure-function relationships of protein polysaccharide complexes: Specific ion-binding properties, *Proc. Natl. Acad. Sci.*, **60**:201–205, 1968.

46. Crockett, D. J.: The protein levels of oedema fluids, *Lancet*, **1**:1179–1182, 1956.

47. Rose, G. A.: A simple and rapid method for the measurement of plasma ultrafiltrable and ionized calcium, *Clin. Chim. Acta*, **37**:343–349, 1972.

48. Gilligan, D. R., M. C. Volk, M. D. Altschule: The diffusibility of plasma calcium following parathormone administration, *J. Biol. Chem.*, **103**:745–756, 1933.

49. Feldstein, A. M., J. Samachson, H. Spencer: Levels of calcium, phosphorus, alkaline phosphatase and protein in effusion fluid and serum in man, *Am. J. Med.*, **35**:530–535, 1963.

50. Chutkow, J. G.: Magnesium and calcium in the cerebrospinal fluid of the rat, *Proc. Soc. Exp. Biol. Med.*, **128**:555–558, 1968.

51. Herbert, F. K.: The total and diffusible calcium of serum and the calcium of cerebrospinal fluid in human cases of hypocalcemia and hypercalcaemia, *Biochem. J.*, **27**:1978–1991, 1933.

52. Palek, J., M. Thomae, D. Ozog: Red cell calcium content and transmembrane calcium movements in sickle cell anemia, *J. Lab. Clin. Med.*, **89**(6):1365–1374, 1977.

53. Hajdu, S., E. J. Leonard: A calcium transport system for mammalian cells, *Life Sci.*, **17**:1527–1534, 1975.

54. Bozler, E.: Distribution and exchange of calcium in connective tissue and smooth muscle, *Am. J. Physiol.*, **205**:686–692, 1963.

55. Robertson, W. G.: Cellular calcium and calcium transport, in B. E. C. Nordin (ed.), *Calcium, Phosphate and Magnesium Metabolism*, Longman, Inc., New York, 1976.

56. Borle, A. B.: Calcium metabolism at the cellular level, *Fed. Proc.*, **32**:1944–1950, 1973.

57. Simkiss, K.: Calcium translocation by cells, *Endeavour*, **23**:119–123, 1974.

58. Carafoli, E., K. Malmström, E. Sigel, M. Crompton: The regulation of intracellular calcium, *Clin. Endocrinol.*, **5**:49s–59s, 1976.

59. Hamilton, J. W., E. S. Holdsworth: The location of calcium during its transport by the small intestine of the chick, *Anst. J. Exp. Biol. Med. Sci.*, **53**:453–468, 1975.

60. Talmage, R. V., S. H. Doppelt, J. H. Postma, Jr.: Observations on the relationship of parathyroid hormone and calcitonin to plasma and liver phosphate, *Proc. Soc. Exp. Biol. Med.*, **153**:131–137, 1976.

61. Rasmussen, H., P. J. Bordier: *The Physiological

and Cellular Basis of Metabolic Bone Disease, The Williams & Wilkins Company, Baltimore, 1974.

62. Keitt, A. S.: Changes in the content and ^{32}P incorporation of glycolytic intermediates during incubation of normal and hereditary spherocytosis erythrocytes, *Br. J. Haematol.*, **11**:177–187, 1965.

63. Tenenhouse, H. S., C. R. Scriver: Orthophosphate transport in the erythrocyte of normal subjects and of patients with x-linked hypophosphatemia, *J. Clin. Invest.*, **55**:644–654, 1975.

64. Lehninger, A. L.: *Biochemistry*, 2d ed., Worth, New York, 1975.

65. Albright, F., E. C. Reifenstein: *The Parathyroid Glands and Metabolic Bone Disease*, The Williams & Wilkins Company, Baltimore, 1948.

66. Baldwin, D., P. K. Robinson, K. L. Zierler, J. L. Lilienthal: Interrelations of magnesium, potassium, phosphorus, and creatinine in skeletal muscle of man, *J. Clin. Invest.*, **31**:850–858, 1952.

67. Nichols, N.: The effect of glycogen deposition on liver phosphorus, *J. Clin. Invest.*, **34**:1719–1718, 1955.

68. Rose, I. A.: The state of magnesium in cells as estimated from the adenylate kinase equilibrium, *Proc. Natl. Acad. Sci., USA.*, **61**:1079–1086, 1968.

69. Veloso, D., R. W. Guynn, M. Oskarsson, R. L. Veech: The concentrations of free and bound magnesium in rat tissues, *J. Biol. Chem.*, **248**:4811–4819, 1973.

70. Petersen, B., M. Schroll, C. Christiansen, I. Transbøl: Serum and erythrocyte magnesium in normal elderly Danish people: Relationship to blood pressure and serum lipids, *Acta Med. Scand.*, **201**:31–34, 1977.

71. Gilbert, D. L.: Magnesium equilibrium in muscle, *J. Gen. Physiol.*, **43**:1103–1118, 1960.

72. Chutkow, J. G.: Lability of skeletal muscle magnesium in vivo. A study in red and white muscle, *Mayo Clin. Proc.*, **49**:448–453, 1974.

73. Bunn, H. F., B. J. Ransil, S. Chao: The interaction between erythrocyte organic phosphates, magnesium ion, and hemoglobin, *J. Biol. Chem.*, **246**:5273–5279, 1971.

74. Wacker, W. E. C., R. J. Williams: Magnesium/calcium balances and steady states of biological systems, *J. Theor. Biol.*, **20**:65–78, 1968.

75. van Rossum, G. D. V.: Net movements of calcium and magnesium in slices of rat liver, *J. Gen. Physiol.*, **55**:18–32, 1970.

76. Lehninger, A. L.: Mitochondria and the physiology of Ca^{2+}, *Trans. Am. Clin. Climatol. Assoc.*, **83**:83–94, 1973.

77. Lehninger, A. L.: Role of phosphate and other proton-donating anions in respiration-coupled transport of Ca^{2+} by mitochondira. *Proc. Natl. Acad. Sci. USA.*, **71**:1520–1524, 1974.

78. Farber, J. L., S. K. El-Mofty, F. A. X. Schanne, J. J. Aleo, Jr., A. Serroni: Intracellular calcium homeostasis in galactosamine-intoxicated rat liver cells, *Arch. Biochem. Biophys.*, **178**:617–624, 1977.

79. Corredor, D. G., G. Sabeh, L. V. Mendelsohn, R. E. Wasserman, J. H. Sunder, T. S. Danowski: Enhanced postglucose hypophosphatemia during starvation therapy of obesity, *Metabolism*, **18**:754–763, 1969.

80. Schrier, S. L.: Transfer of inorganic phosphate across human erythrocyte membranes, *J. Lab. Clin. Med.*, **75**:422–434, 1970.

81. Uchikawa, T., A. B. Borle, R. J. Midgett: Parathyroid hormone and phosphaturia, *Proceedings XI European Symposium on Calcified Tissues*, Fadl's Forlag, Copenhagen, 1976.

82. Brown, K. D., J. F. Lamb: Na-dependent phosphate transport in cultured cells, *J. Physiol. (London)*, **251**:58P–59P, 1975.

83. Straub, R. W., J. Ferrero, P. Jirounek, G. J. Jones, A. Salamin: Transmembrane transport of inorganic phosphate and its implication in some diseases, in L. Bolis, J. F. Hoffman, A. Leaf (eds.), *Membranes and Diseases*, Raven Press, New York, 1976, pp. 219–227.

84. Heaney, R. P.: Calcium kinetics in plasma: As they apply to the measurements of bone formation and resorption rates, in G. H. Bourne (ed.), *The Biochemistry and Physiology of Bone*, vol. IV, *Calcification and Physiology*, Academic Press, New York, 1976.

85. Levenson, S. M., M. A. Adams, H. Rosen, F. H. L. Taylor: Studies in phosphorus metabolism in man. III. The distribution, exchange and excretion of phosphorus in man using radioactive phosphorus (P^{32}) as a tracer, *J. Clin. Invest.*, **32**:497–509, 1953.

86. Ennor, A. H., H. Rosenberg: An investigation into the turnover rates of organophosphates. 1. Extra-

cellular space and intracellular inorganic phosphate in skeletal muscle, *Biochem. J.*, **56**:302–308, 1954.

87. Lax, L. C., S. Sidlofsky, G. A. Wrenshall: Compartmental contents and simultaneous transfer rates of phosphorus in the rat, *J. Physiol. (London)*, **132**:1–19, 1956.

88. MacIntyre, I., S. Hanna, C. C. Booth, A. E. Read: Intracellular magnesium deficiency in man, *Clin. Sci.*, **20**:297–305, 1961.

89. Silver, L., J. S. Robertson, L. K. Dahl: Magnesium turnover in the human studied with Mg[28], *J. Clin. Invest.*, **39**:420–425, 1962.

90. Avioli, L.V., M. Berman: Mg[28] kinetics in man, *J. Appl. Physiol.*, **21**:1688–1694, 1966.

91. Alfrey, A. C., N. L. Miller: Bone magnesium pools in uremia, *J. Clin. Invest.*, **52**:3019–3027, 1973.

92 Brandt, J. L., W. Glaser, A. Jones: Soft tissue distribution and plasma disappearance of intravenously administered isotopic magnesium with observations on uptake in bone, *Metabolism*, **7**:355–363, 1958.

93. Care, A. D., D. B. Ross, A. A. Wilson: The distribution of exchangeable magnesium within the sheep, *J. Physiol. (London)*, **176**:284–293, 1965.

94. Manery, J. F.: Effects of Ca ions on membranes, *Fed. Proc.*, **25**:1804–1810, 1966.

95. Rodan, G. A.: Cellular functions of calcium, in J. T. Irving, *Calcium and Phosphorus Metabolism*, Academic Press, New York, 1973.

96. Berridge, M. J.: Control of cell division: A unifying hypothesis, *J. Cyclic Nucleotide Res.*, **1**:305–320, 1975.

97. MacLennan, D. H., P. C. Holland: Calcium transport in sarcoplasmic reticulum, *Ann. Review Biophys. Bioeng.*, **4**:377–404, 1975.

98. Aikawa, J. K.: *The Relationship of Magnesium to Disease in Domestic Animals and in Humans*, Charles C Thomas, Publisher, Springfield, Ill., 1971.

99. Walser, M.: Magnesium metabolism. *Ergeb. Physiol.*, **59**:185–296, 1967.

100. Parfitt, A. M., H. Duncan: Metabolic bone disease affecting the spine, in R. Rothman, F. Simeone (eds.), *The Spine*, W. B. Saunders Company, Philadelphia, 1976, pp. 599–720.

101. Doty, S. B., R. A. Robinson, B. Schofield: Morphology of bone and histochemical staining characteristics of bone cells, in R. O. Greep, E. B. Astwood, G. D. Aurbach (eds.), *Handbook of Physiology*, vol. VII, American Physiological Society, Washington, D.C., 1976.

102. Glimcher, M. J.: Composition, structure and organization of bone and other mineralized tissues, and the mechanism of calcification, in R. O. Greep, E. B. Astwood, G. D. Aurbach (eds.), *Handbook of Physiology*, vol. VII, American Physiological Society, Washington, D.C., 1976.

103. Vaughn, J. M.: *The Physiology of Bone*, 2d ed., Oxford University Press, London, 1975.

104. Armstrong, W. D., L. Singer: Composition and constitution of the mineral phase of bone, *Clin. Orth.*, **38**:179–190, 1965.

105. Cox, R. W., R. A. Grant: The structure of the collagen fibrie, *Clin. Orthop.*, **67**:172–187, 1969.

106. Urist, M. R.: Biochemistry of calcification, in G. H. Bourne (ed.), *The Biochemistry and Physiology of Bone*, vol. IV, *Calcification and Physiology*, Academic Press, New York, 1976.

107. Nakao, K., R. E. Bashey: Fine structure of collagen filbrils as revealed by Ruthenium Red, *Exp. Mol. Pathol.*, **17**:6–13, 1972.

108. Shim, S. S., S. Mokkhavera, G. D. McPherson, J. F. Schwengel: Bone and skeletal blood flow in man measured by a radioisotopic method, *Can. J. Surg.*, **14**:38–41, 1971.

109. Brookes, M.: Arteriolar blockade: A method of measuring blood flow rates in the skeleton, *J. Anat.*, **106**:557–563, 1970.

110. Talmage, R. V.: Morphological and physiological considerations in a new concept of calcium transport in bone, *Am. J. Anat.*, **129**:467–476, 1970.

111. Parfitt, A. M.: The actions of parathyroid hormone on bone: Relation to bone remodeling and turnover, calcium homeostasis, and metabolic bone disease. I. Mechanisms of calcium transfer between blood and bone and their cellular basis: Morphologic and kinetic approaches to bone turnover, *Metabolism*, **25**:809–844, 1976.

112. Edelman, I. S., A. H. James, H. Baden, F. D. Moore: Electrolyte composition of bone and the penetration of radiosodium and deuterium oxide into dog and human bone, *J. Clin. Invest.*, **33**:127–131, 1954.

113. Neuman, W. F., B. J. Bareham: Further studies on the nature of fluid compartmentalization in chick

calvaria, *Calcif. Tissue Res.,* **17**:249–255, 1975.

114. Owen, M., J. T. Triffitt, R. A. Melick: Albumin in bone, in *Hard Tissue Growth, Repair and Renumeration, Ciba Foundation Symp.,* **11**:263–293, 1973.

115. Arnold, J. S., H. M. Frost, R. P. Buss: The osteocyte as a bone pump, *Clin. Orthop.,* **78**:47–55, 1971.

116. Pellegrino, E. D., R. M. Biltz: The composition of bone in uremia. Observations on the reservoir function of bone and demonstration of a labile fraction of bone carbonate, *Medicine,* **44**:397–418, 1965.

117. Parfitt, A. M.: The actions of parathyroid hormone on bone: Relation to bone remodelling and turnover, calcium homeostasis, and metabolic bone diseases. II. PTH and bone cells: Bone turnover and plasma calcium regulation, *Metabolism,* **25**:904–955, 1976.

118. Canas, F., A. R. Terepka, W. F. Neuman: Potassium and milieu intérieur of bone, *Am. J. Physiol.,* **217**:117–120, 1969.

119. Parfitt, A. M.: The cellular basis of bone turnover and bone loss. A rebuttal of the osteocytic-resorption-bone flow theory, *Clin. Orthop.,* **127**:236–247, 1977.

120. Krempien, B., G. Geiger, E. Ritz, S. Buttner: Osteocytes in chronic uremia. Differential count of osteocytes in human femoral bone, *Virchows Arch. Abt. A. Path. Anat.,* **360**:1–9, 1973.

121. Raisz, L. G.: Mechanisms of bone resorption, in R. O. Greep, E. B. Astwood, G. D. Aurbach (eds.), *Handbook of Physiology,* American Physiological Society, Washington, D.C., 1976.

122. Firschein, H. E.: Collagen and mineral dynamics in bone, *Clin. Orthop.,* **66**:212–225, 1969.

123. Minkin, C.: Mononuclear phagocytes and bone remodelling. Bone mediated macrophage chemotaxis, Poster presentation, *First Scientific Workshop on Localized Bone Loss,* Washington, D.C., 1977.

124. Holtrop, M. E., G. J. King: The ultrastructure of the osteoclast and its functional implications, *Clin. Orthop.,* **123**:177–196, 1977.

125. LeBlond, C. P., M. Weinstock: A comparative study of dentin and bone formation, in G. D. Bourne (ed.), *The Biochemistry and Physiology of Bone,* vol. IV, *Calcification and Physiology,* Academic Press, New York, 1976.

126. Wergedal, J. E., D. J. Baylink: Electron microprobe measurements of bone mineralization rate in vivo, *Am. J. Physiol.,* **226**:345–352, 1974.

127. Richelle, L. J., C. Onkelinx: Recent advances in the physical biology of bone and other hard tissues, in C. L. Comar, F. Bronner (eds.), *Mineral Metabolism: An Advanced Treatise,* vol. III, Academic Press, New York, 1969.

128. Vogel, J. J., B. D. Boyan-Salyers: Acidic lipids associated with the local mechanism of calcification, *Clin. Orthop.,* **118**:230–241, 1976.

129. Pautard, F. G. E.: A biomolecular survey of calcification, in H. Fleisch, H. J. J. Blackwood, M. Owen (eds.), *Calcified Tissues,* Springer-Verlag OHG, Berlin, 1965, pp. 108–121.

130. Mathews, J. L., J. H. Martin: Intracellular transport of calcium and its relationship to homeostasis and mineralization, *Am. J. Med.,* **50**:589–597, 1971.

131. Anderson, H. C.: Matrix vesicles of cartilage and bone, in G. H. Bourne (ed.), *The Biochemistry and Physiology of Bone,* vol. IV, *Calcification and Physiology,* Academic Press, New York, 1976.

132. Howell, D. S.: Current concepts of calcification, *J. Bone Joint Surg.,* **53**A:250–258, 1971.

133. Cuervo, L. A., J. C. Pita, D. S. Howell: Ultramicroanalysis of pH, P_{CO_2} and carbonic anhydrase activity at calcifying sites in cartilage, *Calcif. Tissue Res.,* **7**:220–231, 1971.

134. Engfeldt, B., A. Hjerpe: Glycosaminoglycans and proteoglycans of human bone tissue at different stages of mineralization, *Acta Pathol. Microbiol. Scand.,* Sect. A, **84**:95–106, 1976.

135. Waddell, W. J.: A molecular mechanism for biological calcification, *Biochem. Biophys. Res. Commum.,* **49**:127–132, 1972.

136. Wuthier, R. E.: The role of phospholipids in biological calcification: Distribution of phospholipase activity in calcifying epiphyseal cartilage, *Clin. Orthop.,* **90**:191–200, 1973.

137. Nichols, G., P. Rogers: Bone cell calcium stores: Their size, location, and kinetics of exchange, *Calcif. Tissue Res.,* **9**:80–94, 1972.

138. Aaron, J. E., F. G. E. Pautard: A cell cycle in bone mineralization, in M. Balls, F. S. Billet (eds.),

The Cell Cycle in Development and Differentiation, Cambridge University Press, London, 1973, pp. 325–330.

139. Felix, R., H. Fleisch: Pyrophosphatase and ATPase of isolated cartilage matrix vesicles, *Calcif. Tissue Res.,* 22:1–7, 1976.

140. Termine, J. D., E. D. Eanes: Calcium phosphate deposition from balanced salt solutions, *Calcif. Tissue Res.,* **15**:81–84, 1974.

141. Marotti, G., A. Favia, Z. A. Zambonia: Quantitative analysis of the rate of secondary bone mineralization, *Calcif. Tissue Res.,* 10:67–81, 1972.

142. Neuman, W. F., B. J. Bareham: Evidence for the presence of secondary calcium phosphate in bone and its stabilization by acid production, *Calcif. Tissue Res.,* **18**:161–172, 1975.

143. Fleisch, H., R. G. G. Russell: Pyrophosphate and polyphosphate, in H. Rasmussen (ed.), *International Encyclopedia of Pharmacology and Therapeutics,* Sec. 51, *Pharmacology of the Endocrine System and Related Drugs,* vol. 1, *Parathyroid Hormone, Thyrocalcitonin and Related Drugs,* Pergamon Press, New York, 1970.

144. Jung, A., S. Bisaz, H. Fleisch: The binding of pyrophosphate and two diphosphonates by hydroxyapatite crystals, *Calcif. Tissue Res.,* **11**:269–280, 1973.

145. Minkin, C., L. Blackman, J. Newbrey, S. Pokress, R. Posek, M. Walling: Effects of parathyroid hormone and calcitonin on adenylate cyclase in murine mononuclear phagocytes, *Biochem. Biophys. Res. Commun.,* **76**:875–881, 1977.

146. Harris, W. H., R. P. Heaney: Skeletal renewal and metabolic bone disease, *N. Engl. J. Med.,* **280**:183–202; 253–259; 303–310, 1969.

147. Frost, H. M.: The origin and nature of transients in human bone remodelling dynamics, in B. Frame, A. M. Parfitt, H. Duncan (eds.), *Clinical Aspects of Metabolic Bone Disease,* Excerpta Medica, Amsterdam, 1973.

148. Galasko, C. S. B.: Skeletal metastases and mammary cancer, *Ann. R. Coll. Surg. Engl.,* **50**:3–28, 1972.

149. Duncan, H., C. Mathews, A. M. Parfitt: Cellular basis of bone erosion in rheumatoid arthritis, First Scientific Workshop on Localized Bone Loss, Washington, D.C., November 1977.

150. Parfitt, A. M.: The actions of parathyroid hormone on bone: Relation to bone remodeling and turnover, calcium homeostasis, and metabolic bone disease. III. PTH and osteoblasts, the relationship between bone turnover and bone loss, and the state of the bones in primary hyperparathyroidism, *Metabolism,* **25**:1033–1069, 1976.

151. Groer, P. G., J. H. Marshall: Mechanism of calcium exchange at bone surfaces, *Calcif. Tissue Res.,* **12**:175–192, 1973.

152. Knop, J., K.-H. Reichstein, R. Montz: A ^{47}Calcium kinetic model with two bone compartments, *Eur. J. Nucl. Med.,* **2**:35–41, 1977.

153. Frost, H. M.: Some aspects of the mechanisms and dynamics of blood:bone interchange, *Henry Ford Hosp. Med. Bull.,* **8**:36–51, 1960.

154. Hattner, R., H. M. Frost: Mean skeletal age: Its calculation and theoretical effects on skeletal tracer physiology and on the physical characteristics of bone, *Henry Ford Hosp. Med. Bull.,* **11**:201–216, 1963.

155. Hausmann, E., D. S. Riggs: The effectiveness of negative feedback in regulating plasma calcium in the dog, *J. Theor. Biol.,* **12**:350–363, 1966.

156. DeFronzo, R. A., M. Goldberg, Z. Agus: Reset osmostat—an overlooked cause of hyponatremia, *Proc. Am. Soc. Nephrol.,* **8**:13, 1975.

157. Parsons, J. A.: Parathyroid physiology and the skeleton, in G. H. Bourne (ed.), *Biochemistry and Physiology of Bone,* vol. IV, Academic Press, New York, 1976.

158. Nordin, B. E. C.: Plasma calcium and plasma magnesium homeostasis, in B. E. C. Nordin (ed.), *Calcium, Phosphate and Magnesium Metabolism,* Longman, Inc. New York, 1976.

159. Robertson, W. G., D. B. Morgan: Effect of pyrophosphate on the exchangeable calcium pool of hydroxyapatite crystals, *Biochim. Biophys. Acta,* **230**:495–503, 1971.

160. Neuman, W. F.: Aerobic glycolysis in bone in the context of membrane compartmentalization. *Calcif. Tissue Res.,* **22**(suppl.): 169–178, 1977.

161. Talmage, R. V., S. A. Grubb: A laboratory model demonstrating osteocyteosteoblast control of plasma calcium concentrations, *Clin. Orthop.,* **122**:299–306, 1977.

162. Scarpace, P. J., W. F. Neuman: The blood:bone

disequilibrium. I. The active accumulation of K^+ into the bone extracellular fluid, *Calcif. Tissue Res.*, **20**:137–149, 1976.

163. Scarpace, P. J., W. F. Neumann: The blood:bone disequilibrium. II. Evidence against the active accumulation of calcium or phosphate into the bone extracellular fluid, *Calcif. Tissue Res.*, **20**:151–158, 1976.

164. Triffitt, J. T., A. R. Terepka, W. F. Neuman: A comparative study of the exchange in vivo of major constituents of bone mineral, *Calcif. Tissue Res.*, **2**:165–176, 1968.

165. Neuman, W. F., A. R. Terepka, F. Canas, J. T. Triffitt: The cycling concept of exchange in bone, *Calcif. Tissue Res.*, **2**:262–270, 1968.

166. Zetterström, R.: Renewal of phosphate in bone minerals. I. Renewal rate of phosphate in relation to the solubility of the bone minerals, *Biochim. Biophys. Acta*, **8**:283–293, 1952.

167. Rogers, H. J. S. M. Weidmann, H. G. Jones: Studies on the skeletal tissues. 3. The rate of exchange of the inorganic phosphate in different bones and parts of bone in various species of mammal, *Biochem. J.*, **54**:37–42, 1953.

168. Engfeldt, B., A. Engstrom, R. Zetterström: Renewal of phosphate in bone minerals. II. Radioautographic studies of the renewal of phosphate in different structures of bone, *Biochim. Biophys. Acta*, **8**:375–380, 1952.

169. Falkenheim, M., E. E. Underwood, H. C. Hodge: Calcium exchange. The mechanism of absorption by bone of Ca^{45}, *J. Biol. Chem.*, **188**:805–817, 1951.

170. Copp, D. H.: Calcium and phosphorus metabolism, *Am J. Med.*, **22**:275–285, 1957.

171. Taylor, T. G.: The magnesium of bone mineral, *J. Agric. Sci.*, **52**:207–216, 1959.

172. Neuman, W. F., B. J. Mulryan: Synthetic hydroxyapatite crystals. IV. Magnesium incorporation, *Calcif. Tissue Res.*, **7**:133–138, 1971.

173. Alfrey, A. C., N. L. Miller, R. Trow: Effect of age and magnesium depletion on bone magnesium pools in rats, *J. Clin. Invest.*, **54**:1074–1081, 1974.

174. Breibart, S., J. S. Lee, A. McCoord, G. B. Forbes: Relation of age to radiomagnesium exchange in bone, *Proc. Soc. Exp. Biol. Med.*, **105**:361–363, 1960.

175. Glaser, W., W. D. Gibbs: Localization of radio-

magnesium in puppies: Radioautographic study of heart and bone, *Am. J. Physiol.*, **202**:584–588, 1962.

176. Smith, R. H.: Calcium and magnesium metabolism in calves. 4. Bone composition in magnesium deficiency and the control of plasma magnesium, *Biochem. J.*, **71**:609–614, 1959.

177. Blaxter, K. L.: The magnesium content of bone in hypomagnesaemic disorders of livestock, in G. E. W. Wolstenholme, C. M. O'Connor (eds.), *Bone Structure and Metabolism*, Little, Brown and Company, Boston, 1956, pp. 117–134.

178. Hartsuck, J. M., J. E. Johnson, F. D. Moore: Potassium in bone: Evidence for a nonexchangeable fraction, *Metabolism*, **18**:33–37, 1969.

179. Neuman, W. F., B. J. Mulryan: On the nature of exchangeable sodium in bone, *Calcif. Tissue Res.*, **3**:261–265, 1969.

180. Triffitt, J. T., W. F. Neuman: The uptake of sodium-22 by bone and certain soft tissues, *Calcif. Tissue Res.*, **6**:70–76, 1970.

181. Bergstrom, W. H., W. M. Wallace: Bone as a sodium and potassium reservoir, *J. Clin. Invest.*, **33**:867–873, 1954.

182. Nichols, G., N. Nichols: The role of bone in sodium metabolism, *Metabolism*, **5**:438–446, 1956.

183. Nichols, G., N. Nichols: Effect of parathyroidectomy on content and availability of skeletal sodium in the rat, *Am. J. Physiol.*, **198**:749–753, 1960.

184. Witmer, G., P. Cuisinier-Gleizes, F. Debove, H. Mathieu: Ostéoporose provoquée par la carence en sodium chez le rat en croissance, *Calcif. Tissue Res.*, **7**:114–132, 1971.

185. Rudman, D., W. J. Millikan, T. J. Richardson, T. J. Bixler, II, W. J. Stackhouse, W. C. McGarrity: Elemental balances during intravenous hyperalimentation of underweight adult subjects, *J. Clin. Invest.*, **55**:94–104, 1975.

186. Burnell, J. M.: Changes in bone sodium and carbonate in metabolic acidosis and alkalosis in the dog, *J. Clin. Invest.*, **50**:327–331, 1971.

187. Schaefer, K. E., G. Nichols, Jr., C. R. Carey: Calcium phosphorus metabolism in man during acclimatisation to carbon dioxide, *J. Appl. Physiol.*, **18**:1079–1084, 1963.

188. Kaye, M. A., A. J. Frueh, M. Silverman: A study of vertebral bone powder from patients with

chronic renal failure, *J. Clin. Invest.*, **49**:442–453, 1970.

189. Hirschman, A., A. E. Sobel: Composition of the mineral deposited during in vitro calcification in relation to the fluid phase, *Arch. Biochem. Biophys.*, **110**:237–243, 1965.

190. Lemann, J., J. R. Litzow, E. J. Lennon: The effects of chronic acid loads in normal man: Further evidence for the participation of bone mineral in the defense against chronic metabolic acidosis, *J. Clin. Invest.*, **45**:1608–1614, 1966.

191. Lemann, J., E. J. Lennon: Role of diet, gastrointestinal tract and bone in acid-base homeostasis, *Kidney Int.*, **1**:275–279, 1972.

192. Kildeberg, P., K. Engle, R. W. Winters: Balance of net acid in growing infants, *Acta Paediatr. Scand.*, **58**:321–329, 1969.

193. Barzel, U. S., J. Jowsey: The effects of chronic acid and alkali administration on bone turnover in adult rats, *Clin. Sci.*, **36**:517–524, 1969.

194. Barzel, U. S.: The effect of excessive acid feeding on bone, *Calcif. Tissue Res.*, **4**:94–100, 1969.

195. Hebert, L. A., J. Lemann, J. R. Petersen, E. J. Lennon: Studies of the mechanism by which phosphate infusion lowers serum calcium concentration, *J. Clin. Invest.*, **45**:1886–1894, 1966.

196. Reiss, E., J. M. Canterbury, M. A. Bercovitz, E. L. Kaplan: The role of phosphate in the secretion of parathyroid hormone in man, *J. Clin. Invest.*, **49**:2146–2149, 1970.

197. Eisenberg, E.: Effect of intravenous phosphate on serum strontium and calcium, *N. Engl. J. Med.*, **282**:889–892, 1970.

198. Gersh, I.: The fate of colloidal calcium phosphate in the dog, *Am. J. Physiol.*, **121**:589–594, 1938.

199. Chaudhuri, T. K., T. K. Chaudhuri, R. E. Peterson, J. H. Christie: Effect of phosphate on serum strontium (35499), *Proc. Soc. Exp. Biol. Med.*, **137**:1–4, 1971.

200. Stamp, T. C. B.: The hypocalcaemic effect of intravenous phosphate administration, *Clin. Sci.*, **40**:55–65, 1971.

201. Walton, R. J., R. G. G. Russell, R. Smith, J. A. Kanis, J. S. Woodhead: Effects of a diphosphonate (disodium ethane-1-hydroxy-1, 1 diphosphonate; EHDP) on phosphate transport in man, in L. Avioli, et al. (eds.), Phosphate metabolism, kidney and bone, *Proceedings of the First International Workshop on Phosphate*, Armour Montague, Paris, 1976.

202. Raisz, L. G., J. W. Dietrich, D. Marina: Effects of phosphate on bone formation and resorption in tissue culture, in L. Avioli, et al. (eds.), Phosphate metabolism, kidney and bone, *Proceedings of the First International Workshop on Phosphate*, Armour Montague, Paris, 1976.

203. Parfitt, A. M.: The actions of parathyroid hormone on bone: Relation to bone remodelling and turnover, calcium homeostasis, and metabolic bone disease. IV. The state of the bones in uremic hyperparathyroidism—the mechanisms of skeletal resistance to PTH in renal failure and pseudohypoparathyroidism and the role of PTH in osteoporosis, osteopetrosis, and osteofluorosis, *Metabolism*, **25**:1157–1188, 1976.

204. Haddad, J. G., L. V. Avioli: Comparative effects of phosphate and thyrocalcitonin on skeletal turnover, *Endocrinology*, **87**:1245–1250, 1970.

205. Feinblatt, J., L. F. Belanger, H. Rasmussen: Effect of phosphate infusion on bone metabolism and parathyroid hormone action, *Am. J. Physiol.*, **218**:1624–1631, 1970.

206. Rasmussen, H., J. Feinblatt, N. Nagata, M. Pechet: Effect of ions upon bone cell function, *Fed. Proc.*, **29**:1190–1199, 1970.

207. Cuisinier-Gleizes, P., M. Thomasset, F. Sainteny-Debove, H. Mathieu: Phosphorus deficiency, parathyroid hormone and bone resorption in the growing rat, *Calcif. Tissue Res.*, **20**:235–249, 1976.

208. Bordier, M. J., N. N. Berlois, M. L. Queille, M. F. Kahn, S. DeSize: Phosphate metabolism, hyperparathyroidism and skeletal remodelling in idiopathic hypercalcemia, in L. Avioli, et al. (ed.), Phosphate metabolism, kidney, and bone, *Proceedings of the First International Workshop on Phosphate*, Armour Montague, Paris, 1976.

209. Raisz, L. G., I. Neimann: Effect of phosphate, calcium and magnesium on bone resorption and hormonal responses in tissue culture, *Endocrinology*, **85**:446–452, 1969.

210. McManus, J. M., F. W. Heaton: The influence of magnesium on calcium release from bone in vitro, *Biochim. Biophys. Acta*, **215**:360–367, 1970.

211. McManus, J. M., F. W. Heaton: The effect of

magnesium deficiency on calcium homeostasis in the rat, *Clin. Sci.*, **36**:297–306, 1969.

212. Reddy, C. R., J. W. Coburn, D. L. Hartenbower, R. M. Friedler, A. S. Brickman, S. G., Massry, J. Jowsey: Studies on mechanisms of hypocalcemia of magnesium depletion, *J. Clin. Invest.*, **52**:3000–3010, 1973.

213. Howard, J. E., T. R. Hopkins, T. B. Connor: On certain physiologic responses to intravenous injection of calcium salts into normal, hyperparathyroid and hypoparathyroid persons, *J. Clin. Endocrinol.*, **13**:1–19, 1953.

214. Baylor, C. H., H. E. Van Alstine, E. H. Keutmann, S. H. Bassett: The fate of intravenously administered calcium. Effects on urinary calcium and phosphorus, fecal calcium and calcium-phosphorus balance, *J. Clin. Invest.*, **29**:1167–1176, 1950.

215. Parfitt, A. M., B. Higgins, J. R. Nassim, J. Collins, A. Hilb: Metabolic studies in hypercalciuria, *Clin. Sci.*, **27**:463–482, 1964.

216. Fraser, D., D. W. Geiger, J. D. Munn, P. E. Slater, R. John, E. Liv: Calcification studies in clinical vitamin D deficiency and in hypophosphatemic vitamin D refractory rickets. The induction of calcium deposition in rachitic cartilage without the administration of vitamin D, *Am. J. Dis. Child.*, **96**:460–463, 1958.

217. Bordier, P. H., S. Tun-Chot, J. Martin, M.-L. Queille, D. J. Hioco: Mineralisation en tissu ostéocide chez l'ostéomalacique induite par surcharge phosphorée ou par la vitamine D_3, in D. J. Hioco (ed.), *Phosphate et Metabolisme Phosphocalcique*, L'Expansion Scientifique Française, Paris, 1971.

218. Lever, J. V., C. T. Paterson, D. G. Morgan: Calcium infusion test in osteomalacia: An appraisal, *Br. Med. J.*, **3**:281–282, 1967.

219. Liu, S. H., R. R. Hannon, H. I. Chu, K. L. Chen, S. K. Chou, S. H. Wang: Calcium and phosphorus metabolism in osteomalacia II. Further studies on the response to vitamin D of patients with osteomalacia, *Chim. Med. J. Engl.*, **49**:1–21, 1935.

220. Jackson, W. P. V., L. P. Dancaster: Hypoparathyroidism with bone disease: Use of calciferol and milk in postoperative management, *Metabolism*, **11**:123–135, 1962.

221. Nordin, B. E. C.: Clinical significance and pathogenesis of osteoporosis, *Br. Med. J.*, **1**:571–576, 1971.

222. Malm, O. J.: Calcium requirement and adaptation in adult men, *Scand. J. Clin. Lab. Invest.*, **10**(suppl. 36):1–289, 1958.

223. Parfitt, A. M.: The study of parathyroid function in man by EDTA infusion, *J. Clin. Endocrinol.*, **29**:569–580, 1969.

224. Phang, J. M., M. Berman, G. A. Finerman, R. M. Neer, L. E. Rosenberg, T. J. Han: Dietary perturbation of calcium metabolism in normal man: Compartmental analysis, *J. Clin. Invest.*, **48**:67–77, 1969.

225. Macy, I. G.: *Nutrition and Chemical Growth in Childhood*, Charles C Thomas, Publishers, Springfield, Ill., 1951.

226. Irwin, M. I.: A conspectus of research on calcium requirements of man, *J. Nutr.*, **103**:1019–1095, 1973.

227. Nordin, B. E. C.: Nutritional considerations, in B. E. C. Nordin (ed.), *Calcium, Phosphate and Magnesium Metabolism*, Longman, Inc., New York, 1976.

228. Malm, O. J.: Adaptation to alterations in calcium intake, in R. H. Wasserman (ed.), *The Transfer of Calcium and Strontium across Biological Membranes*, Academic Press, New York and London, 1963.

229. Bronner, F.: Dyamics and function of calcium, in C. L. Comar, F. Bronner (eds.), *Mineral Metabolism: An Advanced Treatise*, Academic Press, New York, 1964, pp. 341–444.

230. Irving, J. T.: *Calcium and Phosphorus Metabolism*, Academic Press, New York, 1973.

231. Wilkinson, R.: Absorption of calcium, phosphorus and magnesium, in B. E. C. Nordin (ed.), *Calcium, Phosphate and Magnesium Metabolism*, Longman, Inc., New York, 1976.

232. Wills, M. R.: Intestinal absorption of calcium, *Lancet*, **1**:820–822, 1973.

233. Harrison, H. E., H. C. Harrison: Calcium, *Biomembranes*, **4**:793–846, 1976.

234. Coburn, J. W., D. L. Hartenbower, A. J. Brickman, S. G. Massry, J. D. Koppel: Intestinal absorption of calcium magnesium and phosphorus in chronic renal insufficiency, in D. J. David (ed.),

Calcium Metabolism and Bone in Renal Failure and Nephrolithiasis, John Wiley & Sons, Inc., New York, 1977.

235. Sunderman, F. W., F. Bremer: *Normal Values in Clinical Medicine,* W. B. Saunders Company, Philadelphia, 1949.

236. Davenport, H. W.: *Physiology of the Digestive Tract,* Year Book Medical Publishers, Chicago, 1966.

237. Code, C. F. (ed.): *Handbook of Physiology,* sec. G., *Alimentary Canal,* vol. II. American Physiological Society, Washington, D. C., 1967.

238. Altman, P. L., D. S. Dittmer: *Blood and Other Body Fluids,* 3d ed., Fed. Am. Soc. Exp. Biol., Bethesda, Md., 1971.

239. Birge, S. J., W. A. Peck, M. Berman, G. D. Whedon: Study of calcium absorption in man, *J. Clin. Invest.,* **48:**1705–1713, 1969.

240. Wensel, R. H., C. Rich, A. C. Brown, W. Volwiler: Absorption of calcium measured by intubation and perfusion of the intact human small intestine, *J. Clin. Invest.,* **48:**1768–1775, 1969.

241. Heaney, R. P., T. G. Skillman: Secretion and excretion of calcium by the human gastrointestinal tract, *J. Lab. Clin. Med.,* **64:**29–41, 1964.

242. Briscoe, A. M., C. Ragan: Bile and endogenous fecal calcium in man, *Am. J. Clin. Nutr.,* **16:**281–286, 1965.

243. Kales, A. N., J. M. Phang: Effect of divided calcium intake on calcium metabolism, *J. Clin. Endocrinol.,* **32:**83–87, 1971.

244. Ireland, P., J. S. Fordtran: Effect of dietary calcium and age on jejunal calcium absorption in humans studied by intestinal perfusion, *J. Clin. Invest.,* **52:**2672–2681, 1973.

245. Spencer, H., I. Lewin, J. Fowler, J. Samachson: Influence of dietary calcium intake on Ca[47] absorption in man, *Am. J. Med.,* **46:**197–205, 1969.

246. Epstein, S., W. Van Mieghem, J. Sage, W. P. U. Jackson: Effect of single large doses of oral calcium levels in the young and the elderly, *Metabolism,* **22:**1163–1173, 1973.

247. Soergel, K. H., K. H. Mueller, R. F. Gustke, J. E. Geenen: Jejunal calcium transport in health and metabolic bone disease: Effect of vitamin D, *Gastroenterology,* **67:**28–34, 1974.

248. Caniggia, A., C. Gennari, M. Bencini, V. Polaz-zouli: Intestinal absorption of radiophosphate in osteomalacia before and after vitamin D treatment, *Calcif. Tissue Res.,* **2:**299–300, 1968.

249. Condon, J. R., J. R. Nassim, A. Rutter: Defective intestinal phosphate absorption in familial and non-familial hypophosphataemia, *Br. Med. J.,* **3:**138–141, 1970.

250. Graham, L. A., J. J. Caesar, A. S. V. Burgen: Gastrointestinal absorption and excretion of Mg[28] in man, *Metabolism,* **9:**646–659, 1960.

251. Trier, J. S.: Functional morphology of the mucosa of the small intestine, in M. D. Armstrong, A. S. Nunn (eds.), *Intestinal Transport of Electrolytes, Aminosugars and Sugars,* Charles C Thomas, Publishers, Springfield, Ill., 1971.

252. Wasserman, R. H.: Calcium transport by the intestine: A model and comment on vitamin D action, *Calcif. Tissue Res.,* **2:**301–313, 1968.

253. Dietschy, J. M., V. L. Sallee, F. A. Wilson: Unstirred water layers and absorption across the intestinal mucosa, *Gastroenterology,* **61:**932–934, 1971.

254. Fordtran, J. S., T. W. Locklear: Ionic constituents and osmolality of gastric and small-intestinal fluids after eating, *Am. J. Dig. Dis.,* **11:**503–520, 1966.

255. Karr, W. G., W. O. Abbott: Intubation studies of the human small intestine. IV. Chemical characteristics of the intestinal contents in the fasting state and as influenced by the administration of acids, of alkalies and of water, *J. Clin. Invest.,* **14:**893–900, 1935.

256. Hurwitz, S., A. Bar: Activity, concentration, and lumen-blood electrochemical potential difference of calcium in the intestine of the laying hen, *J. Nutr.,* **95:**647–654, 1968.

257. Hurwitz, S., A. Bar: Calcium and phosphorus interrelationships in the intestine of the fowl, *J. Nutr.,* **101:**677–686, 1971.

258. Wrong, O., A. Metcalfe-Gibson, R. B. I. Morrison, S. T. Ng, A. V. Howard: In vivo dialysis of faeces as a method of stool analysis. I. Technique and results in normal subjects, *Clin. Sci.,* **28:**357–375, 1965.

259. Metcalfe-Gibson, A., T. S. Ing, J. J. Kuiper, P. Richards, E. E. Ward, O. M. Wrong: In vivo dialysis of faeces as a method of stool anaylsis. II.

The influence of diet, *Clin. Sci.*, **33**:89–100, 1967.

260. Cramer, C. F.: Sites of calcium absorption and the calcium concentration of gut contents in the dog, *Can. J. Physiol. Pharmacol.*, **43**:75–79, 1965.

261. Morgan, D. B.: Calcium and phosphorus transport across the intestine, in R. M. Girdwood, A. W. Smith (eds.), *Malabsorption,* The Williams & Wilkins Company, Baltimore, 1969.

262. Branna, P. G., P. Vergne-Marini, C. Y. C. Pak, A. R. Hull, J. S. Fordtran: Magnesium absorption in the human small intestine, *J. Clin. Invest.*, **57**:1412–1418, 1976.

263. Rao, K. J., M. Miller, A. M. Moses: Hypocalcemic tetany: Result of high-phosphate enema, *N.Y. State J. Med.*, **76**(6):968–969, 1976.

264. Fawcett, Lt. D. W., J. P. Gens: Magnesium poisoning following an enema of epsom salt solution, *JAMA*, **123**:1028–1029, 1943.

265. Juan, D., P. Liptak, T. K. Gray: Absorption of inorganic phosphate in the human jejunum and its inhibition by salmon calcitonin, *J. Clin. Endocrinol. Metab.*, **43**:517–522, 1976.

266. Gray, T. K., J. Walton, R. Lovell, M. E. Williams, D. Dove, R. Shapiro: The absorption of inorganic phosphate in the human small intestine, *Abstracts, Sixth Parathyroid Conference,* Vancouver, 1977.

267. Bergeim, O.: Intestinal chemistry. VII. The absorption of calcium and phosphorus in the small and large intestine, *J. Biol. Chem.*, **35**:51–58, 1926.

268. Schryver, M. F., H. F. Mintz, P. H. Craig: Phosphorus metabolism in ponies fed varying levels of phosphorus, *J. Nutr.*, **101**:1257–1264, 1971.

269. Dempsey, E. F., E. L. Carroll, F. Albright, P. H. Henneman: A study of factors determining fecal electrolyte excretion, *Metabolism*, **7**:108–118, 1950.

270. Schedl, H. P., G. W. Osbaldiston, I. H. Mills: Absorption, secretion and precipitation of calcium in the small intestine of the dog, *Am. J. Physiol.*, **214**:814–819, 1968.

271. Wasserman, R. H., A. N. Taylor: Some aspects of the intestinal absorption of calcium with special reference to vitamin D, in C. L. Comar, F. Bronner (eds.), *Mineral Metabolism. An Advanced Treatise,* Academic Press, New York and London, 1969, pp. 320–403.

272. Helbock, H. J., J. G. Forte, P. Saltman: The mechanism of calcium transport by rat intestine, *Biochim. Biophys. Acta*, **126**:81–93, 1966.

273. Heaney, R. P., P. D. Saville, R. R. Recker: Calcium absorption as a function of calcium intake, *J. Lab. Clin. Med.*, **85**:881–890, 1975.

274. Sampson, H. W., J. L. Matthews, J. H. Martin, A. S. Kunin: An electron microscopic localization of calcium in the small intestine of normal, rachitic, and vitamin-D–treated rats, *Calcif. Tissue Res.*, **5**:305–316, 1970.

275. Warner, R. R., J. R. Coleman: Electron probe anaylsis of calcium transport by small intestine, *J. Cell. Biol.*, **64**:54–74, 1975.

276. Younoszai, M. K., E. Urban, H. P. Schedl: Vitamin D and intestinal calcium fluxes in vivo in the rat, *Am. J. Physiol.*, **2**:287–292, 1973.

277. Birge, S. J., H. R. Gilbert, L. V. Avioli: Intestinal calcium transport: The role of sodium, *Science*, **176**:168–170, 1972.

278. Russell, R. G. G., A. Monod, J. P. Bonjour, H. Fleisch: Relation between alkaline phosphatase and Ca^{2+}-ATPase in calcium transport, *Nature (New Biol.)*, **240**:126–127, 1972.

279. Holdsworth, E. S.: The effect of vitamin D on enzyme activities in the mucosal cells of the chick small intestine, *J. Membrane Biol.*, **3**:43–53, 1970.

280. Birge, S. J., H. R. Gilbert: Identification of an intestinal sodium and calcium-dependent phosphatase stimulated by parathyroid hormone, *J. Clin. Invest.*, **54**:710–717, 1974.

281. Cuisinier-Gleizes, P., H. Mathieu: Effect of low sodium diet on the intestinal absorption of calcium in rats, *Eur. J. Clin. Biol. Res.*, **26**:273–277, 1971.

282. Martin, D. L., H. F. DeLuca: Influence of sodium on calcium transport by the rat small intestine, *Am. J. Physiol.*, **216**:1351–1359, 1969.

283. Chen, T. C., L. Castillo, M. Korychka-Dahl, H. F. DeLuca: Role of vitamin D metabolites in phosphate transport of rat intestine, *J. Nutr.*, **104**:1056–1060, 1974.

284. Kinne, R., W. Berner, N. Hoffmann, H. Myrer: Phosphate transport by isolated renal and intestinal plasma membranes, in S. G. Massry, E. Ritz (eds.), *Phosphate Metabolism,* Plenum Press, New York, 1977.

285. Sampson, H. W., J. L. Matthews: Electron microscope autoradiographic investigation of ^{32}P in

the intestinal epithelium of rachitic, normal and vitamin-D–treated rats, *Calcif. Tissue Res.*, **10**:58–66, 1972.

286. Avioli, L. V., S. J. Birge: Controversies regarding intestinal phosphate transport and absorption, in S. G. Massry, E. Ritz (eds.), *Phosphate Metabolism*, Plenum Press, New York, 1977.

287. Taylor, A. N.: In vitro phosphate transport in chick ileum: Effect of cholecalciferol, calcium, sodium and metabolic inhibitors, *J. Nutr.*, **104**:489–494, 1974.

288. Aldor, T. A. M., E. W. Moore: Magnesium absorption by everted sacs of rat intestine and colon, *Gastroenterology*, **59**(5):745–753, 1975.

289. Coburn, J. W., A. S. Brickman, D. L. Hartenbower, A. W. Norman: Effect of 1,25-(OH)$_2$ and 1 α-OH Vitamin D$_3$ on magnesium absorption in man, *Proceedings of the Second International Symposium on Magnesium*. In press.

290. Heaton, F. W., F. M. Parsons: The metabolic effect of high magnesium intake, *Clin. Sci.*, **21**:273–284, 1961.

291. Briscoe, A. M., C. Ragan: Effect of magnesium on calcium metabolism in man, *Am. J. Clin. Nutr.*, **19**:296–306, 1966.

292. Robertson, W. G.: Urinary excretion, in B. E. C. Nordin (ed.), *Calcium, Phosphate and Magnesium Metabolism*, Longman, Inc., New York, 1976.

293. Sullivan, L. P.: *Physiology of the Kidney*, Lea & Febiger, Philadelphia, 1974.

294. Mudge, G. H., W. O. Berndt, H. Valtin: Tubular transport of urea, glucose, phosphate, uric acid, sulfate, and thiosulfate, in J. Orloff, R. Berliner (eds.), *Handbook of Physiology, Renal Physiology*, 1972, pp. 587–619.

295. Oliver, J., M. MacDowell: The structural and functional aspects of the handling of glucose by the nephrons and the kidney and their correlation by means of structural-functional equivalents, *J. Clin. Invest.*, **40**:1093–1112, 1961.

296. Burgen, A. S. V.: A theoretical treatment of glucose reabsorption in the kidney, *Can. J. Biochem.*, **34**:466–474, 1956.

297. Koushanpour, E.: Tubular reabsorption and secretion: Classification based on overall clearance measurements, in *Renal Physiology, Principles and Functions*, W. B. Saunders Company, Philadelphia, 1976.

298. Kwong, T.-F., C. M. Bennett: Relationship between glomerular filtration rate and maximum tubular reabsorptive rate of glucose, *Kidney Int.*, **5**:23–29, 1974.

299. Harris, C. A., P. G. Baer, E. Chirito, J. H. Dirks: Composition of mammalian glomerular filtrate, *Am. J. Physiol.*, **327**(4):972–976, 1974.

300. Bijvoet, O. L. M.: Kidney function in calcium and phosphate metabolism, in L. V. Avioli, S. M. Krane (eds.), *Metabolic Bone Disease*, vol. 1, Academic Press, New York, 1977.

301. Parfitt, A. M., B. Frame: Phosphate loading and depletion in vitamin D–treated hypoparathyroidism, in L. V. Avioli, et al. (eds.), *Phosphate Metabolism, Kidney and Bone*, Armour Montague, Paris, 1976.

302. Foulks, J. G.: Homeostatic adjustment in the renal tubular transport of inorganic phosphate in the dog, *Can. J. Biochem. Physiol.*, **33**:638–650, 1955.

303. Tröhler, U., J.-P. Bonjour, H. Fleisch: Inorganic phosphate homeostasis—renal adaptation to the dietary intake in intact and thyroparathyroidectomized rats, *J. Clin. Invest.*, **57**:264–273, 1976.

304. Mills, J. M.: Circadian rhythms, *Physiol. Rev.*, **46**:143–153, 1966.

305. Parfitt, A. M.: The effect of cellulose phosphate on plasma and urinary magnesium at different levels of parathyroid function in man, *Clin. Sci. Mol. Med.*, **51**:161–168, 1976.

306. Parfitt, A. M.: A Tm/GFR model for the renal handling of magnesium. Relationship to renal conservation of magnesium and effect of parathyroid hormone. *Proceedings of the Second International Symposium on Magnesium*. In press.

307. Massry, S. G., J. W. Cobrun: The hormonal and non-hormonal control of renal excretion of calcium and magnesium, *Nephron*, **10**:66–112, 1973.

308. Peacock, M., W. G. Robertson, B. E. C. Nordin: Relation between serum and urinary calcium with particular reference to parathyroid activity, *Lancet*, **1**:384–386, 1969.

309. Shaw, W. H.: A study of the renal excretion of calcium by the production of a constant level of hypercalcemia in normal and abnormal human subjects, *Can. J. Physiol.*, **41**:469–478, 1971.

310. Birkenhäger, W. H., H. B. A. Hellendoorn, J. Gerbrandy: Effects of intravenous injections of

calcium laevulinate on calcium and phosphate metabolism, *Clin. Sci.,* **18:**45–53, 1959.

311. Howard, P. J., W. S. Wilde, R. L. Malvin: Localization of renal calcium transport; effect of calcium loads and of gluconate anion on water, sodium and potassium, *Am. J. Physiol.,* **197:**337–341, 1959.

312. Copp, D. H., G. D. McPherson, H. W. McIntosh: Renal excretion of calcium in man; estimation of Tm-Ca, *Metabolism,* **9:**680–685, 1960.

313. Mioni, G., A. D'Angelo, E. Ossi, E. Bertaglia, G. Marcon, G. Maschio: The renal handling of calcium in normal subjects and in renal disease, *Eur. J. Clin. Biol. Res.,* **16:**881–887, 1971.

314. Marshall, D. H.: Calcium and phosphate kinetics, in B. E. C. Nordin (ed.), *Calcium, Phosphate and Magnesium Metabolism,* Longman, Inc., New York, 1976.

315. MacFadyen, J., B. E. C. Nordin, D. A. Smith, D. J. Wayne, S. L. Rae: Effect of variation in dietary calcium on plasma concentration and urinary excretion of calcium, *Br. Med. J.,* **1:**161–164, 1965.

316. Ede, M. C. M., M. H. Faulkner, B. E. Tredre: An intrinsic rhythm of urinary calcium excretion and the specific effect of bedrest on the excretory pattern, *Clin. Sci.,* **42:**433–445, 1972.

317. Jamison, R. L.: Intrarenal heterogeneity: The case for two functionally dissimilar populations of nephrons in the mammalian kidney, *Am. J. Med.,* **54:**281–289, 1973.

318. Burg, M. B.: The renal handling of sodium chloride, in B. M. Brenner, F. C. Rector (eds.), *The Kidney,* W. B. Saunders Company, Philadelphia, 1976.

319. Kinne, R. K. H.: Polarity of the renal proximal tubular cell; function and enzyme pattern of the isolated plasma membranes, *Med. Clin. North Am.,* **59:**615–625, 1975.

320. Scriver, C. R., R. W. Chesney, R. R. McInnes: Genetic aspects of renal tubular transport: Diversity and topology of carriers, *Kidney Int.,* **9:**149–171, 1976.

321. Boulpaep, E. L., H. Sackin: Role of the paracellular pathway in isotonic fluid movement across the renal tubule, *Yale J. Biol. Med.,* **50:**115–131, 1977.

322. Stein, J. H., H. J. Reinerk: The role of the collecting duct in the regulation of excretion of so-dium and other electrolytes, *Kidney Int.,* **6:**1–9, 1974.

323. Knox, F. G., E. G. Schneider, L. R. Willis, J. W. Strandhoy, C. E. Ott: Site and control of phosphate reabsorption by the kidney, *Kidney Int.,* **3:**347–353, 1973.

324. Rouffignac, B. C., N. Roinel, G. Rumrich, K. J. Ullrich: Renal phosphate transport; inhomogeneity of local proximal transport rates and sodium dependence, *Pfluegers Arch.,* **356:**287–297, 1975.

325. Goldberg, M., Z. S. Agus, S. Goldfarb: The renal handling of phosphate, calcium and magnesium, in B. M. Brenner, F. C. Rector (eds.), *The Kidney,* W. B. Saunders Company, Philadelphia, 1976.

326. Quamme, G. A., C. A. Harris, J. H. Dirks: Tubular reabsorption of phosphate during acute phosphate infusion, in L. V. Avioli, et al. (eds), *Phosphate Metabolism, Kidney and Bone,* Armour Montague, Paris, 1976.

327. Amiel, C., H. Kuntziger, G. Richet: Micropuncture study of handling of phosphate by proximal and distal nephron in normal and parathyroidectomized rat: Evidence for distal reabsorption, *Pfluegers Arch.,* **317:**93–109, 1970.

328. Wen, S. -F.: Micropuncture studies of phosphate transport in the proximal tubule of the dog: The relationship to sodium reabsorption, *J. Clin. Invest.,* **53:**143–153, 1974.

329. Kuntziger, H., C. Amiel, C. Gaudebout: Phosphate handling by the rat nephron during saline diuresis, *Kidney Int.,* **2:**318–323, 1972.

330. Murayama, Y., F. Morel, C. Le Grimellec: Phosphate, calcium and magnesium transfers in proximal tubules and loops of Henle, as measured by single nephron microperfusion experiments in the rat, *Pfluegers Arch.,* **333:**1–16, 1972.

331. Greger, R., F. Lang, G. Marchand, F. G. Knox: Site of renal phosphate reabsorption—micropuncture and microinfusion study, *Pfluegers Arch.,* **369:**111–118, 1977.

332. Poujeol, P., D. Chabardes, N. Roinel, C. De Rouffignac: Influence of extracellular fluid volume expansion on magnesium, calcium and phosphate handling along the rat nephron, *Pfluegers Arch.,* **365:**203–211, 1976.

333. Steele, T. H.: Increased urinary phosphate excretion following volume expansion in normal man, *Metabolism,* **19:**129–139, 1970.

334. Schneider, E. G., R. S. Godlsmith, C. D. Arnaud, F. G. Knox: Role of parathyroid hormone in the phosphaturia of extracellular fluid volume expansion, *Kidney Int.*, **7**:317–324, 1975.

335. Baumann, K., Y. -L. Chan, F. Bode, F. Papvassilious: Effect of parathyroid hormone and cyclic adenosine 3′, 5′-monophosphate on isotonic fluid reabsorption: Polarity of proximal tubular cells, *Kidney Int.*, **11**:77–85, 1977.

336. Bank, N., H. S. Aynedjian, S. W. Weinstein: A microperfusion study of phosphate reabsorption in the rat proximal tubule, *J. Clin. Invest.*, **54**:1040–1048, 1974.

337. Eisenberg, E.: Effects of serum calcium level and parathyroid extracts on phosphate and calcium excretion in hypoparathyroid patients, *J. Clin. Invest.*, **44**:942–946, 1965.

338. Davies, M., C. M. Taylor, L. F. Hill, S. W. Stanbury: 1,25 Dihydroxy cholecalciferol in hypoparathyroidism, *Lancet*, **1**:55–59, 1977.

339. Scriver, C. R., T. E. Stacey, M. S. Tenenhouse, W. A. MacDonald: Transepithelial transport of phosphate anion in kidney; potential mechanism for hypophosphatemia, in S. G. Massry, E. Ritz (eds.), *Phosphate Metabolism*, Plenum Press, New York, 1977.

340. Cuche, J. L., C. E. Ott, G. R. Marchand, J. A. Diaz-Buxo, F. G. Knox: Intrarenal calcium in phosphate handling, *Am. J. Physiol.*, **230**:790–796, 1976.

341. Amiel, C., H. Kuntziger, S. Couette, C. Coureau, N. Bergounioux: Evidence for a parathyroid hormone-independent calcium modulation of phosphate transport along the nephron, *J. Clin. Invest.*, **57**:256–263, 1976.

342. Dirks, J. H., G. A. Quamme: Physiology of the renal handling of magnesium, *Proceedings of the Second International Symposium on Magnesium*. In press.

343. Brunette, M. G., B. N. Vigneault, S. Carriere: Micropuncture study of renal magnesium transport in magnesium-loaded rats, *Am. J. Physiol.*, **229**:1695–1701, 1975.

344. Wen, S. -F., N. L. M. Wong, J. H. Dirks: Evidence for renal magnesium secretion during magnesium infusions in the dog, *Am. J. Physiol.*, **220**:33–37, 1971.

345. Walser, M.: Divalent cations: Physicochemical state in glomerular filtrate and urine and renal excretion, in J. Orloff, R. Berliner (eds.), *Handbook of Physiology, Renal Physiology*, American Physiological Society, Washington D.C., 1973.

346. Martin, M., A. H. Aissa, G. Baverel, M. Pellet: Distribution intrarenale de calcium et du magnesium chez le chien: éffet d'une diurèse osmotique, *J. Physiol. (Paris)*, **70**:159–172, 1975.

347. Lennon, E. J., J. Lemann, Jr., W. F. Piering, L. S. Larson: The effect of glucose on urinary cation excretion during chronic extracellular volume expansion in normal man, *J. Clin. Invest.*, **53**:1424–1433, 1974.

348. Dick, M., R. A. Evans, L. Watson: Effect of ethanol on magnesium excretion, *J. Clin. Pathol.*, **22**:152–153, 1969.

349. Sutton, R. A. L., J. H. Dirks: The renal excretion of calcium: A review of micropuncture data, *Can. J. Physiol. Pharmacol.*, **53**:979–988, 1975.

350. Sutton, R. A. L., J. H. Dirks: Renal handling of calcium: Overview, in S. G. Massry, E. Ritz (eds.), *Phosphate Metabolism*, Plenum Press, New York, 1977.

351. Le Grimellec, C., N. Roinel, F. Morel: Simultaneous Mg, Ca, P, K, Na, and Cl analysis in rat tubular fluid. III. During acute Ca plasma loading, *Pfluegers Arch.*, **346**:171–188, 1974.

352. Edwards, B. R., R. A. L. Sutton, J. H. Dirks: Effect of calcium infusion on renal tubular reabsorption in the dog, *Am. J. Physiol.*, **227**:13–18, 1974.

353. Frick, A., G. Rumrich, K. J. Ullrich, W. E. Lassiter: Microperfusion study of calcium transport in the proximal tubule of the rat kidney, *Pfluegers Arch.*, **286**:109–117, 1965.

354. LeGrimellec, C., N. Roinel, F. Morel: Simultaneous Mg, Ca, P, K, Na, and Cl analysis in rat tubular fluid. I. During perfusion of either inulin or ferrocyanide, *Pfluegers Arch.*, **340**:181–196, 1973.

355. Rose, G. A.: The relative importance of the ionized and complexed fractions of calcium in human plasma in control of the urine calcium, *Proc. R. Soc. Med.*, **52**:347–349, 1959.

356. Bernstein, D., C. R. Kleeman, R. E. Cutler, J. T. Dowling, M. H. Maxwell: Comparison of renal clearance of calcium during infusions of calcium

chloride and calcium gluconate, *Proc. Soc. Exp. Biol. Med.*, **110:**671–673, 1962.

357. Schmitt, G. H., M. U. Tsao, J. Tjen, J. R. Claiche, J. T. Cwalina, J. D. Mosson: Dissociation of calciuretic and natriuretic responses to NaCl infusions in adrenalectomized dogs, *Metabolism*, **20:**835–842, 1971.

358. Chen, P. S., W. F. Neuman: Renal excretion of calcium by the dog, *Am. J. Physiol.*, **180:**623–631, 1955.

359. Jamison, R. L., N. R. Frey, F. B. Lacy: Calcium reabsorption in the thin loop of Henle, *Am. J. Physiol.*, **227:**745–751, 1974.

360. Brunette, M., M. Aras: A microinjection study of nephron permeability to calcium and magnesium, *Amer. J. Physiol.*, **221:**1442–1448, 1971.

361. Morrissey, R. L., D. F. Rath: Purification of human renal calcium binding protein from necropsy specimens, *Proc. Soc. Exp. Biol. Med.*, **145:** 699–703, 1974.

362. Sands, H., R. H. Kessler: A calcium binding component of dog kidney cortex and its relationship to calcium transport, *Proc. Soc. Exp. Biol. Med.*, **137:**1267–1273, 1971.

363. Chen, P. S., Jr., W. F. Neuman: Renal reabsorption of calcium through its inhibition by various chemical agents, *Am. J. Physiol.*, **180:**632–636, 1955.

364. Parkinson, D. K., I. C. Radde: Properties of a $Ca^{2}+$ activated ATP-hydrolyzing enzyme in rat kidney cortex, *Biochim. Biophys. Acta*, **242:** 238–246, 1971.

365. Moore, L., D. F. Fitzpatrick, T. S. Chen, E. J. Landon: Calcium pump activity of the renal plasma membrane and renal microsomes, *Biochim. Biophys. Acta*, **345:**405–418, 1974.

366. Gonda, A., N. Wong, J. F. Seely, J. H. Dirks: The role of hemodynamic factors on urinary calcium and magnesium excretion, *Can. J. Physiol.*, **47:**619–626, 1970.

367. Thompson, R. B., C. E. Kaufman, V. A. DiScala: Effect of renal vasodilatation on divalent ion excretion and Tm_{PAH} in anesthetized dogs, *Amer. J. Physiol.*, **221:**1097–1104, 1971.

368. Parfitt, A. M.: The acute effects of mersalyl, chlorothiazide and mannitol on the renal excretion of calcium and other ions in man, *Clin. Sci.*, **36:**267–282, 1969.

369. Better, O. S., S. G. Massry: Effect of chronic bile duct obstruction on renal handling of calcium and magnesium, *J. Lab. Clin. Med.*, **79:**794–800, 1972.

370. Walser, M.: Calcium-sodium interdependence in renal transport, in J. W. Fisher (ed.), *Renal Pharmacology*, Appleton-Century-Crofts, Inc., New York, 1971, pp. 21-41.

371. Schneider, E. G., J. W. Strandhoy, L. R. Willis, F. G. Knox: Relationship between proximal sodium reabsorption and excretion of calcium, magnesium and phosphate, *Kidney Int.*, **4:**369–376, 1973.

372. Walser, M.: Mathematical aspects of renal function: The dependence of solute reabsorption on water reabsorption, and the mechanism of osmotic natriuresis, *J. Theor. Biol.*, **10:**307–326, 1966.

373. Hills, A. G., D. W. Parsons, G. D. Webster, O. Rosenthal, H. Conover: Influence of the renal excretion of sodium chloride upon the renal excretion of magnesium and other ions by human subjects, *J. Clin. Endocrinol.*, **19:**1192–1211, 1959.

374. Lamberg, B.-A., P. Torsti: The dependence of calcium excretion on adrenal steroids; studies with chlorothiazide in patients with impaired adrenal function, *Acta Med. Scand.*, **412:**193–203, 1964.

375. Lemann, J., Jr., W. F. Piering, E. J. Lennon: Studies of the acute effects of aldosterone and cortisol on the interrelationship between renal sodium, calcium and magnesium excretion in normal man, *Nephron*, **7:**117–130, 1970.

376. Paunier, L., M. Borgeaud, M. Wyss: Acute effect of aldosterone on tubular calcium and magnesium reabsorption, *Helv. Med. Acta*, **36:**265–275.

377. Wills, M. R., J. R. Gill, F. C. Bartter: The interrelationships of calcium and sodium excretions, *Clin. Sci.*, **37:**621–630, 1969.

378. Davis, B. B., H. V. Murdaugh: Evaluation of interrelationship between calcium and sodium excretion by canine kidney, *Metabolism*, **19:**439–444, 1970.

379. Knox, F. G., E. G. Schneider, L. R. Willis, J. W. Strandhoy, C. E. Ott, J.-L. Cuche, R. S. Godlsmith, C. D. Arnaud: Proximal tubule reabsorption after hyperoncotic albumin infusion, *J. Clin. Invest.*, **53:**501–507, 1974.

380. Rastegar, A., Z. Agus, T. B. Connor, M. Goldberg: Renal handling of calcium and phosphate

during mineralocorticoid "escape" in man, *Kidney Int.*, **2**:279–286, 1972.

381. Kleeman, C. R., J. Bohannan, D. Bernstein, S. Ling, M. H. Maxwell: Effect of variations in sodium intake on calcium excretion in normal humans, *Soc. Exp. Biol. Med.*, **115**:29–32, 1964.

382. Kirkendall, W. M., W. E. Connor, F. Abboud, S. P. Rastogi, T. A. Anderson, M. Fry: The effect of dietary sodium chloride on blood pressure, body fluids, electrolytes, renal function, and serum lipids of normotensive man, *J. Lab. Clin. Med.*, **87**:418–434, 1976.

383. Meyer, W. J., III, I. Transbol, F. C. Bartter, C. Delea: Control of calcium absorption: Effect of sodium chloride loading and depletion, *Metabolism*, **25**:989–993, 1976.

384. Phillips, M. J., J. N. C. Cooke: Relation between urinary calcium and sodium in patients with idiopathic hypercalciuria, *Lancet*, **2**:1354–1357, 1967.

385. Segre, G. V., H. D. Niall, R. T. Sauer, J. T. Potts Jr.: Edman degradation of radioiodnated parathyroid hormone: Application to sequence analysis and hormone metabolism in vivo, *Biochemistry*, **16**:2417–2427, 1977.

386. Keutmann, H. T., H. D. Niall, J. L. H. O'Riordan, J. T. Potts, Jr.: A reinvestigation of the amino-terminal sequence of human parathyroid hormone, *Biochemistry*, **14**:1842–1847, 1975.

387. Cohn, D. V., J. W. Hamilton: Newer aspects of parathyroid chemistry and physiology, *Cornell Vet.*, **66**:271–300, 1976.

388. Kemper, B., J. F. Habener, J. T. Potts, Jr., A. Rich: Pre-proparathyroid hormone: Fidelity of the translation of parathyroid messenger RNA by extracts of wheat germ, *Biochemistry*, **15**:20–25, 1976.

389. Reaven, E. P., G. M. Reaven: A quantitative ultrastructural study of microtubule content and secretory granule accumulation in parathyroid glands of phosphate- and colchicine-treated rats, *J. Clin. Invest.*, **56**:49–55, 1975.

390. Chertow, B. S., R. J. Buschmann, W. J. Henderson: Subcellular mechanisms of parathyroid hormone secretion; ultrastructural changes in response to calcium, vitamin A, vinblastine, and cytochalasin B, *Lab. Invest.*, **32**:190–200, 1975.

391. Chu, L. L. H., R. R. MacGregor, D. V. Cohn: Energy-dependent intracellular translocation of proparathormone, *J. Cell Biol.*, **72**:1–10, 1977.

392. Hansson, C. G., L. Hamberger: Influence of calcium and magnesium on respiration of isolated parathyroid cells from the rat, *Endocrinology*, **92**:1582–1587, 1973.

393. Dufresne, L. R., C. W. Cooper, H. J. Gitelman: In vivo suppression of parathyroid gland ATP content by hypercalcemia, *Endocrinology*, **90**:291–294, 1972.

394. Mayer, G. P.: Effect of calcium and magnesium on parathyroid hormone secretion in calves, in R. V. Talmage, M. Owen, J. A. Parsons (eds.), *Calcium Regulating Hormones*, Excerpta Medica, Amsterdam, 1975.

395. Blum, J. W., J. A. Fischer, D. Schwoerer, W. Hunziker, U. Binswanger: Acute parathyroid hormone response: Sensitivity, relationship to hypocalcemia and rapidity, *Endocrinology*, **95**:753–759, 1974.

396. Mayer, G. P., J. F. Habener, J. T. Potts, Jr.: Parathyroid hormone secretion in vivo: Demonostration of a calcium-independent, nonsuppressible component of secretion, *J. Clin. Invest.*, **57**:678–683, 1976.

397. Raisz, L. G.: Effects of calcium on uptake and incorporation of amino acids in the parathyroid glands, *Biochim. Biophys. Acta*, **148**:460–468, 1967.

398. Shannon, W. A., Jr., S. I. Roth: An ultrastructural study of acid phosphatase activity in normal, adenomatous and hyperplastic (chief cell type) human parathyroid glands, *Am. J. Pathol.*, **77**:493–501, 1974.

399. Capen, C. C.: Fine structural alterations of parathyroid glands in response to experimental and spontaneous changes of calcium in extracellular fluids, *Am. J. Med.*, **50**:598–611, 1971.

400. Black, H. E., C. C. Capen, C. D. Arnaud: Ultrastructure of parathyroid glands and plasma immunoreactive parathyroid hormone in pregnant cows fed normal and high calcium diets, *Lab. Invest.*, **29**:173–185, 1973.

401. Lee, M. J., S. I. Roth: Effect of calcium and magnesium on deoxyribonucleic acid synthesis in rat parathyroid glands in vitro, *Lab. Invest.*, **33**:72–79, 1975.

402. Jubiz, W., J. M. Canterbury, E. Reiss, F. H. Ty-

ler: Circadian rhythm in serum parathyroid hormone concentration in human subjects: Correlation with serum calcium, phosphate, albumin, and growth hormone levels, *J. Clin. Invest.*, **51**:2040–2046, 1972.

403. Sinha, T. K., S. Miller, J. Fleming, R. Khairi, J. Edmondson, C. C. Johnston, N. H. Bell: Demonstration of a diurnal variation in serum parathyroid hormone in primary and secondary hyperparathyroidism, *J. Clin. Endocrinol. and Metab.*, **41**:1009–1013, 1975.

404. Anast, C. S., J. L. Winnacker, L. R. Forte, T. W. Burns: Impaired release of parathyroid hormone in magnesium deficiency, *J. Clin. Endocrinol. and Metab.*, **42**:707–717, 1976.

405. Kukreja, S. C., G. K. Hargis, E. N. Bowser, W. J. Henderson, E. W. Fisherman, G. A. Williams: Role of adrenergic stimuli in parathyroid hormone secretion in man, *J. Clin. Endocrinol. and Metab.*, **40**:478–479, 1975.

406. Brown, E. M., S. Hurwitz, C. J. Woodard, G. D. Aurbach: Direct identification of beta-adrenergic receptors on isolated bovine parathyroid cells, *Endocrinology*, **100**:1703–1709, 1977.

407. Shah, J. H., G. S. Motto, S. C. Kukreja, G. K. Hargis, G. A. Williams: Stimulation of the secretion of parathyroid hormone during hypoglycemic stress, *J. Clin. Endocrinol. and Metab.*, **41**:692–693, 1975.

408. Kaplan, E. L., G. W. Peskin, B. M. Jaffe: The effects of acute metabolic acid-base changes on secretion of gastrin and parathyroid hormone, *Surgery*, **72**:53–58, 1972.

409. Arnaud, C. D.: Parathyroid hormone: Coming of age in clinical medicine, *Am. J. Med.*, **55**:577–581, 1973.

410. Knights, E. B., S. B. Baylin, G. V. Foster: Control of polypeptide hormones by enzymatic degradation, *Lancet*, **2**:719–723, 1973.

411. Neuman, W. F., M. W. Neuman, P. J. Sammon, G. W. Casarett: The metabolism of labeled parathyroid hormone, *Calcif. Tissue Res.*, **18**:263–270, 1975.

412. Hruska, K. A., R. Kopelman, W. E. Rutherford, S. Klahr, E. Slatopolsky: Metabolism of immunoreactive parathyroid hormone in the dog; the role of the kidney and the effects of chronic renal disease, *J. Clin. Invest.*, **56**:39–48, 1975.

413. Bethune, J. E., R. A. Turpin: A study of urinary excretion of parathyroid hormone in man, *J. Clin. Invest.*, **47**:1583–1589, 1968.

414. Canterbury, J. M., L. A. Bricker, G. S. Levey, P. L. Kozlovskis, E. Ruiz, J. E. Zull, E. Reiss: Metabolism of bovine parathyroid hormone; immunological and biological charactertistics of fragments generated by liver perfusion, *J. Clin. Invest.*, **55**:1245–1253, 1975.

415. Singer, F. R., G. V. Segre, J. F. Habener, J. T. Potts, Jr.: Peripheral metabolism of bovine parathyroid hormone in the dog, *Metabolism*, **24**:139–144, 1975.

416. Blum, J. W., G. P. Mayer, J. T. Potts, Jr.: Parathyroid hormone responses during spontaneous hypocalcemia and induced hypercalcemia in cows, *Endocrinology*, **5**:84–92, 1974.

417. Silverman, R., R. S. Yalow: Heterogeneity of parathyroid hormone; clinical and physiologic implications, *J. Clin. Invest.*, **52**:1958–1971, 1973.

418. Peck, W. A., J. K. Burks, J. Wilkins, S. B. Rodan, G. A. Rodan: Evidence for preferential effects of parathyroid hormone, calcitonin and adenosine on bone and periosteum, *Endocrinology*, **100**:1357–1364, 1977.

419. Luben, R. A., G. L. Wong, D. V. Cohn: Biochemical characterization with parathormone and calcitonin of isolated bone cells; provisional identification of osteoclasts and osteoblasts, *Endocrinology*, **99**:526–534, 1976.

420. Nagata, N., M. Saski, N. Kimura, K. Nakane: The hypercalcemic effect of parathyroid hormone and skeletal cyclic AMP, *Endocrinology*, **96**:725–731, 1975.

421. Froeling, P. G. A. M., O. L. M. Bijvoet: Kidney-mediated effects of parathyroid hormone on extracellular homeostasis of calcium, phosphate and acid-base balance in man, *Neth. J. Med.*, **17**:174–183, 1974.

422. Raisz, L. G., J. D. Wever, C. L. Trummel, J. Feinblatt, W. Y. W. Au: Induction, inhibition and escape as phenomena of bone resortpion, in R. V. Talmage L. P. Munsor (eds.), *Calcium, Parathyroid Hormone and the Calcitonins*, Excerpta Medica, Amsterdam, 1972.

423. Herrmann-Erlee, M. P. M., J. N. M. Heersche, J. W. Hekkelman, P. J. Gaillard, G. W. Tregear, J. A. Parsons, J. T. Potts, Jr.: Effects on bone in vitro of bovine parathyroid hormone and synthetic fragments representing residues 1-34, 2-34, and 3-34, *Endocr. Res. Commun.*, **3**:21–35, 1976.

424. Davis, W. L., J. L. Mathews, J. H. Martin, J. W. Kennedy, R. V. Talmage: The endosteum as a functional membrane, in R. V. Talmage, M. Owen, J. A. Parsons (eds.), *Calcium Regulating Hormone*, Excerpta Medica, Amsterdam, 1975.

425. Norimatsu, H., R. V. Talmage: Rapid ultrastructural changes in the osteocyte lining cell bone units following parathyroid hormone and calcitonin administration to embryonic and reonate rats, in *Abstracts, Sixth Parathyroid Conference*, Vancouver, 1977.

426. Vanderwiel, C., J. L. Mathews, R. V. Talmage: Intracellular calcium localization in cells lining bone surfaces following parathyroid hormone injection, in *Abstracts, Sixth Parathyroid Conference*, Vancouver, 1977.

427. Talmage, R. V., S. H. Doppelt, F. B. Fondren: An interpretation of acute changes in plasma ^{45}Ca following parathyroid hormone administration to thyroparathyroidectomized rats, *Calcif. Tissue Res.*, **22**:117–128, 1976.

428. Parfitt, A. M.: Equilibrium and disequilibrum hypercalcemia: New light on an old concept, in *Metabolic Bone Disease and Related Research.* In press.

429. DiBella, F. P., T. P. Dousa, S. S. Miller, C. D. Arnaud: Parathyroid hormone receptors of renal cortex: Specific binding of biologically active ^{125}I-labeled hormone and relationship to adenylate cyclase activation, *Proc. Natl. Acad. Sci, USA*, **71**:723–726, 1974.

430. Aurbach, G. D., D. A. Heath: Parathyroid hormone and calcitonin regulation of renal function, *Kidney Int.*, **6**:331–345, 1974.

431. Chabardes, D., M. Imbert, A. Clique, M. Montegut, F. Morel: PTH sensitive adenyl cyclase activity in different segments of the rabbit nephron, *Pfluegers Arch.*, **354**:229–239, 1975.

432. Shlatz, L. J., I. L. Schwartz, E. Kinne-Saffran, R. Kinne: Distribution of parathyroid hormone-stimulated adenylate cyclase in plasma membranes of cells of the kidney cortex, *J. Membr. Biol.*, **24**:131–144, 1975.

433. Kurokawa, K., G. Lenchner, S. G. Massry: Interaction between parathyroid hormone and catecholamines on renal cortical cyclic AMP, *Nephron*, **18**:60–67, 1977.

434. Tomlinson, S., G. N. Hendy, J. L. H. O'Riordan: A simplified assessment of response to parathyroid hormone in hypoparathyroid patients, *Lancet*, **1**:62–64, 1976.

435. Kinne, R., L. J. Shlatz, E. Kinne-Saffran, I. L. Schwartz: Distribution of membrane-bound cyclic AMP-dependent protein kinase in plasma membranes of cells of the kidney cortex, *J. Membr. Biol.*, **24**:145–159, 1975.

436. Kaminsky, N. I., A. E. Broadus, J. G. Hardman, D. J. Jones, Jr., J. H. Ball, E. W. Sutherland, G. W. Liddle: Effects of parathyroid hormone on plasma and urinary adenosine 3′, 5′-monophosphate in man, *J. Clin. Invest.*, **49**:2387–2395, 1970.

437. Nordquist, R. E., G. M. A. Palmieri: Intracellular localization of parathyroid hormone in the kidney, *Endocrinology*, **95**:229–237, 1974.

438. Massry, S. G., J. W. Coburn, R. M. Friedler, K. Kurokawa, F. R. Singer: Relationship between the kidney and parathyroid hormone, *Nephron*, **15**:197–222, 1975.

439. Beck, L. H., M. Goldberg: Effects of acetazolamide and parathyroidectomy on renal transport of sodium, calcium and phosphate, *Am. J. Physiol.*, **224**:1136–1142, 1973.

440. Gold, L. W., S. G. Massry, A. I. Arieff, J. W. Coburn: Renal bicarbonate wasting during phosphate depletion; a possible cause of altered acid-base homeostasis in hyperparathyroidism, *J. Clin. Invest.*, **52**:2556–2562, 1973.

441. Vainsel, M., T. Manderlier, H. L. Vis: Proximal renal tubular acidosis in vitamin D deficiency rickets, *Biomedicine*, **22**:35–40, 1974.

442. Kupfer, S., J. D. Kosovsky: Renal intracellular phosphate and phosphate excretion: The effect of digoxin and parathyroid hormone, *Mt. Sinai J. Med.*, **38**:359–374, 1970.

443. Forte, L. R., G. A. Nickols, C. S. Anast: Renal adenylate cyclase and the interrelationship between parathyroid hormone and vitamin D in the regulation of urinary phosphate and adenosine

cyclic 3′, 5′-monophosphate excretion, *J. Clin. Invest.*, **57**:559–568, 1976.

444. Dennis, V. W., E. Bello-Reuss, R. R. Robinson: Response of phosphate transport to parathyroid hormone in segments of rabbit nephron, *Am. J. Physiol.*, **233**:F29–F38, 1977.

445. Egawa, J., W. F. Neuman: Effect of parathyroid extract on the metabolism of radioactive phosphate in kidney, *Endocrinology*, **74**:90–101, 1964.

446. Foulks, J. G., F. A. Perry: Alterations in renal tubular phosphate transport during intravenous infusion of parathyroid extract in the dog, *Am. J. Physiol.*, **196**:567–571, 1959.

447. Meyer, R. A., Jr., M. H. Meyer: Phosphate mobilization from striated muscle following parathyroid hormone administration to thyroparathyroidectomized rats, *Experientia*, **33**:278–280, 1977.

448. Biddulph, D. M.: Influence of parathyroid hormone and the kidney on maintenance of blood calcium concentration in the golden hamster, *Endocrinology*, **90**:1113–1118, 1972.

449. Peacock, M., A. M. Pierides, B. E. C. Nordin: Biochemical changes following parathyroidectomy. Endocrinology, 1971, in S. Taylor (ed.), *Proc. of 3d International Symposium*, W. Heinemann, London, 1972.

450. Talmage, R. V.: Studies on the maintenance of serum calcium levels by parathyroid hormone action on bone and kidney, *Ann. N.Y. Acad. Sci.*, **64**:326–335, 1956.

calcium concentration in the golden hamster, *Endocrinology*, **90**:1113–1118, 1972.

449. Peacock, M., A. M. Pierides, B. E. C. Nordin: Biochemical changes following parathyroidectomy. Endocrinology, 1971, in S. Taylor (ed.), *Proc. of 3d International Symposium*, W. Heinemann, London, 1972.

450. Talmage, R. V.: Studies on the maintenance of serum calcium levels by parathyroid hormone action on bone and kidney, *Ann. N.Y. Acad. Sci.*, **64**:326–335, 1956.

451. Sutton, R. A. L., N. L. M. Wong, J. H. Dirks: Effects of parathyroid hormone on sodium and calcium transport in the dog nephron, *Clin. Sci. Mol. Med.*, **51**:345–351, 1976.

452. Agus, Z. S., P. J. S. Chiu, M. Goldberg: Regulation of urinary calcium excretion in the rat, *Am. J. Physiol.*, **1**:F545–F549, 1977.

453. Parfitt, A. M.: Effect of calcium (Ca) and magnesium (Mg) deprivation on diuretic induced calciuresis in man. Possible clue to site of action of parathyroid hormone (PTH) on the nephron, *Proceedings of the Fourth International Congress on Nephrology*, 1969, pp. 84.

454. Brickman, A. S., S. G. Massry, J. W. Coburn: Calcium deprivation and renal handling of calcium during repeated saline infusions, *Am. J. Physiol.*, **220**:44–48, 1971.

455. Parfitt, A. M.: Tubular reabsorption of calcium in pseudohypoparathyroidism, *Abstracts of the Sixth Parathyroid Conference*, Vancouver, 1977.

456. Vainsel, M., T. Manderlier, J. Vilain, H. His: Study of secondary hyperparathyroidism in vitamin D deficiency rickets. II. Aspects of amino acid metabolism, *Biomedicines*, **20**:404–409, 1974.

457. Birge, S. J., S. C. Switzer, D. R. Leonard: Influence of sodium and parathyroid hormone on calcium release from intestinal mucosal cells, *J. Clin. Invest.*, **54**:702–709, 1974.

458. Vegt, G. B., M. De Ruijter: The effect of parathyroid hormone on the uptake of calcium by fetal rat intestinal tissue and by isolated intestinal epithelial cells, in *Proc. Koninkl. Nederlandse Akademie van Wetenschappen*, Amsterdam, series C, **80**(1), Feb. 18, 1977.

459. Nicolaysen, R., N. Eeg-Larsen: The biochemistry and physiology of vitamin D, *Vitam. Horm.*, **11**:29–60, 1953.

460. Parfitt, A. M., B. Frame: Treatment of rickets and osteomalacia, *Seminars in Drug Treatment*, **2**(1):83–115, 1972.

461. Avioli, L. V., J. G. Haddad: Progress in endocrinology and metabolism. Vitamin D: Current concepts, *Metabolism*, **22**:507–531, 1973.

462. Norman, A. W., H. Henry: The role of the kidney and vitamin D metabolism in health and disease, *Clin. Orthop.*, **98**:258–287, 1974.

463. DeLuca, H. F.: Recent advances in our understanding of the vitamin D endocrine system, *J. Lab. Clin. Med.*, **87**:7–26, 2976.

464. Haussler, M. R., T. A. McCain: Basic and clinical concepts related to vitamin D metabolism and action, *N. Engl. J. Med.*, **297**:974–983, 1041–1050, 1977.

465. Wheatley, V. R., R. P. Reinertson: The presence

of vitamin D precursors in human epidermis, *J. Invest. Derm.*, **31**:51, 1958.

466. Rauschkolb, E. W., H. W. Davis, D. C. Fenimore, H. S. Black, L. F. Fabre: Identification of vitamin D_3 in human skin, *J. Invest. Dern.*, **53**:289–294, 1969.

467. Gaylor, J. L., F. M. Sault: Localization and biosynthesis of 7-dehydrocholesterol in rat skin, *J. Lipid. Res.*, **5**:422–431, 1964.

468. Neer, R., M. Clark, V. Fredman, R. Betsey, M. Sweeney, J. Buonchristiani, J. Potts: Environmental and nutritional influences on plasma. 25 Hydroxyvitamin D concentration and calcium metabolism in man, in A. W. Norman, et al. (eds.), *Vitamin D Biochemical, Chemical, and Clinical Aspects Related to Calcium Metabolism,* W. de Gruyter, Berlin, 1977.

469. Preece, M. A., S. Tomlinson, C. A. Ribot, J. Pietrek, H. T. Korn, D. M. Davies, J. A. Ford, M. G. Dunnigan, J. L. H. O'Riordan: Studies of vitamin D deficiency in man, *Q. J. Med.*, **154**:575–589, 1975.

470. Beadle, P. C.: The epidermal biosynthesis of cholecalciferol (vitamin D_3), *Photochem. Photobiol.*, **25**:519–527, 1977.

471. Gupta, M. M., J. M. Round, T. C. B. Stamp: Spontaneous cure of vitamin-D deficiency in Asians during summer in Britain, *Lancet*, **46**:586–588, 1974.

472. Neer, R. M.: The evolutionary significance of vitamin D, skin pigment and ultraviolet light, *Am. J. Physiol. Anthropol.*, **43**:409–416, 1975.

473. Dale, A. E., M. E. Lowenberg: Consumption of vitamin D in fortified and natural foods and in vitamin preparations, *J. Ped.*, **70**:952–955, 1967.

474. Haddad, J. G., T. J. Hahn: Natural and synthetic sources of circulating 25-hydroxyvitamin D in man, *Nature,* **244**:515–517, 1973.

475. Arnaud, S. B., M. Matthusen, J. B. Gilkinson, R. S. Goldsmith: Components of 25-hydroxyvitamin D in serum of young children in upper midwestern United States, *Amer. J. Clin. Nutr.*, **30**:1082–1086, 1977.

476. Hollander, D.: Mechanism and site of small intestinal uptake of vitamin D_3 in pharmacological concentrations, *Am. J. Clin. Nutr.*, **29**:970–875, 1976.

477. Hollander, D., S. J. Rosenstreich, W. Volwiler: Role of the duodenum in vitamin D_3 absorption in man, *Am. J. Dig. Dis.*, **16**:145–149, 1971.

478. Avioli, L. V.: Current concepts of vitamin D_3 metabolism in man, in H. F. DeLuca, J. W. Sattie (eds.), *The Fat Soluble Vitamins,* The University of Wisconsin Press, Madison, 1970.

479. Olson, E. B., Jr., J. C. Knutson, M. H. Bhattacharyya, H. F. DeLuca: The effect of hepatectomy on the synthesis of 25-hydroxyvitamin D_3, *J. Clin. Invest.*, **57**:1213–1220, 1976.

480. Mawer, E. B., G. A. Lumb, K. Schaefer, S. W. Stanbury: The metabolism of isotopically labelled vitamin D_3 in man: The influence of the state of vitamin D nutrition, *Clin. Sci.*, **40**:39–53, 1971.

481. Mawer, E. B.: Aspects of the control of vitamin D metabolism in man, in A. W. Norman, et al. (eds.), *Vitamin D: Biochemical, Chemical, and Clinical Aspects Related to Calcium Metabolism,* W. de Gruyter, Berlin, 1977.

482. Stamp, T. C. B., J. G. Haddad, C. A. Twigg: Comparison of oral 25-hydroxycholecalciferol, vitamin D and ultraviolet light as determinants of circulating 25-hydroxyvitamin D, *Lancet*, **1**:1341–1343, 1977.

483. Rojanasathit, S., J. G. Haddad: Hepatic accumulation of vitamin D_3 and 25-hydroxyvitamin D_3, *Biochim. Biophys. Acta,* **421**:12–21, 1976.

484. Suda, T., W. Monachi, M. Eukushima, Y. Nishu, E. Ogata: Regulation of the metabolism of vitamin D_3 and 25 hydroxyvitamin D_3, in A. W. Norman, et al. (eds.), *Vitamin D: Biochemical, Chemical, and Clinical Aspects Related to Calcium Metabolism,* W. de Gruyter, Berlin, 1977.

485. Avioli, L. V., S. W. Lee, J. E. McDonald, J. Lund, H. F. DeLuca: Metabolism of vitamin D_3-^{3}H in human subjects: Distribution in blood, bile, feces and urine, *J. Clin. Invest.*, **46**:983–992, 1967.

486. Mawer, E. B., J. Backhouse, C. A. Holman, G. A. Lumb, S. W. Stanbury: The distribution and storage of vitamin D and its metabolites in human tissues, *Clin. Sci.*, **43**:413–431, 1972.

487. Rosenstreich, S. J., C. Rich, W. Volwiler: Deposition in and release of vitamin D_3 from body fat: Evidence for a storage site in the rat, *J. Clin. Invest.*, **50**:679–687, 1971.

488. Lumb, G. A., E. B. Mawer, S. W. Stanbury: The apparent vitamin D resistance of chronic renal

failure. A study of the physiology of vitamin D in man, *Am. J. Med.*, **50**:421–441, 1971.

489. Parfitt, A. M.: The treatment of hypoparathyroidism with 25(OH)D₃: Practical conclusions and metabolic implications, in A. W. Norman, et al. (eds.), *Vitamin D: Biochemical, Chemical, and Clinical Aspects Related to Calcium Metabolism,* W. de Gruyter, Berlin, 1977.

490. Haddad, J. G., L. Hillman, S. Rojanasathit: Human serum binding capacity and affinity for 25-hydroxergocalciferol and 25-hydroxycholecalciferol, *J. Clin. Endocrinol. Metab.*, **43**:86–91, 1976.

491. Imawari, M., K. Kida, D. S. Goodman: The transport of vitamin D and its 25-hydroxy metabolite in human plasma. Isolation and partial characterization of vitamin D and 25-hydroxyvitamin D binding protein, *J. Clin. Invest.*, **58**:514–523, 1976.

492. Bouillon, R., H. Van Baelen, W. Rombauts, P. De Moor: The purification and characterization of the human-serum binding protein for the 25-hydroxycholecalciferol (transcalciferin). Identity with group-specific component, *Eur. J. Biochem.*, **66**:285–291, 1976.

493. Thomas, W. C., Jr., H. G. Morgan, T. B. Connor, L. Haddock, C. E. Bills, J. E. Howard: Studies of antiricketic activity in sera from patients with disorders of calcium metabolism and preliminary observations on the mode of transport of vitamin D in human serum, *J. Clin. Invest.*, **38**:1078–1085, 1959.

494. Balsan, S., I. Antener, P. Royer: Variations de l'activité vitaminique D du serum après injection musculaire d'une dose modérée de vitamine D₂ chez l'enfant normal et dans les rachitismes vitamino-resistants idiopathiques, *Rev. Fr. Etudes Clin. Biol.*, **44**:594–602, 1969.

495. Bec, P., F. Bayard, J. P. Louvet: 25-Hydroxycholecalciferol dynamics in human plasma, *Rev. Eur. Etudes Clin. Biol.*, **107**:793–796, 1972.

496. Gray, R. W., H. P. Weber, J. H. Dominguez, J. Lemann, Jr.: The metabolism of vitamin D₃ and 25-hydroxyvitamin D₃ in normal and anephric humans, *J. Clin. Endocrinol. Metab.*, **39**: 1045–1056, 1974.

497. Haddad, J. G., Jr., S. Rojanasathit: Acute administration of 25-hydroxycholecalciferol in man, *J. Clin. Endocrinol. Metab.*, **42**:284–290, 1976.

498. Weber, H. P., R. W. Gray, J. H. Dominguez, J. Lemann, Jr.: The lack of effect of chronic metabolic acidosis on 25-OH-Vitamin D metabolism and serum parathyroid hormone in humans, *J. Clin. Endocrinol. Metab.*, **43**:1047–1055, 1976.

499. Arnaud, S. B., R. S. Goldsmith, P. W. Lambert, V. L. W. Go: 25-Hydroxyvitamin D₃: Evidence of an enterohepatic circulation in man, *Proc. Soc. Exp. Biol. Med.*, **149**:570–572, 1975.

500. Stamp, T. C. B.: Intestinal absorption of 25-hydroxycholecalciferol, *Lancet*, **2**:121–123, 1974.

501. Hughes, M. R., D. J. Baylink, W. A. Gonnerman, S. U. Toverud, W. K. Ramp, M. R. Haussler: Influence of dietary vitamin D₃ on the circulating concentration of its active metabolites in the chick and rat, *Endocrinology*, **100**:799–806, 1977.

502. Baxter, L. A., H. F. DeLuca: Stimulation of 25-hydroxyvitamin D₃-1-hydroxylase by phosphate depletion, *J. Biol. Chem.*, **251**:3158–3161, 1976.

503. Hughes, M. R., P. F. Brumbaugh, M. R. Haussler: Regulation of serum 1 25-dihydroxyvitamin D₃ by calcium and phosphate in the rat, *Science*, **190**:578–579, 1975.

504. Mawer, E. B., J. Backhouse, L. F. Hill, G. A. Lumb, P. De Silva, C. M. Taylor, S. W. Stanbury: Vitamin D metabolism and parathyroid function in man, *Clin. Sci. Mol. Med.*, **48**: 349–365, 1975.

505. Gray, R. W., D. R. Wilz, A. E. Caldas, J. Lemann, Jr.: The importance of phosphate in regulating plasma 1,25-(OH)₂-vitamin D levels in humans: Studies in healthy subjects, in calcium-stone formers and in patients with primary hyperparathyroidism, *J. Clin. Endocrinol. Metab.*, **45**:299–306, 1977.

506. MacIntyre, I.: Comparative aspects of the biochemistry of the regulation of vitamin D metabolism, in A. W. Norman, et al. (eds.), *Vitamin D: Biochemical, Chemical, and Clinical Aspects Related to Calcium Metabolism,* W. de Gruyter, Berlin, 1977.

507. Gray, R. W., D. R. Wilz, A. E. Caldas, J. Lemann, H. F. DeLuca: Disappearance from plasma of injected ³H-1,25(OH)₂D₃ in healthy humans, in A. W. Norman, et al. (eds.), *Vitamin D: Biochemical, Chemical, and Clinical Aspects Related to Calcium Metabolism,* W. de Gruyter, Berlin, 1977.

508. Brickman, A. S., J. W. Coburn, G. R. Friedman,

W. H. Okamura, S. G. Massry, A. W. Norman: Comparison of effects of 1-hydroxy-vitamin D_3 and 1,25-dihydroxy-vitamin D_3 in man, *J. Clin. Invest.*, **57**:1540–1547, 1976.

509. Haddad, J. G., L. Min, T. Walgate, T. Hahn: Competition by 24,25 dihydroxycholecalciferol in the competitive protein binding radioassay of 25-hydroxycholecalciferol, *J. Clin. Endocrinol.*, **43**:712–715, 1976.

510. Taylor, C. M., P. DeSilva, S. E. Hughes: Competitive protein binding assay for 24,25 dihydroxycholecalciferol, *Calcif. Tissue Res.*, **22**(suppl.):40–44, 1977.

511. Holdsworth, E. S., J. E. Jordan, E. Keenan: Effects of cholecalciferol on the translocation of calcium by non-everted chick ileum in vitro, *Biochem. J.*, **152**:181–190, 1975.

512. Hamilton, J. W., E. S. Holdsworth: The role of calcium binding protein in the mechanism of action of cholecalciferol (vitamin D_3), *Aust. J. Exp. Biol. Med. Sci.*, **53**:469–478, 1975.

513. Wasserman, R. H.: Metabolism, function and clinical aspects of vitamin D, *Cornell Vet.*, **65**:3–25, 1975.

514. Mawer, E. B., J. Backhouse, M. Davies, L. F. Hill, C. M. Taylor: Metabolic fate of administered 1,25-dihydroxycholecalciferol in controls and in patients with hypoparathyroidism, *Lancet*, **1**:1203–1206, 1976.

515. Corradino, R. A.: Cyclic AMP regulation of the 1,25$(OH)_2D_2$-mediated intestinal calcium absorptive mechanism, in A. W. Norman, et al. (eds.), *Vitamin D: Biochemical, Chemical, and Clinical Aspects Related to Calcium Metabolism*, W. de Gruyter, Berlin, 1977.

516. Taylor, A. W., J. E. McIntosh: Light and electron microscopic immunooperosidase localization of chick intestinal vitamin D induced calcium binding protein, in A. W. Norman, et al. (eds.), *Vitamin D: Biochemical, Chemical, and Clinical Aspects Related to Calcium Metabolism*, W. de Gruyter, Berlin, 1977.

517. Lawson, E., R. Spencer, M. Charman, P. Wilson: Recent studies in 1,25$(OH)_2D_3$ action on the intestine, in A. W. Norman, et al. (eds.), *Vitamin D: Biochemical, Chemical, and Clinical Aspects Related to Calcium Metabolism*, W. de Gruyter, Berlin, 1977.

518. Wong, R. G., A. W. Norman: Studies on the mechanism of action of calciferol. VIII. The effects of dietary vitamin D and the polyene antibiotic, filipin, in vitro, on the intestinal cellular uptake of calcium, *J. Biol. Chem.*, **250**:2411–2419, 1975.

519. Birge, S. J., D. H. Alpers: Stimulation of intestinal mucosal proliferation by vitamin D, *Gastroenterology*, **64**:977–982, 1973.

520. Sampson, H. W., E. L. Krawitt: A morphometric investigation of the duodenal mucosa of normal, vitamin D-deficient, and vitamin D-replete rats, *Calcif. Tissue Res.*, **21**:213–218, 1976.

521. Kanis, J. A., G. Heynen, R. G. G. Russell, R. Smith, R. J. Walton, G. T. Wasser: Biological effects of 24,25 dihydroxycholecalciferol in man, in A. W. Norman, et al. (eds.), *Vitamin D: Biochemical, Chemical, and Clinical Aspects Related to Calcium Metabolism*, W. de Gruyter, Berlin, 1977.

522. De Luca, H. F., Y. Tanaka, L. Castillo: Interrelationships between vitamin D and phosphate metabolism, in R. V. Talmage, M. Owen, J. A. Parsons (eds.), *Calcium Regulatory Hormones*, Excerpta Medica, Amsterdam, 1975.

523. Reynolds, J. J.: The role of 1,25-dihydroxycholecalciferol in bone metabolism, *Biochem. Soc. Spec. Publ.*, **3**:91–109, 1974.

524. Reynolds, J. J., H. Pavlovitch, S. Balsan: 1,25-Dihydroxycholecalciferol increases bone resorption in thyroiparathyroidectomised mice, *Calcif. Tissue Res.*, **21**:207–212, 1976.

525. Peck, W. A., I. Dowling: Failure of 1,25 dihydroxycholecalciferol (1,25-$(OH)_2$-D_3) to modify cyclic AMP levels in parathyroid hormone–treated and untreated bone cells, *Endocr. Res. Commun.*, **3**:157–166, 1976.

526. Massry, S. G., R. Stein, J. Garty, A. I. Arieff, J. W. Coburn, A. W. Norman, R. M. Friedler: Skeletal resistance to the calcemic action of parathyroid hormone in uremia: Role of 1,25$(OH)_2D_3$, *Kidney Int.*, **9**:467–474, 1976.

527. Gonnerman, W. A., W. K. Ramp, S. U. Toverud: Vitamin D, dietary calcium and parathyroid hormone interactions in chicks, *Endocrinology*, **96**:275–281, 1975.

528. Liu, C. -C., D. J. Baylink, J. Wergedal: Vitamin D-enhanced osteoclastic bone resorption at vascular canals, *Endocrinology*, **95**:1011–1018, 1974.

529. Weisbrode, S. E., C. C. Capen: Vitamin D–induced hypercalcemia in experimental renal failure, *Nephron*, **18**:26–34, 1977.

530. Bell, N. H., F. C. Bartter, H. Smith: The effect of vitamin D on Ca⁴⁷ metabolism in man, *Trans. Assoc. Am. Phys.*, **526**:163–175, 1963.

531. Nichols, G., Jr., S. Schartum, G. M. Vaes: Some effects of vitamin D and parathyroid hormone on the calcium and phosphorus metabolism of bone in vitro, *Acta Physiol. Scand.*, **57**:51–60, 1963.

532. Kream, B. E., M. Jose, S. Yamada, H. F. DeLuca: A specific high-affinity binding macromolecule for 1,25-dihydroxyvitamin D_3 in fetal bone, *Science*, **197**:1086–1088, 1977.

533. Krempien, B., G. Fredrick, G. Berger, E. Ritz: Ultrastructural studies of bone—influence of vitamin D, PTH and uremia on bone cell ultrastructure and bone cell/bone matrix interaction, in A. W. Norman, et al. (eds.), *Vitamin D: Biochemical, Chemical, and Clinical Aspects Related to Calcium Metabolism*, W. de Gruyter, Berlin, 1977.

534. Fourman, P., D. B. Morgan: Effects of vitamin D in the human, *Biol. Nutr. Dieta*, **13**:30–43, Korger, Basel, 1969.

535. Wells, I. C., D. Gambal: A vitamin D–dependent serum factor promoting calcium uptake by bone, *Proc. Soc. Exp. Biol. Med.*, **127**:1006–1010, 1968.

536. Kodicek, E., G. D. Thompson: Autoradiographic localization in bones of 1 ³H cholecalciferol, in S. Fitton Jackson, et al. (eds.), *Structure and Function of Connective and Skeletal Tissue*, Butterworth & Co. (Publishers), Ltd., London, 1965.

537. Wezeman, F. H.: 25-Hydroxyvitamin D_3: Autoradiographic evidence of sites of action in epiphyseal cartilage and bone, *Science*, **194**:1069–1071, 1976.

538. Edelstein, S., R. Sapir, A. Harell: The action of vitamin D on bone, *Clin. Endocrin.*, **5**:145s–150x, 1976.

539. Ivey, J. L., E. R. Morey, C. C. Liu, J. L. Rader, D. J. Baylink: Effects of vitamin D and its metabolites on bone, in A. W. Norman, et al. (eds.), *Vitamin D: Biochemical, Chemical, and Clinical Aspects Related to Calcium Metabolism*, W. de Gruyter, Berlin, 1977.

540. Bochier, P., A. Ryckwaert, P. More, L. Miravet, A. Norman, H. Rasmussen: Vitamin D metabolites and bone mineralization in man, in A. W. Norman, et al. (eds.), *Vitamin D: Biochemical, Chemical, and Clinical Aspects Related to Calcium Metabolism*, W. de Gruyter, Berlin, 1977.

541. Lumb, G. A., S. W. Stanbury: Parathyroid function in human vitamin D deficiency and vitamin D deficiency in primary hyperparathyroidism, *Am. J. Med.*, **56**:833–839, 1974.

542. Kodicek, E., E. M. Darmady, F. Stranack: The localization of ¹⁴C-labelled vitamin D_2 in the nephron, *Clin. Sci.*, **20**:185–195, 1961.

543. Gekle, D., J. Stroder, D. Rostock: The effect of vitamin D on renal inorganic phosphate reabsorption of normal rats, parathyroidectomized rats and rats with rickets, *Pediat. Res.*, **5**:40–52, 1971.

544. Popovtzer, M. M., J. B. Robinette: Effect of 25(OH)vitamin D_3 on urinary excretion of cyclic adenosine monophosphate, *Am. J. Physiol.*, **229**:907–910, 1975.

545. Puschett, J. B., W. S. Beck, A. Jelonek: Parathyroid hormone and 25-hydroxy vitamin D_3:synergistic and antagonistic effects on renal phosphate transport, *Science,* **190**:473–475, 1975.

546. Bonjour, J. P., M. Fleisch: The effect of vitamin D and its metabolites on the renal handling of phosphate, in A. W. Norman, et al. (eds.), *Vitamin D: Biochemical, Chemical, and Clinical Aspects Related to Calcium Metabolism*, W de Gruyter, Berlin, 1977.

547. Costanzo, L. S., P. R. Sheehe, I. M. Weiner: Renal actions of vitamin D in D-deficient rats, *Am. J. Physiol.*, **226**:1490–1495, 1974.

548. Sutton, R. A. L., C. A. Morris, N. L. M. Wong, J. M. Dirks: Effects of vitamin D on renal tubular calcium transport, in A. W. Norman, et al. (eds.), *Vitamin D: Biochemical, Chemical, and Clinical Aspects Related to Calcium Metabolism*, W. de Gruyter, Berlin, 1977.

549. Birge, S. J., J. G. Haddad: 25-Hydroxycholecalciferol stimulation of muscle metabolism, *J. Clin. Invest.*, **56**:1100–1107, 1975.

550. Wasserman, R. H., R. A. Corradino: Vitamin D, calcium and protein synthesis, *Vitam. Horm.*, **31**:43–103, 1973.

551. Van Baelen, H., R. Bouillon: Are the cytosolic binding proteins for 25 hidyoxycholecalciferol artifacts? in A. W. Norman, et al. (eds.), *Vitamin D: Biochemical, Chemical, and Clinical Aspects Re-*

lated to Calcium Metabolism, W. de Gruyter, Berlin, 1977.

552. Oldham, S. B., J. A. Fischer, L. H. Shen, C. D. Arnaud: Isolation and properties of a calcium-binding protein from porcine parathyroid glands, *Biochemistry,* **13:**4790–4796, 1974.

553. Weckler, W. R., M. L. Menz, A. W. Norman: The subcellular localization of 1,25 dihydroxy vitamin D_3 in the parathyroid glands of chickens, in A. W. Norman, et al. (eds.), *Vitamin D: Biochemical, Chemical, and Clinical Aspects Related to Calcium Metabolism,* W. de Gruyter, Berlin, 1977.

554. Chertow, B. S., D. J. Baylink, J. E. Wergedal, et al.: Decrease in serum immuno-reactive parathyroid hormone in rats and in parathyroid hormone secretion in vitro by 1,25-dihydroxycholecalciferol, *J. Clin. Invest.,* **56:**668–678, 1975.

555. Au, W. Y. W., L. G. Raisz: Effect of vitamin D and dietary calcium on parathyroid activity, *Am. J. Physiol.,* **209:**637–642, 1965.

556. Canterbury, M. J., E. Reiss: Predominance of suppressive effects of D metabolites on PTH secretion, in *Abstracts, Sixth Parathyroid Conference,* Vancouver, 1977.

557. Anast, C. S., H. H. Conaway: Calcitonin, *Clin. Orthop. Rel. Res.,* **84:**207–262, 1972.

558. Queener, S. F., N. H. Bell: Calcitonin: A general survey, *Metabolism,* **24:**555–567, 1975.

559. Gray, T. K., D. A. Ontjes: Clinical aspects of thyrocalcitonin, *Clin. Orthop.,* **3:**238–256, 1975.

560. Avioli, L. V.: Calcitonin, in S. H. Ingbar (ed.), *The Year in Endocrinology,* Plenum Medical Books Company, New York, 1976.

561. Wolfe, H. J., R. A. DeLellis, E. F. Voelkel, A. H. Tashjian, Jr.: Distribution of calcitonin-containing cells in the normal neonatal human thyroid gland: A correlation of morphology with peptide content, *J. Clin. Endocr. Metab.,* **41:**1076–1081, 1975.

562. Moya, F., A. Nieto, J. L. R-Candela: Calcitonin biosynthesis: Evidence for a precursor, *Eur. J. Biochem.,* **55:**407–413, 1975.

563. van der Donk, J. A., R. H. van Dam, J. Goudswaard, W. H. L. Hackeng, C. J. M. Lips: Precursor molecule for calcitonin, *Lancet,* **2:**1133, 1976.

564. Roos, B. D., A. L. Trelinger: Calcitonin biosynthesis and secretion: Isolation, characterization and regulatory studies of procalcitonin and pre-

procalcitonin, in *Abstracts, Sixth Parathyroid Conference,* Vancouver, 1977.

565. Deftos, L. J., B. A. Roos, D. Bronzert, J. G. Parthemore: Immunochemical heterogeneity of calcitonin in plasma, *J. Clin. Endocrinol. Metab.,* **40:**409–412, 1975.

566. Sizemore, G. W., H. Heath, III: Immunochemical heterogeneity of calcitonin in plasma of patients with medullary thyroid carcinoma, *J. Clin. Invest.,* **55:**1111–1118, 1975.

567. Snider, R. H., O. L. Silva, K. L. Becker, C. F. Moore: Heterogeneity of calcitonin, *Lancet,* **4:**49–50, 1975.

568. Parthemore, J. G., L. J. Deftos: The regulation of calcitonin in normal human plasma as assessed by immunoprecipitation and immunoextraction, *J. Clin. Invest.,* **56:**835–841, 1975.

569. Hillyard, C. J., T. J. C. Cooke, R. C. Coombes, I. M. A. Evans, I. MacIntyre: Normal plasma calcitonin: Circadian variation and response to stimuli, *Clin. Endocrinol.,* **6:**291–298, 1977.

570. Rojanasathit, S., J. G. Haddad, Jr.: Human calcitonin radioimmunoassay: Characterization and application, *Clin. Chim. Acta,* **78:**425–437, 1977.

571. Ardaillou, R., P. Sizonenko, A. Meyrier, G. Vallee, C. Beaugas: Metabolic clearance rate of radioiodinated human calcitonin in man, *J. Clin. Invest.,* **49:**2345–2352, 1970.

572. Riggs, B. L., C. D. Arnaud, R. S. Goldsmith, W. F. Taylor, J. T. McCall, A. D. Sessler: Plasma kinetics and acute effects of pharmacologic doses of porcine calcitonin in man, *J. Clin. Endocr.,* **33:**115–127, 1971.

573. Deftos, L. J., B. A. Roos, G. L. Knecht, et al.: Calcitonin secretion, in *Proceedings of the Sixth Parathyroid Conference, 1977.* In press.

574. Kalu, D. N., A. H. Georgopoulos, G. V. Foster: Evidence for physiological importance of calcitonin in the regulation of plasma calcium in rats, *J. Clin. Invest.,* **55:**722–727, 1975.

575. Silva, O. L., K. L. Becker, J. L. Doppman, R. H. Snider, C. F. Moore: Calcitonin levels in thyroid-vein blood of man, *Am. J. Med. Sci.,* **269:**37–41, 1975.

576. Care, A. D., C. W. Cooper, T. Duncan, H. Orimo: A study of thyrocalcitonin secretion by direct measurement of in vivo secretion rates in pigs, *Endocrinology,* **83:**161, 1968.

577. Heynen, G., P. Franchimont: Human calcitonin radioimmunoassay in normal and pathological conditions, *Eur. J. Clin. Invest.*, **4**:213–222, 1974.

578. Gittes, R. F., G. L. Irvin: Thyroid and parathyroid roles in hypercalcemia: Evidence for a thyrocalcitonin-releasing factor, *Science*, **148**:1737–1739, 1965.

579. Deftos, L. J., D. Powell, J. G. Parthemore, J. T. Potts, Jr.: Secretion of calcitonin in hypocalcemic states in man, *J. Clin. Invest.*, **52**:3109–3114, 1973.

580. Heynen, G., P. Franchimont: Human calcitonin and serum-phosphate, *Lancet*, **1**:627, 1974.

581. Selawry, H. P., K. L. Becker, L. E. Bivins, R. H. Snider, O. L. Silva: In vitro studies of calcitonin release in man, *Horm. Metabl. Res.*, **7**:432–437, 1975.

582. Care, A. D., N. H. Bell, R. F. L. Bates: The effects of hypermagnesaemia on calcitonin secretion in vivo, *J. Endocrinol.*, **51**:381–386, 1971.

583. Talmage, R. V., S. H. Doppelt, C. W. Cooper: Relationship of blood concentrations of calcium, phosphate, gastrin and calcitonin to the onset of feeding in the rat, *Proc. Soc. Exp. Biol. Med.*, **149**:855–859, 1975.

584. Reynolds, J. J., J. T. Dingle: A sensitive in vitro method for studying the induction and inhibition of bone resorption, *Calcif. Tissue Res.*, **4**:339–349, 1970.

585. Kallio, D. M., P. R., Garant, C. Minkin: Ultrastructural effects of calcitonin on osteoclasts in tissue culture, *J. Ultrastruct. Res.*, **39**:205–216, 1972.

586. Weisbrode, S. E., C. C. Capen: Ultrastructural evaluation of the effects of calcitonin on bone in thyroiparathyroidectomized rats administered vitamin D, *Am. J. Pathol.*, **77**:455–460, 1974.

587. Mills, B. G., A. M. Haroutinian, P. Holst, P. J. Bordier, S. Tun-Chot: Ultrastructural and cellular changes at the costochondral junction following in vivo treatment with calcitonin or calcium chloride in the rabbit, in S. Taylor (ed.), *Endocrinology 1971*, W. Heinemann, Ltd., London, 1972.

588. Matrajt-Denys, H., S. Tun-Chot, P. Bordier, D. Hioco, M. B. Clark, J. Pennock, F. H. Doyle, G. V. Foster: Effect of calcitonin on vitamin A-induced changes in bone in the rat, *Endocrinology*, **88**:129–137, 1971.

589. Steinetz, B. G., J. R. Matthews, M. C. Butler, S. W. Thompson, II: Inhibition by thyrocalcitonin of estrogen-induced bone resorption in the mouse pubic symphysis, *Am. J. Pathol.*, **73**:735–742, 1973.

590. Wener, J. A., S. J. Gorton, L. G. Raisz: Escape from inhibition of resorption in cultures of fetal bone treated with calcitonin and parathyroid hormone, *Endocrinology*, **90**:752–759, 1972.

591. Evanson, J. M., A. Garner, A. M. Holmes, G. A. Lumb, S. W. Stanbury: Interrelations between thyrocalcitonin and parathyroid hormone in rats, *Clin. Sci.*, **32**:271–278, 1967.

592. Melvin, K. E. W., A. M. Tashjian, P. Bordier: The metabolic significance of calcitonin-secreting thyroid carcinoma, in B. Frame, A. M. Parfitt, H. Cuncan (eds.), *Clinical Aspects of Metabolic Bone Disease*, Excerpta Medica, Amsterdam, 1973.

593. Talmage, R. V., J. L. Matthews, J. H. Martin, J. W. Kenneth, W. L. Davis, J. M. Roycroft: Calcitonin, phosphate and the osteocyte-osteoblast bone cell unit, in R. V. Talmage, M. Owen, J. A. Parsons (eds.), *Calcium Regulating Hormones*, Excerpta Medica, Amsterdam, 1975.

594. Talmage, R. V., J. J. B. Anderson, J. W. Kennedy, III: Separation of the hypocalcemic actions of calcitonin with disodium ethane-1-hydroxy-1, 1-diphosphonate, *Endocrinology*, **94**:413–418, 1974.

595. Thompson, J. S., G. M. A. Palmieri, L. P. Eliel: Dissociation of the lowering effect of calcitonin on plasma Ca and P in cortisone-treated nephrectomized rats, *Endocrinology*, **94**:799–802, 1974.

596. Meyer, R. A., Jr., M. H. Meyer: Thyrocalcitonin injection to rats increases the liver inorganic phosphate, *Endocrinology*, **96**:1048–1050, 1975.

597. Doppelt, S. H., R. V. Talmage: Calcitonin and the bone fluid comparatment; effect of calcitonin and/or parathyroid hormone on plasma radiocalcium changes, *Clin. Orthop.*, **118**:242–250, 1976.

598. Messer, H. H., W. D. Armstrong, L. Singer: Characteristics of calcium uptake by calcitonin-treated mouse calvaria in vitro, *Calcif. Tissue Res.*, **15**:85–92, 1974.

599. Baylink, D., E. Morey, C. Rich: Effect of calcitonin on osteocyte mineral transfer in the rat, in R. V. Talmage, L. Belanger (eds.), *Parathyroid Hormone and Thyrocalcitonin (Calcitonin)*, Excerpta Medica, Amsterdam, 1968.

600. Baud, C. A., J. DeSiebenthal, B. Lauger, M. R. Tupling, R. S. Mack: The effects of prolonged administration of thyrocalcitonin in human senile osteoporosis, in S. Talyor (ed.), *Calcitonin 1969*, W. Heinemann, Educational Books, Ltd. London, 1970.

601. Baron, R., J.-L. Saffar: A quantitative study of the effects of prolonged calcitonin treatment on alveolar bone remodelling in the golden hamster, *Calcif. Tissue Res.*, **22**:265–274, 1977.

602. Baylink, D., E. Morey, C. Rich: Effect of calcitonin on the rates of bone formation and resorption in the rat, *Endocrinology*, **84**:261–269, 1969.

603. Nagata, N., M. Sasaki, N. Kimura, K. Nakane: Effects of porcine calcitonin on the metabolism of calcium and cyclic AMP in rat skeletal tissue in in vivo, *Endocrinology*, **97**:527–535, 1975.

604. Caniggia, A., C. Gennari, A. Vattimo, P. Nardi, R. Nuti: Indirect evidence of calcitonin secretion in man, *Clin. Sci. Mol. Med.*, **51**:281–285, 1976.

605. Ardaillou, R.: Kidney and calcitonin, *Nephron*, **15**:250–260, 1975.

606. Paillard, F., R. Ardaillou, H. Malendin, J.-P. Fillastre, S. Prier: Renal effects of salmon calcitonin in man, *J. Lab. Clin. Med.*, **80**:200–216, 1972.

607. Singer, F. R., N. J. Y. Woodhouse, D. K. Parkinson, G. F. Joplin: Some acute effects of administered porcine calcitonin in man, *Clin. Sci.*, **37**:181–190, 1969.

608. Bijvoet, O. L. M., J. van der Sluys Veer, H. R. De Vries, A. T. J. van Koppen: Natriuretic effect of calcitonin in man, *N. Engl. J. Med.*, **284**:681–688, 1971.

609. Barnett, D. B., I. R. Edwards, A. J. Smith: Antagonism by indomethacin of diuretic response to calcitonin in man, *Br. Med. J.*, **468**:686, 1975.

610. Popovtzer, M. M., M. S. Blum, R. S. Flis: Evidence for interference of 25 (OH)vitamin D_3 with phosphaturic action of calcitonin, *Am. J. Physiol.*, **232**:E515–E521, 1977.

611. Haas, H. G., M. A. Dambacher, J. Guncaga, T. Lauffenburger: Renal effects of calcitonin and parathyroid extract in man. Studies in hypoparathyroidism, *J. Clin. Invest.*, **50**:2689–2702, 1971.

612. Bijvoet, O. L. M., P. G. A. M. Froeling: Renal actions of parathyroid hormone and calcitonin, in *Proceedings of Fourth International Congress of Endocrinology 275*, Excerpta Medica, Amsterdam, 1973.

613. Ardaillou, R., J. P. Faillastre, G. Milhaud, F. Rousselet, F. Dalauney, G. Richet: Renal excretion of phosphate, calcium and sodium during and after a prolonged thyrocalcitonin infusion in man, *Proc. Soc. Exp. Biol. Med.*, **131**:56–60, 1969.

614. Queener, S. F., J. W. Fleming, N. H. Bell: Solubilization of calcitonin responsive renal cortical adenylate cyclase, *J. Biol. Chem.*, **250**:7586–7592, 1975.

615. Kuhn, J. M., J. L. Cazor, R. Isaac, M. P. Nivez, R. Ardaillou, J. P. Fillastre: Etude de la production et de l'éxcretion renale d'AMP$_c$ apres perfusion intraveineuse de calcitonine de saumon chez l'homme, *Compt. Rendu. des Seance Soc. Biol.*, **170**:449–455, 1976.

616. Borle, A. B.: Effects of thyrocalcitonin on calcium transport in kidney cells, *Endocrinology*, **85**:194–199, 1969.

617. Hioco, D., P. L. Bordier, L. Miravet, H. Denys, S. Tun-Chot: Prolonged administration of calcitonin in man: Biological, isotopic and morphologic effects, in S. Taylor (ed.), *Calcitonin, 1969*, William Heinemann, Ltd., London, 1970.

618. Caniggia, A., C. Gennari, M. Bencini, V. Palazzuoli, G. Borrello, F. Lenzi: Action of thyrocalcitonin on intestinal absorption of radiophosphate in man, *J. Nucl. Biol. Med.*, **12**:83–85, 1968.

619. Olson, B., Jr., H. F. DeLuca, J. T. Potts, Jr.: Calcitonin inhibition of vitamin D–induced intestinal calcium absorption, *Endocrinology*, **90**:151–157, 1972.

620. Lorenc, R., Y. Tanaka, H. F. DeLuca, G. Jones: Lack of effect of calcitonin on the regulation of vitamin D metabolism in the rat, *Endocrinology*, **100**:468–472, 1977.

621. Sammon, P. J., R. E. Stacey, F. Bronner: Further studies on the role of thyrocalcitonin in calcium homeostasis and metabolism, *Biochem. Med.*, **3**:252–270, 1969.

622. Anast, C. S., R. A. Guthrie: Decreased calcium tolerance in nongoitrous cretins, *Pediatr. Res.*, **5**:668–672, 1971.

623. Wachman, A., D. S. Bernstein: Parathyroid hormone in metabolic acidosis, *Clin. Orthop.*, **69**:252–263, 1970.

624. Coe, F. L., J. J. Firpo, Jr., D. L. Hollandsworth,

L. Segil, J. M. Canterbury, E. Reiss: Effect of acute and chronic metabolic acidosis on serum immunoreactive parathyroid hormone in man, *Kidney Int.,* **8:**262–273, 1975.

625. Barzel, U. S.: Parathyroid hormone, blood phosphorus, and acid-base metabolism, *Lancet,* **1:**1329–1331, 1971.

626. Wills, M. R.: Fundamental physiological role of parathyroid hormone in acid-base homeostasis, *Lancet,* **2:**802–804, 1970.

627. Thomas, W. C., A. M. Lewis, E. D. Bird: Effect of alkali administration on calcium metabolism, *J. Clin. Endocrinol. Metab.,* **27:**1328–1336, 1967.

628. Perault-Staub, A. M., J. F. Staub, G. Milhaud: A new concept of plasma calcium homeostasis in the rat, *Endocrinology,* **96:**480–484, 1974.

629. Perault-Staub, A. M., J. F. Staub, G. Milhaud: Contrasting and rhythmic a dual concept for homeostasis exemplified by 24-hour plasma calcium regulation in the rat, in R. V. Talmage, M. Owen, J. A. Parsons, (eds.), *Calcium Regulating Hormones,* Excerpta Medica, Amsterdam, 1975.

630. Hill, L. F., S. W. Stanbury: Vitamin D and the kidney, *Nephron,* **15:**369–386, 1975.

631. Massry, S. G.: Effect of phosphate depletion in renal tubular transport, in L. V. Avioli, et al. (eds.), *Phosphate Metabolism, Kidney and Bone,* Armour Montague, Paris, 1976.

632. Aschinberg, L. E., L. M. Solomon, P. M. Zeis: Vitamin D resistant rickets associated with epidermal nevus syndrome: Demonstration of a phosphaturic substance in the dermal lesion, *J. Pediatr.,* **91:**56–60, 1970.

9

Radioisotope techniques

WILLIAM H. BLAHD

Radioisotope techniques have an important role in the study of body fluid and electrolyte metabolism. They have been used to define body compartments, pools, and spaces, and to characterize and estimate electrolyte turnover and volume. In recent years, such studies have been accomplished by application of the techniques described by Moore and his coworkers in 1946, in their classic studies on the measurement of total body water and solids by isotope dilution methods (1). By employing these methods, the various parameters of body water and electrolyte composition can be readily determined with minimum patient discomfort.

PRINCIPLE OF ISOTOPE DILUTION

The principle of isotope dilution is based upon the fundamental principle of dilution: the extent to which a tracer substance is diluted in a solvent constitutes a measure of the volume of the solvent. This simple relationship is expressed by the equation

$$V_2 = \frac{C_1 V_1}{C_2} \qquad (9\text{-}1)$$

where C_1 = concentration of tracer before dilution

V_1 = volume of the tracer before dilution
C_2 = concentration after dilution
V_2 = volume after dilution

The concentration and volume of the tracer before dilution are known, and the concentration after dilution is experimentally measured. The equation is then solved for V_2.

In a simple application of this principle, a known quantity of salt is added to a beaker containing an unknown volume of water. The concentration of salt after complete mixing indicates the volume of water in the beaker (Fig. 9-1).

A three-phase curve of decreasing isotope concentration in the body fluids is characteristic of all isotope dilutions (Fig. 9-2). The preequilibration phase is determined by circulation time, membrane permeability, tissue mass, body temperature, and other variables. The equilibration phase, which is used to calculate dilution, is dependent on the volume or mass in which the dilution has taken place. The postequilibration phase is determined by metabolic turnover or exchange with the environment.

It should be remembered, however, that the hu-

ISOTOPE DILUTION PRINCIPLE

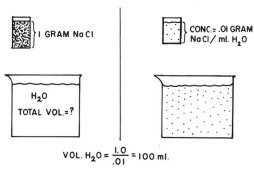

$$VOL. H_2O = \frac{1.0}{.01} = 100 \, ml.$$

Figure 9-1. Example of dilution principle. One gram of NaCl is added to a beaker containing an unknown quantity of water. After complete mixing, a sample is taken which is found to have a concentration 0.1 gram of NaCl. By substituting in the dilution formula the volume of water in the beaker is determined to be 100 mL.

man body, either whole or in part, is not truly analogous to a beaker or tank. It is at all times in dynamic equilibration between liquid and solid phases. It is inhomogenous and multicompartmented. The volume of its compartments may be altered by physiologic changes or disease. In addition, compartmental volume changes may occur when steady-state conditions do not exist, thereby invalidating dilution volume measurements, since such measurements are contingent on the assumption that the subject is in a steady metabolic state during the experimental period.

The validity of dilutional measurements of unknown volumes is also dependent on the injected tracer substance, which must fulfill certain prerequisites: it must be nontoxic; it must mix and equilibrate in the compartment being measured without transfer to another compartment; it must be neither metabolized nor synthesized in the body; the rate of its excretion must be measurable; and it must be available for sampling from the blood or urine and susceptible to precise laboratory measurement. Unfortunately, no tracer substance now used to measure body fluid and electrolyte composition completely fulfills all these requirements. However, the similarity of values obtained by employing multiple tracer substances, as well as comparison with experimental data obtained by direct analytical methods

such as desiccation and tissue sampling, has lent credibility to the results obtained by dilutional measurements.

EXCHANGEABLE MASS

The measurement of body electrolyte mass is closely related to the measurement of body fluid volumes. In measuring total electrolyte, however, the phenomenon of atomic exchange is responsible for the achievement of equilibration from which the dilutional volume is measured and calculated; e.g., radioactive sodium or potassium is diluted by its naturally occurring isotopes within the body. In other words, the mass of a body constituent rather than the volume of a body compartment is measured by this technique.

Some body constituents are in solution and readily equilibrate or exchange with administered tracers. Others are incorporated in muscles, brain, tendons, fascia, bones, and red blood cells and therefore exchange with tracers at varying rates. Because of these variable exchange rates, it is dif-

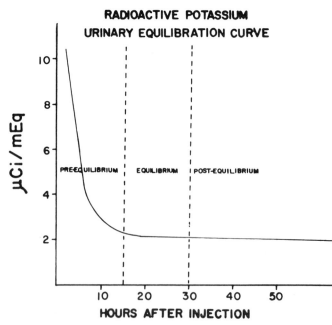

Figure 9-2. Typical three-phase isotope dilution curve.

ficult to obtain a true equilibration value from which to calculate the total body content of any specific constituent. Consequently, the mass, measured by the dilution method, of a body constituent contained in tissues which exchange with the tracer substance slowly or incompletely does not represent total mass but is termed *exchangeable mass*.

SPECIFIC ACTIVITY

Application of the isotope dilution principle to the measurement of the mass of body constituents such as sodium or potassium depends upon the concept of specific activity. Specific activity is a measure of the concentration of radioactivity and is similar to the chemical concept of normality or molarity. It is usually expressed as a ratio—radioactivity per unit weight of stable, or naturally occurring, isotope, e.g., microcuries per milliequivalent:

$$\text{Specific activity} = \frac{\text{radioactive isotope concentration}}{\text{stable isotope concentration}} \quad (9\text{-}2)$$

BODY WATER

The body water may be classified in six main subdivisions: intracellular water and five phases of extracellular water—plasma, interstitial fluid and lymph, connective tissue and cartilage, bone, and transcellular fluid (2). The latter compartment includes a variety of extracellular fluid collections which are not simple transudates of plasma and which have the common property of being formed by the transport activity of secretory cells. These fluids are found in the exocrine glands, the liver and the biliary tree, the kidneys, the eyes, the cerebrospinal fluid, and the gastrointestinal tract. Body water distribution in the normal young adult man is shown in Table 9-1 (3).

A significant difference exists in average body water content of men and women (Table 9-2) (4). After puberty, the mean body water content of men is greater than that of women. This difference persists throughout life and is primarily a consequence of differences in body fat content. Except for a slight increase that occurs in men during adolescence, the percent of body weight which is body water content decreases progressively with age.

The isotopes of water, deuterium (^{2}H) and tritium (^{3}H) oxide, are the tracer substances most frequently employed in the determination of body water by the dilution method. Despite the heavier molecular weight of these compounds, these isotopes behave like ordinary water in the body at low concentrations. The volume of dilution of deuterium and tritium oxide has yielded reliable measures of total body water content in human beings (5). Measurements of body water by desiccation and by tissue sampling techniques compare favorably with results obtained by deuterium and tritium oxide dilution methods. There are no known regions of the body where nonexchangea-

Table 9-1. Body water distribution in a normal young adult man

FLUID	BODY WEIGHT, mL/kg	BODY WEIGHT, %	TOTAL BODY WATER, %
Plasma	45	4.5	7.5
Interstitial fluid and lymph	120	12.0	20.0
Dense connective tissue and cartilage	45	4.5	7.5
Inaccessible bone water	45	4.5	7.5
Transcellular fluid	15	1.5	2.5
Total extracellular water	270	27	45.0
Total intracellular water	330	33	55.0
Total body water	600	60	100.0

Source: After I. S. Edelman.

Table 9-2. Body water compartments: Isotope dilution studies in 20 normal adults

	MEN		WOMEN	
	RANGE	MEAN	RANGE	MEAN
Age, years	23–54	37	23–51	34
Weight, kg	52.7–90.5	72.5	44.5–73.4	59.3
TBW,* L	29.8–50.7	39.0	23.8–31.4	28.5
TBW, %body wt	46.0–59.5	54.3	40.7–55.9	48.6
ECW,† L	14.0–22.8	16.8	11.2–15.2	13.4
ECW, %body wt	20.6–26.6	23.4	19.3–25.6	22.7
ECW, %TBW	39.0–47.0	43.0	44.0–50.0	47.0
ICW,‡ L	15.8–27.9	22.2	12.6–17.4	15.1
ICW, %body wt	25.4–35.9	30.9	20.8–30.3	25.9
ICW, %TBW	53.0–61.1	57.0	50.0–56.0	53.0

* TBW = total body water.
† ECW = extracellular water.
‡ ICW = intracellular water.
Source: After F. D. Moore et al.

ble water exists with respect to the volume of dilution of deuterium or tritium oxide. There is, therefore, a 1:1 correspondence between the volume of dilution of these isotopes and total body water.

Deuterium oxide was first used by von Hevesy and Hofer (6). It is nonradioactive and nontoxic in concentrations below 25%. Deuterium has an atomic mass of 2 and a specific gravity that is about 10 percent greater than that of ordinary water. Although deuterium oxide appears to be the ideal tracer for water, its measurement in body fluids is difficult. The amount of deuterium water which can be injected is small and the dilution factor large; therefore, a relatively small technical error introduces a large error in the final result. Deuterium concentration is usually measured by the densimetric (falling drop technique) or mass spectrometric method. The former technique involves the use of extremely precise and elaborate analytical instrumentation. The latter method requires conversion of deuterium to a gaseous state for analysis.

The accuracy of the deuterium method, despite losses resulting from exchange of deuterium atoms with the labile hydrogen atoms of the solid constituents of the body, mainly proteins, and the difficulties of deuterium analysis, is probably ±1 L of the total body water. In the average adult, a change of less than 1 L of body water is not likely to be biologically significant. The sensitivity of the deuterium method therefore brings it into the realm of clinical usefulness in the management of body fluid and electrolyte disturbances.

Tritium, or radioactive hydrogen with an atomic mass of 3, is widely employed as tritiated water for the measurement of total body water. With the advent of liquid scintillation counting techniques, it has become the method of choice for the determination of body water. This method was first described by Pace and coworkers in 1947 (7). Results with tritium are comparable to those obtained with deuterium. A slight error is also introduced because of exchange with the labile hydrogen atoms of the solid constituents in the body. Tritium has a long half-life of 12.4 years and emits weak beta radiation (0.018 MeV). Tritium is therefore a potential radiation hazard, especially if large numbers of radioactive atoms exchange in the body with labile hydrogen atoms of organic molecules. With the usual dosage levels employed—less than 0.5 millicurie (mCi)—and because of its relatively short biologic half-life of 10 days, the total body radiation dose is well below accepted radiation tolerance levels.

METHODOLOGY (tritium) (Ref. 8)

1. One to two microcuries (μCi) per kilogram of body weight of sterile tritiated water[1] standard solution containing 100 microcuries per milliliter is administered intravenously or orally.
2. Equilibration blood and/or *spot* urine samples are taken after 3 h. In obese or edematous patients, the equilibration time may be prolonged to 6 or 8 h.
3. Five-milliliter samples of serum and/or urine are sublimated by freeze-drying to remove proteins. One-milliliter aliquots of the water so derived are pipetted into counting vials and mixed with 17 to 20 milliliters of scintillation counting solution. All samples are counted together with a diluted aliquot of the tritium standard solution and an internal tritium standard in a liquid scintillation counter.
   a. Internal tritium standard: A commercially available internal tritium standard is employed to determine the counting efficiency of the system.
   b. Liquid scintillation counting solution: Solutions are commercially available, e.g., Biofluor.
4. Calculations:

Total body water, L
$$= \frac{\text{total dose administered, counts/min}}{\text{serum or urine water sample, counts/min/mL}} \times \frac{1}{1000}$$
$$(9\text{-}3)$$

5. Normal ranges: see Table 9-2.

EXTRACELLULAR WATER

Extracellular water constitutes 40 to 45 percent of the total body water. It is, by definition, all water outside the cells. It includes the water of the plasma as well as all other fluids into which ions and small molecules diffuse freely from the plasma. As previously noted, it is composed of five main subcompartments: plasma, interstitial lymph, connective tissue and cartilage, bone, and transcellular fluid (2). These compartments do not behave as a single physiologic unit. The most important extracellular water is plasma and the fluid of other compartments with which it freely exchanges. This physiologically important extracellular water differs from the anatomic extracel-

---

[1] Commercially available in a concentration of 1 mCi/ml.

lular water since it excludes transcellular fluid.

Neither the anatomic nor the physiologic extracellular water can be measured directly; they must be estimated indirectly by the dilution of injected tracer substances. No material has been found which is confined to the physiologic extracellular water compartment. However, since ions and small molecules diffuse rapidly throughout the physiologic extracellular water and relatively slowly into other water compartments of the body, it is possible to make a realistic estimate of the volume of the extracellular water. Estimation of extracellular water is of considerable clinical importance in determining fluid replacement in states of dehydration, since extracellular water is depleted more rapidly in many disease states than is intracellular water.

The volume of the extracellular water can be estimated from the volume of dilution of certain electrolytes and nonelectrolytes. The electrolytes used most often include thiocyanate, sulfate, bromide, and thiosulfate. Among the nonelectrolytes, carbohydrates such as mannitol, inulin, and sucrose have been employed. Inulin and sucrose do not penetrate the connective tissue water, although such water is considered to be a part of the physiologic extracellular water. In addition, inulin is metabolized slowly, so that complete distribution is never reached unless continuous infusion techniques are applied. Most of these carbohydrate agents seem to give similar results, yet they probably underestimate the volume of the extracellular water compartment. In recent years, the radioactive isotopes of sodium, chlorine, bromine, and sulfur have been employed. Sodium 24 was the first radioactive tracer to be used for the determination of extracellular water. Sodium, however, enters the body cells, including those of bone and cartilage, and is therefore not a reliable tracer. More recently, radiosulfate and radiobromide spaces have been used as indices of extracellular water.

Sulfur 35–labeled sulfate equilibrates rapidly within the extracellular water and has a short biologic half-life (9). The disappearance of injected radiosulfate from the plasma is the result of two rates of transfer: the first is completed in 18 to 20 min; the second is a slow exponential which remains unchanged for several hours. It is postulated that the initial rapid disappearance of sulfate represents equilibration with the rapidly circulating extracellular pool that is in dynamic equilibrium with the plasma and that is referred to as the "functional" extracellular water. Reverse extrapolation to zero time of the slow exponential slope of the plasma radioactivity curve yields a volume of extracellular water that is approximately 15 to 19 percent of the body weight (10).

The half-lives of available chlorine isotopes make them unsuitable for human studies: chlorine 36 has a half-life of 4.4×10^5 years, and chlorine 38, 37 min. Furthermore, chloride enters the red cells, pyloric mucosa, salivary glands, and other tissues, so that the space measured is larger than the extracellular volume. However, bromine (as bromide) has essentially the same body distribution as chloride. It is excreted slowly and is not metabolized. Although its volume of distribution is somewhat larger than the extracellular volume, it has proved to be a most useful and reliable tracer for the measurement of extracellular water and is widely accepted (11).

METHODOLOGY (radioactive bromine) (Refs. 12, 13)

1. Two radioactive isotopes of bromine have been employed, [77]Br (half-life, 56 h) and [82]Br (half-life 36 h).
2. Twenty-five microcuries of a sterile solution of sodium bromide—radioactive—is administered intravenously. Radioactive bromine should not be given orally, because of the selectively high concentration of bromide in gastric juice.
3. An equilibrium blood sample is taken at 20 to 24 h. Urine is collected from the time of tracer administration until the time of equilibrium blood sampling.
4. A standard is prepared by diluting an aliquot of the administered dose. The standard, the equilibration serum sample, and an aliquot of the total urine collected are counted in a scintillation well counter.
5. Radioactive bromine volume of distribution is calculated according to the formula[2]

[2] ★Br = radioactive bromine.

$$\star\text{Br volume of distribution} = \frac{\star\text{Br}_i - \star\text{Br}_o}{\star\text{Br}_s} \quad (9\text{-}4)$$

where $\star\text{Br}_i = \star\text{Br}$ injected, μCi
$\star\text{Br}_o = \star\text{Br}$ excreted, μCi
$\star\text{Br}_s = \star\text{Br}/\text{L}$ of serum at equilibrium, μCi

Since bromide enters the red blood cell to a significant extent, the radioactive bromine volume of distribution must be appropriately corrected. The radioactive bromine volume of distribution at 20 to 24 h, corrected for red blood cell bromide concentration, percent of serum volume which is not water, and Donnan effect, is termed *extracellular water*. Corrections are made according to the formula

$$\text{ECW} = \frac{\text{BrV} - \text{PV} - (\text{RCV} \times 0.06)}{1.11} + 0.92\,\text{PV} \quad (9\text{-}5)$$

where ECW = extracellular water, L
BRv = ★Br volume of distribution, L
PV = plasma volume, L
RCV = red cell volume, L

6. Normal ranges: See Table 9-2.

PLASMA AND TOTAL BLOOD VOLUME

The plasma volume represents approximately 7.5 percent of body water and about 18 percent of the extracellular water. Plasma volume can be estimated by measuring the volume of distribution of substances which when injected intravenously are contained largely in the vascular compartment. It is most frequently estimated from the volume of distribution of plasma albumin which has been labeled with radioactive iodine 131 or iodine 125. Since plasma proteins, especially albumin, may escape from the vascular compartment into the lymph and interstitial fluid, this technique may yield inordinately high values, although in normal subjects the actual error is probably less than 5 percent. Plasma volume measurements obtained by these methods are of doubtful validity in patients who have severe burns, ascites, and nephrosis, and in these patients, plasma volume should be derived from the volume of distribution of chromium 51–labeled red cells. The usual limits of plasma volume are 34 to 48 mL/kg body weight, or 1400 to 2000 mL/m² body surface.

Values for the volume of the vascular compartment or the total blood volume vary substantially depending upon the method of determination, ranging from 54 to 80 ml/kg body weight, or 2200 to 3500 ml/m² body surface. The red blood cells usually constitute 42 to 46 percent of the total blood volume. In normal pregnancy, there is an increase in total blood volume with a greater increase in plasma than in red blood cell volume, producing a physiologic decrease in the concentration of red cells and plasma proteins. Primary and secondary polycythemia increase the total blood volume by increasing red cell mass and are usually associated with a normal or sometimes decreased plasma volume. A decrease in total blood volume occurs in hemorrhage, with loss of both plasma and red cells. The plasma volume is quickly restored, however, as water moves from the interstitial compartment to the plasma. Decreased blood volume is also common with water and electrolyte loss, manifested as diarrhea, vomiting, fistulous drainage, excessive sweating, and water restriction.

Radioactive iodinated human serum albumin (^{131}IHSA or ^{125}IHSA) is the tracer most commonly employed for the measurement of plasma volume and total blood volume. Iodination of the albumin molecules does not alter their biologic properties. Once the protein is metabolized, radioactive iodine is excreted, although an insignificant amount is retained by the thyroid. The rate of disappearance of iodinated albumin from the bloodstream is normally 7 to 10 percent per hour, so that within 10 to 15 min of administration the loss is negligible. This rate can vary, however, and in pathologic conditions associated with abnormal albumin loss may be accelerated to 30 percent per hour. In these situations it is advisable to employ radioactive-labeled red cells that will not escape from the vascular system (14).

METHODOLOGY (Ref. 14)

1. Five to ten microcuries of radioiodinated albumin (^{131}IHSA or ^{125}IHSA) is injected into an accessible vein. Commercially available calibrated syringes may be used.

2. A postinjection blood sample is withdrawn at 10 to 15 min from a vein on the opposite limb to avoid contamination. In the presence of shock or severe congestive failure, a longer mixing time is required, and a 20-min venous sample or preferably an arterial sample should be obtained.
3. A standard is prepared by the dilution of an aliquot of the injected radioiodinated albumin.
4. Aliquots of plasma, whole blood, and the standard solution are counted in a scintillation well counter.[3]
5. Calculations:[4]

Plasma volume, mL =

$$\frac{\text{counts/mL standard} \times \text{dilution of standard} \times \text{volume }^{131}\text{IHSA or }^{125}\text{IHSA injected}}{\text{counts/ml postinjection plasma sample}}$$

(9-6)

Whole blood volume, mL =

$$\frac{\text{counts/mL standard} \times \text{dilution of standard} \times \text{volume }^{131}\text{IHSA or }^{125}\text{IHSA injected}}{\text{counts/mL postinjection whole blood sample}}$$

(9-7)

6. Normal ranges:
   Plasma volume:
   Men, 38–48 mL/kg
   Women, 34–44 mL/kg
   Blood volume:
   Men, 64–80 mL/kg
   Women, 54–70 mL/kg

INTRACELLULAR WATER

The volume of the intracellular fluid cannot be measured directly in living subjects but can be calculated as the difference in volume between the extracellular water and the total body water. It is the largest fluid space in the body and represents approximately 55 percent of the total body

---

[3] Semiautomated blood volume computers are available which eliminate preparing standards and simplify the technique.

[4] This method of determination overestimates the whole blood volume by 5 percent as a result of the disparity between the venous and the average body hematocrit, since the ratio of cells to plasma in the vascular system is not constant. There are more cells per unit volume of blood in the peripheral vessels than in the body as a whole.

water. Intracellular water has been estimated from the total amount of body potassium. Since approximately 98 percent of potassium is inside the cells, there should be good correlation between the concentration of whole body potassium and intracellular water (15).

BODY ELECTROLYTES

SODIUM

Measurement of body sodium content may be accomplished by radioisotope dilution. There is a sizable pool of rapidly exchangeable sodium and a smaller pool of slowly exchangeable or probably nonexchangeable sodium, located in the bone. Since bone contains 35 to 40 percent of total body sodium, exchangeable sodium is significantly less than total body quantity.

Following the injection of a tracer dose of radioactive sodium, there is first a rapid disappearance of the tracer from the blood, followed by a slower disappearance phase in 3 to 4 h (Fig. 9-3). Rapid disappearance of radioactive sodium from the blood during the first 30 to 40 min following

injection represents its dilution in the rapidly exchangeable fraction of body sodium, which is primarily extracellular. If an isotope dilution calculation is made during this period, it is possible to estimate the extracellular sodium space (often called simply "sodium space") (16). The later volume of dilution of radioactive sodium between 18 and 24 h, or at 36 h in patients with edema or other disturbances of electrolyte metabolism, is thought to represent penetration of the isotope into the mass of body sodium, principally in bone. After 24 h, there is usually little further exchange. Tissue distribution studies by Forbes and Perley have shown that muscle, skin, kidney, and liver equilibrate rapidly with radioactive sodium within 20 to 60 min (17). Bone and brain, however, are not completely equilibrated at 18 h, although approximately 45 percent of bone sodium will exchange with radioactive sodium during this period. Thus total exchangeable sodium represents about 70 percent of total body sodium.

In contrast to total body water, exchangeable sodium varies little with age and sex (Table 9-3). Edematous patients, i.e., those with liver, kidney, or heart disease, may have 20 to 100 percent in-

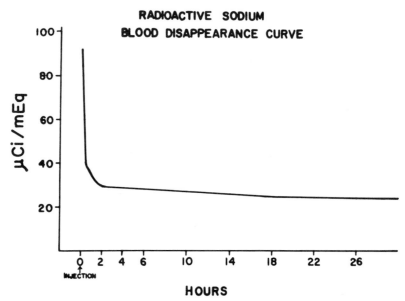

Figure 9-3. Blood radioactivity disappearance curve following the intravenous injection of radioactive sodium.

Table 9-3. Total exchangeable sodium in normal adults

Men			
Age, years	18–33	34–50	51–70
meq/kg body wt	41.4	41.4	40.1
Women			
Age, years	16–33	35–72	
meq/kg body wt	39.2	41.4	

Source: After I. S. Edelman.

creases in total exchangeable sodium. Sodium depletion may occur in some acute disease states, and as much as 20 percent of total body sodium may be lost, mostly from plasma and interstitial fluid. Adrenal cortical insufficiency may be associated with depletion of more than 50 percent of total exchangeable sodium. In such circumstances, there is great distortion of the anatomic relationship between sodium and the various body compartments.

METHODOLOGY (Ref. 17)

1. One to three microcuries per kilogram of body weight of sterile ^{24}Na (half-life, 15.0 h) or ten microcuries ^{22}Na (half-life, 2.6 years)[5] is administered intravenously as sodium chloride. Radioactive sodium may be given orall orally if the patient is fasting.
2. Urine is collected during the subsequent 24-h period. An equilibration blood sample is taken at the end of 24 h.
3. A standard is prepared by diluting an aliquot of the administered dose. The standard, the equilibration serum sample, and an aliquot of the 24-h urine collection are counted in a scintillation well counter. The stable serum sodium concentration is determined by flame photometry.
4. Total exchangeable sodium is calculated according to the following formula:

$$Na_e = \frac{^{24}Na_i - ^{24}Na_o}{^{24}Na_s/^{23}Na_s} \qquad (9\text{-}8)$$

where Na_e = total exchangeable sodium, meq
$^{24}Na_i$ = ^{24}Na injected, μCi
$^{24}Na_o$ = ^{24}Na excreted in the urine prior to equilibrium blood sample, μCi
$^{24}Na_s$ = ^{24}Na in equilibrium serum sample, μCi/L
$^{23}Na_s$ = ^{23}Na in equilibration serum sample, meq/L

[5] Because of its long half-life, sodium 22 is not suitable for repeated use in human beings.

5. Exchangeable sodium may be calculated also from the specific activity of a *spot* urine sample taken at 24 h.
6. Normal ranges: See Table 9-3.

POTASSIUM

The measurement of body potassium content may be accomplished by radioisotope dilution or by means of total body radioactivity counting of naturally occurring potassium 40. The values obtained from the dilution volume of radioactive potassium at 24 h are low because of incomplete exchange of the radioactive tracer with red blood cells, brain, and bone. On the basis of cadaver analyses, total exchangeable potassium at 24 h represents approximately 85 percent of total body potassium (18).

Total body potassium can be measured by whole body counting in a low-level radiation counter which is designed to measure minute quantities of radioactivity in human subjects. The whole body counter is capable of precise measurement of the minute quantity of the naturally occurring radioactive isotope of potassium, potassium 40. Since the isotopic composition of potassium throughout nature is the same irrespective of its source, it is possible to calculate the total body content of potassium from potassium 40 whole body radioactivity. Total body potassium estimations by this method are subject to errors as small as ±5 percent.

Whole body counting methods are most useful for derivation of an average normal total body potassium value from a large group of subjects; in an individual, the random error may be too large for clinical purposes. Only a few acute and chronic disease states manifest deviations of body potassium of such magnitude that they can be measured by the whole body counter. This situation occurs in patients with primary muscle disease, particularly those with muscular dystrophy, and in some unaffected relatives of muscular dystrophy patients (19).

Extensive data have been collected on the body potassium levels of normal subjects. Dependence of body potassium concentrations on age and sex has been well established (Table 9-4) (20). Body mass can be divided into lean and fat portions on

Table 9-4. Total exchangeable potassium in normal adults

Men			
Age, years	18–33	34–50	51–70
meq/kg body wt	48.9	44.9	39.1
Women			
Age, years	16–33	34–81	
meq/kg body wt	37.3	30.9	

Source: After I. S. Edelman.

the basis of body potassium measurements (21). This derivation is important in the study of obesity.

Distortions of body potassium content in disease occur frequently and are often of critical significance. Depletion of total body potassium may result from loss of potassium through the gastrointestinal tract in diarrhea or through the kidney in alkalosis caused by severe vomiting. Depletion may also occur as a result of urinary loss from excessive use of diuretics and adrenal steroids, or from renal disease, such as renal tubular acidosis or chronic pyelonephritis. Potassium is lost primarily from intracellular stores; extracellular potassium concentrations are usually maintained, even though total body potassium is decreased.

METHODOLOGY (Radioactive potassium dilution technique) (Ref. 22)

1. Two radioactive isotopes of potassium have been used in the dilution technique, ^{42}K (half-life 12.5 h) and ^{43}K (half-life 22 h) (12, 24).
2. Two to four microcuries per kilogram of body weight of sterile $*K$ is administered intravenously as potassium chloride.[6] $*K$ may be given orally if the patient is fasting.
3. All urine is collected during the subsequent 24-h period. Since urine specific activity is representative of the mean body specific activity at equilibrium (18 to 24 h), one or more *spot* urine samples are also taken at 24 h.
4. A standard is prepared by diluting an aliquot of the administered dose. The standard, the equilibration spot urine samples, and an aliquot of the total 24-h urine collection are counted in a scintillation well

[6] $*K$ = radioactive potassium.

counter. The stable potassium concentration in the urine spot samples is determined by flame photometry.

5. Total exchangeable potassium is calculated according to the following formula:

$$K_e = \frac{*K_i - *K_o}{*K_u/^{39}K_u} \qquad (9\text{-}9)$$

where K_e = total exchangeable potassium, meq
$*K_i$ = $*K$ administered, μCi
$*K_o$ = $*K$ excreted prior to equilibration urine sample, μCi
$*K_u$ = $*K$ in equilibration urine sample, $\mu Ci/L$
$^{39}K_u$ = ^{39}K in equilibration urine sample, meq/L

6. Normal ranges: See Table 9-4.

MAGNESIUM

The average adult human being has a whole body magnesium content of 21 to 28 g. Magnesium is similar to potassium in its distribution, since it is primarily intracellular. About four-fifths of total body magnesium is present in bone and muscle. Extracellular fluid concentration is approximately 1 percent of total body magnesium.

Following the intravenous administration of a tracer dose of radioactive magnesium (^{28}Mg), there is rapid clearance of radioactivity from the blood during the first 4 h and a more gradual decline up to about 18 h, suggesting that the injected material has equilibrated promptly with stable magnesium in a relatively labile pool and that further exchange occurs very slowly in a less labile pool (23). The size of the labile pool in normal subjects ranges from 135 to 397 meq (2.6 to 5.3 meq/kg body weight) and represents magnesium contained primarily in connective tissue, skin, and the soft tissues of the abdominal cavity. The less labile pool represents magnesium in bone, muscle, and red cells. Since the concentration of body magnesium has been estimated to be 30 meq/kg, it would appear that less than 16 percent of total body content of magnesium is measured by the isotope dilution method.

Computer analyses of magnesium 28 distribution kinetics by Avioli and Berman have confirmed the fact that there are at least three exchangeable magnesium pools with varied rates of turnover (24): a pool with relatively fast turnover, which approximates extracellular fluid in distribution; an intracellular pool containing over 80 percent of exchangeable magnesium, with a turnover which is one-half that of the most rapid pool; and a nonexchangeable or very slowly exchangeable pool representing most of the body magnesium.

METHODOLOGY (Ref. 23)

1. One to one and one-half μCi/kg body weight of sterile ^{28}Mg (half-life, 21.3 h), pH of 4.5 to 5.0, is administered intravenously as magnesium chloride.
2. All urine is collected during the subsequent 24-h period. A 24-h blood sample is drawn.
3. A standard is prepared by diluting an aliquot of the administered dose. The standard, the 24-h serum sample, and an aliquot of the 24-h urine collection are counted in a scintillation well counter. The stable serum magnesium concentration is determined by atomic absorption or fluorometric analysis (25).
4. The 24-h exchangeable magnesium is calculated according to the following formula:

$$Mg_e = \frac{{}^{28}Mg_i - {}^{28}Mg_o}{{}^{28}Mg_s / {}^{24}Mg_s} \qquad (9\text{-}10)$$

where Mg_e = exchangeable magnesium, meq
$^{28}Mg_i$ = ^{28}Mg injected, μCi
$^{28}Mg_o$ = ^{28}Mg excreted at 24 h, μCi
$^{28}Mg_s$ = ^{28}Mg in 24-h serum sample, μCi/L
$^{24}Mg_s$ = ^{24}Mg in 24-h serum sample, meq/L

5. Normal ranges: 2.6 to 5.3 meq/kg.

CALCIUM

Radioisotopes have been used in the study of bone metabolism since the work of Hevesy et al. in 1937 (26). For a long time only the beta-emitting isotopes calcium 45 and phosphorus 32 were available; consequently very few investigations were made in human beings. During the mid-1950s, two gamma-emitting bone mineral tracers, calcium 47 and strontium 85, became available. The gamma rays of these tracers permit the study and assay of calcium 47 and strontium 85 in vivo, and in serum and excreta with standard radiation

detection equipment. Pulse height analysis is required to distinguish between the two isotopes when they are given simultaneously and to differentiate calcium 47 from its daughter isotope scandium 47. Measurement of whole body tracer retention can be accomplished by whole body counting techniques. In addition, regional radioisotope assays can be performed by means of external counting equipment, including automatic scanning devices.

The skeleton does not differentiate between calcium and strontium in tracer amounts, although excretion of strontium is more efficient than that of calcium. Following the intravenous injection of radioactive calcium or strontium, blood radioactivity drops rapidly while the radioactivity in the extravascular fluid reaches a maximum and then drops in parallel with blood radioactivity. Some radioactive tracer is excreted via the kidneys and intestines. Ultimately, a significant portion of the injected tracer will accumulate in bone, especially in areas of active new bone formation (Fig. 9-4). Accumulation of radioactive calcium in bone is due to the exchange of skeletal calcium with circulating calcium. In the

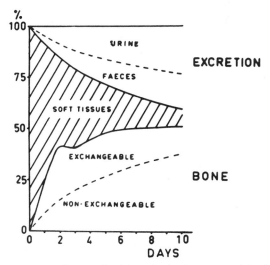

Figure 9-4. Distribution of calcium 47 after intravenous injection in an adult human. [*After G. C. H. Bauer, in W. H. Blahd (ed.), Nuclear Medicine, 2d ed., McGraw-Hill Book Company, New York, 1971, p. 457.*]

adult man, exchangeable calcium of the skeleton represents approximately 0.2 percent of total skeletal calcium.

Analysis of retention, excretion, and blood radioactivity following the injection of radioactive calcium permits the calculation of the amount of exchangeable calcium in the body and the rate at which nonexchangeable bone salt is formed in the skeleton, i.e., the accretion rate. In the normal adult, new bone salt is formed at the rate of about 0.5 g calcium per day, and a corresponding amount is resorbed. The adult skeleton contains between 1000 and 1500 g of calcium, and this is replaced at the rate of approximately 0.05 percent per day. Considerable caution must be exercised in the interpretation of these turnover data, since the rate of turnover varies considerably from area to area within the skeleton. It is higher in the trabecular bone of metaphyses, the vertebrae, and the flat bones of the pelvis than it is in the cortex of long bones.

At present, no accepted model can account for all the data obtained in calcium and strontium tracer studies. Corey et al. have proposed the use of multicompartment models for the precise comparison of studies performed on patients with different calcium excretion rates (27). Marshall believes that the compartmental analysis of calcium tracer kinetics should be supplemented by a method of analysis that treats the body as a continuous system without the assumption of separate pools, such as a power function model (28).

Although there is an extensive literature on the medical applications of calcium tracer kinetics using calcium 47 and strontium 85 (29, 30), the understanding of calcium metabolism is still very limited. There remain numerous problems where the proper application of radioisotope techniques may lead to new and important findings.

CHLORIDE

Total body or total exchangeable chloride has been estimated by the isotope dilution method using bromine 82, chloride 36, chloride 38, or stable bromide as tracers. No regions of nonexchangeable chloride are known. Average values for total exchangeable chloride range from 27.8 to 32.8 meq/kg body weight, or approximately 2100 meq total exchangeable chloride. Total chloride is higher in men. No age-related distribution has been established.

Chloride is predominantly an extracellular ion. Fifty percent of chloride is in the plasma, interstitial fluid, and lymph. Some chloride is present in intracellular fluid, particularly in chloride-secreting cells such as those of the testes, ovaries, gastrointestinal mucosa, and skin. A significant amount of chloride is also found in connective tissue and bone.

Changes in total body chloride content are affected by the same factors and in the same direction as changes in body sodium. In pathologic states, the movement of liquid and electrolytes into the intestine may double or triple the amount of chloride normally found there.

METHODOLOGY

1. Since the half-life of available chlorine isotopes is not suitable for human studies and since chloride and bromide have similar distributions in the body tissues, exchangeable chloride may be calculated from the volume of distribution of radioactive bromide and the stable serum chloride concentration (2):

$$Cl_e = \frac{{}^{\star}Br_i - {}^{\star}Br_o}{{}^{\star}Br_s/{}^{35}Cl_s} \qquad (9\text{-}11)$$

where Cl_e = exchangeable chloride, meq
   ${}^{\star}Br_i$ = ${}^{\star}Br$ injected, μCi
   ${}^{\star}Br_o$ = ${}^{\star}Br$ excreted, μCi
   ${}^{\star}Br_s$ = ${}^{\star}Br$/liter serum, μCi
   ${}^{35}Cl_s$ = ${}^{35}Cl$ in equilibrium serum sample, meq/L

2. Normal range: 27.8 to 32.8 meq/kg.

OTHER ELECTROLYTES

With the possible exception of chloride, suitable radioisotope techniques are not available for the estimation of the anionic electrolytes. Development of techniques for the measurement of bicarbonate, phosphate, and sulfate have been encumbered by the fact that most of the available isotopes are long-lived beta emitters. This property complicates the use of such isotopes in human subjects, since cumbersome and complex assay techniques are required. However, the future availability of gamma-emitting, short-lived carbon 11 (20.5 min) may facilitate studies of the distribution and metabolism of bicarbonate ion.

IN VIVO ACTIVATION ANALYSIS

A technique using whole body neutron activation for the study of the chemical composition of the body has been described (31–33). The technique was developed to measure elements such as calcium that exchange with tracers only to a minor extent. Activation of body elements is achieved by whole body exposure to neutrons from a neutron generator or a cyclotron. Assay of induced body radioactivity is obtained by counting the subject in a whole body counter.

The technique is noninvasive and exposes the subject to a minimal radiation dose (0.28 rem). Although it is an excellent tool for the study of body composition, its application is limited to a few major research centers because of the elaborate and costly facilities required.

REFERENCES

1. Moore, F. D.: Determination of total body water and solids with isotopes, *Science,* **104:**157, 1946.
2. Edelman, I. S., and J. Leibman: Anatomy of body water and electrolytes, *Am. J. Med.,* **27:**256, 1959.
3. Edelman, I. S.: Body water and electrolytes, in J. Brožek and A. Henschel (eds.), *Techniques for Measuring Body Composition,* National Academy of Sciences–National Research Council, Washington, 1961, pp. 140–154.
4. Moore, F. D., et al.: *Body Cell Mass and Its Supporting Environment,* W. B. Saunders Company, Philadelphia, 1963, pp. 532–533.
5. Steele, J. M., E. Y. Berger, M. F. Dunning, and B. B. Brodie: Total body water in man, *Am. J. Physiol.,* **162:**313, 1950.
6. von Hevesy, G., and E. Hofer: Die Verweilzeit des Wassers im Menschlichen Körper, Untersucht mit Hilfe von "Schwerem" Wasser als Indicator, *Klin. Wochenschr.,* **13:**1524, 1934.
7. Pace, N., L. Kline, H. K. Schachman, and M. Harfenist: Studies on body composition. IV. Use of radioactive hydrogen for measurement in vivo of total body water, *J. Biol. Chem.,* **168:**459, 1947.
8. Vaughn, B. E., and E. A. Boling: Rapid assay procedures for tritium-labeled water in body fluids, *J. Lab. Clin. Med.,* **57:**159, 1961.
9. Walser, M., D. W. Seldin, and A. Grollman: An evaluation of radiosulfate for the determination of the volume of extracellular fluid in man and dogs, *J. Clin. Invest.,* **32:**299, 1953.
10. Ryan, R. J., L. R. Pascal, T. Inoye, and L. Bernstein: Experiences with radiosulfate in the estimation of physiologic extracellular water in healthy and abnormal men, *J. Clin. Invest.,* **35:**1119, 1956.
11. Howe, C. T., and R. P. Ekins: The bromide space after the intravenous administration of ^{82}Br, *J. Nucl. Med.,* **4:**469, 1963.
12. Skrabal, F., R. N. Arnot, F. Helus, H. I. Glass, and G. F. Joplin: A method for simultaneous electrolyte investigations in man using ^{77}Br, ^{43}K, and ^{24}Na, *Int. J. Appl. Radiat. Isot.,* **21:**183, 1970.
13. Bauer, F. K.: Radioisotope dilution methods: Measurement of body composition, in W. H. Blahd (ed.), *Nuclear Medicine,* McGraw-Hill Book Company, New York, 1971, pp. 579–581.
14. Albert, S. N.: Blood volume, in W. H. Blahd (ed.), *Nuclear Medicine,* McGraw-Hill Book Company, New York, 1971, pp. 593–619.
15. Novak, L. P.: Total body water in man, in P. E. Bergner and C. C. Lushbaugh (eds.), *Compartments, Pools, and Spaces.* U.S. Atomic Energy Commission, Division of Technical Information, August 1967, pp. 197–216.
16. Kaltreider, N. L., G. R. Meneely, J. R. Allen, and W. F. Bale: Determination of volume of extracellular fluid of body with radioactive sodium, *J. Exp. Med.,* **74:**569, 1941.
17. Forbes, G. B., and A. Perley: Estimation of total body sodium by isotopic dilution. I. Studies on young adults, *J. Clin. Invest.,* **30:**558, 1951.
18. Forbes, G. B., and A. M. Lewis: Total sodium, potassium and chloride in adult man, *J. Clin. Invest.,* **35:**596, 1956.
19. Blahd, W. H., B. Cassen, and M. Lederer: Body

potassium content in patients with muscular dystrophy, *Ann. N.Y. Acad. Sci.,* **110**:282, 1963.

20. Anderson, E. C., and W. H. Langham: Average potassium concentration of the human body as a function of age, *Science,* **130**:713, 1959.

21. Forbes, G. B., J. Gallup, and J. B. Hursh: Estimation of total body fat from potassium-40 content, *Science,* **133**:101, 1961.

22. Corsa, L., Jr., J. M. Olney, Jr., R. W. Steenburg, M. R. Ball, and F. D. Moore: The measurement of exchangeable K in man by isotope dilution, *J Clin. Invest.,* **29**:1280, 1950.

23. Aikawa, J. K.: Magnesium turnover in man, in R. M. Kniseley and W. N. Tauxe (eds.), *Dynamic Clinical Studies with Radioisotopes,* U.S. Atomic Energy Commission, Division of Technical Information, June 1964, pp. 565–579.

24. Avioli, L. V., and M. Berman: Magnesium-28 kinetics in man, *J. Appl. Physiol.,* **21**:1688, 1966.

25. Pruden, E. L., R. Meier, and D. Plaut: Comparison of serum magnesium values by photometric, fluorometric, atomic absorption and flame emission methods, *Clin. Chem.,* **12**:613, 1966.

26. Hevesy, G., J. J. Holst, and A. Krough: Investigations on the exchange of phosphorus in teeth using radioactive phosphorus as indicator, *Kgl. Danske Videnskab. Selskab Biol. Medd.,* **13**:34, 1939.

27. Corey, K. R., D. Weber, M. Merlino, E. Greenberg, P. Kenny, and J. S. Laughlin: Calcium turnover in man, in R. M. Kniseley and W. N. Tauxe (eds.), *Dynamic Clinical Studies with Radioisotopes.* U.S. Atomic Energy Commission, Division of Technical Information, June 1964, pp. 519–536.

28. Marshall, J. H.: Calcium pools and the power function, in P. E. Bergner and C. C. Lushbaugh (eds.), *Compartments, Pools, and Spaces,* U.S. Atomic Energy Commission, Division of Technical Information, August 1967, pp. 451–468.

29. Medical uses of Ca^{47}, *International Atomic Energy Agency Second Panel Rep. Tech. Rep. Ser.,* no. 32, Vienna, 1964 (STI/DOC/10/32).

30. Heaney, R. P.: Evaluation and interpretation of calcium-kinetic data in man, *Clin. Orthop.,* **31**:153, 1964.

31. Chamberlain, M. J., J. H. Fremlin, D. K. Peter, and H. Philip: Total body calcium by whole body neutron activation: New technique for study of bone disease, *Br. Med. J.,* **2**:581, 1968.

32. Palmer, H. E., W. E. Nelp, R. Murano, et al.: The feasibility of in vivo neutron activation analysis of total body calcium and other elements of body composition, *Phys. Med. Biol.,* **13**:269, 1968.

33. Cohn, S. H., A. Vaswani, I. Zanzi, J. F. Aloia, M. S. Roginsky, and K. J. Ellis: Changes in body chemical composition with age measured by total-body neutron activation, *Metabolism,* **25**:85–95, 1976.

10

Total parenteral nutrition and parenteral fluid therapy

JOEL D. KOPPLE / MICHAEL J. BLUMENKRANTZ

SECTION I

Total parenteral nutrition

Total parenteral nutrition (TPN) has decreased mortality, morbidity, and length of convalescence for many diseases and has become an integral part of the recommended therapy for certain illnesses. Two major indications for the use of TPN in attaining and maintaining good nutrition are the inability of patients to receive adequate nutrition through the gastrointestinal (GI) tract and the presence of GI diseases in patients who may benefit from fasting (Table 10-1). Also, it is suggested that in various circumstances TPN can improve recovery and function of certain organs.

A patient's state of nutrition often suffers because food intake is decreased and the stress of illness is catabolic. The prognosis and complications of many diseases may be affected by the state of nutrition. To understand the rationale for TPN, the effects of starvation and physical injury on body nutrition will be briefly reviewed.

EFFECTS OF STARVATION AND PHYSICAL INJURY ON BODY NUTRITION

Energy expenditure can be divided into three types: the basal metabolic expenditure, which in a normal adult may account for 80 percent of en-

ergy consumed each day; energy consumed for the digestion and metabolism of nutrients (the specific dynamic action of foods), which accounts for approximately 8 percent of daily energy ex-

Table 10-1. Indications for total parenteral nutrition

Gastrointestinal disorders
  Mechanical or functional obstruction
  Developmental abnormalities
  Malabsorptive states (short-bowel syndrome)
  Pancreatitis
  Inflammatory bowel disease
  Gastrointestinal fistulas
Hypermetabolic states
  Burns
  Sepsis
  Severe trauma
Other
  Acute renal failure
  Hepatic insufficiency
  Cardiac disorder*
  Psychiatric disturbances (e.g., anorexia nervosa)
  CNS disturbances (e.g., nonterminal coma)
  Malignant disease
  Preparation for surgery (malnourished patients)
  After surgery or any stress which prevents enteral intake of nutrients for more than several days

* Indications are somewhat speculative (see text).

penditure; and physical activity, which in sedentary people accounts for about 12 percent of calories expended each day.

In a healthy individual who is eating normally, carbohydrate and fat are the major sources of energy. Protein catabolism makes a relatively minor contribution to the energy supply, accounting for approximately 15 percent of total calories expended (1). The oxidation of protein and carbohydrates provides approximately 4 kcal/g and oxidation of fat yields about 9 kcal/g.

In early starvation the oxidation of fat provides about 60 percent of the energy consumed (2). There is also a marked breakdown of both protein and glycogen. Approximately 60 to 90 g of protein is degraded a day, primarily from muscle, and this provides about 15 percent of total energy expenditure (1). Oxidation of carbohydrates (glucose and glycogen) accounts for the remaining 25 percent of calories utilized. However, the quantity of carbohydrate available for energy consumption is quite limited. There is probably less than 350 g of glucose and glycogen in a 70-kg man. There is about 10 kg of protein, situated primarily in muscle (3), and during starvation, protein represents a greater source of energy than does carbohydrate. However, protein performs many functions critical to life, and there is a limit to the quantity of protein that may be lost without seriously disrupting metabolic processes. In contrast to a typical man's limited carbohydrate and protein stores, there is approximately 15 kg of fat, primarily as triglyceride (2). Considering its quantity and energy yield and that the major portion is stored as an energy depot, it is obvious that fat represents the main reservoir of energy in the body.

During starvation there is initially a rise in plasma glucagon and then a gradual fall in both insulin and glucagon. The fall in insulin is relatively greater, and the glucagon/insulin ratio remains elevated. Insulin tends to promote anabolic processes, including cellular uptake of glucose, amino acids, and certain minerals and synthesis of glycogen, lipids, and protein. It prevents lipolysis, the release of fatty acids from tissues, and the formation and release of ketone bodies by the liver. With a fall in serum insulin and a relative increase in glucagon, there is increased gluconeogenesis and glycolysis, and fatty acids are mobilized from triglyceride stores in adipose tissue. Fatty acids are converted to ketones, which increase in plasma. As starvation persists over several days, glycogen stores are consumed. Moreover, there are decreased plasma levels of gluconeogenic substrates, principally alanine (4).

During prolonged starvation there is a gradual adjustment in metabolic processes, so that the body maximally utilizes fat and spares carbohydrate and protein. The nervous system is normally a major site where glucose is oxidized completely to carbon dioxide and water. However, with prolonged starvation the brain adapts so as to oxidize ketone bodies, particularly β-hydroxybutyrate and acetoacetate (2, 5). This change spares glucose and decreases dependency on both glycolysis and gluconeogenesis, and fat provides about 80 to 85 percent of energy expended (2).

With prolonged starvation there is also a decrease in the daily metabolic expenditure of energy, which spares carbohydrate, protein, and fats. The adaptive responses of decreased energy expenditure and increased contribution of fat to energy consumption result in a much greater tolerance to starvation in human beings. Hence subjects deprived of food may survive for months. Without these adjustments body stores of carbohydrate and protein would be depleted within weeks to a degree incompatible with life. Since both energy consumption and gluconeogenesis decrease with prolonged fasting, oxidation of protein continues to contribute about 15 percent to the total energy expenditure (1). Patients undergoing extended starvation excrete about 4 to 5 g of nitrogen daily (5). Administration of 100 g of glucose in prolonged starvation will spare protein, and urinary nitrogen may fall to 2 to 3 g a day. Skeletal muscle is the major source of the protein degraded, and certain critical proteins, such as serum immunoglobulins, are relatively spared.

RESPONSE TO PHYSICAL STRESS

Severe physical stress, such as from surgery, infection, or burns, is associated with an increase in the basal metabolic expenditure. Increased energy consumption is related to such factors as altered hormone activity, fever, possibly the release of toxins from pathogens or necrotic tissue, and, in burn patients, heat loss. With physical stress there is an increase in serum insulin, growth hormone, glucagon, cortisol, and catecholamines (6). These changes lead to insulin resistance and enhanced gluconeogenesis, glycolysis, mobilization of fat stores, and oxidation of triglycerides and fatty acids. It has been postulated that enhanced release of amino acids and energy substrates enables the patient to synthesize specific proteins and other compounds and to repair cells and tissues that may be critically needed for the response to stress and for healing (7). In these conditions, the rise in protein catabolism is directly proportional to the rise in basal metabolic energy expenditure (1). Protein continues to contribute approximately 15 to 20 percent to the daily energy requirement. Protein requirements may also be increased because of losses of protein into wounds, inflamed surfaces, or the GI tract. The rise in energy expenditure and protein catabolism is related to the severity of the physical trauma, sepsis, or burn. The basal metabolic rate is also known to increase by approximately 12 percent for each Celsius degree rise in temperature.

Wasting in the physically stressed patient may be markedly enhanced by starvation. If malnutrition is avoided, one may decrease negative nitrogen balance and avoid much of the weight loss and debility which occur after surgery, sepsis, or burns. Indeed, in patients undergoing uncomplicated major abdominal surgery, it may be possible to reverse negative nitrogen balance within 2 to 3 days by providing abundant nutrients (8, 9). However, since the expenditure of energy and protein is typically increased in these conditions, to attain neutral or positive nitrogen balance one may need to increase the energy and protein intake above the patient's usual dietary requirement.

CLINICAL CONSEQUENCES OF POOR NUTRITION

The high prevalence of malnutrition in hospitalized patients is frequently unrecognized (10). Poor nutrition promotes serious complications in the physically injured patient. Weight loss, rate and completeness of wound healing (11), integrity of the immune response, resistance to infection, and surgical mortality rates are adversely affected by malnutrition. Prevention or treatment of malnutrition in sick patients is associated with improved immunologic response and host resistance (12–14). Forty years ago Studley reported that a preoperative weight loss greater than 20 percent was associated with a mortality rate of 33 percent. In contrast, the mortality rate in patients with the same clinical illnesses who had less weight loss was only 3.5 percent (15). Other adverse effects of malnutrition and wasting are prolonged convalescent time and impaired rehabilitation. Since these late consequences of malnutrition are often not apparent until the patient has been discharged from the hospital, they are often overlooked by the physician. Prolonged convalescence caused by poor nutrition may be particularly marked in the elderly or chronically ill patient.

ASSESSMENT OF NUTRITIONAL STATUS

Part of the initial evaluation of the patient should be assessment of nutritional status. Poor nutrition may indicate an increased likelihood of poor response to surgical stress and demonstrate a need for special nutritional therapy. Physical examination of the patient may reveal such signs of malnutrition as muscle atrophy, weakness, decreased adipose tissue, atrophic skin, and changes in hair and nails (16). These signs may be subtle and are often overlooked during a cursory physical examination; a careful search for them may be necessary. Other factors which may indicate undernutrition include steatorrhea, decreased height (in growing patients), low body weight or history of weight loss, anemia, lymphopenia, and decreased serum albumin, phosphorus, and magnesium (17, 18). When available, evaluation of serum transferrin, C_3, retinal-binding protein, carotene, and plasma amino acids (especially the ratios of essential to nonessential amino acids and of valine to glycine) may provide additional information concerning nutritional status (19, 20). A factor of particular importance is the patient's dietary intake. This can be evaluated by interviews and by observing the patient's food intake during hospitalization.

OTHER METHODS OF NUTRITIONAL THERAPY

The maintenance of good nutrition should be a major objective of medical and surgical care. It is easier to maintain good nutritional status than to replete a wasted patient. There are essentially three methods for providing a patient with good nutrition: feeding normal food; administrating nutritional preparations by mouth, feeding tube (21), or alimentary fistula; and giving parenteral nutrition. It is to be emphasized strongly that patients who are not receiving adequate nutrition can often be treated by encouraging them to eat. It is very common for chronically ill, depressed, or elderly patients with well-functioning alimentary tracts to be poorly nourished. Nursing and dietary personnel and family members can often effectively increase the patient's food intake by strongly encouraging or actually feeding him or her. Most patients who will not eat food can be fed with artificial food preparations, including elemental or defined chemical diets (22–24). The latter can frequently be used in patients with GI diseases in whom normal foods may be poorly absorbed, may prevent healing, or may exacerbate the disease process. Patients can also receive nutrition through a feeding tube or esophageal, gastric, or high intestinal fistula. However, a sizable population of patients can be nourished completely only with TPN, and this therapy has been shown to be remarkably effective (25–31).

METHODS OF TOTAL PARENTERAL NUTRITION

TPN should be employed only in patients for whom adequate nutrition cannot be maintained by enteral feeding or for whom such feeding is inadvisable. Parenteral nutrition may also be used to supplement feeding, prepare nutritionally wasted patients for surgery or cancer chemo- or radiation therapy, and treat patients after surgery, physical injury, or infection when there is an in-crease in nutritional requirements or GI malfunction.

Before starting TPN, specific therapeutic goals should be established, such as weight gain, healed wounds, or reestablishment of GI function, so that treatment will not be continued inappropriately. Generally, TPN should not be begun unless it is anticipated that it will be needed for at least 5 to 7 days, as there are major hazards to this therapy. TPN should be replaced by enteral feeding as soon as possible.

ENERGY AND PROTEIN REQUIREMENTS

When planning nutritional therapy, it is important to assess the energy and protein requirements. The energy needs of a nonstressed adult patient living in a hospital are probably similar to the resting metabolic expenditure, about 1900 kcal/day, of a 70-kg man (27 kcal/kg/day). The daily energy requirement will be increased by approximately 10 to 15 percent with uncomplicated major abdominal surgery, 20 percent with major trauma, such as multiple fractures, 50 percent with severe sepsis, such as peritonitis, and 60 to 70 percent or more with major burns (1, 32). The increased energy requirements from stress usually last only a few days. However, with severe stress the requirements may be much greater and last longer.

Both energy and protein requirements should be calculated for the ideal body weight of a patient. The Food and Nutrition Board of the National Research Council has recommended a dietary protein allowance of 0.8 g/kg/day of mixed biologic value protein and 0.6 g/kg/day (42 g/70 kg) of high-quality protein for healthy adults (33). The biologic value of protein is a measure of its utilizability. Animal proteins are generally of higher biologic value. The ratio of essential to nonessential amino acids in solutions for parenteral nutrition is approximately 1:1, and these preparations can be considered of high biologic value. In the stressed or malnourished patient protein requirements may be increased markedly, because of marked catabolism, drainage of wounds or body fluids, blood drawing, and the need for repletion of protein mass. Although, in general, the physically stressed patient should receive a surfeit of protein, restriction of protein may be necessary with hepatic and renal failure (see below).

CHOICE OF NUTRIENTS

There is a risk in proposing standard quantities of nutrients for TPN because of the marked variability in the clinical and metabolic status of patients receiving this therapy. Treatment must be individualized daily for each patient (see discussion of specific diseases). In addition, clinical status, body weight, fluid intake and output, and serum and urinary chemistries will often indicate needed changes in management.

Carbohydrates and alcohols

Dextrose (D-glucose) is the primary carbohydrate used in most TPN solutions. Glucose provides 4.1 kcal/g by in vitro calorimetry, but in vivo, glucose yields 3.75 kcal/g. Moreover, in parenteral solutions, glucose monohydrate is used, which is 91 percent anhydrous glucose and therefore provides only 3.4 kcal/g. Glucose is generally well utilized for energy, and many studies demonstrate that infusions of amino acids and glucose without other carbohydrates, alcohols, or fats can maintain neutral or positive nitrogen balance. Glucose is the closest to ideal carbohydrate available because it is well metabolized by all tissues and stimulates secretion of insulin, the most anabolic hormone. Usually, large quantities of glucose are well tolerated. Surgical stress, sepsis, shock, pancreatitis, uremia, and other conditions that increase catecholamine, glucocorticoid, and glucagon levels can lead to glucose intolerance. Thus, nondiabetic patients can develop hyperglycemia and glycosuria in the postoperative period when given infusions of 5% dextrose (34). Generally, hyperglycemia can be successfully treated by adding crystalline zinc insulin to the infusate, about 1 to 2.5 units per 25 g of glucose. Reactive hypoglycemia may occur if glucose administration is reduced abruptly. The hypertonicity of concentrated glucose solutions can cause thrombophlebitis unless the solution is infused into a large vein.

A number of potential substitutes for glucose have been evaluated, including fructose, sorbitol, xylitol, ethanol, and maltose (35–42). The metabolism of these carbohydrates and alcohols differs from that of glucose and may be semi-independent of insulin. It has been suggested that using these compounds individually or in combination would reduce the need for insulin in states of glucose intolerance, possibly avoiding "overloading" certain metabolic pathways and reducing toxicity. In fact, the metabolism of fructose, sorbitol, and xylitol does require some insulin, and the "insulin-sparing" effects of these carbohydrates have not been an important advantage in clinical use. Moreover, as indicated below, these substances may have clinical toxicity.

After intravenous (IV) infusion, fructose (levulose) is cleared more rapidly from plasma than is glucose, and its urinary excretion is less (43, 44). Fructose may be less irritating to veins than glucose. Fructose has a caloric equivalent of 3.75 kcal/g, and it is phosphorylated to fructose 1-phosphate in the liver and, unlike sorbitol and xylitol, in adipose tissue. Fructose is metabolized by adipose tissue entirely independent of insulin; therefore there is less need for exogenous insulin in the diabetic given fructose as compared with glucose (36). However, if fructose or sorbitol is used in patients with decompensated diabetes, blood glucose will rise (45, 46). With fructose administration, high-energy phosphate and inorganic phosphate become depleted. This results in increased catabolism of adenine nucleotides to uric acid and decreased conversion of lactate to pyruvate (47). Hyperuricemia, increased lactic acid in blood and liver, and a tendency to lactic acidosis occur. Fatal metabolic acidosis has been reported in a child (48). Vacuolization of liver cells and chest pain have also been reported with rapid infusion of fructose. In postoperative patients who received fructose more slowly (0.5 g/kg per h), serum uric acid rose; hyperuricemia was not observed, and the drop in pH and bicarbonate was smaller (49, 50). The formation of lactate from fructose in the liver may be reduced by concomitant infusion of amino acids (51). Fructose should not be administered rapidly and is contraindicated even at lower rates of infusion when lactic or other metabolic acidosis is present or likely such as in hypoxia, hypotension, and diabetic ketoacidosis. Fructose is commercially available in water, polyionic solutions, and protein hydrolysates (Tables 10-3 and 10-13).

Invert sugar is prepared by hydrolyzing sucrose and contains equimolar quantities of glucose and fructose. Because of the method of manufacture, the glucose is not hydrated, and therefore the caloric equivalent of invert sugar is the same as that of fructose (3.75 kcal/g). At similar rates of infusion, considerably less invert sugar than dextrose is lost in the urine. Invert sugar is commercially available in water, saline, polyionic solutions, and protein hydrolysates.

Sorbitol is a hexahydric alcohol which has been extensively used in Europe for parenteral nutrition (38, 41, 52). Unlike glucose or fructose, it will not complex with amino acids in solution to form poorly metabolized glucosamines (see below). Sorbitol is oxidized to fructose in the liver and has the same adverse effects as that sugar. It is not utilized rapidly; hence a relatively large fraction is lost in the urine and can cause osmotic diuresis. When utilized in peritoneal dialysate, it can produce nausea and vomiting, abnormal liver function tests, obtundation, and coma, particularly in diabetic patients (53). Sorbitol is not commercially available for parenteral administration in the United States (54).

Xylitol is a pentiol alcohol which rapidly undergoes glycolysis via the pentose shunt. It has been used in renal failure and other conditions with carbohydrate intolerance and insulin resistance (55). Although formerly it was used in many countries, it has recently been reported to cause metabolic acidosis, hepatic cell injury, hyperuricemia, deposition of calcium oxalate in kidneys, and altered cerebral function (56, 57). Interaction with the 2-mercaptoimidazoline in the rubber stoppers of the infusion bottles has been implicated in xylitol's toxicity (57). Currently xylitol is not recommended for parenteral therapy.

Ethanol provides 7 kcal/g, although all of this energy may not be utilized for normal metabolic functions. It is oxidized by alcohol dehydrogen-

ase to acetaldehyde, which is converted to acetyl-CoA and then enters the tricarboxylic acid cycle. Ethanol has a high calorie/osmotic ratio in solution and produces a mild euphoria. It also produces mild vasodilatation and thus may decrease the incidence of thrombophlebitis at the infusion site (35). Little ethanol is excreted in the urine. Ethanol has toxic effects on the central nervous system, liver, and hematopoietic system and interferes with the action of penicillin (58, 59). Its major uses are probably in temporary situations where a euphoriant effect is desirable, carbohydrate intolerance is present, or high-energy solutions with decreased osmolality are needed. Ethanol is commercially available as a 5% solution in water, with 5% glucose, and in protein hydrolysates (Tables 10-3 and 10-13).

Disaccharides and polysaccharides provide more energy per milliosmole than glucose. Hence, solutions of these carbohydrates are less hypertonic and could be given through a peripheral vein. However, the disaccharides, lactose and sucrose, are poorly utilized when infused IV and are mostly excreted in the urine (60). In contrast, maltose, which is composed of two glucose molecules, appears to be well utilized in rats and humans. After IV infusion of maltose, very little is excreted in the urine, and most is oxidized to CO_2 within 24 h. There are preliminary data indicating that in rats, maltose is poorly tolerated as the sole carbohydrate source. However, other studies indicate successful use of maltose in a variety of patients. In human beings, maltase activity is present in kidney tissue but there is little in serum (42). Hence it is possible that maltose may not be well utilized in patients with advanced renal disease. The metabolism of maltose in diabetes has not been well evaluated. Further studies are necessary to define the potential uses and toxicity of this sugar.

Fats and essential fatty acid deficiency

The advantages of fat solutions include the following: they provide a large quantity of energy relative to their weight and to the volume of solutions; they are present as large particles, so the osmolality is low enough for infusion into low-flow veins, and patients may receive TPN in peripheral veins; they supply the essential fatty acids; they do not present a hyperosmolar load; and they are not lost in urine and do not cause diuresis.

There are three essential fatty acids: linoleic acid, linolenic acid, and arachidonic acid. The last-mentioned can be synthesized in vivo from linoleic acid. When patients receive TPN or synthetic diets free of essential fatty acids, biochemical evidence of essential fatty acid deficiency may develop within 7 days, as evidenced by low levels of plasma linoleic and arachidonic acid (a te-

$$\overset{H}{\underset{|}{}}\overset{H}{\underset{|}{}}$$

traene which has four $-C=C-$ bonds) and increased oleic acid and eicosatrienoic acid (a triene

$$\overset{H}{\underset{|}{}}\overset{H}{\underset{|}{}}$$

which has three $-C=C-$ bonds) (61). Hence the ratio of plasma triene/tetraene (T/T) rises and is a sensitive indicator of essential fatty acid deficiency. Clinical evidence of fatty acid deficiency generally occurs weeks to months later as a characteristic scaly skin eruption, fatty liver with elevated SGOT levels, thrombocytopenia, and hemolysis, possibly related to decreased phospholipids in red cell membranes (62–64). There is some evidence that essential fatty acid deficiency may impair healing of wounds, resistance to infection, utilization of calories, and growth. Manifestation of essential fatty acid deficiency are particularly likely to appear when tissue synthesis is increased, as in premature or newborn infants and children, malnourished or wasted patients, and patients who are hypercatabolic, for example from burns or severe sepsis (65–71).

Although transfusions of plasma and blood can supply some essential fatty acids, they do so inefficiently. The linoleic acid content of 1 mL of Intralipid (see below) is similar to that of 125 mL of stored blood (71). As an alternative to IV lipid, sunflower seed oil and possibly safflower oil applied to the skin may increase serum essential fatty acids (72). Essential fatty acid deficiency may also be prevented by periodically infusing amino acids without carbohydrates (73). (See section, Parenteral Nutrition with Little or No Glucose.)

The IV lipid preparations used in former years

(e.g., Lipomul) often caused fever, dyspnea, thrombocytopenia, defects in coagulation, liver dysfunction, and anemia (74). These complications were probably due to the emulsifying agent, and the lipids were withdrawn from IV use. More recently, soybean oil (Intralipid, Lipofundin S) and cottonseed oil (Lipofundin and Lipophysan) emulsions have become available. Solutions containing soybean lipids, amino acids, and sorbitol or xylitol are also available in Europe (75).

Intralipid is a 10% or 20% emulsion containing in each 1000 mL of solution 100 or 200 g of soybean oil, 12 g of egg yolk phospholipid, and 25 g of glycerol. At present, only the 10% emulsion is available in the United States. The egg yolk phospholipid serves as the emulsifier. The fat in Intralipid is primarily triglycerides, the major lipid in chylomicrons. The 10% Intralipid solution provides 1.1 kcal/mL.

Because 10% and 20% Intralipid are emulsions, osmolality is low, 280 and 330 mosm/kg respectively, and is primarily due to the glycerol present. The mean sizes of the fat particles in 10% and 20% Intralipid are 0.13 and 0.16 μm respectively, and about 99.8 percent of the lipid particles are smaller than 1 μm (75–77). Endogenous chylomicrons are of similar size (mean diameter, 0.096-0.21 μm), and Intralipid appears to be handled similarly in many ways to chylomicrons.

The maximum elimination rate of triglycerides after overnight fasting is 3.8 g/kg per 24 h. The rate is increased by prolonged fasting (76), heparin administration, and in markedly catabolic states (62, 78). In one study, maximum serum triglyceride levels were attained at the end of a 4-h infusion of 10% Intralipid and fell to preinfusion levels within 2 h. Free fatty acid levels were maximal 4 h after the infusion and decreased to basal levels by 6 to 8 h.

The quantity of Intralipid necessary to prevent essential fatty acid deficiency is variably reported to be from 1 to 6 percent of total calories; Jeejeebhoy has recommended a minimum of 25 g/day (79, 80). The discrepancy may be due to individual differences in requirements for maintenance and replacement of essential fatty acids and in criteria for diagnosing deficiency.

The optimum quantity of lipid for TPN is not well defined and may depend on the energy needs.

In patients with severe burns, sepsis, or trauma, it may be difficult to administer the quantity of glucose necessary to provide sufficient calories, particularly because glucose intolerance is common. Lipid solutions may be of special value in these conditions (77, 78), and the 20% emulsion will also provide the needed energy with a smaller water load.

Most investigators recommend that patients receive no more than 40 to 70 percent of total calories from Intralipid (81–83). Some suggest that the distribution among fat, carbohydrate, and amino acids in solutions should be similar to that in the patients' normal diet (i.e., 1.8:5:1 g). Wretlind has suggested proportions of 2 g of fat/2 g of carbohydrate/1 g of amino acids for the usual patient receiving TPN and 3 g of fat/2 g of carbohydrate/1 g of amino acids for the patient with increased energy needs (76, 77). All patients should probably receive no less than 100 g/day of glucose to satisfy the daily glucose requirement and minimize gluconeogenesis.

Some recent reports indicate that in hypercatabolic patients, glucose promotes more positive nitrogen balance than do isocaloric quantities of fat (84, 85). The usual patient requiring TPN, however, is less stressed, and these subjects, particularly when malnourished or fat-depleted, seem well able to utilize lipid infusions to spare nitrogen.

In general, both animals and human beings tolerate infusions of Intralipid for long periods of time with no significant adverse effects except for occasional hypertriglyceridemia. Febrile responses, chills, feelings of warmth, vomiting, and back and chest pains may occur. Impaired liver function occurs rarely in patients receiving Intralipid, although liver biopsies taken after long-term administration of Intralipid show pigment deposition. In animals receiving infusions of Intralipid, microgranulomas in liver are sometimes observed (86). Normal volunteers receiving 500 mL of 10% Intralipid have sometimes developed transient small decreases in pulmonary diffusing capacity. This may be caused by changes in red cell membrane function increased viscosity of blood produced by the lipids, or both and has been prevented by simultaneous administration of heparin (87). Long found no decrease in xenon 133 or carbon monoxide pulmonary diffusion after Intralipid infusion (78). Coagulation is unaffected, and anaphylactic reactions have not been reported.

Lipid emulsions should be administered with caution to patients with primary or secondary hyperlipoproteinemias (i.e., diabetes mellitus) or renal dysfunction (which can impair removal of triglycerides), coagulation disorders, or pulmonary disease.

Amino acids

Amino acids are provided in hydrolysates of casein or fibrin and solutions of free crystalline L-amino acids. Protein hydrolysates tend to be less expensive than the free amino acids. However, the latter may be preferable because hydrolysates contain some peptides that are not well utilized and are excreted in the urine (88). Preparations of free amino acids are reported to maintain slightly more positive nitrogen balance than isonitrogenous quantities of protein hydrolysates (89, 90). There are five commercially available solutions of free L-amino acids in the United States (Table 10-2). Each solution has a high ratio of essential to nonessential amino acids. In general, only L-amino acids are used in these preparations because the D-isomers are less well utilized. Arginine is present in most preparations and may be of particular importance in preventing toxic hyperammonemia when large quantities of amino acids are infused (91). Specific amino acid preparations have also been designed for use in renal and hepatic failure (see below).

Protein hydrolysates currently available are listed in Table 10-3. Certain free amino acids are added to the hydrolysates. However, there is much greater variability in the amino acid composition of these preparations as compared with that of the crystalline amino acid solutions.

Minerals

The daily requirements for water and minerals in patients receiving TPN vary greatly because they may be malnourished, have specific deficiencies

Table 10-2. Approximate composition of amino acid solutions for intravenous use[1]

	AMINOSYN 7%[2]	FREAMINE II 8.5%[3]	NEPHRAMINE 5.35%[3]	VEINAMINE 8%[4]	TRAVASOL 8.5%[5]
Amino acids (mg/dL)					
Essential					
L-Histidine	210	240	none	237	372
L-Isoleucine	510	590	560	493	406
L-Leucine	660	770	880	347	526
L-Lysine[6]	510	870	900	667	492
L-Methionine	280	450[7]	880	427	492
L-Phenylalanine	310	480	880	400	526
L-Threonine	370	340	400	160	356
L-Tryptophan	120	130	200	80	152
L-Valine	560	560	650	253	390
Nonessential					
L-Aspartic acid	none	none		400	none
L-Tyrosine	44	none		none	34
L-Alanine	900	600		none	1760
L-Arginine	690	310		749	880
L-Proline	610	950		107	356
L-Serine	300	500		none	none
L-Glycine	900	1700		3387	1760
L-Cysteine HCl	none	<20		none	none
L-Glutamic acid	none	none		426	none
Electrolytes (meq/L)					
Sodium	—	10	6	—	3
Potassium	5	—	—	—	—
Chloride	—	—	—	—	34
Acetate	88	42	45	50	52
Phosphate	—	20	—	—	—

1. Commercially available in the United States. Data obtained from manufacturers. The usual concentrations of amino acids and electrolytes are those intrinsic to the preparation before addition of dextrose solutions or other substances.
2. Abbott Laboratories, North Chicago, Ill.—also available as 5% and 3.5% with or without added electrolytes
3. McGaw Laboratories, Orange, Calif.
4. Cutter Laboratories, Berkeley, Calif.
5. Baxter-Travenol Laboratories, Deerfield, Ill.—also available as 5.5% with or without added electrolytes
6. Often added as lysine acetate or lysine hydrochloride; "concentrations" refers to the free lysine base.
7. Present as DL-methionine

of certain electrolytes, or sustain excessive losses from urinary excretion, diarrhea, fistula drainage, or gastric aspiration. Also, elderly subjects and patients with impaired heart, liver, and kidney function or certain endocrine disturbances may have decreased tolerance to water or minerals.

The requirement for some minerals will be affected by the volume of solutions administered, particularly for sodium and chloride, which are located primarily extracellularly. In contrast, potassium, phosphorus, and magnesium are incorporated intracellularly; during accretion or loss of protoplasmic mass, requirements for these minerals can increase or decrease. The incorporation or release of calcium, phosphorus, and magnesium from bone can also affect daily needs.

During formation of protoplasm, the ratios of potassium (meq), phosphorus (g), and nitrogen (g) incorporated into tissues is relatively constant, 3:0.07:1 (92), and these relationships persist during TPN (93). There is also a fairly constant ratio of phosphorus (g) to calcium (meq) deposited in bone (0.09) (92). Moreover, during nutritional repletion in wasted patients, there is a constant

Table 10-3. Approximate composition of protein hydrolysate solutions for IV use*

	AMINOSOL 5%†	CUTTER PROTEIN HYDROLYSATE (CPH) 5%‡	HYPROTIGEN 5%§	TRAVAMIN 5%¶
Amino acids, mg/dL				
Essential				
L-Histidine	116	120	119	130
L-Isoleucine	218	240	250	260
L-Leucine	636	415	410	410
L-Lysine	400	350	350	310
L-Methionine	100	220	160	130
L-Phenylalanine	100	230	200	200
L-Threonine	232	180	190	190
L-Tryptophan	50	50	40	35
L-Valine	163	300	300	310
Nonessential				
L-Tyrosine	110	—☆	57	60
L-Alanine		—☆	143	150
L-Arginine	290	—☆	164	180
L-Proline		—☆	602	450
L-Serine		—☆	259	300
L-Glycine	208	2000	93	110
L-Cysteine HCl	30			
L-Glutamic acid			938	1300
L-Aspartic acid			322	350
Electrolytes, meq/L				
Sodium	2	34	25	35
Potassium	17	18	20	19
Calcium	1	6	5	5
Magnesium	2	2	2	2
Chloride	10	14	18	20
Phosphorus	1	14	25	30

* Commercially available in the United States, 1977. The listed concentrations of amino acids and electrolytes are those intrinsic to the preparation before addition of dextrose solutions or additives. Information from the manufacturer. NOTE: Concentrations of nonessential amino acids and electrolytes are not always given in the literature accompanying the product. In addition to the amino acids listed in this table, a large amount of additional amino acids may be present as oligopeptides, possibly up to 40 percent of the total amino acids in the solution.
† Fibrin hydrolysate, Abbott Laboratories.
‡ Casein hydrolysate, Cutter Laboratories (also prepared with 5% dextrose, 6.3% ethanol, and additional electrolytes).
§ Casein hydrolysate, McGaw Laboratories (available with 12.5% fructose, 2.4% ethanol).
¶ Casein hydrolysate, Baxter-Travenol Laboratories (also available as a 10% hydrolysate or prepared with 12.5% fructose, 2.4% ethanol). Same product is marketed as Amigen.
☆ Data not available.

relationship between the increase in extracellular fluid (ECF) (g) and protoplasm (g) of 0.8:1 (93). Rudman and coworkers found that malnourished adults receiving TPN retain nitrogen (g), phosphorus (g), potassium (meq), sodium (meq), and chloride (meq) in ratios of 1:0.08:3.1:3.5:2.7 (93). They also observed that marked deficiencies of one mineral can lead to negative balances for others. Disturbances in mineral metabolism such as hyperaldosteronism, hyperparathyroidism, and

Cushing's disease may affect electrolyte requirements (see Chaps. 14, 19, and 23). During TPN, acid-base disturbances are common because of underlying disorders or infusion of excess chloride. To patients with metabolic acidosis, sodium or potassium acetate may be given. Bicarbonate salts cannot be infused in large amounts because of the formation of insoluble calcium or magnesium carbonate. Patients with metabolic alkalosis, particularly those with large continuing losses of acid, may require more chloride. Chloride can be administered as the sodium or potassium salt, as arginine, lysine, or histidine hydrochloride, and as hydrochloric acid (see Chap. 10B).

During TPN, the daily requirements for minerals may differ from the dietary allowances for oral intake because absorption from the GI tract is incomplete. This is particularly true for calcium, phosphorus, magnesium, iron, zinc, copper, and certain other trace elements.

The daily allowances suggested by different investigators vary greatly because of the variety of clinical disorders in patients receiving TPN and the paucity of studies defining mineral needs with TPN (94–101). A recommended water and mineral intake which can be used in most circumstances in patients with normal ability to regulate mineral and water metabolism is given in Table 10-4.

In general, water intake should be sufficient to allow a urine output of approximately 1500 to 2500 mL/day. Usually, 30 to 50 mL of water per kg daily is adequate. Solutions should contain enough water in excess of sodium salts to prevent hypernatremia. Infusions should be modified according to the clinical condition of the patient and the electrolyte concentrations in plasma, urine, and other outputs. When prescribing minerals, it is important to consider the quantity of electrolytes which are prepared in the amino acids or hydrolysate solutions by the manufacturer. The mineral content of these solutions can vary greatly (Tables 10-2 and 10-3) and may be particularly high for sodium, chloride, potassium, calcium, and phosphorus, in casein hydrolysate. The Aminosyn and Travesol amino acid solutions are also available with sufficient added electrolytes for the needs of many patients. The high concentration of acetate in the amino acid solutions must be taken into account when treating patients with metabolic alkalosis.

Trace elements

There are at least 14 trace elements considered essential for health in mammals. Iron, zinc, copper, manganese, iodine, selenium, chromium, cobalt, and molybdenum have been shown to be essential for human beings. Tin, vanadium, fluorine, silicon, and nickel have not been established as essential for human beings, although they are required by some animals. There are 20 other trace elements for which essentiality has not been excluded (102–104).

There is much concern regarding the occurrence of trace element deficiencies with TPN (105–110). Hankins and coworkers analyzed trace elements in whole blood of eight patients receiving TPN for long periods and found elevated levels of manganese and antimony, low levels of copper, bromine, and rubidium, and near normal levels of zinc, cobalt, selenium, iron, and chromium (111). Although redistribution, increased urinary loss (108, 109), and increased utilization may contribute to lowered plasma trace element levels, the major cause is inadequate quantities in TPN solutions. Several studies indicate that when copper and zinc are not administered during TPN, their concentrations in red cells and plasma fall progressively (107, 109–111). Zinc and copper deficiencies may be of particular importance because these elements are cofactors for many enzymes.

In human beings, zinc deficiency may cause anorexia, impair taste and smell, retard growth and sexual maturation, and impair wound healing (112, 113). Patients receiving TPN with no zinc added have been shown to be in negative zinc balance (109). A zinc deficiency syndrome has been reported during TPN, characterized by diarrhea, mental depression, abdominal pain, an eruption of the skin and oral mucosa with erythema, blisters, and sometimes epidermal necrosis, and alopecia. This syndrome is cured by zinc therapy (109, 112, 114, 115). It resembles the syn-

Table 10-4. Typical composition of solutions for TPN in adults for administration into a large-flow vein[1]

			RDA[5]
Dextrose (D-glucose)	g/L	250[1]	
Amino acids	g/L	42.5[1]	
Energy (approx.)	kcal/L	990[2]	
Electrolytes[3]			
Sodium		35–50	
Potassium		30–40	
Calcium		4–8	
Magnesium	meq/L	4–10	
Phosphate		10–20	
Chloride		25–35	
Acetate		35–40	
Iron		1–4	
Zinc	mg/day	2.5–4.0	
Copper		0.5–1.6	
Other trace elements		4	
Vitamins			
Vitamin A[6]	USP units/day	4000 IU	4000–5000
Vitamin D[6]	USP units/day	400 IU	400
Vitamin K[7]	IU/day	4–10	—[8]
Vitamin E[9]		10	12–15
Niacin		40	12–20
Thiamine HCl (B₁)		5	1–1.5
Riboflavin (B₂)	mg/day	5	1.1–1.8
Pantothenic acid (B₃)		15	5–10[8]
Pyridoxine HCl (B₆)		10	1.6–2
Ascorbic acid (C)		100	45
Biotin		200	150–300[8]
Folic acid[7]		1	0.4
Vitamin B₁₂[7]	μg/day	6	3

1. These nutrients are present in each bottle containing 500 mL of 8.5% crystalline amino acids and 500 ml of 50% dextrose. An exception are the vitamins and trace elements which should be added to only one bottle a day. Typically, 3 L is infused daily.

2. Caloric value of dextrose monohydrate, 3.4 kcal/g; amino acids, 3.5 kcal/g.

3. When adding electrolytes, the amounts intrinsically present in the amino acid or hydrolysate solution should be taken into account (see Tables 10-2 and 10-3).

4. See text.

5. Ranges for nonpregnant nonlactating women and men and boys 11 years or older (33).

6. Quantity may be modified in renal failure.

7. Should be given orally or parenterally and not in solution.

8. RDA is not established; the amounts of pantothenic acid and biotin are considered to be adequate in the usual dietary intake and are listed here.

9. May need to be increased with use of lipid emulsions (see text)

drome of parakeratosis occurring in zinc-deficient swine and acrodermatitis enteropathica, a genetic disorder of zinc deficiency in infants. The fall in plasma zinc levels and the need for zinc may be particularly marked when patients are most anabolic (109).

A copper deficiency syndrome with neutropenia, anemia, and hypoproteinemia which responds to copper therapy has also been reported with TPN (107, 116). Decreased ceruloplasmin may accompany hypocupremia.

Chromium is an integral part of the glucose tolerance factor, which functions as a cofactor for the peripheral action of insulin and is required for the maintenance of normal carbohydrate metabolism in both animals and human beings (102, 104, 117). Chromium deficiency has been reported in a patient receiving long-term TPN and was associated with impaired carbohydrate tolerance (118). Studies in animals have also suggested that carbohydrate tolerance may be impaired with manganese and zinc deficiency, and such mineral deficiencies may contribute to hyperglycemia during TPN.

Human requirements have been established for the oral intake of nine trace elements: iron, zinc, copper, iodide, molybdenum, manganese, selenium, cobalt, and chromium (33). Most trace elements are not absorbed completely from the GI tract, and smaller quantities are probably required for IV nutrition. However, actual studies of trace element requirements during TPN are lacking. Moreover, the effects of disease and poor nutrition on the requirements for these minerals are not defined.

In addition, little is known about the interactions between various trace elements. For example, patients receiving therapeutic doses of zinc may require increased copper. Many trace elements become toxic at high levels, and the difference between toxic and beneficial doses may be small.

Zinc, copper, manganese, calcium, magnesium, and some selenium are present in variable concentrations as contaminants of IV solutions. The rubber stoppers of the IV bottles may be a major source of these elements (121). Jetton and coworkers and Solomon et al. found zinc levels as high as 3 mg/L in IV solutions and point out that variability in concentrations might lead to excessive intake of some trace elements if recommended supplements are added to the infusates (110, 122).

Some workers have suggested that giving plasma, approximately 10 mL/kg at weekly intervals, will provide adequate quantities of trace elements; but infusion of plasma is hazardous and probably will not provide sufficient amounts (107). Shils administers the following quantities IV each day to patients receiving TPN: zinc, 10 mg; copper, 2 mg; manganese, 1 mg; and iodide, 0.28 mg made up in a 5-mL solution (94, 95). Other investigators have suggested different quantities of trace elements (98, 119, 120). Many patients receiving TPN have some GI function, and zinc and copper deficiency has been treated with an oral intake of 40 to 80 mg/day of zinc and 22 mg/day of copper.

Tentative recommendations for daily intake of trace elements in adult patients without marked depletion are as follows: iron, 1 to 4 mg (depending on degree of blood loss and menstruation); zinc, 2.5 to 4 mg; copper, 0.5 to 1.6 mg; manganese, 2 mg; iodine, 120 mg; and chromium, $20\mu g$ (77, 96–101, 118, 120, 121). Their intake should be increased when there are GI losses.

At present there are no trace element preparations for IV use commercially available in the United States. It is anticipated that such preparations will be available in the near future. Solutions of zinc and copper can be prepared by a hospital pharmacist from reagent grade zinc sulfate and cupric chloride dissolved in sterile saline or water for injection and autoclaved and filtered before use.

Vitamins

Vitamins are of critical importance for the metabolism of carbohydrate, fat, protein, and other nutrients. All of the B-complex vitamins function as coenzymes. Thiamin (vitamin B_1) is involved in several steps of carbohydrate metabolism. Riboflavin (vitamin B_2) is contained in two coenzymes, flavin adenine dinucleotide (FAD) and flavin mononucleotide (FMN), which transport electrons and hydrogen in reactions leading to formation of adenosine triphosphate (ATP) and participate in carbohydrate, fat, and amino acid metabolism. Pantothenic acid (vitamin B_3) is a component of coenzyme A. Pyridoxine (vitamin B_6) is particularly important in reactions involving metabolism of amino acids. Niacin is a constituent of nicotinamide adenine dinucleotide (NAD) and nicotinamide adenine dinucleotide phosphate (NADP), which function in hydrogen and electron transport. These are coenzymes for alcohol dehydrogenase and enzymes involved in the Embden-Myerhoff pathway, in a wide variety of cellular processes including respiration and the synthesis of fatty acids. Biotin participates in carboxylation reactions involving cleavage of ATP to adenosine diphosphate (ADP), transference of carboxyl groups essential for fatty acid synthesis, and probably the formulation of carbamyl phosphate, an important step for synthesis of pyrimidines and metabolism of amino acids. Folacin (folic acid) is converted to tetrahydrofolic acid, which is a carrier for single carbon groups. Clinical syndromes of vitamin deficiencies and excesses have been well described in many texts and will not be reviewed here. When there is deficient intake of water-soluble vitamins, manifestations of vitamin deficiency can occur as quickly as within several days to weeks (123–125). In contrast, normal subjects can survive without receiving vitamin B_{12} for 3 to 6 years.

Many patients who need TPN are particularly liable to vitamin deficiency because of chronic underlying illnesses. Diseases of the GI tract, which are common in patients receiving TPN, are often associated with malabsorption of both water-soluble and fat-soluble vitamins and may enhance intestinal losses of B_{12} by interfering with its enterohepatic circulation. Catabolism of pyridoxine may be increased in both liver and renal failure (126). It has been suggested that surgical stress may accelerate the catabolism of ascorbic acid and increase the requirement for this vitamin (127).

Many medicines also promote vitamin deficiencies by causing malabsorption, increased urinary excretion, accelerated degradation, or inhibition of activity. This has been well reviewed by Roe (128). Mineral oil and cholestyramine cause malabsorption of vitamins A, D, and K, and vitamin B_{12} absorption is decreased with this latter drug and with colchicine and paraminosalicyclic acid (PAS) (128). Salicylazosulfapyridine and PAS decrease absorption of folic acid (128). Hydrazides, such as isoniazid, form Schiff bases with pyridoxal phosphate, causing increased excretion of this vitamin. Aspirin may increase urinary excretion of ascorbic acid (129).

Folic acid deficiency may be caused by methotrexate, pyrimethamine, pentamidine, trimethoprim, triamterene, oral contraceptives, diphenylhydantoin, possibly other anticonvulsants, and ethanol. There are reports of increased incidence of seizures when folic acid is administered to epileptic patients receiving anticonvulsant therapy. Drugs which interfere with the actions of vitamin B_6 include isoniazid, hydralazine, iproniazid, cycloserine, pyrazinamide, ethionamide, L- and D-penicillamine, L-dopa, and oral contraceptives. Oral contraceptives may decrease levels of ascorbic acid, riboflavin, and vitamin B_{12}.

Vitamin K deficiency can be produced in patients who are not receiving this vitamin when antibiotics that suppress GI bacteria are administered (130). Drugs such as chloral hydrate, chloramphenicol, clofibrate, phenylbutazone, indomethicin, sulfisoxazole, tolbutamide, and diphenylhydantoin enhance the action of coumarin anticoagulants and increase the antivitamin K effect (128). Barbiturates may enhance enzymatic degradation of coumarin anticoagulants in the liver; when the barbiturate is withdrawn, the anticoagulant effect of the coumarin drugs may increase, causing bleeding. Vitamin D–deficient rickets and osteomalacia have been reported with diphenylhydantoin and barbiturates.

There is preliminary evidence that the daily need for some water-soluble vitamins such as riboflavin and pyridoxine may be greater with TPN because renal excretion is increased (123). Also, excessive carbohydrate or energy intake may increase the need for thiamin and niacin, and the requirement for pyridoxine, riboflavin, and B_{12} may be increased with higher protein intakes (131–133). Conversely, increased tryptophan intake may decrease the requirement for niacin, since approximately 60 mg of this amino acid can be converted to 1 mg of niacin. The requirement for vitamin E, α-tocopherol, is dependent on the intake of polyunsaturated fatty acids. It is suggested that the ratio between dietary intake of α-tocopherol (mg) and polyunsaturated fatty acids (g) should be about 0.4 to 0.6 (33, 134, 135).

There is concern about the potential toxicity of infused vitamins during TPN because the normal safeguards of oral intake are circumvented. It has been questioned whether normal carrier mechanisms for vitamins are operative during IV infusions. The risk of infusing water-soluble vitamins is considered to be relatively small because of their low toxicity and ready excretion in the urine. In contrast, the slower rates of removal of fat-soluble vitamins and the toxicity of excessive vitamins A and D have led workers to be more cautious in the administration of fat-soluble vitamins.

At present, there are few scientific data establishing the vitamin requirements during TPN. A suggested intake for water- and fat-soluble vitamins is given in Table 10-4. Considering the possibly greater requirements for water-soluble vitamins that may occur during TPN, many investigators have suggested a daily intake equal to 1.5 to 3 times the recommended daily allowance (RDA) for normal people (101, 120, 136). Some workers recommend greater amounts of vitamin C, particularly when patients sustain severe physical stress (127), but this has been disputed (136). Large doses of vitamin C may also enhance oxalate formation in some people (137) and possibly impair immune mechanisms (138).

Recommendations for vitamin A and D intake generally call for less than the RDA and range from 2860 to 5000 USP units/day for vitamin A (77, 101, 139, 140) and 100 USP units/week to 500 USP units/day for vitamin D. The requirement for vitamin D in renal failure is increased, in part because of impaired conversion of 25-hydroxycholecalciferol to 1,25-dihydroxycholecalciferol in the diseased kidney (141). Patients with impaired renal function will probably be treated with metabolites of vitamin D when such preparations become commercially available. The suggested dosage of vitamin E also varies widely. Jeejeebhoy and coworkers have recommended about 7 mg/day of α-tocopherol when the intake of polyunsaturated fatty acid is less than 7 g/day and 30 mg for each 500-mL bottle of 10% Intralipid (97, 134).

There are reports of incompatibilities of vitamin K, folate, and vitamin B_{12} in TPN solutions, and these vitamins should probably be given by other routes. They may be given intramuscularly (IM) in the following doses: vitamin K, 4 mg/week; folic acid, 5 mg/twice weekly; vitamin B_{12}, 100 μg/month. Often, patients receiving TPN can take these vitamins orally.

Until vitamin requirements for TPN are better defined, patients receiving long-term therapy with TPN should be evaluated periodically for vitamin excess or depletion.

EXAMPLES OF TPN SOLUTIONS

Typical formulas for TPN solutions are given in Tables 10-4 and 10-5. If IV fat preparations are unavailable or contraindicated, hyperosmolar solutions of glucose and amino acids can be the sole energy sources (Table 10-4). If fat emulsions are available, they may be infused with the hypertonic dextrose and amino acid solutions indicated in Table 10-4 to provide more calories. Alternatively, the energy intake can be kept constant and the glucose concentration reduced. With lower concentrations of glucose, the tonicity of the solutions may be low enough for infusion into a peripheral vein (see below). Table 10-5 illustrates a solution for infusion into a low-flow vein.

ANABOLIC HORMONES AND EXERCISE

In states of severe physical or metabolic stress there often are elevated levels of catabolic hormones that may lead to enhanced gluconeogenesis, glycogenolysis, lipolysis, insulin resistance, and hyperglycemia. Insulin is a potent anabolic hormone and is clearly indicated when there is persistent hyperglycemia. In hypercatabolic states with normal blood glucose, some investigators consider giving insulin for its anabolic effects and administering enough glucose to maintain normoglycemia. Others believe that normoglycemia during TPN with hypertonic glucose indicates that circulating insulin levels are sufficiently high for its anabolic effects and that insulin should be administered only when there is hyperglycemia. Hinton and coworkers infused burn patients with 200 to 600 units/day of insulin and 600 g/day of glucose and found urinary urea excretion to decrease (142).

There are some reports of enhanced anabolism with administration of growth hormone (143). Also, anabolic steroids have been used extensively, especially in patients with renal failure (144, 145). The anabolic effect is only transient;

Table 10-5. Example of an infusate for use with a low-flow vein

	VOLUME	NUTRIENTS	APPROXIMATE ENERGY, KCAL
Amino acids and gluose (Solution 1)			
Crystalline amino acids (7–8.5%)	375	26–32 g	91–112
Dextrose (50%)	100	50 g	170
Additives of minerals & vitamins	25	(see below)	—
Lipid (Solution 2)			
Lipid fat emulsion (10%)	500	50 g	550*
Total	1000		811–832
Electrolytes (added to all bottles of Solution 1)			
Sodium		30–50 meq/L	
Potassium		25–40 meq/L	
Calcium		5–8 meq/L	
Magnesium	meq/L	4–8 meq/L	
Phosphate		10–20 meq/L	
Chloride		20–35 meq/L	
Acetate		30–40 meq/L	

Solution 1 is prepared by mixing 750 mL of 7 to 8.5% crystalline amino acids with 200 mL of 50% dextrose. Because of the relatively long duration of infusion, Solution 1 may be divided into two bottles or bags containing equal volumes (about 500 mL each), and one container is refrigerated until used.

Equal volumes of Solutions 1 and 2 are infused through a "Y" adapter at a constant rate.

These solutions may be administered during each 6-, 8-, or 12-h shift.

Vitamins and trace elements are given as in Table 10-4. They are added to one bottle a day of Solution 1.

Sodium heparin, 1000 IU, is added to each bottle of Solution 1. Osmolality of Solutions 1 and 2, as they enter the vein, is about 900 mosm/L and depends on the quantity of electrolytes (83).

* Some of this represents potential energy from carbohydrates (e.g., glycerol).

however, in wasted or catabolic states there may be benefits to even a temporary enhancement of net protein synthesis or, in patients with acute renal failure, a transient reduction in net urea production. Anabolic steroids are probably ineffective unless appropriate quantities of protein and energy are provided (146).

In patients who are at bed rest, it is suggested that nitrogen balance may be improved with muscle activity. Therefore, patients receiving TPN should undergo planned daily physical exercise whenever possible. The degree to which the sick patient receiving TPN is able to exercise is, of course, variable, and exercise must be carefully designed to meet the specific needs of each patient without exceeding his or her tolerance.

TECHNIQUES OF ADMINISTRATION

When considering TPN, the first step is to establish with certainty the need for it. The incidence of serious complications with TPN is not low, although they may be minimized by meticulous attention to every aspect of this therapy. To minimize complications, it is essential to establish certain policies. First, a committed team of medical workers should be assigned to teach procedures to the medical staff and allied health personnel. Second, the team should establish and disseminate protocols for selection of appropriate nutrients, insertion and maintenance of the catheter and tubing, monitoring of the patient, and control of infection. Examples of such protocols

Table 10-6. Recommendations for placement and maintenance of subclavian catheter and tubing

Placement of Catheter

1. Insertion of the catheter for TPN should be considered a surgical procedure: personnel should wash and should wear gown, mask, and surgical gloves.
2. The skin is shaved, defatted with acetone, and scrubbed with povidone-iodine solution.
3. The patient is placed in a Trendelenburg position to dilate the subclavian vein maximally and to minimize the possibility of air embolism.
4. A local anesthetic is infiltrated into the skin and underlying soft tissue at the junction of the medial and middle third of the clavicle at its inferior border.
5. A 2-in needle is removed from a large radioopaque catheter and attached to a 5-mL syringe. The needle is advanced through the anesthetized area beneath the inferior border of the clavicle. The physician places the fingertips of his free hand firmly in the suprasternal notch, and the needle tip is advanced toward this point.
6. A slightly negative pressure is maintained in the syringe. When the subclavian vein is entered, the patient is asked to hold his breath. The syringe is removed, and the catheter is passed into the superior vena cava. The needle is then removed and the catheter attached to a standard IV administration set connected to a bottle containing an isotonic solution.

7. Verification of the location of the venous catheter is accomplished by lowering the bottle below the patient's chest and observing the backflow of blood.
8. The catheter is sutured to the skin to avoid movement. The entire area is reprepped and povidone-iodine ointment applied to the skin at the exit site of the catheter. A chest x-ray should be obtained immediately to confirm catheter location and to evaluate for pneumothorax. The hypertonic infusate may then be started.

Maintenance of Catheter and Tubing

1. These procedures should be performed only by a physician or nurse trained specifically in techniques of TPN.
2. Cleaning of the catheter and changing of the dressing are performed every 24 to 48 h; IV tubing should be changed daily.
3. Personnel performing catheter maintenance should wash and should wear mask and surgical gloves.
4. The tape and dressing are removed, and gauze pads soaked in acetone are used to scrub loose accumulated debris. Povidone-iodine ointment is applied to the catheter at the cutaneous junction.
5. The dressing is reapplied, using a few 2 × 2 cm sterile gauze pads that are entirely covered with nonporous tape to create an occlusive dressing.

---

are given in Tables 10-6, 10-7, and 10-8. In addition, the team should monitor the therapeutic results and adverse effects of TPN in the patients. The team should be composed of at least one physician, one nurse, a dietitian, and a pharmacist.

Solutions should be prepared by a pharmacist in the "clean" environment of a pharmacy rather than by a busy nurse or doctor on a ward where distractions and microbial contamination are more likely to occur. The pharmacist should be specifically trained in the preparation of TPN solutions. Ideally, fluids should be prepared under a laminar air flow hood, additives injected through a filter, and solutions periodically cultured. Contamination with bacteria or fungi increases when solutions are left standing (147, 148). Moreover, when high concentrations of glucose and amino acids remain in contact for long periods of time, glucosamines may form by the Maillard reaction (149, 150). Glucosamines are particularly likely to form when glucose and amino acid preparations are sterilized by heating.

These compounds are poorly utilized and bind certain trace elements. They are excreted in the urine, and their loss can cause deficiencies of trace elements such as zinc and copper (151). Amino acids may also undergo oxidation in the presence of hypertonic glucose. Solutions should therefore be infused as soon as possible after the glucose and amino acids are mixed. However, storage at 4°C in the dark for up to 48 h is considered safe (150). A single bottle should not be infused for more than 12 h.

A protocol for the placement and day-to-day maintenance of the subclavian catheter and tubing is described in Table 10-6. More detailed protocols have been reported elsewhere (152, 153). Silicone catheters are probably best tolerated; catheters should be radioopaque. The tonicity of solutions containing hypertonic glucose is very high (up to 1600 to 2000 mosm/L), although the use of lipids may allow some reduction in osmotic load. Such solutions must be infused into large-diameter, high-flow veins so that they are diluted by blood and thrombophlebitis will not

Table 10-7. Routine monitoring of the patient receiving TPN

PARAMETER ASSESSED	RECOMMENDED FREQUENCY
Weight	Daily
Fluid intake and output	Daily
Chest x-ray	Initially, to verify central venous catheter placement, then weekly
Temperature	Every 6 h
Urinalysis, urine culture and blood cultures	Initially
Fractional urines for glucose*	Initially after each voiding, then every 6 h
Blood glucose	Initially 2 to 3 times a day, then daily until stable, then twice weekly
Prothrombin time and PTT, serum alkaline phosphatase, glutamic oxaloacetic transaminase, glutamic pyruvic transaminase, bilirubin, total protein, albumin, uric acid, cholesterol, and triglycerides†	Initially, then once weekly
Serum iron and iron-binding capacity	Every 3 weeks
Na, K, Cl, HCO_3, Ca, P, Mg, serum creatinine, and urea nitrogen and complete blood count (observe serum for lipemia)	Daily until stable, then twice weekly
24-h or random urine collections for Na, K, P, and Ca	Daily until stable, then weekly

* In patients with impaired renal function the urine glucose may not reflect the blood sugar and the latter should therefore be monitored more frequently.

† Triglycerides should be monitored more frequently (i.e., daily initially) when lipid emulsions are infused. If no lipid solution is given the triene/tetraene value should be determined about once every two weeks. When fructose or invert sugar is infused, serum lactate should be measured.

NOTE: In the patient receiving long-term ambulatory or home TPN, the frequency of measurements can usually be reduced.

occur. The catheter should not be threaded from a small peripheral vein into a high-flow vein, because thrombophlebitis occurs commonly in the smaller vein within 72 h, possibly because of obstruction to flow or mechanical trauma.

The infusion site of choice is the superior vena cava, with access gained from the subclavian vein. A well-functioning subclavian catheter should usually be changed every 2 to 4 weeks. Other routes of entry should be used only if these veins are unavailable. Other locations for catheterization are the external jugular vein and the vascular access sites used for hemodialysis, including the Quinton-Scribner or Buselmeier arteriovenous shunts and arteriovenous fistulas created from endogenous blood vessels, saphenous veins, or ca-rotid arteries (154–158). These latter access sites may be used for TPN in patients with acute renal failure who require dialysis or for patients with no need for dialysis therapy. In general, the same vascular access should not be used for both long-term maintenance hemodialysis and TPN. For long-term or home TPN, the Broviac right atrial catheter is frequently used (159). The use of femoral veins is associated with a high complication rate. Solutions of low tonicity may be infused into a low-flow peripheral vein (see below).

Most investigators recommend the use of a bacterial filter (160, 161). A 0.45-μm filter will remove particulate contaminants, air bubbles, and most bacteria except for *Pseudomonas*; solutions can still flow by gravity drainage. A 0.22-μm filter

Table 10-8. Guidelines for infection control with total parenteral nutrition*

1. TPN should be administered only when there is a clear indication for such treatment. The need for TPN should be balanced against the significant risks of therapy.
2. TPN should be administered by a team of personnel thoroughly versed in its technique and complications. Such a team should include a nurse, a physician, a dietician and a pharmacist. If possible, a bacteriologist and a physician with an interest in infectious disease should participate.
3. All procedures such as preparation of solutions, placement of catheters, and maintenance of catheters and tubing should be carried out according to well-defined protocols designed to minimize infection.
4. All solutions and additives should be prepared by a pharmacist using aseptic techniques. Ideally, a laminar air flow hood should be employed. The fluid should be used as soon as possible and no later than 48 h after preparation. It should be stored at 4°C until used.
5. With signs of inflammation, thrombosis, or extravasation of fluid, administration of solutions should be discontinued. The catheter and tubing for TPN should not be used to measure central venous pressure, infuse blood, or obtain blood samples. Medications should not be administered through these lines in a "piggy back" manner.
6. Microbial filters are recommended. An 0.22-μm filter excludes virtually all bacteria, including P*seudomonas*, but a pump will usually be necessary to ensure sufficient flow of solutions.
7. If indications of septicemia develop, the IV administration set and solutions should be changed immediately. The infusate and blood from the catheter and peripheral veins should be cultured for bacteria and fungi. Unless another source of infection can be quickly documented, the catheter should be removed and its tip cultured.

* Modified from recommendations of the Hospital Infection Section of the Communicable Disease Center (246)

will block the passage of *Pseudomonas*, but a pump must then be used. An IV pump will deliver nutrients at a controlled rate and may reduce the incidence of thrombosis (161). Care must be taken not to use an infusion device that can pump air. Lipid emulsions should not be infused through bacterial filters. Filters should be changed daily along with all tubing and cultured periodically.

It is generally recommended that fat emulsions not be mixed with other nutrients because these may disturb the stability of the emulsions. They should either be infused through a separate peripheral vein or connected to the dextrose and amino acid solutions with a "Y" adapter. However, Solassol and Joyeux have mixed Intralipid with amino acids, glucose, and other nutrients, and the mixtures are apparently stable at 4°C for at least three months (162). Also, at least two solutions containing lipids, amino acids, and sorbitol or xylitol have been prepared by pharmaceutical firms. The lipid emulsion is less dense than the glucose and amino acid solutions. Hence, if a "Y" adapter is used, the lipid solution should be elevated more than the glucose and amino acid preparation to prevent backflow. During infusion of the fat emulsion, blood drawing for laboratory analyses should be avoided, if possible, as the serum is often lipemic, which may interfere with the measurements.

Usually, on the first day of therapy the patient should receive only 1 L of the hypertonic dextrose and amino acid solution. Patients who have greater water requirements may be given other fluids. The volume infused can be increased gradually over 3 to 5 days to 3 L/day. It has been suggested that lipid emulsions should be infused initially at 1 mL/min for the first day. The quantity of lipids infused may then be increased gradually, depending on the ability of the patient to clear the lipemic serum. Many investigators recommend that patients receive not more than 4 g/kg per day of fat emulsions, although when energy requirements are unusually great others have used larger amounts (76, 78). The infusion rate of Intralipid should not exceed 25 g/h. Heparin stimulates lipoprotein lipase activity, which enhances clearance of triglycerides from plasma. For patients who are hypertriglyceridemic or recieving large doses of emulsified fat, addition of 2500 IU of heparin/100 g of Intralipid may be indicated (76). The routine administration of heparin with Intralipid is not indicated.

Solutions are generally infused continuously in patients who have high energy requirements or are receiving TPN with hypertonic glucose. However, overnight infusions for 12-h periods have been used (see below).

SPECIFIC USES FOR TOTAL PARENTERAL NUTRITION

Although TPN is used in a wide variety of illnesses (Table 10-1), there are certain conditions for which it may have a particular indication or require special formulations.

INTESTINAL FISTULAS

The decrease in morbidity and mortality among patients with intestinal fistulas has been one of the dramatic benefits of TPN. Formerly, intestinal fistulas carried a mortality rate of 40 to 65 percent, and only about 50 percent of surgical closures were successful (163, 164). Deaths associated with intestinal fistulas were usually due to fluid and electrolyte imbalances, malnutrition, or infection. Skin erosion from digestive juices added significantly to the morbidity and impaired the response to surgery. With TPN, these statistics changed radically. In a series of 78 GI fistulas in 62 patients supported with TPN, MacFayden, Dudrick, and Ruberg reported spontaneous closure of fistulas in 75 percent and successful closure in 94 percent of operated patients (165). Others have reported similar results (166, 167, 168).

There are several reasons for this dramatic turnabout with TPN. First, malnutrition is often a very serious complication of intestinal fistulas. Inability to eat, catabolic stress from peritonitis, abdominal abscesses and septicemia, and loss of protein and other nutrients in digestive juices can cause marked wasting with weight losses as high as 1 to 2 kg/day. TPN improves body nutriture and clinical status. Nitrogen balance may become positive in patients with intestinal fistulas who receive TPN (168). In one study, after institution of TPN most patients gained 5 to 25 lb, and serum albumin and total protein became normal (165).

With TPN, enteral intake of nutrients can be completely discontinued. This may be of critical value in patients with fistulas, as it results in marked reduction of alimentary tract secretions (169–171). Hamilton and coworkers gave dogs secretin and pancreozymin and measured gastric and duodenal drainage during infusion of TPN and of lactated Ringer's solution. With TPN, as compared with lactated Ringer's, there was a 50 percent decrease in duodenal fluid, an 86 percent decrease in bile secretion, a 71 percent decrease

in amylase secretion, a 73 percent decrease in duodenal fluid protein content, and an increase in bicarbonate concentration in duodenal fluid of 18 percent (170). Wolfe, Keltner, and Willman studied dogs with enterocutaneous fistulas of the terminal ileum and found reduced loss of fluid, electrolytes, protein, and fat with elemental diets as compared with chow and a further reduction in fistula losses when the dogs were given TPN (171). Hence TPN may decrease fluid and electrolyte losses from fistulas, and since digestive secretion is less, there is less digestive activity in areas of eroded mucosa, fistula tracts, and skin, and fistulas are more likely to close spontaneously.

Before TPN became available, surgical closure was often attempted early. Investigators now feel that surgery should be postponed, because many fistulas heal spontaneously. The likelihood of a fistula's closing spontaneously depends upon its anatomic location and the underlying disease process (166). Even when a fistula is unlikely to close spontaneously, surgery often can be delayed until the patient's nutritional and clinical status has been improved with TPN.

Patients with GI fistulas should generally receive 2000 to 5000 kcal and 80 to 200 g of amino acids a day. Infusions of blood, albumin, and crystalloid, decompression of the bowel by tube, and skin care are also important. TPN is generally begun as soon as possible, even in the presence of sepsis, because of the catabolic status of the patients.

INFLAMMATORY BOWEL DISEASE

Patients with idiopathic inflammatory bowel disease are often malnourished from diminished food intake, bleeding, malabsorption, and protein loss in mucus and purulent exudate. Inflammation and corticosteroids increase wasting (172–174). TPN will improve nutritional status. Moreover, the disease process itself may be ameliorated by avoiding nutrient intake in the GI tract, which stimulates secretions (see above) and may stress the alimentary tract in ways that are poorly defined (175–177).

The response to TPN can depend on the underlying disease. In regional enteritis, enterocutaneous and enteroenteric fistulas may close spontaneously with TPN and cessation of food intake. In one study, surgery was avoided in 70 percent of patients considered to be candidates for operation (177). The best response to TPN was observed in patients who had acute inflammation with segmental involvement, partial bowel obstruction, and no evident scarring or peritonitis. In 16 of 25 prospective surgical patients with granulomatous colitis involving both the small and large intestine, operative procedures were avoided with TPN (177).

When surgery is necessary, TPN may decrease the preoperative and postoperative morbidity and shorten the period of hospitalization and convalescence. It is also suggested that TPN, by reducing inflammation, may allow corticosteroid dosage to be decreased. TPN may also be beneficial when enteritis is complicated by intra-abdominal and perirectal suppuration, short-bowel syndrome, and blind-loop syndrome. Still, early surgery is often of critical importance, particularly when perforation, abscesses, or sepsis are present.

In patients with fulminant ulcerative colitis, TPN does not seem to decrease the need for surgery. However, its use can improve nutritional status and reduce morbidity, mortality, and convalescence time (177). With TPN, patients with ulcerative colitis who would normally require a two-stage colectomy and proctectomy may become healthy enough to tolerate a combined procedure.

Patients with inflammatory bowel disease may have a higher incidence of septic complications with TPN (i.e., 17 percent) than a general population receiving TPN (7 percent) (178). The increased rate of catheter-related septicemia may be due to the use of corticosteroids.

BURNS

Burns may markedly increase the requirements for energy and virtually all nutrients (62, 68, 78, 79, 180). The metabolic rate increases in proportion to the size of the burn area until the latter exceeds 40 to 50 percent of the body surface, after which the metabolic rate remains constant (179).

Weight loss is also proportional to the size of the burn area. With burns exceeding 40 percent of the body surface, weight loss may exceed 20 percent of the initial weight unless vigorous nutritional therapy is instituted. Because of loss of normal integumental function in burns, a disproportionately large amount of energy is expended to maintain body temperature. The metabolic rate is directly related to ambient temperature, and energy expenditure can be reduced by increasing the ambient temperature to at least 25°C (179).

Oral tube feedings can satisfy nutritional requirements in patients with relatively small burn areas. With larger burns, parenteral nutrition may be necessary to satisfy nutritional needs, even in patients who continue to eat. Patients with burns involving more than 40 percent of body surface often require 3000 to 4000 kcal and 15 g of nitrogen (94 g of amino acids) per square meter of body surface per day during the first 10 days of injury. Wilmore et al. have administered up to 8000 kcal/day by combined enteral and parenteral feeding to decrease weight loss and improve wound healing (180). Because water requirements are often increased, the solutions can be made more dilute than in the typical patient receiving TPN.

The increased nitrogen requirement of the burn patient has led some investigators to recommend a high proportion of nitrogen to calories, about 1 g for every 130 kcal (179). Supplementary insulin is often required because of the large quantities of glucose infused and the high circulating levels of insulin-antagonizing hormones, such as catecholamines, glucagon, and corticosteroids.

It is probably best to change the IV catheter every 3 days because of the profusion of bacteria and fungi on the body surface of burn patients and the high incidence of bacteremia and hypercoagulable states.

CANCER

There are several demonstrated and speculative uses for TPN in patients with cancer (181, 182). TPN may prevent or alleviate malnutrition. Cancer results in malnutrition from anorexia, vomiting, diarrhea, interference with normal digestion, and hypercatabolism. Chemotherapy, radiation, surgery, and infections contribute to wasting by enhancing catabolism, decreasing food intake, and interfering with digestion.

Malnutrition is a serious hazard for cancer patients for several reasons. Medical and surgical therapy is often stressful, and marked wasting will often compel a reduction in the intensity of antitumor therapy. Also, when malnutrition is prevented, morbidity may be decreased and convalescence time shortened, which is of particular value for patients with reduced life expectancy. Furthermore, some cancers and many types of cancer therapy cause decreased immune response, which may be hazardous because there is decreased resistance to infection and, possibly, to tumor growth (183). Cell-mediated immunity commonly decreases with malnutrition and may improve with TPN (12, 13). Cancer patients who have skin tests negative to common antigens may develop reactivity after receiving TPN and show an improved response to chemotherapy or radiation (183–185).

It has been suggested that TPN and improved nutrition may accelerate tumor growth (186). However, in growing rats with implanted malignancies, tumor growth is not out of proportion to overall weight gain. Several investigators report improved response to antineoplasia therapy in patients receiving TPN and no augmentation in tumor growth (181, 182).

Immunosuppression in cancer patients has caused concern about a high infection rate with TPN. Copeland and coworkers noted an incidence of only 1.8 percent of catheter-related sepsis among 406 cancer patients receiving TPN for an average of 24 days (182). Special precautions should be taken with tumors of the head, neck, and upper thorax to prevent contamination of the entrance site of the catheter by secretions or draining wounds. Also, the entrance should be placed outside the field of radiation.

It has been suggested that TPN might be used to treat cancer directly (187). Tumor cells may metabolize nutrients differently, and an excess or deficiency of some nutrient might impair tumor growth or increase its susceptibility to chemotherapy. Some reports suggest that tumor size decreases when deficiencies of such nutrients as

amino acids, magnesium, or potassium are created (188–191).

CARDIOVASCULAR DISEASE

Patients with chronic, advanced heart failure are often wasted from multiple causes. One important factor is poor intake caused by anorexia (192). Wasting may be particularly evident in patients with long-standing rheumatic mitral valve disease. Generally, nutritional intake may be improved in such patients without resorting to parenteral therapy. Even patients who have undergone cardiovascular surgery can usually start eating within a short time, so that TPN is not necessary. However, in patients with chronic congestive heart failure, wasting may be so severe as to impair seriously their ability to withstand even minor stress. It has been suggested that nutritional supplements and TPN given to cachetic patients for several weeks before they undergo cardiovascular surgery may reduce morbidity and mortality (193). TPN initiated after cardiovascular surgery in such patients does not seem as beneficial (194, 195). Acute renal failure in these patients is associated with a very high mortality even with TPN (196).

Patients with cardiovascular disease often cannot handle a normal water load; lower volumes of more concentrated solutions are often necessary. The amino acids may be mixed with 70% dextrose, and a diuretic may be administered. Glucose intolerance is common in patients with severe cardiovascular disease, and insulin is often required with TPN. Scrupulous care is particularly important in preventing infection and endocarditis in patients with valvular disease.

TPN may also increase function and survival of cardiac tissue. Under normal conditions, fatty acids are the major energy source of the myocardium. With hypoxia, oxidative phosphorylation decreases, anaerobic glycolysis increases, and glucose becomes the major source of energy (197). When the heart is perfused with either glucose alone or glucose, insulin, and potassium, cardiac glycogen may increase acutely, which improves mechanical function in the isolated anoxic rat heart. Dogs subjected to aortic occlusion or anoxic cardiac arrest who receive infusions of glucose or glucose, potassium, and insulin have better myocardial function than do untreated animals (198, 199).

Pindyck et al. also found that cardiac function improved in critically ill patients after an acute IV infusion of glucose (200). Controlled studies of the effects of such infusions on morbidity and mortality in cardiac patients are clearly necessary before conclusions can be drawn concerning their value (201).

LIVER FAILURE

There are two reasons for administering parenteral nutrition to patients with advanced liver failure. First, these patients often eat poorly and are wasted, and there is evidence that inadequate intake of nutrients promotes liver damage. Second, there is evidence that hepatic encephalopathy may be caused by alterations in the metabolism of certain amino acids (202–204). Patients with chronic cirrhosis of the liver and hepatic encephalopathy have a characteristic plasma amino acid pattern that includes elevated aromatic amino acids (phenylalanine, tyrosine, and tryptophan), increased methionine, and decreased branched chain amino acids (valine, leucine, and isoleucine).

Certain brain neurotransmitters are synthesized from the aromatic amino acids. Tryptophan gives rise to serotonin, and tyrosine is metabolized to dopamine and norepinephrine. In animals with experimental encephalopathy, tryptophan, tyrosine, phenylalanine, serotonin, and false neurotransmitters such as octopamine are increased in the brain, and the catecholamines are decreased (205–208). The increased concentrations of aromatic amino acids, which are probably due to the high ratio of aromatic to branched chain amino acids in plasma, may alter neurotransmitter levels in the brain.

Fischer and coworkers infused glucose solutions containing low concentrations of phenylalanine, tryptophan, and methionine, no tyrosine, and high levels of branched chain amino acids into dogs with hepatic insufficiency. These animals lived longer, with less encephalopathy, than dogs treated with more standard solutions of amino acids or glucose alone (209).

In patients with chronic cirrhosis and hepatic encephalopathy, infusion of Fischer's solution has been associated with improvement in hepatic encephalopathy. The severity of hepatic encephalopathy correlates well with the plasma ratio of the branched chain amino acids to phenylalanine plus tyrosine. As this ratio normalizes with infusion of the amino acid solution, patients become more alert. It is of interest that patients with fulminant viral hepatitis have a different pattern of plasma amino acids, and generally their mentation does not improve with infusion of Fischer's solution.

Although serum ammonia is increased in liver failure, its correlation with encephalopathy has not been established precisely. Nonetheless, keto acid analogues of essential amino acids have been administered in liver failure to "trap" ammonia. The keto acids are aminated, by aminotransferases, forming the corresponding amino acids and binding amino groups that might otherwise be converted to ammonia. Maddrey and coworkers administered four of the essential amino acids (histidine, lysine, threonine, and tryptophan), keto acid analogues of the other five, and arginine to 11 patients with liver failure. The plasma ratio of essential to nonessential amino acids increased, and in 8 of 11 patients, mental function improved. Also, in some patients, arterial blood ammonia decreased (210).

The optimal formulation of amino acids and keto acids for advanced liver failure has not been well defined and is the subject of active investigation. The appropriate intake of other nutrients, such as carbohydrates, fats, and vitamins, must also be determined. Patients with liver failure are often depleted of potassium, magnesium, and phosphorus, and intake of these minerals may need to be increased. Reduced tolerance for sodium and water in liver failure may complicate the use of TPN.

KIDNEY FAILURE

Acute renal failure

Although there have been many advances in the treatment of acute renal failure, the mortality rate remains distressingly high (211, 212). For acute renal failure when associated with major surgery or trauma the mortality rate is about 50 to 70 percent. Patients with acute renal failure are often hypercatabolic and have infection, bleeding, and draining wounds. They may be wasted or malnourished from underlying illnesses and often cannot receive adequate nutrition through the GI tract. Also, the losses of glucose, proteins, amino acids, and water-soluble vitamins during hemodialysis or peritoneal dialysis contribute to wasting (213). Malnutrition may impair wound healing and resistance to infection and may increase mortality (11–14). Two studies indicate that nutritional status may also influence the rate of recovery from acute renal failure (214, 215).

Until recently, the recommended nutritional therapy for acute renal failure was marked or total restriction of protein intake. Small quantities of energy (i.e., 400 to 800 kcal/day) were given as candy or butterballs or IV glucose in order to reduce the rate of protein degradation (216). Dialysis therapy was usually employed only for the specific sequelae of renal failure (i.e., hyperkalemia, acidosis, or congestive heart failure). It is now generally accepted that early and frequent prophylactic dialysis to prevent development of uremic signs and symptoms may decrease morbidity and possibly mortality (217). If patients tolerate food, maintenance of a high intake of primarily high-quality protein (i.e., about 0.5 to 0.6 g/kg per day for a nondialyzed patient and 1 g/kg per day for patients undergoing frequent hemodialysis), energy, and water-soluble vitamins may decrease wasting and improve clinical status.

For patients with acute renal failure who do not tolerate nutrition through the GI tract, TPN may be employed. Experience with TPN in acute renal failure is summarized in Table 10-9. Lee and coworkers administered solutions containing casein hydrolysate, fructose, ethanol, and soya bean oil emulsion (Intralipid) by peripheral vein to patients with acute and chronic renal failure, several of whom were severely ill (218). The investigators reported that there was no marked loss of weight and that convalescence was shortened in these patients. Dudrick et al. infused essential amino acids and hypertonic glucose into the subclavian vein in 10 acutely or chronically uremic patients (219). They reported weight gain, im-

proved wound healing, and stabilization or reduction in blood urea nitrogen (BUN) levels. Serum potassium and phosphorus fell frequently and nitrogen balance was often positive. They also administered essential amino acids and 57% glucose IV to anephric dogs and observed that BUN rose more slowly and that survival was greater as compared with that of animals receiving food or infusions of glucose (5% or 57%) alone (220).

Abel and coworkers treated over 80 patients with acute renal failure with hypertonic glucose and eight essential amino acids, excluding histidine (214, 221–224). They found that serum potassium, phosphorus, and magnesium fell frequently, and BUN remained stable or decreased. These investigators also conducted a prospective double-blind study in 53 patients with acute renal failure who were treated with either a mixture of hypertonic glucose and eight essential amino acids or hypertonic glucose alone (214). The two preparations were isocaloric. Patients who received a mixture of amino acids and glucose lived longer after the episode of renal failure and possibly had a more rapid recovery of renal function. In the patients with more severe renal failure, as indicated by the need for dialysis, and in those with serious complications such as pneumonia, generalized sepsis, or gastrointestinal hemorrhage, survival was significantly greater when amino acids and glucose were infused. However, the hospital mortality was only slightly and not significantly improved in this group.

Leonard, Luke, and Siegel conducted a prospective evaluation of infusions of 1.75% L-essential amino acids and 47% dextrose as compared with 47% dextrose alone (225). Many patients had severe complicating illnesses and most required frequent dialysis. In the group receiving essential amino acids, the BUN rose less rapidly. However, in both groups, nitrogen balance was approximately 10 g/day negative. There was no difference in the rate of survival or recovery of renal function between the two groups.

A comparison of 63 patients with acute renal failure who received a fibrin hydrolysate and hypertonic glucose and 66 patients who were infused with varying quantities of glucose was instituted by Baek and coworkers (226). They found that morbidity and mortality were less in the pa-

Table 10-9. Experience with total parenteral nutrition in acute renal failure

	INFUSATE	NUMBER OF PATIENTS	NITROGEN BALANCE	RATE OF RISE OF BUN	SERUM POTASSIUM	DURATION OF RENAL FAILURE[1]	SURVIVAL FROM ACUTE RENAL FAILURE[2]	OVERALL MORTALITY, %[3]
Dudrick et al. (219)	EAA+G[4]	10[5]	Positive	Stabilized or decreased	Decreased	…	…	…
Abel et al. (214, 221–224)	EAA+G	52	…	Stabilized or decreased	Decreased	…	…	57
	EAA+G as compared with G	53				Decreased	Improved	
Leonard, Luke, Siegel (225)	EAA+G as compared with G	20	10 g/day negative (both groups)	Stabilized or decreased	Stabilized or decreased	No difference	No difference	60
Baek et al. (226)	Fibrin hydrolysate +G as compared with G	129	…	No difference	Stabilized or decreased	…	Improved	58
Blackburn et al. (227)	EAA+G as compared with EAA, NEAA+G or G alone	11	…	No difference	No difference	…	…	…
Sofio & Nicora (228)	EAA+G	192	…	Decreased	Decreased	…	…	60
Abitbol & Holliday (229)	EAA+G as compared with G	6[6]	Positive with EAA+G	Decreased	…	…	…	…
Blumenkrantz et al. (230)	EAA+G as compared with EAA, NEAA+G or G alone	6	Negative (all groups)	No difference	…	No difference	No difference	100

1. Refers to duration of time that patient had acute renal failure.
2. Indicates patients who survived at least until they recovered from acute renal failure.
3. Indicates the percentage of patients who did survive beyond the period of their hospitalization.
4. EAA, essential amino acids; NEAA, nonessential amino acids; G, glucose.
5. Some patients had chronic renal failure.
6. Patients were children, two of whom had chronic renal failure.
Source: After Blumenkrantz et al. (230).

tients receiving the hydrolysate. However, the rise in BUN in the two groups was the same, possibly because of the quantity of nitrogen or nonessential amino acids or peptides in the hydrolysate.

Blackburn and coworkers compared three infusates in a crossover study. Two infusates provided 1550 kcal/L from glucose and either essential amino acids or essential and nonessential amino acids. The third infusate contained 2200 kcal/L from glucose and essential and nonessential amino acids. There was no difference in the rate of rise in BUN and serum potassium with any infusate, but nitrogen balance was less negative with the higher energy intake (227).

The results of treatment with essential amino acids and hypertonic glucose in 192 patients with acute renal failure from 18 centers were reported by Sofio and Nicora (228). BUN rose more slowly, compared with the period before treatment, but there was no effect on recovery of renal function.

Abitbol and Holliday treated six uremic children with IV glucose or glucose, arginine, and essential amino acids (229). Some received both solutions. BUN rose more slowly with glucose and essential amino acids than with glucose alone. Nitrogen balance was positive with the former solution and negative with the latter. Calorie intake was inversely correlated with nitrogen balance. The children were malnourished and their poor nutritional state may have enhanced their response to therapy.

Blumenkrantz and coworkers reported preliminary results of a double-blind study in six patients with acute renal failure who received hypertonic glucose, glucose with 21 g/day of essential amino acids, or glucose with 21 g/day of essential and 21 g/day of nonessential amino acids (230). All infusates were isocaloric. There were no differences in BUN levels, urea appearance rates, or degree of negative nitrogen balances. The similar responses may have been due to the severity of the underlying illnesses and the small sample size.

Differences in the results of the foregoing studies are probably caused by several factors. In some studies, patients were not randomly assigned to different treatment regimens; other studies were conducted retrospectively. Patients were sometimes allowed to eat. The marked variability in the clinical cause of acutely uremic patients is probably also a factor. However, in these studies certain similarities were frequently observed. With infusion of glucose or glucose and essential amino acids, BUN and serum potassium either stabilized or actually decreased. Also, the rise in BUN and potassium was usually less with administration of glucose and essential amino acids as compared with glucose alone. However, the effects of amino acids on recovery of renal function and survival were less conclusive, and mortality was at least 57 to 60 percent, regardless of the composition of the infusates.

The study of Toback on recovery from acute renal failure is pertinent in this regard. He caused acute tubular necrosis in rats by injecting mercuric chloride and then treated the animals with chow or infusion of glucose or essential and nonessential amino acids. The rats receiving IV amino acids had enhanced regeneration of renal cortical cells as indicated by ^{14}C-choline incorporation into phospholipids and lower maximum serum creatinine levels (215).

Several conclusions can be drawn from the current experience with TPN in acute renal failure. First, such patients who are unable to eat have a very high mortality, even with TPN. Second, impaired wound healing, dehiscence, and incidence of infection unrelated to TPN are common and contribute to the high mortality. Third, there is often wasting and markedly negative nitrogen balance, despite the IV administration of 21 to 42 g/day of amino acids. The marked catabolic response in acute renal failure might be decreased by increasing the nitrogen or energy intake, changing the amino acid composition, or giving keto acids or anabolic hormones.

Recommendations concerning TPN in acute renal failure must be considered tentative because of the lack of definitive information. At present, we treat adults with acute renal failure who are unable to eat by infusing about 40 to 42 g/day of approximately equal quantities of essential and nonessential free L-amino acids and 2500 to 3000 kcal, if the water and glucose are tolerated. Although lower quantities (i.e., 12 to 20 g/

day) of essential amino acids may produce less nitrogen waste, we prefer to use those solutions which best nourish the patient and to dialyze as necessary to control uremic symptoms. During an occasional hemodialysis or for each day of peritoneal dialysis, patients are given an additional 40 to 42 g of essential and nonessential amino acids to compensate for amino acid and protein losses during dialysis (213). When patients undergo hemodialysis at frequent intervals (e.g., two to three times a week) they are given about 1 g/kg per day of essential and nonessential acids. Patients with acute renal failure who also have liver failure or for whom dialysis is a particular hazard may be treated with essential amino acids alone.

Chronic renal failure

The chronically uremic patient is also frequently malnourished and wasted from intercurrent illnesses, poor eating (caused by anorexia, associated illnesses, or unpalatable diets), uremic toxicity, increased requirements for certain nutrients, loss of nutrients from dialysis and possibly endocrine disorders (231, 232). When such patients develop intercurrent illnesses, convalescence and rehabilitation are usually slow. Thus, when chronic uremic or dialysis patients become ill and are unable to eat or tolerate tube feeding, early use of TPN may be beneficial.

The chronically uremic patient who is not undergoing maintenance hemodialysis and requires TPN is given about 40 to 42 g/day of essential and nonessential amino acids unless protein losses are excessive. Such patients receive an additional 40 to 42 g for each hemodialysis or each day of peritoneal dialysis. If glucose-free dialysate is used during hemodialysis, 200 g of additional glucose is infused. With dialysate that contains glucose, one may need to reduce the infused glucose to prevent hyperglycemia. When patients undergoing hemodialysis or peritoneal dialysis several times a week require TPN, they are generally given 1 g/kg per day of essential and nonessential amino acids and receive no supplement during dialysis. In some patients, their infusions may increase uremic toxicity or cause overhydration, particularly in those who are hy-

percatabolic, hemodynamically unstable, or have problems with dialysis access. In others, the requirements for amino acids may be even greater. Thus the quantity of amino acids infused should be tailored to individual needs. Insulin may be necessary to control hyperglycemia (see below), particularly during peritoneal dialysis or severe catabolic stress with marked gluconeogenesis.

There is a potential disadvantage to the use of protein hydrolysates as compared with free L-amino acids in renal failure. Peptides in the former solutions are normally excreted in the urine and may accumulate. Also, protein hydrolysates may not be as well utilized as crystalline amino acids (233). Until the metabolic effects of protein hydrolysates in renal failure are better defined, they are probably best avoided. Histidine is an essential amino acid in uremic and normal human beings and should be included in all amino acid preparations (234).

In advanced renal failure many nutritional requirements differ from normal (235, 236). There may be decreased tolerance for sodium, potassium, phosphorus, magnesium, and water. Energy needs may be met in patients who require fluid restriction by adding 70% dextrose to the amino acid solutions. The 20% fat emulsion, where available, will also provide energy in a small volume of fluid. However, uremic patients often have hypertriglyceridemia, and serum triglycerides and cholesterol should be monitored carefully.

When serum electrolyte concentrations are normal and relatively constant, infusion therapy can be started with the following quantities of nutrients: sodium, 50 meq/L; potassium, 35 meq/day; phosphate, 20 meq/day; magnesium, 8 meq/day; and calcium, 10 meq/day. When a serum electrolyte is elevated, it may be prudent not to administer it at the start ot TPN. However, patients must be monitored carefully, as the marked anabolism which often occurs with initiation of TPN may cause serum potassium, phosphorus, or magnesium levels to fall precipitously. We have observed a predialysis serum phosphorus level of 0.5 mg/dL in an anephric patient receiving TPN who inadvertently received no phosphorus. Serum phosphorus is probably best maintained at about

4 meq/L in uremic patients to prevent both phosphate depletion and secondary hyperparathyroidism.

Vitamin A is elevated in chronic renal failure (237), and uremic patients should receive no vitamin A or, at most, only the minimum daily requirement, 4000 and 5000 international units for women and men, respectively. Vitamin D deficiency is common, in part because there is impaired conversion in the kidney of 25-hydroxycholecalciferol to 1,25-dihydroxycholecalciferol (141). 1,25-Dihydroxycholecalciferol should be available for use in the near future. Uremic patients particularly need water-soluble vitamins because the vitamins are lost during dialysis and also may not be metabolized normally (237). Patients with chronic renal failure and those undergoing dialysis should probably have a daily intake of pyridoxine HCl (vitamin B_6), 10 mg; vitamin C, 100 mg; folic acid, 1 mg; and the normal allowances of the other water-soluble vitamins (Table 10-4).

Parenteral nutrition may also be used as a nutritional supplement for patients with acute or chronic renal failure who are malnourished or eat poorly. It is most convenient to administer supplemental IV amino acids during dialysis therapy. Some investigators infuse 20 to 30 g of the nine essential L-amino acids during or near the end of dialysis (238). Patients whose intake of both essential amino acids and total nitrogen is low can be given 40 to 42 g of essential and nonessential amino acids in approximately equal quantities. The amino acids and dextrose, about 200 g, can be infused throughout hemodialysis at a constant rate into the blood leaving the dialyzer. Potassium and phosphorus supplement may also be necessary.

One hazard, reactive hypoglycemia after cessation of the infusion, may be prevented by the following procedures: (1) Infuse the solution at a constant rate throughout the dialysis procedure. (2) Do not stop the infusion before dialysis is completed. (3) Use no more than 200 g of dextrose per dialysis (less if dialysate containing glucose is used). (4) Feed the patient carbohydrate (e.g., two slices of bread) 20 to 30 min before the end of the infusion. Reactive hypoglycemia can also be prevented by administering lower quantities of glucose (5 to 10% dextrose) and adding fat emulsions.

During peritoneal dialysis in normoglycemic patients, about 5 to 18 g of glucose per hour is absorbed when the dialysate contains 1.5% glucose. 25 to 60 g of glucose per hour is absorbed with 4.25% glucose (239, 240). Hence, these patients undergoing peritoneal dialysis can receive amino acid preparations containing smaller quantities of glucose (241).

COMPLICATIONS OF TOTAL PARENTERAL NUTRITION

Although TPN may be lifesaving, complications are frequent and can be fatal. They may be technical, septic, and metabolic (242–244).

TECHNICAL COMPLICATIONS

Most technical complications are related to improper placement of the catheter. These include extravasation of fluid or air into the thorax or mediastinum, injury to the brachial plexus and thoracic duct, penetration or transection of the subclavian artery, and formation of an arteriovenous fistula. Air embolism may occur during insertion of the catheter, during replacement or accidental disruption of the tubing, or when a pump that can infuse air is used (245). It is advisable to have the patient recline when tubing is manipulated and to reinforce all tubing connections with tape.

INFECTIOUS COMPLICATIONS

Infections are a constant risk. Patients who receive TPN often suffer from the following medical conditions predisposing to infection: debility, malnutrition, tissue injury, burns, contaminated wounds, underlying infections, kidney or liver failure, or cancer. They are often receiving broad-spectrum antibiotics, corticosteroids, irradiation, or cancer chemotherapy. These conditions may also mask the usual signs of sepsis. Infection can be minimized only by strict adherence to aseptic techniques and rigid compliance with protocols for infection control (Tables 10-6 to 10-8). In institutions where no uniform protocol is followed, rates of septicemia as high as 27 percent have been reported. However, Goldmann found the incidence of septicemia to be 7 percent in 2078 patients in 31 hospitals using "sound infection control practices" (246). The true rate of infection from TPN may actually be lower, as many infections arise from the underlying illnesses rather than the TPN procedures (247).

Fifty-four percent of TPN-related septicemias are fungal, and *Candida albicans* is the most common pathogen (246). Associated disorders in the patient receiving TPN often predispose to fungal septicemia (see above). Also, *Candida* proliferates more rapidly than most common bacterial pathogens in TPN solutions (248, 249). Moreover, antibacterial ointment containing polymyxin, bacitracin, and neomycin, when applied to the catheter exit site, may predispose to colonization with fungi (250, 251). Growth of bacteria is reported to be enhanced in solutions containing casein or fibrin hydrolysates as compared with those containing free amino acids (252).

METABOLIC COMPLICATIONS

The potential for metabolic complications with TPN is great (Table 10-10), and many of these problems are potentially life-threatening (242, 244). Hyperglycemia is common. Factors predisposing to it include the large glucose load in the infusate, insulin resistance secondary to altered hormone levels in the physically stressed patient, peritoneal dialysis, hypokalemia, increased age, underlying hepatic, renal, pancreatic, or intracranial disease, and possibly trace element deficiencies. Hyperglycemia may cause the hyperosmolar syndrome with dehydration, seizures, coma, and death. Patients may also develop diabetic ketoacidosis. The large glucose load can lead to high serum insulin levels, and sudden cessation of the infusion can result in severe reactive hypoglycemia.

Essential fatty acid deficiency can usually be prevented with infusions of 500 mL of lipid emulsions every 1 to 2 weeks.

Table 10-10. Metabolic complications of total parenteral nutrition

Glucose and fat
  Hyperglycemia*
  Postinfusion hypoglycemia
  Hyperosmolar syndrome
  Ketoacidosis
  Deficiency of essential fatty acids
  Hyperlipidemia
Acid-base and nitrogen
  Metabolic acidosis*
  Hyperammonemia†
  Azotemia*
Fluid and minerals
  Overhydration*–dehydration
  Hypo- hypernatremia*
  Hypo- hyperkalemia*
  Hypo- hyperphosphatemia*
  Hypo- hypermagnesemia*
  Hypo- hypercalcemia
  Trace element deficiency
Vitamins
  Hypervitaminosis A* or D
  Hypovitaminosis D* or K
  Deficiency of the B vitamins,* vitamin C,* and folic acid*
Organ function
  Abnormal liver function

* Particularly prone to occur in patients with impaired renal function
† More likely to occur in patients with liver failure or premature infants

The sulfur-containing amino acids, methionine and cystine, and the hydrochloride salts of amino acids present an acid load to the patient. In patients with impaired ability to excrete acid, such as premature infants, neonates, or patients with renal failure, these infusions have caused acidosis (253, 254). Manufacturers have substituted the free base or acetate salts for the amino acids formerly administered as the hydrochloride, and acidosis is no longer common. Marked alterations in plasma amino acid levels were formerly observed with TPN but are not common with the amino acids now used in infusates, unless liver failure is present (see above). Hyperammonemia may occur, especially in premature infants (255) and patients with severe liver disease. This problem is more likely when protein hydrolysates rather than free amino acids are used, because of the release of ammonia during hydrolysis. Azotemia and uremic toxicity may occur in patients with renal failure who are infused with large quantities of protein hydrolysates or amino acids.

Overhydration and altered serum electrolyte concentrations may occur, particularly in elderly patients, patients undergoing such stress as surgery, and patients with impaired cardiac, hepatic, or renal function. The osmotic effect of hyperglycemia from hypertonic glucose may also lower serum sodium levels by enhancing the extracellular movement of water. Hyperlipidemia from infusion of fat can cause spuriously low serum sodium levels, particularly if blood is drawn while the patient is receiving the lipid IV.

Disorders in serum potassium, phosphorus, and magnesium are particularly likely to occur with TPN. Heart, liver, and kidney failure may impair normal excretion of these minerals. Metabolic acidosis also promotes hyperkalemia. On the other hand, severe deficiencies of potassium, phosphorus, and magnesium may occur with TPN if inadequate quantities are infused. During TPN there are continuing losses of these nutrients, losses that may be greatly increased in certain diseases. Also, TPN promotes anabolism with an intracellular movement of these electrolytes that will further reduce their serum levels. Hypokalemia may cause glucose intolerance. Phosphate depletion may decrease the concentrations of certain intermediary metabolites of the glycolytic pathway and red cell 2,3-diphosphoglycerate (2,3-DPG), a compound which decreases the affinity of red cells for oxygen (256). Low serum phosphorus is also associated with decreased serum phospholipids, and with red cell and brain ATP (257, 258). TPN without adequate phosphorus has been reported to cause phagocytic dysfunction of granulocytes (259), hemolytic anemia (260) with altered platelet Factor 3 weakness, hyperventilation, decreased consciousness, and coma (261–265). Phosphate depletion can also cause marked hypercalciuria and calcium wasting, myopathy, and possibly a fall in cardiac output. Hypomagnesemia can lead to confusion, tremors, seizures, and various other neurologic manifestations, potassium wasting, arrhythmias, and impaired release and action of parathyroid hormone causing refractory hypocalcemia (see Chaps. 8 and 19).

Excessive intake of calcium may cause hypercalcemia (266). Primary or secondary hyperparathyroidism, from such conditions as renal failure or long-standing malabsorption, predisposes to hypercalcemia, especially when serum phosphorus levels are low. Bed rest with mobilization of bone calcium may also lead to hypercalcemia. Vague psychiatric or neuromuscular symptoms or altered consciousness may indicate hypercalcemia. Iron, zinc, copper, chromium, and probably other trace element deficiencies may also occur (see above).

Excessive intake of vitamin A can cause dry skin, headache, blurred vision, nausea, vomiting, and hypoprothrombinemia. Chronic overdosage of vitamin A can cause fatty liver and cirrhosis. Vitamin D intoxication can cause severe, persistent hypercalcemia and soft-tissue calcification. Excessive vitamin K intake can lead to hypoprothrombinemia and, in premature infants, to hemolytic anemia. Large quantities of vitamin C can cause acidosis, particularly in the uremic patient. Deficiencies in water-soluble vitamins are particularly prone to occur because body stores are small, and they are excreted in urine and removed by dialysis (237). In addition, many medications antagonize the effects of certain vitamins, particularly vitamin B_6, vitamin B_{12}, vitamin D, and folic acid (128). Vitamin K deficiency will increase the prothrombin time, and this is more likely to occur in patients who receive antibiotics without vitamin K intake.

In chronic TPN altered liver function with elevated serum glutamic oxaloacetic transaminase may occur. The damage has been ascribed to amino acid imbalance and to excessive deposition of glycogen or fat in the liver (242). Often it can be reversed by decreasing the calorie-to-nitrogen ratio of the infusate.

MONITORING THE PATIENT

The high incidence of potentially dangerous complications with TPN makes careful monitoring mandatory. When TPN is employed, protocols should be established for routine evaluation of patients (Table 10-7). Frequent assessment of the patient is particularly important during the first several days of treatment. Fluid balance must be carefully assessed daily by physical examination and by reviewing intake and output records and body weight. The degree of wasting should also be monitored. In sick patients, changes in body weight often do not reflect altered fat or protoplasmic mass; severely catabolic patients may retain fluid, which can obscure losses of fat and protein.

With unexplained deterioration in a patient's clinical condition, evidence for infection or metabolic disturbance should be sought. An elevation in temperature must be vigorously evaluated. It is not uncommon for uremic, elderly, and chronically ill patients to be hypothermic, and temperatures rising to "normal" in these patients may indicate infection. With clinical deterioration, even in the absence of fever, one should obtain the appropriate specimens for culture, including blood drawn from the catheter (Table 10-8). If there is no obvious source of infection and no metabolic abnormality has been found, the catheter should be removed and the tip cultured.

During the initial stages of therapy, blood glucose levels should be monitored frequently. Urine specimens should be examined for glucose four times daily. Blood glucose should be maintained under 200 mg/dL and ideally should not exceed 140 mg/dL, unless the blood sugar is so labile that careful control is difficult. In general, urine reactions for glucose of 3+ or 4+ require prompt administration of insulin; however, patients with renal failure may have glucosuria with normal blood sugar or elevated blood sugar without glucosuria. Hence, it is important to have an idea of the patient's threshold for glucose. Hyperglycemia may be the initial manifestation of sepsis.

In patients receiving fat emulsions, the serum should be assessed frequently for lipemic appearance and triglycerides, and cholesterol should be measured. This is particularly important with conditions predisposing to lipid intolerance, such as renal failure and diabetes mellitus. When lipid emulsions are not administered, patients should

be evaluated periodically for essential fatty acid deficiency. The serum linoleic acid level and tetraene/triene (T/T) ratio are early indicators of fatty acid deficiency.

Initially, acid-base status should be monitored often, especially in patients with impaired liver or renal function and in premature infants. The volume of blood drawn each day must be carefully monitored, since the quantity removed may cause anemia, particularly in sick patients. Micromethods for laboratory determinations should be used when feasible, particularly for children.

Serum creatinine, urea nitrogen, and electrolytes, including calcium, phosphorus, and magnesium, should be assessed daily until the patient has stabilized. Urinary excretion of water and minerals, particularly potassium and phosphorus, may also be followed to indicate whether intake is inadequate or excessive. In patients with normal renal function not receiving diuretics, excretion of about 40 meq/day of potassium is generally evidence of adequate potassium intake.

Since patients receiving TPN usually defecate infrequently, a comparison of the daily quantity of nitrogen infused and the urinary nitrogen excretion may indicate whether the patient is in positive or negative nitrogen balance. Urea is usually easier to measure than total nitrogen. In patients receiving TPN who do not have significant drainage from fistulas or wounds, total nitrogen output can be estimated by the sum of 1.2 × urinary urea nitrogen (g/day) plus 1 g/day for nitrogen losses from feces and other unmeasured sources. For precise calculation of balance, adjustments must be made for nitrogen losses in feces, wound or fistula drainage, and about 0.4 g/day from routine blood sampling, respiration, and integumentary structures (267).

ALTERNATE METHODS OF PARENTERAL NUTRITION

PARENTERAL NUTRITION WITH LITTLE OR NO GLUCOSE

Blackburn has proposed infusing solutions containing amino acids and no glucose (7, 268). These solutions may be used for patients who are relatively well nourished, not markedly catabolic, and unable to receive adequate nourishment through the alimentary tract for short periods of time. The solutions contain the same high ratio of essential to nonessential amino acids as is used with TPN. Patients usually receive an infusion of 3% amino acids, which is isotonic, although solutions containing up to 5% amino acids have been used. Total intake of amino acids is about 1 to 2 g/kg per day. Minerals and vitamins are given as needed, and lipid emulsions may be administered. Typically, the solutions are infused into a peripheral vein.

This regimen causes marked improvement in nitrogen balance over that in starving patients or those receiving 5% glucose alone (7, 268). With this regimen, nitrogen balance in sick patients is often only 1 to 3 g/day negative and may be positive, particularly when amino acid intake is at least 1.5 to 2 g/kg per day (7, 268–271). In contrast, balance is frequently 8 to 12 g/day negative in similar patients receiving 5% glucose alone (7, 272). Skillman and coworkers reported increased albumin synthesis in postoperative patients receiving a 3.5% amino acid solution as compared with those receiving 5% glucose and no amino acids (273).

Parenteral therapy with amino acids and no glucose can markedly reduce protein losses in catabolic or starving patients who would otherwise receive 5% glucose as the sole source of energy or protein, and it has several advantages over TPN. The treatment is less hazardous as compared with TPN, which must be administered into a high-flow blood vessel and is associated with substantial risks (see below). In comparison with TPN, the regimen is much less expensive and less time-consuming for the medical staff. Since there is less risk, expense, and time required for preparation of infusates, there is no delay in starting treatment, and the infusion can be initiated immediately after surgery. In contrast, TPN is generally recommended only if patients are malnourished or when it is anticipated that they will not receive adequate enteral nutrition for at least several days. In practice TPN is often not initiated until a patient has starved for many days. Also, since with this regimen triglycerides

are mobilized from adipose tissue, signs of essential fatty acid deficiency are less likely to occur (73). This is in contrast to the results with TPN when amino acids, glucose, and no lipid emulsions are used (65, 66, 70).

There are also disadvantages to the administration of amino acids with no glucose. This therapy usually does not promote as positive a nitrogen balance as does TPN, and although it will maintain protein mass with relatively small losses, it generally does not replete protein in patients who are wasted. Patients are glycogen-depleted and continue to consume fat to provide energy. The solution will not meet the increased energy and amino acid requirements of hypercatabolic patients, who can become very wasted with this therapy. Since large quantities of amino acids (1.5 to 2 g/kg per day) are necessary for neutral or positive nitrogen balance, urea or ammonia production is high, and this regimen may be hazardous to patients with renal or liver failure.

It is not clear why infusions of amino acids promote more protein sparing than do isocaloric quantities of glucose. Blackburn et al. have ascribed this effect to the absence of glucose, which leads to hypoinsulinemia and elevated ketone bodies and fatty acids in plasma (7, 268). These investigators suggest that the oxidation of ketone bodies and fatty acids by muscle and other tissues decreases catabolism of amino acids for energy. The infused amino acids thus become available for protein peptide synthesis. The investigators consider that administration of small quantities of glucose (i.e., 5 to 10% dextrose) increase serum insulin, which inhibits lipolysis and reduces ketogenesis but does not provide adequate calories for energy needs. Thus, when small amounts of glucose are added, amino acids are catabolized for energy, and protein breakdown is increased.

The evidence against this proposed mechanism has been reviewed by Felig (274). Greenberg, Freeman, and coworkers have shown that addition of small quantities of either glucose or triglycerides to amino acid infusions does not lead to more negative nitrogen balance, even though plasma insulin rises and plasma glucagon, free fatty acids, and blood β-hydroxybutyrate and acetoacetate fall (275, 276). The addition of even small quantities of glucose to the amino acid infusions will also have a sparing effect on lipid and glycogen stores and thus decrease wasting.

Although the mechanisms by which the infusion of amino acids without glucose spares protein are not known, the effect is well established. In the future, if costs allow, it is likely that patients unable to receive adequate enteral nourishment for periods of several days will be routinely treated with peripheral infusions of amino acids and possibly small quantities of carbohydrates and lipids. Infusion of amino acids without carbohydrates or lipids may also be used to spare body protein in obese patients who are undergoing weight reduction by starvation (277).

PERIPHERAL TOTAL PARENTERAL NUTRITION

Several investigators have reported administration of TPN through peripheral veins (74, 77, 83, 278). This regimen is safer and more convenient than infusions into a central vein. The hypertonicity of typical TPN solutions must be avoided, however, to prevent thrombophlebitis. This is accomplished by using fat emulsions, larger quantities of more dilute solutions, and less abundant quantities of nutrients. A preparation such as described in Table 10-5 may be used which provides 150 g of lipids, 150 g of dextrose, and 80 g of amino acids per day in 3 L of solution. Vitamins and minerals are added as needed. The amino acids, carbohydrates, minerals, and vitamins are mixed in one solution that is infused concurrently with the lipid emulsion through a "Y" connector situated near the infusion site. The lower osmolality of the lipid solution reduces the osmolality of the final infusate as it enters the vein. Care should be taken that the amino acid and glucose solution is not administered without lipids. Otherwise the hypertonicity of the infusate may cause thrombophlebitis.

Ethanol, when added to water, raises the osmolality less than would be expected from the quantity of moles added. Hence, mixtures of amino acids, carbohydrates, and ethanol may also be used in peripheral infusions.

Since these solutions are more dilute than those of conventional TPN, they are not readily used in patients with fluid intolerance. Also, the limited quantity of nutrients which can be administered peripherally restricts this regimen to patients who have relatively low requirements for energy and other nutrients. Even with lowered tonicity, thrombophlebitis in peripheral veins is likely to occur if the needle or cannula is not changed frequently, every 8 to 12 h according to some investigators (77) and 16 to 36 h according to others (278). It has been recommended that after 1 to 3 weeks of peripheral infusion TPN should be administered by central venous catheter, although peripheral TPN has been given for much longer periods. Parenteral nutrition through peripheral veins may also be used to supplement oral nutrition and intermittent parenteral nutrition.

INTERMITTENT OR PARTIAL TPN

For many patients who require long-term or permanent parenteral nutrition and whose nutritional requirements are not excessive, it is possible to restrict infusions to a portion of the day, usually about 10 to 14 h. When solutions are infused at night, patients can lead a more normal daytime life. A heparin lock may be used to prevent clotting when solutions are not being infused. Alternatively, solutions can be infused during the day if nighttime nursing coverage is reduced or when patients wish to sleep without the disturbance of frequent voiding. This regimen is easier to implement when fat emulsions are available. Less glucose can then be given, so that there is less likelihood of hyperglycemia from rapid administration of glucose or of hypoglycemia when the infusion is stopped.

A regimen for intermittent TPN is shown in Table 10-11. Near the end of the infusion, the rate of glucose administration is decreased to prevent reactive hypoglycemia. Heparin may be added to the fat emulsion to reduce hypertriglyceridemia associated with rapid infusion of lipids. When patients are able to eat some food, parenteral nutrition may be administered for shorter periods of time or less often than daily. Adequacy

Table 10-11. A regimen for intermittent total parenteral nutrition* (14 h/day)

HOURS	INFUSION	QUANTITY OF NUTRIENTS	VOLUME
0–7	Glucose 25%	250 g	1000 mL
	Crystalline amino acids 4.25%	42.5 g	
	Electrolytes and multivitamins (Same as Table 10-4)		
7–14†	Glucose 15%	150 g	1000 mL
	Crystalline amino acids 4.25%	42.5 g	
	Electrolytes (same as Table 10-4)		
5–14	Fat emulsion (10%)	100 g	1000 mL
14–24	Fill IV catheter with 3 mL of a solution of 2 mL of heparin 10,000 IU/mL and 18 mL of normal saline. Catheter is again flushed with 2 mL of this solution at 19 h		

TOTAL NUTRIENTS INFUSED	
Glucose	400 g
Fat	100 g
Amino acids	85 g
Energy	2757 kcal
Water	3000 mL

* Modified from Grotte, Jacobson, and Wretlind (77).

† Rate of infusion should be tapered the last two hours to avoid reactive hypoglycemia.

of nutrition should be assessed periodically according to anthropometric and biochemical standards.

AMBULATORY AND HOME TOTAL PARENTERAL NUTRITION

In 1970, Scribner and coworkers introduced the concept of an "artificial gut" for self or home care of patients requiring long-term or permanent parenteral nutrition (279). There is now substantial experience with ambulatory and home parenteral nutrition (162, 280–285). Patients may receive TPN at home during the day or overnight or, with the aid of a wearable apparatus, while they go about their daily activities. Patients who are candidates for home TPN undergo a psychosocial evaluation similar to that used to evaluate feasibility for home dialysis therapy and receive intensive training in techniques of administration and infection control. Individuals may administer their own therapy, often with assistance from their families.

Patients requiring this therapy have insufficient intestinal function to support life. Most often they suffer from such disorders as short-bowel syndrome, congenital disorders of the intestine, radiation enteritis, or regional enteritis. Home TPN is also useful for patients with malignancies who are unable to receive adequate enteral nutrition before cancer therapy or while undergoing long-term chemotherapy or radiation therapy (see above).

The frequency and composition of infusions are determined by the amounts needed to replace nutritional deficiencies and maintain good nutrition. Many patients are able to ingest some food. Depending on their oral intake, most individuals receive infusions 4 to 7 times a week for periods to 8 to 14 h. During recovery from poor nutrition, infusion of nutrients can be kept high. After recovery, patients may adjust the infusion frequency to maintain constant weight. Solutions are infused at a constant rate with a pump, and an alarm system may be used to alert patients when the infusion is nearly complete so that the rate of administration may be tapered to prevent reactive hypoglycemia.

Although arteriovenous shunts and fistulas have been used for vascular access, many physicians employ a cuffed silicone catheter that is implanted in the subclavian vein and threaded into the right atrium (159). The catheter enters through a subcutaneous tunnel in the anterior wall of the chest. A Dacron felt cuff is located at the entrance site in the skin, and fibrous tissue grows into the cuff, fixing it in position and acting as a barrier to infection. The technique of Solassol and Joyeux involves cannulating a tributary of a large-flow vein, such as the subclavian or external iliac, and placing the tip of a Teflon-Scurasil cannula at the junction of the tributary and the large-flow vein. Between infusions the catheter is kept patent by filling it with heparin, and the proximal end is closed with a plastic cap (282). The rate of infection is reported to be low (285), and clotting is uncommon. Metabolic complications are similar to those in patients undergoing TPN in hospitals but are less frequent.

Hundreds of patients have now been treated at home. It is not uncommon for patients whose intestinal function is insufficient to support life to experience restoration of body weight and normal nutritional status, increased energy and sense of well-being, and physical and social rehabilitation.

REFERENCES

1. Duke, J. H., Jr., S. B. Jorgensen, J. R. Broell, C. L. Long, and J. M. Kinney: Contribution of protein to caloric expenditure following injury, *Surgery*, **68:**168, 1970.
2. Cahill, G. F., Jr.: Starvation in man, *N. Engl. J. Med.*, **282:**668, 1970.
3. Keys, A., and F. Grande: Body weight, body composition and calorie status, in R. S. Goodhart and M. E. Shils (eds.), *Modern Nutrition in Health and Disease*, Lea & Febiger, Philadelphia, 1973, pp. 1-27.
4. Felig, P., O. E. Owen, J. Wahren, and G. F. Cahill, Jr.: Amino acid metabolism during prolonged starvation, *J. Clin. Invest.*, **48:**584, 1969.
5. Felig, P., O. E. Owen, A. P. Morgan, and G. F. Cahill, Jr.: Utilization of metabolic fuels in obese subjects, *Am. J. Clin. Nutr.*, **21:**1429, 1968.
6. Ross, H., I. D. Johnston, T. A. Welborn, and A. D. Wright: Effect of abdominal operation on glucose tolerance and serum levels of insulin, growth hormone, and hydrocortison, *Lancet*, **2:**563, 1966.
7. Blackburn, G. L., J. P. Flatt, and T. W. Hensle: Peripheral amino acid infusions, in J. E. Fischer (ed.), *Total Parenteral Nutrition*, Little, Brown and Company, Boston, 1976, pp. 363–394.
8. Vinnars, E., P. Furst, I. L. Hermansson, B. Josephson, and B. Lindholmer: Protein catabolism in the postoperative state and its treatment with amino acid solution, *Acta Chir. Scand.*, **136:**95, 1970.
9. Van Way, C. W., III, H. C. Meng, and H. H. Sandstead: Nitrogen balance in postoperative patients receiving parenteral nutrition, *Arch. Surg.*, **110:**272, 1975.
10. Bistrian, B. R., G. L. Blackburn, J. Vitale, D. Cochran, and J. Naylor: Prevalence of malnutrition in general medical patients, *JAMA*, **235:**1567, 1976.
11. Bozzetti, F., G. Terno, and C. Longoni: Parenteral hyperalimentation and wound healing, *Surg. Gynecol. Obstet.*, **141:**712, 1975.
12. Law, D. K., S. J. Dudrick, and N. I. Abdou: Immunocompetence of patients with protein-calorie malnutrition, *Ann. Intern. Med.*, **79:**545, 1973.
13. Bistrian, B. R., M. Sherman, G. L. Blackburn, R. Marshall, and C. Shaw: Cellular immunity in

adult marasmus, *Arch. Intern. Med.*, **137**:1408, 1977.

14. Neumann, C. E.: Interaction of malnutrition and infection: A neglected clinical concept, *Arch. Intern. Med.*, **137**:1364, 1977.

15. Studley, H. O.: Percentage of weight loss: A basic indicator of surgical risk in patients with chronic peptic ulcer, *JAMA*, **106**:458, 1936.

16. Jelliffe, D. B.: The assessment of the nutritional status of the community, series 53, World Health Organization, Geneva, 1966.

17. Sandstead, H. H., and W. N. Pearson: Clinical evaluation of nutrition status, in R. S. Goodhart and M. E. Shils (eds.), *Modern Nutrition in Health and Disease*, Lea & Febiger, Philadelphia, 1973, pp. 572-592.

18. Waterlow, J. C., and A. E. Harper: Assessment of protein nutrition, in H. Ghadimi (ed.), *Total Parenteral Nutrition*, John Wiley & Sons, Inc., New York, 1975, pp. 231–258.

19. McLaughlan, J. M.: Nutritional significance of alterations in plasma amino acids and serum proteins, Committee on Amino Acids, Food and Nutrition Board, Natl. Research Council, Natl. Academy of Sciences, Washington, 1974.

20. McFarlane H., K. J. Adcock, A. Cooke, M. I. Ogbeide, H. Adeshina, G. O. Taylor, S. Reddy, J. M. Gurney, and J. A. Mordie: Biochemical assessment of protein-calorie malnutrition, *Lancet*, **1**:392, 1969.

21. Davis, L. E., and W. Hofmann: A long-term nasogastric feeding tube made from modified Penrose tubing, *JAMA*, **209**:685, 1969.

22. Russell, R. I.: Progress report: Elemental diets, *Gut*, **16**:68, 1975.

23. McLaughlin, M., A. Price, A. Phillips, R. Bambridge, and G. Feldmanis: Elemental diets, *Lancet*, **2**:767, 1975.

24. Kopple, J. D., and M. J. Blumenkrantz: Nutritional therapy of urologic patient, *Urol. Clin. North Am.*, **3**:403, 1976.

25. Randall, H. T.: Indications for parenteral nutrition in postoperative catabolic states, in H. C. Meng and D. H. Law (eds.), *Parenteral Nutrition*, Charles C Thomas, Publisher, Springfield, Ill., 1970, pp. 113–139.

26. Johnston, I. D. A.: The role of parenteral nutrition in surgical care, *Ann. Coll. Surg. Engl.*, **50**:196, 1972.

27. Van Way, C. W., III, H. C. Meng, and H. H. Sandstead: An assessment of the role of parenteral alimentation in the management of surgical patients, *Ann. Surg.*, **177**:103, 1973.

28. Vinnars, E.: Recent advances in parenteral nutrition, *Crit. Care Med.*, **2**:143, 1974.

29. Dudrick, S. J., E. M. Copeland, III, and B. V. MacFadyen: Long-term parenteral nutrition: Its current status, *Hosp. Pract.*, **10**:47, 1975.

30. Lee, H. A.: Intravenous nutrition: Why, when, and with what? *Ann. R. Coll. Surg. Engl.*, **56**:59, 1970, pp. 113–139.

31. Fleming, C. R., D. B. McGill, H. N. Hoffman II, and R. A. Nelson: Total parenteral nutrition, *Mayo Clin Proc.*, **51**:187, 1976.

32. Kinney, J. M.: Energy requirements for parenteral nutrition, in J. E. Fischer (ed.), *Total Parenteral Nutrition*, Little, Brown and Company, Boston, 1976, pp. 135–142.

33. National Academy of Sciences, Committee on Dietary Allowances, National Research Council Food and Nutrition Board: Recommended dietary allowances, Washington, D.C., 1974.

34. Nuutinen, L., and A. Hollmen: Blood sugar levels during routine fluid therapy of surgical patients, *Ann. Chir. Gynaecol. Fenn.*, **64**:108, 1975.

35. Thoren, L.: Parenteral nutrition with carbohydrate and alcohol, *Acta. Chir. Scand.*, **325**(suppl.):75, 1964.

36. Froesch, E. R., and U. Keller: Review of energy metabolism with particular reference to the metabolism of glucose, fructose, sorbitol and xylitol and of their therapeutic use in parenteral nutrition, in A. W. Wilkinson (ed.), *Parenteral Nutrition*, The Williams & Wilkins Company, Baltimore, 1971, pp. 105–120.

37. Bassler, K. H.: Physiological basis for the use of carbohydrates in parenteral nutrition, in H. C. Meng and D. H. Law (eds.), *Parenteral Nutrition*, Charles C Thomas, Publisher, Springfield, Ill., 1970, pp. 96–111.

38. Mehnert, H., H. Forster, C. A. Geser, M. Haslbeck, and K. H. Dehmel: Clinical use of carbohydrates in parenteral nutrition, in H. C. Meng and D. H. Law (eds.), *Parenteral Nutrition*, Charles C Thomas, Publishers, Springfield, Ill., 1970, pp. 112–130.

39. Bassler, K. H., and H. Bickel: The use of carbohydrates alone and in combination in parenteral

nutrition, in A. W. Wilkinson (ed.), *Parenteral Nutrition*, The Williams & Wilkins Company, Baltimore, 1971, pp. 99–104.

40. Cahill, G. F.: Carbohydrates, in P. L. White and M. E. Nagy (eds.), *Total Parenteral Nutrition*, Am. Med. Assoc., 1974, pp. 147–154.

41. Baessler, K. H., and K. Schultis: Metabolism of fructose, sorbitol, and xylitol and their use in parenteral alimentation, in H. Ghadimi (ed.), *Total Parenteral Nutrition*, John Wiley & Sons, New York, 1975, pp. 65–83.

42. Young, A. E., and E. Weser: The metabolism of infused maltose and other sugars, in A. Jeanes and J. Hodge (eds.), *Physiological Effects of Food Carbohydrates*, Am. Chem. Soc., Symposium Series #15, 1975, pp. 73–99.

43. Weinstein, J. J.: Intravenous infusions of "invert sugar," *Med. Ann. Dist. Columbia,* **19:**179, 1950.

44. Moncrief, J. A., K. B. Coldwater, and R. Elman: Postoperative loss of sugar in urine following intravenous infusion of fructose (levulose), *Arch. Surg.,* **67:**57, 1953.

45. Heuckenkamp, P. U., and N. Zollner: Quantitative comparison and evaluation of utilization of parenteral administered carbohydrates, *Nutr. Metab.,* **18:**209, 1975.

46. Bergstrom, J., E. Hultman, and A. E. Roch-Norlund: Lactic acid accumulation in connection with fructose infusion, *Acta. Med. Scand.,* **184:**359, 1968.

47. Raivio, K. O., M. P. Kekomaki, and P. H. Maenpaa: Depletion of liver adenine nucleotides induced by D-fructose, *Biochem. Parmacol.,* **18:**2615, 1969.

48. Anderson, G., J. Brohult, and G. Starner: Increasing metabolic acidosis following fructose infusion in two children, *Acta Paediatr. Scand.,* **58:**301, 1969.

49. Sahebjami, H., and R. Scalettar: Effects of fructose infusion on lactate and uric acid metabolism, *Lancet,* **1:**366, 1971.

50. Hessov, I.: Effects of fructose and glucose infusions on blood acid-base equilibrium in the postoperative period, *Acta. Chir. Scand.,* **140:**347, 1974.

51. Bergstrom, J., P. Furst, F. Gallyas, E. Hultman, and E. Vinnars: Lactate production during fructose infusion with or without amino acids, *Acta Med. Scand.,* **200:**99, 1976.

52. Lee, H. A., A. G. Morgan, R. Waldram, and J. Bennett: Sorbitol: Some aspects of its metabolism and role as an intravenous nutrient, in A. W. Wilkinson (ed.), *Parenteral Nutrition*, The Williams & Wilkins Company, Baltimore, 1971, pp. 121–137.

53. Blumenkrantz, M. J., D. J. Shapiro, N. Mimura, D. G. Oreopoulus, R. M. Freidler, S. Levin, H. Tenckhoff, and J. W. Coburn: Maintenance peritoneal dialysis as an alternative in the patient with diabetes mellitus and end-stage uremia, *Kidney Int.,* **6**(suppl. 1):108, 1974.

54. Rosen, H. M.: Types of solutions available, in J. E. Fischer (ed.), *Total Parenteral Nutrition*, Little, Brown and Company, Boston, 1976, pp. 15–26.

55. Spitz, I. M., A. H. Rubenstein, I. Bersohn, and K. H. Bassler: Metabolism of xylitol in healthy subjects and patients with renal disease, *Metabolism,* **19:**24, 1970.

56. Schumer, W.: Preliminary report: Adverse effects of xylitol in parenteral alimentation, *Metabolism,* **20:**345, 1971.

57. Thomas, D. W., J. B. Edwards, and R. G. Edwards: Examination of xylitol (letter to ed.), *N. Engl. J. Med.,* **283:**437, 1970.

58. Lieber, C. S.: Hepatic and metabolic effects of alcohol, *Gastroenterology,* **65:**821, 1973.

59. Rydberg, U.: Alcohol metabolism, in H. Ghadimi (ed.), *Total Parenteral Nutrition*, John Wiley & Sons, New York, 1975, pp. 47–56.

60. Young, J. M., and E. Weser: The metabolism of circulating maltose in man, *J. Clin. Invest.,* **50:**986, 1971.

61. Meng, H. C.: Fat emulsions in parenteral nutrition, in J. E. Fischer (ed.), *Total Parenteral Nutrition*, Little, Brown and Company, Boston, 1976, pp. 305–334.

62. Wilmore, D. W., J. A. Moylan, G. M. Helmkamp, and B. A. Pruitt, Jr.: Clinical evaluation of a 10% intravenous fat emulsion for parenteral nutrition in thermally injured patients, *Ann. Surg.,* **178:**503, 1973.

63. Sgoutas, D., R. Jones, and M. F. la Via: The effect of intravenous hyperalimentation on erythrocyte lipids, *Proc. Soc. Exp. Biol. Med.,* **145:**614, 1974.

64. Terry, B. E., and R. L. Wixom: Hemolytic anemia associated with essential fatty acid deficiency

in a normal man on long-term TPN, in H. C. Meng and D. W. Wilmore (eds.), *Fat Emulsions in Parenteral Nutrition*, American Medical Association, Chicago, 1976, pp. 18–24.

65. Connor, W. E.: Pathogenesis and frequency of essential fatty acid deficiency during total parenteral nutrition (editorial), *Ann. Intern. Med.*, **83**:895, 1975.

66. Wene, J. D., W. E. Connor, and L. DenBesten: The development of essential fatty acid deficiency in healthy men fed fat-free diets intravenously and orally, *J. Clin. Invest.*, **56**:127, 1975.

67. Caldwell, M. D.: Human essential fatty acid deficiency: A Review, in H. C. Meng and D. W. Wilmore (eds.), *Fat Emulsions in Parenteral Nutrition*, American Medical Association, Chicago, 1976, pp. 24–28.

68. Beisbarth, H.: Influence of stress on intravenous fat requirements, in H. C. Meng and D. W. Wilmore (eds.), *Fat Emulsions in Parenteral Nutrition*, American Medical Association, Chicago, 1976, pp. 79–81.

69. O'Neill, J. A., Jr., M. D. Caldwell, and H. C. Meng, Essential fatty acid deficiency in surgical patients, *Ann. Surg.*, **185**:535, 1977.

70. Faulkner, W. J., and C. M. Flint, Jr.: Essential fatty acid deficiency associated with total parenteral nutrition, *Surg. Gynecol. Obstet.*, **144**:665, 1977.

71. Caldwell, M. D., H. T. Jonsson, and H. B. Othersen, Jr.: Essential fatty acid deficiency in an infant receiving prolonged parenteral alimentation, *J. Pediatr.*, **81**:894, 1972.

72. Press, M., P. J. Hartop, and C. Prottey: Correction of essential fatty-acid deficiency in man by the cutaneous application of sunflower-seed oil, *Lancet*, **1**:597, 1974.

73. Stegink, L. D., J. B. Freeman, J. Wispe, M. F. Wittine, and W. E. Connor: Absence of the biochemical symptoms of essential fatty acid deficiency (EFAD) during amino acid infusion without glucose, *Fed. Proc.*, **35**:344, 1976.

74. Deitel, M., and V. Kaminsky: Total nutrition by peripheral vein: The lipid system, *Can. Med. Assoc. J.*, **111**:152, 1974.

75. Wretlind, A.: Current status of intralipid and other fat emulsions, in H. C. Meng and D. W. Wilmore (eds.), *Fat Emulsions in Parenteral Nu-*

trition, American Medical Association, Chicago, 1976, pp. 109–122.

76. Wretlind, A.: Current status of intralipid and other fat emulsions, in H. C. Meng and D. W. Wilmore (eds.), *Fat Emulsions in Parenteral Nutrition*, American Medical Association, Chicago, 1976, pp. 109–122.

77. Grotte, G., S. Jacobson, and A. Wretlind: Lipid emulsions and technique of peripheral administration in parenteral nutrition, in J. E. Fischer (ed.), *Total Parenteral Nutrition*, Little, Brown and Company, Boston, 1976, pp. 335–362.

78. Long, J. M. III.: Use of intravenous fat emulsion after trauma and burns, in H. C. Meng and D. W. Wilmore (eds.), *Fat Emulsions in Parenteral Nutrition*, American Medical Association, Chicago, 1976, pp. 76–79.

79. Jeejeebhoy, K. N., G. H. Anderson, A. F. Nakhooda, G. R. Greenberg, I. Sanderson, and E. B. Marliss: Comparison with glucose. Metabolic studies in total parenteral nutrition with lipid in man, *J. Clin. Invest.*, **57**:125, 1976.

80. Jeejeebhoy, K. N., E. B. Marliss, G. H. Anderson, G. R. Greenberg, A. Kuksis, and C. Breckenridge, in H. C. Meng and D. W. Wilmore (eds.), *Fat Emulsions in Parenteral Nutrition*, American Medical Association, Chicago, 1976, pp. 45–54.

81. Yeo, M. T., A. B. Gazzaniga, R. H. Bartlett, and J. B. Shobe: Total intravenous nutrition: Experience with fat emulsions and hypertonic glucose, *Arch. Surg.*, **106**:792, 1973.

82. Hansen, L. M., W. R. Hardie, and J. Hidalgo: Fat emulsion for intravenous administration, *Ann. Surg.*, **184**:80, 1976.

83. Silberman, H., M. Freehauf, G. Fong, and N. Rosenblatt: Parenteral nutrition with lipids, *JAMA*, **238**:1380, 1977.

84. Milne, C. A., L. D. MacLean, and H. M. Shizgal: Casein hydrolysate and intralipid vs. casein hydrolysate and 25% glucose for hyperalimentation, *Surg. Forum*, **52**:000, 1977.

85. Long, J. M., D. W. Wilmore, A. D. Mason, Jr., and B. A. Pruitt, Jr.: Fat-carbohydrate interaction: Effects on nitrogen-sparing in total intravenous feeding, *Surg. Forum*, **25**:61, 1977.

86. Thompson, S. W.: Hepatic toxicity of intravenous fat emulsions, in H. C. Meng and D. W. Wilmore (eds.), *Fat Emulsions in Parenteral Nutrition*,

American Medical Association, Chicago, 1976, pp. 90–95.

87. Greene, H. L., D. Hazlett, and R. Demaree: Relationship between intralipid-induced hyperlipemia and pulmonary function, *Am. J. Clin. Nutr.*, **29:**127, 1976.

88. Jonxis, J. H. P., and T. H. J. Huisman: Excretion of amino acids in free and bound form during intravenous administration of protein hydrolysate, *Metabolism*, **6:**175, 1957.

89. Anderson, G. H., D. G. Patel, and K. N. Jeejeebhoy: Design and evaluation by nitrogen balance and blood aminograms of an amino acid mixture for total parenteral nutrition of adults with gastrointestinal disease, *J. Clin. Invest.*, **53:**904, 1974.

90. Long, C. L., B. A. Zikria, J. M. Kinney, and J. W. Geiger: Comparison of fibrin hydrolysates and crystalline amino acid solutions in parenteral nutrition, *Am. J. Clin. Nutr.*, **27:**163, 1974.

91. Fahey, J. L.: Toxicity and blood ammonia rise resulting from intravenous amino acid administration in man: The protective effect of L-arginine, *J. Clin. Invest.*, **36:**1647, 1957.

92. Reifenstein, E. C., Jr., F. Albright, and S. L. Wells: The accumulation, interpretation, and presentation of data pertaining to metabolic balances, notably those of calcium, phosphorus, and nitrogen, *J. Clin. Endocrinol. Metab.*, **5:**367, 1945.

93. Rudman, D., W. J. Millikan, T. J. Richardson, T. J. Bixler, II, W. J. Stackhouse, and W. C. McGarrity: Elemental balances during intravenous hyperalimentation of underweight adult subjects, *J. Clin. Invest.*, **55:**94, 1975.

94. Shils, M. E.: Guidelines for total parenteral nutrition, *JAMA*, **220:**1721, 1972.

95. Shils, M. E.: Minerals, in P. L. White (ed.), *Total Parenteral Nutrition*, American Medical Association, Chicago, 1974, pp. 257–275.

96. Giovanoni, R.: A suggested profile for selected total parenteral nutrition additives, *Clin. Med.*, **81:**28, 1974.

97. Jeejeebhoy, K. N., G. H. Anderson, I. Sanderson, and M. H. Bryan: Total parenteral nutrition: Nutrient needs and technical tips, *Modern Medicine of Canada*, **29:**000, 1974.

98. Meng, H. C.: Parenteral nutrition: Principles, nutrient requirements, and techniques, *Geriatrics*, **30:**97, 1975.

99. Ellis, B. W., R. de L. Stanbridge, L. P. Fielding, and H. A. Dudley: A rational approach to parenteral nutrition, *Br. Med. J.*, **1:**1388, 1976.

100. Madan, P. L., D. K. Madan, and J. R. Palumbo: Total parenteral nutrition, *Drug Intell. Clin. Pharm.*, **10:**684, 1976.

101. Giovanoni, R.: The manufacturing pharmacy solutions and incompatibilities, in J. E. Fischer (ed.), *Total Parenteral Nutrition*, Little, Brown and Company, Boston, 1976, pp. 27–54.

102. Li, T., and B. L. Vallee: The biochemical and nutritional role of trace elements, in R. S. Goodhart and M. E. Shils (eds.), *Modern Nutrition in Health and Disease—Dietotherapy*, Lea & Febiger, Philadelphia, 1973, pp. 372–399.

103. Schwarz, K.: Recent dietary trace element research, exemplified by tin, fluorine, and silicon, *Fed. Proc.*, **33:**1748, 1974.

104. Tuman, R. W., and R. J. Doisy: The role of trace elements in human nutrition and metabolism, in A. Jeanes and J. Hodge (eds.), *Physiological Effects of Food Carbohydrates*, Symposium Series 15, American Chemical Society, 1975, pp. 156–177.

105. Palmisano, D. J.: Nutrient deficiencies after intensive parenteral alimentation, *N. Engl. J. Med.*, **291:**799, 1974.

106. Dunlap, W. M., G. W. James, III, and D. M. Hume: Anemia and neutropenia caused by copper deficiency, *Ann. Intern. Med.*, **80:**470, 1974.

107. Karpel, J. T., and V. H. Peden: Copper deficiency in long-term parenteral nutrition, *J. Pediatr.*, **80:**32, 1972.

108. Freeman, J. B., L. D. Stegink, P. D. Meyer, L. K. Fry, and L. Denbesten: Excessive urinary zinc losses during parenteral alimentation, *J. Surg. Res.*, **18:**463, 1975.

109. Kay, R. G., C. Tasman-Jones, J. Pybus, R. Whiting, and H. Black: A syndrome of acute zinc deficiency during total parenteral alimentation in man, *Ann. Surg.*, **183:**331, 1976.

110. Solomons, N. W., T. J. Layden, I. H. Rosenberg, K. Vo-Khactu, and H. H. Sandstead: Plasma trace metals during total parenteral alimentation, *Gastroenterology*, **70:**1022, 1976.

111. Hankins, D. A., M. C. Riella, B. H. Scribner, and A. L. Babb: Whole blood trace element concentrations during total parenteral nutrition, *Surgery*, **79:**674, 1976.

112. Halsted, J., J. C. Smith, Jr., and M. I. Irwin: A conspectus of research on zinc requirements of man, *J. Nutr.*, **104:**345, 1974.

113. Henkin, R. I.: Zinc in wound healing, *N. Engl. J. Med.*, **291:**675, 1974.

114. Sandstead, H. H., A. S. Prasad, A. R. Schulert, Z. Farid, A. Miale, Jr., S. Bassilly, and W. J. Darby: Human zinc deficiency, endocrine manifestations and response to treatment, *Am. J. Clin. Nutr.*, **20:**422, 1967.

115. Okada, A., Y. Takagi, T. Itakura, M. Satani, H. Manabe, Y. Iida, T. Tanigaki, M. Iwasaki, and N. Kasahara: Skin lesions during intravenous hyperalimentation: Zinc deficiency, *Surgery*, **80:**629, 1976.

116. Fleming, C. R., R. E. Hodges, and L. S. Hurley: A prospective study of serum copper and zinc levels in patients receiving total parenteral nutrition, *Am. J. Clin. Nutr.*, **29:**70, 1976.

117. Hambidge, K. M.: Chromium nutrition in man, *Am. J. Clin. Nutr.*, **27:**505, 1974.

118. Jeejeebhoy, K. N., R. C. Chu, E. B. Marliss, G. R. Greenberg, and A. Bruce-Robertson: Chromium deficiency, glucose intolerance, and neuropathy reversed by chromium supplementation, in a patient receiving long-term total parenteral nutrition, *Am. J. Clin. Nutr.*, **30:**531, 1977.

119. Hull, R. L.: Use of trace elements in intravenous hyperalimentation solutions, *Am. J. Hosp. Pharm.*, **31:**759, 1974.

120. Prasad, A. S.: Parenteral nutrition in adults, in H. F. Conn (ed.), *Current Therapy 1976*, W. B. Saunders Company, Philadelphia, 1976, pp. 465–475.

121. Dick, W., and W. Seeling: Water and electrolyte requirements during parenteral nutrition, in F. W. Ahnefeld, C. Burri, W. Dick, and Halmaggi (eds.), *Parenteral Nutrition* Springer-Verlag, Berlin, 1976, pp. 99–112.

122. Jetton, M. M., J. F. Sullivan, and R. E. Burch: Trace element contamination of intravenous solutions, *Arch. Intern. Med.*, **136:**782, 1976.

123. Greene, H. L.: Vitamins, in P. L. White and M. E. Naby (eds.), *Total Parenteral Nutrition*, American Medical Association, 1974, p. 241–256.

124. Ballard, H. S., and J. Lindenbaum: Megaloblastic anemia complicating hyperalimentation therapy, *Am. J. Med.*, **56:**740, 1974.

125. Wardrop, C. A. J., G. B. Tennant, R. V. Heatley, and L. E. Hughes: Acute folate deficiency in surgical patients on amino acid/ethanol intravenous nutrition, *Lancet*, **2:**640, 1975.

126. Spannuth, C. L., D. Mitchell, W. J. Stone, S. Schenker, and C. Wagner: Vitamin B_6 nutriture in patients with uremia and liver disease, National Research Council (in press).

127. King, C. C.: Present knowledge of ascorbic acid (vitamin C) in present knowledge in nutrition, The Nutrition Foundation, New York, 1967, pp. 76–79.

128. Roe, D. A.: Drug-induced nutritional deficiencies, AVI Publ., Westport, Conn., 1976.

129. Daniels, A. L., and G. J. Everson: Influence of acetylsalicylic acid (aspirin) on urinary excretion of ascorbic acid, *Proc. Soc. Exp. Biol. Med.*, **35:**20, 1936.

130. Udall, J. A.: Human sources and absorption of vitamin K in relation to anticoagulant stability, *JAMA*, **194:**127, 1965.

131. Bessey, O. A.: Role of vitamins in the metabolism of amino acids, *JAMA*, **164:**1224, 1957.

132. Horwitt, M. K.: Perspectives in nutrition: Nutritional requirements of man, with special reference to riboflavin, *Am. J. Clin. Nutr.*, **18:**458, 1966.

133. Dryden, L. P., and A. M. Hartman: Vitamin B_{12} deficiency in rat fed high protein rations, *J. Nutr.*, **101:**579, 1971.

134. Harris, P. L., and N. D. Embree: Quantitative consideration of the effect of polyunsaturated fatty acid content of the diet upon the requirement for vitamin E, *Am. J. Clin. Nutr.*, **13:**392, 1963.

135. Horwitt, M. K.: Vitamin E and lipid metabolism in man, *Am. J. Clin. Nutr.*, **8:**451, 1960.

136. Van Itallie, T. B., and H. H. Sandstead: Vitamins and minerals colloquium, in P. L. White and M. E. Nagy (eds.), *Total Parenteral Nutrition*, American Medical Association, Chicago, 1974, pp. 276–309.

137. Briggs, M. H., P. Garcia-Webb, and P. Davies: Urinary oxalate and vitamin C supplements (letter), *Lancet*, **1:**201, 1973.

138. Shelotri, P. G., and K. S. Bhat: Effect of megadoses of vitamin C on bactericidal activity of leukocytes, *Am. J. Clin. Nutr.*, **30:**1077, 1977.

139. Shils, M. E.: Total parenteral nutrition, in R. S.

Goodhart and M. E. Shils (eds.), *Modern Nutrition in Health and Disease,* Lea & Febiger, Philadelphia, 1973, pp. 966–980.

140. White, P. L., and M. E. Nagy: Vitamin preparations for parenteral use, in P. L. White and M. E. Nagy (eds.), *Total Parenteral Nutrition,* American Medical Association, 1974, pp. 457–464.

141. Norman, A. W.: Evidence for a new kidney-produced hormone, 1,25-dihydroxycholecalciferol, the proposed biologically active form of vitamin D, *Am. J. Clin. Nutr.,* **24:**1346, 1971.

142. Hinton, P., S. Littlejohn, S. P. Allison, and J. Lloyd: Insulin and glucose to reduce catabolic response to injury in burned patients, *Lancet,* **1:**767, 1971.

143. Richards, P., C. L. Brown, B. J. Houghton, and O. M. Wrong, The incorporation of ammonia nitrogen into albumin in man: The effects of diet, uremia and growth hormone, *Clin. Nephrol.,* **3:**172, 1975.

144. Thaysen, J. H.: Anabolic steroids in the treatment of renal failure, in F. Gross (ed.), *Protein Metabolism, International Symposium,* Springer Verlag, Berlin, 1962, p. 450.

145. Saarne, A., L. Bjerstaf, and B. Ekman: Studies on the nitrogen balance in the human during long-term treatment with different anabolic agents under strictly standardized conditions, *Acta Med. Scand.,* **177:**199, 1965.

146. Thaysen, J. H.: Anabolic steroids in the treatment of renal failure, in F. Gross (ed.), *Protein Metabolism, International Symposium,* Springer Verlag, Berlin, 1962, p. 450.

147. Goldmann, D. A., W. T. Martin, and J. W. Worthington: Growth of bacteria and fungi in total parenteral nutrition solutions, *Am. J. Surg.,* **126:**314, 1973.

148. Melly, M. A., H. C. Meng, and W. Schaffner: Microbial growth in lipid emulsions used in parenteral nutrition, *Arch. Surg.,* **110:**1479, 1975.

149. Rowlands, D. A., W. R. Wilkerson, and N. Yoshimura: Storage stability of mixed hyperalimentation solutions, *Am. J. Hosp. Pharm.,* **30:**436, 1973.

150. Laegeler, W. L., J. M. Tio, and M. I. Blake: Stability of certain amino acids in a parenteral nutrition solution, *Am. J. Hosp. Pharm.,* **31:**776, 1974.

151. Stegink, L. D., J. B. Freeman, P. D. Meyer, L. J.

Filer, Jr., L. K. Fry, and L. DenBesten: Excessive trace metal ion excretion due to sugar-amino acid complexes during total parenteral nutrition, *Fed. Proc.,* **34:**931, 1975.

152. Kaminski, M. W., Jr.: Total parenteral nutrition (hyperalimentation): Prevention and treatment of complications: A policy and procedure manual, hyperalimentation registry, Walter Reed General Hospital, Washington, D.C., 1972.

153. Burke, W. A.: Preparation and guidelines to utilization of solutions, in P. L. White and M. E. Nagy (eds.), *Total Parenteral Nutrition,* American Medical Association, 1974, pp. 329–348.

154. Shils, M. E., W. L. Wright, A. Turnbull, and F. Brescia: A long-term parenteral nutrition through an external arteriovenous shunt, *N. Engl. J. Med.,* **283:**341, 1970.

155. Zincke, H., B. L. Hirsche, D. G. Amamoo, J. E. Woods, and R. C. Andersen: The use of bovine carotid grafts for hemodialysis and hyperalimentation, *Surg. Gynecol. Obstet.,* **139:**350, 1974.

156. Buselmeier, T. J., R. L. Simmons, J. S. Najarian, D. A. Duncan, B. vonHartitzsch, and C. M. Kjellstrand: The clinical application of a new prosthetic arteriovenous shunt: Characteristics and advantages over the standard A-V shunt and the A-V fistula, *Nephron,* **12:**22, 1973.

157. Benotti, P. N., A. Bothe, Jr., J. D. B. Miller, and G. L. Blackburn: Safe cannulation of the internal jugular vein for long term hyperalimentation, *Surg. Gynecol. Obstet.,* **144:**574, 1977.

158. Broviac, J. W., and B. H. Scribner: The problem of circulatory access, in P. L. White and M. E. Nagy (eds.), *Total Parenteral Nutrition,* American Medical Association, 1974, pp. 409–418.

159. Broviac, J. W., J. H. Cole, and B. H. Scribner: A silicone rubber atrial catheter for prolonged parenteral alimentation, *Surg. Gynecol. Obstet.,* **136:**602, 1973.

160. Holland, R. R., J. L. Lamoureux, and D. W. Todd: Filter system for intravenous alimentation, *N. Engl. J. Med.,* **289:**487, 1973.

161. Cooke, J. W.: Pumps and filters, in P. L. White and M. E. Nagy (eds.), *Total Parenteral Nutrition,* American Medical Association, Chicago, 1974, pp. 419–422.

162. Solassol, C., and H. Joyeux: Ambulatory parenteral nutrition, in J. E. Fischer (ed.), *Total Par-*

enteral Nutrition, Little, Brown and Company, Boston, 1976, pp. 285–301.

163. Edmunds, L. H., G. M. Williams, and C. E. Welch: External fistulas arising from the gastrointestinal tract, *Ann. Surg.,* **152:**445, 1960.

164. Chapman, R., R. Foran, and J. E. Dunphy: Management of intestinal fistulas, *Am. J. Surg.,* **108:**157, 1964.

165. MacFadyen, B. V., S. J. Dudrick, and R. L. Ruberg: Management of gastrointestinal fistulas with parenteral hyperalimentation, *Surgery,* **74:**100, 1973.

166. Aguirre, A., and J. E. Fischer: Intestinal fistulas, in J. E. Fischer (ed.), *Total Parenteral Nutrition,* Little, Brown and Company, Boston, 1976, pp. 203–218.

167. Graham, J. A.: Conservative treatment of gastrointestinal fistulas, *Surg. Gynecol. Obstet.,* **144:**512, 1977.

168. Dudrick, S. J., D. W. Wilmore, E. Steiger, J. A. Mackie, and W. T. Fitts, Jr.: Spontaneous closure of traumatic pancreatoduodenal fistulas with total intravenous nutrition, *J. Trauma,* **10:**542, 1970.

169. Towne, J. B., R. F. Hamilton, and D. V. Stephenson: Mechanism of hyperalimentation in the suppression of upper gastrointestinal secretions, *Am. J. Surg.,* **126:**714, 1973.

170. Hamilton, R. F., W. C. Davis, D. V. Stephenson, and D. F. Magee: Effects of parenteral hyperalimentation on upper gastrointestinal tract secretions, *Arch. Surg.,* **102:**348, 1971.

171. Wolfe, B. M., R. M. Keltner, and V. L. Willman: Intestinal fistula output in regular, elemental alimentation, *Am. J. Surg.,* **124:**803, 1972.

172. Clark, R. G., and N. M. Lauder: Undernutrition and surgery in regional ileitis, *Br. J. Surg.,* **56:**736, 1969.

173. Beeken, W. L., H. J. Busch, and D. L. Sylwester: Intestinal protein loss in Crohn's disease, *Gastroenterology,* **62:**273, 1972.

174. Dawson, A. M.: Nutritional disturbances in Crohn's disease, *Proc. Soc. Med.,* **64:**166, 1971.

175. Anderson, D. L., and H. W. Boyce, Jr.: Use of parenteral nutrition in treatment of advanced regional enteritis, *Am. J. Dig. Dis.,* **18:**633, 1973.

176. Vogel, C. M., T. R. Corwin, and A. E. Baue: Intravenous hyperalimentation in the treatment of inflammatory diseases of the bowel, *Arch. Surg.,* **108:**460, 1974.

177. Reilly, J., J. A. Ryan, W. Strole, and J. E. Fischer: Hyperalimentation in inflammatory bowel disease, *Am. J. Surg.,* **131:**192, 1976.

178. Reilly, J.: Inflammatory bowel disease, in J. E. Fischer (ed.), *Total Parenteral Nutrition,* Little, Brown and Company, Boston, 1976, pp. 187–202.

179. Wilmore, D. W., and B. A. Pruitt, Jr.: Parenteral nutrition in burn patients, in J. E. Fischer (ed.), *Total Parenteral Nutrition,* Little, Brown and Company, Boston, 1976, pp. 231–252.

180. Wilmore, D. W., P. W. Curreri, K. W. Spitzer, M. E. Spitzer, and B. A. Pruitt, Jr.: Supranormal dietary intake in thermally injured hypermetabolic patients, *Surg. Gynecol. Obstet.,* **132:**881, 1971.

181. Dudrick, S. J., B. V. MacFadyen, Jr., E. D. Souchon, D. M. Englert, and E. M. Copeland, III: Parenteral nutrition techniques in cancer patients, *Cancer Res.,* **37:**2440, 1977.

182. Copeland, E. M., III, J. M. Daly, and S. J. Dudrick: Parenteral nutrition as an adjunct to cancer treatment in the adult, *Cancer Res.,* **37:**2451, 1977.

183. Eilber, F. R., and D. L. Morton: Impaired immunologic reactivity and recurrence following cancer surgery, *Cancer,* **25:**362, 1970.

184. Bosworth, J. L., N. A. Ghossein, and T. L. Brooks: Delayed hypersensitivity in patients treated by curative radiotherapy, *Cancer,* **36:**353, 1975.

185. Copeland, E. M., B. V. MacFadyen, Jr., and S. J. Dudrick: Effect of intravenous hyperalimentation on established delayed hypersensitivity in the cancer patient, *Ann. Surg.,* **184:**60, 1976.

186. Burke, M., and A. E. Kark: Parenteral feeding and cancer (letter), *Lancet,* **1:**999, 1977.

187. Copeland, E. M., III, and S. J. Dudrick: Intravenous hyperalimentation as adjunctive treatment in the cancer patient, in G. Banks (ed.), *McGaw Clinical Digest,* McGaw Laboratories, Irvine, Calif., 1976.

188. Steiger, E., J. Oram-Smith, E. Miller, L. Kuo, and H. M. Vars: Effects of nutrition on tumor growth and tolerance to chemotherapy, *J. Surg. Res.,* **18:**455, 1975.

189. Demopoulos, H. B.: Effects of reducing the phenylalanine-tyrosine intake of patients with advanced malignant melanoma, *Cancer,* **19:**657, 1966.

190. Parsons, F. M., C. K. Anderson, P. B. Clark, G. F. Edwards, S. Ahmad, C. Hetherington, and G. A. Young: Regression of malignant tumours in magnesium and potassium depletion induced by diet and haemodialysis, *Lancet*, **1**:243, 1974.

191. Martin, G. M.: Nutrition and cancer, *Lancet*, **2**:1014, 1969.

192. Pittman, J. G., and P. Cohen: The pathogenesis of cardiac cachexia, *N. Engl. J. Med.*, **271**:403, 1964.

193. Blackburn, G. L., G. W. Gibbons, A. Bothe, P. N. Benotti, D. E. Harken, and T. M. McEnany: Nutritional support in cardiac cachexia, *J. Thorac. Cardiovasc. Surg.*, **73**:489, 1977.

194. Abel, R. M., J. E. Fischer, M. J. Buckley, G. O. Barnett, and W. G. Austen: Malnutrition in cardiac surgical patients: Results of a prospective, randomized evaluation of early postoperative parenteral nutrition, *Arch. Surg.*, **3**:45, 1976.

195. Abel, R. M.: Parenteral nutrition for patients with severe cardiac illness, in J. E. Fischer (ed.), *Total Parenteral Nutrition*, Little, Brown and Company, Boston, 1976, pp. 171–186.

196. Abel, R. M., M. J. Buckley, W. G. Austen, G. Octo Barnett, C. H. Beck, Jr., and J. E. Fischer: Etiology, incidence, and prognosis of renal failure following cardiac operations: Results of a prospective analysis of 500 consecutive patients, *J. Thorac. Cardiovasc. Surg.*, **71**:323, 1976.

197. Scheuer, J., and S. W. Stezoski: Protective role of increased myocardial glycogen stores in cardiac anoxia in the rat, *Circ. Res.*, **27**:835, 1970.

198. Hewitt, R. L., D. M. Lolley, G. A. Adrouny, and T. Drapanas: Protective effect of glycogen and glucose on the anoxic arrested heart, *Surgery*, **75**:1, 1974.

199. Austen, W. G., J. J. Greenberg, and J. C. Piccinini: Myocardial function and contractile force affected by glucose loading of the heart during anoxia. *Surgery*, **57**:839, 1965.

200. Pindyck, F., M. R. Drucker, R. S. Brown, and W. C. Shoemaker: Cardiorespiratory effects of hypertonic glucose in the critically ill patient, *Surgery*, **75**:11, 1974.

201. Egdahl, R. H.: Hypertonic glucose and improved critical organ performance, *Surgery*, **75**:145, 1974.

202. Soeters, P. B., and J. E. Fischer: Insulin, gluca-gon, amino acid imbalance, and hepatic encephalopathy, *Lancet*, **202**:880, 1976.

203. Munro, H. N., J. D. Fernstrom, and R. J. Wurtman: Insulin, plasma amino acid imbalance, and hepatic coma, *Lancet*, **1**:722, 1975.

204. Fischer, J. E., J. M. Funovics, A. Aguirre, J. H. James, J. M. Keane, R. I. C. Wesdorp, N. Yoshimura, and T. Westman: The role of plasma amino acids in hepatic encephalopathy, *Surgery*, **78**:276, 1975.

205. Lam, K. C., A. R. Tall, G. B. Goldstein, and S. P. Mistilis: Role of a false neurotransmitter, octopamine, in the pathogenesis of hepatic and renal encephalopathy, *Scand. J. Gastroenterol.*, **8**:465, 1973.

206. Mattson, W. J., Jr., V. Iob, M. Sloan, W. W. Coon, J. G. Turcotte, and C. G. Child III: Alterations of individual free amino acids in brain during acute hepatic coma, *Surg. Gynecol. Obstet.*, **130**:263, 1970.

207. Fischer, J. E., N. Yoshimura, A. Aguirre, J. H. James, M. G. Cummings, R. M. Abel, and F. Deindoerfer: Plasma amino acids in patients with hepatic encephalopathy: Effects of amino acid infusions, *Am. J. Surg.*, **127**:40, 1974.

208. James, J. H., J. M. Hodgman, J. M. Funovics, N. Yoshimura, and J. E. Fischer: Brain tryptophan, plasma free tryptophan and distribution of plasma neutral amino acids, *Metabolism*, **25**:471, 1976.

209. Aguirre, A., J. Funovics, R. I. C. Wesdorp, and J. E. Fischer: Parenteral nutrition in hepatic failure, in J. E. Fischer (ed.), *Total Parenteral Nutrition*, Little, Brown and Company, Boston, 1976, pp. 219–230.

210. Maddrey, W. C., F. L. Weber, Jr., A. W. Coulter, C. M. Chura, N. P. Chapanis, and M. Walser: Effects of keto analogues of essential amino acids in portal-systemic encephalopathy, *Gastroenterology*, **71**:190, 1976.

211. Lordon, R. E., and J. R. Burton. Post-traumatic renal failure in military personnel in South Asia, *Am. J. Med.*, **53**:137, 1972.

212. Stott, R. B., J. S. Cameron, C. S. Ogg, and M. Bewick: Why the persistently high mortality in acute renal failure? *Lancet*, **2**:75, 1972.

213. Kopple, J. D.: Dietary requirements, in S. G. Massry and A. L. Sellars (eds.), *Clinical Aspects of Uremia and Dialysis*, Charles C Thomas, Pub-

lisher, Springfield, Illinois, 1976, pp. 453–489.

214. Abel, R. M., C. H. Beck, Jr., W. M. Abbott, J. A. Ryan, Jr., G. O. Barnett, and J. E. Fischer: Improved survival from acute renal failure after treatment with intravenous essential L-amino acids and glucose, *N. Engl. J. Med.*, **288**:695, 1973. 1973.

215. Toback, G. F.: Amino acid enhancement of renal regeneration after acute tubular necrosis, *Kidney Int.*, **12**:193, 1977.

216. Blagg, C. R., F. M. Parsons, and G. A. Young: Effect of dietary glucose and protein in acute renal failure, *Lancet*, **1**:608, 1962.

217. Kleinknecht, O., P. Jungers, J. Chanard, C. Barbanel, and D. Ganeval: Uremic and non-uremic complications in acute renal failure: Evaluation of early and frequent dialysis on prognosis, *Kidney Int.*, **1**:190, 1972.

218. Lee, H. A., P. Sharpstone, and A. C. Ames: Parenteral nutrition in renal failure, *Postgrad. Med. J.*, **43**:81, 1967.

219. Dudrick, S. J., E. Steiger, and J. M. Long: Renal failure in surgical patients. Treatment with intravenous essential amino acids and hypertonic glucose, *Surgery*, **68**:180, 1970.

220. Van Buren, C. T., S. J. Dudrick, K. Dworkin, E. Baumbauer, and J. M. Long: Effects of intravenous L-amino acids and hypertonic dextrose on anephric beagles, *Surg. Forum*, **23**:83, 1972.

221. Abbott, W. M., R. M. Abel, and J. E. Fischer: Treatment of acute renal insufficiency after aortoiliac surgery, *Arch. Surg.*, **103**:590, 1971.

222. Abel, R. M., W. M. Abbott, and J. E. Fischer: Intravenous essential L-amino acids and hypertonic dextrose in patients with acute renal failure, *Am. J. Surg.*, **123**:632, 1972.

223. Abel, R. M., V. E. Shih, W. Abbott, C. H. Beck, Jr., and J. E. Fischer: Amino acid metabolism in acute renal failure: Influence of intravenous essential L-amino acid hyperalimentation therapy, *Ann. Surg.*, **180**:350, 1974.

224. Abel, R. M., W. M. Abbott, C. H. Beck, Jr., J. A. Ryan, Jr., and J. E. Fischer: Essential L-amino acids for hyperalimentation in patients with disordered nitrogen metabolism, *Am. J. Surg.*, **128**:317, 1974.

225. Leonard, C. D., R. G. Luke, and R. R. Siegel: Parenteral essential amino acids in acute renal failure, *Urology*, **6**:154, 1975.

226. Baek, S., G. G. Makabali, C. W. Bryan-Brown, J. Kusek, and W. C. Shoemaker: The influence of parenteral nutrition on the course of acute renal failure, *Surg. Gynecol. Obstet.*, **141**:405, 1975.

227. Blackburn, G. L., P. Rutten, M. Stone, J. P. Flatt, M. Trerice, T. MacKenzie, E. Hallowell, R. Heddle, and G. Page: Muscle synthesis of non-essential amino acids (NEAA) during acute renal failure intravenous feeding. *Proc. Int. Soc. Parenteral Nut.*, Montpellier, France, 1974, p. 625.

228. Sofio, C., and R. W. Nicora: High calorie essential amino acid parenteral therapy in acute renal failure, *Acta Chir. Scand.*, **466**(suppl.):98, 1976.

229. Abitbol, C. L., and M. A. Holliday: Total parenteral nutrition in anuric children, *Clin. Nephrol.*, **5**:153, 1976.

230. Blumenkrantz, M. J., J. D. Kopple, A. Koffler, A. K. Kamdar, M. D. Healy, E. I. Feinstein, and S. G. Massry: Total parenteral nutrition in the management of acute renal failure, *Am. J. Clin. Nutr.*, (in press).

231. Blumenkrantz, M. J., and J. D. Kopple: VA cooperative dialysis study. Participants: Incidence of nutritional abnormalities in uremic patients entering dialysis therapy, *Kidney Int.*, **10**:514, 1976.

232. Kopple, J. D.: Metabolic and endocrine abnormalities: C. nitrogen metabolism, in S. G. Massry and A. Sellars (eds.), *Clinical Aspects of Uremia and Dialysis*, Charles C Thomas, Publisher, Springfield, Ill., 1976, pp. 241–273.

233. Jonxis, J. H. P., and T. H. J. Huisman: Excretion of amino acids in free and bound form during intravenous administration of protein hydrolysate, *Metabolism*, **6**:175, 1957.

234. Kopple, J. D., and M. E. Swendseid: Evidence that histidine is an essential amino acid in normal and chronically uremic man, *J. Clin. Invest.*, **55**:881, 1975.

235. Bergstrom, J., P. Furst and L. O. Noree: Treatment of chronic uremic patients with protein-poor diet and oral supply of essential amino acids. I. Nitrogen balance studies, *Clin. Nephrol.*, **3**:187, 1975.

236. Kopple, J. D., and M. E. Swendseid: Protein and amino acid metabolism in uremic patients undergoing maintenance hemodialysis, *Kidney Int.*, **7**:(suppl. 2):64, 1975.

237. Kopple, J. D., and M. E. Swendseid: Vitamin nutrition in patients undergoing maintenance he-

modialysis, *Kidney Int.*, **7**(Suppl. 2):79, 1975.

238. Heidland, A., and J. Kult: Long-term effects of essential amino acids supplementation in patients on regular dialysis treatment, *Clin. Neprhol.*, **3**:234, 1975.

239. Nolph, K. D., P. S. Rosenfeld, J. T. Powell, and E. Danforth: Peritoneal glucose transport and hyperglycemia during peritoneal dialysis, *Am. J. Med. Sci.*, **259**:272, 1970.

240. Andersson, G., M. Bergquist-Poppen, J. Bergstrom, L. G. Collste, and E. Hultman: Glucose absorption from the dialysis fluid during peritoneal dialysis, *Scand. J. Urol. Nephrol.*, **5**:77, 1971.

241. Blumenkrantz, M. J., C. E. Roberts, B. Card, J. Coburn, and J. D. Kopple: Nutritional management of the adult patient undergoing maintenance peritoneal dialysis, *J. Am. Diet. Assoc.*, (in press).

242. Dudrick, S. J., B. V. MacFadyen, Jr., C. T. van Buren, R. L. Ruberg, and A. T. Maynard: Parenteral hyperalimentation: Metabolic problems and solutions, *Ann. Surg.*, **176**:259, 1972.

243. Ryan, J. A., Jr., R. M. Abel, W. M. Abbott, C. C. Hopkins, T. McChesney, R. Colley, K. Phillips, and J. E. Fischer: Catheter complications in total parenteral nutrition: A prospective study of 200 consecutive patients, *N. Engl. J. Med.*, **290**:757, 1974.

244. Ryan, J. A., Jr.: Complications of total parenteral nutrition, in J. E. Fischer (ed.), *Total Parenteral Nutrition*, Little, Brown and Company, Boston, 1976, pp. 55–100.

245. Green, H. L., and P. Nemir, Jr.: Air embolism as a complication during parenteral alimentation, *Am. J. Surg.*, **121**:614, 1971.

246. Goldmann, D. A., and D. G. Maki: Infection control in total parenteral nutrition, *JAMA*, **223**:1360, 1973.

247. Dillion, J. D., Jr., W. Schaffner, C. W. Van Way, III, and H. C. Meng: Septicemia and total parenteral nutrition: Distinguishing catheter-related from other septic episodes, *JAMA*, **223**:1341, 1973.

248. Brennan, M. F., R. C. O'Connell, J. A. Rosol, and R. Kundsin: The growth of *Candida albicans* in nutritive solutions given parenterally, *Arch. Surg.*, **103**:705, 1971.

249. Curry, C. R., and P. G. Quie: Fungal septicemia in patients receiving parenteral hyperalimentation, *N. Engl. J. Med.*, **285**:1221, 1971.

250. Norden, C. W.: Application of antibiotic ointment to the site of venous catheterization: A controlled trial, *J. Infect. Dis.*, **120**:611, 1969.

251. Jarrard, M. M., and J. B. Freeman: The effects of antibiotic ointments and antiseptics on the skin flora beneath subclavian catheter dressings during intravenous hyperalimentation, *J. Surg. Res.*, **22**:521, 1977.

252. Goldmann, D. A., W. T. Martin, and J. W. Worthington: Growth of bacteria and fungi in total parenteral nutrition solutions, *Am. J. Surg.*, **126**:314, 1973.

254. Heird, W. C., R. B. Dell, J. M. Driscoll, Jr., B. Grebin, and R. W. Winters: Metabolic acidosis resulting from intravenous alimentation mixtures containing synthetic amino acids, *N. Engl. J. Med.*, **287**:943, 1972.

255. Johnson, J. D., W. L. Albritton, and P. Sunshine: Hyperammonemia accompanying parenteral nutrition in newborn infants, *J. Pediatr.*, **81**:154, 1972.

256. Travis, S. F., H. J. Sugerman, R. L. Ruberg, S. J. Dudrick, M. Delivoria-Papadopoulos, L. D. Miller, and F. A. Oski: Alterations of red-cell glycolytic intermediates and oxygen transport as a consequence of hypophosphatemia in patients receiving intravenous hyperalimentation, *N. Engl. J. Med.*, **285**:763, 1971.

257. Derr, R. F., and L. Zieve: Etiology of hyperalimentation coma, *N. Engl. J. Med.*, **288**:1080, 1973.

258. Yawata, Y., P. Craddock, R. Hebbel, R. Howe, S. Silvis, and H. Jacob: Hyperalimentation hypophosphatemia: Hematologic-neurologic dysfunction due to ATP depletion, *Clin. Res.*, **21**:729, 1973.

259. Craddock, P. R., Y. Yawata, L. Van Santen, S. Gilberstadt, S. Silvis, and H. S. Jacob: Acquired phagocyte dysfunction: A complication of hypophosphatemia of parenteral hyperalimentation, *N. Engl. J. Med.*, **290**:1403, 1974.

260. Jacob, H. S., and W. T. Amsden: Acute hemolytic anemia with rigid red cells in hypophosphatemia, *N. Engl. J. Med.*, **285**:1446, 1971.

261. Silvis, S. E., and P. D. Paragas, Jr.: Paresthesias, weakness, seizures and hypophosphatemia in patients receiving hyperalimentation, *Gastroenterology*, **62:**513, 1972.

262. Sand, D. W., and R. A. Pastore: Paresthesias and hypophosphatemia occurring with parenteral alimentation, *Am. J. Dig. Dis.*, **18:**709, 1973.

263. Prins, J. G., H. Schrijver, and J. H. Staghouwer: Hyperalimentation, hypophosphataemia, and coma, *Lancet*, **1:**1253, 1973.

264. Baughman, F. A., Jr., and J. P. Papp: Wernicke's encephalopathy with intravenous hyperalimentation: Remarks on similarities between Wernicke's encephalopathy and the phosphate depletion syndrome, *Mt. Sinai J. Med.*, **43:**48, 1976.

265. Weintraub, M. I.: Hypophosphatemia mimicking acute Guillain-Barré-Strohl syndrome (a complication of parenteral hyperalimentation), *JAMA*, **235:**1040, 1976.

266. Ulstrom, R. A., and D. M. Brown: Hypercalcemia as a complication of parenteral alimentation, *J. Pediatr.*, **81:**419, 1972.

267. Calloway, D. H., A. C. J. Odell, and S. Margen: Sweat and miscellaneous nitrogen losses in human balance studies, *J. Nutr.*, **101:**775, 1971.

268. Blackburn, G. L., J. P. Flatt, G. H. A. Clowes, Jr., T. F. O'Donnell, and T. E. Hensle: Protein sparing therapy during periods of starvation with sepsis or trauma, *Ann. Surg.*, **177:**588, 1973.

269. Freeman, J. B., L. D. Stegink, P. D. Meyer, R. G. Thompson, and L. DenBesten: Metabolic effects of amino acid vs. dextrose infusion in surgical patients, *Arch. Surg.*, **110:**916, 1975.

270. Schulte, W. J., R. E. Condon, and M. A. Kraus: Positive nitrogen balance using isotonic crystalline amino acid solution, *Arch. Surg.*, **110:**914, 1975.

271. Hoover, H. C., Jr., J. P. Grant, C. Gorschboth, and A. S. Ketcham: Nitrogen-sparing intravenous fluids in postoperative patients, *N. Engl. J. Med.*, **293:**172, 1975.

272. Greenberg, G. R., E. B. Marliss, G. H. Anderson, B. Langer, W. Spence, E. B. Tovee, and K. N. Jeejeebhoy: Protein-sparing therapy in postoperative patients: Effects of added hypocaloric glucose or lipid, *N. Engl. J. Med.*, **294:**1411, 1976.

273. Skillman, J. J., V. M. Rosenoer, P. C. Smith, and M. S. Fang: Improved albumin synthesis in postoperative patients by amino acid infusion, *N. Engl. J. Med.*, **295:**1037, 1976.

274. Felig, P.: Intravenous nutrition: Fact and fancy, *N. Engl. J. Med.*, **294:**1455, 1976.

275. Freeman, J. B., L. D. Steginh, M. F. Wittine, and R. C. Thompson: The current status of protein sparing, *Surg. Gynecol. Obstet.*, **144:**843, 1977.

276. Freeman, J. B., L. D. Steginh, M. F. Wittine, M. M. Danney, and R. G. Thompson: Lack of correlation between nitrogen balance and serum insulin levels during protein sparing with and without dextrose, *Gastroenterology*, **73:**31, 1977.

277. Freeman, J. B., L. D. Steginh, R. G. Thompson, E. E. Mason, and L. DenBesten: Infusion of crystalline amino acids with and without dextrose in morbid obesity, *Surg. Forum*, **26:**35, 1975.

278. Wei, P., J. R. Hamilton, and A. E. LeBlanc: A clinical and metabolic study of an intravenous feeding technique using peripheral veins as the initial infusion site, *Can. Med. Assoc. J.*, **106:**969, 1972.

279. Scribner, B. H., J. J. Cole, T. G. Christopher, J. E. Vizzo, R. C. Atkins, and C. R. Blagg: Long-term total parenteral nutrition: the concept of an artificial gut, *JAMA*, **212:**457, 1970.

280. Bergstrom, K., R. Blomstrand, and S. Jacobson: Long-term complete intravenous nutrition in man, *Nutr. Metab.*, **14**(suppl.):118, 1972.

281. Jeejeebhoy, K. N., W. J. Zohrab, B. Langer, M. J. Phillips, A. Kuksis, and G. H. Anderson: Total parenteral nutrition at home for 23 months, without complication, and with good rehabilitation: A study of technical and metabolic features, *Gastroenterology*, **65:**811, 1973.

282. Solassol, C. L., H. Joyeux, L. Etco, H. Pujol, and C. L. Romieu: New techniques for long-term feeding: An artificial gut in 75 patients, *Ann. Surg.*, **179:**519, 1974.

283. Bordos, D. C., and J. L. Cameron: Successful long-term intravenous hyperalimentation in the hospital and at home, *Arch. Surg.*, **110:**439, 1975.

284. Shils, M. E.: A program for total parenteral nutrition at home, *Am. J. Clin. Nutr.*, **28:**1429, 1975.

285. Broviac, J. W., M. C. Riella, and B. H. Scribner: The role of intralipid in prolonged parenteral nutrition. I. As a caloric substitute for glucose, *Am. J. Clin. Nutr.*, **29:**255, 1976.

SECTION II

Parenteral fluid therapy

INTRODUCTION

The use of parenteral infusions for medical therapy has been a subject of speculation for many centuries. It was probably Sir Christopher Wren who first infused medicines intravenously with the use of a goose quill. The first fluid infused seems to have been blood. After an early blood transfusion the urine of one patient was noted to be "as black as soot," apparently the result of hemolysis. With ignorance of blood incompatibilities between different animals or humans, blood transfusions were quickly recognized as hazardous and were discontinued.

In 1831, O'Shaughnessy, in England, described the chemical composition of blood and diarrheal matter in cholera victims in a letter to *Lancet* (1):

Sir, . . . 1) The blood drawn in the worst cases of the cholera is unchanged in its anatomical or globular structure. 2) It has lost a large proportion of its water, 1000 parts of cholera serum having but the average of 860 parts of water. 3) It has lost a great proportion of its neutral saline ingredients. 4) Of the free alkali contained in healthy serum, not a particle is present in some cholera cases, and barely a trace in others. 5) Urea exists in cases where suppression of urine has been a marked symptom. 6) All the salts deficient in blood, especially the carbonate of soda, are present in large quantities in the peculiar white dejected matter. . . . Neither shall I on this occasion offer an observation on the practical inference to which my experiments may lead. . . .

I am, Sir,
Your obedient servant,
W.B. O'Shaughnessy, M.D.
London, 29 December 1831

Thomas Latta (2), reading the report of O'Shaughnessy, gave a patient with cholera intravenous therapy with saline and sodium bicarbonate with the following results:

Leith, May 23, 1832

Sir, . . . I at length resolved to throw the fluid immediately into the circulation. . . . The first subject of experiment was an aged female on whom all the usual remedies had been fully tried, without producing one good symptom; the disease, uninterrupted, holding steadily on its course, she had apparently reached the last moments of her earthly existence, and now nothing could injure her. . . . Having inserted a tube into the basilic vein, cautiously—anxiously, I watched the effects; ounce after ounce was injected, but no visible change was produced. Still persevering, I thought she began to breathe less laboriously, soon the sharpened features, and sunken eye, and fallen jaw, pale and cold, bearing the manifest impress of death's signet, began to flow with returning animation; the pulse, which had long ceased, returned to the wrist. . . . When 6 pints had been injected, she expressed in a firm voice that she was free from all uneasiness, actually became jocular, and fancied all she needed was a little sleep; her extremities were warm, and every feature bore the aspect of comfort and health. . . .

I am, Sir,
Your most obedient servant,
Thomas Latta, M.D.

Subsequently, Lewins reported his experiences in 15 patients with 5 survivals (3). Despite these dramatic efforts, intravenous therapy did not become widely used until well into the twentieth century. In the early 1900s proctoclysis, hypodermoclysis, and gastric tube feeding were employed. Morbidity and mortality from peritonitis, pancreatitis, nonstrangulated intestinal obstruction, or diarrhea at that time were attributed to "toxemia," and the value of fluid therapy was generally considered to lie in its ability to dilute, flush out, or protect from these toxins (4).

Hartwell and Hoguet, in 1912, pointed out the importance of fluid deficits as a cause of death in dogs with experimental intestinal obstruction (5). However, it was not until approximately 10 years later that parenteral fluid therapy for volume replacement gained wide acceptance (6, 7). Gamble and Ross demonstrated the importance of parenteral fluid therapy and saline administration in such conditions as pyloric obstruction and infantile diarrhea (8).

The last 40 years have shown an enormous increase in knowledge of normal fluid and mineral physiology and in understanding and treatment of specific disorders of fluid, electrolyte, and acid-base metabolism. The use of blood, its products, colloidal solutions, and total parenteral nutrition have undergone enormous refinement in the last several decades, and rapid progress is continuing, especially in the areas of total parenteral nutrition and artificial blood.

TREATMENT OF FLUID AND ELECTROLYTE DISORDERS

WATER AND ELECTROLYTE METABOLISM

Water

Total body water accounts for 45 to 70 percent of body weight, the fraction varying with body fat, sex, age, and disease states or injury. In a typical young man, about 30 to 40 percent of body weight consists of intracellular water; 16 percent, interstitial water (including lymph, dense connective tissue, and cartilage); 4.5 percent, plasma water; and 1.5 percent, transcellular water (organ and gastrointestinal secretions, body cavities, and cerebrospinal fluid). In obese individuals, body water as a percentage of body weight is decreased, since the water content of adipose tissue is very low. In men, as compared to women, water generally accounts for a greater proportion of body weight because men usually have relatively more muscle and less fat. Body water accounts for up to 70 to 80 percent of weight in newborn infants, falls to approximately 60 percent in young men and 50 percent in young women, and then remains relatively constant until middle age, when it gradually falls progressively as muscle mass decreases.

In addition to urinary excretion of water, there is a daily loss of about 500 mL from perspiration and insensible skin losses, 400 mL from respiration, and 150 mL in feces. These losses are partially offset by the production of about 350 mL/day of water from oxidation of hydrogen in protein, carbohydrate, and fat. Ingestion of solid foods provides about 750 mL of water per day. During periods of wasting, water is also released from catabolism of protein and glycogen (about 3 mL/g) and from oxidation of fat (about 1.08 mL/g). Nonurinary water loss may be marked under certain conditions. Cutaneous losses can be enormous—greater than 20 L/day—in hot weather, especially in the absence of air movement (9). Perspiration may evaporate so rapidly in a hot, dry environment that the magnitude of water loss is not readily apparent unless body weight or appropriate blood indices are assessed (see below). Cutaneous water loss also increases with fever. Respiratory loss can increase markedly with hyperventilation and may be reduced by respirators which provide nebulized water.

The kidney has great capacity to maintain normal body water. In a healthy individual, the osmolality of urine can vary between 50 and 1200 mosm (9, 10). Normal individuals ingesting limited quantities of water, especially in a hot environment, may excrete only 350 to 500 mL/day of urine (see Chap. 12). With water loading and maximum water diuresis, urinary osmolality can fall to 30 mosm/L and free water clearance (excretion of solute-free water; see Chap. 12) can be as high as 20 mL/min or 1200 mL/h. Low urine volumes can promote formation of urinary calculi, and it has been suggested that water intake in the adult should be sufficient to produce a urinary volume of at least 1200 to 1500 mL/day.

Enhanced antidiuretic hormone (ADH) release, which often accompanies stress and painful stimuli, reduces ability to excrete a water load. ADH secretion may increase in the postoperative state, with drugs which stimulate ADH release, such as narcotics, barbiturates, tranquilizers, and oral hypoglycemic agents, or in the syndrome of inappropriate secretion of ADH (SIADH) (see Chap. 12). Also, diuretics, particularly those such as furosemide and thiazide, which act on the diluting segment in the ascending limb of the loop of Henle, impair urinary dilution and can engender a hypoosmolar state. Renal disease, hypercalcemia, hypokalemia, malnutrition, osmotic diuretics, and drugs inhibiting ADH release or its action on the kidney can impair concentrating ability and predispose to hyperosmolar states (see Chap. 12).

Sodium and osmolality

Sodium is the major extracellular cation. There are approximately 3350 to 4150 meq of sodium in the normal young adult human (11). Half of total body sodium is in extracellular fluid (ECF); another 40 percent is in bone, and only half of this is rapidly exchangeable (12). The intracellular $[Na^+]$ is about 10 meq/kg of water.

Usually sodium is excreted almost entirely in urine. Fecal sodium excretion is about 1 to 3 meq/day, and skin losses are small unless there is excessive sweating. In patients with normal renal function who are not receiving diuretics, urinary sodium excretion can be markedly reduced when intake is restricted. With complete sodium deprivation, urinary sodium excretion can fall to 1 to 2 meq/L within 3 to 5 days. Osmotic or tubular diuretics and impaired renal function can prevent this degree of sodium conservation.

Normally, sodium salts account for about 90 percent of the osmotically active solutes in ECF. Almost all sodium in ECF is dissociated from its anion, and thus each milliequivalent of sodium salt accounts for almost 2 mosm. Since there is normally only a small osmotic effect from other solutes, one can usually estimate the serum osmolality as twice the $[Na^+]$. However, serum glucose or urea also affect serum osmolality, which can be estimated more precisely from the sodium, potassium, urea, and glucose concentrations according to the following equation:

$$\text{Plasma osmolality} = 2.0 \, [\text{Na(meq/L)} + \text{K(meq/L)}]$$
$$+ \frac{\text{SUN(mg/dL)}}{2.8} + \frac{\text{blood glucose (mg/dL)}}{18} \quad (10B\text{-}1)$$

The equation for the osmotic effect of urea is derived as follows: Nitrogen in 1 mmol of urea = 28 mg; 1 mosm of urea nitrogen = 28 mg of urea nitrogen/kg of solution or 2.8 mg/dL. Therefore,

$$\text{mosm of urea nitrogen}$$
$$= \frac{\text{concentration in serum (mg/dL)}}{2.8} \quad (10B\text{-}2)$$

For example, a serum urea nitrogen (SUN) of 140 mg/dL contributes 140/2.8 = 50 mosm/kg to serum osmolality.

It follows from Eq. (10B-1) that when serum glucose or urea is very elevated, sodium salts do not account for all of the osmotic force in ECF. The discordance between serum sodium and osmolality may be particularly great in hyperglycemia and when osmotic diuretics, such as mannitol, are infused. These compounds are not freely distributed intracellularly. Osmotic forces enhance movement of water extracellularly, and serum $[Na^+]$ falls. Urea has no effect on $[Na^+]$ since urea moves freely across the membrane of almost all cells.

Serum Na is spuriously lowered when serum lipids or proteins are elevated, as in the paraproteinemias (e.g., multiple myeloma). Normal human plasma is 93 percent water. Na is not miscible in the protein and lipids which compose the remaining 7 percent of plasma. Thus, Na is limited to plasma water, and its concentration in the water compartment can be estimated by dividing the plasma $[Na^+]$ by 0.93. For example, with a normal plasma $[Na^+]$ of 142 meq/L, the Na level in plasma water is 142/0.93 = 153 meq/L. Elevated lipids or proteins reduce the proportion of water in plasma, and, hence, the volume in which Na is distributed. Spurious hyponatremia causes no symptoms. The importance of recognizing it lies in preventing inappropriate therapy to increase serum sodium and in calling attention to the underlying lipid or protein disorder. Elevated triglycerides is the most frequent cause of spurious hyponatremia and occurs most commonly with diabetic ketoacidosis, pancreatitis, idiopathic hypertriglyceridemia, nephrotic syndrome, uremia, and intravenous infusion of fat emulsions. Spurious hyponatremia should be suspected in patients with lactescent serum or when symptoms are not commensurate with the measured serum Na.

Sodium intake in normal adults can be safely varied over a wide range, because conservation and excretion are so efficient. However, some reports suggest that high sodium intake may predispose to hypertension. Also, sodium ingestion is habit forming. Many diseases require therapeutic restriction of sodium, and people who eat large quantities may have great difficulty reducing sodium intake.

Potassium

Potassium is the primary intracellular ion. Approximately 90 percent of potassium is intracellular, 8 to 9 percent is in bone, connective tissues, and the transcellular space, and 1 to 2 percent is in plasma and interstitial fluid. Homeostatic mechanisms allow potassium (like water and sodium) intake to vary widely in normal adults without causing a deficit or excess. However, potassium cannot be conserved as efficiently as sodium. In a normal individual deprived of potassium for 4 to 5 days, potassium loss is about 25 meq/day, approximately 15 meq in urine and 10 meq in stool. The usual daily urinary potassium loss is at least 40 meq, and this quantity is frequently recommended as the minimum required intake in patients with normal renal function receiving nutrition intravenously. It has been stated that the daily dietary potassium intake for normal adults should be at least 60 to 70 meq (13).

Serum potassium frequently varies independently of total body potassium, and it is the most critical compartment to control because relatively small changes in serum levels can severely alter myocardial and skeletal muscle function. Serious hyperkalemia has a variety of causes, such as oliguric renal failure, the hyporenin hypoaldosterone syndrome, use of spironolactone or triamterene, and rapid administration of potassium, particularly intravenously.

Potassium deficiency and hypokalemia are most frequently caused by excessive urinary potassium excretion from diuretics, loss of gastrointestinal fluids, and diabetic ketoacidosis. Hypokalemia may also accompany renal tubular acidosis, hyperaldosteronism, Bartter's syndrome, cirrhosis, metabolic alkalosis, ileostomy, colostomy, external biliary drainage, and parenteral nutrition with inadequate potassium intake.

Serum potassium can be altered by movement of potassium in and out of cells. Alkalosis, insulin, glucose, and anabolism enhance intracellular movement of potassium. Conversely, acidosis and catabolic stress such as trauma, surgery, or starvation promote extracellular movement of potassium and can cause severe hyperkalemia if renal function is reduced.

Water imbalance

Water deficit. Dehydration can be classified into three types, depending on the relative deficits of salt and water: hypernatremic, normonatremic, and hyponatremic. The most common type of dehydration is hypernatremic, where water is lost in excess of sodium; some degree of sodium depletion is often present. Hypernatremic dehydration is commonly found in patients who, because of impaired mental or physical ability, do not experience thirst normally or do not have access to water. Causes of hypernatremic dehydration include water deprivation, enhanced sweating, excessive urine flow due to osmotic or tubular diuretics, diabetic ketoacidosis, nonketotic hyperosmolar coma, a high-protein, low-water diet (with enhanced formation and excretion of urea), vasopressin-sensitive and nephrogenic diabetes insipidus, diuresis following relief of urinary tract obstruction, excessive salt intake, peritoneal dialysis with high glucose solutions, and selective impairment of thirst (see also Chap. 12).

Normonatremic dehydration occurs most commonly with loss of gastrointestinal fluids from vomiting or diarrhea, although if water is ingested in excess of salt, hyponatremia can develop.

Hyponatremic dehydration occurs in salt-wasting renal diseases, nonoliguric chronic renal failure with excessive salt loss, and adrenocortical insufficiency. Salt-wasting may occasionally occur with mild renal failure. Although it may occur in virtually any type of nonoliguric chronic renal failure, salt-wasting is particularly prevalent in diseases affecting the renal interstitium, such as polycystic disease, analgesic nephropathy, medullary cystic disease, or pyelonephritis. In patients with diabetic ketoacidosis or nonketotic hyperosmolar coma, serum sodium may be high, normal, or low (see Chap. 24).

Water excess. Water excess, like dehydration, can be associated with increased, normal, or decreased serum [Na+]. Elevated total body water is not infrequently associated with some degree of hyponatremia and hypoosmolality. Water excess and hyponatremia are usually caused by reduced ability to excrete free water, as occurs in (1) conditions in which there is decreased delivery of fluid to the diluting segment of the renal tubule, such as decreased glomerular filtration rate, congestive heart failure, cirrhosis with ascites, nephrotic syndrome, and myxedema; (2) treatment with "loop" diuretics such as furosemide or thiazides, or Bartter's syndrome, which decrease solute reabsorption in the diluting segment; (3) enhanced water absorption in the distal tubule and collecting duct due to increased antidiuretic hormone or to glucocorticoid deficiency. Primary polydipsia can lead to hyponatremia with fluid excess, although this usually occurs only when a coincidental factor impairs free water clearance.

Water excess with normal serum [Na+] is common, particularly in heart, liver or kidney failure or the nephrotic syndrome. Water excess with hypernatremia is uncommon but may occur with intravenous infusion of large quantities of normal or hypertonic saline in patients with impaired renal function.

Hyponatremia cannot occur unless intake of water is high relative to that of sodium. The [Na+] in fluids lost from the body is virtually always less than that in plasma (Table 10-12), even with hyponatremia. Hence, it is virtually impossible to develop hyponatremia in the absence of water intake.

We emphasize that total body sodium is usually not depleted in hyponatremia; rather, there is usually normal or increased body sodium and a greater excess of body water. Conversely, hypernatremia is often associated with decreased total body sodium and a greater loss of water.

ASSESSMENT OF WATER AND ELECTROLYTE DISORDERS

Fluid and electrolyte disturbances, even if complex, are usually readily diagnosed if approached systematically. The history should be reviewed, the patient examined, and the hemodynamic and biochemical data evaluated. Armchair diagnoses made solely from laboratory data subject the patient to unnecessary risks. It is helpful to make the following assessments: (1) the character of the disorder (e.g., hyponatremic dehydration), (2) the cause of the disorder, (3) the magnitude of the deficits or excesses, (4) the rate of continuing loss or gain of fluid or electrolytes. The syndromes caused by sodium, potassium, calcium, phosphorus, and magnesium disorders are discussed in Chaps. 3, 4, 8, and 19. Evaluation of disturbances in water and osmolality will be discussed.

Medical history

Evidence for abnormal fluid loss or gain can often be elicited from the history (i.e., vomiting, diarrhea, heat exposure, or polydipsia). A psychiatric disturbance may suggest covert polydipsia or excessive serum ADH levels. Thirst may indicate hyperosmolality, but it may be absent with cerebral injury, mental obtundation, hot ambient temperatures, or, rarely, selective disorders of the brain. The magnitude of a fluid disorder can often be estimated from the history, e.g., change in body weight, severity of vomiting or diarrhea.

Physical examination

Dehydration is suggested by a dry, shrunken tongue with deep furrows, dry mucous mem-

Table 10-12. Electrolyte content of body fluids

FLUID	Na$^+$, meq/L	K$^+$, meq/L	Cl$^-$, meq/L	HCO$_3$, meq/L
Plasma				
Mean	142	4.5	102	26
Normal range	135–150	3.5–5.0	98–106	22–30
Saliva				
Mean	33	20	34	
Normal range	20–46	16–23	24–44	
Gastric juice				
Mean	60	9	84	0
Normal range	30–90	4.3–12	52–124	
Bile				
Mean	149	4.9	101	45
Normal range	120–170	3–12	80–120	30–50
Pancreatic juice				
Mean	141	4.6	77	92
Normal range	113–153	2.6–7.4	54–95	70–110
Small bowel				
Mean	105	5.1	99	50
Normal range	72–158	3.5–6.8	70–127	20–40
Ileal fluid				
Mean	129	11.2	116	29
Normal range	90–140	6–30	82–125	25–30
Fecal fluid				
Mean	80	21	48	22
Normal range	50–116	11–28	35–70	15–30
Cerebrospinal fluid				
Mean	141	2.9	127	23
Normal range	135–147	2.5–3.4	116–132	21–25
Sweat				
Mean	45	4.5	58	0
Normal range	18–97	1–15	18–97	
Aqueous humor				
Mean	143	4.7	108	
Normal range	142–145	. . .	106–110	

branes, decreased skin turgor, soft and contracted eyes, and flattened neck veins. Dry buccal mucous membranes may be misleading in patients who mouth breathe. Also, skin turgor may be decreased from loss of subcutaneous tissue in wasted patients. The skin over the sternum and forehead tends to be most reliable for assessing tissue dehydration.

Low blood pressure is more likely to occur when dehydration is associated with loss of sodium or albumin. For example, when the water lost contains sodium, 140 meq/L, plasma volume decreases by approximately 25 percent of the total fluid loss. In contrast, in pure water depletion without loss of sodium or albumin, plasma volume is only decreased by about 7.5 percent of the total water lost, and blood pressure is better maintained. Postural changes in blood pressure and pulse may be sensitive indicators of low intravascular volume. Also, increased sensitivity of blood pressure to hypotensive medicines and exaggerated postural changes with these agents may indicate depleted intravascular volume; however, these findings may also occur with pericardial effusions.

When water excess is accompanied by proportional increases in salt, volume expansion is primarily extracellular. Neck vein distention, edema, and ascites or frank congestive heart failure may occur. In contrast, when there is positive water balance with little or no gain in sodium, the excess water is distributed in the large intracellular as well as the extracellular compartment. In the latter case, water gain is usually better tolerated, and when symptoms occur, signs of hyponatremia and water intoxication may predominate.

Laboratory tests

With dehydration, there may be a low urine volume, a high urine osmolality and specific gravity, an increased ratio of urine/plasma osmolality, creatinine and urea, and an elevated serum osmolality. With low urine flow, fractional reabsorption of urea by the distal nephron is increased. Hence, in oliguria, there is a disproportionate decrease in urea clearance relative to creatinine or inulin clearance, and SUN levels and SUN/serum creatinine ratios are elevated. In overhydration, the urine volume is often of no diagnostic value because there is usually some degree of functional or organic impairment in renal function. The urine/plasma osmolality ratio is usually elevated in SIADH, but even a hypotonic urine may be inappropriately hypertonic for the degree of overhydration. For example, in patients with psychogenic polydipsia, water intoxication may occur because of slightly increased ADH secretion or impaired function of the diluting segment of the nephron. Urine osmolality may fall to 70 to 140 mosm/L, whereas normally it would be less than 50 to 60 mosm/L.

Hematocrit and serum proteins may be elevated in dehydration and reduced with increased body water. However, the usefulness of these measurements is limited by the multiplicity of factors affecting their concentrations, particularly when values are low. Previous measurements of hematocrit and proteins may be helpful for comparison. Serum protein concentrations are affected by posture and can increase because of hemoconcentration after several hours of standing.

Central venous pressure is usually reduced with dehydration, and may or may not be elevated with overhydration. It is a less reliable indicator of left heart-filling pressure than the pulmonary capillary wedge pressure as measured with a Swan-Ganz catheter. In the absence of heart failure, central venous and pulmonary wedge pressures depend on intravascular volume; when total body water is increased and intravascular volume is normal or low (e.g., with hypoalbuminemia, the nephrotic syndrome, cirrhosis, or blood loss), the venous or wedge pressure is not increased.

THERAPY OF WATER AND ELECTROLYTE DISORDERS

A standard fluid and electrolyte composition for intravenous therapy is difficult to define because patients requiring such therapy often have disorders which profoundly affect requirements. A 70-kg patient who has no fluid and electrolyte disorder or severe impairment of heart, liver, or kidney function, and is able to handle normally a load of sodium, potassium, and water may be administered the following preparations during a 24-h period:

1.0 L 5% dextrose in Ringer's acetate or normal saline
1.5 to 2.0 L 5% dextrose in water
Potassium chloride or potassium acetate, 60 to 80 meq/day administered in concentrations of 20 to 40 meq/L
Total fluid intake of 2.5 to 3 L/day

These recommendations must be modified by underlying fluid and electrolyte disorders or losses from nasogastric suction, diarrhea, or fistula drainage. Water and electrolyte needs should be reassessed on the basis of the patient's clinical condition and serum electrolyte concentrations. It is emphasized that the foregoing solutions are lacking in many minerals and in amino acids, vitamins, lipids, and sufficient energy. These nutrients should also be administered as indicated (Chap. 10, Sec. I).

During the postoperative state, there is an antidiuretic effect, and urine volume often decreases to 500 to 700 mL/day, even in the presence of a substantially greater fluid intake. Under these conditions, it may be of value to restrict water to prevent hyponatremia. During and after surgery there is frequently decreased effective intravascular volume from blood loss, sequestration of fluid in wounds or injury sites, and vasodilation, and the water and sodium intake may have to be increased. If the patient is hypotensive or has marked hypoalbuminemia, colloid solutions may be infused (see below). During heart or liver failure, the ability to excrete a sodium load or free water may be impaired, and both sodium and water intake may need to be reduced. Potassium intolerance may be reduced in severe heart failure. Hypokalemia is common in liver failure, and potassium supplements may be necessary. In acute renal failure with oliguria, excretion of sodium, potassium, and water are markedly reduced. Hypercatabolism often leads to a marked release of phosphorus and potassium from intracellular sites, and hyperkalemia and hyperphosphatemia may occur rapidly. The breakdown of protein, glycogen, and fat may increase the endogenous release of water, and the fluid requirements are often as little as 300 to 500 mL per 24 h plus urinary and other measured losses. Sodium intake may need to be restricted to about 40 to 70 meq/L. In nonoliguric chronic renal failure, there is usually an inability both to excrete a large sodium and water load and to conserve sodium and water normally. If possible, salt and water intake should be sufficient to maintain a urine output of at least 1500 mL every 24 h and to maintain normal serum sodium concentrations. Not infrequently, patients with nonoliguric chronic renal failure may be depleted in salt and water. This depletion may be manifested by a decrease in the patient's usual blood pressure, postural hypotension, and decreased skin turgor. Such patients may benefit from a trial of loading with normal saline infusion until maximum improvement in renal function occurs or hypertension, edema, or heart failure supervenes. Saline loading should be performed with great caution in these patients.

In patients who are unable to receive adequate nourishment via the gastrointestinal tract, total parenteral nutrition (TPN) may be instituted (Chap. 10, Sec. I). In general, TPN is not recommended unless it is anticipated that adequate enteral intake will not be tolerated for at least 5 to 7 days, malnutrition is present, or there are specific metabolic requirements. Infusion of amino acids with little or no glucose through a peripheral vein may be initiated as soon as enteral intake is reduced. More detailed discussions of fluid and electrolyte metabolism in the heart, liver, kidney, in gastrointestinal diseases and postoperative states are given in Chaps. 16, 21, and 22.

When managing patients with fluid and electrolyte disorders, it is important to maintain flow sheets and serially tabulate body weight, input and output of water and electrolytes, and the response to therapy (i.e., blood pressure, pulse, skin turgor, serum and urine electrolytes).

Once water and electrolyte abnormalities are corrected, a patient should normally be maintained in balance; that is, intake and output of fluid and minerals should be equal. Catabolic patients form water and release potassium, phosphorus, and magnesium as carbohydrate, protein, and fat are consumed. Hence, they should be in negative water and electrolyte balance. Generally, a starving patient should lose 0.2 to 0.5 kg/day of body weight to prevent an increase in his water compartment. When starvation is complicated by severe infection, burns, or tissue injury, weight loss will be even greater. Conversely, when patients are anabolic, as in growth, pregnancy, or convalescence, water and mineral balance should be positive and weight allowed to increase. Nonetheless, weight gain during anabolism is usually slow, and rapid increases often reflect a positive water balance. This is particularly common when starving or wasted patients are refed.

Patients may have large quantities of water and electrolytes sequestered in a "third space," where they are relatively unavailable to other physiological compartments. This occurs most commonly in the peritoneal cavity with ascites, peritonitis, or pancreatitis, in surgical wounds and burn sites, and in the intestinal lumen with inflammation, obstruction, or paralysis of the intestine. In these conditions, the total body water and sodium may be increased, but the patient may suffer from intravascular and sometimes interstitial dehydration and require colloid solutions. During recovery from burn injuries there may be marked mobilization of extravascular fluid with movement of large quantities of salt and water into the intravascular space. If the patient cannot readily excrete this load, pulmonary edema may occur.

In patients who have symptoms from ascites, ascitic fluid can generally be safely removed with salt and water restriction and diuretics (see Chap. 21). Removal should be carried out slowly, at about 0.5 to 1.0 kg/day to allow for equilibration between peritoneal and intravascular spaces. Alternatively, more aggressive paracentesis may be combined with intravenous infusions of ascitic fluid and vigorous diuretic therapy. Not all ascitic fluid can be safely removed in every patient, and attempts to do so may result in depletion of intravascular volume with prerenal azotemia.

When planning fluid and electrolyte therapy, the rapidity with which a disorder is corrected should depend upon the severity of the deficit and the clinical condition of the patient. In general, disorders which occur rapidly or are more severe are less well tolerated and require more rapid correction. For example, in severe depletion due to cholera, the initial 1000 mL of replacement may need to be infused over 10 min. On the other hand, infants with hypernatremia who receive dextrose and water too rapidly may convulse. With chronic alterations in fluid and electrolyte status, rapid correction can be hazardous, and fluid and electrolyte replacement should be more gradual. The goal is to correct disorders *toward* normal and to reassess frequently the clinical response of the patient to judge how vigorous further therapy should be. Disturbances in osmolality are generally well treated by returning plasma osmolality halfway to normal within 24 h.

Treatment of fluid and electrolyte losses from the gastrointestinal tract may be designed more rationally if the mineral content of the fluid output is known (Table 10-12). Electrolyte concentration in gastrointestinal fluids varies widely, and losses are most precisely assessed in an individual patient by measuring concentrations in aliquots of the total daily fluid output. Fluid and electrolyte metabolism in the gastrointestinal tract is discussed in Chap. 22.

WATER AND SODIUM

When calculating the quantity of water or sodium necessary to correct hypernatremic or hyponatremic states, it is important to recognize that although sodium is distributed primarily in ECF and bone, water is freely diffusible intracellularly and extracellularly. It follows from this that the osmolality in the intravascular and extravascular spaces is maintained equal. For example, when sodium loss from the body exceeds water loss, hyponatremia and hypoosmolality occur. Water then moves into cells along an osmotic gradient until the intracellular and extracellular osmotic pressures become equal. This movement of water will tend to raise serum and extracellular sodium. The final serum sodium concentration will be equivalent to that which would occur if sodium had been distributed in total body water. The reverse situation occurs when water is lost in excess of sodium; serum sodium then rises, and water moves out of cells. Again, the serum sodium level responds as if sodium were distributed in total body water. Thus, the changes in serum sodium or osmolality following a gain or loss of sodium or water can be calculated by assuming that the sodium concentration and osmolality are distributed in total body water and not in extracellular fluid.

A 44-year-old man with polycystic kidney disease developed nausea, vomiting, diarrhea, and fever. Food intake stopped, but he continued to drink large quantities of water. His usual obligatory urinary sodium loss was 3.5 g (152 meq)/day. After 4 days, he developed progressive malaise, somnolence, and had a grand mal convulsion. At the time of examination he was comatose. His weight had changed from 80.8 to 79.8 kg, serum sodium was 105 meq/L, chloride 70 meq/L, HCO_3 20 meq/L, creatinine 11 mg/dL, and SUN 140 mg/dL.

The total sodium deficit can be estimated from the following equation:

$$TBW_d (SNa_d) + Na_{balance} = TBW_p (SNa_p) \quad (10B-3)$$

where TBW = total body water (L)
SNa = serum sodium concentration (meq/L)
d = normal or desired state
p = pathologic state

The sodium deficit is 140 − 105 = 35 meq/L. In this patient it is assumed that the 1.0-kg decrease in body weight represents primarily a loss of fat, carbohydrate, and protein since he did not eat for 4 days but continued his usual intake of water. Hence, his total body water was essentially unchanged, and $TBW_d = TBW_p$. The total body water is estimated as 0.54 (80) = 43 L (Table 10-13). Thus, the following values can be substituted in Eq. (10B-3):

$$(43\,L)(140\,meq/L) + Na_{balance} = (43\,L)(105\,meq/L)$$
$$Na_{balance} = 4515\,meq - 6020\,meq$$
$$Na_{balance} = -1505\,meq$$

Thus, the patient sustained a sodium deficit of approximately 1505 meq. Because of the acute nature and severity of the hyponatremia, it was decided to raise his serum sodium rapidly to 120 meq/L. The intake necessary to raise the serum sodium to this level is calculated from Eq. (10B-3).

$$(43\,L)(120\,meq/L) + Na_{balance} = (43\,L)(105\,meq/L)$$
$$Na_{balance} = 4515\,meq - 5160\,meq$$
$$Na_{balance} = -645\,meq$$

Due to the severity of his symptoms, the patient was given an infusion of hypertonic saline, 5 g NaCl/dL (855 meq Na/L, Table 10-14). The volume of 5% saline which contains the desired 645 meq of Na was determined from the following equation:

$$\frac{855\,meq}{1000\,mL} = \frac{645\,meq}{X\,mL} \quad (10B-4)$$

He received 754 mL of 5% saline during a 12-h period. The remainder of the calculated sodium deficit was repleted more gradually with normal saline during the next 3 days.

In addition to calculating the quantity of sodium necessary for replacement of the deficit, the patient should receive enough sodium to satisfy his maintenance requirements. This patient has a relatively high obligatory sodium loss, 3.5 g/day (152 meq/day) due to the nature of his renal disease, so he will require about 1 L of normal saline (154 meq) per day for maintenance.

Table 10-13. Body water compartments throughout life span (as percent of body weight)

AGE	SEX	BODY WEIGHT, kg	TOTAL BODY WATER, PERCENT	EXTRA-CELLULAR WATER, PERCENT	INTRA-CELLULAR WATER, PERCENT
0–11 days			76.4	41.6	34.8
11–180 days			72.8	34.9	37.9
½–2 years			62.2	27.5	34.7
2–7 years			65.5	25.6	36.9
7–14 years			64.2	17.5	46.7
23–54 years	Men	72.5	54.3 ±1.39*	23.4 ±0.64	30.9 ±0.89
23–51 years	Women	59.3	48.6 ±1.47	22.7 ±0.54	25.9 ±0.96
71–84 years	Men	68.1	50.8 ±1.55	25.4 ±1.36	25.4 ±0.58
61–74 years	Women	63.9	43.4 ±1.32	21.4 ±0.45	22.4 ±0.97

* Standard error of the mean.
Source: Modified from H. V. Parker, K. H. Olesen, J. McMurrey, and B. Friis-Hansen, in *Ciba Foundation, Colloquia on Ageing*, vol. 4, Little, Brown and Company, Boston, 1958.

Table 10-14. Approximate electrolyte content in meq/L of carbohydrate and saline solutions

SOLUTION	pH[1]	Na$^+$	K$^+$	Cl$^-$	mosm/L[2]	ENERGY, cal/L
Dextrose[3] in water						
2.5%	5.1				126	85
5%	5.0				253	170
10%	4.9				505	340
20%	4.6				1010	680
50%	4.2				2526	1700
70%	. . .				3536	2380
Fructose in water[4]						
10%	3.8				555	375
Invert sugar in water						
5%	3.8				277	190
10%	4.0				555	375
Alcohol in 5% dextrose[5]						
5%	4.9				1114	450
Saline solution						
0.45%	6.0	77		77	154	
0.9%	6.1	154		154	308	
3%	6.0	513		513	1026	
5%	5.9	855		855	1710	
Dextrose in saline[6]						
5% in 0.11%	4.7	19		19	292	170
5% in 0.22%	4.7	38		38	330	170
5% in 0.45%	4.8	77		77	406	170
5% in 0.9%	4.8	154		154	559	170
Potassium chloride in 5% dextrose[7]						
20	4.5		20	20	293	170
40	. . .		40	40	333	170

[1] pH values represent the average pH.
[2] Refers to calculated osmolality which may differ in some instances from actual osmolality.
[3] Glucose monohydrate.
[4] Also available in 0.9% saline.
[5] Also available 10% alcohol in 5% dextrose.
[6] Also available 3.3% in 0.3%, 5% in 0.3%, 2.5% in 0.45%, 2.5% in 0.9%, and 10% in 0.9%.
[7] Also available D$_5$W with 10, 27, and 30 meq KCl and with 0.2 and 0.45% NaCl.

The foregoing calculations of sodium and water imbalances and requirements for replacement and maintenance represent a gross over-simplification of the patient's pathophysiology and homeostatic mechanisms. The precise sizes of the water compartments, the distribution of sodium between extracellular, intracellular and bone pools, the degree of potassium depletion and intracellular osmotic forces, and the effect of replacement therapy on continuing losses, to mention some of the variables, make precise calculation of the deficits and requirements for replacement and maintenance impossible. For example, with infusion of hypertonic saline in a patient without severe cardiac or renal failure, there is usually a large sodium and water diuresis. This is particularly likely to occur in conditions with volume expansion such as in SIADH (see Chap. 12). Thus, it is very important to reassess continually the fluid and electrolyte status and requirements of all patients.

Equation (10B-3) can be used to calculate a patient's water deficit or excess.

A 50-year-old woman living in a nursing home whose normal weight was 60 kg stopped eating and became dehydrated. On presentation to the hospital, her weight was 56 kg; serum sodium, 158 meq/L; and serum osmolality, 321 mosm/L. The patient's usual total body water is estimated from Table 10-13 to be 48.6 percent of body weight. Thus, her normal total body water is estimated to be $(0.486)(60) = 29.2$ L. Her normal serum sodium is taken as 140 meq/L. Total body sodium was considered to be essentially unchanged (i.e., sodium balance = 0). Her present total body water can be calculated from Eq. (10B-3) as follows:

$$(29.2\,L)(140\,meq/L) + 0\,Na_{balance} = TBW_p(158\,meq/L)$$
$$TBW_p = \frac{(29.2\,L)(140\,meq/L)}{158\,meq/L}$$
$$= 25.9\,L$$

The estimated water deficit is $29.2 - 25.9 = 3.3$ L. Equation (10B-3) can be modified to calculate body water from the serum osmolality:

$$(TBW_d)(osm_d) + osmolar\ balance = (TBW_p)(osm_p)$$

Normal or desired serum osmolality is taken as 285 osm/L. Substituting in this equation,

$$(29.2\,L)(285\,mosm/L) + 0 = TBW_p(321\,mosm/L)$$
$$TBW_p = \frac{(29.2\,L)(285\,mosm/L)}{321\,mosm/L}$$
$$= 25.9\,L$$

Again, the calculated water deficit is
$$29.2 - 25.9 = 3.3\ L$$

The incidence and severity of symptoms with hyponatremia appear to be related to the magnitude and the acuteness of the hyponatremia. Arieff and coworkers reported that the mean serum sodium levels in patients with acute or chronic hyponatremia who developed abnormal mentation or convulsions was 112 ± 2 meq/L and 115 ± 1 meq/L, respectively. In the 14 patients with acute hyponatremia, greater survival followed treatment with hypertonic saline as compared to normal saline (14). However, infusion of hypertonic saline is not without hazard, especially since hyponatremia is often associated with normal or increased total body sodium with a proportionately greater excess in water. Under these conditions, the use of hypertonic or even normal saline can precipitate cardiac or respiratory distress. If serum sodium is 120 meq/L or greater, or if the serum sodium is somewhat lower and the patient is asymptomatic, it is often prudent to treat primarily by restricting water.

Schrier's group has treated hyponatremia and SIADH with intravenous furosemide and replacement of urinary electrolyte losses (15). During therapy, the urine/plasma osmolality ratio fell below 1.0, and mean serum sodium rose from 120 to 133 meq/L within 6 to 8 h. In volume-expanded patients who have good renal function, this procedure may be less hazardous than infusion of hypertonic saline. In patients who have symptomatic hyponatremia and volume expansion, it may be of value to administer either isotonic or hypertonic saline and furosemide. Hyponatremia with impaired renal function can be treated with peritoneal dialysis or hemodialysis with or without saline. It is generally not necessary to treat patients with asymptomatic hyponatremia due to a "reset osmostat."

As previously indicated, hypernatremia is usually associated with dehydration and Na depletion. Patients with severe hypernatremia are frequently critically ill because hypotension due to depletion of intravascular volume and neurological disorders are present. Macaulay and Watson report that 22 percent of children with serum [Na⁺] of 160 meq/L or greater had neurological signs (16). Children may be more sensitive to the neurological results of hypernatremia; neurological signs include lethargy, tremor, increased deep tendon reflexes, stupor, opisthotonus, coma, and convulsions. There may be permanent brain damage due to hemorrhage, and death may occur. Marked hyperglycemia may also be present because hypertonicity impairs insulin release and glucose uptake by tissues.

When hypernatremia with hypotension is present, normal and half normal saline should be infused vigorously until the blood pressure is restored. Reduction of hypertonicity with hypotonic solutions and insulin should not be too rapid as cerebral edema and worsening of central nervous system function may occur.

POTASSIUM

Because patients receiving parenteral fluid therapy almost invariably have continuing outputs of potassium, potassium is generally administered with intravenous infusions. However, intravenous potassium therapy requires caution because of the severe risks of hyperkalemia. The hazards of hyperkalemia are discussed in Chaps. 4 and 15; disturbances in cardiac conduction are the greatest risk. In the Boston Collaborative Drug Surveillance Program reported by Lawson in which 4900 consecutive patients received oral and/or intravenous potassium, hyperkalemia occurred in 3.6 percent (17). Hyperkalemia was considered the major cause of death in 7 patients, and it created a life-threatening condition in another 21. Hyperkalemia is particularly likely to occur in patients with renal failure, advanced age, diabetes mellitus, and those receiving spironolactone or triamterene. Burchell has suggested somewhat facetiously, "... more lives may have been lost than saved by potassium therapy...." (18). It is pertinent that acidosis, hypercalcemia, and hypernatremia may enhance the effects of hyperkalemia while alkalosis, hypocalcemia, and hyponatremia may decrease the effects.

The quantity of potassium for intravenous therapy may be difficult to ascertain because serum potassium may not reflect total body potassium, and the potassium requirement may change with the magnitude of losses and alterations in the relative rates of anabolism and catabolism. Also, serum potassium can change markedly if insulin or glucose is administered, such as during parenteral nutrition, or if the blood pH varies. For example, in diabetic ketoacidosis serum potassium may be normal or high despite profound potassium deficits; with therapy, the serum potassium may fall precipitously. Hence, in diabetic ketoacidosis, infusion of potassium is usually begun when the blood glucose begins to decrease or when serum potassium is either low or falling significantly. When renal failure is also present, potassium infusions may be initiated later and administered less aggressively.

As a guide to intravenous therapy, there are several rough correlations between the serum K and acidosis and between serum K and the magnitude of K deficit: (1) with every 0.1 unit change in plasma pH, there is an inverse change in serum $[K^+]$ of 0.6 meq/L (19); (2) in metabolic alkalosis with paradoxical aciduria (urine pH 6 to 6.5), there is usually a K deficit of at least 400 meq; (3) if the serum K is less than 3 meq/L, an infusion of 200 to 400 meq of K is generally necessary to raise the serum K by 1 meq/L; (4) if the serum K is between 3 and 4.5 meq/L, an infusion of 100 to 200 meq will raise the serum K by 1 meq/L.

Although 60 to 90 meq/day of potassium is usually sufficient for maintenance, there are many conditions when potassium must be given aggressively. Rapid infusion of potassium may be necessary in the diuretic phase of acute renal failure, in the treatment of diabetic ketoacidosis, and when the plasma or total body potassium deficit is severe, especially if excessive losses continue. If serum potassium is greater than 2.5 meq/L and the electrocardiographic disturbances of hypokalemia are absent, potassium should not be administered at rates greater than 10 meq/h or in concentrations above 30 meq/L. Not more than 100 to 200 meq/day should be given. If there are indications for urgent therapy, such as serum potassium less than 2.0 meq/L, abnormal electrocardiogram, or paralysis, potassium may be infused at rates up to 40 meq/h in concentrations not greater than 60 meq/L.

Whenever potassium is infused, it must first be determined that the patient is not hyperkalemic or oliguric, and adequacy of renal function should be established (e.g., by serum creatinine levels). If the patient receives potassium at rates of 120 meq/day or 20 meq/h for more than 2 h, the electrocardiogram should be monitored continuously (20) and the serum potassium measured with each 50 to 100 meq infused. With severe hypokalemia, potassium should be infused in saline if there are no contraindications rather than in dextrose and water because infusion of glucose may further depress the serum potassium. Potassium should never be infused as a bolus. Hemodialysis and peritoneal dialysis may be used to treat both hypokalemia and hyperkalemia. Treatment of hypokalemia with high dialysate concentrations of potassium (21) may be indicated for hypokalemic patients who have increased body water or congestive heart failure, subjects with poor vascular access, and uremic patients. Treatment of hyperkalemia is discussed in Chaps. 4 and 15.

There are several potassium preparations available for intravenous infusion (Table 10-15). In hypochloremic alkalosis with hypokalemia, it is important to administer potassium as the chloride salt. Administration of an alkaline potassium salt in this condition can result in excessive urinary losses of potassium and impede replacement of the potassium deficit. With acidosis or hypophosphatemia, potassium acetate or potassium phosphate may be administered.

When potassium is added to an intravenous container, particularly a plastic nonrigid one, it may not mix well; and during intravenous administration it may enter the bloodstream as a bolus and cause potassium intoxication (22, 23). Better mixing is obtained by administering potassium directly into the container rather than into the injection port. Also, instilling the potassium before the container is inverted seems to promote mixing.

ACID-BASE

Normal and pathologic acid-base physiology is discussed extensively in Chaps. 6 and 24. This section therefore considers acid-base metabolism mainly as it relates to parenteral therapy. There are four primary disturbances in acid-base metabolism, respiratory acidosis and alkalosis, and

Table 10-15. Approximate concentration of electrolytes in meq/mL of additives

SOLUTIONS	Na+	K+	Ca^{2+}	Mg^{2-}	NH$_4^+$	Cl$^-$	HPO$_4^-$	SO$_4^{2-}$	HCO$_3^-$ PRECURSOR
Potassium chloride		1–3				1–3			
Potassium acetate		2–4							2–4
Potassium phosphate		2					2		
Sodium bicarbonate	1								1
Sodium acetate	3								3
Sodium lactate	2.5–4.0								2.5–4.0
Sodium phosphate	4						4		
Sodium chloride	2.5–4.0					2.5–4.0			
Ammonium chloride					4	4			
Magnesium sulfate				2				2	
Calcium gluconate			0.5						1
Calcium chloride			1.5			3			
Multiple electrolyte meq/25 mL Hyperlyte, McGaw Labs	25	40.5	5	8		33.5			45.6

metabolic acidosis and alkalosis. There is usually some degree of compensation for these disorders which partially corrects the pH. However, complete compensation is rare, because as the pH becomes more normal, the stimulus for compensation diminishes. Hence, if complete compensation—i.e., fully normal pH—is seen, more than one primary acid-base disorder is probably present, as is not infrequently the case in a sick patient.

Respiratory acidosis occurs from CO_2 retention due to poor pulmonary perfusion, shunting of blood, decreased movement of the chest wall, or reduced activity of the respiratory centers in the central nervous system. It is best treated by improving exchange of CO_2. In severe respiratory acidosis unresponsive to assisted ventilation, as in severe asthma, it may be necessary to treat the acidosis directly. Infusion of tris-(hydroxymethyl)-aminomethane (TRIS) buffer has been used (see below), but sodium bicarbonate is considered preferable.

Primary respiratory alkalosis results from hyperventilation, which may be caused by hypoxia, pain, anxiety, hysteria, hypermetabolic states, salicylate intoxication, central nervous system diseases, hypotension, hepatic insufficiency, pulmonary embolism, and gram-negative infections. Treatment of the underlying disorder is usually effective. Occasionally, a rebreathing bag or 5% CO_2 may be needed.

Metabolic acidosis may result from the following: (1) loss of intestinal fluid bicarbonate from diarrhea, intestinal intubation or fistulas, or renal bicarbonate losses associated with either renal tubular acidosis or acetazolamide, (2) increased production of acid, as in diabetic ketoacidosis, lactic acidosis, or intoxication from salicylate, paraldehyde, or methanol, (3) impaired renal excretion of acid, as in renal failure or renal tubular acidosis, and (4) excessive intake of acid.

The metabolism of 128 g of infused crystalline amino acids or protein hydrolysates produces an acid load of about 60 to 70 meq which is due primarily to the oxidation of the sulfur-containing amino acids methionine and cystine. If some of the amino acids, such as lysine, histidine, or arginine, are present as the hydrochloride salt, the acid load can be much greater. This acid intake is readily handled if renal function is normal and there are no other causes for acidosis. Most amino acid solutions now contain acetate, histidine, and arginine as the free base and lysine as lysine acetate to reduce the acid load (Chap. 10, Sec. I).

The pH of almost all intravenous solutions is acidic (Table 10-14). However, they are unbuffered, and the low pH represents a very minor quantity of acid. Infusion of large quantities of normal saline can cause a mild hyperchloremic acidosis because of the high concentration of chloride (154 meq/L) and dilution of plasma bicarbonate. This can be avoided by providing less chloride and substituting bicarbonate or alkalinizing salts such as lactate or acetate which are metabolized to bicarbonate.

The cause of acidosis may be evident from inspection of serum chloride, bicarbonate, and the anion gap. For example, hyperchloremic acidosis occurs with bicarbonate loss or, less importantly, dilution and is associated with a normal serum anion gap [sodium − (chloride + bicarbonate)] of 8 to 12. An increased anion gap in metabolic acidosis occurs with accumulation of phosphate, sulfate, or organic acids, such as lactic acid and ketoacids.

Metabolic alkalosis can be classified according to whether there is (1) depletion of sodium chloride and extracellular volume or (2) sufficient amounts of sodium chloride and water but excessive losses of hydrogen and potassium by the kidney. The first (sodium chloride–responsive) type of metabolic alkalosis can be caused by (1) loss of gastric acid (vomiting, gastric drainage), (2) diuretic-induced renal loss of sodium, potassium, and chloride, (3) rapid correction of chronic hypercapnia, and (4) large fecal losses of sodium, potassium, and chloride from villous adenoma or chloride diarrhea.

Causes of metabolic alkalosis of the second type, which is relatively unresponsive to sodium chloride replacement, include (1) excessive endogenous or exogenous mineralocorticoids or glucocorticoids, as in hyperaldosteronism, Cushing's syndrome, and Bartter's syndrome, (2) excessive licorice (glycyrrhizic acid) intake, and (3) severe potassium depletion. Also, excessive intake of alkali, particularly in patients with impaired renal function, can cause metabolic alkalosis.

Sodium chloride–responsive and –resistant alkaloses can generally be distinguished by the clinical history of the patient and the urinary chloride concentration, which is usually less than 10 meq/L in the former case and greater than 20 meq/L in the latter.

Principles of treatment of metabolic acidosis and alkalosis

When treating acidosis or alkalosis, it is important to assess the severity of the disorder. Mild disturbances may have little clinical significance and require no corrective therapy. If the underlying cause can be treated effectively, there is often no need for specific therapy of acid-base disorder (e.g., mild to moderate diabetic ketoacidosis). When specific treatment is indicated, complete correction of the disturbance is usually not necessary. The goal is generally to correct the disorder toward normal and allow the body to make the fine adjustments itself. The acuteness and severity of the disorder often determines the rapidity and aggressiveness with which it should be corrected. The acid-base status must be monitored frequently and the treatment modified according to the patient's response.

Severe acidosis (pH less than 7.20) can lead to widespread metabolic disorders, increased pulmonary vascular resistance, peripheral vasodilatation, decreased myocardial contractility, pulmonary edema, shock, and refractoriness to endogenous catecholamines and pressor and bronchodilator drugs. Shock can lead to intracellular hypoxia, enhanced anaerobic metabolism, production of lactic acid, and metabolic acidosis. In shock with severe acidosis, the blood pressure may not respond effectively to pressor medications. Hence, severe acidosis should be treated with bicarbonate.

The use of alkali in diabetic ketoacidosis is frequently recommended when the arterial blood pH is less than 7.15 or the serum bicarbonate is 8 meq/L or less. It has been suggested that such acid-base disorders should not be corrected aggressively with bicarbonate because it diffuses more slowly than carbon dioxide across the blood-brain barrier (24). When severe metabolic acidosis is rapidly correlated with bicarbonate, hyperventilation decreases and arterial P_{CO_2} rises. Since CO_2 diffuses into the cerebrospinal fluid (CSF) more rapidly than does bicarbonate, the pH of this fluid may decrease further, and obtundation, convulsions, or coma have been reported (24).

Rapid correction of acidosis may be associated with intracellular movement of potassium, and correction of extracellular alkalosis can result in movement of potassium out of cells. Moreover, acid-base disorders are often associated with potassium excess or depletion. Hence, it is critical to monitor serum potassium levels when acid-base disorders are corrected. When acidosis is corrected rapidly in a patient who is normokalemic or even hyperkalemic, hypokalemia may occur. Thus, during treatment of acidosis, potassium is often administered, sometimes in large quantities.

Metabolic acidosis. The quantity of base needed to correct acidosis can only be estimated because the buffering capacity and the rate of generation of acid in patients vary widely. In lactic acidosis in which there is continuing production of large amounts of lactic acid, massive quantities of bicarbonate are often needed. Inadequate treatment is generally more common in this condition than in other types of acidosis. With methanol intoxication, the rate of production of formic acid may also be great, and large quantities of bicarbonate may be required. In contrast, in severe acidosis in uncomplicated chronic renal failure, the rate of acid production may be approximately 50 to 70 meq/day, and acidosis may be corrected more easily.

The following formula, in which the bicarbonate space is taken as 50 percent of body weight, may also be used to estimate the bicarbonate required for correction of acidosis:

$$(HCO_{3d} - HCO_{3p})$$
$$\times \ 0.5 \ \text{body weight} = HCO_3 \ \text{deficit} \quad (10B-5)$$

where d and p equal the desired and pathologic bicarbonate concentrations (meq/L), respectively, and body weight is given in kilograms. Some investigators estimate bicarbonate space as 40 percent of body weight. One-half of the calculated deficit may be replaced in 3 to 4 h. Further correction of acidosis should always be modified according to the preceding response and should be conducted more slowly to prevent paradoxical shifts in CSF pH, marked falls in serum potassium or ionized calcium, and development of alkalosis.

In acidosis with hypocalcemia, as may occur in uremia, bicarbonate should be administered cautiously, because alkalosis induced by the bicarbonate increases the binding of calcium to albumin, and tetany can occur. When bicarbonate is administered to a hypocalcemic patient, the Q-T interval of the electrocardiogram should be monitored continuously.

In contrast to acute or severe acidosis, chronic mild or moderate metabolic acidosis can often be treated more slowly, particularly when acid production is not increased, as in chronic renal failure or renal tubular acidosis. In these conditions it is frequently just as effective to give a safe amount of bicarbonate and formulate further therapy on the basis of the patient's blood pH, P_{CO_2}, and electrolytes. Oral medications such as sodium bicarbonate, calcium carbonate, or Shohl's solution may be used. A number of alkalinizing compounds are currently available (Table 10-16). These include bicarbonate, acetate, lactate, citrate, and gluconate, which are used as additives for intravenous infusion or for direct injection. Bicarbonate, acetate, or lactate are also present in certain polyelectrolyte solutions, such as Darrow's solution and lactated or acetated Ringer's.

Lactate was introduced as an alkali for intravenous therapy by Hartmann and coworkers because of the technical problems of preparing bicarbonate for intravenous injection (27). Also, they believed that the less abrupt alkalinizing effect of lactate as compared to bicarbonate might have metabolic advantages. Technical problems with the preparation of bicarbonate have now been largely overcome, and as Schwartz and Waters have indicated, the degree of alkalinization from bicarbonate can be easily controlled (28).

The alkalinizing effects of lactate are dependent on its conversion in vivo to bicarbonate with concurrent taking up of one hydrogen ion.

Table 10-16. Approximate concentration of electrolytes in alkalinizing and acidifying solutions

SOLUTIONS	APPROX. pH	H^+	Na^+	K^+	NH_4^+	Cl^-	HCO_3^-*	mosm
Alkalinizing								
Sodium lactate								
$\frac{1}{6}M$	6.9		167				167	334
Sodium bicarbonate			167				167	334
$\frac{1}{6}M$								
5%	7.8		595				595	1190
7.5%			893				893	1786
THAM (0.3M)	8.6		30	5		35	297	
Acidifying								
Ammonium chloride								
0.9%†					169	169		
2.14%					400	400		
Arginine HCl								
10%	6.5	100				100		

* HCO_3^- or equivalent
† Also available in 0.9% sodium chloride

Lactate may also be converted to glucose and glycogen, which binds one hydrogen ion per molecule of lactate (28, 29). These reactions are dependent on cellular oxidative mechanisms. The first step in the metabolism of lactate is its conversion to pyruvate. This reaction requires the transformation of NAD (nicotinamide-adenine dinucleotide) to $NADH_2$ as follows:

$$\text{Pyruvate } (CH_3COCOO^-) + NADH + H^+ \rightleftharpoons$$
$$\text{lactate } (CH_3CHOHCOO^-) + NAD^+ \quad (10B\text{-}6)$$

Normally, oxygen is an electron acceptor for $NADH_2$, allowing NAD to be regenerated. However, during hypoxia, glycolysis leads to an accumulation of electrons, which results in accumulation of $NADH_2$ (30). Thus, lactate is not readily converted to pyruvate and accumulates. Lactate is primarily metabolized in the liver, but the kidneys and possibly the heart and skeletal muscle may also contribute. During severe acidosis, the capacity of the liver to metabolize lactate is reduced. Thus, the administration of lactate is generally contraindicated when there is altered liver function, hypotension, poor circulatory perfusion (e.g., in prolonged shock), hypoxia, severe anemia, or lactic acidosis. Fifty to 200 mg/day of lactate is normally excreted in the urine, and the amount may rise with increased blood levels.

Acetate is metabolized more effectively in peripheral tissues (31). Its use in intravenous solutions is becoming more popular, as it may be converted to bicarbonate more readily than lactate in the foregoing conditions. Dialysate solutions used for hemodialysis or peritoneal dialysate usually contain acetate. Patients undergoing dialysis usually receive a large load of acetate, which generally is rapidly metabolized to bicarbonate (32). A very small percentage seems to be converted into a variety of fats. Sometimes, patients receiving large loads of acetate during hemodialysis may become acidotic transiently because of the rapid dialysis of bicarbonate from blood and a delay in the conversion of acetate to bicarbonate. Some investigators have implicated acetate as a cause of hypotension and other symptoms which not uncommonly occur during dialysis (33).

Sodium bicarbonate is an excellent alkalinizing agent. As with lactate and acetate, it presents a sodium load (1 meq of sodium per milliequivalent of alkali) and can cause congestive heart failure in patients with impaired cardiac, pulmonary, or renal function. Sodium bicarbonate is usually the alkalinizing agent of choice for metabolic acidosis. The main advantage of acetate and lactate over bicarbonate is that the latter compound in vitro tends to form insoluble salts with calcium and magnesium, and its high pH inactivates certain medications. If the patient is potassium-deficient, potassium acetate may also be administered, either intravenously or orally. Sodium citrate binds calcium and cannot be administered intravenously in large doses. Peritoneal dialysis and hemodialysis are very effective therapies for severe metabolic acidosis in patients who are intolerant of sodium.

TRIS or THAM is an organic amine buffer which has been used for the treatment of respiratory and metabolic acidosis. It is a stronger base than bicarbonate, with a higher pK (7.84 versus 6.10). TRIS can combine with carbonic acid and release bicarbonate and thereby corrects acidosis in two ways. However, it depresses ventilation, leading to accumulation of carbon dioxide. With modern techniques of artificial ventilation, TRIS probably has no role in the treatment of respiratory acidosis.

It has been suggested that TRIS is preferable to bicarbonate because it corrects intracellular acidosis more rapidly, but this may be undesirable (see above). Since TRIS contains no sodium, it has been advocated for acidotic patients with sodium intolerance. However, TRIS presents an osmotic load. Also, the high alkalinity of TRIS may cause venous spasm, phlebitis, or thrombosis. Extravasation of TRIS may lead to necrosis and sloughing of the overlying skin. It is excreted primarily by the kidneys and therefore is contraindicated in renal failure. In general, TRIS seems to have few or no advantages over sodium bicarbonate for treatment of metabolic acidosis (34).

Metabolic alkalosis. Most cases of metabolic alkalosis are associated with depletion of sodium chloride and ECF and respond to volume expansion with sodium chloride. Since volume contraction enhances renal tubular reabsorption of bicarbonate, infusion of albumin may be helpful in hypoalbuminemic states. Potassium depletion frequently accompanies both sodium chloride–responsive and –resistant metabolic alkalosis, and administration of potassium chloride is generally necessary, sometimes in massive amounts.

In some conditions of metabolic alkalosis, administration of sodium and potassium and volume expansion may be poorly tolerated, as when heart, liver, and kidney failure are present or may be insufficient to replace massive continued gastric losses of hydrochloric acid. In these cases, other acidifying compounds may be used, such as ammonium chloride, hydrochloric acid, and hydrochloride salts of the amino acids, arginine and lysine.

L-Arginine monohydrochloride is commercially available (R-Gene, Cutter) as a 10% solution for intravenous use. The solution is hypertonic (950 mosm/L) and contains 47.5 meq of chloride ion per 100 mL. Arginine monohydrochloride gives rise to equimolar quantities of hydrochloric acid. It contains nitrogen, most of which is ultimately incorporated into urea and may be poorly tolerated in renal failure. Arginine hydrochloride can cause flushing, nausea, vomiting, headache, numbness, and local irritation at the infusion site. An allergic erythematous macular eruption has been reported.

L-Lysine hydrochloride can be obtained from chemical supply firms, and, if other acidifying agents are contraindicated or unavailable, it can be prepared for intravenous use by a hospital pharmacy. It also presents a nitrogen load.

Ammonium chloride is available for infusion as an isotonic (160 meq/L) or hypertonic (400 meq/L) solution, and in a number of polyionic, e.g., "gastric replacement," solutions (about 70 meq/L) (Table 10-17). Ammonium chloride ionizes in solution into ammonium and chloride, and the former dissociates further into ammonia and hydrogen ion. Ammonium can be excreted in the urine or participate in the formation of urea in the liver, leaving hydrogen and chloride ions. The hydrogen ion combines with bicarbonate to form CO_2 and water. Thus, the chloride essentially replaces bicarbonate, and the metabolic products of ammonium chloride result in little solute load. The urea is distributed in total body water so there is little extracellular volume expansion from the ammonium load.

Ammonium chloride can cause serious toxicity. Pallor, sweating, vomiting, and respiratory and mental depression have been reported. These symptoms may be related to the rate of infusion. Severe parenchymal liver disease is an absolute contraindication to the administration of ammonium chloride, as hepatic encephalopathy can be precipitated. In renal failure its use may also increase serum urea levels.

There have been a number of reports pointing out the value of hydrochloric acid for correction of severe metabolic alkalosis (35–37). Hydrochloric acid has been used in severely alkalotic patients with renal or liver failure who are intolerant to sodium, intravascular volume expansion, and nitrogen, and have continuing losses of large quantities of acid, particularly from the stomach.

A simplified description of its action is as follows:

$$HCl + HCO_3^- \rightarrow CO_2 + H_2O + Cl^- \quad (10B\text{-}7)$$

Thus, as with ammonium chloride, the chloride in hydrochloric acid primarily replaces bicarbonate. The volume of infused fluid is distributed through the total body water which is better tolerated than expansion of the intravascular or extracellular space. The reaction described in Eq. (10B-7) should occur virtually at the moment of contact of hydrochloric acid with plasma. Thus, some investigators suggest administering hydrochloric acid in normal saline or 5% dextrose, so that when the acid is metabolized, pure water will not be formed and cause hemolysis (37).

Hydrochloric acid can be prepared by diluting the concentrate with distilled water for injection and passing the solution through a 0.22-μm filter. It may then be added to dextrose or saline to form the appropriate solution. Hydrochloric acid is generally administered as a 0.1 to 0.2 N solution (100 to 200 meq/L HCl) over 6 to 24 h into a large-diameter, high-flow vein. Necrosis and sloughing of tissue at the infusion site, and coagulation of blood at the catheter tip have been reported; but these complications seem to occur with higher rates of infusion or more concentrated solutions. When hydrochloric acid is administered, it is particularly important to frequently monitor the vital signs, serum electrolytes, arterial blood pH and P_{CO_2}, hemoglobin and hematocrit, and the condition of the infusion site.

The amount of protons or acid necessary to correct the metabolic alkalosis can be estimated by calculating the chloride deficit:

$$(Cl_d - Cl_p) [0.2 \text{ (body weight)}]$$
$$= \text{chloride deficit} \quad (10B-8)$$

where Cl_d = desired or normal chloride concentration (meq/L)

Cl_p = current or abnormal chloride concentration (meq/L)

Body weight is given in kilograms.

0.2 reflects the extracellular fluid space (L/kg), which is the major compartment for chloride. In general, about half of the deficit should be replaced during the first 24 h. Also, the ongoing chloride losses should be replaced each day. Since alkalotic patients often continue to lose large quantities of acid, it is important to measure the volume and chloride concentrations of the fluids lost.

A 70-kg man with acute renal failure is severely alkalotic and loses 2000 mL of gastric fluid per 24 h. The chloride concentration of his gastric aspirate averages 100 meq/L. Serum chloride is 78 meq/L, and pH is 7.56. The chloride deficit is calculated as:

$$(103 \text{ meq/L} - 78 \text{ meq/L}) [0.2(70 \text{ kg}) = 25(14) = 350 \text{ meq/L}]$$

The patient's daily chloride loss is

$$(2000 \text{ mL})(100 \text{ meq/L}) = 200 \text{ meq}$$

He should therefore be given approximately the following quantities of chloride in the first 24 h:

$$[\tfrac{1}{2}(350 \text{ meq})] + 200 \text{ meq} = 375 \text{ meq}$$

Peritoneal dialysis and hemodialysis can also be effective for correcting severe metabolic alkalosis, especially in patients with heart, liver, or kidney failure. Dialysis is useful in several ways. Bicarbonate is readily removed by dialysis. Thus, patients with very high serum bicarbonate levels may have a net loss of base during dialysis even though they receive acetate from the dialysate. Also, the concentration of acetate in dialysate can be reduced or omitted entirely and replaced with chloride. Moreover, dialysis can remove sodium and water, enabling the patient to tolerate intravenous infusions of large quantities of isotonic or hypertonic saline. In an edematous alkalotic patient who is intolerant of saline, arginine monohydrochloride, and lysine hydrochloride, ammonium chloride, or hydrochloric acid may be infused during dialysis.

INTRAVENOUS SOLUTIONS

DEXTROSE IN WATER

Dextrose (D-glucose) is present in a variety of concentrations ranging from 2.5 to 70% (Table 10-14). These solutions provide 3.4 kcal/g dextrose. Since dextrose is normally metabolized to carbon dioxide and water, administration of a solution of dextrose and water is equivalent to providing the same volume of free water. The water in these solutions is distributed in total body water; thus dextrose and water is a poor volume expander; only about 7.5 percent of the water remains in the intravascular space. The main indications for the use of dextrose and water are to supply energy or to provide free water in cases where the patient's osmolality or the tonicity of the combined fluids administered is greater than desired.

The more concentrated dextrose solutions are used primarily as an energy source and are discussed in Chap. 10, Sec. I. Hypertonic dextrose can also be administered with insulin to lower serum potassium or may be infused as a bolus to treat hyperkalemia. Because of the high osmolality of solutions containing 20% or more dextrose, they should be infused into a high-flow vein unless administered as a bolus.

SALINE SOLUTIONS

Isotonic sodium chloride has been termed "physiologic" or "normal" saline. Each liter contains 9.0 g of sodium chloride or 154 meq each of sodium and chloride. Isotonic saline is probably the most widely used electrolyte solution. Since the concentration of chloride is greater than in plasma and saline does not contain other electrolytes, it may best be used in patients whose chloride loss is equal to or greater than their sodium loss (e.g., as in vomiting or nasogastric suction). In other conditions requiring volume replacement or correction of electrolyte disorders, other preparations may be more suitable (see Table 10-17). The use of saline as the sole electrolyte solution may lower the concentration of other electrolytes by dilution. Normal saline can cause metabolic acidosis by dilution of bicarbonate ("expansion acidosis"), and this may be prevented by infusing a solution which contains approximately 27 meq/L of bicarbonate or a bicarbonate precursor (38).

Normal saline is available with concentrations of dextrose ranging from 2.5 to 10% (see Table 10-14). Hypotonic saline is prepared in concentrations of 0.11, 0.20, 0.22, 0.33 and 0.45% sodium chloride and is usually combined with various concentrations of glucose. Hypotonic saline provides free water and is most useful when water has been lost in excess of salt.

Hypertonic saline is available in 3% and 5% solutions (Table 10-14). The sodium and chloride concentrations are each 513 meq/L and 855 meq/L in the 3% and 5% saline, respectively. These solutions are useful for correction of symptomatic hyponatremia. They may cause volume overload or severe hypernatremia and hyperchloremia. They should be given slowly in relatively small quantities, and serum sodium and chloride concentrations should be measured frequently.

POLYIONIC SOLUTIONS

Polyionic solutions have been used for intravenous therapy for many decades. In addition to sodium and chloride, these solutions may contain potassium, calcium, magnesium, ammonium, phosphate, and bicarbonate precursors such as lactate, acetate, citrate or gluconate. D-

Glucose, fructose, invert sugar, and alcohol may also be present, and their use is discussed in Chap. 10, Sec. I. Certain polyionic solutions are listed in Table 10-17.

There are several important advantages to polyionic solutions as compared to solutions of dextrose and water or saline: (1) the concentrations of electrolytes may more closely approximate the actual fluid and electrolyte needs of the patient, and the kidney can more readily adjust for differences between the replacement solution and the actual deficit; there are solutions designed specifically for replacement of gastric, small-intestinal, and diarrheal losses; (2) they can be obtained more quickly than solutions which must be prepared by the addition of specific electrolytes; (3) there is less risk of contamination because there are fewer additives.

There are also hazards to such solutions. They often do not satisfy the specific needs for correction of an electrolyte disorder. The electrolyte composition of fluids lost varies widely (Table 10-12). Also, patients may have superimposed acid-base, respiratory, cardiac, hepatic, or renal disorders which complicate fluid and electrolyte requirements. Most importantly, the use of these solutions may give a false sense of security to a busy physician, who may then evaluate and monitor the needs of an individual patient less carefully. The most precise way to manage fluid and electrolyte requirements is to measure the volume and electrolyte concentration of fluid losses (including urine) and frequently monitor the clinical status and plasma electrolyte concentrations of the patient. When possible, the electrolyte composition of the fluids lost should be determined from an aliquot of the *total* 24-h volume, because the content of a randomly obtained "spot" collection may not be indicative of the concentration in the total output.

Some of the better known traditional polyionic solutions are discussed below. With the exception of Ringer's acetate and lactate, they are no longer commonly used. Ringer's solution is similar to normal saline but contains small amounts of calcium and potassium. However, like saline, it contains an excess of chloride relative to serum. Lactated Ringer's saline, or original

Hartmann's solution, was designed to correct the chloride excess in isotonic saline. Lactate has replaced part of the chloride in this preparation. In lactated Ringer's or modified Hartmann's solution, some of the chloride is replaced with lactate, and there is less sodium than in Ringer's solution. Dextrose may be included, and a half-strength lactated Ringer's solution is also available. It is a standard replacement solution which does not cause acidosis. Acetated Ringer's solution differs only in that acetate is used instead of lactate. The potential advantages of acetate over lactate have been discussed (see above).

Darrow's solution is similar to the original Hartmann's solution except that some of the sodium has been replaced with potassium, 35 meq/L. It was designed for treatment of diarrhea.

Within recent years, dozens of newer polyionic solutions have been developed (Table 10-17). Space does not permit a comprehensive discussion of these preparations. The newer solutions have certain advantages over the older ones. They contain a greater variety of cations and anions in concentrations similar to those present in specific physiological fluids, and some of the electrolytes may be more readily metabolized or more suitable for specific disorders.

pH of solutions

The vast majority of water, electrolyte, and dextrose solutions are acidic, with the pH usually varying from 3.5 to 6.7. The pH of the same preparation actually can vary from batch to batch, and the United States Pharmacopiea gives a range of pH values for many intravenous solutions. The acidity of solutions is due to several factors. First, "pure" water is itself acidic because of dissolved carbon dioxide and formation of carbonic acid. Second, preparations of dextrose are acidic because of formation of sugar acids (i.e., glucuronic and levulinic acid). Moreover, with sterilization by heating, acid may be added to minimize caramelization. Third, additives to stabilize a drug may be very acidic (e.g., tetracycline hydrochloride, which is buffered with ascorbic acid to a pH of 1.8 to 2.8). Alternatively, other additives may be basic, such as sodium diphenylhydantoin, which may be alkalinized with sodium hydroxide to pH 10.0 to 12.3, in order to maintain solubility. Thrombophlebitis has been attributed to the acid pH of solutions (39, 40) and can reportedly be reduced by adding buffers to raise the pH. It has also been suggested that the acidity of solutions may predispose to acidosis. However, despite their relatively low pH, the titratable acidity and therefore the acid load of these solutions are very low, e.g., 0.003 to 0.303 meq/L (41).

Drug incompatibilities

Incompatibilities between drugs and intravenous solutions are a serious problem in patients receiving parenteral fluid therapy and unfortunately are infrequently recognized by the physi-

Table 10-17. Concentration of ions in meq/L of polyionic solution

SOLUTIONS*	APPROX. pH†	Na⁺	K⁺	Ca²⁺	Mg²⁺	NH₄⁺	Cl⁻	HPO₄⁻	HCO₃⁻‡ PRECURSOR
Ringer's	5.9	147	4	5	—	—	156	—	—
Lactated or acetated Ringer's (Hartmann's)	6.7	130	4	3	—	—	109	—	28
Darrow's	—	121	35	—	—	—	103	—	53
"Gastric" replacement	—	63	17	—	—	70	150	—	—
"Duodenal" replacement	6.1	80	36	5	3		64	—	60
"Maintenance" solutions	5.6	40–55	13–35	0–5	0–6	—	40–55	12–15	16–26
"Extracellular" replacement	—	140	5–10	5	3	—	98–103		50–55

* A variety of modifications of multiple electrolyte solutions, many with carbohydrates, are commercially available.
† pH is lower when carbohydrate is present.
‡ HCO₃⁻ equivalent may be bicarbonate, lactate, acetate, gluconate, citrate, or combinations of these.

cian. Physicians would do well to periodically familiarize themselves with these incompatibilities. Several texts are available (42, 43, 44). A study by Ho and Rosero in a major teaching hospital indicated that 70 percent of all intravenous infusates contained additives: 30 percent contained one drug; 24 percent, two drugs; 14 percent, three drugs; 18 percent, four drugs; and 14 percent, five or more drugs (45). Hence, there is a critical need for careful monitoring of drug additives.

Drug interactions may be caused by the preservatives, stabilizers, buffers, antioxidants, or vehicles in which the drugs are prepared. Incompatibilities can lead to altered physical-chemical states or loss of pharmacological properties. Also, interacting drugs can form potentially harmful new products. Incompatibilities may lead to visible changes, such as altered color or clarity of a solution or formation of a frank precipitate; however, changes are frequently not visible, as when drug inactivation occurs (46).

Changes in pH are a major cause of drug inactivations, and many additives will alter acidity. For example, the optimum pH for buffered potassium penicillin G in 5% dextrose in water solution is 6.0 to 7.0. A pH less than 5.5 or greater than 8.0 will cause significant inactivation of the penicillin. Additives which can lower the pH include aramine, ascorbic acid, and tetracycline, while aminophylline, sodium bicarbonate, or TRIS will raise the pH. Many antibiotics are incompatible in solution, such as gentamycin mixed with cephalothin or carbenicillin. Gentamycin and ampicillin in the same solution may lose 50 percent of their activity in less than 2 h. Incompatibility is also a function of time, and some drugs may be stable for several hours but lose activity over a period of 6 to 72 h. Some medicines lose stability in solution even in the absence of other additives. The rate of degradation of ampicillin in solution is directly related to its concentration, the degree of alkalinity (ampicillin is basic), the ambient temperature, and the presence of dextrose. Ampicillin, 1%, in 5% and 10% dextrose, loses 14% and 19% of its activity, respectively, in 7 h (47).

There are advantages to having the pharmacy service, rather than nurses or physicians, prepare additives for intravenous solutions. Pharmacists often have more knowledge concerning drug incompatibilities and have ready access to publications concerning this problem. They are frequently better trained to avoid contamination of solutions. Also, they are often able to work in a less distracting environment than a nurse on a busy hospital ward.

Contamination of solutions

A fact poorly recognized by many physicians and nurses is that intravenous solutions are not infrequently contaminated with particulate matter, chemicals, or microbial organisms (48, 49). Contamination can occur during manufacture of the product or during administration to the patient. Particulate matter may originate from glass fragments, cellulose fibers released from filters, crystals and chemical precipitates, and most commonly from rubber closures which can release rubber particles, carbon black, zinc oxide, chalk, and clay. Studies in both animals and humans have demonstrated pulmonary microemboli, thrombi, and granuloma after prolonged intravenous infusion. More recently, awareness of contamination has lead to improved techniques of manufacturing, and the incidence and severity of particulate contamination has lessened. Also, the use of plastic containers has reduced the incidence of particulate contamination because the container is made from one material and there are no rubber closures or glass. Also, the absence of an airway in the plastic containers has reduced the risk of air embolism which can occur when fluid is pumped.

Chemical contamination can occur from solutions, additives, rubber closures, and the containers themselves. Rubber closures can release trace elements (see Chap. 10, Sec. I). Potentially toxic chemicals, which are used in the manufacture of polyvinyl chloride (PVC) bags, can be leached out, particularly when the bags contain blood. Regulations concerning the manufacture of bags and the use of higher quality PVC or other materials have reduced this problem.

Some drugs may be adsorbed onto the wall of the container, and patients may receive only an unpredictable fraction of the amount prescribed. This has been described for vitamin A and sodium warfarin for plastic bags and for insulin in glass and plastic containers (50, 51).

Microbial contamination remains a serious problem and may originate from the intravenous solutions, the infusion equipment, or during insertion of the needle or catheter. In recent years there have been well-publicized epidemics caused by bacterial contamination during manufacturing (52). Autoclaved bottles have been spray-cooled with unsterile water, and the contraction of the rubber closure and negative pressure within the bottle which occur during cooling may draw unsterile water into the solution. Plastic bags can reduce contamination because there is no rubber closure and air does not enter the bag during infusion. Improved techniques of production have probably reduced the incidence of contamination. Recently, endotoxin-type material has been discovered in peritoneal dialysate by the limulus test which was not detected by standard methods of monitoring, and it is possible that endotoxin may also contaminate intravenous solutions (53).

Most microbial contamination is believed to occur in the hospital from additives, unfiltered air, contamination of connectors, stopcocks, and injection ports or at the needle or cannula sites (46, 54, 55). During insertion of needles or connectors breaks in the seal may occur allowing microbes to enter. The incidence of microbial contamination of intravenous fluids is not low, from 3.3 to 27 percent (46). Once contamination occurs, the nutrients in the solution may foster rapid growth of bacteria and fungi, particularly if dextrose, protein hydrolysates, or amino acids are present. The risk of contamination increases with the duration of time in which a solution is administered, an infusion set is used, or an intravenous cannula or needle remains in place. There is an increased incidence of infection with intravenous plastic cannulas as compared to needles because cannulas tend to be used for longer periods and a fibrin sheath forms around the cannula and may become a source for bacterial growth and sequestration. The incidence of positive cultures from the plastic cannulas ranges from 3.8 to 57 percent, and rates of associated septicemia from zero to 8 percent (55). The incidence of positive cultures from catheters and related septicemias increased from 11 percent and none, respectively, at 1 day, to 33 percent and 3 percent, respectively, at 4 or more days (55).

Many investigators have recommended filters in all intravenous lines to remove particulate matter and bacteria and fungi. Filters of 0.45 μm will remove most particles, bacteria, and fungi, although *Pseudomonas*, *E. coli*, and other gram-negative bacilli may start to traverse the filter after 6 h of continuous use (56). Filters of 0.22 μm will remove all bacteria; however, obstruction of fluid by these filters is common, and infusion pumps may be necessary, especially with viscous solutions. It should be stressed that no prospective controlled studies have definitely shown a lower incidence of infection with the use of filters. Moreover, the filters themselves may become contaminated and sources of infection.

The following techniques can be used to decrease the incidence of particulate and microbial contamination:

1. All drugs should be added to parenteral solutions in a pharmacy by specially trained personnel under a laminar flow hood.
2. An intravenous therapy team should be constituted which ideally should institute intravenous therapy and also monitor the techniques of preparation and administration of solutions and the incidence of adverse reactions.
3. The entire delivery system including the cannula should be changed every 24 to 48 h.
4. Particulate and microbial filters should probably be used routinely.

PLASMA VOLUME EXPANDERS

In 1915, Hogan published the first report on the use in humans of a plasma volume expander, gelatin. Many different products have since been used for volume expansion. These include (1) whole blood and its derivatives, such as packed red cells, plasma, albumin, and plasma protein fraction; (2) chemically modified proteins, such as gelatin; (3) polymerized carbohydrates, such as dextran, hydroxy-starch, and pectin; (4) crystalloid solutions, such as polyvinylpyrrolidone (PVP). Under current development are artificial blood replacements containing fluorocarbons or free or complexed hemoglobin.

Ideally, a plasma volume expander should have the following properties: it should be confined to the intravascular compartment for a clinically useful period of time, have a relatively large colloid osmotic pressure, have a low enough viscosity to allow rapid administration intravenously, and be completely removed from the body by excretion or degradation, so that it does not accumulate in tissues. Also, it should be pyrogen-free, nontoxic, nonallergenic, and should not cause hemolysis, agglutinate red blood cells, impair hemostasis, or interfere with cross-matching. It should be easily sterilized, stable in storage and at widely varying temperatures, readily available, and inexpensive. In general, substances have been sought with a molecular weight and colloid osmotic pressure similar to that of albumin (MW 66,000 daltons). Although some plasma expanders satisfy many of these criteria, all have some shortcomings (57–61).

Plasma volume expanders have a critical and growing role in the treatment of many severe illnesses. Blood and its products are in increasingly short supply. Blood cannot be stored for extended periods, causes sensitization and transfusion reactions, and, as with plasma, can transmit hepatitis and other infections. In remote areas and during military activity or civilian emergencies, blood and plasma may not be available.

Plasma volume expanders may be as beneficial as whole blood when there is hypotension or decreased effective circulating blood volume, and oxygen-carrying capacity is not severely diminished. In many conditions, plasma volume expanders may have specific advantages over blood and plasma; they can decrease blood viscosity, or at least prevent increased viscosity, and low-molecular-weight dextran may possibly improve the microcirculation. In hypoproteinemic states with edema, colloidal volume expanders may be of specific value for mobilizing extravascular fluid and increasing urinary output.

Dextran

Dextrans have been known since the last half of the nineteenth century as a carbohydrate slime generated by bacterial action during the commercial preparation of sucrose. Dextrans are polymers of glucose produced enzymatically by the action of the bacteria *Leuconostoc mesenteroides,* which enzymatically splits sucrose to form polymers of fructose and glucose. Dextrans are prepared for clinical use by purifying, hydrolyzing, and fractionating these polymers. There is considerable overlap in the molecular size of dextrans, and this is reflected in their clinical properties.

Three preparations of dextran have been available for clinical use. Low-molecular-weight (LMW) dextran has a mean molecular weight of 40,000. Ninety percent of the molecules have a molecular weight between 10,000 and 80,000. Medium-molecular-weight (MMW) dextran has an average molecular weight of 75,000. Ninety percent of the molecules have a molecular weight between 25,000 and 200,000. High-molecular-weight dextran has a mean molecular weight of 150,000. Ninety percent of the molecules have a molecular weight between 25,000 and 1,000,000. The last preparation is not available in the United States for clinical use.

Low-molecular-weight dextran. LMW dextran is a hyperoncotic solution. Each gram of LMW dextran exerts the colloid osmotic pressure of 25 mL of plasma. Hence, 500 mL of a 10% solution will draw approximately 750 mL of additional fluid into the plasma compartment. Although LMW dextran is used as a plasma volume expander, its effectiveness for this purpose is quite limited. The low molecular size of much of the LMW dextran leads to its rapid egress from the intravascular space. About 80 percent of LMW dextran molecules have a molecular weight of less than 50,000 (62). Since the glomerular filtration threshold for dextran is about 50,000 daltons, about 50 percent of a dose of LMW dextran is excreted in the urine in 3 h, and 70 percent in 24 h (62). LMW dextran can cause an osmotic diuresis, and urine concentrations as high as 42 g/L have been reported (63). The plasma half-life of dextran is only 15 min for molecular weights between 14,000 and 18,000 daltons, 7.5 h for 44,000 to 55,000 daltons, and several days for more than 55,000 daltons (64). The mean molecular weight of the dextran molecules in the circulation increases rapidly after an infusion of LMW dextran as the smaller molecules are excreted, and the average molecular size and clinical properties become more similar to those of MMW dextran. In a normal individual after 24 h, the average molecular weight of dextran in plasma is about 80,000. Most of the plasma expansion from LMW dextran abates within about 90 min after infusion. In shock, plasma volume expansion may last somewhat longer. During continuous infusion, larger dextran molecules accumulate in plasma for several days. LMW dextran which is not excreted by the kidney is taken up by the reticuloendothelial system and oxidized over the ensuing 3 to 14 days (65, 66).

LMW dextran has been advocated for plasma volume expansion in such conditions as shock and burns, pump priming for extracorporeal circulation, prevention of thromboembolic disease (67–70), frostbite (71), and other conditions associated with vascular insufficiency. The therapeutic effects of LMW dextran have been attributed to several mechanisms: (1) rapid, although transient, volume expansion (72, 73); (2) decrease in blood viscosity by hemodilution, reduction of factor VII and fibrinogen (74) and formation of dextran-fibrinogen complexes (75); (3) altering red cell surface, increasing the negative charge and decreasing sludging of red cells (76); (4) coating platelets (77) and injured walls of blood vessels (78), altering the surface charge of platelets (79), decreasing platelet adhesiveness and aggregation (80); (5) decreasing platelet factor III (81); (6) promoting lysis of fibrin clots. It is noteworthy that many of these effects are due to the larger size molecules in LMW dextran.

The most specific therapeutic results attributed to LMW dextran are related not to volume expansion but to its effects on the microcirculation and on coagulation. The pathophysiology of shock is related to decreased organ perfusion due to diminished blood flow through the capillaries and sludging and agglutination of red cells and platelets. These alterations lead to formation of thrombi and coagulation in the capillaries and tissue ischemia. Studies indicate that LMW dextran decreases erythrocyte sludging and blood viscosity and improves capillary flow (see above).

However, as pointed out by Data and Nies (82), in almost all conditions for which LMW dextran has been recommended, controlled clinical studies demonstrating its efficacy are either lacking or conflicting. Exceptions are its use as a plasma volume expander and to prevent thromboembolism in high-risk surgical patients. However, there are other plasma volume expanders which are at least as effective as LMW dextran, and it is not clear that LMW dextran prevents thromboembolic disease more effectively than does warfarin (83, 84).

Moreover, LMW dextran has a number of adverse effects; mild urticaria, nausea, chills, fever, dyspnea, anaphylaxis, and death have occurred (85–87). During periods of oliguria, LMW dextran can precipitate in the renal tubules, causing obstruction and acute renal failure which may not be reversible (88, 89). Thus, its use in shock may significantly increase the risk of renal failure unless high renal blood flow and urine volume are maintained. There is also a risk of bleeding, particularly with administration in amounts greater than 1 L of LMW dextran (59, 74), and doses should be lowered when the two drugs are administered concurrently. LMW dextran can cause excessive volume expansion in patients with heart failure. LMW dextran also interferes with certain laboratory procedures, such as cross-matching of blood by enzymatic methods and determination of glucose (causing false elevations), bilirubin, and total protein.

Recommended dosages vary. Thomas and Silva recommend that the rate of infusion of LMW dextran should be adjusted to the hourly output and specific gravity of urine. If urine volume is greater than 25 mL/h and specific gravity is less than 1.030, the rate of infusion can be gradually increased to 50 mL/h (90). Atik suggests doses of up to 10 to 15 mL/kg per day for 3 to 5 days administered over 12 to 24 h (91). The manufacturers state that 20 mL/kg per day can be administered and that the first 500 mL may be given rapidly. Maximum dose on subsequent days should be 10 mL/kg per day for not more than 5 consecutive days. The *Medical Letter on Drugs and Therapeutics* recommends that infusions be less than 1000 mL/day (92). Evarts and Feil report a greater effect in preventing thromboembolic disease when 1000 mL of LMW dextran was infused during surgery and then for each of the following 10 days, rather than when 500 mL was first administered after surgery and then daily for 10 to 12 days (68).

LMW dextran is provided in 500-mL containers as a 10% solution in either normal saline or 5% dextrose in water. It is stable for long periods at a constant temperature under 25°C. Elevated or fluctuating temperatures can cause crystallization.

Medium-molecular-weight dextran. Many effects of MMW dextran on volume expansion and coagulation are similar to those of the larger compounds of LMW dextran (see above). Solutions of MMW dextran have a colloidal osmotic pressure equivalent to that of plasma (91). Since the average molecular size of MMW dextran is larger than that of LMW dextran, extravascular movement and renal excretion are slower, and plasma volume expansion lasts longer, approximately 4 h after the end of infusion. About 40 percent of MMW dextran is lost in the urine in 12 h, and in contrast to LMW dextran, it exerts little osmotic diuretic effect. A substantial fraction of MMW dextran is oxidized gradually by the reticuloendothelial system.

MMW dextran has been used primarily for volume expansion and antithrombogenic effects. It is useful in such emergency situations as hypovolemic shock and burns. It has been used in lieu of albumin to increase intravascular volume and promote diuresis in patients with hypoalbuminemia. MMW dextran has many of the same anticoagulant effects as LMW dextran (93). It has been used to prevent thrombophlebitis (94, 95) and reclotting of arteriovenous shunts for hemodialysis. However, controlled studies of the efficacy of MMW dextran as compared to oral anticoagulants, dextrose, or saline in preventing thrombophlebitis or thromboembolism have given variable results (59). MMW dextran promotes rouleau formation (in vivo) and platelet aggregation and is not used to improve microcirculation.

MMW dextran has generally the same adverse effects as does LMW dextran. These include allergic reactions, heart failure, and interference with the same laboratory measurements. Clinical episodes of bleeding have also been reported (74) and are particularly likely to occur when more than 1 L is given. Blood samples for typing and cross-matching should be obtained before administering MMW dextran. Coagulopathies and heart failure are contraindications to its use. Sludging in the renal tubules and development of acute renal failure is not reported with MMW dextran. The recommended dose of MMW dextran for volume expansion is up to 20 mL/kg in 6 h; the usual dose for adults is about 500 mL/day. For antithrombotic effects, 10 to 15 mL/kg per day may be infused for 3 to 5 days (91). MMW dextran is available in the United States in 500-mL containers as a 6% solution in normal saline.

Hydroxyethyl starch

Hydroxyethyl starch (HES) (Volex, McGaw Laboratories) is a colloid which is widely used as a plasma volume expander in certain countries (96). HES also increases sedimentation of red cells (97) and is used for leukophoresis. HES is derived from the starch amylopectin, which is structurally more similar to glycogen than are the dextrans. The glucose molecules in amylopectin, as in glycogen, are primarily bound by α-1,4 linkages. For medical use, amylopectin is modified by adding hydroxyethyl groups to glucose by an ether linkage so that 90 percent of the glucose molecules contain hydroxyethyl ($-CH_2CH_2OH$) groups on the sixth carbon atom. Whereas amylopectin is rapidly degraded in serum by α_1-amylases, the hydroxyethyl substitution reduces the rate of degradation. HES has an average molecular weight of about 450,000, and the sizes of 90 percent of the molecules are between 10,000 and 1,000,000 daltons. Its mean molecular weight is larger than that of the more linear MMW dextran. However, HES has a compact, bushlike structure, and therefore exerts a colloidal osmotic force per gram similar to that of MMW dextran (98). HES seems at least as effective as MMW dextran in the treatment of hypovolemic shock (99–103).

Infusion of HES into humans expands plasma volume by approximately 110 percent of the volume administered. Plasma volume expansion falls to about 42 percent of the infused load at 6 h, 29 percent at 24 h, and 7 percent at both 48 and 72 h. The amount of the infused dose remaining in the circulation is 48 percent at 12 h, 38 percent at 24 h, and 22 percent at 72 h (97). The distribution and excretion of HES and MMW dextran are similar. In animals, HES is removed by the kidney and taken up by the reticuloendothelial system (104). HES molecules with a molecular weight less than 50,000 are rapidly excreted in the urine, and a moderate diuresis may occur after infusion.

Probably the major advantage of HES over MMW dextran is its lower immunological reactivity (105, 106) and lower incidence of sensitivity reactions. HES is retained in plasma longer than MMW dextran, and expansion of plasma volume with HES may be slightly greater (96, 107). Swelling and vacuolization have been observed in the renal tubular cells with large doses of HES as well as with MMW dextran and mannitol (107). The comparative merits of HES and dextran have been well reviewed by Thompson (59, 107).

HES is stable with storage. It has a shelf life of about 3 years and, unlike dextran, does not readily crystallize with fluctuations in temperature. Although abnormalities in coagulation have been observed with HES, particularly with high doses (98, 108, 109), in clinical use bleeding problems have been infrequent (110). In Japan, HES of MW 30,000 to 40,000 daltons has been used. Clinical studies with a LMW HES are currently under way in the United States. HES is available in 500-mL containers as a 6% solution in normal saline. It may be administered in doses of up to 1.2 g/kg body weight per day.

Gelatins

Gelatin solutions are not available in the United States, but they are used in Europe and elsewhere. There are three types of gelatins: oxypolygelatin, which has a mean molecular weight of approximately 30,000; modified fluid gelatin, which has a mean molecular weight of 20,000 to 35,000; and Haemaccel, which has a mean molecular weight of 35,000 to 45,000.

The molecular weights of the molecules in these preparations vary from 5,000 to 50,000. Their half-life in plasma is about 8 to 10 h, and after 48 h they have been completely removed from the circulation. After infusion of gelatin, plasma volume remains increased by 30 percent after 2 to 4 h, and a diuresis may occur from excretion of the smaller molecules. The duration of volume expansion depends upon the blood volume before the infusion; volume expansion is considered to last longer when gelatin is infused in the hypovolemic condition as compared to the normovolemic state (61). Approximately 85 percent of administered gelatin (Haemaccel) is excreted through the kidney, 10 percent in the feces, and about 3 percent is degraded in the body (61). Gelatin solutions containing electrolytes tend to be slightly hypertonic (350–390 mosm/L) and have an oncotic pressure similar to that of plasma.

Gelatin is used for plasma volume expansion, replacement of blood loss, and priming for cardiopulmonary bypass (111, 112). Two major advantages of gelatin solutions are their minimal effect on coagulation and bleeding (111) and the relatively low incidence of hypersensitivity reactions as compared with blood. Patients have received more than 100 g of gelatin during periods of active bleeding with no evidence of altered coagulation (113, 114). However, the 0.12 percent incidence of mild allergic reactions and an 0.028 percent incidence of severe allergic reactions to gelatin is higher than for plasma protein solutions, hydroxyethyl starch, or dextran.

Other plasma volume expanders. Pectin, polyvinyl alcohol, polyvinylpyrrolidine (PVP), and acacia (gum arabic) are no longer used as plasma volume expanders. The major disadvantage to their use is their very long retention time in tissues.

BLOOD AND ITS PRODUCTS

Blood

Whole blood provides colloidal osmotic pressure, electrolytes, and oxygen-carrying capacity. It is used for replacement of blood loss, exchange transfusions, extracorporeal circulation, and advanced anemia and debility. Packed red cells may be used instead of whole blood in most circumstances requiring blood transfusions; they have approximately twice the oxygen-carrying capacity per milliliter, with less likelihood of causing circulatory overload and nonhemolytic transfusion reactions. The colloidal osmotic properties of whole blood are greater, and it is usually the preferred source of red cells for the prevention or treatment of hypovolemia or shock. Packed red cells have a shorter shelf life than whole blood, and therefore there may be greater wastage of packed cells.

Fresh whole blood retains the active clotting factors V, VIII, and fibrinogen and viable platelets, although these deteriorate with storage. It is therefore used to replace blood lost in consumption coagulopathy and for massive transfusions (equivalent to one or two times the blood volume).

Although whole blood has been considered the ideal plasma volume expander, there are many problems associated with its use. These have been well reviewed by Collins (115). Whole blood transmits infectious agents, such as hepatitis virus, cytomegalovirus, Epstein-Barr and various respiratory viruses, and malaria parasites. It has been speculated that tumor-causing viruses may be transmitted. With storage of whole blood, clotting factors and platelets decrease rapidly within hours. Transfusion of large quantities of stored blood can lead to coagulation abnormalities from hemodilution of endogenous clotting factors and platelets. With storage, there is a fall in blood pH and 2,3-diphosphoglycerate (DPG) content and a rise in potassium, phosphate, ammonia, lactate, pyruvate, and hemoglobin for oxygen. The acid pH of stored blood tends to counteract the increased oxygen binding associated with reduced 2,3-DPG. After transfusion, the pH rises rapidly from buffering and the metabolism of citrate and lactate; the red cell resynthesizes 2,3-DPG within hours, and the oxyhemoglobin dissociation curve becomes normal (116, 117).

In the usual patient, transfusion of a small amount of blood does not cause acidosis. However, in patients who receive massive quantities of blood and are hypotensive, acidosis may develop. In general, when such subjects have adequate perfusion of tissues, acidosis is mild and transient, and the routine administration of bicarbonate is not indicated. When acidosis does not resolve, hypoperfusion is usually the cause (118).

With transfusion of large quantities of blood, a transient acidosis may be followed by a mild metabolic alkalosis caused by the metabolism of citrate and lactate. Approximately 135 meq of citrate is necessary to produce a mild alkalosis (119). This amount of citrate is contained in about 4000 mL of whole blood. Severe metabolic alkalosis (arterial pH, 7.58) has been reported in a patient undergoing maintenance hemodialysis who received large quantities of whole blood and was unable to excrete excess citrate or bicarbonate in the urine (120).

The relatively large quantities of citrate in blood can also cause symptomatic hypocalcemia. This generally occurs only with rapid transfusion of large volumes of citrated blood, particularly in hypotension, liver disease, or hypothermia.

Hypothermia may result from transfusion of large quantities of unwarmed blood. Hypothermia tends to increase energy and oxygen consumption, impair metabolism of citrate and lactate, promote extracellular movement of potassium, and decrease oxyhemoglobin dissociation. Blood must be warmed cautiously because of the danger of hemolysis from heating (121).

Pulmonary microemboli can occur from the considerable quantities of clots and debris which can pass through the blood filters. It has been suggested that these emboli may sometimes contribute to hypoxia.

Adenosine triphosphate (ATP) decreases in stored red cells, and the cells change concomitantly to a more spherical and rigid shape (115). It is speculated that this may impair red cell movement through the capillaries. ATP is regenerated rapidly after transfusion, and it is not known whether increased red cell rigidity is a clinical problem in the transfused patient.

Plasma potassium in blood rises progressively with storage; it may increase from 12 meq/L at 7 days' storage in acid-citrate-dextrose (ACD) at 4°C to as high as 40 meq/L at 28 days (122). The typical range of plasma potassium in transfused blood is 10 to 25 meq/L. However, this represents only 6 to 15 meq of plasma potassium in a liter of whole blood; and when blood volume is expanded by transfusion, the excess potassium is only about 2 to 11 meq. Moreover, potassium tends to move back into viable red cells after transfusion. There is evidence that hypokalemia is more common than hyperkalemia after massive blood transfusions because of the alkalosis which often develops. In patients with poor tissue perfusion, metabolic acidosis, soft tissue injuries, marked catabolism, or renal failure, hyperkalemia is more likely to occur. The combination of citrate-produced hypocalcemia and hyperkalemia is hazardous, as their adverse effects on the heart are additive.

Plasma ammonia levels rise markedly in stored blood, from 50 μg/dL at the beginning of storage to as high as 680 μg/dL at 21 days. Some investigators recommend fresh blood for patients with advanced liver failure to minimize hyperammonemia (115).

With storage of blood for 3 weeks, plasma phosphate may also rise to about 9 mg/dL, and plasma sodium may fall from 150 to 142 meq/L. Hemolysis during storage may have adverse effects. Plasma hemoglobin may increase from 0 to 10 mg/dL to about 100 mg/dL from hemolysis (117); free hemoglobin appears to be well tolerated, but the lipids in red cell stroma can lead to intravascular coagulation (115). With modern methods of blood banking, hemolysis is generally mild and not a clinical problem.

In addition to transfusion of incompatible red cells, white cells, and platelets, there has been concern that transfusion of stored blood may cause adverse effects from vasoactive substances, such as serotonin (123) and denatured proteins, impairment of reticuloendothelial function, and graft versus host reactions from administered lymphocytes.

For many years blood for transfusion has been prepared with ACD. In general, the citrate is for anticoagulation, dextrose provides substrate for energy utilization, and acidification with citric acid retards glycolysis. Recently, the preservative citrate-phosphate-dextrose (CPD) has begun to replace ACD for the following reasons: CPD contains 20 percent less citrate, has a higher pH, keeps red cells viable somewhat longer, and there is less efflux of potassium from red cells. Whole blood remains viable (as determined by 70 percent red cell survival in vivo 24 h after transfusion) for 21 days of storage with ACD and 28 days with CPD (115, 124).

Crystalloid solutions are usually administered at the start of blood transfusions, and there is often some mixing of these solutions with blood. Only normal saline or 5% dextrose and normal saline should be used to start a blood transfusion. When administered with 5% dextrose in water, clumping and hemolysis may occur; with lactated Ringer's solution, small clots may form (125).

Blood derivatives

Increasingly, blood derivatives are used for treatment of specific disorders. Although whole blood is a versatile therapeutic agent, the problems and expense associated with its use and the frequent need for only one or a few of the components of whole blood have led to the development of many blood derivatives. These include packed cells (see above), fresh platelets, fresh or fresh-frozen plasma (for bleeding conditions associated with decreased labile clotting factors), antihemophilic factor, fibrinogen, thrombin, gamma globulin, plasma, albumin, and plasma protein fraction (126).

Plasma

Plasma has been used as a volume expander, but it can transmit viral hepatitis. The use of pooled human plasma is particularly risky and is not recommended (126). As with blood or packed cells, transfusion of single donor plasma is safer but can still transmit hepatitis, even when donors are screened for hepatitis-associated antigen.

Human serum albumin

Normal subjects have about 4 to 5 g/kg body weight of exchangeable albumin, approximately one-third of which is intravascular. Albumin has a half-life of 18 to 21 days; 6 to 10 percent (10 to 20 g) is degraded per day. Albumin synthesis is inversely related to colloid osmotic pressure or extravascular albumin levels, and decreases with poor nutritional intake. Albumin synthesis is also affected by many hormones, liver failure, and numerous physical stresses. Albumin catabolism is also affected by similar factors including infection, trauma, and such hormonal disorders as deficiency or excess of corticosteroids and hyperthyroidism. Administration of dextran or serum globulin decreases albumin synthesis, while excessive infusion of albumin may lead to an increased catabolic rate (127, 128).

Albumin provides 80 percent of the colloid osmotic pressure of plasma (129, 130). However, plasma oncotic pressure is not linearly related to albumin concentration, and when serum albumin is decreased by half, the oncotic pressure is decreased by one-third. When hypoalbuminemia is present, systemic or pulmonary edema may develop at relatively low filling pressures of the right or left ventricles. Interestingly, however, analbuminemic individuals have little or no edema, probably because of elevated plasma globulins.

Intravenous administration of human albumin has increased rapidly and has threatened to cause shortages. According to aforementioned criteria (see introduction in section on plasma volume expanders), albumin is the best available volume expander. Its major disadvantages are its relative scarcity, its expense, and the occasional occurrence of mild side effects, primarily hyperpyrexia. Pooled human albumin is treated by heating and filtering, and it will not transmit hepatitis.

When patients require fluid as well as albumin, 5% albumin or plasma protein fraction (see below) can be administered. The 25% albumin solution, which is hyperoncotic, is often used in patients who should not receive additional fluid. Twenty-five percent of albumin will rapidly draw three to four times its volume of interstitial fluid into the intravascular space (i.e., 300 to 400 mL per 25 g of albumin in 100 mL of solution). If a patient is dehydrated, 25% albumin should not be administered without crystalloid solutions or further depletion of extravascular and intracellular fluid compartments may occur.

Albumin has been used for the treatment of disorders associated with hypoalbuminemia and hypovolemia. In patients who are hypotensive, albumin can expand intravascular volume and increase blood pressure and cardiac output. The hyperoncotic effect of 25% albumin can mobilize edema fluid; however, this effect is transient since albumin distributes in the extracellular space.

Albumin has been used for the treatment of shock, burns, and adult respiratory distress syndrome, and as a pump prime during cardiopulmonary bypass. The goal is often to increase serum albumin to about 2.5 g/dL or the total protein concentration to 5.2 g/dL, which is equivalent to a plasma oncotic pressure of approximately 20 mmHg (131, 132). There are occasional indications for its use in patients with hepatic failure or nephrotic syndrome with symptomatic hypovolemia, during extensive transfusion with packed red cells, and during removal of ascitic fluid. Albumin may be administered to previously stable hypoalbuminemic patients who sustain a superimposed stress which decreases circulating blood volume such as abdominal surgery or infection. It may also be indicated in patients with acute protein loss following radical abdominal resection of tumors. Albumin has been given in association with diuretics to promote diuresis in hypoalbuminemic patients with cirrhosis or nephrotic syndrome, although other methods are available.

Albumin serves as a transport protein because of its binding affinities for many compounds including drugs, hormones, fatty acids, enzymes, and trace elements and vitamins. Its ability to bind reversibly may enable it to transiently inactivate substances and prolong their duration of action. Its affinity for bilirubin is used for the treatment of kernicterus. It has been suggested that albumin infusions may be used to treat certain drug intoxications (132).

Albumin is often used when crystalloid solutions, other volume expanders, or no treatment at all would suffice. It is not indicated in stable chronic nephrosis or asymptomatic cirrhosis with ascites. It should not be used as a nutrient because its breakdown is slow and its content of certain essential amino acids, particularly tryptophan, is low. Total parenteral nutrition with protein hydrolysates or crystalline amino acids and an energy source provides more effective nutrition (see Chap. 10, Sec. I).

It is noteworthy that hypoalbuminemia in malnourished patients can often be treated by increasing protein and energy intake. Even in advanced liver disease, oral administration of amino acids may increase albumin synthesis, although care must be taken to avoid development of hepatic encephalopathy (Chap. 10, Sec. I).

Human albumin is available as a 5% concentration in a polyionic solution and as a salt-poor 25% solution. It is relatively nonviscous and can be given rapidly in emergency situations. Albumin is more stable than other plasma proteins and can be stored for 3 years at room temperature or up to 10 years if refrigerated. Bovine albumin is an effective plasma expander but can cause both immediate and delayed allergic reactions.

Plasma protein fraction

The hazard of hepatitis from pooled human plasma led to the development of plasma protein fraction (PPF). This is an isotonic solution containing about 4.4% albumin, 0.35% α globulin and 0.25% β globulin. PPF contains approximately 110 to 112 meq of sodium, 0.25–0.5 meq/L of potassium, and 50 meq/L of chloride. The proteins are prepared from pooled human plasma by precipitating out other proteins in cold ethanol (126). The resulting solution is heated at 60°C for 10 h, which inactivates hepatitis virus. Anti-α and anti-β globulins are removed, and thus PPF can be given to patients of any blood type. Untoward reactions are very uncommon, even with repeated administration for many weeks.

PPF is used as a plasma volume expander, to replace protein losses, and to treat hypoproteinemia. Blood volume may remain expanded for up to 48 h after infusion. PPF is as effective a volume expander as plasma, does not transmit hepatitis, and is less expensive than albumin. It may be safely mixed with carbohydrate and electrolyte solutions but not with amino acids.

Disadvantages to the use of PPF are its relative diluteness and high sodium concentration, which restrict its use in patients who are intolerant to water and sodium. Also, it contains no coagulation factors or γ globulin.

PPF can be administered intravenously at rates up to 1 L/h; if shock and hypovolemia are severe, it can probably be infused more rapidly. It should be administered cautiously to normovolemic patients or to patients with heart or kidney disease. PPF is prepared by several companies under different brand names [Plasmanate (Cutter), Plasmatein (Abbott), Plasma-Plex (Armour), and Protenate (Hyland)].

ARTIFICIAL SUBSTITUTES FOR BLOOD

Hemoglobin solutions

Investigators have been intrigued for over 40 years with the use of free hemoglobin as a substitute for blood. The potential advantages of free hemoglobin are that it can exert colloidal osmotic pressure (MW 68,000), can transport and exchange oxygen and carbon dioxide, and does not require typing or cross-matching (133, 134).

Free hemoglobin is often used experimentally in polyionic solutions. During preparation it is separated from erythrocyte stroma, which may cause a hypercoagulable state and renal damage (133). In vivo studies demonstrate that free hemoglobin solutions can transport and exchange oxygen fairly effectively and possibly improve blood flow in the capillary circulation. Rats or dogs subjected to partial exchange transfusions with plasma, dextran, saline, or free hemoglobin survive longer with the latter solution (135). Baboons rendered free of erythrocytes have been kept alive for 3 h with solutions of free hemoglobin and saline (136). Renal function and histology appear to be unaffected by free hemoglobin solutions. Preliminary reports of humans subjected to trauma or thoracic surgery who received solutions containing 3% free hemoglobin indicate that the solutions were effective oxygen carriers and did not affect creatinine or urea clearances. Conversion to methemoglobin appears limited (133, 134).

A disadvantage to free hemoglobin is its rapid clearance from plasma (approximate half-life in humans, 3 h) (137) and removal by the kidney. To increase the residence time of hemoglobin in plasma, the possibility of linking hemoglobin molecules has been assessed (138). A covalent complex of dextran and hemoglobin has been evaluated (139). These complexes may also increase the effectiveness of hemoglobin as a plasma volume expander. Further clinical experience with these promising preparations seems assured.

Synthetic oxygen carriers

A number of artificial compounds have been developed which can carry oxygen and carbon dioxide. Chief among these are the perfluorinated compounds called fluorocarbons (140, 141). They are composed of carbon and fluorine and sometimes contain a nitrogen, oxygen, or sulfur atom. Oxygen and carbon dioxide dissolve in these compounds. They have been used to perfuse isolated brain, kidney, lung, and liver in rats, dogs, and rabbits for up to several hours with little evidence of tissue damage (142).

Animals from whom most or all red cells have been removed have been kept alive for many hours to days with solutions of artificial blood containing perfluorinated compounds. Geyer maintained bloodless rats alive and in apparent good health with these compounds for 5 to 7 days, until their serum proteins and red blood cells regenerated (143, 144). Experience with these compounds in humans has not been reported.

Perfluorinated compounds are generally emulsified to 0.1-μm particles for use. They appear to be nonreactive and well tolerated; however, in some studies, animals developed thrombocytopenia, clotting abnormalities, and hypoxia, presumably due to pulmonary intravascular thromboembolism. It has been suggested that the emulsified perfluorocarbons stimulate platelet aggregation and/or intravascular coagulation. In many animal experiments, this problem has not been observed, possibly because of removal of clotting factors during exsanguination or administration of anticoagulants. Perfluorinated hydrocarbons are rapidly excreted in the urine and must be given repetitively in studies of more than 36 hours' duration.

A disadvantage to the use of perfluorinated hydrocarbons is that oxygen is dissolved in these compounds, so that, in contrast to hemoglobin, there is a linear relationship between oxygen carrying capacity and P_{O_2}. Consequently, to attain levels of oxygenation similar to blood, animals perfused with fluorocarbons must be maintained in an atmosphere containing about 100 percent oxygen. In this regard, recent studies with non-hemoglobin compounds which bind oxygen by chelation are of interest. These chelates have oxygen-binding capacities which are more similar to that of hemoglobin, and high oxygen tensions should therefore not be required (145).

Artificial blood

Concurrently with the development of artificial carriers of oxygen and carbon dioxide, there has been considerable interest in artificial blood (146, 147). The impetus for its development has been the hazards, cost, and relative scarcity of blood and its products. Potentially, artificial blood could be safer, more economical, and more readily available than blood. Also, it could be designed to satisfy more effectively the specific needs of the sick patient, such as enhanced capillary perfusion and tissue oxygenation.

Artificial blood substitutes have been used in animal studies with promising results. The tested solutions have contained emulsified perfluorinated carbons, poloxames, polyols, hydroxyethyl starch, and multiple electrolytes, including bicarbonate. Their viscosity, oncotic and osmotic pressure, and pH are made similar to those of the animal's blood. They transport oxygen and carbon dioxide and maintain colloidal osmotic pressure. Theoretically, specific enzymes, antibodies, and other compounds of normal blood could be added to these solutions.

Artificial blood has potential use in the treatment of refractory anemias, acute blood loss, shock, local ischemia, anaerobic infections and other conditions in which there is a need to increase oxygenation at the cellular level, and might be used for extracorporeal circulation (148).

USE OF NONCOLLOIDAL SOLUTIONS FOR PLASMA VOLUME EXPANSION

Many investigators are currently evaluating the conditions under which crystalloid solutions could replace blood or plasma volume expanders. Solutions which have been most thoroughly evaluated are normal saline, lactated Ringer's and other polyionic solutions (Tables 10-14 and 10-17). Crystalloid solutions are safer, cheaper, more readily available, and have a longer shelf life than colloid solutions. They are often effective in the treatment of shock or hypotension, because volume expansion and tissue perfusion are frequently more critical problems than oxygen-carrying capacity. In shock, burns, and trauma, there is often a decrease in interstitial and intracellular fluid as well as in intravascular volume, and infusion of whole blood may result in an abnormally high hematocrit from subsequent hemoconcentration. Indeed, studies in patients with bleeding peptic ulcers have shown fewer complications with Ringer's lactate replacement than with blood transfusion (149–153).

Crystalloid solutions have high sodium concentrations and are essentially isotonic so that the infusate is distributed in the extracellular volume. Ringer's lactate is often chosen as a replacement solution because it contains several of the electrolytes lost in shock, burns, or trauma. It is also an alkalinizing solution which counteracts the metabolic acidosis which often accompanies hemorrhage, shock, or severe catabolism. Acetated polyionic solutions are coming into wider use because lactate may be poorly metabolized with poor tissue perfusion and hypoxia (see above). However, any crystalloid solution which improves capillary perfusion will usually correct metabolic acidosis from hypoxia.

Addition of glucose to these solutions may be advantageous if the patient is not intolerant to glucose. The glucose provides a needed energy source and will lower the rate of lipolysis and fatty acid oxidation; glucose is not, however, a substitute for more complete intravenous nutrition.

Although the hematocrit falls when lost blood is replaced with crystalloid solution, it is generally accepted that the oxygen-carrying capacity of blood with a hematocrit of 30 percent is not much lower than that with a value of 40 percent. Approximately 1 L of lost blood can usually be replaced with crystalloid solution without lowering the hematocrit below 30 percent. Blood is generally not necessary unless the hematocrit falls below this level.

In past practice, mild to moderate degrees of blood loss were not treated at all, and the patient would be allowed to "stabilize," or replace his deficit. In actuality, the lost intravascular volume was replaced by creating a deficit in another compartment (i.e., the extracellular). Crystalloid replacement of lost volume is preferable. Serum protein concentrations may fall with this therapy, but they usually remain within normal limits and, if continuing stress or poor nutrition is not present, return to their previous levels.

Since crystalloid solutions are dispersed in the extracellular space, about three to four volumes must be administered to replace each volume of blood lost. However, even greater quantities of crystalloid solution may be necessary because of tissue edema, pooling of fluid in a "third space" (i.e., body cavities or organ lumina), and movement of water into cells. Under experimental conditions in animals, ratios as high as 58:1 of crystalloid solutions administered/blood lost have been required to prevent hypovolemia and hypotension.

The patient must be monitored carefully when blood loss or hypotension is treated with crystalloid solution. Signs of hypoxia, cardiac ischemia, persisting hypotension, progressive anemia, or actual or threatened continued bleeding may indicate the need for blood or colloidal-osmotic expanders (154). In patients with heart, kidney, or liver failure, debility, or advanced age, the large volumes of crystalloid solutions which may be necessary to replace lost blood must be administered with great caution.

REFERENCES

1. O'Shaughnessy, W. B.: Experiments on the blood in cholera, *Lancet,* **1:**490, 1831–32.

2. Latta, T.: Relative to the treatment of cholera by the copious injection of aqueous and saline fluids into the veins (letter), *Lancet*, **2**:274, 1832.

3. Lewins, R.: Letter to editor, *Lancet*, **2**:280, 1832.

4. Mengoli, L. R.: Excerpts from the history of post-operative fluid therapy, *Am. J. Surg.*, **121**:311, 1971.

5. Hartwell, J. A., and J. P. Hoguet: Experimental intestinal obstruction in dogs with especial reference to the cause of death and the treatment by large amounts of normal saline solution, *JAMA*, **59**:82, 1912.

6. Penfield, W. G., and D. Teplitsky: Prolonged intravenous infusion and the clinical determination of venous pressure, *Arch. Surg.*, **7**:111, 1923.

7. Matas, R.: The continued intravenous drip, *Ann. Surg.*, **79**:643, 1934.

8. Gamble, J. L., and S. G. Ross: The factors in the dehydration following pyloric obstruction, *J. Clin. Invest.*, **1**:403, 1924–25.

9. Gamble, J. L.: *Chemical Anatomy Physiology and Pathology of Extracellular Fluid*, vol. 1 Harvard University Press, Cambridge, Mass., 1954, p. 164.

10. Harrington, J. T., and J. J. Cohen: Clinical disorders of urine concentration and dilution, *Arch. Intern. Med.*, **131**:810, 1973.

11. Edelman, I. S., and J. Leibman: Anatomy of body water and electrolytes, *Am. J. Med.*, **27**:256, 1959.

12. Widdowson, E. M., and J. W. T. Dickerson: Chemical composition of the body, in C. L. Comar and F. Bronner (eds.), *Mineral Metabolism*, vol. 2, part A, Academic Press, Inc., New York, 1964.

13. *Recommended Dietary Allowances,* National Academy of Sciences, Committee on Dietary Allowances, National Research Council Food and Nutrition Board, Washington, D.C., 1974.

14. Arieff, A. I., F. Llach, and S. G. Massry: Neurological manifestations and morbidity of hyponatremia: Correlation with brain water and electrolytes, *Medicine (Baltimore)*, **55**:121, 1976.

15. Hantman, C., B. Rossier, R. Zohlman, and R. Schrier: Rapid correction of hyponatremia in the syndrome of inappropriate secretion of antidiuretic hormone, *Ann. Intern. Med.*, **78**:870, 1973.

16. Macauley, D., and M. Watson: Hypernatraemia in infants as a cause of brain damage, *Arch. Dis. Child.*, **42**:485, 1967.

17. Lawson, D. H.: Adverse reactions to potassium chloride, *Q. J. Med.*, **171**:433, 1974.

18. Burchell, H. B.: Dilemmas in potassium therapy, *Circulation*, **47**:1144, 1973.

19. Burnell, J. M., M. F. Villamil, B. T. Uyeno, and B. H. Scribner: The effect in humans of extracellular pH change on the relationship between serum potassium concentration and intracellular potassium, *J. Clin. Invest.*, **35**:935, 1956.

20. Soler, N. G., M. A. Bennett, M. G. Fitzgerald, and J. M. Malins: Electrocardiogram as a guide to potassium replacement in diabetic ketoacidosis, *Diabetes*, **23**:610, 1974.

21. Lawson, D. H.: The clinical use of potassium supplements, *J. Maine Med. Assoc.*, **66**:166, 1975.

22. Williams, R. H. P.: Potassium overdose: A potential hazard of non-rigid parenteral fluid containers, *Br. Med. J.*, **24**:714, 1973.

23. Lankton, J. W., J. N. Scher, and J. L. Neigh: Hyperkalemia after administration of potassium from non-rigid parenteral fluid containers, *Anesthesiology*, **39**:660, 1973.

24. Posner, J. B., and F. Plum: Spinal-fluid pH and neurologic symptoms in systemic acidosis, *N. Engl. J. Med.*, **277**:605, 1967.

25. Hems, R., B. D. Ross, M. N. Berry, and H. A. Krebs: Gluconeogenesis in the perfused rat liver, *Biochem. J.*, **101**:284, 1966.

26. Ohman, J. L., Jr., E. B. Marliss, T. T. Aoki, C. S. Munichoodappa, V. V. Kahnna, and G. P. Kozak: The cerebrospinal fluid in diabetic ketoacidosis, *N. Engl. J. Med.*, **284**:382, 1971.

27. Hartmann, A. F., and J. J. E. Senn: Studies in the metabolism of sodium r-lactate. I. Response of normal human subjects to the intravenous injection of sodium r-lactate, *J. Clin. Invest.*, **11**:327, 1932.

28. Schwartz, B. W., and W. C. Waters: Lactate versus bicarbonate: A reconsideration of the therapy of metabolic acidosis, *Am. J. Med.*, **32**:831, 1962.

29. Cohen, R. D., and R. Simpson: Lactate metabolism, *Anesthesiology*, **43**:661, 1975.

30. Harken, A. H.: Lactic acidosis, *Surg. Gynecol. Obstet.*, **142**:593, 1976.

31. Lundquist, F.: Production and utilization of free acetate in man, *Nature*, **193**:579, 1962.

32. Novello, A., R. C. Kelsch, and R. E. Easterling:

Acetate intolerance during hemodialysis, *Clin. Nephrol.,* **5**:29, 1976.

33. Graefe, U., J. Milutinovich, W. Follette, J. Vizzo, A. Babb, and B. Schribner: Less dialysis-induced morbidity and vascular instability with bicarbonate in dialysate, *Ann. Intern. Med.,* **88**(3):332, 1978.

34. Bleich, H. L., and W. B. Schwartz: TRIS buffer (Tham): An appraisal of its physiologic effects and clinical usefulness, *N. Engl. J. Med.,* **274**:282, 1966.

35. Abouna, G. M., P. R. Veazey, and D. B. Terry, Jr.: Intravenous infusion of hydrochloric acid for treatment of severe metabolic alkalosis, *Surgery,* **75**:194, 1974.

36. Shavelle, H. S., and R. Parke: Postoperative metabolic alkalosis and acute renal failure: Rationale for the use of hydrochloric acid, *Surgery,* **78**:439, 1975.

37. Harken, A. H., R. A. Gabel, V. Fencl, and F. D. Moore: Hydrochloric acid in the correction of metabolic alkalosis, *Arch. Surg.,* **110**:819, 1975.

38. Garella, S., B. S. Chang, and S. I. Kahn: Dilution acidosis and contraction alkalosis: Review of a concept, *Kidney Int.,* **8**:279, 1975.

39. Elfving, G., and K. Saikku: Effect of pH on the incidence of infusion thrombophlebitis, *Lancet,* **1**:953, 1966.

40. Vere, D. W., C. H. Sykes, and P. Armitage: Venous thrombosis during dextrose infusion, *Lancet,* **1**:627, 1960.

41. Lebowitz, M. H., J. Y. Masuda, and J. H. Beckman: The pH and acidity of intravenous infusion solutions, *JAMA,* **215**:1937, 1971.

42. Martin, E. W. (ed.): *Hazards of Medication, A Manual on Drug Interactions, Incompatibilities, Contraindications and Adverse Effects,* J. B. Lippincott Company, Philadelphia, 1971.

43. *Parenteral Drug Information Guide,* American Society of Hospital Physicians, 1974.

44. Williams, J. T., and D. F. Moravec (eds.): *Intravenous Therapy,* Clissold Publishing Company, North State Press, Inc., Hammond, Indiana, 1967.

45. Williams, J. T., and D. F. Moravec: The extent of incompatible drug combinations, in J. T. Williams and D. F. Moravec (eds.), *Intravenous Therapy,* Clissold Publishing Company, North State Press, Inc., Hammond, Indiana, 1967.

46. D'Arcy, P. F.: Additives—An additional hazard? in I. Phillips, P. D. Meers, and P. F. D'Arcy (eds.), *Microbiological Hazards of Infusion Therapy,* Publishing Sciences Group, Inc., Littleton, Massachusetts, 1976.

47. Raffanti, E. F. Jr., and J. C. King: Effect of pH on the stability of sodium ampicillin solutions, *Am. J. Hosp. Pharm.,* **31**:745, 1974.

48. Hambleton, R., and M. C. Allwood: Containers and closures, in I. Phillips, P. D. Meers, and P. F. D'Arcy (eds.), *Microbiological Hazards of Infusion Therapy,* Publishing Sciences Group, Inc., Littleton, Massachusetts, 1976.

49. Garvan, J. M., and B. W. Gunner: Particulate contamination of intravenous fluids, *Br. J. Clin. Prac.,* **25**:119, 1971.

50. Moorhatch, P., and W. L. Chiou: Interactions between drugs and plastic intravenous fluid bags, part i: Sorption studies on 17 drugs, *Am. J. Hosp. Pharm.,* **31**:72, 1974.

51. Chou, W. L., and P. Moorhatch: Interaction between vitamin A and plastic intravenous fluid bags (letter to editor), *JAMA,* **223**:328, 1973.

52. Felts, S. K., W. Schaffner, M. A. Melly, and M. G. Koenig: Sepsis caused by contaminated intravenous fluids, *Ann. Intern. Med.,* **77**:881, 1972.

53. Karanicolas, S., D. G. Oreopoulos, Sh. Izatt, A. Shimizu, R. F. Manning, H. Sepp, G. A. DeVeber, and T. Darby: Epidemic of aseptic peritonitis caused by endotoxin during chronic peritoneal dialysis, *N. Engl. J. Med.,* **296**:1336, 1977.

54. Maki, D. G.: Preventing infection in intravenous therapy, *Hosp. Prog.,* **11**:95, 1976.

55. Maki, D. G.: Sepsis arising from extrinsic contamination of the infusion and measures for control, in I. Phillips, P. D. Meers, and P. F. D'Arcy (eds.), *Microbiological Hazards of Infusion Therapy,* Publishing Sciences Group, Inc., Littleton, Massachusetts, 1976.

56. Maki, D. G.: Final filters, *Hosp, Inf. Control,* **3**:22, 1976.

57. Kliman, A.: Presently useful plasma volume expanders, *Anesthesiology,* **27**:419, 1966.

58. Mendelson, J. A.: The selection of plasma volume expanders for resuscitation following trauma: A review, *Milit. Med.,* **140**:258, 1975.

59. Thompson, W. L.: Rational use of albumin and plasma substitutes, *Johns Hopkins Med. J.,* **136**:220, 1975.

60. Moffitt, E. A.: Blood substitutes, *Can. Anaesth. Soc. J.,* **22**:12, 1975.

61. Rudowski, W., and E. Kostrzewska: Blood substitutes, *Ann. R. Col. Surg. Engl.,* **58**:115, 1976.

62. Arturson, G., K. Granath, L. Thorén, and G. Wallenius: The renal excretion of low molecular weight dextran, *Acta. Chir. Scand.,* **127**:543, 1964.

63. Arturson, G., and G. Wallenius: The renal clearance of dextran of different molecular sizes in normal humans, *Scand. J. Clin. Lab. Invest.,* **1**:81, 1964.

64. Arturson, G., and G. Wallenius: The intravascular persistence of dextran of different molecular sizes in normal humans, *Scand. J. Clin. Lab. Invest.,* **1**:76, 1964.

65. Atik, M.: Dextrans, their use in surgery and medicine, *Anesthesiology,* **27**:425, 1966.

66. Atik, M.: The uses of dextran in surgery: A current evaluation, *Surgery,* **65**:548, 1969.

67. Evarts, C. M.: Prevention of thromboembolism, *Arch. Surg.,* **106**:134, 1973.

68. Evarts, C. M., and E. J. Feil: Prevention of thromboembolic disease after elective surgery of the hip, *J. Bone Joint Surg. [Am.],* **53-A**:1271, 1971.

69. Gruber, U. F., R. Fridrich, F. Duckert, J. Torhorst, and J. Rem: Prevention of postoperative thromboembolism by dextran 40, low doses of heparin, or xantinol nicotinate, *Lancet,* **1**:207, 1977.

70. Gilroy, J., M. I. Barnhart, and J. S. Meyer: Treatment of acute stroke with dextran 40, *JAMA,* **210**:293, 1969.

71. Mundth, E. D., D. M. Long, and R. B. Brown: Treatment of experimental frostbite with low molecular weight dextran, *J. Trauma,* **4**:246, 1964.

72. Matsuda, H., and W. C. Shoemaker: Cardiorespiratory responses to dextran 40: Hemodynamic and oxygen transport changes in normal subjects and critically ill patients, *Arch. Surg.,* **110**:296, 1975.

73. Mohr, P. A., D. O. Monson, C. Owczarski, and W. C. Shoemaker: Sequential cardiorespiratory events during and after dextran-40 infusion in normal and shock patients, *Circulation,* **39**:379, 1969.

74. Karlson, K. E., A. A. Garzon, G. W. Shaftan, and C. J. Chu: Increased blood loss associated with administration of certain plasma expanders: Dextran 75, dextran 40, and hydroxyethyl starch. *Surgery,* **62**:670, 1967.

75. Langsjoen, P. H., and R. A. Murray: Treatment of postsurgical thromboembolic complications, *JAMA,* **218**:855, 1971.

76. Wells, R. E.: Comparison of effects of low molecular weight dextran on blood viscosity and the sludging phenomenon in vitro and in vivo, *Circulation,* **31**:217, 1965.

77. Ponder, E., and R. V. Ponder: Age and molecular weight of dextrans, their coating effects, and their interaction with serum albumin, *Nature,* **190**:277, 1961.

78. Bloom, W. L., D. S. Harmer, M. F. Bryant, and S. S. Brewer: Coating of vascular surfaces and cells. A new concept in prevention of intravascular thrombosis, *Circulation,* **26**:690, 1962.

79. Ross, S. W., and R. V. Ebert: Microelectrophoresis of blood platelets and the effects of dextran, *J. Clin. Invest.,* **38**:155, 1959.

80. Bygdeman, S., and R. Eliasson: Effect of dextrans on platelet adhesiveness and aggregation, *Scand. J. Clin. Lab. Invest.,* **20**:17, 1967.

81. Ewald, R. A., J. W. Eichelberger, Jr., A. A. Young, H. J. Weiss, and W. H. Crosby: The effect of dextran on platelet factor 3 activity: In vitro and in vivo studies, *Transfusion,* **5**:109, 1965.

82. Data, J. L., and A. S. Nies: Dextran 40, *Ann. Intern. Med.,* **81**:500, 1974.

83. Salzman, E. W., W. H. Harris, and R. W. DeSanctis: Reduction in venous thromboembolism by agents affecting platelet function, *N. Engl. J. Med.,* **284**:1287, 1971.

84. Rothermel, J. E., J. B. Wessinger, and F. E. Stinchfield: Dextran 40 and thromboembolism in total hip replacement surgery, *Arch. Surg.,* **106**:135, 1973.

85. Bailey, G., R. L. Strub, R. C. Klein, and J. Salvaggio: Dextran-induced anaphylaxis, *JAMA,* **200**:185, 1967.

86. Brisman, R., L. C. Parks, and J. A. Haller, Jr.: Anaphylactoid reactions associated with the clinical use of dextran 70, *JAMA,* **204**:166, 1968.

87. Michelson, E.: Anaphylactic reaction to dextrans, *N. Engl. J. Med.,* **278**:552, 1968.

88. Feest, T. G.: Low molecular weight dextran: A

continuing cause of acute renal failure, *Br. Med. J.*, **2:**1300, 1976.

89. Mailloux, L., C. D. Swartz, R. Capizzi, K. E. Kim, G. Onesti, O. Ramirez, and A. N. Brest: Acute renal failure after administration of low-molecular-weight dextran, *N. Engl. J. Med.*, **277:**1113, 1967.

90. Thomas, J. M., and J. R. Silva: Dextran 40 in the treatment of peripheral vascular diseases, *Arch. Surg.*, **106:**138, 1973.

91. Atik, M.: Dextran 40 and dextran 70: A review, *Arch. Surg.*, **94:**664, 1967.

92. Dextran 40 and other dextrans, *Med. Lett. Drugs Ther.*, **10:**3, 1968.

93. Sawyer, R. B., and J. A. Moncrief: Dextran specificity in thrombus inhibition, *Arch. Surg.*, **90:**562, 1965.

94. Bonnar, J., and J. Walsh: Prevention of thrombosis after pelvic surgery by British dextran 70, *Lancet*, **1:**614, 1972.

95. Carter, A. E., and R. Eban: The prevention of postoperative deep venous thrombosis with dextran 70, *Br. J. Surg.*, **60:**681, 1973.

96. Solanke, T. F.: Clinical trial of 6% hydroxyethyl starch (a new plasma expander), *Br. Med. J.*, **3:**783, 1968.

97. Metcalf, W., A. Papadopoulos, R. Tufaro, and A. Barth: A clinical physiologic study of hydroxyethyl starch, *Surg. Gynecol. Obstet.*, **130:**255, 1970.

98. Banks, W., C. T. Greenwood, and D. D. Muir: The structure of hydroxyethyl starch, *Br. J. Pharmacol.*, **47:**172, 1973.

99. Ballinger, W. F., T. F. Solanke, and W. L. Thompson: The effect of hydroxyethyl starch upon survival of dogs subjected to hemorrhagic shock, *Surg. Gynecol. Obstet.*, **122:**33, 1966.

100. Gollub, S., D. C. Schechter, T. Hirose, and C. P. Bailey: Use of hydroxyethyl starch solution in extensive surgical operations, *Surg. Gynecol. Obstet.*, **128:**725, 1969.

101. Thompson, W. L., J. J. Britton, and R. P. Walton: Persistence of starch derivatives and dextran when infused after hemorrhage, *J. Pharmacol. Exp. Ther.*, **136:**125, 1962.

102. Kinoshita, T., C. Watanuki, M. Shinozaki, K. Kita, S. Oku, Y. Ueyama, Y. Ohta, H. Tamura, N. Nishimoto, Y. Izawa, and H. Ueyama: A clin-ical evaluation of a new plasma expander "hydroxyethyl starch," *Wakayama Med. Rept.*, **15:**53, 1971.

103. Kitamura, Y., A. Yamada, N. Sha, R. Hamai, K. Nishimura, and M. Fujimori: A clinical study of hydroxyethyl starch, *Osaka City Med. J.*, **18:**21, 1972.

104. Thompson, W. L., T. Fukushima, R. B. Rutherford, and R. P. Walton: Intravascular persistence, tissue storage, and excretion of hydroxyethyl starch, *Surg. Gynecol. Obstet.*, **131:**965, 1970.

105. Brickman, R. D., G. F. Murray, W. L. Thompson, and W. F. Ballinger: The antigenicity of hydroxyethyl starch in humans: Studies in seven normal volunteers, *JAMA*, **198:**139, 1966.

106. Maurer, P. H., and B. Berardinelli: Immunologic studies with hydroxyethyl starch (HES): A proposed plasma expander, *Transfusion*, **8:**265, 1968.

107. Thompson, W. L.: Plasma proteins and substitutes in critically ill patients, Scientific Exhibit, American College of Surgeons, Sixtieth Annual Clinical Congress, Miami, Florida, October 21–25, 1974.

108. Garzon, A. A., C. Cheng, B. Lerner, S. Lichtenstein, and K. E. Karlson: Hydroxyethyl starch (HES) and bleeding: An experimental investigation of its effect on hemostasis, *J. Trauma*, **7:**757, 1967.

109. Alexander, B., K. Odake, D. Lawlor, and M. Swanger: Coagulation, hemostasis, and plasma expanders: A quarter century enigma, *Fed. Proc.*, **34:**1429, 1975.

110. Gollub, S., C. Schaefer, and A. Squitieri: The bleeding tendency associated with plasma expanders, *Surg. Gynecol. Obstet.*, **124:**1203, 1967.

111. Moyes, D. G.: Haemodilution with a plasma expander as priming solution in cardiopulmonary bypass, *S. Afr. Med. J.*, **48:**1615, 1974.

112. Solanke, T. F., M. S. Khwaja, and E. I. Madojemu: Plasma volume studies with four different plasma volume expanders, *J. Surg. Res.*, **11:**140, 1971.

113. Pessereau, G., J. Migne, P. Piccard, P. Radiguet de la Bastaie, G. G. Nahas, and D. V. Habif: The use of a balanced fluid gelatin for fluid replacement, in Fox (ed.), *Body Fluid Replacement in the Surgical Patient*, Grune & Stratton, Inc., New York, 1970, pp. 115–124.

114. Tschirren, B., and P. Lundsgaard-Hansen: The

use of fluid gelatin in the surgical patient: Report of 120 cases receiving 2 liters or more, in Fox (ed.), *Body Fluid Replacement in the Surgical Patient*, Grune & Stratton, Inc., New York, 1970, pp. 125–136.

115. Collins, J. A.: Problems associated with the massive transfusion of stored blood, Presented at Coll. of Phy. and Surg. Col. Univ., New York, Fenwal Labs, Morton Grove, Ill. 1973.

116. Schechter, D. C., and H. Swan: Biochemical alterations of preserved blood, *Arch. Surg.*, **84:**17, 1962.

117. Bunker, J. P.: Metabolic effects of blood transfusion, *Anesthesiology*, **27:**446, 1966.

118. Collins, J. A., R. L. Simmons, P. M. James, C. E. Bredenberg, R. W. Anderson, and C. A. Heisterkamp: Acid-base status of seriously wounded combat casualties: II. Resuscitation with stored blood, *Ann. Surg.*, **173:**6, 1971.

119. Litwin, M. S., L. L. Smith, and F. D. Moore: Metabolic alkalosis following massive transfusion, *Surgery*, **45:**805, 1959.

120. Barcenas, C. G., T. J. Fuller, and J. P. Knochel: Metabolic alkalosis after massive blood transfusion, correction by hemodialysis, *JAMA*, **236:**953, 1976.

121. Arens, J. F., and G. L. Leonard: Danger of overwarming blood by microwave, *JAMA*, **218:**1045, 1971.

122. Mollison, P. L.: *Blood Transfusion in Clinical Medicine*, chap. 13, Other unfavorable effects of transfusion, Blackwell Scientific Publications, London, 1972.

123. Strauss, H. W., R. B. Smith, P. Polimeni, A. C. Schenker, V. J. Schenker, and J. H. Stuckley: Plasma serotonin levels in stored human blood, *Angiology*, **18:**535, 1967.

124. Gibson, J. G., C. B. Gregory, and L. N. Button: Citrate-phosphate-dextrose solution for preservation of human blood, *Transfusion*, **1:**280, 1961.

125. Ryden, S. E., and H. A. Oberman: Compatibility of common intravenous solutions with CPD blood, *Transfusion*, **15:**250, 1975.

126. Huestis, D. W., J. R. Bove, and S. Busch: Blood components, fractions, and derivatives, in *Practical Blood Transfusion*, Little, Brown and Company, Boston, 1969.

127. Peters, T.: Serum albumin, in O. Bodansky and C. P. Stewart (eds.), *Advances in Clinical Chemistry*, Academic Press, New York and London, 1970.

128. Rothschild, M. A., M. Oratz, and S. S. Schreiber: Albumin metabolism, *Gastroenterol.*, **64:**324, 1973.

129. Reiff, T. R.: Colloid osmotic homeostasis in humans—I. Theoretical aspects and background, *J. Theor. Biol.*, **28:**1–14, 1970.

130. Armstrong, S. H., and J. C. Kukral: Significance of plasma proteins in surgical practice, in L. M. Zimmerman and R. Levine (eds.), *Physiologic Principles of Surgery*, W. B. Saunders Company, Philadelphia, 1964.

131. Tullis, J. L.: Albumin, background and use, *JAMA*, **237:**355, 1977.

132. Tullis, J. L.: Albumin, guidelines for clinical use, *JAMA*, **237:**460, 1977.

133. Rabiner, S. F., J. R. Helbert, H. Lopas, and L. H. Friedman: Evaluation of a stroma-free hemoglobin solution for use as a plasma expander, *J. Exp. Med.*, **126:**1127, 1967.

134. Rabiner, S. F.: Hemoglobin solution as a plasma expander, *Fed. Proc.*, **34:**1454, 1975.

135. Kaplan, H. R., and V. S. Murthy: Hemoglobin solution: A potential oxygen transporting plasma volume expander, *Fed. Proc.*, **34:**1461, 1975.

136. Moss, G. S., R. DeWoskin, A. L. Rosen, H. Levine, and C. K. Palani: Transport of oxygen and carbon dioxide by hemoglobin-saline solution in the red cell-free primate, *Surg. Gynecol. Obstet.*, **142:**357, 1976.

137. Bonhard, K.: Acute oxygen supply by infusion of hemoglobin solutions, *Fed. Proc.*, **34:**1466, 1975.

138. Mok, W., D. Chen, and A. Mazur: Cross-linked hemoglobins as potential plasma protein extenders, *Fed. Proc.*, **34:**1458, 1975.

139. Tam, S-C., J. Blumenstein, and J. T-F. Wong: Soluble dextran-hemoglobin complex as a potential blood substitute. *Proc. Natl. Acad. Sci. U.S.A.*, **73:**2128, 1976.

140. Dixon, D. D., and D. G. Holland: Fluorocarbons: Properties and syntheses, *Fed. Proc.*, **34:**1444, 1975.

141. Sloviter, H. A.: Perfluoro compounds as artificial erythrocytes, *Fed. Proc.*, **34:**1484, 1975.

142. Hall, C. A.: Perfluorocarbon emulsion in the perfusion of canine organs, *Fed. Proc.*, **34:**1513, 1975.

143. Geyer, R. P.: Fluorocarbon-polyol artificial blood substitutes, *N. Engl. J. Med.,* **289:**1077, 1973.

144. Geyer, R. P.: "Bloodless" rats through the use of artificial blood substitutes, *Fed. Proc.,* **34:**1499, 1975.

145. Baldwin, J. E.: Chelating agents as possible artificial blood substitutes, *Fed. Proc.,* **34:**1441, 1975.

146. New blood substitutes (editorial), *Lancet,* **1**(848):125, 1974.

147. Geyer, R. P.: Summary of workshop, *Fed Proc.,* **34:**1529, 1975.

148. Geyer, R. P.: Potential uses of artificial blood substitutes, *Fed. Proc.,* **34:**1525, 1975.

149. Rigor, B., P. Bosomworth, and B. F. Rush: Replacement of operative blood loss of more than 1 liter with Hartmann's solution, *JAMA,* **203:**111, 1968.

150. Rush, B. F., J. D. Richardson, P. Bosomworth, and B. Eiseman: Limitations of blood replacement with electrolyte solutions, a controlled clinical study, *Arch. Surg.,* **98:**49, 1969.

151. Carey, L. C., C. T. Cloutier, and B. D. Lowery: The use of balanced electrolyte solution for resusciation, in C. L. Fox, Jr., and G. G. Nahas (eds.), *Body Fluid Replacement in the Surgical Patient,* Grune & Stratton, Inc., New York, 1970.

152. Lund, B., D. Benveniste, J.-E. P. Pedersen, and M. Hebjørn: Replacement of blood loss with physiological saline in major surgery, *Acta Chir. Scand.,* **141:**461, 1975.

153. Cervera, A. L., and G. Moss: Dilutional re-expansion with crystalloid after massive hemorrhage: Saline versus balanced electrolyte solution for maintenance of normal blood volume and arterial pH, *J. Trauma,* **15:**498, 1975.

154. Laks, H., N. E. O'Connor, W. Anderson, and R. N. Pilon: Crystalloid versus colloid hemodilution in man, *Surg. Gynecol. Obstet.,* **142:**506, 1976.

11

Signs and symptoms of electrolyte disorders

FRANKLIN H. EPSTEIN

A genuine understanding of the functions of sodium, potassium, calcium, magnesium and their salts in the organism would necessitate a comprehension of the nature of protoplasm and its behavior in living cells, something we have not begun to attain.

> J. P. Peters and D. D. Van Slyke,
> *Quantitative Clinical Chemistry*, 1st ed.,
> vol. I. p. 764, The Williams & Wilkins Company,
> Baltimore, 1931.

Since Peters and Van Slyke published their classic text, there has been an enormous increase in understanding of the processes governing the transport of ions across cell membranes. It is chastening, nevertheless, to reflect on the fact that the major clinical manifestations of electrolyte disorders observed at the bedside by history and physical examination were known well to clinicians 40 and more years ago.

For the most part, disturbances of the distribution and concentration of body electrolytes affect cellular function rather than structure. Exceptions to this rule are seen in the nephropathy and myocarditis of severe potassium deficiency and in the well-marked lesions of calcium intoxication. But the predominant effect of alterations in electrolyte concentration is likely to be detected in their influence on chemical and electric gradients across cell membranes. Hence the symptomatology of electrolyte disorders has much to do with changes in the behavior of *excitable tissues*. Neurologic disturbances are prominent (see Table 11-1), as are changes in cardiovascular function and in skeletal muscle. Most important of all from the standpoint of the clinician, a feature of most of the symptoms described in this chapter is that they are *reversible with proper therapy*.

HYPERNATREMIA

The sense of thirst is so strong a defender of the serum sodium in normal individuals that hypernatremia is never encountered unless thirst is impaired or rendered ineffective because the patient is comatose or is denied access to water. Even in patients with diabetes insipidus, in whom water losses may amount to gallons per day, the intake of water usually keeps pace with its excretion. Serum sodium is elevated minimally or not at all as long as the patient is awake and able to drink. When thirst is no longer permitted to operate, however, the serum sodium increases. Hyperna-

Table 11-1. Neurologic manifestations of electrolyte disturbances

DISTURBANCE	LETHARGY, CONFUSION, DELIRIUM, PSYCHOSIS, COMA	SEIZURES	MUSCLE WEAKNESS	PARALYSIS	MUSCLE CRAMPS	PARESTHESIS	MYOCLONUS	ASTERIXIS	TETANY	DEEP TENDON REFLEXES	CEREBROSPINAL FLUID PRESSURE	CEREBROSPINAL FLUID PROTEIN
Hypernatremia	+*	+	+	−	−	−	+	−	±	I	D	I
Hyponatremia	+	+	+	−	+	−	+	±	−	ID	I	U
Hyperkalemia	−	−	+	+	−	+	−	−	−	UD	U	U
Hypokalemia	±	±	+	+	+	+	−	−	±	U	U	U
Hypercalcemia	+	±	+	−	+	−	−	−	−	UD	U	I
Hypocalcemia	+	+	+	−	+	+	−	−	+	U	I	U
Hypermagnesemia	+	−	+	+	−	−	±	−	−	D	?	?
Hypomagnesemia	+	+	+	−	+	+	±	−	+	I	?	?
Acidosis	+	±†	−	−	−	−	±	+	−	UI	I†	U
Alkalosis	+	+	+	−	+	+	±	±	+	UI‡	U	I‡

* +, common; ±, occasional; −, absent; I, increased; D, decreased; U, unchanged.

† Respiratory acidosis only.

‡ Respiratory alkalosis only.

tremia is especially likely to become a problem when water losses are enhanced.

Hypernatremia is commonly seen under the following circumstances:

1. *The desiccation of a semicomatose patient.* A good example is the elderly patient who has a stroke and is unable to drink normally. After a week of gradually decreasing responsiveness and lethargy, complicated during the last few days by a low-grade fever, she is admitted from the nursing home to a general hospital where the serum sodium is found to be elevated. In such patients CNS depression induced by hypernatremia further reduces the desire and ability to drink, thus initiating a vicious circle.

2. *Greatly increased urinary losses of water, when intake is restricted.* Examples include neurosurgical patients with diabetes insipidus occurring postoperatively, patients in whom high-protein feedings are dissolved in minimal amounts of water and fed by stomach tube, producing a large urea diuresis, and patients with diabetes mellitus in whom prolonged glucose diuresis has resulted in losses of water

which exceed those of salts. Some of the most striking instances of hypertonicity we have seen have been in patients in whom relief of urinary obstruction has resulted in the sudden diuresis of large volumes of dilute urine which could not be adequately replaced by water taken by mouth because the patient was comatose or lethargic.

3. *Large evaporative losses from the skin.* When the normal vapor barrier of the skin is destroyed by extensive second- and third-degree burns and especially when the burns are treated by the "open method," hypernatremia commonly ensues.

4. *Salt poisoning.* A greatly increased intake of salt in a constant inadequate volume of water may produce severe hypernatremia, as occurred in the infants described by Finberg and his collaborators (1).

5. *Peritoneal dialysis with hypertonic glucose solutions* (2).

6. *Selective depression or elimination of the sense of thirst.* Hypernatremia characterizes a special group of patients in whom the sense of thirst

has been selectively depressed or eliminated. In all these cases, neurons of the thirst center in the hypothalamus have presumably been damaged or destroyed. The most common cause is a cerebral tumor, such as a glioma, a craniopharyngioma, a pinealoma, or a metastatic tumor (3), but a similar syndrome has been reported in poliomyelitis of the bulbar type and in meningitis. In some patients, like the microcephalic and mentally retarded boy with hypernatremia described by Segar (4), a specific neurologic diagnosis is difficult to define; in others (those with "essential hypernatremia"), no lesion in the central nervous system is demonstrable (5, 6). Destruction of the thirst center seems the more plausible explanation for chronic hypernatremia, but "resetting" of the osmoreceptors has been suggested as a possibility. In the case reported by Segar (4) the threshold for water diuresis appeared elevated, from a serum [Na$^+$] of 140 to 150 meq/L, thus providing evidence for "resetting" of the osmoreceptors governing the release of antidiuretic hormone.

The most important symptoms and signs associated with hypernatremia are referable to the *nervous system*; indeed, it is sometimes difficult to decide whether neurologic signs are a result of the hypertonicity or of the primary disease (8, 9). The degree of neurologic disturbance is roughly related to the rate at which hypernatremia has appeared. One reason for this is apparent when one considers the pathology of the brain in experimental hypertonicity in animals. If severe hypernatremia is rapidly induced in kittens by the injection of hypertonic saline solution, the sudden shrinkage of the brain tears dural blood vessels, producing cerebral hemorrhages and subdural hematomas (10). When hypertonicity is produced more gradually, however, cerebral hemorrhages are not seen, and functional changes are less pronounced. Thus, an occasional patient has been reported whose consciousness appeared unimpaired with the serum sodium level as high as 170 to 180 meq/L. There is some evidence that the intracellular solute content of brain tissue increases in chronic hypernatremia so that cellular volume can be better preserved (8, 11).

The earliest effect of hypernatremia is depression of the central nervous system, producing lethargy that progresses to coma. In children signs of irritability are usual, and a high-pitched cry is heard (12), similar to that characteristic of meningitis. The reflexes are sometimes hyperactive but are usually normal. Muscle rigidity and tremor may occur and myoclonus may be seen. Hyperreflexia and spasticity may be present; in such cases cerebral bleeding may contribute to the picture. Transient generalized chorea has been reported (13), and epileptiform seizures may occur. Paradoxically, these are sometimes exaggerated when the level of serum sodium is rapidly brought down to normal by the administration of water (14). Convulsions are probably best explained by focal hemorrhages in the brain, but they may also find an analogy in the fact that when concentrated solutions of sodium salts are injected locally over the cortex of the brain, seizure activity is evoked (15). Such activity, interestingly enough, is not elicited by hypertonic solutions of mannitol.

Cerebrospinal fluid protein is often increased (without pleocytosis) to a higher level than might be expected on the basis of dehydration alone, and the electroencephalogram may be abnormal. Abnormalities due specifically to hypernatremia are often difficult to define because of the frequent clinical association of other cerebral lesions. In rabbits in which hypernatremia has been induced experimentally, the electroencephalogram shows a generalized reduction in voltage, disappearance of fast activity, and 4 to 5 bursts of spindlelike activity per second, progressing to high-voltage waves at a frequency of 1 to 3 per second (16). Electroencephalograms (EEGs) obtained on hypernatremic patients are usually either normal or they show minor slowing of background frequencies. However, some patients have generalized slow-wave activity and about 7 percent demonstrate characteristic epileptic activity. In most cases, these EEG changes are no longer present 4 to 6 weeks after successful therapy.

Permanent brain damage may result from severe hypernatremia, especially in children. Spasticity, seizures, and retardation of growth and mental development have all been recorded. Persistent neurologic abnormalities were present in one-third of 32 children examined 1 to 5 years after an episode of hypernatremia associated with dehydration 17). It seems likely that these are the late effects of subdural effusions, subarachnoid hemorrhages, and intracerebral bleeding.

The symptom of muscular weakness is usually overshadowed by disorientation and coma, but sometimes it may dominate the clinical picture (6, 7). In one patient with an optic glioma which had produced diabetes insipidus as well as loss of thirst, quadriceps weakness was found to be the most disabling symptom as well as the most reliable predictor of his hypernatremia. The patient was unable to mount the stairs when his serum sodium was 170 meq/L but promptly gained strength to climb normally when water was administered so as to reduce serum sodium to normal levels. In another patient, rhabdomyolysis with myoglobinuria was attributed to hypernatremia (18).

While hypernatremia per se does not appear to damage renal function, the loss of body water that usually accompanies it is usually reflected in moderate *prerenal azotemia*. In order for the serum sodium to increase from 140 to 170 meq/L, more than 20 percent of the body water must be lost. Under these circumstances the blood pressure is often depressed and glomerular filtration rate decreases. The blood urea nitrogen may increase to three or four times normal. The reduction in glomerular filtration rate consequent to dehydration may enable the patient to concentrate the urine up to or slightly beyond the osmolarity of plasma, so that an underlying state of diabetes insipidus may not be appreciated.

A low-grade *fever* occasionally accompanies hypernatremia, disappearing when proper hydration returns the serum sodium to normal.

The *cardiovascular effects* of hypernatremia are largely related to the decrease in blood volume secondary to dehydration. The electrocardiogram is usually unchanged, though infusions of hypertonic sodium chloride tend to correct certain electrocardiographic abnormalities seen in hyperkalemia (19) and quinidine intoxication (20). Hypernatremia does not appear to affect cardiac performance in the intact dog (21).

Hypocalcemia was reported by Finberg and Harrison in hypernatremic infants accidentally poisoned with sodium chloride (12). It is not clear what the mechanism of the fall in serum calcium level was. Hypocalcemia has not been a constant feature of other patients with an elevated serum sodium level.

HYPONATREMIA

The subjective manifestations of sodium chloride deficiency in humans have never been more vividly described than by R. A. McCance, who in 1936 produced sodium deficiency in himself and other normal volunteers by a salt-free diet combined with sweating and ad libitum water intake (22). The low-sodium regimen lasted for 11 days. During this time serum sodium decreased from 147 to 131 meq/L and serum chloride from 100 to 83 meq/L. Blood urea nitrogen increased from 15 to 42 mg/dL. The net negative balance of sodium was about 800 meq, and weight loss averaged 2 to 3 kg. Their experience is quoted below:

The sense of flavor and taste was affected. E. interpreted this aberration or lack of sensation as thirst. She complained of it constantly and drank freely but without obtaining any relief . . . R. A. M. recognized the feeling as distinct from thirst. His mouth was not unduly dry but food was tasteless, even highly flavored food, and this was the more noticeable because such foods were eagerly sought to make the meals more appetizing. The distaste however was not confined to meals and was a feature of every waking hour. "Even cigarettes don't taste." . . . On the whole all slept well but R. A. M. and R. B. N. were apt to be roused by attacks of nocturnal diuresis and both were troubled by nightmares. R. A. M. was "never hungry." . . . Nausea accompanied almost every meal . . . R. A. M. suffered considerable abdominal discomfort. . . .

Both the male subjects suffered considerably from cramps . . . not of the very localized type which are said to affect stokers and miners but were widespread, frequent, not very painful, and generally controllable. Any muscle in the body was liable to go into spasmodic contraction, especially if some little effort was demanded of it. . . . Perhaps the most characteristic of all were the manual cramps. R. A. M. experienced "constant mild cramps of the fingers and thumb when using forceps at the balance." . . .

A mild breathlessness at first and sense of fatigue gave place later to general exhaustion and distress on the least exertion. R. A. M. found that going up two flights of stairs to the laboratory was a serious undertaking causing a sense of breathlessness and the most unpleasant feeling of constriction across the sternum which compelled him to stop and rest. Throughout the experiment he used to go for a measured walk for about a mile after breakfast. Toward the end of the deficient period the breathlessness and sense of constriction forced him to sit down and rest two or three times at a hill for which he would ordinarily not have slackened pace. Little acts of the daily routine produced a localized sense of fatigue; his "arm got tired shaving" and finally his "jaw got tired eating."

Mentally R. A. M. felt normal but R. B. N. felt "slow in the head" and showed it in his behavior. For several days he experienced at frequent intervals sensations of "déjà vu." He became apathetic and his mental processes appeared to be dulled....

In both subjects the resting pulse rate remained normal but the volume became very small. Both subjects had normal blood pressure and maintained them within narrow limits throughout the experiment....

Recovery was quite dramatic. R. A. M. found his sense of flavor returned before he had finished his first salt meal. In a few hours he was much more comfortable in mounting the stairs and by evening was "no longer aware of his legs as he moved about the room." R. B. N. ate his first meal containing salt in the evening . . . after 48 hours he "jumped off the bus while it was going and ran up the stairs"—simple pleasures but keenly enough appreciated to make him record that he had "had a grand day."

CARDIOVASCULAR AND RENAL EFFECTS

The hemodynamic changes and the deterioration of renal function caused by sodium depletion are largely explained by the effects of a concomitant depletion of plasma volume on the cardiovascular system. It is doubtful whether sodium depletion can itself produce marked circulatory effects if it is not accompanied by a reduced plasma volume. In the syndrome of inappropriate secretion of antidiuretic hormone, in which plasma volume is usually normal or increased despite hyponatremia, there is no hypotension and no reduction in glomerular filtration rate. On the other hand, there is evidence that in the presence of a contracted plasma volume the sodium concentration per se may influence the severity of the circulatory changes (23, 24). Such an influence might be exerted through effects of the sodium ion on the tone of vascular smooth muscle and its responsiveness to pressor substances (25).

In the range of serum sodium commonly encountered, down to 100 meq/L, hyponatremia does not appear to affect the electrocardiogram in any consistent way. In hyponatremia due to sodium depletion, there is usually a reduced cardiac output and a tendency toward arterial hypotension (26). Coronary flow, left ventricular work, and cardiac output are all reduced. Pulse rate may be normal at rest but may rise sharply with slight exertion. There is a tendency to fainting because of postural hypotension. Vasoconstriction in the renal vascular bed leads to reduction in the renal plasma flow and glomerular filtration rate (27). In experimental animals, sodium restriction leads to a preferential restriction of blood flow through cortical nephrons (28). Urea clearance tends to be reduced proportionately more than filtration rate because of the low urine flow and the increased fractional resorption of glomerular filtrate in the proximal tubule; hence the blood urea nitrogen tends to rise rather rapidly. It is unusual to see increases of blood urea nitrogen greater than 100 mg/dL, however, unless the depletion has been severe enough to produce vascular collapse and anuria with tubular necrosis (29).

In the typical patient with moderately severe salt depletion, urine volume is scanty, and the osmolar concentration of urine is equal to or greater than that of plasma. There is sometimes slight proteinuria, and the urinary sediment may contain numerous hyaline and granular casts. The normal diurnal variation in urine volume is reversed: renal blood flow, GFR, water and solute excretion decrease during the day and increase at night, so that nocturia may be present even though the total daily urine volume is low. Because of the circulatory impairment induced by depletion of extracellular and plasma volume, water diuresis is impaired in spite of the fact that body fluids are hypotonic. Water without salt given to a salt-depleted patient may, therefore, merely accentuate the hyponatremia, as in the following illustrative case:

A 48-year-old man underwent bilateral lumbodorsal sympathectomy for malignant hypertensive cardiovascular disease. Before the operation his blood urea nitrogen was 20 mg/dL, and repeated urinalysis revealed only a trace of albumin. Serum sodium was normal.

After the operation he vomited on several occasions and was unable to take nourishment by mouth. There was profuse sweating from the upper half of the body associated with a low-grade fever. Several liters of glucose and water were administered each day. Urine output was always greater than 1 L/day. It was noted that the blood urea nitrogen was increasing steadily. On the eighth postoperative day he was confused and somnolent. There were no signs of dehydration. The blood pressure was 140/80, the blood urea nitrogen 63 mg/dL, the serum sodium 119 meq/L, chloride 80 meq/L, bicarbonate 32 meq/L, and potassium 3.7 meq/L.

In the course of the next 2 days 50 g (862 meq) sodium chloride was given intravenously in a total volume of 2 L. The patient's condition rapidly improved thereafter despite the transient appearance of dyspnea, tachycardia, and pulmonary rales. Blood pressure rose, urinary output increased, and the mental confusion cleared. The blood urea began a steady decline. Six days later the blood urea nitrogen was 25 mg/dL, serum sodium was 142 meq/L, chloride, 101 meq/L, and bicarbonate, 32 meq/L. Signs and symptoms of congestive heart failure had disappeared, and the blood pressure was stabilized at moderately high levels.

GASTROINTESTINAL SYMPTOMS

Loss of appetite, nausea, and vomiting frequently accompany hyponatremia. A low serum sodium level should therefore be immediately suspected when, for example, anorexia follows administration of a diuretic or nausea appears in a patient with impaired renal function who has been instructed to go on a low-salt diet. Abdominal cramps may occur. Nausea, vomiting, and abdominal pains often combine to limit the further ingestion of water, as was the case when Jaenicke and Waterhouse tried to produce hyponatremia by excessive water intake combined with injections of long-acting vasopressin in human subjects (30). Gastric emptying time is said to remain normal despite moderately severe sodium depletion, which may produce paralytic ileus of the rest of the bowel (31). Diarrhea is not a usual symptom of hyponatremia or sodium depletion, although it is occasionally seen in acute instances of severe water intoxication. When diarrhea is present with hyponatremia, therefore, it is likely to be a cause rather than a result. The peculiar thirst described

in many instances of salt depletion is probably due to contraction of body fluids, since it is not seen in most cases of inappropriate secretion of antidiuretic hormone, where serum sodium is low but body water increased. Intense salivation is a rare accompaniment of massive water intoxication.

NEUROMUSCULAR AND CENTRAL NERVOUS SYSTEM SIGNS

Neurologic symptomatology in acute hyponatremia is related to rapid swelling of the brain owing to overhydration of cells. Swelling of brain cells is mitigated in chronic hyponatremia by loss of intracellular sodium and potassium, but this may have secondary effects on brain function that are not yet clear (32). The symptoms are correlated with the level of serum sodium and the rapidity of its fall rather than with the presence or absence of contraction of the plasma volume. They therefore appear with equal frequency in hyponatremia due to sodium depletion and hyponatremia due primarily to dilution of body fluids with water. A rapid fall of serum sodium level to, say, 128 to 130 meq/L may be associated with distinct and disturbing neurologic signs, as in the experiments of McCance quoted above. On the other hand, when hyponatremia has developed slowly, the serum sodium may decrease to as little as 110 meq/L before neurologic symptoms are obvious.

Light-headedness and headaches may be prominent. The cerebrospinal fluid pressure is often elevated, and papilledema may be seen (33). Nevertheless, the cerebrospinal fluid protein is usually normal. Chronic headache may be the only manifestation of persistent hyponatremia.

Weakness, lethargy, restlessness, confusion, and delirium usually mark the progressive deterioration of cerebral function as hyponatremia develops and worsens. The ability to perform simple tasks like mental arithmetic is impaired. The patient may be unable to recognize his physician or his relatives even though he is able to carry on a conversation.

Psychosis may be the result and dominant feature of hyponatremia, but it can also be the cause. Inappropriate secretion of antidiuretic hormone can be induced by psychosis and by certain psychotropic drugs; excessive drinking may be psychogenic, caused by a dry mouth from tricyclic antidepressants. Hence, hyponatremia may also exacerbate a preexisting psychosis.

Muscular twitches and tremors may be particularly troublesome in certain cases of hyponatremia (34). These need not be accompanied by muscle cramps that sometimes mimic the jacitations of uremia. "Miners' cramps" are classical symptoms of acute hyponatremia, and the muscle cramps following hemodialysis can often be relieved by raising the serum sodium.

Hyponatremia predisposes to convulsions. The seizures are occasionally heralded by muscular twitches but more often appear explosively *de novo* as the first warning of a low serum sodium level. They may be generalized or focal. The electroencephalogram usually shows diffuse abnormalities, including an irregular slow pattern (35), low-frequency activity, and increased excitability (36), but it is sometimes normal (37).

Because hyponatremia may complicate diseases of the central nervous system, it is important to remember that symptoms and signs referable to the low serum sodium level alone include a wide variety of focal as well as diffuse manifestations. For example, aphasia (38), hyporeflexia (38), hyperreflexia (34), generalized rigidity (39), ataxia (40), and staggering (41) may all occur. Focal signs suggesting a localized lesion, including hemiparesis (42), focal weakness, and unilateral Babinski's sign (39), have all been reported. The importance of correcting hyponatremia before making a final judgment about the nature and extent of neurologic deficits is obvious.

Permanent brain damage may ensue if severe symptomatic hyponatremia is left untreated (32).

HYPOKALEMIA

Neuromuscular symptoms are prominent in severe hypokalemia but are not usually seen before the serum potassium has decreased to the neighborhood of 2.5 meq/L. Below this level, some degree of muscular weakness is common. The weakness follows a distinctive pattern. Muscles innervated by cranial nerves are almost never affected (43). The weakness is most prominent in the legs, especially the quadriceps muscles (44). In a case of chronic potassium depletion due to laxative addiction with a serum potassium of 1.7 meq/L, the grip was said to be remarkably good, and flexion of the elbows and dorsiflexion of the wrists surprisingly strong. The legs, however, were so weak that the patient was unable to lift them or to flex her hips (45). With profound potassium depletion the respiratory muscles become involved. The diaphragm becomes paralyzed before the intercostal and accessory muscles of respiration (46). As respiratory function is progressively impaired, "fishmouth" breathing, characterized by pursing of the lips, occurs (47). Death may be caused by respiratory failure.

Despite the prominence of muscle weakness, deep tendon reflexes are usually present. The abdominal and cremasteric reflexes are not impaired (43).

Muscle cramps and paresthesias may be extraordinarily troublesome even when weakness is not marked. Muscular pains may so dominate the clinical picture as to prompt a mistaken diagnosis of "arthritis" or "rheumatism." The muscles are often tender. In familial periodic paralysis, but not in other forms of hypokalemia, the muscles sometimes appear to swell and have a firm, rubbery consistency (48). Chronic, long-standing potassium depletion can result in muscle atrophy (49, 50). Presumably this reflects pathologic changes of the same kind that are seen in the skeletal muscles of experimental animals—patchy or diffuse necrosis, with a variable degree of regeneration (51).

The signs of latent tetany (Chvostek's and Trousseau's signs) can be elicited in certain patients with severe potassium depletion. The tetany is not due to concomitant deficiencies of magnesium and calcium, since serum levels of these ions may be normal (52). Interestingly, signs of tetany often become more prominent during the first 24 to 48 h after potassium repletion has begun (53). When serum calcium is low, potassium replacement may "uncover" tetany, a reflection of the antagonistic effects on neuromuscular excitability of potassium and calcium (54).

RESTING CONDITIONS	NORMAL	K DEFICIENCY		K INTOXICATION	
		ACUTE	CHRONIC	ACUTE	CHRONIC
$\dfrac{[K]_i}{[K]_e}$	$\dfrac{160}{4.5}$	$\dfrac{140}{2.0}$	$\dfrac{90}{2.0}$	$\dfrac{160}{12.5}$	$\dfrac{170}{8}$
	35	70	45	13	21
K equil. pot. E_k $= -61.5 \log \dfrac{[K]_i}{[K]_e}$	−95 mV	−113 mV	−102 mV	−68 mV	−82 mV
Membrane pot., E_m $= -61.5 \log \dfrac{[K]_i + 0.01[Na]_i}{[K]_e + 0.01[Na]_e}$	−88 mV	−100 mV	−88 mV	−65 mV	−77 mV
Excitability $= E_m - E_t$	$\dfrac{88 - 65}{23 \text{ mV}}$	$\dfrac{100 - 65}{35 \text{ mV}}$	$\dfrac{88 - 65}{23 \text{ mV}}$	$\dfrac{65 - 65}{0}$	$\dfrac{77 - 65}{12}$
Electrochemical excitation	Normal	Hyper-polarization block: paralysis	Normal	Depolarization block: paralysis	Partial depolarization: hyperexcitability

Figure 11-1. Neuromuscular excitability as a function of intracellular and extracellular concentrations of potassium. The values given for $[K]_i$ and $[K]_e$ under various circumstances are illustrative only and do not represent actual data. (*From Seldin, Carter, and Rector*)

Potassium depletion exerts its effects on muscle and nerve through at least two mechanisms. The first is through changes in the resting membrane potential. Since this is proportional to the logarithm of the ratio of the external potassium concentration to the internal potassium concentration, small changes in the concentration of potassium in extracellular fluid will obviously be more important than small changes in the already high concentration of potassium inside of cells (see Fig. 11-1). Secondly, changes in the intracellular concentration of potassium probably influence cellular function by altering the operation of intracellular enzymes. Small decreases in intracellular potassium greatly affect the rate of synthesis of macromolecules, including protein, ribonucleic acid (RNA), and deoxyribonucleic acid (DNA) (55).

Changes in cerebral function in potassium-deficient patients include lethargy, apathy, drowsiness, confusion, and irritability (56). Coma, delirium, and hallucinations are rarer. Potassium depletion may occasionally present as an acute brain syndrome with memory impairment, disorientation, and confusion (57). It is interesting that cerebral symptoms are not usually part of the picture of familial periodic paralysis, despite profound hypokalemia in this disease. Since potassium balance is usually normal in periodic paralysis but markedly negative in other forms of hypokalemia, it is possible that depletion in the central nervous system is partly responsible for cerebral symptoms when the serum potassium level is low; whether a potassium deficit in the brain accompanies whole body potassium depletion is uncertain, however (58, 196). It is conceivable that stupor or coma responding dramatically in certain patients to potassium replacement is

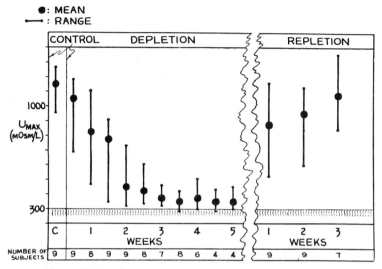

Figure 11-2. Reduction in concentration ability (U_{max}) in normal subjects maintained on a diet deficient in potassium. (*From Rubini.*)

due in part to effects of potassium upon the circulation, or, in patients with cirrhosis of the liver, on the metabolism of ammonia (see below).

The electroencephalogram is usually unaffected by hypokalemia, but rarely an abnormal electroencephalogram has been observed to be associated with potassium depletion, with restoration to normal following the administration of potassium (59).

RENAL FUNCTION

The most important abnormality of renal function is an inability to concentrate the urine (60). When potassium is restricted in the diet of normal young individuals, significant hyposthenuria is apparent as early as the fourth day in occasional subjects and is present in all by the second week (61). Impairment of concentrating ability is usually slight until approximately 200 meq potassium has been lost (Figs. 11-2 and 11-3). By the time 400 to 600 meq has been lost, it is difficult for the kidneys to concentrate urine above the osmolality of plasma. Nocturia, polyuria, and polydipsia are consequently among the most common symptoms of potassium deficiency. The mecha-

nism of the reduction in concentrating ability involves a decrease in the transport and trapping of sodium in the interstitium of the medulla (63); the ability of the kidneys to dilute the urine, however, is well maintained. Resistance to antidiuretic hormone (ADH) may be induced by an in-

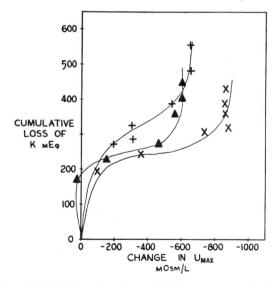

Figure 11-3. Relation of cumulative K deficit to concentrating ability in human subjects. (*From Rubini.*)

crease in prostaglandin produced by cells of the renal papilla (64).

In certain patients, thirst appears to be present out of proportion to the water loss, and it has been proposed that in such patients the hypothalamic centers for thirst are affected (62); perhaps, however, they are responding to the circulatory instability induced by a deficit of potassium.

Potassium deficiency also reduces the ability of the kidneys to excrete an acid load and to establish maximal concentration gradients of hydrogen ion between urine and plasma (65) (see Chap. 4). It is therefore unusual for a potassium-depleted patient to excrete urine with a pH lower than 5.5.

Prolonged potassium depletion produces some fall in glomerular filtration rate, reflected in a reduction in creatinine clearance and an increase in serum creatinine and blood urea nitrogen. Severe impairment of concentrating ability may exist, however, with a normal glomerular filtration rate. The lowering of filtration rate and the diminished renal blood flow are probably caused by swelling, vacuolation, necrosis, and subsequent scarring of cells lining the renal tubules (66). In rats with potassium deficiency the collecting ducts seem most heavily involved (66), whereas in humans with severe potassium depletion the proximal tubules are the site of intense water-clear vacuolation (60).

Aminoaciduria has been found in a few patients with potassium depletion but is absent in many others; hence the significance of this observation is uncertain.

The urinary sediment is usually benign. Slight proteinuria is occasionally present, but this is not common. Potassium depletion does not impair the ability of the kidneys to conserve potassium. If extrarenal losses of potassium have caused the deficit, the concentration of potassium in the urine is usually below 10 meq/L.

The muscular paralysis associated with abrupt falls in serum potassium, as seen in the familial periodic paralysis, sometimes affects the bladder. Patients in the grip of an attack of periodic paralysis are often unable to void and require catheterization.

In humans and animals, potassium deficiency is associated with an increase in the output of ammonia into the urine and in some species with an increase in the concentration of glutaminase in the kidney. At low urine flow rates, the increased ammonia may diffuse from the cells backwards into venous blood. The result in patients who are unable to clear ammonia rapidly from the circulation, e.g., with hepatic cirrhosis or portal shunting, may be an increase in blood ammonia. This may lead to rapid clinical deterioration when potassium deficiency induced by diarrhea or by a diuretic is superimposed upon an already precarious state of hepatic insufficiency (67).

CARDIOVASCULAR CHANGES

Electrocardiographic changes are noted in the majority of patients with a serum potassium of less than 3 meq/L. Virtually all changes in the electrocardiogram are rapidly reversed when the potassium deficit has been corrected (Fig. 11-4). Electrocardiographic abnormalities include (20, 68–70):

1. Depression of the ST segment.
2. Lowering, flattening, or inversion of the T wave.
3. Presence of an elevated (greater than 1 mm) U wave.
4. Prolongation of the QT interval may appear to occur because of T-wave flattening with a large U wave, the QU interval thus seeming to be the QT interval, resembling hypocalcemia.
5. Rarely, tall narrow peaked U waves may be seen in the precordial leads.
6. Increase in P-wave amplitude.
7. Prolongation of PR interval.
8. Severe hypokalemia may prolong the QRS period by 0.1 to 0.3 s, without changes in QRS configuration.

Severe hypokalemia may produce arrhythmias which can be detected at the bedside. A sinus bradycardia is sometimes seen, accentuated by increased sensitivity to vagal stimulation. Prolongation of the PR interval and dropped beats can sometimes be abolished by atropine; however, atropine does not affect the abnormal T waves

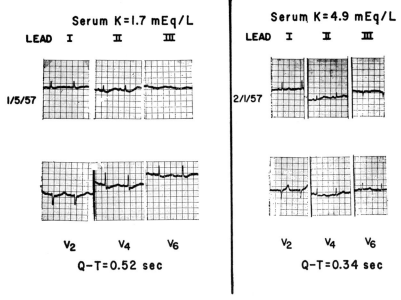

Figure 11-4. Electrocardiogram before and after correction of hypokalemia. Note prolongation of the QT interval and flattening of the T wave in all leads, which disappeared after treatment of potassium depletion.

(71). Second-degree atrioventricular (AV) block with the Wenckebach phenomenon has also been observed, presumably due also to increased vagal tone (20). Atrial arrhythmias include atrial flutter and paroxysmal atrial tachycardia with block (20, 72). Atrioventricular dissociation and even ventricular fibrillation have been observed. These arrhythmias, commonly associated with digitalis toxicity, may be observed in the absence of digitalis when severe potassium deficiency with hypokalemia is present.

Although myocardial necrosis is a constant finding in severe potassium depletion in rats, the electrocardiographic changes just enumerated probably reflect changes in serum potassium rather than in the intracellular stores of potassium in the myocardium. Electrocardiographic changes are prominent in familial periodic paralysis, where the body stores of potassium are not depleted (73). Congestive heart failure is not encountered in the vast majority of patients with potassium depletion, although scattered areas of necrosis in the myocardium have been described in

patients dying with severe potassium deficiency. An increase in cardiac size, sometimes accompanied by a systolic murmur, has been noted in certain patients with hypokalemia due to periodic paralysis or severe potassium deficiency, disappearing when potassium was given (74, 75).

Postural hypotension, by contrast, is common. The normal blood pressure overshoot in response to the Valsalva maneuver is abolished (76). Dizziness and a tendency to fainting are common symptoms (Fig. 11-5). An important consequence of this effect of potassium deficiency on blood pressure is the susceptibility of patients depleted of potassium to postoperative shock. The hypotensive effect is not due to hypokalemia alone, since hypotension is not a feature of periodic paralysis. The vascular response to catecholamines and other pressor substances is reduced in potassium deficiency possibly owing to increased production of prostaglandins (64).

The tendency to edema formation noticeable in many patients with potassium depletion is probably an expression of the cardiovascular effects of

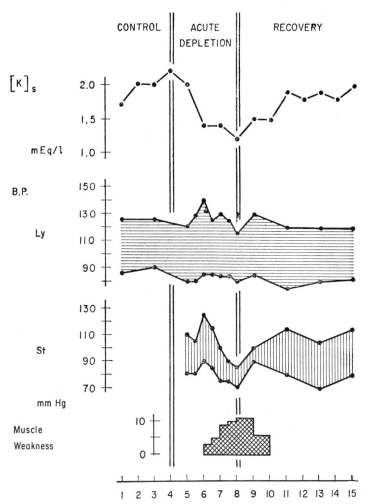

Figure 11.5 Severe postural hypotension and muscular weakness associated with acute depletion of potassium disappeared when partial repletion of potassium was accomplished. (*From E. J. Huth and R. D. Squires, Circulation,* **14**:60, 1953.)

potassium deficiency (see Chap. 5). Gross pitting edema is uncommon, but mild degrees of ankle swelling are frequently seen, and the tendency to accumulate fluid in the upright position and excrete it when supine probably contributes to the nocturia that troubles many patients.

The hyperemic response to exercise is impaired in potassium-depleted muscles. Perhaps for

this reason potassium depletion appears to predispose to rhabdomyolysis, particularly after prolonged exercise (77).

CARBOHYDRATE METABOLISM

Potassium depletion tends to impair carbohydrate tolerance, causing mildly elevated fasting blood sugar levels and glucose tolerance curves which are diabetic in type (78). The secretion of insulin by pancreatic islets is reduced (79). The mild diabetes sometimes induced by diuretics can in many instances be partly or completely reversed by providing potassium supplements.

GASTROINTESTINAL SYMPTOMS

Evaluation of abdominal symptoms is difficult when the serum potassium level is low. Loss of gastrointestinal fluids often causes hypokalemia (see Chap. 22), and since potassium depletion itself produces ileus and vomiting, a vicious circle may aggravate electrolyte deficits.

Anorexia and nausea, progressing to vomiting, are common. The motility of the bowel is decreased. Prolonged gastric emptying, failure to pass stools or gas, distention, abdominal cramps, and paralytic ileus may all be produced by potassium depletion alone. The clinical signs, including x-ray evidence of dilated bowel, are easy to confuse with those of intestinal obstruction or peritonitis. The abdominal distention is usually unresponsive to neostigmine (80), while decompression by nasal gastric suction is often ineffective and may accelerate the process of potassium depletion. Weakness of the smooth muscles of the gastrointestinal tract and impairment of the

response to parasympathetic stimulation are the basis of the symptoms. Replacement of potassium prompts immediate return of bowel sounds with frequent voluminous bowel movements and subsidence of distention (81).

HYPERKALEMIA

The effect of hyperkalemia that overshadows all others in clinical importance is its influence on the initiation and conduction of the electric impulse propagating the heartbeat. The danger of hyperkalemia is that patients will die of cardiac standstill or arrhythmia.

The effects of an elevated serum potassium level on the heart are usually unimportant below 7 meq/L but are almost always present above 8 meq/L. They are heralded by characteristic changes in the electrocardiogram, illustrated in Fig. 11-6. The initial change is the appearance of high, peaked T waves, especially pronounced in the chest leads (82). These may be differentiated from other disorders causing an increase in the amplitude of the T wave by the presence of a normal or decreased QT interval (20). As the serum potassium level rises, the PR interval becomes prolonged (83). This is followed by disappearance of the P waves, and finally decomposition and prolongation of the QRS complex (84). Complete

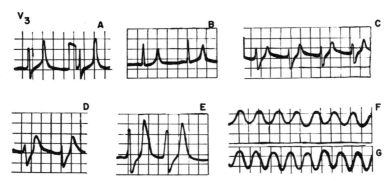

Figure 11-6. Rpresentative electrocardiograms in potassium intoxication. In general, the changes are sequential. The earliest change is the development of peaked T waves (A and B). The S wave may increase in depth and the S-T segment become depressed (C). The P wave disappears and the QRS complex lengthens (D). Ventricular flutter of tachycardia supervenes (F and G). (From J. P. Merrill, *The Treatment of Renal Failure*, Grune & Stratton, Inc., New York, 1965.)

heart block may accompany an increase in serum potassium and disappear when hyperkalemia is relieved. Occasionally an apparent elevation of the R-ST junction and a coved RS-T segment may simulate an acute injury pattern suggesting myocardial infarction or pericarditis (85). Ectopic premature or escape beats may also appear (86). At levels of serum potassium above 9 or 10 meq/L, the QRS complex becomes smooth, wide, and sinuous, joining with the T wave and resulting in a continuous sine wave appearance. This is thought to represent a form of ventricular flutter and progresses to ventricular fibrillation or standstill (87).

The electrocardiographic changes of hyperkalemia are exaggerated by a low serum sodium level and a low serum calcium level, as well as by acidosis and an elevated level of serum magnesium. They are counteracted by a high serum calcium level. Calcium infusion is therefore a useful measure in the emergency treatment of severe hyperkalemia.

Although the electrocardiographic changes of hyperkalemia are frequently helpful, they cannot be directly correlated with serum potassium levels (see Chap. 5). Figure 11-7 demonstrates the

Acute renal failure

NPN = 227 mg %
K = 5.8 mEq /L
Na = 122 mEq /L
CO_2 = 18 mEq /L
CL = 82 mEq /L

V_2 Day 7

R_x : Hypertonic NaCL
and $NaHCO_3$

NPN = 253 mg %
K = 6.8 mEq /L
Na = 133 mEq /L
CO_2 = 19 mEq /L
CL = 87 mEq /L

V_2 Day 9

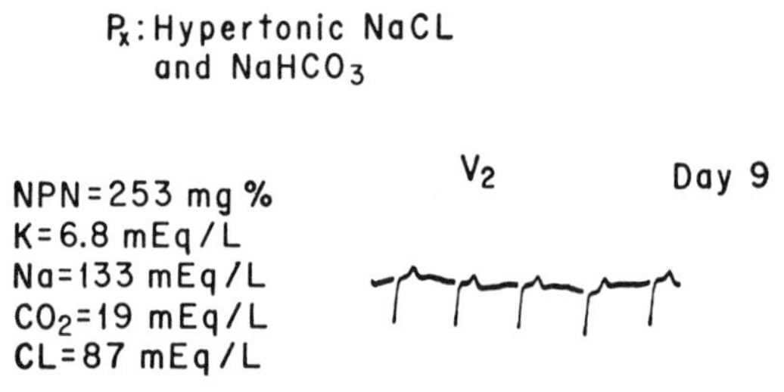

Figure 11-7. In this patient with acute renal failure, peaked T waves in leads V_2 and V_3 on the seventh day became normal on the ninth day, despite a rise in serum potassium. "Normalization" of the electrocardiogram was associated with a rise of 11 meq/L in serum sodium.

regression of the electrocardiographic signs of hyperkalemia (peaked T waves) in a patient with renal failure, despite a rise in the level of serum potassium. The improvement shown in the electrocardiogram occurred in conjunction with treatment of acidosis and hyponatremia.

Although cardiac performance may be altered because of arrhythmias and conduction changes, hyperkalemia per se does not appear to interfere with cardiac contractility. Goodyer et al. found that in intact dogs an increase in serum potassium to the range of 8.4 to 11.5 meq/L had no significant effect upon ventricular contractile strength, even in the presence of marked electrocardiographic abnormalities (21).

NEUROMUSCULAR SIGNS

A Landry type of rapidly ascending muscular weakness that leads to flaccid quadriplegia but tends to preserve cerebration and cranial nerve function is occasionally observed with the very high serum potassium levels that sometimes accompany either renal insufficiency or Addison's disease (88). In such patients, the serum potassium is greater than 7 and usually greater than 8.5 meq/L. The cerebrospinal fluid is normal. The muscle weakness may be associated with tremor. Paresthesias are sometimes present (89). Vibratory and position sense as well as cutaneous sensory perception may be diminished or absent; usually, however, no objective sensory abnormalities are noted. The deep tendon reflexes may be elicited early, when weakness is present but before paralysis has occurred. Respiratory paralysis and involvement of the muscles of phonation have been described.

In the rare inherited condition of hyperkalemic periodic paralysis (90), stiffness and weakness occur most often after exercise and during sleep. The spontaneously occurring episodes of weakness can be provoked by potassium loads taken orally. The serum potassium level in such patients is normal or only slightly elevated during an attack, and the condition appears to be due to some special susceptibility to levels of serum potassium that are borne with equanimity by normal people.

The mechanism of the effects of both hyperkalemia and hypokalemia on neuromuscular excitability can best be understood by reference to Fig. 11-1 (91). The excitability of neuromuscular tissue is defined as the difference between the membrane potential E_M and the threshold potential E_T. Alterations in potassium change membrane excitability only through changes in the resting membrane potential E_M and do not alter the threshold potential E_T. During excitation the discharge of acetylcholine at neural junctions and motor end plates depolarizes the membrane and decreases E_M toward threshold. When E_M reaches about -65 mV (the threshold potential), the tissue is activated. Therefore, any factor which increases E_M or decreases E_T will render the tissue less excitable, while factors which decrease E_M or increase E_T will enhance excitability. Severe acute hyperkalemia brings E_M close to the level of E_T and thereby induces a depolarization block with paralysis and also slows ventricular conduction.

HYPERCALCEMIA

NEUROLOGIC AND PSYCHIATRIC SIGNS AND SYMPTOMS

The records of patients with hyperparathyroidism or vitamin D intoxication leave a forcible impression of the large number and variety of psychiatric disturbances. In general, the symptoms are proportional to the degree of elevation of the serum calcium level. Certain patients, however, become profoundly disturbed when the serum calcium is only 12 mg/dL while others behave perfectly normally with a serum calcium of 16 mg/dL.

Tiredness, listlessness, lethargy, apathy, and depression are frequently observed. Other patients are agitated and nervous, and complain of insomnia. Decreased memory, poor calculation, and decreased attention span are common defects. As hypercalcemia becomes more severe, delirium, confusion, somnolence, and even coma may occur. Neurotic behavior, slow mentation, psychomotor retardation, agitated depression, hallucinations, and paranoia have all been documented in hypercalcemia and shown to be re-

versible when the hypercalcemia was controlled (92–95).

Headache occurs frequently; it was reported, for example, in one-fifth of a large series of patients with hyperparathyroidism (93). The headache may be particularly severe in hypercalcemic crisis, where it is exacerbated by the vomiting and dehydration that regularly accompany this disorder. Hypercalcemia alone may cause an increase in cerebrospinal fluid protein (96). Thus, when hypercalcemia complicates cancer, the combination of disturbed consciousness, headache, and increased cerebrospinal fluid protein may wrongly suggest a cerebral metastasis, when in fact the symptoms are due to hypercalcemia and are reversible.

Convulsions sometimes occur in hypercalcemia, but they are rare. Focal seizures have been ascribed to thrombosis in small blood vessels within the brain (97). Acute hypercalcemia is attended by a generalized tendency to thrombosis, due in part to rapid dehydration (98).

Easy fatigability and muscular weakness are common, especially in hyperparathyroidism, and less often in other hypercalcemic states (99). The patient complains of aches, pains, and heaviness in the legs and of difficulty in climbing stairs and getting out of a chair or a bathtub. Muscle aches are so prominent in a few patients as to raise the suspicion of periarteritis nodosa. The proximal muscles of the legs are most often involved, though in severe cases the deltoid and biceps are also affected. Upper extremity weakness does not occur without involvement of the lower extremities. Weakness in hyperparathyroid patients is not clearly related to the level of serum calcium or phosphorus. The level of muscle enzymes in serum is usually normal. Muscle biopsy shows moderate atrophy affecting few or many muscle fibers, but no inflammatory cells and none of the hallmarks of ordinary myopathy such as necrotic, phagocytosed, or regenerating muscle.

Hyperreflexia is often pronounced, and in some cases Babinski's sign is present. Abnormal tongue movements resembling fasciculations may also be seen. The clinical picture thus sometimes recalls amyotrophic lateral sclerosis, though it is reversible with control of hypercalcemia. Muscle tone is decreased, sometimes strikingly so in relation to the hyperreflexia; occasional patients are said to have hyperflexible limbs (100). The conduction time in motor nerves is normal and the electromyogram is often abnormal but not diagnostic. Mild sensory impairment is sometimes present.

GASTROINTESTINAL MANIFESTATIONS

Loss of appetite, nausea, and vomiting usually accompany hypercalcemia. Anorexia and loss of weight, for example, are early signals of overdosage with vitamin D in the treatment of hypoparathyroidism. Abdominal pain may be so severe that patients are admitted to the hospital as abdominal emergencies to undergo laparotomy (101). Severe hypercalcemic crisis may be complicated by abdominal distention and ileus. With more moderate hypercalcemia, constipation is commonly noted; it occurred in 7 of 35 patients with vitamin D poisoning reported by Anning and his coworkers (102) and probably results from a reduction in tone of the smooth muscle of the bowel and from dehydration. Loose stools and diarrhea are unusual. Increased salivation and difficulty in swallowing are occasionally encountered.

There appears to be an association between hyperparathyroidism and pancreatitis, although pancreatitis is rarely associated with hypercalcemia from other causes (103). Hemorrhagic pancreatitis is found postmortem in one-third of patients dying from acute hyperparathyroid crisis (104).

Hypercalcemia increases the secretion of acid and pepsin by the stomach (105), probably by stimulating the secretion of gastrin. It is therefore not surprising that symptoms similar to those of peptic ulcer occur in a sizable minority of all patients with chronic elevation of the serum calcium level. The incidence of peptic ulcers in hyperparathyroidism varies from 8 to 25 percent (106). Conversely, 1.3 percent of 300 patients with peptic ulcer were shown to have a parathyroid adenoma (107).

CARDIOVASCULAR SYSTEM

Acute hypercalcemia induced, for example, by the infusion of calcium salts in the usual Howard test results in a systolic blood pressure rise of at least 30 mmHg in about half of the patients (108). A local action of calcium on peripheral blood vessels to increase vascular resistance is probably partly responsible (109); more important may be the effect of calcium to promote the release of catecholamines (110). Hypercalcemic crisis is therefore sometimes associated with hypertension that disappears when the serum calcium returns to normal (111). Hypertension is present in one-third to one-half of all patients with chronic hypercalcemia of any cause, but in most cases it is caused by renal scarring secondary to hypercalcemic nephropathy, and it persists when the hypercalcemia is cured (112).

The most notable electrocardiographic change is shortening of the QT interval (113). The distance from the Q wave to the origin of the T wave is said to be inversely proportional to the level of serum calcium up to levels as high as 20 mg/dL (20, 114). The PR interval is sometimes prolonged. A variety of arrhythmias may complicate hypercalcemia, especially when the serum calcium level rises abruptly (115, 116).

The positive inotropic effect of digitalis is enhanced by calcium, but more important, digitalis toxicity is aggravated by hypercalcemia (117). It may be necessary to give calcium intravenously to certain patients who are already digitalized, as in renal insufficiency, but great care should be taken to avoid a rise in the serum calcium level above 10 mg/dL.

OCULAR MANIFESTATIONS (REF. 118)

A diagnosis of chronic hypercalcemia can sometimes be made at the bedside from the characteristic corneal and conjunctival deposits of calcium. Small, glasslike, crystal-clear particles are seen within the ocular conjunctiva in the region of the palpebral fissure. In the cornea there are hazy, grayish or whitish granular opacities in the form of a crescent running concentrically with the limbus on the nasal or temporal side or both, densest at the periphery, and fading out centrally (119). These resemble band keratitis ordinarily seen in association with intraocular inflammation. They are superficially similar to arcus senilis, except that the latter is most prominent at the superior and inferior borders of the cornea whereas corneal calcification is most marked at the lateral and medial margins (Fig. 11-8). The opacities can be seen with the naked eye and with a strongly positive lens correction on the ophthalmoscope but are most easily delineated by slit lamp examination. They represent precipitates of calcium phosphate salts. Precipitation occurs at the surface of the eye because the P_{CO_2} here is low and the pH alkaline. The conjunctival deposits sometimes produce intense irritation with redness and watering of the eyes. The lesions have been detected within only 2 weeks after vitamin D was given in toxic doses. They disappear extremely slowly (often over several years) after the hypercalcemia has been controlled. A similar lesion may frequently be seen in severe secondary hyperparathyroidism, where the product of the calcium and phosphorus concentrations is markedly elevated but the serum calcium is normal.

ITCHING

This is an annoying problem in a few patients with chronic hypercalcemia. It may be related in some cases to calcium deposits in the epidermis,

but it disappears so rapidly when the serum calcium is controlled that it seems more likely to be related to the hypercalcemia itself (120).

CALCIUM NEPHROPATHY

Perhaps the most dramatic clinical example of the deleterious effect of hypercalcemia on the kidneys is hyperparathyroid crisis, where serum calcium concentrations as high as 18 or 20 mg/dL may be associated with initial polyuria, followed by dehydration, oliguria, and rapidly advancing azotemia (92, 102, 121). In contrast, prolonged hypercalcemia and/or hypercalcinuria, associated with vitamin D intoxication, extensive paralysis, sarcoidosis, excessive ingestion of calcium and alkali, hyperthyroidism, or hyperparathyroidism, may result in diffuse nephrocalcinosis and present as renal insufficiency insidious in onset and only slowly progressive. In such cases, severe impairment in renal function need not be associated with stones or even with radiologic evidence of calcification in the kidneys.

Of 45 patients with hyperparathyroidism reported by Hellstrom (112), 37 had renal impairment as evidenced by an elevated blood nonpro-

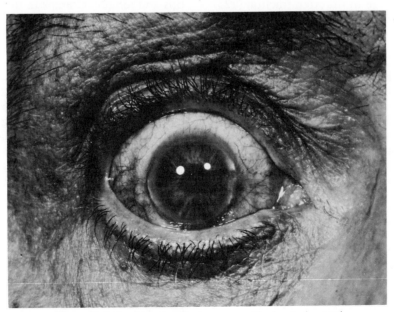

Figure 11-8. Band keratopathy in a man with chronic hypercalcemia and the milk-alkali syndrome.

tein nitrogen level or diminished ability to concentrate the urine. Polyuria and polydipsia may be so striking in hypercalcemic patients that diabetes insipidus is suspected (100, 122). These symptoms are often out of proportion to the degree of azotemia. In fact azotemia need not be present at all. Frequently, the magnitude of the polyuria and polydipsia cannot be explained by the severity of the hypercalcemic-induced concentrating defect. This suggests that at times there may be an associated primary disturbance of thirst (62). However, it is clear that hypercalcemia can cause a form of acquired nephrogenic diabetes insipidus in which the urine is persistently hypotonic to the plasma, despite water restriction or administration of ADH. Impairment of maximum urinary concentration is usually an early sign of calcium nephropathy. Certain hypercalcemic patients seem to retain the ability to concentrate urine normally; this is especially likely to be the case, in our experience, when the serum calcium level is below 13 mg/dL, although an elevated serum calcium level is not a prerequisite for the concentrating defect.

In more severe cases, there is usually a depression in glomerular filtration rate and renal plasma flow, without a change in filtration fraction (123). The urinary sediment may contain red blood cells, as well as leukocytes and white blood cell casts, even when urine cultures are repeatedly sterile. Calcium phosphate casts are sometimes seen. In many patients, however, the urine is remarkably free of abnormal formed elements. Unless congestive heart failure is present, proteinuria is slight. Moderate anemia, normocytic and normochromic in type, often appears in association with renal impairment.

The ability of the kidneys to secrete an acid urine and to manufacture ammonium in response to acidifying salts was noted to be diminished in some hypercalcemic patients by Wrong and Davies (124). With the appearance of azotemia, the ability to conserve sodium may be impaired. However, this is not a prominent accompaniment of mild calcium nephropathy.

Extensive deposition of calcium in the renal substance with subsequent scarring results in persistent hypertension. Even if hypercalcemia is cured, such patients may eventually die from the effects of progressive vascular disease, although renal insufficiency may remit temporarily when the serum calcium is returned to normal.

HYPOCALCEMIA

TETANY

Tetany, the cardinal manifestation of hypocalcemia, is the expression of excessive irritability of the motor nervous system. Hypocalcemia increases the threshold potential (E_T), thus decreasing the difference between E_T and the resting membrane potential (E_M) (125). In its mildest forms tetany can be detected only by determination of the electric reactions of muscles or by the presence of certain abnormal reflexes. In overt cases active spasms, varying from typical contractions of the extremities to generalized convulsions, are observed.

The earliest symptoms of hypocalcemia are frequently not motor, but sensory. Numbness of the fingers is often the first complaint. Tingling and burning are felt in the extremities and about the lips and tongue. Cramps in the muscles of the extremities may be felt before tetanic spasm is actually seen. This parallels the sequence seen in the development of the Trousseau phenomenon, in which the regular order of occurrence is tactile paresthesias, fasciculation, sensation of the spasm, and finally the spasm itself (126). In typical carpal spasm (accoucheur's sign) the fingers are flexed at the metacarpophalangeal joints and forcibly extended at the interphalangeal joints. The thumb is extended midway between opposition and adduction, tightly pressing against the other fingers. In severe cases, the lower extremities become involved with the thigh adducted, the hip and the knee extended, and the foot and toes plantarflexed (true "carpopedal" spasm). With tetany of the facial musculature the corners of the mouth are drawn down, the nasolabial folds accentuated, the eyes widely opened, the forehead transversely wrinkled, and the mouth pursed.

When tetany is latent, the spasm can be elicited by placing a blood pressure cuff around the arm and occluding arterial flow. Spasm occurring within 5 min is considered a positive Trousseau test. Chvostek noted in 1876 that latent tetany of the facial musculature could be uncovered by tapping over the facial nerve in front of the ear. When Chvostek's sign is fully positive, this results in contraction of the muscles of the eyelid, upper lip, alae nasi, and corner of the mouth, but in less pronounced cases the corner of the mouth with or without the alae nasi are affected alone.

Laryngeal stridor frequently accompanies hypocalcemia. After neck surgery it is easily mistaken for vocal cord paralysis. Spasm of the laryngeal muscles producing hypoxia with dyspnea and cyanosis is probably the most common cause of death from severe hypocalcemia.

Because neural excitability is influenced by many factors in addition to the level of ionized calcium in extracellular fluid, the level of serum calcium at which tetany occurs is extremely variable. Children are more susceptible than adults. Intra-arterial injection of epinephrine produces a marked local increase in the intensity of tetany, and small amounts of epinephrine may produce laryngeal stridor in hypocalcemic patients (127). For this reason catecholamines should be given with the greatest caution when hypocalcemia is present.

Convulsions frequently occur without the preliminary warning of tetany. The seizures are usually generalized, but they may be focal; in analysis of 43 patients with hypocalcemic fits, 5 had some focal element (128). The predominant finding in the electroencephalogram is the presence of slow waves at a frequency of 2 to 5 per second, which may dominate the entire record or alternate with the basic normal rhythm (129).

IMPAIRMENT OF MENTAL FUNCTION

This is an underemphasized consequence of hypocalcemia. Severe intellectual and emotional changes may occur in the absence of other signs or symptoms (130). Chronic hypocalcemia in childhood may produce mental retardation as seen in certain cases of idiopathic and pseudohypoparathyroidism (126). Severe psychosis may be seen 3 or 4 months after neck surgery with postoperative hypoparathyroidism simulating idiopathic schizophrenia or manic-depressive psychosis (131, 132). Emotional lability, apprehension, and depression disappear when hypocalcemia is corrected. Any or all of these symptoms may occur in the absence of overt or latent tetany (131, 132). Interestingly, patients with postoperative hypocalcemia appear to have an increased susceptibility to the production of "visual afterimages" by complex visual stimuli (133). This may play a role in the production of hallucinations.

Profound hypocalcemia that develops suddenly, as with pancreatitis, may occasionally produce coma without tetany; the diagnosis may be suggested by the prolonged Q-T interval in the electrocardiogram (134).

CEREBROSPINAL FLUID PRESSURE

This may be elevated in chronic hypocalcemia, and papilledema may be present (135, 136), producing the clinical picture of pseudotumor cerebri. The cerebrospinal fluid protein is normal (135).

INTRACEREBRAL CALCIFICATION

This is most frequently associated with idiopathic hypoparathyroidism and pseudohypoparathyroidism, probably because both these conditions produce unrecognized chronic hypocalcemia in childhood (122). It occurs but is rarer in postoperative hypoparathyroidism (138). The mechanism of this interesting phenomenon is entirely unexplained. While it is not seen in other hypocalcemic disorders, it is not known whether this is due simply to the long duration of hypoparathyroid hypocalcemia or whether some other factor in these cases contributes to the cerebral calcification (see Chap. 26). The calcification is localized to the basal ganglia and is usually most prominent in the head of the caudate nucleus. The dentate nucleus of the cerebellum may also be calcified. The deposits of calcium are heaviest in perivascular areas. It may be pertinent that the basal ganglia seem particularly prone to calcification after nonspecific injury to the brain produced by carbon monoxide, anoxia, kernicterus, encephalitis, tuberous sclerosis, or toxoplasmosis.

In the majority of instances, calcification of the basal ganglia produces few or no symptoms, but chorea, athetosis, and parkinsonism are severe and sometimes disabling in certain cases (139). Patients with hypoparathyroidism are unusually susceptible to dystonic reactions to phenothiazine drugs even when they are normocalcemic; this may reflect subclinical changes in the function of the basal ganglia (195).

OCULAR MANIFESTATIONS

A distressing complication of chronic hypocalcemia due to hypoparathyroidism is lenticular cataract. Cataracts may grow rapidly, over a period of 2 to 3 months after parathyroidectomy, or appear very slowly, after several years. Calcium is deposited underneath the anterior and posterior capsule as discrete opacities that later extend from the periphery of the lens toward the center. As the cataracts develop, the lenses become more completely involved, and the condition becomes indistinguishable from senile cataracts (140). A less common manifestation of early lenticular involvement is sagittal flattening of the lens (141).

Keratitis and conjunctivitis producing photophobia and blepharospasm may also occur (142) (see Chap. 8). Conjunctival changes are seen particularly in the syndrome of moniliasis, Addison's disease, and hypocalcemia (143).

EFFECTS ON THE INTEGUMENT

Thinning and loss of hair in all parts of the body are especially characteristic of untreated patients with idiopathic hypoparathyroidism (144). The skin becomes dry, keratotic, and scaly, with a dermatitis resembling eczema, and appears particularly susceptible to infection with Monilia (145). Growth of the nails is slowed, and the nails are shortened (142). They become thickened, white, brittle, and chipped (141). Transverse or longitudinal grooves may appear (144). The nails sometimes become atrophic and overgrown by skin.

When hypocalcemia is present in childhood, secondary to pseudohypoparathyroidism or the idiopathic variety, the teeth usually show marked dystrophic changes (141). The deciduous teeth erupt in a delayed and irregular fashion, and the permanent teeth are retarded in growth and development. Blunting of the roots of the molar teeth is especially characteristic. In adults, dental changes are less common, although the teeth may become loose and fall out (146).

CARDIOVASCULAR MANIFESTATIONS

The major electrocardiographic feature is prolongation of the QT interval owing to a widened isoelectric ST segment. The QRS complex is usually normal (147).

Cardiac contractility is impaired by hypocalcemia. Rapid falls in serum calcium to low levels may produce heart failure, with enlargement of the heart and hypotension (148–150). Pulmonary edema is a special danger if at the same time the patient is being given a rapid infusion of sodium salts. This may occur, for example, in acute pancreatitis or as a complication of treating hypercalcemia with intravenously administered sodium phosphate.

Sudden falls in serum calcium induced by sodium edetic acid (EDTA) infusion produce severe orthostatic hypotension in normal subjects (151) (see Chap. 8). In addition to a direct action on the heart, the mechanism may involve impairment of the contractility of peripheral blood vessels and of catecholamine release. The secretion of renin is unaltered by acute or chronic hypocalcemia.

GASTROINTESTINAL MANIFESTATIONS

Disorders of bowel function usually cause hypocalcemia, rather than the reverse. An occasional patient has diarrhea, steatorrhea, and hypocalcemia; in these patients intestinal absorption seems to be improved when the hypocalcemia is properly treated (152, 153).

HYPOMAGNESEMIA

Magnesium depletion is not commonly encountered after simple dietary restriction, because of the exceedingly efficient mechanisms of renal and gastrointestinal conservation. Symptomatic magnesium deficiency is therefore likely to be seen only when decreased intake or absorption of magnesium is present together with increased losses.

It is not entirely clear whether the symptoms commonly ascribed to hypomagnesemia reflect the level of the serum magnesium alone, the concentration of magnesium in cerebrospinal fluid, or the intracellular concentration of magnesium in the tissue of nerves, brain, and muscles. Certain patients whose renal conservation of magnesium is impaired can experience a rapid fall in the concentration of magnesium in plasma from the normal level of 2 meq/L to as low as 0.3 meq/L without symptoms (154). In other patients, serum magnesium levels of 1 or 1.2 meq/L are associated with dramatic neurologic manifestations.

The most careful studies of magnesium deficiency in humans are those reported by Shils, who observed several patients in whom magnesium deficiency developed after they were fed for several months with a diet low in magnesium (155, 156). Hypomagnesemia was associated with episodic confusion. The patients became surly and irritable. Anorexia developed, and they sometimes vomited. In one patient, paralytic ileus appeared. Tremors and muscle fasciculations were observed in association with positive Trousseau and Chvostek signs. Urinary incontinence in one man seemed to be associated with magnesium depletion, since it disappeared when magnesium was given. Dependent purpura was seen in some patients. In these studies the serum magnesium level fell to as low as 0.5 meq/L. There was a consistent fall in serum potassium level as well. Serum calcium decreased to 5 to 6 mg/dL, although the diet was not deficient in calcium or vitamin D.

NEUROMUSCULAR MANIFESTATIONS (REF. 157)

Tremors and seizures are classic signs of magnesium deficiency. The deep tendon reflexes are increased, and clonus may be present. Difficulty with fine movements, muscular fasciculations, and irregular handwriting may appear (158). Insomnia is sometimes prominent and annoying.

Convulsive seizures, usually generalized but sometimes focal, serve most often as the dramatic event that calls attention to the magnesium deficit. The electroencephalogram is usually abnormal, but the seizure patterns and diffuse dysrhythmias are not specific (159).

Signs of tetany, including Chvostek's and Trousseau's signs, may be present, but Trousseau's sign is less commonly seen. Frank carpal spasm is unusual. The tetany, like the convulsions, does not respond to intravenous infusion of calcium.

Other neurologic changes less consistently associated with hypomagnesemia include vertigo, ataxia, rigidity and cogwheeling, nystagmus, and dysarthria (160, 161). Bizarre involuntary muscular movements, with athetoid and choreiform movements of the extremities and twitching of the face, were described by Flink et al. as a characteristic clinical feature of magnesium depletion (162).

Changes in personality attributable to loss of magnesium run the gamut from mild depression and nervousness to delirium, hallucinations, and psychosis (158).

Although the picture of magnesium deficiency superficially resembles that of patients with chronic alcoholism and delirium tremens, in whom serum magnesium may sometimes be low, magnesium replacement does not appear to be effective in treating most cases of delirium tremens. It is unlikely that magnesium deficiency is primarily responsible for this disorder (163, 164).

CARDIOVASCULAR SIGNS

Sinus or nodal tachycardia is common in magnesium deficiency (159). Premature atrial or ventricular beats may occur. Flattening or inversion of the T waves, reversible when magnesium is administered, is especially prominent in children with protein-calorie malnutrition, in whom magnesium deficiency rapidly develops when they are refed (165). Cutaneous flushing is a prominent sign of magnesium deficiency in rats (166), though not in man, but it may have its analogy in the tendency toward hypotension sometimes seen in human patients (158).

GASTROINTESTINAL SIGNS

In patients with malabsorption syndromes like sprue or enteritis, absorption appears to be affected by the state of magnesium stores. Malabsorption is intensified by hypomagnesemia and improved when magnesium is repleted (167). When adequate body stores of magnesium are maintained in such patients, the improvement in weight gain and general health may be striking.

CHANGES IN OTHER SERUM ELECTROLYTES

Magnesium deficiency in humans is associated with a tendency toward hypocalcemia (198). The latter is probably due to both an inappropriately low secretion of parathyroid hormone and an end organ resistance to the hormone (see Chap. 19). Both are corrected by giving magnesium.

The tendency toward mild hypokalemia seen in patients who are magnesium-deficient remains unexplained.

An illustrative case follows:

A 44-year-old man was admitted after a generalized convulsion. He had had regional enteritis for 15 years. Twelve years before admission an ileocolostomy had been performed. Persistent diarrhea and spiking fever had prompted his recent admission to another hospital, where diseased bowel was resected 3 weeks before his convulsion. During convalescence from this operation, diarrhea continued, but food intake was poor.

On admission he seemed confused, and grimaced continually, jerking his left arm in what seemed like focal seizures. Chvostek's and Trousseau's signs were positive, and the serum calcium was measured and found to be 7.5 mg/dL. Calcium was infused, raising the serum calcium level to 13 mg/dL the next day and to 10 mg/dL on the following day. Despite this, the

state of consciousness did not improve, the positive Chvostek's sign persisted, and the patient had another convulsion 2 days after admission, even though the serum calcium was now normal.

Magnesium deficiency was now belatedly suspected, and the concentration of magnesium was measured in the serum. It was 0.8 meq/L—half the normal level.—During the next 12 h he was given 120 meq of magnesium as a 1% solution by intravenous infusion in glucose. By the next day he was awake, lucid, and responsive. The serum magnesium was maintained at a normal level by injections of 32 meq of $MgSO_4 \cdot 8H_2O$ per day. Neuromuscular irritability disappeared. The patient's appetite returned. Interestingly enough, the diarrhea improved. He soon was discharged from the hospital to the care of his private physician, who gave him weekly injections of magnesium at home. In 3 months he had gained 30 lb and felt better and stronger than at any time in the previous 10 years.

HYPERMAGNESEMIA

An elevated level of magnesium (168) in the serum occurs almost exclusively in patients who have renal insufficiency, either when renal failure is far-advanced or when patients are being treated with magnesium-containing salts or antacid mixtures. An excess of magnesium ions blocks neuromuscular transmission mainly by decreasing the amount of acetylcholine liberated at the neuromuscular function (182).

At levels of serum magnesium between 3 and 5 meq/L, there is a tendency to low blood pressure because of peripheral vasodilatation. Intractable hypotension sometimes dominates the clinical picture at higher magnesium levels (169). Facial flushing is sometimes seen, often accompanied by a sensation of heat and thirst (170). Nausea and vomiting may occur but are by no means constant (Fig. 11-9). At levels of serum magnesium between 5 and 7 meq/L, patients become lethargic, dysarthric, and drowsy, progressing to coma at 12 to 15 meq/L. Intravenously administered magnesium sulfate has been used to produce surgical anesthesia. An analeptic such as pentamethylenetetrazol can reverse the central effects but has no effect on the peripheral manifestations.

The deep tendon reflexes are regularly lost

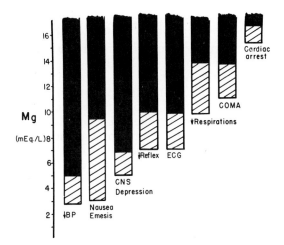

Figure 11-9. Signs and symptoms of magnesium intoxication. The hatched areas represent the variable serum concentrations at which the toxic phenomena may occur during the infusion of magnesium and the solid areas imply uniform occurrence of the phenomena at the concentrations represented. (*From Randall*)

when serum magnesium increases to about 7 meq/L. Weakness and finally paralysis of all muscles supervene with progressively increasing concentration of magnesium. A curarelike effect, the paralysis may be counteracted with physostigmine (171, 172). The pupils are sometimes dilated and react poorly to light (173). The respiratory center is depressed at levels of magnesium greater than 10 meq/L producing shallow respirations, irregular brief apneic periods, and finally, prolonged apnea. Deep tendon reflexes disappear before respirations are depressed. Thus, the presence of knee jerks can usually be relied on to indicate that there is not a life-threatening hypermagnesemia. Conversely, magnesium should not be administered intravenously or orally to patients with impaired renal function if the deep tendon reflexes are absent.

Hypermagnesemia produces a variety of disturbances in the electrocardiogram in animals (174, 175). In humans the QT interval may be prolonged and AV and intraventricular (IV) conduction depressed. Cardiac arrest may be expected when the magnesium level exceeds 15 to 20 meq/L. Magnesium sulfate injected intravenously into normal humans produces sinus bradycardia, pro-

longed PR interval, and increased sensitivity to vagal stimuli induced by carotid massage.

The association of elevated serum magnesium levels with uremia raises the possibility that some symptoms of renal insufficiency are secondary to the accumulation of magnesium. Infusions of magnesium into uremic patients (a time-tested method of treating uremic convulsions) caused in some an accentuation of nausea and malaise with increased drowsiness, lethargy, and ataxia (168). Postural hypotension became troublesome, and it was difficult for some patients to void. Dialysis with subsequent lowering of the magnesium level relieved these symptoms. The mildly elevated levels of serum magnesium in most patients with uremic symptoms, however, do not suggest that magnesium intoxication plays an important part in symptomatology of renal failure.

ACIDOSIS AND ALKALOSIS

ACIDOSIS

The classic sign of systemic acidosis is the state of "fearful dyspnea" described by Kussmaul. The characteristic deep, sighing respirations reflect intense stimulation of the respiratory center. At a pH of 7.2, pulmonary ventilation increases about four times; at a pH of 7.0, about eight times (176). The hyperpnea appears to affect the depth before the rate of respiration. With lesser degrees of metabolic acidosis the increase in depth of breathing may be overlooked except by an experienced observer, and the patient experiences no dyspnea at rest, although he or she becomes breathless on exertion. The intensity of respiration is related to the pH of blood and cerebrospinal fluid rather than to their bicarbonate content. Patients with chronic compensated metabolic acidosis, as, for example, in chronic renal insufficiency, may have easy respiration even with a serum bicarbonate level below 10 meq/L, while Kussmaul breathing is prominent in other patients with a higher blood bicarbonate level in whom acidosis has developed abruptly and compensation has not yet taken place. When acidosis is extremely severe, the function of the central nervous system is disrupted to such a degree that the respiratory center itself is depressed. An arterial pH less than about 6.8 is not compatible with life.

With progressive acidosis, consciousness is depressed, and lethargy, disorientation, and stupor appear. These can usually be reversed promptly by infusions of alkali. Seizures are uncommon.

There is considerable evidence that the depression of the central nervous system seen in acidosis is related more closely to the pH of the spinal fluid than the pH of blood (177). For example, neurologic symptoms are much more frequent and more profound in respiratory acidosis than in metabolic acidosis. In the former, acidosis regularly involves the brain as well as the blood, since CO_2 diffuses readily across the blood-brain barrier. In metabolic acidosis, on the other hand, cerebrospinal fluid pH is better defended (see Chap. 26).

Severe uncompensated respiratory acidosis produces a characteristic syndrome referred to as CO_2 narcosis (178–180). Early symptoms are fatigue and weakness, followed by irritability, lethargy, and confusion. Headache is common, sometimes associated with blurred vision. Mental derangements vary from depression and anxiety through somnolence to combative delirium. Abnormalities in the electroencephalogram include an abundant slow-frequency activity, prominent theta waves, and slow alpha activity with increased or decreased voltage (181). Tremors, jerking of the extremities, and clonic movements may occur (182). Asterixis is characteristic. The cerebrospinal fluid pressure is often increased, perhaps as a reflection of the increase in cerebral blood flow induced by CO_2 (183). Papilledema and engorged retinal vessels may be seen on funduscopic examination (181).

Systemic acidosis of any type causes peripheral vasodilatation (184). The skin may be warm and flushed, the heart rate rapid, and the pulse pressure wide. The cardiac output may be elevated initially, but with profound acidosis it falls as hypotension becomes pronounced. In experimental animals, as pH is reduced toward 6.8, cardiac output is reduced because of a decrease in cardiac contractility (199) and slowing of the heart rate (200). Bradycardia is probably the result of en-

hanced vagal effect during acidosis; the lowering of blood pH produces an inhibition of cholinesterase activity and consequent decrease in hydrolysis of acetylcholine (201). Both the peripheral vessels and the heart are less responsive to catecholamines (202). Patients who are acidotic have a similarly decreased responsiveness to catecholamines, and restoring the pH to normal reduces the amount of vasopressor substance necessary to support the blood pressure (203–205).

Acute reduction of pH, usually due to rapid elevation of the P_{CO_2}, is often associated with cardiac arrhythmia (185). Other electrocardiographic changes that are found include ST depression and changes in the height of the R and T waves.

Mild degrees of metabolic acidosis associated, for example, with a decrease in the serum bicarbonate to less than 20 meq/L are often accompanied by loss of appetite, nausea, headache, and lethargy. Such symptoms are common in patients with renal insufficiency, and can be combated by the prescription of small amounts of sodium bicarbonate. Chronic metabolic acidosis as severe as that present in diabetic coma interferes with carbohydrate metabolism and the action of insulin (186). When blood pH is below 7, therefore, early infusion of sodium bicarbonate may be important not only in reversing coma but in allowing insulin to take effect.

ALKALOSIS

The predominant effect of a fall in hydrogen ion concentration in the extracellular fluid is an increase in irritability of the central and peripheral nervous systems. Because changes in P_{CO_2} are more rapidly and directly reflected in the cerebrospinal fluid than changes in blood bicarbonate, respiratory alkalosis is likely to be accompanied by much more dramatic symptoms than metabolic alkalosis of the same degree.

Tetany caused by alkalosis is indistinguishable from that occurring in hypocalcemia. It is preceded by numbness and tingling of the extremities and the face around the mouth, and sometimes by tinnitus, cramps in the arms and legs, and a warm feeling in the abdomen. Spontaneous contractions of the facial and mouth muscles, with dysarthria, have been reported (187). Patients with chronic hyperventilation, many of whom are hysterical, often complain of headache, dry mouth, inability to take a deep breath, chest pressure and pain, anxiety, and apprehension. Some of these symptoms reflect their psychiatric difficulties; others may be intensified by the respiratory alkalosis.

Convulsive tendencies are aggravated by alkalosis; hence petit mal or grand mal epilepsy may be provoked by hyperventilation (188). Paroxysmal or continuous slow waves of high voltage are seen in the electroencephalogram, though the changes correlate poorly with arterial pH (189).

Metabolic alkalosis tends to depress respiration, although this is often not apparent at the bedside. The ventilatory response to inhalations of carbon dioxide is decreased (190).

Changes in the electrocardiogram produced by alkalosis resemble those of hypokalemia and may be produced in part by the shift of potassium from an extracellular to an intracellular position. The T wave is usually flattened. The ST segment may be prolonged and the delayed T wave closely followed by a P wave, producing the "TP" phenomenon (191, 192).

Severe metabolic alkalosis is produced in patients with compensated hypercapnia secondary to chronic lung disease when ventilatory function is suddenly improved, with rapid lowering of the P_{CO_2} and consequent elevation of blood pH. Mental confusion and delirium, with focal or generalized seizures, cardiac arrhythmias, and hypotension may complicate the systemic alkalosis. The symptoms are reversible if the P_{CO_2} is allowed to rise (193). Chronic alkalosis produced by repeated vomiting can also be associated with delirium, obtundation, and seizures, but in such cases depletion of sodium and potassium and some degree of renal insufficiency also contribute to the picture.

Both respiratory and metabolic alkalosis regularly cause a fall in the concentration of phosphorus in serum and urine. This is particularly pronounced in the case of respiratory alkalosis (194). Intracellular alkalosis enhances the activity of phosphofructokinase, a key enzyme regulating

glycolysis (195). The resulting increase in the three-carbon phosphorylated compounds within cells causes inorganic phosphate to move into cells and out of the extracellular fluid. As far as is known, the resulting hypophosphatemia does not cause any symptoms, but the chemical finding may stimulate an unnecessary search for hyperparathyroidism.

REFERENCES

1. Finberg, L., J. Kiley, and C. N. Luttrell: Mass accidental salt poisoning in infancy, *JAMA*, **184**:187, 1963.
2. Boyer, J., G. N. Gill, and F. H. Epstein: Hyperglycemia and hyperosmolality complicating peritoneal dialysis, *Ann. Intern. Med.*, **67**:568, 1967.
3. Kustin, A. J., M. B. Lipsett, A. K. Ommaya, and J. M. Moser: Asymptomatic hypernatremia, *Am. J. Med.*, **38**:306, 1967.
4. Segar, W. E.: Chronic hyperosmolality, *Am. J. Dis. Child.*, **112**:318, 1961.
5. DeRubertis, F. R., M. F. Michelis, and B. B. Davis: "Essential" hypernatremia: Report of three cases and review of the literature, *Arch. Intern. Med.*, **134**:889, 1974.
6. Alford, F. P., and B. A. Scoggins: Symptomatic normovolemic essential hypernatremia. A clinical and physiologic study, *Am. J. Med.*, **54**:359, 1973.
7. Maddy, J. A., and W. W. Winternitz: Hypothalamic syndrome with hypernatremia and muscular paralysis, *Am. J. Med.*, **51**:394, 1971.
8. Arieff, A. I., and R. Guisado: Effects on the central nervous system of hypernatremic and hyponatremic states, *Kidney Int.*, **10**:104, 1976.
9. Ross, E. F., and S. B. M. Christie: Hypernatremia, *Medicine*, **48**:441, 1969.
10. Finberg, L., C. Luttrell, and H. Redd: Pathogenesis of lesions in the nervous system in hypernatremic states. II. Experimental studies of gross anatomic changes and alterations of chemical composition of the tissues. *Pediatrics*, **23**:46, 1959.
11. Hogan, G. R., et al.: Pathogenesis of seizures occurring during restoration of plasma tonicity to

normal animals previously chronically hypernatremic, *Pediatrics,* **43:**54, 1969.

12. Finberg, L., and H. E. Harrison: Hypernatremia
in infants, *Pediatrics,* **16:**1, 1955.

13. Sparacio, R. R., B. Anziska, and H. S. Schutta:
Hypernatremia and chorea. A report of two cases,
Neurology, **26:**46, 1976.

14. Skinner, A. L., and F. C. Moll: Hypernatremia
accompanying infant diarrhea, *Am. J. Dis. Child.,*
92:562, 1956.

15. Glaser, G. H.: Sodium and seizures, *Epilepsia,*
5:97–111, 1964.

16. Sotos, J. F., P. R. Dodge, P. Mears, and N. B.
Talbot: Studies in experimental hypertonicity. I,
Pediatrics, **26:**925, 1960.

17. Morris-Jones, P. H., I. B. Houston, and R. C. Evans: Prognosis of the neurological complications
of acute hypernatremia, *Lancet,* **2:**1385, 1967.

18. Ulvila, J. M., and V. J. Nessan: Hypernatremia
with myoglobinuria, *Am. J. Med. Sci.,* **265:**79,
1973.

19. Surawicz, B.: Arrhythmias and electrolyte disturbances, *Bull. N.Y. Acad. Med.,* **43:**1160, 1967.

20. Surawicz, B.: Relation between the ECG and
electrolytes, *Am. Heart J.,* **73:**814, 1967.

21. Goodyer, A. V. N., M. J. Goodkind, and E. J.
Stanley: The effects of abnormal concentrations
of the serum electrolytes on left ventricular function in the intact animal, *Am. Heart J.,* **67:**779,
1964.

22. McCance, R. A.: Experimental sodium chloride
deficiency in man, *Proc. R. Soc. Med.,* **119:**245,
1936.

23. Elkinton, J. R., A. W. Winkler, and T. S. Danowski: Importance of volume and tonicity of body
fluids in salt depletion shock, *J. Clin. Invest.,*
26:1002, 1947.

24. Elkinton, J. R., A. W. Winkler, and T. S. Danowski: Transfers of cell sodium and potassium in
experimental and clinical conditions, *J. Clin. Invest.,* **27:**74, 1948.

25. Friedman, S. M., C. L. Friedman, and M. Na-
kashima: Sodium and the regulation of peripheral
vascular resistance, in "Hypertension," *Am.
Heart Ass. Monogr.,* **13:** 178, 1965.

26. Leiter, L., R. Weston, and J. Grossman: The low
sodium syndrome, its origins and varieties, *Bull.
N.Y. Acad. Med.,* **29:**833, 1953.

27. Chasis, H., et al.: Salt and protein restriction: Effects on blood pressure and renal hemodynamics
in hypertensive patients, *JAMA,* **142:**711, 1950.

28. Pomeranz, B. H., A. G. Birtch, and A. C. Barger:
Neural control of intrarenal blood flow, *Am. J.
Phys.,* **215:**1067, 1968.

29. Relman, A. S., and W. B. Schwartz: Effects of
electrolyte disorders on renal structure and function, in D. A. K. Black (ed.), *Renal Disease,*
Blackwell Scientific Publications, Ltd., Oxford,
1967.

30. Jaenicke, J. J., and C. Waterhouse: The renal response to sustained administration of vasopressin
and water in man, *J. Clin. Endocrinol. Metab.,*
21:231, 1961.

31. Krnjevic, K., R. Kilpatrick, and P. G. Aungle: A
study of some aspects of nervous and muscular
activity during experimental human salt deficiency, *Q. J. Exp. Physiol.,* **40:**205, 1955.

32. Arieff, A. I., F. Llack, and S. G. Massry: Neurological manifestations and morbidity of hyponatremia: Correlations with brain water and electrolytes, *Medicine,* **55:**121, 1976.

33. Scott, J. C., J. S. Welch, and I. B. Berman: Water
intoxication and sodium depletion in surgical patients, *Obstet. Gynecol.,* **26:**168, 1965.

34. Saphir, W.: Chronic hypochloremia simulating
psychoneurosis, *JAMA,* **129:**510, 1945.

35. Grant, J. L., A. MacDonald, S. R. Brovender, and
N. Yankopoulos: Hypoadrenocorticotropism with
hyponatremia resembling antidiuretic hormone
excess, *Ann. Intern. Med.,* **63:**486, 1965.

36. Cohn, R., L. C. Kolb, and D. W. Mulder: EEG
changes induced by water intoxication, *J. Nerv.
Ment. Dis.,* **106:**513, 1947.

37. Grumer, H. A., W. Derryberry, A. Dubin, and
S. S. Waldstein: Idiopathic episodic inappropriate
secretion of antidiuretic hormone, *Am. J. Med.,*
32:954, 1962.

38. Goldberger, E.: *A Primer of Water, Electrolyte
and Acid Base Syndromes,* Lea & Febiger, Philadelphia, 1965.

39. Schwartz, E., R. L. Fogel, W. V. Chokas, and
V. A. Panariello: Unstable osmolar homeostasis
with and without renal sodium wastage, *Am. J.
Med.,* **33:**39, 1962.

40. Wynn, V.: Water intoxication and serum hypotonicity, *Metabolism,* **5:**590, 1956.

41. Weir, J. F., E. E. Larson, and L. G. Rowntree: Studies in diabetes insipidus: Water balance and water intoxication, *Arch. Intern. Med.*, **29**:306, 1922.

42. Schwartz, W. B., W. Bennett, S. Curelop, and F. C. Bartter: A syndrome of renal sodium loss and hyponatremia probably resulting from inappropriate secretion of antidiuretic hormone, *Am. J. Med.*, **23**:529, 1957.

43. Streeten, D. H. P.: Periodic paralysis, in J. B. Stanbury, J. B. Wyngaarden, and D. S. Fredrickson, *The Metabolic Basis of Inherited Disease*, 2d ed., McGraw-Hill Book Company, New York, 1966.

44. Duggin, G. G., and M. A. Price: Hypokalaemic muscular paresis in migratory Papua/New Guineas, *Lancet*, **1**:649, 1974.

45. Houghton, B. J., and M. A. Pears: Chronic potassium depletion due to purgation with cascara, *Br. Med. J.*, **1**:1328, 1958.

46. Holler, J. W.: Potassium deficiency and diabetic acidosis, *JAMA*, **131**:1186, 1946.

47. Nicholson, W., and W. Spaeth: Some clinical manifestations of abnormal potassium metabolism, *South. Med. J.*, **42**:77, 1944.

48. MacLachlan, T. K.: Familial periodic paralysis: A description of six cases occurring in three generations of one family, *Brain*, **55**:47, 1932.

49. Mohamed, S. D., R. S. Chapman, and J. Crowley: Hypokalemic, flaccid, quadriparesis and myoglobinuria with carbenoxalone, *Br. Med. J.*, **1**:1581, 1966.

50. Gross, E. G., et al.: Hypokalemic myopathy and myoglobinuria associated with liquorice ingestion, *N. Engl. J. Med.*, **274**:602, 1966.

51. Cohen, J., R. Schwartz, and R. M. Wallace: Lesions of epiphyseal cartilage and skeletal muscle in rats on a diet deficient in potassium, *AMA Arch. Path.*, **54**:119, 1952.

52. Fourman, P.: Experimental observations on the tetany of potassium depletion, *Lancet*, **2**:525, 1954.

53. Stephens, F. I.: Paralysis due to reduced serum potassium during treatment of diabetic acidosis, *Ann. Intern. Med.*, **30**:1272, 1942.

54. Engel, F. L., S. P. Martin, and H. Taylor: On relation of potassium to neurologic manifestations of hypocalcemic tetany, *Bull. Johns Hopkins Hops.*, **84**:285, 1949.

55. Lubin, M.: Intracellular potassium and macromolecular synthesis in mammalian cells, *Nature*, **213**:451, 1967.

56. Elman, R., et al.: Intracellular and extracellular potassium deficits in surgical patients, *Ann. Surg.*, **136**:111, 1952.

57. Mitchell, W., and F. Feldman, Neuropsychiatric aspects of hypokalemia, *Can. Med. Assoc. J.*, **98**:48, 1968.

58. Ziegler, M., J. A. Anderson, and I. McQuarrie: Effect of desoxycorticosterone acetate on water and electrolyte content of brain and other tissue, *Proc. Soc. Exp. Biol. Med.*, **56**:242, 1944.

59. Foye, I. V., and T. V. Feichtmeir: Adrenal cortical carcinoma producing solely mineralocorticoid effect, *Am. J. Med.*, **19**:966, 1955.

60. Relman, A., and W. B. Schwartz: The kidney in potassium depletion, *Am. J. Med.*, **24**:764, 1958.

61. Rubini, M.: Water excretion in potassium deficient man, *J. Clin. Invest.*, **40**:2215, 1961.

62. Fourman, P., and P. M. Leeson: Thirst and polyuria: With a note on the effects of potassium deficiency and calcium excess, *Lancet*, **1**:268, 1959.

63. Manitius, A., H. Levitin, D. Beck, and F. H. Epstein: On the mechanism of impairment of renal concentrating ability in potassium deficiency, *J. Clin. Invest.*, **39**:684, 1960.

64. Galvez, O. G., B. W. Roberts, W. H. Bay, and T. F. Ferris: Studies of the mechanism of polyuria with hypokalemia, *Proc. Am. Soc. Nephrol.*, 1976, p. 97.

65. Clarke, E., B. M. Evans, I. MacIntyre, and N. D. Milne: Acidosis in experimental electrolyte depletion, *Clin. Sci.*, **14**:421, 1955.

66. Muehrcke, R. C., and S. Rosen: Hypokalemic nephropathy in rat and man: A light and electron microscopic study, *Lab. Invest.*, **13**:1359, 1964.

67. Reed, A. E., J. Laidlaw, R. M. Haslam, and S. Sherlock: Neuropsychiatric complications following chlorothiazide therapy in patients with hepatic cirrhosis: Possible relation to hypokalemia, *Clin. Sci.*, **18**:409, 1959.

68. Huth, E. J., and R. D. Squires: The relation of cardiovascular phenomena to metabolic changes in a patient with chronic hypokalemia, *Circulation*, **14**:60, 1956.

69. Windsor, T.: Electrolyte abnormalities and the ECG, *JAMA*, **203**:347, 1968.

70. Sarina, R. N.: Unusually tall and narrow U waves simulating hyperkalemic T waves, *Am. Heart J.*, **70**:397, 1965.

71. Earle, D. P., S. Sherry, L. W. Eichna, and N. S. Conan: Low potassium syndrome due to defective renal tubular mechanisms for handling potassium, *Am. J. Med.*, **11**:283, 1951.

72. Bellet, S., W. A. Steiger, et al.: ECG features in hypokalemia, *Am. J. Med. Sci.*, **219**:542, 1950.

73. Grob, D., R. J. Johns, and A. Liljestrand: Potassium movement in patients with familial periodic paralysis: Relation to the defect in muscle function, *Am. J. Med.*, **23**:356, 1957.

74. Bender, J. A.: Family periodic paralysis in a girl aged seventeen, *Arch. Neurol. Psychiat.*, **35**:131, 1936.

75. Surawicz, B., H. A. Braun, W. B. Crum, R. L. Kemp, S. Wagner, and S. Bellet: Clinical manifestations of hypopotassemia, *Am. J. Med. Sci.*, **233**:603, 1957.

76. Biglieri, E. G., and M. B. McIlroy: Abnormalities of renal function and circulatory reflexes in primary aldosteronism, *Circulation*, **33**:78, 1966.

77. Knochel, J. P., and E. M. Schlein: On the mechanism of rhabdomyolysis in potassium depletion, *J. Clin. Invest.*, **51**:1750, 1972.

78. Eliel, L. P., D. H. Pearson, and F. C. White: Postoperative potassium deficit and metabolic alkalosis: The pathogenic significance of operative trauma and of potassium and phosphorus deprivation, *J. Clin. Invest.*, **31**:419, 1952.

79. Mondon, C. E., S. D. Burton, G. M. Grodsky, et al.: Glucose tolerance and insulin response of potassium-deficient rat and isolated liver, *Am. J. Physiol.*, **215**:779, 1968.

80. Keele, K. D., and N. M. Matheson: *Intra-abdominal Crises*, Butterworth Inc., Washington, 1961, p. 46.

81. Lans, H. S., et al.: Diagnosis, treatment and prophylaxis of potassium deficiency in surgical patients: Analysis of four hundred and four patients, *Surg. Gynecol. Obstet.*, **95**:321, 1952.

82. Bellet, S.: *Clinical Disorders of the Heart Beat*, Lea & Febiger, Philadelphia, 1963, p. 802.

83. Finch, C. A., C. G. Sawyer, and J. M. Flynn: Clinical syndromes of potassium intoxication, *Am. J. Med.*, **1**:377, 1946.

84. Herndon, R., W. Meroney, and C. Pearson: The ECG effects of alteration in concentration of plasma chemicals, *Am. Heart J.*, **50**:188, 1955.

85. Levine, H. D., S. H. Wanger, and J. P. Merrill: Dialyzable currents of injury in potassium intoxication resembling acute myocardial infarction or pericarditis, *Circulation*, **13**:29, 1956.

86. Pick, A.: Arrhythmias and potassium in man, *Am. Heart J.*, **72**:295, 1966.

87. Levine, H. D.: Electrolyte imbalance and the ECG, *Mod. Conc. Cardiov. Dis.*, **23**:246, 1954.

88. Pollen, R. H., and R. H. Williams: Hyperkalemic neuromyopathy in Addison's disease, *N. Engl. J. Med.*, **263**:273, 1960.

89. Emanuel, M., and R. G. Metcalf: Quadriplegia in hyperkalemia, *J. Maine Med. Assoc.*, **157**:134, 1966.

90. Layzer, B. B., R. E. Lovelace, and L. P. Rowland: Hyperkalemic periodic paralysis, *Arch. Neurol.*, **16**:455, 1967.

91. Seldin, D. W., N. W. Carter, and F. C. Rector: Consequences of renal failure and their management, in M. B. Strauss and L. G. Welt (eds.), *Diseases of the Kidney*, Little, Brown and Company, Boston, 1963.

92. Albright, F., J. C. Aub, and W. Bauer: Hyperparathyroidism, *JAMA*, **102**:1276, 1934.

93. Karpati, G., and B. Frame: Neuropsychiatric disorders in primary hyperparathyroidism, *Arch. Neurol.*, **10**:387, 1964.

94. Dent, C. E.: Some problems of hyperparathyroidism, *Br. Med. J.*, **2**:1419, 1495, 1962.

95. Fitz, T. E., and B. C. Hallman: Mental changes associated with hyperparathyroidism, *Arch. Intern. Med.*, **89**:547, 1952.

96. Edwards, G. A., and S. M. Daum: Increased spinal fluid protein in hyperparathyroidism and other hypercalcemic states, *Arch. Intern. Med.*, **104**:29, 1959.

97. Bauermeister, D. E., E. R. Jennings, D. R. Cruse, and V. deM. Sedgwich: Hypercalcemia with seizures: A clinical paradox, *JAMA*, **201**:132, 1967.

98. Thomas, W. C., Jr., J. G. Wiswell, T. B. Connor, and J. E. Howard: Hypercalcemic crisis due to hyperparathyroidism, *Am. J. Med.*, **24**:229, 1958.

99. Patten, B. M., J. P. Bilezikan, L. E. Mallette, A. Prince, W. K. Engel, and G. D. Auerbach: Neuromuscular disease in primary hyperparathyroidism, *Annals Intern. Med.*, **80**:182, 1974.

100. Snapper, I.: *Bone Disease in Medical Practice,* Grune & Stratton, Inc., New York, 1957.

101. Waife, S. O.: Parathyrotoxicosis, *Am. J. Med. Sci.,* 218:624, 1949.

102. Anning, S. T., J. Dawson, D. E. Dolby, and J. T. Ingram: The toxic effects of calciferol, *Q. J. Med.,* 17:203, 1948.

103. Kleppel, N. Y., M. H. Goldstein, and H. H. Leveen: Hypercalcemic crisis and pancreatitis in primary hyperparathyroidism, *JAMA,* 192:916, 1965.

104. Fink, W. J., and J. D. Finfrock: Fatal hyperparathyroid crisis associated with pancreatitis, *Am. J. Surg.,* 27:424, 1961.

105. Spiro, H. M.: Hyperparathyroidism, parathyroid "adenomas" and peptic ulcer, *Gastroenterology,* 39:544, 1960.

106. Wilder, W. T., B. Frame, and W. S. Haubrich: Peptic ulcer in primary hyperparathyroidism, *Ann. Intern. Med.,* 55:885, 1961.

107. Frame, B., and W. S. Haubrich: Peptic ulcer and hyperparathyroidism: A review of 300 ulcer patients, *Arch. Intern. Med.,* 105:536, 1960.

108. Moore, W. T., and L. H. Smith: Experience with a calcium infusion test in parathyroid disease, *Metabolism,* 12:447, 1963.

109. Haddy, F. J., et al.: Local vascular effects of hypokalemia, alkalosis, hypercalcemia, and hypomagnesemia, *Am. J. Phys.,* 204:202, 1963.

110. Douglas, W. W.: The mechanism of the release of catecholamines from the adrenal medulla, *Pharmacol. Rev.,* 18:471, 1966.

111. Earll, J. M., N. A. Kurtzman, and R. H. Moser: Hypercalcemia and hypertension, *Ann. Intern. Med.,* 64:378, 1966.

112. Hellstrom, J.: Primary hyperparathyroidism: Observations in a series of 50 cases, *Acta. Endocrinol.,* 16:30, 1954.

113. Bradlow, B. A., and N. Segal: Acute hyperparathyroidism with ECG changes, *Br. Med. J.,* 2:197, 1956.

114. Paul, N. G.: The ECG changes associated with hypercalcemia and hypocalcemia, *Am. J. Med. Sci.,* 224:413, 1952.

115. Voss, D. M., and E. H. Drake: Cardiac manifestations of hyperparathyroidism with presentation of a previously unreported arrhythmia, *Am. Heart J.,* 73:235, 1967.

116. Wilson, R. E., W. F. Bernhard, H. Polet, and F. D. Moore: Hyperparathyroidism, *Ann. Surg.,* 159:79, 1964.

117. Gold, H., and D. J. Edwards: The effects of ouabain on the heart in the presence of hypercalcemia, *Am. Heart J.,* 3:45, 1927.

118. Wagener, H. P.: The ocular manifestations of hypercalcemia, *Am. J. Med. Sci.,* 321:218, 1956.

119. Walsh, F. B., and J. E. Howard: Conjunctival and corneal lesions in hypercalcemia, *J. Clin. Endocrinol.,* 7:644, 1947.

120. McMillan, D. E., and R. B. Freeman: The milk alkali syndrome, *Medicine (Baltimore),* 44:486, 1965.

121. Thomas, W. C., J. G. Wiswell, T. B. Connor, and J. E. Howard: Hypercalcemia crisis due to hyperparathyroidism, *Am. J. Med.,* 24:229, 1958.

122. Allen, F. N.: Hyperparathyroidism: Report of a case, *Proc. Staff Meetings Mayo Clinic,* 6:684, 1931.

123. Edvall, C. A.: Renal function in hyperparathyroidism. A clinical study of 30 cases with special reference to selective renal clearance and renal vein catheterization. *Acta Chir. Scand. (suppl.)* 229, 1958.

124. Wrong, O., and H. E. F. Davies: The excretion of acid in renal disease, *Q. J. Med.,* 28:259, 1959.

125. Shanes, A. M.: Electrochemical aspects of physiological and pharmacological action in excitable cells. II. The action potential and excitation, *Pharmacol. Rev.,* 10:165, 1958.

126. Simpson, J. A.: Neurologic manifestations of hypoparathyroidism, *Brain,* 75:76, 1952.

127. Harvey, A. M., and J. L. Lilienthal: Observations on the nature of tetany: The effect of adrenalin, *Bull. Johns Hopkins Hosp.,* 71:163, 1942.

128. Blanchard, B. M.: Focal hypocalcemic seizures 33 years after thyroidectomy, *Arch. Intern. Med.,* 110:382, 1962.

129. Roth, B., and O. Newsimal: EEG study of tetany and spasmophilia, *Electroencephalogr. Clin. Neurophysiol.,* 17:36, 1964.

130. Denko, J. D., and R. Kaelbling: The psychiatric effects of hypoparathyroidism, *Acta Psychiatr. Scand. (suppl.)* 38:164, 1962.

131. Clark, J. A., L. J. Davidson, and H. C. Ferguson: Hypoparathyroidism, *J. Ment. Sci.,* 108:811, 1963.

132. Barrett, A. M.: Mental symptoms of tetany, *Am. J. Insan.,* 76:373, 1920.

133. Katz, G. G.: An investigation of eidetic imagery

in conditions of hypocalcemia with and without latent tetany *Dissertation Abstracts*, **17**:889, 1957.

134. Kreisler, B., A. Dinbar and D. B. Tulcinsky: Postoperative atetanic hypocalcemic coma: Report of a case, *Surgery*, **65**:916–918, 1969.

135. Walsh, F. B., and R. G. Murray: Ocular manifestations of disturbances in calcium metabolism, *Am. J. Ophthal.*, **36**:1657, 1953.

136. Barr, D. P., C. M. MacBride, and T. E. Sanders: Tetany with increased intracranial pressure and papilledema: Results from treatment with dihydrotachysterol, *Trans. Assoc. Am. Physicians*, **53**:227, 1938.

137. Levin, P., et al.: Intracranial calcification and hypoparathyroidism, *Neurology (Minneap.)*, **11**:1076, 1961.

138. Frame, B.: Parkinsonism in post-operative hypoparathyroidism, *Arch. Intern. Med.*, **116**:424, 1965.

139. Levin, P.: Intracranial calcification associated with hypoparathyroidism, *Bull. N.Y. Acad. Med.*, **38**:632, 1962.

140. Svane-Knudsen, P.: Severe secondary ocular changes in a patient suffering from idiopathic hypoparathyroidism, *Acta Ophthalmol. (Kbh)*, **37**:560, 1959.

141. Dietrich, F. S., M. L. Rice, and E. F. Lutton: Clinical manifestations of idiopathic hypoparathyroidism, *Ann. Intern. Med.*, **37**:1052, 1952.

142. Emerson, K., F. B. Walsh, and J. E. Howard: Idiopathic hypoparathyroidism: A report of two cases, *Ann. Intern. Med.*, **14**:1256, 1941.

143. McGass, J. D.: The syndrome of keratoconjunctivitis, superficial moniliasis, idiopathic hypoparathyroidism and Addison's disease, *Am. J. Ophthal.*, **54**:660, 1962.

144. Wells, G. C.: Skin disorders in relation to malabsorption, *Br. Med. J.*, **2**:937, 1962.

145. Dent, C. E., and M. Garretts: Skin changes in hypocalcemia, *Lancet*, **1**:142, 1960.

146. Albright, F., and E. C. Reifenstein: *Parathyroid Glands and Metabolic Bone Disease,* The Williams & Wilkins Company, Baltimore, 1948.

147. Bronsky, D., et al.: The relationship of the intervals of the ECG to the level of the serum calcium, *Am. J. Cardiol.*, **7**:840, 1960.

148. Demath, W. E., and H. S. Rottenstein: Death associated with hypocalcemia after small bowel short circuiting, *N. Engl. J. Med.*, **270**:1239, 1964.

149. Edge, W. E. B.: Hypocalcemia in infancy with special reference to cardiac failure, *S. Afr. Med. J.*, **37**:262, 1963.

150. Falko, J. M., C. A. Bush, M. Tzagournis, and F. B. Thomas: Congestive heart failure complicating the hungry bone syndrome, *Am. J. Med. Sci.*, **271**:85, 1976.

151. Llack, F., P. Weidmann, R. Reinhart, M. H. Maxwell, J. W. Coburn, and S. G. Massry: Effect of acute and long-standing hypocalcemia on blood pressure and plasma renin activity in man, *J. Clin. Endocrinol. Metab.*, **38**:841, 1974.

152. Kusin, A. S., B. R. Mackay, S. L. Burns, and M. J. Halberstam: A syndrome of hypoparathyroidism and adrenocortical insufficiency, *Am. J. Med.*, **34**:856, 1963.

153. Clarkson, B., et al.: Clinical and metabolic study of a patient with malabsorption and hypoparathyroidism, *Metabolism*, **9**:1093, 1960.

154. Gitelman, H. J., J. B. Graham, and L. G. Welt: A new familial disorder characterized by hypokalemia and hypomagnesemia, *Trans. Assoc. Am. Physicians*, **71**:235, 1966.

155. Shils, M. E.: Experimental human magnesium depletion. I. Clinical observations and blood chemistry alterations, *Am. J. Clin. Nutr.*, **15**:133, 1964.

156. Shils, M. E.: Experimental human magnesium depletion, *Medicine (Baltimore)*, **48**:61, 1969.

157. Fishman, R. A.: Neurological aspects of magnesium metabolsim, *Arch. Neurol.*, **12**:562, 1965.

158. Flink, E. B., et al.: Evidences for clinical magnesium deficiency, *Ann. Intern. Med.*, **47**:956, 1957.

159. Randall, R. E., M. Ross, and K. M. Bleifer: Magnesium depletion in man, *Ann. Intern. Med.*, **50**:257, 1959.

160. MacIntyre, I.: An outline of magnesium metabolism in health and disease, *J. Chronic Dis.*, **16**:201, 1963.

161. Greenwald, J. H., A. Dubin, and L. Cardon: Hypomagnesemic tetany due to excessive lactation, *Am. J. Med.*, **35**:854, 1963.

162. Flink, E. B., et al.: Magnesium deficiency after prolonged parenteral fluid administration and after chronic alcoholism complicated by delirium tremens, *J. Lab. Clin. Med.*, **43**:169, 1954.

163. Smith, W. O., and J. E. Hammarsten: Intracellular magnesium in delirium tremens and uremia, *Am. J. Med. Sci.*, **237**:413, 1959.

164. Fankuchen, D., et al.: The significance of hy-

pomagnesemia in alcoholic patients, *Am. J. Med.*, **37**:802, 1964.

165. Caddell, J. L.: Studies in protein-calorie malnutrition. I. A double blind clinical trial to assess magnesium therapy, *N. Engl. J. Med.*, **276**:535, 1967.

166. Wacker, W. E. C., and B. L. Vallee: Magnesium metabolism, *N. Engl. J. Med.*, **259**:431–438, 475–482, 1958.

167. Peterson, V. P.: Potassium and magnesium turnover in magnesium deficiency, *Acta Med. Scand.*, **174**:595, 1963.

168. Randall, R. E., M. D. Cohen, C. C. Spray, Jr., and E. C. Rossmeisl: Hypermagnesemia in renal failure, *Ann. Intern. Med.*, **61**:73, 1967.

169. Mordes, J. P., R. Swartz, and R. A. Arky: Extreme hypermagnesemia as a cause of refractory hypotension, *Ann. Intern. Med.*, **83**:657, 1975.

170. Fawcett, D. W.: Magnesium poisoning following an enema of epsom salt solution, *JAMA*, **123**:1028, 1943.

171. Joseph, R., and S. J. Meltzer: The life saving action of physostigmine in poisoning by magnesium, *J. Pharmacol. Exp. Ther.*, **1**:369, 1910.

172. Brosnan, J. J., and J. E. Boyd: Agents which antagonize the curare-like action of magnesium, *Am. J. Physiol.*, **119**:281, 1937.

173. Alfrey, A. C., D. S. Terman, L. Brettschneider, K. M. Simpson, and D. A. Ogden: Hypermagnesemia after renal homotransplantation, *Ann. Intern. Med.*, **73**:367, 1970.

174. Haury, V. G.: The effect of intravenous injection of magnesium sulfate on the vascular system, *J. Pharmacol. Exp. Ther.*, **65**:453, 1939.

175. Smith, P., A. W. Winkler, and H. E. Hull: ECG changes and concentration of magnesium in serum following intravenous injection of magnesium salts, *Am. J. Physiol.*, **126**:720, 1939.

176. Davenport, H. W.: *The ABC of Acid Base Chemistry*, The Univeristy of Chicago Press, Chicago, 1950.

177. Posner, J. B., and F. Plum: Spinal fluid pH and neurologic symptoms in acidosis, *N. Engl. J. Med.*, **277**:605, 1967.

178. MacDonald, F.: Respiratory acidosis, *Arch. Intern. Med.*, **116**:689, 1965.

179. Dufano, M., and S. Ishikawa: Hypercapnia: Mental changes and extra-pulmonary complications, *Ann. Intern. Med.*, **63**:829, 1965.

180. Kilburn, K. H.: Neurologic manifestations of respiratory failure, *Arch. Intern. Med.*, **116**:409, 1965.

181. Austen, F., et al.: Neurologic manifestations of chronic pulmonary insufficiency, *N. Engl. J. Med.*, **257**:579, 1957.

182. Sieker, H. O., and J. B. Hickam: CO_2 intoxication, *Medicine (Baltimore)*, **35**:389, 1956.

183. Rich, M., P. Scheinber, and M. S. Belle: Relationship between cerebrospinal fluid pressure change and cerebral blood flow, *Circ. Res.*, **1**:389, 1953.

184. Haddy, F. J., and J. B. Scott: Metabolically linked vasoactive chemicals in local regulation of blood flow, *Physiol. Rev.*, **48**:688, 1968.

185. MacDonald, F. M., and E. Simson: Human ECG during and after inhalation of 30% CO_2, *J. Appl. Physiol.*, **6**:304, 1953.

186. Guest, G. H., B. Mackler, and H. C. Knowles, Jr.: Effects of acidosis on insulin action and on carbohydrate and mineral metabolism, *Diabetes*, **1**:276, 1952.

187. Grant, S. B., and A. Goldman: A study of forced respiration: Experimental production of tetany, *Am. J. Physiol.*, **52**:209, 1920.

188. Brown, E. B.: Physiologic effects of hyperventilation, *Physiol. Rev.*, **33**:445, 1953.

189. Saltzman, H. A., A. Heyman, and H. O. Sieker: Correlation of clinical and physiologic manifestations of sustained hyperventilation, *N. Engl. J. Med.*, **268**:143, 1963.

190. Stone, D.: Respiration in man during metabolic alkalosis, *J. Appl. Physiol.*, **17**:33, 1962.

191. Thompson, W. P.: The ECG in the hyperventilation syndrome, *Am. Heart J.*, **25**:372, 1943.

192. Carter, C. P., and E. C. Andrus: QT interval in human ECG in absence of cardiac disease, *JAMA*, **78**:1922, 1922.

193. Rotheram, E., P. Safar, and E. P. Robin: Central nervous system disorder during mechanical ventilation in chronic pulmonary disease, *JAMA*, **189**:993, 1964.

194. Mostellar, M. E., and E. P. Tuttle: Effects of alkalosis on plasma concentration and urinary excretion of inorganic phosphate in man, *J. Clin. Invest.*, **43**:138, 1964.

195. Ui, M.: A role of phosphofructokinase in pH-dependent regulation of glycolysis, *Biochim. Biophys. Acta*, **124**:310, 1966.

196. Schaaf, M., and C. A. Payne: Dystonic reactions

to prochloperazine in hypoparathyroidism, *N. Engl. J. Med.*, **275:**991, 1966.

197. Hoagland, H., and D. Stone: Brain and muscle potassium in relation to stressful activities and adrenal cortex function, *Am. J. Physiol.*, **152:**423, 1948.

198. Estep, H., W. A. Shaw, C. Watlington, R. Hobe, W. Holland, and St. G. Tucker: Hypocalcemia due to hypomagnesemia and reversible parathyroid hormone unresponsiveness, *J. Clin. Endocrinol.*, **29:**842, 1969.

199. Thrower, W. B., T. D. Darby, and E. E. Aldinger: Acid-base derangements and cardiac contractility, *Arch. Surg.*, **82:**56, 1961.

200. Silberschmid, M., S. Saito, and L. L. Smith: Circulatory effects of acute lactic acidosis in dogs prior to and after hemorrhage, *Am. J. Surg.*, **112:**176, 1966.

201. Campbell, G. S.: Cardiac arrest: Further studies on the effect of pH on vagal inhibition of the heart, *Surgery*, **38:**615, 1955.

202. Bygdeman, S.: Vascular reactivity in cats during induced changes in the acid-base balance of the blood, *Acta Physiol. Scand. (suppl)*:222, 1963.

203. Campbell, G. S., D. B. Houle, N. W. Crisp, Jr., M. H. Weil, and E. B. Brown: Depressed response to intravenous sympathomimetic agents in humans during acidosis, *Dis. Chest.*, **33:**18, 1958.

204. Oliva, P. B.: Lactic acidosis, *Am. J. Med.*, **48:**209, 1970.

205. Mitchell, J. H., K. Wildenthal, and R. L. Johnson, Jr.: The effects of acid-base disturbances on cardiovascular and pulmonary function, *Kidney Int.*, **1:**375, 1972.

12

Water metabolism and the neurohypophyseal hormones*

Richard Weitzman / Charles R. Kleeman

GENERAL CONCEPTS OF WATER METABOLISM

In normal individuals, osmolality, or the concentration of osmotically active solutes in body fluids, is maintained remarkably constant despite large variations in water and solute intake and excretion. Every kilogram of body water contains 285 to 290 mosm of solute, consisting primarily of salts of sodium in ECF (extracellular fluid) and of potassium in ICF (intracellular fluid). The identical osmolality of ICF and ECF is produced by free movement of water across all cellular and subcellular membranes, governed only by the physical forces of osmosis and diffusion. A gain or loss of free water will be shared by all major body compartments (vascular, interstitial, intracellular) in proportion to their relative sizes. The single exception to this free movement is the control of water permeability of the distal portion of the mammalian nephron by antidiuretic hormone AVP (arginine vasopressin). Among all the vertebrates, only the mammals (and to a certain extent, the birds) possess the unique ability to excrete a hyperosmotic urine and thus conserve free

water when the supply of available water is limited. It has been suggested by Homer Smith that this concentrating ability of the mammalian kidney may have played an important role in our ultimate domination over the dinosaurs and other reptiles at the end of the Mesozoic era. There is a continuous decrease in the proportion of total body water (and particularly the extracellular compartment) with growth and aging, as well as a difference between men and women (Table 12-1).

The day-to-day fluctuations in total body water in a normal individual are very small, amounting to approximately 0.2 percent of body weight per 24 h. Although the infant has a relative "excess" of body water and extracellular volume as related to total body weight, the surface area, oxygen consumption, cardiac output, insensible water loss, renal water excretion, and overall metabolism are all high in relation to total body water. When one compares these fundamental metabolic parameters to total body water, the infant and young child are seen to be more vulnerable to water deficit and dehydration than the adult (1).

The average daily water turnover of a normal individual is shown in Table 12-2. Even with maximal renal conservation of water, the body is unable to prevent the continuous loss of insensi-

*Supported by Los Angeles County Affiliate of American Heart Association, National Institute of Child Health and Human Development (grant no. HD-06335), and James Fleming Fund.

Table 12-1. Body water compartments throughout life span
(As percent of body weight)

AGE	SEX	BODY WEIGHT, kg	TOTAL BODY WATER, PERCENT	EXTRA-CELLULAR WATER, PERCENT	INTRA-CELLULAR WATER, PERCENT
0–11 days			76.4	41.6	34.8
11–180 days			72.8	34.9	37.9
½–2 years			62.2	27.5	34.7
2–7 years			65.5	25.6	36.9
7–14 years			64.2	17.5	46.7
23–54 years	Men	72.5	54.3 ±1.39*	23.4 ±0.64	30.9 ±0.89
23–51 years	Women	59.3	48.6 ±1.47	22.7 ±0.54	25.9 ±0.96
71–84 years	Men	68.1	50.8 ±1.55	25.4 ±1.36	25.4 ±0.58
61–74 years	Women	63.9	43.4 ±1.32	21.4 ±0.45	22.4 ±0.97

* Standard error of the mean.
Source: Modified from H. V. Parker, K. H. Olesen, J. McMurrey, and B. Friis-Hansen, in *Ciba Foundation, Colloquia on Ageing,* vol. 4, Little, Brown and Company, Boston, 1958.

ble fluid through the skin, lungs, and gastrointestinal tract. For the replacement of this extrarenal loss, the individual must rely on adequate water ingestion. Man and other mammals vary considerably in their need for an exogenous source of water in the diet during maximal renal conservation (Fig. 12-1). Of all mammals, only certain desert rodents can so minimize their renal and extrarenal water losses that they are able to maintain water balance from that available in the preformed and oxidative water of the desert plants they ingest. These rodents can concentrate their urine to a level of four to five times that of humans, and by living in underground burrows they reduce to a minimum their insensible pulmonary and cutaneous water loss (2). Humans, in contrast, even when forming maximally concentrated urine, require some exogenous source of free water to replace continued insensible and minimal renal losses of water.

The day-to-day regulation of body water is dependent, therefore, on the kidneys and on a receptor system for signaling the relative need for water ingestion. This signal, thirst, plays an essential

Table 12-2. Average daily water turnover of a normal individual

	WATER INTAKE, g			WATER OUTPUT, g	
SOURCE OF WATER	OBLIGATORY	FACULTATIVE		OBLIGATORY	FACULTATIVE
Drink	650	1000	Urine	700	1000
Preformed	750		Skin	500	
Oxidative	350		Lungs	400	
			Feces	150	
Subtotals	1750	1000	Subtotals	1750	1000
Total	2750		Total	2750	

Source: A. V. Wolf, *Thirst,* Charles C Thomas, Springfield, Ill., 1958.

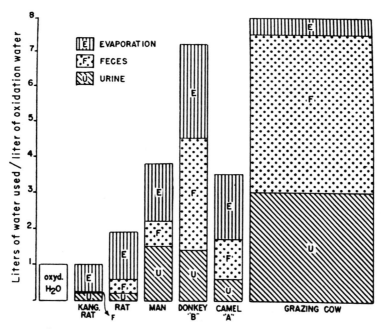

Figure 12-1. Minimum water expenditure in various mammals presented as liters of water expended per liter of water formed by metabolic oxidation. The base of the column for the cow has been made four times as wide as the others. Thus, the values are represented by the areas of the columns and the figures read on the ordinate should, in this case, be multiplied by four. [*Courtesy of B. Schmidt-Nielsen (2).*]

role in the regulation of the volume and tonicity of the body fluids. The sensation of thirst is dependent on excitation of the cortical centers of consciousness. Although the sensation of thirst may be modified somewhat by stimuli arising in the oropharynx or gastrointestinal tract, it is doubtful that in humans these local stimuli are of great importance (3).

HYPOTHALAMIC THIRST CENTERS

Although thirst is a cortical or conscious sensation, it has been clearly established that there exist in the hypothalamus specific nuclear centers essential for the integration of various types of signals altering water ingestion (3–5). Andersson and his associates have contributed greatly to our knowledge of the location of these centers (4, 5).

Figures 12-2 and 12-3, adapted from Andersson's data, show that these centers are located in the ventromedial and anterior area of the hypothalamus. The local instillation of hypertonic solutions of chloride or direct electrical stimulation of this area in the goat leads to profound polydipsia culminating in severe water intoxication, with an increase in body weight of as much as 40 percent (Fig. 12-4). Destruction of these same centers causes marked hypodipsia or complete adipsia. The animal then develops profound hypertonic dehydration, but shows no distinct inclination to drink. Stimulating and inhibitory impulses are transmitted from these centers to the cerebral cortex and consciousness, thus transforming the need, or lack of need, for water into appropriate behavior. Furthermore, impulses of cortical or voluntary origin can readily condition the sensation of thirst and create what might appropriately

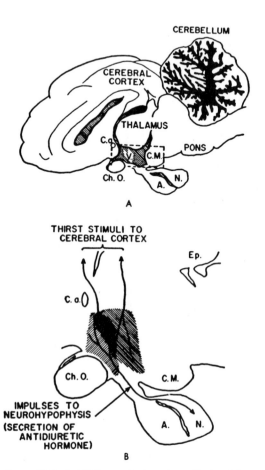

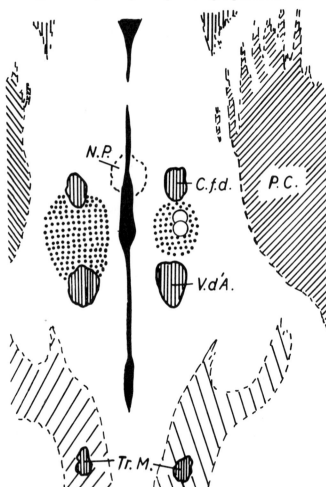

The proximity of the thirst centers to the hypothalamic nuclei which regulate the production and release of ADH (antidiuretic hormone) or AVP is immediately evident. In view of this proximity, it is surprising that pathologic processes do

Figure 12-2. *A.* Midline sagittal section of brain of the goat. The rectangle indicated by the broken lines approximates the extent of the hypothalamus. (Key below.) *B.* Hypothalamus and hypophysis of the goat, illustrating overlap of the "thirst center" (hatched area to the right) and the probable center of regulation of the ADH of the neurohypophysis (hatched area to the left.) A., Adenohypophysis; C.a., commissura anterior; C.M., corpus mammillare; Ch. O., chiasma opticum; Ep., epiphysis; N., neurohypophysis; V., third ventricle. [*After B. Andersson (4, 5).*]

Figure 12-3. Diagram of a horizontal section of the hypothalamus of the goat. The dotted area on the left side represents the region where microinjections of hypertonic sodium chloride solutions produced polydipsia. The dotted area on the right side represents the area where electrical stimulation caused drinking. (The white circles within this area mark the points where the most obvious polydipsic effect was obtained by electrical stimulation. C.f.d., Columna fornicis descendens; P.C., pedunculus cerebri; V. d'A., tract of Vicq d'Azyr; Tr.M., tract of Meynert; N.P., nucleus paraventricularis. (*From B. Andersson et al.,* Acta Physiol. Scand., *33:336, 1955.*)

be called the thirst "appetite," or voluntary habits of drinking. These vary greatly from individual to individual, psychogenic polydipsia representing the extreme form of excessive ingestion (see later). Conversely, in humans, injury to these centers, or the failure of hypothalamocortical impulses to stimulate thirst in the stuporous or unconscious patient, will cause inadequate water ingestion despite need.

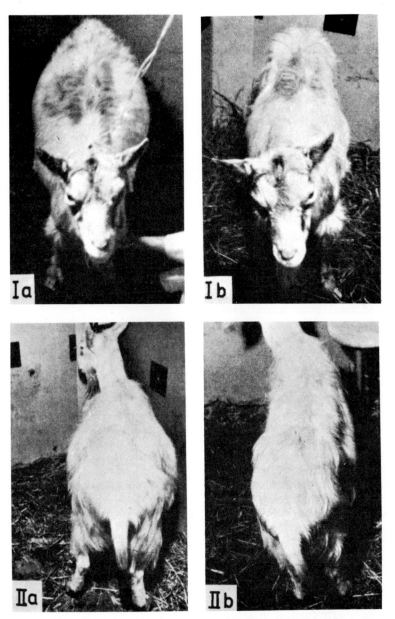

Figure 12-4. Contrast between the appearance of two goats after overhydration induced by electrical stimulation and their appearance 15 h later, when most of the water had been excreted. (*From B. Andersson et al.,* Acta Physiol. Scand., *33:339, 155.*)

not produce more frequently simultaneous disturbances in thirst regulation and AVP release (Fig. 12-2). Physiologically, these centers must be carefully integrated in the maintenance of normal total body water. It is not surprising, therefore, that the major stimuli for thirst also cause the release of AVP and the renal conservation of water, the "water repletion reaction." Those stimuli which inhibit thirst also inhibit the release of AVP and therefore initiate water diuresis, the "water depletion reaction" (6).

THIRST STIMULI AND INHIBITORS

The major physiologic stimulus for thirst is a decrease in total body water, with or without cellular dehydration (Table 12-3). The usual daily sensation of thirst, and its subcortical stimulus, in the normal individual is the result of a 1 to 2 percent contraction of total body water with a comparable rise in the osmolality of the body fluids and slight cellular dehydration. In more severe degrees of water depletion, or water loss in excess of sodium, marked cellular dehydration and hyperosmolality of all body fluids will occur. Cellular dehydration with marked thirst will also occur, even with an increased total body water, if hypertonic solutions of sodium chloride, glucose, mannitol, etc., are given to the point of producing hyperosmolality of the body fluids. Of equal importance, the decrease in total body water may be due to a primary isosmotic contraction of the extracellular phase, i.e., hemorrhage, vomiting, diarrhea, massive saline diuresis, a rapid accumulation of ascites or intraluminal gastrointestinal fluid ("third space").

Under these circumstances, thirst may be induced even in the face of hyponatremia and cellular overhydration and, in fact, may aggravate the latter. In experimental studies in animals, Stricker has shown that cellular overhydration in association with, or at the expense of, extracellular volume will frequently produce severe thirst in rats (6, 7). This hypovolemic thirst is permanently satisfied only when the extracellular or intravascular volume is repleted. Stricker also demonstrated that a pronounced and permanent decre-

Table 12-3. Known stimuli and inhibitors of thirst and/or the release of AVP

STIMULI

1. Osmotic
   Contracted intracellular volume of osmoreceptor neurons due to hyperosmolality of extracellular fluids [water loss or infusions of hypertonic solutions of molecules that do not freely permeate the blood-brain barrier (sodium chloride, mannitol)]
2. Nonosmotic
   a. Decreased arterial pressure (? pulse pressure) in carotid and possibly aortic baroreceptors, resulting from vascular or extracellular volume contraction or fall in cardiac output
   b. Decrease in tension in the left atrial wall and great pulmonary veins, because of reduced intrathoracic blood volume (such as blood loss, quiet standing, upright position, and positive-pressure breathing)
   c. Pain
   d. Psychosis
   e. Increased temperature of blood perfusing hypothalamus
   f. Drugs (acetylcholine and other cholinergic drugs, morphine, barbiturates, nicotine, adrenergic agents), ?chlorpropamide, clofibrate, carbamazepine, cytoxan, vincristine
   g. Carotid body chemoreceptor stimulation by hypoxia or hypercapnea
   h. Stimulation of the renin-angiotensin system

INHIBITORS

3. Osmotic
   Expansion of intracellular volume of the neurons of supraoptic hypophyseal nuclei secondary to hypoosmolality of extracellular fluids (water ingestion)
4. Nonosmotic
   a. Increased arterial pressure (? pulse pressure) in carotid and possibly aortic baroreceptors secondary to vascular or extracellular volume expansion, with rise in cardiac output
   b. Increase in tension in left atrial wall and great pulmonary veins secondary to increased intrathoracic blood volume (hypervolemia, reclining position, negative-pressure breathing, immersion in water up to neck, acute cold exposure with peripheral vasoconstriction, and shift of blood centrally)
   c. Occasionally, emotional stress
   d. Decreased temperature of blood perfusing the hypothalamus
   e. Drugs [alcohol, diphenylhydantoin, ? norepinephrine, narcotic antagonists (oxilorphan, butorphanol), ? anticholinergic drugs, and atropine]
   f. ? Inhibition of the renin-angiotensin system

ment in hypovolemic thirst is observed in rats with bilateral lesions of the lateral hypothalamus or the thirst centers. He used two experimental procedures to bring about the contraction of intravascular volume (Fig. 12-5): (1) Subcutaneous injection of 2.5 mL of 1.5% formalin, which causes diminished intravascular volume, stimulated thirst, and excessive water ingestion, which in turn caused expanded intracellular volume associated with hyponatremia. The decrease in intravascular volume was due to the sequestration of protein-rich plasma at the site of the injection, resulting from increased permeability of the local capillary walls. (2) In addition, subcutaneous injection of 5 mL of 10, 20, or 30% solutions of polyethylene glycol decreased intravascular volume by raising the oncotic pressure of the local interstitium, thereby causing the loss of a protein-free fluid from the intravascular compartment. Since with this technique the sequestered fluid is isosmotic with the plasma, there is no alteration of intracellular volume. Similarly, thirst may occur despite massive expansion of total body water or of interstitial fluid volume and despite hyponatremia, when "effective" circulating blood volume, blood pressure, and cardiac output are reduced, e.g., in severe congestive heart failure, cirrhosis of the liver during the rapid accumulation of ascites, or edema and the nephrotic syndrome. Whenever a patient complains of thirst despite adequate ingestion of water or when a deficit of water per se does not seem to exist, one must immediately think of the possible presence of a diminished vascular or extracellular volume and/or a reduced cardiac output and blood pressure.

Such "inappropriate" stimulation of thirst in eu- or hypoosmolar patients may also occur with normal or elevated blood pressure. In these situations there is overactivity of the renin-angiotensin system which in turn stimulates thirst. For example, intense thirst has been seen in patients with malignant hypertension or in hypertensive patients overtreated with diuretic therapy (vide infra).

McCance (8) first suggested that thirst was not exclusively related to hyperosmolality and cellular dehydration when he demonstrated increased water intake in humans that was associated with salt depletion secondary to rigid salt restriction and mercurial diuretics. Here we see thirst in association with a contracted extracellular volume, overhydration of all body cells as water enters to restore transcellular osmotic equilibrium, and hypoosmolality of all body fluids. It is most reasonable to consider the major inhibitors of thirst as simply the opposite of those stimuli described above and listed in Table 12-3, i.e., expansion of total body water and hypoosmolality of body fluids, and isosmotic expansion of intravascular and/or extracellular volume.

The exact mechanism(s) by which a reduction in vascular and extracellular volume stimulates the hypothalamic thirst centers is unknown. Although it is probable that pure water depletion with its accompanying hyperosmolality of the body fluids and contraction of intracellular volume would affect the receptor cells of the hypothalamus directly, it is not obvious that isosmolar or hypoosmolar or osmolal contraction of the extracellular volume would do the same. However, in view of the clear demonstration that the latter can cause the release of AVP by stimulation of intrathoracic and carotid sinus baroreceptors (Table 12-3) (9–14), these same receptors may well represent the receptors initiating the reflex arc responsible for the nonosmolar stimulation of thirst. In addition, recent excellent studies have strongly implicated the renin-angiotensin system in the control of hypovolemic (hypotensive) thirst (15–22) and in the release of AVP (17, 19, 23–29a). The drinking produced by isosmotic depletion of intravascular volume (15), by hypotension accompanying β-adrenergic activation with isoproterenol, and by constriction of the aorta above the renal arteries (20) is abolished by nephrectomy but survives sham nephrectomy and ureteral ligation

Effects of Formalin or polyethylene glycol on water intake and urine output

	No. of Rats	Intake, ml		Output, ml	
		Pretreatment	Treated	Pretreatment	Treated
Formalin	8	0.70	8.63	2.68	0.93
Formalin vehicle	8	0.93	1.50	2.63	2.74
PG	10	0.36	5.49	3.01	0.55
PG vehicle	10	0.69	0.31	2.94	3.68

Figure 12-5. (*From E. M. Stricker, Am. J. Physiol., 211:235, 1966.*)

(15, 20). In the nephrectomized hypotensive rat, renin administered systemically and angiotensin II intracranially (anterior hypothalamus) restore drinking (15, 16, 18, 20). It thus seems possible that low cardiac output, hypovolemia, and/or hypotension, by stimulating renin release from the kidney and the formation of angiotensin II, may cause thirst by a direct effect of the angiotensin II on the thirst regulatory centers in the hypothalamus.

As a corollary to these studies, Andersson and associates (17, 19) not only confirmed the dipsogenic effect of angiotensin II when infused into the hypothalamic region of the normally hydrated, trained goat, but also demonstrated that this effect was markedly potentiated by the simultaneous infusion of hypertonic NaCl. The ability of the latter to stimulate drinking in these animals was also greatly augmented by the angiotensin II. These authors suggested the possibility that angiotensin facilitates the transport of sodium into the brain cells regulating thirst and the release of AVP (see below), and that the concentration of intracellular sodium rather than strictly osmotic forces determines the activity of these cells. The earliest suggestion that the kidney is involved with thirst regulation was made by Linazasoro et al. in 1954 (30). They found that nephrectomized rats provided with water lost weight and that this loss could be prevented by giving the animals glycerine extracts of pig kidney. The authors concluded that nephrectomized rats lost weight because the sensation of thirst was impaired owing to the absence of a renal thirst factor. From all the aforementioned studies (15–19, 30), it is clear that any physiologic or pathologic change that causes the renal release of renin and the generation of angiotensin will stimulate or contribute to the stimulation of thirst and probably the release of AVP (see below). We do not know the exact neurohumoral mechanisms or chemical transmitters responsible for the activation of the hypothalamic component of thirst regulation. However, several experiments have demonstrated that the local hypothalamic application of heat and cold and cholinergic and adrenergic agents in animals can profoundly influence their relative drives for food and water and their water excretion (31–34) (Fig. 12-6A and B).

Recently, local administration of PGE (prostaglandin E) has also been used to stimulate both thirst and AVP release (35). Furthermore, PGE potentiates the action of either angiotensin or hypertonic saline on central release of AVP (36, 37). These data suggest a possible central role for PGE in the modulation of thirst and AVP release.

Warming of the hypothalamus leads to a decrease in food intake, in increase in water intake, and a decrease in urinary output, the water repletion reaction. Cooling of the hypothalamus does the reverse (Fig. 12-6C and D). In addition, systemic administration of norepinephrine directly inhibits the action of AVP on the nephron (see later discussion). Of extreme importance are the recent observations that, in contrast to norepinephrine, β-adrenergic agents such as Isuprel, when applied locally, stimulate the classic water repletion reaction, which can be completely inhibited by the simultaneous application of the β-adrenergic blocking drugs. Finally, Fitzsimons and Setler (38) have clearly demonstrated that interference with catecholaminergic systems in the diencephalon (preoptic region) by local instillation of catecholamine antagonists markedly inhibited angiotensin-induced drinking but had little effect on cholinergic (carbachol)-induced drinking. The latter was completely inhibited by atropine. These findings suggest that the final common pathway for the central effect of angiotensin on the thirst mechanism involves stimulation of the adrenergic (?β) neurotransmitters of this area of the hypothalamus.

These experimental observations should be considered when the eating, drinking, or urinary flow patterns of a given patient seem to be altered while the patient is under the influence of cholinergic or adrenergic drugs or their inhibitors or in a clinical setting in which the renin-angiotensin II system is stimulated. It is most reasonable to consider the major inhibitors of thirst as simply the opposite of those stimuli described previously and listed in Table 12-3, i.e., expansion of total body water and hypoosmolality of body fluids, isosmotic expansion of intravascular or extracellular volume. Various organic hypothalamic lesions may alter thirst to the point at which adipsia, severe hypertonic dehydration, and sustained

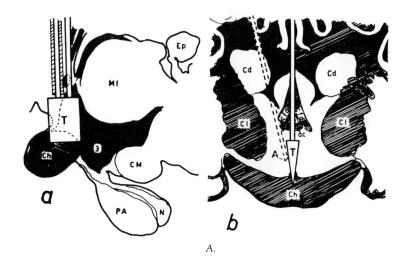

A.

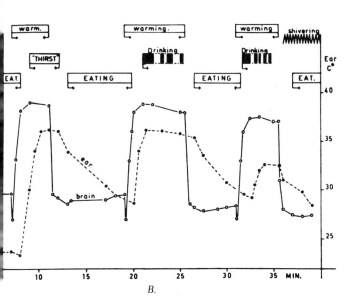

B.

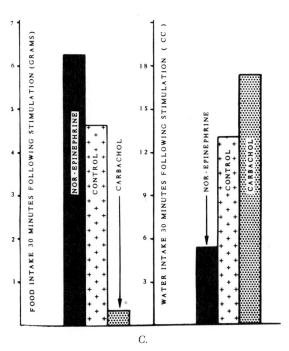

C.

Figure 12-6. *A.* Medial sagittal section through the hypothalamus (a) and a transverse section through the preoptic area of the goat (b) showing the positions of the thermode (T) and the needle applicator (A). ac. Commissura anterior; Cd, nucleus caudatus; cfd. columna fornicis descendens; Ch, chiasma opticum; Cl, capsula interna; CM, corpus mammillare; Ep, epiphysis; MI, assa intermedia; N, neurohypophysis; PA, adenohypophysis; 3, third ventricle. (*Ref. 31.*) *B.* Results of warming the preoptic area and rostral

hypothalamus in the previously hungry animal. Brain temperature was recorded close to the surface of the thermode. The goat was fed hay at the beginning of the experiment and had free access to water except during the first period of central warming. During the periods of warming eating stopped simultaneously with the onset of peripheral vasodilatation (rise of ear temperature) and started again when ear surface temperature had begun to fall after discontinuation of central warming. The perfusion of the thermode

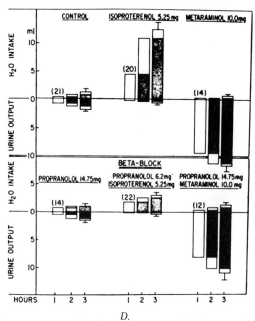

D.

with warm water induced a strong urge to drink. During the first period of central warming, when the water container was temporarily removed, it was evidenced by the animal's licking of the drops of water coming out of the outlet tubing of the thermode ("thirst") and later on by the repeated drinking of large amounts of water during the periods of central warming. (*Ref. 31.*) *C.* Effects of adrenergic and cholinergic stimulation of the hypothalamus on food and water intake of 24-h food- or water-deprived animals, during a 30-min observation period beginning 10 min after stimulation. Control levels were determined on a preceding control test without central stimulation. (*Ref. 32.*) *D.* The influence of β-adrenergic blockade upon modification of water balance by α- and β-adrenergic stimulation. All doses are in milligrams per kilogram of body weight. The blank parts on the top and bottom of the bars represent the water intake and urine output, respectively, of a particular hour, whereas the uniform shaded and black parts of the bars (water and urine, respectively) denote the total volume accumulated from all preceding periods of measurement. All values represent milliliters per animal. The figures in parentheses indicate the number of animals. The T bars represent S.E.M. (standard error of the mean). (*Ref. 34.*)

hypernatremia may occur (38, 39, 41). These lesions may be traumatic, inflammatory (i.e., encephalitis), eosinophilic granuloma, histiocytosis, internal hydrocephalus, craniopharyngioma, pinealoma, and, in rare cases, so-called essential hypernatremia with a defect in thirst regulation in which no specific lesion may be found. In some

of these patients diabetes insipidus and/or anterior pituitary insufficiency is also present. DeRubertis and his associates (39) studied a patient with a hypothalamic mass resulting from histiocytosis which had caused not only anterior pituitary insufficiency, but also an unusual pattern of posterior pituitary insufficiency. Their patient presented with sustained hypernatremia, indicating some defect in thirst regulation, but they also demonstrated that AVP was not released by changes in osmolality, but appeared to be controlled by alterations in effective blood volume (see below). They classified this disorder as "essential" hypernatremia, because mechanisms in addition to defective thirst were operative in maintaining sustained hyperosmolality. However, when a conscious individual develops hypernatremia without a desire to drink, a defect in the thirst regulatory mechanism must exist.

Polydipsia and polyuria are common symptoms in patients with chronic hypercalcemia or hypokalemic syndromes. Although a significant renal concentrating defect may contribute to the polyuria, we have noted that the polydipsia may be present despite the patient's ability to form a moderately hypertonic urine (400 to 700 mosm/L), and that the polydipsia may disappear after correction of hypercalcemia and hypokalemia long before any basic improvement in the concentrating abnormality has occurred. These observations suggest that the electrolyte disorder may cause a primary disturbance in thirst regulation. Recently, Berl et al. have confirmed this clinical observation by noting that in the potassium-depleted rat a primary polydipsia was responsible for the polyuria rather than the concentrating defect (40). Since potassium depletion now has been shown to be a strong stimulus to enhanced PGE synthesis, it is possible that this polydipsia is PGE induced. As calcium ion is a specific biologic antagonist of potassium, it would not be surprising to find that hypercalcemia also stimulates PGE synthesis.

ANTIDIURETIC HORMONE (AVP)

Through its action on the renal tubule, AVP has a fundamental role in the homeostatic regulation of the volume and osmolality of the body fluids in mammals. The integration of AVP release with the thirst mechanism is necessary to assure the maintenance of a normal water content and osmolality in the body fluids. It is readily apparent that a distortion in the thirst mechanism without a corrective response in the renal handling of water, or a primary disorder in the renal handling of water without an appropriate corrective response in the thirst mechanism, will result in a serious distortion of the volume and osmolality of body fluids.

The neurohypophyseal system

In the mammal the neurohypophyseal system responsible for the synthesis, storage, and release of AVP consists of a group of specialized hypothalamic nuclei (the supraoptic and the paraventricular) and the neurohypophyseal tract, made up of the axons originating from these nuclei and terminating in the pars nervosa or posterior lobe of the pituitary.

A discrete neural lobe with its systemic blood supply first appears phylogenetically in the amphibia (Fig. 12-7). This semiterrestrial vertebrate required a carefully regulated system for the retention and elimination of water. Its neural lobe supplies the hormone arginine vasotocin for this purpose. The neural lobe in the earlier vertebrates appeared to be a structure totally surrounded by the anterior pituitary (Fig. 12-7), and the peptides formed in this area probably served primarily as releasing factors for anterior pituitary hormones.

Neurohypophyseal peptides

Despite the absence of a distinct neural lobe, biologically active octapeptides have been identified in the neurohypophyseal extracts of lower vertebrates; these are listed in Table 12-4, reproduced from Sawyer's excellent review (42, 44). Only three of these principles were considered by Sawyer, and others, to be antidiuretic hormones: arginine vasopressin, lysine vasopressin, and arginine vasotocin. All three contain a basic amino acid in the penultimate position of the side chain, a molecular configuration responsible for their

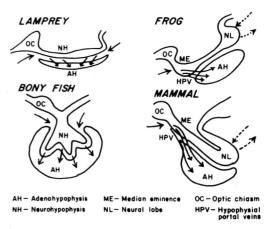

AH – Adenohypophysis   ME – Median eminence   OC – Optic chiasm
NH – Neurohypophysis   NL – Neural lobe   HPV – Hypophysial portal veins

Figure 12-7. Highly schematic diagrams of the hypophyseal circulation in four vertebrate types. Solid arrows represent blood flow from neurohypophysis to adenohypophysis. Broken arrows represent the blood flow to and from the neural lobe. [*From W. H. Sawyer et al.*, Circulation (suppl.), *21(2):1028, 1960. By permission of the American Heart Association, Inc.*]

strong antidiuretic and vasopressor properties. The remaining natural peptides resemble oxytocin more closely in that they contain a neutral amino acid in the 8-position of the side chain. These have relatively weak vasopressor and antidiuretic effects. The exact chemical structure of arginine and lysine vasopressin was determined by du Vigneaud and his associates after they defined the structure of oxytocin. As in the case of oxytocin, they confirmed the exactness of the chemical configuration by synthesizing peptides with biological properties identical to those of the natural principles which they isolated from beef and hog posterior pituitaries. Arginine vasopressin appears to be present in representative species from most of the major groups of mammals, including the egg-laying monotremes and the marsupials. Lysine vasopressin has been found only in pituitaries from members of one suborder, the Suina, which contains pigs, peccaries, and the hippopotami. All members of the other suborder of artiodactyls that have been examined, the ruminants, appear to secrete arginine vasopressin. Although lysine vasopressin occurs in all three living families of the Suina, it has not entirely replaced arginine vasopressin. One of five pituitaries from the wild boar contained arginine vasopressin as well as lysine vasopressin. This spe-

Table 12-4. The known active neurohypophyseal hormones of vertebrates

Common structure with variable amino acids in positions 3, 4, and 8 denoted by X				$1 \quad 2 \quad 3 \quad 4 \quad 5 \quad 6 \quad 7 \quad 8 \quad 9$ $Cys\text{-}Tyr\text{-}(X)\text{-}(X)\text{-}Asn\text{-}Cys\text{-}Pro\text{-}(X)\text{-}Gly\text{-}NH_2$

	AMINO ACIDS IN POSITIONS			
PRINCIPLES	3	4	8	PROBABLE PHYLETIC DISTRIBUTION
Antidiuretic vasopressor (basic) principles				
Arginine vasopressin	Phe	Gln	Arg	Most mammals
Lysine vasopressin	Phe	Gln	Lys	Suina
Arginine vasotocin	Ile	Gln	Arg	All (?) vertebrates
Oxytocinlike ("neutral") principles				
Oxytocin	Ile	Gln	Leu	Mammals, ratfish
Mesotocin	Ile	Gln	Ile	Nonmammalian tetrapods, lungfishes
Isotocin	Ile	Ser	Ile	Ray-finned fishes
Glumitocin	Ile	Ser	Gln	Rays
Valitocin	Ile	Gln	Val	Spiny dogfish, (? other sharks)
Aspartocin	Ile	Asn	Leu	Spiny dogfish, (? other sharks)

Source: W. H. Sawyer (42a).

cies is believed to be ancestral to the domestic pig, suggesting that the ability to synthesize arginine vasopressin may have been lost by domestic pigs as an indirect result of selective breeding. Since the synthesis of vasopressin is almost certainly genetically determined, this implies that the gene allowing lysine vasopressin synthesis originated by mutation, occurring in a species ancestral to the Suina. Figure 12-8 from Sawyer (42) shows the distribution of antidiuretic-vasopressor neurohypophyseal hormone among the various groups of vertebrates. In general, the bony fishes as well as the teleosts have only one neurohypophyseal hormone, that is, vasotocin. Some teleosts and holocephalians contain a second active principle, called isotocin (Table 12-4). This peptide may also be present in the lungfish. The elasmobranchs may have two different neutral peptides: (1) arginine vasotocin and (2) glumitocin (Table 12-4). Vasotocin, having the ring of oxytocin and side chain of vasopressin, produces both antidiuretic and milk-ejection effects when injected into mammals, but it is not nearly so potent in this regard as vasopressin. Vasotocin enhances water transport in the nephrons of birds, reptiles, and amphibians but not in bony fishes, cartilaginous fishes, or cyclostomes; it appears to enhance sodium excretion in these latter vertebrates (42) (Table 12-5). Extraordinarily low doses of vaso-

tocin (10^{-16} mol) have been shown to have potent effects on the contraction of the oviduct of the mud puppy (*Necturus maculosus*) during the spring of the year (44). This action of vasotocin

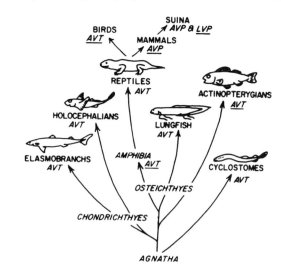

Figure 12-8. The distribution of antidiuretic-vasopressor neurohypophyseal principles among the various major groups of vertebrates. AVP, Arginine vasopressin; LVP, lysine vasopressin; AVT, arginine vasotocin. Underlining of the abbreviation indicates that the peptide has been chemically identified in at least one member of the phyletic group. (*From W. H. Sawyer, Am. J. Med., 42:678–686, 1967.*)

Table 12-5. Responses to synthetic arginine vasotocin described as occurring in representatives of the major phyletic groups of vertebrates

GROUP	URINE FLOW	FILTRATION RATE	SODIUM EXCRETION	PERMEABILITY TO WATER	
				SKIN	BLADDER
Mammals	−	0	0, +		
Birds	−	0			
Reptiles	−	−	−	. . .	0
Amphibians	−, 0	0, −	0, −	+, 0	+, 0
Lungfish	+	+	+	0	
Teleosts	+	+	+	0	
Cyclostomes	0	. . .	+	0	

Note: + means an increase; −, a decrease; 0, no change. Where two signs appear, species differ in their responses to arginine vasotocin.
Source: W. H. Sawyer (42).

reflects its oxytocic as opposed to its vasopressor properties.

Vasotocin has also been identified in the posterior pituitary of fetal mammals as well as in the pineal glands and subcommissural organs of adult mammals (45–47). The function of AVT in mammals is not known, although it has been shown to have potent antigonadotrophic and prolactin-releasing effects after intravenous or intracerebroventricular injection (48, 48a).

Osmoreceptors for AVP release

For sometime it had been felt that the magnocellular neurons in the hypothalamus were capable of sensing changes in plasma osmolality and releasing vasopressin. There is now evidence that there are multiple osmosensitive areas outside the supraoptic and paraventricular nuclei. Using microinjections of hypertonic solutions into various locations in the central nervous system. Peck and Blass (49) identified separate osmoreceptors mediating thirst and vasopressin release. The osmoreceptor centers were diffusely located within the preoptic areas and anterior hypothalamus. The electrophysiologic studies of Hayward and colleagues (vide infra) have suggested that there are different functional types of osmosensitive cells (specific and nonspecific) and that these cells are one synapse removed from the neurosecretory neurons. Van Gemert and coworkers (50) have demonstrated that lesions placed in the medial preoptic area and sparing the supraoptic nuclei resulted in polyuria and impaired vasopressin release. These observations pointed to regulatory centers for thirst and AVP release outside the neurosecretory nuclei.

Formation and storage of AVP

The posterior lobe of the pituitary is the storage site for the AVP and oxytocin formed in the nerve cell bodies in the supraoptic and paraventricular nuclei. Although the oxytocin and AVP content of the posterior pituitary are approximately equal and frequently both hormones are released together, selective release appears to occur when some physiologic stimuli are applied, i.e., hemorrhage causes AVP release, whereas distention of the cervix and suckling cause the release of oxytocin per se (see Oxytocin). In autopsy material we have found the AVP content of the posterior pituitary in humans to be 85 ± 15 U/mg relative to the U.S.P. International Standard, and others have reported approximately 15 U.S.P. units per whole human gland.

Electron microscopic and other histologic studies of the neurohypophyseal system strongly suggest that the membrane-bound neurosecretory granules which are formed by the nerve cell bodies of the supraoptic nuclei are carried by axoplasmic streaming down the axons which terminate as bulbous expansions on the basement membranes of the capillaries in the posterior lobe

(Fig. 12-9). The granules containing the peptide hormones and their carrier proteins gradually enlarge as they descend along their intra-axonal path to their storage site in the posterior lobe (Fig. 12-9).

In 1940, Rosenfeld (43), and in 1942, van Dyke et al. (51) isolated a protein from the posterior lobe of the ox pituitary gland which on bioassay showed constant oxytocic pressor and antidiuretic activities. This material often is called the "van Dyke" protein and was considered to contain the biologically active principles of the posterior lobe. In the mid-1950s, Acher and his associates (52, 53) demonstrated the relationship between the peptide hormones oxytocin and vasopressin and the cystine-rich "van Dyke" protein (extracted from bovine pituitaries). They found that oxytocin and vasopressin could be reversibly separated from the larger binding proteins, and they suggested the name neurophysin for the hormone-free proteins. The results of Acher and his associates were confirmed by Ginsburg and Ireland (54). These latter investigators, as well as Dean and Hope (55), found that the neurophysins were stored in the same subcellular organelles (neurosecretory granules) as oxytocin and vasopressin, and they have come to be regarded as the physiologic "carrier proteins" for the intraneuronal transport of the hormones from their site of synthesis the hypothalamus to the neurohypophysis. The neurophysins, isolated from the rat (56), porcine (57), bovine (57, 58), and human (59) posterior glands, are relatively small protein molecules, containing 18 different amino acids per mole and varying in molecular weight from 9500 to 10,500 g. The evidence is quite conclusive that there is a specific oxytocin- as well as a specific vasopressin-binding neurophysin (56, 57, 59–62), each mole of protein binding 1 mol of vasopressin or oxytocin. It is of considerable interest that neurohypophyseal extracts from homozygous rats with hereditary hypothalamic diabetes insipidus (Brattleboro strain) contain normal amounts of oxytocin and oxytocin-binding neurophysin, but no vasopressin or its neurophysin (56). The finding of hormone-specific neurophysins may contribute significantly to our understanding of the selective release of oxytocin and vasopressin (see below).

Sachs et al. (63), utilizing ^{35}S cysteine injections into the hypothalamus and subsequent in vitro isolation of ^{35}S-labeled vasopressin and neurophysin, have clearly documented that the biosynthesis of labeled vasopressin is paralleled by the formation of labeled neurophysin. More recently, Sachs et al. (64) confirmed these observations, utilizing supraoptic neurosecretory neurons of the guinea pig in organ culture, thus suggesting that protein and hormonal peptide might arise from a common precursor (see below). On the basis of these observations and their own studies, Burford et al. (56) have suggested that the relationship of each neurohypophyseal hormone and its relevant neurophysin is analo-

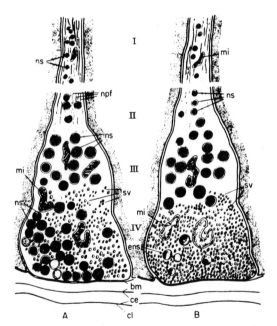

Figure 12-9. Diagram of the different regions (I, II, III, and IV) of a neurosecretory axon. *A.* A control animal. *B.* A chronically dehydrated toad. Note the release of neurosecretory material (ns) from region IV and the increase in number of synaptic vesicles (sv); npf indicates neuroprotofibrils, and mi, mitochondria. The relative size of the granules and synaptic vesicles in the different regions is maintained; bm, basement membrane; ce, capillary endothelium; cl, capillary lumen. (*From H. M. Gershenfeld et al.,* Endocrinology, 66:741, 1960.)

gous to that of insulin and peptide C. By this analogy, whereas in the β-cell of the pancreatic islet, proinsulin is split to give insulin and peptide C, in the hypothalamo-neurohypophyseal cell, provasopressin and prooxytocin would give rise to vasopressin and vasopressin neurophysin and oxytocin and oxytocin neurophysin, respectively. In 1967, Friesen and Astwood (65) suggested that these binding proteins might be secreted into the circulation because after dehydration or hypertonic saline administration in the rat, they observed a parallel decrease in the vasopressin and neurophysin content of the extracted posterior pituitary glands. Shortly thereafter, Fawcett et al. (66) were able to extract neurophysinlike proteins from cavernous sinus blood following hemorrhage. Because of the development in a number of laboratories (61, 62, 67–69) of sensitive and specific radioimmunoassays for the neurophysins, the evidence is now indisputable that neurophysin is not confined to the neurohypophysis but is released into the circulation in response to various physiologic stimuli which cause the release of vasopressin and oxytocin (see below).

In recent years, Sachs and his associates have attempted to delineate the steps in the biosynthesis of vasopressin in the hypothalamo-neurohypophyseal complex of the dog and guinea pig by use of isotope-labeling techniques (70, 71). They have proposed a precursor model for vasopressin biosynthesis in which the biosynthesis would occur solely in the perikaryon of the neurons or nerve cell body of the supraoptic nucleus. Hormone synthesis is presumably initiated on the ribosomes via pathways common to the biosynthesis of other proteins and peptides, involving transfer RNA (ribonucleic acid), messenger RNA, etc. However, Sachs et al. propose that the biosynthesis of vasopressin first leads to a bound biologically inactive form (?provasopressin) as part of a precursor molecule, and that the appearance of the biologically active nonapeptide occurs at a time and place removed from the initial biosynthetic events.

Conceivably, the release of the nonapeptide from the precursor molecule would take place during the formation and maturation of the neurosecretory granule. The most convincing evidence in favor of the "precursor molecule model" has come from labeling experiments carried out in vitro with guinea pig hypothalamo-median eminence tissue. As in the case of the in vivo isotope experiments, the incorporation of ^{35}S- and ^{3}H-labeled amino acids into vasopressin was preceded by a lag period of about 1-h duration. If the slices were removed from the initial incubation medium after the first hour of incubation, and reincubated in fresh buffer, labeled hormone appeared under conditions which precluded further de novo peptide bond synthesis. Furthermore, the release of labeled vasopressin from a labeled precursor can take place in a cell-free system. Although the biosynthesis of labeled precursor formed during the first hour of slice incubation was inhibited by puromycin, the release of hormone from precursor was not inhibited by this drug.

Figure 12-10, reproduced from Sachs's article, is a schematic representation of his concept of the intermediate stages involved in the neurosecretory function of the vasopressin-producing cells of the mammalian neurohypophysis. Using the radioisotope-labeling model of hormone biosynthesis, Sachs and his associates demonstrated that if prolonged water deprivation (4 days) were applied to the intact guinea pig prior to the removal of the neurohypophyseal tissues, it was the consistent finding that the neurohypophyseal tissue incorporated two to five times more radioactivity in the newly synthesized vasopressin than these same tissues from guinea pigs with free access to water, thus suggesting that the prolonged maintenance of nerve impulses effective in the release of vasopressin is probably also translated into sustained synthesis of the hormone. It is probable, therefore, that all stimuli which enhance release of AVP also enhance its synthesis (Table 12-3). It is of great interest that a species of rat (Brattleboro strain) with congenital vasopressin-sensitive diabetes insipidus has enormously enlarged supraoptic nuclei which, on chemical analysis, contain little or no AVP (72). Therefore, although the hormone-forming neurons exist, some specific chemical defect prevents their synthesis of AVP.

The posterior lobe receives its blood supply

from and secretes its hormone directly into the systemic circulation.

Neurophysiology of AVP secretion

The introduction of methods capable of recording electrical activity in a single magnocellular neuron and of confirming the identity of these cells by antidromic stimulation has provided many insights into the regulation of neurosecretion (73). Hayward and coworkers identified two distinct cell types on the basis of their response to infusion of hypertonic saline (74). Cells with a monophasic pattern of activity that were stimulated by hyperosmolality, but were not affected by noxious stimuli, were thought to be the specific osmore-

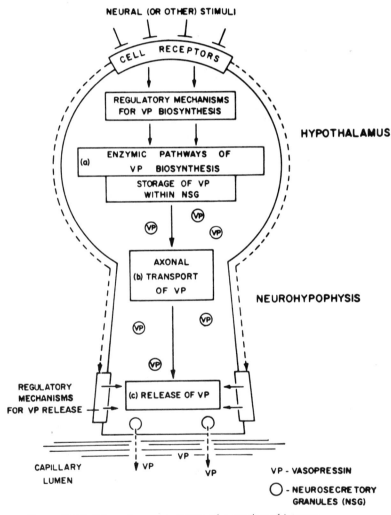

Figure 12-10. Schematic representation of a number of intermediate stages involved in the neurosecretory function of the vasopressin-producing cells of the mammalian hypothalamo-neurohypophyseal complex. [*From H. Sachs et al. (70).*]

ceptors of Verney which are involved in AVP release; cells with a similar specificity, but having a biphasic response pattern, were felt to be the magnocellular neurons. Alternately, cells that responded to either osmotic or noxious stimuli were designated osmoreceptors of Sawyer (Fig. 12-11*a* and 11*b*). It was speculated that these were important in the drinking and behavioral aspects of osmoregulation. In other studies, the magnocellular neurons were characterized on the basis of their firing pattern into three groups: silent, phasic (bursting), or continuously active. Several groups have described modification in the firing patterns of these neurons in response to various stimuli (75, 76, 76a). This suggests that the firing pattern. is in part a reflection of the state of activity of the

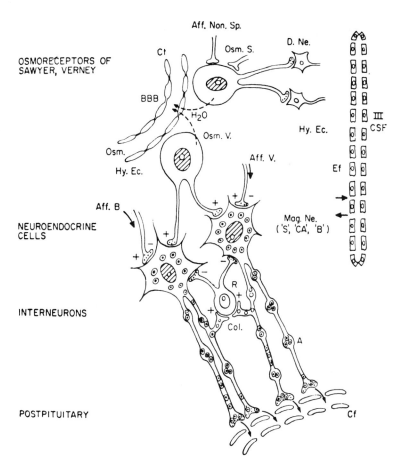

Figure 12-11. Schematic drawing of the hypothalamo-neurohypophyseal system. The osmoreceptors of Verney (Osm. V.) are seen as anatomically discrete cells whose axons project to the magnocellular neurons (Mag. Ne.) in the hypothalamus. The latter cells then project to the posterior pituitary. Also shown are the osmoreceptors of Sawyer (Osm. S.) which respond not only to changes in osmolality but also to noxious stimuli (Aff. Non. Sp.). Axons from afferent neurons sensing changes in blood volume (Aff. V.) and axons from afferents related to behavioral stimuli (Aff. B.) are shown projecting to the magnocellular neurons. [*From J. N. Hayward, Neurohumoral regulation of neuroendocrine cells in the hypothalamus, in K. Lederis (ed.), Recent Studies of Hypothalamic Function, S. Karger, AG Basel, 1974, pp. 166–179. (Reproduced with permission.)*]

neuron. There is evidence, however, that a phasic firing pattern appears to be associated with vasopressin-secreting cells and a random firing pattern with oxytocin-secreting cells (76a). Data from such neurophysiologic studies have suggested that the specific neurons which synthesize and secrete vasopressin and oxytocin are distributed in both the supraoptic and paraventricular nuclei (Fig. 12-11a). At the present time, no specific functions can be attributed totally to one or the other nucleus.

Considerable progress in unraveling the physiology of AVP secretion has come about in recent years through utilization of techniques for histochemical identification of neurosecretory neurons. The use of specific antibodies to arginine vasopressin, oxytocin, and neurophysins has facilitated histologic identification not only of magnocellular (secretory) neurons but has also resulted in delineation of additional pathways of AVP secretion in the hypothalamus. Immunohistochemical studies of hypothalamic nuclei have confirmed the intermingling of vasopressin- and oxytocin-secreting neurons in both the supraoptic and paraventricular nuclei as described above (76b). The bulk of the evidence from such studies seems to support the concept of one neurosecretory neuron producing either vasopressin and its neurophysin or oxytocin and its neurophysin (76b, 77). These studies have also permitted identification of fiber tracts (Fig.12-11a) from the neurosecretory nuclei other than those traversing the

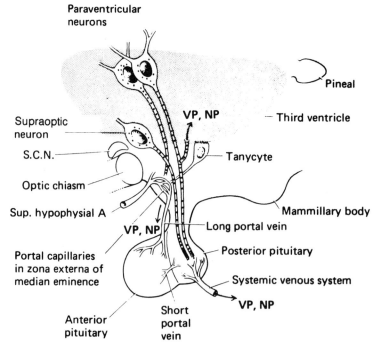

Figure 12-11a. Anatomic drawing of the mammalian hypothalamus and pituitary, sagital view, depicting pathways secreting vasopressin (VP) and neurophysin (NP). Pathways are seen from the hypothalamic nuclei to the posterior pituitary, the zona externa of the median eminence, and the third ventricle. [*From E. A. Zimmerman and A. G. Robinson (76b).*]

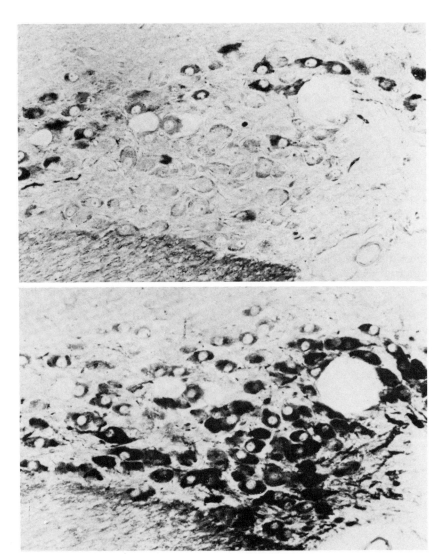

Figure 12-11b. Adjacent 5-μmol coronal sections of the supraoptic nucleus of a normal rat reacted for oxytocin (A) and vasopressin (B) by immunoperoxidase technique. Oxytocin-containing cells are concentrated in one dorsal part of the nucleus whereas vasopressin cells are found diffusely distributed throughout the nucleus with most intense staining seen in the ventral portion. Some cells are reactive for both hormones. ($\times$ 260). (*From E. A. Zimmerman and R. Defendini, Hypothalamic pathways containing oxytocin vasopressin and associated neurophysins,* International Conference on the Neurohypophysis, *Key Biscayne, Florida, S. Karger, AG Basel, Nov. 14–19, 1976. In press.*)

pituitary stalk. One of these tracts projects to the zona externa of the median eminence and appears to be responsible for the very high concentration of AVP found in hypophyseal portal blood (78).

Staining in this area was greatly increased in adrenalectomized rats who also had significant elevations of plasma AVP (79). These observations suggest a possible role for AVP along with other hypothalamic factors in modulating corticotrophin secretion. There is also evidence suggesting transport of AVP from the neurosecretory neurons to the third ventricle. Studies in our laboratory have shown that hemorrhage provokes a significant rise in both plasma and CSF (cerebrospinal fluid) AVP concentrations, albeit to a lesser extent in the latter (80). Such elevations did not occur after intravenous administration of AVP which suggests that AVP was actively secreted into the CSF. This is supported by the failure of intravenously administered tritiated oxytocin to cross the blood-CSF barrier (81). The vasopressin present in the CSF may play some role in memory consolidation. Van Wimersma Greidanus et al. have demonstrated that injection of vasopressin into the third ventricle increased resistance to the extinction of a conditioned avoidance response. Memory consolidation was inhibited by injection of antivasopressin antiserum into the third ventricle (82). They suggested that hypothalamic pathways can transport AVP to the infundibular recess of the third ventricle where it can be released into the CSF and influence memory processes related to behavioral homeostasis.

Secretion or release of AVP

The release of AVP into the circulation, regardless of the stimulus, is dependent on depolarizing impulses arising in the supraoptic nuclei and propagated down the axon to its hormone-storing terminal ending in the posterior lobe (10). The "pores" in the capillaries of the neural lobe have a diameter of approximately 30 to 74 μm or 300 to 750 Å, whereas the intact neurosecretory granules in the neural lobe have a diameter of from 1600 to as large as 5000 Å (10). This difference in size suggests that the intact granule cannot be released as such into the circulation. However, the elegant electron microscopic and biochemical studies of Douglas and his associates (83–86) have clearly reconciled this difference as well as defined the nature of the cellular events involved in the secretion of posterior pituitary hormones.

Earlier studies (83, 87, 88) suggested that on stimulation of the neurohypophysis the granules stored in the nerve ending (Fig. 12-9) release their contents in the form of a molecular dispersion which allows the hormones to traverse the cytoplasm and the plasma membrane of the nerve ending to reach the extracellular space and from there the capillary lumen. Douglas and associates (83–86) point out that all previously proposed schemes have had in common this concept of an "intracellular" mechanism responsible for the dissociation of the hormones from their intracellular sites of storage or binding and the subsequent transport, possibly by molecular diffusion across the various plasma membrane barriers, into the circulation. Douglas et al. (83–86) have convincingly concluded from their electron microscopic evidence that the neurosecretory granules discharge their contents directly on the cell exterior by the process of exocytosis (Figs. 12-12 and 12-13), beginning with fusion of the granules with the plasma membrane, and the subsequent formation of an opening which communicates with the extracellular space. This mode of secretion is most consistent with the observations (61, 62, 67–69) that the hormone-binding protein neurophysin, in the neurosecretory granules, escapes into the circulation with the hormones when the posterior pituitary gland is stimulated.

From their excellent studies these investigators (83–86) have further proposed that the "synaptic vesicles," which accumulate at the nerve endings after the release of AVP and oxytocin (Fig. 12-9), arise as byproducts of secretion by exocytosis. These electron-lucent structures, about one-fifth to one-fourth the diameter of the neurosecretory granules, were called synaptic vesicles by Paley (89), since their size, appearance, and distribution were similar to those of the synaptic vesicles in ordinary neurons. Paley and others suggested that they participate in hormone release. Douglas has conclusively shown that the "synaptic vesicles" form by inward-budding endocytosis of the cell surface, mainly at the base of the exocytotic pit. The microvesicles so formed are thought to move away from the membrane, aggregate, and migrate centripetally in the fiber away from the terminal region of membrane engaged in hormone extrusion (Figs. 12-12 and 12-13). Through this mechanism "surplus" plasma membrane, made available by the incorporation of the membrane of the neurosecretory granule into that of the axon terminal (Fig. 12-12), can be disposed of.

Douglas and Poisner have shown that when the neural lobe is incubated in vitro and stimulated (depolarized) electrically or by high extracellular concentrations of potassium, the actual release of the hormone is strongly calcium ion dependent (90). Depolarization caused an increased uptake of ^{45}Ca by the neural lobe, and the secretion rate waned with the calcium content of the extracel-

lular environment. They proposed the following steps: (1) propagation of impulse, after specific stimulus, down the neurohypophyseal stalk from supraoptic nuclei; (2) depolarization of neurosecretory axon terminals by impulses; (3) influence of calcium ion across the axon's plasma membrane; and (4) activation of some calcium-dependent exocytotic process leading to hormone extrusion.

An extremely important concept relative to the

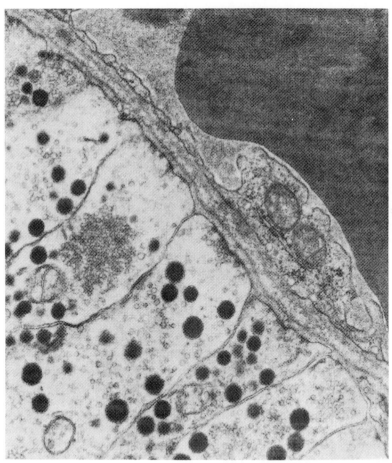

Figure 12-12. Neurosecretory terminals abutting on a capillary containing (upper right) a red blood cell. The arrangement is conventional, with the terminal regions of the neurons separated from the fenestrated capillary wall by the parenchymal and endothelial basement membranes. The terminals show evidence of secretory activity: paucity of large electron-dense neurosecretory granules and abundance of microvesicles ("synaptic vesicles"). Note (1) the absence of large electron-lucent vesicles; (2) the depressions and dense "thickenings" of the plasma membrane of the terminals facing the capillary, sometimes associated (see central neuron) with clusters of microvesicles. Hamster. ($\times$ 30,000). [*From W. W. Douglas, J. Nagasawa, and R. Schulz (83)*.]

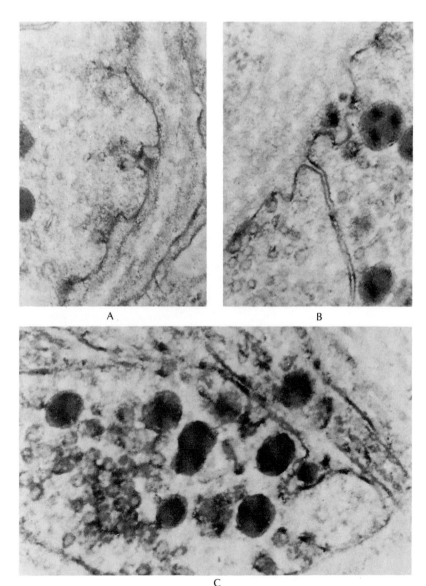

Figure 12-13. Higher-power views of neurosecretory terminals, showing pits in the plasma membranes and extracellular dense material. *A,* An ending with four distinct pits, each associated with a cluster of microvesicles and one containing electron-dense material lying extracellularly between plasma membrane and parenchymal basement membrane. Hamster. ($\times$ 60,000). *B,* Two neurosecretory terminals. The lower shows a small caveolus and adjacent to it a cluster of microvesicles subjacent to a region of the membrane showing increased density. The upper terminal shows a pit containing electron-dense material. The pit has a small caveolus at its base. This, in conjunction with the subjacent mi-crovesicle (of the coated variety), is suggestive of inward budding (endocytosis) at the base of the exocytotic pit. Hamster. ($\times$ 58,000). *C,* A small nerve terminal with several features believed characteristic of secreting neurons. Note (1) exocytotic pit containing electron-dense material. The base of the pit is budding inward and shows a coated caveolus; (2) above and to the left of this a coated pit; (3) below, on the nerve membrane opposed to the parenchymal basement membrane, two regions associated with clusters of microvesicles. Hamster. ($\times$ 88,000). [*From W. W. Douglas, J. Nagasawa, and R. Schulz (83).*]

characteristics of the release of large amounts of AVP from the neurohypophysis is that derived from the experiments of Sachs and associates (91). Acute hemorrhagic hypotension is one of the most powerful stimuli for the immediate release of antidiuretic hormone. Within a few minutes after reduction of blood pressure of dogs to 50 mmHg by bleeding, there is a rapid discharge of arginine vasopressin into the blood. In the presence of a maintained stimulus of hemorrhagic hypotension, the initial secretory response is not sustained beyond the first few minutes of hemorrhage. Reinfusion of the shed blood, after 30 min of hemorrhage, restored the arterial pressure and the blood AVP concentration to relatively normal values. A second hemorrhage 1 h later failed to raise the concentration of blood AVP beyond the level observed just prior to blood reinfusion. Direct analysis of the pituitary gland showed that the decline in the release of AVP during hemorrhage could not be attributed to exhaustion of the pituitary content of AVP. Furthermore, AVP release did not appear to be a simple function of the total hormone content of the gland. Nevertheless, this attenuation of AVP release appears to reside, in part, at the level of the pituitary. Pituitaries taken from bled dogs released much less AVP in vitro in response to electrical or potassium stimulation than pituitaries from nonbled animals. Electron microscopic studies showed that the fine structure of the neural lobe from intact and bled dogs was similar in appearance, and there was no difference in the isolated specimen. Analogous results were obtained under circumstances (carotid perfusion and section of the vagi) in which hemorrhage failed to elicit an appreciable discharge of AVP.

It is suggested as a working hypothesis that the pool of neurohypophyseal AVP is heterogenous and that there is a readily releasable pool which comprises about 10 to 20 percent of the total hormone content of the gland (91). Once this readily releasable pool of hormone has been discharged, the neurohypophysis continues to release arginine vasopressin in response to appropriate stimuli, but at a greatly reduced rate. Analysis of the amount of hormone·remaining in the pituitary at the termination of these experiments showed values which ranged from 2500 to 7000 mU of vaso-

pressin per gland. There was no apparent correlation between the amount of AVP released during the second hemorrhage and the amount of hormone found in the gland.

Quantitative aspects of secretion

From studies utilizing bioassay of the hormone or its infusion at varying rates in water-loaded humans (92–94), one may conclude that in the normal ambulatory adult human, the mild, sustained osmotic and nonosmotic stimuli cause the release of approximately 150 μU/min per m^2 or 200 mU per 24 h/m^2 of AVP into the circulation. This is associated with a urinary osmolality of 500 to 1000 mosm/L. During sustained dehydration (24 to 48 h), with maximally concentrated urine, this probably increases at least three to five times (11–13, 92, 94, 95). Therefore, in a 24-h period a normal dehydrated human (1.73 m^2) will secrete between 1 and 2 units while maintaining a maximally concentrated urine. Stimuli such as severe pain, hemorrhage, or an acute decrease in cardiac output may cause a 50- to 100-fold increase in the rate of secretion (9, 93). For orientation it may be recalled that the commercially available aqueous Pitressin contains 20 U/mL, whereas Pitressin tannate in oil contains 5 U/mL; 1 mg of the pure nonapeptide contains approximately 400 to 450 U.

The direct assay of antidiuretic hormone in the plasma of normal subjects in various states of hydration and the simultaneous measurement of plasma and urinary osmolality allow one to determine the relationship between concentrating ability and a given level of AVP in the circulation (9, 11, 13, 92, 94). Segar and Moore (13) and Moore (12) graphed this relationship in a large number of subjects, from undetectable levels during water diuresis to values as high as 20 μU/mL during 24 to 48 h of dehydration. They found that in the state of normal hydration, at AVP concentrations around 1.5 to 2.0 μU/mL, the U/P (urinary-to-plasma) osmolar ratio varied from 1 to a high of 4. The sigmoid nature of their entire curve (Fig. 12-14) suggests that between 1 and 3 μU/mL small changes in plasma AVP will cause relatively large changes in the U/P osmolar ratio,

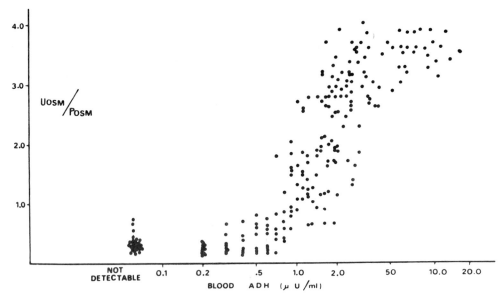

Figure 12-14. Relationship between blood ADH concentration and U_{osm}/P_{osm} in humans; 203 pairs of data are shown. [*From W. W. Moore, (12).*]

whereas above 4 μU/mL urinary concentration will change only slightly as circulating AVP levels approach their highest value during dehydration (13). A similar plot of plasma AVP versus urine osmolality by Thomas and Lee (96) shows that urine osmolality varies as a linear function of log plasma AVP. This is in keeping with the log dose response curve for AVP versus renal medullary adenylate cyclase. Thus, from this curve and other available data (11–13, 92, 94, 97), it is apparent that maximal renal conservation of water can be achieved by the release of only moderate amounts of AVP. Higher rates of secretion, which would increase the plasma AVP concentration above 4 μU/mL, would not influence further the maximal concentrating capacity in the dehydrated subject. This ability to produce the most concentrated urine at rates of AVP secretion far below maximal is due to the increased "efficiency" of the vascular and countercurrent mechanisms in the kidney responsible for the production of the hypertonicity of the renal medulla. This intrarenal "adaptation" allows for a further renal conservation of water without the need for further secretion of AVP. This is strik-

ingly apparent in the experiments of Valtin (72) and Miller and Moses (97) in rats with congenital diabetes insipidus that are unable to form AVP, yet in which progressive dehyration causes the urine osmolality to rise from its usual hypotonic level of 150 to 200 mosm/L to a peak of 1100 to 1200 mosm/L, thus emphasizing the importance of nonhormonal factors in the production of a maximally concentrated urine (see below).

Osmotic and nonosmotic stimuli to AVP secretion

In Table 12-3 are listed the known stimuli and inhibitors of the release of AVP. The final common pathway for all these, regardless of their nature, is the nerve cell bodies of the hypothalamic supraoptic nuclei. The rate of hormone release at any moment will be controlled by the algebraic sum of the stimulating and inhibiting impulses impinging on the final common pathway. From this concept it is easy to understand how the same osmotic stimulus, i.e., a given increase in effective plasma osmolality, can be associated with different rates of secretion of AVP, depending on the other impulses of nonosmotic origin impinging on the supraoptic nuclei. The most common physiologic factor altering the osmolality of the blood is water depletion or water excess. The former causes a rise in the tonicity of all body fluids and cellular hydration, whereas the latter causes the reverse. The osmoreceptor neurons, in com-

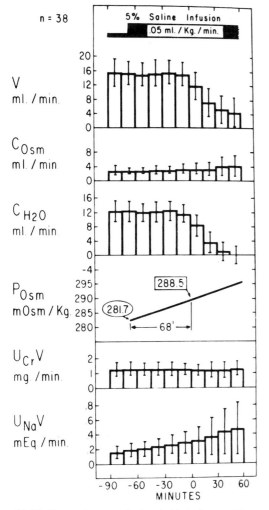

Figure 12-15. Composite osmotic threshold studies on 38 normal subjects. Mean osmotic threshold in mosm per kg is entered in rectangle and mean plasma osmolality at the beginning of the rapid saline solution infusion is entered in ellipse. Bars and brackets represent mean ± standard deviation for urinary volume, osmolal clearance, free water clearance, creatinine excretion, and sodium excretion. Time intervals are expressed in relation to the time of the osmotic threshold. [*From A. M. Moses et al. (98).*]

mon with all body cells, share in this change in intracellular volume. The latter is probably responsible for altering the electrical activity of these neurons and thus the release of AVP. If the tonicity or osmolality of all body fluids is chronically increased by the administration of a solute such as urea that freely penetrates all body cells, no change in intracellular volume will occur and AVP release will not be stimulated. In contrast, an increase in the osmotic pressure of only 2 percent, caused by the administration of hypertonic saline during a water diuresis, will cause the immediate release of a quantity of AVP sufficient to cause a marked antidiuresis (Fig. 12-15) (98, 99), whereas a comparable decrease in osmotic pressure, secondary to a water load, will stop the release of AVP and produce a maximal water diuresis *unless AVP release is maintained by some nonosmotic stimulus* (Fig. 12-16). The concept of the osmotic control of AVP and its subsequent effect on the nephron was painstakingly developed in the dog experiments of Verney and his associates, presented in his outstanding Croonian lectures (100). These represent the most fundamental work in this field and are a lucid, exciting description of the scientific approach to the clarification of a complicated physiologic feedback system.

Robertson and coworkers have plotted concomitant levels of plasma AVP and osmolality in a large number of subjects or experimental animals and showed that they were related by the function plasma AVP = k (plasma osmolality − X), where k was the slope of the regression line and X was the X intercept (Fig. 12-17) (101, 101a). They proposed that the X intercept represented the "osmotic threshold" which was the critical level of osmolality at which AVP secretion would be stimulated (101, 101a). The threshold concept had been proposed earlier by Moses et al. on the basis of the abrupt onset of a decrease in free water clearance in water-loaded subjects undergoing an infusion of hypertonic saline (99).

Alternative theories on the osmotic control of AVP secretion have been proposed. Studies in our laboratory have suggested that instead of a discrete level of plasma osmolality above which AVP secretion would be initiated, there was rather a continuous relationship between the logarithm of

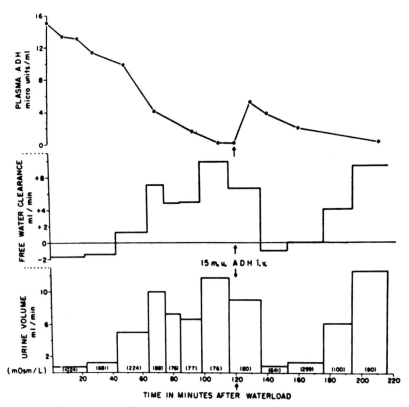

Figure 12-16. Effect of a sustained oral water load (2000 mL), followed by the intravenous injection of AVP, on the plasma level of ADH and the parameters of a maximal water diuresis. (*From J. W. Czaczkes and C. R. Kleeman, J. Clin. Invest., 43:1625–1640, 1964.*)

plasma AVP and plasma osmolality (Fig. 12-18 *a* and *b*) (102). This type of relationship also appears to exist between log plasma AVP and blood volume after hemorrhage (101a).

Several Scandinavian investigators have raised the question of whether a nonspecific alteration in osmolality was the factor responsible for initiation of thirst or AVP release. Eriksson and coworkers showed that intracarotid injection of hypertonic glycerol or galactose failed to produce an antidiuresis comparable to that occurring after injection of hypertonic saline or sucrose (103). Similarly, injections of hypertonic saline into the lateral ventricles of the brain produced intense hyperdipsia and antidiuresis, while hypertonic solutions of sucrose, D-glucose, or glycerol brought about increased free water clearance (104, 105).

This effect of cerebroventricular infusion of sodium on thirst and antidiuresis could be potentiated by concomitant administration of angiotensin II (104). These results suggested the presence of a central sensitive receptor near the third ventricle which was capable of controlling both thirst and AVP secretion. It appeared that angiotensin enhanced sodium transport to the regulatory structures or sensitized them in some fashion. The contradictions between this hypothesis and the more general osmoreceptor hypothesis have not been resolved.

The osmotic stimulation of AVP secretion can be significantly modified by changes in body fluid volumes. Both the apparent osmotic threshold and the sensitivity (slope) of the osmolality-plasma AVP relationship were shown to be altered by modification of ECF or plasma volumes (Fig. 12-19). Hypovolemia in experimental animals resulted in lowering of the osmotic threshold, while the slope of the response relationship became steeper (101a). In later studies in humans, upright posture was shown to lower the osmotic threshold compared to the recumbent posture (106). In these studies there was no significant change in the slope. Intravenous infusion of angiotensin II in dogs significantly steepened the slope of the relationship between plasma osmolality and plasma AVP and served to potentiate osmotically stimulated AVP release (107). These

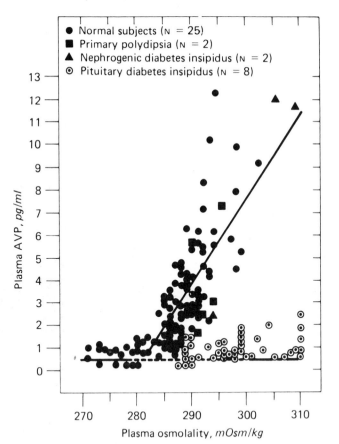

Figure 12-17. Plot of plasma AVP and plasma osmolality in a series of normal subjects as well as those with primary polydipsia, nephrogenic diabetes insipidus, and pituitary diabetes insipidus. The best-fit regression line is shown with the solid line. (*From G. L. Robertson, R. L. Shelton, and S. Athar, Kidney Int., 10:25–37, 1976.*)

observations suggested an interaction of osmolar and volume factors so that AVP secretion at any moment is controlled by the algebraic sum of the stimulating and inhibiting impulses impinging on the final common pathway (Fig. 12-20).

From the above, the importance of volume as well as osmolality of the body fluids in the control of the secretion of AVP is immediately apparent. A change in vascular and/or extracellular volume exerts its effect through baro- or pressor receptor mechanisms somewhere in the circulation. In Table 12-3, under 2a and 2b, these receptors have been listed. In recent years, an increasing number of investigators have devoted their attention to delineating the nature of the reflex arcs activated by these receptors (9, 10–14, 17, 19, 23–25, 27, 39, 108–110).

These receptors are located in the carotid sinus, the aortic arch, the left atrium and great pulmonary veins, and probably the juxtaglomerular apparatus of the kidney (17, 19, 23–25, 110). As baroreceptors they respond to tension developed in the wall of the receptor organ rather than to the volume of blood per se; in other words, the higher the compliance (less change in mural tension for any given change in volume), the less will be the stimulation or inhibition of the receptor. The afferent limbs of the first three of these neurohumoral arcs are the ninth or glossopharyngeal nerves from the carotid sinus, the aortic nerves for the aorta, and the tenth or vagus nerve from the wall of the left atrium and great veins. Their impulses ascend from the medulla by way of the reticular formation of the midbrain and diencephalon to the supraoptic nuclei in the hypothalamus. A *decrease* in afferent impulses from these baroreceptors, caused by the stimuli listed in Table 12-3 under 2a and 2b, brings about an *increase* in the secretion of AVP; conversely, an *increase* in the afferent impulses caused by the inhibitors listed in 4a and 4b will *decrease* the secretion of AVP.

Section of the thoracic or cervical vagi, and denervation of the carotid sinus, will completely block these nonosmotic stimuli to the release of ADH. Similarly, denervation of the vagus will lead to a more exaggerated rise in the circulating level of AVP when a stimulus is applied which lowers pressure in the carotid sinuses as well as

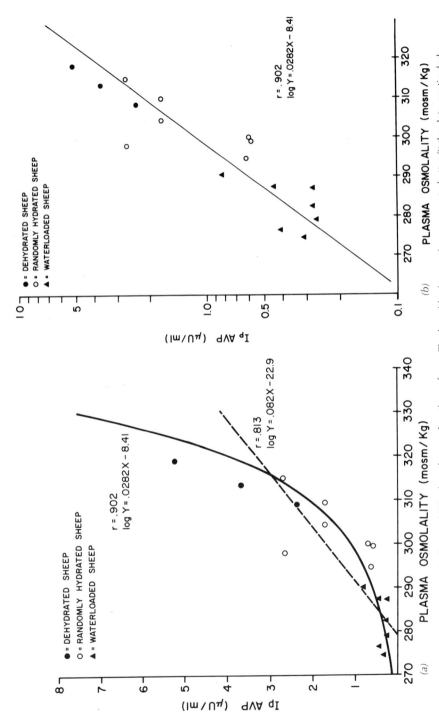

Figure 12-18. Integrated plasma AVP plotted as a function of plasma osmolality in sheep. (a) Each point represents the mean or integrated plasma AVP concentration determined from 10 samples collected at 3-min intervals. The best fit for the equation AVP = $k_1 P_{osm} + b$ is shown with the dashed line, while the best fit for the equation log AVP = $k_2 P_{osm} + b$ is shown with the solid line.

The logarithmic equation appears to better fit the data, particularly at the extremes of plasma osmolality. (b) The data are replotted in a similar fashion except that log AVP is shown as a function of plasma osmolality. (*From R. E. Weitzman and D. A. Fisher, Am. J. Phys., 233:E36–E40, 1977.*)

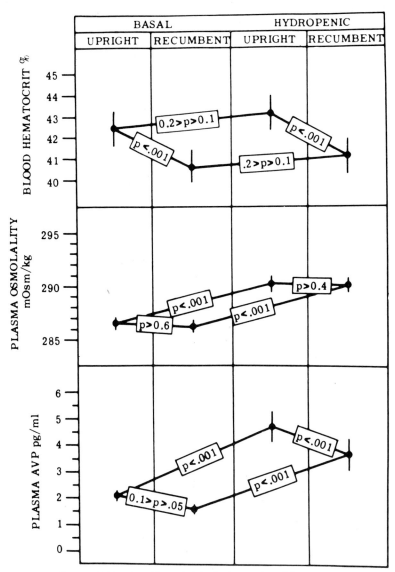

Figure 12-19. The effect of dehydration and upright posture on plasma AVP, osmolality, and hematocrit in humans. A significant rise in plasma AVP in the upright posture compared to the recumbent posture is only seen when the subjects were hydropenic. [*From G. L. Robertson and S. Athar (106).*]

the great veins of the thorax and the left atrium (Fig. 12-21). Conversely, if the pressure in the carotid sinus is maintained despite a fall in cardiac output or blood volume, there will be a significantly lesser increment or a prevention of rise in the circulating level of antidiuretic hormone. Share, in his classic studies, has shown that within a few minutes after reduction of blood pressure of dogs to 50 mmHg by bleeding, there is a rapid discharge of vasopressin AVP into the

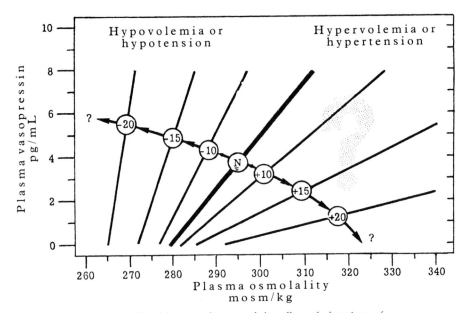

Figure 12-20. Schematic diagram of the effect of alterations of blood volume or pressure on the relationship between plasma osmolality and plasma AVP. Decreased blood volume or blood pressure appear to enhance vasopressin release at any particular level of plasma osmolality, while increased blood volume has the opposite effect. (*From G. L. Robertson, R. L. Shelton, and S. Athar, Kidney Int., 10:25–37, 1976.*)

blood (9, 109). Carotid perfusion to maintain a high pulse pressure, in the vagotomized dog, prevented this discharge (Fig. 12-22).

Independent of its effect on renal hemodynamics, contraction of the extracellular or plasma volume without an alteration in the tonicity of the body fluids may cause a striking release of AVP. Positive-pressure breathing, which decreases the intrathoracic blood volume, causes a significant release of AVP. Similarly, negative-pressure breathing with a rise in intrathoracic volume is followed by a typical water diuresis. This volume receptor, or more correctly baroreceptor, in the left atrium or great pulmonary veins, appears to be extremely sensitive to small shifts in volume or tension.

Alterations in posture have been thought to modify AVP secretion in humans. Moore and co-workers demonstrated significant elevation in plasma AVP in humans upon assumption of upright posture (12, 13). The large changes in

bioassayable AVP concentration that they observed have not been confirmed in more recent studies using radioimmunoassay. Robertson and Athar were able to show an increase in upright plasma AVP compared to supine only in dehydrated subjects (Fig. 12-19) (106). They did show that upright posture influenced the relationship between plasma osmolality and plasma AVP by lowering the apparent osmotic threshold (vide supra). In contrast, upright posture produced by head-up tilting produced significant elevations of plasma AVP (111). This occurred in a biphasic pattern with a small initial increase after 10 min of 85° of tilt followed by a substantially larger increase after 45 min. The initial hypovolemic stimulus appeared to be due to venous pooling which led to transudation of protein-free fluid through dependent vascular beds and the later decline in plasma volume. Therefore, it appears that posture (the upright position) exerts a tonic nonosmotic stimulus to the sustained neurohypophy-

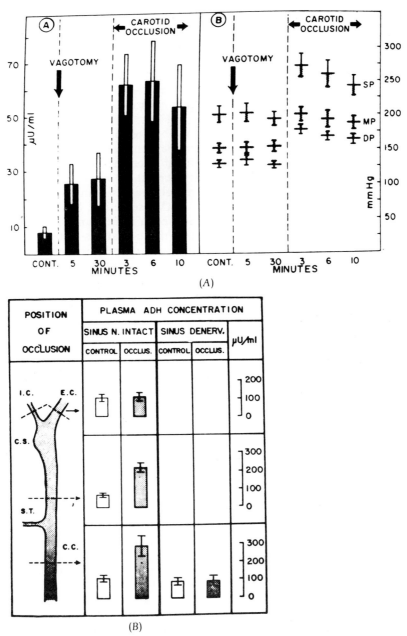

Figure 12-21. *A.* Effect of bilateral cervical vagotomy followed by occlusion of both common carotid arteries on (A) blood titer of ADH, and (B) femoral arterial systolic (SP), mean (MP), and diastolic (DP) pressures. Means ± S.E. for seven experiments in (A), six experiments in (B), (*Ref. 9.*) *B.* The effect of partial ligation of the carotid artery, above and below the carotid sinus, on plasma ADH with and without sinus denervation. (*From S. Chien, et al., The reflex nature of release of antidiuretic hormone upon common carotid occlusion in vagotomized dogs, Proc. Soc. Exptl. Biol. Med., 111:193–196, 1962.*)

seal-released AVP, and, when one reclines, this stimulus is lessened, AVP secretion decreases, and a mild diuresis of more dilute urine occurs. Recently, Epstein and his associates have clearly demonstrated that head-out immersion in humans creates an antigravity model whose cardiovascular (and renal) effects closely simulate those of the reclining position. In one of their studies they determined urinary AVP excretion in 10 normal subjects undergoing immersion after 14 h

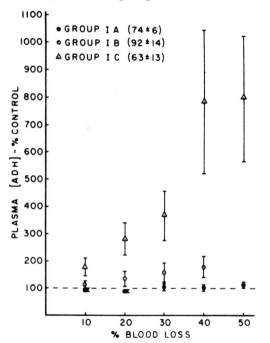

Figure 12-22. Effect of hemorrhage on the concentration of ADH in plasma, when the carotid sinuses were perfused with a high pulse pressure. The concentration of ADH in the first plasma sample of each experiment is taken as 100 percent. The ADH concentrations in subsequent samples are expressed as percent of the concentration in this first sample. These values are indicated on the ordinate. The abscissa is the degree of blood loss, expressed as percent of the initial blood volume, which was estimated to be 8 percent of the body weight. The lines extending above and below the symbols indicate ± S.E. The figures in parentheses are the concentrations of ADH in the initial blood samples in microunits per milliliter plasma (mean ± S.E.). There were 6 experiments in group 1A, 8 in group 1B, and 8 in group 1C. Group 1A, control group; group 1B, perfused, with high pulse pressure during hemorrhage; group 1C, hemorrhage. [*From L. Share (109).*]

of overnight water restriction. The immersion resulted in a progressive decrease in AVP secretion from 80 ± 7 to 37 ± 6 μU/min during the recovery hour (112).

Zehr, et al. (14), by carrying out detailed studies on normal, unanesthetized sheep, concluded that senstive osmo- and volume (baro-) receptors exist that are concerned with the regulation of AVP secretion. At the stimulus levels employed in their studies, neither receptor system was dominant over the other and under normal circumstances they act in concert to maintain the osmolality and volume of the ECF via their effect on AVP secretion. Similar conclusions have been arrived at in humans (112a). It is of great interest that those changes in the circulation and the volume and distribution of body fluids which stimulate the baroreceptors of the carotid sinus and left atrium (Table 12-3) are also the changes that bring about the release of renin by stimulating the juxtaglomerular apparatus of the kidneys, and thereby the production of angiotensin. If angiotensin, through its direct action on hypothalamic centers, cannot only stimulate thirst but can also augment the release of AVP (17, 19, 23–25, 110), we now must consider an additional regulatory system making its contribution to the modulating impulses impinging on the final common pathway, the supraoptic neurons. The tonic nature of the stimuli arising from the upright position can be readily demonstrated by observing the increase in flow of a more hypotonic urine which almost invariably follows the assumption of a reclining position. From this, one would expect a similar diuresis to develop after the subject has retired for the night. However, this is not observed and, on the contrary, the sleeping hours are fortunately accompanied by a period of antidiuresis associated with an elevated plasma concentration of AVP (113). The mechanism responsible for the nocturnal antidiuresis obviously overrides the inhibitory stimulus of the reclining position per se. This nocturnal antidiuresis is only in part explained by the nocturnal decrease in glomerular filtration rate and solute excretion.

Many disease states, particularly those associated with a tendency toward salt and water retention (i.e., cirrhosis, cardiac failure, nutritional edema, nephrosis), are almost invariably associated with a reversal of the normal diurnal pattern of water excretion. These disorders, accompanied by an alteration or redistribution of the vascular volume, also exaggerate the postural effect on the release of AVP. Therefore, it is probable that while exercising or in the upright position, these patients, despite their expanded extracellular volume, have a far greater release of AVP than the normal subject. The assumption of the reclining position during the night may actually decrease the amount of AVP and lead to a nocturnal water diuresis. This is suggested by the classic studies of Borst and de Vries (114). It is probable that the improved renal hemodynamics, reduced secretion of aldosterone and AVP, and increase in circulating natriuretic factor (115, 116) all contribute to the nocturnal polyuria that is so characteristic of the previously mentioned disease states. That this reversal is also seen in states of primary or secondary adrenal insufficiency suggests a role of the glucocorticoids in the maintenance of the normal diurnal pattern. However, no clear-cut relationship has been established. One might well ask why in the aforementioned edematous states, especially those like congestive heart failure and cirrhosis in which blood volume is also increased, we do not see a raised osmotic threshold for AVP release as described in the volume-expanded normal human (99, 100) and animal (14). The most likely explanation is that the impaired circulation and/or redistribution of blood seen in those states cause an "abnormal" response of the baroreceptors of the carotid sinus, left atrium, and juxtaglomerular apparatus. Strong support for this explanation comes from the study of decompensated cirrhotics by Epstein and associates (117) utilizing water immersion to the neck, a procedure that redistributes blood volume with concomitant central hypervolemia. This model assessed the role of "effective volume" in the impairment of sodium and water handling in cirrhosis. They demonstrated a striking rise in C_{H_2O} and a drop in minimal urinary osmolality (Figs. 12-23A and B) which were most consistent with the interpretation that both avid reabsorption of filtrate proxi-

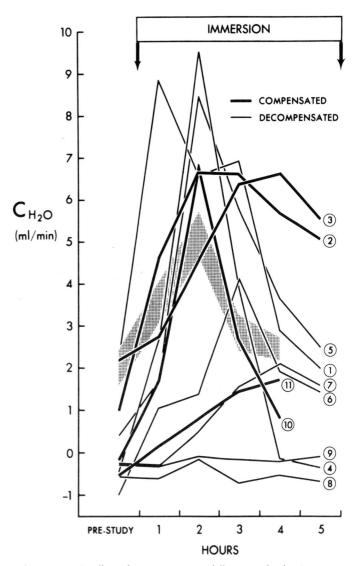

Figure 12-23A. Effect of water immersion following 1 h of quiet sitting (prestudy) on free water clearance (C_{H_2O}) in 11 patients with alcoholic liver disease. Shaded area represents the mean ± S.E. for C_{H_2O} for 18 normal control subjects undergoing immersion while in balance on a 150-meq sodium diet. These controls received a water load (1700 mL) which was twice as great as that utilized in the present study. Immersion resulted in a significant increase in C_{H_2O} ($P < 0.01$) which equalled or exceeded that of the controls on the higher sodium intake. [From M. Epstein et al. (117).]

mal to the diluting site and increased levels of AVP may participate to varying degrees in mediating the impaired water excretion of cirrhosis.

It is well recognized that during very rigid salt restriction in normal individuals the early negative salt balance during the first few days, before

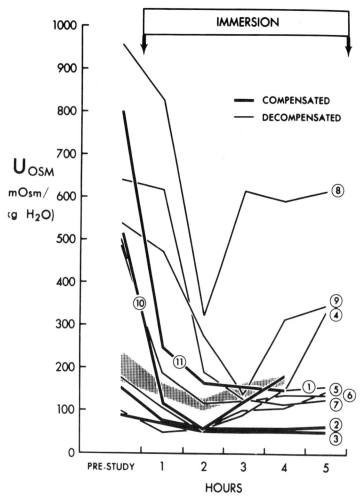

Figure 12-23B. Effect of water immersion following 1 h of quiet sitting (prestudy) on total urinary solute concentration (U_{osm}) in 11 patients with alcoholic liver disease. Shaded area represents the mean ± S.E. for U_{osm} for 18 normal subjects undergoing immersion. These controls received a water load twice as great as that utilized in the present study. All patients diluted their urine impressively, attaining levels of minimal U_{osm} equal to or less than that of the controls. [*From M. Epstein et al. (117).*]

there is maximal renal conservation of sodium, is associated with weight loss ranging from 0.5 to 2.0 kg. During this period, water ingested is readily excreted in isotonic proportions with salt. Furthermore, negative salt balance and loss of extracellular volume may significantly impair the water diuresis and urinary dilution. This was clearly demonstrated in the early human experiments of McCance (8) (Fig. 12-24) and the dog and human studies of Leaf and his associates (118, 119) (Fig. 12-25). Studies in our laboratory have shown that mild salt restriction for 3 days in normal subjects produced a statistically insignificant rise in plasma AVP. At the same time there was a significant fall in plasma tonicity (112a). In this setting, AVP secretion was inappropriate for the concomitant level of plasma osmolality. Under these conditions, volume factors were responsible for the relative elevation of plasma AVP. There is no doubt that the reduction in renal blood flow and GFR, the marked conservation of sodium, and the sustained nonosmotic release of AVP all contribute to the magnitude of the impaired water diuresis. In many disorders associated with extensive loss of vascular or extracellular volume, the nonosmotic stimulus to the release of AVP may be of such a magnitude and duration that it may override the inhibitory effect of hypoosmolality and cellular overhydration. When this occurs, hypotonic retention of water and hyponatremia invariably follow. This might be considered an "inappropriate" secretion of AVP, but it is apparent that the body is merely sacrificing a small change in tonicity to buffer a larger change in volume.

Major surgery, with its accompanying premedication, anesthesia, abdominal incision, traction on viscera, decrease in blood volume and cardiac output, and finally, the postoperative pain, creates a constellation of nonosmotic stimuli which lead to sustained operative and postoperative release of AVP (Fig. 12-26). This, more than any reduction in renal blood flow or nonhormonal impairment in water excretion, is responsible for the relative or absolute impairment of water excretion in the postoperative period and the extremely common symptomatic or asymptomatic hyponatremia observed so frequently after major surgery.

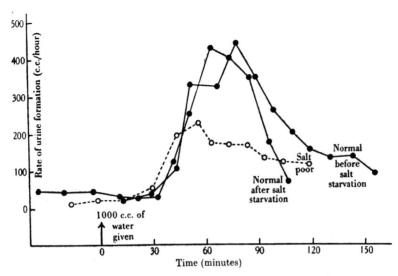

Figure 12-24. The effect of salt starvation on the rate of urine formation. [*From R. A. McCance (8).*]

From our earlier discussion on thirst, it was evident that hypothalamic centers regulating the third sensation could be stimulated by impulses from the cerebral cortex. This also holds true for the release of AVP. It is known that pain can bring about a sudden release of AVP and antidiuresis. Demerol, barbiturates, and morphine are all capable of stimulating AVP release when given in large amounts. This effect may be mediated through the baroreceptor mechanisms (Table 12-3) rather than through a direct pharmacologic effect on the neurohypophyseal system.

In an earlier section, we discussed the effect of various pharmacologic agents (chemicals) on the regulation of thirst and their role as possible neurohumoral transmitters in the hypothalamus. These drugs, or their analogues, also alter the release of AVP or the activity of the supraoptic neurons (Table 12-3) (120–122). The cholinergic agents acetylcholine, mecholyl, or carbachol, when injected systemically or into the carotid artery, or applied locally to the supraoptic nuclear area, stimulate the immediate release of AVP (Fig. 12-6C and D). It is of great interest that at the same time as these drugs cause a "water repletion reaction," they inhibit food ingestion (32). Ingestion of food at a time when water must be con-

served would simply tend to enhance solute and water excretion. Possibly acting through these neurochemical transmitters are the effects created by warm blood perfusing the hypothalamus. Overheating the animal or direct heating of the hypothalamus creates a sensation of thirst, a stimulation of the release of AVP, antidiuresis, and inhibition of food intake, the "water repletion reaction" (Fig. 12-6A and B). However, the sensation of thirst and the release of AVP after exposure to a hot environment may also be due to stimulation of the baroreceptor mechanism listed in Table 12-3. The peripheral vasodilatation and the associated redistribution of blood with a decrease in central blood volume could stimulate the receptors. This is the interpretation of Segar and Moore (13), who found that exposure of normal subjects for 2 h at 50°C caused a four- to fivefold increase in plasma AVP. The critical importance of this "water repletion reaction" when an individual is in a hot environment is readily apparent.

Recent studies have indicated that the β-adrenergic agent isoproterenol (Isuprel), when infused systemically into normal human volunteers (see below), anesthetized (123), and trained unanesthetized dogs (124) all undergoing a maximal sustained water diuresis, and into rats with congenital diabetes insipidus (125), causes an antidiuresis that is indistinguishable from that caused by AVP. However, a direct renal arterial injection of isoproterenol had no antidiuretic effect (123, 126). It is still unclear whether this β-adrenergic antidiuresis is primarily due to the release of AVP or to the circulatory effects of the drug or both. The antidiuresis can be completely inhibited by the α-adrenergic agent norepinephrine (124). The latter inhibits the action of antidiuretic hormone at the renal tubule (124, 127) and it also appears to inhibit the electrical activity of the supraoptic neurons (120) and the release of AVP. Norepinephrine also suppresses AVP release via elevation of blood pressure and stimulation of baroreceptors. These studies on the interrelationship of catecholamines with AVP and water metabolism make it necessary, as with the renin-angiotensin system, to consider still another set of neurohumoral regulators which may influence the hypothalamic centers controlling thirst and the release of AVP.

Osmotic and nonosmotic inhibitors of AVP secretion

The physiologic inhibitors of the release of AVP (Table 12-3) are (1) cellular overhydration and (2) expansion of the plasma or ECF volume. Water diuresis with the production of a very dilute urine reflects the inhibition of the neurohypophyseal system. Cellular overhydration accompanies reduction in the osmolality of the body fluids secondary to water ingestion. When the effective osmotic pressure is reduced by 1 or 2 percent, expansion of ICF volume completely inhibits the release of AVP (128) unless maintained by some

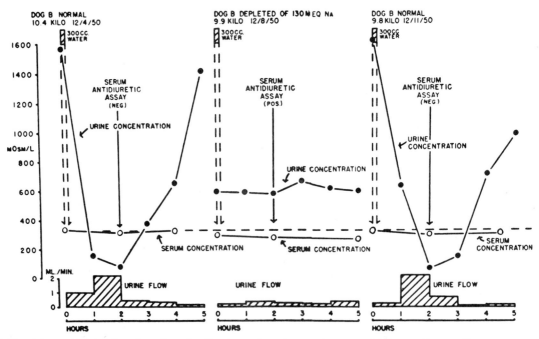

Figure 12-25. The right- and left-hand portions show the diuretic pattern before and following depletion. These are entirely normal diuretic patterns. The middle section shows conversion to the abnormal antidiuretic pattern following removal of 130 meq sodium by peritoneal dialysis. In this section we see again a dilute serum but a hypertonic urine and failure of dilution of the urine or diuresis following water administration. Antidiuretic activity was demonstrated in the serum during depletion but not in the controls. [*From A. Leaf et al. (118, 119).*]

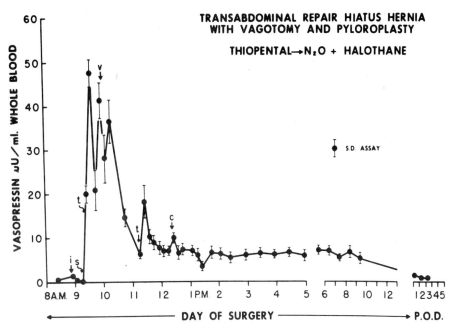

Figure 12-26. Changes in blood levels of AVP during and after a major surgical procedure. (*From B. Zimmerman,* Surg. Clin. N. Amer., *45:310, 1965.*)

nonosmotic stimulus (Fig. 12-27). It is generally felt that the cells of the neurohypophyseal nuclei share the cellular overhydration with the other body cells and that this inhibits the release of AVP. This is the first step in a normal water diuresis. As long as a sustained water load is continued and cellular overhydration persists, the release of AVP will be reduced to a minimal level and a maximal diuresis will be maintained. This state, often used in experimental studies, has been termed "physiologic diabetes insipidus."

When a subject is in the reclining position and the extracellular or plasma volume is expanded with such solutions as isotonic saline or isooncotic albumin, a characteristic water diuresis occurs. These solutions, although expanding the plasma and extracellular volume, do not alter intracellular volume or the osmolality of the body fluids. It is therefore apparent that volume expansion per se can influence the baroreceptor impulses from the carotid sinus and left atrium (Ta-

ble 12-3) and inhibit the renin-angiotensin system, thereby inhibiting the release of AVP.

We have mentioned earlier the experiments by Moses and his associates (98, 99) in humans and Zehr et al. (14) in the unanesthetized sheep, both clearly demonstrating that the osmotic release of AVP can be significantly attenuated by prior isotonic expansion of plasma and/or extracellular volume. Furthermore, when 400 to 500 mL of hypertonic saline (5%) is administered to a subject who is under the influence of a sustained positive water load, e.g., 1300 to 1500 mL, the subject may not develop a typical antidiuresis in spite of a marked hyperosmolality which causes withdrawal of water from the cells. This is due not only to the fact that the further expansion of the extracellular volume which occurs in these subjects after the hypertonic salt administration is great enough to blunt the stimulatory effect of the hyperosmolality and therefore decrease the release of AVP. Also, on occasion, the increase in salt ex-

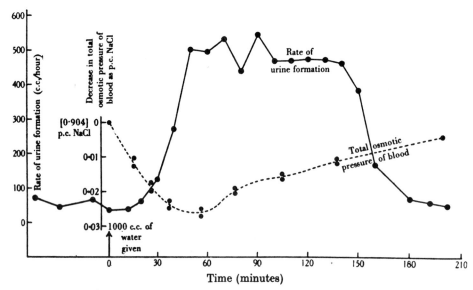

Figure 12-27. The relationship between the total osmotic pressure of the blood and the rate of urine formation after giving water.

cretion and osmolar clearance (see later) may be so great that despite a significant decrease in free water clearance (see later), indicating an approximate inhibition of the water diuresis, the rate of urine flow may not decrease (Fig. 12-28).

Nonosmotic stimulation of the baroreceptors, and their inhibition of AVP release, may be produced clinically by an episode of paroxysmal atrial arrhythmia in an individual with a basically normal heart. This will cause a sudden increase in cardiac output and, possibly, left atrial tension. The inhibition of AVP secretion causes a water diuresis (129) (Fig. 12-29). The polyuric syndrome that may accompany sudden cardiac arrhythmias which do not significantly impair myocardial function has been known for years. We have had the opportunity to study one such polyuric patient who, despite moderate dehydration and *a rise in plasma osmolality of approximately 20 percent,* excreted a persistently hypotonic urine; no AVP could be detected in his plasma.

We see here an example of a rise in the osmotic threshold for the release of AVP caused by stimulation of the cardiac baroreceptors which in turn led to a nonosmotic inhibition of AVP secretion

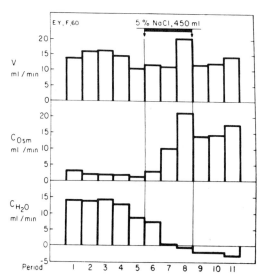

Figure 12-28. Effect of 5% saline solution infusion, 0.125 mL/kg per min, on urinary volume, osmolal clearance, and free water clearance in a patient with hypopituitarism treated with hydrocortisone. Note the apparent lack of antidiuretic response when the volume alone is considered. The decrease in free water clearance is masked by the marked increase in osmolal clearance. (*From A. M. Moses, et al., Am. J. Med., 42:368–377, 1967.*)

and hyperosmolality (hypernatremia). This is analogous to the effect of isotonic plasma and/or extracellular volume expansion on the osmotic threshold (14, 100). From these clinical and experimental observations it is possible to explain the mild hyperosmolality and hypernatremia seen in many patients with primary hyperaldosteronism. The excess mineralocorticoid secretion causes sodium retention and sustained steady-state expansion of the plasma and extracellular volume. The latter elevates the osmotic threshold, and hypernatremia must be present to allow the osmotic release of AVP. The hypernatremia may lead to thirst, a not uncommon symptom in these patients, but when water is drunk and the plasma hyperosmolality decreases slightly, AVP secre-

tion is again inhibited and a water diuresis ensues; thus, the hypernatremia is sustained. Such suppression of plasma AVP has been confirmed experimentally in our laboratory (112a). The administration of 9α-fluorohydrocortisone (Florinef) to normal volunteers produced a significant fall in plasma AVP.

The converse of the "water repletion reaction," which follows the administration of heat, cholinergic, and β-adrenergic agents, is the water depletion reaction, which accompanies the local hypothalamic application or intracarotid or systemic injection of anticholinergic or α-adrenergic drugs such as norepinephrine. The latter may inhibit thirst and the release of AVP (120), stimulate food intake, and antagonize the action of AVP on the

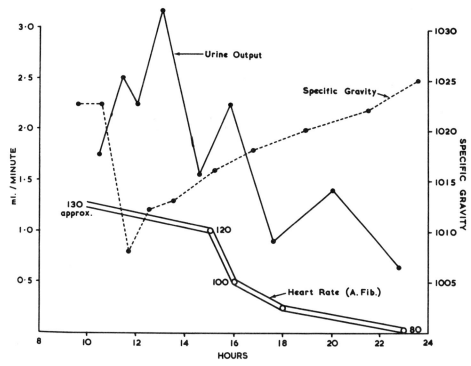

Figure 12-29. Chart of a 63-year-old man, with an otherwise normal heart, showing the increased volume and diminished specific gravity of the urine during a paroxysm of atrial fibrillation that started at 9:50 A.M. Though the paroxysm lasted 31 h, the patient ceased to be aware of it after about 4 h when the ventricular rate fell from 120 and over toward 100/min. As in most of his attacks, the diuresis came early, occurred mostly in the first 4 h, and finished in 7 h. The peak of the volume output was at 3 h, and the nadir of the specific gravity at 2 h. His attacks had recurred for 7 years and had been more frequent, almost once a week, for 3 years. [*From P. Wood (129).*]

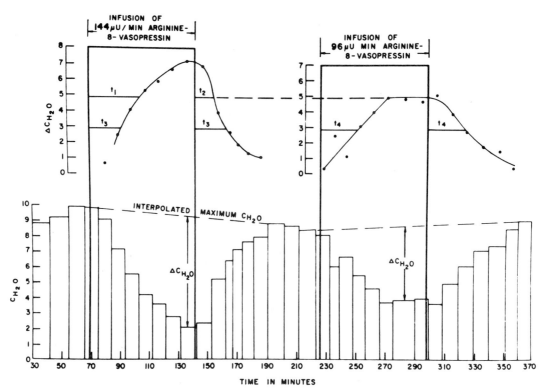

Figure 12-30. A typical experiment with infusions of 144 and 96 $\mu U/min$ arginine-8 vasopressin. The C_{H_2O} is graphed for each period. The change in C_{H_2O} (ΔC_{H_2O}) is determined by the difference between the interpolated maximum C_{H_2O} and the actual C_{H_2O} for each period. [*From L. Miller et al. (93).*]

distal nephron (124, 127). As would be expected, exposure of the animal to cold or cooling of the blood perfusing the hypothalamus will cause a decrease in thirst, a water diuresis (the classic "cold" diuresis), and an increase in food intake. Segar and Moore (13) found that exposure of normal subjects for 1 h at 13°C caused a definite inhibition of AVP release and a fall in its concentration in the plasma. They concluded that this was due to a rise in central blood volume and blood pressure stimulating the left atrial and carotid baroreceptors.

It has been frequently demonstrated that ethyl alcohol is a potent chemical inhibitor of the release of AVP (10). This inhibition occurs during a rising level of alcohol in the blood after its oral or intravenous administration, but in humans, at least, the maintenance of a constant blood level does not assure the continued inhibition of AVP release. Alcohol appears to block stimuli which would ordinarily cause the release of AVP such as hypertonic saline, reduction in blood volume, or prolonged venous congestion of the lower extremities. Therefore, the water diuresis that frequently follows the administration of ethyl alcohol, or the ingestion of one or two cocktails, probably represents the inhibition of certain tonic stimuli continuously reaching the neurohypophyseal nuclei. Alcohol has been used in certain clinical states, i.e., cirrhosis and congestive heart failure, to determine whether the observed oliguria and hypertonic urine are due to continued release of AVP. Usually, between 1 and 3 oz of 100 proof whiskey, or its equivalent, is necessary for maximal temporary inhibition of AVP release. Unfortunately, alcohol in these amounts has not proved to be especially useful in investigation of the vast majority of states associated with inappropriate or sustained nonosmotic release of AVP (see later). Recently, diphenylhydantoin (Dilantin) has also been demonstrated in humans to inhibit the release of AVP when administered intravenously (130). This inhibition, as with alcohol, is quite transient and nonsustained. This also limits its usefulness in clinical states associated with inappropriate release of AVP.

Metabolism of AVP

AVP turnover can also be assessed by determining the biologic half-life of AVP in vivo. Such studies have given a value of 16 to 20 min for the half-life of AVP (92, 93). AVP is infused intravenously into subjects undergoing a maximal sustained water diuresis. This will cause a reproducible degree of antidiuresis in a given individual under carefully controlled conditions. When the infusion is stopped, the rate of return of the urine flow to its maximal level reflects the rate of disappearance of the hormone from the circulation. An example of this is shown in Fig. 12-30. The half-time calculated by this indirect technique (93) correlates quite well with that determined by direct bioassay of the hormone in the circulation (92, 94), but is somewhat slower than those determined by immunoassay in separate studies cited above. Once secreted, AVP is rapidly cleared from the circulation. In humans, the plasma half-life of AVP, estimated by radioimmunoassay after pulse injection or after termination of a constant infusion of hormone, ranges from 6 to 9 min (131–133). Plasma disappearance follows a biexponential pattern with a rapid first phase and somewhat slower second phase (Fig. 12-31). AVP is cleared in approximately equal fractions by kidney and liver (94). Renal clearance persists after ureteral ligation and thus appears to take place largely in the postglomerular circulation (134). Total clearance declines as the plasma concentration of AVP rises above the physiologic range (135). These and

other data have suggested a role of high-affinity plasma membrane receptors in mediating AVP clearance (136). It is postulated that the receptors bind the biologically active hormone and facilitate its transfer from the vascular compartment to an extravascular compartment where enzymatic degradation occurs (136).

AVP can be degraded directly in plasma at a rate of 11 percent per hour (137), but this is relatively

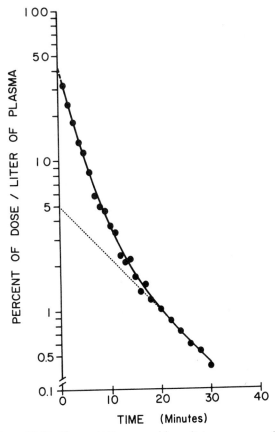

Figure 12-31. Plasma AVP measured by radioimmunoassay after pulse injection of unlabeled hormone. Two exponentials can be identified. The metabolic clearance rate is calculated as the area under the curve and the volume of distribution as the reciprocal of the fractional dose per liter extrapolated to the time of injection. The MCR for six dogs studied in this fashion was 35.5 ± (S.E.M.) 0.6 mL/kg per min and the volume of distribution was 12.7 ± 0.9 percent body weight. (*From R. Weitzman and D. A. Fisher, unpublished data.*)

insignificant compared to total body clearance. It is sufficiently great to warrant special handling of plasma samples for AVP assay. During pregnancy in humans and other primates, the placenta produces a circulating enzyme, cystine aminopeptidase (vasopressinase), which considerably augments plasma degradation. The impact of this enzyme on overall hormonal clearance is not known.

Bioassays for AVP have, for many years, been of great value in experimental and clinical studies of normal and abnormal physiology of AVP. However, they are very time consuming and lack the sensitivity of the newer and more specific RIA (radioimmunoassays) (131–133, 138). The latter have permitted detection of as little as 0.2 to 0.5 μU/mL of plasma. In either RIA or bioassays, it is necessary to extract AVP from plasma to separate out substances in plasma which nonspecifically interfere with the assay. In some bioassays, it is necessary to utilize chemical tests such as inactivation by thioglycollate or pregnancy plasma to exclude the presence of other substances that could evoke either a pressor or antidiuretic response. In the few studies where both types of assays have been used, they generally correlate well; however, the RIA may give higher readings due to the presence of immunologically but not biologically reactive "hormone" fragments. Such

fragments may lead to an artifactual overestimation of AVP concentrations by immunoassay compared to bioassay.

Some laboratories express their data in μU/mL, using bioassayed USP posterior pituitary extract as a standard. This material is widely available and quite stable so that results from different laboratories may easily be compared. Other laboratories use synthetic AVP as a standard and express their results in pg/mL. Unfortunately, commercially available synthetic AVP is of widely variable potency, as determined by bioassay, so that there may be considerable variation in the normal range in different laboratories—1 pg/mL is roughly equivalent to 0.4 μU/mL.

Blood samples for AVP measurement must be quickly chilled after collection and the plasma rapidly frozen to minimize enzymatic degradation. Even so, progressive loss of immunoreactive AVP content of plasma can be demonstrated with prolonged freezer storage. Extraction prevents further degradation.

AVP, like many other hormones, is secreted episodically (Fig. 12-32) (139). Thus, a solitary sample may not accurately reflect neurohypophyseal secretion in a given patient. Collection of multiple samples, with pooling of the plasma prior to assay, has been suggested to minimize such variation.

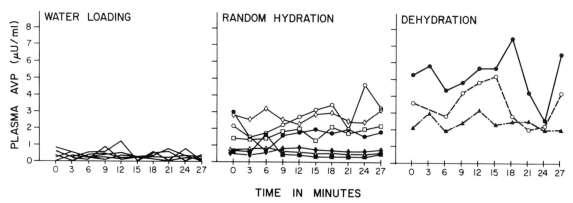

Figure 12-32. Plasma AVP concentration sampled ever 3 min for ½ h in sheep. The panel on the left shows only minimal variation in sequential samples collected in water-loaded sheep with low overall mean plasma AVP concentration. Mean AVP levels are higher in the randomly hydrated sheep (center panel) and higher still in the dehydrated animals (panel on the right). A tendency for pulsatile secretion can be observed in some of the randomly hydrated sheep and in the dehydrated sheep. (*R. E. Weitzman and D. A. Fisher, unpublished data.*)

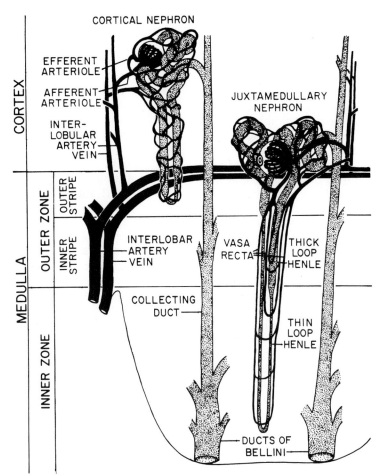

Figure 12-33. Diagrammatic representation of the cortical and juxtamedullary nephrons and their vascular supply. (*From R. F. Pitts, Physiology of the Kidney and Body Fluids, Year Book Medical Publishers, Chicago, 1963. Used by permission.*)

RENAL REGULATION OF WATER

The anatomic and physiologic concepts upon which we based our earlier discussion (140) of the kidney's maximal concentrating and diluting capacity have been confirmed and broadened by continuing investigations and the latter have been analyzed and summarized in recent excellent reviews (141–145). The improved microdissection, microperfusion, micropuncture, and microchemical techniques, combined with transmission and scanning electron microscopy used in these in-

vestigations, have contributed to a better understanding of water excretion in normal humans and in diseased states.

Physiologic anatomy

The nephrons of the mammalian kidney arise from the intralobular arteries and their afferent arterioles at varying depths within the cortex of the kidney, and they are of varying lengths. The latter is dependent on the length of the loop of Henle (Fig. 12-33). The loop of Henle consists of the straight portion of the proximal tubule (pars recta), the thin limb, descending and ascending segment, the ascending thick segment, and a short straight portion of the distal tubule (pars recta) proximal to the macula densa. Basically, all the nephrons in the mammalian kidney can be divided into two populations: the outer cortical with the short loop of Henle consisting of abbreviated, thin limb segments penetrating, at most, to the inner strip of the outer zone of the medulla (Fig. 12-33), and the juxtamedullary with the long loop of Henle, the well-developed descending and ascending thin segments which traverse the entire medulla and form their hairpin loops at varying depths within the inner medullary zone. The larger the number of these nephrons and the longer their loops of Henle, the greater is the concentrating capacity of the animal.[1] In the human (141, 143), it has been estimated that approximately 15 percent of the nephrons have long loops of Henle (141, 145). Of course, as we descend from outer cortex to juxtamedullary zone, we may encounter gradations or variations between the two basic types depending on their relative positions in the cortex (145). In general, the pars recta changes to the thin descending limb at the outer strip of the outer medullary zone and the thick segment of the ascending limb is located in the outer medullary zone. The segment of the thick ascending limb of Henle's loop, which begins at the point where it crosses from outer medulla to the cortex and extends to the macula densa, is called the cortical diluting segment, the cortical portion of the thick ascending limb, or the straight (pars recta) segment of the distal tubule. The proximal and distal *convoluted* tubules of all nephrons are confined to the isotonic cortex where the distal convoluted tubule terminates or becomes the unbranched cortical collecting duct. The latter traverses the cortex to the junction with other cortical collecting tubules near the corticomedullary or outer strip of the outer medullary zone to form here the medullary collecting duct

which traverses the entire medulla and enlarges to terminate at the duct of Bellini near the tip of the medullary pyramid.

The blood supply of the renal medulla is composed entirely of postglomerula vessels derived from the juxtamedullary glomeruli. These vessels (vasa recta) descend into the medulla, take a hairpin turn, and ascend to their level of origin. These vascular loops (capillaries) lie in the closest proximity with the loop of Henle and collecting ducts (Fig. 12-33). However, Kriz and Lever (146) described a tubulovascular relationship that must be of functional significance. The descending limb is juxtaposed to both descending and ascending vasa recta, while the ascending thin limb is adjacent to the collecting duct. The descending vasa recta, at various levels in the medulla, gives off branches that form a capillary plexus which surrounds the ascending limb and collecting duct, with blood flowing in a descending direction concurrent to collecting duct and countercurrent to the ascending limb. As emphasized by Rector (141), this juxtaposition of limbs, collecting ducts, and capillaries suggests that various elements are not exchanging equally with well-mixed interstitium, and, furthermore, that none of the current models takes full consideration of these unique anatomic features.

The loop of Henle (functioning as a countercurrent multiplier system) *creates* the hypertonicity of the renal medulla, essential to the production of a hypertonic urine, whereas the vascular loop (acting as a countercurrent exchanger) *prevents* the dissipation of the hypertonic gradient of the medulla. Throughout the entire nephron, the fundamental processes involved in the production of a dilute and concentrated urine are the active reabsorption of sodium chloride and the variable permeability of the nephron to the passive back-diffusion of water and urea along their concentration gradients (Fig. 12-34), the only possible exception being the passive permeability of the thin ascending segment of Henle's loop to salt (see below).

Solute and water reabsorption in the nephron

In the average adult approximately 100 mL of glomerular filtrate is presented to the proximal

---

[1]While this relationship holds for most mammalian kidneys (141), there are some striking exceptions. The macaque monkey, while capable of forming concentrated urine well above 1000 mosm/kg during fluid deprivation, has virtually no inner medulla or long loops of Henle. Other exceptions are the mountain beaver and the chinchilla (141).

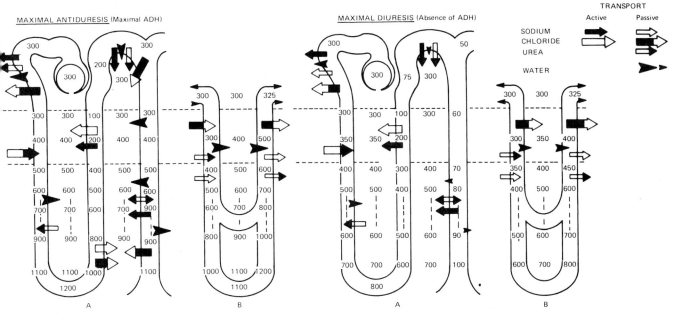

Figure 12-34. Countercurrent mechanism as it is believed to operate in the juxtamedullary nephron (*A*) and vasa recta (*B*). The numbers represent illustrative osmolality values during maximal antidiuresis (left) and maximal diuresis (right). No quantitative significance is to be attached to the number of arrows; only net movements are indicated. As with the vascular loops, not all loops of Henle reach the tip of the papilla and, hence, the fluid in them does not become as concentrated as that of the final urine, but rather only as concentrated as the medullary interstitial fluid at the same level. (*Modified from Gottschalk and Mylle, Am. J. Physiol., 196:927, 1959.*)

tubules every minute. During its passage through this water-permeable segment (proximal convoluted and pars recta), approximately two-thirds to three-fourths of the glomerular ultrafiltrate is reabsorbed into the bloodstream. In this reabsorption process, the tubule fluid remains isosmotic with respect to plasma and there is usually no transepithelial concentration gradient for sodium. Therefore, the amount of isosmotic fluid delivered into the loop of Henle is dependent upon the filtered solute load and on the amount of solute resorbed in the proximal tubule. The fluid entering the descending limb of the loop of Henle becomes progressively more concentrated as it approaches the tip of the loop; as it ascends in the ascending limb it becomes increasingly dilute until it enters the distal convoluted tubule as a distinctly hypotonic (150 to 200 mosm/L) fluid (Fig. 12-34). These basic changes in the loop of Henle, while they may be modified (see below) from a quantitative point of view, occur under all circumstances regardless of the volume and composition of the final urine. This is the consequence of the unique transport and permeability characteristics of the loop of Henle which allow it to function as an efficient countercurrent multiplier system, the latter being primarily responsible for our capacity to produce a maximally hypertonic urine.

In the past few years, the countercurrent hypothesis as applied to the mammalian nephron has been subjected to the most rigorous experimental verification and new models have been formulated to reconcile the observed facts. Many reviews have been forthcoming (141–145) and we have drawn most heavily on the very lucid and recent one of Jamison and Maffly (143) for our discussion.

Before presenting a description of the newer knowledge that has, in recent years, greatly enhanced our understanding of the function of the loop of Henle, it will be of help to review the concepts of countercurrent flow that enabled the physical chemist Werner Kuhn to recognize the fundamental implications of the U-shaped configuration of the long loops in which fluid flows in opposite directions in adjacent limbs (143). With respect to heat exchangers, he was well aware that large temperature gradients can be established in the longitudinal axis of such channels while the temperature differences between them at any given horizontal level can be very small. He applied this concept to the concentration or osmotic pressure differential in the loop of Henle and concluded that here too small differences in concentrations between ascending and descending limbs, at any given transverse level, could be responsible for great differences in solute concentration along the long axis of the tubules and in the surrounding adjacent interstitial tissue.

For such a system to function as a countercurrent multiplier, Kuhn proposed three basic requirements: (1) countercurrent flow, (2) differences in permeability between tubules carrying fluid in opposite directions, and (3) a source of energy. The loop of Henle provides the countercurrent flow, the descending limb has a very high level of permeability to water while the thin and thick ascending limb is almost impermeable to water (141, 147), and the active transport of NaCl out of the thick ascending limb to surrounding interstitium provides the basic energy source (141, 143).

The impermeability of this latter segment to water means that the concentrations of NaCl transported into the surrounding interstitium must be distinctly hypertonic while the intraluminal NaCl concentration, at this level of the ascending limb, will be hypotonic. As the isotonic fluid from the pars recta of the proximal tubule enters the highly water-permeable descending limb of Henle's loop, it becomes hypertonic as it loses water to the more concentrated (hypertonic NaCl) surrounding medullary interstitium. As it rounds the bend of the loop, and ascends, this intraluminal fluid, now considerably more concentrated (hypertonic) with respect to NaCl, is presented to the active transport site and pumped into the surrounding medullary interstitium and elevates the NaCl concentration and osmolality of the interstitial

tissue to an even higher degree of hypertonicity. Thus, the active transport process in the water-impermeable thick ascending limb, when augmented or *multiplied* by the countercurrent flow in the loop and the continued osmotic flow of water out of the descending limb, results in the very large concentration difference in the longitudinal axis of the medulla between the isosmotic fluid entering the descending limb and the most hypertonic fluid at the tip of the loop and adjacent papillary interstitium (Fig. 12-34). Note that this whole process, initiated by the active transport of NaCl into the outer medulla, occurs without the need to create a transepithelial concentration gradient for NaCl exceeding 100 meq or 200 mosm in the horizontal plane at any level of the medulla. "One of the most compelling features of the countercurrent mechanism is its biologic economy. When the urine is hyperosmotic, at no point along the renal tubule does the transepithelial osmotic gradient exceed 200 mosm per kilogram of water" (143).

As noted in Fig. 12-34, the newly created hypotonic fluid (150 to 200 mosm/L) in the thick ascending limb enters the distal convoluted tubule. As it flows from this cortical segment into the cortical and medullary collecting ducts, its concentration is primarily determined by the level of AVP in the surrounding capillaries. When the amount is sufficient to create maximal permeability of the collecting ducts and, probably, the terminal portion of the distal convoluted tubule, the luminal fluid is reabsorbed until osmotic equilibrium is achieved with the surrounding isotonic cortical or increasingly hypertonic medullary interstitium. Thus, the most concentrated urine equal to the osmolality of the interstitial fluid of the innermost medulla or papillary tip is created. Lesser amounts of AVP, acting on the nephron, create less than maximally concentrated urine.

Essential prerequisites of the process described above would appear to be active salt reabsorption *throughout* the ascending limb and that fluid in this segment be rendered definitely hypoosmotic to the adjacent interstitium. The low-level permeability to the osmotic flow of water has been clearly demonstrated for both the thin and thick ascending limbs (141, 147) and there is unquestioned active reabsorption of salt in the thick ascending limb (141, 143). However, studies in vitro of the thin segment have failed to disclose any evidence of active transport of sodium or chloride (147). The contrast between the organelle-rich cuboidal epithelium of the thick ascending limb and the organelle-poor squamous epithelium of the thin ascending limb is consistent with this difference in active salt transport (145).

If the in vitro studies of the transport and permeability characteristics of the *entire* ascending limb do not fulfill the essential prerequisites, how then can we explain the highly efficient countercurrent multiplier system obviously existing in the inner medulla and producing the most hypertonic interstitium at the tip of the pyramid?

This dilemma may have been solved by the proposed models of Stephenson (148, 149) and Kokko and Rector (150) which demonstrated that *passive* transport of salt from lumen to interstitium of the thin ascending limb in the inner medulla could be brought about if certain assumptions about relative impermeabilities of various nephron segments to water, salt, and urea were made. These impermeabilities have been demonstrated (147, 151–153) and are presented in Table 12-6, modified from Britton et al. (153).

Furthermore, the models allowed the active transport of NaCl to be confined to the thick ascending limb, they provided a clear explanation for the role of urea in augmenting the urinary concentrating ability, and they explained the early important observations of Ullrich and Jarausch (154) that the sodium concentration gradient rose

steeply along the axis of the outer medulla but only slightly along the axis of the inner medulla, whereas the urea gradient rose much more steeply along the axis of the inner medulla. These findings are inconsistent with the hypothesis that active salt transport is the local driving force in the inner medulla, favoring instead an important role for urea. The details of the Stephenson–Kokko-Rector models are presented in Fig. 12-35. The chloride pump (155) in the thick ascending limb of the loop of Henle, in the outer medulla, is the active source of energy for the whole medulla (153). The active transport of salt from the lumen of the water- and urea-impermeable thick ascending limb leaves behind a hypotonic fluid rich in urea which flows into the distal convoluted tubule and the cortical and outer medullary collecting ducts; segments which actively reabsorb salt are impermeable to urea and freely permeable to water (at least the cortical collecting duct) in the presence of AVP or hydropenia. Here the urea becomes progressively more concentrated in a smaller volume of fluid which enters the inner medullary collecting ducts. As the collecting ducts join they become increasingly permeable to urea, especially in the presence of AVP (141, 143, 150, 151), allowing the urea to flow along its concentration gradient and approach equilibrium with the adjacent interstitium of the inner medulla. The increase in medullary osmolality thus created draws water out of the adjacent tubules, the terminal collecting ducts, and especially the descending limb of the loop. The NaCl in this relatively salt-impermeable descending limb becomes progressively more concentrated as the fluid ap-

Table 12-6. Simplified summary of permeability characteristics of different parts of the nephron (rabbit)

PART OF NEPHRON	WATER	SODIUM IONS	UREA
Descending	Very permeable	Impermeable*	Impermeable*
Thin ascending	Impermeable	Very permeable	Moderately permeable
Thick ascending	Impermeable	Very permeable active Cl⁻ pump	Impermeable
Distal tubule (and/or cortical collecting duct)	Permeable with AVP	Partial Na–K exchange	Impermeable
Medullary collecting duct	Permeable with AVP	Moderately permeable*	Impermeable except at collecting duct junctions in inner medulla

* Varies with different species.

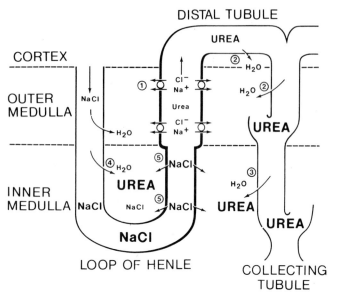

Figure 12-35. Recent modifications of the countercurrent hypothesis by Stephenson and Kokko and Rector. Both the thin ascending limb in the inner medulla and the thick ascending limb in the outer medulla, as well as the first part of the distal tubule, are impermeable to water, as indicated by the thickened lining. In the thick ascending limb, active chloride reabsorption, accompanied by passive sodium movement (1), renders the tubule fluid dilute and the outer medullary interstitium hyperosmotic. In the last part of the distal tubule and in the collecting tubule in the cortex and outer medulla, water is reabsorbed down its osmotic gradient (2), increasing the concentration of urea that remains behind. In the inner medulla both water and urea are reabsorbed from the collecting duct (3). Some urea reenters the loop of Henle (not shown). This medullary recycling of urea, in addition to trapping of urea by countercurrent exchange in the vasa recta (not shown), causes urea to accumulate in large quantities in the medullary interstitium (indicated by the large type), where it osmotically extracts water from the descending limb (4) and thereby concentrates sodium chloride in descending-limb fluid. When the fluid rich in sodium chloride enters the sodium chloride–permeable (but water-impermeable) thin ascending limb, sodium chloride moves passively down its concentration gradient (5), rendering the tubule fluid relatively hypoosmotic to the surrounding interstitium. [*From R. L. Jamison and R. H. Maffly (143).*]

proaches the hairpin turn, while the salt concentration in the adjacent interstitium is somewhat reduced by dilution. As the luminal fluid with its highest concentration of NaCl rounds the tip of the loop, it enters the water-impermeable, salt-permeable thin ascending limb and immediately sodium and chloride ions diffuse down their concentration gradient into the surrounding interstitium, thus increasing its osmolality. The luminal fluid left behind becomes relatively hypotonic to the adjacent interstitial fluid (Figs. 12-34 and 12-35). The rise in osmolality of the latter tends to draw more water into the interstitium from the collecting ducts and tends to dilute the interstitial urea. This process reestablishes the urea gradient from the terminal and inner medullary collecting ducts to interstitium. Urea now diffuses down its gradient from these ducts, thus increasing the osmolality of the interstitium; more water moves in from the descending limbs, and in so doing, reestablishes the salt gradient and so on. The osmolality of the interstitium continues to rise and water reabsorption from the collecting duct is thus enhanced. Water that has entered the medulla from the descending limb and collecting ducts is carried away by the ascending avas recta. Quoting from Britton and associates (153):

The crux of the matter is that the osmolality of the interstitium depends on the *sum* of the salt and urea contributions whereas the diffusion of urea depends only on the passive gradient of urea from collecting duct to interstitium; and the diffusion of salt depends only upon the passive gradient of the ions from thin ascending limbs to interstitium. The model demonstrates how these two gradients are continuously but alternately reformed in an escalating manner as the diffusion of specific solute and water due to one gradient recreates the other. This is an example of the bootstrap concept because the energy of the chloride pump in the cortex and outer medulla is transduced to the high urea concentration in the collecting ducts which primes the solute gradient interaction to increase the osmolality in the interstitium. The situation may be visualized as salt raising its own concentration by hauling on urea's bootstraps and vise versa.

Two recent studies from Jamison's laboratory (156, 157) lend added weight to the passive models of Stephenson (148, 149) and Kokko and Rector (141, 150). In one study (156), they examined the contents of the collecting tubule, loop of Henle, and vasa recta before and after an infusion of urea to protein-deprived rats and compared the results to similar studies in animals not given urea. Not only did urinary osmolality increase significantly in the urea-infused animals, but water extraction from the descending limb also increased significantly. An additional finding of importance was that the urea concentration in the fluid at the end of the descending limb was appreciably higher than could be explained by simple osmotic flow of water from lumen to interstitium. This strongly suggests that part of the medullary "recycling" of urea involved its movement from interstitium to urine somewhere in the nephron segment between the end of the proximal tubule and the end of the descending limb. However, Rector (144) has stressed that if a significant amount of urea is added to the thin descending limb, it will diminish water abstraction from this segment and actually impair the efficiency of the postulated passive model. To the extent that osmotic equilibrium in the thin descending limb occurs by solute entry, the ability of urea to enhance urine concentration will be diminished. The greater the solute urea entry, the less the water abstraction and the lower the NaCl concentration in the loop fluid delivered to the thin ascending limb.[2] An additional way in which urea may enter the papillary tips and inner medulla was suggested by

[2] Very recently, Jamison (R. L. Jamison: Urinary concentration and dilution, in Kurtzman and Martinez-Maldonado (eds.), *Pathophysiology of the Kidney*, Charles C Thomas, Springfield, Ill., 1977, p. 213) addressed himself to the reservations referred to above by Rector. He asked the question, how can urea simultaneously extract water from the descending limb *and* be "secreted" into the descending limb? He and his associates devised a computerized model to examine this question. They determined transtubular water and urea flux in the descending limb with their model utilizing available data of this segment's permeability to water and urea, and the surrounding medullary concentrations of urea and NaCl. They found that the greater majority of the water transport from lumen to medullary interstitium took place in the first half of the descending limb while, on the other hand, urea *entry* took place as a function of distance, little urea entering over the early portion of the descending limb. Urea concentration therefore remains low in this early portion of the descending limb, but continues to rise throughout owing to both increasing entry of urea and additional water extraction. Jamison and his associates concluded that in this manner urea in the medullary interstitium can extract water from the descending limb and also diffuse into the descending limb, i.e., undergo medullary recycling. Thus, their findings (156) are consistent with the passive model of countercurrent multiplication in the renal medulla.

Gertz et al. (158) and confirmed by Schütz and Schnermann (159). Since the papillary tips are bathed by pelvis urine containing the highest concentration of urea, the latter could diffuse across the pelvis epithelium into the adjacent medulla. Schütz and Schnermann found, in rats, that when the renal pelvis was opened and maintained free of urine, the osmolality of urine emerging from the collecting ducts fell from 1400 to 800 mosm/kg. However, if they bathed the exposed papillae in increasingly hypertonic urea solutions, the urinary osmolality rose simultaneously to 2000 to 2500 mosm/kg. Thus, the pelvis urine appears to be an important source of urea, and the absence of this intimate contact between papillae and pelvis urine could impair the function of the countercurrent system.

Rector, in his excellent analysis of the renal-concentrating mechanisms (141), concluded that not all the available micropuncture studies in rats, hamsters, and Psammomys are consistent with the passive model for the production of a maxillary concentrated urine, derived primarily from the permeability characteristics of the isolated perfused rabbit nephron. It may well be that there are important species differences in the intimate mechanism(s) responsible for the optimum function of the renal medullary countercurrent system.

In the other study from Jamison's laboratory (157), the differences in sodium concentration between fluid in Henle's thin limb and that in adjacent vasa recta plasma in normal hydropenic rats were examined. Assuming that the vasa recta plasma was an accurate indicator of the sodium concentration in the interstitial fluid, they found a clear-cut gradient favoring passive reabsorption or diffusion of sodium. The results of both of these studies fulfill key requirements of the passive models.

The anatomic arrangement of the vasa recta and their function as a countercurrent exchanger imminently facilitates the function of the loop in the maintenance of the hypertonic interstitium (Figs. 12-33, 12-34, and 12-36) and, at the same time, allows water from the descending limb and collecting duct to be removed from the medulla by way of the ascending vasa recta. The endothelium of the vasa recta is freely permeable to water, much less permeable to plasma proteins, and its permeability to smaller solutes, such as electrolytes, lies between these extremes.

As blood in the vasa recta descends in the capillary loop, it approaches osmotic equilibrium with the surrounding hypertonic environment by the

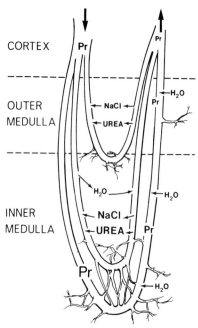

Figure 12-36. Countercurrent exchange by the vasa recta. The medullary circulation, unlike the loops of Henle, consists of a network of channels with main thoroughfares (the vasa recta) and branch connections. Pr denotes plasma protein. The size of type indicates the relative concentrations of each solute with respect to its location in the medulla but not necessarily with respect to other solutes. The progressive rise in the concentration of sodium chloride and urea in the medullary interstitium is due to the loop of Henle and collecting tubule. Since the capillaries are permeable to sodium chloride and urea, these solutes enter descending vasa recta and leave ascending vasa recta. This transcapillary exchange helps "trap" the solutes in the medulla. Conversely, water leaves the descending vasa recta, causing the plasma protein concentration to increase. In the ascending vasa recta the sum of oncotic (that due to plasma protein) and osmotic (that due to nonprotein solutes) pressures results in capillary fluid uptake. Thus, water reabsorbed from the collecting tubule and Henle's descending limb is removed from the medulla and returned to the general circulation. Vasa recta function is a dual capacity, trapping solute and removing water, to preserve the hyperosmolality of the renal medulla. [*From R. L. Jamison and R. H. Maffly (143).*]

passive diffusion of sodium salts and other solutes, notably urea, *into* the capillary lumen while water diffuses *out* along its osmotic and hydrostatic pressure gradient. The rapidity of blood flow creates an osmotic disequilibrium in which the osmotic pressure of the interstitial fluid and the hydrostatic pressure in the capillary together oppose the oncotic pressure exerted by the plasma proteins. This generates the net force. As the blood doubles back on itself and flows toward the corticomedullary junction in the ascending vasa recta, urea and sodium salts return to the interstitium while water diffuses into the blood. In the ascending limb plasma, the concentration of the small solutes now exceeds that in the adjacent interstitium and this osmotic force, plus the now additive oncotic pressure of the proteins, causes a net fluid entry into the blood. The quantity of water entering exceeds that lost from the descending vasa recta and is equal to the volume of fluid reabsorbed from the collecting tubule and descending limb of the loop of Henle. The net effect is the free diffusion of salt and urea from ascending to descending, and of water from descending to ascending limb of the vascular loop, and return to the bloodstream of the water that has diffused into the medulla from the descending limb of the loop of Henle and the collecting ducts. Thus, the vascular loop, as a countercurrent exchanger, minimizes the loss of excess sodium and urea from the medulla and maintains the hypertonic gradient which would be dissipated if the vasa recta blood did not double back on itself (Figs. 12-33, 12-34, and 12-36).

The "trapping" and recycling of urea in the medulla creates the surprising phenomenon in which the *net* resorption of urea *into the bloodstream* (normally 40 to 50 percent of the filtered urea) occurs only in the cortical parts of the nephron. The urea which is resorbed from the collecting ducts, and which approaches the same concentration in medullary water and collecting duct fluid, is trapped in the medullary interstitium from which an amount approximating proximal resorption diffuses into the loop (?descending limb) of Henle (Figs. 12-34 and 12-36). As urea, during antidiuresis, approaches diffusion equilibrium across the collecting duct (equal concentration in medullary water and collecting duct fluid), it contributes equally to the total osmolality of the medulla and urine. Therefore, it increases the osmotic pressure of the urine beyond that attained by the osmotic equilibrium of collecting duct fluid with the hypertonic sodium chloride in the interstitium.

In summary, the hypertonicity in the medulla and the magnitude of the hypertonic gradient from corticomedullary junction to papilla at any given moment during both diuresis and antidiuresis will be *directly proportional* to the number and length of the loops of Henle, the rate of salt delivered to and actively transported across the ascending limb, and the load of urea presented to the collecting duct; they will be *inversely proportional* to the velocity of medullary blood flow, the flow of tubular fluid in the loop of Henle, and the rate of water transport into the medulla from the collecting ducts and descending limb of the loop.

ROLE OF AVP AND THE CONTROL OF URINE CONCENTRATION AND DILUTION

Although solutes are actively resorbed in the distal part of the distal convoluted tubule and the cortical segment of the collecting duct, the resorption of water in these segments is dependent primarily on the presence of AVP (Fig. 12-34). In the absence of AVP, there is a minimal transport of water into the surrounding capillary beds, and the dilute fluid from the ascending limb and the more proximal segment of the distal convoluted tubule is made progressively more hypotonic by continued active solute resorption. Therefore, when AVP is absent, the fluid in the distal portion of the cortical collecting duct approaches the lowest osmolality observed throughout the nephron, possibly between 15 and 20 mosm/L. This is the situation seen during maximal sustained water diuresis, in diabetes insipidus, or in any physiologic state that prevents AVP from acting on this segment of the nephron. Although the medullary collecting ducts are also relatively impermeable to water in the absence of AVP, the marked gradient between the hypotonic luminal fluid and hypertonic interstitium allows some back-diffusion of

water, the magnitude of which is determined by the volume per minute delivered to the collecting duct during water diuresis. If this volume is small enough, a moderately hypertonic urine can be formed in the absence of AVP (160).

When a maximal amount of AVP is available, the cortical collecting duct is freely permeable to water and, as the solutes are actively resorbed, the tubular fluid in this segment will approach isotonicity. If less than maximal amounts of AVP are available, the permeability of this segment will be proportionately decreased, lesser amounts of water will back-diffuse with the solute, and the tubular fluid will not reach isotonicity. AVP therefore simply permits the back-diffusion of water to occur along established concentration gradients. Since approximately 90 percent of the solute delivered into the distal convoluted tubule and cortical collecting duct is resorbed, at least 90 percent of the water delivered to it will back-diffuse. It is apparent that a reduction in the resorption of solutes in these segments, such as may occur during an osmotic diuresis, will increase the volume of residual isosmotic tubular fluid delivered into the medullary collecting tubules during the maximal AVP activity. As a consequence of the alterations taking place in the thick ascending limb, distal convoluted tubule, and cortical collecting duct, the fluid delivered into the medullary collecting duct may be of minimal osmolality and approximately the same volume as that delivered into the distal convoluted tubules, or the luminal fluid may decrease to the smallest volume necessary to excrete the remaining urinary solutes in isotonic or isosmotic concentration.

The isotonic fluid entering the medullary collecting duct courses down through the hypertonic medulla. In the hydropenic animal (maximal AVP activity), this small volume of fluid is maximally concentrated by the back-diffusion of water along its osmotic gradient into the hypertonic interstitium. The maximal concentration of urine that is usually achieved in the moderately hydropenic human is approximately 1000 to 1100 mosm/L. However, in prolonged water deficit, such as may occur during complete abstinence from water for a 72-h period, the urinary concentration may attain values of 1300 to 1400 mosm/L. As stated earlier, the attainment of these maximal values is not due to a further increase in circulating AVP or in the permeability of the collecting duct, but rather to the continued decrease in medullary blood flow and increase in medullary tonicity. The volume abstracted in the final concentrating process is ordinarily quite small, being below 1.5 mL/min. This water is returned to the circulation via the vasa recta.

The exact cellular mechanism(s) by which AVP creates a physicochemical change in certain epithelial membranes to allow the differential passage of water, urea, and salt is still unknown. However, the recent reviews by Andreoli and Schafer (142, 161) and Hays (162) have added greatly to our understanding.

It is of great interest that in the mammalian cortical medullary collecting ducts AVP enhances the transcellular movement of water without any effect on urea or sodium transport (142, 161). This is in contrast to its effect on amphibian skin and bladder where all three are influenced by the hormone and where water, urea, and sodium permeate the hormone-responsive apical membranes through what appears to be parallel but dissociable routes (142, 161). In fact, there may even be separate membrane-bound adenyl cyclases controlling the hormone's stimulation of water and sodium transport.

In both species, the initial step in the action of AVP is its binding to receptors in the basal lateral membrane of the responsive cells. As mentioned earlier, this receptor-hormone interaction may not only initiate the cellular processes responsible for water and solute transport, but its magnitude and saturation may also determine the metabolic turnover and degradation of the hormone. Exactly how the spatial configuration and physicochemical structure of AVP determine its binding to the receptor is beyond the scope of this chapter, but an in-depth analysis of the available information can be found in the review of Walter and associates (163).

Once AVP is bound to its receptor on the basal (peritubular) surface of the cell, it initiates a series of reactions which lead to the increased apical (luminal) permeability to water and enhanced transcellular hydraulic flow along osmotic gra-dients. First in this series is the activation of the membrane-bound adenyl cyclase. The latter stimulates the conversion of ATP (adenosine triphosphate) to $3'5'$-cAMP (adenosine monophosphate), the intracellular concentration of which is regulated by phosphodiesterase. The more active or the greater the amount of the latter, the greater the inactivation and breakdown of cAMP. These initial steps proposed by Handler and Orlof (164) to be fundamental to the action of AVP have been widely confirmed and accepted. The subsequent intracellular steps are actively being investigated. These are discussed in detail by Dousa and Valtin (165) and Andreoli and Schafer (161). Based on the current concepts of the intracellular role of cAMP in various tissues (166), it appears that cAMP in turn activates one or more protein kinases in the cell, thus regulating the level of phosphorylation of specific cell proteins which may be bound or involved in the intracellular formation, aggregation, and translocation of certain unique intracellular organelles, known as microtubules and microfilaments, the formation of which accompanies and may be essential for the hydroosmotic effect of AVP (167). Whatever the role of microtubules and microfilaments in the action of AVP, it is clear that acute and chronic administration of colchicine (the classic antimitotic agent) and the related plant alkaloid, vinblastine, can significantly impair the hormone's hydroosmotic effect on the mammalian collecting duct (Fig. 12-37) without themselves altering GFR (glomerular filtration rate), solute excretion, or urine flow. Furthermore, this inhibitory effect did not involve an action of these alkaloids on the activity of the enzymes involved in cAMP metabolism and cAMP-dependent protein phosphorylation (168). It is well established that these antimitotic agents interfere with intracellular microtubule assembly in vitro and exert disruptive effects on cytoplasmic microtubules in vivo (167). Numerous morphologic studies have demonstrated a temporal and spatial relationship between the presence of microtubules and/or microfilaments and a variety of cell processes involving the movement of cellular components, i.e., pigment granules, phagocytosis, release of secretions, mobility of membrane receptors, pinocytosis, and exocyto-

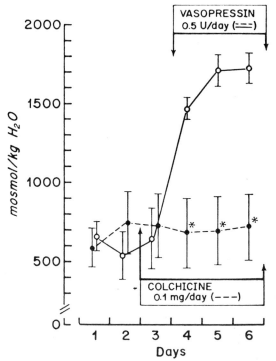

Figure 12-37. Response of urine osmolality to vasopressin in control rats (O——O) and in rats treated with colchicine on 3 to 6 experimental days (● - - - ●). Each group consisted of six animals. Asterisk indicates value significantly different from controls at $P<0.05$ or more (t test). [*From T. P. Dousa and L. D. Barnes (168).*]

sis (167). How this tubular aggregation and assembly can be related to water transport across AVP-responsive epithelium is unknown. As suggested by Taylor (167), it is possible that it can be related to the dramatic structural or organizational change in the (epithelial cell) luminal membranes of amphibian bladders in response to AVP as recently described by Kachadorian and associates (169, 170). By utilizing freeze fracture electron microscopy, they were able to consistently demonstrate that, in the presence or absence of an osmotic gradient, vasopressin and dibutyrl cAMP induced a reversible organized aggregation of intramembranous particles (presumably representing intramembranous proteins) in epithelial cell luminal membranes (Figs. 12-38a and 12-38b). Taylor speculated that microtubules and microfilaments may play a role in determin-

ing the distribution of intramembranous particles in the amphibian bladder. These organelles might play an anchorage role and/or be the effectors of movement of intramembranous particles in the plane of the plasma membrane, thus controlling the surface topography of the luminal membrane and, in turn, its permeability characteristics. In summary, AVP binds to high-affinity receptors on the basolateral or contraluminal surface of responsive epithelial cells which results in an adenyl cyclase–mediated generation of cAMP from ATP. The cAMP in turn mediates the kinetics of apical or luminal membrane-bound protein phosphorylation-dephosphorylation reactions which somehow interact with the formation and assembly of the microtubules. These permeability steps are associated with or followed by the permeability change(s) in the luminal membrane which cause the increased hydroosmotic flow of water, antidiuresis, and a more concentrated urine. The luminal surfaces of the cortical and medullary collecting ducts constitute the rate-limiting site for water transport and the final locus of action of AVP-mediated effects on transepithelial water permeation (142). Schafer and Andreoli (142, 161) most recently reviewed in depth the various studies contributing to an understanding of the physicochemical factors involved in the hormone-regulated movement of water across the luminal membrane, i.e., the way in which water traverses this hormone-regulated membrane. A brief summary of their conclusions will be presented and the reader is referred to their excellent analysis for additional information. (1) Water probably traverses the luminal membrane through hydrophilic sites having the characteristics of narrow aqueous channels (effective radius 1.8 to 2.0 Å) and AVP increases water permeability by increasing the number of such hydrophilic sites ("pores") in these membranes rather than increasing "pore" radii. (2) The primary process for hormone-dependent water movement is diffusion rather than laminar net volume flow, i.e., bulk flow through aqueous channels, pores, or cylinders as originally proposed by Koefoed-Johnson and Ussing (171). (3) The experimental observation that AVP enhances not only the diffusion of water but also certain small lipophilic (high oil/water partition

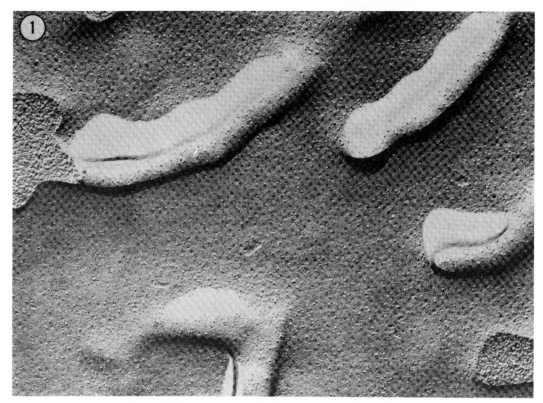

Figure 12-38a. Fracture face *P* of the luminal membrane of a granular cell from toad urinary bladder not stimulated with vasopressin. Ridgelike microvilli are prominent and intramembranous particles are distributed randomly over the entire membrane face. (× 47,500). [*From W. A. Kachadorian et al. (170).*]

ratios) molecules such as butyramide, isobutyramide, and antipyrine across the isolated, perfused, cortical collecting duct of the rabbit is best explained by assuming parallel diffusion pathways influenced by the hormone. (4) The water permeation pathways virtually exclude the diffusion of small hydrophilic molecules such as urea and thiourea as well as the electrolytes sodium and chloride.

Under normal physiologic conditions, the maximal urinary osmolality is determined by the magnitude of the hypertonicity of the medullary interstitial fluid bathing the collecting tubules and their permeability to water. The available data suggest that in certain circumstances the concentrating process is limited by a maximal rate at which free water can be abstracted from the tubular urine. Since the volume of the water resorbed ordinarily can considerably exceed the volume delivered to the collecting tubule, it is obvious that the maximal rate of back-diffusion of free water can be measured only when a large volume of isotonic fluid is delivered to this segment in the hydropenic animal. This can be achieved by the administration of an osmotic diuretic.

Figure 12-39 demonstrates the effects of increasing solute excretion on maximal urinary osmolality in the hydropenic human being administered a continuous infusion of vasopressin. It is readily apparent that, as the solute load increases, the maximum concentration of the urine falls in an asymptotic fashion toward the plasma osmolality (285 mosm/L). Under these circumstances, increasing amounts of isosmotic fluid are delivered to the concentrating segment of the nephron, and it can be calculated that the maximal amounts of free water abstracted from these relatively large volumes as they pass through the collecting tubule approach 5 to 8 mL/min. As will be subsequently shown, this rate may be altered by many factors, including, of course, renal functional mass.

Minimal osmolality and maximal volume of the urine during a water diuresis (absence of AVP) may also be influenced by the rate of solute excre-

tion. Figure 12-39 illustrates that, as solute excretion is increased during a maximal water diuresis, the osmolality of the urine increases in an asymptotic manner toward isotonicity. These alternations would, of course, be the result of the decreased fractional solute resorption in the diluting segment of the nephron (thick ascending limb and distal convoluted tubule). The residual urine leaving this segment during maximal water diuresis would approach isotonicity as proportionately less and less of the solute delivered to it is resorbed.

If the back-diffusion of free water in the cortical and medullary collecting tubule is a passive process, what are the factors limiting its maximal

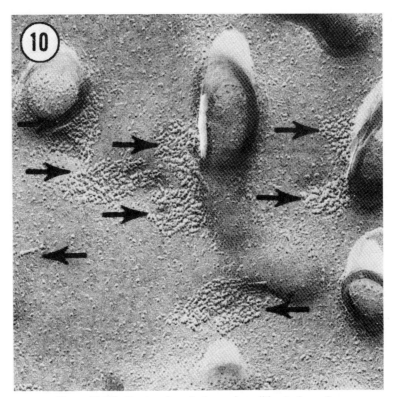

Figure 12-38b. Fracture face *P* of granular cell luminal membrane from toad bladder stimulated with vasopressin (20 mU/mL) in the absence of an osmotic gradient. Aggregates (arrows) appear identical to those found after vasopressin stimulation in the presence of an osmotic gradient. (×60,000). [*From W. A. Kachadorian et al. (170).*]

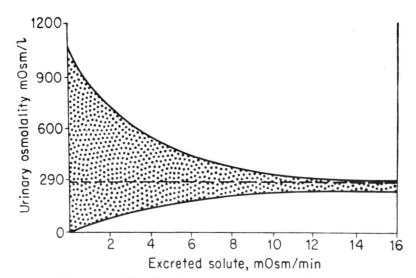

Figure 12-39. The effect of a progressive increase in solute excretion on the maximal urinary osmolality in the hydropenic animal (above horizontal line which represents plasma osmolality), and minimal urinary osmolality during water diuresis (below horizontal line).

rate? During osmotic diuresis the back-diffusion of increasing quantities of water into the hypertonic interstitium would, of course, reduce the hypertonicity of the interstitium, and this in turn would decrease the maximal concentration of the urine if the interstitial fluid and urine are in osmotic equilibrium. The model earlier described for the production of maximal medullary hypertonicity requires that urea be progressively concentrated in the distal convoluted tubule and collecting duct and, thus, in medullary interstitium, and, in turn, that sodium chloride be maximally concentrated by water abstraction in the descending limb of Henle's loop. As progressively more water is obligated or held back in the lumen during an increasing osmotic diuresis, it would progressively lower tubular urea concentration in the distal nephron and NaCl concentration in the descending limb, further reducing the medullary interstitial concentration of those solutes responsible for its hypertonicity. Also of importance in limiting the final back-diffusion of free water is the fact that the volume and velocity of flow of the fluid passing down the medullary collecting duct progressively increase during osmotic diuresis,

leaving less and less time for contact between the tubular urine and the cells of the collecting tubule. It also should be pointed out that efficiency of any countercurrent multiplier (including the loop of Henle) is inversely related to the velocity of flow. Osmotic diuretics may also reduce the hypertonicity of the renal medulla by increasing medullary blood flow (see previous discussion) which, in turn, decreases the "trapping" efficiency of the countercurrent exchange function of the medullary circulation. Therefore, during an osmotic diuresis maximal hypertonicity of the medullary interstitium cannot be achieved because of the decreased efficiency of the countercurrent exchange and multiplier mechanisms. This would contribute materially to limiting the maximal rate of free water resorption and urinary concentration during osmotic diuresis.

It is apparent from the previous discussion that active reabsorption of water need not be invoked to explain its movement anywhere in the nephron. Water diffuses passively along osmotic gradients, its movement being limited only by the magnitude of the gradient and the relative permeability of various segments of the nephron.

Therefore, the maximal U/P concentration ratios during oliguria and the maximal rate of back-diffusion of free water during osmotic diuresis, although of marked physiologic importance in the homeostatic regulation of water, do not denote any form of tubular maxima limited by an active transport process.

Although the collecting tubule is relatively impermeable to water in the absence of AVP, if the volume of fluid delivered to this segment is small enough, a moderately hypertonic urine can be produced. This phenomenon is most strikingly seen in the production of a significantly hypertonic urine during hydropenia in rats with congenital diabetes inspidus (172, 173).

In Tables 12-7 and 12-8 we have summarized the physiologic events responsible for a maximal water diuresis and antidiuresis after an acute water load or a period of hydropenia.

Concept of free water clearance

For functional purposes, Homer Smith and his associates conceived of the urinary water as being divided into two moieties: that volume necessary to excrete all the urinary solutes in isosmotic proportion, and that volume resorbed from the urine without solute during the concentrating process or "freed" of solute during the diluting process. Homer Smith called these two moieties of urinary water the C_{osm} (osmolar clearance) and the C_{H_2O} (free water clearance), respectively.

As mentioned, the osmolar clearance repre-

Table 12-7. Sequence of events in water diuresis

1. Ingestion of water load 1000 to 1500 mL
2. Dilution of all body fluids, hydration of cells of supraoptic nuclei, inhibition of secretions of ADH (AVP) from the neurohypophysis
3. Destruction of circulating AVP (half-life approximately 9 to 16 min) requires 60 to 90 min to reach peak water diuresis
4. No action of AVP in distal nephron (cortical and medullary collecting ducts) → maximal impermeability of these segments to water so that almost all the water delivered to them appears in the urine (approximately 10 to 15 percent of the filtered water)
5. Continued normal resorption of salts; therefore, urine of minimal solute concentration and maximal volume

Table 12-8. Sequence of events in maximal antidiuresis

1. Moderate negative water balance, i.e., rigid water restriction for 24 h →
2. Negative water balance of approximately 1500 mL or 1 to 2 percent of body weight →
3. Hyperosmolality of all body cells, with dehydration of cells of the supraoptic nuclei →
4. Release of impulses down neurohypophyseal stalk to posterior pituitary gland → AVP release into circulation on sustained basis
5. AVP acts on cortical and medullary collecting duct to make these segments freely permeable to water and the latter flows along concentration gradients established by continued solute resorption
6. Approximately 80 to 90 percent of solute reaching distal convoluting tubule is actively resorbed here and 80 to 90+ percent water resorbed, leaving small volumes of isotonic fluid to deliver into medullary collecting duct
7. In collecting duct water continues to passively back-diffuse into hypertonic interstitial tissue of medulla until urine and medulla reach maximal and equal concentrations; small volume reaching collecting duct reduced from one-third to one-fourth its volume and maximally concentrated (1100 to 1300 mosm/L; sp gr, 1.037)

sents the volume of urine necessary to excrete all the urinary solutes in an isosmotic solution. This would include the solutes remaining after all segments in proximal and distal nephron had acted upon them. It is calculated as follows:

$$C_{osm} = \frac{U_{osm} \, V}{P_{osm}}$$

where U_{osm} = urinary osmolality, mosm/L
V = urinary flow, mL/min
P_{osm} = plasma osmolality, mosm/L
$U_{osm} \, V$ = solute excretion, mosm/min

When U_{osm} is hypertonic to plasma, the ratio U_{osm}/P_{osm} will exceed 1. Therefore, $(U_{osm}/P_{osm}) \times V$ will exceed urinary volume, or C_{osm} will exceed urinary volume. Thus:

$$V = C_{osm} + C_{H_2O} \qquad C_{H_2O} = V - C_{osm}$$

Therefore, the free water clearance will have a negative value when the urine is hypertonic and a positive value when the urine is hypotonic. Expressed another way, free water clearance is that quantity of water excreted which is virtually "freed" of solutes during the process of urinary dilution.

An example of the calculation of osmolar clearance and positive and negative free water clearance will assist in clarifying these terms. Assume that 100 mL of glomerular filtrate is being formed per minute and that 80 percent of this filtrate is resorbed in isosmotic proportions by the beginning of the descending limb of the loop of Henle. In the descending limb, an additional 5 mL of water is reabsorbed. Assuming no water resorption in the ascending limb, 15 mL of hypotonic (150 mosm/L) fluid is delivered into the distal convoluted tubule. If during maximal AVP activity 90 percent of the remaining solutes were resorbed and enough water back-diffused to bring the urine to isotonicity by the end of the cortical collecting duct, 1.5 mL of isotonic fluid would be delivered to the medullary collecting duct. Here fluid would be withdrawn until 0.3 mL maximally concentrated urine of 1400 mosm/L were formed. If we assume plasma osmolality to be 285 mosm/L, then

$$\frac{1400 \times 0.3}{285} = \frac{420}{285} = 1.5 \text{ mL/min} = C_{\text{osm}}$$

$$V - C_{\text{osm}} = C_{\text{H}_2\text{O}}$$

$$0.3 - 1.5 = -1.2 \text{ mL/min}$$

The magnitude of the negative free water clearance, or the fluid back-diffusing in the ultimate concentrating process, equals 1.2 mL/min.

Conversely, if 15 mL of hypotonic fluid were delivered into the distal tubule in the absence of AVP and 90 percent of the solute were reabsorbed without water, approximately 15 mL of a dilute fluid (osmolality of 28.5 mosm/L) would be delivered into the final segment. Here a minimal amount of fluid would be removed in the absence of AVP (2 mL/min), leaving 14 mL of urine with a final concentration of 30 mosm/L.

$$C_{\text{H}_2\text{O}} = V - C_{\text{osm}}$$

$$C_{\text{osm}} = \frac{14 \times 30}{285} = 1.5 \text{ mL/min}$$

$$C_{\text{H}_2\text{O}} = 14 - 1.5 = 12.5 \text{ mL/min}$$

In recent years, the generation of a positive $C_{\text{H}_2\text{O}}$ during a maximal sustained water diuresis in dog and humans has been used as an index of NaCl reabsorption in the diluting segment of the nephron (174) and maximal urine volume (V), under these conditions, has been used as an index of NaCl delivery to this site(s). The exact anatomic location of this segment is not actually designated. In the state of physiologic diabetes insipidus (no apparent circulating AVP), it includes at least the thick ascending limb, the distal convoluted tubule, the cortical collecting duct, and some have even included the medullary collecting duct. To use $C_{\text{H}_2\text{O}}$ and V in this manner as an approximation of distal nephron NaCl reabsorption, one must assume little or no back-diffusion of water in this segment. It is clear from the micropuncture study of Jamison et al. (175) in rats with hereditary DI (diabetes insipidus) that even in the absence of AVP at least 2 percent of the filtered load of water is reabsorbed in the medullary collecting duct.

In Table 12-9 are listed the physiologic factors altering the maximal renal-concentrating capacity during hydropenia or when there is a maximal effect of AVP on the kidney.

Solute excretion rate

The effect of the rate of solute, excretion, or osmotic diuresis has been described earlier in the chapter.

GFR glomerular filtration rate

When the GFR is functionally decreased by more than 25 percent, insufficient sodium chloride and urea are delivered to the ascending limb and col-

Table 12-9. Physiologic factors altering the maximal concentrating capacity (presence of maximal AVP)

1. Rate of solute excretion or osmotic diuresis (sodium chloride, urea, glucose, mannitol, etc.)
2. GFR
3. Rate of medullary blood flow
4. Protein content of the diet
5. Water intake and the state of hydration
6. Salt (NaCl) intake and salt depletion
7. Presence or absence of an adequate amount of adrenal glucocorticoid and mineralocorticoid
8. Altered renal medullary prostaglandin synthesis by interstitial cells of the renal medulla
9. Diuretics with the exception of aminophylline

lecting duct, respectively, to provide maximal interstitial hypertonicity and, therefore, maximal urinary concentration. However, a decrease in GFR of less than 25 percent has been demonstrated to actually enhance slightly the maximal urinary osmolality of the hydropenic animal.

Medullary blood flow rate

The effect of change in medullary blood flow has been discussed earlier. However, it may be emphasized that if other factors remain relatively constant, a decrease in medullary blood flow increases maximal urinary concentration; an increase will decrease the maximal osmolality.

Dietary protein

An increase in the protein content of the diet increases the maximal capacity of the concentrating mechanism. Although it is possible that a low-protein diet impairs slightly the ability of the kidney to concentrate nonurea urinary solutes, the primary effect of protein on the concentrating mechanism is actually due to the resultant variations in urea excretion. It has been demonstrated that increased urea excretion enhances the concentrating mechanism (141, 143). From micropuncture studies and analysis of the medullary tissues of the hydropenic animal, it is evident that urea exists in equal and high concentration in the urine, in the tip of the vascular loop, and in the interstitium of the surrounding medulla (141, 143). Thus, in the hydropenic animal under the maximal influence of AVP, urea appears to be freely diffusible across the cells of the collecting tubule; as water is resorbed in this segment, urea follows it passively along its own concentration gradient. This, of course, adds to the hypertonicity of the interstitium and enhances the maximum concentrating ability of the nephron. The protein content or the urea formed from the diet does not appear to alter the maximal diluting capacity except by its effect on total solute excretion. The greater the protein content of the diet, therefore, the greater would be the back-diffusion of urea during the concentrating process, and the more hypertonic the medullary interstitium.

Hydration

Prolonged overhydration impairs the concentrating mechanism, whereas chronic dehydration enhances it (176). This effect of chronic overhydration may be of clinical significance, particularly in patients with psychogenic polydipsia. A mild concentrating defect may be evident after a few days of chronic overhydration. However, polydipsia of months or years duration may impair the concentrating mechanism markedly. These individuals may be unable to form urine with a concentration greater than isotonicity. The demonstration of this concentrating defect may lead to the mistaken diagnosis of polyuria and polydipsia secondary to a primary renal tubular lesion. Rigid water restriction for a number of days in these individuals, although difficult to maintain, will definitely enhance the maximal concentrating capacity. These individuals are capable of producing a normal maximal water diuresis, and their kidneys respond to the administration of AVP with the production of an isotonic or only slightly hypertonic urine. There is evidence that this concentrating defect is due to a reduction in medullary hypertonicity rather than any decrease in tubular responsiveness to AVP (177). The prolonged water ingestion in some way diminishes the efficiency of the countercurrent exchange and multiplier mechanisms. The augmentation in concentrating capacity associated with prolonged water restriction, conversely, is associated with an increase in medullary tonicity. The impaired responsiveness to AVP and the production of an increasingly concentrated urine in congenital diabetes insipidus rats during water restriction is a most striking example of this phenomenon.

Sodium chloride balance

It is readily apparent from the discussion of the function of the loop of Henle and the production of a hypertonic interstitium that if the active reabsorption of chloride accompanied by passive reabsorption of sodium in the thick ascending limb is defective or altered, or the amount of sodium chloride delivered to this site is diminished, the critical force for initiating a hypertonic medullary interstitium will be inadequate and the "bootstrap" effect mentioned earlier will be blunted, water will not adequately diffuse out of the descending limb, and the build-up of the NaCl concentration in the loop and ascending thin limb essential for the passive step of the countercurrent multiplier will not occur. Thus, for pathologic or physiologic reasons, we are left with a less hypertonic inner medulla and an inability to form a maximally concentrated urine in the terminal collecting ducts. It is often observed clinically that subjects who are severely salt depleted may, in spite of their marked oliguria, continue to produce an isotonic or only slightly hypertonic urine. This phenomenon may be secondary to a reduced sodium content of the interstitial tissues of the medulla.

Adrenal corticoids

Both glucocorticoid (cortisol) and mineralocorticoid (aldosterone) seem necessary for the production of a maximally concentrated urine during hydropenia (178). A distinct concentrating defect has been repeatedly demonstrated in the patient with adrenal insufficiency. This defect is probably due to a decrease in the delivery of NaCl to the loop of Henle and impaired active resorption of NaCl in the ascending limb of the loop. The possibility that glucocorticoids, through their permissive role, are essential for the normal action of AVP on the nephron has not been ruled out as a factor contributing to the concentrating defect of adrenal insufficiency. Recent studies suggest that glucocorticoids may enhance the hydroosmotic effect of AVP on epithelial membranes by inhibiting the generation of prostaglandins (179).

Prostaglandins

Prostaglandin (PGE) secretion by the interstitial cells of the renal medulla or the cells of the medullary collecting duct clearly modulates the action of AVP on the mammalian nephron (180–182). A local increase in PGE concentration inhibits the action of AVP (decreases maximal urinary concentration) while a decrease in PGE enhances the antidiuretic effect of AVP (181, 182). This modulating capacity of PGE appears to be exerted through its ability to alter the AVP activation of adenyl cyclase. The concentrating defect caused by potassium depletion is associated with an increased renal medullary generation of PGE and the defect can be markedly ameliorated by PGE synthesis inhibition in dogs (183). These observations on the AVP-PGE interrelationship indicate that any physiologic or pathophysiologic change which alters the renal response to AVP must engender the possibility that the deviation from normal is caused by a change in the synthesis of PGE. It is also of great interest that recent studies have shown that vasopressin can increase renal PGE biosynthesis in the rabbit, normal rat, and the Brattleboro rat (180).

Diuretics

Diuretic agents impair maximal concentrating capacity by inhibiting active chloride resorption in the thick ascending limb of Henle's loop (ethacrynic acid, furosemide, mercurials) and by producing chronic potassium depletion (184). It is of great interest that the xanthine diuretic aminophylline actually enhances both maximal diluting *and* maximal concentrating capacity of the mammalian nephron (185). It seems to act by increasing the delivery of sodium and water to the loop of Henle and distal nephron without interfering with NaCl resorption in any segment other than the proximal tubule. It is obvious that the concentrating capacity of the kidney cannot be evaluated while the patient is receiving a "loop" diuretic.

PATHOLOGIC FACTORS ALTERING MAXIMAL CONCENTRATING CAPACITY

All the clinical syndromes listed in Table 12-10 impair the kidney's ability to form a concentrated, or maximally concentrated, urine by producing singly or in combination the following lesions: (1) A progressive destruction of renal mass, leaving a reduced number of functional nephrons, which would cause an increased GFR and/or an increased osmotic (primarily urea and NaCl) load per nephron. The ensuing osmotic diuresis in each tubule could reach enormous proportions,

Table 12-10. Clinical states which impair maximal concentrating capacity

1. Chronic renal failure (pyelonephritis, glomerulonephritis, nephrosclerosis, gout, polycystic and medullary cystic kidneys, analgesic nephropathy, and other causes of interstitial nephritis)
2. Diuretic phase of acute tubular necrosis of any etiology
3. Hypokalemic nephropathy
4. Hypercalcemic nephropathy
5. Hyperaldosteronism (primary)
6. Multiple myeloma, amyloid disease, and Sjogren's syndrome
7. Postobstructive uropathy
8. Postrenal transplantation
9. Sickle cell anemia
10. Congenital nephrogenic diabetes insipidus (failure to respond to AVP)
11. High-dose chronic lithium ingestion
12. Methoxyflurane anesthesia
13. Psychogenic polydipsia
14. Chronic glucocorticoid and mineralocorticoid deficiency (Addison's disease)
15. Dichlormethyltetracycline (Declomycin)

thus causing the same "defect" in concentrating capacity that we see during an osmotic diuresis in normal animals and humans (Fig. 12-39), and for the same reasons. (2) Organic lesions of the renal medulla which disrupt the anatomic arrangement of the loop of Henle and the vasa recta or produce a specific defect in the active transport capacity of the thick ascending limb of the loop, which would seriously interfere with the countercurrent exchange and multiplier function of this part of the kidney. The maximal osmolality of the urine would be equal to or less than the reduced hyperosmolality of the medullary (or papillary) interstitium. (3) Organic lesions in the cortical and/or medullary collecting ducts which would impair their response to AVP. Such lesions would cause a polyuric syndrome associated with the persistence of a *hypotonic* urine despite hydropenia with high circulating levels of AVP or the administration of Pitressin.

DIABETES INSIPIDUS

Diabetes insipidus is a syndrome which results from failure of the neurohypophyseal system to produce or to release a quantity of AVP sufficient to bring about the normal homeostatic renal conservation of free water. In recent years this disorder has been called vasopressin-sensitive DI to distinguish it from the rare congenital and familial disorder NDI (nephrogenic diabetes insipidus), in which greater than normal amounts of AVP are produced; the latter has no observable effect upon the diluting segments of the nephron. It is obvious that the disturbance in water metabolism would be identical in both states, each characterized by the continuous production of an inappropriately large volume of hypotonic urine (specific gravity usually less than 1.005, osmolality less than 200 mosm/L). Diabetes insipidus may be complete or partial, permanent or temporary, and these forms will be discussed in greater detail.

This syndrome has been produced experimentally in many mammals over a number of decades. In general, to produce a persistent abnormality in the production or release of AVP, it has been necessary to destroy either the supraoptic nuclei or a major part of the neurohypophyseal tract or pituitary stalk. The simple removal of the posterior lobe, although at times associated with a short period of DI, has never been capable of producing the sustained disorder. This is strong evidence in favor of the currently accepted view that the neural lobe, although the major site for storage and release of the hormone, is not involved in its synthesis, and that in the absence of the posterior pituitary the newly formed hormone can still be released into the circulation.

PATHOPHYSIOLOGY

All the clinicopathologic lesions associated with DI involve the supraoptic and paraventricular nuclear areas or a major portion of the stalk.

It is generally concluded today that a primary functional abnormality in the thirst mechanism is not a significant factor in the polydipsia, but that the latter is a response to the profound renal water loss. However, it is not inconceivable that the associated hypothalamic lesions might at times produce a specific disorder of the thirst mechanism. In fact, the authors have had the opportunity of observing a patient with well-documented DI who, on recovery from this illness, was left with a severe thirst in spite of the fact that his renal-conserving mechanism for water was perfectly normal. Over the period of a year there was a gradual reduction in the thirst of this patient, and he was able to do well with increasingly smaller oral intakes of water. This could possibly be considered a conditioning defect of the thirst center, secondary to the excessive water ingestion of DI.

After experimental injury to the neurohypophyseal system, the development of the DI syndrome frequently follows a characteristic triphasic pattern (Fig. 12-40). This pattern, which may also occur clinically after acute surgical or traumatic injury to this area, is as follows: After the acute injury the initial effect is the immediate development of a polyuric, polydipsic syndrome indistinguishable from the full-blown disorder. Within hours to days this polyuric syndrome is replaced by a progressive reduction in urinary volume approaching the control level in terms of both concentration and value, and the animal appears to be normal once again. During this "normal interphase," however, the administration of an acute or sustained water load will not cause a normal water diuresis. The animal will continue to excrete little and inappropriately concentrated urine. If one persists in the water administration, a state of profound hypoosmolality and water intoxication will ensue. In a matter of days the "normal interphase" is replaced by a progressive increase in polyuria and polydipsia until a sustained state of DI is attained. The latter may be permanent or temporary, complete or partial. It is difficult to be certain about the exact cause of the first and second phases of this triphasic response. The initial temporary DI-like state probably represents a physiologic lesion comparable to spinal shock, that is, as a consequence of the sudden injury to the axons or nerve cell bodies, all impulses re-

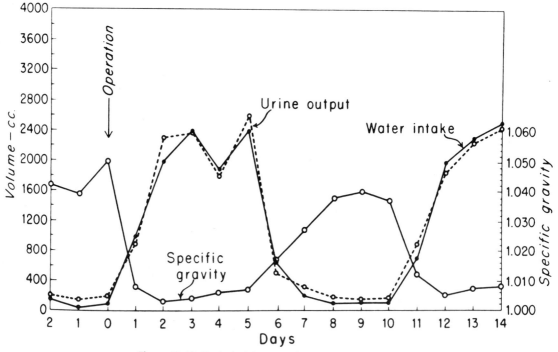

Figure 12-40. Typical triphasic cycle produced by section of the hypophyseal stalk and damage to the median eminence. The interphase extends from day 6 to day 10 or 11. (*From W. H. Hollinshead*, Proc. Mayo Clin., *39:95, 1964.*)

Table 12-11A. Weight and antidiuretic hormone (ADH) content of the posterior lobe of stalk-lesioned rats and intact controls (means ± S.E.)

DAYS AFTER OPERATION	WEIGHT OF POSTERIOR LOBE, mg	ADH CONTENT OF POSTERIOR LOBE, μmol PER GLAND	ADH CONTENT OF HYPOTHALAMUS, μmol PER WHOLE HYPOTHALAMUS
Control rats			
0	0.90 ± 0.05	1120 ± 55	111 ± 15
Stalk-lesioned rats			
1	0.89 ± 0.04	1050 ± 45	98 ± 7.5
3	0.61 ± 0.03	480 ± 25	57 ± 11
5	0.46 ± 0.05	135 ± 15	18 ± 2.5
7	0.35 ± 0.03	120 ± 12	16 ± 2.5
	Eight animals in each group		

Source: From F. A. Laszlo and D. de Wied (186).

sponsible for discharge of the hormone from the neurohypophysis are eliminated and the hormone is not discharged into the circulation. On the basis of chemical analysis of the hypothalamus and neural lobe, it appears that during the "normal interphase" there is a slow "leak" of AVP from the injured axons and the neurohypophysis itself into the circulation as the neurohypophysis undergoes atrophy and its hormone content disappears (186) (Table 12-11). Extensive lesions also produce progressive disappearance of the hormone content of the hypothalamus itself (186). If at the time of the initial experimental injury the stalk, posterior lobe, and median eminence are removed, the "normal interphase" will not develop (187). Finally, in the third phase the sustained state of DI is attained.

In those instances in which the lesion does not destroy or lead to the degeneration of the supraoptico-hypophyseal nuclei, the animal or patient may be left with the incomplete DI syndrome. The latter may manifest itself as a less severe polyuria (3000 to 6000 mL/day), with an impaired but not necessarily absent response to various osmotic and nonosmotic stimuli. At times this type of patient may fail to respond to hypertonic saline, but will develop a distinct antidiuresis after acetylcholine or mecholyl administration (39, 188, 189). The triphasic response may be seen in many instances of pituitary stalk section, total hypophysectomy, cryohypophysectomy, or even yttrium implantation. Figure 12-41 is an example of a patient who developed water intoxication and severe hyponatremia during the

Table 12-11B. Water intake, urine output, excretion of AD (antidiuretic) activity, weight of the posterior lobe, and ADH content in the hypothalamo-neurohypophyseal system of intact control and stalk-lesioned rats operated upon 2 months previously (means ± S.E.)

GROUP	BODY WEIGHT, g	WATER INTAKE, mL PER 24 h	URINE OUTPUT, mL PER 24 h	AD ACTIVITY EXCRETED IN URINE, μmol PER 24 h	WEIGHT OF POSTERIOR LOBE, mg	ADH CONTENT OF POSTERIOR LOBE, μmol PER GLAND	ADH CONTENT OF HYPOTHALAMUS, μmol PER WHOLE HYPOTHALAMUS
Intact rats	196.0 ± 6.1	27.0 ± 1.6	13.6 ± 1.0	0.47 ± 0.06	0.90 ± 0.05	1123.7 ± 49.4	112.6 ± 13.5
Stalk-lesioned rats with manifest diabetes insipidus	254.5 ± 11.2	166.9 ± 18.8	128.8 ± 16.2	0.05 ± 0.01	0.43 ± 0.03	17.7 ± 3.7	12.5 ± 1.6
Stalk-lesioned rats with "regression" of diabetes insipidus	261.0 ± 9.3	56.2 ± 4.1	23.9 ± 2.1	0.22 ± 0.05	0.48 ± 0.04	90.7 ± 6.9	73.4 ± 8.3
	Eight animals in each group						

Source: From F. A. Laszlo and D. de Wied (186).

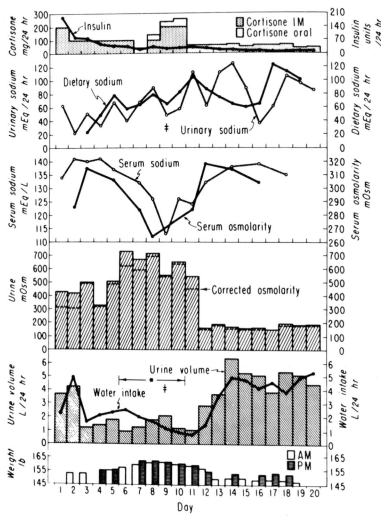

Figure 12-41. Metabolic changes after pituitary stalk section in a 39-year-old woman. *Asterisk* shows period of confusion, headache, and lethargy. *Double dagger* indicates intravenous administration of 385 meq of sodium chloride as 5% solution. (*From C. F. Gastineau et al.,* Proc. Mayo Clin., *42:406, 1967.*)

"normal interphase" of a mild DI which followed pituitary stalk section. This syndrome can be quickly differentiated from the impaired water excretion of acute glucocorticoid deficiency by giving the patient liberal amounts of cortisol or its equivalent. This therapy will immediately correct the water retention and hyponatremia if a glucocorticoid deficit exists. If it does not, the water retention of the "normal interphase" will persist and only rigid water restriction will correct it.

ETIOLOGY

The following are the major causes of DI in their relative order of frequency: (1) idiopathic (approximately 50 percent), which may appear in a congenital and familial form; (2) posthypophysectomy (surgical, yttrium implants, cryohypophysectomy, or stalk section); (3) basal skull fractures; (4) supra- and intrasellar tumors, either primary or metastatic, i.e., suprasellar cysts, craniopharyngioma, pinealoma, carcinoma of the breast, leukemia; (5) histiocytosis, i.e., eosinophilic granuloma and Schüller-Christian disease; (6) granulomatous disease, i.e., sarcoidosis and tuberculosis; (7) vascular lesions, i.e., aneurysms, atherosclerotic thrombosis; (8) encephalitis or meningitis; and (9) intraventricular hemorrhage (190).

Idiopathic or primary DI may be a familial disease; the hereditary form has been described as autosomal dominant with incomplete female penetrance, or else an x-linked recessive. This form may appear at any time during the lifetime of an individual. Although few postmortem studies have

been carried out, a recent study by Braverman and his associates has demonstrated that this disorder was due to a marked decrease in the nerve cells of the supraoptic and paraventricular nuclei with increased gliosis (Fig. 12-42) and decreased size of the posterior pituitary (191). The histologic changes observed in the patients with idiopathic DI are in striking contrast to the intact and enlarged supraoptic nuclei without gliosis seen in the rats with hereditary congenital DI. In rats there is a defect in hormone synthesis and in the human, a degeneration of the hormone-producing cells. The cause of this degeneration and gliosis is completely unknown. These cases do not dem-

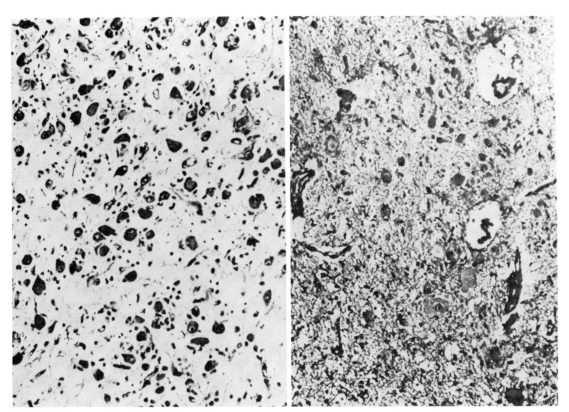

Figure 12-42. Photomicrograph of supraoptic nucleus of a normal 52-year-old male (*left*) and of a patient with diabetes insipidus (*right*). Note, in the normal, the large number of nerve cells with prominent peripheral distribution of Nissl substance. In the patient with diabetes insipidus there are loss of nerve cells, loss of Nissl substance, and moderate gliosis. (× 200). [*From L. E. Braverman et al. (191).*]

onstrate any associated abnormality of anterior pituitary function.

The various types of therapeutic hypophysectomy are becoming an increasingly common iatrogenic cause of DI. Of the primary tumors, in the region of the neurohypophysis, the adenomas of the anterior pituitary almost never cause DI. This is consistent with the experimental observation that removal of the posterior lobe per se does not result in DI. Those tumors that do create such a state must do so by involving the supraoptic and paraventricular nuclei or a major part of the neurohypophyseal stalk. The most classic examples of this are craniopharyngiomas and suprasellar cysts. On rare occasions, an acute DI state will develop as a result of metastases to the neurohypophyseal system. By far the most common such malignancy is carcinoma of the breast. Usually the DI develops late in the course of the disease and is almost always associated with other metastatic lesions. However, it may be the first subjective evidence of metastases. With this or other malignant tumors metastasizing to the area, DI always precedes the development of anterior pituitary insufficiency if the latter occurs. The tumor involves the anterior pituitary by contiguous spread from the neurohypophyseal system rather than by direct bloodstream metastasis to the adenohypophysis. As illustrated in Fig. 12-43 from the excellent study by Duchen (189), the anterior lobe receives its blood supply through a portal circulation, whereas the neurohypophyseal system is supplied by the systemic circulation. Tumor cells would not readily gain entrance to this portal circulation. When DI develops in a given patient, every effort should be made to determine its cause, since it may be amenable to specific therapy. The DI may be accompanied by symptoms of the causative disorder, such as sarcoidosis, central nervous system tumor, or xanthomatosis.

CLINICAL FEATURES

Diabetes insipidus may occur at any age, and there is no sexual predilection. Because of the rare familial nature of the disorder, other family members should be evaluated if a patient develops the idiopathic type. Almost all cases of true DI are of abrupt onset. These patients often recall that the polyuria and thirst started suddenly and reached a peak in a day or two. The history of a gradually increasing urinary flow, over weeks to months, generally suggests some other polyuric disorder. Continuous thirst is, of course, a classic symptom of the disease, the patient showing a predilection for very cold or iced water. This desire for very cold water is not characteristic of other polyuric syndromes, including psychogenic polydipsia. The urinary volume may range between 3000 and 15,000 mL daily, and a prominent nocturia is almost invariably present.

The patient with psychogenic polydipsia is rarely bothered with nocturnal polyuria. It must be remembered, however, that with DI of long duration the patient may develop an incredibly large calyceal, ureteral, and bladder capacity with frank hydronephrosis and hydroureter. The muscular wall of the bladder becomes thinned and decreased in tone. These patients may void as much as 1000 mL at a time, and the absence of nocturia, or the presence of only a mild nacturia, may be due to these alterations in the character and capacity of the urinary drainage system. On rare occasions the hydronephrosis may lead to definite impairment in kidney function with elevated BUN and creatinine (193). Diabetes insipidus may occasionally present in an atypical fashion. In one instance, the earliest symptom of diabetes insipidus in a young boy was the presence of severe night sweats. Nocturia did not occur becaue of dilatation of the urinary collecting system (192).

Characteristically, the withdrawal of water from a patient with severe DI will lead to an extremely rapid weight loss, profound thirst, and the rapid development of hypertonic dehydration. As long as the patient can satisfy this thurst, the patient will experience little but the inconvenience of the polyuria and the state of hydration will remain close to normal.

DIAGNOSIS

One must differentiate DI from all other important polyuric syndromes (Table 12-12). In DI, with the exception of mild plasma hyperosmolal-

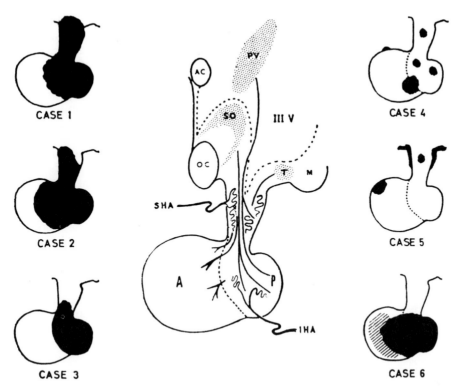

Figure 12-43. Diagram of neural and vascular connections between hypothalamus and pituitary gland (center) and of the location of carcinomatous deposits (solid black) in cases 1 to 6. The metastases are mainly in neural tissue at the sites of the primary capillary beds. In case 6 the stalk had been transected and the hatched area indicates the extent of infarction of the anterior lobe.

A, Anterior lobe; AC, anterior commissure; IHA, inferior hypophyseal artery; M, mammillary body; OC, optic chiasma; P, posterior lobe; PV, paraventricular nucleus; SHA, superior hypophyseal artery; SO, supraoptic nucleus; T, tuberal nucleus; III V, third ventricle. [*From G. W. Duchen (189).*]

ity (5 percent above normal) and unless significant dehydration is present, the blood and urinary chemistries are normal. This will not be the case in many of the syndromes listed in Table 12-12. A knowledge of the physiologic basis for polyuria is most helpful when one is confronted with this symptom.

True polyuria invariably means a decrease in the percentage of the filtered water that is absorbed by the renal tubules. This decrease may be secondary to an alteration in the tubular handling of water per se, to an impaired resorption of solutes with the development of an osmotic type of diuresis, or, finally, as in most acquired renal disease, to a combination of both these functional

abnormalities. The classification in Table 12-12 is relatively self-explanatory, and when the physician is confronted with a polyuric syndrome, the physician must think of most of the disorders listed. Polyuria may be the consequence of excessive water ingestion. Compulsive water drinking may be seen as a reflection of an underlying psychiatric disorder. Severe water intoxication to the point of death has been seen on occasion in severely disturbed or psychotic patients. The precise etiology of this disturbance is not known. It is also possible that selective lesions in the hypothalamus can produce enhanced thirst such as those which occur after experimental stimulation of the hypothalamus in goats (see earlier discus-

Table 12-12. Major polyuric syndromes due to a decrease in tubular reabsorption of water, solutes, or both

WATER	
Excessive H$_2$O ingestion—minimal circulatory AVP	Psychogenic polydipsia
	Polydipsia due to injury to hypothalamic thirst centers (rare)
	Potassium depletion and hypercalcemia
	Marked hyperreninemia (uncommon)
Inability to reabsorb adequate amounts of filtered H$_2$O	Inadequate circulatory AVP (complete or partial AVP-responsive diabetes insipidus)
	Renal tubular failure to respond normally to AVP
	A. Nephrogenic diabetes insipidus (congenital and familial)
	B. Nephrogenic diabetes insipidus (acquired): (1) Chronic renal diseases not primarily involving the glomerulus, i.e., pyelonephritis, polycystic kidneys, analgesic nephropathy, gouty nephropathy, medullary cystic disease, acute and chronic interstitial nephropathies; (2) Obstructive uropathy; (3) Multiple myeloma; (4) Amyloid disease; (5) Sjögren's syndrome; (6) Potassium deficiency; (7) Hyperaldosteronism or mineralocorticoid excess; (8) Nephrocalcinosis or renal damage secondary to hypercalcemia; (9) Unilateral renal artery occlusion (acute) with marked hyperreninemia; (10) Diuretic phase of ATN or nonoliguric ATN; (11) Postrenal transplantation; (12) PGE excess acting on distal nephron may contribute to any of the above; (13) Sickle cell anemia; (14) High-dose Lithium ingestion; (15) Methoxyflurane anesthesia; (16) Dichlormethyltetracycline (Declomycin).

SOLUTES: INABILITY TO REABSORB ADEQUATE QUANTITIES OF FILTERED SOLUTES (OSMOTIC-TYPE DIURESIS)	
Glucose—diabetes mellitus	1. Various types of chronic renal disease, particularly chronic pyelonephritis
Salts—primarily sodium chloride	2. After various diuretics, including mannitol
Urea—tissue catabolism or excess production of urea from hyperalimentation	

sion). Indeed, primary polydipsia has been reported in a patient with histiocytosis which may reflect the influence of an organic lesion on water balance (194). Alternatively, endogenous dipsogens such as angiotensin II (195) or PGE (see earlier discussion) may play a role in some of these patients. Thus, compulsive water drinking could have a psychologic, structural, or neurochemical etiology.

Nephrogenic DI or vasopressin-resistant DI is a rare congenital and familial disorder in which, in the homozygous form, the renal tubules are totally refractory to the antidiuretic effect of vasopressin (196–199). It is fascinating that although spontaneous mutation may rarely be the cause of this disorder (197, 198), all the affected individuals may have been of common genetic origin, descendants of an Ulster Scotsman (199). In the heterozygous form or in the absence of complete penetrance, there may be varying degrees of responsiveness to AVP and, in turn, varying degrees of polyuria. When basal plasma AVP and osmolality are measured in these patients, they are usually found to be above normal (92, 200) suggesting a state of mild water depletion. The patient with NDI is clinically indistinguishable from one with DI until a complete, or almost complete, lack of response to Pitressin is demonstrated. The exact cause of this defect in the nephron is unknown. Any step, from the initial binding of vasopressin to its receptor sites to the final metabolic event responsible for the maximum increase in the permeability of the distal nephron to water, could be defective. When the GFR and renal blood flow of NDI patients are reduced to a degree comparable to that of the DI patient, the former are unable to produce a urine hypertonic to the plasma (196). This suggests that in NDI either the collecting duct is truly impermeable to water or the renal medulla of these patients is either isotonic or even less hypertonic than the reduced medullary osmolality observed in the animal with DI.

The diagnosis of acquired nephrogenic diabetes insipidus should be restricted to the patient with an acquired renal disorder whose polyuria is associated with a *persistently hypotonic* urine unresponsive to Pitressin or hydropenia. In general, these disorders (Table 12-12) do not attain the degree of polyuria observed in DI or NDI, because, in most, the overall functioning renal mass is reduced by the basic disease process.

In DI a moderate concentration defect is usually present which will be corrected by the continuous administration of Pitressin. Valtin (72) found that the correction of the defect in congenital DI rats receiving Pitressin was associated with a return of the medulla to its maximally hyperosmolar state. The latter was due especially to a rise in urea concentration and, to some extent, NaCl. Invariably in the DI patient or animal, urine volume will decrease markedly following a single injection of Pitressin even though urinary osmolality, at first, may only slightly exceed isotonicity, i.e., 450 mosm/L.

The diagnosis of DI is assured when it has been demonstrated that one or more of the major stimuli to the release of AVP, such as carefully controlled water restriction, hypertonic saline infusions, and nicotine administration (rapidly smoking three or four cigarettes), do not cause a significant antidiuresis or the production of hypertonic urine, and that the kidney is responsive to exogenous AVP or Pitressin. Probably the most important and reliable test to demonstrate endogenous secretion of AVP is simple water restriction. This will lead to mild or moderate dehydration, and, if complete DI is present, a hypotonic urine (specific gravity below 1.005) or osmolality significantly below the simultaneously measured plasma osmolality will continue to be formed in spite of the dehydration. Restriction of water intake in a patient with probable DI should be done only with great care while the patient is observed closely. A patient with a severe case may lose as much as 0.5 kg of body water, per hour, and the test should be terminated if the patient loses 3 percent of body weight. It must be remembered that if the dehydration causes a major drop in GFR and solute excretion, oliguria and a slightly hypertonic urine may be formed even in the absence of AVP secretion. If a sensitive bio- or immunoassay for AVP is available, it is possible to demonstrate that during water restriction the rise in plasma osmolality does not cause an appropriate rise in the level of AVP in the plasma (92, 200, 201) (Fig. 12-17).

It had been generally thought that DI was an "all or nothing" disorder and that mild to moderate forms of DI did not exist. However, over 15 years ago Lipsett and Pearson (202) clearly demonstrated that incomplete failure of production or release of AVP occurred clinically. Their patients developed DI after surgery in the region of the neurohypophyseal system. This form is most apt to be seen after surgery in the region of the neurohypophyseal system. Figure 12-44 shows the maximal concentration of the urine as contrasted with the simultaneous plasma osmolality in subjects with varying degrees of posthypophysectomy DI following mild dehydration (10-h period of water withdrawal). It is apparent that a hypertonic urine can be formed by some of these patients, although they are not capable of producing a urine with an osmolality in the normal range for this test. The diagnosis of DI is obvious in those subjects whose urine was distinctly hypotonic at the end of the water restriction, but the presence of a moderately hypertonic urine after this period of water restriction does not rule out the diagnosis of partial DI. These subjects, therefore, had a quantitative decrease in the release or production of AVP.

Recently, Miller and his associates (203) studied the maximal concentrating capacity, during standardized conditions of dehydration, or normal volunteers, hospitalized "normals," and a wide variety of patients with diabetes insipidus. They clearly confirmed the observations of Lipsett and Pearson (202) and further demonstrated that the patients with partial and complete DI, after attaining their maximal but subnormal urinary concentration, still responded with a further increase in urinary osmolality after an injection of AVP (Fig. 12-45). The normal subjects and patients with psychogenic polydipsia did not demonstrate this response to exogenous AVP at the end of their period of dehydration. Thus, the production of a mildly to moderately hypertonic urine during water restriction, followed by a further significant increase in urinary osmolality (greater

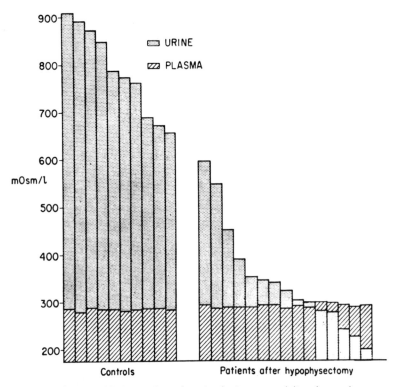

Figure 12-44. Comparison of maximal urinary osmolality of normal subjects with that from patients with varying degrees of diabetes insipidus following 10 h of water restriction. [*From M. B. Lipsett and O. H. Pearson (202).*]

than 9 percent) with an injection of Pitressin, indicates the presence of incomplete DI. As we will see below, the response of patients with DI to the sulfonylurea chlorpropamide now indicates that incomplete DI is far more common than ever suspected.

A rare patient with a syndrome indistinguishable from DI may be unable to form a concentrated urine during simple dehydration or after the administration of hypertonic salt, but is able to produce a hypertonic urine after the administration of nicotine, a strong nonosmotic stimulus to the release of AVP. This would suggest that the subject is incapable of responding to an osmotic stimulus but may respond to a nonosmotic one. However, it should be stressed that nicotine frequently produces a marked reaction with nausea,

vomiting, and, at times, a significant drop in blood pressure. Such an intense nonosmotic stimulus to the neurohypophyseal system would be quantitatively a far greater signal to its receptor and releasing capacity than the standard dehydration or hypertonic saline test. Thus, we may not be dealing with a truly qualitative difference but rather degrees of quantitative unresponsiveness. Furthermore, this marked reaction to nicotine certainly may produce a considerable alteration in renal hemodynamics. If the patient does have such a subjective reaction in association with a definite antidiuretic response, a significantly concentrated urine (> 450 mosm/L) might also be formed even if the patient had not released AVP with this stimulus.

This type of patient will still be polyuric because the total daily secretion of AVP is less than that necessary to bring about normal homeostatic renal conservation of free water, and would be classified as incomplete DI with the ability to release AVP in response to a strong nonosmotic stimulus. It is possible that if every patient with DI were tested for his or her response to various *nonosmotic* (Table 12-3) as well as the usual osmotic stimuli (dehydration and hypertonic saline), we would find many more patients with qualitative as well as quantitative defects in the release of AVP. DeRubertis and his associates (39) described in remarkable detail another type of qualitative abnormality in AVP secretion in which the patient had little or no response to osmotic stimuli, but an excellent response to various nonosmotic volume or baroreceptor stimuli. Enough

AVP was secreted to prevent polyuria, but the patient had sustained hypernatremia and a deficit in thirst regulation. This syndrome will be described in greater detail in the section below on hyperosmolar syndromes.

The vast majority of patients with DI will not develop an antidiuresis during or after the administration of hypertonic saline (5g/dL NaCl) (Fig. 12-46). For reasons cited earlier, during this test the subject should not have too great a prior·positive water load (not in excess of 500 mL) and probably should not receive more than 300 mL of 5% saline. The normal subject develops a distinct antidiuresis with hypertonic urine within 30 to 60 min after starting the hypertonic saline infusion. Although the absence of an antidiuresis strongly suggests DI, it must be remembered that on rare

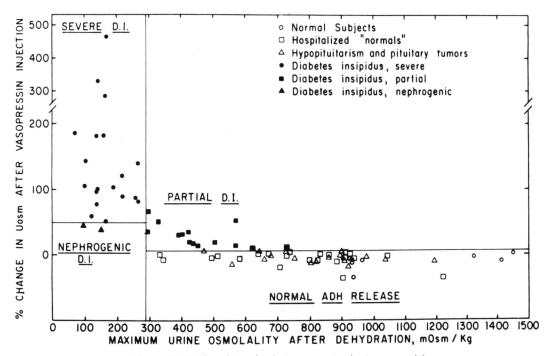

Figure 12-45. The relationship between maximal urinary osmolality after dehydration in normal subjects and patients with vasopressin-sensitive (pituitary) diabetes insipidus and vasopressin-insensitive (nephrogenic) diabetes insipidus, and the change in urinary osmolality after an injection of ADH. [*From M. Miller et al. (203).*]

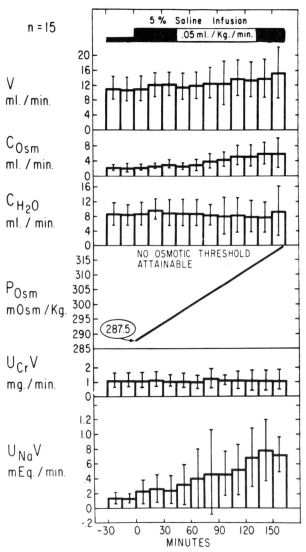

Figure 12-46. Composite of 15 osmotic threshold studies in 10 subjects with diabetes insipidus, of whom 6 had combined pituitary deficiency. No osmotic threshold was attainable even though the experiments were continued until the highest plasma osmolality in each instance ranged from 298 to 332 mosm/kg. Time intervals are expressed in relation to the beginning of the rapid saline infusion. (*From A. M. Moses et al.,* Am. J. Med., *42:368–377, 1967.*)

occasions if a given individual develops a marked augmentation of salt excretion, the osmotic diuresis may be so great that there may be little or no drop in total urinary volume despite a distinct fall in free water clearance. The drop in free water clearance, with the production of a hypertonic urine, is a true measure of a significant increase in permeability of the distal nephron or the presence of an effective amount of circulating AVP. The failure of a normal response to hypertonic saline, simple water withdrawal, or nicotine (rapid smoking of three or four cigarettes) should be followed by the intravenous Pitressin test over a 2- to 3-h period (described later). If a hypertonic urine is now formed, the diagnosis of DI is assured. A failure to produce a hypertonic urine after Pitressin administration does not absolutely rule out the diagnosis of DI, but suggests the possible presence of some functional or organic disorder of the renal tubules as the primary diagnosis.

The absence of significant polyuria does not necessarily rule out the diagnosis of DI. When GFR and solute excretion are significantly reduced (e.g., combined anterior and posterior pituitary insufficiency, severe water and salt depletion), and back-diffusion of water occurs even in the absence of AVP, the urinary volume may be less than 3000 mL per 24 h, and urinary osmolality may approach or slightly exceed isotonicity.

In recent years a number of attempts to devise more simplified tests for the diagnosis of DI have appeared (204). Basically, these have consisted of a standard period of rigid water restriction, varying from 6 to 8 h, with a measure of plasma and urinary osmolality at the beginning and end of this period. Normal individuals will have little or no change in their plasma osmolality; they will frequently begin with a moderately hypertonic urine which will become more concentrated by the end of the period of water restriction, that is, the U/P osmolality ratio will always significantly exceed 1 and, frequently, 2. The patient with complete DI will initiate the test with a plasma osmolality which on a random specimen *usually exceeds that of the normal subject*; the patient's initial urine osmolality is less concentrated than plasma, and, after the 6- to 8-h period of water restriction, plasma osmolality may rise significantly with little or no change in urinary osmolality. Therefore, the U/P ratio does not go up and may actually fall. This test, if unequivocally positive, is strong presumptive evidence for the diagnosis of DI, but the authors prefer in any given case to carry out the more extensive procedures described earlier. Too many patients have been misdiagnosed as having DI and have needlessly taken injections of Pitressin for months or sometimes years.

In the patient with psychogenic polydipsia, as a consequence of the profound and sustained primary ingestion of water, *the random plasma osmolality is usually significantly below that of the normal person and certainly lower than that of the patient with DI.* The patient with psychogenic polydipsia, when water is restricted under careful observation for a period of 12 to 18 h, will always reduce urine volume to a low level (1 to 2 mL/min) and increase urinary osmolality at least to isotonicity. On occasion, however, a compulsive water drinker may be so overhydrated that it may require longer than 24 h to excrete the positive water load and therefore a longer time to reduce urine volume to a low level. This patient can usually be suspected from an initial plasma osmolality and sodium concentration considerably below normal. Patients with psychogenic polydipsia when given an infusion of hypertonic saline will respond like the normal subject with the single exception that maximal urinary osmolality will be less hypertonic. In the author's experience, despite the concentrating defect resulting from months and years of excessive water ingestion, the patient with psychogenic polydipsia can invariably concentrate at least to isotonicity. This response to dehydration and hypertonic saline administration readily differentiates this patient from the one with complete DI. Incomplete DI may cause a problem in differential diagnosis, but the clinical picture, as described previously, the response to Pitressin after a period of dehydration (198), and the progressive improvement in concentrating ability with modest water restriction in the patient with psychogenic polydipsia usually confirm the true diagnosis.

The authors have observed that subjects with DI, under the influence of a maximal sustained water diuresis, do not generally produce a urine quite so dilute or so high in volume as a normal subject under similar circumstances, and random samples of their urine obtained when they are not receiving AVP are usually less dilute than during a sustained intravenous water load. This suggests that the patient with DI develops some new mechanism for either delivering a smaller volume of salt and water to the diluting segments of the nephron, or, less likely, allowing a greater degree of back-diffusion of water in these segments even in the absence of AVP.

TREATMENT

Once the diagnosis of DI has definitely been established, every effort should be made to find and treat the underlying causative disorder. Although newer modes of therapy are now available to treat DI (see below), some form of AVP frequently remains the mainstay of treatment. The most common form at the present time is Pitressin Tannate-in-Oil (5 units/mL). There is a general tendency among most physicians to use an excessive dose of this drug. As little as 0.5 mL every 2 days, given as a deep intramuscular injection, is usually adequate for optimal control. Unfortunately, Pitressin Tannate is packed in 1-mL ampules. The residual 0.5 mL may be covered with an alcohol sponge and adhesive and stored in the refrigerator. If an ampule of Pitressin Tannate is looked at carefully, a patch of dirty-brown material will be seen on the bottom of the ampule. This is the hormone. The ampule must be warmed in the hand and thoroughly mixed until this material is suspended in a slightly discolored emulsion. The importance of this cannot be too greatly emphasized. A small percentage of subjects will have an occasional allergic or local reaction to this preparation. If this occurs, a period of desensitization may be instituted, beginning with doses of 0.01 mL/day or less, and gradually increasing in stepwise fashion. Antihistaminics may be simultaneously administered. During the first days of treatment, and for emergency or acute use, aqueous Pitressin (20 U/mL) may be administered subcutaneously, particularly when DI complicates an acute disorder such as basal skull fracture or surgical or nonsurgical hypophysectomy. Use of the Pitressin Tannate-in-Oil, with its 24- to 48-h effect, makes it difficult to follow the unpredictable course of this DI complication. Also, the patient is prone to the development of water intoxication with the combination of the long-acting preparation and parenteral water administration. Recently the authors observed a 30-year-old male patient who was started on Pitressin Tannate-in-Oil (*1 mL three times a day*) for acute DI associated with a basal skull fracture, who continued to take this dose for 2 years. On admission to the hospital, his serum sodium was 120 meq/L with a proportionate decrease in plasma osmolality; urine osmolality was 300 mosm/L. When the Pitressin Tannate was stopped, the patient had a profound diuresis of very hypotonic urine and lost 20 lb in 24 h, with a return of serum sodium and osmolality to normal. He was shown on subsequent testing to have recovered completely from the DI, and the only abnormality was a functional concentrating defect resulting from the prolonged overhydration. This defect was corrected after 4 days of moderate water restriction (1000 mL/day).

The usual dose of aqueous Pitressin is 0.1 to 0.3 mL ever 4 to 6 h. One should be careful in administering these amounts to subjects with known coronary artery disease because of the vasoconstrictive effect of this hormone.

A nasal spray of synthetic lysine-8-vasopressin, 50 U/mL, in isotonic saline (Diapid) has been available for clinical use for almost a decade. In contrast to arginine-8-vasopressin, lysine-8-vasopressin is remarkably stable, and therefore this antidiuretic hormone, although not quite as potent as arginine-8-vasopressin, lends itself admirably to use as a nasal spray. The studies indicate that this preparation is both stable and nontoxic, and when used approximately every 4 h may cause a 50 to 75 percent reduction in urinary flow in the average case of DI. The nonirritating saline solution is sprayed deeply into the nasal passages from a plastic squeeze bottle, one to two sprays in each nostril. In the most severe cases of DI, it has been necessary to combine this nasal spray with the far less frequent use of Pitressin Tannate-in-Oil. A synthetic analogue of vasopressin is dDAVP (1-desamino, 8-D-arginine vasopressin), in which the L-arginine in position 8 has been replaced by D-arginine, and the free amino group in position 1 has been removed. This remarkable analogue has greater antidiuretic degree and duration potency than the natural hormone or any

other known analogue, whereas pressor activity in therapeutic doses has been reduced to very low values. The reduced pressor activity of this compound permits administration of high doses via the nasal passages without the smooth-muscle constricting effects of either AVP or LVP which often led to abdominal cramps or hypertension. It appears to be 6 to 10 times more potent than aqueous Pitressin, depending on dose, and it is very stable and can be administered as nasal drops. Five to twenty micrograms of dDAVP given as a nasal spray results in 8 to 20 h of antidiuresis in patients with central DI. The introduction of this highly potent, long lasting AVP analogue dramatically changes the therapeutic options for patients with DI. It is certain that it will become the drug of choice for this disorder, avoiding the necessity for the nonhormonal forms of therapy discussed below.

Recent years have also seen the development of two nonhormonal forms of therapy in the treatment of DI: (1) various diuretics, primarily thiazides and (2) oral hypoglycemic agents such as chlorpropamide (Diabinese). The former has also made a major contribution to the treatment of nephrogenic DI, because no other successful treatment for this disorder has existed in the past. Crawford and Kennedy (209) first demonstrated that the chronic administration of thiazide diuretics to patients with NDI and DI could cause approximately a 50 percent reduction in 24-h urinary volume and a comparable amelioration of thirst. The reduced urine volume, although less hypotonic, was never hypertonic. This suggested that thiazides did not act by significantly increasing the permeability of the distal convoluted tubule or collecting duct. Recent studies have clearly demonstrated, however, that other diuretics, as well as rigid sodium restriction, can cause a comparable degree of antidiuresis in these patients and, conversely, when the thiazide or the other diuretic is administered with enough sodium chloride to prevent a negative salt balance or a reduction in extracellular volume, the antidiuretic effect does not occur (10, 196). This implies that the mild negative salt balance and reduction in GFR, created by the diuretic, lead to enhanced reabsorption of isosmotic fluid in the proximal nephron. This in turn leads to a decrease in the amount of fluid delivered to the water-impermeable segments and therefore the reduced urinary volume. Although diuretic therapy, particularly thiazides, is now the specific form of therapy for NDI, it is at most an adjunct in the treatment of DI. The authors would recommend this form of therapy in DI, either alone or in combination with the sulfonylureas, when a significant sensitivity to the available vasopressins is present or the polyuria is so severe that the AVP preparation must be administered too frequently to be practical as a form of therapy in itself. It is important to instruct the patient to restrict oral sodium intake while on diuretics since the antidiuretic effectiveness of these agents is markedly reduced by ad libitum sodium.

While treating diabetes mellitus with the sulfonylurea chlorpropamide (Diabinese) in a patient with DI, Arduino and associates (210) noted that the nonglycosuric polyuria was significantly ameliorated. They clearly demonstrated that this compound had an AVP-like effect and could be used successfully in the treatment of vasopressin-sensitive DI. It had no effect in nephrogenic DI. Since these astute observations, numerous investigators have confirmed the antidiuretic effect of chlorpropamide that mimics small to moderate doses of AVP, and the therapeutic efficacy of chlorpropamide in many patients with DI (211–218). Chlorpropamide acts through a mechanism(s) distinctly different from that of the thiazides or other diuretics. The antidiuresis caused by the diuretics is secondary to their effect on sodium metabolism, and it is never accompanied by the production of a *hypertonic* urine. In contrast, when effective, a mild to moderate hypertonic urine is almost always produced by chlorpropamide and it has no known effects on sodium metabolism. It also does not alter the polyuria of nephrogenic DI, and the diuretics are as effective in NDI (210, 211) as in DI. The use of another sulfonylurea hypoglycemic agent, tolbutamide, has, on rare occasions, also been associated with hyponatremia, but it is not as effective as chlorpropamide for the treatment of DI (219).

An interesting clinical observation that may bear directly on the mechanism of action of chlorpropamide is the demonstration that some patients with DI do not respond to oral or parenteral administration of chlorpropamide. These patients appear to be those with the most severe or "complete" DI (patients who release no AVP from their neurohypophysis and therefore have none in their circulation). This suggests that the antidiuretic effect of these agents requires a minimal concentration of AVP in the circulation, a level which by itself has little, if any, antidiuretic action in the DI patient. In most clinical studies (210–218), 50 to 80 percent of the patients with DI respond in varying degrees to chlorpropamide therapy. Many of these patients, from the magnitude of their polyuria and failure to respond to antidiuretic stimuli, were considered to be patients with "complete" DI. Chlorpropamide responsiveness greatly broadens the spectrum and numbers of patients with incomplete DI. It further indicates that a "maximal" sustained water diuresis may be present in these patients and water-loaded, normal subjects (218), despite the presence of minimal amounts of AVP in the circulation. These observations and the fact that chlorpropamide has no antidiuretic effect, but potentiates the action of nonantidiuretic doses of AVP in congenital DI rats (220), indicate that chlorpropamide acts through a mechanism that potentiates or enhances the action of AVP on the distal nephron.

Ingelfinger and Hays (221) have carried out in vitro experiments on the toad bladder that strongly suggest this conclusion. They found that chlorpropamide alone at concentrations as high as 3×10^{-3} mol had no effect on water movement across the toad bladder. This concentration is almost six times the mean blood level attained in patients on long-term therapy with 0.5 g chlorpropamide. However, when vasopressin in low concentration (6 mU/mL) was added to the bladders that had been incubated with the chlorpropamide, water movement was significantly greater than that of the paired controls receiving vasopressin alone. This enhancement was not seen when a high concentration of vasopressin (60 mU/mL) was used. Although chlorpropamide enhanced the action of vasopressin, it did not augment the effect of cAMP on water movement across the toad bladder. These observations led Ingelfinger and Hays to question whether the sulfonylureas exert a direct AVP-like effect on the kidney in DI, and to suggest that they acted by increasing the sensitivity of the distal tubule to trace amounts of vasopressin or vasopressinlike peptides that persist in some patients with DI. They concluded from their observations that vasopressin and chlorpropamide share at least one site of action, and that this common site may precede cAMP within the receptor cell. This is supported by several in vitro studies in which chlorpropamide was shown to increase the activation of adenylate cyclase in the presence of submaximal concentrations of AVP (222, 223). However, more recently Brooker and Fichman (224) in an in vitro system have found that sulfonylureas inhibit the cAMP phosphodiesterase, and thereby could increase the steady-state level of cAMP in tissues, depending upon the tissue concentration achieved after oral or parenteral administration. As might have been anticipated from the present state of the art, Zusman and associates (180) most recently demonstrated that chlorpropamide enhances the hydroosmotic effect of AVP by inhibiting the AVP-stimulated tissue synthesis of PGE, a step proximal to and independent of the stimulation of the adenyl cyclase–cAMP system. As mentioned earlier, PGE appears to modulate the action of AVP on the nephron, i.e., a rise in local PGE decreases the effectiveness of AVP while a fall increases the antidiuretic response to AVP. Conversely, AVP stimulates PGE synthesis from the kidney of the rabbit, normal rat, the Brattleboro rat, and in the toad urinary bladder (180) by increasing the rate of release of the PGE precursor arachidonic acid from intracellular storage pools (180). That the chlorpropamide has no antidiuretic effect in patients with congenital nephrogenic DI (210, 211), despite the presence of elevated plasma levels of AVP (92, 200), is consistent with Ingelfinger and Hays' (221) concept that vasopressin and chlorpropamide share a common site of action. In the NDI patients, this site in the tubular epithelium is nonresponsive to these agents.

Miller and Moses (218) found a significant correlation between the ability of the patients with DI to reduce free water clearance in response to water deprivation and the ability to reduce the free water clearance in response to subsequent chlorpropamide treatment. Both ethanol and water loading were able to overcome the chlorpropamide-induced antidiuresis. Water deprivation while the patients were receiving chlorpropamide resulted in a further increase in urine concentration. Their data lend further insight to the concept that for chlorpropamide to produce an antidiuresis, some low level of endogenous antidiuretic hormone must be present. The single best explanation for its action is that chlorpropamide is capable of potentiating the action of non-antidiuretic or low submaximal levels of endogenous or exogenous AVP. No evidence for direct AVP-like action of chlorpropamide has been found, because the ability to respond to the drug appears to depend on the presence of the residual AVP-releasing capacity of the neurohypophyseal system. The available data to date have not ruled out the additional possibility that chlorpropamide can enhance the release of AVP from the normal or an abnormal neurohypophyseal system. Such a central action is suggested by the effect of chlorpropamide in restoration of thirst in patients with adipsia (173a). Miller and Moses (218) concluded from their observations that the response to water deprivation in a patient with DI may serve as a useful test to predict which patients are most likely to be benefited by treatment with chlorpropamide.

In the adult the dose would be 250 mg once or twice per day and in the child, one-half to one-third these doses, depending on the age of the child. The antidiuretic effect should begin within the first day after ingestion of the drug, reaching peak effectiveness within 3 to 4 days (210–218). However, the authors have observed an occasional patient who requires as long as 7 days to attain maximal antidiuretic benefit. Urine flow may fall to as little as one-third of the predrug level with the production of a moderately (300 to 600 mosm/L) hypertonic urine. When the response is optimal, chlorpropamide can be used as the sole form of therapy. In other patients it may be an important adjunct to the various forms of vasopressin. Because its mechanism of action differs from the thiazides, the two drugs will have additive effects and thereby complement each other therapeutically. An occasional patient, primarily one of those who appear to have complete DI, will not respond to maximal doses (500 to 750 mg/day) of chlorpropamide, and the drug should not be continued in such a patient. It is extremely important to remember that hypoglycemia may accompany the antidiuretic dose, especially during periods of fasting. The patient must be made aware of the hypoglycemic symptoms, and it is recommended that small between-meal and bedtime feedings be taken. Excess water ingestion in the patient with DI and even in the non-DI patient with diabetes mellitus ingesting sulfonylureas may cause hyponatremia and water intoxication (68, 216, 225); this is because of the sustained effect of those agents on the distal nephron.

Clofibrate (Atromid) has also been shown to exert an antidiuretic action in patients with DI who have some residual neurohypophyseal function (226). This action appears to be mediated by enhanced secretion of endogenous AVP (227). Clofibrate has the advantage of having considerably fewer side effects than chlorpropamide. Carbamazepine (Tegretol), a potent anticonvulsant also used for the treatment of tic douloureux, has been shown to be very effective in the oral therapy of DI (228). Rado has shown that this agent has a synergistic action when used along with chlorpropamide in patients who show an inadequate response to chlorpropamide alone (229). Combined use of both agents permits lower doses to be used of each agent with less likelihood of dose-related toxicity. Kimura and coworkers have shown significant increases in bioassayable plasma AVP that were not fully suppressed by oral water loading after treatment with carbamazepine (230). This suggested that the drug acted centrally to release AVP independently of osmotic stimulation. In contrast, Meinders and coworkers were unable to detect plasma AVP by immunoassay during the period of maximal antidiuresis after carbamazepine therapy in both patients with DI and in control subjects (231). The explanation for this discrepancy is unclear. Carbamazepine does not appear to have any intrinsic antidiuretic activity or does it augment submaximal doses of AVP (232).

Needless to say, the well-treated patient with DI may lead a normal life in every respect. In the untreated, as long as water is available and can be taken ad libitum, despite the inconvenience of the frequent day and night voidings, these patients suffer no basic ill effects and do remarkably well. However, if for any reason they are unable to ingest water or have it readily available, profound dehydration, water depletion, and hyperosmolar syndrome may develop in a very short period of time.

The patient with DI receiving adequate amounts of vasopressin and/or other forms of therapy need not alter his or her diet in any manner. During the first few days or weeks of treatment the patient should be warned against continued excessive habitual water ingestion because of the danger of water intoxication. In those cases in which the DI is frequently of a temporary nature, the therapy should be discontinued at intervals to note the patient's water turnover and possible recovery.

THE WATER DEPLETION (HYPEROSMOLAR) AND WATER EXCESS (HYPOOSMOLAR) SYNDROMES

HYPEROSMOLAR SYNDROMES

Table 12-13 shows those situations in which the effective osmolality of the body fluids is increased above normal. This is most often due to a loss of water from the body in excess of NaCl (a hypotonic solution), or the addition of a solute that does not freely penetrate cells, i.e., hypertonic glucose or mannitol, or a combination of both. In almost all instances in which there is a net hypotonic loss of water, hypernatremia occurs. Diabetes mellitus and prolonged administration of hypertonic mannitol solution are the only common clinical situations in which profound hypertonic dehydration may occur in the presence of normal or low serum sodium. In the uncontrolled diabetic with progressive hyperglycemia (and in the patient receiving hypertonic mannitol), osmotic withdrawal of water from all body cells will cause severe cellular dehydration and dilution of the residual sodium in the ECF. The extent of the lowering of plasma sodium by hyperglycemia per se can be estimated by multiplying 1.6 meq/L times each 100 mg/dL the plasma glucose is elevated above normal. At times, however, especially in the syndrome of nonketotic hyperglycemic diabetic coma (233), the magnitude of the water depletion may be so great that despite the profound hyperglycemia (> 1000 mg/dL), which is so characteristic of this syndrome, the serum sodium is normal or, more frequently, significantly elevated (> 145 meq/L) (see Chap. 24).

We have been increasingly aware of the hypernatremic hyperosmolar syndrome associated with hypertonic (glucose) peritoneal dialysis (234). The latter (4.5% glucose added to the isotonic dialysis fluid) is commonly used to treat intractable edematous states, especially in association with severe renal failure. When this hypertonic solution is put in the peritoneal cavity, water moves along its osmotic gradient into the peritoneal cavity, and extracellular electrolytes follow by diffusion. However, the glucose at 4500 mg/dL in the dialysis fluid diffuses rapidly into the bloodstream, elevating blood glucose to values of 500 to 1000 mg/dL. The marked extracellular hyperglycemia and hyperosmolality rapidly draw water out of all cells and dilute the salts of the ECF. The concentration of sodium in the blood and the ECF during this continuing unsteady state will fall below the sodium concentration in the dialysis fluid, thus establishing a gradient for sodium and chloride to diffuse from peritoneal cavity into ECF. The net effect of this process at the end of the peritoneal dialysis is the removal of water in excess of isotonic proportions of sodium. When the hypertonic glucose in the ECF is metabolized by the patient, usually over a 12- to 14-h period, the blood sugar returns to normal, the osmotic effect of the hyperglycemia disappears, water moves back into the dehydrated cells, and the sodium and chloride concentrations in the blood and the ECF rise to hypernatremic levels. It is apparent that this hypernatremia will prevent the complete rehydration of all body cells. This whole syndrome can be prevented or minimized by using the least hypertonic dialysis fluid necessary to achieve the desired negative fluid balance, i.e., 1½% alternating with 3 to 4% glucose, and giving the patient orally or parenterally adequate free water to take care of all insensible and renal losses occurring during the dialysis.

Hypertonic dehydration is particularly prone to occur in the elderly or the unconscious patient who cannot respond to the thirst stimulus, or cannot adequately request water when it is needed. Furthermore, these subjects are often tube fed a high-protein-containing mixture or given parenteral hyperalimentation. Very often a large part of the administered protein or amino acids is not retained but is converted to urea, and the excretion of the latter causes a sustained osmotic diuresis. This, like any other osmotic diuresis, will produce large urinary volumes that are hypotonic with respect to sodium. The relatively high rate of urine flow falsely assures the physician that the patient is getting an adequate intake of fluid. In reality, a progressive contraction of body water is taking place. Peters referred to the pathophysiologic events accompanying profound water loss as the "dehydration reaction." This consists of a low urinary water volume, a high urinary concentration and excretion of potassium, and, in spite of hypernatremia, a low concentration and excretion of urinary sodium.

The fascinating group of patients with hypernatremia and hyperosmolality with supposedly normal hydration, and their differentiation from other sustained hyperosmolar states (Table 12-13), has been reviewed in detail by DeRubertis and his associates (39). They investigated, in a most illuminating manner, a patient with this syndrome resulting from histiocytosis involvement of the hypothalamus. Abnormalities in water metabolism associated with lesions in this area appear to result from (1) impaired thirst, (2) impaired AVP production and secretion (DI), and (3) altered regulation of AVP secretion. These disturbances may occur either singly or in combination. DeRubertis has outlined the physiologic characteristics of those patients with hypernatremia and possibly normal hydration as follows.

The sustained hypernatremia is usually unassociated with a significant deficit of ECF volume as reflected by an absence of oliguria, azotemia, or decreased urinary sodium content. The spontaneous fluid intake is generally low relative to the elevated plasma osmotic pressure, indicating defective thirst. In addition, the release of ADH in response to osmotic stimuli appears impaired.

Table 12-13. Primary water depletion and other hyperosmolar states

A. Hypernatremia and hyperosmolality with dehydration secondary to water loss in excess of sodium:
  1. Polyuric states with failure of renal conservation of water in association with inadequate water intake.
    a. DI, nephrogenic DI (congenital and acquired).
    b. Osmotic diuresis, with unreplaced loss of hypotonic urine; marked glycosuria, mannitol diuresis (may be hyperosmolar and hyponatremic), high-protein gavage to comatose patients (urea diuresis), chronic renal failure.
  2. Primary water depletion in excess of sodium, with normal renal-concentrating mechanisms; comatose or disoriented patients with inadequate water intake, primary disorder of thirst regulation, diabetic coma, excess sweating and diarrheal disorders in children, hypothalamic lesions causing adipsia or hypodipsia in which forced fluid administration corrected the hyperosmolar syndrome.
  3. Hypertonic peritoneal dialysis.
B. Hypernatremia and hyperosmolality with possible normal hydration:
  Reset of osmoregulatory center with or without hypodipsia (idiopathic, hydrocephalus, brain tumor, histiocytosis X, postconcussive hyperosmolality).
C. Hypernatremia and hyperosmolality with overhydration:
  Primary aldosteronism, Cushing's syndrome, congestive heart failure with tracheostomy, pneumonia, etc., hypertonic saline, enemas to infants, hypertonic saline orally to infants, iatrogenic hypertonic saline administration to patients with chronic renal failure, inadvertent dialysis with hypertonic sodium solution, hypertonic (glucose) peritoneal dialysis.

However, endogenous ADH production is at least partially intact as implied by concentration of urine under certain circumstances. In a number of these patients hyperosmolality was not completely corrected by acute or chronic fluid loading, excluding inadequate fluid intake as the predominant factor in the disruption of osmotic homeostasis. It has been suggested that the sustained hyperosmolality in this group is the result of an elevated osmotic threshold for release of ADH. With such a disturbance in the osmotic regulation of ADH secretion, urine would be concentrated and water conserved only at very high levels of plasma osmolality (P_{osm}). Thus, a new steady state at a high plasma osmolality would be maintained by this proposed upward "resetting of the hypothalamic osmostat."

This hypothesis for the cause of the hypernatremia appeared to be substantiated in the patient studied by DeRubertis and his associates. During 23 days of observation, on normal diet and ad libitum water intake, plasma sodium fluctuated between 148 and 160 meq/L and plasma osmolality between 298 and 323 mosm/L. Endogenous AVP release was indicated by urine osmolalities as high as 710 mosm/L during water restriction, but only after a rise in plasma osmolality to 326 mosm and a weight loss of 1.4 kg. Fluid intakes as high as 6 L/day did not lower plasma osmolality, but merely led to a prompt water diuresis, indicating that simple water deficiency was not the cause of the hypernatremia. Hypertonic saline infusion during water diuresis, while causing a marked increase in plasma osmolality, resulted in the excretion of an increased volume of hypotonic urine (Fig. 12-47). An isotonic saline infusion, initiated during hydropenia, resulted in a water diuresis which continued despite a rise in the plasma osmolality from 302 to 320. The diuresis was terminated by orthostasis and resumed with return to the recumbent position (Fig. 12-48). Antecedent alcohol ingestion blocked the antidiuresis of orthostasis (Fig. 12-48).

These experimental observations indicated that the neurohypophysis was unresponsive to osmotic stimuli, but responded promptly and normally to nonosmotic volume changes or baroreceptor stimuli. In the steady state, the patient's extracellular volume (inulin space) was slightly below normal (11.2 L with a predicted normal of 12), as was her blood volume of 3.3 L with a standard normal of 3.7, corrected to height and lean body weight. DeRubertis suggested that the wide abnormal swings in random plasma osmolality (between 298 and 323 mosm/L) indicated that the altered AVP was not simply due to a resetting of the "osmostat," but was the consequence of (1) the loss of the sensitive osmotic regulation of AVP secretion, which normally maintains plasma osmolality at a relatively constant value, and (2) intact volume (baroreceptor) modulation of AVP secretion, which would result in relatively normal overall water balance but a less stable plasma osmolality.

The response to 250 mg/day, orally, of chlor-

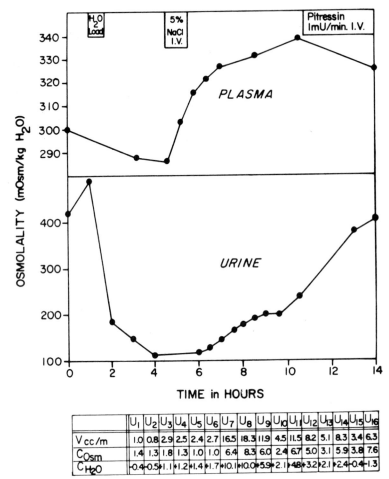

		U_1	U_2	U_3	U_4	U_5	U_6	U_7	U_8	U_9	U_{10}	U_{11}	U_{12}	U_{13}	U_{14}	U_{15}	U_{16}
V cc/m		1.0	0.8	2.9	2.5	2.4	2.7	16.5	18.3	11.9	4.5	11.5	8.2	5.1	8.3	3.4	6.3
C_{Osm}		1.4	1.3	1.8	1.3	1.0	1.0	6.4	8.3	6.0	2.4	6.7	5.0	3.1	5.9	3.8	7.6
C_{H_2O}		-0.4	-0.5	+1.1	+1.2	+1.4	+1.7	+10.1	+10.0	+5.9	+2.1	+4.8	+3.2	+2.1	+2.4	-0.4	-1.3

Figure 12-47. Response to hypertonic saline infusion. After establishment of a water diuresis with an oral water load (H_2O load), 20 mL/kg body weight, infusion of intravenous hypertonic saline (5% NaCl intravenously), 0.1 mL/kg of body weight per minute, did not result in urinary concentration despite a marked acute rise in plasma osmolality (52 mosm/kg of water, 18 percent in 6 h). Rather, urine flow (maximum 18.3 mL/min) increased with saline infusion. The maximum values were noted 90 min after cessation of the infusion. Water diuresis, still in progress at hour 10, was terminated with exogenous vasopressin (Pitressin, 1 mU/min intravenously). Table, at bottom, depicts V, C_{osm}, and C_{H_2O} in milliliters per minute, for individual determinations corresponding in sequence to points plotted for urine osmolality. (*From F. R. DeRubertis, M. F. Michelis, N. Beck, J. B. Field, and B. B. David, J. Clin. Invest., 50:97–111, 1971.*)

propamide is shown in Fig. 12-49, with a return of plasma osmolality to a normal level after 8 to 10 days of therapy. Mahoney and Goodman (220) also successfully employed chlorpropamide in a remarkably similar patient with chronic hypernatremia Bode et al. described a restoration of thirst with subsequent enhancement of oral water intake and amelioration of hypernatremia in patients with hypodipsia and DI (173a). This effect upon thirst suggests a possible CNS (central nervous system) site for action for chlorpropamide.

Chlorpropamide could be completely effective in this syndrome for two reasons, both based on its ability to markedly potentiate the presence of small amounts of AVP in the circulation: (1) A rise above normal in plasma osmotic pressure in these patients may still have caused a minimal release of AVP into the circulation, which in the presence of the chlorpropamide effectively increased water transport in the distal nephron, but was ineffective in the absence of the drug. (2) Despite the complete absence of osmotic release of AVP in these patients, chlorpropamide so enhanced the action of minimal amounts of AVP in the circulation that the smallest volume deviations from normal were *adequate* to supply this minimal necessary amount of hormone when chlorpropamide was present, but *not adequate* in its absence. These effects would complement any enhancement of thirst that might occur. The continued lethargy and clouded sensorium observed in these patients cleared completely when plasma sodium and osmolality returned to normal with therapy. DeRubertis and coworkers have subsequently described additional cases of essential hypernatremia (235). In these cases and in others from the literature, there was evidence for

"normovolemia," intact nonosmolar secretion of AVP, and defective osmolar stimulation of AVP. The absence of thirst seemed to play a significant role in the pathogenesis of the hypernatremia. This could not be the entire explanation since oral water loading failed to correct the disorder. They pointed out that exogenous vasopressin did return plasma sodium to normal, which suggested that AVP deficiency had a significant role in the perpetuation of the hypernatremia.

It is not clear, however, that such patients are truly normovolemic. Hypernatremia must be due to either renal water loss in excess of water intake with normal total body sodium or sodium excess. There is no evidence for the latter. Under conditions of water deficiency one would assume that both cellular and extracellular dehydration would be present and body fluid volumes reduced.

In recent years there have been several well-

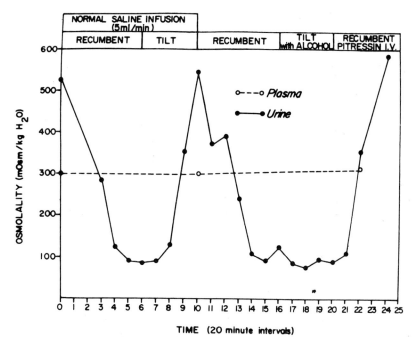

Figure 12-48. Interruption with orthostasis of a water diuresis induced by normal saline infusion. After overnight dehydration, a water diuresis was established during recumbency with normal saline infusion (5 mL/min). Tilting to 75° for 90 min resulted in urinary concentration with urine osmolality rising from 87 to 543 mosm/kg of water. Water diuresis resumed with recumbency. Tilt-

ing was repeated 15 min after administration of ethanol alcohol orally. Urinary concentration was not observed. During this study urine was collected at 20-min intervals by an indwelling bladder catheter. (*From F. R. DeRubertis, M. F. Michelis, N. Beck, J. B. Field, and B. B. David, J. Clin. Invest., 50:97–111, 1971.*)

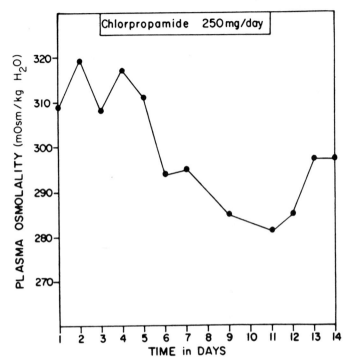

Figure 12-49. Response to chlorpropamide. A significant fall in plasma osmolality (P$_{osm}$) was noted on the fourth day of therapy with 250 mg of chlorpropamide daily. Response persisted for 2 days after cessation of the drug. Subsequent readministration of chlorpropamide resulted in a sustained lowering of P$_{osm}$ (*From F. R. DeRubertis, M. F. Michelis, N. Beck, J. B. Field, and B. B. David, J. Clin. Invest., 50:97–111, 1971.*)

documented case reports of hypernatremia in a setting of severe plasma volume contraction (236, 237). These patients may represent a more severe involvement of the hypothalamic–posterior pituitary system with simultaneous impairment of both osmolar and volume stimulation of thirst and AVP secretion. Urine volumes are kept normal because of both renal and extrarenal factors that contribute to water retention in this setting. The low level of residual circulating AVP, when combined with (1) a decreased GFR and renal blood flow, (2) enhanced reabsorption of solutes and water proximal to the collecting duct, (3) enhanced medullary tonicity over that observed in the nondehydrated state, and (4) enhanced vaso-

pressin-independent water reabsorption in the collecting duct as a consequence of the low rate of water flow through this segment, will result in the absence of polyuria observed in these cases.

Sridhar et al. (238) described a case of a 17-year-old girl who had originally manifested transient polydipsia and polyuria 2 years earlier and then presented with severe hyponatremia and hypovolemia unresponsive to oral water loading. When the U/P osmolar ratio was plotted as a function of serum sodium, it became apparent that the patient was capable of concentrating her urine if the serum osmolality were sufficiently elevated. They felt that the data did not support the concept of an elevated osmotic threshold for AVP release but rather suggested impaired AVP release at all levels of serum osmolality. A similar conclusion can be reached from the data of Grubb et al. from a unique case of a patient with adipsia following an episode of tuberculosis meningitis who also developed vasopressin-resistant hyposthenuria from streptomycin therapy (239). Plasma AVP was determined under varying conditions of hydration and was plotted as a function of plasma osmolality (Fig. 12-50a). In some instances, plasma AVP levels were well within normal range but this only occurred under circumstances of extreme hyperosmolality. As in the case described by Sridhar et al. (238), there was significant impairment of AVP secretion at all levels of plasma osmolality. In such patients what little AVP release is observed after dehydration could be stimulated in part by relative hypovolemia. Halter et al. (240) studied a patient with chronic hypernatremia and hypodipsia and found that although plasma AVP levels were inappropriately low for the given level of plasma osmolality, the patient was capable of substantially elevating plasma AVP after hypovolemic stimulation (Fig. 12-50b). As in the case described earlier, there was a significant correlation between plasma AVP and osmolality but with distinctly subnormal values for any degree of osmolality. The hypernatremia in these cases could be due to dysfunction of osmoreceptor stimulation of thirst and AVP release with sparing of magnocellular neurons for AVP synthesis. One might speculate that subsequent involvement of the supraoptic and paraventricular nuclei could eliminate even hypovolemic-stimulated AVP release with a resultant deterioration in volume homeostasis and profound hypovolemia. Thus, there may be a spectrum of disorders due to qualitative and quantitative defects in the separate components regulating thirst and AVP release (Table 12-14). There is evidence for a functional and anatomic separation of the osmoreceptors for thirst and those for AVP release as well as the neurosecretory neurons (Fig. 12-10). One could envisage a disease process selectively involving the magnocellular neurons in the hypothalamus or the axons traversing the pituitary stalk but sparing the thirst centers in the anterior hypothalamus. In this situation, renal water losses would produce hypertonicity of ECF which would in turn result in osmotically stimulated polydipsia and polyuria. The same clinical syndrome could also be produced by a disease process directly involving the osmoreceptors for AVP release but not those for thirst. If the disease then extended to impair the osmoregulation of thirst, then polydipsia would

cease and urine volumes would be reduced despite the continuing deficiency of AVP secretion. Renal water loss and impaired thirst would result in hypernatremia while nonosmolar stimulation of AVP would tend to minimize volume contraction. Finally, if the nonosmotic regulation of AVP secretion is impaired (probably by involvement of the magnocellular neurons themselves), then severe hypovolemia would ensue.

The proposed mechanism for the hypernatremia associated with overhydration syndromes, such as primary hyperaldosteronism, was described earlier.

Clinical manifestations of the hyperosmolar syndrome

If the patient is conscious, thirst may be extreme, unless there is a hypothalamic lesion causing defective thirst regulation. Severe hyperpnea may be present which does not resemble the deep respirations of Kussmaul respiration. Invariably there are significant alterations in the sensorium, with confusion, stupor, and eventually coma. Almost any type of focal CNS neurologic syndrome may accompany the altered sensorium. Convulsions may occur rarely, and xanthochromic or sanguineous spinal fluid may be found, confusing the diagnosis. The latter is due to the marked increase in permeability or even rupture of the fine capillaries of the brain and subarachnoid space caused by the marked contraction of the brain, secondary to its osmotic water loss. Macaulay and Watson have shown that some children with no antecedent neural disorder, surviving from severe hypertonic dehydration, may be left with a state of generalized cerebral dysfunction characterized by impairment of intellect, clumsiness, hyperactivity, and difficulty in social adjustment (241). The most severe CNS dysfunction is seen at both ends of the age spectrum and the more rapidly the hyperosmolality develops. Arieff and associates (242) have clearly demonstrated that, given time, the brain protects itself from dehydration by generating osmotically active substances, "idiogenic osmoles," which minimize the degree of water

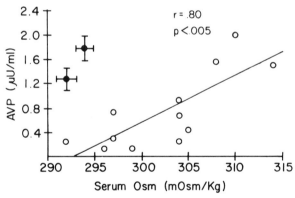

Figure 12-50a. Plasma AVP values plotted as a fucntion of plasma osmolality in a patient with adipsia and hypernatremia (open circles). The mean values for plasma, AVP, and osmolality for 24 normal subjects after 12 and 18 h of water deprivation (solid circles) are shown for comparison. Plasma AVP rose progressively with increasing plasma osmolality in this patient but always remained inappropriately low relative to plasma tonicity. Plasma AVP did eventually approach the normal range, but only at the expense of substantial hyperosmolality. [*Replotted from data of S. R. Grubb et al. (239) and R. Weitzman, unpublished data.*]

loss from the brain for any given increase in the osmolality of the blood (see Chap. 24).

The skin and mucous membranes are extremely dry and usually erythematous. In contrast to dehydration associated with salt depletion, the actual skin turgor may remain fairly normal. However, hypotension, tachycardia, and, at times, even hyperthermia without a discernible cause may be seen. Oliguria may be present, unless an osmotic diuresis is simultaneously occurring or a polyuric syndrome (Table 12-2) with hypotonic urine prevents renal water conservation. The concentration of hemoglobin and plasma proteins, as well as the hematocrit, will be elevated.

Water replacement using hypotonic solutions is the basic therapy of hyperosmolar states associated with water depletion. As the loss of water in this form of dehydration is derived proportionately from all the fluid spaces, it is possible to calculate the magnitude of the deficit from the observed serum sodium concentration and the assumed normal total body water (243). For example, a 20 percent increment in the concentration of sodium (assuming no significant loss of the total body solutes) will indicate a 20 percent reduction in the total body water. Therefore, the ratio of the normal serum sodium over the observed serum sodium multiplied by the assumed normal body water (60 percent of the usual body weight) will approximate the total volume of free water to be replaced. This can be administered parenterally in the form of 2.5 to 5% glucose in water or hypotonic (75 meq/L) saline, in an amount calculated to return the serum osmolality to normal.

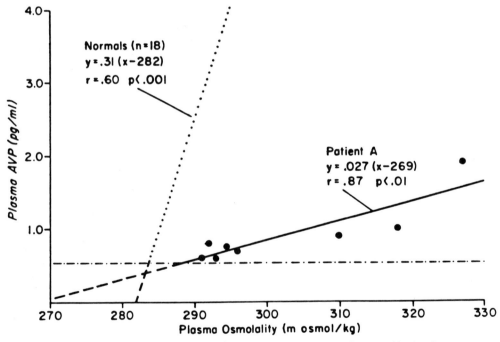

Figure 12-50b. Regression analysis of plasma AVP versus P_{osm} during hypertonic saline infusion in a patient with essential hypernatremia compared with the regression line for the plasma AVP–P_{osm} relationship during hypertonic saline infusion in normal subjects (data from Robertson and Athar, *J. Clin. Endocrinol. Metab.*, *42:613*, 1976). The horizontal broken line represents the sensitivity limit of the plasma AVP assay (0.5 pg/mL). (*From J. B. Halter, A. P. Goldberg, G. L. Robertson, and D. Porte, Jr., J. Clin. Endocrinol. Metab., 44(4):609–616, 1977.*)

Table 12-14. Evolution of hypernatremia owing to progressive disease of the hypothalamic centers for the regulation of thirst and AVP release

	POLYURIC DI*	"NORMOVOLEMIC" HYPERNATREMIA	HYPOVOLEMIC HYPERNATREMIA
Osmolar regulation of AVP secretion	−	−	−
Thirst	+	−	−
Nonosmolar regulation of AVP secretion, hypovolemia, hypotension	+	+	−
Serum sodium	+ ↑ −	↑	↑

* This syndrome could also be produced by selective destruction of the neurosecretory neurons or their axons in traversing the pituitary stalk, in which case nonosmolar stimulation of AVP secretion would be absent.

Tap water can of course be taken by mouth, if possible, and tap-water enemas will be very rapidly absorbed from the rectosigmoid colon. It is critical not to correct the hyperosmolar state too rapidly. When the rehydration and reexpansion of the brain is excessively rapid, convulsions and coma may ensue. Forty-eight to seventy-two hours would be a reasonably safe interval to achieve return to an euosmolar state. The cause of the hypertonic dehydration should, of course, be corrected, if possible, and measures taken to avoid its occurrence. Any undiagnosed comatose, stuporous, or confusional state in a dehydrated-appearing child or adult should suggest this hypertonic dehydration syndrome.

HYPOOSMOLAR SYNDROMES

As water moves freely across all cell membranes along established concentration (osmolal) gradients, any lowering of ECF osmolality results in an osmotic disequilibrium which produces a net flux of water from the ECF into the cells until osmotic equilibrium is reestablished. The resultant expansion of intracellular volume may alter cellular function and lead to definite symptoms. This is particularly marked in the CNS where lethargy, seizures, and coma may ensue (vidae infra).

In general, hypoosmolality and hyponatremia are synonymous or reflect each other. However, the presence of a lower than normal serum sodium concentration does not always imply the presence of hypoosmolality. In patients having marked elevations of either serum lipid or serum protein concentration, there is an artifactual reduction in the measured serum sodium concentration (Table 12-15). This is because the sodium, of course, is dissolved only in the water phase of the plasma. This phase normally amounts to 93 to 94 percent of a given unit volume of plasma. When in each milliliter there is a very large proportion of lipid or protein, the water phase is proportionately reduced. While the concentration of sodium in *plasma water* would be normal, the concentration per milliliter or per liter of *plasma* would be artifactually low. One can calculate the depression in measured serum sodium under these circumstances by multiplying the concentration of lipid in mg/dL by 0.002 or the elevation in serum protein concentration greater than 8 g/dL by 0.25. In contrast, the osmolality or freezing-point depression of the plasma is not influenced by its fat or protein content. Therefore, osmolality will be correctly measured and we will be alerted to this laboratory abnormality by finding a disproportionate reduction in sodium concentration relative to osmolality in the lipemic or markedly hyperproteinemic plasma.

A pathophysiologic situation in which hyponatremia is not associated with hypoosmolality of ECF occurs when there are high concentrations of low-molecular-weight solutes that are localized in the ECF compartment (Table 12-15). This would occur after intravenous infusion of large amounts of mannitol or glucose, or in diabetes mellitus with severe hyperglycemia. Under these conditions, the accumulation of osmoles in the ECF draws water from the cells and results in dilution of the sodium (in the serum or ECF). This type of hyponatremia has been designated cellular dehydration hyponatremia and the magnitude of the depression of serum sodium can be calculated by multiplying the elevation in plasma glucose greater than 100 mg/dL by 0.016, that is, for every 100-mg/dL increase in plasma glucose, the sodium will be diluted 1.6 meq/L (244). Under most other conditions, hyponatremia usually signifies hypoosmolality. This does not imply, however, that a single disease process or entity is responsible. The hypoosmolar states can be subdivided into three subcategories according to the status of the body sodium and water compartments (Table 12-15). The first category, which probably accounts for less than 30 percent of the patients with hyponatremia, we have designated *hypovolemic hyponatremia or hypotonic dehydration*. In this situation there is a significant deficit of total body water, but there is an even larger deficit of total body sodium, the latter occurring by either renal or extrarenal routes. Clinically, the patients are observed to have signs of ECF volume depletion coexistent with ICF expansion (see Chap. 3). Under these circumstances there is a marked reduction in ECF volume which is a stimulus to the renin-angiotensin system, to thirst, and to the nonosmolar or volume stimulus to AVP release. This is combined with a reduction in GFR, enhanced tubular reabsorption of salt, and a sodium and chloride concentration in the urine of usually less than 10 meq/L (unless the sodium loss occurred through the kidneys). The laboratory findings in this disorder are shown in Tables

Table 12-15. Differential diagnosis of hyponatremia

| | HYPEROSMOLAR HYPONATREMIA | EUOSMOLAR HYPONATREMIA | HYPEROSMOLAR HYPONATREMIA | | |
	CELLULAR DEHYDRATION (HYPERGLYCEMIA, MANNITOL INFUSION)	ARTIFACTUAL (PROFOUND HYPERLIPIDEMIA OR HYPERPROTEINEMIA)	HYPOVOLEMIC (SALT DEPLETION, THIRD SPACE)	MINIMAL HYPERVOLEMIA (SYNDROMES OF INAPPROPRIATE SECRETION OF ADH, MYXEDEMA)	HYPERVOLEMIC (CIRRHOSIS, CHF NEPHROSIS)
ECF	↑ or ↓	N	↓	nl or sl ↑	↑
ICF	↓	N	↑	↑	↑
"Effective blood volume"	↑ or ↓	N	↓	sl ↑	↓
AVP	↑ or ↓*	N	↑ †	↑ †	↑ †
PRA	N	N	↑	↓	↑
U_{Na}^+	N	N	↓	↑	↓
Treatment					
Mild (asymptomatic)	R_x underlying condition	R_x underlying condition	Normal saline	H$_2$O restriction or Declomycin	H$_2$O restriction R_x underlying condition
Severe (symptomatic)	R_x underlying condition	R_x underlying condition	Hypertonic saline	Hypertonic saline with furosemide, or peritoneal dialysis	Hypertonic saline with furosemide

* Hyperglycemia produced by intravenous infusion of dextrose in water has been reported to lower plasma AVP while mannitol stimulates AVP secretion.

† AVP is elevated in relation to the concomitant level of plasma osmolality.

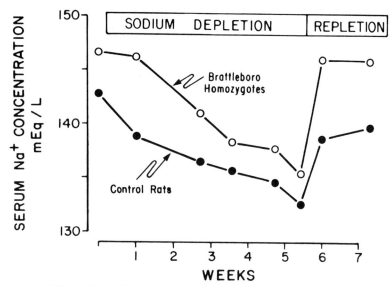

Figure 12-51. Development of hyponatremia during NaCl depletion in 7 control rats and 8 Brattleboro homozygotes. Similarity of
responses suggests that vasopressin is not required for selective
retention of water seen during sodium depletion. (*Abstracted from
A. R. Harrington, Am. J. Physiol., 222:768–774, 1972 and reproduced from H. Valtin et al., Rec. Prog. Horm. Res., 31:447–486,
1975.*)

12-15 and 12-16. This syndrome can occur at
times even in the absence of AVP, although AVP
levels are frequently elevated in hypotonic dehydration. We discussed earlier the fact that moderately hypertonic urine and oliguria can be produced in the absence of AVP if the volume of salt
and water delivered to the ultimate segments of
the nephron is markedly reduced. In fact, the severely sodium-depleted, congenital (Brattleboro)
DI rat may develop a degree of hyponatremia and
oliguria almost indistinguishable from that of a
salt-depleted non-DI rat when both are allowed
free access to water (Fig. 12-51) (245).

The second category probably accounts for at
least 60 percent of the patients with hyponatremia that we see in the hospital setting. It is due
basically to a primary excess of total body water
associated with a normal or slightly decreased total body sodium. This condition we have designated *hyponatremia with minimal hypervolemia.*
Under these conditions there is an "across the

board" expansion of intravascular, interstitial, and
ICF compartments proportional to their relative
sizes, i.e., each compartment is increased by the
same fractional amount. These patients have a
primary defect in the renal excretion of free water.
The clinical and laboratory characteristics of these
patients are described in Tables 12-15 and 12-16.

Excluding patients with chronic renal failure in
whom impaired water excretion may result simply from the marked reduction in renal mass (246),
we are left with the patient who fails to excrete
water in adequate amounts despite a structurally
intact kidney. This failure could be due to (1) an
alteration in renal function, which prevents the
delivery of an adequate volume of water to the diluting segments of the nephron (ascending limb
of the loop of Henle, distal convoluted and collecting tubules) (Table 12-17); (2) an abnormal
permeability of these segments to water despite the
absence of circulating ADH (AVP), or a substance such as oxytocin which in high concentra-

Table 12-16. Diagnostic and therapeutic approach to hyponatremia

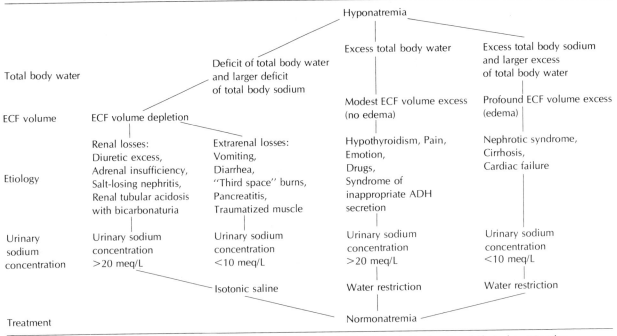

			Hyponatremia	
Total body water		Deficit of total body water and larger deficit of total body sodium	Excess total body water	Excess total body sodium and larger excess of total body water
ECF volume	ECF volume depletion		Modest ECF volume excess (no edema)	Profound ECF volume excess (edema)
Etiology	Renal losses: Diuretic excess, Adrenal insufficiency, Salt-losing nephritis, Renal tubular acidosis with bicarbonaturia	Extrarenal losses: Vomiting, Diarrhea, "Third space" burns, Pancreatitis, Traumatized muscle	Hypothyroidism, Pain, Emotion, Drugs, Syndrome of inappropriate ADH secretion	Nephrotic syndrome, Cirrhosis, Cardiac failure
Urinary sodium concentration	Urinary sodium concentration >20 meq/L	Urinary sodium concentration <10 meq/L	Urinary sodium concentration >20 meq/L	Urinary sodium concentration <10 meq/L
Treatment		Isotonic saline	Water restriction / Normonatremia	Water restriction

Source: From R. Schrier and T. Berl, Disorders of water metabolism, in R. W. Schrier (ed.), *Renal and Electrolyte Disorders*, Little, Brown and Company, Boston, 1976, p. 36.

tion can mimic the effect of AVP on the nephron; such an abnormal permeability *may* be present in patients or animals with a deficiency of adrenal glucocorticoids, i.e., cortisol; or (3) a sustained level of circulating AVP which causes an increased permeability to water of the distal convoluted tubule and collecting duct.

Each of the above could make the urine more concentrated and low in volume than *appropriate for a given solute and water intake*, thus resulting in abnormal water retention and hypoosmolality of body fluids. While (2) may be confined to adrenal cortical insufficiency (247), (1) and (3) may frequently be present together and result in a greater impairment in water excretion than either alone (246, 247). In fact, all three may at times contribute to the defect in water excretion almost invariably present in primary or secondary adrenal insufficiency (246, 247). The abnormalities in renal function mentioned could prevent a *necessary* water diuresis, the urine being relatively low

in volume and *less* hypotonic than it should be, and even moderately hypertonic. Confronted with this situation, one would be unable to determine whether the impaired diuresis were the result of an "inappropriate" circulating level of AVP or some other antidiuretic material, the altered renal function, or a combination of both. Bartter and Schwartz, in their original critical review of hypoosmolar syndromes (248), stressed the importance of a critical evaluation of the nonhormonal factors presented previously and the need for a more specific identification of the antidiuretic activity detected in the biologic fluids of certain of these patients.

Appropriate and inappropriate release of AVP

At this point, clarification of the term "inappropriate" is indicated. In Table 12-3 are listed the known regulators of AVP secretion.

Table 12-17. Physiologic and pathologic factors altering maximal water diuresis and urinary dilution independent of AVP

Rigid sodium restriction or sodium depletion impairs water diuresis:
a. Decreased filtered load of sodium and water
b. Enhanced proximal tubular reabsorption of sodium and water
c. Decreased delivery of sodium and water to distal tubule
d. Decreased velocity of flow to loop of Henle
e. Decreased medullary blood flow
GFR
   Decreased GFR may impair maximal water diuresis by above mechanisms; increased does converse
Medullary blood flow
   Decreased medullary blood flow impairs maximal water diuresis by increasing hypertonicity of medulla which allows increased back-diffusion of water in descending limb and collecting duct in absence of AVP; increased medullary blood does converse
Osmotic diuresis
   Increases water diuresis (free water clearance) but causes increase (less dilute) in minimal urinary osmolality because of increased delivery of solute and water to diluting segments
Diuretics
   Impair maximal urinary dilution and water diuresis
a. Induce sodium depletion with resultant changes
b. Selectively block sodium resorption by the cortical diluting segment (thiazides) or also in the ascending limb (furosemide, ethacrynic acid, ? mercurials)
Chronic renal failure
   Impairs maximal diuresis and urinary dilution by:
a. Decrease in number of functioning nephrons
b. Increase in osmotic load per nephron
Primary or secondary adrenal glucocorticoid deficiency
   Impairs maximal water diuresis and urinary dilution:
a. Decrease in GFR and (?) medullary blood flow
b. Enhancement of back-diffusion of water in the diluting segments of the nephron in absence of AVP
c. Inappropriate secretion of AVP on basis of volume depletion or ? stress
Hypothyroidism
   Impairs water diuresis by:
a. Decrease in GFR and (?) renal medullary blood flow
b. (?) Inappropriate secretion of AVP
Prostaglandin "deficiency"
   Administration of PGE synthatase inhibitors such as indomethacin

These have been discussed in detail in an earlier section. The final common pathway is the nerve cell bodies of the hypothalamic supraoptic nuclei, and the rate of hormone release at any moment will be the algebraic sum of its stimulatory and inhibitory impulses. We have stressed the continuous delicate balance that exists between the osmotic and nonosmotic (i.e., baroreceptor, chemoreceptor, thermoreceptor, etc.) stimuli impinging on this final common pathway. We know that normally a positive water balance, with its consequent drop in the osmolality of the blood perfusing the hypothalamic osmoreceptors, will inhibit the release of AVP to a degree necessary to establish normal water diuresis (Table 12-7). As mentioned earlier, small amounts of AVP may continue to be released into the circulation at this time owing to the tonic stimulation of the nonosmotic baroreceptors (Table 12-3). However, if a significant fall in blood pressure or cardiac output, and/or a decrease or redistribution of blood volume, caused a sustained change in impulses from these receptors, AVP release would be maintained at a higher level despite the positive water balance, and the necessary water diuresis would not occur.

Table 12-18 is designed to indicate the distinction between *appropriate* yet nonosmotic stimuli and truly *inappropriate* release of antidiuretic peptides, whether derived from the neurohypophysis or from an ectopic source such as a malignant tumor producing AVP. It is also important to emphasize that the states listed in Table 12-17 which also lead to hyponatremia are also those in which the functional alterations in renal hemodynamics and the renal handling of solutes and water may impair water diuresis *in the absence of any circulating antidiuretic material.*

The sustained release of AVP in these syndromes is due to one or more of the following: (1) An abnormal stimulation, by CNS dysfunction or disease, pain, drugs, or psychosis (Table 12-3) of those areas of the reticular formation, limbic system, or cerebral cortex which have neural connections with the hypothalamic, supraoptic, and paraventricular nuclei. (2) The stimulation of the nonosmotic mechanisms listed in Table 12-3 under 2a–2c. (3) Tumors of varied causes that have been demonstrated by analysis of the tumor, the plasma, or the urine to contain an antidiuretic material biologically indistinguishable from AVP (Table 12-18). The group of disorders, in which AVP is secreted independently of known osmotic

Table 12-18. Clinical hypoosmolar states associated with measured or probable increased secretion of AVP

A. States in which AVP may be released (appropriately) in response to the nonosmotic stimuli listed in Table 12-3, 2a and 2b
  1. Hypovolemia or hypotension secondary to blood loss, or loss of extracellular volume of any cause
  2. Intrinsic myocardial disease with reduced cardiac output or edematous states (enhanced proximal tubular resorption of salt and water in either of these two conditions may at times be more important than increased AVP secretion in the impaired water excretion)
    a. Cirrhosis with ascites or after large paracentesis.*
    b. Nephrotic syndrome with hypoalbuminemia and hypovolemia
    c. Congestive heart failure
    d. Postmitral valvulotomy, with relief of distention of left atrial receptors (Table 12-3, 2b)*
  3. Stimulation of other pathways for AVP secretion: chemoreceptors,* thermoreceptors,* pain,* nausea,* hormones,* etc.
B. States in which AVP secretion may be increased despite the absence of appropriate stimuli (Table 12-3) ("inappropriate" AVP syndrome): bronchogenic carcinoma,* adenocarcinoma of the pancreas,* lymphosarcoma, duodenal adenocarcinoma,* pulmonary tuberculosis, pulmonary abscess,* subdural hematoma,* brain tumors,* subarachnoid hemorrhage,* cerebral vascular thrombosis,* skull fractures,* cerebral atrophy,* central pontine myelinolysis,* paroxysmal seizure disorders, acute psychoses,* herpes simplex encephalitis, administration of large quantities of oxytocin and water to obstetrical patients, Guillain-Barré syndrome, tuberculosis meningitis, purulent meningitis, acute intermittent porphyria,* myxedema,* postoperative ADH release due to morphine, barbiturates,* cyclophosphamide, vincristine,* carbanazepine,* anesthesia or surgical stress,* and transient "idiopathic" hyponatremia (secondary to diuretics, especially thiazides*), ADH release after surgery* and after hypophysectomy*
C. Hyponatremic states with absolute or relative overhydration in which factors other than sustained inappropriate ADH secretion may be responsible for impaired water excretion
  1. Primary and secondary adrenal (glucocorticoid insufficiency)
  2. Chlorpropamide* and rarely tolbutamide ingestion (both enhanced renal sensitivity to AVP and possibly increased AVP release)

* Increased levels of AVP have been measured in serum, urine, or tumor extracts by bioassay or immunoassay.

or nonosmotic pathways (Nos. 1 and 3), are called SIADH, or syndromes of inappropriate secretion of ADH.

In Table 12-18, paragraph B, we have placed asterisks after those clinical states in which antidiuretic activity has been detected in plasma, urine, or tissue extracts by bioassay (249) and/or radioimmunoassay (249, 250). The references to some of these studies are given in the review by Bartter and Schwartz (248). Table 12-19 presents our findings in neoplastic disease with the hypoosmolar syndrome (249). In five of the patients, significant quantities of antidiuretic activity were extracted from the original tumor and/or its metastases. This activity was identified as arginine vasopressin by immunoassay in four, and by complete inactivation of the antidiuretic activity by human pregnancy plasma (vasopressinase) and rabbit vasopressin antisera in all five. Although the concentration of AVP per milligram of dried powder (47 to 763 μU) is only a fraction of that in the human neurohypophysis (85 mU/mg dried powder), the total mass of the tumor is so great that it is capable of releasing enough hormone to cause a sustained inappropriate AVP syndrome. It should be emphasized that in five patients (Table 12-19), despite the classic hypoosmolar syndrome, no antidiuretic activity was detected in their tumors. Either the syndrome in these cases was due to sustained nonosmotic release of AVP from the neurohypophysis, or the concentration of the hormone in the tumor at the time of extraction was too low to be detected by the assay procedures.

The presence of AVP in tumor extracts, blood, and urine, although strongly suggestive that the tumor is the source of the inappropriate AVP "secretion," is not final proof. The latter requires the demonstration that the tumor is actually capable of producing the hormone. This has been achieved by George et al. (251). They extracted bronchogenic carcinoma that had been removed from a patient with the classic syndrome of inappropriate secretion of AVP and found 23.5 mU of vasopressin per gram of wet weight by radioimmunoassay. Slices of this tumor were incubated with phenylalanine-^{3}H and arginine-vasopressin-^{3}H was purified from the incubate, thus demonstrating in vitro biosynthesis of vasopressin by the tumor. On electron microscopy the small undifferentiated cells of the tumor had well-developed endoplasmic reticulum and ribosomes. "Secretion" granules surrounded by limiting mem-

Table 12-19. Characteristics of tissue, plasma, and tumor antidiuretic principle from patients with inappropriate ADH syndrome

SPECIMEN	ANTIDIURETIC ACTIVITY, μU/mg POWDER				MILK-EJECTION ACTIVITY, μU/mg POWDER	
			AFTER INCUBATION			AFTER INCUBATION
	BIOASSAY	IMMUNOASSAY	H.P.P.	V.A.R.		V.A.R.
1. Bronchogenic carcinoma	763 ± 53*	610	⊖	⊖	169 ± 7	⊖
Normal lung	⊖				⊖	
2. Bronchogenic carcinoma	16 ± 13	116	⊖	⊖	57 ± 8	⊖
Hepatic metastasis	⊖	10			⊖	
Normal lung	⊖	<3			⊖	
Normal liver	⊖	<4			⊖	
Plasma	15/mL		⊖			
3. Bronchogenic carcinoma	150 ± 14		⊖	⊖		
Liver metastasis	⊖	<4				
Plasma	⊖					
4. Bronchogenic carcinoma	130 ± 10		⊖	⊖	⊖	⊖
Breast metastasis	740 ± 76	1540	⊖	⊖	124 ± 11	⊖
Mediastinal metastasis	283 ± 19	120	⊖	⊖	48 ± 2	
Brain metastasis	307 ± 72		⊖	⊖		
Kidney metastasis	⊖				⊖	
Normal lung	⊖				⊖	
5. Adenocarcinoma of pancreas	⊖				⊖	
Hepatic metastasis	47 ± 7	24	⊖	⊖	⊖	
Plasma	8/mL					
6. Bronchogenic carcinoma	⊖	<20			⊖	
Hepatic metastasis	⊖	<1			⊖	
Normal lung	⊖	<5			⊖	
Normal liver	⊖	<3			⊖	
7. Bronchogenic carcinoma						
Biopsy	⊖				⊖	
Autopsy	⊖				⊖	
Plasma	⊖				⊖	
8. Bronchogenic carcinoma	⊖	<4			⊖	
9. Bronchogenic carcinoma	⊖	<4			⊖	
Plasma	10/mL		⊖			
10. Bronchogenic carcinoma	⊖	<5			⊖	

Source: From H. Vorherr, S. G. Massry, R. D. Utiger, and C. R. Kleeman: *J. Clin. Endocrinol.*, **28**:162, 1968.

* Mean values ± standard error were calculated from values obtained in three to five rats. For each rat the average of several assays was used.

Abbreviations: H.P.P. = human pregnancy plasma, V.A.R. = vasopressin antiserum from rabbit, ⊖ = <10 to 20 μU/mg powder for vasopressin and <12.5 to 25 μU/mg powder for oxytocin.

branes were present which resembled those seen in polypeptide hormone-secreting cells (Fig. 12-52). Vorherr (252) has recently added additional proof that the malignant tumor is the source of the AVP.

Chronic pulmonary tuberculosis was one of the earliest described causes of the hypoosmolar syndrome, being referred to as "pulmonary salt wasting" (248). Vorherr and his associates (253) have clearly demonstrated the presence of vasopressin in tuberculosis lung tissue from a patient with advanced pulmonary tuberculosis and a typical syndrome of inappropriate secretion of AVP. The extracted tissue contained 22 μU of vasopressin

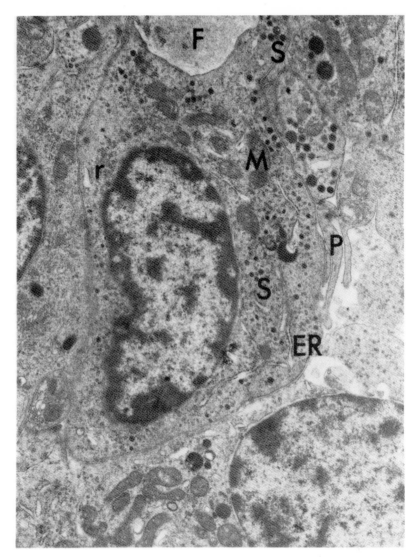

Figure 12-52. Neoplastic cell with numerous intracytoplasmic secretory granules (S) and long profiles of endoplasmic reticulum (ER) with attached ribosomes. These cells were observed less frequently than the poorly differentiated neoplastic cells (at left and bottom). In addition to the secretion granules, large mitochondria (M) and aggregations of free ribosomes (r) were present in the cytoplasm. Cytoplasmic projections (P) extended into the prominent intercellular spaces which often contained a network of intermeshed fibrils (F). (× 11,300). [*From J. M. George, C. C. Capen, and A. S. Phillips (251).*]

per milligram of dried extract. The uninvolved lung tissue, and suspension of *Mycobacterium tuberculosis*, and the culture media with its metabolites failed to show antidiuretic activity. This is the first case in which a relationship between AVP

and hyponatremia in a patient with pulmonary tuberculosis has been demonstrated. Pulmonary diseases of other etiologies have been associated with SIADH. These include chronic obstructive pulmonary disease with emphysema, acute lobar pneumonia, and empyema. In some of these syndromes it has been suggested that AVP release might be provoked by impaired pulmonary compliance and some diminished stretch on great pulmonary vein or left atrial receptors.

Pathophysiology of water retention in minimal hypervolemic hyponatremia

The hypoosmolar syndromes may or may not be associated with overt edema or reduction in the renal hemodynamics, neither of which is essential to the development of the water retention and hypoosmolar state. The mechanism in the nonedematous cases is identical to that which results from the continuous administration of exogenous Pitressin to normal subjects ingesting a constant and liberal amount of water (Fig. 12-53) (254).

The patient is found to have hyponatremia, hypochloremia, normal or low blood urea and creatinine (unless a separate cause for renal impairment exists), mild to moderate oliguria, and a urinary excretion of sodium in excess of 25 meq per 24 h, or approximating intake. Note that although the dose of Pitressin was constant throughout the experiment, urinary osmolality and oliguria were considerably greater in the first few days of its administration (Fig. 12-53). Subsequently, urine volume rose and the concentration of the urine, although still hypertonic, approached the pre-Pitressin period. This "escape" from the maximal renal effect of the hormone must be related to the intra- and extrarenal response to the progressive expansion of total body water. It is referred to by Bartter and Schwartz (248) as a new "steady state" in which the degree

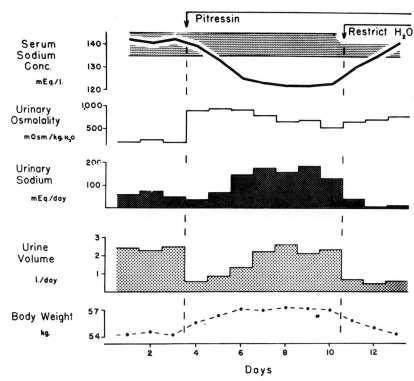

Figure 12-53. Diagrammatic summary of the effects of Pitressin and water administration to normal subjects. (*From M. Goldberg, Med. Clin. N. Am., 47:915, 1963. See also Ref. 254.*)

of hypoosmolality or hyponatremia may range from slight to as low as 100 to 110 meq/L. At this period urinary sodium usually reflects intake. Although it is evident that the new steady state protects the patient from even more severe degrees of oliguria and water retention, the hypoosmolar syndrome will persist as long as a normal water diuresis cannot occur or the patient remains in positive water balance.

Rigid restriction of water (negative water balance) returns the serum sodium to normal in association with a prompt and marked reduction in sodium excretion (Fig. 12-44). The cause of the relatively high urinary sodium or the sodium loss has been attributed in part to hypervolemic inhibition of aldosterone secretion in assocation with an actual increase in the GFR and the filtered load of sodium (248). However, in some patients urinary aldosterone excretion and GFR have been within the normal range despite the continued urinary loss of sodium, indicating that some additional mechanism must be present (115, 116). It is true that in many cases there is a relative inhibition of aldosterone secretion, but the most reasonable explanation for the enhanced loss of sodium is that expanded total body fluid with expansion of the plasma and extracellular volume causes an inhibition of tubular reabsorption of sodium which may cause enhanced excretion of sodium despite continued secretion of aldosterone (115, 116).

Nolph and Schrier (255) carried out a careful and accurate balance study on a patient with cerebrovascular disease and the syndrome of inappropriate secretion of AVP. The results of their study are most helpful in explaining some of the unusual biochemical features of the syndrome. Weight gain and decreased plasma sodium always occurred when the daily fluid intake was 25 mL/kg, causing gradual expansion of body fluids; 30 mL/kg led to a rapid expansion. The latter caused a sudden increase in sodium excretion, whereas with gradual expansion there was minimal, if any, increase in sodium excretion. Aldosterone excretion rates were normal during the control and volume-expansion periods. The authors concluded that negative sodium balance, owing to renal loss of sodium, did not contribute significantly to the hyponatremia with either gradual or rapid expansion. During both states estimated net positive water balance greatly exceeded the actual weight gain. We also have observed this phenomenon. Since the patient was on an isocaloric diet throughout the study, these results suggested that the positive water balance in this syndrome may enhance pulmonary and cutaneous insensible water loss so that more water is retained by balance than actually calculated from weight gain. During water restriction and recovery from hyponatremia, sodium excretion was well below the control level. This was associated with a rapid return of the plasma sodium concentration to normal over several days *with only slight weight loss relative to weight gain* during the previous water-expansion period. Aldosterone excretion increased during this recovery period and together with increased proximal resorption may have been responsible for the positive sodium balance. During a period of gradual expansion (fluid intake 25 mL/kg), if the patient were on a high sodium intake, isonatremic volume expansion occurred. Positive sodium balance protected against the development of hyponatremia. Thus, an inappropriate retention of water can occur in this syndrome *without* the development of hyponatremia if the rate of fluid ingestion is not too great and the patient is on a relatively high sodium intake.

It should be stressed that to develop a water intoxication syndrome the patient need only be unable to achieve a water diuresis when hypoosmolality of the body fluids exists. Although hypertonic urine is frequently present, the patient may be excreting an isotonic or even slightly hypotonic (200 to 250 mosm/L) urine. At this point acute expansion of the ECF with *isotonic* saline (which is actually hypertonic to the patient) may paradoxically cause a mild water diuresis, with the urine becoming even more hypotonic. This has been observed when the "inappropriate AVP syndrome" is due to a bronchogenic carcinoma (248). If the latter is "secreting" AVP, it is unlikely that volume expansion would inhibit release of the hormone from the tumor. Therefore, the paradoxical water diuresis is probably due to a renal "escape" from the antidiuretic effect. As mentioned by Bartter and Schwartz, "an analogous 'escape' is seen in normal dogs given infusions of saline and vasopressin and has been attributed to an increase in tubular flow of a magnitude such that there is inadequate time for osmotic equilibration in the distal portion of the nephron" (248).

At times, however, when a sustained nonosmotic release of AVP from the neurohypophysis is the cause of the hypoosmolar syndrome, the patient may respond to a water load with a normal water diuresis. This suggests that the patient is now able to regulate the release of AVP but only in the presence of the expanded total body water and hyponatremia. At this point the subject may respond in a normal fashion to a test load of water. This phenomenon might be anticipated from our earlier discussion of the continuous sensitive interrelationship between osmolar and nonosmolar stimuli controlling the release of AVP. There is a "resetting" of the "osmostat" created by the nonosmotic impulses impinging on the final common pathway or the magnocellular neurons of the neurohypophyseal system. For example, the cirrhotic patient with hyponatremia with a markedly expanded total body water may have a distinct water diuresis when a sustained water load (1000 to 1500 mL) causes a further decrease in the osmolality of the patient's body fluids. During this diuresis, if hypertonic saline is infused, an antidiuresis with the production of a hypertonic urine will occur as the serum becomes less hypoosmotic. This indicates that the normal osmotic stimuli now produce an appropriate homeostatic response of the neurohypophyseal system. It is evident therefore that a normal water diuresis in this new steady state does not rule out the possibility that the initial water retention was produced by sustained nonosmotic release of AVP. The edematous patient who develops this water-excess syndrome (*hypervolemic hypernatremia*, see below and Table 12-15), in association with severe congestive heart failure, the nephrotic syndrome, cirrhosis of the liver, or some other disorder which functionally reduces GFR, enhances the release of aldosterone, and inhibits the humoral natriuretic "third factor" (115, 116), may have a urine that is free of sodium rather than demonstrate the "salt wasting" phase described above.

A most unusual example of the conversion of the "salt wasting" to a "salt retaining" state was described by Heinemann and Laragh (256). Two patients with neoplastic disease (oat cell carcinoma of the lung and adenocarcinoma of the stomach) and the syndrome of hyponatremia, with excessive renal sodium loss, were studied. Both had normal renal and adrenal function, which in one was unquestionably due to a sustained inappropriate secretion of AVP. While under observation both patients developed occlusion of the vena cava, and the hyponatremic "salt wasting" state was converted to one of progressive sodium retention and edema formation. In the one with superior vena caval occlusion, the salt retention occurred without an increase in aldosterone secretion; in the other with occlusion of the inferior vena cava, the edema formation occurred in association with hypersecretion of aldosterone. The disease of these two patients then closely resembled the hypoosmolar syndrome seen in other edematous states.

Most recently an increasing number of reports of diuretic- (especially thiazide) and chlorpropamide-induced hyponatremic water intoxication syndromes have appeared (130, 225, 257–260). Fichman et al. (130) studied 25 cases of severe hyponatremia secondary to the use primarily of thiazide diuretics in nonedematous patients without signs of dehydration and with normal creatinine clearances. These cases could be distinguished from other hyponatremic syndromes (Tables 12-16 and 12-20) by the presence of hypokalemia and alkalosis, the return of serum sodium to normal and unimpaired excretion of a water load within 3 to 10 days after withdrawing the diuretic, and the recurrence of hyponatremia within 2 to 12 days of readministering the drug (Fig. 12-54). Bioassay of the plasma while the patients were severely hyponatremic showed elevated AVP levels in all 10 patients studied. In Fig. 12-55, the concentration of AVP in these patients is compared with that in the plasma of 23 cases

Table 12-20. Differential diagnosis of hyponatremia with normal hydration

	INAPPROPRIATE ADH SECRETION	HYPOPITUITARISM	HYPOTHYROIDISM	DIURETIC-INDUCED	CHLORPROPAMIDE-INDUCED	POLYDIPSIC VOMITING
Creatinine clearance	Normal or ↑	Normal or slightly ↓	Normal or slightly ↓	Normal or slightly ↓	Normal or ↑	Normal or ↓
Serum K	Normal	Normal	Normal	↓	Normal	↓
Serum HCO₃	Normal	Normal	Normal	↑	Normal	↑
Urine Na⁺	↑	↑	↓	↑ Early ↓ Later	↑	↓
Urine osmolality	↑	↑	↑	↑ Early ↓ Later	↑	↑
Metapyrone response	Normal	↓	Normal	Normal	Normal	Normal
H₂O load response	↓	↓	Delayed	Normal	Delayed	Normal
Correction	H₂O restriction	Cortisol	Thyroid	Discontinue diuretics or ↑ K⁺ intake	Discontinue chlorpropamide	NaCl HCl H₂O restriction

Source: From M. P. Fichman, H. Vorherr, C. R. Kleeman, and N. Telfer, *Ann. Intern. Med.*, **75:**853–863, 1971.

of the typical syndrome of inappropriate secretion of AVP of varied cause, and of 10 patients with secondary adrenal insufficiency associated with pituitary disease. Simultaneous isotope dilution studies in 10 of the patients with diuretic-induced hyponatremia disclosed a marked decrease in exchangeable potassium, but only a borderline decrease in exchangeable sodium. Increasing potassium intake improved the hyponatremia or prevented its development. The authors concluded that these patients represented a small proportion of those ingesting diuretics who rapidly developed potassium depletion after relatively small doses of the drug. The minimal and usual diuretic-induced sodium loss, when associated with the hypokalemia and potassium depletion, possibly caused an exaggerated and sustained stimulation of the baroreceptor mechanism controlling the release of AVP. The persistent high level of AVP in the circulation was then primarily responsible for the impaired water excretion and its consequences. Other explanations for the abnormal AVP release include a direct effect of potassium deficiency on the neurohypophyseal system or indirectly by PGE enhancement of AVP release (35–37, 183). Finally, an impairment of the ability to excrete free water may occur in the absence of circulating AVP as thiazide diuretics prevent the reabsorption of sodium salts in the distal convoluted tubule and, possibly, the cortical collecting duct (260).

In the section on DI we discussed in detail the mechanism by which chlorpropamide can cause antidiuresis and thereby impair water excretion. Once this effect of the oral hypoglycemic agent was realized, it was not long before hyponatremia and water intoxication were reported, owing to its use in the treatment of diabetes mellitus (225, 258, 259). Garcia et al. (258), after observing two elderly diabetics (ages 71 and 76) with this syndrome, gave chlorpropamide to six additional adult-onset diabetics, studying the response to an oral water load before and after drug administration. All showed markedly impaired water diuresis with chlorpropamide. Twenty-three normal subjects, studied in a similar manner, also demonstrated a decrease in their maximal water diuresis, but the decrease was significantly less than that observed in the diabetic patients. It is possible that chlorpropamide is capable of greater inhibition of AVP-stimulated renal PGE synthesis in the adult-onset diabetic than it is in the nondiabetic subject and therefore any residual AVP remaining in the circulation in a water-loaded or water-excess state can cause a greater degree of antidiuresis or impaired water excretion in the diabetic (see earlier discussion of AVP-PGE interrelationships).

The reason why relatively few patients using chlorpropamide develop hyponatremia and water intoxication is unclear. Theoretically in all patients and normal subjects receiving chlorpropamide, water retention and hyponatremia should be minimal. The drug should initially cause an inappropriate antidiuresis, leading to a mild positive water balance and hypoosmolality. This should inhibit the release of AVP on an osmotic basis, initiate a water diuresis, and return water balance *almost* to normal. The data reported by Garcia and his associates (258) and others (225, 259) strongly suggest that in some patients with

diabetes mellitus, particularly the elderly, a sustained nonosmotic stimulus to the release of AVP persists despite the marked positive water balance. The frequent degenerative changes in the cardiovascular system of the diabetic may cause abnormal function of those baroreceptor mechanisms modulating the secretion of AVP (Table 12-3). Alternatively, in these patients AVP secretion could be the result of a direct action of chlorpropamide on the CNS.

Two unusual groups of patients with water intoxication have recently been reported. One was a group of patients with beer potomania, each ingesting high quantities (many gallons per day) of beer (261). Coma and other neurologic signs were present, and serum sodium ranged between 98 and 120 meq/L. The authors concluded that low so-

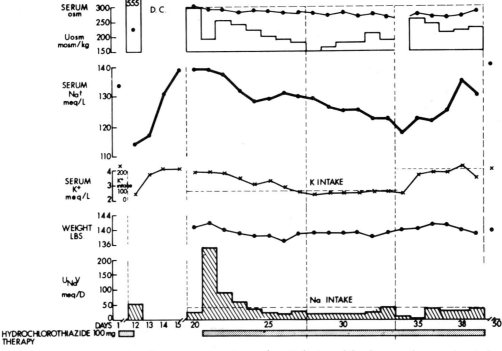

Figure 12-54. Improvement in diuretic-induced hyponatremia with potassium loading. The crosshatched bars on the bottom of the figure represent the 24-h urine Na$^+$; the horizontal dashed line at the bottom, the Na$^+$ intake; and the horizontal dashed line in the center, the K$^+$ intake, which was changed from 80 to 210 meq/ day. At the top of the diagram, the open bars indicate the urine osmolality; the circles, the serum osmolality; the dashed line, the normal serum osmolality of 290 mosm/kg body weight. [*From M. P. Fichman, H. Vorherr, C. R. Kleeman, and N. Telfer (130).*]

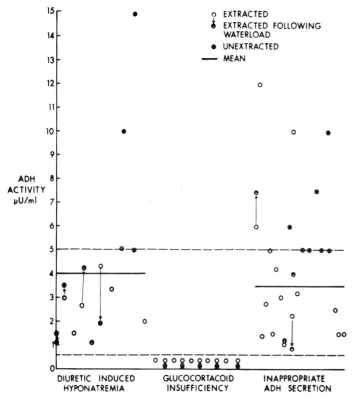

Figure 12-55. Results of bioassay for vasopressin activity in plasma samples of 43 patients with hyponatremia caused by diuretics (left), hypopituitarism (middle), or inappropriate ADH secretion (right). The solid circles represent ADH activity in unextracted samples, the open circles ADH activity in extracted samples before water load, and the semisolid circles ADH activity in extracted samples after a 20-mL/kg-body-weight water load, with arrows connecting specimens from the same patient before and after the water load. The dashed lines represent the lower limit of sensitivity of the assay for unextracted (5 μU/mL) and extracted (0.5 μU/mL) samples; the solid horizontal lines represent the mean values for each group. [*From M. P. Fichman, H. Vorherr, C. R. Kleeman, and N. Telfer (130).*]

consisted of psychotic patients who appeared to actually "drink themselves" into water intoxication without a known cause for impaired water excretion (262). It is clear that despite their striking polyuria even those cases of profound polydipsia associated with severe emotional illness that develop a hypoosmolar syndrome must have some relative defect in water excretion. If we assume that at normal rates of solute excretion the maximal free water clearance is at least 10 percent of the simultaneous GFR, then a patient with a GFR of 120 mL/min could excrete 12 mL/min of free water or C_{H_2O} would equal 17,280 mL per 24 h. It is almost inconceivable, therefore, that patients could "drink themselves" into a severe hyperosmolal state if inhibition of AVP secretion and renal water excretion were normal. However, the brain dysfunction of these psychotic patients and/or the drugs they are therapeutically ingesting may well cause a sustained release of AVP that cannot be homeostatically inhibited by hypoosmolality of their body fluids. Raskind and co-workers (263, 264) have recently reported that plasma AVP levels are elevated in randomly selected untreated psychotic patients (Table 12-21). However, the mean plasma osmolality of these patients was normal. For dilution of body fluids to occur there must be impairment of water excretion as well as enhanced water intake (in excess of obligatory and insensible losses). The relative infrequency of severe hyponatremia in psychotic patients may be a reflection of normal or reduced water intake. Conversely, enhanced water intake by itself (up to 20 L/day) is rarely associated with severe hyponatremia.

In recent years, the number of drugs that have been implicated in the production of a hypoos-

dium intake (the "beer diet"), absorption of large quantities of water, and possibly some form of inappropriate secretion of AVP accounted for the syndrome. It is of interest that a number of the patients were also ingesting various types of diuretic drugs for hypertension, possible heart failure, or steroid-induced edema. The other group

Table 12-21. Elevated plasma AVP in psychosis

VARIABLE ± S.E.M.	AVP, μU/mL, STANDING	AVP, μU/mL, SUPINE	P_{OSM}, mosm/kg	N
Psychotic	3.47 ± 0.45*	2.49 ± 0.56	288 ± 2.04	8
Anxious	1.6 ± 0.23	1.65 ± 0.22	288 ± 1.36	8
Normal control	1.71 ± 0.29	1.39 ± 0.31	290 ± 1.60	8

* $p < 0.05$.
Source: From M. A. Raskind, et al. (264).

molar water retention state have increased strikingly. In Table 12-22 we have listed these drugs and the probable mechanism by which they impair water excretion. We are certain that the list will grow longer with each passing year.

The last major category of the hyponatremic states may be designated *hypervolemic hyponatremia*. In this situation there is marked expansion of total body sodium with even further expansion of total body water. In spite of these elevations, there is a substantial diminution in effective plasma volume. This is usually the result of decreased cardiac output and high venous pressure

Table 12-22. Drugs associated with hyponatremia

PRINCIPAL MECHANISMS

1. Augmented thirst
    Mellaril (thioridazine)
2. Augmented renal action of AVP

    Chlorpropamide
    Tolbutamide
    Acetominaphen*
    Phenformin
    Indomethacin*

3. Impaired renal water excretion independent of AVP

    Oxytocin
    Thiazide diuretics

4. Enhanced hypothalamic release of AVP

    Chlorpropamide
    Clofibrate
    Carbamazepine
    Vincristine
    Vinblastine
    Cyclophosphamide
    Opiates
    Histamine

5. Nonosmolar stimulation of AVP release (baroreceptor-mediated)

    Thiazides (?)
    Isoproterenol
    Nicotine
    Barbiturates (?)

* Enhances AVP action but is not associated with hyponatremia.

as in heart failure, sequestration of ECF volume to the interstitial fluid compartment as in nephrosis, or sequestration of ECF volume in the form of ascitic fluid as in cirrhosis. In all these states there is diminished effective renal blood flow which produces substantial sodium retention by both the renin-angiotensin system and renal autoregulatory mechanisms.

The symptoms and signs associated with these syndromes will depend, of course, on the underlying disorder which causes the impaired water excretion. The specific manifestations of the hypoosmolar state will depend on the rapidity with which it develops and the severity of the hyponatremia. The old and the very young are most susceptible to its adverse effects. If we are dealing with a state of pure water retention that has developed slowly over weeks to months, it is surprising how asymptomatic the patient may be despite concentrations of sodium well below 120 meq/L (osmolality usually less than 240 mosm/L). However, when hypoosmolality of this degree develops rapidly over days to a week or so, the manifestations of disturbed brain function, owing to overhydration of the CNS, may be profound. In addition to progressive depression of the sensorium (confusion, lethargy, headache, stupor, and coma), any type of focal neurologic brain syndrome may occur including, finally, focal or generalized convulsions. Recently, Arieff and his associates (265) in a prospective study of a large number of patients with acute (days) and chronic (weeks) hypoosmolality stressed the danger to life of the acute production of water intoxication with concentrations of sodium below 120 meq/L. In addition to an in-depth review of this subject, they presented new experimental data on acute and chronic water intoxication in the rabbit. The more acutely the same degree of severe hyponatremia (< 100 meq/L) was produced, the higher the mortality. Similar degrees of hypoosmolality were very well tolerated by the animals when produced over a number of days. By analysis of brain tissue for its water, electrolytes, and osmole content, Arieff et al. were able to demonstrate that the chronic animals had significantly less edema or overhydration of the brain, when severely hyponatremic, than was observed in the acute preparations at the same level of serum sodium. This difference was due to the fact that the brain compensated by losing osmoles (sodium, chloride, and potassium) when water intoxication was produced more slowly and therefore less water moved into the brain of these animals on an osmotic differential basis. They "sacrificed" brain solute to prevent brain swelling and death (see Chap. 26).

Therapy of the hyponatremic state

Once we have decided into which category our hyponatremic patient belongs, we can then plan a rational therapeutic approach. The patient's history preceding the detection of the hypoosmolality, symptoms and physical signs, and finally certain critical chemical analyses in blood and urine when combined with the patient's change in weight and approximated water balance allow us to categorize the patient (Tables 12-14 and 12-15).

The salt- and volume-depleted patient (hypovolemic hyponatremia), when supplied with adequate amounts of isotonic, or occasionally hypertonic saline solution, will make whatever final renal adjustments are necessary to maintain ICF and ECF volume and tonicity at a normal level. This, of course, implies a neurohypophyseal system *appropriately* responsive to the removal of nonosmotic stimuli, and basically normal kidneys that can respond to the neurohumoral adjustments which follow the salt and water replacement. This is the usual situation associated with an extrarenal cause for the salt and water depletion. Unfortunately, when a functional (excess diuretics, adrenal insufficiency) or organic (salt-losing nephropathy) disorder of the kidney is responsible, the renal adjustment may not be completely appropriate. Therefore, the functional causes must be corrected, and the impact of the organic lesion on the homeostatic excretion of salt and water must be taken into consideration during the replacement therapy.

In patients in our second category [hyponatremia with minimal hypervolemia (Table 12-15)], a primary excess of total body water with normal or minimally decreased total body sodium, once diagnosed, must be corrected by the creation of a negative water balance and, at times, the administration of hypertonic saline to restore the osmolality of body fluids to normal. At the same time that the hypoosmolality is being treated, we must make every effort to remove or correct the underlying cause of the impaired water excretion (Tables 12-15 and 12-16). Given a patient with a "water excess" syndrome our choice of therapy will depend on the severity of the hypoosmolality, the rapidity of its development, and the magnitude of "water intoxication" (see earlier discussion and Chap. 26). Basically, a negative water balance must be created and our first therapeutic maneuver is to restrict water intake to the lowest possible level. The drier the diet, the better. In the great majority of cases, this will be adequate until the underlying cause can be corrected. Serum sodium and osmolality should be returned to a normal level. Urine volume will, of course, decrease further under this therapy, but this will be of no consequence as long as the patient remains in negative water balance through renal and extrarenal routes. The only exception to this approach may be the patient with so called "asymptomatic" hyponatremia. This patient is usually one with inappropriate or ectopic secretion of AVP, who has slowly developed a hypoosmolar state over many weeks or even longer, whose serum sodium is between 120 and 130 meq/L, and whose CNS and other tissues have "adjusted" to their hypotonic environment (265). The patient may not necessarily look or feel better when the osmolality of the body fluids is normal. Furthermore, because the underlying cause for the SIADH often cannot be readily removed, hyponatremia will rapidly return when water intake is liberalized.

In striking contrast to this patient is the one who is truly "water intoxicated." The impaired water excretion relative to intake, from the causes listed in Table 12-18, has developed over hours to days and often reaches a point where serum sodium is below 120 meq/L. All the symptoms and signs described earlier and in Chap. 26 may present and seriously threaten the recovery and life of the patient. In this situation our foremost objective is to correct the severe cellular overhydration, particularly of the cells of the CNS. This can be accomplished by rapidly (hours) increasing the *effective* osmolality of the ECF while continuing the water-restriction regimen. Hypertonic saline (5%) or hypertonic mannitol (10% to 20%) comprises the effective osmotic solutes. One can estimate the approximate expansion of total B. W. (body water) in these patients by calculating the volume of total B. W. required to dilute the serum sodium concentration to its observed level. Total B. W. is estimated as 60 percent of total weight in females and 65 percent of total weight in males of average body composition. One then multiplies the patient's normal total B. W. times a normal total serum sodium concentration and then divides this by the observed serum sodium concentration to get the total B. W. in the hypotonic state. As mentioned above, such calculations frequently overestimate the true amount of weight gain from the premorbid state. For example, this estimate is for a 70-kg female:

$$B.W. = (70 \text{ kg})(0.60) = 42 \text{ L}$$
$$(x)(120 \text{ meq/L}) = (42)(140 \text{ meq/L})$$
$$x = 49 \text{ L}$$

Therefore, total B.W. in the abnormal state is approximately 49 L or 7 L greater than normal. The amount of sodium in milliequivalents required for correction of the hyponatremia can then be calculated by multiplying the difference between the observed sodium concentration and a desired concentration times the total B. W. While it is clear that the salt is actually distributed in ECF, the rise in osmolality that it creates at any given point continuously draws water out of the cells along the newly established osmotic gradient until at any given new steady state the rise in osmolality or sodium concentration is as though the salt were distributed in a volume equivalent to total body water. The serum sodium should be elevated approximately 10 to 15 percent over the first 8 to 10 h of therapy.

The correction of cellular overhydration will almost always be associated with a marked improvement in the CNS symptoms and signs during the first 24 h if they are due to the water intoxication. Occasionally in the older age group (above 65 years), the rate of recovery may be delayed an additional 24 to 48 h. It is also in this age group that the large salt load and the rapid expansion of the extracellular volume, over and above that created by the original water retention, may precipitate acute congestive heart failure. It is for this reason, and the desire to greatly increase the rate of salt *and* water excretion, that Hantman and associates (266) first suggested the combined use of hypertonic saline and a potent diuretic such as furosemide (Lasix) at an initial dose of approximately 1 mg/kg IV. This approach is illustrated in Fig. 12-56. This "loop" diuretic by inhibiting the active reabsorption of NaCl in the thick ascending limb (see earlier discussion and Chap. 3) (1) prevents excessive ECF volume expansion during and immediately following the saline infusion, (2) markedly impairs the function of the medullary countercurrent multiplier system so that concentrated urine cannot be produced despite the excess circulating AVP, and (3) causes the excretion of large amounts of water and sodium in a concentration below that of the plasma, and, of course, greatly below that of the administered hypertonic saline. The net effect of this therapy is a large negative water balance produced in a matter of hours associated with a rapid (hours) return of plasma osmolality to normal (Fig. 12-56). An adverse "trade off" of this approach is the simultaneous diuretic-induced renal loss of potassium and magnesium ions. This may cause the rapid development of hypokalemia and hypomagnesemia. The former may have immediate deleterious effects which should be anticipated and prevented by simultaneous administration of 150 to 200 meq of potassium during the first 24 h of therapy. The excretion of this amount of potassium (in 24 h) would not be unusual during the diuretic-induced natriuresis. Magnesium excretion may reach 15 to 20 meq or 180 to 240 mg at the same time. Its rapid development depends on the development of any degree of hypomagnesemia. In any event, it is wise to simultaneously measure serum magnesium and potassium when serum osmolality and sodium are determined, and the rate of excretion of these ions (Mg^{2+} and K^+) during the diuresis.

Hypertonic mannitol has been suggested as an alternative to hypertonic sodium chloride for the treatment of hypoosmolar states, but it offers no

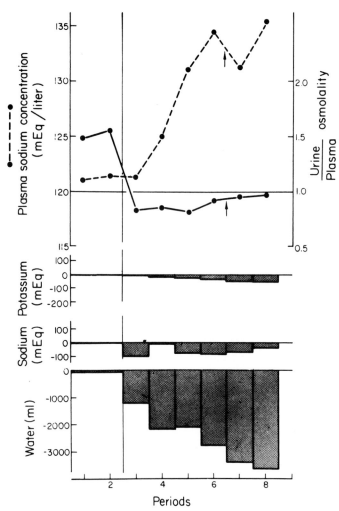

Figure 12-56. Use of furosemide and hypertonic saline in the rapid correction of hyponatremia in patient C.H. with the syndrome of inappropriate secretion of ADH. The control periods in this and subsequent figures are separated from the periods collected after furosemide administered by the vertical line. The arrow indicates the last dose of furosemide. Each period indicates 1-h duration of time. Furosemic administration was associated with hypotonic urine and an increase in plasma sodium concentration in the absence of either a positive sodium or potassium balance. The cumulative potassium, sodium, and water balances are shown in the bottom three panels on the figure.

particular advantages and has several possible disadvantages compared to hypertonic saline (243, 267).

Three drugs which specifically inhibit the se-

cretion or renal effect of AVP have been used in the treatment of SIADH syndrome. These are diphenylhydantoin (Dilantin) which when administered intravenously can block the release of AVP from the neurohypophysis (268), dichlormethyltetracycline (Declomycin, Demeclocycline) (267), and lithium (270). Both of these latter compounds act by directly blocking the renal tubular effect of AVP. They would seem to have a role in those patients in whom the syndrome is not self-limited and the underlying cause cannot be removed. In this setting, e.g., AVP-secreting bronchogenic carcinoma, a drug that could be taken by mouth and for a prolonged period would be most desirable. While both have untoward and toxic effects, the antibiotic dechlormethyltetracycline in doses of 1 to 2 g/day would be least objectionable. With greater experience in the use of this drug, we will be better able to define the practical limits of its use.

GLUCOCORTICOIDS AND WATER EXCRETION

The inability to excrete a water load in a normal manner is a characteristic of primary and secondary adrenal insufficiency. This defect is due to a deficiency of hydrocortisone, and it continues to be demonstrable in the presence of a normal extracellular volume and adequate mineralocorticoid (247). These subjects are unable to form a maximally dilute urine or to attain a maximal rate of water diuresis after either an acute or chronic water load and therefore are particularly prone to the development of water intoxication. The continued production of a hypertonic urine relatively low in volume during a sustained positive water load suggests the possible presence of continued circulating AVP. However, to date the evidence is still inconclusive in both humans and animals as to the exact role of AVP in the impaired water excretion of primary and secondary adrenal insufficiency. It is clear that if the patient with primary or secondary adrenal insufficiency has hypovolemia, hypotension, or reduced cardiac output (Table 12-3), these could cause a sustained release of AVP which would contribute to an impaired water excretion caused by a nonhormonal mechanism. Share and Travis (271) demonstrated in trained unanesthetized adrenalectomized dogs that if blood and extracellular volume were maintained normal by a liberal intake of NaCl, basal plasma AVP concentration was not increased. However, the concentration of AVP in the plasma rose progressively if the NaCl were withdrawn. Giving the animal at this time a large dose of cortisol only slightly reduced the elevated AVP level, whereas an infusion of saline, without steroid administration, returned the plasma AVP almost to normal. Additional experimental evidence against a *primary* role of AVP in the impaired water diuresis of the adrenal-insufficient human or animal is the observation of Green et al. (271a) that the diuresis is equally impaired in the adrenalectomized rat with hereditary DI (Brattleboro strain). AVP *cannot* participate in the defect in water excretion in these adrenal-insufficient animals. Our studies utilizing a sensitive bioassay indicated a normal disappearance of AVP from the circulation of untreated patients with adrenal insufficiency despite impaired diuresis (130, 247). These patients showed no delay in inactivation of, or increased sensitivity to, exogenously administered AVP. Although their peak water diuresis is subnormal, the rate at which this level is attained is comparable to that observed in normal individuals (247). Ahmed and his associates (272) and recently others (273, 274) have implicated sustained circulating AVP in the impaired water diuresis of primary or secondary adrenal insufficiency. However, it is reasonable to conclude that the sustained circulating AVP is not essential for this defect in water excretion.

If the latter is correct, why do these subjects demonstrate this physiologic abnormality? Certainly, any reduction in GFR or renal blood flow would impair the attainment of a maximal water diuresis (see earlier discussion). GFR and renal blood flow have both been found to be moderately reduced in subjects with adrenal insufficiency, and hemodynamic abnormalities are corrected by adequate therapy with glucocorticoids. However, hydrocortisone administered acutely during impaired water diuresis can markedly improve the rate of urinary flow and the production of a maximally dilute urine with little or no acute alteration in renal hemodynamics (275) (see below). Nonhormonal techniques that considerably im-

prove renal blood flow and GFR, such as aminophylline administration, do not appreciably enhance the water diuresis (275). These observations suggest that the glucocorticoids improve water diuresis through some intrarenal mechanism that ultimately causes a decrease in the back-diffusion of water in the diluting segments of the nephron. It is also possible that these steroids allow these segments to become maximally impermeable to water in the absence of AVP. This could be considered a "permissive" role of the glucocorticoids.

The pure water excess syndrome secondary to the sustained release of AVP can be almost mimicked by primary and secondary adrenal insufficiency (glucocorticoid deficiency). In the latter circumstances the hyponatremia and relative or absolute excess of total body water can be quickly corrected by the oral or intravenous administration of glucocorticoids; in contrast, the syndrome of inappropriate secretion of AVP not associated with glucocorticoid deficiency will not be corrected by steroid administration (130, 276).

REFERENCES

1. Kerpel-Fronius, E.: Clinical consequences of the water and electrolyte metabolism peculiar to infancy, *Ciba Foundation Colloquia on Aging,* vol. 4, Little, Brown and Company, Boston, 1958, pp. 154–162.

2. Schmidt-Nielsen, B.: The resourcefulness of nature in physiological adaptation to the environment, *Physiologist,* **1**(2):4–20, 1958.

3. Wayner, M. J. (ed.): *Thirst—First International Symposium on Thirst in the Regulation of Body Water,* The Macmillan Company, New York, 1964.

4. Andersson, B.: Polydipsia caused by intrahypothalamic injections of hypertonic NaCl solutions, *Experientia,* **8**:157, 1952.

5. Andersson, B., and S. M. McCann: The effect of hypothalamic lesions on the water intake of the dog, *Acta Physiol. Scand.,* **35**:312–320, 1965.

6. Stricker, E. M.: Behavioral control of intravascular fluid volume: Thirst and sodium appetite, *Ann. N.Y. Acad. Sci.,* **157**:553–568, 1969.

7. Stricker, E. M.: Osmoregulation and volume reg-

ulation in rats: Inhibition of hypovolemic thirst by water, *Am. J. Physiol.*, **217**:98–105, 1969.

8. McCance, R. A.: Experimental sodium chloride deficiency in man, *Proc. R. Soc. London Biol.*, **119**:245–268, 1936.

9. Share, L.: Vasopressin, its bioassay and the physiological control of its release, *Am. J. Med.*, **42**:701–712, 1967.

10. Kleeman, C. R., and R. Cutler: The neurohypophysis, *Ann. Rev. Physiol.*, **25**:385–432, 1963.

11. Nash, F. D.: Introductory remarks—control of antidiuretic hormone secretion, *Fed. Proc.*, **30**:1376–1377, 1971.

12. Moore, W. W.: Antidiuretic hormone levels in normal subjects, *Fed. Proc.*, **30**:1387–1394, 1971.

13. Segar, W. E., and W. W. Moore: The regulation of antidiuretic hormone release in man, *J. Clin. Invest.*, **47**:2143–2141, 1968.

14. Zehr, J. E., J. A. Johnson, and W. W. Moore: Left atrial pressure, plasma osmolality, and ADH levels in the unanesthetized ewe, *Am. J. Physiol.*, **217**:1672–1680, 1969.

15. Fitzsimons, J. T., and B. J. Simons: The effect on drinking in the rat of intravenous infusion of angiotensin, given alone or in combination with other stimuli of thirst, *J. Physiol.*, **203**:45–57, 1969.

16. Epstein, A. N., J. T. Fitzsimons, and B. J. Rolls: Drinking induced by injection of angiotensin into the brain of the rat, *J. Physiol.*, **210**:457–474, 1970.

17. Andersson, B., L. Eriksson, and R. Oltner: Further evidence for angiotensin-sodium interaction in central control of fluid balance, *Life Sci.*, **9**:1091–1096, 1970.

18. Fitzsimons, J. T.: The effect of drinking of peptide precursors and of shorter-chain peptide fragments of angiotensin II injected into the rat's diencephalon, *J. Physiol.*, **214**:295–303, 1971.

19. Andersson, B., and L. Eriksson: Conjoint action of sodium and angiotensin on brain mechanisms controlling water and salt balances, *Acta Physiol. Scand.*, **81**:18–29, 1971.

20. Fitzsimons, J. T.: The role of a renal thirst factor in drinking induced by extracellular stimuli, *J. Physiol.*, **201**:349–368, 1969.

21. Severs, W. B., and A. E. D. Severs: Effects of angiotensin on the central nervous system, *Pharmacol. Rev.*, **415**:448, 1973.

22. Reid, I. A., and D. J. Ramsay: The effects of intracerebroventricular administration of renin on drinking and blood pressure, *Endocrinology*, **97**:536, 1975.

23. Mouw, D., J.-P. Bonjour, R. L. Malvin, and A. Vander: Central action of angiotensin in stimulating ADH release, *Am. J. Physiol.*, **220**:239–242, 1971.

24. Bonjour, J.-P., and R. L. Malvin: Stimulation of ADH release by the renin-angiotensin system, *Am. J. Physiol.*, **218**:1555–1559, 1970.

25. Nicoll, R. A., and J. L. Barker: Excitation of supraoptic neurosecretory cells by angiotensin II, *Nature [New Biol.]*, **233**:172–173, 1971.

26. Bonjour, J.-P., and R. L. Malvin: Plasma concentrations of ADH in conscious and anesthetized dogs, *Am. J. Physiol.*, **218**:1128–1132, 1970.

27. Malvin, R. L.: Possible role of the renin-angiotensin system in the regulation of antidiuretic hormone secretion, *Fed. Proc.*, **30**:1383–1386, 1971.

28. Keil, L. C., J. Summy-Long, and W. B. Severs: Release of vasopressin by angiotensin II, *Endocrinology*, **96**:1063–1065, 1975.

29. Sirois, P., and D. J. Gagnon: Increase in cyclic AMP levels and vasopressin release in response to angiotensin I in neurohypophyses: Blockade following inhibition of the converting enzyme, *J. Neurochem.*, **25**:727–729, 1975.

29a. Uhlich, E., P. Weber, J. Elgler, and U. Grö shel-Stewart: Angiotensin stimulated AVP-release in humans, *Klin. Wochenschr.*, **53**:177–180, 1975.

30. Linazasoro, J. M., C. Jimenez-Diaz, and H. Castro-Mendoza: The kidney and thirst regulation, *Bull. Inst. Med. Res. Madrid*, **7**:53–61, 1954.

31. Andersson, B., and B. Larsson: Influence of local temperature changes in the preoptic area and rostral hypothalamus on the regulation of food and water intake, *Acta Physiol. Scand.*, **52**:75–89, 1961.

32. Grossman, S. P.: Direct adrenergic and cholinergic stimulation of hypothalamic mechanisms, *Am. J. Physiol.*, **202**:872–882, 1962.

33. Levitt, R. A., and A. E. Fisher: Anticholinergic blockade of centrally induced thirst, *Science*, **154**:520–521, 1966.

34. Lehr, D., J. Mallow, and M. Krukowski: Copious drinking and simultaneous inhibition of urine flow elicited by beta adrenergic stimulation and

contrary effect of alpha adrenergic stimulation, *J. Pharmacol. Exp. Ther.*, **158**:150–163, 1967.

35. Leksell, L. G.: Influence of PGE_2 on cerebral mechanisms involved in control of fluid balance, *Acta Physiol. Scand.*, **98**:85, 1976.

36. Andersson, B., and L. G. Leksell: Effects on fluid balance of intraventricular infusions of prostaglandin E_1, *Acta Physiol. Scand.*, **93**:286, 1975.

37. Yamamoto, M., L. Share, and R. E. Shade: Vasopressin release during ventriculocisternal perfusion with prostaglandin E_2, *J. Endocrinol.*, **71**:325, 1976.

38. Fitzsimons, J. T., and P. E. Setler: Catecholaminergic mechanisms in angiotensin induced drinking, *J. Physiol.*, **218**:43P–44P, 1971.

39. DeRubertis, F. R., M. F. Michelis, N. Beck, J. B. Field, and B. B. David: "Essential" hypernatremia due to ineffective osmotic and intact volume regulation of vasopressin secretion, *J. Clin. Invest.*, **50**:97–111, 1971.

40. Berl, T., R. G. Anderson, G. A. Aisenbray, S. L. Linas, and R. W. Schrier: On the mechanisms of the polyuria in potassium depletion: The role of polydipsia, *Clin. Res.*, **25**:136A, 1977.

41. Schrub, J. C. L., M. Dubuisson, B. Hillemand, and J. C. L. Leroy: L'hypernatrémie neurogène (neurogenic hypernatremia—a case noted during development of a pinealoma), *Sem. Hop. Paris*, **46**:2084–2089, 1970.

42. Sawyer, W. H.: Active neurohypophysial principles from a cyclostome and two cartilaginous fishes, *Am. J. Med.*, **42**:678–686, 1967.

42a. Sawyer, W. H.: Evolution of active neurohypophyseal principles among the vertebrates, *American Zoologist*, **17**:727, 1977.

43. Rosenfeld, M.: The native hormones of the posterior pituitary glands: The pressor and oxytocic principles, *Bull. Johns Hopkins Hosp.*, **66**:398–403, 1940.

44. Sawyer, W. H.: Evolution of neurohypophysial hormones and their receptors, *Fed. Proc.*, **36**:1842–1847, 1977.

45. Pavel, S., R. Goldstein, and M. Calb: Vasotocin content in the pineal gland of foetal, newborn and adult male rats, *J. Endocrinol.*, **66**:283–284, 1975.

46. Rosenbloom, A. A., and D. A. Fisher: Radioimmunoassayable AVT and AVP in adult mammalian brain tissue: Comparison of normal and Brat-

tleboro rats, *Neuroendocrinology*, **17**:354–361, 1975.

47. Skowsky, W. R., and D. A. Fisher: Fetal neurohypophysial arginine vasopressin and arginine vasotocin in man and sheep, *Pediatr. Res.*, 1977. In press.

48. Vaughan, M. K., D. E. Blask, G. M. Vaughan, and R. V. Reiter: Dose dependent prolactin releasing activity of arginine vasotocin in intact and pinealectomized estrogen-progesterone treated adult male rats, *Endocrinology*, **99**:1319, 1976.

48a. Cheesman, D. W., R. B. Osland, and P. H. Forsham: Suppression of the preovulatory surge of luteinizing hormone and subsequent ovulation in the rat by arginine vasotocin, *Endocrinology*, **101**:1194–1202, 1977.

49. Peck, J. W., and E. M. Blass: Localization of thirst and antidiuretic osmoreceptors by intracranial injections in rats, *Am. J. Physiol.*, **228**:1501–1509, 1975.

50. Van Gemert, M., M. Miller, R. J. Carey, and A. M. Moses: Polyuria and impaired ADH release following medial preoptic lesioning in the rat, *Am. J. Physiol.*, **228**:1293–1297, 1975.

51. van Dyke, H. B., B. F. Chow, R. O. Greep, and A. Rothen: The isolation of a protein from pars neuralis of the ox pituitary with constant oxytocic, pressor, and diuresis inhibiting activities, *J. Pharmacol. Exp. Ther.*, **74**:190–209, 1942.

52. Acher, R., J. Chauvet, and G. Olivry: Sur l'existence éventuelle d'une hormone unique neurohypophysaire. I. Relation entre l'ocytocine, la vasopressine et la protéine de van Dyke extraites de la neurohypophyse du boeuf, *Biochim. Biophys. Acta*, **22**:421–427, 1956.

53. Acher, R., and C. Fromageot: The relationship of oxytocin and vasopressin to active proteins of posterior pituitary origin. Studies concerning the existence or non-existence of a single neurohypophysial hormone, in H. Heller (ed.), *The Neurohypophysis*, Butterworth & Co. (Publishers), Ltd., London, 1957, pp. 34–37.

54. Ginsburg, M., and M. Ireland: The role of neurophysin in the transport and release of neurohypophysial hormones, *J. Endocrinol.*, **35**:289–298, 1966.

55. Dean, C. R., and D. B. Hope: The isolation of neurophysin I and II from bovine pituitary neurosecretory granules separated on a large scale

from other subcellular organelles, *Biochem. J.*, **106**:565–573, 1968.

56. Burford, G. D., C. W. Jones, and B. T. Pickering: Tentative identification of a vasopressin-neurophysin and an oxytocin-neurophysin in the rat, *Biochem. J.*, **124**:809–813, 1971.

57. Cheng, K. W., and H. G. Friesen: Isolation and characterization of a third component of porcine neurophysin, *J. Biol. Chem.*, **246**:7656–7665, 1971.

58. Hollenberg, M. D., and D. B. Hope: The isolation of the native hormone binding proteins from bovine posterior pituitary lobes, *Biochem. J.*, **106**:557–564, 1968.

59. Cheng, K. W., and H. G. Friesen: The isolation and characterization of human neurophysin, *J. Clin. Endocrinol. Metab.*, **34**:165–176, 1972.

60. Ranch, R., M. D. Hollenberg, and D. B. Hope: Isolation of a third bovine neurophysin, *Biochem. J.*, **115**:476–479, 1969.

61. Robinson, A. G., E. A. Zimmerman, and A. G. Frantz: Physiologic investigation of posterior pituitary binding. Proteins neurophysin I and neurophysin II, *Metabolism*, **20**:1148–1155, 1971.

62. Robinson, A. G., E. A. Zimmerman, E. G. Engleman, and A. G. Frantz: Radioimmunoassay of bovine neurophysin: Specificity of neurophysin I and neurophysin II, *Metabolism*, **20**:1138–1147, 1971.

63. Sachs, H., C. P. Fawcett, Y. Takabatake, and R. Portanova: Biosynthesis and release of vasopressin and neurophysin, *Rec. Progr. Horm. Res.*, **25**:447–491, 1969.

64. Sachs, H., R. Goodman, J. Osinchak, and J. McKelvy: Supraoptic neurosecretory neurons of the guinea pig in organ culture. Biosynthesis of vasopressin and neurophysin, *Proc. Natl. Acad. Sci. U.S.A.*, **68**:2782–2786, 1971.

65. Frieson, H. G., and E. B. Astwood: Changes in neurohypophysial proteins induced by dehydration and ingestion of saline, *Endocrinology*, **80**:278–287, 1967.

66. Fawcett, C. P., A. E. Powell, and H. Sachs: Biosynthesis and release of neurophysin, *Endocrinology*, **83**:1299–1310, 1968.

67. Cheng, K. W., and H. G. Friesen: Physiological factors regulating secretion of neurophysin, *Metabolism*, **19**:876–890, 1970.

68. Cheng, K. W., and H. G. Friesen: A radioimmunoassay for vasopressin binding proteins—neurophysin, *Endocrinology*, **88**:608–619, 1971.

69. Legros, J. J., and P. Franchimont: The radioimmunoassay of bovine neurophysin: Evidence of a cross-reaction with a substance in human plasma, in K. E. Kirkham and W. M. Hunter (eds.), *Radioimmunassay Methods*, Churchill, Livingston, Edinburgh, 1971, p. 98.

70. Sachs, H., R. Portanova, E. W. Haller, and L. Share: Cellular processes concerned with vasopressin biosynthesis, storage, and release, in F. Stutinsky (ed.), *Neurosecretion, Fourth International Symposium on Neurosecretion*, Springer-Verlag OHG, Berlin, 1967, p. 146.

71. Sachs, H.: Biosynthesis and release of vasopressin, *Am. J. Med.*, **42**:687–700, 1967.

72. Valtin, H.: Hereditary hypothalamic diabetes insipidus in rats (Brattleboro strain). A useful experimental model, *Am. J. Med.*, **42**:814–827, 1967.

73. Cross, B. A., R. E. J. Dyball, R. G. Dyer, C. W. Janes, D. W. Lincoln, J. F. Morris, and B. T. Pickering: Endocrine neurons, *Rec. Progr. Horm. Res.*, **31**:243–294, 1975.

74. Hayward, J. N.: Neural control of the posterior pituitary, *Ann. Rev. Physiol.*, **37**:191–210, 1975.

75. Arnauld, E., J. D. Vincent, and J. J. Dreifus: Firing patterns of hypothalamic supraoptic neurons during water deprivation in the monkey, *Science*, **185**:535–537, 1974.

76. Wakerley, J. B., D. A. Poulain, R. E. J. Dyball, and B. A. Cross: Activity of phasic neurosecretory cells during hemorrhage, *Nature*, **258**:82–84, 1975.

76a. Dreifus, J. J., M. E. Harris, and E. Tribollet: Excitation of phasically firing hypothalamic supraoptic neurons by carotid occlusion in rats, *J. Physiol.*, **257**:337–354, 1976.

76b. Zimmerman, E. A., and A. G. Robinson: Hypothalamic neurons secreting vasopressin and neurophysin, *Kidney Int.*, **10**:12–24, 1976.

77. Zimmerman, E. A.: Localization of hypothalamic hormones by immunocytochemical techniques, in L. Martini and W. F. Ganong (eds.), *Frontiers in Neuroendocrinology*, vol. 4, Raven Press, New York, 1976.

78. Zimmerman, E. A., P. W. Carmel, M. K. Husain, M. Ferin, M. Tannenbaum, A. G. Frantz, and A. G. Robinson: Vasopressin and neurophysins. High concentrations in monkey hypophysial portal blood, *Science*, **182**:925–927, 1973.

79. Seif, S. M., A. B. Huellmantel, M. Shullman, L. Recht, and A. G. Robinson: Neurophysin and

vasopressin in the plasma and hypothalamus of adrenalectomized and normal rats, *Endocrinology,* **96**:186A, 1975.

80. Vorherr, H., M. W. B. Bradbury, M. Hoghoughi, and C. R. Kleeman: Antidiuretic hormone in cerebrospinal fluid during endogenous and exogenous changes in its blood level, *Endocrinology,* **33**:246, 1968.

81. Zaid, S. M., and H. Heller: Can neurohypophysial hormones cross the blood-cerebrospinal fluid-barrier? *J. Endocrinol.,* **60**:195–196, 1974.

82. Van Wimersma Greidanus, T. B., J. Dogterom, and D. de Wied: Intraventricular administration of antivasopressin serum inhibits memory consolidation in rats, *Life Sci.,* **16**:637–644, 1975.

83. Douglas, W. W., J. Nagasawa, and R. Schultz: Electron microscopic studies on the mechanism of secretion of posterior pituitary hormones and significance of microvesicles ("synaptic vesicles"): Evidence of secretion by exocytosis and formation of microvesicles as a by-product of this process, in H. Heller and K. Lederis (eds.), *Memoirs of the Society for Endocrinology—Subcellular Organization and Function in Endocrine Tissues,* Cambridge University Press, London, 1971, pp. 353–378.

84. Nagasawa, J., W. W. Douglas, and R. A. Schulz: Ultrastructural evidence of secretion by exocytosis and of "synaptic vesicle" formation in posterior pituitary gland, *Nature,* **227**:407–409, 1970.

85. Nagasawa, J., W. W. Douglas, and R. A. Schulz: Micropinocytotic origin of coated and smooth microvesicles ("synaptic vesicles") in neurosecretory terminals of posterior pituitary glands demonstrated by incorporation of horseradish peroxidase, *Nature,* **232**:341–342, 1971.

86. Douglas, W. W., J. Nagasawa, and R. A. Schulz: Coated microvesicles in neurosecretory terminals of posterior pituitary glands shed their coats to become smooth "synaptic" vesicles, *Nature,* **232**:340–341, 1971.

87. Barer, R., H. Heller, and K. Lederis: The isolation, identification and properties of the hormonal granules of the neurohypophysis, *Proc. R. Soc. London Biol.,* **158**:388–416, 1963.

88. Gerschenfeld, H. M., J. H. Tramezzani, and E. DeRobertis: Ultrastructure and function in the neurohypophysis of the toad, *Endocrinology,* **66**:741–762, 1960.

89. Paley, S.: The fine structure of the neurohypophysis, in H. Waelsch (ed.), *Ultra-structure and Cellular Chemistry of Neural Tissue, Progress in Neurobiology 2,* Paul B. Hoeber, Inc., New York, 1957, pp. 31–49.

90. Douglas, W. W., and A. M. Poisner: Stimulus-secretion coupling in a neurosecretory organ. The role of calcium in the release of vasopressin from the neurohypophysis, *J. Physiol. (London),* **172**:1–18, 1964.

91. Sachs, H., L. Share, J. Osinchak, and A. Carpie: Capacity of the neurohypophysis to release vasopressin, *Endocrinology,* **81**:755–770, 1967.

92. Czaczkes, J. W., and C. R. Kleeman: The effects of various states of hydration and the plasma concentration on the turnover of antidiuretic hormone in mammals, *J. Clin. Invest.,* **43**:1625–1640, 1964.

93. Miller, L., L. Fisch, and C. R. Kleeman: Relative potency of arginine-8-vasopressin and lysine-8-vasopressin in humans, *J. Lab. Clin. Med.,* **69**:270–291, 1967.

94. Lauson, H.: Metabolism of antidiuretic hormones, *Am. J. Med.,* **42**:713–744, 1967.

95. Sawyer, W. H.: Biological assays for neurohypophysis principles in tissues and in blood, in G. W. Harris and B. T. Donovan (eds.), *The Pituitary Gland,* vol. 3, University of California Press, Berkeley, 1966, pp. 288–306.

96. Thomas, T. H., and M. R. Lee: The specificity of antisera for the radioimmunoassay of arginine vasopressin in human plasma and urine during water loading and dehydration, *Clin. Sci. Mole. Med.,* **51**:525–536, 1976.

97. Miller, M., and A. M. Moses: Radioimmunoassay of urinary antidiuretic hormone with application to study of the Brattleboro rat, *Endocrinology,* **88**:1389–1396, 1971.

98. Moses, A. M., D. H. P. Streeten, and M. D. Streeten: Differentiation of polyuric states by measurement of responses to changes in plasma osmolality induced by hypertonic saline infusions, *Am. J. Med.,* **42**:368–377, 1967.

99. Moses, A. M., M. Miller, and D. H. P. Streeten: Quantitative influence of blood volume expansion on the osmotic threshold for vasopressin release, *J. Clin. Endocrinol.,* **27**:655–662, 1967.

100. Verney, E. B.: The antidiuretic hormone and the

factors which determine its release, *Proc. R. Soc. London Biol.*, **135**:25–106, 1947–1948.

101. Robertson, G.L., E.A. Mahr, S. Athar, and T. Sinha: Development and clinical application of a new method for the radioimmunoassay of arginine vasopressin in human plasma, *J. Clin. Invest.*, **52**:2340–2352, 1973.

101a. Dunn, F. L., T. J. Brennan, A. E. Nelson, and G. L. Robertson: The role of blood osmolality and volume in regulating vasopressin secretion in the rat, *J. Clin. Invest.*, **52**:3212–3219, 1973.

102. Weitzman, R. E., and D. A. Fisher: Log linear relationship between plasma arginine vasopressin and plasma osmolality, *Am. J. Physiol.*, **233**:E37–E40, 1977.

103. Eriksson, L., O. Fernandez, and K. Olsson: Differences in the antidiuretic response to intracarotid infusions of hypertonic solutions in the conscious goat, *Acta Physiol. Scand.*, **83**:554–562, 1971.

104. Anderson, G., and L. Eriksson: Conjoint action of sodium and angiotensin on brain mechanisms controlling water and salt balances, *Acta Physiol. Scand.*, **81**:18–29, 1971.

105. Eriksson, L.: Effect of lowered CSF sodium concentration on the central control of fluid balances, *Acta Physiol. Scand.*, **91**:61–68, 1974.

106. Robertson, G. L., and S. Athar: The interaction of blood osmolality and blood volume in regulating plasma vasopressin in man, *J. Clin. Endocrinol. Metab.*, **42**:613–620, 1976.

107. Shimizu, K., L. Share, and J. R. Claybaugh: Potentiation by angiotensin II of the vasopressin response to an increased plasma osmolality, *Endocrinology*, **93**:42–50, 1973.

108. Gauer, O. H., and J. P. Henry: Circulatory basis of fluid volume control, *Physiol. Rev.*, **43**:423–481, 1963.

109. Share, L.: Role of peripheral receptors in the increased release of vasopressin in response to hemorrhage, *Endocrinology*, **81**:1140–1146, 1967.

110. Travis, R. H., and L. Share: Vasopressin-renin-cortisol interrelations, *Endocrinology*, **89**:246–253, 1971.

111. Davies, R., J. D. H. Slater, M. L. Forsling, and N. Payne: The response of arginine and plasma renin to postural change in normal man with observations on syncope, *Clin. Sci. Mole. Med.*, **51**:267–274, 1976.

112. Epstein, M.: Cardiovascular and renal effects of head out water immersion in man, *Circ. Res.*, **39**:619–628, 1976.

112a. Weitzman, R., L. Farnsworth, R. MacPhee, C. C. Wang, and C. M. Bennett: The effect of opposing osmolar and volume stimuli on plasma arginine vasopressin (pAVP) in man, *Mineral and Electrolyte Metabolism*, **1**:43–47, 1978.

113. George, P. L., F. H. Messenli, J. Genest, et al.: Diurnal variation of plasma AVP in man, *J. Clin. Endocrinol. Metab.*, **41**:332–338, 1975.

114. Borst, J. G. G., and L. A. de Vries: The three types of "natural" diuresis, *Lancet*, **2**:1–6, 1950.

115. Cirksena, W. J., J. H. Dirks, and R. W. Berliner: Effect of thoracic cava obstruction in response of proximal tubule sodium reabsorption to saline infusion, *J. Clin. Invest.*, **45**:179–186, 1966.

116. Rector, F. C., Jr., J. C. Sellman, M. Martinez-Maldonado, and D. W. Seldin: The mechanisms of suppressions of proximal tubular reabsorption by saline infusions, *J. Clin. Invest.*, **46**:47–56, 1967.

117. Epstein, M., D. S. Pins, R. Schneider, and R. Levinson: Determinants of deranged sodium and water homeostasis in decompensated cirrhosis, *J. Lab. Clin. Med.*, **87**:822–839, 1976.

118. Leaf, A., and A. R. Mamby: An antidiuretic mechanism not regulated by extracellular fluid, *J. Clin. Invest.*, **31**:60–71, 1952.

119. Leaf, A., and H. S. Frazier: Some recent studies on the actions of neurohypophyseal hormones, *Progr. Cardiovasc. Dis.*, **4**:47–64, 1961.

120. Barker, J. L., J. W. Crayton, and R. A. Nicoll: Noradrenaline and acetylcholine responses of supraoptic neurosecretory cells, *J. Physiol.*, **218**:19–32, 1971.

121. Berl, T., P. Cadnaphornchai, J. A. Harbottle, and R. W. Schrier: Mechanisms of suppression of vasopressin during alpha adrenergic stimulation with norepinephrine, *J. Clin. Invest.*, **53**:219–227, 1974.

122. Shimamoto, K., and M. Miyahara: Effect of norepinephrine infusion on plasma vasopressin levels in normal human subjects, *J. Clin. Endocrinol. Metab.*, **43**:201–204, 1976.

123. Schrier, R. W., R. Lieberman, and R. C Ufferman: Mechanism of antidiuretic effect of beta-adrenergic stimulation, *J. Clin. Invest.*, **51**:97–111, 1972.

124. Klein, L. A., B. Liberman, M. Laks, and C. R. Kleeman: Interrelated effects of antidiuretic hormone and adrenergic drugs on water metabolism, *Am. J. Physiol.*, **221**:1657–1665, 1971.

125. Levi, J., J. Grinblat, and C. R. Kleeman: Effect of isoproterenol on water diuresis in rats with congenital diabetes insipidus, *Am. J. Physiol.*, **221**:1728–1732, 1971.

126. Gill, J. R., Jr., and A. C. T. Casper: Depression of proximal sodium reabsorption in the dog in response to renal beta-adrenergic stimulation by isoproterenol, *J. Clin. Invest.*, **50**:112–118, 1971.

127. Fisher, D. A.: Norepinephrine inhibition of vasopressin antidiuresis, *J. Clin. Invest.*, **47**:540–547, 1968.

128. Baldes, E. J., and F. H. Smirk: The effect of water drinking, mineral starvation and salt administration on the total osmotic pressure of the blood in man, chiefly in relation to the problems of water absorption and water diuresis, *J. Physiol.*, **82**:62–74, 1934.

129. Wood, P.: Polyuria in paroxysmal tachycardia and paroxysmal atrial flutter and fibrillation, *Br. Heart J.*, **25**:273–282, 1963.

130. Fichman, M. P., H. Vorherr, C. R. Kleeman, and N. Telfer: Diuretic-induced hyponatremia, *Ann. Intern. Med.*, **75**:853–863, 1971.

131. Skowsky, W. R., A. A. Rosenbloom, and D. A. Fisher: Radioimmunoassay measurement of arginine vasopressin in serum; development and application, *J. Clin. Endocrinol. Metab.*, **38**:278–287, 1974.

132. Beardwell, C. G., G. Geelen, H. M. Palmer, D. Roberts, and L. Salamonson: Radioimmunoassay of plasma vasopressin in physiological and pathological states in man, *J. Endocrinol.*, **67**:189–202, 1975.

133. Morton, J. J., P. L. Padfield, and M. L. Forsling: A radioimmunoassay for plasma arginine vasopressin in man and dog, applications to physiological and pathological states, *J. Endocrinol.*, **65**:411–424, 1975.

134. Rabkin, R., J. Young, J. Crofton, and R. Shade: The renal handling of arginine vasopressin, *Clin. Res.*, **25**:62A, 1977.

135. Levi, J., S. Rosenfeld, and C. R. Kleeman: Inactivation of arginine vasopressin by the isolated perfused rabbit kidney, *J. Endocrinol.*, **62**:1–10, 1974.

136. Weitzman, R. E., and D. A. Fisher: Arginine vasopressin metabolism in dogs, I: Evidence for a receptor mediated mechanism, *Amer. J. Physiol.*, in press.

137. Wilson, K. C., R. E. Weitzman, and D. A. Fisher: Arginine vasopressin metabolism in dogs, II: Modeling and systems analysis, *Amer. J. Physiol.*, in press.

138. Robertson, G. L., E. A. Mahr, S. Athar, and ·T. Sinha: Development and clinical application of a new method for the radioimmunoassay of arginine vasopressin in human plasma, *J. Clin. Invest.*, **52**:2340–2352, 1973.

139. Weitzman, R. E., D. A. Fisher, J. J. Di Stefano, IV, and C. M. Bennett: Episodic secretion of AVP, *Am. J. Physiol.*, **233**:E32–E36, 1977.

140. Kleeman, C. R., and H. Vorherr: Water metabolism and the neurohypophysial hormones, in P. K. Bondy and L. Rosenberg (eds.), *Duncan's Diseases of Metabolism,* vol. 2, chap. 22, W. B. Saunders Company, Philadelphia, p. 1459.

141. Rector, E. C., Jr.: Renal concentrating mechanisms, in T. E. Andreoli, J. J. Grantham, and F. C. Rector, Jr. (eds.), *Disturbances in Body Fluid Osmolality,* chap. 8, American Physiology Society, Bethesda, Maryland, 1977, p. 179.

142. Schafer, J. A., and T. E. Andreoli: Action of antidiuretic hormone on water and nonelectrolyte transport processes in mammalian collecting tubules, in T. E. Andreoli, J. J. Grantham, and F. C. Rector, Jr. (eds.), *Disturbances in Body Fluid Osmolality,* chap. 3, American Physiology Society, Bethesda, Maryland, 1977, p. 57.

143. Jamison, R. L., and R. H. Maffly: The urinary concentrating mechanism, *N. Engl. J. Med.*, **295**:1059–1067, 1976.

144. Hays, R. M., and S. D. Levine: Pathophysiology of water metabolism, in B. M. Brenner and F. C. Rector, Jr. (eds.), *The Kidney,* W. B. Saunders Company, Philadelphia, 1976, p. 553.

145. Tisher, C. C.: Anatomy of the kidney, in B. M. Brenner and F. C. Rector, Jr. (eds.), *The Kidney,* chap. 1, W. B. Saunders Company, Philadelphia, 1976.

146. Kriz, W., and A. F. Lever: Renal countercurrent mechanisms: Structure and function, *Am. Heart J.*, **78**:101–118, 1969.

147. Kokko, J. P.: Membrane characteristics govern-

ing salt and water transport in the loop of Henle, *Fed. Proc.*, **33**:25–30, 1974.

148. Stephenson, J. L.: Concentration of urine in a central core model of the renal counterflow system, *Kidney Int.*, **2**:85–94, 1972.

149. Stephenson, J. L.: Concentrating engines and the kidney: I and II, *Biophys. J.*, **13**:512–546, 1973.

150. Kokko, J. P., and F. C. Rector, Jr.: Countercurrent multiplication system without active transport in inner medulla, *Kidney Int.*, **2**:214–223, 1972.

151. Rocha, A. S., and J. P. Kokko: Sodium chloride and water transport in the medullary thick ascending limb of Henle, *J. Clin. Invest.*, **52**:612, 1973.

152. Grantham, J. J., and M. B. Burg: Effect of vasopressin and cyclic AMP on permeability of isolated collecting tubules, *Am. J. Physiol.*, **211**:255, 1966.

153. Britton, K. E., E. R. Carson, and P. E. Cage: A "bootstrap" model of the renal medulla, *Postgrad. Med. J.*, **52**:279–284, 1976.

154. Ullrich, K. J., and K. H. Jarausch: Untersuchungen zum problem der harn knonzentrierung und verdünnung, *Pflügers Arch. Gesamte Physiol.*, **262**:537, 1956.

155. Burg, M. B.: Tubular chloride transport and the mode of action of some diuretics, *Kidney Int.*, **9**:189–197, 1976.

156. Pennell, J. P., V. Sanjana, and N. R. Frey: The effect of urea infusion on the urinary concentrating mechanism in protein depleted rats, *J. Clin. Invest.*, **55**:399–409, 1975.

157. Johnston, P. A., C. A. Battilana, F. B. Lacy, and R. L. Jamison: Evidence for a concentration gradient favoring outward movement of sodium from the thin loop of Henle, *J. Clin. Invest.*, **59**:234–240, 1977.

158. Gertz, K. H., B. Schmidt-Nielsen, and D. Pagel: Exchange of water, urea and salt between mammalian renal papilla and the surrounding urine (abstract), *Fed. Proc.*, **25**:327, 1966.

159. Schütz, W., and J. P. Schnermann: Pelvic urine composition as a determinant of inner medullary solute concentration and urine osmolality, *Pflügers Arch.*, **334**:154, 1972.

160. Berliner, R. W., and C. M. Bennett: Concentration of urine in the mammalian kidneys, *Am. J. Med.*, **42**:777–789, 1967.

161. Andreoli, T. E., and J. A. Schafer: Mass transport across cell membranes: The effects of antidiuretic hormone on water and solute flows in epithelia, in E. Knobil, R. R. Sonnenschein, and I. S. Edelman (eds.), *Annual Review of Physiology*, vol. 38, Annual Reviews, Inc., Palo Alto, California, 1977, p. 451.

162. Hays, R. M.: Antidiuretic hormone, *N. Engl. J. Med.*, **295**:659, 1976.

163. Walter, R., W. S. Clark, P. K. Mehta, S. Boonjdrern, J. A. L. Arruda, and N. A. Kurtzman: Conformational considerations of vasopressin as a guide to development of biological probes and therapeutic agents, in T. E. Andreoli, J. J. Grantham, and F. C. Rector, Jr. (eds.), *Disturbances in Body Fluid Osmolality*, chap. 1, American Physiology Society, Bethesda, Maryland, 1977, p. 1.

164. Handler, J. S., and J. Orloff: The mechanism of action of antidiuretic hormone, in J. Orloff and R. W. Berliner (eds.), *Handbook of Physiology: Renal Physiology*, sec. 8, chap. 24, American Physiology Society, Washington, D.C., 1973, pp. 791–814.

165. Dousa, T. P., and H. Valtin: Cellular actions of vasopressin in the mammalian kidney, *Kidney Int.*, **10**:55–72, 1976.

166. Kuo, J. F., and P. Greengard: Cyclic nucleotide dependent protein kinases. IV. Widespread occurrence of adenosine 3′5′ monophosphate dependent protein kinase in various tissues and phyla of the animal kingdom, *Proc. Natl. Acad. Sci. U.S.A.*, **64**:1349–1355, 1969.

167. Taylor, A.: Role of microtubules and microfilaments in the action of vasopressin, in T. E. Andreoli, J. J. Grantham, and F. C. Rector, Jr. (eds.), *Disturbances in Body Fluid Osmolality*, chap. 5, American Physiology Society, Bethesda, Maryland, 1977, p. 97.

168. Dousa, T. P., and L. D. Barnes: Effects of colchicine and vinblastine on the cellular action of vasopressin in mammalian kidney. A possible role of microtubules, *J. Clin. Invest.*, **54**:252–262, 1974.

169. Kachadorian, W. A., J. B. Wade, and V. A. Di Scala: Vasopressin induced structural change in toad bladder luminal membrane, *Science*, **190**:67–69, 1975.

170. Kachadorian, W. A., J. B. Wade, C. C. Viterwyk,

and V. A. Di Scala: Membrane structural and functional responses to vasopressin in toad bladder, *J. Membr. Biol.*, **30**:381–401, 1977.

171. Koefoed-Johnsen, V., and H. H. Ussing: The contributions of diffusion and flow to the passage of D₂O through living membranes, *Acta Scand. Physiol.*, **28**:60, 1953.

172. Valtin, H.: Hereditary hypothalamic diabetes insipidus in rats (Brattleboro strain). A useful experimental model, *Am. J. Med.*, **42**:814–827, 1967.

172a. Valtin, H.: Genetic models for hypothalamic and nephrogenic diabetes insipidus, in T. E. Andreoli, J. J. Grantham and F. C. Rector, Jr. (eds.), *Disturbances in Body Fluid Osmolality*, The American Physiology Society, Bethesda, Maryland, 1977, pp. 197–216.

173. Miller, M., and A. M. Moses: Radioimmunoassay of urinary antidiuretic hormone with application to study of the Brattleboro rat, *Endocrinology*, **88**:1389–1396, 1971.

173a. Bode, H. H., B. M. Harley, and J. D. Crawford: Restorational normal drinking behavior by chlorpropamide in patients with hypodipsia and diabetes insipidus, *Amer. J. Med.*, **51**:304–313, 1971.

174. Eknoyan, G., W. N. Suki, F. C. Rector, Jr., and D. W. Seldin: Functional characteristics of the diluting segment of the dog nephron and the effect of extracellular volume expansion on its reabsorptive capacity, *J. Clin. Invest.*, **46**:1178, 1967.

175. Jamison, R. L., J. Buerkert, and F. Lacy: A micropuncture study of collecting tubule function in rats with hereditary diabetes insipidus, *J. Clin. Invest.*, **50**:2444, 1971.

176. Epstein, F. H., C. R. Kleeman, and A. Hendrikx: The influence of bodily hydration on the renal concentrating process, *J. Clin. Invest.*, **36**:629, 1957.

177. Miller, L., L. Fisch, and C. R. Kleeman: Relative potency of arginine-8-vasopressin and lysine vasopressin in humans, *J. Lab. Clin. Med.*, **69**:270–291, 1967.

178. Kleeman, C. R., J. Levi, and O. Bettor: Kidney and adrenocortical hormones, *Nephron*, **15**:261–278, 1975.

179. Zusman, R. M., H. R. Keiser, and J. S. Handler: Adrenal steroids enhance vasopressin stimulated water flow in the toad bladder by inhibiting prostaglandin E biosynthesis, *Proc. Am. Soc. Neph. Mtg.*, Washington, D.C., 1977, p. 127A.

180. Zusman, R. M., H. R. Keiser, and J. S. Handler: A hypothesis for the molecular mechanism of action of chlorpropamide in the treatment of diabetes mellitus and diabetes insipidus, *Fed. Proc.*, **36**:2728–2729, 1977.

181. Anderson, R. J., T. Berl, K. M. McDonald, and R. W. Schrier: Evidence for an *in vivo* antagonism between vasopressin and prostaglandin in the mammalian kidney, *J. Clin. Invest.*, **56**:420–426, 1975.

182. Berl, T., A. Raz, J. Horowitz, and C. W. Czaczkes: Prostaglandin synthesis inhibition and the action of vasopressin: Studies in man and rat, *Am. J. Physiol.*, **232**:F529–F537, 1977.

183. Galvez, O. G., B. W. Roberts, W. H. Bay, and T. F. Ferris: Studies of the mechanism of polyuria with hypokalemia, *Proc. Am. Soc. Neph. Mtg.*, Washington, D. C., 1976, p. 97.

184. Goldberg, M.: The renal physiology of diuretics, in J. Orloff and R. W. Berliner (eds.), *Handbook of Physiology*, American Physiology Society, Washington, D.C., 1973, pp. 1003–1031.

185. Kleeman, C. R., and R. Cutler: The neurohypophysis, *Ann. Rev. Physiol.*, **25**:385–432, 1963.

186. Laszlo, F. A., and D. de Wied: Antidiuretic hormone content of the hypothalamo-neurohypophysial system and urinary excretion of antidiuretic hormone in rats during the development of diabetes insipidus after lesions in the pituitary stalk, *J. Endocrinol.*, **36**:125–137, 1966.

187. Kovacs, K., F. A. Laszlo, and M. A. David: The antidiuretic phase of water metabolism in rats after lesions of the pituitary stalk. II. The role of the antidiuretic hormone, *J. Endocrinol.*, **25**:397–401, 1962.

188. Vejjajiva, A., V. Sitprija, and S. Shuangshoti: Chronic sustained hypernatremia and hypovolemia in hypothalamic tumor. A physiologic study, *Neurology*, **19**:161–166, 1969.

189. Duchen, G. W.: Metastatic carcinoma in the pituitary gland and hypothalamus, *J. Pathol. Bacteriol.*, **91**:347–355, 1966.

190. Adams, J. M., J. D. Kenny, and A. J. Rudolph: Central diabetes insipidus following intraventricular hemorrhage, *J. Pediatr.*, **88**:292–294, 1976.

191. Braverman, L. E., J. P. Mancini, and D. P. M. McGoldrick: Hereditary idiopathic diabetes insipidus. A case report with autopsy findings, *Ann. Intern. Med.,* **63:**504–508, 1965.

192. Raff, S. B., and H. Greenberg: Night sweats, a dominant symptom in diabetes insipidus, *JAMA,* **234:**1252–1253, 1975.

193. Friedland, G. W., M. M. Axman, M. F. Russi, and W. R. Fair: Renal back pressure atrophy with compromised renal function due to diabetes insipidus. Case report. *Radiology,* **98:**359–360, 1971.

194. Helbock, H., W. Krivit, and M. E. Nesbit: Patterns of antidiuretic function in diabetes insipidus caused by histiocytosis X, *J. Lab. Clin. Med.,* **78:**194–202, 1971.

195. Rogers, P. W., and N. A. Kurtzman: Renal failure, uncontrollable thirst and hyperreninemia, *JAMA,* **225:**1236–1238, 1973.

196. Cutler, R., C. R. Kleeman, M. H. Maxwell, and J. T. Dowling: Physiologic studies in nephrogenic diabetes insipidus, *J. Clin. Endocrinol.,* **22:**827–838, 1962.

197. Feigin, R. D., D. L. Rimoin, and R. L. Kaufman: Nephrogenic diabetes insipidus in a Negro kindred, *Am. J. Dis. Child.,* **120:**64–68, 1970.

198. Kaplan, S. A., A. M. Yuceoglu, and J. Strauss: Vasopressin-resistant diabetes insipidus, *Am. J. Dis. Child.,* **97:**308–313, 1959.

199. Bode, H. H., and J. D. Crawford: Nephrogenic diabetes insipidus in North America: The Hopewell hypothesis, *N. Engl. J. Med.,* **280:**750–754, 1969.

200. Robertson, G. L.: Immunoassay of plasma vasopressin in man, *Proc. Natl. Acad. Sci.,* **66:**1298–1305, 1970.

201. Beardwell, C. G.: Radioimmunoassay of arginine vasopressin in human plasma, *J. Clin. Endocrinol. Metab.,* **33:**254–260, 1971.

202. Lipsett, M. B., and O. H. Pearson: Further studies of diabetes insipidus following hypophysectomy in man, *J. Lab. Clin. Med.,* **49:**190–199, 1957.

203. Miller, M., T. Dalakos, A. M. Moses, H. Fellerman, and D. H. T. Streeten: Recognition of partial defects in antidiuretic hormone secretion, *Ann. Intern. Med.,* **73:**721–729, 1970.

204. Dashe, A. M., R. E. Cramm, C. A. Crist, J. F. Habener, and D. H. Solomon: A water deprivation test for differential diagnosis of polyuria, *JAMA,* **185:**699–703, 1963.

205. Dahse, A. M., C. R. Kleeman, J. W. Czaczkes, H. Rubinoff, and I. Spears: Synthetic vasopressin nasal spray in the treatment of diabetes insipidus, *JAMA,* **190:**1069–1071, 1964.

206. Vavra, G., A. Machova, and V. Holecek: Effect of synthetic analogue of vasopressin in animals and in patients with diabetes insipidus, *Lancet,* **1:**948–952, 1968.

207. Robinson, A. G.: DDAVP in the treatment of diabetes insipidus, *N. Engl. J. Med.,* **294:**507–511, 1976.

208. Lee, W. P., B. M. Lippe, S. H. La Franchi, and S. A. Kaplan: Vasopressin analog DDAVP in the treatment of diabetes insipidus, *Am. J. Dis. Child.,* **130:**166–169, 1976.

209. Crawford, J. D., and G. Kennedy: Chlorothiazide in diabetes insipidus, *Nature,* **183:**891–892, 1959.

210. Arduino, F., F. P. J. Ferraz, and J. Rodrigues: Antidiuretic action of chlorpropamide in idiopathic diabetes insipidus, *J. Clin. Endocrinol. Metab.,* **26:**1325–1328, 1966.

211. Reforzo-Membrines, J., L. I. Moledo, A. E. Lanaro, and A. Megias: Antidiuretic effect of 1-propyl-3-p-chlorobenzene-sulfonylurea (chlorpropamide), *J. Clin. Endocrinol. Metab.,* **28:**332–336, 1968.

212. Kunstadter, R. H., E. C. Cabana, and W. Oh: Treatment of vasopressin-sensitive diabetes insipidus with chlorpropamide, *Am. J. Dis. Child.,* **117:**436–441, 1969.

213. Zgliozynski, S.: Antidiuretic effect of sulfonylureas in idiopathic diabetes insipidus, *Helvet. Med. Acta.,* **34:**478–485, 1969.

214. Vallet, H. L., M. Prasad, and R. B. Goldbloom: Chlorpropamide treatment of diabetes insipidus in children, *Pediatrics,* **45:**246–253, 1970.

215. Meinders, A. E., J. L. Touber, and L. A. de Vries: Chlorpropamide treatment in diabetes insipidus, *Lancet,* **2:**544–546, 1967.

216. Webster, B., and J. Bain: Antidiuretic effect and complications of chlorpropamide therapy in diabetes insipidus, *J. Clin. Endocrinol. Metab.,* **30:**215–227, 1970.

217. Berndt, W. O., M. Miller, W. M. Kettyle, and H. Valtin: Potentiation of the antidiuretic effect of

vasopressin by chlorpropamide, *Endocrinology*, **86:**1028–1032, 1970.

218. Miller, M., and A. M. Moses: Mechanism of chlorpropamide action in diabetes insipidus, *J. Clin. Endocrinol. Metab.*, **30:**488–496, 1970.

219. Hagen, G. A., and T. F. Frawley: Hyponatremia due to sulfonylurea compounds, *J. Clin. Endocrinol. Metab.*, **31:**570, 1970.

220. Mahoney, J. H., and D. A. Goodman: Hypernatremia due to hypodipsia and elevated threshold for vasopressin release. Effects of treatment with hydrochlorthiazide, chlorpropamide and tolbutamide, *N. Engl. J. Med.*, **279:**1191–1196, 1968.

221. Ingelfinger, J. R., and R. M. Hays: Evidence that chlorpropamide and vasopressin share a common site of action, *J. Clin. Endocrinol. Metab.*, **29:**738–740, 1969.

222. Lozada, E. S., J. Gouaux, N. Franki, G. B. Appel, and R. M. Hays: Studies of the mode of action of the sulfonylureas and phenylacetamides in enhancing the action of vasopressin, *J. Clin. Endocrinol. Metab.*, **34:**704–712, 1972.

223. Beck, N., K. S. Kim, and B. B. Davis: Effect of chlorpropamide on cyclic AMP in rat renal medulla, *Endocrinology*, **95:**771–774, 1974.

224. Brooker, G., and M. Fichman: Chlorpropamide and tolbutamide inhibition of adenosine 3′5′ cyclic monophosphate phosphodiesterase, *Biochem. Biophys. Res. Commun.*, **42:**824–828 1971.

225. Weissman, P. N., L. Shenkman, and R. I. Gregerman: Chlorpropamide hyponatremia. Drug-induced inappropriate antidiuretic-hormone activity, *N. Engl. J. Med.*, **284:**65–71, 1971.

226. de Gennes, J. L., C. Bertrand, B. Bigorie, and J. Trufert: Études préliminaires de l'action antidiurétique du clofibrate (ou Atromid S) dans le diabéte insipide pH ressosensible, *Ann. Endocrinol.*, **31:**300–308, 1970.

227. Moses, A. M., J. Howanitz, M. Van Gemert, and M. Miller: Clofibrate induced antidiuresis, *J. Clin. Invest.*, **52:**535–542, 1973.

228. Braunhoter, J., and L. Zicha: Eröffnet tegretol neve therapie möglichkeitan bei best immten neurologischen und endokrinen krankheits bildern? *Med. Welt.*, **17:**1875–1880, 1966.

229. Rado, J. P.: Combination of carbamazepine and chlorpropamide in the treatment of "hyporesponder" pituitary diabetes insipidus, *J. Clin. Endocrinol. Metab.*, **38:**1–7, 1974.

230. Kimura, T., K. Matsui, T. Sato, and K. Yoshinaga: Mechanism of carbamazepine (Tegretol) induced antidiuresis: Evidence for release of antidiuretic hormone and impaired excretion of a water load, *J. Clin. Endocrinol. Metab.*, **38:**356–362, 1974.

231. Meinders, A. E., V. Cejka, and G. L. Robertson: The antidiuretic action of carbamazepine in man, *Clin. Sci. Mole. Med.*, **47:**289–299, 1974.

232. Moses, A. M., and M. Miller: Drug induced dilutional hyponatremia, *N. Engl. J. Med.*, **291:**1234–1239, 1974.

233. Arieff, A. I., and H. J. Carroll: Nonketotic hyperosmolar coma with hyperglycemia: Clinical features, pathophysiology, renal function, acid-base balance, plasma-cerebrospinal fluid equilibria and the effects of therapy in 37 cases, *Medicine*, **51:**73–94, 1972.

234. Boyer, J., G. N. Gill, and F. H. Epstein: Hyperglycemia and hyperosmolality complicating peritoneal dialysis, *Ann. Intern. Med.*, **67:**568–572, 1967.

235. DeRubertis, F. R., M. F. Michelis, and B. B. Davis: Essential hypernatremia. Report of three cases and review of the literature, *Arch. Intern. Med.*, **134:**889–895, 1974.

236. Trust, P. M., J. J. Brown, R. H. Chinn, A. C. Lener, J. J. Moston, P. A. Padfield, J. I. S. Robertson, J. T. Ireland, I. D. Melville, and W. S. T. Thompson: A case of hypopituitarism with diabetes insipidus and loss of thirst. Role of antidiuretic hormone and angiotensin II in the control of urine flow and osmolality, *J. Clin. Endocrinol. Metab.*, **41:**346–353, 1975.

237. Schalekamp, M., S. Donker, A. Jansen-Goemans, T. D. Fawz, and A. Muller: Dissociation of renin and aldosterone during dehydration: Studies in a case of diabetes insipidus and adipsia, *J. Clin. Endocrinol. Metab.*, **43:**287–294, 1976.

238. Sridhar, C. B., G. D. Calvert, and H. K. Ibbertson: Syndrome of hypernatremia, hypodipsia and partial diabetes insipidus: A new interpretation, *J. Clin. Endocrinol. Metab.*, **38:**890–901, 1974.

239. Grubb, S. R., C. O. Watlington, and W. G. Blackard: Osmoreceptor dysfunction, chronic hyperna-

tremia, adipsia and vasopressin resistant diabetes insipidus, *Clin. Res.*, **25**:13a, 1977.

240. Halter, J., A. Goldberg, G. Robertson, and D. Porte: Selective osmoreceptor dysfunction in the syndrome of chronic hypernatremia and hypodipsia, *Endocrinology*, **98**(suppl.):159, 1976.

241. Macaulay, D., and M. Watson: Hypernatremia in infants as a cause of brain damage, *Arch. Dis. Child.*, **42**:485–491, 1967.

242. Arieff, A. I., R. Guisada, and V. C. Lazarowitz: Pathophysiology of hyperosmolar states, in T. E. Andreoli, J. J. Grantham, and F. C. Rector, Jr. (eds.), *Disturbances in Body Fluid Osmolality*, chap. 11, American Physiology Society, Bethesda, Maryland, 1977, pp. 227–250.

243. Covey, C. M., and A. I. Arieff: Disorders of sodium and water metabolism and their effects on the central nervous system, in B. M. Brenner and J. H. Stein (eds.), *Sodium and Water Homeostasis*, chap. 9, Churchill-Livingston, New York, 1978, pp. 212–241.

244. Katz, M. A.: Hyperglycemia-induced hyponatremia—calculation of expected serum sodium depression, *N. Engl. J. Med.*, **289**:843–844, 1973.

245. Valtin, H.: Genetic models for hypothalamic and nephrogenic diabetes insipidus, in T. E. Andreoli, J. J. Grantham, and F. C. Rector, Jr. (eds.), *Disturbances in Body Fluid Osmolality*, American Physiology Society, Bethesda, Maryland, 1977, pp. 197–215.

246. Kleeman, C. R., D. A. Adams, and M. H. Maxwell: An evaluation of maximal water diuresis in chronic renal disease. I. On normal solute intake, *J. Lab. Clin. Med.*, **58**:169–184, 1961.

247. Kleeman, C. R., J. W. Czaczkes, and R. Cutler: Mechanisms of impaired water excretion in adrenal and pituitary insufficiency. IV. Antidiuretic hormone in primary and secondary adrenal insufficiency, *J. Clin. Invest.*, **43**:1641–1648, 1964.

248. Bartter, F. C., and W. B. Schwartz: The syndrome of inappropriate secretion of antidiuretic hormone, *Am. J. Med.*, **42**:790–806, 1967.

249. Vorherr, H., S. G. Massry, R. D. Utiger, and C. R. Kleeman: Antidiuretic principle in malignant tumor extracts from patients with inappropriate ADH syndrome, *J. Clin. Endocrinol. Metab.*, **28**:162–168, 1968.

250. Utiger, R. D.: Inappropriate antidiuresis and carcinoma of the lung. Detection of arginine-vasopressin in tumor extracts by radioimmunoassay, *J. Clin. Endocrinol. Metab.*, **26**:970–974, 1966.

251. George, J. M., C. C. Capen, and A. S. Phillips: Biosynthesis of vasopressin in vitro and ultrastructure of a bronchogenic carcinoma, *J. Clin. Invest.*, **51**:141–148, 1972.

252. Vorherr, H.: Paraendocrine tumor activity with emphasis on ectopic production of ADH secretion, *Oncology*, **29**:382–416, 1974.

253. Vorherr, H., S. G. Massry, R. Fallet, L. Kaplan, and C. R. Kleeman: Antidiuretic principle in tuberculous lung tissue of a patient with pulmonary tuberculosis and hyponatremia, *Ann. Intern. Med.*, **72**:383–387, 1970.

254. Leaf, A., F. C. Bartter, R. F. Santos, and O. Wrong: Evidence in man that urinary electrolyte loss induced by Pitressin is a function of water retention, *J. Clin. Invest.*, **32**:868–878, 1953.

255. Nolph, K. D., and R. W. Schrier: Sodium, potassium and water metabolism in the syndrome of inappropriate antidiuretic hormone secretion, *Am. J. Med.*, **49**:534–545, 1970.

256. Heinemann, H. O., and J. H. Laragh: Inappropriate renal sodium loss reverted by vena cava obstruction, *Ann. Intern. Med.*, **65**:708–718, 1966.

257. Beresford, H. R.: Polydipsia, hydrochlorothiazide, and water intoxication, *JAMA*, **214**:879–883, 1970.

258. Garcia, M., M. Miller, and A. M. Moses: Chlorpropamide-induced water retention in patients with diabetes mellitus, *Ann. Intern. Med.*, **75**:549–554, 1971.

259. Hagen, G. A., and T. F. Frawley: Hyponatremia due to sulfonylurea compounds, *J. Clin. Endocrinol. Metab.*, **31**:570–576, 1970.

260. Kennedy, R. M., and L. E. Earley: Profound hyponatremia resulting from a thiazide-induced decrease in urinary diluting capacity in a patient with primary polydipsia, *N. Engl. J. Med.*, **282**:1185–1186, 1970.

261. Demanet, J. C., M. Bonnyns, H. Bleiberg, and C. Stevens-Rocmans,: Coma due to water intoxication in beer drinkers, *Lancet*, **2**:1115–1117, 1971.

262. Hobson, J. A., and J. T. English: Case study of a chronically schizophrenic patient with physiological evidence of water retention due to inappropriate release of antidiuretic hormone, *Ann. Intern. Med.*, **58**:324–332, 1963.

263. Raskind, M. A., H. Orenstein, and G. Christo-

pher: Acute psychosis, increased water ingestion and inappropriate antidiuretic hormone secretion, *Am. J. Psychol.*, **132:**407–410, 1975.

264. Raskind, M. A., R. E. Weitzman, D. A. Fisher, H. Orenstein, and N. Courtney: Antidiuretic hormone is elevated in psychosis, *Biol. Psychiatry,* **13:**385–390, 1978.

265. Arieff, A. I., F. Llach, and S. G. Massry: Neurological manifestations and morbidity of hyponatremia: Correlation with brain water and electrolytes, *Medicine,* **55:**121–129, 1976.

266. Hantman, D., B. Rossier, R. Zohlman, and R. Schrier: Rapid correction of hyponatremia in the syndrome of inappropriate secretion of antidiuretic hormone, *Ann. Intern. Med.,* **78:**870–875, 1973.

267. Maclean, D., M. Champion, and D. B. Trash: Pulmonary edema during treatment of acute water intoxication, *Postgrad. Med. J.,* **52:**532–535, 1976.

268. Fichman, M. P., C. R. Kleeman, and J. E. Bethune: Inhibition of antidiuretic hormone secreted by diphenylhydantoin, *Arch. Neurol.,* **22:**45, 1970.

269. Cherrill, D. A., R. M. State, J. R. Birge, and I. Singer: Demeclocycline treatment in the syndrome of inappropriate antidiuretic hormone secretion, *Ann. Intern. Med.,* **83:**654–656, 1975.

270. White, M. E., and C. D. Fetner: Treatment of the syndrome of inappropriate secretion of antidiuretic hormone with lithium carbonate, *N. Engl. J. Med.,* **292:**390–392, 1975.

271. Share, L., and R. H. Travis: Interrelations between the adrenal cortex and the posterior pituitary, *Fed. Proc.,* **30:**1378–1382, 1971.

271a. Green, H. H., A. R. Harrington, and H. Valtin: On the role of antidiuretic hormone in the inhibition of acute water diuresis in adrenal insufficiency and the effects of gluco- and mineralocorticoids in reversing the inhibition, *J. Clin. Invest.,* **49:**1724–1736, 1970.

272. Ahmed, A. B. J., B. C. George, C. Gonzalez-Auvert, and J. F. Dingman: Increased plasma arginine vasopressin in clinical adrenocortical insufficiency and its inhibition by glucosteroids, *J. Clin. Invest.,* **46:**111–123, 1967.

273. Seif, M., A. G. Robinson, E. A. Zimmerman, and J. Wilkins: Plasma neurophysin and vasopressin in the rat: Response to adrenalectomy and steroid replacement, *Endocrinology,* 1978. In press.

274. Boykin, J., A. McCool, K. McDonald, G. Robertson, and R. Schrier: Mechanism of effect of glucocorticoid deficiency on renal water excretion in the conscious dog (abstract), *Clin. Res.,* **24:**269A, 1976.

275. Kleeman, C. R., M. H. Maxwell, and R. E. Rockney: Mechanism of impaired water excretion in adrenal and pituitary insufficiency. 1. The role of altered glomerular filtration rate and solute excretion, *J. Clin. Invest.,* **37:**1799–1812, 1958.

276. Fichman, M. P., and J. E. Bethune: The role of adrenocorticoids in the inappropriate antidiuretic hormone syndrome, *Ann. Intern. Med.,* **68:**806–820, 1968.

13

Pathogenesis and treatment of edema with special reference to the use of diuretics

GEORGE J. KALOYANIDES

INTRODUCTION

Edema is an excessive accumulation of interstitial fluid. It may be localized and confined to a circumscribed area as occurs with venous, lymphatic, or inflammatory disease, or it may be generalized so that interstitial fluid accumulates in virtually every organ and tissue of the body and in most serous cavities. Regardless of whether it is localized or generalized, edema formation ultimately can be explained by one or more of the factors (Table 13-1) that influence the distribution of extracellular fluid (ECF) between the intravascular and interstitial compartments. However, generalized edema carries important clinical implications not shared by localized edema in that it signals the presence of a major disturbance in the normal regulation of extracellular volume characterized by renal retention of sodium and water with expansion of interstitial and frequently of plasma volume.

The objective of this chapter is to review current concepts of generalized edema formation and to outline general theraupeutic principles including the use of diuretic agents in the treatment of edema.

CONCEPT OF VOLUME REGULATION

To understand the pathogenesis of edema formation requires a general appreciation of the normal regulation of extracellular volume. In normal subjects the volume of ECF is regulated within rather narrow limits. This fact can be readily appreciated by the observation that despite wide fluctuation in daily sodium and water intake, the body weight of an individual in caloric balance is kept remarkably constant. Figure 13-1A illustrates the response to a sudden increase in sodium intake in a normal subject previously in sodium balance. In response to the increased intake of sodium, urinary sodium excretion increases over the next several days until a new steady state is achieved, at which time sodium excretion equals sodium intake. Before the new steady state is achieved, there is an increase in body weight, re-

Table 13-1. Factors causing expansion of interstitial fluid volume

1. Increase in capillary hydrostatic pressure
2. Decrease in plasma colloid osmotic pressure
3. Increase in interstitial fluid colloid osmotic pressure
4. Increase in capillary permeability
5. Impaired lymphatic flow

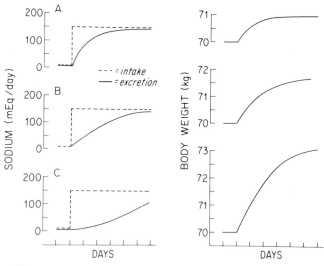

Figure 13-1. Pattern of sodium balance in response to a sustained increase in sodium intake in normal subjects (A) and in subjects with mild (B) and severe (C) congestive heart failure. See text for details. (*After Strauss et al. and Braunwald et al.*)

flecting a gain in body sodium along with water in isotonic proportions and expansion of extracellular volume. Figure 13-1B illustrates the response to a sudden and sustained increase in sodium intake in a patient with compensated heart failure. The main points deserving emphasis are that the time required to establish a new steady state is prolonged and the degree of positive sodium balance as reflected by the gain in body weight exceeds that of the normal subject. Figure 13-1C depicts the response to an acute and sustained increase in sodium intake in a patient with severe heart failure. Note that during the period of observation a new steady state is not achieved and progressive positive sodium balance ensues manifested by the continuing rise in body weight and the failure of sodium excretion to approximate sodium intake. In the last illustration the continuing positive sodium balance would lead to progressive circulatory congestion and edema.

The renal response to sodium loads provides a useful tool for assessing the overall integrity of the control system for regulating extracellular fluid volume. In normal subjects the ECF volume appears to be regulated within ± 5 percent of what

may be termed the normal or optimal extracellular volume measured during a sodium intake of 150 meq/day. This conclusion may be deduced from average changes in body weight measured under steady-state conditions in individuals whose sodium intake is varied between 10 and 150 meq/day (1).

Excessive weight gain in response to sodium loading as depicted in Figs. 13-1B and 13-1C implies a derangement in one or more elements of the control system which regulates ECF volume. This conclusion is obvious in the individual with clinically apparent edema. Perhaps less well appreciated is the fact that subtle abnormalities in the regulation of sodium metabolism, insufficient to cause clinically evident edema, can be detected by assessing the response to sodium loading (2). Moreover, the response patterns to sodium loading illustrated in Figs. 13-1B and 13-1C are not specific for mild and severe heart failure; indeed similar abnormalities are seen in all conditions associated with generalized edema. The more severe the underlying disorder, the greater the impairment in excreting a sodium load and the greater the deviation in extracellular volume from normal. Although the response to sodium loading is a sensitive index of the integrity of the control system for regulating extracellular volume, it obviously is not a discriminating index because by itself it provides no insight into the nature of the underlying abnormality. This requires an assessment of the functional status of the various elements constituting the control system.

EFFECTIVE CIRCULATING BLOOD VOLUME

Although it is customary to speak of regulation of *extracellular fluid volume,* most of the available evidence supports the concept that *plasma volume* is the dimension of ECF volume that is regulated (3). *Interstitial fluid volume* is regulated secondarily by the balance of Starling forces operating across the capillaries. Moreover, it is obvious that the control system is not tuned to maintain a constant intravascular volume; rather, plasma volume is regulated so as to achieve a functionally effective blood volume adequate to meet the metabolic requirements of the peripheral tissues. Given the present state of knowledge, the definition of effective blood volume cannot be reduced to a precise mathematical equation. Nevertheless it is evident that effective blood volume is related to some derivative of cardiac output and peripheral vascular resistance or circulatory capacitance (3). In order to give appropriate emphasis to the dynamic aspects of blood volume the expression *effective circulating blood or plasma volume* is frequently used.

The response to upright posture illustrates the dynamic relationship between plasma volume, circulatory capacitance, and cardiac output (4). On changing from the recumbent to the upright position a person's cardiac output falls due to venous pooling of blood in the lower extremities and the consequent decrease in venous return to the heart. Central blood volume has been estimated to fall by 500 mL most of which, under the influence of gravity, shifts to the lower extremities. The reflex adjustments to upright posture include baroreceptor-mediated increases in heart rate and peripheral vascular resistance; the latter maintains arterial blood pressure in the face of a decreased cardiac output. The contribution of venoconstriction to the circulatory adjustments to upright posture remains controversial (3). In any event, since cardiac output remains depressed, it is obvious that the reflex adjustments to upright posture are insufficient to decrease venous capacitance and restore venous return to the level that existed during recumbency unless the pumping action of the leg muscles is engaged. Thus, upright posture simulates a decrease in effective circulating blood volume due to an increase in the holding capacity of the venous circulation that is incompletely compensated for by reflex vasoconstriction. Renal conservation of sodium and water, a response detected within minutes of assuming the upright posture, represents a compensatory mechanism for conserving and eventually restoring effective circulating blood volume (5).

In all conditions characterized by generalized edema formation, with the exception of circulatory congestion associated with acute renal failure, *the primary stimulus for renal retention of sodium and water is a decrease in effective circulating blood volume*. To the extent that renal retention of sodium and water restores an effective circulating blood volume, a new state of sodium balance will be established, but interstitial and, frequently, plasma volume will be higher than normal.

AFFERENT LIMB

If a decrease in effective circulating blood volume is the common denominator for stimulating renal conservation of sodium and water, what elements constitute the sensory or afferent limb of the arc? It has long been recognized that maneuvers which decrease *central* blood volume without changing absolute blood volume, such as upright posture, positive pressure breathing, and lower-body negative suction, stimulate renal conservation of sodium and water, whereas maneuvers which increase central blood volume promote sodium and water excretion (6). The thoracic volume receptor hypothesis received considerable support from subsequent studies which established a role for left atrial stretch receptors in the modulation of antidiuretic hormone (ADH) secretion (7–12) (see Chap. 12) and, thus, stimulated the search for receptors in the low-pressure circuit of the heart and lungs that might modulate renal sodium excretion. Identification of the sites and elucidation of the physiological function of these postulated receptors has proved to be a challenging problem that remains to a large extent unresolved (13). Nevertheless, from such studies has emerged increasing evidence that receptors in the cardiopulmonary circuit, in particular the left atrium, exert a strong influence on renal nerve activity (14–19) and thus could modulate renal function and sodium excretion through changes in renal hemodynamics. Renal nerve traffic is decreasd by maneuvers which increase left atrial volume or pressure; whereas renal nerve traffic is augmented by maneuvers which decrease left atrial volume or pressure. Moreover, appropriate changes in renal hemodynamics have been observed in response to these maneuvers (20–22).

Receptors in the right atrium have been implicated in the control of renin secretion. Elevation of right atrial pressure elicits a decrease in plasma renin activity (23), whereas low atrial pressure appears to increase plasma renin activity (24). Whether the efferent limb of the reflex limb is neurogenically (25) or humorally (26) mediated remains uncertain.

Several lines of evidence suggest that receptors in the portal circulation may also participate in the reflex regulation of sodium and water excretion (27–31).

The carotid and aortic baroreceptors are not thought of as classical volume receptors. However, it is evident that these receptors influence renal function both indirectly by their dominant effect on cardiovascular and circulatory reflexes (14) and directly by influencing renal sympathetic nerve activity (32–34). It is also evident, however, that the carotid baroreceptors exert a greater influence on muscle resistance vessels than on renal resistance vessels (17, 35–39) due to the tonic inhibitory influence or cardiopulmonary receptors on the vasomotor center. Thus, the net effect of these cardiopulmonary receptors is to oppose renal vasoconstriction associated with withdrawal of carotid baroreceptor input to the vasomotor center (40, 41). In addition to influencing renal nerve discharge, the carotid baroreceptors have been implicated in ADH (42, 43) and renin secretion (44–46).

Although the kidney is usually thought of as being part of the efferent limb of the volume control system, it is also an important element of the afferent limb. For example it is well established that renin secretion is modulated by both a renal vascular and the macula densa receptor (47) (see also Chap. 14). Moreover, the kidney is also the source of centrally directed nerve impulses whose frequency is augmented by increasing intrarenal pressure (48–51). The location and function of the receptors which give rise to the afferent impulses have not been elucidated. Electrical stimulation of afferent renal nerves has been reported to cause a decrease (52, 53), no change (54), or an increase (55) in systemic arterial blood pressure.

Finally, studies from several laboratories have provided evidence for the existence of brain receptors which influence renal sodium and water excretion and renin secretion (56–63).

The present state of knowledge leads to the conclusion that the afferent limb of the volume control system is composed of multiple receptors, some of which undoubtedly are yet to be identified, distributed throughout the circulation and in various organs which provide input as to the effectiveness of intravascular and possibly interstitial volume. The relative importance of these receptors and the order in which they are engaged in the control of ECF volume are questions that remain unresolved. Although major emphasis has been placed on the importance of the cardiopulmonary receptors in initiating reflex adjustment for maintaining an effective circulating blood volume (3), it is difficult to conceive of a change in volume in the low-pressure circuit that would not influence circulatory adjustments in the high-pressure circuit and, thereby, engage receptors in this circuit as well.

The question also arises whether disorders characterized by edema formation might be related to an aberration in the afferent limb of the control system. Greenberg et al. (64) have suggested that a reduced sensitivity of atrial receptors may be responsible, at least in part, for the reduction in renal electrolyte and water excretion in congestive heart failure. The evidence in support of this concept is far from compelling (13). It should be noted that in experimental animals subjected to cardiac denervation, the abnormalities in sodium and water metabolism are rather modest (65–68). This undoubtedly reflects the fact that regulation of extracellular volume is mediated by the complex interplay of feedback loops involving multiple afferent and efferent mechanisms which endow the contol system with a remarkable degree of stability even when one or more loops are inoperative or function abnormally (69).

EFFERENT LIMB

The kidney, by virtue of its capacity to alter the rate of sodium and water excretion in response to neurogenic, humoral, and hemodynamic stimuli, functions as a final common pathway through which the efferent limb of the volume control system is expressed. In recent years considerable progress has been made in elucidating the various forces (Table 13-2) that modulate sodium and water excretion by the kidney. A detailed discussion of these factors is given in Chaps. 3, 7, and 12 and will not be covered here. Less clear, however, is the quantitative contribution of these forces to the renal regulation of sodium and water or the order in which they are recruited for the defense of ECF volume. Despite these gaps in our knowledge, it is still possible operationally to define a scheme by which these various effector mechanisms interact.

Neurogenic reflexes

As previously discussed, the renal nerves provide an efferent pathway for modulating renal sodium and water excretion in response to activation of volume receptors. Increased renal sympathetic tone has been implicated in the renal conservation of sodium observed during upright posture, sodium deprivation, hemorrhage, and various edema-forming states (70). A particularly convincing demonstration of neurogenically mediated sodium retention is provided by the study of Gill and Casper (71). These investigators examined the renal response to hemorrhage in dogs with one kidney perfused in situ by a second dog

Table 13-2. Factors which influence renal sodium excretion

I. HEMODYNAMIC
A. Glomerular filtration rate
B. Renal blood flow
C. Renal vascular resistance
D. ? Blood flow distribution

II. PHYSICAL
A. Renal perfusion pressure
B. Peritubular capillary hydraulic and colloid osmotic pressures
C. Plasma colloid osmotic pressure
D. Hematocrit

III. NEUROGENIC
A. Renal sympathetic nerve activity

IV. HORMONAL
A. Aldosterone
B. Renin-angiotensin
C. Catecholamines
D. Natriuretic hormone
E. ? Prostaglandins

such that the renal nerves remained intact. Hemorrhage promoted a sharp decrease in sodium excretion in the perfused kidney in the absence of a detectable decrease in glomerular filtration rate (GFR). Since the renal nerves provided the only communication between the isolated kidney and the hemorrhaged dog, it follows that the decrease in sodium excretion must have been mediated by reflex nerve stimulation.

Several mechanisms have been proposed to explain the decrease in sodium excretion associated with increased renal nerve activity. The most widely accepted theory is that an increase in renal adrenergic tone due to increased nerve traffic or possibly increased circulating levels of catecholamines causes a rise in filtration fraction due to a preferential vasocontriction at the efferent arteriole (70–72). Thus renal blood flow (RBF) may decrease prior to a fall in GFR. The resultant rise in peritubular capillary plasma colloid osmotic pressure and fall in hydrostatic pressure would favor an increase in net reabsorption of sodium along the proximal tubule and possibly the distal nephron as well (73). This mechanism presumably contributed to the decrease in sodium excretion observed in the study of Gill and Casper (71) since RBF was consistently depressed in response to hemorrhage whereas GFR did not change.

Redistribution of RBF from outer to inner cortical nephrons has also been proposed as a mechanism by which renal nerve stimulation or catecholamines may promote renal conservation of sodium in normal and pathologic states (74–81). However, in these studies RBF and blood flow distribution were measured by the inert gas technique. Other studies, particularly those employing the radiolabeled microsphere technique, have failed to confirm significant redistribution of intrarenal blood flow under similar experimental conditions (82, 83). Although the theory is attractive, convincing evidence that redistribution of cortical blood flow is an important determinant of sodium excretion is lacking.

In addition, several lines of evidence suggest that renal nerve activity may modulate sodium excretion by a direct effect on tubular transport. Direct or reflex renal nerve stimulation was shown to decrease sodium excretion in the absence of significant changes in GFR, RBF or blood flow distribution (84). This effect was rapid in onset, rapidly reversible, and could be blocked by sympatholytic agents. Surgical denervation has been shown to depress proximal tubular reabsorption of filtrate (85), whereas it was increased in response to direct renal nerve stimulation (86). These responses could not be explained by changes in systemic or intrarenal hemodynamics, again suggesting a direct effect of renal nerve transmission on tubular sodium transport. Additional support for this concept derives from the findings of Müller and Barajas (87) that renal nerve endings make contact with the basement membrane of proximal and distal tubular cells. Although an effect of the renal nerves on distal tubular sodium transport has not been shown, it is of interest that norepinephrine stimulates sodium transport in the isolated toad bladder (88), a membrane that in many respects resembles the collecting duct of the mammalian kidney.

Finally the renal nerves have also been shown to be an important mediator of renal renin secretion (47). Indeed, under circumstances in which reflex renal nerve stimulation occurs, increased renin secretion also is observed. To what extent the alterations in sodium excretion and intrarenal hemodynamics observed in response to sodium restriction or in edema-forming states reflect the direct influence of renal sympathetic activity per se or reflex activation of the renin-angiotensin system remains uncertain. For example sodium restriction leads to an increase in renin secretion thought to be mediated in part by the renal nerves (89, 90). Hollenberg and colleagues (91), however, reported that alpha adrenergic blockade achieved with intrarenal arterial infusions of phentolamine failed to reverse the decrease in RBF observed in human subjects maintained on a low-sodium diet. In contrast, intrarenal arterial infusions of an angiotensin II antagonist in animals maintained on a low-sodium diet restored RBF toward normal (92, 93). These observations suggest that the alterations in intrarenal hemodynamics associated with sodium restriction are mediated by angiotensin II rather than by a direct effect of the renal nerves.

Constriction of the thoracic inferior vena cava,

an animal model of edema formation, is associated with increased sympathetic activity and renin secretion (94). Slick and colleagues (95) found that intrarenal arterial infusions of an angiotensin II antagonist failed to block the renal hemodynamic changes that accompany acute constriction of the thoracic inferior vena cava, suggesting that the influence of the nerves was dominant in this setting. However, opposite results have been reported by other investigators (92, 96).

The available evidence does not permit any definitive conclusion as to what extent changes in sodium excretion and intrarenal hemodynamics seen in sodium-retaining states are mediated by the renal nerves directly or indirectly via activation of the renin-angiotensin system. Regardless, it is evident that the renal nerves provide an efferent pathway for accomplishing rapid, reflex adjustments in renal sodium excretion. The intensity of reflex renal nerve stimulation will be proportional to the severity of the stress imposed by the decrease in effective circulating blood volume.

Renin-angiotensin system. The renin-angiotensin system constitutes another rapidly acting mechanism for effecting adjustments in the renal excretion of sodium and water in response to a reduction in effective circulating blood volume. In addition angiotensin stimulates aldosterone secretion, which can be classified as a more slowly adapting mechanism for promoting renal sodium conservation.

Multiple factors influence renin secretion (47) (see also Chap. 14). Neurogenic reflex control of renin secretion has been mentioned. However, despite interruption of the renal nerves, appropriate compensatory increases in renin secretion occur in response to decreases in effective plasma volume. Activation of the macular densa receptor, the renal baroreceptor, and possibly circulating catecholamines may mediate renin secretion in the absence of the renal nerves. Indeed, the multiple loops involved in renin secretion ensure that this critically important system can be recruited to the defense of extracellular volume.

Angiotensin has been shown to have important effects on systemic as well as renal hemodynamics. Thus, angiotensin II participates in the maintenance of systemic arterial blood pressure when effective circulating blood volume is reduced by sodium depletion or in animal models of heart failure (24, 92, 93, 96). The immediate effect of angiotensin on renal function and sodium excretion appears to be related to its effects on intrarenal hemodynamics. Although a direct action of angiotensin II on distal tubular sodium transport has been suggested, the data on which this concept rests are inconclusive (97). Intrarenal arterial infusion of angiotensin II decreases RBF out of proportion to GFR, causing a rise in filtration fraction. These observations indicate a preferential efferent arteriolar vasoconstrictor action which has been confirmed by direct micropuncture of surface glomeruli (98). In addition a decrease in glomerular capillary ultrafiltration coefficient was detected. If intra-arterial infusions of angiotensin II mimic the action of the endogenously formed peptide, it suggests that angiotensin may mediate renal conservation of sodium by alterations in peritubular capillary Starling forces. The similarity of renal hemodynamic effects seen with angiotensin and sympathetic stimulation is obvious. In addition redistribution of intrarenal blood flow has also been suggested by studies in which the inert gas technique was used. However, this finding has not been confirmed with other techniques (83). Although the acute antinatriuresis observed with angiotensin infusions has been attributed to its effects on intrarenal hemodynamics, it is of interest that in several studies restoration of RBF by infusing an inhibitor of angiotensin II did not augment sodium excretion (92, 93, 99).

Aldosterone. Whereas the renal nerves and angiotensin II comprise efferent mechanisms for accomplishing rapid adjustments in the renal excretion of sodium, aldosterone provides a mechanism for more long-term regulation. Through its stimulatory effects on sodium transport along the terminal nephron, aldosterone functions as the fine tuner in regulating sodium excretion. Under the influence of aldosterone, the urine can be rendered virtually free of sodium; in the absence of aldosterone, renal sodium wasting may progress until vascular collapse ensues.

That changes in aldosterone secretion are im-

portant for the normal regulation of sodium balance and ECF volume can be appreciated from the recent study of Young et al. (100). Adrenalectomized dogs were maintained on a fixed daily replacement dose of glucocorticosteroid and aldosterone and then fed low- and high-sodium diets to determine to what extent ECF volume regulation was impaired. Compared to normal dogs, the adrenalectomized dogs exhibited wider fluctuations in sodium balance, arterial pressure, plasma renin activity, and sodium space. Extracellular fluid volume was estimated to have increased by 12 percent in adrenalectomized dogs whose sodium intake was increased from 10 meq/day to 200 meq/day. In normal dogs extracellular volume increased only 2 percent. This study demonstrates that in the absence of an intact aldosterone feedback loop the precision of ECF volume regulation is greatly impaired.

The importance of aldosterone in mediating sodium retention in response to restricted sodium intake or in edema-forming states is beyond question. However, *hyperaldosteronism* is neither a sufficient nor even a necessary condition for sodium retention and edema to occur. That hyperaldosteronism is not a sufficient condition is readily apparent from studies of sodium balance in subjects with primary hyperaldosteronism or subjects given exogenous mineralocorticosteroid (101). Positive sodium balance proceeds in these individuals until the point is reached when expansion of effective circulating blood volume activates other natriuretic mechanisms that exceed the sodium-retaining influence of aldosterone. These mechanisms probably include withdrawal of sympathetic tone, suppression of angiotensin, renal vasodilatation, increased RBF and GFR, decreased filtration fraction, elevated renal perfusion pressure, and possibly activation of natriuretic hormone. Regardless of the precise contribution of these various factors to the escape phenomenon, the essential observation is that *aldosterone by itself does not promote sodium and water retention of sufficient magnitude to cause clinically evident edema.*

That increased mineralocorticosteroid is not a necessary condition for sodium retention to occur is supported by the studies of Davis and col-

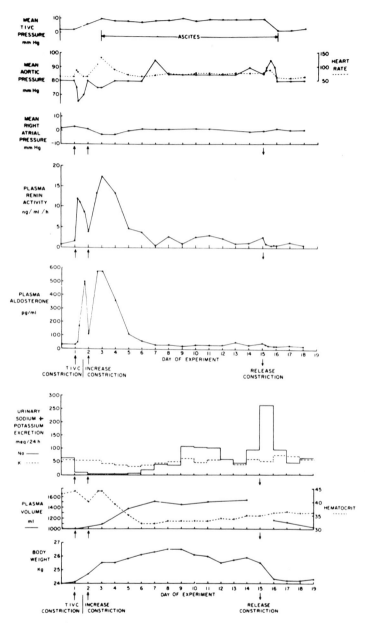

Figure 13-2. Dynamics of the renin-angiotensin-aldosterone system in dogs with experimental congestive heart failure induced by constriction of the thoracic inferior vena cava. Note sharp rise in plasma renin activity and aldosterone following acute caval constriction and the subsequent return to normal levels as sodium and water retention repair the deficit in effective circulating plasma volume. Release of the caval constriction is followed by a diuresis of the retained fluid. (*From Watkins et al.*)

leagues (102). These investigators demonstrated in adrenalectomized dogs with constriction of the thoracic inferior vena cava and fed a normal sodium diet that the rate of sodium retention and ascites formation was a direct function of the daily dose of mineralocorticosteroid. However, as little as 0.5 mg/day of deoxycorticosterone was sufficient to maintain positive sodium balance and ascites formation in these animals. When this minimal maintenance dose of mineralocorticosteroid was discontinued, negative sodium balance developed and the dogs lost their ascites. These studies support the obvious conclusion that some other antinatriuretic mechanism operating in concert with mineralocorticosteroid is essential to promote chronic renal sodium retention and edema formation and that the continuing influence of this other antinatriuretic factor prevents the escape phenomenon. Since renal sympathetic activity and the renin-angiotensin system would be stimulated in all edema-forming disorders associated with a decrease in effective plasma volume, either or both may be the other antinatriuretic factor.

In subjects with an intact adrenal-renal axis, increased aldosterone secretion undoubtedly participates in the renal retention of sodium at some point in the course of edema formation. The finding that plasma renin activity or aldosterone levels are not consistently elevated in some patients with edema formation (103–105) is not surprising. If the retention of sodium and water is sufficient to restore and maintain an effective plasma volume, then the stimulus for continued sodium retention would be removed and the activity of the renin-angiotensin-aldosterone system would decrease appropriately as sodium balance was reestablished. The recent study of Watkins and colleagues (24) provides an excellent demonstration of the dynamic changes in the activity of the renin-angiotensin-aldosterone system in dogs with acute constriction of the thoracic inferior vena cava (Fig. 13-2). During the first few days after caval constriction, plasma renin activity and aldosterone levels were markedly elevated in response to the decrease in plasma volume and arterial pressure. Sodium excretion was severely depressed, and positive sodium balance occurred. Over the course of the next two weeks, as plasma volume was gradually reexpanded to preconstriction levels, plasma renin activity and aldosterone declined to control levels and a new state of sodium balance was established at the expense of an expanded extracellular volume. However, if the retained sodium and water did not expand plasma volume to normal due to continuous trapping of fluid in the peritoneal cavity, the hyperactivity of the renin-angiotensin-aldosterone system persisted along with progressive positive sodium balance and weight gain. Similar derangements are seen in patients with severe congestive heart failure, nephrotic syndrome, or portal hypertension with ascites formation. In addition, however, the possibility cannot be excluded that the normal aldosterone levels observed in some patients actively retaining sodium may indicate heightened end-organ responsiveness to aldosterone or that in these patients other antinatriuretic mechanisms (such as increased renal sympathetic tone) may be dominant in mediating sodium retention.

Natriuretic hormone. In recent years a growing body of evidence has implicated the existence of a "natriuretic hormone" (106, 107). The source of the factor, its biochemical structure, and its role in the regulation of extracellular volume and sodium excretion remain to be defined. Present knowledge suggests that "natriuretic hormone" may be an adaptive mechanism for regulating sodium excretion in chronic renal failure and in states of sustained expansion of extracellular and intravascular volume. The contribution of this mechanism to the day-to-day adjustments in sodium excretion remains unclear. Nevertheless, it is of some interest that "natriuretic hormone" was not detectable in the urine of subjects with edema. (108)

Prostaglandins. Despite an ever expanding literature, the role of renal prostaglandins in the regulation of extracellular volume and sodium excretion remains uncertain (109). Some studies suggest that renal prostaglandins are natriuretic; other studies support the opposite conclusion. It is also unclear whether the influence of prostaglandins on sodium excretion is mediated primarily by alterations in intrarenal hemodynamics or by a more direct effect on tubular sodium transport. While these issues remain unresolved, the data supporting a role for renal prostaglandins in

the regulation of renal blood flow are more secure. A number of observations support the concept that renal prostaglandins through their vasodilator effect antagonize renal ischemia elicited by a variety of stimuli and stresses (109). Vatner (110) has demonstrated that renal prostaglandins contribute to the maintenance of RBF in conscious dogs subjected to moderate hemorrhage. That prostaglandins may play a similar role in edema-forming disorders is suggested by the preliminary report of Zipsen and colleagues (111). Elevated plasma and urinary prostaglandin E levels were observed in patients with liver disease and ascites. Inhibition of prostaglandin synthesis led to a sharp decline in creatinine clearance. Although these observations suggest a role for renal prostaglandins in maintaining RBF and GFR, they provide no insight concerning the contribution of prostaglandins in regulating renal sodium excretion.

Physical factors

Renal perfusion pressure has long been recognized to influence sodium and water excretion. Raising renal perfusion pressure causes natriuresis and diuresis unrelated to changes in RBF, GFR, humoral, or neurogenic factors (112). Recent evidence suggests that the pressure-related increase in sodium excretion derives from a decrease in sodium reabsorption along segments distal to the proximal tubule (113, 114). Although the renal mechanisms mediating the response remain obscure, it is obvious that renal perfusion pressure constitutes another feedback loop for regulating extracellular volume. The salient features of this loop are that expansion of extracellular and intravascular volume leads to a rise in arterial blood pressure secondary to an increase in cardiac output augmented by a rise in venous pressure. The rise in arterial blood pressure promotes an increase in sodium and water excretion until intravascular volume and arterial pressure are returned to their set points. Conversely, a decrease in intravascular volume leads to a fall in arterial pressure and a reduction in urinary sodium and water excretion. This basic loop permits regulation of extracellular volume even in the absence of neurogenic and humoral efferent mechanisms, although the efficiency of the control system would obviously be greatly reduced.

Changes in plasma colloid osmotic pressure and packed cell volume have also been shown to influence renal sodium and water excretion (73). Indeed Nizet et al. (115), using an isolated perfused dog kidney preparation, has shown that addition of saline to the perfusate leads to the quantitative excretion of the sodium load by the isolated kidney, presumably as a consequence of hemodilution. Thus, it is possible that compositional changes related to dilution or concentration of plasma protein may constitute yet another basic loop for regulating sodium excretion and extracellular volume. However, the quantitative contribution of this loop as well as the pressure loop in the day-to-day regulation of extracellular volume remains speculative.

ADH and thirst reflex

It is obvious that volume regulation is intimately linked with regulation of the tonicity of the body fluids. Since sodium and its accompanying anion account for the bulk of osmotically active solute in ECF, it follows that addition of sodium to or loss of sodium from ECF must entail a proportional addition or loss of water in order to maintain tonicity of the body fluids within normal limits. These adjustments are accomplished by the interaction of antidiuretic hormone and the thirst mechanism. This subject is reviewed in Chap. 12. The reader should appreciate that ADH is not required for sodium retention and edema formation.

Summary

The efferent limb of the control system for regulating ECF volume comprises neurogenic, humoral, and hemodynamic elements through which reflex adjustments in renal sodium excretion are effected. Although the integration of these elements is not completely understood, the available evidence suggests that the sympathetic nervous system functions in concert with the renin-angiotensin-aldosterone system to accomplish rapid and long-term adjustments in sodium excretion in response to changes in effective circulating blood volume. The mechanisms operating in edema-forming states are not different from those which mediate renal sodium conservation in normal subjects. As will be discussed, sodium retention progressing to edema formation occurs because of failure of the retained sodium and water to restore effective circulating blood volume to normal.

PATHOPHYSIOLOGY OF EDEMA

HEART FAILURE

A state of heart failure exists when the heart, due to an abnormality of myocardial contractility, is unable to pump blood at a rate commensurate with the requirements of the peripheral tissues. This broad definition encompasses both high and low cardiac output failure but excludes states of circulatory insufficency such as hemorrhagic shock, cardiac tamponade, or circulatory congestion associated with acute renal failure in which myocardial function is not primarily impaired. Regardless of the etiology of heart failure, it is accompanied by renal retention of sodium and water which, depending on the severity of the disease, may progress to massive edema and/or pulmonary congestion.

The onset of clinical heart failure may be heralded by a sudden catastrophic insult to the heart such as acute myocardial infarction in which failure of the left ventricle may be so severe that cardiac output is inadequate to maintain a normal blood pressure despite intense vasoconstriction and reduced flow to virtually all peripheral beds. Not uncommonly the consequent damming of blood behind the left ventricle precipitates acute pulmonary edema. Conversely, heart failure may develop insidiously as a consequence of arteriosclerosis, hypertension, valvular heart disease, or the various cardiomyopathies. The first clinical sign of heart failure may be a decrease in tolerance to moderate exercise, whereas during lesser degrees of exercise the patient is asymptomatic. As the heart disease progresses and cardiac output cannot be augmented sufficiently to meet the requirements of the peripheral tissues, the subject exhibits easy fatigability and dyspnea during normal daily activities. Signs of pedal edema may be evident towards the end of the day whereas by morning the swelling has subsided. Nocturia may become a troublesome complaint, and episodes of paroxysmal nocturnal dyspnea may occur. With further progression of heart failure dyspnea is evident even during mild exertion. The edema that was evident towards the end of the day is now present throughout the day. The attacks of paroxysmal nocturnal dyspnea occur more frequently, and the patient has learned to sleep with his head elevated on several pillows.

This sequence of signs and symptoms is not atypical for the individual who develops chronic congestive heart failure over a period of months to years. Irrespective of whether heart failure is acute or chronic, clinicians have long recognized that such patients avidly retain sodium and water; indeed a high sodium intake may be lethal to these patients. In acute heart failure as described above, the avid retention of sodium and water by the kidney can be readily explained on the basis of a sustained decrease in cardiac output causing hypoperfusion of the kidneys, high renal sympathetic tone, high levels of angiotensin II and aldosterone and depressed RBF and GFR. Similar mechanisms undoubtedly participate in the renal retention of sodium and water evidenced by patients who present in the end stages of chronic congestive heart failure. The questions that have puzzled physiologists and clinicians alike are: What is the primary stimulus for sodium retention? At what stage in the course of heart failure do the abnormalities in the renal handling of sodium and water become manifest? What are the renal mechanisms involved? Consideration of volume control theory leads to the inescapable conclusion that the primary stimulus for sodium and water retention in heart failure, as in all edema-forming states, is a decrease in effective circulating blood volume, and that sodium retention occurs during the very early stages of heart failure mediated by the same renal mechanisms that regulate sodium excretion in normal subjects.

Circulatory adjustments to heart failure

In the early stages of heart failure, cardiac output and measurements of myocardial mechanics are frequently normal at rest. However, in response to exercise cardiac output fails to increase appropriately and indirect measurements of myocardial contractility reveal an abnormal rise in ventricular end-diastolic pressure with little or no change in stroke volume (116). The failure of cardiac output to increase commensurate with peripheral demands must in some manner signal that effective circulating blood volume is decreased. Whether the signal derives from the underperfused tissues per se or whether it originates from receptors in the low- or high-pressure circuits remains unclear. In any event sympathetic reflexes are initiated to augment myocardial contractility and cardiac output. Depending on the level of exercise, redistribution of peripheral blood flow also occurs in an attempt to meet the increased blood flow requirements of muscle. Studies in humans (117) and experimental animals with heart failure (118–120) indicate that this redistribution of blood flow is accomplished in part by a reduction in flow to the kidneys mediated by neurogenic reflexes (119). Nevertheless RBF is relatively well preserved compared to other vascular beds and may reflect the tonic inhibitory influence of receptors in the left atrium on renal nerve activity (40, 41). Obviously sodium excretion would be decreased during periods of exercise which induce a fall in RBF. However, it should be apparent from the predictable behavior of the control system that even during less strenuous exercise the kidney might be exposed to a higher than normal level of renal nerve activity or circulating catecholamines (121) sufficient perhaps to stimulate sodium reabsorption directly or indirectly through the renin-angiotensin-aldosterone system. In the early stages the degree of sodium retention may be so trivial that during periods of rest, when cardiac output is adequate to meet the demands of the peripheral tissues, the stimulus for sodium retention would be withdrawn and the retained sodium would be eliminated in the course of the same day. However, as heart disease progresses to the point that cardiac output cannot be augmented sufficiently to meet the requirements of normal activity, the stimulus for sodium retention becomes more intense and sustained for longer periods of time so that the sodium retained during the day is incompletely eliminated during the evening. During this phase modest gain in body weight becomes evident, reflecting expansion of interstitial and plasma volume. Measurement of myocardial mechanics reveals an increase in ventricular end-diastolic pressure even at rest although resting cardiac output is still normal (116). The rise in ventricular end-diastolic pressure at rest signifies that the heart is functioning along a depressed Frank-Starling curve where a higher filling pressure is required to maintain the same stroke volume (Fig. 13-3). More-

over the increment in stroke volume as a function of filling pressure is also depressed.

The renal retention of sodium and water with the consequent rise in plasma volume and venous pressure, therefore, subserves a basic compensatory mechanism for sustaining cardiac output in the presence of depressed myocardial contractility. If adequate cardiac compensation occurs, then the stimulus for further sodium and water retention is withdrawn and sodium balance is reestab-

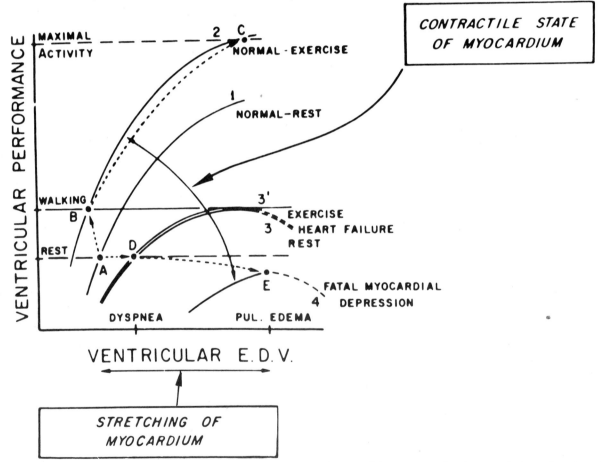

Figure 13-3. Diagram showing the interrelations between influences on ventricular end-diastolic volume (E.D.V.) through stretching of the myocardium and the contractile state of the myocardium. Levels of ventricular E.D.V. associated with filling pressure that result in dyspnea and pulmonary edema are shown on the abscissa. Levels of ventricular performance when the subject is at rest, while walking, and during maximal activity are designated on the ordinate. The dotted lines are the descending limbs of the ventricular performance curves which are rarely seen during life but which show the level of ventricular performance if end-diastolic volume could be elevated to very high levels. (*From Braunwald et al.,* N. Engl. J. Med., *277:1012, 1967.*)

lished but at a higher than normal extracellular and intravascular volume. It should be emphasized, however, that although sodium balance is established, subtle abnormalities in sodium metabolism would still be evident. If challenged with a sustained increase in sodium intake, these patients would exhibit a greater than normal positive sodium balance and weight gain before augmentation of sodium excretion to match sodium intake (Fig. 13-1B). That patients with compensated heart failure exhibit a depressed natriuretic response to sodium loading unexplained by reduction in GFR or RBF is well recognized (2, 122). Theoretical considerations suggest that the depressed natriuretic response is directly related to the depression in myocardial contractility. For a given degree of volume expansion and rise in venous pressure, the patient whose heart is functioning on a depressed Frank-Starling curve would experience less of a rise in cardiac output, i.e., effective circulating plasma volume, than would the individual with normal myocardial contractility. Consequently a greater increase in absolute plasma volume and venous filling pressure is sustained by the patient with a failing heart before achieving the level of effective circulating plasma volume required to activate natriuretic reflexes and reestablish sodium balance.

The abnormalities in myocardial function and sodium metabolism outlined above occur in the early stage of heart failure. As heart disease progresses, cardiac output becomes inadequate to meet the demands of even minimal activity. Further sodium and water retention occurs, resulting in further expansion of plasma volume and elevation in venous pressure. During this phase peripheral edema becomes evident as interstitial volume also increases consequent to the rise in plasma volume and venous pressure which promotes translocation of fluid from the intravascular to the interstitial space. The clinical picture may be dominated by symptoms of dyspnea due to the increase in pulmonary interstitial fluid or by signs of right-sided failure. Although cardiac output may still be normal at rest, it may fail to increase or may even decrease during minimal exercise (Fig. 13-3). At this stage assessment of renal function reveals more serious impairment in

handling of a sodium load along with the typical findings of a decrease in RBF and increase in filtration fraction (123, 124). Whether the changes in renal hemodynamics are mediated primarily by increased sympathetic activity, which is well known to occur in heart failure (70, 72, 74, 121, 124), via the renin-angiotensin-aldosterone system or, as is likely to be the case, by the interaction of the two mechanisms remains to be clarified. In any event the abnormalities in sodium metabolism and renal function observed in a patient with heart failure at a given time in the evolution of the disease are directly related to the severity of myocardial dysfunction and the degree to which effective circulating blood volume is compromised.

In end-stage congestive heart failure cardiac output is below normal even at rest. Persistent generalized peripheral vasoconstriction occurs with further diversion of blood flow from the kidneys as well as other vascular beds in order to maintain perfusion of vital organs. Consequently GFR and RBF are reduced, and intense, unrelenting sodium retention ensues leading to further expansion of an already congested circulation.

Summary

When analyzed from the perspective of volume control theory, renal sodium retention in heart failure is seen as a predictable and inevitable consequence of impaired myocardial function and the resultant decrease in effective circulating blood volume. Retention of sodium and water leading to plasma volume expansion may be viewed, at least in the initial stages, as a compensatory mechanism for sustaining cardiac output. Emphasis has been placed on the role of the sympathetic nervous system and the renin-angiotensin-aldosterone system in mediating the renal conservation of sodium in heart failure primarily because they constitute the major efferent limbs for accomplishing reflex adjustments in sodium excretion in normal humans. As our understanding of the renal mechanisms controlling sodium excretion improves, particularly with respect to the role of natriuretic hormone and prostaglandins, this scheme will have to be expanded accordingly. However, it should be emphasized that there is not cogent evidence to suggest that sodium retention in heart failure or in any edematous state reflects a primary aberration in one or more of the efferent limbs that normally regulate sodium excretion. Rather the kidney is responding appropriately to stimuli generated as a consequence of a decrease in effective circulating blood volume. The implications of this analysis for the therapy of heart failure are obvious. Therapy should be directed at improving myocardial function, which is the basic pathophysiologic derangement that initiates renal sodium and water retention.

Figure 13-4 summarizes the major pathogenetic mechanisms leading to renal sodium retention and edema formation in congestive heart failure.

ARTERIOVENOUS FISTULA

Arteriovenous fistula denotes a direct communication between an artery and vein that provides a low-resistance pathway for the rapid egress of blood from the arterial tree. The severity of the derangements in systemic hemodynamics and sodium metabolism observed in patients with arteriovenous fistula is directly related to the magnitude of the flow through this shunt pathway.

Studies in humans and animals (125–131) have

provided insight into the pathophysiology of this disorder. Opening an arteriovenous shunt in experimental animals causes an immediate fall in diastolic and systolic pressure due to the accelerated egress of blood from the arterial tree through the low-resistance pathway. The immediate circulatory adjustments include reflex peripheral vasoconstriction and an increase in cardiac output mediated by an increase in stroke volume and heart rate. In anesthetized dogs Frank and colleagues (128) observed that the reflex augmentation in cardiac output was commensurate with the rate of flow through the fistula so long as shunt flow did not exceed 20 percent of the resting cardiac output. At high shunt flows, however, the immediate compensatory rise in cardiac output was consistently less than the flow through the shunt, indicating that basal flow to peripheral tissues must have decreased. The resultant decrease in effective circulating blood volume initiates renal conservation of sodium and expansion of plasma volume which facilitates a further compensatory rise in cardiac output through the Frank-Starling mechanism. Thus, sodium retention in this disorder, as in heart failure, provides an important compensatory mechanism for reestablishing an effective circulating blood volume, albeit at the expense of an expanded plasma and interstitial volume. With large fistulas the circu-

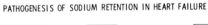

PATHOGENESIS OF SODIUM RETENTION IN HEART FAILURE

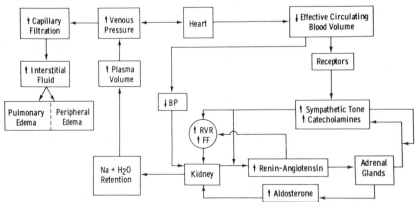

Figure 13-4. Summary of the major factors leading to edema formation in heart failure.

latory stress may be so severe that adequate cardiac compensation may not be achieved and progressive sodium retention ensues, leading to edema, circulatory congestion, and death.

In patients with arteriovenous fistulas the clinical course is usually more protracted. During the early phase adequate cardiac compensation is accomplished by an increase in stroke volume secondary to plasma volume expansion but without evidence of circulatory congestion or renal dysfunction. However, with time the chronic stress of maintaining an elevated cardiac output may lead to progressive cardiac dilatation, hypertrophy, and eventually the appearance of high-output congestive heart failure.

PORTAL HYPERTENSION

Sodium retention and ascites formation commonly occur in association with portal hypertension secondary to intra- or extrahepatic obstruction of blood flow (Table 13-3) (132, 133). Although ascites may occur with infrahepatic obstruction of portal blood flow, the incidence is lower than that seen with intra- or suprahepatic obstruction, supporting the notion that liver involvement is an important factor in the genesis of ascites.

In the United States the most common cause of portal hypertension and ascites formation is cirrhosis of the liver secondary to chronic alcoholism. Disruption of the normal architecture by fibrous tissue and regenerating nodules impedes hepatic blood flow. The conclusion that the obstruction is postsinusoidal is based on the common finding of an elevated wedged hepatic vein pressure. Increased hepatic arterial blood flow has also been reported in patients with acute alcoholic liver disease (134), but it remains unclear to what extent the increase in blood flow contributes to portal hypertension. In chronic liver disease with cirrhosis, total hepatic blood flow is usually reduced (135, 136); this supports the conclusion that obstruction to portal blood flow is the major factor causing portal hypertension.

The preeminent factor giving rise to ascites is the increase in hydrostatic pressure not only at the

Table 13-3. Classification of portal hypertension

I. EXTRA HEPATIC

A. Obstruction to venous outflow above the liver
   1. Budd-Chiari syndrome (hepatic vein thrombosis, e.g., primary hepatic or metastatic tumors, polycythemia, thrombophlebitis migrans)
   2. Obstruction of venous outflow through the suprahepatic vena cava (e.g., constrictive pericarditis, tricuspid insufficiency, chronic congestive heart failure, tumors, congenital abnormality of the vena cava)
B. Obstruction to portal venous inflow below the liver
   1. Congenital (cavernomatous transformation, atresia, stenosis)
   2. Thrombosis (e.g., pylephlebitis due to neonatal omphalitis or intra-abdominal infection, trauma, polycythemia)
   3. Compression (e.g., tumors, pancreatitis)
C. Arterioportal fistula (e.g., hepatic artery–portal vein or splenic artery–splenic vein fistula following trauma or ruptured aneurysm)

II. INTRAHEPATIC

A. Cirrhosis
   1. Laennec's (alcoholic, nutritional)
   2. Postnecrotic (posthepatic)
   3. Biliary (following chronic bile duct obstruction)
B. Other forms of fibrosis (congenital cystic liver, sarcoidosis, polycystic disease, syphilis, schistosomiasis, hemochromatosis)
C. Tumors (neoplasm or granuloma)

level of the liver sinusoids but throughout the capillaries of the splanchnic bed. The resultant imbalance of Starling forces promotes accelerated loss of fluid from the intravascular space. In the liver the increased filtration of protein-rich fluid across the sinusoids is removed by the lymphatic channels located in close proximity to the hepatocytes and sinusoids and is returned to the circulation by way of the thoracic duct. A similar sequence of events occurs throughout the splanchnic bed. When the capacity of the lymphatic system for removing the increased volume of lymph is exceeded, the excess lymph leaks across the liver capsule and splanchnic bed and accumulates in the peritoneal cavity as ascites. In addition, formation of ascites in liver disease with portal hypertension is also facilitated by the presence of hypoalbuminemia which reflects both accelerated egress from the intravascular space, primarily within the liver, and a variable degree of impaired synthesis (137). Finally the coexistence of lymphatic obstruction will also facilitate accumulation of ascites in liver disease by limiting the rate at which lymph can be returned to the intravascular space. Some investigators have argued that relative obstruction at the thoracic duct ostium impeding return of lymph to the circulation is a significant factor in ascites formation since following venting of the thoracic duct ostium so as to facilitate lymph flow ascites frequently subsides (138, 139). However, enthusiasm for this concept waned when careful measurements of thoracic duct and subclavian venous pressures failed to document a significant pressure gradient (140).

Ascites represents an extension of interstitial fluid volume that ultimately is derived from intravascular fluid. Obviously if this fluid were not replaced by adjustments in the renal reabsorption of sodium and water, intravascular volume depletion and circulatory collapse would ensue. Implied by the above formulation is the notion that renal conservation of sodium and water occurs in response to a decrease in absolute plasma volume consequent to the rise in portal hydrostatic pressure with or without an associated fall in plasma colloid osmotic pressure. However, plasma volume in patients with portal hypertension and ascites is usually increased, not decreased (141, 142). Moreover, spontaneous loss of ascites is not accompanied by an increase in plasma volume; this suggests that plasma volume is not contracted as a consequence of ascites formation (142).

This apparent paradox can be explained by analyzing the evolution of events occurring early in the course of liver disease and portal hypertension. It should be remembered that the veins, due to their thin walls, are highly compliant vessels. Thus, when venous outflow from the liver is impeded, the immediate consequence is distention of the portal circulation with blood before a major rise in portal pressure occurs. The capacity of the liver and splanchnic bed to sequester blood when hepatic venous pressure is raised has been documented experimentally (143, 144). Moreover the development of venous collaterals during the course of chronic portal hypertension also contributes to the increase in plasma volume by increasing the holding capacity of the circulation.

Expansion of portal blood volume occurs at the expense of decreased venous return to the heart and a predictable fall in cardiac output. Renal conservation of sodium is stimulated by the same mechanisms operative in heart failure or any other circumstance of decreased effective circulating blood volume. Initially expansion of plasma volume will lead to a rise in portal pressure until the resistance to flow across the hepatic bed is overcome and venous return to the heart is restored. Although the rise in portal pressure will promote increased capillary filtration, compensation is accomplished by augmented lymph flow, which has been documented in the early stages of portal hypertension prior to the appearance of ascites (133). Increased lymph flow, therefore, provides another mechanism for overcoming the obstruction to venous return to the heart. Once effective circulating blood volume is restored, sodium balance is reestablished at an expanded extracellular and plasma volume. Although during this compensated phase, prior to the appearance of ascites, renal function defined in terms of GFR, RBF, diluting ability, and concentrating capacity may be normal, these patients frequently exhibit a decreased capacity to excrete a sodium load (145, 146). The explanation relates to the hemodynamic alteration within the portal bed. It can be predicted that in these patients effective circulating blood volume would be expanded to a lesser degree in response to a given sodium load, whether administered orally or intravenously, due to increased sequestration of fluid within the portal circulation. Thus, the pattern of sodium balance would be similar to that illustrated in Fig. 13-1B.

As liver disease progresses and intrahepatic resistance to blood flow increases, the resultant decrease in effective circulating blood volume promotes further sodium and water retention, most of which, however, is confined to the portal circulation. Portal pressure rises and augments further the rate of fluid filtration throughout the portal bed until the point is reached when the capacity of the lymphatics is exceeded and the excess fluid accumulates in the peritoneal cavity as ascites. During the decompensated phase of liver disease with ascites formation, abnormalities in renal hemodynamics ranging from mild to severe reductions in RBF and GFR are commonly seen (78, 147, 148). Nevertheless, in a number of such patients sodium retention with ascites formation continues in the face of a normal GFR and RBF. At the present time there is no convincing evidence to support the notion that sodium retention in this disorder is related to a unique derangement of intrarenal blood flow.

Aldosterone and plasma renin activity are usually elevated at this stage of the disease (148, 149). Both increased secretion as well as decreased degradation secondary to reduced hepatic blood flow are responsible for the elevated plasma levels.

In the advanced stage of liver disease with ascites, marked deterioration in RBF and GFR with oliguria, commonly referred to as functional renal failure (150), may occur and signifies a further reduction in effective circulating blood volume. Paradoxically cardiac output may be elevated in some of these patients (134, 151), presumably as a consequence of multiple arteriovenous shunts. However, effective blood flow to the peripheral tissues is inadequate, leading to intense peripheral vasoconstriction of the renal as well as other vascular beds. Plasma volume expansion may improve renal function and systemic hemodynamics in some patients, but the effect is usually transient (151, 152).

Although ascites is the most striking evidence of an expanded extracellular volume in patients with liver disease, peripheral edema also may be present. Peripheral edema may develop as a consequence of hypoalbuminemia, or an increase in inferior vena caval pressure due to mechanical compression by an enlarged left lobe of the liver (153) or tense ascites (154). In addition patients with alcoholic liver disease are also prone to develop myocardial failure, which compounds the derangements in portal and systemic hemodynamics, promoting further sodium and water retention.

Summary

The stimulus for sodium retention in liver disease with portal hypertension is a decrease in effective circulating blood volume consequent to obstruction of blood flow through the liver with sequestration of blood volume within the portal bed. The kidneys are stimulated to retain sodium and water by the same mechanisms which mediate renal sodium and water conservation in normal subjects. The retained sodium and water leads to expansion of plasma volume, most of which, however, is trapped in the splanchnic bed. Portal pressure rises, promoting increased filtration of fluid across the splanchnic capillaries. When the rate of filtration exceeds the capacity of the lymphatic drainage system, the excess fluid accumulates in the peritoneal cavity as ascites. Figure 13-5 outlines the major pathogenetic mechanisms leading to sodium retention and ascites formation in patients with liver disease and portal hypertension.

NEPHROTIC SYNDROME

The nephrotic syndrome is a clinical entity of diverse etiologies characterized by albuminuria, hypoalbuminemia, and generalized edema (155). The central pathophysiologic lesion common to the diseases (Table 13-4) giving rise to the nephrotic syndrome is an increase in glomerular capillary permeability to serum albumin. When the loss of albumin in the urine exceeds the rate of albumin synthesis by the liver, hypoalbuminemia ensues. The variability in albumin synthesis rate (156) as well as the possibility that albumin may be lost from the circulation through other capillary beds besides the kidney may explain why the degree of hypoalbuminemia cannot be precisely correlated with the severity of albuminuria. With the onset of hypoalbuminemia, plasma colloid osmotic pressure falls and leads to an imbalance in Starling forces across the capillary bed which favors the egress of fluid from the intravascular to the interstitial space. The resultant contraction of plasma volume activates neurogenic and humoral reflexes to conserve sodium and water and repair the volume deficit. However, the retained fluid tends to further dilute the plasma protein concentration, leading to further egress of fluid from the intravascular to the interstitial space and progressive edema.

In contrast to that for heart failure and liver disease, the primary stimulus for renal retention

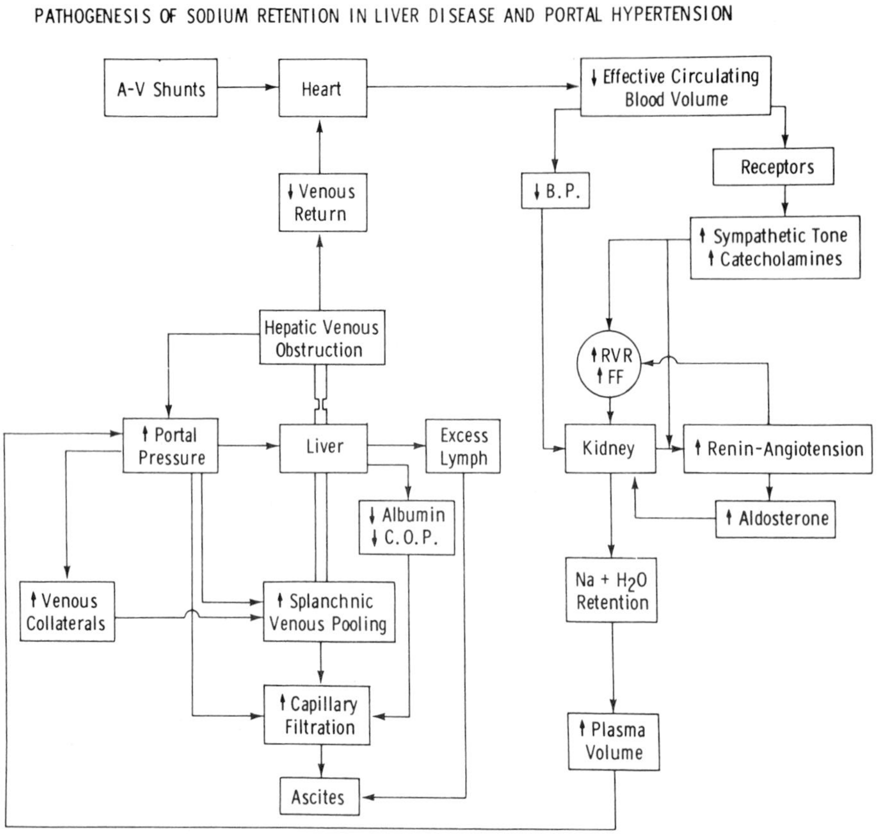

PATHOGENESIS OF SODIUM RETENTION IN LIVER DISEASE AND PORTAL HYPERTENSION

Figure 13-5. Summary of the major factors leading to ascites formation in portal hypertension.

of sodium and water in the nephrotic syndrome is a reduction in absolute plasma volume. The extent of plasma volume contraction is quite variable (157–159). In some patients plasma volume may be within normal limits, indicating that to a large extent compensation has occurred. In others, plasma volume may be so contracted as to produce orthostatic hypotension and circulatory collapse (157).

The renal mechanisms mediating sodium and water retention are basically the same in the nephrotic syndrome as in heart failure and liver disease. Heightened activity of the sympathetic nervous system (160) and the renin-angiotensin-aldosterone system (161) have been documented. Increased renal vascular resistance with decreased GFR and RBF occurs in proportion to the degree of hypoalbuminemia and plasma volume

contraction. However, interpretation of renal hemodynamic changes may be complicated to the extent that the underlying disease process causes renal parenchymal damage and loss of nephrons. In some patients, particularly those with lipoid nephrosis, GFR may be greater than normal due to the fact that the hypoalbuminemia and reduced plasma colloid osmotic pressure favor increased filtration across the glomerular capillaries as in other capillary beds. Moreover, proximal tubular sodium reabsorption may be depressed, presumably as a result of the low plasma colloid osmotic pressure within the peritubular capillaries (162). Nevertheless sodium retention and edema formation still occur in these patients despite the increased filtered sodium load which serves to emphasize the important role of augmented distal tubular sodium reabsorption in mediating sodium

Table 13-4. Classification of nephrotic syndrome

1. Idiopathic
   a. Lipoid nephrosis (minimal change or "nil" disease)
   b. Focal glomerulosclerosis
   c. Membranous glomerulonephritis
   d. Proliferative glomerulonephritis
2. Associated with heavy metals, drugs, toxins (mercury, gold, bismuth, pencillamine, probenecid, paradione, trimethadione, heroin)
3. Associated with infections
   a. Bacterial (poststreptococcal, endocarditis, shunt nephritis, syphilis, leprosy)
   b. Viral (hepatitis B, cytomegalovirus, Epstein-Barr, herpes zoster)
   c. Protozoal (malaria, toxoplasmosis)
   d. Helminthic (schistosomiasis, trypanosomiasis, filariasis)
4. Associated with malignancies
   a. Solid tumors (stomach, breast, lung, colon, ovary, melanoma, cervix, kidney)
   b. Lymphoma (Hodgkin's, reticulum cell, chronic lymphatic leukemia, lymphosarcoma)
5. Associated with systemic diseases (systemic lupus erythematosus, Henoch-Schönlein syndrome, polyarteritis, Goodpasture's syndrome, cryoglobulinemia, serum sickness)
6. Associated with metabolic and heredofamilial diseases (diabetes mellitus, amyloidosis, Alport's syndrome, Fabry's syndrome, congenital and familial nephrotic syndrome)

retention and edema formation. Figure 13-6 summarizes the major pathogenetic mechanisms mediating sodium retention and edema formation in the nephrotic syndrome.

IDIOPATHIC EDEMA

Idiopathic edema, also referred to as cyclic or periodic edema, is a syndrome characterized by irregular, intermittent bouts of generalized edema seen almost exclusively in adult females in whom by definition there is no evidence of cardiovascular, liver, renal, endocrine, lymphatic, or venous disease (163–167). The onset of edema appears after the menarche but before the menopause; however once established the syndrome may persist after the meopause. Early symptoms may suggest premenstrual tension, but further study reveals no consistent relationship of the attacks to the menstrual cycle.

Typically these patients exhibit a greater than normal diurnal weight gain which reflects reten-

tion of sodium and water during upright posture. Failure to completely lose at night the sodium and water gained during the day leads to a stepwise expansion of the extracellular volume until the patient is conscious of puffiness of the hands and face on waking in the morning and abdominal distention and swelling of the legs towards the end of the day. Warm weather and prolonged standing aggravate the severity of edema. Spontaneous diuresis may ensue or the edema may wax and wane dramatically yet never completely disappear. Emotional lability, nervousness, irritability, depression, somnolence, and headache are prominent symptoms in some but not all patients, raising the possibility that idiopathic edema may be a somatic expression of a deep-rooted psychological disorder.

The stereotype of this disorder is an attractive middle-aged woman, excessively concerned with her appearance, frequently overweight and "desperately" trying to reduce. The patient complains of swelling of the face, hands, breasts, abdomen, and thighs and claims to have unpredictable sudden increases in weight. Often she has been taking a variety of diuretic agents, each of which in turn seems to lose its effectiveness. Physical examination, particularly if performed early in the day, often fails to reveal edema or swelling. The absence of obvious cardiovascular, hepatic, renal, or endocrine abnormalities leads the physician to attribute the patient's complaints to manifestation of an underlying emotional disorder which in some cases may be true. However, careful monitoring of intradiem weight gain over a period of several weeks reveals a group of patients whose daily fluctuation in weight exceeds 1.4 kg, and when they are examined towards the end of the day demonstrate evidence of pedal edema.

The prevalence of this disorder is difficult to determine. Many women in response to direct questioning will admit to episodic swelling of the hands and feet which they accept as a natural phenomenon of life; they do not seek medical attention unless the swelling is severe or persistent. The so-called stereotype of idiopathic edema may represent that portion of the population who, being overly concerned with their appearance, seek out medical attention for complaints most women dismiss as trivial.

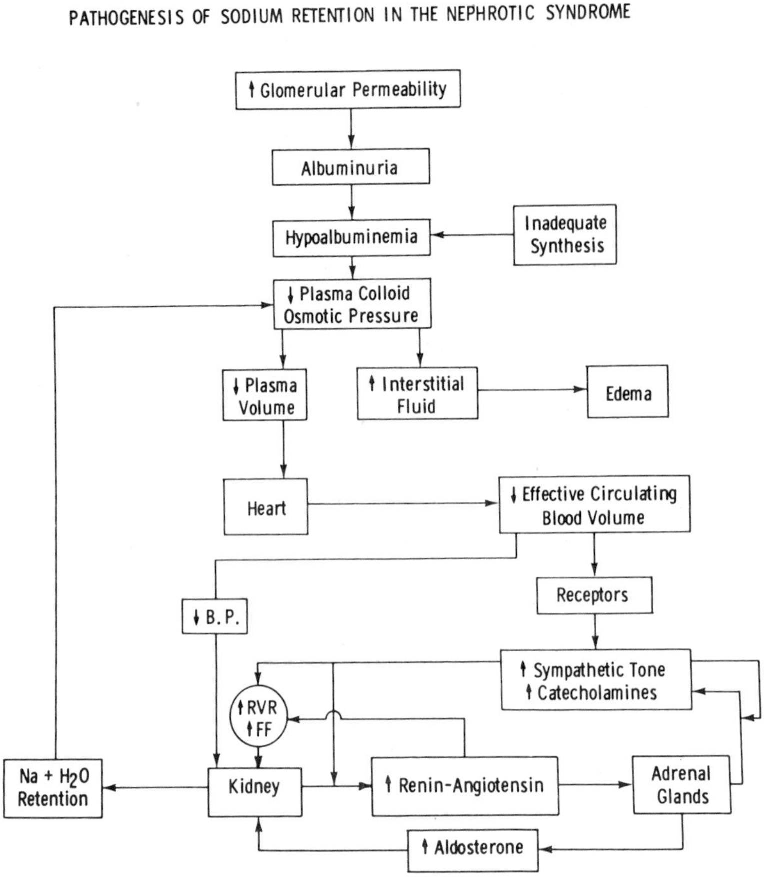

PATHOGENESIS OF SODIUM RETENTION IN THE NEPHROTIC SYNDROME

Figure 13-6. Summary of major factors leading to edema formation in the nephrotic syndrome.

The diagnosis of idiopathic edema should be reserved for those patients in whom other causes of edema formation have been excluded by thorough evaluation. In particular an occult cardiomyopathy must be sought since these patients may respond to cardiac glycosides (168, 169). When the common causes of edema formation have been excluded, there emerges a seemingly homogenous group of patients who exhibit excess sodium retention during upright posture, whereas in the recumbent position they lose their edema and respond normally to sodium loading. In some cases normal escape from mineralocorticosteroid has been demonstrated (167, 170, 171).

Thus, upright posture appears to unmask an abnormality in volume regulation the causes of which, however, may be multiple. In some patients an increase in capillary permeability to protein appears to be the basic mechanism. The tendency for plasma volume to decrease during upright posture (166, 167) as well as the accelerated egress of labeled albumin from the intravascular space (167) is consistent with this interpretation. However, the structural or functional basis for the increase in capillary permeability to protein is far from clear. In a few patients idiopathic edema may be an unusual manifestation of a systemic disease such as diabetes mellitus (172, 173) or systemic lupus erythematosus (174). In the vast majority of cases the cause is obscure. Since this syndrome is confined almost exclusively to women, attention has been focused on the possible role of estrogens and progesterone in altering capillary permeability. Although increased capillary permeability to protein has been reported to occur in normal women during the luteal phase (175), Edwards and Bayliss (176) found no correlation between postural fluid retention and the phase of the menstrual cycle in their patients with idiopathic edema. The possible role of other vasoactive substances, such as bradykinin, in this syndrome has not been evaluated.

The study of Gill and colleagues (177) indicates that subtle abnormalities in albumin metabolism giving rise to mild hypoalbuminemia and contracted plasma volume may underlie the expression of idiopathic edema. In some of their patients the hypoalbuminemia was due to decreased synthesis or increased catabolism of albumin; in others an imbalance in the ratio of albumin synthesis to fractional catabolic rate was detected. Increased egress of albumin from the intravascular space was also evident, although the cause was not determined. The prevalence of abnormal albumin metabolism in patients with idiopathic edema is not clear since similar studies have not been performed by other investigators actively pursuing this problem. However, as has been emphasized (166), hypoalbuminemia is distinctly uncommon as judged from the cases reported in the literature.

Autonomic dysfunction with excessive venous pooling during upright posture may also cause idiopathic edema (178). Venous pooling might promote increased filtration across an expanded capillary surface area or autonomic dysfunction might cause an imbalance between pre- and postcapillary resistance leading to an abnormal rise in capillary hydrostatic pressure (170).

Idiopathic edema appears to be a syndrome of multiple etiologies. Although exaggerated sodium and water retention during upright posture is a feature common to most if not all patients, the basic underlying mechanism may be quite different. (The reader should appreciate that upright posture will augment sodium and water retention in all patients with generalized edema from whatever cause.) The frequent observation that plasma renin activity or aldosterone excretion is elevated in patients with idiopathic edema is wholly consistent with an appropriate compensatory response to a reduced effective circulating blood volume. In several studies exaggerated postural increments in plasma renin activity, aldosterone secretion, or urinary catecholamine excretion have been clearly documented (166, 170, 178). The renal mechanisms which mediate sodium and water retention in idiopathic edema are identical to those seen in other edematous states, although perhaps less pronounced. In some patients exaggerated falls in RBF and GFR may become evident during quiet standing (166), presumably as a consequence of a greater reduction in effective or absolute circulating blood volume. In the recumbent posture renal function is normal.

HYPONATREMIA AND EDEMA

Hyponatremia is a common complication in the advanced stages of heart failure, liver disease with ascites, and the nephrotic syndrome. The presence of generalized edema signifies that total body sodium and water are increased above normal. The presence of hyponatremia and edema signifies that total body water is increased out of proportion to total body sodium, i.e. water is being retained in excess of sodium, resulting in dilution of the body fluids and a state of hypoosmolality. The pathogenesis of hyponatremia in edema-forming states is multifactorial, but in the final analysis hyponatremia develops because of excessive water intake in the presence of an impairment in renal free water excretion. In most patients with edema the dominant factor in the genesis of hyponatremia is impaired renal excretion of free water so that even though the level of absolute water intake is considered normal, it may still exceed the capacity of the kidney to form a dilute urine and excrete the excess water. In some patients, however, the absolute level of water intake is consistently higher than normal and may reflect stimulation of the thirst reflex elicited by a low effective circulating blood volume, possibly mediated by angiotensin (179).

Several factors contribute to impaired free water

excretion in these patients. As previously discussed, a decrease in GFR and/or RBF and an elevated filtration fraction are commonly seen in patients with congestive heart failure. These hemodynamic changes facilitate an increase in reabsorption of filtrate along the proximal tubule with a reduced volume of filtrate delivered to the water-clearing segments of the distal nephron. Several studies in patients with congestive heart failure have provided indirect evidence for augmented proximal reabsorption of filtrate (180, 181). The reduced volume of filtrate delivered to the distal tubule sets an upper limit to the volume of free water that can be generated and would be manifested by a reduced free water clearance. Support for this concept is provided by studies of patients with congestive heart failure (182) or cirrhosis (183) who, in response to mannitol infusion, exhibited increased free water excretion. Presumably mannitol decreased proximal tubular reabsorption of filtrate and increased filtrate delivery to the water-clearing segments of the distal nephron.

This mechanism by itself, however, does not completely explain impaired water excretion in these patients. For example in the study of Bell et al. (182), patients with congestive heart failure given a standard water load achieved a minimum osmolality of 88 mosm/kg compared to 55 mosm/kg by normal subjects. These data implicate a defect in urine dilution as well. The inability to achieve a maximally dilute urine may reflect failure to completely suppress ADH even though plasma osmolality is significantly reduced. In the clinical setting of a reduced absolute or effective circulating blood volume, the threshold for ADH release may be lowered due to the influence of volume receptors on ADH secretion (184). In addition, it should be emphasized that under conditions of low distal tubular flow rates, increased back-diffusion of water across the distal tubular epithelium can occur even in the absence of ADH (185). In other words, the epithelium of the distal nephron is not completely impermeable to water despite the lack of ADH, and this finite permeability becomes accentuated under conditions in which distal flow rates are reduced, as in congestive heart failure and cirrhosis of the liver.

Whereas ADH has been implicated in the genesis of hyponatremia in congestive heart failure (186–188), its role in the hyponatremia observed in cirrhotic patients is less well established (146, 189). In general the severity of the diluting defect in cirrhosis parallels the degree to which RBF and GFR are depressed (190–192), which in turn reflects the degree to which effective circulating blood volume is compromised. Since the secretion threshold for ADH would be expected to be reduced when effective circulating blood volume is severely compromised, it is likely that the markedly impaired water excretion seen in the advanced stages of liver disease as well as in heart failure and nephrotic syndrome is mediated both by intrarenal hemodynamic factors and ADH. Finally, impaired free water excretion and hyponatremia can be induced in these patients by excessive diuretic therapy, causing a relative or absolute contraction of plasma volume and depression of RBF and GFR.

The therapeutic approach to hyponatremia associated with edema-forming states is basically the same, namely restriction of water intake and treatment directed at the underlying cause of the edema in order to improve renal hemodynamics and free water excretion.

Before considering the therapeutic approach to the treatment of the various edema-forming disorders, the pharmacology of diuretic drugs will be reviewed.

DIURETICS

PHARMACOLOGY OF DIURETICS

Over the past twenty years the pharmaceutical industry has expanded the therapeutic arsenal of the clinician with an impressive, some might argue bewildering, number of potent diuretic agents. While there can be no disputing the fact that these agents, when properly prescribed, have proved to be of inestimable value in the management of complex edematous and nonedematous disorders alike, it cannot be denied that these agents, when prescribed indiscriminately due to inadequate understanding of their action as well as the basic pathophysiologic derangements for which diuretic therapy may be indicated, have given rise to a distressing number of serious, sometimes fatal, complications.

This section will review current understanding of how diuretics act—which is limited primarily to a description of where they act in the nephron—their clinical application, and common complications.

Tubular sites of action of diuretics

Although knowledge of how diuretics impair tubular transport of electrolytes and water at the membrane level is limited, it has been possible to deduce from clearance and micropuncture studies (193–195) where they act along the nephron. This information has contributed greatly to our understanding of the potency of diuretic drugs as well

as the synergistic effect seen with certain combinations of diuretic agents.

Figure 13-7 is a schematic of the nephron which defines the major sites of action of diuretic agents. Site 1 drugs act along the proximal tubule where 60 to 70 percent of the filtered load of sodium together with chloride and bicarbonate is reabsorbed in isotonic proportion with water. Approximately 90 percent of the bicarbonate is reabsorbed along this segment coupled to hydrogen ion secretion and is dependent on the enzyme carbonic anhydrase. Inhibition of net proximal tubular reabsorption of filtrate does not increase urine flow to the extent that might be expected due to the fact that more distal nephron segments, particularly the ascending limb, have a reserve capacity that permits increased reabsorption of filtrate in proportion to the increased rate of filtrate delivery (glomerulotubular balance). Thus, inhi-

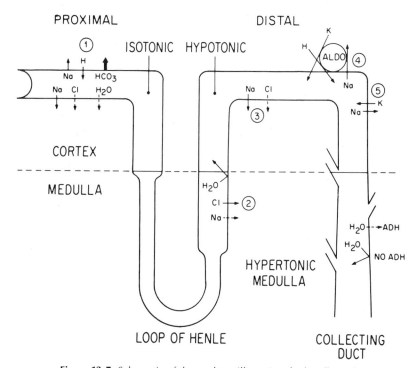

Figure 13-7. Schematic of the nephron illustrating the handling of water and electrolytes by the differing segments and the major nephron sites of diuretic action. The solid arrows signify active transport, interrupted arrows passive transport.

bition of distal tubular transport mechanisms elicits a greater diuresis that can be induced by proximal inhibition.

The ascending limb of Henle's loop, site 2, reabsorbs approximately 15 to 25 percent of the filtered sodium and chloride. Recent studies in the isolated perfused rabbit tubule indicate that chloride is the actively transported species along this segment (196). The thick ascending limb is impermeable to water under all conditions independent of the presence of ADH. Consequently, fluid exiting from the ascending limb is made hypotonic by the reabsorption of electrolytes without water. Accumulation of electrolytes with urea in the medulla provides the osmotic driving force for the reabsorption of water from the collecting duct in the presence of ADH. Inhibition of electrolyte transport along the ascending limb impairs the urine-concentrating and -diluting mechanisms.

The precise anatomical boundaries and functional characteristics of the distal convoluted tubule (site 3) are undergoing reexamination. At present it remains unclear where the cortical segment of the ascending limb ends and the cortical segment of the collecting duct begins. From a functional point of view the distal convoluted tubule can be classified as part of the cortical diluting segment since inhibition of sodium chloride along this segment impairs free water clearance with little effect on urine concentration. Approximately 5 to 10 percent of the filtered load of sodium is reabsorbed along this segment.

The remaining sodium reaching the distal tubule and collecting duct is reabsorbed in part under the influence of aldosterone (site 4), which also stimulates potassium and hydrogen secretion, and by a non-aldosterone-sensitive transport system (site 5).

Site 1 diuretics

The discovery that the enzyme carbonic anhydrase is important in the renal tubular secretion of hydrogen ion and that sulfanilamide, a carbonic anhydrase inhibitor, produces acidosis and causes a diuresis and natriuresis in patients with congestive heart failure led to the systematic search for less toxic and more potent inhibitors

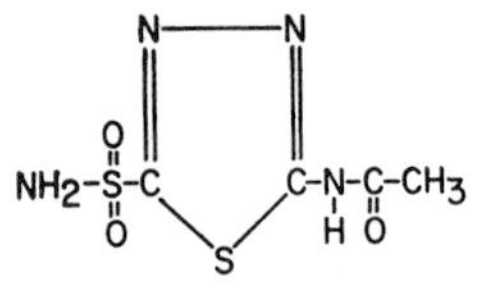

Figure 13-8. Acetazolamide (Diamox).

of this enzyme (197). Of these acetazolamide (Diamox) has been found most practical for clinical use (see Fig. 13-8). This drug is effective whether given orally or intravenously in inhibiting proximal tubular reabsorption of bicarbonate and sodium chloride. The urine becomes alkaline and contains an excess of sodium bicarbonate and potassium. The kaliuresis is related to the effect of bicarbonate, a poorly reabsorbable anion in the distal tubule, in stimulating potassium secretion. Little change in chloride excretion occurs due to increased reabsorption of sodium and chloride by more distal nephron segments. The effectiveness of acetazolamide is blunted by the development of metabolic acidosis consequent to the bicarbonaturia.

Acetazolamide by itself is of little therapeutic value in the management of edema. It may be useful in combination with more distally acting agents. In addition the bicarbonaturia and alkaline urine caused by acetazolamide may be of advantage in conditions where high uric acid excretion may be anticipated.

A number of diuretic drugs (thiazides, furosemide) exhibit carbonic anhydrase inhibitory activity, but, as will be discussed, the natriuretic potency of these agents is related to inhibition of non-carbonic-anhydrase-dependent transport processes in the distal nephron.

Site 2 diuretics

Organomercurials. The organomercurials (193, 198) are substituted mercuripropyl compounds which require parenteral administration; oral compounds are unpredictable in their effects due to variable intestinal absorption. Following administration the drug circulates in the plasma bound to albumin and then accumulates in proximal tubular cells with subsequent secretion as the cysteine and acetyl derivatives (193). Although organomercurials may have a modest proximal tubular effect, their predominant site of action as judged by clearance and micropuncture studies (193, 195, 198) appears to be the ascending limb of Henle's loop where they, along with ethacrynic acid and furosemide, have been shown to inhibit active chloride transport (199). In addition to in the ascending limb, organomercurials have been shown to act in the distal tubule when they inhibit potassium secretion (200).

Following parenteral administration, the onset of diuretic action is delayed for 30 to 60 min and may not reach peak levels for 2 to 4 h. Typically these agents cause marked chloruresis and slightly less natriuresis which under optimal conditions of hydration and pH may exceed 10 percent of the filtered load. Generally there is little increase in bicarbonate excretion. The effects on potassium are variable, but overall the kaliuretic effect of organomercurials appears to be less than that of other loop diuretics. Repeated administration of these compounds produces hypochloremic metabolic alkalosis at which point refractoriness to the drug becomes evident. Administration of acidifying agents, such as ammonium chloride, to correct the alkalosis and raise serum chloride concentration will reverse the refractoriness. If the agent is combined with a xanthine compound, the diuretic potency is augmented, presumably by raising GFR and RBF, although a direct effect of the xanthine compound on tubular sodium transport has not been excluded (193).

Organomercurials are used less frequently today due to the availability of other agents of equal or greater potency which do not require parenteral administration. Nevertheless, they are still useful in the therapy of occasional patients with congestive heart failure or incipient pulmonary edema who cannot take an oral agent.

These drugs are contraindicated in patients with renal insufficiency. The risk of complications increases with dose and frequency of administration. Renal failure, hemorrhagic cystitis, stomatitis, colitis, and dermatitis are manifestations of mercurialism, a form of heavy metal poisoning. Extracellular volume depletion, metabolic alkalosis, and hypokalemia are predictable consequences of excessive diuresis. Failure to achieve

the desired diuretic response with an organomercurial should signal the physican to discontinue the drug, search for the reason for the therapeutic failure, and consider other diuretic agents.

Furosemide (Fig. 13-9). Furosemide is an extremely potent sulfonamide diuretic which, although not a benzothiadiazine, like the thiazides exhibits mild carbonic anhydrase inhibitory activity (193). Its major diuretic action, however, is independent of its carbonic anhydrase inhibitory effect. Like ethacrynic acid, it has a rapid onset of action, occurring within 15 min after intravenous administration, and a peak effect in 30 to 60 min. By 3 h the diuretic effect is largely spent. Following oral administration, diuresis begins in 30 to 60 min, reaches a peak effect within 2 h, and subsides over 6 to 8 h (193, 201, 202).

In contrast to ethacrynic acid, furosemide has been reported to cause a slight initial increase in urinary pH and bicarbonate excretion, presumably reflecting mild carbonic anhydrase inhibition, with a return to control values after the first 15 min (202). Moreover, unlike ethacrynic acid, it also produces a slight increase in phosphorus excretion and only a modest decrease in free water clearance during maximal water diuresis, suggesting inhibition of proximal tubular sodium transport as well as ascending limb transport (193). Inhibition of active chloride transport in the ascending limb has been demonstrated in isolated perfused tubules (203).

Furosemide, like ethacrynic acid, causes an increase in RBF and GFR following acute administration (193). These hemodynamic effects may contribute to the initial natriuretic response, but are short lived as the decrease in plasma volume elicits reflex reduction in RBF and GFR.

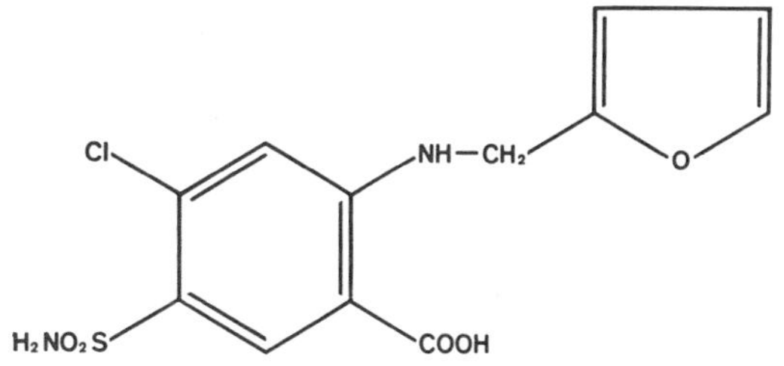

Figure 13-9. Furosemide (Lasix).

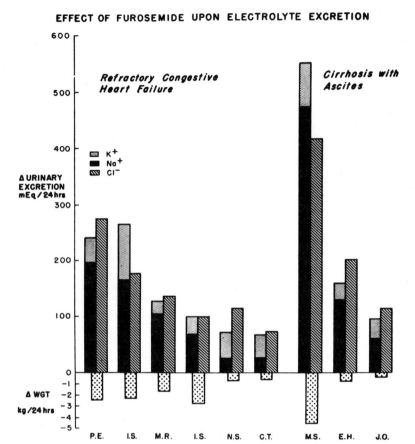

Figure 13-10. Diuretic effects of furosemide (40 mg four times daily, orally) in patients with refractory edema due to congestive heart failure or hepatic cirrhosis. (*From Stason et al.*)

Extensive clinical and laboratory animal studies have established that furosemide, like ethacrynic acid, is much more potent at maximal doses than the mercurial or site 3 diuretics, producing marked chloruresis and natriuresis with weight loss, often in otherwise totally diuretic-resistant patients and despite very low filtration rates, hypoalbuminemia, and marked electrolyte disturbances such as metabolic alkalosis, acidosis, hypochloremia, or hyponatremia (204–206).

In salt-retaining subjects furosemide, like murcurials, thiazides, and ethacrynic acid produces greater excretion of chloride than sodium due to augmented sodium transport along the terminal nephron segments under the influence of aldosterone (Fig. 13-10). The combined influence of al-

dosterone and augmented distal sodium loads and flow rates accelerates potassium secretion along the distal convoluted tubule and collecting duct. Consequently, if the chloride and potassium losses are not replaced, potassium depletion and metabolic alkalosis may develop during continuous daily use of furosemide.

In well-digitalized patients with cardiac disease, during the profuse diuresis and kaliuresis seen with intravenous administration of furosemide, sudden shifts in extracellular potassium as well as accelerated loss of potassium from the myocardium (207) may provoke serious cardiac arrhythmias, which may be prevented by intravenous or oral administration of potassium chloride. It should be emphasized that cardiac arrhythmias may occur even in noncardiac patients after intravenous administration of furosemide or ethacrynic acid. In patients taking furosemide or ethacrynic acid chronically, combined therapy with spironolactone or triamterene (see below), agents which block potassium secretion and sodium reabsorption along the terminal nephron, may minimize potassium losses as well as potentiate sodium diuresis. However, in some patients who require larger doses of furosemide several times daily, such distal tubular blocking agents may not adequately reduce potassium losses, and *cautious* oral administration of potassium chloride is occasionally necessary to prevent potassium depletion. In such circumstances, frequent determinations of serum electrolyte concentration are mandatory to guide such therapy.

The remarkable potency of both furosemide and ethacrynic acid makes it necessary to determine the effective oral dose empirically in every patient by starting with the minimum dose. Occasionally, even this will produce a massive diuresis with severe volume contraction in an unpredictably susceptible subject. Patients with little or no depression in GFR are most likely to experience excessive diuresis even with 40 mg of furosemide. Because of the potent action of the loop diuretics, they generally should be reserved for situations where other less potent agents are ineffective. These situations include acute pulmonary edema, intractable edema of heart failure, and chronic renal failure. Their value in the treatment of acute hypercalcemia and intoxications is also well established (208).

In patients with chronic renal failure it is possible to induce a natriuresis even when GFR is less than 10 mL/min, but it often requires administration of very large doses, sometimes in excess of 1 g per day (209). The renal clearance of furosemide is obviously depressed in these patients so that the major route of excretion is via the liver (210). Consequently plasma levels are greatly increased and the half-life of furosemide is prolonged. The possibility that chronically elevated levels of furosemide may cause undesirable metabolic effects in nonrenal tissue has not been carefully evaluated. In patients with chronic renal failure and liver disease, the risk would be magnified due to the fact that the reduced hepatic clearance in the face of reduced renal clearance would further prolong the half-life of the drug (210).

Ototoxicity is a well-recognized complication of furosemide therapy, particularly when administered intravenously to patients with chronic renal failure (211, 212). Ototoxicity is probably related to excessively high peak levels caused by too-rapid intravenous infusion. In one report, infusion of 1000 mg at a rate of 25 mg/min produced a temporary hearing loss in 9 of 15 uremic patients, whereas no toxicity occurred when the same dose was infused at less than 5.6 mg/min (213).

Other side effects, besides those related to the hemodynamic and electrolyte abnormalities mentioned above, include hyperuricemia and hyperglycemia.

Ethacrynic acid (Fig. 13-11). The search for a nonorganometallic inhibitor of sulfhydryl-catalyzed systems which might prove to be more effective than mercurial diuretics led to the synthesis of aryloxyacetic acid derivatives. Ethacrynic acid proved to be the most effective of these compounds and more potent that the organomercurials. The drug is equally effective when given intravenously or orally. After intravenous administration a diuretic effect is evident within 15 min. Onset of action after oral administration occurs in 30 to 60 min; the peak effect is reached within 2 h, and its action is complete within 6 h (214). Circulating ethacrynic acid is largely bound to protein, and it gains access to the lumen by secretion by the organic acid transport system in the proximal tubule. The active form of the drug appears to be ethacrynic cysteine (214, 215). Its mechanism of action does not seem to involve sulfhydryl inhibition. The drug inhibits sodium- and potassium-activated adenosine triphosphatase (194), but the relationship of this effect to its diuretic potency and its inhibition of active chlo-

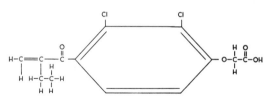

Figure 13-11. Ethacrynic acid (Edecrin).

ride transport in the thick ascending limb remains unclear (194, 196). In addition, ethacrynic acid has been shown to have other metabolic effects including inhibition of sodium transport, respiration, and glycolysis in renal and nonrenal tissue (196).

Ethacrynic acid, like furosemide, induces a marked chloruresis, natriuresis, and kaliuresis (193, 201, 202). Under appropriate experimental conditions, a proximal site of action not dependent on carbonic anhydrase inhibition can be demonstrated (195) but is of little clinical significance. Ethacrynic acid's major site of action is the ascending limb, where it inhibits active chloride transport (215) and impairs both urine concentration and dilution (193, 201, 202). The marked kaliuresis seen with this agent is related to the effect of increased sodium delivery and volume flow, enhancing potassium secretion along the distal nephron, as well as decreased reabsorption of potassium along the ascending limb of Henle's loop.

The clinical indications for this drug are identical to those enumerated above for furosemide (216, 217). Like that of furosemide, the dose of ethacrynic acid can be increased in patients with chronic renal failure until the desired diuretic effect is achieved (218) but not without risk.

The complications with respect to acute volume depletion, hypokalemia, metabolic alkalosis, glucose intolerance, and hyperuricemia are similar in frequency and severity to those occurring with furosemide. Irreversible ototoxicity appears to be more common with ethacrynic acid (219). Although it was thought that ototoxicity occurred only with high-dose drug therapy, particularly in renal failure, transitory deafness has been reported in two nonuremic patients after intravenous administration of 50 mg of ethacrynic acid (220), possibly due to an interaction between the diuretic and an aminoglycoside antibiotic.

Site 3 diuretics

Benzothiadiazines. The obvious deficiencies of acetazolamide as a diuretic stimulated a search for a better carbonic anhydrase inhibitor to which refractoriness might not develop so rapidly. The

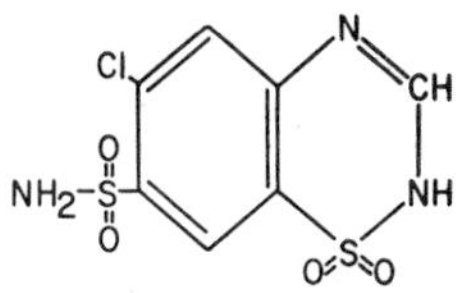

Figure 13-12. Chlorothiazide (Ciuril).

unexpected byproduct of this research was another sulfonamyl derivative, chlorothiazide, which revolutionized diuretic therapy (see Fig. 13-12). This compound is a weak carbonic anhydrase inhibitor, but it significantly decreases tubular sodium reabsorption by some other mechanism and promotes increased urinary excretion of chloride rather than bicarbonate as the principal anion (221, 222). It was quickly recognized that chlorothiazide could well be the ideal diuretic, being effective orally and producing both natriuresis and chloruresis, thereby mobilizing excess ECF without the development of the refractory state which ultimately renders the pure carbonic anhydrase inhibitors ineffective.

The discovery of chlorothiazide inspired the synthesis of a series of compounds (Table 13-5), all possessing the same benzothiadiazine ring characteristic of the so-called thiazide diuretics. Although these compounds are effective at lower doses than chlorothiazide, their maximal diuretic effect is not significantly different from that which can be achieved with chlorothiazide. Thus, a patient resistant to one thiazide will not respond to another member of the same class. The benzothiadiazines do differ in one important respect among themselves, namely their duration of action. The older thiazides (chlorothiazide and hydrochlorothiazide) have their main diuretic effect within 4 to 6 h after oral administration, and it is largely dissipated by 10 to 12 h. The compounds synthesized subsequently (methyclothiazide, polythiazide, and cyclothiazide) have a more prolonged diuretic effect lasting for at least 24 h. The prolonged action of these compounds appears to be conferred by their greater lipid solubility so that they have a larger volume of distribution and are eliminated more slowly than the more water-soluble compounds which are confined primarily to extracellular water.

The main route of excretion of the benzothiadiazines is secretion by the organic acid transport system of the proximal tubule. Although a slight proximal tubular effect has been identified (195), their main site of action is along the cortical diluting segment as judged by a depression in maximal free water clearance with no depression of free water reabsorption (193). Micropuncture studies have demonstrated an effect along the distal convoluted tubule (223). Direct evidence for an action along the cortical segment of the ascending limb is lacking.

Potassium secretion is accelerated along the distal convoluted tubule and collecting duct during thiazide therapy by the same mechanism described for furosemide, namely increased distal delivery of sodium and augmented distal tubular fluid flow rate. Consequently chronic daily administration of these agents will promote hypokalemia and hypochloremic metabolic alkalosis. This complication should be routinely anticipated and supplemental potassium chloride or a potassium-sparing diuretic should be added in sufficient quantities to maintain a normal serum potassium.

Table 13-5. Diuretics used in clinical practice

TYPE OF AGENT	GENERIC NAME	COMMERCIAL PREPARATION	USUAL DAILY DOSAGE, ORAL
Carbonic anhydrase inhibitor	Acetazolamide	Diamox	250–500 mg
Loop diuretics			
Anthranilic acid derivative	Furosemide	Lasix	40–160 mg (higher in chronic renal failure)
Phenoxyacetic acid derivative	Ethacrynic acid	Edecrin	50–200 mg (higher in chronic renal failure)
Organomercurial	Mercaptomerin	Thiomerin	1–2 mL (IM)
Thiazide and related sulfonamide derivatives			
Benzothiadiazine compounds	Chlorothiazide	Diuril	250–1500 mg
	Hydrochlorothiazide	Esidrix HydroDiuril Oretic	25–150 mg
	Bendroflumethiazide	Naturetin	
	Methyclothiazide	Aquatensen Enduron	5–150 mg
	Hydroflumethiazide	Diucardin Saluron	25–150 mg
	Benzthiazide	Exna	25–150 mg
	Polythiazide	Renese	2–8 mg
	Cyclothiazide	Anhydron	2–6 mg
	Trichlormethiazide	Metahydrin Naqua	2–8 mg
Phthalimidine compound	Chlorthalidone	Hygroton	50–100 mg
Quinazoline compounds	Metolazone	Zaroxolyn	2.5–10 mg
	Quinethazone	Hydromox	50–150 mg
Potassium-sparing agents (distal tubule diuretics)	Spironolactone	Aldactone	50–200 mg
	Triamterene	Dyrenium	100–200 mg

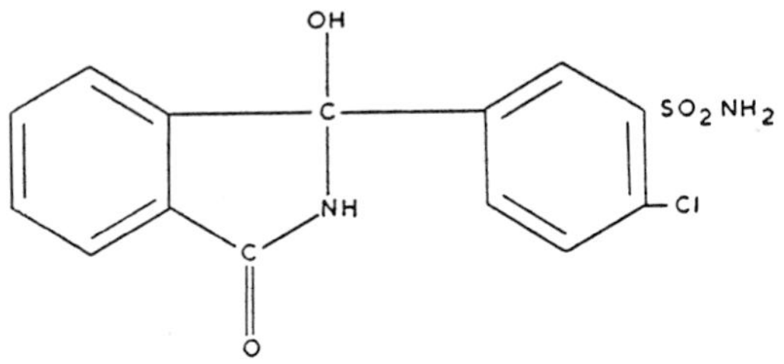

Figure 13-13. Chlorthalidone (Hygroton).

The thiazides or one of the other site 3 drugs should be considered as first choice drugs in the chronic management of most patients with edema or hypertension not complicated by chronic renal insufficiency. Thiazides are usually ineffective when the GFR falls below 25 mL/min. In addition to treatment of edema and hypertension, the thiazides have been employed in the therapy of diabetes insipidus, proximal renal tubular acidosis, and idiopathic hypercalciuria with nephrolithiasis (208).

Although these agents are generally well tolerated during chronic administration, a number of side effects occur. Sodium depletion with symptomatic extracellular volume contraction can occur during thiazide therapy but is less severe than that induced by the loop diuretics. Profound hypokalemia can occur during chronic therapy. Although thiazides impair maximal free water clearance, this effect by itself does not usually lead to hyponatremia except when associated with excessive water ingestion (224).

Thiazide-induced carbohydrate intolerance was recognized shortly after the agents were introduced. Depression of insulin secretion secondary to hypokalemia, diuretic inhibition of phosphodiesterase, or altered cation exchange as well as catecholamine stimulation of glycogenolysis and decreased peripheral glucose utilization have been advanced as explanations for the carbohydrate intolerance (225, 226). In nondiabetics the hyperglycemia is mild and is generally easily controlled with diet and correction of hypokalemia. In diabetics or prediabetics a higher incidence of hyperglycemia is seen with thiazides and may require specific drug therapy.

Hyperuricemia is a very common finding in patients on chronic thiazide therapy and reflects decreased uric acid clearance by the kidney as a consequence of extracellular volume contraction promoting increased proximal tubular reabsorption of uric acid and possibly decreased uric acid secretion (227). The vast majority of patients with diuretic-induced hyperuricemia remain asymptomatic. Except for the patients with known gout, there is no established rationale as to when antihyperuricemic therapy should be initiated.

Other idiosyncratic toxic effects attributed to thiazides include thrombocytopenia, neutropenia, skin rashes, photosensitivity, necrotizing vasculitis, gastrointestinal ulceration, and acute hemorrhagic pancreatitis. More recently allergic pneumonitis (228) and allergic interstitial nephritis (229) have also been attributed to thiazides.

Phthalimidines. These are heterocyclic compounds which lack the thiadiazine ring but, like the benzothiadiazines, have substituted sulfamyl and halogen in the ortho position of a benzine ring. Chlorthalidone is the most popular example of these (see Fig. 13-13). It has gained wide use because it produces natriuresis for as long as 72 h following an oral dose of 100 mg (230). With the exception of its more prolonged diuretic action, which reflects slow absorption from the gastrointestinal tract plus selective fixation in renal tissue, chlorthalidone acts pharmacologically and clinically exactly as does any benzothiadiazine with the same mode and site of action in the nephron and the same toxic potential with respect to carbohydrate, uric acid, and potassium metabolism.

Quinazolinones. Metolazone and quinethazone are representative of this class of diuretics (see Fig. 13-14). Metolazone, similar to the thiazides, inhibits reabsorption of sodium in the cortical diluting segments (231) with a lesser effect in the proximal tubule (232). It is not an inhibitor of carbonic anhydrase; thus, its action in the proximal tubule appears to differ from that of the thiazides.

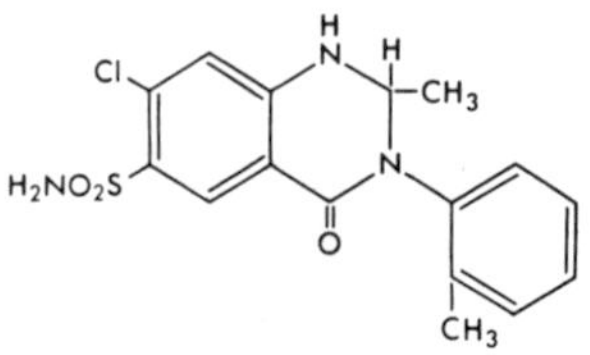

Figure 13-14. Metolazone (Zaroxolyn).

In man metolazone is well absorbed from the gut and is excreted in the urine unchanged (233). After an oral dose, diuresis begins in 1 h, reaches a maximum between 2 to 3 h, and continues for 12 to 24 h. With intravenous administration, peak natriuresis occurs in 60 min and continues for 3 to 5 h. Although studies in animals suggest that the drug is less kaliuretic than thiazides and loop diuretics (234), clinical experience indicates that hypokalemia does occur.

Site 4 diuretics

Recognition of the importance of aldosterone in mediating sodium retention in edema-forming states led to the synthesis of a series of compounds which are specific competitive inhibitors of aldosterone (235, 236). Spironolactone (Aldactone) is the most widely used aldosterone antagonist in clinical medicine. This agent, structurally similar to aldosterone, inhibits binding of aldosterone and other mineralocorticosteroids to their specific receptors not only in the cells of the distal nephron but in other target tissues, such as the gastrointestinal tract, sweat glands, and salivary glands, as well (237). Aldosterone stimulates sodium reabsorption and secretion of potassium and hydrogen along the terminal nephron (238). Thus, inhibition of aldosterone action leads to an increase in sodium chloride excretion and a decrease in potassium and hydrogen excretion (235). The magnitude of the natriuresis induced by these antagonists is relatively slight due to the fact that aldosterone normally regulates less than 2 percent of the filtered sodium load. Consequently the maximal natriuretic effect of aldosterone antagonists will not exceed this level. Nevertheless, the spironolactones have an important role to play in the chronic management of edema-forming states, particularly cirrhosis of the liver and the nephrotic syndrome in which secondary hyperaldosteronism is commonly present. When combined with more proximally acting agents, such as the thiazide or loop diuretics, they potentiate the natriuretic effect of these drugs while reducing the amount of potassium lost in the urine.

The usual dose of Aldactone is 25 mg four times daily. In some patients the desired effect, particularly in terms of reducing potassium excretion, may be achieved with a lower dose. In others a higher dose schedule is required. It should be emphasized that the effectiveness of this agent is limited to the extent that it inhibits aldosterone. In patients with marked elevation of aldosterone, larger doses may be required to achieve the desired effect. In addition the natriuretic effect will be limited to the extent that compensatory increased reabsorption of sodium by more proximal nephron sites together with a decrease in GFR limits the delivery of sodium to the terminal nephron; both decreased delivery and augmented aldosterone secretion contribute to the refractoriness observed with these agents.

In an occasional patient supplemental potassium chloride may be required in addition to spironolactone in order to correct severe hypokalemia. This must be done under close supervision to avoid hyperkalemia. In patients with advanced chronic renal failure this drug is contraindicated because of the risk of inducing fatal hyperkalemia.

A number of nonspecific side effects have been reported with the chronic administration of spironolactone including lethargy, drowsiness, skin rash, and epigastric distress. Endocrine dysfunction characterized by impotence and gynecomastia in men and menstrual irregularities and painful breast enlargement in women may appear during chronic administration of this agent (239). Finally aspirin has been shown to antagonize the natriuresis of spironolactone (240).

Site 5 diuretics

Investigation of the potential diuretic properties of a series of synthetic pteridines led to the development of triamterene (Dyrenium), a triaminopteridine (Fig. 13-15) (241–243). This agent inhibits sodium reabsorption and potassium and hydrogen secretion along the distal tubule (193,

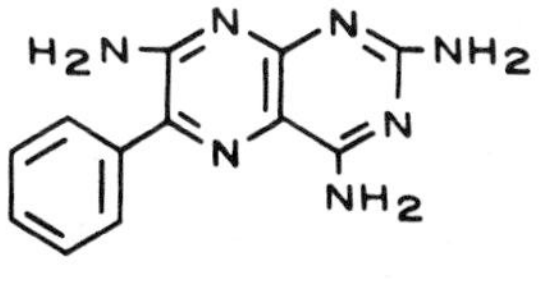

Figure 13-15. Triamterene (Dyrenium).

243). Its potency is equivalent to that of spirono-lactone but, unlike spironolactone, triamterene is not an aldosterone antagonist. It is effective in the presence or absence of aldosterone (242), and its effect is additive to that of spironolactone.

Following oral administration in humans triamterene's diuretic effect is seen in approximately 2 h, increases to a maximum by 6 to 8 h, and subsides by 16 h.

The major clinical application of triamterene is in combination with site 3 or site 2 drugs to augment their natriuretic effect and minimize urinary potassium excretion. The major risk of triamterene, like spironolactone, is hyperkalemia.

INDICATIONS AND PRINCIPLES OF DIURETIC THERAPY IN EDEMA

Generalized edema is a sign, and not a disease. It is a sign signaling the presence of an underlying derangement in the regulation of extracellular volume. It reflects an attempt of the body to compensate for an ineffective circulating blood volume. Rational therapy must be based on an understanding of all the factors, both primary and secondary, contributing to edema in a given patient, and where possible therapy should be directed at reversing the underlying cause of edema formation. In the patient with heart disease, primary therapy should be directed at improving myocardial function and cardiac output. In the patient with cirrhosis and ascites, effective primary therapy is lacking. In patients with nephrotic syndrome effective primary therapy is also lacking with the exception of steroid-responsive idiopathic nephrotic syndrome. Nevertheless by careful attention to measures designed to mobilize edema, such as restriction of activity and supportive stockings, as well as evaluating the adequacy of nutrition and instituting appropriate restriction of sodium and water intake, it is frequently possible to reduce significantly ascites and edema in these patients without causing them harm or discomfort.

Diuretics as a rule should be employed only as adjunctive therapy to the above measures. The basic indications for diuretic therapy in edema-tous disorders are (1) to alleviate or prevent acute and chronic pulmonary congestion and circulatory overload; (2) to mobilize excess fluid that may severely limit activity, cause discomfort or, in the patient with recurrent tense ascites, respiratory embarrassment, and (3) to encourage adequate nutrition while avoiding further sodium retention.

Having decided on the need for diuretic therapy, the physician should establish clearly defined therapeutic goals and employ the diuretic agent which will accomplish those goals with minimum risk of complications to the patient. During the initial stages of diuresis this demands frequent and thorough evaluation of the primary disease process together with monitoring of serum electrolytes and renal function. Symptoms of weakness, dizziness, orthostatic hypotension together with laboratory findings of a rising blood urea nitrogen (BUN) and serum creatinine in a patient losing weight on diuretic therapy are obvious clues that excessive or too-rapid diuresis has been induced. With the exception of the treatment of acute pulmonary edema, slow diuresis is always preferable to rapid diuresis in order to minimize rapid shifts in volume or electrolytes. In some patients intermittent diuretic therapy is preferable to continuous daily therapy.

If a patient escapes from diuretic control, re-evaluation of the underlying disease process, i.e., whether progression or deterioration of cardiac, liver, or renal function has occurred, the effectiveness of the primary therapy, e.g., adequacy of digitalization, together with reassessment of activity, nutrition, and sodium and water intake should be undertaken before adjustments in diuretic drug or dosage are made. For example, a patient who is reaccumulating edema and excreting 150 meq of sodium per day is obviously ingesting too much sodium. Restricting sodium intake may be all that is required to restore sodium balance and control of edema. In contrast, if a patient is gaining weight while on therapy and has a low urinary sodium concentration (less than 10 meq/L) and/or excretion rate (less than 20 meq/day) it usually signals progression of the primary disease or escape from primary therapy.

The appearance of diuretic refractoriness before the therapeutic goal is reached is also a sign to pause and reevaluate all aspects of the disease and therapy. Diuretic refractoriness will occur eventually in all patients as effective circulating blood volume becomes depleted and renal compensation occurs via stimulation of the sympathetic nervous system and the renin-angiotensin-aldosterone system. Depending on the degree of volume depletion, a variable rise in the BUN and serum creatinine and fall in the creatinine clearance are usually evident. These changes in renal function signify excessive diuresis with resultant depletion of effective circulating blood volume. Further attempts to mobilize edema or ascites by increasing the diuretic should be abandoned and attention should be focused on preventing reaccumulation of edema fluid.

The notion that effective therapy, particularly of ascites in the cirrhotic or edema in the nephrotic syndrome is judged by the extent to which these patients are rendered free of edema fluid without due regard for the consequences of such therapy on systemic hemodynamics, renal function, and electrolyte balance must be discouraged.

In the sections that follow, the application of these principles to the management of the major edematous disorders will be discussed.

TREATMENT OF EDEMA

TREATMENT OF CONGESTIVE HEART FAILURE

Congestive heart failure is a symptom complex of multiple etiologies. Effective therapy ultimately must be directed towards correcting the underlying cause of myocardial failure such as hypertensive cardiovascular disease, valvular heart disease, thyrotoxicosis, arteriovenous fistula, anemia, etc. However, there are certain general therapeutic measures that are applicable to most, if not all, forms of congestive heart failure.

Limitation of activity

Limitation of activity immediately reduces the work load of the heart. During rest cardiac output

and effective circulating blood volume may become adequate to meet the metabolic requirements of the peripheral tissues so that the stimulus for renal sodium retention is withdrawn and a spontaneous diuresis ensues. The common complaint of nocturia by patients in heart failure reflects this phenomenon. Restriction of physical activity is adjusted to the severity of heart failure. In some patients complete bed rest, especially during the acute phase of heart failure, may be required; in others, symptoms may subside by eliminating moderate activity and scheduling periods of rest during the day. The objective is to maintain the requirements of the peripheral tissues within the work capacity of the failing heart until myocardial performance can be improved with more specific measures.

Digitalis

The cardiac glycosides are the only available therapeutic agents for correcting the primary defect in heart failure, depressed myocardial contractility. The contractile response to digitalis is directly proportional to the dose administered, as is its toxicity. Digitalization may increase cardiac reserve sufficiently to permit resumption of normal activity. In recent years the appropriateness of digitalis therapy in a number of cardiac disease states has been questioned, as has been the need for maintaining therapy once it has been started (244–246). In addition it has been suggested that diuretics may be preferable to digitalis as primary therapy in congestive heart failure (247). While this may be true for certain high-risk patients, in the vast majority of patients with congestive heart failure due to depressed myocardial contractility, digitalis remains the initial therapy of choice, and when combined with appropriate sodium restriction it often obviates the need for diuretic therapy. Diuretic therapy, by itself, does not correct the basic pathophysiological derangement of heart failure.

The variety of available digitalis preparations includes drugs satisfactory for almost every specific clinical situation. Information concerning the pharmacology, clinical application, advantages and disadvantages of the various glycosides is available in several recent reviews (244, 245) and will not be further considered here.

The point to be emphasized is that the physician should ascertain that optimal therapeutic levels of digitalis have been achieved before committing the patient to long-term diuretic therapy. In some patients the risk of digitalis toxicity may dictate prescribing a suboptimal dose of drug and initiating diuretic therapy earlier than would otherwise be necessary. In many patients with cardiac disease, particularly if vigorous diuretic therapy has been employed, depletion of myocardial potassium may lead to the appearance of electrocardiographic manifestations of digitalis toxicity, such as premature contractions, long before therapeutically effective digitalization has been achieved. The consequent bigeminy and other abnormal cardiac rhythms are erroneously attributed to excessive digitalization, and digitalis is withheld. Under these circumstances, administration of potassium chloride may lead to prompt disappearance of the cardiac arrhythmias and permit cautious administration of additional digitalis. It should be emphasized that serum potassium levels do not always reflect the intracellular potassium stores, particularly when acid-base disturbances are present. When in doubt as to the presence of digitalis toxicity, plasma levels should be determined, and if they are below the usual toxicity levels, a trial of increased potassium chloride supplementation should be instituted despite a normal serum potassium.

In a previously stable patient who shows signs of decompensation the possibility of escape from adequate digitalization should be evaluated by determining plasma levels before resorting to or augmenting diuretic therapy.

Low-sodium diet

Restriction of sodium intake remains an essential aspect of therapy not only in heart failure but in all edematous disorders. As discussed in the section on pathogenesis, these patients have an impaired ability to excrete sodium even in the early stages of their disease before overt clinical failure becomes evident. The availability of potent diuretics should not persuade the physician to neglect this important aspect of therapy. By limiting sodium intake it is frequently possible to effectively manage these patients with digitalization alone. In other patients restriction of sodium intake may permit a reduction in diuretic therapy from a daily to an intermittent schedule or to reduce the daily dose of diuretic required to maintain sodium balance. The degree of sodium restriction will depend on the severity of the heart failure. During the decompensated phase rigid sodium restriction is required to obviate further expansion of an already congested circulation. Once the patient's condition is stabilized and compensation achieved, the appropriate level of sodium intake is defined by monitoring changes in body weight and urinary sodium excretion during adjustments in dietary sodium intake. Even the patient with mild compensated heart failure should be placed on restricted sodium intake. By simply eliminating the addition of salt to food and avoiding high-sodium foods, sodium intake can be reduced to 2000 mg/day. Most patients when educated to the rationale behind the therapy and properly instructed as to what constitutes a sodium-restricted diet will acquiesce. Having the patient record his weight each morning is particularly effective in alerting the patient and physician to a change in sodium balance. All too often the gain in weight and reappearance of pedal edema or dyspnea signifies dietary indiscretion with excessive sodium intake rather than a deterioration in myocardial function. Measurements of urinary sodium excretion will usually resolve the issue.

Diuretic therapy

In view of the fact that sodium retention and plasma volume expansion is a compensatory mechanism for augmenting cardiac output in the presence of depressed myocardial contractility and that diuretics by decreasing plasma volume and ventricular filling pressure will impair this important compensatory mechanism, careful consideration should be given to the indications and potential complication of diuretic therapy. In my opinion, diuretic therapy should be reserved for the patient who continues to manifest pulmonary congestion and edema that is unresponsive to optimal digitalization and sodium restriction.

The choice of diuretic will be dictated by the degree of heart failure and level of renal function. In the absence of primary parenchymal renal disease most patients will respond to a site 3 diuretic. With the exception of duration of action, there is no particular advantage of one drug over another. The dose of drug should be adjusted to the minimal amount required to keep the patient free of pulmonary symptoms. Minimal pedal edema per se in the absence of pulmonary congestion is not an indication for initiating or increasing diuretic therapy. Whenever diuretic therapy is started, supplemental potassium chloride, 40 to 60 meq/day, should be prescribed initially and adjusted as necessary to maintain serum potassium within normal limits. Serum potassium concentration should be monitored at least monthly during the early period of diuretic therapy to establish that the potassium chloride supplement is adequate. Once the patient's condition has been stabilized on therapy, serum potassium concentration can be monitored at less frequent intervals of 3 to 4 months. Renal function should also be monitored frequently. An elevated BUN out of proportion to the serum creatinine in a patient who is free of edema and pulmonary congestion is usually a sign of excessive diuretic therapy.

If pulmonary congestion and edema is unresponsive to full doses of a site 3 diuretic in conjunction with optimal digitalization, limitation of activity, and restricted sodium intake, a more advanced degree of heart failure is obviously signified. These patients usually exhibit evidence of increased activity of the sympathetic nervous system and the renin-angiotensin-aldosterone system along with mild to moderate depression in RBF and GFR. The enhanced reabsorption of sodium along the proximal tubule and ascending limb reduces the volume of filtrate reaching the distal tubule, thereby limiting the effect of inhibiting sodium transport along the distal convoluted tubule, site 3. Moreover, to a large extent the sodium which escapes reabsorption along site 3 is reclaimed under the influence of aldosterone. Augmented potassium excretion is evident in this situation. In some patients addition of spirono-lactone or triamterene may increase the diuretic effectiveness of a site 3 drug and control pulmonary congestion. In most patients, however, it is usually necessary to resort to furosemide or ethacrynic acid. Because of the unpredictably excessive diuretic response of some patients, it is always advisable to start with the minimum dose and increase the dose as necessary to achieve the desired effect. Accelerated potassium losses may occur requiring adjustments in potassium chloride supplements or addition of a potassium-sparing diuretic. Again it should be emphasized that the objective of diuretic therapy in these patients is to decrease plasma volume and pulmonary capillary pressure to the point where the patient is relieved of symptoms. Attempts to render these patients edema-free may seriously compromise cardiac output, leading to symptoms of orthostatic hypotension and signs of deteriorating renal function manifested by a rise in BUN out of proportion to the rise in serum creatinine. In this situation further stimulation of the renin-angiotensin-aldosterone system occurs and promotes further potassium wasting.

In patients with predominant right-sided failure, peripheral edema of sufficient magnitude to cause discomfort and limitation of activity is a valid indication for diuretic activity. Again, diuretic therapy should be tailored to alleviate the symptoms to the extent possible without compromising cardiac output and renal function.

Patients with congestive heart failure complicated by chronic renal failure may be unresponsive to site 3 drugs particularly if GFR is below 25 mL/min. Depending on the severity of heart failure and the level of renal function it may be advisable to initiate therapy with a loop diuretic. If a diuretic response is not achieved with 40 mg of furosemide or 50 mg of ethacrynic acid, then increasing the frequency of the same dose will also prove ineffective. The diuretic response to a given dose of furosemide or ethacrynic acid should be determined by recording the urinary output before and for 8 h after the drug is administered. Once the effective dose is established for a given patient, that dose may be administered as frequently as necessary, whether every other day or twice daily, to achieve the desired result. The need

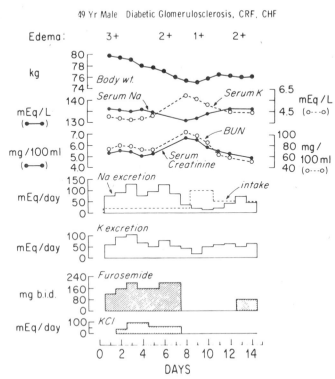

Figure 13-16. This figure illustrates the potential problems that may arise when chronic renal failure is complicated by congestive heart failure. This patient was diagnosed as having chronic renal failure secondary to diabetic glomerulosclerosis with mild nephrotic syndrome. Prior to the onset of congestive heart failure the patient had been managed on furosemide, 80 mg, b.i.d. and sodium restriction; the serum creatinine was 4.0 mg/dL. At the time of admission he demonstrated moderate pulmonary congestion, 3+ peripheral edema, and a weight gain of 4.5 kg. Bed rest, sodium restriction, digitalization, and diuretic therapy were initiated with rapid clearing of pulmonary symptoms and improvement of edema and renal function over the subsequent 5 days. On day 8 the serum creatinine, BUN, and serum potassium were noted to have increased dramatically in association with a further weight loss of 2 kg. Although the patient still exhibited edema, the deterioration in renal function with hyperkalemia is best explained on the basis of a contracted effective circulating blood volume due to excessive diuresis. Interruption of diuretic therapy and potassium chloride supplements together with liberalization of sodium intake permitted reexpansion of effective circulating blood volume and restoration of renal function to the level observed prior to the onset of heart failure. Although peripheral edema was still present, for this patient it represents the optimal level of extracellular volume to maintain stable renal function while keeping the patient free of symptoms from pulmonary congestion.

for potassium chloride supplements in these patients is variable and depends on the severity of the heart failure as well as the degree of renal insufficiency. If potassium supplements are required, frequent determinations of serum potassium concentration should be performed to guard against hyperkalemia. Excessive diuresis in these patients may precipitate a sudden deterioration in renal function causing hyperkalemia. Thus frequent monitoring of creatinine clearance, serum creatinine, and BUN is also advisable during the initial stages of therapy until the patient's condition has stabilized. Rapid progression of chronic renal failure in a patient who exhibits unequivocal improvement in terms of symptoms and signs of heart failure usually signifies excessive diuresis (Fig. 13-16). The diuretic should be temporarily discontinued or reduced until effective circulating blood volume is restored to a level that is optimal for maintaining renal function while preventing pulmonary congestion.

Intravenous diuretic therapy should be reserved for the patient with life-threatening pulmonary edema or the patient with intractable edema who may exhibit unresponsiveness to oral agents due to impaired absorption across an edematous bowel. Both furosemide and ethacrynic acid have been demonstrated to be particularly effective in managing acute pulmonary edema (248, 249). Their potent and rapid onset of action following intravenous administration facilitates mobilization of fluid from the lungs by decreasing plasma volume and reducing left ventricular end-diastolic pressure (250–252).

However, Dikshit and colleagues (251) have reported that the initial improvement seen with intravenous furosemide administration is probably due to an extrarenal hemodynamic effect of this agent. These authors studied both renal and central hemodynamic changes occurring after intravenous administration of furosemide to patients with acute myocardial infarction and left ventricular failure. Onset of renal hemodynamic changes, diuresis, and natriuresis were detected within 15 min of drug administration; peak diuresis and natriuresis occurred between 30 and 60 min (Fig. 13-17). Measurements of left ventricular filling pres-

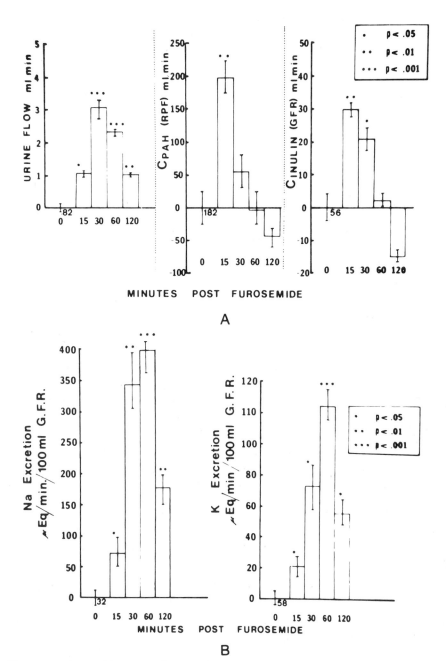

Figure 13-17. Effect of intravenous furosemide on urine flow, renal plasma flow (RPF) and glomerular filtration rate (GFR) in patients with acute myocardial infarction and left ventricular failure. RPF increased by 197, and GFR by 30 mL/min respectively from control values at 15 min (A). Changes in sodium and potassium excretion expressed in microequivalents per minute per 100 mL GFR were maximum at 60 min (B). The numbers listed to the right of the control period are the mean control values for each measurement. Bars indicate the standard error. CPAH represents PAH clearance, and CIN inulin clearance. (*From Dikshit et al.*)

Table 13-6. Central hemodynamic effects of furosemide*

PERIOD OF OBSERVATION	HR	BP PER MIN	RA	LVFP, mmHg	CI, L/(min)(m²)
Control	90±3	90± 6	7.0±0.6	20.4±1.4	2.1±0.2
After furosemide					
5 min	90±2	90±10	7.0±0.7	17.0±1.8†	
10 min	91±3	88± 9	6.0±0.7†	17.3±1.7†	
15 min	89±3	90± 8	6.0±0.7†	14.9±1.3†	2.3±0.3
30 min	89±3	90± 6	6.0±0.7†	15.1±1.6†	2.1±0.4
60 min	90±2	90± 7	6.0±0.6†	14.8±1.2†	2.2±0.3

* Values are means ± SEM (HR represents heart rate, BP blood pressure, RA right atrial pressure, LVFP left ventricular filling pressure, and CI cardiac index). No significant changes were observed in heart rate, blood pressure, or cardiac index, whereas there was a significant drop (<0.0001) in left ventricular filling pressure, most of which occurred in the first 15 min. The change in right atrial pressure was significant but of no biologic importance.

† <p 0.01.
From Dikshit et al.

sure revealed a significant decrease prior to the onset of the peak natriuresis, as shown in Table 13-6. The decrease in left ventricular filling pressure coincided temporally with an increase in peripheral venous capacitance (Fig. 13-18). Thus, the initial beneficial effect of intravenously administered furosemide appears to be related to a direct action of this agent in decreasing venous tone, and this effect is subsequently magnified by the increase in urine output and reduction in absolute plasma volume.

It should be emphasized, however, that if ventricular function is dependent on a high filling pressure, a precipitous decline in cardiac output, often out of proportion to the magnitude of the diuresis, may occur in response to the sudden decrease in venous pressure and plasma volume induced by these agents. Similar hemodynamic effects may occur even when these agents are administered orally for the treatment of pulmonary congestion or peripheral edema. Figure 13-19 illustrates the appearance of hypotension out of proportion to the diuresis induced by oral administration of furosemide to a patient with chronic congestive heart failure and pulmonary congestion. Presumably this patient's myocardium required a high ventricular filling pressure to maintain cardiac output. With adequate digitalization the patient became responsive to intermittent oral diuretic therapy.

Persistent and intractable pulmonary congestion and edema resistant even to loop diuretics often develops in the terminal stages of heart failure. Careful evaluation for complicating factors such as unsuspected pulmonary emboli, rhythm disturbances, electrolyte imbalance, adequacy of digitalization, hypoxia, hypertension, anemia, endocrine factors, diet, alcohol, etc., must be sought and corrected where possible. If heart failure remains refractory, then consideration should be given to vasodilator therapy. Peripheral vasodilatation by decreasing impedance to left ventricular ejection may lead to significant increases in cardiac output with simultaneous decreases in pulmonary and systemic venous pressures (253). A significant diuresis with clearing of pulmonary symptoms may ensue. Long-term improvement with oral vasodilator therapy in an outpatient setting has been reported (254). On rare occasions, removal of excess fluid by peritoneal or hemodialysis may improve cardiopulmonary function sufficiently that a new state of compensation can

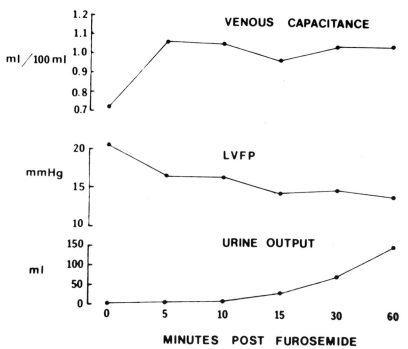

Figure 13-18. Temporal changes in mean left ventricular filling pressure within the first 15 min are accompanied by a simultaneous increase in calf venous capacitance, during which time there was insignificant urine output. At 1 h there was, in addition, a significant volume diuresis that may further have reduced intravascular volume.

be maintained with drug therapy. In most cases, however, the benefit is transient.

TREATMENT OF ASCITES IN LIVER DISEASE AND PORTAL HYPERTENSION

Some of the most challenging and perplexing problems of fluid and electrolyte imbalance are presented by patients with cirrhosis of the liver and ascites. Unrelenting sodium and water retention, with resistant hyponatremia, hypokalemia and acid-base disturbances in association with hypoproteinemia, malnutrition, cardiopulmonary disease, and functional renal failure are commonly seen in the same patient. While ascites may be the most prominent sign of liver disease, it should not be the physician's primary focus of concern in determining therapy. Rather the appearance or progression of ascites in a patient with

cirrhosis of the liver should alert the physician to undertake a thorough evaluation of all possible factors—hepatic, cardiovascular, renal, and nutritional—that may be contributing to the development of ascites. The only absolute indication for therapy of ascites per se is when pulmonary function is compromised due to elevation of the diaphragms causing atelectasis. Discomfort and limitation of activity is a relative indication for therapy, which should be undertaken only to the extent that mobilization of ascites does not compromise cardiovascular and renal function.

The same general principles apply to the treatment of edema and ascites as were outlined for the treatment of edema in congestive heart failure.

Limitation of activity

As in congestive heart failure, placing the patient at bed rest will often result in a spontaneous di-

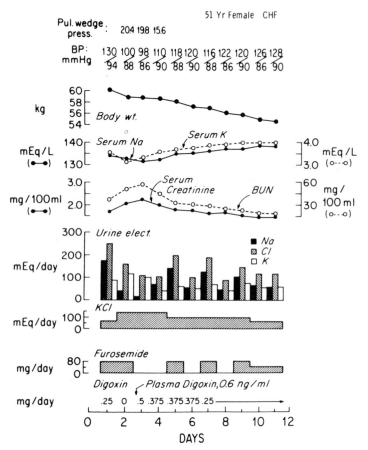

Figure 13-19. This patient illustrates the abrupt deterioration in cardiovascular and renal function that may attend the institution of diuresis in patients whose ventricular function is dependent on a high filling pressure. This patient carried a diagnosis of hypertensive cardiovascular disease with compensated heart failure treated with digoxin, hydrochlorothiazide, and Aldomet. She presented to the hospital with a history of increasing dyspnea and swelling of the ankles. Physical examination revealed pulmonary congestion, cardiomegaly, an S3 gallop and 3+ peripheral edema. An electrocardiogram revealed left ventricular hypertrophy with an occasional ectopic ventricular contraction; there was no evidence of acute myocardial infarction. Therapy was initiated with furosemide, 80 mg orally as a single dose, to which the patient responded with a moderate diuresis and weight loss of 1.4 kg with subjective and objective improvement of pulmonary congestion. However, a disturbing fall in blood pressure (BP) was noted. Furthermore, the serum creatinine and BUN had increased sharply. Concern for digitalis toxicity, due to hypokalemia, prompted withholding of digoxin while potassium chloride supplements were increased. The pulmonary wedge pressure was found to be elevated to 20.4 mmHg. A second dose of furosemide, 80 mg orally, promoted only a slight diuresis with a further decline in BP and deterioration of renal function. When subsequently it was determined that the patient was underdigitalized, further attempts to promote diuresis were withheld until digitalization could be accomplished. Thereafter, the patient responded to intermittent oral furosemide therapy with improvement in cardiovascular and renal function and clearing of edema.

uresis resulting in significant weight loss with mobilization of both peripheral edema fluid and ascitic fluid (Fig. 13-20) (255). The mechanism relates to the improvement in cardiac output and effective circulating blood volume that attends assumption of the supine position. In the patient with tense ascites the lateral recumbent position is usually better tolerated. This therapeutic approach by itself has obvious limitations but when combined with a program of diet control and judicious diuretic therapy is often effective in mobilizing ascites.

Sodium restriction

When the patient exhibits evidence of weight gain and ascites, it is always advisable to measure the urinary excretion of sodium as a guide to determining the level of sodium restriction. If urinary sodium excretion exceeds 100 meq/day, it obviously indicates dietary indiscretion in a patient with an impaired ability to handle a sodium load. Reducing sodium intake to 50 meq/day when combined with limitation of activity may prove adequate in mobilizing ascites. Many patients, however, will not tolerate this level of sodium restriction or it may be incompatible with the goal of improving nutrition. Thus, the physician may elect to institute diuretic therapy to prevent progression of ascites. If the patient is accumulating

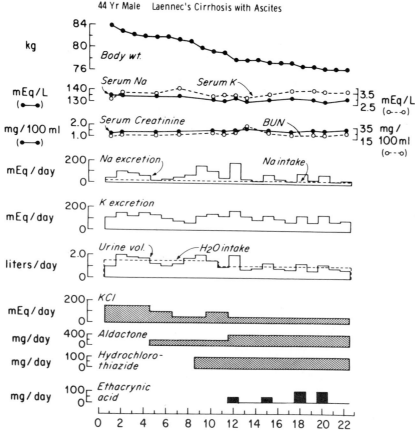

Figure 13-20. Effect of bed rest, sodium restriction, and combination diuretic therapy in a patient with cirrhosis of the liver and ascites. With bed rest and sodium restriction alone the patient experienced a 2-kg weight loss. Addition of Aldactone induced a further reduction in weight without significant change in renal function. Hydrochlorothiazide was then added to the regimen and supplemented with the intermittent administration of ethacrynic acid. Note the decreasing natriuretic response to hydrochlorothiazide and ethacrynic acid which signifies the appearance of diuretic refractoriness; compensatory mechanisms for protecting effective circulating blood volume are intensified reflected by the rise in serum creatinine and BUN and the persistent kaliuresis requiring supplemental KCl to prevent hypokalemia. By using combination drug therapy together with a program of bed rest and sodium restriction this patient was rendered free of ascites while in the hospital. Following discharge, however, despite the continued use of diuretics, ascites reappeared as the patient resumed his usual lifestyle.

ascites and the urine sodium excretion is less than 10 meq/day, progression of the basic disease process is usually signified, most commonly due to continued alcohol abuse. Hospitalization with enforced abstinence together with a program of bed rest, diet and sodium restriction may temporarily interrupt the cycle and allow compensation to be achieved during a sodium intake of 25 to 50 meq/ day. In others unrelenting sodium retention continues and ascites progresses unless sodium intake is severely restricted or diuretic therapy is instituted.

Diuretic therapy

Various diuretic regimens have been proposed for the treatment of ascites (256–259). In general diuretic therapy should not be instituted until a thorough evaluation of all aspects of the patient's disease has been completed and the patient has been shown to be unresponsive to bed rest and sodium restriction. A spontaneous diuresis during bed rest and sodium restriction usually signifies a favorable response to diuretic therapy. Diuretic therapy should be initiated with a distally acting diuretic, spironolactone or triamterene, administered in low doses at first and then increased to maximal doses depending on the magnitude of the response (Fig. 13-20). As has been emphasized by others (255), the reabsorption of ascitic fluid occurs slowly, usually less than 1000 mL/day. Consequently, attempts to induce fluid loss in excess of 1 L/day will inevitably lead to depletion of intravascular volume with serious consequences for renal and hepatic function. Precipitation of hepatic encephalopathy by excessive diuresis is well recognized and may be related to a further decline in hepatic blood flow as well as the development of hypokalemia. The rate of diuresis should be adjusted to prevent deterioration in renal function. Frequent monitoring of serum creatinine, BUN, and serum electrolytes is mandatory. If hypokalemia persists or progresses despite the use of a potassium-sparing diuretic, potassium chloride supplements may be required. The appearance or progression of hyponatremia in this setting usually indicates inadequate fluid restriction.

If a satisfactory diuresis is not induced by the potassium-sparing diuretic, then cautious addition of a site 3 diuretic is suggested beginning with the minimum dose and gradually increasing the dose to achieve the desired effect. It should be obvious that the patient who requires multiple diuretics to mobilize ascitic fluid is in a more advanced stage of liver disease and more susceptible to the multiple complications of excessive diuretic therapy (Fig. 13-21).

Other measures

The goal of therapy is to reduce the symptoms related to ascitic fluid and not simply to eliminate ascites. In many instances even this goal cannot be achieved despite the use of loop diuretics. Prior to the availability of effective diuretics, recurrent ascites was managed by paracentesis. This method has been largely abandoned. The complications of infection, protein depletion, volume depletion, and electrolyte imbalance that often attend this procedure have been well documented. At present paracentesis is reserved for diagnostic purposes or to relieve respiratory distress in the patient with tense ascites. Occasionally the slow removal of several liters of ascitic fluid will be followed by a spontaneous diuresis or increased diuretic responsiveness. Other methods have included hemodialysis, intravenous infusion of ascitic fluid, or more recently the reinfusion of protein concentrate obtained by ultrafiltration of ascitic fluid (260).

These methods are of little long-term benefit. Enthusiasm for portacaval shunt procedures for the treatment of intractable ascites has faded due to the unacceptably high morbidity and mortality of this therapy. More recently, intractable ascites has been managed by peritoneovenous shunting of ascites through a chronically implanted catheter with a pressure-sensitive valve (261).

TREATMENT OF THE NEPHROTIC SYNDROME

Therapy for the primary disorder, increased glomerular capillary permeability to albumin, is limited but should not be neglected. The diagnosis

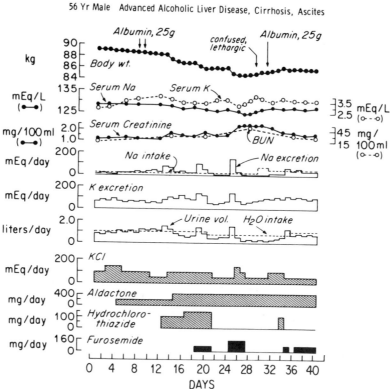

Figure 13-21. Refractory ascites in a patient with advanced cirrhosis of the liver due to chronic alcoholism. The indication for diuretic therapy in this patient was tense ascites which severely restricted his activity. Bed rest, sodium restriction, and Aldactone were ineffective in promoting a diuresis and weight loss. Infusion of salt-poor albumin to expand effective circulating blood volume was also unsuccessful in promoting a diuresis. A slight natriuresis was induced with hydrochlorothiazide. Addition of furosemide led to a further loss of 1 kg of body weight, but note the rise in BUN and serum creatinine reflecting contraction of intravascular volume leading to reduced GFR. Diuretic therapy was withheld for 3 days in order to allow time for intravascular volume to be repleted from the ascitic fluid. Note the persisting hypokalemia, despite larger potassium supplements combined with Aldactone and note the increasing hyponatremia which necessitated further water restriction. Attempts to mobilize additional ascitic fluid with larger doses of furosemide led to further decline in renal function as manifested by the rise in serum creatinine and BUN and appearance of impending hepatic encephalopathy. Sodium intake was liberalized and diuretic therapy was withheld; this led to the gradual improvement in the patient's mental status and renal function. Subsequently diuretic therapy was adjusted to prevent reaccumulation of ascites. This therapeutic goal was achieved only while the patient remained in the hospital.

of "nil disease" established by immunofluorescent and electron microscopic examination of renal tissue warrants a trial of steroid therapy. Steroid therapy has not been documented to be effective in the treatment of other causes of nephrotic syndrome. When the nephrotic syndrome is related to an allergen, toxin, or drug, elimination of the offending agent will frequently lead to clearing or reduction in proteinuria. In patients with nephrotic syndrome associated with infec-

tion, such as shunt nephritis, treatment of the infection may lead to remission. Similarly, in nephrotic syndrome associated with malignancy, regression of the malignancy during therapy may be accompanied by improvement of the nephrotic syndrome. In the vast majority of patients, however, therapy is limited to controlling those factors which contribute to or aggravate sodium retention and edema formation. Since the nephrotic syndrome is often part of a systemic disease, attention must be given to the possibility that cardiovascular disease or liver disease may be contributing to the development or progression of edema.

The same principles of decreased activity with elevation of the lower extremities, support stockings to reduce venous pooling and fluid accumulation, and restriction of sodium intake apply to the management of edema in the nephrotic syndrome. In addition particular attention should be given to nutrition. Although hypoalbuminemia is primarily a consequence of excessive urinary losses, impaired albumin synthesis by the liver due to chronic protein deficiency may be a significant factor. A high-protein diet is advisable in most patients unless contraindicated by advanced chronic renal failure. Diuretic therapy is indicated only for the relief or control of symptomatic edema. Attempts to render these patients edema-free with diuretics leads inevitably to further contraction of effective circulating blood volume and increases the risks of hypotension, impairment of renal function, and electrolyte imbalance (Fig. 13-22).

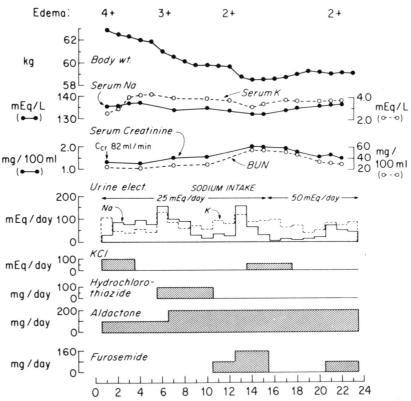

Figure 13-22. Diuretic therapy in a patient with nephrotic syndrome. This patient was found to have idiopathic membranous glomerulonephritis established by light and immunofluorescent microscopy. Proteinuria ranged between 5 and 9 g/day. Serum albumin was 2.3 g/dL. Bed rest, sodium restriction, and Aldactone led to the mobilization of only 1 L of edema fluid. Addition of hydrochlorothiazide together with Aldactone promoted further weight loss and reduction of peripheral edema. Attempts to further reduce edema, however, by adding furosemide led to symptomatic hypotension and deterioration in renal function. Diuretic therapy was withheld and sodium intake liberalized until renal function as assessed by the serum creatinine and BUN returned toward baseline. Subsequently diuretic therapy was tailored to keep the patient from reaccumulating peripheral edema.

TREATMENT OF IDIOPATHIC EDEMA

The problem of idiopathic edema often proves as frustrating to the physician as to the patient. Having established that the patient does experience edema or excessive weight gain, the physician faces the frequently challenging task of trying to determine the cause. A thorough history and physical examination aided by appropriate blood and urine tests will usually identify the major causes of generalized edema. The decision to proceed with more sophisticated studies will be dictated in large measure by the severity of the edema and the extent to which the patient is incapacitated. Having excluded the more obvious causes of edema, the physician prescribes support stockings, periods of rest during the day with elevation of the legs, and restricted sodium intake. Many persons will not adhere to this regimen, and intermittent diuretic therapy may be required. Diuretic abuse by these patients is common and may compound their symptoms by inducing wide fluctuations in weight. Diuretic-induced edema has been reported in these patients (262). Presumably the diuretic activates compensatory mechanisms for retaining sodium and water that exceed the natriuretic effect of the drug, thereby promoting further edema formation.

CONCLUSION

It is evident that edema formation is an expression of a basic derangement in ECF regulation. The fundamental abnormality common to the major edema syndromes is an ineffective circulating blood volume. The renal mechanisms which mediate sodium and water retention in these syndromes are the same. The clinical expression of the syndromes varies depending on the distribution of the retained fluid which is determined by the basic disease process. Appropriate therapy depends upon proper diagnosis and understanding of the pathogenesis of these disorders.

REFERENCES

1. Strauss, M. B., E. Lamdin, W. P. Smith, and D. J. Bleifer: Surfeit and deficit of sodium: A kinetic concept of sodium excretion, *Arch. Intern. Med.,* **102:**527, 1958.
2. Braunwald, E., W. H. Plauth, Jr., and A. G. Morrow: A method for the detection and quantification of impaired sodium excretion, *Circulation,* **32:**223, 1965.
3. Gauer, O. H., J. P. Henry, and C. Behn: The regulation of extracellular volume, *Ann. Rev. Physiol.,* **32:**547, 1970.
4. Gauer, O. H., and H. L. Thron: Postural changes in the circulation, *Handbook of Physiology,* sec. 2, vol. 3, American Physiol. Soc., Washington, D.C., 1965, p. 2409.
5. Epstein, F. H., A. V. N. Goodyer, F. D. Lawrason, and A. S. Relman: Studies on the antidiuresis of quiet standing: The importance of changes in plasma volume and glomerular filtration rate, *J. Clin. Invest.,* **30:**63, 1951.
6. Gauer, O. H., and J. P. Henry: Circulatory basis of fluid volume control, *Physiol. Rev.,* **43:**423, 1963.
7. Henry, J. P., O. H. Gauer, and J. L. Reeves: Evidence of the atrial location of receptors influencing urine flow, *Circ. Res.,* **4:**85, 1956.
8. Henry, J. P., and J. W. Pearce: The possible role of cardiac atrial stretch receptors in the induction of changes in urine flow, *J. Physiol. (London),* **131:**572, 1956.
9. Ledsome, J. R., and R. J. Linden: The role of left atrial receptors in the diuretic response to left atrial distention, *J. Physiol. (London),* **198:**487, 1968.
10. Share, L.: Effects of carotid occlusion and left atrial distention on plasma vasopressin titer, *Am. J. Physiol.,* **208:**219, 1965.
11. Paintal, A. S.: Vagal sensory receptors and their reflex effects, *Physiol. Rev.,* **53:**159, 1973.
12. DeTorrente, A., G. L. Robertson, K. M. McDonald, and R. W. Schrier: Mechanism of diuretic response to increased left atrial pressure in the anesthetized dog, *Kidney Int.,* **8:**355, 1975.
13. Goetz, K. L., G. C. Bond, and D. D. Bloxham: Atrial receptors and renal function, *Physiol. Rev.,* **55:**157, 1975.
14. Oberg, B.: Overall cardiovascular regulation, *Ann. Rev. Physiol.,* **38:**537–570, 1976.
15. Shepherd, J. T.: Intrathoracic baroreceptors, *Mayo Clin. Proc.,* **48:**426–437, 1973.

16. Clement, D. L., C. L. Pelletier, and J. T. Shepherd: Role of vagal afferents in the control of renal sympathetic nerve activity in the rabbit, *Circ. Res.*, **31**:824–830, 1972.

17. Pelletier, C. L., A. J. Edis, and J. T. Sheperd: Circulatory reflex from vagal afferents in response to hemorrhage in the dog, *Circ. Res.*, **29**:626–634, 1971.

18. Oberg, B., and P. Thoren: Circulatory responses to stimulation of left ventricular receptors in the cat, *Acta Physiol. Scand.*, **88**:8–22, 1973.

19. Karim, F., C. Kidd, C. M. Malpus, and P. E. Penna: The effects of stimulation of the left atrial receptors on sympathetic efferent nerve activity, *J. Physiol. (London)*, **227**:243–260, 1972.

20. Lydtin, H., and W. E. Hamilton: Effect of acute changes in left atrial pressure on urine flow in unanesthetized dogs, *Am. J. Physiol.*, **207**:530–536, 1964.

21. Gorfinkel, H. J., J. P. Szidow, L. J. Hirsch, and A. P. Fishman: Renal performance in experimental cardiogenic shock, *Am. J. Physiol.*, **22**:1260–1268, 1972.

22. Kahl, F. R., J. F. Flint, and J. P. Szidon: Influence of left atrial distention on renal vasomotor tone, *Am. J. Physiol.*, **226**:240–246, 1974.

23. Brennan, L. A., Jr., R. L. Malvin, K. E. Jochim, and D. E. Roberts: Influence of right and left atrial receptors on plasma concentrations of ADH and renin, *Am. J. Physiol.*, **221**:273–278, 1971.

24. Watkins, L., Jr., J. A. Burton, E. Haber, J. R. Cant, F. W. Smith, and A. C. Barger: The renin-angiotensin-aldosterone system in congestive failure in conscious dogs, *J. Clin. Invest.*, **57**:1606–1617, 1976.

25. Mancia, G., J. C. Romero, and J. T. Shepherd: Continuous inhibition of renin release in dogs by vagally innervated receptors in the cardiopulmonary region, *Circ. Res.*, **36**:529–535, 1975.

26. Schrier, R. W., E. A. Reid, T. Berl, and L. E. Earley: Parasympathetic pathways, renin secretion and vasopressin release, *Clin. Sci. Mol. Med.*, **48**:83–89, 1975.

27. Haberisch, F. J.: Osmoregulation in the portal circulation, *Fed. Proc.*, **27**:1137–1141, 1968.

28. Daly, J. J., J. Roe, and P. Horrocks. A comparison of sodium excretion following the infusion of saline into systemic and portal veins in the dog, *Clin. Sci.*, **33**:481–487, 1967.

29. Strandhoy, J. W., and H. E. Williamson: Evidence for an hepatic role in the control of sodium excretion, *Proc. Soc. Exp. Biol. Med.*, **33**:419–422, 1970.

30. Passo, S. S., J. R. Thornborough, and S. R. Rothballer: Hepatic receptors in control of sodium excretion in anesthetized cats, *Am. J. Physiol.*, **224**:373–375, 1972.

31. Niijima, A.: Baroreceptor effects on renal and adrenal nerve activity, *Am. J. Physiol.*, **230**:1733–1736, 1976.

32. Iriuchijima, J., and M. F. Wilson: Sympathetic vasoconstrictor activity to the kidney in carotid occlusion pressor reflex, *Proc. Soc. Exp. Biol. Med.*, **131**:189–192, 1969.

33. Ninomiya, I., and H. Irisawa: Summation of baroreceptor reflex effects on sympathetic nerve activities, *Am. J. Physiol.*, **216**:1330–1336, 1969.

34. Kezdi, P., and E. Geller: Baroreceptor control of postganglionic sympathetic nerve discharge, *Am. J. Physiol.*, **214**:427–435, 1968.

35. Kendrick, E., B. Oberg, and G. Wennergren: Extent of engagement of various cardiovascular effectors to alteration of carotid sinus pressure, *Acta Physiol. Scand.*, **86**:410–418, 1972.

36. Kendrick, E., B. Oberg, and G. Wennergren: Vasoconstrictor fiber discharge to skeletal muscle, kidney, intestine and skin at varying levels of arterial baroreceptor activity in the cat, *Acta Physiol. Scand.*, **85**:464–476, 1972.

37. Oberg, B., and S. White: Role of vagal cardiac nerves and arterial baroreceptor in the circulatory adjustments to hemorrhage in the cat, *Acta Physiol. Scand.*, **80**:395–403, 1970.

38. Kendrick, J. E., and G. L. Matson: Effects of carotid occlusion on the renal and iliac vascular resistance during constant flow and constant perfusion pressure, *Proc. Soc. Exp. Biol. Med.*, **142**:1306–1309, 1973.

39. Mancia, G., J. T. Shepherd, and D. E. Donald: Role of cardiac, pulmonary and carotid mechanoreceptors in the control of hind-limbs and renal circulation in dogs, *Circ. Res.*, **37**:200–208, 1975.

40. Mancia, G., D. E. Donald, and J. T. Shepherd: Inhibition of adrenergic outflow to peripheral blood vessels by vagal afferents from the cardi-

opulmonary region in the dog, *Circ. Res.*, **33**:713–721, 1973.

41. Oberg, B., and S. White: Circulatory effects of interruption and stimulation of cardiac vagal afferents, *Acta Physiol. Scand.*, **80**:383–394, 1970.

42. Rocha e Silva, M., Jr., and M. Rosenberg: The release of vasopressin in response to hemorrhage and its role in the mechanism of blood pressure regulation, *J. Physiol. (London)*, **202**:535–557, 1969.

43. Share, L., and J. R. Claybaugh: Regulation of body fluids, *Ann. Rev. Physiol.*, **34**:235–260, 1972.

44. Skinner, S. L., J. W. McCubbin, and I. H. Page: Control of renin secretion, *Circ. Res.*, **15**:64–76, 1964.

45. Bunag, R. D., I. H. Page, and J. W. McCubbin: Neural stimulation of renin, *Circ. Res.*, **19**:851–858, 1966.

46. Hodge, R. L., R. D. Lowe, and J. R. Vane: Increased angiotensin formation in response to carotid occlusion in the dog, *Nature*, **211**:491–493, 1966.

47. Davis, J. O. and R. H. Freeman: Mechanisms regulating renin release, *Physiol. Rev.*, **56**:1, 1976.

48. Astrom, A., and J. Crafoord: Afferent activity recorded in the kidney nerves of rats, *Acta Physiol. Scand.*, **70**:10–15, 1967.

49. Beacham, W. S., and D. L. Kunze: Renal receptors evoking a spinal vasomotor reflex. *J. Physiol.*, **201**:73–83, 1969.

50. Niijima, A.: Afferent discharges from arterial mechanoreceptors in the kidney of the rabbit, *J. Physiol.*, **219**:477–485, 1971.

51. Niijima, A.: Observations on the localization of mechanoreceptors in the kidney and afferent nerve fibers in the renal nerves in the rabbit, *J. Physiol.*, **245**:81–90, 1975.

52. Ueda, H., Y. Uchida, and K. Kamisaka: Mechanism of reflex depressor effect by kidney in dog, *Jap. Heart J.*, **8**:597–606, 1967.

53. Aars, H., and S. Akra: Reflex changes in sympathetic activity and arterial pressure evoked by afferent stimulation of the renal nerve, *Acta Physiol. Scand.*, **78**:184–188, 1970.

54. Astrom, A., and J. Crafoord: Afferent and efferent activity in the renal nerves of cats, *Acta Physiol. Scand.*, **74**:69–78, 1968.

55. Calaresu, F. R., A. Stella, and A. Zanchetti: Hemodynamic responses and renin release during stimulation of afferent renal nerves in the cat, *J. Physiol. (London)*, **255**:687–700, 1976.

56. Andersson, B., M. F. Dallman, and K. Olsson: Evidence for hypothalamic control of renal sodium excretion, *Acta Physiol. Scand.*, **75**:496–510, 1969.

57. Andersson, B., and L. Eriksson: Conjoint action of sodium and angiotensin on brain mechanisms controlling water and salt balance, *Acta Physiol. Scand.*, **81**:18–29, 1971.

58. Andersson, B., M. Jobin, and K. Olsson: A study of thirst and other effects of an increased sodium concentration in the third brain ventricle, *Acta Physiol. Scand.*, **69**:29–36, 1967.

59. Dorn, J. B., H. Levin, G. Kaley, and A. B. Rothballer: Natriuresis induced by injection of hypertonic saline into third cerebral ventricle of dogs, *Proc. Soc. Exp. Biol. Med.*, **131**:240–242, 1969.

60. Dorn, J., and J. C. Porter: Diencephalic involvement in sodium excretion in the rat, *Endocrinology*, **86**:1112–1117, 1970.

61. Mouw, D. R., and A. J. Vander: Evidence for brain Na receptors controlling renal Na excretion and plasma renin activity, *Am. J. Physiol.*, **219**:822–832, 1970.

62. Mouw, D. R., and A. J. Vander: Evidence for hormonal mediation of the renal response to low-sodium stimulation of the brain, *Proc. Soc. Exp. Biol. Med.*, **137**:179–182, 1971.

63. Mouw, D. R., S. F. Abraham, J. R. Blair-West, J. P. Coghlan, D. A. Denton, J. S. McKenzie, M. J. McKinley, and B. A. Scoggins: Brain receptors, renin secretion, and renal sodium retention in conscious sheep, *Am. J. Physiol.*, **226**:56–62, 1974.

64. Greenberg, T. T., W. N. Richmond, R. A. Stocking, P. D. Gupta, J. P. Meehan, and J. P. Henry: Impaired atrial receptor responses in dogs with heart failure due to tricuspid insufficiency and pulmonary artery stenosis, *Circ. Res.*, **32**:424–433, 1973.

65. Gilmore, J. P., and W. M. Daggett: Response of the chronic cardiac denervated dog to acute volume expansion, *Am. J. Physiol.*, **210**:509–512, 1966.

66. Willman, V. L., L. P. Mujavy, R. Pennell, and C. R. Hanlon: Response of the autotransplanted heart to blood volume expansion, *Ann. Surg.*, **166**:513–517, 1967.

67. Knox, F. G., B. B. Davis, and R. W. Berliner: Effect of chronic cardiac denervation on renal response to saline infusion, *Am. J. Physiol.*, **213:**174–178, 1967.

68. McDonald, K. M., A. Rosenthal, R. W. Schrier, J. Galicich, and D. P. Lauler: Effect of interruption of neural pathways on renal response to volume expansion, *Am. J. Physiol.*, **218:**510–517, 1970.

69. Guyton, A. C., T. G. Coleman, and H. J. Granger: Circulation: Overall regulation, *Ann. Rev. Physiol.*, **34:**13–46, 1972.

70. Gill, J. R., Jr.: The role of the sympathetic nervous system in the regulation of sodium excretion by the kidney, in W. F. Ganong and L. Martini (eds.), *Frontiers in Neuroendocrinology,* Oxford University Press, New York, 1969, p. 289.

71. Gill, J. R., Jr., and A. G. T. Casper: Role of the sympathetic nervous system in the renal response to hemorrhage, *J. Clin. Invest.*, **48:**915, 1969.

72. Schrier, R. W.: Effects of adrenergic nervous system and renal hemodynamics, sodium and water excretion and renin secretion, *Kidney Int.*, **6:**291, 1974.

73. Schrier, R. W., and H. E. DeWardener: Tubular reabsorption of sodium ion; influence of factors other than aldosterone and glomerular filtration rate, *N. Engl. J. Med.*, **285:**1231, 1971.

74. Barger, A. C.: Renal hemodynamic factors in congestive heart failure, *Ann. N.Y. Acad. Sci.*, **139:**276, 1966.

75. Pomeranz, B. H., A. G. Birtch, and A. C. Barger: Neural control of intrarenal blood flow, *Am. J. Physiol.*, **214:**1067, 1968.

76. Kilcoyne, M. M., and P. J. Cannon: Influence of thoracic caval occlusion on intrarenal blood flow and sodium excretion, *Am. J. Physiol.*, **220:**1220, 1971.

77. Kilcoyne, M. M., and P. J. Cannon: Neural and humoral influence on intrarenal blood flow distribution during thoracic caval occlusion, *Am. J. Physiol.*, **220:**1231, 1971.

78. Kew, M. C., P. W. Brunt, R. R. Varma, K. L. Harrigan, H. S. Williams, and S. Sherlock: Renal and intrarenal blood-flow in cirrhosis of the liver, *Lancet*, **2:**504, 1971.

79. Truniger, B., S. M. Rosen, A. Grandchamp, H. Strebel, and H. R. Kriek: Redistribution of renal blood flow in hemorrhagic hypotension. Role of renal nerves and circulating catecholamines, *Eur. J. Clin. Invest.*, **1:**277, 1971.

80. Sparks, H. V., H. H. Kopald, S. Carriere, J. E. Chimoskey, M. Kinoshita, and C. A. Barger: Intrarenal distribution of blood flow with chronic congestive heart failure, *Am. J. Physiol.*, **223:**840, 1972.

81. Kilcoyne, M. M., D. H. Schmidt, and P. J. Cannon: Intrarenal blood-flow in congestive heart failure, *Circulation*, **47:**786, 1973.

82. Stein, J. H., S. Boojarern, C. B. Wilson, and T. F. Ferris: Alteration in intrarenal blood flow distribution, *Circ. Res.*, **32, 33** (suppl. I): I-61, 1973.

83. Aukland, K.: Renal blood flow, in K. Thurau (ed.), *Kidney and Urinary Tract Physiology II*, vol. 11, *International Review of Physiology*, University Park Press, Baltimore, 1976, p. 23.

84. Slick, G. L., A. J. Aguilera, E. J. Zambraski, G. F. DiBona, and G. J. Kaloyanides: Renal neuroadrenergic transmission, *Am. J. Physiol.*, **229:**60, 1975.

85. Bello-Reuss, E., R. E. Colindres, E. Pastoriza-Munoz, R. A. Mueller, and C. W. Gottschalk: Effects of acute unilateral renal denervation in the rat, *J. Clin. Invest.*, **56:**208, 1975.

86. Bello-Reuss, E., D. L. Trevino, and C. W. Gottschalk: Effect of renal sympathetic nerve stimulation on proximal water and sodium reabsorption, *J. Clin. Invest.*, **57:**1104, 1976.

87. Müller, J., and L. Barajas: Electron microscopic and histochemical evidence for a tubular innervation of the renal cortex of the monkey, *J. Ultrastruct. Res.*, **41:**533, 1972.

88. Handler, J. S., R. Bensinger, and J. Orloff: Effect of adrenergic agents on toad bladder response to ADH and theophylline, *Am. J. Physiol.*, **214:**1024, 1968.

89. Vander, A. J., and J. R. Luciano: Neural and humoral control of renin release in salt depletion, *Circ. Res.*, **20, 21** (suppl. II): II-69, 1967.

90. Zanchetti, A., and A. Stella: Neural control of renin release, *Clin. Sci. Mol. Med.*, **48:**215S, 1975.

91. Hollenberg, N. K., D. F. Adams, A. Rashid, M. Epstein, H. L. Abrahms, and J. P. Merrill: Renal vascular response to salt restriction in normal man, *Circulation*, **43:**845, 1971.

92. Freeman, R. H., J. O. Davis, S. J. Vitale, and J. A.

Johnson: Intrarenal role of angiotensin II: Homeostatic regulation of renal blood flow in the dog, *Circ. Res.*, **32**:692, 1973.

93. Mimran, A. L., L. Guiod, and N. K. Hollenberg: The role of angiotensin in the cardiovascular and renal response to salt restriction, *Kidney Int.*, **5**:348, 1974.

94. Whitty, R. T., J. O. Davis, R. E. Shade, J. A. Johnson, and R. L. Prewitt: Mechanisms regulating renin release in dogs with thoracic caval constriction, *Circ. Res.*, **31**:339, 1972.

95. Slick, G. L., G. F. DiBona, and G. J. Kaloyanides: Renal blockade to angiotensin II in acute and chronic sodium-retaining states, *J. Pharmacol. Exp. Ther.*, **195**:185, 1975.

96. Taub, K. J., W. J. H. Caldicott, and N. K. Hollenberg: Angiotensin antagonists with increased specificity for the renal vasculature, *J. Clin. Invest.*, **59**:528, 1977.

97. Blair-West, J. R.: Renin angiotensin system and sodium metabolism, in K. Thurau (ed.), *Kidney and Urinary Tract Physiology II*, vol. 11, *International Review of Physiology*, University Park Press, Baltimore, 1976, p. 95.

98. Blantz, R. C., K. S. Konnen, and B. J. Tucker: Angiotensin II effects upon glomerular microcirculation and ultrafiltration coefficient of the rat, *J. Clin. Invest.*, **57**:419, 1976.

99. Freeman, R. H., J. O. Davis, W. S. Spielman, and T. W. Lohmeieri: High-output heart failure in the dog: Systemic and intrarenal role of angiotensin II, *Am. J. Physiol.*, **229**:474, 1975.

100. Young, D. B., R. E. McCaa, Y. Pen, and A. C. Guyton: Effectiveness of the aldosterone sodium and potassium feedback control system, *Am. J. Physiol.*, **231**:945, 1976.

101. August, J. T., D. H. Nelson, and G. W. Thorn: Response of normal subjects to large amounts of aldosterone, *J. Clin. Invest.*, **37**:1549, 1958.

102. Davis, J. O., D. S. Howell, and J. L. Southworth: Mechanisms of fluid retention in experimental preparations in dogs. III. Effect of adrenalectomy and subsequent desoxycorticosterone acetate administration on ascites formation, *Circ. Res.*, **1**:260, 1953.

103. Laragh, J. H.: Hormones and the pathogenesis of congestive heart failure: Vasopressin, aldosterone and angiotensin II, *Circulation*, **25**:1015, 1962.

104. Wolff, H. P.: Aldosterone in congestive heart failure, *Acta Cardiol. (Brux.)*, **20**:424, 1965.

105. Ayers, C. R., R. E. Bowden, and J. E. Schrank: Mechanisms of sodium retention in congestive heart failure, *Adv. Exp. Med. Biol.*, **17**:227, 1972.

106. Klahr, S., and H. J. Rodriguez: Natriuretic hormone, *Nephron*, **15**:387, 1975.

107. Bricker, N. S., R. W. Schmidt, H. Favre, L. Fine, and J. J. Bourgoignie: On the biology of sodium excretion: The search for a natriuretic hormone, *Yale J. Biol. Med.*, **48**:293, 1975.

108. Bourgoiognie, J. J., K. H. Hwang, E. Ipakchi, and N. S. Bricker: The presence of a natriuretic factor in urine of patients with chronic uremia: The absence of the factor in nephrotic uremic patients, *J. Clin. Invest.*, **53**:1559, 1974.

109. Anderson, R. J., T. Berl, K. M. McDonald, and R. W. Schrier: Prostaglandins: Effect on blood pressure, renal blood flow, sodium and water excretion, *Kidney Int.*, **10**:205, 1976.

110. Vatner, S. F.: Effects of hemorrhage on regional blood flow distribution in dogs and primates, *J. Clin. Invest.*, **54**:225, 1974.

111. Zipser, R., J. Hoefs, P. Speckart, P. Zia, and R. Horton: Evidence for a critical role of prostaglandins in renin release, vascular reactivity, and renal function in liver disease, *Clin. Res.*, **25**:305A, 1977.

112. Kaloyanides, G. J., G. F. DiBona, and P. Raskin: Pressure natriuresis in the isolated kidney, *Am. J. Physiol.*, **220**:1660, 1971.

113. Schnermann, J.: Physical forces and transtubular movements of solutes and water, in K. Thurau (ed.), *MTP International Review of Science, Physiology Series One*, vol. 6, *Kidney and Urinary Tract Physiology*, University Park Press, Baltimore, 1974, p. 157.

114. Kunau, R. T., and N. H. Lamiere: The effect of an acute increase in renal perfusion pressure on sodium transport in the rat kidney, *Circ. Res.*, **5**:689, 1976.

115. Nizet, A., J. P. Godon, and P. Mahieu: Comparative excretion of water and sodium load by isolated dog kidney, autonomous renal response to blood dilution factors, *Pfluegers Arch.*, **304**:30, 1968.

116. Braunwald, E., J. Ross, Jr., and E. H. Sonnenblick: *Mechanisms of Contraction in the Normal*

and Failing Heart, Little, Brown and Company, Boston, 1968.

117. Werko, L., E. Varnauskas, H. Eliasch, H. Bucht, B. Thomason, and J. Bergstioni: Studies on the renal circulation and renal function in mitral valvular disease. 1. Effect of exercise, *Circulation,* **9:**687, 1954.

118. Higgins, C. B., S. F. Vatner, D. Franklin, and E. Braunwald: Effects of experimentally produced heart failure on the peripheral vascular response to severe exercise in conscious dogs, *Circ. Res.,* **31:**186, 1972.

119. Millard, R. W., C. B. Higgins, D. Franklin, and S. F. Vatner: Regulation of the renal circulation during severe exercise in normal dogs and dogs with experimental heart failure, *Circ. Res.,* **31:**881, 1972.

120. Higgins, C. B., S. F. Vatner, D. Franklin, and E. Braunwald: Pattern of differential vasoconstriction in response to acute and chronic low-output states in the conscious dog, *Cardiovasc. Res.,* **8:**92, 1974.

121. Chidsey, C. A., D. C. Harrison, and E. Braunwald: Augmentation of the plasma norepinephrine response to exercise in patients with congestive heart failure, *N. Engl. J. Med.,* **267:**650, 1962.

122. Chobanian, A. V., B. A. Burrows, and W. Hollander: Body fluids and electrolyte composition in cardiac patients with severe heart disease but without peripheral edema, *Circulation,* **24:**743, 1961.

123. Vander, A. J., R. L. Malvin, W. S. Wilder, and L. P. Sullivan: Re-examination of salt and water retention in congestive heart failure: Significance of renal filtration fraction, *Am. J. Med.,* **25:**497, 1958.

124. Barger, A. C., F. P. Muldowney, and M. R. Liebowitz: Role of the kidney in the pathogenesis of congestive heart failure, *Circulation,* **20:**273, 1959.

125. Van Loo, A., and E. C. Heringman: Circulatory changes in the dog produced by acute arteriovenous fistula, *Am. J. Physiol.,* **158:**103, 1947.

126. Epstein, F. H., R. S. Post, and M. McDowell: Effects of arteriovenous fistula on renal hemodynamics and electrolyte excretion, *J. Clin. Invest.,* **32:**233, 1953.

127. Hilton, G. H., D. M. Kantar, D. R. Hays, E. H. Bowen, J. R. Golub, J. H. Keating, and R. Wegira: The effects of acute arteriovenous fistula on renal functions, *J. Clin. Invest.,* **34:**732, 1955.

128. Frank, C. W., H. Wang, J. Lammerant, R. Miller, and R. Wegria: An experimental study of the immediate hemodynamic adjustments to acute arteriovenous fistulas of various sizes, *J. Clin. Invest.,* **34:**722, 1955.

129. Guyton, A. C., and K. Sagawa: Compensation of cardiac output and other circulatory functions in areflex dogs with large A-V fistulas, *Am. J. Physiol.,* **200:**1157, 1961.

130. Holman, E.: Contribution to cardiovascular physiology gleamed from clinical and experimental observation of abnormal arteriovenous communications, *J. Cardiovasc. Surg.,* **3:**48, 1962.

131. Taylor, R. R., J. W. Covell, and J. Ross, Jr.: Left ventricular function in experimental aorto-caval fistula with circulatory congestion and fluid retention, *J. Clin. Invest.,* **47:**1333, 1968.

132. Reynolds, T.: Portal hypertension, in Schiff (ed.), *Diseases of the Liver,* 3d ed., J. B. Lippincott Co., Philadelphia, 1969.

133. Liebowitz, H. R.: Pathogenesis of ascites in cirrhosis of liver, *N.Y. State J. Med.,* **69:**1895, 1969.

134. Cohn, J. N., I. M. Khatri, R. J. Groszmann, and B. Kotelanski: Hepatic blood flow in alcoholic liver disease measured by an indicator dilution technique, *Am. J. Med.,* **53:**704, 1972.

135. Bradley, S. E., F. J. Ingelfinger, and G. P. Bradley: Hepatic circulation in cirrhosis of the liver, *Circulation,* **5:**419, 1952.

136. Redeker, A. G., H. M. Geller, and T. B. Reynolds: Hepatic wedge pressure, blood flow, vascular resistance and oxygen consumption in cirrhosis before and after end-to-side portacaval shunt, *J. Clin. Invest.,* **37:**606, 1958.

137. Rothchild, M. A., M. Oratz, D. Zimmon, S. S. Schreiber, I. Weiner, and A. Van Canegheim: Albumin synthesis in cirrhotic subjects with ascites studied with carbonate—^{14}C, *J. Clin. Invest.,* **48:**344, 1969.

138. Dumont, A. E., and M. N. Witte: Significance of excess lymph in the thoracic duct in patients with hepatic cirrhosis, *Am. J. Surg.,* **112:**401, 1966.

139. Zotti, E., A. Lisage, R. Bradham, R. Nignoni, W. Sealy and W. Young, Jr.: Prevention and treatment of experimentally induced ascites in dogs by thoracic duct to vein shunt, *Surgery,* **60:**28, 1966.

140. Warren, W. D., J. J. Fomon, and C. A. Leite: Critical assessment of the rationale of thoracic duct drainage in the treatment of portal hypertension, *Surgery, 63*:7, 1968.

141. Lieberman, F. L., and T. B. Reynolds: Plasma volume in cirrhosis of the liver: Its relation to portal hypertension, ascites and renal failure, *J. Clin. Invest., 46*:1297, 1967.

142. Lieberman, F. L., S. Ito, and T. B. Reynolds: Effects of plasma volume in cirrhosis with ascites. Evidence that a decreased value does not account for renal sodium retention, a spontaneous reduction in GFR and a fall in GFR during drug-induced diuresis, *J. Clin. Invest., 48*:975, 1969.

143. Greenway, C. V., and W. W. Lautt: Effects of hepatic venous pressure on transsinusoidal fluid transfer in the liver of the anesthetized cat, *Circ. Res., 26*:697, 1970.

144. Lautt, W. W., and C. V. Greenway: Hepatic venous compliance and role of liver as a blood reservoir, *Am. J. Physiol., 231*:292, 1976.

145. Papper, S., and L. Saxon: Abnormalities in the excretion of water and sodium in compensated cirrhosis of the liver, *J. Lab. Clin. Med., 40*:423, 1952.

146. Wolff, H. P., K. R. Koczorek, and E. Buchborn: Aldosterone and antidiuretic hormone in liver disease, *Acta. Endocrinol., 27*:45, 1958.

147. Papper, S., and C. A. Vaamonde: The kidney in liver disease, in M. B. Strauss and L. G. Velt (eds.), *Diseases of the Kidney*, Little, Brown and Company, Boston, 1971, p. 1139.

148. Vecsei, P., G. Dusterdieck, J. Johnecke, L. Lommer, and H. P. Wolff: Secretion and turnover of aldosterone in various pathological states, *Clin. Sci., 36*:241, 1969.

149. Schroeder, E. T., R. H. Eich, H. Smulyan, A. B. Gould, and G. J. Gobuzda: Plasma renin level in hepatic cirrhosis, *Am. J. Med., 49*:187, 1970.

150. Manier, J. W., and R. B. Shafer: Renal functional failure associated with cirrhosis, *Am. J. Med. Sci., 262*:276, 1971.

151. Tristani, F. E., and J. N. Cohn: Systemic and renal hemodynamics in oliguric hepatic failure: Effect of volume expansion, *J. Clin. Invest., 46*:1894, 1967.

152. Reynolds, T. B., F. L. Lieberman, and A. G. Rederker: Functional renal failure with cirrhosis.

The effect of plasma expansion therapy, *Medicine (Baltimore), 46*:191, 1967.

153. Mullane, J. F., and M. L. Gliedman: Elevation of the pressure in the inferior vena cava as a cause of hepatorenal syndrome in cirrhosis, *Surgery, 59*:1135, 1966.

154. Robinson, R. M., J. S. Vasko, J. L. Doppman, and A. G. Morrow: Inferior vena caval obstruction from increased intra-abdominal pressure. Experimental and angiographic observations, *Arch. Surg., 91*:935, 1965.

155. Glassock. R. J., and C. M. Bennett: The glomerulopathies, in B. M. Brenner and F. C. Rector, Jr. (eds.), *The Kidney*, W. B. Saunders Company, Philadelphia, 1976, p. 941.

156. Rothschild, M. A., M. Oratz, and S. S. Schreiber: Albumin synthesis, *N. Engl. J. Med., 286*:816, 1972.

157. Yamauchi, H., and J. Hopper, Jr.: Hypovolemic shock and hypotension as a complication in the nephrotic syndrome, *Ann. Intern. Med., 60*:242, 1964.

158. Garnett, E. S., and C. E. Webber: Changes in blood-volume produced by treatment in the nephrotic syndrome, *Lancet, 2*:798, 1967.

159. Hopper, J., Jr., P. Ryan, J. C. Lee, and W. Rosenau: Lipoid nephrosis in 31 adult patients: Renal biopsy study by light electron and fluorescence microscopy with experience in treatment, *Medicine (Baltimore), 49*:321, 1970.

160. Oliver, W. J., R. C. Kelch, and J. P. Chandler: Demonstration of increased catecholamine excretion in the nephrotic syndrome, *Proc. Soc. Exp. Biol. Med., 125*:1176, 1967.

161. Leutscher, J. A., Jr., and B. B. Johnson: Observations on the sodium retaining corticoid (aldosterone) in the urine of children and adults in relation to sodium balance and edema, *J. Clin. Invest., 33*:1441, 1954.

162. Grauz, H., R. Lieberman, and L. E. Earley: Effect of plasma albumin on sodium reabsorption in patients with nephrotic syndrome, *Kidney Int., 1*:47, 1972.

163. Thorn, G. W.: Cyclical edema, *Am. J. Med., 23*:407, 1957.

164. Thorn, G. W.: Approach to the patient with idiopathic edema or periodic swelling, *JAMA, 206*:333, 1968.

165. Streeten, D. H. P.: The role of posture in idiopathic edema, *S. Afr. Med. J.*, **49**:462, 1975.

166. Streeten, D. H. P., T. G. Dalakos, M. Souma, H. Fellerman, G. V. Clift, F. E. Schletter, C. T. Stevenson, and P. J. Speller: Studies of the pathogenesis of idiopathic edema: The roles of postural changes in plasma volume, plasma renin activity, aldosterone secretion rate and glomerular filtration rate in the retention of sodium and water, *Clin. Sci. Mol. Med.*, **45**:347, 1973.

167. Edwards, O. M., and R. I. S. Bayliss: Idiopathic edema of women, *Q. J. Med.*, **45**:125, 1976.

168. Gill, J. R., Jr., D. T. Mason, and F. C. Bartter: Idiopathic edema resulting from occult cardiomyopathy, *Am. J. Med.*, **38**:475, 1965.

169. Obeid, A. I., D. H. P. Streeten, R. H. Eich, H. Smulyan, F. E. Schletter, and G. V. Clift: Cardiac function in idiopathic edema, *Arch. Intern. Med.*, **134**:253, 1974.

170. Gill, J. R., Jr., J. Cox, C. S. Delea, and F. C. Bartter: Idiopathic edema. II Pathogenesis of edema in patients with hypoalbuminemia, *Am. J. Med.*, **52**:452, 1972.

171. Marieb, M. J., and P. J. Mulrow: Failure to escape. A mechanism in idiopathic edema, *J. Clin. Invest.*, **43**:1279, 1964.

172. Coleman, M., M. Horwith, and J. L. Brown. Idiopathic edema. Studies demonstrating protein-leaking angiopathy, *Am. J. Med.*, **49**:106, 1970.

173. Sims, E. A. H., B. R. MacKay, and T. Shira: The relation of capillary angiopathy and diabetes to idiopathic edema, *Ann. Intern. Med.*, **63**:972, 1965.

174. Weinbren, I, P. I. Taggart, and H. I. Glass: Edema due to abnormal distribution of protein, *Lancet*, **3**:512, 1965.

175. Jones, E. M., R. H. Fox, P. W. Ferrow, and A. W. Asscher: Variations in capillary permeability to plasma proteins during the menstrual cycle, *J. Obstet. Gynaec. Br. Commonw.*, **73**:666, 1966.

176. Edwards, O. M., and R. I. S. Bayliss: Postural fluid retention in patients with idiopathic edema: Lack of relationship to the phase of the menstrual cycle, *Clin. Sci. Mol. Med.*, **48**:331, 1975.

177. Gill, J. R., Jr., T. A. Waldmann, and F. C. Bartter: Idiopathic edema. I. The occurrence of hypoalbuminemia in women with unexplained edema, *Am. J. Med.*, **52**:444, 1972.

178. Fisher, D. A., and M. D. Morris: Idiopathic edema and hyperaldosteronuria: Postural venous pooling, *Pediatrics*, **35**:413, 1965.

179. Epstein, A. N.: The physiology of thirst, *Can. J. Physiol. Pharmacol.*, **54**:639, 1976.

180. Bennett, W. M., C. B. Grover, Jr., J. N. Antonovic, and G. A. Porter: Influence of volume expansion on proximal tubular reabsorption in congestive heart failure, *Am. Heart J.*, **85**:55, 1973.

181. Gibson, D. G., J. C. Marshall, and E. Lockey: Assessment of proximal tubule sodium reabsorption during water diuresis in patients with heart disease, *Br. Heart J.*, **32**:399, 1970.

182. Bell, N. H., H. P. Schedl, and F. P. Bartter: An explanation for abnormal water retention and hypo-osmolality in congestive heart failure, *Am. J. Med.*, **36**:351, 1964.

183. Schedl, H. P., and F. C. Bartter: An explanation for an experimental correction of the abnormal water diuresis in cirrhosis, *J. Clin. Invest.*, **39**:248, 1970.

184. Robertson, G. L., R. L. Shelton, and S. Athar: The osmoregulation of vasopressin, *Kidney Int.*, **10**:25, 1976.

185. Berliner, R. W., and P. G. Davidson: Production of hypertonic urine in the absence of pituitary antidiuretic hormone, *J. Clin. Invest.*, **36**: 1416, 1957.

186. Lamdin, E., C. R. Kleeman, M. Rubini, and F. H. Epstein: Studies on alcohol diuresis. III. The response to ethyl alcohol in certain disease states characterized by impaired water tolerance, *J. Clin. Invest.*, **35**:386, 1956.

187. Murdaugh, H. V., Jr.: Production of diuresis in hyponatremic states with alcohol, *J. Clin. Invest.*, **35**:726, 1956.

188. Yamani, Y.: Plasma ADH levels in patients with congestive heart failure, *Jap. Circ. J.*, **32**:745, 1968.

189. Chaudhury, R. R., H. K. Chuttani, and V. Ramalingswani: The antidiuretic hormone and liver damage, *Clin. Sci.*, **21**:199, 1961.

190. Papper, S., and L. Saxon: The diuretic response to administered water in patients with liver disease. II. Laennec's cirrhosis of the liver, *Arch. Intern. Med.*, **103**:750, 1959.

191. Baldus, W. P., R. N. Feichter, and W. H. J. Summerskill: The kidney in cirrhosis. I. Clinical and biochemical features of the azotemia of hepatic failure, *Ann. Intern. Med.*, **60**:600, 1964.

192. Shear, L., P. W. Hall, and G. J. Gabuzda: Renal failure in patients with cirrhosis of the liver. II. Factors influencing maximal urinary flow rate, *Am. J. Med.*, **39**:198, 1965.

193. Goldberg, M.: The renal physiology of diuretics, in *Handbook of Physiology*, sec. 8, *Renal Physiology*, American Physiol. Soc., Washington, D.C., 1973, p. 1003.

194. Suki, W. N., G. Eknoyan, and M. Martinez-Maldonado: Tubular sites and mechanisms of diuretic action, *Ann. Rev. Pharmacol.*, **13**:91, 1973.

195. Seely, J. F., and J. H. Dirks: Site of action of diuretic drugs, *Kidney Int.*, **11**:1, 1977.

196. Burg, M. B.: Mechanisms of action of diuretic drugs, in B. M. Brenner and F. C. Rector, Jr. (eds.), *The Kidney*, W. B. Saunders Company, Philadelphia, 1976, p. 737.

197. Maren, T. H.: Carbonic anydrase: Chemistry, physiology and inhibition, *Physiol. Rev.*, **47**:595, 1967.

198. Cafruny, E. J.: The site and mechanism of action of mercurial diuretics, *Pharmacol. Rev.*, **20**:89, 1968.

199. Burg, M., and N. Green: Effect of mersalyl on the thick ascending limb of Henle's loop, *Kidney Int.*, **4**:245, 1973.

200. Evanson, R. L., E. A. Lockart, and J. H. Dirks: Effect of mercurial diuretics on the tubular sodium and potassium transport in dogs, *Am. J. Physiol.*, **222**:282, 1972.

201. Stein, J. H., C. B. Wilson, and W. M. Kirkendall: Differences in the acute effects of furosemide and ethacrynic acid in man, *J. Lab. Clin. Med.*, **71**:654, 1968.

202. Puschett, J. B., and M. Goldberg: The acute effects of furosemide on acid and electrolyte excretion in man, *J. Lab. Clin. Med.*, **71**:666, 1968.

203. Burg, M., L. Stoner, J. Cardinal, and N. Green: Furosemide effect on isolated perfused tubules, *Am. J. Physiol.*, **225**:119, 1973.

204. Stason, W. B., P. J. Cannon, H. O. Heinemann, and J. H. Laragh: Furosemide: Clinical evaluation of its diuretic action, *Circulation*, **34**:910, 1966.

205. Stewart, J. H., and K. D. G. Edwards: Clinical comparisons of furosemide with bendrofluazide, mersalyl and ethacrynic acid, *Br. Med. J.*, **2**:1277, 1965.

206. Barnett, A. J., and D. G. Robertson: Treatment of resistant edema with new diuretics, ethacrynic acid and furosemide, *Med. J. Aust.*, **2**:531, 1965.

207. Seller, R. H., S. Banach, T. Namey, M. Neff, and C. Swartz: Cardiac effect of diuretic drugs, *Am. Heart J.*, **89**:493, 1975.

208. Martinez-Maldonado, M., G. Eknoyan, and W. N. Suki: Diuretics in non-edematous states, *Arch. Intern. Med.*, **121**:797, 1973.

209. Muth, R. G.: Diuretic properties of furosemide in renal disease, *Ann. Intern. Med.*, **69**:249, 1968.

210. Huang, C. M., A. J. Atkinson, Jr., M. Levin, N. W. Levin, and A. Quintanilla: Pharmocokinetics of furosemide in advanced renal failure, *Clin. Pharmacol. Ther.*, **16**:659, 1974.

211. Schwartz, G. H., D. S. David, R. R. Riggio, K. H. Stenzel, and A. L. Rubin: Ototoxicity induced by Frusemide, *N. Engl. J. Med.*, **282**:1413, 1970.

212. Wigand, M. E., and A. Heidland: Ototoxic side-effects of high doses of Frusemide in patients with uremia, *Postgrad. Med. J.*, **47** (suppl. Apr): **54** 1971.

213. Heidland, A., and M. E. Wigand: Einslus hoher Furosemiddosen auf die Gehörfunktion bie Uramie, *Klin. Wochenschr.*, **48**:1052, 1970.

214. Beyer, K. H., J. E. Baer, J. F. Michaelson, and H. F. Russo: Renotropic characteristics of ethacrynic acid: A phenoxyacetic saluretic-diuretic agent, *J. Pharmacol. Exp. Ther.*, **147**:1, 1965.

215. Burg, M., and N. Green: Effect of ethacrynic acid on the thick ascending limb of Henle's loop, *Kidney Int.*, **4**:301, 1973.

216. Cannon, P. J., H. O. Heinemann, W. B. Stasson, and J. H. Laragh: Ethacrynic acid: Effectiveness and mode of diuretic action in man, *Circulation*, **31**:5, 1965.

217. Maher, J. F., and G. E. Schreiner: Studies on ethacrynic acid in patients with refractory edema, *Arch. Intern. Med.*, **62**:15, 1965.

218. Hagedorn, C. W., A. M. Kaplan, and W. H. Hulet: Prolonged administration of ethacrynic acid in patients with chronic renal disease, *N. Engl. J. Med.*, **272**:1152, 1965.

219. Matz, G. J., D. D. Beal, and L. Krames: Ototoxicity of ethacrynic acid, *Arch. Otolaryngol.*, **90**:152, 1969.

220. Meriwether, W. D., R. J. Mangi, and A. A. Serpick: Deafness following standard intravenous dose of ethacrynic acid, *JAMA*, **216**:795, 1971.

221. Beyer, K., and J. Baer: Physiological basis for the action of newer diuretic agents, *Pharmacol. Rev.,* **13:**517, 1961.

222. Pitts, R., F. Kruch, R. Lozano, D. Taylor, O. Heindenreich, and R. Kessler: Studies on the mechanism of diuretic action of chlorothiazides, *J. Pharmacol. Exp. Ther.,* **123:**89, 1958.

223. Kunau, R., D. Weller, and H. Webb: Clarification of the site of action of chlorothiazide in the rat nephron, *J. Clin. Invest.,* **56:**401, 1975.

224. Fichman, M. P., H. Vorherr, C. R. Kleeman, and N. Telfer: Diuretic-induced hyponatremia, *Ann. Intern. Med.,* **75:**853, 1971.

225. Dollery, C. T.: Diuretic drugs, in Meyler and Herxheimer (eds.), *Side Effects of Drugs,* Excerpta Medica, Amsterdam, 1971, p. 307.

226. Gordon, P.: Glucose intolerance in hypokalemia, *Diabetes,* **22:**544, 1973.

227. Steele, T. H., and S. Oppenheimer: Factors affecting urate excretion following diuretic administration in man, *Am. J. Med.,* **47:**564, 1969.

228. Beaudry, C., and L. Laplante: Severe allergic pneumonitis from hydrochlorothiazide, *Ann. Intern. Med.,* **78:**251, 1973.

229. Lyons, H., V. W. Pinn, S. Cortell, J. J. Cohen, and J. T. Harrington: Allergic interstitial nephritis causing reversible renal failure in four patients with idiopathic nephrotic syndrome, *N. Engl. J. Med.,* **288:**124, 1973.

230. Fuchs, M., J. H. Moyer, and B. E. Newman: Human clinical pharmacology of the newer diuretics: Benzothiadiazine and phthalimidine, *Ann. N.Y. Acad. Sci.,* **88:**795, 1960.

231. Suki, W. N., F. Dawoud, G. Eknoyan, and M. Martinez-Maldonado: Effects of metolazone on renal function in normal man, *J. Pharmacol. Exp. Ther.,* **180:**6, 1972.

232. Fernandez, P. C., and J. B. Puschett: Proximal tubular actions of metolazone and chlorothiazide, *Am. J. Physiol.,* **225:**954, 1973.

233. Tilstone, W. J., H. Dargie, E. N. Dargie, H. G. Morgan, and A. C. Kennedy: Pharmacokinetics of metolazone in normal subjects and in patients with cardiac or renal failure, *Clin. Pharmacol. Ther.,* **16:**322, 1974.

234. Puschett, J. B., and A. Rastegar: Comparative study of the effects of metolazone and other diuretics on potassium excretion, *Clin. Pharmacol. Exp. Ther.,* **15:**397, 1974.

235. Liddle, G.: Specific and non-specific inhibition of mineralocorticoid activity, *Metabolism,* **10:**1021, 1961.

236. Liddle, G.: Aldosterone antagonists and triamterene, *Ann. N.Y. Acad. Sci.,* **139:**466, 1966.

237. Edelman, I., and G. Fimognari: *On the Biochemical Mechanism of Action of Aldosterone. Recent Progress in Hormone Research,* Academic Press, Inc., New York, 1968, p. 1.

238. Sharp, G. W. G., and A. Leaf: Effects of aldosterone and its mechanism of action on sodium transport, *Handbook of Physiology,* sec. 8, *Renal Physiology,* American Physiol. Society, Washington, D.C., 1973, p. 815.

239. Loriaux, D. L., R. Menard, A. Taylor, J. C. Pita, and R. Santen: Spironolactone and endocrine dysfunction, *Ann. Intern. Med.,* **85:**630, 1976.

240. Tweeddale, M. G., and R. I. Olgivie: Antagonism of spironolactone-induced natriuresis by aspirin in man, *N. Engl. J. Med.,* **289:**198, 1973.

241. Weibelhaus, V. D., J. Weinstock, A. R. Maas, F. T. Brennan, G. Sosnowski, and T. Larsen: The diuretic and natriuretic activity of triamterene and several related pteridines in the rat, *J Pharmacol. Exp. Ther.,* **149:**397, 1965.

242. Baba, W. I., G. R. Tudhope, and C. M. Wilson: Triamterene, a new diuretic drug. I. Studies in normal men and in adrenalectomized rats, *Br. Med. J.,* **2:**756, 1962.

243. Baba, W. I., G. R. Tudhope, and G. M. Wilson: Site and mechanism of action of the diuretic, triamterene, *Clin. Sci.,* **27:**181, 1964.

244. Smith, T. W.: Drug therapy: Digitalis glycosides, *N. Engl. J. Med.,* **288:**719, 942, 1973.

245. Smith, T. W., and E. Haber: Digitalis, *N. Engl. J. Med.,* **289:**945, 1010, 1063, 1125, 1973.

246. Cohn, J. N.: Indications for digitalis therapy: A new look, *JAMA,* **229:**1911, 1974.

247. Rubin, I. L., S. R. Arbeit, and H. Gross: Diuretics versus digitalis in the treatment of congestive heart failure, *J. Clin. Pharmacol.,* **12:**121, 1972.

248. Rosenberg, B., G. Dobkin, and R. Rubin: The intravenous use of ethacrynic acid in the management of acute pulmonary edema, *Am. Heart J.,* **70:**333, 1965.

249. Davidov, M., N. Kakaviatos, and F. Finnerty, Jr.:

Intravenous administration of furosemide in heart failure, *JAMA,* **200:**824, 1967.

250. Scheinman, M., M. Brown, and E. Rapaport: Hemodynamic effects of ethacrynic acid in patients with refractory acute left ventricular failure, *Am. J.Med.,* **50:**291, 1971.

251. Dikshit, K., J. V. Vyden, J. S. Forrester, K. Chatterjee, R. Prakash, and H. J. C. Swan: Renal and extrarenal hemodynamic effects of furosemide in congestive heart failure after acute myocardial infarction, *N. Engl. J. Med.,* **288:**1087, 1973.

252. Tattersfield, A. E., M. W. McNicol, and R. W. Sillet: Hemodynamic effects of intravenous frusemide in patients with myocardial infarction and left ventricular failure, *Clin. Sci. Mol. Med.,* **46:**253, 1974.

253. Guiha, N. H., J. N. Cohn, E. Mikulic, J. A. Franciosa, and C. J. Limas: Treatment of refractory heart failure with infusion of nitroprusside, *N. Engl. J. Med.,* **291:**587, 1974.

254. Chaterjee, K., D. Drew, W. W. Parmley, S. C. Klausner, J. Polansky, and B. Zacherle: Combined vasodilator therapy for severe chronic congestive heart failure, *Ann. Intern. Med.,* **85:**467, 1977.

255. Shear, L., S. Ching, and G. J. Gabuzda: Compartmentalization of ascites and edema in patients with hepatic cirrhosis, *N. Engl. J. Med.,* **282:**1391, 1970.

256. Lieberman, F. L., and T. B. Reynolds: The use of ethacrynic acid in patients with cirrhosis and ascites, *Gastroenterol.,* **49:**531, 1965.

257. Vesin, P.: Diuretic therapy in hepatic cirrhosis, *Lancet,* **2:**1424, 1966.

258. Sherlock, S., B. Senewiratne, A. Scott, and J. G. Walker: Complications of diuretic therapy in hepatic cirrhosis, *Lancet,* **1:**1050, 1966.

259. Arroya, V., and J. Rodes: A rational approach to the treatment of ascites, *Postgrad. Med. J.,* **51:**558, 1975.

260. Parbhoo, S. P., and A. Ajdukiewicz: Treatment of ascites by continuous ultrafiltration and reinfusion of protein concentrate, *Lancet,* **1:**949, 1974.

261. Leveen, A. H., G. Christoudias, I. P. Moon, R. Luft, G. Falk, and S. Grosberg: Peritoneo-venous shunting for ascites, *Ann. Surg.,* **180:**580, 1974.

262. MacGregor, G. A., P. R. W. Tasker, and H. E. DeWardener: Diuretic-induced edema, *Lancet,* **3:**489, 1975.

14

Fluid electrolyte and acid-base abnormalities in hypertensive disease

GORDON H. WILLIAMS / ROBERT G. DLUHY

INTRODUCTION

Hypertension is a common cause of altered electrolyte and water homeostasis. The mechanism(s) by which hypertension is produced is incompletely understood. Since an elevated blood pressure may result from a derangement in volume homeostatic forces the kidneys and cardiovascular system are critical components in maintaining blood pressure in the normal range. Cardiovascular and renal responses are modulated by a variety of agents, such as aldosterone, ADH (antidiuretic hormone), angiotensin II, and the catecholamines.

Most investigators describing abnormalities in patients with hypertension have studied their subjects in a chronic or basal state. More recently, however, with sensitive assay techniques available, the acute responsiveness of a number of parameters determining volume, electrolyte balance, and blood pressure in patients with hypertension has been under intensive investigation. These studies revealed a number of differences between certain groups of patients with hypertension and normotensive subjects. This chapter will deal with the normal regulation of blood pressure and the changes that occur in various hypertensive states which can produce electrolyte or volume abnormalities.

BASIC CONSIDERATIONS

In other chapters (14 to 20) the role of the heart and kidney in the overall regulation of fluid and electrolyte metabolism is outlined. In this section, we will briefly review some of these concepts and then discuss the relationship of cardiovascular, renal, and hormonal factors to the control of blood pressure.

The cardiovascular system comprises two elements: a system of channels for the distribution of fluid to supply the metabolic needs of the body's tissues, and a pump which induces flow in this system. Derangement of the normal status of either element can change electrolyte, acid-base, and water balance. The changes result directly from deficiencies in the cardiovascular system and indirectly from the impact of these deficiencies on the function of other organ systems.

ROLE OF THE HEART AS A PUMP IN MAINTAINING NORMAL ELECTROLYTE BALANCE

The physiologic functions of the various organ systems of the body depend on the flow of blood bringing nutrients and other agents and removing waste and active products of the organ. This flow is ultimately dependent on cardiac output. Cardiac output in turn is dependent on four interrelated factors: (1) myocardial contractile state (contractility, inotropic state, or the position of the heart's force-velocity curve); (2) preload (the length of cardiac muscle at the onset of contraction); (3) afterload (the tension which the muscle is called upon to develop during contraction); and (4) heart rate. The contractile force can be defined in terms of the maximal velocity of shortening of the muscle fiber; the maximal velocity of shortening with zero load is a sensitive index of contractility. Those agents which increase this maximal velocity and thereby increase myocardial contractility are termed *positive inotropic agents*. Starling in 1918 (1) showed that the strength of contraction of myocardium also depends on the degree of stretch of the muscle fiber prior to contraction. The Starling relationship is an intrinsic regulatory system which can permit the heart to respond with increased contractile force to an increased work load which increases the stretch on the myocardial fibers. This is an effective way to maintain circulatory integrity. However, when the load increases beyond the ability of the ventricle to respond, end-diastolic ventricular pressure rises and cardiac output falls.

Myocardial contractility can be altered by a variety of extrinsic factors. The cardiac sympathetic innervation is probably the single most important mechanism available to the heart for increasing myocardial contractility. Exogenous inotropic agents similarly improve the basic myocardial force-velocity relationship. They include the cardiac glycosides, isoproterenol, calcium, and caffeine. Normal hydrogen ion concentration in conjunction with normal P_{O_2} and P_{CO_2} is necessary for optimal myocardial contractility. Acidosis, hypercapnia, and hypoxia depress myocardial contractility. Loss of function of part of the myocardium, e.g., postmyocardial infarction, will result in depression of overall myocardial contractility. Also, in congestive heart failure the fundamental mechanism necessary for optimal contractility is depressed. The cause of this depression is not known.

CARDIOVASCULAR EFFECTS ON WATER AND ELECTROLYTE METABOLISM MEDIATED THROUGH THE KIDNEY

The kidney is the major organ maintaining electrolyte and water homeostasis. Sodium is the predominant osmotically active ion in the extracellular fluid; therefore, regulation of extracellular fluid volume is achieved by regulating the sodium content. This is determined by the amount of sodium presented to and resorbed by the renal tubules. The first step in the formation of urine is the filtration of blood at the glomerulus. The rate of filtration can be controlled within certain limits by intrinsic renal mechanisms, i.e., afferent and efferent arteriolar resistances, but it is ultimately dependent on the amount of blood pumped to the kidney. When cardiac output decreases, the kidney bears a proportionately greater decrease in flow than other organs. However, intrinsic renal mechanisms maintain a near-normal glomerular filtration rate until the renal blood flow is severely restricted; as the renal blood flow decreases, there is an increase in the postglomerular resistance, which maintains the glomerular filtration rate. This intrinsic regulation is independent of nervous stimuli, as the denervated kidney shows a similar response. The maintenance of a normal filtration rate with a decreased plasma flow increases the filtration fraction; this change may be significant in congestive heart failure.

The bulk of the sodium in the glomerular filtrate is resorbed in the proximal tubule, where fractional resorption usually parallels the filtered load. This phenomenon is termed *glomerular-tubular balance* (see Chaps. 3 and 15). Distal sodium transport involves a much smaller fraction of filtered sodium, and it is modulated by hormones. In the distal collecting duct sodium resorption is rate-limited, and if the quantity of sodium entering the duct is not too large, virtually all of it can be removed from the urine.

Because only a small fraction of the sodium filtered by the glomerulus is finally excreted in the urine, a slight increase in the filtration rate could supply enough additional sodium to double or triple the sodium excretion if no alterations in tubular handling of sodium occurred.

In the normal state, changes in filtration rate have little effect on sodium excretion, because a concomitant change in the tubular resorption of sodium occurs to maintain sodium homeostasis. The exact balance achieved has been amply illustrated by Mueller et al. (2) in experiments on dogs, in which urine was collected separately from each kidney. If a constricting band is placed around one renal artery, there is a marked decrease in the amount of sodium that is excreted by the constricted kidney. Sodium balance is maintained by the contralateral normal kidney, which increases its sodium excretion. However, if the normal kidney is then removed, adjustments take place in the experimental kidney which permit sodium resorption to fully compensate for the decrease in glomerular filtration. Several extrarenal factors, for example, the adrenal cortical hormones, may play a role in this process.

Potassium profoundly affects cardiac contractility and rhythm. The level of serum potassium is regulated in part by the kidney. Tubular resorption of potassium occurs largely in the proximal tubule. Then, distally, under the influence of aldosterone, potassium is secreted in exchange for sodium. Secretion obviously depends on how much sodium is delivered to the distal site for exchange. It is also dependent on the capacity of the exchange mechanism itself, as well as on the rate of secretion of hydrogen ion by the tubule; increased hydrogen ion secretion tends to decrease tubular excretion of potassium and vice versa.

The ability to excrete a water load is dependent on the integrity of the diluting mechanism of the kidney. This is in part a function of hormonal factors and in part a function of intrinsic renal factors. A dilute urine can be formed only if adequate amounts of sodium and water are delivered to the diluting segments of the nephron (see Chap. 5).

REGULATION OF THE RENIN-ANGIOTENSIN-ALDOSTERONE AXIS

The renin-angiotensin-aldosterone axis is the hormonal system most extensively studied in relation to hypertension, since this axis can modulate both sodium and volume homeostasis and vasoconstrictor activity. Thus, an abnormal increase in the responsiveness or the level of activation of this system can raise blood pressure by altering either volume or vasoconstriction or both. Abnormal function of this system may also derange potassium balance.

Renin-angiotensin physiology

Renin is a proteolytic enzyme with an approximate molecular weight of 35,000 to 40,000. It has been partially purified. It is produced and stored in granules in the juxtaglomerular cells surrounding the afferent arterioles of the cortical glomeruli (3). Various inhibitors of intrarenal renin formation are believed to exist. The juxtaglomerular appatus consists of both the juxtaglomerular cells and the cells of the macula densa; the latter area also contains some renin. Renin acts on the basic substrate angiotensinogen, a circulating α_2-globulin made in the liver, to form the decapeptide angiotensin I (Fig. 14-1). Angiotensin I is then converted by angiotensin-converting enzyme to the octapeptide angiotensin II by the splitting off of the two C-terminal amino acids. Angiotensin II is the most potent pressor compound (on a mole for mole basis) made in the body (4–7), acting directly on arteriolar smooth muscle. In addition, angiotensin II stimulates the zona glomerulosa of the adrenal cortex to produce aldosterone. Various peptidases, collectively termed "angiotensinases," in organ tissue, vessel walls, and circulating plasma are responsible for the ultimate biochemical degradation of circulating angiotensin II. Angiotensinases rapidly destroy angiotensin II (half-life approximately 1 min); the half-life of renin is longer (10 to 20 min).

A number of studies have documented that other tissues, such as uterus, vascular tissue, brain, and salivary glands, also produce reninlike substances. The significance of these so-called "isorenins" is not known.

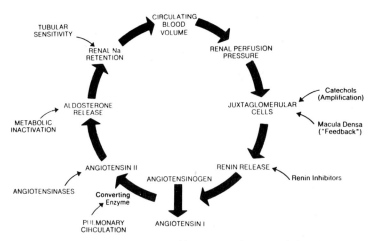

Figure 14-1. Renin-angiotensin-aldosterone volume regulation in normal man. [*From G. H. Williams et al., Harrison's Principles of Internal Medicine, 8th ed., McGraw-Hill, New York, pp. 520–557, 1977.*]

Renin release has four major controls. For the most part, these are interdependent, and the amount of renin released reflects the input of all four (3, 7). The *juxtaglomerular cells,* which are specialized myoepithelial cells cuffing the afferent arterioles, act as miniature pressure transducers, sensing renal perfusion pressure through corresponding changes in afferent arteriolar perfusion pressures. The changes in pressure are perceived as distortions in the stretch on the arteriolar walls. For example, if circulating blood volume is reduced, there will be a corresponding reduction in renal perfusion pressure, and therefore, in afferent arteriolar pressure (Fig. 14-1). This is perceived by the juxtaglomerular cells as a decreased stretch exerted on the afferent arteriolar walls. The juxtaglomerular cells will then release increasing quantities of renin into the kidney circulation, leading to the formation of angiotensin I. Angiotensin I leaves the kidney by both renal lymphatic and renal venous outflow. It is converted into angiotensin II and stimulates aldosterone release from the adrenal cortex. Increasing plasma levels of aldosterone increase renal sodium retention and thus result in expansion of extracellular fluid volume, which, as it is

completed, dampens the initiating signal for renin release. Within this context, the renin-angiotensin-aldosterone system is subserving volume control by appropriate modifications of renal tubular sodium transport.

A second control mechanism for renin release centers in the *macula densa* cells. These are a group of special-staining, distal convoluted tubular epithelial cells found in direct opposition to the juxtaglomerular cells. It has been suggested that they may function as chemoreceptors, monitoring the sodium load presented to the distal tubule and to the juxtaglomerular cells, where appropriate modifications in renin release take place. Such an intrarenal renin-release mechanism is postulated to operate independently of changes in renal perfusion pressure. If increased filtered sodium were delivered to the macula densa, feedback would occur to the juxtaglomerular apparatus, which would result in the release of increasing quantities of renin. This would act to decrease glomerular filtration rate, thereby reducing the filtered load of sodium. The evidence for this hypothesis is conflicting (9–13).

The *sympathetic nervous system* is also a significant regulator (9–13) of renin release. Infusion of catecholamines directly into the renal artery or electrical stimulation of renal nerves increases renin release (14). Conversely, α- or β-adrenergic blockade can block the renin response to upright posture or acute volume depletion (15). The mechanism by which sympathetic activity alters renin secretion is not known. It may act directly on the juxtaglomerular cells to increase adenyl cyclase generation, or it may influence either the juxtaglomerular or the macula densa cells indirectly by constricting the afferent arteriole.

Finally, a number of circulating factors may alter renin release. Increasing dietary *potassium* can decrease renin release; decreasing potassium intake increases renin release (16, 17). These effects are not secondary to potassium-stimulated aldosterone secretion with an alteration in sodium balance, because similar renin responses occur with subjects on a low-sodium intake (17). In addition, direct infusion of potassium into the renal artery also decreases renin release (18). The significance of this potassium effect is unclear. *Angiotensin* itself can exert a negative feedback control on renin release, independent of alterations in renal blood flow, pressure, or aldosterone secretion (19, 20). There is also some evidence that both adrenocorticotropic hormone (ACTH) and vasopressin can increase renin release. Thus, the control of renin release is complex, consisting of both *intrarenal* (pressoreceptor and macula densa) and *extrarenal* (sympathetic nervous system, potassium, angiotensin, etc.) mechanisms. Renin secretion at any moment probably reflects the interaction of all these factors, with the intrarenal mechanism predominating.

Mineralocorticoid physiology

The major mineralocorticoid produced by the human adrenal cortex is aldosterone (21). Other mineralocorticoids are produced, i.e., 11-desoxycorticosterone and 18-hydroxy-11-desoxycorticosterone, but because of differences in potency they are far less important than aldosterone.

It is thought that aldosterone begins to act after it passively diffuses into a target cell and combines with a specific high-affinity cytoplasmic receptor protein. It is then transferred to specific acceptor sites on nuclear chromatin, inducing an increase in ribonucleic acid (RNA) synthesis and later in protein synthesis (23, 24). Under normal circumstances, aldosterone has two important activities: (1) it is a major regulator of extracellular fluid volume, and (2) it is a major determinant of potassium metabolism. It regulates volume through a direct effect on the renal tubular transport of sodium. Aldosterone acts predominantly in the distal convoluted tubule, where it decreases the urinary excretion of sodium with an increase in urinary excretion of potassium (6). The net result appears to be a reabsorption of sodium from the filtrate, while potassium is secreted into the urine. The reabsorbed sodium ions are then transported out of the tubular epithelial cells into the interstitial fluid of the kidney and from there into the renal capillary circulation. Water will passively follow the transported sodium.

The action of aldosterone on the kidney is commonly referred to as distal sodium-potassium exchange. A number of studies, however, cast doubt on the validity of this simplistic concept. Much evidence suggests that potassium is not actively secreted by the tubular epithelium but rather simply follows a change in the transtubular electric gradient (22). The reabsorption of positively charged sodium ions causes a fall in the transmembrane potential, thus producing an environment favorable for the flow of positive ions out of the cell into the lumen. The major singly charged positive ion in the cell is potassium. Since its concentration in the cell is 40- to 80-fold greater than in the lumen, it will passively follow this electric gradient in order to restore the normal positive charge to the lumen.

Hydrogen ion is also abundant in the tubular epithelial cell. Since its concentration in the lumen is still greater than in the cell, it must be actively secreted; however the reduced intraluminal positivity produced by sodium reabsorption would allow more hydrogen to be secreted for the same amount of energy expended.

Aldosterone and other mineralocorticoids also act on the epithelium of the salivary ducts and sweat glands and on the epithelial cells of the gastrointestinal tract to cause reabsorption of sodium and secretion of potassium ions.

When normal individuals are given a long-term course of aldosterone (or a comparable mineralocorticoid, such as parenteral desoxycorticosterone acetate), an initial period of sodium retention is followed by a natriuresis, and sodium balance is reestablished after 3 to 5 days albeit at a higher body fluid volume. As a result, clinical edema formation does not develop. This phenomenon is referred to as the "escape phenomenon," signifying an "escape" by the renal tubules from the sodium-retaining action of chronically administered aldosterone (25). The mechanism responsible for the escape phenomenon has remained elusive. "Escape" is exhibited by patients with hypertension but is characteristically absent in patients with edema disorders.

There are three well-defined controls of aldosterone release—the renin-angiotensin system, potassium, and ACTH (6, 26–30). The renin-angiotensin system is the major control of extracellular fluid volume, via regulation of aldosterone secretion. In effect, the renin-angiotensin system attempts to maintain the circulating blood volume constant by causing aldosterone-induced sodium retention during periods registered as volume deficiencies, and by decreasing aldosterone-dependent sodium retention under conditions in which volume is registered as being ample. Our understanding of the renin-angiotensin-aldosterone relationship in normal subjects has deepened over the last several years with the development of sensitive assays for plasma aldosterone and angiotensin II. Michelakis and Horton were the first to correlate these parameters in normotensive subjects. They demonstrated significant increments in both plasma aldosterone and renin activity in response to sodium restriction and upright posture (31). Other investigators have confirmed these findings and have documented that there is a close inverse correlation between dietary intake of sodium and posturally induced changes in plasma renin activity and aldosterone (32–34). Tuck et al. (35) have documented the sequential response of the three components of this axis to acute volume depletion induced by standing. The levels of plasma renin activity, angiotensin II, and aldosterone were assessed frequently following acute postural alteration (assumption of the upright position or return to the supine) on both a low (10 meq) and a high (200 meq) sodium intake. Within 5 to 20 min of standing there was a significant increment in both plasma renin activity and angiotensin II with a peak occurring within 90 min and a tendency to plateau until the end of the study at approximately 240 min. The increment in plasma aldosterone was delayed 20 to 30 min, but the peak level was also achieved by 90 min (Fig. 14-2). These studies also documented that sodium intake influences the responsiveness of the axis to upright posture. Sodium restriction enhanced the rate and magnitude of the increase in each of the components of the axis and changed the slope of the regression relationship between plasma renin activity and plasma aldosterone. It is apparent from this study that dietary sodium intake can markedly influence the relative responses of the various components of the renin-angiotensin-aldosterone axis—a factor which needs to be considered to interpret properly studies performed in hypertensive subjects.

Like volume depletion, volume expansion also has a significant effect on aldosterone secretion and the activity of the renin-angiotensin system. With expansion of extracellular fluid volume, there will be a decrease in renal renin release, a decrease in circulating plasma renin activity, and a decrease in aldosterone secretion and/or excretion. This would be the appropriate "normal" response.

Volume expansion has been produced by a number of techniques, including oral or intravenous administration of sodium chloride (36–39), intramuscular administration of desoxycorticosterone acetate (DOCA) (40–42), and partial immersion (43, 44). These procedures have been used to attempt mineralocorticoid suppression, specifically to assess whether primary aldosteronism is present.

Tests differ in the rate at which extracellular fluid volume is expanded. The normal saline suppression test involves the intravenous administration of 2 L of normal saline solution over a

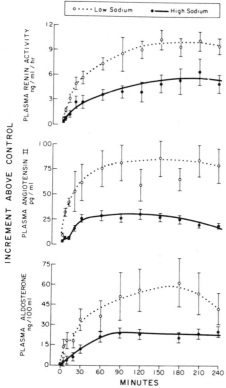

Figure 14-2. Increments (mean ± standard error of the mean) above control of plasma renin activity, angiotensin II, and plasma aldosterone after the assumption of upright posture in 10 normal subjects on low (10 meq) or high (200 meq) sodium intake. In both studies, plateau levels were reached within 90 min of assuming the upright position. Significant increments in renin activity and angiotensin II occurred within 5 min on the sodium-restricted diet and within 10 min on the sodium-loaded diet. All three parameters were significantly correlated with each other. [*From M. L. Tuck et al. (35).*]

4-h period from 9 A.M. until 1 P.M. on two consecutive days (39, 45). Aldosterone secretion or excretion rate is measured the day before and on the second day of saline loading; plasma aldosterone levels are measured before and at the end of each saline infusion day (32, 45). The patient previously has been permitted to equilibrate on a 10 meq sodium and 100 meq potassium diet. Normally, aldosterone secretion should be suppressed by this maneuver to less than 200 μg/day (excretion less than 15 μg/day and supine postinfusion plasma levels less than 5 ng/dL). The oral salt-loading suppression test is conveniently carried out by abruptly increasing the patient's sodium intake from a constant level of 10 meq/day to 200 meq/day for a period of 3 to 5 days, with measurement of aldosterone levels on the fourth or fifth day, at which time they should be similar to those for the saline suppression test. Potassium intake is held constant throughout the test, since potassium affects aldosterone secretion independently of the renin-angiotensin system. The DOCA suppression test is carried out by placing the patient on a normal (100 meq) or high (200 meq) sodium intake (40). After the patient is in sodium balance, desoxycorticosterone acetate is administered intramuscularly (10 mg every 12 h) for a period of 3 to 5 days. Normal subjects on a sodium intake of 100 meq daily demonstrate a 70 percent decrease in aldosterone levels, which means that the aldosterone secretory value should be less than 250 μg/day (excretion less than 15 μg/day and supine morning plasma levels less than 5 ng/dL).

Recently, the rate of response of the axis following acute volume expansion induced by the intravenous administration of either saline, dextran, or glucose has been assessed (46). Studies were performed in normal subjects in balance on a 10 meq sodium and 100 meq potassium intake. Plasma renin activity, angiotensin II, aldosterone and cortisol, and serum sodium and potassium were measured at frequent intervals after the initiation of the infusions.

During saline infusion (500 mL/h for 6 h) mean plasma renin activity and angiotensin II levels declined rapidly, with significant decrements observed 10 min after the initiation of the infusion and a 50 percent fall by 60 min. Thereafter, the rate of fall was more gradual, with levels reaching a nadir at 360 min. Aldosterone levels declined in a parallel fashion after an initial lag; significant decrements did not occur until 30 min after the initiation of the infusion (Fig. 14-3). Despite equivalent volume expansion (Fig. 14-3) dextran infusion (250 mL/h for 4 h) did not produce a sig-

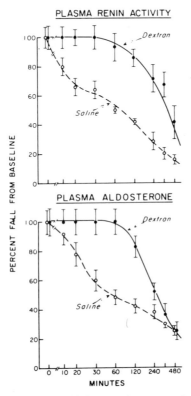

Figure 14-3. Comparison of the rate of response of plasma renin activity and aldosterone to saline and dextran infusions in 12 normotensive subjects. Results are expressed as percent fall from the baseline (mean ± standard error of the mean) plotted against time on the log axis. Note the rapid, early response to saline infusion of both parameters with the delayed response to intravascular volume expansion with dextran. Also, note that the saline response curve appears to have two phases: a rapid, early response with a plateau; and then a second decrement occurring at the same time as the suppression of these two parameters with dextran [*From M. L. Tuck et al. (46).*]

nificant fall in plasma renin activity, angiotensin II, or plasma aldosterone until 4 h after the start of the infusion. Infusion of 5% glucose in water at 500 mL/h for 6 h had no significant effect on plasma renin activity, angiotensin II, or aldosterone. Although the rates of response of plasma renin activity, angiotensin II, and aldosterone were different in each of the three infusion studies, these parameters were always significantly

correlated within each study. The results demonstrate that the rate of responsiveness of plasma renin activity, angiotensin II, and aldosterone is dependent on the volume-expanding agent employed. Saline produces a more rapid suppression than dextran in sodium-depleted subjects, supporting a specific role for the sodium ion itself in the regulation of renin and aldosterone secretion.

Potassium ions can regulate aldosterone secretion independently of the renin-angiotensin system. In normal humans, oral potassium loading increases the secretion and plasma levels of aldosterone (47–49). In addition, systemic infusion of potassium ions may significantly increase plasma aldosterone levels with as small as a 0.1 meq/L increase in serum potassium (Fig. 14-4)(50). That this is secondary to a direct action of the potassium ion is supported by a number of facts: potassium suppresses renin secretion (Fig. 14-5); the effect of potassium on aldosterone excretion is independent of reciprocal changes in

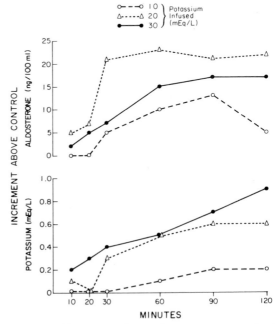

Figure 14-4. Aldosterone and potassium responses to potassium chloride infusion in five normotensive sodium-restricted subjects (mean ± standard error of the mean).

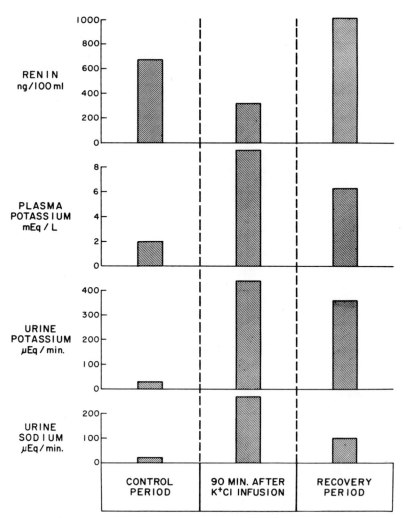

Figure 14-5. The response of renal vein renin activity to an acute
renal arterial infusion of potassium chloride in the dog.

intravascular volume; the infusion of potassium ions directly into the adrenal artery produces an immediate increase in adrenal venous aldosterone levels; and finally, increasing the potassium content of incubation medium containing adrenal tissue results in an increase in aldosterone production (51–54). How potassium alters aldosterone secretion is not known. The effect may be due to small changes in serum potassium levels, to changes in intracellular potassium concentration, or to a change in the flux of potassium across the adrenal cortical cell membrane. This potassium control mechanism may operate clinically to minimize the hazard of potassium intoxication. For example, high-potassium intake increases plasma potassium, which leads to an increase in aldosterone secretion and thus to an increase in renal potassium excretion.

The exact degree of participation of ACTH and the glucocorticoids in the normal regulation of aldosterone secretion is still uncertain. Acute ACTH infusion induces a marked increase in aldosterone secretion (55, 56), despite an increase in body weight (due to retained water), presumably secondary to contaminant antidiuretic hormone present in the ACTH infusion. However, aldosterone secretion begins to fall if the infusion is continued for 48 h or longer (57). The mechanism underlying this cutback is not understood. Decreasing salt intake enhances the response to ACTH (57). In contrast, the abnormal response of an individual with panhypopituitarism is shown in Fig. 14-6. A normal level of aldosterone secretion is reached in response to salt restriction, but this takes approximately 40 to 50 percent longer than in normal humans. Remarkably, ACTH stimulation produces little if any increase in aldosterone secretion in these patients (58).

These results have been shown by Palmore and Mulrow (59) and Ganong et al. (60) to be true in the experimental animal. It is interesting that this failure does not seem to be secondary to a chronic lack of ACTH. If a similar ACTH infusion is performed in a patient who has been on long-term steroid therapy for asthma or in an experimental animal placed on high-dose glucocorticoids, the response is similar to that of normal humans (58). It has been postulated that somatotropin is the non-ACTH factor of the pituitary gland which is needed for enhanced aldosterone secretion.

Finally, the prior dietary intake of both potassium and sodium can alter the magnitude of the aldosterone response to acute stimulation. Increasing potassium intake or decreasing sodium intake sensitizes the glomerulosa cells to acute stimulation by ACTH, angiotensin II, and/or potassium (57, 61–64). In vitro studies in animals indicate that aldosterone-stimulating substances may act on the late (corticosterone to aldosterone) as well as the early (cholesterol to pregnenolone)

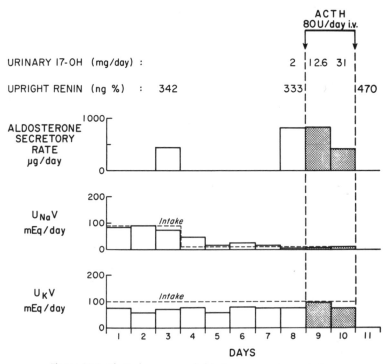

Figure 14-6. Blunted response of aldosterone secretory rate to an acute ACTH infusion in a patient with hypopituitarism.

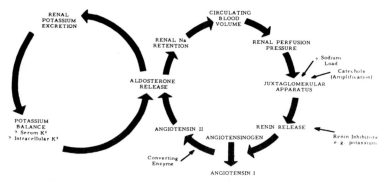

Figure 14-7. The interrelationship of the volume and potassium feedback loops on aldosterone secretion. Integration of signals from each loop determines the level of aldosterone secreted. [*From G. H. Williams and R. G. Dluhy (6).*]

steps in aldosterone biosynthesis (51–54, 65). Since all acute stimuli increase the activity of the early steps in the pathway, an attractive unifying hypothesis that could explain the sensitizing effects of dietary sodium restriction and potassium loading is that these conditions maintain the final step of aldosterone biosynthesis.

In summary, the renin-angiotensin system and potassium may be of equal importance in the regulation of aldosterone secretion in humans (Fig. 14-7), and the interaction of dietary sodium and potassium can sensitize the response of aldosterone secretion following acute stimulation. How dietary changes might alter the late pathway, and whether sodium and potassium manipulations are acting on the same cells or receptor sites, is not clear from the information presently available. While physiologic levels may stimulate aldosterone secretion under certain circumstances, ACTH seems to be less important than potassium and the renin-angiotensin system in the control of aldosterone production.

FACTORS CONTROLLING BLOOD PRESSURE

In order to understand the pathophysiology of hypertension, a brief description of those factors which play a role in the maintenance of normal blood pressure is necessary. Arterial pressure is the product of cardiac output and peripheral re-

sistance. Cardiac output is equal to the stroke volume times the heart rate. Stroke volume depends on the venous return and myocardial contractility. Peripheral resistance is determined by the intrinsic physical characteristics of the resistance vessels (i.e., the ratio of lumen to wall thickness) as well as the neurohumoral influences that act on vascular smooth muscle. These influences include the neurotransmitters norepinephrine, which is a vasoconstrictor, and in some vessels acetycholine, which is a vasodilator. Humoral and locally acting substances include angiotensin II (vasoconstriction) and prostaglandins and kinins (vasodilators). Hypoxia and products of metabolism such as adenosine, H^+, and lactic acid also exert potent *local* vasodilating influences.

For arterial pressure to rise, there must be either an increase in cardiac output or peripheral resistance, or both. Theories of the pathogenesis of essential hypertension have suggested increases in either cardiac output or peripheral resistance as the initiating events.

Renal factors

Goldblatt et al. in 1934 (66) produced hypertension in the dog by constriction of the renal artery. It has been demonstrated that a number of renal diseases—pyelonephritis, glomerulonephritis, tuberculosis, carcinoma, as well as vascular changes—produce hypertension. The exact mechanism involved in renal hypertension is not known, but its occurrence implicates the kidney in the control of blood pressure.

One of the determinants of cardiac output is the venous return, which is dependent on total blood volume. As discussed above, the renin-angiotensin-aldosterone system causes retention of salt and water, increasing the total blood volume. It is in this way that the system helps maintain blood pressure. In addition, angiotensin II is a potent vasoconstrictor (67). This effect, which may be exerted directly on the peripheral vasculature or may possibly potentiate the effect of adrenergic stimulation, may be a second renal factor in the control of blood pressure. Third, it has been postulated that the kidney, functioning as an excretory and detoxifying organ, may help control the level of extrarenal pressor substances and thereby help prevent hypertension. A fourth and more recently postulated renal mechanism for control of blood pressure is the production of a vasodilator substance. The postulated vasodilator substance is one of the prostaglandins, which is found in high concentration in the medulla of the normal kidney. A second potential vasodilator is kallikrein synthesized and secreted by the kidney. Kallikreins are enzymes which have the potential for acting on certain substrates to form a group of potent vasodilator polypeptides called kinins (68). Further investigations with these compounds are needed in order to determine their role, if any, in the normal maintenance of blood pressure.

Endocrine factors

Pheochromocytoma and primary aldosteronism, both of which are due to tumors of the adrenal gland, are two surgically correctable causes of hypertension. Because of this and other evidence, it has been postulated that epinephrine, norepinephrine, and aldosterone play significant roles in the regulation of normal blood pressure.

The difficulties in trying to ascertain the exact role of the catecholamines in blood pressure regulation are three. First, it is difficult to quantitate these compounds in biologic fluids. Second, they come from two different sources, the adrenal medulla and the postganglionic sympathetic axones. Third, the axones not only synthesize norepinephrine but also take up free norepinephrine from the tissues around them. Therefore, even if precise quantitative measurements of serum catecholamines could be determined, the relationship of these values to the quantity secreted would always be in doubt.

Catecholamines manufactured in the postganglionic sympathetic axone are stored bound to adenosine triphosphate (ATP) in granular sacs. The propagated nerve impulse causes the release of norepinephrine from these granules into the synapse, across which it diffuses to the receptor organs. Some of the discharged norepinephrine is resorbed by the axone, and there it is either detoxified by monoamine oxidases or stored in new granules. The norepinephrine which escapes from the vicinity of the axone is inactivated by methyltransferase enzymes present in the peripheral circulation and elsewhere. The fine balance of this system plays a significant role in the determination of blood pressure. The discharged norepinephrine regulates not only arterial resistance but also cardiac contractility and rate. When more precise measurements of catecholamines become available and the relationship between these measurements and actual activity is determined, a more sophisticated understanding of how this complex system interacts with others in the maintenance of blood pressure will be possible.

Aldosterone is a potent salt-retaining hormone. It helps regulate blood pressure by maintaining blood volume through salt and accompanying water retention. The significance of the renin-angiotensin-aldosterone system in normal volume control has been stressed. This role may be significant in patients with various forms of hypertension, as will be discussed below.

The role of cortisol in maintaining blood pressure is related to its maintenance of normal vascular reactivity, a feature not shared by the mineralocorticoids. Goldstein and his associates (69) have demonstrated this in a series of studies on adrenalectomized dogs. In response to stimulation of the gastrocnemius muscles, normal dogs maintain work performance and blood pressure for 12 h, while adrenalectomized dogs show a regressive decline in blood pressure within 1 to 4 h despite treatment with DOCA. The failure of blood pressure maintenance is interpreted as a defect in the neurocirculatory system. It has also been shown that the pressor response to infused norepinephrine cannot be maintained in adrenalectomized animals. Normal vascular reactivity can be restored through the injection of C_{11} oxysteroids, presumably cortisol, but not by DOCA (70). Clinically, we see that the hypotensive, volume-contracted state of the person in adrenal crisis can be corrected by saline and glucocorticoids, but only with difficulty, by mineralocorticoids and saline. Whether excesses or abnormal metabolism of the glucocorticoids, aside from Cushing's syndrome, are responsible for any hypertensive states is difficult to determine. Cortisol secretory rates, response to ACTH, and suppression with dexamethasone are all within normal limits in patients with nonadrenal forms of hypertension. Thus it seems improbable that glucocorticoids play more than a permissive role in hypertension, although they appear to be essential for the normal regulation of blood pressure.

The role of thyroid hormone in the normal maintenance of blood pressure is disputed. Certainly, the hyperkinetic circulatory state of the thyrotoxic patient can produce systolic hypertension. However, hypertension is also found in patients with hypothyroidism. The interesting interrelations of thyroid hormone with both catecholamines and the myocardium have been extensively investigated without agreement as to their physiologic significance. There is a diminished vascular reactivity to epinephrine and norepinephrine in the hypothyroid state; yet there appear to be no lasting effects on the blood pressure in patients with hypertension when hypothyroidism is induced. Thyroid hormone produces peripheral vasodilation, but it has also been shown to augment the normal response of tissues to sympathetic stimulation and might be expected thereby to increase blood pressure. This augmented reactivity may be due to an increase in angiotensin secretion or to a decrease in a detoxifying enzyme.

Ivy and his associates at the Mayo Clinic (71) have reported a mean decrease in arterial pressure of 21 mmHg in patients with both hyperthyroidism and hypertension after the thyroid condition is corrected. From their extensive studies, they concluded that hypertension, both systolic and diastolic, may be found in patients with hyperthyroidism and that it may be due either entirely to the thyroid hormone or to the exaggeration of underlying hypertension by the hyperthyroid state.

Other hormones may play a role in blood pressure control. Antidiuretic hormone also has pressor activity, but only in high doses. Both its antidiuretic and pressor effects could be important in the regulation of blood pressure through determining changes in blood volume and peripheral resistance. The role of vasopressin will be clarified when more precise and rapid methods of determining its activity are available. The androgens, estrogen, and progesteronelike compounds all affect sodium balance. However, it is doubtful that pathologic changes in these hormones or their sodium-retaining capacity have significant effects except on rare occasions.

Approximately 30 to 50 percent of patients with acromegaly also have hypertension. The role of growth hormone in the production of this hypertension and whether growth hormone is important in regulating blood pressure have not been extensively investigated. Acromegalic subjects are reported to be sodium expanded and hypervolemic (72). Rarely, these patients may also have aldosterone-producing adenomas (72). In general, renin and aldosterone levels are suppressed in hypertensive acromegalic subjects, and in normotensive subjects, renin responsiveness is normal (73). Thus, it is unclear why hypervolemia and hypertension are commonly observed in acromegaly; an effect of growth hormone per se has been postulated, because the renin-angiotensin-aldosterone system seems to respond normally to the sodium-expanded state. However, Lee and de-Wied (74) have shown that growth hormone is essential in the normal aldosterone response to ACTH of the hypophysectiomized rat.

Primary vascular factors

Many factors influence the level of peripheral resistance; one of them is the structure of the vessels. For example, blood pressure tends to rise with increasing age, paralleling the increasing rigidity of the arteries. Pulsatile flow entering a rigid rather than a flexible tube results in an increased pressure because of the inability of vessel walls to absorb part of the energy by mechanical stretch.

Sensitivity of the vessel to pressor agents may vary under different conditions. The addition of sodium to a bath containing a rat aortic strip will increase its responsiveness to angiotensin II; conversely, removal of sodium will decrease the responsiveness. Potassium may also have a direct effect on vascular responses. It has been well documented that modest increases in the plasma potassium concentration evokes vasodilatation. It has been postulated that this effect is related to the role played by potassium in the excitation phase of vascular smooth muscle contraction (75).

ETIOLOGY AND CHARACTERISTICS OF HYPERTENSION

The clinical manifestations of hypertension can be divided into two major categories: (1) the effect of the elevated blood pressure on the vessels and (2) the effect of the elevated blood pressure on the various organ systems. In hypertension of various causes, peripheral arterioles are often observed to be occluded or conspicuously tortuous, particularly in the optic fundi. These vascular changes may be the cause of many of the common symptoms; cerebral symptoms, such as headaches, usually of the pounding nature, vertiginouslike attacks, and episodes of cerebral vascular disease, such as minor strokes and cerebral hemorrhages, are probably all secondary to vascular changes. Similar changes in the renal vascular system lead to the pathologic changes of nephrosclerosis and may finally lead to renal insufficiency. The increase in pressure work induces myocardial hypertrophy, which may be so severe that the myocardium outgrows its blood supply. This leads to myocardial infarction and congestive heart failure with their sequelae. Likewise, ocular manifestations, such as papilledema, and cerebral manifestations, such as hypertensive encephalopathy, are probably the result of the increased pressure.

In most cases, the pathophysiology underlying the hypertensive state is not understood. Defects in any of the normal regulatory mechanisms could produce hypertension.

Borst and Borst de Geus in 1963 proposed that "hypertension is part of a homeostatic reaction of deficient renal sodium output" (76). The renal function abnormality, i.e., reduced sodium excretion at normal arterial pressure, might be secondary to (1) mild increases in mineralocorticoid activity; (2) local increases in vasoconstrictor activity (angiotensin II or sympathetic nervous system) reducing renal blood flow and thereby reducing sodium excretion; (3) decreased renal kallikrein-kinin or prostaglandin activity; or (4) a primary (perhaps genetic) tubular defect. According to this hypothesis, regardless of the mechanism of salt retention initially because of the decreased sodium excretion, blood volume rises, raising central venous pressure and preload, and thereby, cardiac output, i.e., systemic blood flow. However, peripheral tissues have the intrinsic capacity to regulate this overperfusion, by increasing local vascular resistance. When resistance is decreased in many vascular beds, arterial pressure rises, cardiac afterload increases, and stroke volume and cardiac output are thereby depressed. The elevated arterial (renal perfusion) pressure also increases the urinary excretion of sodium, thereby serving as a second negative feedback reducing blood volume, central venous pressure, preload, and ultimately cardiac output (77). Thus, the end result of this process would be increased peripheral resistance and arterial pressure with all other parameters, including blood volume, cardiac output, and renal sodium excretion remaining normal. Indeed, this sequence has been documented in experimental human (desoxycorticosterone) and animal (renal artery stenosis) hypertension. However, patients with essential hypertension have been reported to have a normal cardiac output and elevated peripheral resistance, suggesting either that the studies have not been performed early enough in the course of the disease or that this theory is incorrect in that a change in peripheral resistance is actually a *primary* not a secondary event.

Such a primary elevation in peripheral resistance can occur either because of an increase in factors tending to produce vasoconstriction, a reduction in factors producing vasodilation, or a

Table 14-1. Classification of arterial (systolic and diastolic) hypertension

A. Renal
　　1. Chronic pyelonephritis
　　2. Acute and chronic glomerulonephritis
　　3. Polycystic renal disease
　　4. Renovascular stenosis and renal infarction
　　5. Renin producing tumors
　　6. Most other severe renal disease (arteriolar nephrosclerosis, diabetic nephropathy, etc.)
B. Endocrine
　　1. Oral contraceptives
　　2. Adrenocortical hyperfunction
　　　　a. Cushing disease and syndrome
　　　　b. Primary hyperaldosteronism
　　　　c. Congenital or hereditary adrenogenital syndromes (17α-hydroxylase and 11β-hydroxylase defects)
　　3. Acromegaly
　　4. Pheochromocytoma
　　5. Myxedema
C. Neurogenic
　　1. Psychogenic
　　2. Diencephalic syndrome
　　3. Familial dysautonomia (Riley-Day syndrome)
　　4. Poliomyelitis (bulbar)
　　5. Polyneuritis (acute porphyria, lead poisoning)
　　6. Increased intracranial pressure (acute)
　　7. Spinal cord section
D. Miscellaneous
　　1. Coarctation of aorta
　　2. Increased intravascular volume (excessive transfusion)
　　3. Polyarteritis nodosa
　　4. Hypercalcemia
E. Unknown etiology
　　1. Essential hypertension (>90% of all cases of hypertension)
　　2. Toxemia of pregnancy
　　3. Acute intermittent porphyria

change in the arterial smooth muscle, i.e., an increase in muscle mass or an increase in its responsiveness and/or sensitivity to vasoconstrictor stimuli. Each theory has its advocates. Thus, the hypertension associated with some neurologic disorders, emotional stress, and perhaps early essential hypertension may be accompanied by increased plasma or urine levels of norepinephrine. Presumably, this reflects augmented neural release of the vasoconstrictive adrenergic neurotransmitter which is responsible for the increased arterial pressure. Secondly, many patients with essential hypertension have increased vascular response to vasoconstrictor agents (e.g., angioten-

sin II, norepinephrine). Finally, hypertensive patients since the early 1930s have been noted to exhibit a decrease in the urinary excretion of kinins and thus it is possible that reduced vasodilator activity could also result in increased arterial pressure.

The "deficient renal sodium output" theory and the "primary increase in peripheral resistance" hypothesis are not necessarily mutually exclusive. For example, an increased retention of sodium enhances vascular reactivity, at least to angiotensin II, even in normotensive subjects. Thus, a primary defect of sodium excretion could simultaneously increase both cardiac output and peripheral resistance. It appears that all of the above mentioned factors play some role in the development of essential hypertension; individual patients may differ in the relative importance of each. Thus, essential hypertension might be best regarded as a multifactorial disease related to abnormalities of the regulatory mechanisms normally concerned with the control of systemic vascular resistance, sodium excretion, blood volume, cardiac output, and ultimately of arterial pressure.

The causes of hypertension can be broken down into five large categories, as outlined in Table 14-1. The electrolyte and water disturbances in endocrine, renal, and essential hypertension will be discussed.

ELECTROLYTE DISTURBANCES IN HYPERTENSION CAUSED BY ENDOCRINE DISEASE

The electrolyte disturbances in Cushing's syndrome, thyroid diseases, acromegaly, and other forms of endocrine diseases that give rise to hypertension are discussed elsewhere (Chap. 23). This section will deal specifically with disturbances in primary aldosteronism and pheochromocytoma.

ALDOSTERONISM

Aldosteronism is a syndrome associated with hypersecretion of the major adrenal mineralocorticoid aldosterone. *Primary* aldosteronism signifies that the stimulus for the excessive aldosterone production resides within the adrenal gland; in *secondary* aldosteronism the stimulus is of extra-adrenal origin.

Primary aldosteronism

The constellation of signs and symptoms of excessive inappropriate aldosterone production was first summarized by Conn in 1955 (79). In the original case and in the majority of the subsequent cases, the disease was the result of an *aldosterone-producing adrenal adenoma* (Conn's syndrome). The majority of cases (75 percent) involved a unilateral adenoma, usually small and occurring with equal frequency on either side (80–83). Rarely primary aldosteronism has been reported in association with adrenal carcinoma. It is twice as common in women as in men, presenting between the ages of 30 and 50 (Fig. 14-8). In recent years, a number of cases have been reported with clinical and biochemical characteristics previously considered diagnostic of primary aldosteronism, but a solitary adenoma was not found at surgery. Instead, these patients had *bilateral cortical nodular hyperplasia* (84–86). The cause of this hyperplasia is unknown. In the lit-

erature this disease has been alternatively termed "pseudo" primary aldosteronism (PPA), idiopathic hyperaldosteronism (IHA), or nodular hyperplasia.

Incidence. Primary aldosteronism is an uncommon disease. The incidence in unselected hypertensive patients is between 0.5 and 2 percent (80). Because of special diagnostic procedures involved, diagnosis has been largely restricted to symptomatic patients. With greater availability of these procedures an increased incidence may be seen.

Signs and symptoms. (See also Chap. 11.) Almost all patients have diastolic hypertension, usually not of marked severity, and complain of headaches (Fig. 14-8). The hypertension is related in some unknown manner to the increased sodium reabsorption and extracellular volume expansion. The continual hypersecretion of aldosterone increases the renal distal tubular exchange of intratubular sodium for secreted potassium and hydrogen ions, with progressive depletion of body potassium and development of hypokalemia. *Potassium depletion* is responsible for the major complaints of muscle weakness and fatigue, which are related to the effect of intra- and extracellular potassium ion depletion on muscle mem-

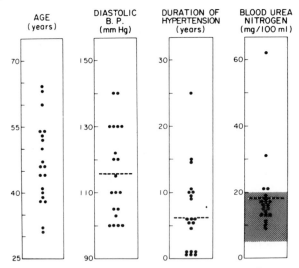

Figure 14-8. Clinical characteristics of 20 patients with proven primary aldosteronism (shaded area represents the normal range).

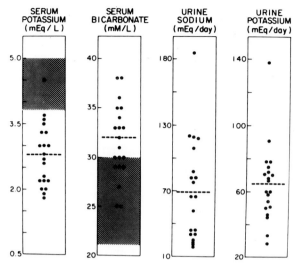

Figure 14-9. Electrolyte status of 20 patients with primary aldosteronism on admission to the hospital (shaded area represents the normal range).

brane potentials. The muscle weakness is most striking in the legs and may progress to transient paralysis. Muscles innervated by cranial nerves are usually spared. Frank tetany may also occur. Electrocardiographic signs of potassium depletion such as prominent U waves are often present, and cardiac arrhythmias and premature contractions are not uncommon. These patients may have electrocardiographic and roentgenographic signs of left ventricular enlargement, which is secondary to their hypertension. Hypertensive retinopathy is often seen but papilledema is usually absent (83). In the absence of associated congestive heart failure, renal disease, or preexisting local abnormalities (such as thrombophlebitis), edema is characteristically absent (80–84). Polyuria results from hypokalemic impairment of concentrating ability and is often associated with polydipsia.

In cases of long duration, potassium-depletion nephropathy becomes manifest, with azotemia, often with superimposed bacilluria, and in some instances with congestive heart failure and edema.

Laboratory findings. Laboratory findings are dependent on both the duration and the severity of the potassium depletion. On examination of the urine, negative to trace amounts of protein are found, sometimes with superimposed pyuria and bacilluria, presumably because of the predilection of potassium-depleted kidneys for infection. Urine specific gravity is low (less than 1.015), and an overnight concentration test with simultaneous vasopressin administration reveals impaired ability to concentrate the urine. Urine pH is often neutral to alkaline, because of excessive secretion of ammonium and bicarbonate ions. Potassium depletion also increases the capacity of the proximal convoluted tubule to reabsorb filtered bicarbonate. Urine 17-hydroxycorticosteroid and 17-ketosteroid excretion levels are always within the normal range in patients with aldosteronomas but may occasionally be elevated in those rare instances of primary aldosteronism due to adrenal carcinoma. Mild azotemia is an inconstant finding (Fig. 14-8).

Serial blood sampling usually reveals *hypokalemia* and sometimes hypernatremia (Fig. 14-9). Serial blood sampling is stressed. The hypokalemia may be severe (less than 3 meq potassium/L) and reflects significant body potassium depletion, usually in excess of 300 meq. *Hypernatremia* is due to both sodium retention and concomitant water loss from polyuria. The serum bicarbonate level may be elevated as a result of increased renal bicarbonate reabsorption and migration of hydrogen ions into potassium-depleted cells, with alkalosis then developing. In the absence of azotemia, serum uric acid concentration is normal.

Salivary sodium-potassium ratios are reduced in the majority of cases, as is thermal sweat sodium concentration.

Total body sodium content is increased, but not to the degree seen in edematous states. Total exchangeable sodium is moderately elevated, and total exchangeable body potassium is usually, but not invariably, reduced. The volume of extracellular fluid is expanded in most cases, with expansion of plasma volume in many. The expanded extracellular fluid volume is thought to be responsible for the reversed diurnal excretory pattern for salt and water that many of these patients exhibit, with predominant salt and water excretion occurring during the night. The decreased proximal resorption of sodium incident to the volume-expanded state is accompanied by decreased proximal magnesium resorption, which may exceed the magnesium resorptive capacity of the distal tubule, resulting at times in hypomagnesemia.

Diagnosis of primary aldosteronism. The major criteria which permit the clinician to derive an unequivocal diagnosis of primary aldosteronism are (1) diastolic hypertension without edema; (2) hypersecretion of aldosterone which is not suppressed appropriately during volume expansion (salt loading); (3) hyposecretion of renin (as judged by low plasma renin activity levels) which fails to increase appropriately during volume depletion (upright posture); (4) hypokalemia and/or inappropriate urine potassium loss.

Diastolic hypertension is a prerequisite for the diagnosis of primary aldosteronism, even though transient periods of blood pressure within the normal range may be observed during long-term evaluation. The diastolic hypertension exhibited by patients with primary aldosteronism does not differ from that of essential hypertension (Fig. 14-8). Blood pressure readings characteristically fall after hospitalization, but moderate to severe rises may occur in hospital and are often related to emotional situations. Accelerated diastolic hypertension is uncommon, but it has been reported (87).

Patients with primary aldosteronism and normal renal function characteristically *do not have edema*, since they are in a chronic state of escape from the sodium retention of mineralocortocoids. For the same reason, they characteristically excrete an administered salt load faster than do normotensive subjects, a characteristic which is shared by patients with essential hypertension (see below). Only limited sodium retention occurs when patients with primary aldosteronism are given sodium-retaining hormones parenterally.

Estimation of plasma renin activity helps to separate (88) patients with primary aldosteronism from those with other causes of hypertension (Table 14-1). The failure of plasma renin activity to rise normally during volume-depletion maneuvers (e.g., sodium depletion, diuretic administration, hemorrhage, ambulation) has been a major diagnostic criterion for primary aldosteronism; it is in contrast to what occurs in those hypertensive patients in whom hyperaldosteronism is secondary to *increased* renin levels. However, suppressed renin activity is not diagnostic of primary aldosteronism, as it occurs in about 25 percent of patients with essential hypertension, in patients with hyperaldosteronism secondary to idiopathic bilateral nodular adrenal hyperplasia, and in other mineralocorticoid excess syndromes, including desoxycorticosterone-secreting adrenal tumors (see below).

The most commonly used screening test for primary aldosteronism is a serum potassium, since a major criterion for the diagnosis of primary aldosteronism is the demonstration of *hypokalemia* associated with an inappropriately high urine potassium excretion (Fig. 14-10). To judge the significance of a given degree of hypokalemia for a given rate of urine potassium excretion, one must take into account the patient's potassium and sodium intake. Patients with hypokalemia secondary to diuretics, laxatives, etc., will generally have a 24-h urine potassium excretion of less than 40 meq/day, and often the value is markedly less. Most patients with primary aldosteronism, on the other hand, with a potassium intake of 100 meq/day will have a 24-h urine potassium excre-

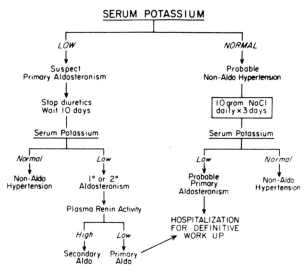

Figure 14-10. Flow sheet for office screening of hypertensive patients for hyperaldosteronism. [*From G. H. Williams and R. G. Dluhy*, Practical Management of Hypertension, *Futura Publishing Co., Inc., Mount Kisco, N.Y. 1975, p. 47.*]

tion of greater than 40 meq/day. Since potassium excretion can be modified by sodium intake, the latter must be considered. During periods of high-sodium intake, delivery of sodium ions to the distal tubular sodium-potassium exchange site will be increased, resulting in a rise in potassium excretion over control values. Contrariwise, potassium excretion can be minimized by restriction of sodium intake, which limits the amount of sodium reaching the distal tubular exchange site. Patients with primary aldosteronism will always exhibit inappropriate urine potassium losses during saline or oral salt-loading procedures.

Determination of plasma renin responsiveness and hypokalemia are not definitive, and demonstration of lack of suppression of aldosterone secretion is necessary to diagnose primary aldosteronism properly. Appropriate suppression testing may be carried out by saline loading, oral salt loading, or DOCA administration. Aldosterone tumors are autonomous only in their resistance to suppression during volume expansion; the tumors can and do respond either in normal or supernormal fashion to the stimuli of potassium loading or ACTH infusion. Patients with primary aldosteronism do not respond to volume expan-

sion because their renin-angiotensin system is already suppressed.

It is obvious that there is an inherent hazard in performing these tests in patients who indeed have primary aldosteronism. The test itself induces a greater than normal kaliuresis. If the patient begins the test with a low serum potassium level, a significant decrease in serum potassium may occur and precipitate a number of uncomfortable, even disastrous events. It is therefore important before initiating the sodium loading that the patient's potassium stores be repleted by means of a low-salt, high-potassium diet until a normal serum potassium level is achieved.

The autonomy of these tumors to volume expansion is not necessarily complete; many patients with primary aldosteronism will demonstrate some decrease of secretion during volume expansion, but the decrease is always significantly less than the expected normal response. In some patients apparent suppression of plasma or urinary levels of aldosterone in response to saline loading may be produced by the associated kaliuresis and hypokalemia.

Aldosterone-producing adenomas may be precisely localized preoperatively in many cases by the technique of percutaneous transfemoral bilateral adrenal vein catheterization with simultaneous adrenal arteriography and venography (89–91). This technique permits radiologic localization; in addition, the adrenal vein sampling may demonstrate a two- to threefold increase in plasma aldosterone concentration on the involved side compared with the uninvolved side.

A flow chart for evaluation of patients with suspected primary aldosteronism is presented in Fig. 14-11.

Differential diagnosis. All patients with *accelerated hypertension* and hypokalemia must be evaluated for unilateral renal disease. If this diagnosis is confirmed, the simultaneous occurrence of primary aldosteronism is unlikely, although in rare instances it has been recorded. A useful maneuver in distinguishing between secondary aldosteronism due to accelerated hyper-

tension and primary aldosteronism is the measurement of plasma renin activity (Fig. 14-12). In patients with accelerated hypertension and secondary aldosteronism, the aldosteronism is secondary to elevated plasma renin levels. In contrast, patients with primary aldosteronism have suppressed plasma renin levels. A maneuver which is sometimes useful is based on the observation of Melby that the majority of patients with primary aldosteronism become normotensive and normokalemic when treated with the aldosterone antagonist, spironolactone, in a dose of 50 to 100 mg every 6 to 8 h over a period of 2 to 5 weeks (92). Some patients with essential hypertension also become normotensive, so a positive response to spironolactone is not diagnostic of primary aldosteronism. Most of the responsive patients with essential hypertension have "low-renin hypertension." Spironolactone therapy in patients with

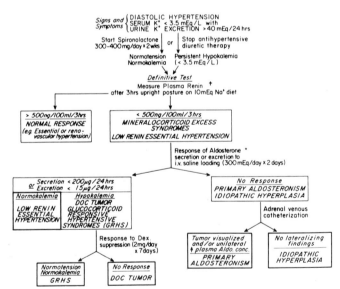

Figure 14-11. Diagnostic flow chart for evaluating patients with suspected primary aldosteronism. Identification of the hydroxylase deficiency in glucocorticoid-responsive hypertensive syndromes (GHRS) is the measurement of increased excretion of certain urinary metabolites of the intermediates of cortisol biosynthesis. [*From G. H. Williams et al., Harrison's Principles of Internal Medicine, 8th ed., McGraw-Hill, New York, 1977, pp. 520–557.*]

* Alternative methods producing comparable suppression of aldosterone secretion include oral sodium loading (200 meq/day × 5 days) or 10 mg desoxycorticosterone acetate (DOCA) intramuscularly q 12 h × 3 days.

† An alternative outpatient method is the response of plasma renin activity to 3 h of upright activity following 80 mg furosemide given the day before.

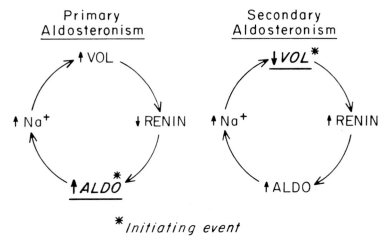

Figure 14-12. Comparison of the volume feedback loops in primary and secondary aldosteronism. [*From G. H. Williams et al.,* Harrison's Principles of Internal Medicine, *8th ed., McGraw-Hill, New York, 1977, pp. 520–557.*]

accelerated hypertension and secondary aldosteronism often will correct the electrolyte abnormalities, but hypertension will persist. It is of interest that patients with primary aldosteronism have been successfully managed medically for years with chronic spironolactone therapy (93), but therapy with spironolactone is limited in male patients by the common occurrence of gynecomastia, decreased libido, and impotence (92).

Primary aldosteronism must also be distinguished from other *hypermineralocorticoid states.* The most common problem is to distinguish between hyperaldosteronism due to an adenoma and that due to idiopathic bilateral nodular hyperplasia. This distinction is of considerable importance, since it is now generally agreed that the hypertension associated with idiopathic hyperplasia is often not affected by bilateral adrenalectomy (86). In contrast, the hypertension associated with aldosterone-producing tumors is usually improved or cured following removal of the adenoma (83). Although patients with idiopathic bilateral nodular hyperplasia tend to have less severe hypokalemia, lower aldosterone secretion, and higher plasma renin activity than patients with primary aldosteronism, differentiation is dif-

ficult, if not impossible, solely on clinical and biochemical grounds. An anomalous postural decrease in plasma aldosterone has been reported in the majority of patients with a unilateral lesion, but this test is of limited diagnostic value in the individual patient (94). Sometimes a definitive diagnosis can be made only at laparotomy, but preoperative cannulation of the adrenal veins may be diagnostic. Cases of primary aldosteronism will demonstrate unilateral increments in plasma aldosterone concentration and/or tumor visualization on the involved side (89–91).

In a few instances, hypertensive patients with hypokalemic alkalosis have been found to have desoxycorticosterone (DOC)-secreting adenomas (94). Such patients will have reduced plasma renin activity levels, but aldosterone measurements will be either normal or reduced. Rare cases of hypermineralocorticoidism due to a defect in cortisol biosynthesis, specifically 11- or 17-hydroxylation, have also been reported (94). ACTH levels are increased, with a resultant increase in the production of the mineralocorticoid 11-desoxycorticosterone. *Hypertension and hypokalemia can be corrected in these patients by glucocorticoid administration.* The definitive diagnosis is made by demonstrating an elevation of urinary metabolites of precursors of cortisol biosynthesis. Occasionally, glucocorticoid administration will produce normotension and normokalemia although a hydroxylase deficiency cannot be identified.

Licorice ingestion produces a syndrome mimicking primary aldosteronism. Licorice contains a sodium-retaining compound, glycyrrhizinic acid, which causes sodium retention, expansion of the extracellular fluid volume, hypertension, depressed plasma renin levels, and suppressed aldosterone levels. The diagnosis is excluded by a careful history.

Secondary aldosteronism

Secondary aldosteronism refers to an appropriately increased production of aldosterone in response to stimuli from outside the adrenal gland (Fig. 14-12). In all reported cases, the stimulus has been the renin-angiotensin system. The rate of aldosterone production is often higher in patients with secondary aldosteronism than in those with primary aldosteronism (95). In most patients, secondary aldosteronism is associated with either the accelerated phase of hypertension (regardless of the primary disease) or an underlying edema disorder. Secondary aldosteronism in pregnancy is a normal physiologic response to estrogen-induced increases in circulating levels of renin substrate and plasma renin activity as well as the antialdosterone actions of the progestins.

Secondary aldosteronism is found in hypertensive states secondary to either primary overproduction of renin (primary reninism) (96) or overproduction of renin in response to a decrease in renal blood flow or perfusion pressure. Secondary hypersecretion of renin can be due to narrowing of one or both of the major renal arteries either by an atherosclerotic plaque or by fibromuscular hyperplasia. Over production of renin from both kidneys also occurs in association with severe arteriolar nephrosclerosis (malignant hypertension) or profound renal vasoconstriction (accelerated phase of hypertensive disease). These patients are characterized by hypokalemic alkalosis, absence of edema, moderate to severe increases in plasma renin activity, and moderate to marked increases in aldosterone secretion/excretion rates (see below).

Secondary aldosteronism with hypertension is also associated with the rare renin-producing tumor, so-called primary reninism (96). These patients have all the biochemical characteristics of renovascular hypertension; however, the primary defect is not a decrease in renal blood flow or perfusion pressure, but renin secretion by a juxtaglomerular-cell tumor. The diagnosis can be made by renal arteriography, which demonstrates either no change in the renal vasculature or the presence of a space-occupying lesion, with a unilateral increase in renal vein renin activity. A second differential test is the change in renin activity when the patient assumes the upright posture. Patients with primary reninism characteristically have a very brisk increase in renin activity in contrast to patients with other forms of secondary aldosteronism, associated with hypertensive disorders (96).

PHEOCHROMOCYTOMA

Pheochromocytomas are tumors arising from the chromaffin cells of the sympathoadrenal system. They secrete catecholamines and are perhaps the rarest of all causes of hypertension. They account for less than 1 in 1000 cases of hypertension in most series (97). However, like tumors of the adrenal cortex, they are extremely important as a cause of curable hypertension. Most of these tumors originate unilaterally from adrenal medullary tissue. However, they may be found in any area in the midline region from neck to sacrum. They are usually benign. Most cases appear to be sporadic, although there is some familial incidence (98). The combination of a parathyroid adenoma or hyperplasia, medullary thyroid carcinoma, and pheochromocytoma, usually bilateral, has an especially high familial incidence (so-called Sipple's syndrome or multiple endocrine neoplasia, type 2A) (99).

The usual disturbance in electrolyte and fluid

homeostasis in these patients is a decrease in plasma and total blood volumes. When the blood pressure is increased by norepinephrine, vasoconstriction occurs not only on the arterial side but also on the venous side of the capillary bed. This increases capillary pressure and causes transudation of fluid from the intravascular to the extracellular space. If one infuses norepinephrine into normal subjects, the loss of fluid results in a rise in serum protein concentration and hematocrit. However, with a sustained release of norepinephrine, readjustments may occur in the bone marrow and the liver so that hematocrit and total proteins return to normal concentrations within a decreased total blood volume. Nevertheless, a high hematocrit is still seen in some patients with pheochromocytoma. The high hematocrit probably reflects a contracted plasma volume, but polycythemia has also been reported secondary to erythropoietin production by a pheochromocytoma.

Because of their decreased blood volume, these patients may experience postural hypotension. The reduction of blood volume probably also accounts for the occasional catastrophic fall in blood pressure during surgical treatment, despite relatively minor blood loss prior to removal of the tumor. Pressor agents are usually ineffective; the treatment of choice is infusion of plasma expanders and whole blood to replace operative losses. Preoperative treatment of the hypertension with diuretics or sodium restriction can increase this risk.

Treatment of the disease is surgical removal of the chromaffin tumor, if at all possible. It is mandatory to restore normal blood volume preoperatively by controlling the blood pressure with orally administered phenoxybenzamine. Preoperatively, twice daily phenoxybenzamine should be increased slowly over a 5- to 7-day period until blood pressure is controlled. During this treatment phase, the hematocrit and total protein concentration will fall as fluid volume increases.

In certain cases of malignant pheochromocytoma, medical treatment can be continued indefinitely with a fair degree of success in controlling symptoms and the elevated arterial blood pressure.

ELECTROLYTE DISTURBANCES IN PATIENTS WITH RENAL HYPERTENSION

BACKGROUND

Acute and chronic renal disease including renal vascular abnormalities, is the most common secondary cause of hypertension, accounting for 7 to 10 percent of the total hypertensive population (100). How renal disease produces hypertension is still uncertain. The mechanisms have been divided into two major groups: vasoconstrictor (angiotensin)-dependent and volume-mediated. It is assumed that vasoconstrictor-mediated hypertension is secondary to renal ischemia or reduced blood flow due to injury or constriction of the vascular supply to the kidney. In volume-dependent hypertension there is loss of renal mass; the kidney is less able to excrete sodium, and a derangement in volume homeostasis results. There is also evidence that in some anephric individuals with hypertension, the lack of a renal vasodepressor substance(s) may contribute to the elevated blood pressure; prostaglandins and/or tissue kallikreins are the suggested vasodepressors. The electrolyte and volume abnormalities associated with loss of kidney mass are similar in any form of chronic renal disease, and are covered in detail in Chaps. 15 and 16. In this section, we will primarily discuss the electrolyte disturbances and pathophysiology associated with angiotensin-dependent hypertension.

The studies reported by Goldblatt and colleagues in 1934 (66) serve as a reference point in assessing the role of the kidney in producing hypertension. While renin had been characterized years before, the development of hypertension in dogs with renal artery constriction was needed to establish renin's potential role in hypertension. The role of renin (and angiotensin II) in the development and maintenance of hypertension with renal artery stenosis is still disputed. Part of the confusion is the result of the different physiology of the dog, the animal used by Goldblatt, and the human or rat. In Goldblatt's original studies hypertension could only be produced by clipping one renal artery and removing the contralateral kidney. On the other hand, in rats hypertension can be produced by clipping one renal artery alone. Confusion has also arisen because the same model has been called by different names. In the following discussion, one kidney hypertension will refer to the model in which one renal artery is clipped and the contralateral kidney removed. Two kidney hypertension will refer to the model in which one renal artery is clipped and the contralateral left intact.

It has been suggested that one kidney hypertension is produced by sodium retention and is volume-dependent hypertension similar to that of chronic renal disease, while two kidney hypertension is similar to the hypertension of renal artery stenosis in humans. These hypotheses are supported by the following evidence: (1) increased renin content in the clipped kidney in two kidney hypertension, with decreased renin content in the clipped kidney in one kidney hypertension (101); (2) significant reduction of blood pressure in two kidney hypertension with an angiotensin II competitive inhibitor, which reduces blood pressure minimally or not at all in one kidney hypertension (102); (3) increase in exchangeable sodium in the one kidney versus the two kidney model (103); and (4) restoration of normal blood pressure in one kidney (but not two kidney hypertensive rats) by elimination of dietary sodium (104).

One difficulty with ascribing the entire hypertensive process in renovascular disease to increased levels of angiotensin II is that normal subjects fail to increase their blood pressure when infused with enough angiotensin II to produce the plasma levels seen in patients with renal artery stenosis. However, two groups have suggested that part of the hypertensive effect of angiotensin II may be to sensitize vascular tissue to other vasoconstrictor agents, e.g., norepinephrine (105, 106). These studies reported the vascular effects of infusing subpressor doses of angiotensin II into either rabbits or dogs for several days. While at first there were no changes in blood pressure, after 3 or more days arterial pressures began to rise and eventually reached hypertensive levels. Additionally, it was found that when tyramine was given to these animals, they had a much more marked response than did animals not pretreated with angiotensin.

This indirect action of angiotensin on the sensitivity of the postganglionic sympathetic nerve fibers may help explain the role of the kidney in normal blood pressure regulation as well as in renal hypertension. The difficulty in studying the direct action of this hormone is that the sensitivity of the blood vessels to it depends on sodium balance, and angiotensin itself, by its effect on aldosterone secretion, alters the state of sodium balance. It may be that the heightened reactivity to tyramine observed by Page and his group (105) is due to changes in sodium balance induced by the small infusions of angiotensin.

The initiating event in the development of hypertension with renal artery stenosis is presumably the release of renin in response to a decrease in flow or pressure or the development of renal ischemia. Angiotensin II levels would then increase (Fig. 14-1). The increase in angiotensin II would have two significant effects: an increase in aldosterone secretion and an increased peripheral resistance leading to an increase in blood pressure. The increased aldosterone secretion would, initially at least, produce sodium retention and increased cardiac output; then, by autoregulation, peripheral resistance would be further increased and cardiac output lowered. With the sodium retention initiated by aldosterone's effect, extracellular fluid volume would expand, which would be expected to reduce renin release. However, for the level of volume expansion, renin and angiotensin II levels would still be inappropriately elevated (107). These theoretical considerations have in part been substantiated by observation and experiment. Cardiac output is above normal in some patients with renovascular hypertension (107) but presumably is not as important as the increased peripheral resistance in raising the blood pressure (108). Animal studies suggest that at least initially there is an increase in aldosterone secretion in renovascular hypertension (109).

DIAGNOSIS OF RENOVASCULAR HYPERTENSION

The most useful procedures to screen for and definitively diagnose those patients who have surgically correctable renal hypertension are not agreed upon. There are two major problems: (1) to determine if unilateral renal disease is present; and (2) to prove that the hypertension is secondary to the renal disease. The rapid sequence intravenous pyelogram remains the cornerstone of any screening approach. Using the three variables of difference in renal length, difference in appearance in time of contrast material, and hyperconcentration, the number of intravenous pyelograms positive for unilateral renal disease has varied from 22 to 93 percent in patients with proven renovascular hypertension and 8 to 17 percent in patients with essential hypertension (110a, 110b). In order to improve their overall accuracy, some centers have combined the intravenous pyelogram with a radioisotopic renogram and/or renoscan. While each of these procedures is less accurate than an intravenous pyelogram (the incidence of false positives is approximately 20 percent, and that of false negatives 14 percent), the combination of both procedures can improve the accuracy of diagnosis to better than 85 to 90 percent (111). If a unilateral renal lesion can be documented, it still must be proven functionally significant. Early investigators used split renal function studies to assess the significance of a renovascular lesion. However, these have been replaced in nearly all centers by bilateral renal vein renin determinations. Theoretically, if a vascular lesion is functionally significant, there should be increased renin secretion from the involved kidney; simultaneously obtained renin measurements should predict renal ischemia, and therefore response to therapy. In most studies a renin ratio (involved to uninvolved) of 1.6 or greater has been required (112). However, with this requirement, the number of false negative results has remained substantial (100). While an abnormal ratio is highly predictive of a good response to surgery, a normal ratio does not mean that a good response will not occur. A number of studies have suggested that patients who have normal ratios and a good response to surgery probably were not studied under optimal conditions. Renal ischemia should be more apparent if renins are determined after volume depletion (Fig. 14-1). Therefore, many centers have suggested

that renin measurements should only be performed after volume or sodium depletion. In one study, prognostic accuracy increased from 35 to 90 percent using this approach (113).

It has been recently proposed that a more accurate way of screening for renovascular hypertension is to assess the blood pressure response to an agent that inhibits angiotensin II. Saralasin (1-sar,8-ala-angiotensin II) is a competitive antagonist which under certain circumstances will block vascular response to angiotensin II (114a). When saralasin is infused into patients with hypertension, those who show a fall in blood pressure are presumed to have angiotensin-dependent hypertension, and would then undergo angiography with bilateral renal vein renins to document the presence of surgically correctable disease. The false positive rate of saralasin infusion varies from 20 to 50 percent (114b). The false negative rate is unclear from the available studies but may be as low as 5 percent (114c).

ELECTROLYTE AND VOLUME ABNORMALITIES

Fluid and electrolyte changes in renovascular hypertension are secondary to the underlying renal disease and to the occasional secondary hyperaldosteronism induced by this disease. The interaction of these two broadens the range of electrolyte and water disturbances that can occur. In some patients, there may be a biochemical picture indistinguishable from that of primary aldosteronism.

The renin-angiotensin-aldosterone system does not account for all the disturbances observed in salt and water metabolism in renal hypertension. It has been shown that a decrease in renal perfusion pressure also causes increased salt and water resorption from tubule sites that are not aldosterone-dependent. On the other hand, this resorption may be countered by the contralateral uninvolved kidney, in which a rise in perfusion pressure decreases fractional salt and water reabsorption proximally and thereby increases sodium excretion. The variable balance of these three factors, i.e., increased perfusion pressure in the uninvolved kidney, decreased perfusion pressure in the involved kidney, and occasional secondary aldosteronism, accounts for the variable volume and electrolyte picture observed in patients with renovascular hypertension.

If the hypertension is severe enough to cause renal failure, the electrolyte pattern changes to that of renal insufficiency. It is then characterized by renal acidosis, sodium wasting, hyperkalemia, and abnormalities in calcium and phosphate. These patients can neither concentrate the urine properly nor excrete a water load normally, and so are prone both to dehydration if an adequate intake of fluid is not maintained, and to water intoxication if large loads of water are given.

TREATMENT

The treatment of choice for renovascular hypertension remains surgical correction of the lesion, since this therapy carries a potential for cure. However, with increasing experience, enthusiasm for surgical procedures has decreased, notably for those individuals with atherosclerotic lesions. Thus, older patients with aortic atherosclerosis who have a reasonable response to medical therapy may not be candidates for surgery. On the other hand, young individuals with fibromuscular disease of one renal artery are still excellent candidates for surgery.

Part of the change in emphasis results from improved medical therapy. There are a variety of agents (including α-methyldopa and the β-blocker, propranolol), which block or reduce renin release and are therefore effective and specific forms of therapy (100).

ELECTROLYTE DISTURBANCES IN PATIENTS WITH ESSENTIAL HYPERTENSION

Most patients with nonmalignant essential hypertension appear to have normal serum electrolyte levels, pH, and plasma and extracellular fluid volumes. However, several factors may alter this satisfactory state and produce marked abnormalities. Certain abnormalities in salt and water balance have been uncovered in patients with this disease. An early finding is an exaggerated natriuresis with which some hypertensive subjects respond to hypertonic or isotonic saline infusions (115a). This exaggerated natriuresis occurs regardless of the pretreatment sodium balance, of whether the infusion is hypo-, iso-, or hypertonic, of the response of the blood pressure to the infusion, or of simultaneous changes in renal hemodynamics. However, it is often associated with a marked increase in central venous pressure before the natriuresis occurs. Whether the abnormal natriuresis is due simply to elevated blood pressure or is intrinsic to the disease is difficult to state. A number of studies have shown that the same exaggerated natriuresis does occur in other forms of hypertension. However, Aviram and his associates (115b) have shown that patients with labile hypertension or normotensive women who have recovered from toxemia of pregnancy react to an infusion of hypertonic salt solution in much the same manner as those who have various forms of hypertension even though the former groups are normotensive during the period of testing. Confusion exists because the exaggerated natriuresis can be induced in experimental animals and in humans with appropriate vasoconstrictive stimuli (115b, 116). This has led some to postulate that the natriuresis is a response to hypertension per se rather than a basic physiologic defect. However, the exaggerated response in normotensive subjects, such as those studied by Aviram, goes unexplained if an elevated blood pressure is assumed to be the sole requirement. This phenomenon suggests a problem in the volume-sensing or volume-regulating mechanism in these individuals, which may be etiologically significant in both the production of essential hypertension and the natriuretic response.

Recently, it has been suggested that the basal renin secretion may play a role in the response of hypertensive patients to sodium loading. Low-renin essential hypertensive patients and patients with primary aldosteronism invariably had an exaggerated natriuresis. However, patients with normal-renin essential hypertension had a normal natriuresis. This difference may explain some of the discrepancies in the response of hypertensive patients in previous studies.

A second volume aberration seen in some patients with essential hypertension is a decrease in the plasma volume. This decrease reportedly is greater the higher the diastolic pressure and becomes significant when the diastolic pressure reaches 105 mmHg (117). This finding is in contrast to that seen in primary aldosteronism (118).

Measurements of sodium content of the arterial walls of experimental animals with hypertension have repeatedly shown increased values (119). This could be due to muscular contraction causing cellular potassium efflux and sodium influx or could be secondary to some factor significant in the pathogenesis of the disease. In any case, it has been shown that sensitivity of a perfused aortic strip to angiotensin increases as the sodium content of the bath is increased (120). While this response has not been conclusively shown with catecholamines, some studies have suggested a similar type of enhanced responsiveness in the sodium-loaded state as opposed to the sodium-depleted state. The enhanced sensitivity could be due to a Starling type of phenomenon in the vessel wall; on the other hand, sodium and volume depletion may decrease the stretch on the vessel wall, thereby decreasing its responsiveness to any stimulus. However, the increased sensitivity of the aortic strip when increased sodium is present makes it equally probable that the sodium ion itself is etiologically significant.

THE RENIN-ANGIOTENSIN-ALDOSTERONE SYSTEM IN ESSENTIAL HYPERTENSION

Because of the key role of the kidney-adrenal axis in maintaining both sodium balance and blood volume, many groups have studied the renin-angiotensin-aldosterone system in patients with essential hypertension. In the late 1950s, two groups reported that some patients with malignant hypertension had increased levels of urinary aldosterone (95, 121). Since then, it has been demonstrated that some individuals with hypertension and renal artery stenosis also have an increased secretion of aldosterone. Thus, patients with hypertension and elevated aldosterone secretion may have primary or secondary aldosteronism (malignant hypertension, renal artery stenosis, etc.) (Fig. 14-12).

Considerable disagreement still exists as to whether aldosterone secretion is normal in patients with essential hypertension. Some of the differences between reports may reflect different definitions of the disease, inadequate selection of controls, variation in the control of the factors known to alter aldosterone secretion and methodologic differences. To achieve greater uniformity, most recent studies have assessed the dynamic response of the renin-angiotensin-aldosterone axis under controlled conditions. While the significance of these studies is still uncertain, it seems clear that a large number of patients with essential hypertension may have an altered volume- or sodium-sensing mechanism which is particularly evident in studies investigating acute suppression of the renin-angiotensin-aldosterone axis. Also, a significant fraction of patients seems to have decreased responsiveness of the renin-angiotensin system following acute and chronic volume depletion. These studies all provide evidence that the volume- or sodium-sensing mechanism is abnormal in patients with essential hypertension. The abnormalities and their possible relationship to alterations in volume electrolyte patterns in patients with essential hypertension will be reviewed.

Acute suppression of the renin-angiotensin-aldosterone axis in essential hypertension

Several groups have examined the suppression of aldosterone secretion or excretion in patients with essential hypertension following chronic dietary sodium loading. Most studies have found no significant differences between normals and hypertensive subjects (45, 122, 123). However, Collins and his colleagues (124), using a higher sodium load, i.e., 300 meq/day, have reported that some patients with essential hypertension have a significantly greater rate of aldosterone excretion than do normal controls. Increased aldosterone excretory rates occurred both in patients who had a normal and those who had a subnormal suppression of renin activity with sodium loading. None had signs of primary aldosteronism.

A recent study also indicates that a substantial proportion of patients with essential hypertension have abnormalities in the acute suppression of the renin-angiotensin-aldosterone axis. This study assessed the acute suppression of plasma renin activity, angiotensin II, and plasma aldosterone at frequent intervals in sodium-restricted hypertensive subjects during the infusion of isotonic saline at a rate of 500 mL/h for 6 h (125). All subjects had normal plasma renin activity in response to sodium restriction and upright posture. In contrast to normotensive subjects, 60 percent of the hypertensive subjects showed no significant decline in plasma renin activity or plasma aldoste-

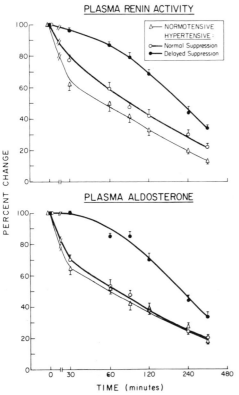

Figure 14-13. The mean ± standard error of the mean percent change from control of plasma renin activity and plasma aldosterone following infusion of 0.9% sodium chloride (500 mL/h for 6 h) in 60 hypertensive patients with a normal renin response to sodium restriction. The response of normal subjects (mean ± standard deviation) is also presented. The renin response patterns were divided into those with normal suppression and those with a delayed suppression. A delayed suppression occurred in two-thirds of the patients studied. [*From M. L. Tuck et al. (125).*]

rone until 120 and 240 min after the beginning of the infusion (Fig. 14-13). Normotensive subjects, as noted earlier, show a significant fall in these parameters by 20 to 30 min (Fig. 14-3). In addition, while there were no significant differences between normotensive subjects and two hypertensive subgroups in control plasma renin activity or plasma aldosterone levels, the plasma aldosterone levels at 30 to 240 min during the saline infusion were significantly higher ($P < 0.01$) in the hypertensive subjects with delayed suppression (Fig. 14-13). There were two distinct populations in the hypertensive group: one group demonstrated suppression of plasma renin activity at 30 min and the other group at 240 min (Fig. 14-14). Neither group had an exaggerated natriuresis in response to sodium loading; on the other hand, the delayed-suppression group excreted sodium at half the rate of normotensive subjects. The delayed suppression had two further notable consequences: first, the delayed-suppression group had a significantly greater kaliuresis than the normally suppressed group; and second, there was a significant increase in blood pressure in the delayed-suppressed group. These studies indicate an abnormality in the acute suppression of the renin-angiotensin-aldosterone axis in a substantial portion of patients with so-called normal-renin essential hypertension.

Since previous studies in normal subjects have reported that the early response to saline infusion is related to the sodium ion per se and not to intravascular volume expansion (46), the above data are consistent with the hypothesis that the delayed-suppression hypertensive group have a diminished ability to respond to the sodium ion. Two other explanations are possible. The first and most obvious is that those with the delayed suppression have a greater volume deficit prior to the infusion of saline; therefore, greater volume repletion needs to be accomplished before the system is suppressed. This is unlikely, because plasma renin activity was similar in both the delayed and the normally suppressed essential hypertensive groups. Furthermore, a recent study on normal subjects suggests that volume depletion actually enhances the acute early fall in renin activity in response to saline infusion. In this study

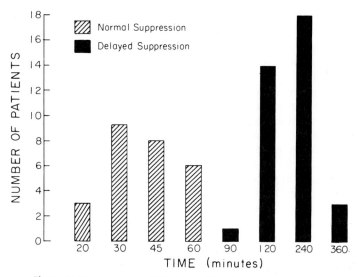

Figure 14-14. Frequency distribution of the time necessary to produce a significant (30 percent) decrement in plasma renin activity in response to saline infusion (500 mLh for 6 h) in 62 subjects with normal-renin essential hypertension. [*From M. L. Tuck et al. (125).*]

saline was infused at a rate of 500 ml per hour for 2 h in two groups of normal subjects, one group in balance on a 10-meq diet and the other on a 200-meq intake. The patients on the high sodium intake had much less suppression of the renin-angiotensin-aldosterone axis. Thus, the hypertensive patients with the delayed-response pattern behave like volume-expanded rather than volume-depleted normal subjects. A second possibility is that the delayed-suppression group is simply less sensitive to a comparable degree of volume expansion. This could occur if there is a higher receptor threshold or a sluggish response system. If so, a similar sluggish response to sodium restriction in these subjects might be anticipated. Because none was found, either the response system is not altered or the chronicity of the stimulus from sodium restriction was able to overcome the deficiency. Finally, the data could be explained by an altered response to the infusion of sodium per se. As noted earlier, recent studies on normal humans provided evidence for sodium-dependent suppression of renin and aldosterone secretion independent of changes in vascular volume (46). While this study does not distinguish between renin regulation by sodium-dependent intrarenal mechanisms versus a change in extracellular fluid volume, it does suggest that sodium has a role independent of its ability to expand intravascular volume in altering renin release. Therefore, the delayed suppression of patients with normal-renin essential hypertension may reflect a loss of sensitivity of this sodium-sensing mechanism. While these changes are not enough to produce significant alterations in serum concentrations of sodium or volume in a chronic state, they may be enough to produce or sustain an elevated blood pressure.

Renin response to acute stimulation in essential hypertension

The most frequently evaluated component of the renin-angiotensin axis in patients with hypertension is the plasma renin response to acute stimulation. Helmer in 1965 reported that 29 percent of the patients he studied with hypertension had values below those of normal controls (126). Numerous studies have confirmed these findings, and the terms "low renin" and "hyporesponsive renin essential hypertension" have been coined to characterize this subgroup of the essential hypertensive population (127–133).

A number of stimuli have been used to define the low-renin group. In most studies, plasma renin activity has been determined, although a few have measured plasma renin concentration. The majority of studies have used low-sodium intake and upright posture to define renin responsiveness. However, this requires hospitalization and rigorous dietary control, so it is impractical for screening large numbers of hypertensive patients. Two outpatient procedures have been developed in recent years. The first is the renin response to acute administration of a potent diuretic. One variant (45) of this test is the renin response 30 to 90 min after the IV administration of furosemide, a modification of a procedure originally used by Rosenthal et al. in normal subjects (134). A second variant is to give oral furosemide,

either in divided doses over a 12-h period or as a single dose, testing the renin response to upright posture 4 h later (129, 133). The second outpatient procedure is to correlate 24-h sodium excretion with upright plasma renin activity. A nomogram can be developed to assess whether plasma renin activity is high, low, or appropriate for any given sodium intake (130).

The cause of low-renin hypertension is controversial. However, a number of factors seem to be consistently associated with this condition. Nearly all studies in which a significant number of hypertensive subjects have been studied have reported that the low-renin group is significantly older than the normal-renin subgroup (129–131, 135, 136). In the more than 500 patients in the literature in whom renin responsiveness and age have been correlated, the mean age of the low-renin subgroup is 47.1 years whereas the mean age of the normal-renin subgroup is 39.5 years (Fig. 14-15). However, correlation between duration of hypertension and the incidence of low-renin activity has not been found (Fig. 14-15). This discrepancy between age and duration may reflect the inability to determine the onset of hypertension because of its relatively asymptomatic course for variable periods. Most studies have also suggested that there is a higher incidence of low-renin hypertension in black subjects; however, this may be related to the lower range of renin activity observed in normotensive black subjects (137). Thus, in defining the incidence of low-renin hypertension in the black population, a pool of black normotensives is necessary. Finally, Schalekamp and his colleagues have suggested that renin release may be suppressed in hypertensive patients because of the increase in intravascular pressure at the level of the juxtaglomerular cell (136). This postulate would predict that those individuals with higher blood pressures would have lower levels of renin activity. While some studies have suggested that such a correlation does exist, most have reported no simple relation between renin responsiveness and the level of blood pressure (Fig. 14-15).

Because of the similarity between low-renin essential hypertension and primary aldosteronism in terms of suppression of renin activity and blood pressure responsiveness to volume depletion, a

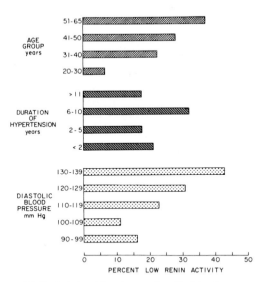

Figure 14-15. Relationship of age, diastolic blood pressure, and known duration of hypertension to the incidence of low-renin essential hypertension. One-hundred patients with essential hypertension were studied on a 10 meq sodium/100 meq potassium diet, and renin activity determined after 4 h of upright activity. There was a significant positive correlation between the incidence of low-renin activity and age and diastolic blood pressure. However, there was no correlation between known duration of hypertension and the incidence of low-renin essential hypertension. [*From M. L. Tuck et al. (131).*]

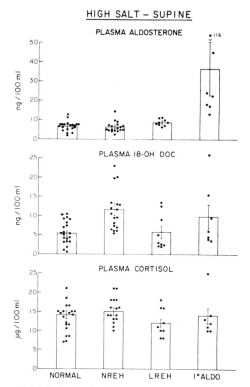

Figure 14-16. Individual and mean ± standard error of the mean plasma levels of aldosterone, 18-OH-DOC, and cortisol in 20 normal controls, 18 patients with normal-(NREH) and 9 patients with low-renin essential hypertension (LREH), and 7 patients with primary aldosteronism (1° ALDO) in balance on a 200 meq sodium/100 meq potassium intake. All samples were obtained supine at 8 A.M. [*From G. H. Williams et al. (148).*]

number of studies have looked for volume expansion, secondary to a nonaldosterone mineralocorticoid, as the cause of low-renin hypertension. Several steroids have been suggested, most commonly 11-desoxycorticosterone (DOC) and 18-hydroxy-11-desoxycorticosterone (18-OH-DOC) (138, 139). Scattered reports have also suggested that 16, α-18-dihydroxy-11-desoxycorticosterone 16, α-18-diOH-DOC), 16, β-hydroxydehydroepiandosterone (16, β-OH-DHEA), and dehydroepiandosterone sulfate (DHEA-S) may produce the low-renin state (140–142). However, there is no conclusive evidence that patients with low-renin activity are volume expanded. While early reports suggested that there was an increase in exchangeable sodium and extracellular volume in patients

with low-renin essential hypertension (128, 143, 144), recent reports have not documented a difference in exchangeable sodium, plasma volume, or extracellular fluid volume (145, 146). Furthermore, elevated levels of any of the various nonaldosterone mineralocorticoids have not been consistently found. In one report, only 6 out of 21 patients had elevated DOC levels (138). In another, DOC secretion and excretion was normal in low-renin essential hypertension (144). 18-Hydroxy-DOC excretion has been reported to be elevated in the majority of patients with low-renin essential hypertension (139); however, other studies have suggested that patients with low-renin essential hypertension do not have greater secretion rates or plasma levels of 18-OH-DOC than those with normal-renin essential hypertension (147, 148). In fact, on a high-salt diet, the latter have higher 18-OH-DOC levels (Fig. 14-16). There have been reports of increased mineralocorticoid activity in extracts of urine from low-renin patients (149), and yet increased binding of plasma extracts to mineralocorticoid receptors has not been found (150).

The most consistent finding in low-renin hypertensives is the favorable response of their blood pressure to volume depletion. Initially, it was felt that this was specifically induced by spironolactone; however, recent reports indicate that other diuretics can have beneficial effects (133). Another consistent response is normalization of blood pressure with adrenal inhibitors (144).

There are a number of lines of evidence suggesting that low-renin essential hypertension is not a hypermineralocorticoid state; one of the most compelling arguments is the failure to document alterations in potassium homeostasis. Almost invariably, serum potassium levels and potassium balance are within the normal range in these patients, unlike the findings in primary aldosteronism. If another mineralocorticoid were acting upon the aldosterone receptor, one would expect sodium retention and potassium wasting to occur together. While potassium wasting is not a universal finding in hypermineralocorticoid states (151), the weight of evidence suggests that volume expansion on the basis of excess mineralocorticoid activity should be accompanied by potassium depletion.

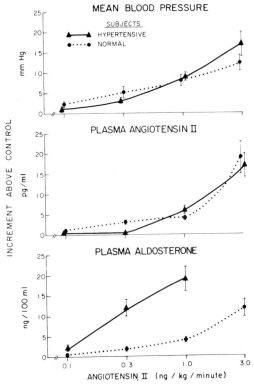

Figure 14-17. Increments in plasma angiotensin II, plasma aldosterone, and mean blood pressure in response to graded infusions of angiotensin II in 7 normotensive and 12 hypertensive subjects (mean ± standard error of the mean). All subjects were studied supine, in balance, on a 200 meq sodium/100 meq potassium intake. There were no significant differences in the plasma angiotensin II concentrations. Threshold sensitivity for blood pressure was similar (between 0.3 and 1 ng/kg per min) in both groups; however, the increment in blood pressure at 3 ng/kg per min was significantly greater ($P < 0.05$) in the hypertensive group. On the other hand, both threshold sensitivity and peak response for aldosterone secretion were significantly greater in the hypertensive group ($P < 0.01$). [From E. S. Kirsch et al.]

A recent intriguing suggestion is that the suppressed renin levels are due to an increase in the adrenal sensitivity to angiotensin II (152a). If so, then the volume-renin-aldosterone feedback loop could be closed with lower levels of angiotensin II, an appropriate adaptive mechanism in the face of an elevated blood pressure. Increased adrenal sensitivity to angiotensin II has also been reported in hypertensive patients with normal

plasma renin levels (152b). Twelve patients with essential hypertension were studied on a high (200 meq)-sodium intake. Adrenal responsiveness to the graded infusion of angiotensin II from 0.1 to 3 ng/kg per min was assessed. A significant increment in plasma aldosterone occurred at an infusion rate of 0.3 ng/kg per min in the patients with hypertension; this change was not seen in the normotensive controls until the infusion rate reached 1 ng/kg per min. Even at an angiotensin II infusion rate of 1 ng/kg/ per min, the increment in plasma aldosterone in normotensive subjects (4.2 ± 0.6 ng/dL) was significantly less than that in patients with essential hypertension (19 ± 3 ng/dL) ($p < 0.001$) (Fig. 14-17).

Enhanced adrenal sensitivity to angiotensin II could also explain the variable reports regarding volume spaces, exchangeable sodium, potassium, or other features of hypermineralocorticoidism in patients with low-renin hypertension. Renin release is controlled by a number of factors in addition to volume and sodium. A floor exists below which renin secretion cannot be reduced by volume or sodium alone. With an enhanced adrenal response to angiotensin II, the potential exists for transient hypermineralocorticoidism even during volume-expanded states.

As noted earlier, several studies have reported a decreased plasma volume in patients with hypertension, usually correlated with the level of blood pressure. It has generally been assumed that these volume changes result from a pressure natriuresis. However, some studies have suggested that relative hypoaldosteronism may be present in some patients with hypertension. Streeten and his colleagues were the first to report that some patients with normal-renin essential hypertension have abnormal aldosterone secretory responses to volume depletion (153). Forty-five percent of their patients had a smaller increment in aldosterone excretion in response to sodium restriction than did normal subjects. Studies performed in our laboratory on patients with essential hypertension have also documented that many have an abnormality in the relative responsiveness of the various components of the renin-angiotensin-aldosterone axis. In half of 40 patients with normal-renin essential hypertension studied on low (10 meq)-sodium intake, plasma aldosterone failed to increase in response to acute volume depletion induced by diuretics or venous hemorrhage, even though a sharp increment in plasma renin activity occurred (154, 155). Weinberger and his colleagues have reported similar findings (156). Furthermore, a discrepancy between renin-angiotensin and aldosterone responsiveness to volume depletion has been documented by assessing the incremental response of renin or angiotensin II and aldosterone to upright posture (157). Sixty patients with essential hypertension who were previously documented as having normal renin responses to sodium restriction and upright posture were studied on a restricted sodium intake. Two-thirds of the patients had responses within the normal range. However, one-third showed normal increments in plasma renin activity in association with subnormal increments in plasma aldosterone (Fig. 14-18). Since patients with low-renin activity had been excluded, the abnormality appears to be an altered relationship between the renin-angiotensin system and the adrenal cortex. It is unlikely that there is a deficiency in converting-enzyme activity since plasma angiotensin II and renin activity increased in parallel. A primary adrenal biosynthetic defect also seems unlikely since aldosterone responses to ACTH infusion were normal (154). Thus, the most likely explanation is a change in the action of angiotensin II at its glomerulosa cell receptor. This hypothesis has been tested by infusing angiotensin II at rates of 0.1 to 3 ng/kg per min into patients with essential hypertension on a 10 meq sodium intake. In those hypertensive subjects with a normal renin-aldosterone response to volume depletion, aldosterone levels began to rise at an infusion rate between 0.3 and 1 ng/kg per min. On the other hand, no significant increment in plasma aldosterone occurred even at an infusion rate of 3 ng/kg per min in those subjects who had appeared to have a decreased adrenal response to angiotensin II based on volume-depleting procedures (157).

DIFFERENTIAL DIAGNOSIS

Any screening tests performed must separate curable from noncurable forms of hypertension. The curable causes include unilateral renal disease, renal artery stenosis, pheochromocytoma, diseases of adrenal cortex, such as primary aldosteronism and Cushing's syndrome, and, less commonly other endocrine disorders such as thyroid dysfunction and acromegaly. The minimally effective screening procedure consists of obtaining values for serum electrolytes, blood urea nitrogen (BUN), 24-h urine catecholamines and vanilmandelic acid or metanephrine (the urine preferably being collected during the time the patient is hypertensive), rapid-sequence intravenous pyelogram, urine culture with urinalysis, and measurement of renin activity with the patient in supine and upright positions on a low-salt diet. The use of analogues which act as competitive inhibitors of angiotensin II (e.g., saralasin) is a promising technique for screening for angiotensin-mediated hypertension such as renal artery stenosis. The extensive studies necessary for the diagnosis of primary aldosteronism should be reserved for those hypertensive patients who present with hypokalemia and suppressed plasma renin activity (Fig. 14-11). If abnormalities in any of the

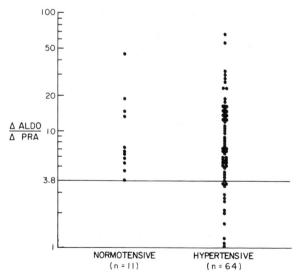

Figure 14-18. Comparison of normotensive and hypertensive subjects classified according to their ΔALDO/ΔPRA ratios which represent the increment in plasma aldosterone (ΔALDO) divided by the increment in plasma renin activity (ΔPRA) when the subjects changed from the supine to the upright position (10 meq sodium diet). [*From T. J. Moore et al. (157).*]

screening tests seem to warrant further investigation, then a specific protocol designed to bring out the basic defect should be carried out as described above.

TREATMENT

A particular form of antihypertensive therapy is chosen empirically to lower blood pressure, or specifically, to treat a known type of secondary hypertension. In secondary forms of hypertension, an important decision to be made is the choice between medical management and surgical intervention. In most instances, surgery will be recommended, since it may be curative; however, elderly patients or subjects with advanced vascular disease, who are major operative risks, can often be managed successfully with drug therapy. Some drug therapies are specific, such as spironolactone for primary aldosteronism or phenoxybenzamine for pheochromocytoma. Renin-lowering agents are often successful in patients with renal artery stenosis if peripheral levels are significantly elevated. However, combination therapy on an empirical basis may still be necessary in some patients with secondary hypertension who are managed by medical means.

The role of dietary sodium restriction in the management of hypertension was established by Allen and Sherrill in 1922 (158) and by the success of Kempner's fruit-and-rice diet (159). Although severe sodium restriction is definitely beneficial, many physicians have abandoned dietary measures in favor of sodium-depleting diuretic agents. However, it is suggested that modest sodium restriction (2 to 4 g daily) be attempted as initial therapy in patients with mild essential hypertension. Sodium restriction will also reduce the potassium-wasting effects of thiazide diuretic therapy and will lower blood pressure beyond the level obtainable through diuretic therapy alone (160, 161).

Many favor a thiazide diuretic as the initial agent in an antihypertensive regimen. Thiazides not only produce a sustained contraction of plasma and extracellular fluid volume, but also lower peripheral resistance. Moreover, the volume contraction associated with diuretic therapy appears to enhance the antihypertensive effect of other drugs, such as hydralazine and guanethidine, which produce sodium retention. It has recently been questioned whether diuretics should invariably form the base of the antihypertensive regimen, because complications are possible in certain patients. Hypokalemia, hyperuricemia, glucose intolerance, and hyperlipidemia are recognized side effects of thiazide diuretic therapy; plasma volume contraction may also further elevate renin levels in patients with angiotensin-mediated hypertension. Although alternative diuretic agents (e.g., spironolactone) can minimize certain complications of thiazides (such as hypokalemia), these compounds have their own side effects (gynecomastia and impotence in male patients). Diuretic agents have a particularly favorable effect in patients with low-renin essential hypertension.

The other major types of drugs that are used in therapy include peripheral vasodilators (hydralazine, prazosin), adrenergic blocking drugs (α-methyldopa, clonidine, reserpine, guanethidine), and β-adrenergic blocking agents (propranolol). Choice of a drug regimen for the individual patient should be guided by a number of considerations, including severity of hypertension, age, sex, compliance, associated cardiovascular and other medical disorders, and cost (100).

SUMMARY OF ELECTROLYTE AND WATER DISTURBANCES IN HYPERTENSION

Hyponatremia. Hyponatremia associated with hypertension is usually related to diuretic therapy, renal disease, or accelerated hypertension with secondary aldosteronism. The hyponatremia produced by renal disease is usually present only when the renal disease is obvious.

Hypernatremia. The most common cause of hypernatremia associated with hypertension is increased aldosterone secretion, specifically in primary aldosteronism. It is unusual to find elevated sodium levels in secondary aldosteronism. The level of serum sodium depends on the degree of autonomy of aldosterone secretion.

Hypokalemia. A decrease in serum potassium occurs in two common conditions associated with hypertension: diuretic therapy and increased aldosterone secretion. Kaliuresis is quite common with thiazide-type diuretics. It can usually be corrected with supplemental potassium chloride. Either a primary or secondary increase in aldosterone secretion will produce a kaliuresis. Some patients with essential hypertension also have borderline hypokalemia without a known cause.

Hypomagnesemia. This may occur in primary aldosteronism. (See Chap. 19.)

Metabolic alkalosis. Metabolic alkalosis is due to diuretics which increase the amount of sodium chloride presented to the distal tubules and thereby induce increased bicarbonate resorption and chloride loss. Metabolic alkalosis is also produced by excess aldosterone (or cortisol) secretion via the mechanism of hydrogen and potassium ion exchange for sodium at the distal sites with resultant increased serum bicarbonate levels. (See Chaps. 4 and 6.)

Total body water. Total body water is increased in primary aldosteronism (increased extracellular and plasma volume) and in hypertension associated with acromegaly (increased extracellular, intracellular, and plasma volume). In renal vascular hypertension, there is often a decrease in plasma volume, while in essential hypertension it may be normal or decreased.

Metabolic acidosis. Metabolic acidosis does not occur in uncomplicated hypertension. If present, it is usually secondary to renal failure.

REFERENCES

1. Starling, E. H.: *The Law of the Heart Beat: Linacre Lecture*, Longmans, Green & Co., Ltd., London, 1918.
2. Mueller, C. B., A. Surtshin, M. R. Carmen, and H. A. White: Glomerular and tubular influence of sodium and water excretion, *Am. J. Physiol.*, **165:**411, 1951.
3. Vander, A. J.: Control of renin release, *Physiol. Rev.*, **47:**359, 1967.
4. Blair-West, J., J. P. Coughlin, D. A. Denton, J. R. Golding, J. A. Monroe, R. E. Peterson, and M. Winter: Humoral stimulation of adrenal cortical secretion, *J. Clin. Invest.*, **41:**1606, 1960.
5. Davis, J. O., J. Urquhart, and J. T. Higgins, Jr.: Effects of alterations of plasma sodium and potassium concentration on aldosterone secretion, *J. Clin. Invest.*, **42:**597, 1963.
6. Williams, G. H., and R. G. Dluhy: Aldosterone biosynthesis: Interrelationship of regulatory factors, *Am. J. Med.*, **53:**595, 1972.
7. Davis, J. O.: The control of renin release, in *Hypertension Manual*, Dun-Donnelley Publishing Corp., New York, 1974, p. 163.
8. Ganten, D., P. Granger, U. Ganten, R. Boucher, and J. Genest: An intrinsic renin-angiotensin system in the brain, in *Hypertension, 1972*, Springer-Verlag Inc., New York, 1972, p. 423.
9. Vander, A. J., and R. Miller: Control of renin secretion in the anesthetized dog, *Am. J. Physiol.*, **207:**537, 1964.
10. Thurauk, K., J. Schnermann, W. Nagle, M. Horster, and M. Wohl: Composition of tubular fluid in the macula densa segment as a factor regulating the function of the juxtaglomerular apparatus, *Circ. Res.*, **21**(suppl. II):79, 1967.
11. Cooke, C. R., T. C. Brown, B. J. Zacherle, and W. G. Walker: Effect of altered sodium concentration in the distal nephron segments on renin release, *J. Clin. Invest.*, **49:**1630, 1970.
12. Nash, F. D., H. H. Rostorfer, M. D. Bailie, R. L. Wathen, and E. G. Schneider: Renin release: Relation to renal sodium load and dissociation from hemodynamic changes, *Circ. Res.*, **22:**473, 1968.
13. Thurau, K. W. C., H. Dahlheim, A. Gruner, J. Mason, and P. Granger: Activation of renin in the single juxtaglomerular apparatus by sodium chloride in the tubular fluid at the macula densa, *Circ. Res.*, **30, 31** (suppl. II):182, 1972.
14. Vander, A. J.: Effect of catecholamines and the renal nerves on renin secretion in anesthetized dogs, *Am. J. Physiol.*, **209:**659, 1965.
15. Assaykeen, T. A., P. L. Clayton, A. Goldfien, and W. F. Ganong: Effect of alpha- and beta-adrenergic blocking agents on the renin response to hypoglycemia and epinephrine in dogs, *Endocrinology*, **87:**1318, 1970.
16. Sealey, J. E., I. Clark, M. B. Bull, and J. H. Laragh: Potassium balance and the control of renin secretion, *J. Clin. Invest.*, **49:**2119, 1970.

17. Dluhy, R. G., J. P. Cain, and G. H. Williams: Influence of dietary potassium on the renin and aldosterone responses to diuretic-induced volume depletion, *J. Lab. Clin. Med.*, **83**:249, 1974.

18. Dluhy, R. G., G. L. Wolf, A. R. Christlieb, R. B. Hickler, and D. P. Lauler: Suppression of plasma renin activity by acute potassium chloride loading, *Circulation*, **38** (suppl. 6):VI-66, 1968.

19. Vander, A. J., and G. W. Geelhoed: Inhibition of renin secretion by angiotensin II, *Proc. Soc. Exp. Biol. Med.*, **120**:399, 1965.

20. Shade, R. E., J. O. Davis, J. A. Johnson, R. W. Gotshall, and W. S. Spielman: Mechanism of action of angiotensin II and antidiuretic hormone on renin secretion, *Am. J. Physiol.*, **224**:926, 1973.

21. Simpson, S. A., J. F. Tait, A. Wettstein, R. Neherr, J. Von Euw, and T. Reichstein: Isolieurung eines neyen Kristablisierten Hormons aus Nebennieren mit besonders Noher Wirksamkeit auf dem Mineralstoffwechsel, *Experientia*, **9**:333, 1953.

22. Thorn, G. W., R. H. Sheppard, W. I. Morse, W. J. Reddy, P. M. Beigelman, and A. E. Renold: Comparative action of aldosterone and 9-alpha-fluorohydrocortisone in man, *Ann. N.Y. Acad. Sci.*, **61**:609, 1955.

23. Sharp, G. W., and A. Leaf: The central role of pyruvate in the stimulation of sodium transport by aldosterone, *Proc. Natl. Acad. Sci. U.S.A.*, **52**:1114, 1964.

24. Edelman, I. S., R. Bogoroch, and G. A. Porter: On the mechanism of action of aldosterone on sodium transport: The role of protein synthesis, *Proc. Natl. Acad. Sci. U.S.A.*, **50**:1169, 1963.

25. August, J. T., D. H. Nelson, and G. W. Thorn: Response of normal subjects to large amounts of aldosterone, *J. Clin. Invest.*, **37**:1549, 1958.

26. Gross, F.: The regulation of aldosterone secretion by the renin-angiotensin system under various conditions, *Acta Endocrinol.*, **124** (suppl.):41, 1967.

27. Ganong, W. F., E. G. Biglieri, and P. J. Mulrow: Mechanism regulating adrenocortical secretion of aldosterone and glucocorticoids, *Recent Prog. Horm. Res.*, **22**:381, 1966.

28. Blair-West, J. R., J. P. Coghlan, D. A. Denton, J. R. Golding, M. Wintour, and R. D. Wright: The control of aldosterone secretion, *Recent Prog. Horm. Res.*, **19**:311, 1963.

29. Müller, J.: *Regulation of Aldosterone Biosynthesis*, Springer-Verlag Inc., New York, 1971.

30. Laragh, J. H., and H. C. Stoerk: A study of the mechanism of secretion of the sodium-retaining hormone (aldosterone), *J. Clin. Invest.*, **36**:383, 1957.

31. Michelakis, A. M., and R. Horton: The relationship between plasma renin and aldosterone in normal man, *Circ. Res.*, **26, 27** (suppl.):1, 1970.

32. Williams, G. H., M. L. Tuck, L. I. Rose, R. G. Dluhy, and R. H. Underwood: Studies of the control of plasma aldosterone concentration in normal man. III. Response to sodium chloride infusion, *J. Clin. Invest.*, **51**:2645, 1972.

33. Balikian, H. M., A. H. Brodie, S. L. Dale, J. C. Melby, and J. F. Tait: Effect of posture on the metabolic clearance rate, plasma concentration and blood production rate of aldosterone in man, *J. Clin. Endocrinol. Metab.*, **28**:1630, 1968.

34. Boyd, G. W., A. R. Adamson, M. Arnold, V. H. T. James, and W. S. Peart: The role of angiotensin II in the control of aldosterone in man, *Clin. Sci.*, **42**:91, 1972.

35. Tuck, M. L., R. G. Dluhy, and G. H. Williams: Sequential responses of the renin-angiotensin-aldosterone axis to acute postural change: Effect of dietary sodium, *J. Lab. Clin. Med.*, **86**:754, 1975.

36. Bartter, F. C., G. W. Liddle, L. E. Duncan, J. K. Barbour, and C. Delea: Regulation of aldosterone secretion in man. Role of fluid volume, *J. Clin. Invest.*, **35**:1306, 1956.

37. Williams, G. H., J. P. Cain, R. G. Dluhy, and R. H. Underwood: Studies of the control of plasma aldosterone concentration in normal man. I. Response to posture, acute and chronic volume depletion and sodium-loading, *J. Clin. Invest.*, **51**:1731, 1972.

38. Crabbe, J., E. J. Ross, and G. W. Thorn: Significance of secretion of aldosterone during dietary sodium deprivation in normal subjects, *J. Clin. Endocrinol. Metab.*, **18**:1159, 1958.

39. Espiner, E. A., J. R. Tucci, P. I. Jagger, and D. P. Lauler: Effect of saline infusions on aldosterone secretion and electrolyte excretion in normal subjects and patients with primary aldosteronism, *N. Engl. J. Med.*, **277**:1, 1967.

40. Biglieri, E. G., P. I. Slaton, and S. J. Kronfield, et al.: Diagnosis of an aldosterone-producing adenoma in primary aldosteronism, *JAMA*, **201**:510, 1967.

41. Horton, R.: Stimulation and suppression of aldosterone in plasma of normal men and in primary aldosteronism, *J. Clin. Invest.*, **48**:1230, 1969.

42. Shade, R. E., and C. E. Grim: Suppression of renin and aldosterone by small amounts of DOCA in normal man, *J. Clin. Endocrinol. Metab.*, **40**:652, 1975.

43. Epstein, M., and T. J. Saruta: Effect of water immersion on renin aldosterone and renal handling in normal man, *J. Appl. Physiol.*, **31**:368, 1971.

44. Crane, M. G., and J. J. Harris: Suppression of plasma aldosterone by partial immersion, *Metabolism,* **23**(4):359, 1974.

45. Kem, D. C., M. H. Weinberger, D. M. Mayes, and C. A. Nugent: Saline suppression of plasma aldosterone in hypertension, *Arch. Intern. Med.*, **128**:380, 1971.

46. Tuck, M. L., R. G. Dluhy, and G. H. Williams: A specific role for saline or the sodium ion in the regulation of renin and aldosterone secretion, *J. Clin. Invest.*, **53**:988, 1974.

47. Veyrat, R., H. R. Brunner, E. L. Mannine, and A. F. Mueller: Inhibition de l'activite de la renine plasmatique par le potassium, *Urol. Nephrol.*, **73**:271, 1967.

48. Dluhy, R. G., R. H. Underwood, and G. H. Williams: Influence of dietary potassium on plasma renin activity in normal man, *J. Appl. Physiol.*, **28**:299, 1970.

49. Brunner, H. R., L. Baer, J. E. Sealey, J. G. G. Ledingham, and J. H. Laragh: The influence of potassium administration and of potassium deprivation on plasma renin in normal and hypertensive subjects, *J. Clin. Invest.*, **49**:2128, 1970.

50. Himathongkam, T., R. G. Dluhy, and G. H. Williams: Potassium-aldosterone-renin interrelationships, *J. Clin. Endocrinol. Metab.*, **41**:153, 1975.

51. Kaplan, N. M.: The biosynthesis of adrenal steroids. Effects of angiotensin II, adrenocorticotropin and potassium, *J. Clin. Invest.*, **44**:2029, 1965.

52. Haning, R., S. A. S. Tait, and J. F. Tait: *In vitro* effects of ACTH, angiotensins, serotonin and potassium on steroid output and conversion of corticosterone to aldosterone by isolated adrenal cells, *Endocrinology,* **87**:1147, 1970.

53. Williams, G. H., L. M. McDonnell, S. A. S. Tait, and J. F. Tait: The effect of medium composition and *in vitro* stimuli on the conversion of corticosterone to aldosterone in rat glomerulosa tissue, *Endocrinology,* **91**:948, 1972.

54. Müller, J., and R. Huber: Effects of sodium deficiency, potassium deficiency, and uremia upon the steroidogenic response of rat adrenal tissue to serotonin, potassium ions, and adrenocorticotropin, *Endocrinology,* **85**:43, 1969.

55. Venning, E. H., I. Dyrenfurth, and J. C. Beck: Effect of corticotropin and prednisone on the excretion of aldosterone in man, *J. Clin. Invest.*, **35**:1299, 1956.

56. Crabbe, J., W. J. Reddy, E. J. Ross, and G. W. Thorn: The stimulation of aldosterone secretion by adrenocorticotropic hormone (ACTH), *J. Clin. Endocrinol Metab.*, **19**:1185, 1959.

57. Tucci, J. R., E. A. Espiner, P. I. Jagger, G. L. Pauk, and D. P. Lauler: ACTH stimulation of aldosterone secretion in normal subjects and in patients with chronic adrenocortical insufficiency, *J. Clin. Endocrinol. Metab.*, **27**:568, 1967.

58. Williams, G. H., L. I. Rose, R. G. Dluhy, J. F. Dingman, and D. P. Lauler: Aldosterone response to sodium restriction and ACTH stimulation in panhypopituitarism, *J. Clin. Endocrinol. Metab.*, **32**:27, 1971.

59. Palmore, W. P., and P. J. Mulrow: Control of aldosterone secretion by the pituitary gland, *Science,* **158**:1482, 1967.

60. Ganong, W. F., D. L. Pemberton, and E. E. Banbrunt: Adrenal cortical responsiveness to ACTH and angiotensin II in hypophysectomized dogs and dogs treated with large doses of glucocorticoids, *Endocrinology,* **81**:1147, 1967.

61. Hollenberg, N. K., W. R. Chenitz, D. F. Adams, and G. H. Williams: Reciprocal influence of salt intake on adrenal glomerulosa and renal vascular responses to angiotensin II in normal man, *J. Clin. Invest.*, **54**:34, 1974.

62. Oelkers, W., J. J. Brown, R. Fraser, A. L. Lever, J. J. Morton, and J. I. S. Robertson: Sensitization of the adrenal cortex to angiotensin II in sodium-depleted man, *Circ. Res.*, **34**:69, 1974.

63. Ganong, W. F., and A. T. Boryczka: Effect of a low sodium diet on aldosterone-stimulating activ-

ity of angiotensin II in dogs, *Proc. Soc. Exp. Biol. Med.*, **124**:1230, 1967.

64. Hollenberg, N. K., G. H. Williams, B. Burger, and I. Hooshmand: Potassium's influence on the renal vasculature, the adrenal, and their responsiveness to angiotensin II in normal man, *Clin. Sci.*, **49**:527, 1975.

65. Williams, G. H., N. K. Hollenberg, and L. M. Braley: Influence of sodium intake on vascular and adrenal angiotensin II receptors, *Endocrinology*, **98**:1343, 1976.

66. Goldblatt, H., J. R. F. Lynch, R. Hazal, and W. W. Summerville: Studies on experimental hypertension. I. The production of persistent elevation of systolic blood pressure by means of renal ischemia, *J. Exp. Med.*, **59**:347, 1934.

67. Ames, R. P., A. J. Brokowski, A. M. Sicinski, and J. H. Laragh: Prolonged infusion of angiotensin II and norepinephrine on blood pressure and electrolyte balance, aldosterone and cortisol secretion in normal man and in cirrhosis with ascites, *J. Clin. Invest.*, **44**:1171, 1965.

68. Colman, R. W.: Formation of human plasma kinin, *N. Engl. J. Med.*, **291**:509, 1974.

69. Goldstein, M. S., E. R. Ramey, and R. Levine: Relation of muscular fatigue in adrenalectomized dog to inadequate circulatory adjustments, *Am. J. Physiol.*, **163**:561, 1950.

70. Fritz, I., and R. Levine: Action of adrenocortical steroids and norepinephrine on vascular responsiveness in stress in adrenalectomized rats, *Am. J. Physiol.*, **165**:456, 1951.

71. Ivy, H. K., A. Schirger, H. Fuller, and W. M. McConahey: Hypertension associated with hyperthyroidism, in William M. Manger (ed.), *Hormones and Hypertension*, Charles C Thomas, Publisher, Springfield, Ill., 1966.

72. Strauch, G., M. B. Vallotton, Y. Touitou, and H. Bricaire: The renin-angiotensin-aldosterone system in normotensive and hypertensive patients with acromegaly, *N. Engl. J. Med.*, **287**:795, 1972.

73. Cain, J. P., G. H. Williams, and R. G. Dluhy: Plasma renin activity and aldosterone secretion in patients with acromegaly, *J. Clin. Endocrinol. Metab.*, **34**:73, 1972.

74. Lee, T. C., and D. deWied: Somatotropin as the non-ACTH factor of anterior pituitary origin for the maintenance of enhanced aldosterone secre-

tory responsiveness of dietary sodium restriction in chronically hypophysectomized rats, *Life Sci.*, **7**:35, 1968.

75. Overbeck, H. W., R. S. Derifield, M. B. Pamnani, and T. Sozen: Attenuated vasodilator responses to K⁺ in essential hypertensive men, *J. Clin. Invest.*, **53**:678, 1974.

76. Borst, J. G. G., and A. Borst de Geus: Hypertension explained by Starling's theory of circulatory homeostasis, *Lancet*, **1**:677, 1963.

77. Guyton, A. C.: *Textbook of Medical Physiology*, 5th ed., W. B. Saunders Company, Philadelphia, 1976, pp. 265–294.

78. Conn, J. W., and I. H. Lewis: Primary aldosteronism: A new entity, *Ann. Intern. Med.*, **44**:1, 1956.

79. Conn, J. W.: Presidential address. II. Primary aldosteronism: A new clinical syndrome, *J. Lab. Clin. Med.*, **45**:3, 1955.

80. Kaplan, N. M.: Commentary on incidence of primary aldosteronism: Current estimations based on objective data, *Arch. Intern. Med.*, **123**:152, 1969.

81. Conn, J. W., R. F. Knopf, and R. M. Nesbit: Clinical characteristics of primary aldosteronism from an analysis of 145 cases, *Am. J. Surg.*, **107**:159, 1964.

82. George, J. M., L. Wright, N. H. Bell, F. C. Bartter, and R. Brown: The syndrome of primary aldosteronism, *Am. J. Med.*, **48**:343, 1970.

83. Cain, J. P., M. L. Tuck, G. H. Williams, R. G. Dluhy, and S. H. Rosenoff: The regulation of aldosterone secretion in primary aldosteronism, *Am. J. Med.*, **53**:627, 1972.

84. Davis, W. W., H. H. Newsome, L. D. Wright, W. G. Hammond, J. Easton, and F. C. Bartter: Bilateral adrenal hyperplasia as a cause of primary aldosteronism with hypertension, hypokalemia and suppressed renin activity, *Am. J. Med.*, **42**:642, 1967.

85. Ferris, J. B., J. J. Brown, R. Fraser, A. W. Kay, A. F. Lever, A. M. Neville, I. G. O'Muirchearthaigh, J. I. S. Robertson, and T. Symington: Hypertension with aldosterone excess and low plasma renin: pre-operative distinction between patients with and without adrenocortical tumor, *Lancet*, **2**:995, 1970.

86. Baer, L., S. C. Sommers, L. R. Krakoff, M. A. Newton, and J. H. Laragh: Pseudo-primary aldo-

steronism: An entity distinct from true primary aldosteronism, *Circ. Res.*, **26, 27** (Suppl. 1):203, 1970.

87. Kaplan, N. M.: Primary aldosteronism with malignant hypertension, *N. Engl. J. Med.*, **269**:1282, 1963.

88. Conn, J. W., E. L. Cohen, D. R. Rovner, and R. M. Nesbit: Normokalemic primary aldosteronism: A detectable cause of curable "essential" hypertension, *JAMA*, **193**:200, 1965.

89. Scoggins, B. A., C. H. Oddie, W. S. C. Hare, and J. P. Coghlan: Pre-operative lateralisation of aldosterone-producing tumors in primary aldosteronism, *Ann. Intern. Med.*, **76**:891, 1972.

90. Nicolis, G. L., H. A. Mitty, R. S. Modlinger, and J. L. Gabrilove: Percutaneous adrenal venography, *Ann. Intern. Med.*, **76**:899, 1972.

91. Melby, J. C., R. F. Spark, S. L. Dale, R. H. Egdahl, and P. C. Kahn: Diagnosis and localization of aldosterone-producing adenomas by adrenal-vein catheterization, *N. Engl. J. Med.*, **277**:1050, 1967.

92. Spark, R. F., and J. C. Melby: Aldosteronism in hypertension: The spironolactone response test, *Ann. Intern. Med.*, **69**:685, 1968.

93. Fraser, R., J. J. Brown, R. Chinn, A. F. Lever, and J. I. S. Robertson: The control of aldosterone secretion and its relationship to the diagnosis of hyperaldosteronism, *Scot. Med. J.*, **14**:420, 1969.

94. Biglieri, E. G., J. R. Stockigt, and M. Schambelan: Adrenal mineralocorticoids causing hypertension, *Am. J. Med.*, **52**:623, 1972.

95. Laragh, J. H., S. Ulick, V. Januszewicz, Q. B. Deming, W. G. Kelly, and S. Lieberman: Aldosterone excretion and primary and malignant hypertension, *J. Clin. Invest.*, **39**:1091, 1960.

96. Conn, J. W., E. L. Cohen, C. P. Lucas, W. J. McDonald, G. H. Mayor, W. M. Blough, W. C. Eveland, J. J. Bookstein, and J. Lapides: Primary reninism, *Arch. Int. Med.*, **130**:682, 1972.

97. Sjoerdsma, A., K. Engleman, and T. A. Waldman, et al.: Pheochromocytoma: Current concepts of diagnosis and treatment, *Ann. Intern. Med.*, **65**:1203, 1966.

98. Steiner, A. L., A. D. Goodman, and S. R. Powers: Study of a kindred with pheochromocytoma, medullary thyroid carcinoma, hyperparathyroidism, and Cushing's disease: Multiple endocrine

neoplasia, type 2, *Medicine*, **47**:371, 1968.

99. Sarosi, G., and R. P. Doe: Familial occurrence of parathyroid adenomas, pheochromocytoma, and medullary carcinoma of the thyroid with amyloid stroma (Sipple's syndrome), *Ann. Intern. Med.*, **68**:1305, 1968.

100. Kaplan, N. M.: *Clinical Hypertension*, Medcom Press, Inc., New York, 1973.

101. Regoli, D., H. Brunner, G. Peters, and F. Gross: Changes in renin content in kidneys of renal hypertensive rats, *Proc. Soc. Exp. Biol. Med.*, **109**:142, 1962.

102. Brunner, H. R., J. D. Kirschman, J. E. Sealey, and J. H. Laragh: Hypertension of renal origin: Evidence for two different mechanisms, *Science*, **174**:1344, 1971.

103. Tobian, L., K. Coffee, and P. McCrea: Contrasting exchangeable sodium in rats with different types of Goldblatt hypertension, *Am. J. Physiol.*, **217**:458, 1969.

104. Swales, J. D., H. Turston, F. P. Queiroz, and A. Medina: Sodium balance during the development of experimental hypertension, *J. Lab. Clin. Med.*, **30**:539, 1972.

105. McCubbin, J. W., and I. H. Page: Renal pressor system in neurogenic control of arterial pressure, *Circ. Res.*, **12**:553, 1963.

106. Dickinson, C. J., and J. R. Lawrence: Slowly developing pressor response to small concentrations of angiotensin, *Lancet*, **1**:1354, 1963.

107. Frohlich, E. D., M. Ulrych, R. C. Tarazi, H. P. Dustan, and I. H. Page: A hemodynamic comparison of essential and renovascular hypertension. Cardiac output and total peripheral resistance in supine and tilted patients, *Circulation*, **35**:289, 1967.

108. Tarazi, R. C., E. D. Frohlich, and H. P. Dustan: Contribution of cardiac output to renovascular hypertension in man. Relation to surgical treatment, *Am. J. Cardiol.*, **31**:600, 1973.

109. Blair-West, J. R., J. P. Coglan, D. A. Denton, E. Orchard, B. A. Scoggins, and R. D. Wright: Renin-angiotensin-aldosterone system and sodium balance in experimental renal hypertension, *Endocrinology*, **83**:1199, 1968.

110a. Maxwell, M. H., H. C. Gonick, R. Wiita, and J. J. Kaufman: Use of the rapid sequence intravenous pyelogram in the diagnosis of renovascular hypertension, *N. Engl. J. Med.*, **270:**213, 1964.

110b. Bookstein, J. J., H. L. Abrams, R. E. Buenger, J. Lecky, S. S. Franklin, M. D. Reiss, K. H. Bleifer, E. C. Klatte, P. D. Varady, and M. H. Maxwell: Radiologic aspects of renovascular hypertension. Part 2, The role of urography in unilateral renovascular disease, *JAMA,* **220:**1225, 1972.

111. Page, I. H., and J. W. McCubbin (eds.): *Renal Hypertension,* Year Book Medical Publishers, Inc., Chicago, 1968, p. 316.

112. Stockigt, J. R., C. A. Noakes, R. D. Collins, and M. Schambelan: Renal-vein renin in various forms of renal hypertension, *Lancet,* **1194,** June 3, 1972.

113. Strong, C. S., J. C. Hunt, S. G. Sheps, R. M. Tucker, and P. E. Bernatz: Renal venous renin activity enhancement of sensitivity of lateralization by sodium depletion, *Am. J. Cardiol.,* **27:**602, 1971.

114a. Hollenberg, N. K., G. H. Williams, B. Burger, I. Ishikawa, and D. F. Adams: Blockade and stimulation of renal, adrenal and vascular angiotensin II receptors with 1-sar, 8-ala angiotensin II in normal man, *J. Clin. Invest.,* **57:**39, 1976.

114b. Streeten, D. H. P., G. H. Anderson, and J. M. Freiberg, et al.: Use of an angiotensin II antagonist (saralasin) in the recognition of "angiotensinogenic" hypertension, *N. Engl. J. Med.,* **292:**657, 1975.

114c. Williams, G. H., and N. K. Hollenberg: 1-Sar, 8-Ala Angiotensin II's effect on renal, adrenal and vascular receptors in man: Its usefulness in screening for renal and adrenal diseases, in M. P. Sambhi (ed.), *Systemic Effects of Antihypertensive Agents,* Stratton Intercontinental Medical Book Corp., New York, 1976.

115a. Baldwin, D. S., A. W. Biggs, W. Goldring, W. H. Hulet, and H. Chasis: Exaggerated natriuresis in essential hypertension, *Am. J. Med.,* **24:**893, 1958.

115b. Aviram, A., W. J. Czaczkes, and T. D. Ullmann: Diuretic and natriuretic response to a salt load in hypertensive and prehypertensive subjects, *Nephron,* **2:**82, 1965.

116. Eisinger, R. P.: Augmented natriuretic response to infusion of saline in dogs rendered acutely hypertensive with metaraminol, *Proc. Soc. Exp. Biol. Med.,* **122:**804, 1966.

117. Tarazi, R. C., E. D. Frohlich, and H. P. Dustan: Plasma volume in men with essential hypertension, *N. Engl. J. Med.,* **278:**762, 1968.

118. Tarazi, R. C., M. M. Ibrahim, E. L. Bravo, and H. P. Dustan: Haemodynamic characteristics of primary aldosteronism, *N. Engl. J. Med.,* **289:**1330, 1973.

119. Tobian, L., and J. Benion: Artery wall electrolytes in renal and DOCA hypertension, *J. Clin. Invest.,* **33:**1407, 1954.

120. Napondano, R. J., F. S. Caliva, C. Lyons, J. DeSimone, and R. H. Lyons: The reactivity to angiotensin of rabbit aorta strips after either alterations of external sodium environment or direct addition of benzydroflumethiazide, *Am. Heart J.,* **64:**498, 1962.

121. Genest, J., E. Koiw, W. Nowaczynski, and G. Leboeuf: Further studies on urinary aldosterone in human arterial hypertension, *Proc. Soc. Exp. Biol. Med.,* **97:**676, 1958.

122. Espiner, E. A., A. R. Christlieb, E. A. Amsterdam, P. I. Jagger, S. J. Dobrzinsky, D. P. Lauler, and R. B. Hickler: The pattern of plasma renin activity and aldosterone secretion in normal and hypertensive subjects before and after saline infusions, *Am. J. Cardiol.,* **27:**585, 1971.

123. Coghlan, J. P., A. E. Doyle, G. Jerums, and B. A. Scoggins: The effects of sodium loading and deprivation on plasma renin and plasma and urinary aldosterone in hypertension, *Clin. Sci.,* **42:**15, 1972.

124. Collins, R. D., M. H. Weinberger, A. J. Dowdy, G. W. Nokes, C. M. Gonzales, and J. A. Luetscher: Abnormally sustained aldosterone secretion during salt loading in patients with various forms of benign hypertension: Relation to plasma renin activity, *J. Clin. Invest.,* **49:**1415, 1970.

125. Tuck, M. L., G. H. Williams, R. G. Dluhy, M. Greenfield, and T. J. Moore: A delayed suppression of the renin-aldosterone axis following saline infusion in human hypertension, *Circ. Res.,* **39:**711, 1976.

126. Helmer, O. M.: The renin-angiotensin system and its relation to hypertension, *Prog. Cardiovasc. Dis.,* **8:**117, 1965.

127. Creditor, M. C., and U. K. Loschky: Plasma renin

activity in hypertension, *Am. J. Med.*, **43**:371, 1967.

128. Jose, A., J. R. Crout, and N. M. Kaplan: Suppressed plasma renin activity in essential hypertension. Role of plasma volume, blood pressure, and sympathetic nervous system, *Ann. Intern. Med.*, **72**:9, 1970.

129. Carey, R. M., J. G. Douglas, J. R. Schweikert, and G. W. Liddle: The syndrome of essential hypertension and suppressed plasma renin activity. Normalization of blood pressure with spironolactone, *Arch. Intern. Med.*, **130**:849, 1972.

130. Brunner, H. R., J. H. Laragh, L. Baer, M. A. Newton, F. T. Goodwin, L. R. Krakoff, R. H. Bard, and F. R. Buhler: Essential hypertension: Renin and aldosterone, heart attack and stroke, *N. Engl. J. Med.*, **286**:441, 1972.

131. Tuck, M. L., G. H. Williams, J. P. Cain, J. M. Sullivan, and R. G. Dluhy: Relation of age, diastolic pressure and known duration of hypertension to presence of low renin essential hypertension, *Am. J. Cardiol.*, **22**:637, 1973.

132. Crane, M. G., J. J. Harris, and J. J. Varner: Hyporeninemic hypertension, *Am. J. Med.*, **52**:457, 1972.

133. Spark, R. F., and C. M. O'Hare: Low-renin hypertension. Restoration of normotension and renin responsiveness, *Arch. Intern. Med.*, **133**:205, 1974.

134. Rosenthal, J., R. Boucher, W. Nowaczynski, and J. Genest: Acute changes in plasma volume, renin activity, and free aldosterone levels in healthy subjects following furosemide administration, *Can. J. Physiol. Pharmacol.*, **46**:85, 1968.

135. Padfield, P. L., J. J. Brown, A. F. Lever, and M. A. D. Schalekamp, et al.: Is low-renin hypertension a stage in the development of essential hypertension or a diagnostic entity? *Lancet*, **ii**:548, 1975.

136. Schalekamp, M. A. D. H., X. H. Krauss, M. P. A. Schalekamp-Kuyken, G. Kolsters, and W. H. Birkenhager: Studies on the mechanism of hyper-natriuresis in essential hypertension in relation to measurements of plasma renin concentration, body fluid compartments and renal function, *Clin. Sci.*, **41**:219, 1971.

137. Creditor, M. C., and U. K. Loschky: Incidence of suppressed renin activity and of normokalemic

primary aldosteronism in hypertensive negro patients, *Circulation*, **37**:1027, 1968.

138. Brown, J. J., J. B. Ferriss, and R. Fraser, et al.: Apparently isolated excess deoxycorticosterone in hypertension, *Lancet*, **2**:243, 1972.

139. Melby, J. C., S. L. Dale, and T. E. Wilson: Secretion of 18-hydroxydeoxycorticosterone (18-OH DOC) in human hypertensive disease, *Circ. Res.*, **28, 29**(suppl. 2):143, 1971.

140. Liddle, G. W., and J. A. Sennett: New mineralocorticoids in the syndrome of low-renin essential hypertension, *J. Steroid Biochem.*, **6**:751, 1974.

141. Dale, S. L., and J. C. Melby: Isolation and identification of 16, α 18-dihydroxydeoxycorticosterone from human adrenal gland incubations, *Steroids*, **21**:617, 1973.

142. Sekihara, H., N. Ohsawa, and K. Kosaka: Serum dihydroepiandrosterone sulfate and dehydroepiandrosterone levels in essential hypertension, *J. Clin. Endocrinol. Metab.*, **40**:156, 1975

143. Helmer, O. M., and W. E. Judson: Metabolic studies on hypertensive patients with suppressed plasma renin activity not due to hyperaldosteronism, *Circulation*, **38**:965, 1968.

144. Woods, J. W., G. W. Liddle, and E. G. Stant, et al.: Effect of an adrenal inhibitor in hypertensive patients with suppressed renin, *Arch. Intern. Med.*, **123**:366, 1969.

145. Schalekamp, M. A., D. G. Beevers, and G. Kolsters, et al.: Body-fluid volume in low-renin hypertension, *Lancet*, **1**:310, 1974.

146. Lebel, M., J. J. Brown, and D. Kremer, et al.: Sodium and the renin-angiotensin system in essential hypertension and mineralocorticoid excess, *Lancet*, **1**:308, 1974.

147. Messerli, F. H., O. Luchel, and W. Nowaczynski, et al.: Mineralocorticoid secretion in essential hypertension with normal and low plasma renin activity, *Circulation*, **53**:406, 1976.

148. Williams, G. H., L. M. Braley, and R. H. Underwood: The regulation of plasma 18-hydroxy-11-deoxycorticosterone in man, *J. Clin. Invest.*, **58**:221, 1976.

149. Sennett, J. A., and G. W. Liddle: New mineralocorticoids in patients with low-renin essential hypertension (abstract), *Clin. Res.*, **23**:45A, 1975.

150. Baxter, J. D., M. Schambelan, and T. Matulich, et al.: Aldosterone receptors and the evaluation of

plasma mineralocorticoid activity in normal and hypertensive states, *J. Clin. Invest.*, **58**:579, 1976.

151. Ulick, S.: Adrenocortical factors in hypertension. 1. Significance of 18-hydroxy-11-deoxycorticosterone, *Am. J. Cardiol.*, **38**:814, 1976.

152a. Wisgerhof, M., and R. D. Brown: Increased adrenal sensitivity to angiotensin II in low renin essential hypertension, *J. Clin. Invest.*, **61**:1456-1462, 1978.

152b. Kisch, E. S., R. G. Dluhy, and G. H. Williams: Enhanced aldosterone response to angiotensin II in human hypertension, *Circ. Res.*, **38**:502, 1976.

153. Streeten, D. H. P., F. E. Schletter, G. V. Clift, C. T. Stevenson, and T. G. Dalakos: Studies of the renin-angiotensin-aldosterone system in patients with hypertension and in normal subjects, *Am. J. Med.*, **46**:844, 1969.

154. Williams, G. H., L. I. Rose, R. G. Dluhy, D. McCaughn, P. I. Jagger, R. B. Hickler, and D. P. Lauler: Abnormal responsiveness of the renin aldosterone system to acute stimulation in patients with essential hypertension, *Ann. Intern. Med.*, **72**:317, 1970.

155. Tuck, M. L., J. M. Sullivan, N. K. Hollenberg, R. G. Dluhy, and G. H. Williams: Hemodynamic and endocrine response patterns in young patients with normal renin essential hypertension, *Clin. Res.*, **21**:505, 1973.

156. Weinberger, M. H., A. J. Dowdy, G. W. Nokes, and J. A. Luetscher: Plasma renin activity and aldosterone secretion in hypertensive patients during high and low sodium intake and administration of diuretics, *J. Clin. Endocrinol. Metab.*, **28**:359, 1968.

157. Moore, T. J., G. H. Williams, and R. G. Dluhy, et al.: Altered renin-angiotensin-aldosterone relationships in normal renin essential hypertension, *Circ. Res.*, **41**:167, 1977.

158. Allen, F. M., and J. W. Sherrill: Treatment of arterial hypertension, *J. Metab. Res.*, **2**:429, 1922.

159. Kempner, W.: Treatment of kidney disease and hypertensive vascular disease with rice diet, *N. Carolina Med. J.*, **5**:125, 1944.

160. Winer, B. M.: The antihypertensive mechanisms of salt depletion induced by hydrochlorothiazide, *Circulation*, **24**:788, 1961.

161. Kirkendall, W. M., and M. L. Overturf: Thiazide diuretics and salt consumption in the treatment of hypertension, in M. P. Sambhi (ed.), *Systemic Effects of Antihypertensive Agents*, Stratton Intercontinental Medical Book Corp., New York, 1976.

15

Acute renal failure

STANLEY S. FRANKLIN / MORTON H. MAXWELL

INTRODUCTION

The term acute renal failure refers to the clinical syndrome of an abrupt, frequently reversible impairment or cessation of renal function which is usually manifested by oliguria or anuria. This syndrome encompasses many different disease entities. The taxonomy of acute renal failure will be enumerated in order to clarify terminology:

1. *Abrupt impairment of renal function.* Acute renal failure most commonly presents as a sudden onset of azotemia with prior documentation of normal renal function. It can occur as a rapid, progressive worsening of renal function without known previous renal disease. Occasionally acute impairment of renal function will be superimposed on well-documented chronic renal failure, so-called acute-on-chronic renal failure. Infrequently, a patient with acute renal failure may present with what is mistaken as end stage chronic renal disease.
2. *Urine output.* Although decreased urine volume is most characteristic of acute renal failure, urine output varies from total anuria to polyuria. Specific categories are defined as follows: oliguria less than 400 mL/day; anuria, less than 50 to 100 mL/day; total anuria, zero urine output; nonoliguria, from 400 to 1000 mL/day; and polyuric renal failure, greater than 1000 to 2000 mL/day.
3. *Anatomical site of involvement.* Prerenal refers to renal hypoperfusion which results in acute azotemia without associated renal parenchymal damage. Postrenal refers to outflow obstruction distal to the tubular site of urine formation. Renal sites of involvement may be subdivided into primary vascular, glomerular, interstitial, and tubular with some overlap of pathologic involvement occurring as a secondary event.
4. *Clinical setting.* This is a useful method of classifying acute renal failure. Although incidence will vary widely depending on the type of referral population, an average breakdown is as follows: surgery, 40 percent, trauma, 10 percent, pregnancy, 10 percent, nephrotoxins, 10 percent, and miscellaneous medical causes, 30 percent.

This chapter will deal chiefly with one form of acute renal failure, namely acute tubular necrosis (ATN). Other etiologies of acute renal failure will be considered as they relate to differential diagnosis. ATN is a pathologic term and may not accurately reflect underlying pathogenesis. The term ATN will be used in this chapter, however, because other names such as lower nephron nephrosis, tubulointerstitial nephritis, and vasomotor nephropathy have not gained general acceptance.

Acute tubular necrosis is also a syndrome rather than a distinct clinical entity. Variability in the syndrome of ATN will be briefly mentioned:

1. *Initiation of ATN.* Although there are multiple etiologies of ATN, only a few underlying pathogenic events initiate renal damage. These include ischemia, disseminated intravascular coagulation, abnormal proteinuria, pigmenturia, and nephrotoxins.
2. *Maintenance of ATN.* The persistence of reduced renal function, often with associated oliguria, may be ascribed to many possible causes: vasomotor shunting of blood away from the glomerulus, altered glomerular permeability, abnormal back diffusion through injured tubular epithelium, obstructed tubules, or a combination of these events. One hallmark of ATN is inviolate: the inability to restore renal function by manipulating extrarenal factors such as fluid volume, neurogenic tone, or vasoactive substances.
3. *Clinical course.* Typically, the oliguria of acute tubular necrosis lasts 1 to 2 weeks followed by the onset of diuresis and the return of renal function to almost normal values. However, the oliguric phase may be absent, permanent, or may last from 1 day to 6 weeks before the onset of diuresis. Similarly, renal function may return only partially or remain totally absent, requiring permanent hemodialysis therapy.

ETIOLOGY AND PATHOGENESIS

The major causes of acute tubular necrosis (ATN) are summarized in Table 15-1. Despite the apparent diversity of clinical settings, the main causes of ATN can be divided into two categories, nephrotoxic injury and renal ischemia, each of which results in a distinctive pathologic lesion.

NEPHROTOXIC INJURY

Under this category are drugs, solvents, heavy metals, and a wide variety of chemicals which are directly toxic to the renal tubular cells (1). The kidney is extremely vulnerable to damage from a large number of compounds because of its unique characteristics of (1) a large renal blood flow which exposes the renal parenchyma to a high proportion of the toxic substance; (2) a high oxygen consumption, which makes the kidney especially susceptible to agents which produce cellular anoxia; (3) the characteristic of concentrating certain nonresorbable solutes within the tubule lumen as water resorption takes place along the length of the nephron; (4) the vascular rete mirabile, which serves as a countercurrent mechanism resulting in the hypertonicity of the medullary interstitium, so that local concentrations of specific compounds may be highly concentrated in this area; and (5) the high permeability of the proximal tubules, which allows these cells to resorb high-molecular-weight molecules.

Potential toxic compounds enter the kidney by one of three general routes: (1) those which are solely filtered and because of water resorption are subject to progressive concentration along the luminal cell surfaces of the nephron; (2) those which are filtered and also undergo tubular resorption, involving penetration of the tubular cell, interaction with carrier systems, and local concentration on the capillary cell border; and (3) those which are actively secreted, interacting with enzyme systems and carriers, and finally concentrated in the luminal fluid.

Since the toxins are distributed by the bloodstream, the two kidneys are generally affected equally. The lesion most commonly seen is that of nephrotoxic tubular necrosis, affecting the proximal tubules of all nephrons. If there is no accompanying circulatory disturbance, the tubular basement membranes remain intact and can

Table 15-1. Classification of causes of acute tubular necrosis

I. ACUTE ISCHEMIC RENAL FAILURE

A. Surgery
  1. Major abdominal surgery (2)*(1)
  2. Aortic surgery (1) (2)
  3. Open-heart surgery (1) (2) (3)
  4. Transureteral prostatectomy (water irrigation) (3)
B. Diagnostic radiology (2)
C. Obstetrics
  1. Septic abortion (5) (2) (4)
  2. Postpartum hemorrhage (1) (2)
  3. Placenta previa (1) (2)
  4. Abruptio placentae (1) (2)
  5. Uterine rupture (1) (2)
  6. Intrauterine fetal death (1) (2) (4)
  7. Severe toxemia (1) (2) (4)
D. Trauma
  1. Crush injuries (2) (3) (1) (4)
  2. Fractures (1) (2)
E. Pigment release (3)
  1. Hemoglobin
    a. Infections
      1. Septicemia, endotoxins, Clostridium welshii (1) (2) (4) (5)
      2. Epidemic hemorrhagic fever (2) (4) (5)
      3. Malaria (blackwater fever) (1) (4) (5)
    b. Mismatched transfusion (3) (4)
    c. Hemolytic-uremic syndrome (4)
    d. Glucose 6-phosphate dehydrogenase deficiency (2) (1) (5)

    e. Valvular heart disease (2) (4)
    f. Venomous snake bites (2) (1) (4)
    g. Glycerol therapy (3) (4)
    h. Fresh water submersion (1) (2) (3)
  2. Myoglobin
    a. Rhabdomyolysis
      1. Excessive exercise (march myoglobinuria, anterior tibia syndrome, karate, etc.) (2) (1) (4)
      2. Crush injury (2) (1) (4)
      3. Electric shock
      4. Burns (2) (3) (1) (4)
      5. Heat stroke (2) (4)
      6. Hoff's disease (epidemic myoglobinuria) (2)
      7. Potassium depletion (2)
      8. Idiopathic, primary, paroxysmal (2)
      9. Acute polymyositis (2)
    b. McArdle's syndrome (2)
F. Proteinuria
  1. Multiple myeloma with BenceJones proteinuria (2) (1)
  2. Waldenström's macroglobulinemia (2) (1)
  3. Nephrotic syndrome (2) (1)
  4. Low-molecular-weight dextran therapy (2) (1)
G. Miscellaneous
  1. Major hemorrhage (internal or external) (2)
  2. Vomiting or diarrhea (severe) (2)
  3. Myocardial infarction (1)
  4. Hepatorenal syndrome (?) (2) (4)

II. ACUTE NEPHROTOXIC RENAL FAILURE

A. Heavy metals and their compounds
  Mercury (organic and inorganic), bismuth, uranium, cadmium, arsenic, and arsine, lithium
B. Organic solvents
  Carbon tetrachloride, tetrachloroethylene, ethoxyethanol, methanol, toluene, chloroform, trichlormethane, trichlorethylene
C. Glycols
  Ethylene glycol, diethylene glycol, diglycolic acid, oxalic acid, diglycolic acid

D. Antibiotics
  Neomycin, kanamycin, gentamicin, polymyxin, colistin, bacitracin, phenazopyridine, cotrimoxazole, amphotericin, rifampin
E. Pesticides
  Chlorinated hydrocarbons—chlordane, paraquat
F. Miscellaneous
  Carbon monoxide, mushroom poison, creasol, aniline and other methemoglobin-producing chemicals, phenylbutazone, Lysol, phenols, sodium chlorate, diesel fuel, and methoxyflurane

* Numbers in parentheses indicate contributing factors in order of importance: (1) hypotension, (2) extracellular fluid loss, (3) release of pigments (hemoglobin, myoglobin), (4) disseminated intravascular coagulation, (5) infection.

provide a scaffolding for the epithelial regeneration, which starts within a few days after the initial injury. With this type of lesion, therefore, regeneration may result in entirely normal kidneys, anatomically and functionally, and indeed the prognosis with conservative therapy is quite good (3, 4). The prototype of this lesion is bichloride of mercury or carbon tetrachloride poisoning (1). In contrast, other toxins such as glycols and oxalic acid may produce irreversible renal failure with evidence of extensive cortical necrosis and crystalline calcium oxalate deposition within tubules and interstitial spaces (1, 5). Some nephrotoxic antibiotics such as kanamycin, gentamicin, neomycin, polymyxin, and amphotericin may produce ATN which is reversible or irreversible depending on the total dose and duration of administration (1, 6).

RENAL ISCHEMIA

Many of the clinical situations causing ATN are associated with decreased effective blood volume, hypotension, or severe dehydration. Thus, oliguria may result from traumatic shock after an automobile accident, from the plasma loss of extensive burns, from salt and water loss associated with prolonged vomiting or diarrhea, or

from the loss of whole blood incident to surgical treatment or internal bleeding. All these situations set off a chain of homeostatic reactions which, if prolonged or extensive, can result in renal damage (Fig. 15-1). With hypovolemia or a decreased cardiac output from any cause, vasoconstriction occurs in the kidney, resulting in a marked reduction in renal blood flow.

Concomitantly, the intense renal ischemia and anoxia, if prolonged, may cause tubulorrhexis. As described by Oliver, this consists of widespread and random necrosis in any portion of the renal tubule, with disruption of the basement membrane (2, 3). When there is a predominance of tubulorrhexis, it is likely that permanent kidney damage will result. With loss of the tubular basement membrane to act as a scaffolding, epithelial regeneration occurs in a random, haphazard fash-

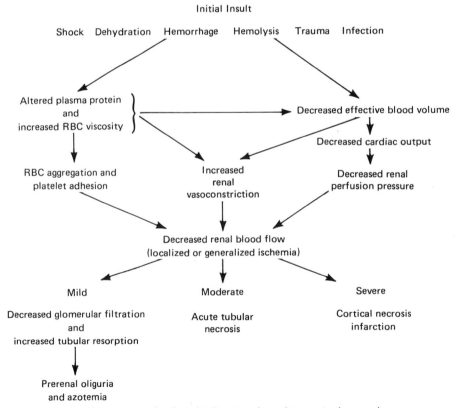

Figure 15-1. Role of renal ischemia in the pathogenesis of prerenal azotemia and acute renal failure.

ion, frequently leading to total obstruction of the lumen at the site of tubulorrhexis (2, 3). Since the intact nephron can never be reconstituted in its entirety, return of renal function must come from reparative processes in nephrons which have escaped this type of damage. The prognosis in any given patient, therefore, depends on the extent of tubulorrhexic necrosis. It must be recognized that tubulorrhexic and nephrotoxic lesions often coexist. Many patients with carbon tetrachloride intoxication, for example, have severe vomiting and dehydration with attendant renal ischemia. Since it is often impossible, in an anuric or oliguric patient, to assess the degree of permanent renal damage, the clinician must always treat the patient on the assumption that the lesion is reversible.

Unfortunately, it is difficult in specific instances to correlate the development of ATN with the degree or duration of clinical shock or hypotension (7). This is attributable to the multiple factors which can contribute to renal vasoconstriction, to the prior condition of the patient (age, state of hydration, circulatory status, etc.), and to the wide individual variability in vascular reactivity. In addition, renal ischemia may occur in the absence of clinical shock or hypotension because of a localized change in the renal microcirculation.

Renal blood flow is determined by both arterial blood pressure and the sum of pre- and postglomerular resistance in series. Glomerular resistance is influenced by (1) inherent myogenic vasomotor tone, (2) autonomic vasomotor impulses, (3) vasoactive substances, and (4) changes in blood viscosity. Therefore, decreased renal blood flow can occur secondary to changes in renal vascular resistance when systemic arterial blood pressure is well within the normal range. Similarly there is often a poor correlation between renal ischemia, decreased glomerular filtration rate (GFR), and the diminution or cessation of urine flow. Glomerular ultrafiltration is determined by (1) renal plasma flow rate, (2) mean transcapillary hydrostatic pressure difference, and (3) glomerular capillary permeability and surface area. Thus, there can be a reduction in glomerular filtration with resulting oliguria or anuria secondary to a decrease in factor (2) or factor (3) in the absence of

a significant reduction in factor (1), renal plasma flow, and, therefore, an absence of ischemic damage to the tubular epithelium. Similarly, nonoliguric ATN or polyuric ATN may occur because of the combination of persistent reduction in glomerular filtration and associated tubular defects in sodium and water reabsorption.

An understanding of the rheology of blood in the microvasculature is basic to the full understanding of the pathogenesis of tissue ischemia (8, 9). Whereas vasomotor control of the circulation occurs principally in the arteriolar vessels, most of the circulating blood volume is contained within the vessels of the microcirculation (lumen 100 μm or less), which consists chiefly of the capillary bed. Because of the small limiting diameter of the capillary vessels, impairment of flow with resultant ischemia may be caused by cell aggregates. Cell aggregation is influenced by the concentration and nature of the plasma proteins, especially under conditions of low flow rates. In major trauma or extensive burns, fibrinogen levels may exceed 1000 mg/dL, and plasma albumin values significantly decrease; it is in these conditions that diffuse aggregation and abnormal microcirculatory flows have been observed. It may be postulated that the localized areas of tubulorrhexic necrosis may represent areas of ischemia induced by these excessive red blood cell aggregates.

In recent years, the above concepts have been expanded to encompass the syndromes of disseminated intravascular coagulation (10–18). This biologic process begins with the entry of a procoagulant material or activity into the circulating blood and then progresses to platelet aggregation and fibrin formation, with or without the production of thrombosis of the capillaries, arterioles, and venules. It is associated with the composition of platelets, fibrinogen, and other blood-clotting factors during the process of coagulation and with the activation of the fibrinolytic enzyme system, with the subsequent dissolution of fibrin and fibrinogen and the release of fibrin split products into the plasma. Disordered activation of the fibrinolytic enzyme system, responsible for dissolution of fibrin and fibrinogen, may be responsible for perpetuation of the coagulation cascade which ultimately results in disseminated or local intravascular coagulation. The mesangial cells of the glomerulus, rich in plasminogen activator, may play a key role in normal fibrinolysis (17, 18). Tissue trauma or sepsis can initiate disordered fibrinolytic activity throughout the body and specifically in the kidney with the resultant development of ATN.

The major etiologic factors leading to intravascular coagulation are (1) release of tissue thromboplastin, as in abruptio placentae; (2) intravascular hemolysis, as in transfusion reactions, burns, and tissue trauma; (3) bacterial endotoxins, as in gram-negative sepsis; and (4) release of proteolytic enzymes, as in acute pancreatitis. All these conditions may lead to ATN.

Each of the above disease processes has unique clinical and pathologic changes in addition to those associated with intravascular clotting. The damage to the kidney from red blood cell aggregation, fibrin deposition, and severe anoxia can lead to ischemic ATN when the insult is mild to moderate and to bilateral renal cortical necrosis when the insult is severe.

The role of circulating blood and muscle pigments (burns, transfusion reactions, severe trauma) in the pathogenesis of ATN has long

been controversial (19). The accumulated evidence, however, both in animals and humans, tends to discredit a direct nephrotoxic effect of these substances. The intravenous administration of hemoglobin to normal animals or humans does not result in ATN (20). As demonstrated by Castle and his coworkers, incompatible red blood cells in vivo first agglutinate before hemolyzing (21); therefore, it is probable that the agglutination within the capillary system, as described above, rather than the hemolysis which follows, is the explanation for ATN following the administration of incompatible blood. It would appear likely, therefore, that blood and muscle pigments are not nephrotoxic substances per se. When they are associated with ATN, their main etiologic role may be their contribution to renal ischemia, i.e., the effect of the release of high-molecular-weight proteins into the plasma with a resulting change in plasma viscosity.

The multifactoral pathogenesis of ischemic nephron damage can be pictured as occurring in three distinct stages (see Table 15-2). The first stage is mild ischemia without injury. Host factors are favorable and the clinical setting is one

Table 15-2. Pathogenesis of ischemic renal damage

STAGE	PREDISPOSING HOST FACTORS	CLINICAL SETTING, ACUTE INSULT	PATHOPHYSIOLOGY	CLINICO PATHOLOGIC MANIFESTATIONS
I. Mild ischemia without injury	None	Dehydration Hemorrhagic shock Myocardial shock Adrenal crisis Hepatic failure	↓Renal perfusion pressure ±Mild ↑ renal vascular resistance	Na-H$_2$O Retention Oliguria Anuria Prerenal azotemia
II. Severe ischemia with tubular cell injury	Aging Nephrosclerosis Diabetes mellitus Jaundice Proteinuria	Surgery Trauma Radiopaque contrast material Hemolysis Rhabdomyolysis Endotoxemic shock	Severe ↑ renal vascular resistance ± ↓ Renal perfusion pressure ± Local or general intravascular coagulation	Tubular cell injury Acute tubular Necrosis (ATN)
III. Severe ischemia and endothelial injury with impaired fibrinolysis	Pregnancy Infancy Estrogens Abnormal reticuloendothelial system	Severe and prolonged shock Specific infectious agents Hyperacute transplant rejection Malignant hypertension	Severe ↑ renal vascular resistance Local or general intravascular coagulation with defective fibrinolysis Endothelial injury	Patchy or confluent renal cortical necrosis Hemolytic-uremic syndrome

of uncomplicated hypovolemia. This results in a decreased renal perfusion pressure and only a mild increase in renal vascular resistance. The resultant clinical picture is one of sodium and water retention, oligoanuria, and prerenal azotemia.

The second stage is severe renal ischemia with tubular cell injury. Predisposing host factors of nephrosclerosis, jaundice, or heavy proteinuria may be present. In addition to the presence of hypovolemia, there may be other associated insults such as pigmenturia, endotoxemia, or the introduction of radiopaque contrast material. Ischemia now progresses to injury with associated marked increased intravascular resistance, with or without local intravascular coagulation, and frequently results in acute tubular necrosis.

The third stage consists of intense ischemia, endothelial injury, and impaired fibrinolysis. Predisposing host factors may be pregnancy, early infancy, or alterations in the reticuloendothelial system. The precipitating insult may be severe or prolonged shock, infectious agents, or hyperacute transplant rejection. There is a resulting severe increase in vascular resistance, localized or generalized intravascular coagulation, and defective fibrinolysis resulting in patchy or confluent cortical necrosis.

MECHANISMS OF IMPAIRED RENAL FUNCTION AND OLIGURIA

Intensive investigation of the maintenance of ATN over the past two decades has not resulted in a unitary hypothesis. Instead, two major points of view have emerged. One emphasizes tubular necrosis and the other normal tubular function. Within these alternate concepts are a variety of distinct or interrelated mechanisms which may play a role in pathogenesis (Table 15-3).

CLASSIC THEORY OF TUBULAR NECROSIS

This concept assumes that the syndrome of ATN is the result of organic renal parenchymal damage which occurs after a period of renal ischemia or nephrotoxicity and consists of acute tubular necrosis, interstitial edema, tubular ob-

Table 15-3. Proposed pathophysiologic mechanisms in acute renal failure

A. Tubular injury or necrosis
 1. Abnormal back-diffusion
 2. Obstructing tubular casts or debris
 3. Impaired-reflow phenomenon
 4. Tubuloglomerular feedback
B. Normal renal tubules
 1. Vasomotor nephropathy
 2. Efferent arteriolar dilation
 3. Altered glomerular permeability
 4. Obstructing tubular casts or debris

struction by casts, and abnormal back-diffusion of glomerular filtrate through damaged tubular epithelium. This theory was originally proposed by Bywaters and Beall (22) and Lucke (23), and later championed by Merrill (24, 25). It presupposes that the glomerular filtrate leaks through the damaged tubular basement membrane into the renal interstititium and accounts for the tense, swollen kidneys seen at postmortem examination. The resulting interstitial edema is thought to exert sufficient pressure to collapse and mechanically obstruct the remaining unaffected functioning tubules, furthering the oliguria in this manner.

CLINICOPATHOLOGIC CORRELATION

There seems to be little doubt as to the existence of tubular necrosis in most cases of nephrotoxic-induced ATN. In ischemic ATN, however, the clinicopathologic correlation is not as clear. At times, ATN may develop with little or no pathologic evidence of tubular necrosis. In the past, this poor clinicopathologic correlation has been ascribed to (1) examination of renal tissue only after regeneration of renal epithelium has commenced, i.e., kidney biopsies obtained late in the oliguric phase or at postmortem examination, (2) the presence of only minor lesions on light microscopy, whereas the electron microscope may reveal pronounced cellular lesions (3, 26), and (3) the finding that only one severe tubulorrhexic lesion can interfere with urine formation within that nephron although the majority of the nephron epithelium may appear normal (3).

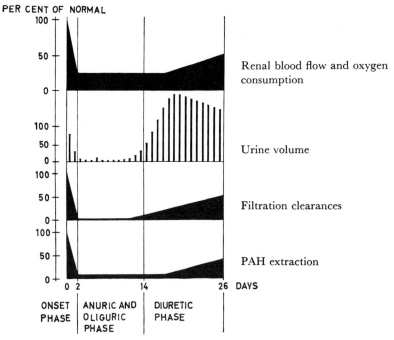

PER CENT OF NORMAL

Figure 15-2. Diagram showing the circulatory and some other functional disturbances in the course of acute renal failure. Urine flow and PAH extraction and filtration clearances are much more reduced than renal blood flow and oxygen consumption. (*From C. Brun and O. Munck,* Prog. Surg., *4:1, 1964.*)

There are several physiologic observations which tend to support the persistence of glomerular filtration, although at a much reduced rate. Although renal blood flow was formerly thought to be almost negligible as measured by conventional clearance techniques (27), more recent studies using radioactive krypton (^{85}Kr) and an indirect Fick method of analysis showed that renal blood flows are one-third to one-half of normal values in patients during the oliguric phase (Fig. 15-2). This level of renal blood flow could be compatible with a substantial glomerular filtration rate. Observations made during infusion urography in patients with oliguric ATN are strongly supportive of the concept of continuing glomerular filtration (28, 29). The typical finding is that of the prompt appearance of a nephrogram which is of normal intensity in most patients with ATN. Furthermore, the nephrogram ususally persists unchanged for hours or even days. Because iodinated contrast media are almost exclusively excreted by filtration and not secretion, the finding of an early and persistent nephrogram is strong evidence for continued glomerular filtration.

Strong experimental evidence in favor of leakage of filtrate back through damaged tubular epithelium has been shown in a number of nephrotoxic animal models (30–33) as well as in postischemic ATN (34–39). Reabsorption would then occur, as in any capillary bed, by the osmotic force of the postglomerular blood. Both the experimental and clinical finding of a substantial increase in kidney weight in association with a swollen, edematous cut surface would be consistent with damaged tubular epithelium, continued glomerular filtration, and excessive back-diffusion of filtrate.

The role of mechanical obstruction to urine flow by cast formation has long been controversial (19). Although casts are not a prominent feature in the usual microscopic preparation, microdissection techniques of the entire nephron reveal them with great frequency, particularly in those cases associated with transfusion reactions or crush injuries. It is easy to visualize how one strategically placed cast in a large collecting duct could effectively block urine formation from many nephrons which drain into it. As mentioned above, hemoglobin or myoglobin does not appear to be intrinsically toxic to the renal tubules and seems to be associated with the production of ATN only when there is renal ischemia and a decreased renal tubular flow rate.

There is substantial experimental evidence favoring tubular obstruction in both experimental nephrotoxic and postischemic ATN (30, 34, 35, 38, 40). In contrast, some investigators have found that intratubular pressure is low in nephrons that appear to contain tubular casts or impacted debris (41, 42). This finding implies that the tubular plugging is secondary to reduced tubular flow rather than the cause of it. Recent studies by Finn, Arendshorst, and Gottschalk (43, 44), working in postischemic rats, suggest that tubular obstruction is prominent throughout the first 24 h after arterial occlusion. Thereafter, normal intratubular pressures and collapsed proximal tubules were noted, consistent with preglomerular vasoconstriction and cessation of glomerular filtration. At this point in time acute volume expansion reversed the reduced pressures and renal blood flow, yet the experimental kidneys remained oliguric. These findings strongly suggest that tubular obstruction and passive back flow of tubular fluid are the cardinal reasons for maintenance of ATN; the mechanism by which obstruction of a tubule decreases blood flow to its glomerulus is unknown.

An alternative mechanism for the persistence of ischemia and renal failure in the face of tubular injury was proposed by Leaf and his associates (45, 46). They found that renal blood flow remained low after release of arterial obstruction (impaired-reflow phenomenon). These experiments suggest that intrarenal capillaries must have been narrowed during ischemia, possibly by swollen ischemic vascular endothelial or tubular epithelial cells. When arterial pressure is restored, swollen endothelium and impacted red blood cells impede capillary flow. However, additional studies from both the same investigators in rats and by others in dogs indicate that the no-reflow phenomenon is at most a transient event and cannot explain persistent renal failure after arterial occlusion (47, 48).

An alternative hypothesis has been put forward by Thurau and Boylan (49). They postulate that acute tubular necrosis to the macula densa cells results in persistent vasoconstriction and reduced glomerular filtration secondary to the local release of angiotensin II at the site of the juxtaglomerular apparatus and acting in situ. Thus a tubuloglomerular feedback is operating to prevent excessive loss of salt and water which would otherwise occur if a damaged tubular epithelium is exposed to a normal volume of filtrate. This hypothesis, however, does not adequately explain polyuric ATN, the persistence of oliguria after normalization of renal blood flow in experimental ischemic ATN of rats, or the occasionally low urine sodium chloride concentration that is present in hypovolemic ATN patients.

FUNCTIONAL THEORIES

In order to account for the many inconsistencies of the classic organic theory of ATN, Finckh has proposed that there is a disturbance of intrarenal vascular tone persisting throughout the oliguric and even into the diuretic phase which causes a decrease in glomerular filtration rate out of proportion to the observed decrease in renal blood flow (50). This implies an inordinate degree of preglomerular arteriolar vasoconstriction or relative postglomerular vasodilation (50). Thus nonuniformity of the disturbance of vascular tone and local reaction may account for the patchy evidence of tubular necrosis observed. Recovery with the onset of a sudden diuresis can then be explained on the basis of a normalization of intrarenal tone. Schnermann and his associates proposed that local vasoconstriction, in association with renal ischemia, may persist due to local continued activation of the renin-angiotensin system (51). According to this hypothesis a wide variety of initiating events such as hypotension, hemorrhage, sepsis, nephrotoxins, or autoimmune vascular damage predispose to the development of acute renal failure and are potent stimuli for renin release. Renal ischemia, then, would activate the renin-angiotensin system and perpetuate cortical ischemia after the initiating stimulus has disappeared. The following observations would be consistent with this hypothesis: (1) absence of an early rapid component in the xenon washout curve in patients with acute renal failure, suggestive of a preferential renal cortical ischemia (52), (2) failure to demonstrate intralobular arteries in selective arteriograms in patients with ATN (46), and (3) the finding of elevated levels of plasma renin and angiotensin activity in the oliguric phase of ATN with a subsequent decrease in plasma renin during the diuretic phase (53–55).

Indirect evidence supporting this concept comes from the studies of Oken and his associates (41, 42, 56–58) in mercury- and glycerol-induced hemoglobinuric ATN. In these experimental models using micropuncture studies they found greatly decreased proximal tubular fluid flow rates and normal or low intratubular pressure in association with oliguria. This was interpreted as being consistent with an extreme reduction in GFR in the absence of significant transtubular leakage or cast obstruction. Furthermore, rats with chronic salt loading which resulted in depletion of plasma and tissue renin were largely protected from glycerol-induced ATN (59). This protection was not related to expansion of blood volume, polyuria, or low urine osmolality. In contrast, rats with hereditary diabetes insipidus were not spared from glycerol-induced renal failure, which suggests that polyuria is not a protective feature (60). In clinical ATN most patients show an increase in plasma renin activity during the period of renal insufficiency which returns to normal as renal function improves (53–55). Thus there are data supporting the role of the renin-angiotensin excess and the development of ATN although one cannot separate cause and effect.

More recently strong evidence has accumulated which suggests that renin-angiotensin activation is not necessary for the production of ATN. There is no protection from the experimental production of acute renal failure after active or passive immunization to angiotensin (61–63). Moreover, angiotensin II blocking agents are without effect in protecting from experimental ATN (64). Infusion of vasodilators such as acetylcholine, hydralazine, and prostaglandins into the renal artery markedly increased renal blood flow in patients with both nephrotoxic and ischemic ATN, but oliguria and impaired renal function persisted (65, 66). Thus this data as well as previous studies quoted above would suggest that intense afferent arteriolar vasoconstriction, so-called vasomotor nephropathy, is not a necessary or sufficient cause of acute renal failure.

The possible role of altered glomerular permeability in the pathogenesis of acute renal failure, with or without associated renal tubular necrosis, has only recently come into focus. Baehler et al. (67), investigating oliguric renal failure in mercuric chloride–infused dogs, found that infusions of Ringer's solution reversed renal vasoconstriction but had no significant effect on urine flow. Microscopic observation of the surface of the kidney showed tubules to be collapsed and devoid of fluid both before and after renal blood flow was increased by volume expansion. Two mechanisms could explain a marked reduction in GFR in association with an increase in renal plasma flow and no tubular obstruction. Glomerular capillary pressure could be reduced because of disparate alterations in afferent and efferent arteriolar resistance, i.e., the coexistence of afferent arteriolar constriction and efferent arteriolar vasodilation. There is no direct evidence for this hypothesis, and futhermore afferent and efferent resistance have been shown to rise proportionately in ischemic ATN (68). The alternative explanation is that there is a derangement in glomerular capillary permeability, and indeed transmission and scanning electron microscopy demonstrated mild abnormalities in glomerular epithelial morphology in the mercuric chloride-treated dogs. It should be noted that glomerular permeability (glomerular capillary ultrafiltration coefficient, K_F) is the product of the glomerular capillary surface area and the hydrolic conductivity across the capillary membrane. Even more marked alterations in glomerular epithelial morphology have been described in uranyl nitrate ATN as well as in a model of oliguric renal failure produced by intrarenal administration of norepinephrine (69–71). Recent reviews of the mechanisms regulating glomerular filtration have alluded to a variety of vasoactive endogenous substances and drugs which can affect glomerular permeability (72, 73). It is quite possible that changes in glomerular permeability play a significant role in both experimental and clinical ATN.

The role of renal tubular obstruction by cast formation in the absence of acute tubular necrosis must also be considered as a possible mechanism for acute renal failure. The most important product of tubular epithelium, Tamm-Horsfall urinary mucoprotein, has been identified in the collecting tubules of patients with acute renal failure (74). Administration of contrast media can precipitate Tamm-Horsfall urinary mucoprotein and contribute to intratubular obstruction. Excessive proteinuria of the nephrotic syndrome, abnormal proteinuria of multiple myeloma, and other dysproteinemias may cause renal tubular obstruction by cast formation which is precipitated within tubules when dehydration is present (75–77). Similarly, the administration of low-molecular-weight dextran in association with dehydration or hypovolemia can also produce acute renal failure, presumably by a tubular obstructive process (78, 79). Experimental folic acid acute renal failure in animals is likewise thought to represent an obstructive rather than ischemic model (80, 81). Acute renal failure associated with acute severe hyperuricemia, hypercalcemia, and excessive oxalate excretion may produce renal impairment by their tendency to produce obstructive uropathy in the distal tubule and collecting system of the nephron (82–85). Intratubular obstruction, with or without associated tubular injury, must be distinguished from extrarenal obstruction which by and large has a different natural history and clinical course. Until a more definitive pathophysiologic classification can be established, the term ATN appears preferable to obstructive uropathy in describing intratubular obstruction.

From the above data the following tentative conclusions can be made regarding the pathogenesis of acute renal failure. ATN is the hallmark of nephrotoxic acute renal failure and is frequently seen with postischemic acute renal failure. The consequences of ATN are intratubular obstruction, abnormal back-diffusion through damaged tubular epithelium resulting in swollen, edematous kidneys and a continuation of glomerular filtration although at a reduced rate. The finding of a diminished renal blood flow is not a primary event but secondary to tubular obstruction or an abnormal tubuloglomerular feedback mechanism which reduces the single-nephron GFR. The mechanism by which renal blood flow is reduced is probably not dependent on the intact renin-angiotensin mechanism, although it could be contributory. Where acute tubular necrosis cannot be demonstrated, the oliguric syndrome may be secondary to a change in glomerular membrane permeability and/or primary obstruction at the site of the intratubular and collecting duct level.

The apparent discrepancy in the etiologic mechanisms for ATN as described above is caused by (1) differences in etiologic agents, (2) variations in dosages and routes of administration, (3) differences in the stage of the process studied, and (4) possible differences between animal models and clinical ATN. From the present evidence it is concluded that the oliguria of ATN results from several different mechanisms, operating either independently or in consort. The relative importance of these mechanisms varies with the situation and is dependent upon the evolution of the disease process as well as the severity of pathologic damage. One can therefore speak of a variety of acute renal failures with varying pathophysiology, a varying clinical picture from total anuria to nonoliguric ATN, and varying degrees of residual damage from failure of recovery to complete restoration of renal function.

DIAGNOSIS

Prompt recognition of ATN and its differentiation from other types of acute renal and urinary tract disorders are of particular importance, since early recognition may help to prevent or attenuate severe renal failure and oliguria. Moreover, once complete ATN has developed, proper management during the first few days often determines the eventual outcome. Following any of the numerous conditions listed above that are reported to cause ATN (Table 15-1), diagnosis is usually not difficult if the physician is aware of this possibility. After restoration of blood pressure and replacement of blood, water, and electrolytes, the response of the urinary flow to fluid administration is the principal guide. It is essential for diagnosis, even in the face of incontinence, coma, or delirium, to obtain accurate volumes at intervals as short as every 1 to 2 h.

It should be remembered that ATN usually occurs in a previously healthy individual; that during the first few days after onset one should not see stigmata of chronic renal failure (muscle wasting, pallor, pigmentation of the skin), periorbital edema (except after carbon tetrachloride intoxication), severe diastolic hypertension, retinopathy, flank pain, costovertebral angle tenderness, or dysuria; that the specific gravity of the urine is close to 1.010 with a pH of 5.5 to 7.5 and radiologically the kidneys are observed to be equal and normal in size, without calculi; and that oliguria, but not anuria, is usually present.

Early diagnosis of prerenal oliguria is essential, for therapy properly directed at preventing the development of ATN may become detrimental once it has appeared. The usual homeostatic response in a normal subject to pure water depletion is an increased secretion of antidiuretic hormone, resulting in a urine of small volume, high specific gravity, and high urea content. The extent of the oliguria will depend largely upon the water requirements for obligatory solute excretion. On an ordinary intake of salt and protein, for example, a urine volume of 400 mL/day will be required for the excretion of approximately 600 mosm solute at a maximum specific gravity of 1.032, or an osmolality of 1200 mosm/L. The minimum urinary volume may be even smaller if the intake of protein and salt has been low and a high rate of tissue breakdown is not present.

When hypertonic dehydration has become severe enough to cause hypovolemia or when circulatory insufficiency and reduced effective blood volume have developed incident to the loss of extracellular fluid or hypotension (hemorrhage, diarrhea, severe sweating, myocardial infarction, burns, or sepsis), other factors come into play. Aldosterone secretion occurs in response to increased renin and angiotensin II levels, and the concentration of sodium in the urine diminishes markedly. In addition, the decreased renal blood flow resulting from renal vasoconstriction is associated with further diminution in the excretion of sodium and water. Because of the virtually complete tubular resorption of salt, urinary osmolality is largely accounted for by urea.

When renal ischemia is severe enough to cause a measurable reduction in the glomerular filtration rate, there is a decreased filtered load and an increased tubular resorption of urea, so that azotemia results. In most clinical situations in which this occurs, the patient is usually hypotensive or shows clinical evidence of severe dehydration, i.e., poor skin turgor, dry axillae, shriveled tongue, and soft eyeballs.

It is obvious that the causes and mechanisms of prerenal azotemia are identical with some of those which result in true acute tubular necrosis (Fig. 15-1); the only difference is the lack of organic parenchymatous kidney damage and the rapid reversibility of the former syndrome. When the renal ischemia resulting from dehydration or circulatory insufficiency is prolonged and/or severe, then ATN may ensue. Frequently, however, in the transition of prerenal oliguria to complete ATN there is an intermediate phase which is called partial ATN. In this transitional phase there may be sufficient reduction of renal blood flow and glomerular filtration rate to impair concentrating ability significantly as well as to cause varying degrees of azotemia. The reason for making this distinction is that proper therapy during the transition phase may prevent further progression to complete ATN with its obligatory period of severe oliguria unresponsive to therapy. Successfully treated incipient or partial ATN can be likened to nonoliguric ATN, in which there is a modest rise in BUN and serum creatinine levels, indicating parenchymal renal damage despite a normal or even increased urine output.

SEQUENTIAL DIAGNOSTIC EVALUATION OF OLIGOANURIA

The clinical strategy for the diagnosis of oligoanuria makes use of a sequential list of questions to be answered (see Table 15-4):

1. Is there true oligoanuria?

This requires a bladder catheterization to rule out outlet obstruction, determine bladder content, and thereafter determine urinary flow rate.

2. Is there physiologic oliguria?

As described above, antecedent history of fluid and solute intake along with measurement of urine flow rate and concentration can rule out possible physiologic forms of oliguria.

3. Is there renal circulatory insufficiency, and what is the cause? (See Table 15-5.)

It is well to remember that renal circulatory insufficiency can arise from a number of clinical states including diminished perfusion pressure secondary to shock, absolute hypovolemia with or without normal blood pressure, diminished cardiac function secondary to congestive heart failure and/or low cardiac output, diminished adrenal function in the setting of a hypovolemic

Table 15-4. Sequential diagnostic evaluation of oligoanuria

1. Is there true oligoanuria?
2. Is there physiologic oliguria?
3. Is there renal circulatory insufficiency and what is the cause?
4. Is there acute renal failure?
5. What is the anatomical localization and cause of acute renal failure?
6. Is the cause of acute tubular necrosis apparent or hidden?
7. Is there an atypical clinical course for acute tubular necrosis?

Table 15-5 Renal circulatory insufficiency without acute renal failure

	CLINICALLY PRESENT, IN GENERAL	
	DIAGNOSTIC PARAMETERS	THERAPEUTIC CHALLENGE
	$\uparrow$ BUN/creatinine	Mannitol
	$\uparrow$ U/P creatinine	
	$\uparrow$ U/P osmolality	
	$\uparrow$ PSP excretion	
	$\downarrow$ U_{Na} excretion	
	SPECIFIC CAUSE	
1. $\downarrow$ Perfusion pressure'	$\downarrow$ BP, $\uparrow$ pulse rate	Correct systemic hypotension
2. Absolute hypovolemia	Normal or $\downarrow$ BP	Fluid, crystalloid, colloid or blood administration
	Weight Loss	
	Negative fluid balance	
	Fluid sequestration	
	Tissue turgor $\downarrow$	
	Hematocrit change	
3. $\downarrow$ Cardiac function	$\uparrow$ Central venous or Swan-Ganz pressures	Loop diuretic
		Digitalis
	Edema, S_3 gallop	Decrease afterload
4. $\downarrow$ Adrenal function	$\downarrow$ BP, weight loss	Cortisone
	$\downarrow P_{Na}$, $\uparrow P_K$	Volume replacement
	$\uparrow U_{Na}$, $\downarrow U_K$	
	$\downarrow$ P cortisol	
5. $\downarrow$ Hepatic function	Normal or $\downarrow$ BP	Volume and/or vasopressors
	Ascites	
	Abnormal liver function tests	

U = Urine
P = Plasma
$\downarrow$ = Decreased
$\uparrow$ = Increased

crisis and the hepatorenal syndrome where there is shunting of blood away from the kidney because of factors as yet unknown. These diagnoses can usually be made clinically with the occasional aid of central venous or pulmonary wedge pressure monitoring.

4. Is there acute renal failure? (see Table 15-6)

A variety of simple renal function tests may be helpful in distinguishing between renal circulatory insufficiency and acute renal failure:

Table 15-6. Laboratory aids in the diagnosis of acute renal failure*

	PRERENAL OLIGURIA	PARTIAL ACUTE RENAL FAILURE	COMPLETE ACUTE RENAL FAILURE
1. U/P osmolality	> 2:1	1.1:1–1.9:1	<1.1:1
2. Urine sodium concentration, meq/L	<20	20–40	>40
3. U/P urea	>20:1	20:1–10:1	<10:1
U/P creatinine	>40:1	20:1–15:1	<15:1
4. 1-h PSP excretion, percent	>5	1–5	Zero to trace
5. U_{Na}/U/P creatinine	<1.0	1–5	>5

* Characteristic of ATN but also indistinguishable from obstructive, vascular, or interstitial disease. Only acute glomerulopathies may present with urinary findings suggestive of prerenal oliguria during the early phase; later, the urinary findings may merge with those of acute renal failure.

a. The urine/plasma (U/P) osmolality ratio is usually greater than 2:1 in prerenal oliguria and decreases toward a ratio of 1.1:1 with varying degrees of partial acute renal failure. In contrast, complete acute renal failure has a ratio of less than 1.1:1 (86).

b. Urine sodium concentration is usually below 20 meq/L in prerenal oliguria and above 40 meq/L in complete acute renal failure, frequently as high as 60 to 80 meq/L (87).[1]

c. The U/P urea concentration ratio is usually more than 20:1 in prerenal oliguria and much below this value in acute renal failure (90). Similarly, the U/P creatinine concentration ratio is usually more than 40:1 in prerenal oliguria. In our experience, the U/P creatinine ratio is somewhat more reliable than the U/P urea ratio, because creatinine does not back-diffuse and therefore is a truer estimate of water resorption across the nephron.

d. The 1-h phenolsulfonphthalein (PSP) excretion test is carried out in a manner similar to the conventional test, except that only a 1-h

[1]Persistently lower urinary sodium concentrations despite all the other stigmata of acute renal failure have been noted in nonoliguric renal failure and renal failure associated with severe hypovolemia (88, 89). This finding would suggest that tubular function is relatively intact in the nephrons which are forming urine and that they are responding to a hypovolemic stimulus or congestive heart failure.

specimen is obtained via a catheter and the bladder is irrigated with saline solution to minimize bladder-residual error (91). PSP excretion requires both adequate renal blood flow and tubular secretion. Therefore, negligible excretions suggest acute renal failure, whereas a 5 percent or more excretion may be associated with severe prerenal oliguria but intact tubular function.

Misleading results are occasionally obtained when urine that has remained in the bladder for several hours is examined. Moreover, the prior use of diuretics may render the urine sodium concentration invalid. Because some of the above tests can occasionally give an erroneous value and because of the simplicity of these maneuvers, it is our general practice to do these four tests together as a profile of renal function. In addition, in the absence of concomitant diuretic administration, a superior diagnostic separation of renal circulatory insufficiency from acute failure can be obtained by calculating the excretory fraction of sodium, i.e., urine sodium concentration divided by U/P creatinine ratio (92–95).

Specific therapy directed at correcting systemic hypotension, correcting absolute hypovolemia, improving cardiac function, or replacing glucocorticoid hormones may be instrumental in correcting oligoanuria. If these maneuvers fail, one may wish to proceed with a mannitol provocative test. This is potentially useful because of the possible therapeutic value of mannitol in preventing acute tubular necrosis and as an aid in diagnosis (96, 97). A trial dose of mannitol, 12.5 g (50 mL of 25% mannitol), is given rapidly intravenously over a 3-min period. If within 2 h the urine output increases to greater than 40 mL/h, this is suggestive evidence of good tubular function and prerenal oliguria. With questionable increases in urine volume, a second provocative dose of mannitol should be tried.[2]

Three different responses have been encountered with mannitol. First, there may be no significant increase in urine output, which would suggest that complete acute renal failure is present. Second, there may be an immediate and marked increase in urine output with a resumption of normal renal function, suggesting prerenal azotemia. Third, there may be an increase in urine output, but creatinine clearance may remain low. The third response would suggest that there is already partial acute renal failure and the action of the diuretic has been to prevent complete renal failure and to convert the process into a more mild form of nonoliguric renal failure.

Although loop diuretics such as ethacrynic acid or furosemide have been advocated as a provocative test of renal function in oliguric states (98), there are reasons for proceeding with a mannitol challenge prior to using diuretics:

1. A diuretic response does not necessarily distinguish hypovolemia from normal or excessive fluid retention; therefore a brisk diuresis may aggravate hypovolemia and predispose to the development of possible tubular damage.
2. A diuretic response may occur in patients with both prerenal oliguria and partial acute renal failure and thus not be of diagnostic value. (This is in contrast to mannitol, where only a

very limited increase in urine output occurs with partial acute renal failure.)
3. A weak diuretic response in the presence of severe hypovolemia may obscure diagnostic urinary findings and erroneously suggest a diagnosis of acute renal failure.

However, there may be a role for loop diuretics when given prior to an insult in order to prevent the development of acute renal failure (see below). Moreover, diuretics, when used after the onset of ATN, may make fluid management easier by converting oliguric renal failure into a nonoliguric state.

5. What is the anatomical localization and cause of acute renal failure? (see Table 15-7)

In a majority of cases of established acute renal failure the site of nephron involvement can be determined by careful consideration of (1) urinary sediment, (2) degree of proteinuria, (3) presence and severity of hypertension, and (4) clinical characteristics. The urinary sediment in 70 to 80 percent of patients with acute tubular necrosis will have a characteristic composition: abundant epithelial cells, epithelial cell casts along with a few degenerating cell casts and coarsely granular casts (99). These cells have not undergone fatty degeneration, as is frequently seen in the tubular epithelial shed in the nephrotic syndrome. If there is associated hemoglobinuria or myoglobinuria, the casts may be pigmented. These findings must be contrasted with those of patients with prerenal oliguria where only a few hyaline and finely granular casts and infrequent epithelial cell are noted.

A full differential diagnosis of acute renal failure is shown in Table 15-8. The following brief discussion will characterize some of the causes of acute renal failure which are often confused with acute tubular necrosis.

Postrenal obstruction. Both ureters are occasionally obstructed simultaneously. More often, because of disease or agenesis, there is only one functioning kidney, which can be obstructed by a variety of conditions. With acute obstructive uropathy, the nature of urine flow is often dis-

[2]If the mannitol is administered too slowly or if prerenal oliguria is associated with excessive volume depletion with or without hypotension, there may be no significant increase in urine output. Therefore, if there is clear or suggestive evidence of intravascular and/or extracellular volume depletion, attempts should be made to return hydration to normal prior to the administration of mannitol.

Table 15-7. Anatomical location of acute renal failure

LOCATION	SEDIMENT	PROTEINURIA	HBP	MISCELLANEOUS
Postrenal (obstruction)	Scanty	±	±	Total anuria, irregular flow, renal colic, known cancer, calculi disease, single kidney, unequal size kidneys, mass on pelvic-rectal examination
Vascular	Scanty or RBC	2-4 +	3-4 +	Abdominal and/or flank pain, neurological symptoms, cardiovascular disease, embolization, DIC syndrome
Glomerular	RBC, RBC-Hgb casts Oval fat bodies Fat droplets	3-4 +	0-4 +	Edema, nephrotic syndrome, systemic symptoms and signs
Interstitial	Scanty WBC, WBC casts Bacilluria Necrotic papilla	± − 2 +	0-2 +	Fever, chills, rash, eosinophilia, dysuria, back and/or flank pain
Tubular	Epithelial cells Epithelial casts ± pigmentation	± − 2 +	±	Clinical setting for ATN, necrosis, nephrotoxins

tinctive. Total anuria, although occasionally associated with vascular insults or acute tubular necrosis, is the hallmark of acute obstruction. Another characteristic pattern of postrenal obstruction is intermittent anuria or oliguria alternating with widely fluctuating rates of urine output. With acute obstruction, symptoms such as flank pain, fever, chills, dysuria, and costovertebral angle tenderness may be present. At times, however, the obstruction may be asymptomatic. The finding of a rectal or pelvic mass would suggest neoplastic obstruction to the distal ureters.

There are a variety of useful laboratory aids in the diagnosis of postrenal obstruction. Oliguria appearing in the presence of unequal kidney sizes demonstrated radiologically is suggestive of an obstructive cause. The renal sonogram characteristically may demonstrate a dilated collecting system diagnostic of obstruction. Renal pyelocalyceal system opacification by renal scanning or intravenous pyelography which fails to disappear with time is characteristic of obstructive uropathy. It should be noted that intratubular obstruction, for example from acute uric acid precipitation, may give a false negative response for obstruction by the usual diagnostic tests. When there is any uncertainty about the possibilty of upper or lower urinary tract obstruction, it is our

practice to ask the urologist to insert cautiously a small-lumen ureteral catheter into the pelvis of the kidney on one side only.

Renal vascular disease. Included in this category are acute bilateral renal vein thrombosis, bilateral renal artery occlusion by embolism or thrombosis, dissecting aneurysm, and malignant nephrosclerosis.

When renal vein thrombosis is bilateral, complete and acute, oliguria and renal failure may develop (100). Clinically there may be severe lumbar, low abdominal, and flank pain, fever, and leukocytosis. Tender, swollen flank masses may result from hemorrhagic infarction of the kidneys. Either microscopic or gross hematuria is common, as well as marked proteinuria. Thrombectomy and anticoagulant therapy may be instrumental in preserving renal function and may result in partial or complete recovery. The renal biopsy in early renal vein thrombosis may show basement membrane thickening, glomerular leukocyte stasis, and interstitial edema. A definitive diagnosis can usually be made by roentgenographic examination (101). The intravenous pyelogram shows no opacification, and increased renal size may be demonstrated by a plain film of the abdomen. The inferior venacavogram may show filling defects. Selective renal phlebography may reveal renal vein obstruction. The renal

Table 15-8. Differential diagnosis of acute renal failure

A. Preglomerular
  1. Low perfusion pressure (shock or hypotension)
  2. Absolute hypovolemia (dehydration, hemorrhage, trauma, burn)
  3. Defective cardiac function (congestive heart failure, myocardial infarction, tamponade)
  4. Acute hypoadrenal crises
  5. Hepatorenal syndrome
B. Postrenal Obstructive
  1. Low ureteral obstruction (cancer, calculi, ligation, hematoma, edema)
  2. Mid ureteral obstruction (retroperitoneal fibrosis, aneurysm)
  3. High ureteral obstruction (hyperuricemia, hypercalcemia, calculi)
C. Vascular
  1. Bilateral renal vein thrombosis (dehydration, sickle cell disease, hypernephroma)
  2. Bilateral renal artery occlusion (thrombosis, embolism, aneurysm)
  3. Malignant nephrosclerosis (essential hypertension, renal hypertension, renovascular hypertension)
  4. Scleroderma
  5. Hemolytic-uremic syndrome, renal cortical necrosis
D. Glomerular
  1. Acute proliferative glomerulonephritis
  2. Rapidly progressive glomerulonephritis
  3. Lupus nephritis
  4. Polyarteritis nodosa
  5. Allergic vasculitis
  6. Wegener's granulomatosis
  7. Henoch-Schönlein syndrome
  8. Goodpasture's syndrome
  9. Infectious nephritis (bacterial endocarditis, AV shunt infections, visceral abscesses)
E. Interstitial
  1. Fulminant pyelonephritis ± abscess formation
  2. Papillary necrosis (phenacetin, alcoholic, diabetes, obstruction)
  3. Acute interstitial nephritis (leptospirosis, idiopathic, drugs: Methicillin, other penicillins, rifampin, sulfa, antileptics, anti-inflammatory agents)
F. Tubular: acute tubular necrosis
  1. Nephrotoxic
  2. Ischemic

arteriogram may be characterisitc with delayed flow and decreased renal artery caliber, accompanied by stretching and splaying of the interlobular arteries. The venous phase is absent with no signs of renal vein opacification. Predispos-

ing factors which should alert the physician to the possibility of acute renal vein thrombosis are local injury, thromboembolic disease, known amyloid disease, hypernephroma, or membranous glomerulonephritis.

The clinical signs and symptoms of bilateral renal artery occlusion are generally indistinguishable from those of acute bilateral renal vein thrombosis. There are no characteristic urinary findings, although proteinuria and hematuria are less marked than in renal vein thrombosis with infarction. The diagnosis may be suspected with the finding of poor uptake on renal scintiangiography and confirmed by renal arteriography (102).

The more recently described entity of atheroembolic renal disease frequently is associated with severe oliguria or anuria (103, 104). Because of the large number and small size of these cholesterol emboli there may be no characteristic arteriographic findings, except for a patchy decreased nephrographic phase. Of more diagnostic value is a renal biopsy which may show cholesterol crystals and amorphous debris within the lumina of the involved vessels. With the passage of time, foreign-body giant cells appear, and ultimately concentric fibrosis predominates.

It should be noted that anuria is not necessarily indicative of irreversible complete arterial occlusion. Reflex vasospasm may account for lack of function in portions of remaining parenchyma which show normal perfusion on arteriography. This may account for the occasional spontaneous improvement in renal function after renal artery occlusion. Once diagnosed, prompt arterial endarterectomy has been shown to be effective in improving renal impairment (105).

Glomerular disease. In rare instances, acute glomerulonephritis causes anuria or marked oliguria (106). There is general agreement that a high mortality rate results from this form of the disease especially in the adult and older age group. There is, however, an occasional patient who survives and enters the chronic stage of glomerulonephritis with moderate to marked renal impairment or who may even make a complete clinical recovery. The history and physical examination may reveal a recent streptococcal infection, bacterial endocarditis, abdominal visceral abscesses (107), or gram-negative sepsis (108); periorbital edema or dark urine may be noted prior to oliguria. Since glomerular filtration is diminished in the face of relatively intact tubular function during the early phase, the urine specific gravity is usually high (1.020 or greater), the urinary urea and creatinine concentrations are high, and the urinary sodium concentration is low (109). In contrast to other forms of acute glomerulonephritis, it has been observed that some patients with rapidly progressive glomerulonephritis have little or no evidence of hypertension. In general, the urinary findings of oliguric disseminated vasculitis are more characteristic of what is observed in acute glomerulonephritis than in acute tubular necrosis (110). A definitive diagnosis of glomerular disease can best be established by renal biopsy (111).

The oliguria following renal homotransplantation must be carefully evaluated to distinguish the cause. The presence of a preformed, circulating antibody against the transplant kidney may result in so-called hyperacute rejection, with little or no kidney function from the time of surgical intervention, and a pathologic picture which is consistent with bilateral cortical necrosis (112). An intense primary rejection, in contrast, usually occurs in the first few days after transplantation and is characterized by a decrease in cortical blood flow with a high filtration fraction, oliguria, and a urine with a high specific gravity and a lowered sodium concentration (113). Further progression of the ischemic process facilitates the appearance of direct tubular damage and eventual excretion of an isotonic urine that contains high sodium concentrations and, therefore, is indistinguishable from acute tubular necrosis. The acute rejection phenomenon may occasionally be associated with evidence of autoimmune damage to the tubular epithelium. When this occurs, there may be accompanying hyperchloremic systemic acidosis, aminoaciduria, and renal glycosuria (114). Autoimmune processes which produce oliguria in the transplant patient must be distinguished from the true development of acute tubular necrosis. This is especially true with cadaveric transplantation, where acute renal necrosis is not uncommon.

Interstitial disease. The entity of acute, diffuse, interstitial nephritis has recently been defined and can be clearly differentiated from acute glomerulonephritis (115–117). Although a large number of inciting agents have been described, the largest number of cases have occurred in association with the use of methicillin. The clinical picture suggests an autoimmune reaction with the features of fever, rash, peripheral eosinophilia, and the development of acute impairment in renal function frequently associated with severe oliguria or anuria. Characteristically, the urinalysis shows a low specific gravity with prominent hematuria and with little proteinuria. Hypertension is usually minimal or absent. An abdominal x-ray discloses bilaterally swollen kidneys which on renal biopsy show intense, diffuse interstitial infiltrate of lymphocytes, plasma cells, and eosinophils with a moderate degree of interstiital edema. The glomeruli and arterioles are not involved. There may be other signs of autoimmune disease such as exfoliative dermatitis and Coombs' positive hemolytic anemia. Further confirmation of the autoimmune nature of this disease is the finding by immunofluorescent methods of a penicilloyl haptene bound to the interstitial kidney tissue of patients with this entity (116) and demonstration of antitubular basement-membrane antibodies by indirect fluorescence (118). The prompt diagnosis by biopsy is of great importance, because discontinuation of the offending agent and/or prompt treatment with corticosteroids may result in complete recovery.

Acute interstitial nephritis has been described following streptococcal or leptospiral infections as well as from an exposure to a variety of drugs including the penicillin antibiotics and rifampin (116, 119, 120). Recently, Chazan et al. (121) have described five patients with probable idiopathic acute interstitial nephritis who presented with severe renal failure. Two patients improved spontaneously and three improved in association with the introduction of corticosteroid therapy. No ideologic agent was incriminated in any of these patients although an immunologic mechanism was suspected. The diagnosis of this form of interstitial nephritis can only be diagnosed by exclusion after proceeding with a renal biopsy.

Necrotizing papillitis often occurs in patients with diabetes or chronic analgesic ingestion with partial urinary tract obstruction or with preexisting lower urinary tract infection (122, 123). The usual signs of pyelonephritis may be present (fever, chills, flank pain, dysuria, bacteriuria), and at times shreds of necrotic papillary tissue may be found in the urine. The clinical course may be that of severe oliguria, progressive azotemia, and death. With a large dose of contrast media, the intravenous pyelogram may reveal definite "ring" changes in the renal papilla, formation of cavities in the pyramids or at the papilla, and the outline of concretions formed around necrotic fragments. If recognized promptly, antibiotic therapy, adequate hydration, and drainage with an indwelling ureteral catheter may preserve renal function and prevent death from sepsis or renal failure.

6. Is the cause of ATN apparent or hidden?

If the oligoanuric patient shows a distinctive clinical setting and apparent etiology for ATN, no further diagnostic tests are necessary or desirable. If on the other hand, there appears to be a tubular localization by urinary sediment and an absence of other apparent anatomical sites of disease, one must investigate for hidden causes of acute tubular necrosis. Among the most common occult etiologies are (1) hidden hemolysis from glucose 6-phosphate dehydrogenase deficiency (124) or delayed transfusion reaction (125), etc. (see Table 15-9); (2) nontraumatic rhabdomyolysis secondary to potassium depletion (126, 127), ethanolism (128), heroin addiction (129, 130), amphetamines (131), or specific viral infections (132, 133), etc. (see Table 15-10); (3) paraproteinemias such as multiple myeloma, lymphoma, or carcinoma presenting with Bence Jones proteinuria (75–77) (see Table 15-11). It is

Table 15-9. Occult hemoglobinuric ATN

1. Delayed transfusion reaction
2. Glucose 6-phosphate dehydrogenase deficiency (oxidant drug ingestion)
3. Microangiopathic hemolytic anemia
4. Paroxysmal nocturnal hemoglobinuria
5. Acute autoimmune hemolytic anemia
6. Toxins (arsine, aniline, chlorate)

Table 15-10. Occult myoglobinuric ATN

A. Metabolic
  1. Hypokalemia
  2. Hypophosphatemia
  3. Diabetic nonketotic coma
  4. Diabetic ketotic coma
B. Drug induced
  1. Heroin
  2. Ethanolism
  3. Amphetamine
  4. Carbon monoxide
  5. Prolonged drug coma
  6. Succinylcholine
C. Physical
  1. Heat stroke
  2. Hyperpyrexia
  3. Grand mal seizures
  4. Vascular occlusions
  5. Strenuous exercise in presence of:
    a) poor conditioning
    b) sickle cell trait
    c) McCardle's syndrome
    d) heat excess
    e) potassium depletion

estimated that 18 percent of myeloma kidneys are first diagnosed when they present with acute renal failure in association with dehydration; (4) nephrotoxins such as carbon tetrachloride (134), ethylene glycol (135, 136), paraquat intoxication (137), solvent sniffing (138), poison mushroom ingestion (139), and heavy metal poisoning, etc. (see Table 15-12). Each of these nephrotoxins may be difficult to diagnose because of a latent period between exposure and the development of acute tubular necrosis.

The diagnosis of these hidden causes of ATN requires a careful historical review, specifically inquiring as to addictions, hobbies, unusual occupations, and homocidal or suicidal intent. Certain laboratory studies give some clue as to the

Table 15-11. Occult dysproteinemia and paraproteinemia associated with acute tubular necrosis

1. Myeloma
2. Lymphoma
3. Pancreatic acinar cell carcinoma
4. Medullary thyroid carcinoma
5. Macroglobulinemia
6. Cryoglobulinemia
7. Amyloidosis
8. Nephrotic syndrome

Table 15-12. Occult nephrotoxic acute tubular necrosis

1. Carbon tetrachloride and other chlorinated hydrocarbons
2. Ethylene glycol
3. Solvent sniffing
4. Arsenic
5. Bromates and chromates
6. Paraquat
7. Mushroom poisoning

presence of occult ATN. The triad of a low blood urea nitrogen (BUN) creatinine ratio, a high serum creatinine phosphokinase, and a positive urine orthotolidin (hematest) without hematuria is characteristic of nontraumatic rhabdomyolysis (140, 141). Acidosis with an unexplained anion gap or unexplained Fanconi renal tubular acidosis syndromes, may give a clue to specific nephrotoxins (140).

7. Is there an atypical clinical course for ATN?

If an initial diagnosis of ATN was made on the basis of an apparent etiology and clinical setting but the onset of a diuretic phase and improvement in renal function is not apparent after four weeks, reevaluation is in order. Often initial or subsequent anuria may be present. The causes of this prolonged period of oliguric renal failure could be a misdiagnosis secondary to vascular, glomerular, interstitial, or obstructive etiologies often presenting with an atypical clinical picture and misleading urinary sediment. In addition, unresolved acute renal failure may result from overwhelming ischemic or nephrotoxic insults to the kidney, the superimposition of acute on chronic renal failure, or cortical necrosis.

Renal cortical necrosis (Table 15-13) may occur from a variety of causes with complications of late pregnancy making up the majority of adult cases. The diagnosis of cortical necrosis may be suspected on the basis of clinical features but can be confirmed only by specific studies. The characteristic pattern of bilateral and symmetrical renal cortical calcification may be observed on plain films within a few weeks of the onset of renal cortical necrosis. Calcification may be extensive, scattered or patchy, "tram-line," or in the

form of a calcified renal cortical shell. The intravenous pyelogram shows very poor uptake of contrast media (absent nephrogram) in contrast to the excellent uptake but poor excretion seen in acute tubular necrosis (28, 29).

The use of the renal biopsy in patients whose oliguria is persistent and prolonged can be useful both in making a diagnosis and in establishing prognosis (111). In this regard, however, even the finding of cortical necrosis with involvement of most of the glomeruli can lead one astray. It is frequently very difficult to correlate pathologic damage with the ultimate ability of the kidney to function. In general, however, one would expect a much poorer prognosis with extensive involvement and destruction of glomeruli and an ultimately good prognosis where there are reversible histologic changes largely affecting the tubules and interstitial tissue rather than the glomeruli. Perhaps the least invasive quantitative measure of renal prognosis is the 30-min Hippuran ^{131}I renal scan (143). If renal uptake is absent or minimal, there is a very poor chance of the ultimate recovery of significant renal function.

PREVENTION

GENERAL MEASURES

A steady decline in the incidence of ATN paralleling improved patient care during surgical treatment and in traumatic injuries suggests that supportive measures may play an important role in prevention. Convincing evidence for increased

Table 15-13. Unresolved acute renal failure: bilateral renal cortical necrosis

1. Toxemia of pregnancy
2. Complications of pregnancy (septic abortions, retained placental fragments, concealed hemorrhage)
3. Postpartum renal failure
4. Contraceptive pill accelerated hypertension
5. Gram-negative septicemia
6. Hemorrhagic pancreatitis
7. Severe traumatic or burn shock
8. Viral infections (Coxsackie, influenza, mumps)
9. Altered host immunity (infections, vaccinations)
10. Hyperacute transplant rejection

prevention has been observed in military casualties. ATN developed in 1 out of 10 casualties during World War II (144), 1 in 200 during the Korean War (145) and 1 in approximately 600 in the Vietnam conflict (146). This diminished incidence of ATN in military casualties is undoubtedly due to many factors, including more rapid evacuation by helicopter, prompt restoration of volume depletion, and early and aggressive wound debridement.

An optimal plan of prevention must include (1) the maintenance of tissue perfusion by ensuring adequate circulating blood volume, renal blood flow, and urinary volume, (2) the recognition of the inherently poor-risk patient who may develop ATN, and (3) the recognition of clinical settings associated with an increased incidence of ATN (Table 15-4).

MAINTENANCE OF OPTIMAL TISSUE PERFUSION

Surgical treatment is the prime example of a clinical setting frequently associated with suboptimal tissue perfusion (Chap. 30). The use of anesthetic agents (147), preoperative fluid restrictions, and desiccation dehydration (pure water loss) (148), surgical blood loss (149); and third-spacing of extracellular fluid at the site of surgical trauma (150, 151) all predispose to decreased tissue perfusion. The main determinant of surgical and postsurgical oliguria is hypovolemia together with the secondary responses invoked by hypovolemia: increased elaboration of antidiuretic hormone, aldosterone, angiotensin, and catecholamines. The pathophysiologic changes in renal function during surgical treatment (diminished renal blood flow, diminished glomerular filtration rate, antidiuresis, and antinatriuresis) are generally reversible. If, on the other hand, during the ischemia and oliguria of surgical treatment there is a transfusion reaction, endotoxin shock, direct kidney trauma, or excessive circulation of potential renal toxins, ATN may develop, i.e., as an additive, or multifactorial, event.

Decreased renal perfusion in oliguria is not a necessary consequence of surgical procedures. Barry et al. have shown that operative and post-operative decreases in renal blood flow can be prevented or minimized by adequate prehydration with salt-containing parenteral solutions (152). In contrast, once renal blood flow has been decreased after the induction of anesthesia, the same parenteral solutions will have minimal effect in increasing renal blood flow to normal values, because of secondary humoral and neurogenic mechanisms which are brought into play (152). Using these principles and utilizing Ringer's lactate solution preoperatively, Terry and Trudnowski showed a statistically significant correlation with the use of prehydration and a decreased incidence of recovery-room hypotension; decreased transfusion requirements were also demonstrated with this approach (153). Treatment, however, should be adapted to each patient according to kidney function, preoperative hydration, cardiac status, and the amount of trauma or hemorrhage associated with the surgical procedure (154).

It has been recommended that intravenously administered fluid should be started and an adequate urinary output demonstrated before the induction of anesthesia (155). In order to accomplish this, it is strongly recommended that the anesthetist monitor urine flow from the catheter in complicated major surgical cases. The urine output should be at least 50 mL/h, rates of 75 to 100 mL/h being preferable. In patients with poor cardiovascular reserve, the use of mannitol and/or potent diuretic agents in conjunction with prehydration may be utilized to achieve and maintain adequate urinary outputs and thereby lessen the danger of cardiovascular overload (156).

Similarly, a better understanding of the *shock syndrome* with resultant improved therapy has improved the mortality rate and the incidence of ATN in military casualties (157). Shock is defined as an inadequate flow of blood to vital capillaries, with blood pressure low, normal, and high. A necessary part of the management of all types of severe shock is the placement of a central venous or Swan-Ganz catheter for pressure measurements and fluid administration (90). Regardless of the cause of shock, the finding of a low central venous or pulmonary wedge pressure is an indication for the administration of fluid volume.

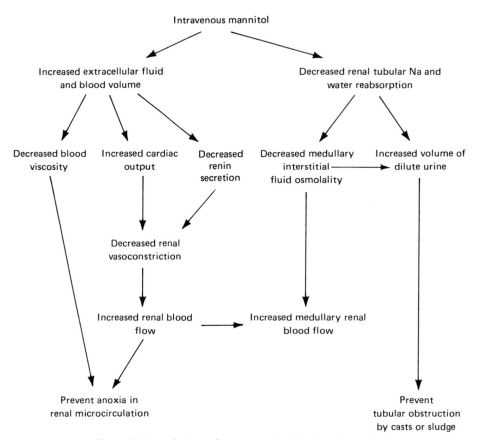

Figure 15-3. Mechanism of intravenously administered mannitol in preventing acute renal failure.

In the presence of acute blood loss, adequate blood replacement can be administered on the basis of the central venous pressure measurement. In the absence of acute blood loss and with a normal red cell mass, parenteral fluid and colloid administration should be given. The early recognition and treatment of acute respiratory failure with resultant anoxia and respiratory acidosis are also important in preventing renal failure and ultimate mortality in the shock syndrome (158). The use of cardiac glycosides and vasodilator agents may be important measures in improving tissue perfusion in some patients with the shock syndrome (157).

Since *mannitol therapy* may play a role in the diagnosis (see above) and prevention of ATN

(159, 160), its properties, function, and effects on renal hemodynamics warrant further consideration. Mannitol is the reduced form of the sugar mannose, an inert hexitol with no known biologic or metabolic activity. Because mannitol does not readily penetrate cells, upon intravenous infusion it is distributed throughout extracellular fluid. It is readily filtered across the renal glomerulus into the tubular lumen but is not resorbed. Figure 15-3 summarizes some of the potential benefits of mannitol in protecting the kidney from ATN. The renal excretion of mannitol and its obligated fluid constitutes an osmotic diuresis which may prevent excessive cast formation (161). Perhaps of more importance is the increase in plasma volume and associated decrease in blood viscosity and tissue resistance (162, 163). Since renal blood flow is proportional to perfusion pressure and tissue resistance, a lowering of the latter with mannitol may allow a decrease in afferent arterial constriction with resultant increase in renal blood flow and glomerular filtration rate.

The main principle in the clinical use of mannitol in prevention of ATN is to administer the smallest continual or intermittent dose of mannitol which will maintain urine volume from 50 to 100 mL/h or more (159). It is recommended that a maximum of 100 g of mannitol, or 500 mL of 20% mannitol, be administered over a 24-h period (159). The volume of the hourly urine output is replaced with 0.5% saline solution containing 10 to 20 meq of potassium per liter. In the presence of excessive extracellular volume or hyperkalemia, the replacement of urinary electrolyte losses is withheld until a more normal balance is achieved. Urinary sodium and potassium concentrations are determined on spot urines in order more accurately to estimate losses and replacement of these ions.

Excessive mannitol administration may result in an abrupt increase in plasma volume with precipitation of pulmonary edema. A sudden increase in plasma volume following mannitol administration is most likely when there is a minimal or absent diuretic response. On the other hand, if there is a brisk diuresis in association with the mannitol administration, this indicates that a much larger proportion of mannitol is being excreted into the urine, and it is unlikely that a significant increase in plasma volume will develop. Hyponatremia may occur if an excessive amount of mannitol accumulates as a result of poor urine excretion or excessive administration (164). The osmotic activity of mannitol causes water to move from the intracellular to the extracellular compartment, thereby decreasing extracellular sodium concentration. Hypernatremia may result if there is both excessive administration of mannitol and a brisk urine output (hypotonic urine) in association with inadequate fluid replacement (165).

The use of potent loop diuretics, such as ethacrynic acid or furosemide, may also be used to maintain optimal renal blood flow and urinary volume. Unlike mannitol, however, these agents tend to decrease plasma volume, increase renin secretion, and further reduce the GFR (Table 15-15). Loop diuretics would be preferable to the use of mannitol in oliguric states associated with cardiovascular overload.

During the past several years, experimental animal studies have shown that both mannitol and furosemide administration are effective in decreasing the incidence of ATN when given before or within a few minutes of the insult (160, 166, 167); when given later, there is no improvement in survival or renal function (168, 169). In man there is suggested evidence that mannitol when used in high-risk surgery may decrease the incidence of ATN although no convincing control studies have yet been reported (154–156). Other studies suggest that a saline diuresis is as protective as mannitol (59, 153). Despite the absence of convincing proof, it would appear advisable to use mannitol and intravenous fluids to maintain high urine flows in both poor-risk patients and clinical settings which predispose to ATN. There is less evidence that loop diuretics are protective, and it is our current policy not to use these agents unless there is evidence of cardiovascular overload.

RECOGNITION OF POOR-RISK PATIENTS

Although no person is exempt from the development of ATN when there is exposure to severe predisposing factors, certain patients appear to have a greater propensity to the development of this syndrome (see Table 15-4). The presence of diminished renal blood flow in association with a

Table 15-15. Comparison of mannitol and loop diuretics in prevention of ATN

ACTION	MANNITOL	LOOP DIURETIC
1. Vasodilation of arterioles	+	+
2. Tubular washout of casts	+	+
3. Decrease renin secretion	+	−
4. Overcome no-reflow phenomenon	+	−
5. Volume expansion effect on GFR	+	−

relatively normal concentration mechanism, produced experimentally (170) and as present in the aged with nephrosclerosis, predisposes to the development of ATN.

The presence of *severe proteinuria* from a variety of disease entities is associated with a substantial incidence of ATN. As long known, in patients with multiple myeloma and Bence Jones proteinuria reversible or irreversible ATN may develop in association with intravenous pyelography (171). From a review of reported cases Morgan and Hammack concluded that the ATN is more likely due to dehydration than secondary to the contrast medium itself (172), although both factors are probably operative. Another factor predisposing to ATN is increased plasma viscosity in Waldenström's macroglobulinemia where a low-molecular-weight protein leakage into the glomerular filtrate is not observed (173). As a group patients with a nephrotic syndrome in association with severe proteinuria appear to be more susceptible to ATN (174). In addition to the heavy proteinuria which may predispose to cast formation and obstructing uropathy, these patients have a tendency toward low plasma volumes. ATN has been described in elderly patients after the administration of large quantities of low-molecular-weight dextran (118). Specific gravities reaching 1.132 have been observed in patients receiving low-molecular-weight-dextran therapy. In susceptible patients the presence of highly concentrated urinary filtrate may predispose to cast formation and obstructive uropathy. In the great majority of patients receiving low-molecular-weight dextran, however, no impairment of renal function develops (175).

For many years surgeons have been aware that *obstructive jaundice* predisposes to acute postoperative renal failure. Dawson has shown that there is a significant correlation between the preoperative serum bilirubin level and the percentage postoperative fall in creatinine clearance (176, 177). The postoperative decrease in creatinine clearance was prevented by the prophylactic administration of mannitol (177). The explanation of why obstructive jaundice predisposes to impaired renal function remains obscure.

There are a variety of clinical conditions associated with the liberation of *pigments from blood or muscle* which predispose to the development of ATN in association with dehydration, hypovolemia, or trauma (see Table 15-1). ATN has been described in primary atypical pneumonia with resulting cold agglutination syndrome (178), rickettsial infections in patients with glucose 6-phosphate dehydrogenase deficiency (179), and idiopathic paroxysmal myoglobinuria (180). In the presence of known myopathies or hemoglobinopathies special precautions should be taken to prevent excessive exertion or hypovolemia.

RECOGNITION OF PREDISPOSING CLINICAL SETTINGS
(See Table 15-14.)

In a review of 100 cases of *postoperative renal failure*, Sawyer et al. found the highest incidence in cardiac, aortic aneurysm, biliary, and gastrointestinal surgical treatment (181). In aortic surgical treatment the kidney is especially vulnerable to injury, because cross clamping of the aorta is associated with tremendous increase in renovascular resistance and ischemia (182, 183). In addition, aortic cholesterol plaque embolization to the kidneys constitutes a potential hazard. In open-heart surgical procedures, the use of a pump oxygenator has been associated with a significant incidence of acute renal failure. Here the absence of a pulsatile blood flow, excessive intravascular cell agglutination, sludging, and hemolysis lead to excessive tissue hypoxia and metabolic acidosis. In recent years the incidence of ATN in association with cardiopulmonary bypass has been greatly diminished by the use of pulsatile flow techniques, hypothermia, mannitol, and hemodilution (184, 185).

Diagnostic radiology has been incriminated as predisposing to ATN (186). This has been described in cholecystography, cholangiography, renal angiography, and rarely after intravenous pyelography. Renal failure has been observed with a wide variety of radiopaque agents all having in common a triiodinated aeromatic nucleus (187). Undoubtedly, the amount of agent used is an important predisposing factor, the greatest incidence of renal damage occurring after double-

Table 15-14. Prevention of acute tubular necrosis

CLINICAL SETTING	PREDISPOSING FACTORS	PREVENTIVE MEASURES
A. Diagnostic radiology		
1. Cholecystographic examination	Advanced age	Avoidance of dehydration
	Nephrosclerosis	Proper spacing of procedures
	Jaundice	
	Repeat examinations with double dose	
2. Renal angiography, intravenous urography, and computerized axial tomography (CAT) scans	Nephrosclerosis and hypertension, diabetes mellitus	Limitation of amount of contrast material
	Renal insufficiency	
B. Surgical procedures		
1. Aortic surgical treatment	Cross clamping of aorta	Correction of hypovolemia
2. Open-heart surgical treatment	Cholesterol emboli	Measures prior to, during, and after surgical treatment with maintenance of adequate urine output
	Excess hemodialysis with extracorporeal circulation	
	Hypovolemia from surgical trauma and blood loss	Careful typing and cross matching of transfusions
3. Biliary surgical treatment	Obstructive jaundice	
	Poor hepatic function	
C. Pregnancy		
1. Abortions	Infections, hypovolemia, and nephrotoxic abortifacients	Adequate antibiotics
		Early radical hysterectomy
		Heparinization
2. Toxemia	Disseminated intravascular coagulation	
3. Pre- and postpartum hemorrhage	Abruptio placentae	Early recognition of hemorrhage and adequate transfusion of blood
	Placenta previa	
D. Pigment released		
1. Transfusion reactions	Renal ischemia: anesthesia, surgical treatment, dehydration, hypovolemia	Careful major and minor cross matching
		Early diagnosis of reaction
2. Intravascular hemolysis	Paroxysmal cold hemaglobinuria	Early diagnosis and recognition
	Glucose 6-phosphate dehydrogenase deficiency	
3. Myoglobinuria	Predisposing muscle disorder	
	Excessive exertion with poor physical condition	
	Tissue trauma	
E. Proteinuric states		
1. Nephrotic syndrome	Dehydration	Adequate hydration and prevention of hypovolemia and adequate urine volume
	Hypotension	
2. Multiple myeloma	Dehydration with use of radiographic contrast media	
3. Dysproteinemias		
4. Low-molecular-weight dextran	Nephrosclerosis	

dose gallbladder series following initial failure to visualize on a single-dose procedure, and after multiple injections of contrast media during renal arteriography (188). The presence of obstructive jaundice appears to predispose to ATN in association with oral or intravenous cholangiography or cholecystography. Patients with severe nephrosclerosis and impaired renal blood flow are especially susceptible to renal damage from angiography. The presence of preexisting renal disease with impaired concentrating ability does not appear to predispose to acute renal injury following radiographic procedure, as evidenced by the very low incidence of nephrotoxicity from drip-infusion pyelography in the presence of renal insufficiency (189). In striking contrast to overall statistics there is a significant incidence of complicating ATN in long-standing diabetics with prior chronic renal insufficiency (190, 191). This increased risk of ATN in long-standing diabetic patients may pertain to any radiographic or scanning procedure where large doses of contrast substances are administered.

The mechanism of renal damage would not appear to be direct nephrotoxicity, but rather the hypertonicity of the contrast substances which result in crenation of red cells and subsequent agglutination, capillary thrombosis, and ischemia (192). The prevention of renal failure during diagnostic radiology can best be achieved by proper spacing of diagnostic procedures, avoidance of dehydration, and the use of mannitol infusions and/or diuretic agents in particularly high-risk patients.

Acute obstetric renal failure results largely from septic abortions during the first trimester of pregnancy and hemorrhage or toxemia of pregnancy late in the third trimester or at the time of delivery (193). The etiologic factors leading to ATN in septic abortions are bacterial infections, hypovolemia, and nephrotoxic abortifacient chemicals. Prevention of ATN in this clinical setting requires early diagnosis, adequate antibiotic therapy, and, often, early radical hysterectomy (especially if there is a history of a chemical abortion) (194). Major blood loss is frequently an important predisposing factor in ATN of late pregnancy. In accidental antepartum hemorrhage much of the blood loss may be concealed as retroperitoneal clot. Therefore, early recognition and treatment with adequate blood replacement is an important factor in preventing ATN.

In a significant number of patients with toxemia of pregnancy renal failure develops in the absence of bleeding. In this group of patients, as well as those with gram-negative septicemia after abortion, disseminated intravascular coagulation (DIC) represents the main cause in the development of acute renal failure (10, 12). Clinical manifestations can include hypotension, a bleeding tendency, oliguria, convulsions and coma, abdominal or back pain, dyspnea, and cyanosis. Intravascular coagulation produces a characteristic sequence of changes in the components of the hemostatic mechanism which can best be diagnosed by obtaining a battery of the common coagulation tests, as well as specialized fibrin split product or fibrin monomer tests (195). The spectrum of damage to the kidney in DIC varies from no disease to mild focal tubular necrosis, complete tubular necrosis with oliguria, or bilateral renal cortical necrosis. Early diagnosis is crucial, because vigorous therapy with intravenous heparin may reverse DIC and prevent or minimize acute renal damage from this disorder (196, 197).

CLINICAL COURSE

The course of ATN can usually be divided into four stages: oliguria, early diuresis, late diuresis, and the recovery phase (4).

OLIGURIA

The clinical picture at the onset is determined to a large extent by the severity of the acute injury or the illness which precipitated the renal failure. Indeed, the oliguria is often unnoticed by the physician because of preoccupation with the associated illness. Oliguria usually starts within a few hours of the initial insult with a progressive reduction in urine flow over the next 24- to 48-h period; the onset may not occur, however, for several days after exposure to nephrotoxic chemicals such as carbon tetrachloride, ethylene glycol, or paraquat. The period of severe oliguria (50 to 400 mL/day) may last from 1 day to 6 weeks, the average duration being from 7 to 12 days (198). In addition to the more common oliguric pattern, ATN may occasionally present with anuria (less than 50 mL of urine per day). Anuria can occur in those patients who continue to be volume-depleted, hypotensive, or in heart failure. The presence of anuria after correction of these problems may signify a massive insult to the kidney with involvement of the majority of nephron units; however, an anuric course is not incompatible with total recovery of renal function. If anuria exists or oliguria lasts longer than 3 weeks, one must consider other diagnoses in the differential diagnosis of acute renal failure (see above).

ATN may occur without oliguria or anuria (nonoliguric or polyuric ATN) in association with progressive azotemia. The incidence of nonoliguric ATN, once thought to be rare, has been noted between 30 to 60 percent in recent series (95, 199, 200). The etiology varies widely with a large percentage secondary to nephrotoxins, such as gentamicin (201, 202), methoxyflurane (203), or lithium (204). Other causes of nonoliguric ATN include radiocontrast media toxicity, hypercalcemia, hyperuricemia, endotoxemia, rhabdomyolysis, trauma, and miscellaneous operative procedures (95). The use of prophylactic mannitol, loop diuretics, and vasodilators in conjunction with high-risk surgery, trauma and burns explains in part but not fully the high incidence of nonoliguric ATN with these insults. The nonoliguric form of ATN is generally associated with a lesser degree of renal injury and azotemia, a briefer duration of azotemia and a better overall prognosis.

ATN may also be superimposed on chronic renal insufficiency. Examples on acute-on-chronic renal failure are contrast media toxicity in diabetes mellitus (190, 191), and aminoglycoside (202), cotrimoxaside (205), and phenazopyridine (206) administration in standard dosages in patients with significant impairment in renal function.

Various tubular syndromes (Fanconi, renal tubular acidosis, nephrogenic diabetes insipidus, etc.) may accompany ATN in association with a number of specific nephrotoxins such as amphotericin (207), streptozotocin (208), methoxyflurane (203), paraquat (137), lithium (204), and heavy metal intoxication (1).

The formation of urine during the oliguric period most likely emanates from a few minimally damaged functioning nephrons undergoing an osmotic diuresis secondary to increased blood levels of nitrogenous products. Although it was long thought that urine formed during the oliguric phase was essentially unaltered glomerular filtrate, the presence of substantial tubular function is demonstrated by the finding of a urine so-

dium concentration considerably lower than that of the plasma (209), the absence of glycosuria (210, and an acid urine (211).

The main signs and symptoms during the oliguric phase are related to disturbances in the gastrointestinal, cardiovascular, and neuromuscular systems, and any of the manifestations usually associated with "uremia" may appear. For a detailed discussion of the manifestations of uremia, the reader is referred to the discussion of chronic renal failure in Chap. 18. The rapidity of the development of uremic symptoms depends upon the rate of tissue catabolism, which in turn is dependent upon (1) the age and muscle mass of the patient, (2) the degree of associated tissue trauma, (3) the presence or absence of complicating infection, and (4) the use of special measures to reduce endogenous protein catabolism (see Nutrition, under Conservative Therapy, later in the chapter). In general, patients with ATN tend to develop uremic symptoms at a lower level of urea nitrogen retention than patients with chronic renal failure, who probably develop some degree of tolerance to uremic toxins in association with the slow rate of deterioration of renal function.

The changes in renal function and in fluid and electrolyte balance which occur during the oliguric phase will be discussed later in the chapter, under Fluid and Electrolyte Changes.

EARLY DIURESIS

The onset of the diuretic phase may be defined arbitrarily as a daily urine volume of 400 mL or more. Although a profound diuresis may start abruptly, in most cases there is an acceleration of a slowly progressive increase in urine flow begun some days earlier. In the early reports of ATN, maximal daily urine flows of 5 to 10 L, lasting for several days or weeks, were frequently seen during diuresis (4). These enormous volumes were largely iatrogenic, resulting from excessive fluid administration during the oliguric period and from attempts to replace salt and water losses quantitatively during the diuresis. With adequate fluid restriction during oliguria, peak urine volumes during diuresis will seldom exceeed 4 L, and the early diuretic phase lasts only a few days. Moreover, the diuresis can be further attenuated or even eliminated by the removal of retained nitrogenous products and excess extracellular fluid with frequent dialysis treatment. Under these conditions, the early diuretic phase is recognized by finding increased urea and creatinine U/P ratios rather than by the presence of polyuria.

With the onset of the diuretic period it is not uncommon to see a continual increase in BUN for several days, largely because glomerular filtration rate remains minimal, and urea clearance does not keep up with endogenous urea production. Therefore, the clinical symptoms of uremia (vomiting, mental changes, epistaxis, convulsions) may persist or even increase during the first few days of the diuresis. The mean duration of the early diuretic stage is between 4 and 7 days (198).

LATE DIURESIS

This is the period between the initial decrease in BUN and the disappearance of azotemia. It represents a period of rapid improvement in renal function. On the average, the BUN becomes normal within approximately 15 to 20 days after the onset of the diuretic period (16). Most patients show considerable clinical improvement by the second week of diuresis.

RECOVERY PHASE

The clinical signs and symptoms of uremia subside rapidly, although it may be at least 2 or 3 months from the start of the illness before the patient is well enough to resume full activities. The associated anemia, which is resistant to iron therapy, improves gradually over a period of months (4). Characteristically, urine-concentrating defects remain for several months, implying a long delay in the restitution of the normal hypertonicity of the medullary interstitium, a defect in tubular function, or both (212). Although the vast majority of patients appear clinically well without evident urinary abnormalities within 2 to 3 months, discrete tests reveal that maximal restitution of renal function may not occur for a period of up to 1 year (213).

Whereas recovery from ATN is usually adequate for maintenance of homeostasis, several investigators have noted approximately a 30 percent permanent reduction in inulin and para-aminohippuric acid (PAH) clearances in a significant number of patients (213–216). This reduction in renal function would be consistent with the irreversible damage of tubulorrhexic lesions in ischemic ATN. Since the reduction in glomerular filtration rate was in most cases not associated with proteinuria, it likely results from the total nonfunctioning of some nephrons rather than the formation of urine by some partially damaged nephrons. There is no relation between the duration of oliguria and the degree of renal function in those patients who survive the acute phase. Although there appears to be an increased incidence of urinary tract infections during the course of ATN which is perhaps related to indwelling urinary catheters, long-term follow-up studies do not show a significant incidence of bacteriuria or hypertension (213).

In contrast to the substantial recovery from ATN observed in the majority, there are a number of well-documented patients who permanently remained in a severe oliguric or anuric state; others, after starting a diuresis, continued to have marked impairment of renal function (217–219). An occasional patient, after a long anuric period and slow resolution of the diuretic phase, will develop further deterioration in renal function (216, 225). Significant permanent renal damage following ATN can occur following a variety of insults. Nephrotoxins such as methoxyflurane (203, 219), ethylene glycol (221), heavy doses of aminoglycosides (202) or arsine (222) characteristically are associated with a significant incidence of permanent renal damage. ATN following heat stroke (220), severe or prolonged septic shock, dehydration and contrast media administration (191) often results in permanent renal damage. The underlying etiology of irreversible or poorly reversible renal impairment may be secondary to (1) a specific toxin, (2) overwhelming ischmeic tubulorrhexic injury, (3) subsequent development of interstitial nephropathy, or (4) associated confluent renal cortical necrosis.

Acute renal failure in cadaver transplants may also have a variable recovery of renal function. Perfusion preservation may be associated with a significant incidence of intravascular coagulation which leads to permanent renal impairment (223). Similarly, in cadaver kidneys harvested from patients where the heart has been allowed to stop, there is a high incidence of permanent ischemic damage sometimes progressing on to large artery thromboses (224). In contrast, when the cadaver kidney is harvested from a patient with brain death and a beating heart, there is an eventful clinical course with good recovery from ATN (225). A small number of these patients, however, may undergo rapid necrosis of the transplanted kidney secondary to hyperacute rejection or arterial thromboses.

Acute renal failure in pregnancy has a variable clinical course (see Table 15-16). During the first half of pregnancy, acute renal failure is secondary to unskilled abortions, nephrotoxic abortifacients, intrauterine sepsis, intravascular hemolysis, or intrauterine hemorrhage (226). If these patients survive, they almost invariably recover good renal function with only occasional, patchy cortical necrosis. During the second half of pregnancy (most frequently the four weeks prior to delivery) acute renal failure is secondary to toxemic complications and intrauterine hemorrhage (226). A few patients develop acute renal failure without antecedent toxemia in association with concealed retroperitoneal bleeding. Although the majority of these patients will have reversible acute tubular necrosis, a significant minority will have patchy or confluent renal cortical necrosis with some permanent impairment in renal function. In contrast, when acute renal failure develops in the immediate postpartum period, frequently without antecedent toxemia, the accompanying clinical picture is one of microangiopathic hemolytic anema, thrombocytopenia with an associated high incidence of irreversible confluent renal cortical necrosis (142). A similar syndrome of disseminated intravascular coagulation often associated with severe or malignant hypertension and progressing to permanent renal failure secondary to confluent cortical necrosis has been observed occasionally in women on contraceptive hormone therapy.

Patients with jaundice and acute renal failure also have a variable clinical course (see Table 15-17). Many systemic diseases produce acute renal failure and hepatic involvement with the underlying prognosis for recovery depending on the type and severity of the disease process. The association of jaundice and ATN has been noted in a variety of infectious diseases and toxic exposures. In obstructive jaundice there is a high incidence of ATN in association with ascending cholangitis (227), biliary surgery (228) and the use of radiopaque contrast media (178). There is also a significant incidence of ATN in patients with the hepatorenal syndrome (functional renal failure) when complicated by hypovolemia or terminal cardiovascular collapse (229–231). The overall recovery from ATN with jaundice is generally poor because of a higher mortality rate from the underlying disease process and a worsening

Table 15-16. Acute renal failure in pregnancy

		MANIFESTATIONS		
			BRCN‡	
STAGE	ETIOLOGY	ATN†	PATCHY	CONFLUENT
1st Half	Unskilled abortion	4+	±	0
2d Half	Toxemia, concealed hemorrhage	3+	+	±
Postpartum	DIC*	0	+	3+
Contraceptive pill	DIC with malignant hypertension	0	+	3+

* DIC = disseminated intravascular coagulation (with microangiopathic hemolytic anemia).

† ATN = acute tubular necrosis.

‡ BRCN = bilateral renal cortical necrosis.

Table 15-17 Acute renal failure in association with jaundice

A. Prerenal
  1. Hepatorenal syndrome (functional renal failure, FRF)
  2. Hepatic failure with hypovolemia
B. Vascular
  1. Polyarteritis nodosa†
  2. Hemolytic-uremic syndrome†
C. Glomerular
  1. Lupus†
  2. Autoimmune glomerulonephritis associated with hepatitis, cirrhosis*
D. Interstitial
  1. Leptospirosis*
  2. Heat stroke*
E. Tubular (acute tubular necrosis)
  1. Infections (malaria,* septicemia*)
  2. Toxins (carbon tetrachloride, methoxyflurane,† phosphorus, mushroom poisoning, phenols,† paraquat)
  3. Obstructive jaundice (ascending cholangitis, pancreatitis,* postradiocontrast media,* postbiliary surgery)
  4. Hepatorenal syndrome (FRF) (dehydration, terminal event)

* Occasional permanent renal damage.
† Frequent permanent renal damage.

of hepatic failure in association with uremic complications. If the patient survives the underlying illness, recovery of renal function may be complete or may result in permanent damage secondary to confluent cortical necrosis or from specific nephrotoxins.

FLUID AND ELECTROLYTE CHANGES

As a consequence of oliguria or anuria, there is disruption of the two main functions of the kidneys: maintenance of a constant composition and volume of the body water and electrolytes, and the excretion of the catabolic end products of protein breakdown. The role of the kidneys in other metabolic functions, such as glucose and fat metabolism, or in the normal regulation of blood pressure is poorly understood and will not be discussed. Since the aim of therapy in acute tubular necrosis is to maintain the internal environment in as normal a state as possible until the kidneys resume function, it is necessary to delineate and understand the changes which occur in the untreated patient.

Fluid balance

As discussed in Chap. 7, in the normal individual insensible water loss by vaporization from the skin and lungs is 12 mL/kg body weight, or about 850 mL/day in a 70-kg man. This is a fixed loss which entails no loss of accompanying electrolytes and is modified by rate and depth of respiration, fever and ambient temperature, humidity, and active sweating. In the absence of water intake, insensible water loss will be partially compensated by endogenous water of oxidation formed from the catabolism of body fat and protein (1.07 mL of water per gram of fat; 0.41 mL of water per gram of protein). The water of oxidation made available in this manner in a 70-kg man in the fasting state is ordinarily about 300 mL/day, or one-third of the insensible loss; in calculations of water balance, water of oxidation must be considered as intake (232).

In the oliguric patient with ATN, a concatenation of events, physiologic and iatrogenic, usually results in a large relative excess of body water. This has been verified by measurement of total body water with deuterium oxide (heavy water) (233). The setting in which renal damage occurs is usually a very stressful situation, and in the acutely ill or traumatized patient the catabolism of both fat and protein is markedly increased. It has been shown, for example, that fat utilization in the patient with ATN, as in the postoperative or traumatic injury patient, may be twice normal: these patients therefore produce far more endogenous water of oxidation than the normal individual (234).

Biochemical changes

The major biochemical abnormalities of acute renal failure result from the retention of products of protein metabolism: (1) *nitrogenous compounds*, such as urea, creatinine, uric acid, and many other intermediary products, (2) *nonvolatile acids*, chiefly resulting from the breakdown of protein with the liberation of sulfuric and phosphoric acid, and (3) *magnesium and potassium*. The rate at which these metabolites accumulate is variable and is dependent on the rate of endogenous protein catabolism. This in turn is influenced by the intensity of the "stress response," size of muscle mass, prior state of nutrition, extent of necrotic tissue or collections of blood within the body, and presence of infection or fever (235). In addition, carbohydrate depletion accentuates tissue breakdown and also permits the accumulation of ketone bodies from the oxidation of fat.

During the oliguric period, caloric intake is seldom adequate, so that most patients lose 0.3 to 0.4 kg lean body mass per day (22). In maintaining a normal ratio between water and decreasing fat-free solids, a proportionate amount of tissue water is freed, providing still another source of endogenous fluid. Unfortunately, excessive ingestion or administration of fluids is the rule rather than the exception during the first few days of acute renal failure. Voluntary fluid intake is largely a matter of habit rather than thirst, and patients often continue to drink the usual amount of water, coffee, and other beverages in the face of the diminished urine volume. There may also be an element of increased thirst which is brought about by the stimulus of hypovolemia, frequently present during the initiating events associated with acute renal failure. Furthermore, the physicians may administer parenteral fluids in a vain attempt to "flush out the kidneys." If no salt is given, this excess water is distributed between extracellular and intracellular fluid compartments, decreasing the osmolality of the body fluids. If saline solution is given, it remains largely extracellular. Thus, intracellular and/or extracellular edema may be produced.

The state of fluid balance during diuresis is variable, depending on the previous state of hydration and on replacement therapy during diuresis. By this time the excessive endogenous water production associated with the stress response of the initiating episode is terminated. Because tubular resorption of water may be impaired and the functioning nephrons are under a high osmotic load, large volumes of hypotonic urine are excreted (4). The danger, therefore, is from rapid contraction of body fluid compartments and unrestricted loss of individual electrolytes.

Azotemia, or the accumulation in the blood (and other extracellular fluid) of nonprotein nitrogens, progresses most rapidly during the first few days of oliguria (82). Urea, the major substance of this group, is freely diffusible. It is therefore distributed in equal concentration throughout the total body water, causing no disturbance in osmotic relationships between the intracellular and extracellular compartments.

Blood urea nitrogen, representative of other nitrogenous products, has a rapid rate of rise (between 25 and 35 mg/dL per day) for the first 3 to 5 days of the anuric period. This rapid phase of urea nitrogen rise reflects the underlying catabolic events that may have precipitated ATN. In young muscular males undergoing severe trauma the rate of catabolism may produce a daily rise in blood urea nitrogen of 50mg/dL or more. In this first stage, urea production may be as great as 30g day and correspond to the destruction of 90 g of protein or some 400 g of tissue. Following the third to fifth day of anuria, there is usually a reduction in the rate of urea accumulation conforming to a decrease in tissue catabolism. Blood urea nitrogen may now increase from 10 to 20 mg/dL per day in association with the production of an average of 5 to 6 g of urea per day. A diet which contains abundant carbohydrate calories may produce a distinct slowing in the rate of rise of urea nitrogen, but intercurrent infection, resorption of hematoma, or the persistence of devitalized tissue may increase the daily rise in blood urea nitrogen.

Metabolic acidosis is caused by the failure of the kidneys to excrete hydrogen ions. The metabolism of ingested foods and the increased breakdown of body tissue, chiefly protein, in the face of renal shutdown results in the rapid accumulation of acids. The increased extracellular hydrogen ion is buffered by serum bicarbonate in an effort to maintain normal pH (see Chap. 8). The net result is a lower concentration of bicarbonate, a higher concentration of carbonic acid (and temporarily an increase of P_{CO_2}), and a minimal lowering of pH. Respiration is stimulated to blow off carbonic acid in order to maintain the low compensatory serum bicarbonate level; when the metabolic acidosis is extreme, the deep, labored, slow respiration known as Kussmaul's respiration ensues.

The hydrogen ions are retained to a large extent in the form of sulfuric, phosphoric, and organic acids (236, 237). The serum levels of anions, phosphate, and sulfate are therefore elevated, as is the concentration of "undetermined anion." From the therapeutic viewpoint, it is well to remember that the metabolic acidosis of acute renal failure results from retention of acids, not from "loss of sodium," and that the low level of serum bicarbonate (carbon dioxide combining power) is a compensatory mechanism to retard a fall in the more important parameter, pH.

The increased concentration of serum phosphate often is accompanied by *hypocalcemia*. The hypocalcemia is seldom so marked as in chronic renal insufficiency but on occasion may be extreme. The cause of hypocalcemia in acute renal failure is not altogether clear. Hypoalbuminemia is usually not present. There is an associated increase in serum phosphate, but this correlates poorly with hypocalcemia which can reach levels as low as 6.5 to 8.5 mg/dL within 2 days of oliguria. In association with hypocalcemia there is a demonstrable increase in circulating parathormone which is ineffective in the homeostatic regulation of serum calcium, perhaps because of associated vitamin D resistance or increased circulating calcitonin (238). Because severe hypocalcemia occurs rapidly in association with the ATN of rhabdomyolysis, it is postulated that low serum calcium is secondary to deposition of calcium within necrotic muscle tissue. Moreover, hypercalcemia is not an uncommon finding during the diuretic period of rhabdomyolysis ATN (239). This is best explained by the rapid dissolution of dystrophic calcifications in traumatized skeletal muscle in association with a falling serum phosphate and improved skeletal responsiveness to parathormone (239).

The rarity of frank hypocalcemic tetany in uremia is usually attributed to the concomitant acidosis, which increases the proportion of ionized calcium, the physiologically active form. By the same reasoning, the appearance of tetany during correction of acidosis with alkali therapy has been attributed to decreased ionization of serum calcium accompanying the rise in pH. Studies on changes in ultrafiltrable calcium (used as an index of ionized calcium) caused by changes in plasma pH tend to discredit this hypothesis, since even extreme changes in pH alter the ultrafiltrable calcium by less than 5 percent (130). However, it is difficult to explain the alleviation of alkali-induced tetany by calcium administration in any other way.

The various forms of serum calcium and the fact that the concentrations of diffusable and ionized calcium are influenced by such variables as pH, phosphate, sulfate, bicarbonate, citrate and other organic acids, and the serum proteins compound the problem (see Chaps. 9 to 11).

It may be that the heightened neuromuscular irritability of hypocalcemia is partially offset by the central nervous system effects of hypermagnesemia. At the present time, the benignity of hypocalcemia associated with acute uremia cannot be entirely explained. Of more importance in acute renal failure is the worsening of the cardiac effects of hyperkalemia by concomitant hypocalcemia (see below).

The majority of patients with acute renal failure exhibit some degree of *hyponatremia*. In the absence of prior sodium loss (vomiting, diarrhea, etc.), this decrease in sodium concentration is almost invariably secondary to dilution, from excessive administration of sodium-free fluids and/or increased production of endogenous water (233). The clinical fact that drastic water restriction usually results in an increase in sodium concentration during oliguria favors dilution as a primary mechanism; in addition, total exchangeable sodium, measured by the isotope technique, has been found to be normal or increased.

Moderate hyponatremia, per se, is usually asymptomatic. Since sodium is the main determinant of extracellular osmolality, when the serum concentration is markedly reduced (below 120 meq/L), enough water may be shifted intracellularly in response to osmotic demands to cause the signs and symptoms of water intoxication (see Chap. 7). When mannitol has been administered in large amounts and cannot be excreted, hypotonicity results from shift of water from the intracellular to the extracellular compartment in response to osmotic demands. Hypochloremia usually accompanies the hyponatremia. If there has not been excessive loss of chloride, either by vomiting or via another route, then the depressed chloride concentration can also be attributed to dilution.

Serum magnesium increases progressively during the oliguric phase of acute renal failure and decreases during the diuretic phase with hypomagnesemia being occasionally noted. In the majority of patients, hypermagnesemia is not extreme; the serum concentration increases from the normal value of 2 meq/L to 3 or 4 meq/L. Experimental magnesium intoxication causes central nervous system and cardiac depression, but this usually only occurs when serum levels reach 7 to 8 meq/L (241), values seldom if ever reached during acute renal failure. The toxic effects of magnesium may be more pronounced in uremic patients than in normal individuals, but the evidence that hypermagnesemia causes central nervous system depression in acute renal failure is not decisive. Similarly, the hypomagnesemia occurring during the diuretic phase is seldom, if ever, associated with enhanced neuromuscular irritability, as has been described in experimental magnesium deficiency.

Potassium intoxication is one of the main causes of death in acute renal failure. With cessation of the usual obligatory potassium excretion by the kidneys concomitant with continuous breakdown of muscle protein, an accumulation of released potassium in the extracellular fluid is to be anticipated. This is accelerated by the increased catabolic response of trauma or infection, by the resorption of blood or necrotic tissue, by negative caloric balance and depletion of carbohydrate depots (most of the available glycogen in the body is utilized within 24 h), by transfusions of (bank) blood,[3] by the hemolysis of transfusion reactions,

and by the tendency of acidosis to cause transfer of potassium from the intracellular to the extracellular space (see Chap. 4). All the foregoing are common circumstances in acute renal failure, and, indeed, in the majority of such patients significant hyperkalemia develops during the oliguric phase; this becomes life-threatening in about one-third of the cases in the absence of specific preventive therapy. Loss of potassium from the gastrointestinal tract before or during oliguria (vomiting, nasal gastric suction, diarrhea) tends to prevent an increase in its serum level and may thus be beneficial if concomitant sodium is replaced. Although there is a rough clinical correlation between the rapidity and extent of hyperkalemia in relation to the factors cited above, this relationship is variable and sometimes unpredictable.

The untoward effects of alterations of potassium on neuromuscular contraction and, more important, on the myocardium are better correlated with serum levels than with total body content, although it may be the concentration ratio on both sides of the cell membrane which is critical. It also must be emphasized that cardiac changes, as reflected in the electrocardiogram, represent a summation of the influence of various other extracellular electrolytes and of pH (242). Hyponatremia, hypocalcemia, and acidosis enhance the deleterious effects of hyperkalemia. It often has been noted that a serum potassium concentration of 8.5 meq/L when the sodium concentration is 140 meq/L may be more benign than a level of 7meq/L with a serum sodium level of 120 meq/L. For these reasons, the electrocardiogram is a better clinical index of serious potassium intoxication than is the serum level, although both should be obtained when possible.

Progressive electrocardiographic changes follow a fairly definite pattern (Fig. 15-4) (243). In sequence, these are (1) tall, peaked T waves with a relatively narrow base (the amplitude of the T wave must be correlated with the amplitude and configuration of the QRS complex in a specific lead under consideration), (2) depressed RST segment, (3) decreased amplitude of the R wave and increased depth of the S wave, (4) prolonged PR interval, followed by the disappearance of the

---

[3]Potassium migrates from the red blood cells into the plasma of banked blood, the plasma concentration increasing with the age of the blood. Potassium concentrations of over 30 meq/L have been reported in banked blood over 10 days old. In addition, red cell survival is shortened in aged blood, with the eventual potassium release from hemolysis in the recipient.

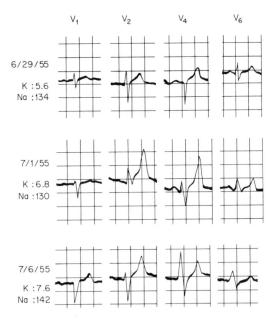

Fig. 15-4. Electrocardiographic changes of hyperkalemia. The typical alterations are best seen in leads V_2 and V_4. With increasing serum potassium, the following occur in sequence: T-wave peaking, prolonged PR interval, prolonged QRS complex.

P waves, (5) progressive widening of the QRS complex with prolongation of the QT interval, eventually merging with the T wave into an undulating, sine-wave configuration. These changes are most apparent in the precordial leads. Ectopic ventricular beats, bradycardia, or other arrhythmias may appear at this time. Death is usually from ventricular standstill or fibrillation.

Although a "syndrome" of potassium intoxication has been described, in our experience clinical symptoms are preceded by electrocardiographic changes, are minor, are atypical, or are difficult to attribute specifically to hyperkalemia. Sometimes present, however, are parasthesias or numbness, particularly of the mouth, hands, and feet; progressive increase in generalized weakness resulting in severe paresis of the extremities or muscles of respiration; restlessness, apprehension, and sweating; and faint heart sounds, falling blood pressure, bradycardia, or arrhythmia (see Chap. 1).

During early diuresis, for reasons cited previously, there may be copious loss of fluids and electrolytes. The kidneys at this stage exhibit a negligible or blunt response to salt or water loading, so that increased or decreased concentrations of sodium and other electrolytes can result from injudicious therapy. In most patients there is a relative excess of salt and water in the body at the end of the oliguric period. Moderate weight loss and polyuria therefore represent a return of fluid volumes toward normal and should be tolerated for this reason (4).

MORTALITY

With the recognition that the syndrome of ATN is the common end product of diverse diseases and traumatic insults and with greater understanding of the ensuing physiologic disturbances, the mortality rate in well-treated patients during the past three decades has decreased from over 90 to 50 percent (244). These therapeutic advances have been largely the result of (1) cognizance of positive water and salt balance, often iatrogenic in origin, and the general use of drastic fluid restriction, (2) abandonment of various maneuvers aimed at abruptly causing a diuresis, such as "flushing out" the kidneys with intravenously administered saline solution, renal decapsulation, caudal anesthesia, and the use of vasodilating drugs, (3) earlier recognition and more effective means of preventing hyperkalemia, and (4) the availability and earlier use of artificial dialysis to remove various metabolites and/or fluid when their accumulation becomes life-threatening, and (5) the availability of critical care units where a multidiscipline approach can be focused on upgrading patient care.

Despite these advances, the mortality rate remains at approximately 50 percent (226). Two-thirds of these deaths occur during the oliguric period and one-third during diuresis, with an occasional patient dying during the late recovery phase. There is general agreement that the mortality rate is related to the causal background, the prognosis being worse in patients who have sustained marked tissue destruction. Thus, in cases following incompatible transfusions, carbon tetrachloride intoxication, or obstetric complications the mortality is 25 percent or less. This may be contrasted with a 65 to 70 percent mortality in patients in whom oliguria develops after major surgical treatment, crush injuries, or battle trauma.

What are the reasons for the persistently high mortality of approximately 50 percent in dialysis centers throughout the world? Of some importance is the method of case selection. Many patients with mild, reversible renal failure of lesser severity are treated in neighborhood hospitals and not referred to dialysis centers. Because of improved surgical technique, a larger number of older patients with many risk factors are being subjected to more complicated operative procedures; open heart, aortic, and biliary surgery are associated with a higher incidence of ATN and greater overall mortality (245). In contrast, there has been a steady decline in low-risk obstetric ATN. With these changes in case selection it is not surprising that the overall mortality of ATN has not significantly improved despite multiple advances in acute care medicine and surgery.

An important factor which may contribute to mortality is the severity of renal failure. Patients with nonoliguric ATN of multiple etiology have milder renal disease with a smaller daily rise in blood urea nitrogen and a decrease dialysis requirements (95). In postoperative ATN there was an overall mortality rate of 21 to 26 percent in nonoliguric ATN as compared to the usual mortality rate of 60 to 70 percent in oliguric ATN (95, 246). This association of mortality with degree of renal failure was observed by Bhat et al. in a series of 490 patients undergoing open-heart surgery (247). The duration of cardiopulmonary bypass correlated with the incidence of hypotension, hemoglobinemia and postoperative renal failure. There was a 0.9 percent mortality rate in 340 of the 490 patients undergoing open-heart surgery who had no evidence of renal failure. In those patients whose serum creatinine peaked out at less than 5 mg/dL the mortality rate was 8 percent. In the 21 patients whose serum creatinine increased above 5 mg/dL there was an overall mortality rate of 67 percent; In this group 48 percent had nonoliguric ATN with an overall mor-

tality rate of 50 percent whereas the patients with oliguric ATN had an increased mortality rate of 83 percent. Postoperative renal failure was correlated with the underlying severity of cardiovascular disease and resulted in early death from cardiopulmonary complications. However, approximately one-half of the mortality was associated with late infectious complications despite early institution of dialysis therapy. It can be tentatively concluded, therefore, that the coexistence of oliguric renal failure in catabolic postsurgical patients introduces added risk to the original injury. Current dialysis therapy may reduce but cannot eliminate this risk.

Controversy exists regarding the cause of high mortality in posttrauma and postsurgical ATN. Are patients dying primarily from the serious complications of their disease state, or also because of other factors which alter metabolic, nutritional, and immunological integrity? For example, case selection cannot explain the absence of improvement in the mortality rate of battle trauma ATN during the past 25 years. Here the victims were primarily young, healthy men who sustained multiple fragment or gunshot wounds; when they developed ATN the overall mortality rate was 60 to 70 percent as opposed to 2.5 percent in the absence of ATN (248, 249). The risk of dying was related directly to the wound site, accounting for a 78 percent mortality rate in abdominal wounds, 40 percent in head, face, and extremity wounds and 25 percent in chest wounds (248).

The correlation of high mortality with abdominal injuries reflects two major problems. First, there is difficulty in eradicating infection from deep-lying traumatized tissues, often with the development of abscesses, fistulas, and peritonitis. Secondly, patients with abdominal injuries have a high rate of catabolism, are unable to take oral nourishment, and require frequent dialysis treatment which further depletes essential body nutriments. The end result is a rapid occurrence of protein-caloric malnutrition which leads to defective host immunity toward infection and poor wound healing.

This concatenation of events was borne out by military ATN statistics. Of those who did not die early of their wounds, the most frequent cause of death was infection, present in 89 percent of battle trauma ATN and directly responsible for death in 72 percent (248). Frequent masked complications of infection were jaundice, hemorrhage, and wound dehiscence; when present, these complications accounted for an overall mortality rate of greater than 80 percent. There is some evidence that treatment of posttraumatic ATN with adequate parenteral nutriments may prevent malnutrition, reduce infectious complications, and result in a lower mortality rate (see below).

MANAGEMENT

TREATMENT OF THE OLIGURIC PHASE

After reversible causes of acute renal failure have been eliminated, hypotension has been corrected, and gross water and electrolyte losses have been restored, therapy resolves itself into maintenance of as normal a *milieu intérieur* as possible until spontaneous diuresis takes place. Therapy can be divided into conservative measures and dialysis treatment.

Conservative therapy

Fluids. In calculating fluid balance, the production of endogenous water (see above) must be taken into account, so that replacement of insensible loss requires a total fluid intake of only 400 mL/day in the average 70-kg man (22, 250). When there is excessive tissue catabolism, as in traumatic injury or superimposed sepsis, the acceptable total fluid intake may be less than 400 mL/day. Unusual circumstances, such as severe sweating or diarrhea, will, of course, modify the required intake accordingly. If one is to err in calculating fluid intake, it should be in the direction of too little rather than too much. Inadvertent mild dehydration does not prevent or delay the onset of diuresis. The most accurate and simplest check on overall fluid balance is the daily weight of the patient; there should be a weight loss of 0.2 to 0.5 kg/day. In centers with a policy of early and frequent artificial dialysis resulting in net fluid loss, a more liberal fluid intake is permissible.

Electrolytes. Acute renal failure may be one of the few clinical situations in which the widespread use of the flame photometer and "treating the electrolyte abnormalities present" have done more actual harm than good. The slow development of acidosis, manifested by a low serum bicarbonate level, is a regular feature of acute renal failure. Plasma carbon dioxide content usually decreases by 1 to 3 mmol/L per day in uncomplicated acute renal failure. Acidosis may develop more rapidly in association with marked tissue trauma or uncontrolled infection. Moderate acidosis (carbon dioxide contents of 15 mmol or more per liter) ordinarily does not require treatment, and infusion of sodium bicarbonate or lactate may precipitate pulmonary edema or may cause clinical tetany in the presence of hypocalcemia. More severe acidosis may be treated cautiously with sodium bicarbonate solutions, although artificial dialysis treatment is preferable in the majority of cases.

When hyponatremia is present, it usually represents serum dilution from excess body water. The proper treatment for the usual low serum sodium concentration is water restriction, not the administration of sodium salts. There are, however, definite indications for the administration of sodium-containing solutions. As has been emphasized, any abnormal electrolyte loss (except for potassium) from the gastrointestinal tract or via severe sweating should be quantitatively replaced with the appropriate solutions. Except for the rare patient who maintains a urine volume of 400 to 800 mL/day for a prolonged period without progressing to a diuretic phase, the sodium losses in the urine need not be replaced until the daily urine output is greater than 1 L. When dangerous water intoxication is present, it may be necessary to partially correct the low serum sodium level and, by thus increasing the extracellular osmolality, to mobolize water from within the cells. For this purpose, parenteral hypertonic solutions of 3 or 5% sodium chloride are used. Dialysis therapy, however, is frequently the treatment of choice for this complication.

Since *symptomatic hypocalcemia* is rare in acute renal failure, the routine prophylactic use of calcium is not necessary. Anorexia and nausea often

Table 15-18. Treatment of hyperkalemia

SEVERITY	AGENT	ONSET	DURATION	MECHANISM
Mild	1. Decreased intake	Variable	Variable	Restriction
(S_K 5.5–6.5 meq/L)	2. K exchange resin	1–2 h	4–6 h	Excretion
Moderate	3. Glucose and insulin	10–30 min	2–4 h	Redistribution
(S_K 6.5–7.5 meq/L				
Severe	4. NaHCO$_3$	1 h or <	1–2 h	Redistribution
(S_K >7.5 meq/L)				Antagonism
	5. Calcium gluconate	< 5 min	30–60 min	Antagonism
	6. Dialysis	< 5 min	Variable	Excretion

prevent the oral administration of aluminum hydroxide gel, which binds phosphates in the intestinal tract, preventing the rise in serum phosphate level that is ultimately responsible for the low calcium level. When jerky movements, twitchings, or overt tetany are thought to be the result of hypocalcemia, the response to 30 mL calcium gluconate[4] intravenously given slowly will usually temporarily ameliorate these symptoms. A lack of response suggests that these symptoms are not caused by hypocalcemia but are more likely manifestations of uremia. If symptoms are ameliorated, then calcium should be infused continuously (100 mL of calcium gluconate per day or 30 mL of calcium chloride per day), or given intramuscularly, (100 mL of calcium gluconate per 6 h). Since the administration of alkalinizing solutions, when necessary, may cause tetany from the abrupt decrease of ionized calcium some writers advocate the prophylactic use of calcium prior to alkali therapy; the transfusion of citrated bank blood may cause tetany by the same mechanism. As will be discussed, calcium is also used in the treatment of potassium intoxication.

Potassium intoxication (see Table 15-18) often requires immediate, and at times heroic, therapy. It has been previously stressed that the immediate cause of death from hyperkalemia is disruption of cardiac conduction and that the electrocardiogram, which reflects the summated effects of various ions on the heart, is a better guide to therapy than any single serum electrolyte determination (132, 133). Daily, or even twice daily, electrocardiograms should be obtained and left in the patient's room for comparison with the preceding day's tracings. In addition, when feasible, daily serum potassium and sodium levels should be obtained. Potassium accumulation may be prevented or retarded by meticulous attention to the prophylactic measures already discussed: treatment of infections, debridement of necrotic tissue, drainage of accumulations of blood, prohibition of potassium intake, and provisions of nonprotein calories in the form of glucose and fat.

Additional prophylaxis against potassium intoxication may be accomplished by the use of ion-exchange resins (Kayexalate) (251). When feasible, these exchange resins may be given by mouth in doses of 15 gm twice or three times daily. Since obstruction and even intestinal obstruction has been reported with the use of exchange resins, the use of sorbitol, a poorly absorbed osmotically active alcohol, can be combined with the resin in sufficient quantity to produce mild diarrhea (251). If the resin cannot be taken by mouth, it is often useful to combine it with sorbitol and administer it as a high-retention enema. This should be retained for at least 1 to 2 h for effective removal of potassium. Thereafter, a Harris flush can be given to facilitate the removal of the previously administered resin prior to installation of another retention enema.

The most effective means of removing excess potassium from the body and preventing or reversing hyperkalemia is the use of artificial dialysis. This should be used if hyperkalemia recurs, or is accompanied by other indications for

[4]It often is not realized that calcium gluconate contains only 9% calcium; i.e., a 10-mL vial of 10% solution has 90 mg of calcium. The usual daily oral intake of 1 g calcium would therefore be equivalent to over 100 mL calcium gluconate given intravenously. Calcium chloride contains 36% calcium.

dialysis, or if ion-exchange resins are not effective.

In the presence of advanced hyperkalemia, i.e., with a serum level of 7 meq/L or greater and/or significant changes on the electrocardiogram (see above), treatment that produces rapid lowering of the serum potassium level is indicated. Several therapeutic measures are available for the emergency treatment of severe hyperkalemia:

1. *Dextrose and insulin* lowers extracellular levels by transferring potassium into the cells during gluconeogenesis. If the patient is not already receiving continuous 50% dextrose intravenously (see below), this procedure is instituted, and crystalline insulin is added to the infusate in a ratio of 1 unit insulin per 5 gm dextrose. This form of treatment may take from 30 to 60 min but is usually effective for several hours (133). Once begun, dextrose-insulin therapy should not be discontinued until total body potassium has been reduced by other means because of the danger of rapid in-

tracellular to extracellular potassium shifts and the return of dangerous levels of hyperkalemia.

2. *Intravenously administered calcium* (see Fig. 15-5) is a rapidly effective potassium and antagonist (235). With continuous electrocardiographic monitoring, 50 to 100 mL calcium gluconate can be given by syringe at a rate of 2 mL/min, followed by addition of calcium to the infusion of hypertonic glucose in insulin.

3. *Hypertonic sodium* solutions have not been very effective in our hands.

4. *Correction of acidosis* by the rapid infusion of 7½% sodium bicarbonate (1 ampul of sodium bicarbonate contains 44 meq sodium and bicarbonate) not only provides sodium ion for antagonizing the cardiac effects of potassium but also deposits potassium intracellularly as a result of corrective acidosis. It must be remembered that these effects are short-lived (1 to 2 h) and must be reinforced by exchange resins and artificial dialysis. The foregoing emergency measures have been lifesaving at

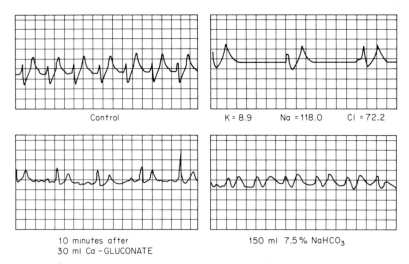

Control

K = 8.9   Na = 118.0   Cl = 72.2

10 minutes after
30 ml Ca – GLUCONATE

150 ml 7.5% NaHCO₃

Figure 15-5. Rapid movement seen in electrocardiogram following intravenous administration of calcium in the presence of hyperkalemia: *upper left,* 10 A.M.; *upper right,* 1 P.M.; *lower left,* 1:10 P.M.; *lower right,* 2:25 P.M. Intravenous calcium gluconate rapidly reversed the sine-wave configuration caused by hyperkalemia. Hypertonic sodium was not as effective.

times, and they must temporarily take precedence over all other considerations, such as fluid restriction and sodium overload.

Nutrition. One of the chief aims of the conservative treatment of acute renal failure is to decrease or prevent protein catabolism. This is important not only because the products of protein catabolism retained within the body include nitrogenous metabolites (the most likely causes of uremic symptoms), hydrogen ions, and potassium ions but also because excessive protein catabolism may lead to malnutrition which serves as an additional threat to recovery from acute renal failure.

It is well recognized that *nonprotein calories* have a protein-sparing action and that if other sources of calories are inadequate, protein is utilized in providing calories. Although earlier studies suggested that the daily ingestion of 100 g of carbohydrate produced maximal protein-sparing action (22), recent investigations have suggested that a larger carbohydrate intake can further increase the protein-sparing effect, even in patients with a severe catabolic response following injury (252). To be effective, the carbohydrate intake should be spaced evenly over the entire 24-h period, i.e., by frequent feedings or continuous intravenous administration.

When possible, carbohydrates should be given by mouth. One popular preparation of high carbohydrate content consists of equal parts Karo syrup and ginger ale, flavored with lemon juice and served chilled. A preparation, not yet available in the United States, which shows promise is Caloreen; this is a glucose-polymer mixture which has the desirable quality of being less sweet and therefore more palatable than glucose (253). When a patient's injuries preclude oral administration, it becomes necessary to use the intravenous route. Since calories must be given in a manner which does not exceed the fluid limit of 400 mL daily, they are provided by 50% dextrose in water. Peripheral venous thrombosis by this hypertonic solution is prevented by the insertion of an indwelling catheter via the saphenous vein into the vena cava, where the slow drip of hypertonic glucose will be diluted by a large

blood flow; when a "medical cutdown" is not feasible, the catheter is inserted by means of a surgical cutdown. The 50% dextrose is administered as a continuous drip and once started should not be discontinued until diuresis occurs or hemodialysis is performed (see above). The slow rate of the intravenous infusion requires the addition of 10 mg aqueous heparin per 250 mL 50% dextrose to prevent thrombosis at the catheter tip.

The importance of a *protein-free diet* in the treatment of acute renal failure was first emphasized by Borst in 1938 (254) and Bull et al. in 1949 (135). The elimination of protein in the diet along with adequate caloric administration reduces the rate of protein catabolism and the rate at which azotemia develops. With this type of dietary management, serum urea nitrogen increases by approximately 15 to 20 mg/dL per day. More rapid increase suggests excessive protein intake, inadequate caloric intake, damaged tissue, infection, or a combination of these factors.

The effect of androgenic hormones in decreasing protein catabolism has been well documented. Testosterone and testosterone proprionate have been advocated in the treatment of uremic patients, although their virilizing action may outweigh their anabolic effect (255). The synthetic androgenic steroids, with a greater anabolic/androgenic ratio, appear to be more effective in acute renal failure. McCracken and Parsons showed that norethandrolone was effective in decreasing urea formation in patients with postpartum renal failure, as well as renal failure from other causes (256). Those patients with high rates of protein catabolism from trauma or infection demonstrated a negligible anabolic response to this androgenic steroid. It is possible that anabolic steroids cannot prevent breakdown of devitalized tissue or are antagonized by excessive production of corticosteroids in the clinical setting of tissue trauma and/or infection.

There is evidence that protein restriction may not be the treatment of choice in acute renal failure. Giordano, treating chronic renal failure patients with a diet composed largely of essential amino acids and carbohydrates, showed a decrease in azotemia and a positive nitrogen balance (257). Similarly, Berlyne and his associates, by administering 14 g of animal protein (high in essential amino acids) daily and adequate calories to patients with acute renal failure, were able to show a smaller daily increase in urea nitrogen as compared to protein-free isocaloric therapy (258). Thus, urea hydrolized to ammonium ion in the gut by bacteria served as a source of α-amino nitrogen for the synthesis of nonessential amino acids.

Gallina and Dominquez have recently defined the prerequisites for the metabolism of endogenous urea into nonessential amino acids as follows: (1) hydrolysis into ammonium ion by bacteria, (2) incorporation of ammonium ion into α-ketoglutarate to yield glutamate, (3) availability of α-keto precursors of nonessential amino acids and (4) transamination of the α-keto acid from glutamate (259). They suggested that the rate-limiting step was the availability of carbon fragments for the synthesis of α-keto acids. Therefore, the synthesis of nonessential amino acids requires carbon fragments in the form of carbohydrates to serve as α-keto acid analogues.

Because of associated injuries, many patients with acute renal failure are unable to take nourishment by mouth. The recent development of total parenteral nutrition by Dudrick and his associates has proven beneficial in postsurgical or posttraumatic acute renal failure patients who cannot tolerate oral alimentation (260). This approach utilizes a subclavian or external carotid catheter through which large amounts of dextrose, essential amino acids, and vitamins are administered in small volumes of fluid (261). In order to provide for a longer period of parenteral administration, a Silastic catheter (Broviac catheter) can be inserted through a subcutaneous tunnel into the cephalic vein and threaded into the right atrium (262). With careful aseptic placement of catheters and local wound care, septic complications have decreased from 30 percent to less than 5 percent (263). However, total parenteral nutrition in the acute renal failure patient is maximally effective only when concurrent frequent hemodialysis is used to prevent fluid overload and uremia-induced catabolism (see below).

The specific composition of total parenteral nutrition in patients with acute renal failure must reflect high energy needs, insulin resistance, and negligible free water and urea clearance of these patients. Therefore, patients with acute renal failure require hypertonic solutions with a caloric/nitrogen ratio in excess of 450:1 and approximately one-third of the usual protein requirements in the form of essential amino acids. Since protein hydrolysate available in the United States contains only 60 to 70 percent of available nitrogen as free amino acid, this solution is not desirable for patients with renal failure; when given, there may be a rapid rise in blood urea nitrogen and increasing uremic symptoms. A mixture of synthetic essential and nonessential amino acids (Freamine, Aminosyn, Travamin) is superior to protein hydrolysate as a source of readily metabolizable amino acids, but even small quantities of nonessential amino acids may worsen azotemia in the presence of severe renal failure. Thus, a mixture of eight essential L-amino acids in concentrations recommended by Rose (Freamine E) is the most efficacious parenteral preparation now in use for the treatment of renal failure.

Although intravenously administered fat emulsions are available for parenteral nutrition, there is evidence that dextrose is a superior source of calories for patients in acute renal failure (264, 265). This suggests that the availability of carbon fragments to serve as α-keto acid analogues of nonessential amino acids is rate limiting (258). Thus, intravenous feedings of isotonic amino acid solutions with endogenous fatty acids or exogenous intravenous fats as a source of calories is not suitable for the specific needs of patients in acute renal failure although it is efficacious in reversing catabolism in postoperative patients (266–268).

Using the optimal techniques of parenteral hyperalimentation as outlined above, Abel et al. were able to show in a prospective, double-blind, matched series of patients with postoperative ATN that essential amino acid administration significantly decreased infectious complications and reduced overall mortality to 25 percent as compared to a significantly higher mortality of 66 percent in the control patients receiving intravenous glucose (269–271). Furthermore, the group treated with essential amino acids had a shorter overall duration of renal functional impairment, suggesting that improved nutrition contributed to enhanced regeneration of renal tubular cells. These findings were confirmed by Tobak using amino acid infusions in rats with mercuric chloride–induced ATN (272). The amino acid–treated rats showed increased synthesis of phospholipid tubular cell membranes, enhanced regeneration of tubular cells, and an improvement in renal function as compared to the glucose-treated controls (272). Baek et al., using a similar treatment protocol as Abel and his colleagues, observed in 122 consecutive postoperative ATN patients a reduced mortality of 46 percent in a protein hydrolysate–treated group (inferior to synthetic essential amino acid solutions) as compared to a 70 percent mortality in the glucose-treated control patients (273). Kleinknecht et al., using total parenteral nutrition and hemodialysis therapy, have reported an improved mortality rate of 38 percent in postsurgical and 33 percent in posttraumatic ATN patients (274). However, Asbach et al. showed an overall mortality rate of 78 percent in hypercatabolic ATN patients treated with parenteral nutrition and hemodialysis (275). Certain clinical settings, such as ruptured abdominal aneurysm with anuria, are associated with an almost 100 percent mortality rate (276). The type and severity of trauma in any reported series, therefore, may in part determine mortality even with optimal medical management.

Treatment of infection. The most frequent cause of death and morbidity in acute renal failure is infection, (277–281), most commonly pulmonary, wound, peritoneal, urinary tract, or septicemic infection. The distinguishing features of infection may be difficult to interpret; since hypothermia is a well-recognized complication of renal failure, fever is frequently absent in the presence of infection. Not only is the acutely uremic patient more susceptible to infections, but once started the bacterial invasion is extremely difficult to control. Meticulous care in the intravenous use of catheters and the avoidance of urethral catheters are helpful in preventing infections. Prophylactic antibiotics have not reduced the incidence of infections in acute renal failure. If infections occur, however, prompt treatment

should be instituted, agents being chosen with due consideration of excretory route, nephrotoxicity, as well as efficacy (282). Kanamycin, polymyxin, and gentamicin should be given in markedly reduced maintenance doses. Sulfonamides, nitrofurantoin, and tetracycline should not be used. Erythromycin, chloramphenicol, penicillin, and the penicillin derivatives can be used with only slight reduction in dosage.

Miscellaneous measures. The treatment of such uremic manifestations as vomiting, hypertension, heart failure, changes in the sensorium, and pruritis is discussed in Chap. 3.

Anemia is treated with packed red blood cells when it is symptomatic or contributing to heart failure. It has been our practice not to transfuse patients until their packed cell volume falls below 20 to 25 percent, because clinical effects attributable to anemia do not develop until this stage.

It has been our impression that there is a significant risk of serious bleeding from stress ulcers, especially in acute renal failure following trauma. Therefore, antacid therapy by mouth or by nasogastric tube may be of value in these patients.

Stomatitis, thrush, and acute parotitis are occasional complications of acute renal failure. These complications can be largely prevented with good oral hygiene and proper nursing care. Orally administered nystatin (Mycostatin) and mouthwashes are effective treatment for superinfection.

The routine use of an indwelling urethral catheter is to be condemned unless one is dealing with an outlet obstruction. Surveillance of hourly urine volumes is needed only during the mannitol-challenge stage (see above). Thereafter, once the diagnosis of acute oliguric renal failure has been made and obstructive uropathy has been excluded, the indwelling bladder catheter should be removed, for it serves no useful purpose and predisposes to acute and chronic pyelonephritis.

Artificial dialysis therapy

The principles, techniques, and complications of artificial dialysis are discussed in detail in Chap.

20. It is appropriate at this time, however, to discuss the indications for dialysis in acute renal failure. Until recently it was believed that the majority of patients with acute renal failure could be successfully treated by the conservative methods described in the preceding sections. The previous indications for the use of artificial dialysis were severe uremia, potassium intoxication, acidosis, and salt and water overload. In contrast, many dialysis centers now begin early treatment with peritoneal dialysis or hemodialysis in order to prevent the development of clinical symptoms of uremia. Improved techniques of peritoneal dialysis have made this a clinically useful procedure (283). Specific indications favoring peritoneal dialysis as the treatment of choice in acute renal failure are as follows: (1) small children, (2) severe fluid overload, (3) gastrointestinal bleeding, (4) cardiovascular instability (shock or acute myocardial infarction), (5) acute pancreatitis or peritonitis, and (6) lack of availability of hemodialysis therapy.

The technique of frequent hemodialysis has been made possible by the development of chronic cannulation techniques (284, 285). Prophylactic hemodialysis has been advocated by Teschan et al. (280), Parsons et al., (286), and Kleinknecht et al. (274), whose studies suggest (but do not conclusively prove) a decreased mortality with early and frequent dialysis in poor-risk patients with acute renal failure.

The use of frequent hemodialysis not only prevents uremia with its attendant complications but permits the oliguric patient to consume sufficient fluid, calories, and high-quality protein to avoid complications of malnutrition. It is our feeling, therefore, that patients with acute renal failure should be transferred at the earliest possible time to dialysis centers, where this more optimal therapy can be provided.

One unsolved problem is the patient with postsurgical and posttraumatic acute renal failure; the mortality rate still remains at approximately 70 percent. Although this high death rate is often attributed to concurrent organ damage, there is evidence that another important factor is the development of malnutrition. Frequent peritoneal or hemodialysis can prevent or reverse uremia but simultaneously removes significant amounts of valuable nutrients such as albumin (peritoneal dialysis) (287) and amino acids (hemodialysis) (288). Because adequate oral alimentation is contraindicated for an extended period of time in this type of problem and because protein has traditionally been omitted during the oliguric period, protein malnutrition is a frequent occurrence and may contribute to poor wound healing and infection. The use of prophylactic dialysis together with parenteral hyperalimentation with amino acids and adequate calories (as described above) may prove to be of great value in preventing malnutrition and reducing the mortality in this high-risk acute renal failure group.

TREATMENT DURING THE DIURETIC PHASE

During early diuresis the kidneys have, in effect, lost all flexibility. Because of a continued high osmotic load and effective tubular resorption of water and sodium, there is a fairly fixed and constant concentration of electrolytes in the urine which is relatively independent of serum levels or of intake. The urine is generally hypotonic, with concentrations of sodium, chloride, and potassium in the neighborhood of 50 meq/L.

Because of this inability to conserve water or electrolytes by the usual mechanisms and a common tendency by the physician to continue salt and protein restriction, severe dehydration, salt depletion, hypokalemia, or combinations of these abnormalities have been reported. The ideal way to determine replacement therapy is to measure urinary electrolyte concentrations. This need not be done daily, since the concentrations remain relatively constant during the early diuretic period, and if accurate records of urine volume are maintained, the electrolyte losses can be calculated from the preceding day. Serum electrolyte levels and electrocardiograms are of ancillary value and should be obtained when possible.

It has already been pointed out that for various reasons most patients have an excess of salt and

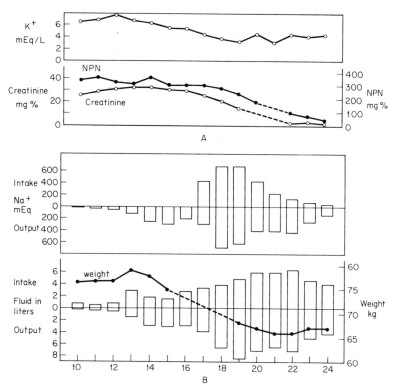

Figure 15-6. Diuretic phase of acute renal failure following carbon tetrachloride poisoning. Despite lack of edema, the patient lost over 10 kg during early diuresis, which started on the thirteenth day. Fluid and sodium intake during the diuretic phase was purposely restricted to less than that excreted in the urine. *A.* Changes in serum potassium, creatinine, and nonprotein nitrogen. *B.* Fluid and sodium balance.

water at the end of the oliguric period. Unless rigid fluid restriction has been maintained from the time of the initial episode or a fluid excess has been prevented by the removal of fluids by repeated dialysis procedures, quantitative replacement will serve to perpetuate the obligatory water and salt loss. We therefore seldom allow more than 3500 mL of fluid intake daily and expect a weight loss of several pounds during the diuresis (Fig. 15-6). On the other hand, when salt and water overload, as well as inordinate elevations in the blood urea level, have been prevented by repeated dialysis therapy, it is not unusual to see a gradual improvement in renal function in the ab-

sence of a large diuresis. Creatinine clearances and creatinine U/P ratios reflect the improvement in renal function although urine output may be no greater than 1000 to 1500 mL per 24 h.

REFERENCES

1. Schreiner, G. E., and J. F. Maher: Toxic nephropathy, *Am. J. Med.*, **38**:409, 1965.
2. Oliver, J., M. MacDaniell, and A. Tracy: The pathogenesis of acute renal failure associated with traumatic and toxic injury: Renal ischemia,

nephrotoxic damage and the ischemuric episode, *J. Clin. Invest.*, **30**:1307, 1951.

3. Oliver, J.: Correlations of structure and function and mechanisms of recovery in acute tubular necrosis, *Am. J. Med.*, **15**:535, 1953.

4. Swann, R. C., and J. P. Merrill: The clinical course of acute renal failure, *Medicine (Baltimore)*, **32**:215, 1953.

5. Friedman, E. A., J. B. Greenberg, J. P. Merrill, and G. J. Dammin: Consequences of ethylene glycol poisoning, *Am. J. Med.*, **32**:891, 1962.

6. Kunin, C. M.: Nephrotoxicity of antibiotics, *JAMA*, **202**:204, 1967.

7. Brun, C., and O. Munck: Pathophysiology of the kidney in shock and in acute renal failure, *Prog. Surg.*, **4**:1, 1964.

8. Wells, R. E.: Rheology of blood in the microvasculature, *N. Engl. J. Med.*, **270**:832, 1964.

9. Merrill, E. W.: Rheology of blood, *Physiol. Rev.*, **49**:863, 1969.

10. Hjort, P. F., and S. I. Rapoport: The Shwartzman reaction: Pathogenetic mechanisms and clinical manipulations, *Annu. Rev. Med.*, **16**:135, 1965.

11. Rodriguez-Erdmann, F.: Medical progress: Bleeding due to increased intravascular blood coagulation, *N. Engl. J. Med.*, **273**:1370, 1965.

12. McKay, D. G.: Progress in disseminated intravascular coagulation, *Calif. Med.*, **111**:186, 279, 1969.

13. Colman, R. W., S. J. Robbay, and J. D. Minna: Disseminated intravascular coagulation (DIC): An approach, *Am. J. Med.*, **52**:679, 1972.

14. Owens, C. A., and E. J. W. Bowie: Chronic intravascular coagulation syndromes, a summary, *Mayo Clin. Proc.*, **49**:673, 1974.

15. Lieberman, E.: Hemolytic-uremic syndrome, *J. Pediatr.*, **80**:1, 1972.

16. Gianantonia, C. A., M. Vitacco, F. Mendilaharzu, G. E. Gallo, and E. T. Sojo: The hemolytic-uremic syndrome, *Nephron*, **11**:174, 1973.

17. Wardle, E. N.: Endotoxin and acute renal failure, *Nephron*, **14**:321, 1975.

18. Wardle, E. N.: Renal failure in obstructive jaundice—pathogenic factors, *Postgrad. Med. J.*, **51**:512, 1975.

19. Franklin, S. S., and J. P. Merrill: Acute renal failure, *N. Engl. J. Med.*, **262**:711, 761, 1960.

20. Conn, H. L., Jr., J. C. Wood, and J. C. Rose: Cir-

culatory and renal effects following transfusion of human blood and its components to dogs, *Circ. Res.*, **4**:18, 1956.

21. Castle, W. B., T. H. Ham, and S. C. Shen: Observations on mechanisms of hemolytic transfusion reactions occurring without demonstrable hemolysin, *Trans. Assoc. Am. Physicians*, **63**:161, 1950.

22. Bywaters, E. G. J., and D. Beall: Crush injuries with impairment of renal function, *Br. Med. J.*, **1**:427, 1941.

23. Lucke, B.: Lower nephron nephrosis, *Milit. Surg.*, **99**:371, 1946.

24. Merrill, J. P.: *The Treatment of Renal Failure*, Grune & Stratton, Incorporated, New York, 1955.

25. Merrill, J. P.: Kidney disease: Acute renal failure, *Annu. Rev. Med.*, **11**:127, 1960.

26. Dalgaard, O. Z., and K. J. Pedersen: Renal tubular degeneration, *Lancet*, **2**:484, 1959.

27. Bull, G. M., A. M. Joekes, and K. G. Lowe: Renal function studies in acute tubular necrosis, *Clin. Sci.*, **9**:379, 1950.

28. Fry, I. K., and W. R. Cattell: Radiology in the diagnosis of renal failure, *Br. Med. Bull.*, **27**:148, 1971.

29. Cattell, W. R., C. S. McIntosh, and I. F. Moseley: Excretion urography in acute renal failure, *Br. Med. J.*, **2**:575, 1973.

30. Bank, N., B. F. Mutz, and H. S. Aynedjian: The role of "leakage" of tubular fluid in anuria due to mercury poisoning, *J. Clin. Invest.*, **46**:695, 1967.

31. Biber, T., M. Mylle, and A. D. Baines: A study by micropuncture and microdissection of acute renal damage in rats, *Am. J. Med.*, **44**:664, 1968.

32. Steinhausen, M., G. Eisenbach, and V. Helmstädter: Concentration of lissamine green in proximal tubules of antidiuretic and mercury poisoned rats and the permeability of these tubules, *Pfluegers Arch.*, **311**:1, 1969.

33. Blantz, R. C.: The mechanism of acute renal failure after uranyl nitrate, *J. Clin. Invest.*, **55**:621, 1975.

34. Jaenike, J. R.: The renal lesion associated with hemoglobinemia: A study of the pathogenesis of the excretory defect in the rat, *J. Clin. Invest.*, **46**:378, 1967.

35. Jaenike, J. R.: Micropuncture study of methemoglobin-induced acute renal failure in the rat, *J. Lab. Clin. Med.*, **73**:459, 1969.

36. Eisenbach, G. M., and M. Steinhausen: Micropuncture studies after temporary ischemia of rat kidneys, *Pfluegers Arch.*, **343**:11, 1973.

37. Tanner, G. A., K. L. Sloon, and S. Sophoson: Effects of renal artery occlusion on kidney function in the rat, *Kidney Int.*, **4**:377, 1973.

38. Henry, L. N., C. E. Lane, and M. Kashgarian: Micropuncture studies of the pathophysiology of acute renal failure in the rat, *Lab. Invest.*, **19**:309, 1968.

39. Eisenbach, G. M., B. Kitzlinger, and M. Steinhausen: Renal blood flow after temporary ischemia of rat kidneys, *Pfluegers Arch.*, **347**:223, 1974.

40. Donohue, J. F., M. A. Venkatachalam, and D. B. Bernard: Tubular leakage and obstruction in acute ischemic renal failure, *Kidney Int.*, **10**:567, 1976.

41. Falnigon, W. J., and D. E. Oken: Renal micropuncture study of the development of anuria in the rat with mercury-induced acute renal failure, *J. Clin. Invest.*, **44**:449, 1965.

42. Oken, D. E., M. L. Arce, and D. R. Wilson: Glycerol-induced hemoglobinuric acute renal failure in the rat. I. Micropuncture study of the development of oliguria, *J. Clin. Invest.*, **45**:724, 1966.

43. Finn, W. F., W. J. Arendshorst, and C. W. Gottschalk: Pathogenesis of oliguria in acute renal failure, *Circ. Res.*, **36**:675, 1975.

44. Arendshorst, W. J., W. F. Finn, and C. W. Gottschalk: Pathogenesis of acute renal failure following temporary renal ischemia in the rat, *Circ. Res.*, **37**:558, 1975.

45. Leaf, A.: Regulation of intracellular fluid volume and disease, *Am. J. Med.*, **49**:291, 1970.

46. Flores, J., D. R. DiBona, and C. H. Beck: The role of cell swelling in ischemic renal damage and the protective effect of hypertonic solute, *J. Clin. Invest.*, **51**:118, 1972.

47. Frega, N. S., D. R. DiBona, and B. Guertler: Ischemic renal injury, *Kidney Int.*, **4**(Suppl. 6): S-17, 1976.

48. Riley, A. L., E. A. Alexander, and S. Migdal: The effect of ischemia on renal blood flow in the dog, *Kidney Int.*, **7**:27, 1975.

49. Thurau, K., and J. W. Boylan: Acute renal success—the unexpected logic of oliguria in acute renal failure, *Am. J. Med.*, **61**:308, 1976.

50. Finckh, E. S.: The pathogenesis of uremia in acute renal failure, *Lancet*, **2**:330, 1962.

51. Schnermann, J., W. Nagel, and K. Thurau: Die frühdistale Natriumkonzentration in Rattennieren nach renaler ischämie und hämorrhagischer Hypotension, *Pfluegers Arch.*, **287**:296, 1966.

52. Hallenberg, N. K., M. Epstein, S. M. Rosen, R. I. Basch, D. E. Oken, and J. P. Merrill: Acute oliguric renal failure in man: Evidence for preferential renal cortical ischemia, *Medicine (Baltimore)*, **47**:455, 1968.

53. Tu, W. H.: Plasma renin activity in acute tubular necrosis and other renal diseases associated with hypertension, *Circulation*, **31**:686, 1965.

54. Kakot, F., and J. Kuska: Plasma renin activity in acute renal insufficiency, *Nephron*, **6**:115, 1969.

55. Brown, J. J., R. I. Gleadle, D. H. Lawson, A. F. Levers, A. L. Linton, R. F. Macadam, E. Prentice, J. I. S. Robertson, and M. Tree: Renin and acute renal failure: Studies in man, *Br. Med. J.*, **1**:253, 1970.

56. Thiel, G., D. R. Wilson, M. L. Arce, and D. E. Oken: Glycerol induced hemoglobinuric acute renal failure in the rat. II. The experimental model predisposing factors and pathophysiologic features, *Nephron*, **4**:276, 1967.

57. Wilson, D. R., G. Thiel, M. L. Arce, and D. E. Oken: Glycerol induced hemoglobinuric acute renal failure in the rat. III. Micropuncture study of the effects of mannitol and isotonic saline on individual nephron function, *Nephron*, **4**:337, 1967.

58. Oken, D. E.: On the passive back flow theory of acute renal failure, *Am. J. Med.*, **58**:77, 1975.

59. McDonald, F. D., G. Thiel, D. R. Wilson, G. F. DiBona, and D. E. Oken: The prevention of acute renal failure in the rat by long-term saline loading: A possible role of the renin-angiotensin axis, *Proc. Soc. Exp. Biol. Med.*, **131**:610, 1969.

60. Wilson, D. R., G. Thiel, M. L. Arce, and D. E. Oken: The role of the concentration mechanism in the development of acute renal failure: Micropuncture studies using diabetes insipidus rats, *Nephron*, **6**:128, 1969.

61. Flamenbaum, W., T. A. Kochen, and D. E. Oken: Effect of renin immunization on mercuric chlo-

ride and glycerol-induced renal failure, *Kidney Int.*, 1:406, 1972.

62. Powell-Jackson, J. D., J. MacGregor, and J. J. Brown: The effect of angiotensin II antisera and synthetic inhibitors of the renin-angiotensin system on glycerol-induced acute renal failure in the rat, in E. A. Friedman and H. E. Eliahou (eds.), *Proceedings of the Acute Renal Failure Conference,* Department of Health, Education, and Welfare Publication NIH 74-608, 1973, p. 281.

63. Matthews, P. G., T. O. Morgan, and C. I. Johnston: The renin-angiotensin system in acute renal failure in rats, *Clin. Sci. Mol. Med.*, 47:79, 1974.

64. Baranowski, R. I., G. U. O'Connor, and N. A. Kurtzman: The effect of 1-sarcosine; 8-leucyl angiotensin II on glycerol-induced acute renal failure, *Arch. Int., Pharmacodyn, Ther.*, 217:322, 1975.

65. Ladefoged, T., and K. Winkler: Effect of dihydralazine and acetylcholine on renal blood flow, mean circulation time for plasma and renal resistance in acute renal failure, in V. Gessler, K. Schroder, and H. Weideiger (eds.), *Pathogenesis and Clinical Findings with Renal Failure,* George Thieme Verlag Stuttgart, 1971, pp. 7–15.

66. Reubi, F. C.: The pathogenesis of anuria following shock, *Kidney Int.*, 5:106, 1974.

67. Baehler, R. W., T. A. Kotchen, J. A. Burke, J. H. Galla, and D. Bhathena: Considerations on the pathophysiology of mercuric chloride-induced acute renal failure, *J. Lab. Clin. Med.*, 90 (2):330, 1977.

68. Daugharty, T. M., I. F. Ueki, and P. F. Mercer: Dynamics of glomerular ultrafiltration in the rat. V. Response to ischemic injury, *J. Clin. Invest.*, 53:105, 1974.

69. Blantz, R. C.: The mechanism of acute renal failure after uranyl nitrate, *J. Clin. Invest.*, 55:621, 1975.

70. Cox, J. W., R. W. Boehler, and H. Sharma: Studies on the mechanism of oliguria in a model of unilateral acute renal failure, *J. Clin. Invest.*, 53:1546, 1974.

71. Stein, J. H.: The glomerulus in acute renal failure, *J. Lab. Clin. Med.*, 90:227, 1977.

72. Brenner, B. M., and H. D. Humes: Mechanics of glomerular ultrafiltration, *N. Engl. J. Med.*, 297 (3):148, 1977.

73. Maddox, D. A., and B. M. Brenner: Glomerular filtration of fluid and macromolecules: The renal response to injury, *Annu. Rev. Med.*, 28:91, 1977.

74. Patel, R., J. K. McKenzie, and E. G. McQueen: Tamm-Horsfall urinary microprotein and tubular obstruction by casts in acute renal failure, *Lancet*, 1:457, 1964.

75. Defronzo, R. A., R. L. Humphrey, J. R. Wright, and C. R. Cooke: Acute renal failure in multiple myeloma, *Medicine (Baltimore)*, 54 (3):209, 1975.

76. Min, K.-W., G. D. Cain, P. Györkey, and F. Györkey: Myeloma-like lesions of the kidney, *Arch. Intern. Med.*, 136:1299, 1976.

77. Burke, J. F. Jr., R. Flis, N. Lasker, and M. Simenhoff: Malignant lymphoma with "myeloma kidney" acute renal failure, *Am. J. Med.*, 60:1055, 1976.

78. Mailloux, L., C. D. Swartz, R. Capizzi, K. E. Kim, G. Onesti, O. Ramirez, and A. N. Brest: Acute renal failure after administration of low-molecular-weight dextran, *N. Engl. J. Med.*, 277 (21):1113, 1967.

79. Matheson, N. A., and P. Diomi: Renal failure after the administration of dextran 40, *Surg. Gynecol. Obstet.*, 131:661, 1970.

80. Schmidt, U., and U. C. Dubach with the technical assistance of B. Funj and E. Engeler: Acute renal failure in the folate-treated rat: Early metabolic changes in various structures of the nephron, *Kidney Int.*, 10 (4)(suppl. 6):S-39, 1976.

81. Schubert, G. E.: Folic acid-induced acute renal failure in the rat: morphological studies, *Kidney Int.*, 10 (4)(suppl. 6):S-46, 1976.

82. Warren, D. J., A. G. Leitch, and R. J. E. Leggett: Hyperuricaemic acute renal failure after epileptic seizures, *Lancet*, 2:385, 1975.

83. Robinson, R. R., and W. E. Yarger: Acute uric acid nephropathy (editorial), *Arch. Intern. Med.*, 137:839, 1977.

84. Duffy, J. L., Y. Guzuki, and J. Chung: Acute calcium nephropathy, *Arch. Pathol.*, 91:340, 1971.

85. Frascino, J. A., P. Varamee, and P. P. Rosen: Renal oxalosis and azotemia after methoxyflurane anesthesia, *N. Engl. J. Med.*, 283:676, 1970.

86. Eliahou, H. E., and A. Bota: The diagnosis of acute renal failure, *Nephron*, 2:287, 1965.

87. Bull, G. M., A. M. Joekes, and K. G. Lowe:

Renal function studies in acute tubular necrosis, *Clin. Sci.,* **9:**379, 1950.

88. Vertel, R. M., and J. P. Knochel: Nonoliguric acute renal failure, *JAMA,* **200:**118, 1967.

89. Graber, I. G., and S. Sevitt: Renal function in burned patients and its relationship to morphological changes, *J. Clin. Pathol.,* **12:**25, 1959.

90. Perlmutter, M., S. L. Grossman, S. Rottenberg, and G. Dobkin: Urine-serum urea nitrogen ratio, *JAMA,* **170:**1533, 1959.

91. Lyon, R. P.: Nonobstructive oliguria, *Calif. Med.,* **99:**83, 1963.

92. Handa, S. P., and P. A. F. Morrin: Diagnostic indices in acute renal failure, *Can. Med. Assoc. J.,* **96:**78, 1967.

93. Swenson, R. S., W. F. Corell, and G. J. Redding: Differential diagnostic indices in early acute renal failure (ARF), *Clin. Res.,* **23:**122A, 1975.

94. Espinel, C. H.: The FE$_{Na}$ test—use in the differential diagnosis of acute renal failure, *JAMA,* **236** (6):579, 1976.

95. Anderson, R. J., S. L. Linas, A. S. Berns, W. L. Henrich, T. R. Miller, P. A. Gabow, and R. W. Schrier: Nonoliguric acute renal failure, *N. Engl. J. Med.,* **296** (20):1134, 1977.

96. Barry, K. G., A. Cohen, J. P. Knochel, T. J. Whelon, Jr., W. R. Beisel, C. A. Vargas, and P. C. LeBlanc, Jr.: Mannitol infusion. II. The prevention of acute functional renal failure during resection of an aneurysm of the abdominal aorta, *N. Engl. J. Med.,* **264:**967, 1961.

97. Eliahou, H. E.: Mannitol therapy in oliguria of acute onset, *Br. Med. J.,* **1:**807, 1964.

98. Augur, R., D. Dayton, C. E. Harrison, R. M. Tucker, and C. F. Anderson: Use of ethacrynic acid in mannitol-resistant oliguric renal failure, *JAMA,* **206:**891, 1968.

99. Levinsky, N. G., and E. A. Alexander: Acute renal failure, in R. Breimer and F. Rector (eds.), *The Kidney,* W. B. Saunders Company, Philadelphia, 1976, p. 809.

100. Rosenmann, E., V. E. Pollak, and C. L. Pirani: Renal vein thrombosis in the adult: A clinical and pathologic study based on renal biopsies, *Medicine (Baltimore),* **47:**269, 1968.

101. Wegner, G. P., A. B. Crummy, T. T. Flaherty, and F. A. Hipona: Renal vein thrombosis, *JAMA,* **209:**1661, 1969.

102. Long, E. K., J. H. O. Mertz, and M. Nourse: Renal arteriography in the assessment of renal infarction, *J. Urol.,* **99:**506, 1968.

103. Harrington, J. T., S. C. Sommers, and J. P. Kassirer: Atheromatous emboli with progressive renal failure, *Ann. Intern. Med.,* **68:**152, 1968.

104. Kassirer, J. P.: Atheroembolic renal disease, *N. Engl. J. Med.,* **280:**812, 1969.

105. Goldsmith, E. I., F. W. Fuller, C. T. Lambrew, and V. F. Marshall: Embolectomy of the renal artery, *J. Urol.,* **99:**366, 1968.

106. Lemieux, G., A. A. Cuvelier, and R. Lefebure: The clinical spectrum of renal insufficiency during acute glomerulonephritis in the adult, *Can. Med. Assoc. J.,* **96:**1129, 1967.

107. Beaufils, M., L. Morel-Maroger, J.-D. Sraer, A. Kanfer, O. Kourilsky, and G. Richet: Acute renal failure of glomerular origin during visceral abscesses, *N. Engl. J. Med.,* **295** (4):185, 1976.

108. Zappacosta, A. R., and B. L. Ashby: Gram-negative sepsis with acute renal failure, *JAMA,* **238** (13):1389, 1977.

109. Hilton, P. J., N. F. Jones, M. A. Barraclough, and R. W. Lloyd-Davies: Urinary osmolality in acute renal failure due to glomerulonephritis, *Lancet,* **1:**655, 1969.

110. Ladenfoged, J., B. Nielsen, F. Raaschou, and A. W. Sorensen: Acute anuria due to polyarteritis nodosa, *Am. J. Med.,* **46:**827, 1969.

111. Kark, R. M.: Renal biopsy, *JAMA,* **205:**270, 1968.

112. Myburgh, J. A., J. Cohen, L. Gecelter, A. M. Meyers, C. Abrahams, K. I. Furman, B. Goldberg, and P. J. von Blerk: Hyperacute rejection in human-kidney allografts—Shwartzman vs. Arthus reaction? *N. Engl. J. Med.,* **281:**131, 1969.

113. Clapp, J. R., and R. R. Robinson: Functional characteristics of the transplanted kidney, *Arch. Intern. Med.,* **123:**531, 1969.

114. Massry, S. G., H. G. Preuss, J. F. Maher, and G. E. Schreiner: Renal tubular acidosis after cadaver kidney homotransplantation: Studies on mechanism, *Am. J. Med.,* **42:**284, 1967.

115. Simenhoff, M. L., W. R. Guild, and G. J. Dammin: Acute diffuse interstitial nephritis, *Am. J. Med.,* **44:**618, 1968.

116. Baldwin, D. S., B. B. Levine, R. T. McCluskey, and G. R. Gallo: Renal failure and interstitial ne-

phritis due to penicillin and methicillin, *N. Engl. J. Med.*, **279**:1245, 1968.

117. Knepshield, J. H., P. H. B. Carstens, and D. E. Gentile: Recovery from renal failure due to acute diffuse interstitial nephritis, *Pediatrics*, **43**:533, 1969.

118. Bergstein, J., and N. Litman: Interstitial nephritis with anti-tubular-basement-membrane antibody, *N. Engl. J. Med.*, **292** (17):875, 1975.

119. Bain, B. J., N. T. Ribush, P. Nicoll, H. M. Whitsed, and T. O. Morgan: Renal failure and transient paraproteinemia due to *Leptospira pomona*, *Arch. Intern. Med.*, **131**:740, 1973.

120. Nessi, R., G. L. Bonoldi, B. Redaelli, and G. di Filippo: Acute renal failure after rifampin: A case report and survey of the literature, *Nephron*, **16**:148, 1976.

121. Chazan, J. A., S. Garella, and A. Esparza: Acute interstitial nephritis—a distinct clinico-pathological entity? *Nephron*, **9**:10, 1972.

122. Lauler, D. P., G. E. Schreiner, and A. David: Renal medullary necrosis, *Am. J. Med.*, **29**:132, 1960.

123. Hellebusch, A. A.: Renal papillary necrosis, *JAMA*, **210**:1098, 1969.

124. Owusu, S. K., J. H. Addy, A. K. Foli, M. Janosi, F. I. D. Konotey-Ahulu, and E. B. Larbi: Acute reversible renal failure associated with glucose-6-phosphate-dehydrogenase deficiency, *Lancet*, **1**:1255, 1972.

125. Meltz, D. J., J. F. Bertles, D. S. David, and A. C. deCiutiis: Delayed haemolytic transfusion reaction with renal failure, *Lancet*, **2**:1348, 1971.

126. Hamilton, R. W.: Acute tubular necrosis caused by exercise-induced myoglobinuria, *Ann. Intern. Med.*, **77**:77, 1972.

127. Knochel, J. P., and E. M. Schlein: On the mechanism of rhabdomyolysis in potassium depletion, *J. Clin. Invest.*, **51**:1750, 1972.

128. Koffler, A., R. M. Friedler, and S. G. Massry: Acute renal failure due to nontraumatic rhabdomyolysis, *Ann. Intern. Med.*, **85**:23, 1976.

129. Richter, R. W., Y. B. Challenor, J. Pearson, L. J. Kagen, L. L. Hamilton, and W. H. Ramsey: Acute myoglobinuria associated with heroin addiction, *JAMA*, **216** (7):1172, 1971.

130. Klock, J., and M. J. Sexton: Rhabdomyolysis and acute myoglobinuric renal failure following heroin use, *Calif. Med.*, **119**:5, 1973.

131. Kendrick, W. C., A. R. Hull, and J. P. Knochel: Rhabdomyolysis and shock after intravenous amphetamine administration, *Ann. Intern. Med.*, **86** (4):381, 1977.

132. Minow, R. A., S. Gorbach, B. L. Johnson, Jr., and L. Dornfeld: Myoglobinuria associated with influenza A infection, *Ann. Intern. Med.*, **80** (3):359, 1974.

133. Shenouda, A., and F. E. Hatch: Influenza A viral infection associated with acute renal failure, *Am. J. Med.*, **61**:697, 1976.

134. Neu, P. S., G. D. Lubash, and L. Scherr: Acute renal failure associated with carbon tetrachloride intoxication, *JAMA*, **181**:903, 1962.

135. Collins, J. M., D. M. Hennes, C. R. Holzgang, R. T. Gourley, and G. A. Porter: Recovery after prolonged oliguria due to ethylene glycol intoxication—the prognostic value of serial, percutaneous renal biopsy, *Arch. Intern. Med.*, **125**:1059, 1970.

136. Parry, M. F., and R. Wallach: Ethylene glycol poisoning, *Am. J. Med.*, **57**:143, 1974.

137. Fisher, H. K., M. Humphries, and R. Bails: Paraquat poisoning, recovery from renal and pulmonary damage, *Ann. Intern. Med.*, **75**:731, 1971.

138. Baerg, R. D., and D. V. Kimberg: Centrilobular hepatic necrosis and acute renal failure in solvent sniffers, *Ann. Intern. Med.*, **73**:713, 1970.

139. Grossman, C. M., and B. Malbin: Mushroom poisoning, *Ann. Intern. Med.*, **40**:249, 1954.

140. Grossman, R. A., R. W. Hamilton, B. M. Morse, A. S. Penn, and M. Goldberg: Nontraumatic rhabdomyolysis and acute renal failure, *N. Engl. J. Med.*, **291** (16):807, 1974.

141. Olerud, J. E., L. D. Homer, and H. W. Carroll: Serum myoglobin levels predicted from serum enzyme values, *N. Engl. J. Med.*, **293** (10):483, 1975.

142. Finkelstein, F. O., M. Kashgarian, and J. P. Hayslett: Clinical spectrum of postpartum renal failure, *Am. J. Med.*, **57**:649, 1974.

143. Harwood, T. H., Jr., D. R. Hiesterman, R. G. Robinson, D. E. Cross, F. C. Whittier, Jr., D. A. Diederich, and J. J. Grantham: Prognosis for recovery of function in acute renal failure—value of the renal image obtained using iodohippurate sodium I 131, *Arch. Intern. Med.*, **136**:916, 1976.

144. Board for the Study of the Severely Wounded: *Surgery in World War II: The Physiologic Effects*

of Wounds, Office of the Surgeon General, Department of the Army, 1952.

145. Teschan, P. E., R. S. Post, and L. H. Smith, Jr.: Post-traumatic renal insufficiency in military casualties, *Am. J. Med.,* **18**:172, 1955.

146. Whelton, A., and J. A. Donadio: Post-traumatic acute renal failure in Vietnam, *Johns Hopkins Med. J.,* **124**:95, 1969.

147. Papper, S., and E. M. Papper: The effects of preanesthetic, anesthetic, and postoperative drugs on renal function, *Clin. Pharmacol. Ther.,* **5**:205, 1964.

148. Hayes, M. A.: Water and electrolyte therapy after operation, *N. Engl. J. Med.,* **278**:1054, 1968.

149. Moore, F. D.: The effects of hemorrhage on body composition, *N. Engl. J. Med.,* **273**:567, 1965.

150. Fountain, S. S., and P. R. Schloerb: The dynamics of post-traumatic intestinal fluid sequestration, *Surg. Gynecol. Obstet.,* **123**:1237, 1966.

151. Mouridsen, H. T., and M. Faber: Accumulation of serum-albumin at the operative wound site as a cause of postoperative hypoalbuminuria, *Lancet,* **2**:723, 1966.

152. Barry, K. G., A. Cohen, J. P. Knochel, T. J. Whelon, W. R. Beisel, C. A. Vargas, and P. C. LeBlanc: Mannitol infusion, *N. Engl. J. Med.,* **264**:967, 1961.

153. Terry, R. N., and R. J. Trudnowski: Intraoperative fluid therapy, *New York State J. Med.,* **64**:2646, 1964.

154. Parry, W. L.: Consideration of acute renal failure for the surgeon, *Surg. Clin. North Am.,* **45**:6, 1965.

155. Powers, S. R., Jr., A. Boba, W. Hostnik, and A. Stein: Prevention of postoperative acute renal failure with mannitol in 100 cases, *Surgery,* **55**:15, 1964.

156. Silverberg, D. S., and W. J. Johnson: The use of mannitol in oliguric renal failure, *Med. Clin. North Am.,* **50**:1159, 1966.

157. Hardaway, R. M.: Clinical management of shock, *Milit. Med.,* **134**:643, 1969.

158. Weil, M. H., and H. Shubin: The "VIP" approach to the bedside management of shock, *JAMA,* **207**:337, 1969.

159. Barry, K. G.: Post-traumatic renal shutdown in humans: Its prevention and treatment by the intravenous infusion of mannitol, *Milit. Med.,* **128**:224, 1963.

160. Stremple, J. F., E. H. Ellison, and L. C. Carey: Osmolar diuresis: Success and/or failure: A collective review, *Surgery,* **60**:924, 1966.

161. Parry, W. L., J. A. Schaefer, and C. B. Mueller: Experimental studies of acute renal failure. I. The protective effect of mannitol, *J. Urol.,* **80**:1, 1963.

162. Hoff, H. E., S. Deavers, and R. A. Huggins: Effects of hypertonic glucose and mannitol on plasma volume, *Proc. Soc. Exp. Biol. Med.,* **122**:630, 1966.

163. Goldberg, A. H., and L. S. Lilienfield: Effects of hypertonic mannitol on renal vascular resistance, *Proc. Soc. Exp. Biol. Med.,* **119**:635, 1965.

164. Golombos, J. T., E. G. Herndon, Jr., J. L. Achord, and J. H. Christy: Effect of osmotic (mannitol) diuresis on electrolyte and water excretion in ascitic, cirrhotic patients, *Clin. Res.,* **11**:69, 1963.

165. Gann, D. S., H. K. Wright, and H. H. Newsome: Prevention of sodium depletion during osmotic diuresis, *Surg. Gynec. Obstet.,* **119**:265, 1964.

166. Cantarovich, F., A. Locatelli, J. C. Fernandez, J. P. Loredo, and J. Christhot: Furosemide in high doses in the treatment of acute renal failure, *Postgrad. Med. J.,* April Suppl.:13, 1971.

167. Montoreano, R., M. T. Mouzet, J. Cuñarro, and A. Ruiz-Guinazú: Prevention of the initial oliguria of acute renal failure by the administration of furosemide, *Postgrad. Med. J.,* April Suppl.:7, 1971.

168. Epstein, M., N. S. Schneider, and B. Befeler: Effect of intrarenal furosemide on renal function and intrarenal hemodynamics in acute renal failure, *Am. J. Med.,* **58**:510, 1975.

169. Kleinknecht, D., D. Ganeval, L. A. Gonzalez-Duque, and J. Fermanian: Furosemide in acute oliguric renal failure—a controlled trial, *Nephron,* **17**:51, 1976.

170. Owen, K., R. Desautels, and C. W. Walter: Experimental renal tubular necrosis. Effect of Pitressin, *Surg. Forum,* **4**:459, 1953.

171. Bartels, E. D., G. C. Brun, A. Gammeltoft, and P. A. Gjørup: Acute anuria following intravenous pyelography in patients with myelomatosis, *Acta Med. Scand.,* **150**:297, 1954.

172. Morgan, C., and W. J. Hammack: Intravenous urography in multiple myeloma, *N. Engl. J. Med.,* **275**:77, 1966.

173. Argani, I., and G. F. Kipkie: Macroglobulinemic nephropathy, *Am. J. Med.,* **36**:151, 1964.

174. Conolly, M. E., O. M. Wrong, and N. F. Jones: Reversible renal failure in idiopathic nephrotic syndrome with minimal glomerular changes, *Lancet,* **1:**665, 1968.

175. Matheson, N. A., and J. W. Robertson: Effects of dextran 40 on postoperative renal hemodynamics, *Lancet,* **2:**251, 1966.

176. Dawson, J. L.: Jaundice and anoxic renal damage: Protective effect of mannitol, *Br. Med. J.,* **1:**810, 1964.

177. Dawson, J. L.: Post-operative renal function in obstructive jaundice: Effect of a mannitol diuresis, *Br. Med. J.,* **1:**82, 1965.

178. Lawson, D. H., R. M. Lindsay, J. D. Sawers, R. G. Luke, J. F. Davidson, C. J. Wardrop, and A. L. Linton: Acute renal failure in the cold-agglutination syndrome, *Lancet,* **2:**704, 1968.

179. Whelton, A., J. V. Donadio, Jr., and B. L. Elisberg: Acute renal failure complicating rickettsial infections in glucose-6-phosphate dehydrogenase-deficient individuals, *Ann. Intern. Med.,* **69:**323, 1968.

180. Tavill, A. S., J. M. Evanson, S. B. de C. Baker, and V. Hewitt: Idiopathic paroxysmal myoglobinuria with acute renal failure, *N. Engl. J. Med.,* **271:**283, 1964.

181. Sawyer, K. C., Jr., R. B. Sawyer, and W. C. Robb: Postoperative renal failure, *Am. J. Surg.,* **106:**668, 1963.

182. Wheeler, C. G., J. E. Thompson, M. M. Kartchner, D. J. Austin, and R. D. Patman: Massive fluid requirement in surgery of the abdominal aorta, *N. Engl. J. Med.,* **275:**320, 1966.

183. Payne, J. H., D. L. Wood, and J. A. Goethel: Oliguria and renal failure in abdominal aortic surgery, *Am. Surg.,* **29:**713, 1963.

184. Etheredge, E. E., H. Levitin, K. Nakamura, and W. W. Glenn: Effect of mannitol on renal function during open-heart surgery, *Ann. Surg.,* **161:**53, 1965.

185. Mielke, J. E., J. C. Hunt, F. T. Maher, and J. W. Kuklin: Renal performance during clinical cardiopulmonary bypass with and without hemodilution, *J. Thorac. Cardiov. Surg.,* **51:**229, 1966.

186. Schreiner, G. E.: Nephrotoxicity and diagnostic agents, *JAMA,* **196:**413, 1966.

187. Malt, R. A., H. G. Olken, and W. J. Goade, Jr.: Renal tubular necrosis after oral cholecystography, *Arch. Surg.,* **87:**743, 1963.

188. Sanen, F. J., R. M. Myerson, and J. G. Teplick: Etiology of serious reactions to oral cholecystography, *Arch. Intern. Med.,* **113:**133, 1964.

189. Schencker, B.: Drug infusion pyelography, *Radiology,* **83:**12, 1964.

190. Diaz-Buxo, J. A., R. D. Wagoner, R. R. Hattery, and P. J. Palumbo: Acute renal failure after excretory urography in diabetic patients, *Ann. Intern. Med.,* **83** (2):155, 1975.

191. Ansari, Z., and D. S. Baldwin: Acute renal failure due to radio-contrast agents, *Nephron,* **17:**28, 1976.

192. Deon, R. E., J. H. Andrew, and R. C. Read: The red cell factor in renal damage from angiographic media, *JAMA,* **187:**127, 1964.

193. Smith, K., J. C. Browne, R. Shackman, and O. M. Wrong: Renal failure of obstetric origin, *Br. Med. Bull.,* **24:**49, 1968.

194. Bartlett, R. H., and C. Yahia: Management of septic chemical abortion with renal failure, *N. Engl. J. Med.,* **281:**747, 1969.

195. Brodsky, I., and N. H. Siegel: The diagnosis and treatment of disseminated intravascular coagulation, *Med. Clin. North Am.,* **54:**555, 1970.

196. Clarkson, A. R., R. E. Sage, and J. R. Lawrence: Consumption coagulopathy and acute renal failure due to gram-negative septicemia after abortion, *Ann. Intern. Med.,* **70:**1191, 1969.

197. Green, D., R. A. Seeler, and N. Allen: The role of heparin in the management of consumption coagulopathy, *Med. Clin. North Am.,* **56:**193, 1972.

198. Loughridge, L. W., M. D. Milne, R. Shackman, and J. D. P. Woolton: Clinical course of uncomplicated acute tubular necrosis, *Lancet,* **1:**351, 1960.

199. Villazon, A., J. Portos, and A. Sierra: Polyuric syndromes in the critically ill patient, *Crit. Care Med.,* **4** (1):24, 1976.

200. Meyers, C., D. M. Roxe, and J. E. Hano: The clinical course of nonoliguric acute renal failure, *Cardiovascular Med.,* July:669, 1977.

201. Appel, G. B., and H. C. Neu: The nephrotoxicity of antimicrobial agents, *N. Engl. J. Med.,* **296** (12):663, 1977.

202. Milman, N.: Renal failure associated with gentamicin therapy, *Acta. Med. Scand.,* **196:**87, 1974.

203. Churchill, D., J. Knaack, E. Chirito, P. Barré, C. Cole, R. Muehrcke, and M. H. Gault: Persisting

renal insufficiency after methoxyflurane anesthesia, *Am. J. Med.*, **56**:575, 1974.

204. Lavender, S., J. N. Brown, and W. T. Berrill: Acute renal failure and lithium intoxication, *Postgrad. Med. J.*, **49**:277, 1973.

205. Kalowski, S., R. S. Nanra, T. H. Mathew, and P. Kincaid-Smith: Deterioration in renal function in association with co-trimoxazole therapy, *Lancet*, **1**:394, 1973.

206. Eybel, C. E., K. F. W. Armbruster, and T. S. Ing: Skin pigmentation and acute renal failure in a patient receiving phenazopyridine therapy, *JAMA*, **228** (8):1027, 1974.

207. Burgess, J. L., and R. Birchall: Nephrotoxicity of amphotericin B, with emphasis on changes in tubular function, *Am. J. Med.*, **53**:77, 1972.

208. Sadoff, L.: Nephrotoxicity of Streptozotocin (NSC-85998), *Cancer Chemother. Rep.*, **54** (6):457, 1970.

209. Meroney, W. H., and M. E. Rubini: Kidney function during acute tubular necrosis: Clinical studies and theory, *Metabolism*, **8**:1, 1959.

210. Lowe, K. G., G. Moodie, and M. B. Thomson: Glycosuria in acute tubular necrosis, *Clin. Sci.*, **13**:187, 1954.

211. DeLuna, M. B., A. Metcalfe-Gibson, and O. Wrong: Urinary excretion of hydrogen-ion in acute oliguric renal failure, *Nephron*, **1**:3, 1964.

212. Ward, E. E., P. Richards, and O. Wrong: Urine concentration after acute renal failure, *Nephron*, **3**:289, 1966.

213. Briggs, J. D., A. C. Kennedy, L. N. Young, R. G. Luke, and M. Gray: Renal function after acute tubular necrosis, *Br. Med. J.*, **3**:513, 1967.

214. Finkenstaedt, J. T., and J. Merrill: Renal function after recovery from acute renal failure, *N. Engl. J. Med.*, **254**:1023, 1956.

215. Hall, J. W., W. J. Johnson, F. T. Maher, and J. C. Hunt: Immediate and long-term prognosis in acute renal failure, *Ann. Intern. Med.*, **73** (4):515, 1970.

216. Lewers, D. T., T. H. Mathew, J. F. Maher, and G. E. Schreiner: Long-term follow-up of renal function and histology after acute tubular necrosis, *Ann. Intern. Med.*, **73** (4):523, 1970.

217. Levin, M. L., N. M. Simon, P. B. Herdson, and F. del Greco: Acute renal failure followed by protracted, slowly resolving chronic uremia, *J. Chronic Dis.*, **25**:645, 1972.

218. Siegler, R. L., and A. Bloomer: Acute renal failure with prolonged oliguria, *JAMA*, **225** (2):133, 1973.

219. Hollenberg, N. K., F. D. McDonald, R. Cotran, E. G. Galvanek, M. Warhol, L. D. Vandam, and J. P. Merrill: Irreversible acute oliguric renal failure, *N. Engl. J. Med.*, **286** (16):877, 1972.

220. Kew, M. C., C. Abrahams, and H. C. Seftel: Chronic interstitial nephritis as a consequence of heatstroke, *Q. J. Med.*, **39** (154):189, 1970.

221. Collins, J. M., D. M. Hennes, C. R. Holzgang, R. T. Gourley, and G. K. Porter: Recovery after prolonged oliguria due to ethylene glycol intoxication, *Arch. Intern. Med.*, **125**:1059, 1970.

222. Uldall, P. R., H. A. Khan, J. E. Ennis, R. I. McCollum, and T. A. L. Grimson: Renal damage from industrial arsine poisoning, *Br. J. Ind. Med.*, **27**:372, 1970.

223. Spector, D., C. Limas, J. L. Frost, J. B. Zachary, S. Sterioff, G. M. Williams, R. T. Rolley, and J. H. Sadler: Perfusion nephropathy in human transplants, *N. Engl. J. Med.*, **295** (22):1217, 1976.

224. Baxby, K., R. M. R. Taylor, and M. Anderson: Assessment of cadaveric kidneys for transplantation, *Lancet*, **2**:977, 1974.

225. Kjellstrand, C. M., R. E. Casali, R. L. Simmons, J. R. Shideman, T. J. Buselmeier, and J. S. Najarian: Etiology and prognosis in acute post-transplant renal failure, *Am. J. Med.*, **61**:190, 1976.

226. Smith, R., J. C. McClure Browne, R. Sharkman, and O. M. Wrong: Acute renal failure of obstetric origin, *Lancet*, **2**:351, 1965.

227. Burden, R. P., D. V. Ash, W. N. Boyd, J. G. Gray, and G. M. Aber: Acute reversible renal failure in patients with acute cholecystitis and cholangitis, *Q. J. Med.*, **44** (173):65, 1975.

228. Wardle, E. N.: Renal failure in obstructive jaundice—pathogenic factors, *Postgrad. Med. J.*, **51**:512, 1975.

229. Conn, H. O.: Progress in hepatology—a rational approach to the hepatorenal syndrome, *Gastroenterology*, **65** (2):321, 1973.

230. Wilkinson, S. P., B. Portmann, D. Hurst, and R. Williams: Pathogenesis of renal failure in cirrhosis and fulminant hepatic failure, *Postgrad. Med. J.*, **51**:503, 1975.

231. Vesin, P., and H. Traverso: Functional renal failure (FRF) in cirrhosis of the liver and liver carcinoma, *Postgrad. Med. J.*, **51**:489, 1975.

232. Ashley, B. C., and H. M. Whyte: Practical methods for estimating the basic water requirements during oliguric renal failure, *Aust. Ann. Med.*, **12**:127, 1963.

233. Bluemle, L. W., Jr., H. P. Potter, and J. R. Elkinton: Changes in body composition in acute renal failure, *J.Clin. Invest.*, **35**:1094, 1956.

234. Teschan, P. E., R. S. Post, L. H. Smith, Jr., R. S. Abernathy, J. H. Davis, D. M. Gray, J. M. Howard, K. E. Johnson, E. Klopp, R. L. Mundy, M. P. O'Meara, and B. F. Rush, Jr.: Post-traumatic renal insufficiency in military casualties. I. Clinical characteristics, *Am. J. Med.*, **18**:172, 1955.

235. Meroney, W. H., and R. F. Herndon: The management of acute renal insufficiency, *JAMA*, **155**:877, 1954.

236. Relman, A. S., E. J. Lennon, and J. Lemann, Jr.: Endogenous production of fixed acid and the measurement of the net balance of urea in normal subjects, *J. Clin. Invest.*, **40**:1621, 1961.

237. Lemann, H., Jr., D. O. Goodman, E. J. Lemmon, and A. S. Relman: Production, excretion and balances of fixed acid in patients with renal acidosis, *J. Clin. Invest.*, **42**:951, 1963.

238. Ardaillou, R., M. Beaufils, M.-P. Nivez, R. Isaac, C. Mayaud, and J.-D. Sraer: Increased plasma calcitonin in early acute renal failure, *Clin. Sci.*, **49**:301, 1975.

239. de Torrente, A., T. Berl, P. D. Cohn, E. Kawamoto, P. Hertz, and R. W. Schrier: Hypercalcemia of acute renal failure—clinical significance and pathogenesis, *Am. J. Med.*, **61**:119, 1976.

240. Walser, M.: The separate effects of hyperparathyroidism, hypercalcemia of malignancy, renal failure and acidosis on the state of calcium phosphate and other ions in plasma, *J. Clin. Invest.*, **41**:1454, 1962.

241. Randall, R. E., Jr., M. D. Cohen, C. C. Spray, Jr., and E. C. Rossmeisl: Hypermagnesium in renal failure, *Ann. Intern. Med.*, **61**:73, 1964.

242. Surawicz, B.: Electrolytes and the electrocardiogram, *Mod. Concepts Cardiovasc. Dis.*, **33**:875, 1964.

243. Merrill, J. P., H. D. Levine, W. Somerville, and S. Smith, III: Clinical recognition and treatment of acute potassium intoxication, *Ann. Intern. Med.*, **33**:797, 1950.

244. Bolslov, J. T., and H. E. Jorgensen: A survey of 489 patients with acute anuric renal insufficiency: Causes, treatment, complications and mortality, *Am. J. Med.*, **34**:753, 1963.

245. Stott, R. B., J. S. Cameron, C. S. Ogg, and M. Bewick: Why the persistently high mortality in acute renal failure? *Lancet*, **2**:75, 1972. In Vietnam, *Clin. Nephrology*, **2** (5):186, 1974.

246. Brooks, D. H., and J. W. Schulhoff: Acute nonoliguric renal failure in the postoperative patient, *Crit. Care Med.*, **4** (4):193, 1976.

247. Bhat, J. G., M. C. Gluck, J. Lowenstein, and D. S. Baldwin: Renal failure after open heart surgery, *Ann. Intern. Med.*, **84** (6):677, 1976.

248. Lordon, R. E., and J. R. Burton: Post-traumatic renal failure in military personnel in Southeast Asia—experience at Clark USAF Hospital, Republic of the Philippines, *Am. J. Med.*, **53**:137, 1972.

249. Stone, W. J., and J. H. Knepshield: Post-traumatic acute renal insufficiency

250. Bull, G. M., A. M. Joekes, and K. G. Lowe: Conservative treatment of anuric uremia, *Lancet*, **2**:229, 1949.

251. Flinn, R. B., J. P. Merrill, and W. R. Welzant: Treatment of the oliguric patient with a new sodium-exchange resin and sorbital, *N. Engl. J. Med.*, **264**:111, 1961.

252. Wolthus, F. H.: Balance studies on protein metabolism in normal and uremic man, *Acta Med. Scand.* [Suppl.] 373, 1961.

253. Berlyne, G. M., R. A. L. Brewis, E. M. Booth, and N. P. Mallick: A soluble glucose polymer for use in renal failure and calorie-deprivation states, *Lancet*, **1**:689, 1969.

254. Borst, J. G. G.: Protein katabolism in uremia: Effects of protein-free diet, infection and blood transfusion, *Lancet*, **1**:824, 1948.

255. Freeman, P., and A. G. Spencer: Testosterone propionate in the treatment of renal failure, *Clin. Sci.*, **16**:11, 1957.

256. McCracken, B. H., and F. M. Parsons: Use of Nilevar (17-ethyl-19-norteseosterone) to suppress protein catabolism in acute renal failure, *Lancet*, **2**:885, 1958.

257. Giordano, C.: Use of exogenous and endogenous urea for protein synthesis in normal and uremic subjects, *J. Lab. Clin. Med.*, **62**:231, 1963.

258. Berlyne, G. M., F. J. Bazzard, E. M. Booth, K.

Janabi, and A. B. Shaw: The dietary treatment of acute renal failure, *Q. J. Med.*, **36:**59, 1967.

259. Gallina, D. L., and J. M. Dominquez: Human utilization of urea nitrogen in low caloric diets, *J. Nutr.*, **101:**1029, 1971.

260. Wilmore, D. W., and S. J. Dudrick: Treatment of acute renal failure with intravenous essential L-amino acids, *Arch. Surg.*, **99:**669, 1969.

261. Wilmore, D. W., and S. J. Dudrick: Safe long-term venous catheterization, *Arch. Surg.*, **98:**256, 1969.

262. Scribner, B. H., J. W. Broviac, and M. I. Ivey: *Patient Instruction Manual for Home Use of the Artificial Gut System*, University of Washington Press, Seattle, 1975.

263. Sanders, R. A., and G. F. Sheldon: Septic complications of total parenteral nutrition—a five year experience, *Am. J. Surg.*, **132:**214, 1976.

264. Van Buren, C. T., S. J. Dudrick, L. Dworkin, E. Baumbauer, and J. M. Long: Effects of intravenous essential L-amino acids and hypertonic dextrose in anephric beagles, *Surg. Forum*, **23:**83, 1972.

265. Coran, A. G., and C. M. Herman: The use of parenteral alimentation in renal failure: The effects of an intravenous fat emulsion and essential amino acids on dogs undergoing bilateral nephrectomy, *J. Pediatr. Surg.*, **7:**21, 1972.

266. Blackburn, G. L., S. P. Flott, G. H. A. Clowes, and T. E. O'Donnell: Peripheral intravenous feeding with isotonic amino acid solutions, *Am. J. Surg.*, **125:**447, 1973.

267. Blackburn, G. L., J. P. Flatt, G. H. A. Clowes, T. E. O'Donnell, and T. E. Hensle: Protein-sparing therapy during periods of starvation with sepsis or trauma, *Ann. Surg.*, **177:**588, 1973.

268. Jeejeebhoy, K. N., G. H. Anderson, A. F. Nakhooda, G. R. Greenberg, I. Sanderson, and E. B. Marliss: Metabolic studies in total parenteral nutrition with lipid in man—comparison with glucose, *J. Clin. Invest.*, **57:**125, 1976.

269. Abel, R. M., C. H. Beck, Jr., W. M. Abbott, J. A. Ryan, Jr., G. O. Barnett, and J. E. Fischer: Improved survival from acute renal failure after treatment with intravenous essential L-amino acids and glucose—results of a prospective, double-blind study, *N. Engl. J. Med.*, **288:**695, 1973.

270. Abel, R. M., W. M. Abbott, C. H. Beck, Jr., J. A. Ryan, Jr., and J. E. Fischer: Essential L-amino acids for hyperalimentation in patients with disordered nitrogen metabolism, *Am. J. Surg.*, **128:**317, 1974.

271. Abel, R. M., V. E. Shik, W. M. Abbott, C. H. Beck, Jr., and J. E. Fischer: Amino acid metabolism in acute renal failure: Influence in intravenous essential L-amino and hyperalimentation therapy, *Ann. Surg.*, **180:**350, 1974.

272. Toback, F. G.: Amino acid enhancement of renal regeneration after acute tubular necrosis, *Kidney Int.*, **12:**193, 1977.

273. Baek, S., G. G. Makabali, C. W. Bryan-Brown, J. Kusik, and W. C. Shoemaker: The influence of parenteral nutrition on the course of acute renal failure, *Surg. Gynecol. Obstet.*, **141:**405, 1975.

274. Kleinknecht, D., P. Jungers, J. Chanard, C. Barbanel, and D. Ganeval: Uremic and non-uremic complications in acute renal failure: Evaluation of early and frequent dialysis on prognosis, *Kidney Int.*, **1:**190, 1972.

275. Asbach, H. W., H. Stoeckel, H. W. Schüler, R. Conradi, K. Wiedemann, K- Möhring, and L. Röhl: The treatment of hypercatabolic acute renal failure by adequate nutrition and haemodialysis, *Acta Anaesthesiol. Scand.*, **18:**255, 1974.

276. Tilney, N. L., G. L. Bailey, and A. P. Morgan: Sequential system failure after rupture of abdominal aortic aneurysms: An unsolved program in post-operative care, *Ann. Surg.*, **178:**117, 1973.

277. Parsons, F. M., and B. H. McCracken: Artificial kidney, *Br. Med. J.*, **1:**740, 1959.

278. Bluemle, L. W., G. D. Webster, Jr., and J. R. Elkinton: Acute tubular necrosis: Analysis of 100 cases with respect to mortality, complications and treatment with and without dialysis, *Arch. Intern. Med.*, **104:**180, 1959.

279. Montgomerie, J. Z., G. M. Kalmonson, and L. B. Guze: Renal failure and infection, *Medicine (Baltimore)*, **47:**1, 1968.

280. Teschan, P. E., C. R. Baxter, T. F. O'Brien, J. N. Freyhof, and W. H. Hall: Prophylactic hemodialysis in the treatment of acute renal failure, *Ann. Intern. Med.*, **53:**992, 1960.

281. Law, D. K., S. J. Dudrick, and N. I. Abdou: The effects of protein calorie malnutrition on immune competence of the surgical patient, *Surg. Gynecol. Obstet.*, **139:**257, 1974.

282. Kunin, C. M.: A guide to use of antibiotics in patients with renal disease, *Ann. Intern. Med.*, **67**:151, 1967.

283. Maxwell, M. H., R. E. Rockney, C. R. Kleeman, and M. R. Twiss: Peritoneal dialysis. I. Technique and applications, *JAMA*, **170**:917, 1959.

284. Scribner, B. H., J. E. Z. Coner, R. Buri, and W. Quinton: The technique of continuous hemodialysis, *Trans. Am. Soc. Artif. Intern. Organs*, **6**:88, 1960.

285. Quinton, W., D. Dillard, and B. H. Scribner: Cannulation of blood vessels for prolonged hemodialysis, *Trans. Amer. Soc. Artif. Intern. Organs*, **8**:315, 1962.

286. Parsons, F. M., S. M. Hobson, C. R. Blogg, and B. H. McCracken: Optimum time for dialysis in acute reversible renal failure, *Lancet*, **1**:129, 1961.

287. Berlyne, G. M., V. Hewitt, J. H. Jones, and M. B. Nilwarangkur: Protein loss in peritoneal dialysis, *Lancet*, **1**:738, 1964.

288. Young, G. A., and F. M. Parsons: Amino nitrogen loss during haemodialysis: Its dietary significance and replacement, *Clin. Sci.*, **31**:299, 1966.

16

The pathophysiology of
chronic renal failure

NEAL S. BRICKER / LEON G. FINE

Normal humans are born with approximately 2 million nephrons. They probably can survive, albeit with difficulty, with less than 20,000 nephrons. This reserve capacity is fortunate indeed, for there are a large number of different diseases with a predilection for nephron destruction. These processes vary in their pathogenetic and histologic detail and in their rate of progression, but they all evoke common alterations in renal function and ultimately a common constellation of chemical and physiologic abnormalities. This chapter is addressed to the changes in the economy of a human being that evolve in the course of the chronic progressive renal diseases as the nephron population is reduced relentlessly from 2 million to less than 20,000.

The story as it unfolds today is very different than it was as recently as two decades ago. The change unfortunately is not because the means have become available either to prevent or to halt the progression of the various forms of chronic renal disease, for with few exceptions they have not. However, it has become possible to trace with increasing accuracy the sequential events in pathologic physiology that transpire during the natural history of chronic renal disease, and from such knowledge to develop more effective principles of conservative treatment. A second and major difference focuses on the end of the natural history of chronic renal disease. Due to the advent of chronic hemodialysis and renal transplantation, death, the end point of chronic renal disease since the beginning of humanity, is no longer inevitable when the nephron population falls below the minimum number compatible with unassisted life. The importance of in-depth knowledge about the sequential events in the natural history of chronic Bright's disease is, if anything, accentuated by the existence of these techniques for life sustenance and potential rehabilitation. The more effective conservative treatment is, the more satisfying will be the patient's life prior to the initiation of "end-stage" treatment, and the fewer will be the stigmata of chronic uremia which can prejudice the opportunity for rehabilitation after these procedures are initiated.

CHRONIC PROGRESSIVE RENAL DISEASE: A PERSPECTIVE

The kidney's major contribution to well-being is the selective excretion of various solutes and water into the urine in amounts which will prevent either their retention or loss from body fluids (i.e., the maintenance of *balance*). Any excretion rate thus must be balanced against the total acquisition from diet, parenteral administration (if applicable), and metabolic production, and it must reflect any excretion via extrarenal routes or any metabolic utilization or degradation. The contributions of the kidney, however, extend beyond solute and water excretion. For example, as is discussed in Chap. 7, the kidneys synthesize bicarbonate, ammonia, and a number of hormones or hormone precursors. They also detoxify certain compounds, degrade others, contribute to blood pressure regulation, etc. But the maintenance of the external balance of multiple solutes and of water constitutes the *primary* functional obligation of the kidneys. In general, the amounts of most substances that must be excreted do not decrease as chronic renal disease advances, but the number of nephrons available to do the excretions decreases progressively.

The challenge to survival posed by the loss of nephrons is met in a variety of ways and through a variety of these adaptive mechanisms. The overall success of these adaptations is attested to most vividly by the fact that life persists until well over 95 percent of the original nephron population has been destroyed. From a more quantitative point of view, the excretion rates of some of the principal solutes of body fluids (including sodium, chloride, and potassium) typically are regulated, down to very low levels of GFR (glomerular filtration rate), with sufficient precision to permit the maintenance of external balance without any appreciable rise in their serum concentrations. However, the adaptations are not this effective for all solutes. Indeed, for urea and creatinine there appear to be no adaptations. Thus, following each permanent reduction in GFR, both solutes are retained in the body; and the restitution of balance is achieved only after the serum level has risen sufficiently to affect the necessary increase in the filtered load, and more critically in the excretion rate per nephron. The progressive increments in serum urea (or urea nitrogen) and creatinine concentrations as GFR falls account for the fact that the blood levels of those two solutes can be used clinically to estimate the value for GFR.

For a host of other solutes, the degree of regulation (i.e., the magnitude of the adaptive increase in excretion rate per nephron as GFR falls) varies between that of sodium and that of urea. When and to what extent a solute is retained in body fluids in the course of chronic progressive renal disease is determined by the extent of the adaptation in relation to the amount requiring excretion.

THE "TRADE-OFF" HYPOTHESIS

The possibility that some of the adaptations are mediated by hormonal messengers, that the circulating levels of these hormones rise each time GFR falls and the excretion rate per surviving nephron must increase, and that these same hormonal agents may ultimately become "uremic toxins" has recently been suggested (1). As an example, PTH (parathyroid hormone) levels increase strikingly in advancing renal disease, an adaptation which contributes importantly to the progressive increments in phosphate excretion per nephron and thus to the maintenance of external phosphate balance. However, PTH also stimulates bone resorption and it recently has been suggested that high levels of PTH may produce central nervous system abnormalities, abnormalities of nerve conduction, pruritus, impotence, and several other symptoms or signs of the uremic state (2–5). A substance also appears to be present in the blood and urine of uremic patients which inhibits sodium transport and which may be a part of the adaptation of the sodium control system that assures an increasing rate of sodium excretion per nephron (6–10). But in advanced uremia, this material could conceivably inhibit sodium transport in extrarenal structures such as red blood cells, the central nervous system, or the gastrointestinal tract. Hence a natriuretic hormone, which might serve a salutory and physiologic role in modifying sodium excretion, could also contribute to the overall abnormalities of the uremic syndrome.

"PROPORTIONAL REDUCTION" OF SOLUTE INTAKE

The therapeutic implications of the above hypothesis may be of importance. If a given abnormality of uremia is attributable to an adaptation in solute excretion, it should be possible to prevent the abnormality by preventing the adaptation (11, 12). Since the adaptation is necessary only if the requirements for solute excretion *per nephron* increase as the nephron population diminishes, the adaptation can be obviated by decreasing the rate of entry of the solute into the body fluids in *exact proportion* to the reduction in renal function. The necessity for adaptation would then be removed, no increase in "messenger" activity would occur, and "trade-off" abnormalities should be prevented. The implications and use of this approach will be described more fully later in the chapter.

The loss of synthetic functions of the kidneys may also contribute to the abnormalities of uremia. For example, a decrease in erythropoietic hormone precursor may play a role in the anemia of uremia (13), the altered production of blood pressure controlling factor(s) may conceivably contribute to the high incidence of hypertension in chronic renal disease (14, 15), and the reduced ability to contribute to the synthesis of the most potent metabolite of vitamin D [1,25-$(OH)_2D_3$](16) may contribute to the calcium, phosphorous, and bone abnormalities of uremia (17, 18). (See Chaps. 19 and 20.)

BIOLOGIC COMMITMENTS OF THE NEPHRONS IN CHRONIC RENAL DISEASE AND THE ROLE OF CONTROL SYSTEMS

If the dietary intake of a solute such as sodium or potassium remains unchanged as chronic renal disease advances, the first requisite for survival is that the average rate of excretion per nephron *increase* as the nephron population diminishes. But the charge to the nephrons is not confined to increasing basal rates of excretion, for the patient with advancing renal disease may vary the intake of sodium, potassium, and other solutes from day to day just as does a normal person. Thus, the residual nephrons must respond to these variations in intake with sensitive and precise variations in excretion. *But with every reduction in nephron mass, the dimensions of this added responsibility become increasingly formidable; the fewer*

the number of nephrons, the greater must be the *change* in excretion rates per nephron with any given change in solute intake (19).

THE "MAGNIFICATION PHENOMENON"

The "magnification phenomenon" (20) refers to the fact that the excretory response of individual nephrons to the acquisition of a fixed amount of sodium or potassium or any other solute must increase progressively as the underlying disease advances and GFR falls if permanent solute retention is to be prevented.

A fixed perturbation of the extracellular fluid thus will evoke an end-organ response that varies inversely with the number of nephrons if there is a regulatory system governing the excretion of the solute. Figure 16-1 depicts in schematic form the two components of the magnification phenomenon using sodium as a prototypic solute. The number of sodium ions excreted per 100 filtered (i.e., the percentage of filtered sodium excreted) is depicted for a normal person with a GFR of 120 mL/min and for a patient with uremia with a GFR of 4 mL/min. The patterns are shown for both a 3.5- and a 7-g/day salt intake. At both levels of salt intake, the diseased kidneys must excrete a very much larger percentage of filtered so-

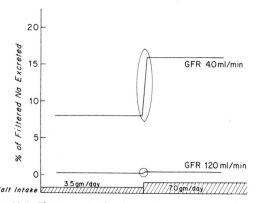

Figure 16-1. The patterns of sodium excretion, expressed as the percentage of filtered sodium excreted, are shown at a normal GFR (glomerular filtration rate) and at a GFR of 4 mL/min. The graph depicts the difference in base-line rates of excretion on both a 3.5-g salt diet and a 7.0-g salt diet; it also emphasizes the striking difference in the change in excretory patterns occasioned by the transition from the lower to the higher salt intake.

dium than the normal person in order to maintain sodium balance. Thus, for any given level of salt intake, the lower the GFR, the greater must be the fractional sodium excretion rate. The second part of the adaptation is depicted by the *change* in fractional excretion in the transition from the lower to the higher salt intake. For the patient with normal renal function, the increment in fractional excretion is so small as to be barely discernible in the figure. On the other hand, for the patient with advanced renal disease, the increment is very large. The lower the GFR, the greater must be the *change* in excretion per nephron to maintain external balance in the face of modest changes in solute intake.

THE CONTRIBUTION OF CONTROL SYSTEMS

In Chap. 7, the concept of control systems and their contribution to the maintenance of solute balance in health is discussed. A control system for any solute must monitor the amount of the substance that enters body fluids, and must modulate its rate of excretion in a manner that will assure the maintenance of balance. A control system must first be *solute specific*. It must have a *detector* element capable of perceiving very small dislocations from the steady state; it may very well have an *integrating element* capable of collating multiple stimuli if more than one detector element exists for any solute. Finally, it must have an *effector element* which is capable of influencing excretion of the specific solute by the end organ of the system, the kidney.

The requirements imposed upon a control system in advancing renal disease include one dimension that is never encountered in health. In health, the number of nephrons remains a constant. In renal disease the number of nephrons falls progressively. Thus, as described above, the degree to which the control system affects excretion rate per nephron in response to a fixed amount of solute acquired must vary inversely with GFR. The forces which increase excretion rate per nephron of key solutes therefore must be augmented increasingly as chronic renal disease advances. How this increased responsivity, or

magnification, occurs for each of the biologic control systems is still incompletely understood.

The characterization of individual biologic control systems assumes added complexity when the requirements for the simultaneous excretion of two or more solutes are considered. Assume, for example, that the intake of sodium remains constant at 120 meq/day and that of potassium at 80 meq/day. At a GFR of 120 mL/min, the amount of sodium excreted is equal to approximately 0.5 percent of the amount filtered, and the amount of potassium secreted is equal to approximately 12 percent of the amount filtered (assuming serum sodium and potassium concentrations of 140 and 4.0 meq/L respectively). From these calculations it may be deduced that for every potassium ion secreted, approximately 300 sodium ions are resorbed, and if 30 percent of the filtered sodium enters the distal sites where potassium is secreted, the ratio of distal sodium resorption to potassium secretion approaches 100:1.

Next consider the transformations that are required to maintain balance for both ions at a GFR of 4 mL/min. Now 15 percent of the filtered sodium is excreted. In this setting, for every potassium ion secreted[1] approximately eight sodium ions are resorbed. If 50 percent of the sodium is resorbed proximally, the ratio of distal sodium resorption to distal potassium secretion is reduced to 4:1. The sodium control system therefore must *decrease* fractional sodium resorption from 99.5 to 85 percent, while simultaneously the potassium control system must *increase* potassium secretion from 12 to 350 percent of the filtered load (Fig. 16-2). And despite the fact that there is some form of coupling between sodium resorption and potassium secretion, the ratio between the two processes changes in a very striking manner. Thus in the face of a constant intake of sodium and potassium, nephron reduction, in some manner, leads to dramatic changes in the response of the residual nephrons characterized by a decrease in fractional sodium transport and a great increase

---

[1] The simplifying assumptions are made in these calculations that the serum potassium value is 4.0 meq/L, that all filtered potassium is resorbed, and that all excreted potassium is delivered by tubular secretion.

GFR	% Filtered Na Resorbed	% Filtered K Secreted
120	99.5	12
4	85	350

Figure 16-2. Calculation for the percentage of filtered sodium resorbed and potassium excreted expressed as a fraction of the amount filtered in a normal patient with a GFR of 120 mL/min and a uremic patient with a GFR of 4.0 mL/min. These calculations are based upon an intake and excretion rate of sodium of 120 meq/day and an intake and excretion rate of potassium of 80 meq/day.

in potassium transport. If one adds to the equation a decrease in phosphate resorption, an increase in ammonia secretion, a decrease in fractional magnesium resorption, and an increase in hydrogen ion secretion, with all the transport rates geared closely to the homeostatic needs of the organism and with a variable percentage of the functioning nephrons altered structurally, the fact that a patient with advancing renal disease can remain alive and reasonably well must be regarded as an extraordinary phenomenon.

THE NATURE OF THE INTRARENAL ADAPTATIONS

One of the qualitative intrarenal adaptations to nephron loss is a rise in single-nephron GFR (SNGFR) similar to that which occurs in the remaining kidney following unilateral nephrectomy. This adaptation has been documented in the experimental animal with pyelonephritis and following marked nephron reduction (21–23). In experimental glomerular disease, mean values for SNGFR are normal or decreased (24–26). It is not known, however, whether SNGFR increases with time, ultimately reaching supernormal values, in slowly progressing chronic glomerulopathies in man. To whatever extent SNGFR does rise, the excretory capacity of the nephrons, for all filtered solutes, should be enhanced. This change, however, would be nonspecific and would be unlikely to contribute to the fine control of excretion rates of any specific solute or solutes.

A second intrarenal adaptation consists of compensatory hypertrophy of the nephrons, another change which is reminiscent of the response to unilateral nephrectomy (27). The length and tortuosity of the proximal tubules increase, due presumably to both an increase in the number of cells and in the size of individual cells. These changes must contribute to the capacity of individual nephrons to perform greater than normal amounts of transport and greater than normal amounts of metabolism (28). However, the actual rates of transport of each of the key solutes must nevertheless remain responsive to the needs for homeostasis, and therefore to any humoral or other regulatory factors that serve to modulate actual transport rates.

LIMITATIONS IN RENAL FUNCTION

Brief reference has already been made to the limitations in the range of solute excretion achievable in advanced chronic renal disease. Although the range of excretion *per nephron* may be increased in chronic renal disease, progressive reduction in the total number of nephrons must, in the final analysis, define the upper limit of total urinary excretion for any specific solute. For some solutes, there appears to be a lower limit of excretion (i.e., a limitation in the ability to conserve maximally) in advanced disease, and at least for sodium and water the elevated "floor" may assume clinical significance. The patterns of potassium excretion illustrate the significance of the reduced "upper limit" of excretion. As indicated previously, the smaller the population of residual nephrons, the higher must be the rate of excretion of potassium per nephron. Thus if only 10 percent of the nephron population remains, an average of 10 times as much potassium must be secreted per tubule (discounting any decrease in resorption) for the maintenance of balance. Consequently, the nephrons in disease are presumably functioning far closer to the maximum velocity of transport for potassium than in health, and any sudden requirement for additional excretion imposed by an acute increase in potassium intake may be difficult or impossible to achieve.

There also is a limitation, more marked in degree, for ammonia secretion. The reasons supporting the view that this "defect" occurs as a consequence of nephron loss, and in the face of supernormal excretion rates per nephron, will be considered in the discussion of acid-base regulation later in this chapter.

The upper limit of sodium excretion generally remains high enough so that sodium retention does not often occur on an average salt intake. Nevertheless, there is a limit to the maximum amount of sodium that may be excreted, and if this is exceeded, edema formation will occur. A more detailed discussion of the ceiling for sodium excretion will also be considered later in the chapter.

The limitation in sodium conservation becomes manifest in patients with relatively far advanced disease; when salt intake drops below 1 to 2 g/day, negative sodium balance typically will ensue. The basis of this inability to conserve sodium maximally and its potential reversibility also will be discussed in the section on the control of sodium excretion.

A major restriction in renal function in uremia relates to the range of water excretion. There is a progressive impairment in the urinary concentrating ability in advancing renal disease (29–32). Whereas in health the urine may be excreted at an osmolality about four times as great as that of plasma, as renal disease advances, the maximum osmolality falls, and ultimately approaches that of plasma. If total solute excretion remains normal, as it typically does in uremia, some 400 to 600 mosm of solute will be excreted per day. Hence if the maximal urinary osmolality is fixed at slightly over 300 mosm/kg water, 1 L of water will be excreted with every 300 mosm solute, and obligatory water excretion will approximate 1½ to 2 L/day. The fact that urine enters the bladder at a rate of about 1 mL/min not only during the day, but at night, explains the occurrence of nocturia in chronic renal disease.

There also is a restriction on the upper limit of water excretion which is imposed by the reduction in the nephron population. Although diluting ability [expressed as milliliters of solute-free water (C_{H_2O}) excreted per 100 mL GFR] is normal or even slightly increased in uremia (29), the total number of milliliters of free water added to the urine must decrease as the nephron population (and GFR) diminishes. For example, if sustained water diuresis is induced in both a normal person and a uremic patient and both excrete 10 mL free water/dL glomerular filtrate, urine volume will increase in both. But the increments will be quite different in amount. In the normal person (GFR 120/mL per min), 24-h urine volume will increase from 2 L of isosmotic urine to 19.3 L of dilute urine/day; in the uremic patient (GFR 4 mL/min), the increase will be from 2 to 2.6 L/day.

SUMMARY OF THE LIMITATIONS IN RENAL FUNCTION

As the nephron population diminishes and GFR falls, solutes that are excreted primarily by glomerular filtration without regulated and active tubular transport, such as urea and creatinine, will be retained in the blood. Indeed, the degree of retention of these two solutes provides a rough index of the percentage reduction in GFR. As GFR decreases below approximately 25 percent of normal, other solutes which are either filtered and resorbed or secreted may also be retained in body fluids. These include phosphate, sulfate, urate, and, in some patients, magnesium. Finally, a host of other solutes including organic acids, guanidium compounds, etc., accumulates in the blood when the renal disease is far advanced. Although the range of solute excretion *per nephron* for most regulated solutes increases with advancing disease, the fewer the number of nephrons, the smaller is the *total* range of excretion achievable by the composite nephron population. Thus the upper limit of excretion for many solutes and for water is less than that achieved by normal subjects, and for sodium (and perhaps other solutes) and water there is an inability to reduce the amounts excreted to levels as low as those achieved in health. The overall effect is that of decreased flexibility in responding to wide changes in dietary intake of solutes which are actively transported by the renal tubular epithelial cells and water.

In an occasional patient unusual limitations in renal function may be observed. These include massive salt losing wherein the obligatory sodium excretion may range from 5 to over 30 g/day (33), hyperchloremic acidosis (34), and ADH (antidiuretic hormone)-unreponsive hyposthenuria (30). The last is characterized by the continued excretion of urine which is hypotonic to the serum even when the homeostatic requirements for water would best be subserved by more avid water retention.

THE UREMIC SYNDROME

When GFR falls below 15 to 20 percent of normal, the untoward consequences of nephron reduction begin to appear and to alter the overall economy of the organism. The greater the subsequent fall in GFR, the more serious and extensive are the symptoms and signs; and in far-advanced renal insufficiency, virtually no organ or organ system escapes unscathed. A partial list of the abnormalities, illustrating the multiple-system nature of the uremic syndrome, is shown in Table 16-1.

The central nervous system and peripheral nerves are affected with diverse consequences. Nerve conduction time characteristically is prolonged, and overt signs of peripheral neuropathy may ultimately develop in advanced uremia; sleep patterns are disturbed and asterixis, convulsions, and psychosis all may occur. The cardiovascular system may be modified through the intervention of diastolic hypertension, and the combination of hypertension, anemia, and acidosis all contribute to the increased propensity for congestive heart failure. The musculoskeletal system may be involved, in part through the peripheral neuropathy and in part through muscle wasting and weakness. There is wasting of adipose tissue. Cutaneous manifestations of uremia include pigmentation of the skin, pruritus, and a variety of changes in the nails. Menstrual abnormalities may develop, and potency may be impaired in the male. Gastrointestinal abnormalities include anorexia, nausea, and vomiting, and gastrointestinal bleeding from multiple and diffuse small ulcerations. The skeleton is afflicted with uremic osteodystrophy (a combination of osteitis fibrosa, osteomalacia, and osteopenia) (see Chap. 20). Serous membranes do not escape, and pleuritis, peritonitis, and pericarditis all may occur. The latter may be complicated by bloody pericardial effusions and car-

Table 16-1. Systemic involvement in uremia

1. Nervous
   a. Central—sleep, asterixis, convulsions, psychosis, abnormal electroencephalogram
   b. Peripheral—neuropathy, prolonged conduction time
2. Cardiovascular
   a. Hypertension
   b. Congestive heart failure
   c. Pericarditis
3. Musculoskeletal
   a. Weakness
   b. Osteodystrophy
4. Cutaneous
   a. Pigmentation, purpura, "frost"
   b. Pruritus, nail changes
5. Genitourinary
   a. Menstruation, potency, libido
   b. Nocturia, polyuria, diurnal rhythm
6. Gastrointestinal
   a. Nausea, emesis
   b. Bleeding, diarrhea
   c. Parotitis
7. Ocular
   a. Conjunctivitis, calcium deposition
   b. Intraocular pressure
8. Hematopoietic
   a. Anemia
   b. Bleeding tendency, platelet abnormality
   c. Erythropoiesis
   d. Hemolysis
9. Intermediary metabolism
   a. Carbohydrate—tolerance impaired
   b. Fat-wasting
   c. Protein—synthesis impaired, abnormal enzymes

diac tamponade. Intraocular pressure may decrease, presumably due to inhibition of sodium transport by the ciliary body. Anemia may be profound due to a combination of decreased erythropoiesis, decreased red cell survival time, and blood loss. In far-advanced uremia, a diffuse hemorrhagic tendency may develop with bleeding into the skin and serous cavities, as well as the gastrointestinal tract. This appears to be due to a combination of events including a platelet defect. Salivary glands may be altered, and parotitis may become a painful complication of uremia. Genitourinary function is altered by virtue of nocturia, which contributes to altered sleep patterns; by relative polyuria by day, which is particularly noticeable in hot weather when a normal person produces a highly concentrated urine; and by autonomic dysfunction, which can interfere with normal emptying of the urinary bladder. Impairment of both protein synthesis and protein degradation occurs. Finally, there are abnormalities in both carbohydrate and lipid metabolism.

Surprisingly little is known about the basis of the multiple-system abnormalities of the uremic syndrome. Retention of certain solutes in the blood is a hallmark of uremia and traditionally has been thought to contribute to at least certain of the abnormalities, but the specific compounds that are responsible for most of the abnormalities are unknown. Less conspicuous than the retention of solutes is the absence of normal substances from body fluids, but the latter may also contribute to the uremic syndrome. An example of such a deficiency is the decrease in erythropoietic hormone precursor synthesized normally by the kidneys. Finally, the possibility that normal hormones may increase markedly in concentration and contribute to the genesis of uremic abnormalities (i.e., the "trade-off" hypothesis) has been alluded to previously.

Chronic dialysis is an imperfect excretory system and does not replace any of the synthetic functions of the kidneys. However, it can produce marked symptomatic improvement in chronically uremic patients. Consequently, it is reasonable to assume that one or many low-molecular-weight solutes which are dialyzable contribute to the reversible abnormalities. These so-called "middle molecules" (MW 500 to 5000) (35, 36) have received much attention in recent years as being potentially important "uremic toxins." Nevertheless, their precise nature and specific toxic effects have thus far escaped elucidation.

SPECIFIC FUNCTIONAL SYSTEMS

Certain of the different forms of chronic progressive renal disease have relatively distinctive features which relate to their etiology, pathogenesis, or morphologic characteristics. For example, in the glomerulonephritides, the pathologic involvement of the glomeruli permits the passage of red blood cells and protein into the tubular lumina and urine in increased quantities, and if protein-uria becomes marked, the nephrotic syndrome may develop. In some forms of interstitial nephritis, concentrating ability may be lost at a relatively higher GFR than in glomerular diseases; in analgesic nephritis there may be advancing renal disease with a benign urine sediment and little or no proteinuria; in medullary cystic disease there may be a tendency toward early loss of concentrating ability and an exaggerated salt-losing state; in polycystic renal disease, concentrating ability may be lost early, etc.

Yet from a functional point of view, the most striking feature of all the various forms of chronic Bright's disease relates, not only to their unique facets or unusual characteristics, but rather to the common sequence of changes in renal function and thus the common effects on the economy of the host. *At any given GFR*, the setting of glomerular-tubular balance for a variety of different solutes must be the same regardless of the type of underlying renal disease, if external balance is being maintained at a uniform rate of acquisition of the solute. This means that the percentage of a filtered solute, such as sodium, that must be excreted *is the same* in glomerulonephritis as in pyelonephritis at the same GFR and serum sodium concentration, if intake is equal and balance is maintained. The residual nephrons in all forms of chronic Bright's disease tend to undergo comparable adaptations which better enable them to maintain homeostasis (19, 20). Finally, as was indicated previously, the residual nephrons and their extrarenal control systems exhibit a remarkable capacity to adjust to the changing needs of the organism throughout the natural history of chronic progressive renal disease. Because of these common functional patterns, it is possible to consider the events in pathologic physiology of chronic renal disease on a generic basis, rather than on a disease-by-disease basis.

THE SODIUM CONTROL SYSTEM

The basic features of sodium excretion in renal disease have already been covered. There is an increase in excretion rate per nephron as the nephron population diminishes; the range over which excretion per nephron varies in response to a given change in intake *increases* with advancing disease (20), but the *total range of excretion* by all the constituent nephrons *diminishes* as disease advances.

Perhaps the best way to examine the biology of sodium excretion in chronic progressive renal disease is to consider the sequential events that evolve beginning with the earliest loss of nephrons.

The sodium control system is believed to monitor some property of ECF (extracellular fluid) volume (37, 38) (see Chap. 13). When sodium is added to body fluids, a finite expansion of ECF volume occurs, and the detector element(s) of the sodium control system monitors this increase; the information is then presumably transmitted to an integrating element in the central nervous system, and natriuretic forces are mobilized. The latter lead to a decrease in sodium resorption which will effect the excretion of the sodium that was added to the body fluids. If salt intake remains relatively constant from day to day, the activity of the natriuretic forces will increase and decrease during each 24-h interval in a reproducible and uniform manner.

However, following the onset of a nephron-destroying renal disease, the biology of sodium control must be modified. With the very first loss of nephrons, the natriuretic forces, which previously were appropriate, will prove inadequate; there will be fewer nephrons excreting sodium, and if intake remains constant and the excretion rate per nephron does not increase, total sodium excretion must fall in proportion to the number of nephrons destroyed. Thus, immediately upon the destruction of nephrons a period of sodium retention will follow as well as an associated period of expansion of ECF volume. The expansion would be perceived by the detector elements of the sodium control system and the control system through its effector mechanisms will initiate an increase in the rate of sodium excretion in the remaining nephrons. The natriuretic forces hence will be increased in activity from their predisease level. When the excretion rate of sodium in the residual nephrons rises sufficiently to compensate for the decrease in the number of nephrons, ECF volume will stabilize or decrease toward the previous level and balance can once again be maintained. But to preserve balance on a continuing basis on the same salt intake, natriuretic stimuli must remain at a higher level than in health, for sodium excretion per nephron must remain permanently increased.

The next phase of nephron destruction will reinitiate the entire cycle; transient sodium retention will occur, and sodium excretion per surviving nephron must once again increase. Thus there will follow a second increment in the activity of the natriuretic forces. With each wave of nephron reduction, the cycle should repeat itself, and thus with each successive fall in GFR natriuretic forces should rise to a new level of activity. In accordance with this view, the activity of the natriuretic forces should be very great indeed in far-advanced renal disease, perhaps greater than ever exists even under the most extreme conditions of salt loading in normal individuals. This schema is depicted in Fig. 16-3.

A stepwise increase in natriuretic forces will theoretically contribute to the progressive increment in basal sodium excretion rates per nephron

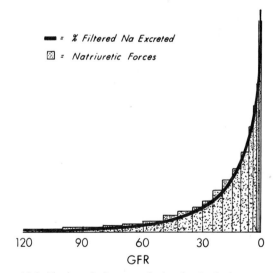

Figure 16-3. The hyperbolic curve depicts the rise in the percentage of filtered sodium excreted with decreasing GFR in the course of chronic progressive renal disease on any given salt intake. The vertical bars depict the theoretical parallel increments in the total "natriuretic forces" that effect the progressive increase in fractional sodium excretion.

that occurs in advancing renal disease, but the explanation for the ever larger fluctuations about the basal rates that are required to maintain balance in the face of normal daily variations in intake is far less obvious. The intake of a specific quantity of NaCl should not induce any greater expansion of ECF volume in a uremic patient than in a normal individual; yet in the uremic patient the response (per nephron) must increase progressively as GFR falls (20). Thus the sensitivity of the control system must be continually heightened. Whether this involves an increase in the responsivity of the detector element, an increase in the natriuretic factors released in response to a given stimulus, or an augmented responsivity of the tubular epithelial cells to the natriuretic factors remains to be established (20).

Considerable interest has been engendered in the sodium control system in uremia, both because the requirements imposed upon it change so markedly with time and because it responds to these changing requirements with great precision under most conditions. Because the expressions of the system become ever more pronounced, the opportunity exists for examination of its component parts in a manner that might not be possible in normal subjects. Moreover, it is not necessary to subject the uremic patient or animal to large sodium loads to elicit the excretion of a high percentage of the filtered sodium, for at low filtration rates a very small sodium load will initiate large changes in fractional sodium excretion. Consequently, the uremic model has been studied intensively not only to learn more about uremia, but in the hope of elucidating elements of the sodium control system that might also be relative to the physiology of sodium regulation in the normal state (38–40).

In Chap. 13 various possible effector elements currently considered to play a role in the modulation of sodium excretion were discussed. These include changes in GFR, changes in mineralocorticoid hormone activity, the "physical factors" (which include peritubular capillary oncotic pressure and peritubular capillary hydrostatic pressure), and finally "natriuretic hormone."

A rise in GFR per nephron which is believed to occur as an adaptive phenomenon in at least some forms of advancing renal disease could contribute to the capacity of nephrons to excrete greater quantities of sodium. However, it seems most unlikely that hyperfiltration per se could explain the "magnification phenomenon" (20) for sodium. Thus appropriate patterns of sodium excretion persist in the animal with renal disease when the adaptive increase in SNGFR is prevented or reversed experimentally (39). Moreover, in chronic glomerulonephritis where SNGFR is normal or low (24–26), sodium balance is maintained with precision. Finally, even if hyperfiltration could be invoked as a partial explanation for the progressive increment in fractional sodium excretion, it would not seem to offer a suitable explanation for the very large and precise short-term changes that occur in uremia with modest changes in salt intake.

A redistribution of glomerular filtrate between superficial and deep nephrons could play a supporting role in the advancing natriuresis per nephron, but there is no evidence that this factor plays a major regulatory role in modulating sodium excretion in advancing chronic renal disease.

Changes in aldosterone activity also do not appear to explain adequately the modulation of sodium excretion in uremia. To account for the type of progressive reduction in fractional sodium resorption (i.e., increase in fractional excretion) that occurs throughout the natural history of chronic renal disease, mineralocorticoid hormone activity would probably have to diminish with time,[2] but the available measurements suggest that aldosterone activity is normal or increased in most uremic patients (41, 43). Moreover, in dogs subjected to experimental reduction of the nephron population by approximately 75 percent, the residual nephrons exhibit the appropriate increments in sodium excretion rate on a chronic basis and

---

[2] This is a complicated issue, because while *fractional* sodium resorption decreases with time, *absolute* sodium resorption in individual nephrons may increase in advancing renal disease. The explanation for this is that GFR per nephron, and thus the filtered load of sodium per nephron, may increase adaptively by as much as 50 to 100 percent while fractional sodium excretion rarely exceeds 30 to 40 percent. Thus the increase in filtered sodium exceeds the increase in excreted sodium, and net sodium resorption must increase.

the appropriate changes in short-term excretion rates following acute sodium loads despite the fact that mineralocorticoid hormone activity is maintained constant at very high (or very low) levels (40). In chronic uremia, administration of large doses of mineralocorticoid hormone in no way interferes with the precise regulation of sodium balance in the face of changing levels of salt intake (39). Although the foregoing considerations suggest that aldosterone is not of central importance in the regulation of sodium excretion in patients with chronic uremia, there is evidence that it does play a supportive or contributory role (43).

Changes in "physical factors" are known to influence sodium resorption, particularly in the proximal tubule (44, 45) (see Chap. 13). However, it also seems unlikely that this mechanism alone can account for the modulation of sodium excretion in uremia. Each time GFR diminishes in the course of chronic progressive renal disease, either filtration fraction or peritubular capillary blood pressure (or some other intrarenal physical factor) would have to be clearly evident. No consistent correlation exists between changes in filtration fraction and changes in sodium excretion in advancing nephron reduction; nor does there appear to be any quantitative correlation between sodium excretion per nephron and systemic blood pressure (40) or hydrostatic pressure in the peritubular capillaries. Finally, no consistent change in any of these physical parameters capable of producing large variations in fractional sodium excretion has been found in uremic dogs with short-term variations in salt intake (39).

Site-specific damage to functioning nephrons also could contribute to a natriuresis per nephron owing to imposed defects in the capacity of the tubules to resorb sodium. But the regulation of sodium excretion in accordance with salt intake would have to occur despite such defects and not because of them.

A final effector mechanism that could play a role in the regulation of sodium excretion is a natriuretic hormone (46). Such a hormone would act by inhibiting sodium resorption by the tubular epithelial cells. It would be present in a finite concentration under normal conditions of living in health; it would be decreased in activity in most salt-retaining states; and it would be increased in activity in most natriuretic states including uremia. Its activity in theory should rise in a stepwise fashion as the nephron population diminishes. Thus the lower the steady-state GFR, the greater should be the activity of the natriuretic hormone (for any given level of salt intake); the activity also should vary with short-term changes in sodium intake about the steady-state level.

Conceptually, the existence of such a hormone is attractive because (1) it could provide a biochemical mechanism for altering one or more rate-limiting steps in sodium transport and thus make it possible to exercise fine control over transepithelial sodium movements, (2) it could have a rapid onset of action, and (3) it could have a short biologic half-life. Evidence has recently been accumulated which supports the existence of such a circulating inhibitor of sodium transport in uremia. In chronically uremic patients and animals with high fractional sodium excretion rates, a factor has been isolated from serum and urine which inhibits sodium transport by the frog skin, toad bladder, and isolated mammalian collecting tubules and is natriuretic in the rat (6–10). The fact that this substance is not only increased in activity in uremic serum but is excreted in greater quantity in uremic than in normal urine suggests either that its production is increased or that it has a prolonged half-life in uremia. Using existing bioassay systems, the presence of this factor appears to correlate well with patterns of sodium excretion rather than with the uremic state per se (47). Furthermore, a factor with apparently identical biologic and chemical characteristics has been isolated from the urine of nonuremic dogs subjected to a high salt intake and large doses of a mineralocorticoid hormone and which were exhibiting "escape" natriuresis (48). In addition, this same inhibitor has been found in normal humans undergoing water-immersion natriuresis (49).

At present, the chemical nature of this natriuretic substance is under investigation (50). Its biologic characteristics include (1) a rapid onset of action (51); (2) sodium transport inhibitory activity only when applied to the serosal surface of anuran membranes or the peritubular surface of the collecting tubule (6, 8, 10); (3) inhibition of pyruvate oxidation in isolated epithelial cells together with a rise in intracellular sodium concentration suggesting an action at the site of active sodium transport (8); (4) inhibition of net fluid reabsorption in the proximal tubule of the rat kidney; and, more importantly, (5) inhibition of active sodium transport with no effect or passive back-leak in the isolated perfused mammalian collecting tubule (10). Although the above evidence suggests an important role of a natriuretic hormone in the ability of the chronically diseased kidney to maintain external sodium balance, it does not exclude the participation of any of the other modulators of sodium excretion already discussed.

Recent in vivo studies have examined the responsivity of the residual nephrons to the natriuretic factor in uremic rats. The results demonstrated an enhanced end-organ responsiveness to the natriuretic factor in uremic versus nonuremic rats (51). It appears, therefore, that the adaptive natriuresis per nephron in uremia may involve a "resetting" of one or more of the component parts of the control system for sodium.

The biologic control system for sodium appears to be "detector oriented." This means that the addition of a given amount of sodium to the body fluids will set into motion a series of events that will culminate in the augmentation of the basal rate of sodium excretion. The natriuresis which ensues causes the ECF volume to return to its original state and in fact may result in an "overshoot" in the direction of minimal volume contraction. At this point the detector-oriented system will sense the need to retain sodium and the appropriate signals are provided to the kidneys, probably in the main by turning off natriuretic forces. Such an oscillating system, similar in operation to a thermostat, would control the volume and composition of the extracellular fluid on a day-to-day basis with fluctuations which are too small to measure by conventional methods.[3] Since, in chronic renal failure, the overall sensi-

---

[3] Changing rates of aldosterone secretion will not contribute to short-term oscillations in sodium excretion, which are implicit in the above model of the "detector-oriented" control system.

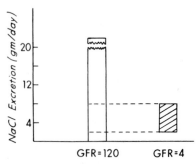

Figure 16-4. The range of sodium excretion in a normal person (GFR 120 mL/min) compared with a uremic patient (GFR 4.0 mL/min). Whereas the normal individual is capable of varying salt excretion from essentially zero to values well in excess of 20 g (salt) per day, the range in the uremic patient is finite but restricted. In the average patient with a GFR below 10 mL/min, the floor for sodium excretion is approximately 2 g salt/day and the ceiling may not exceed 7 to 8 g/day.

tivity and responsivity of the system is greatly magnified, it is anticipated that important insights into the normal control system will accrue from the study of control systems in uremia.

THE RESTRICTION IN RANGE OF SODIUM EXCRETION

The restriction in range for the whole kidney involves both a "ceiling" and a "floor." The maximal rate of excretion is reduced, and there is an obligatory sodium loss even when salt intake is curtailed (see Fig. 16-4).

THE CEILING FOR SODIUM EXCRETION

The ceiling rarely is a problem until the GFR reaches very low levels and then only if the salt intake is greater than 7 to 8 g/day. However, if hypoalbuminemia (secondary to high rates of protein excretion), congestive heart failure, or acute glomerulitis supervene, the upper limit of sodium excretion may diminish below the intake on an average or even moderately restricted salt intake. Edema formation then will follow. Occasionally a patient with advanced renal disease who does not have an obvious basis for an edema-forming state will have a low ceiling and will retain salt unless sodium intake is reduced below 5 to 6 g of salt/day. It is more characteristic, however, for a patient with a GFR as low as 2 to 3 mL/min, who is not yet on dialysis, to be able to excrete up to 7 or 8 g of salt/day, and edema formation in uncomplicated chronic progressive renal disease, contrary to popular opinion, is unusual.

The inability to increase sodium excretion above the ceiling, whatever the level of the latter, occurs interestingly enough in the face of the continued tubular resorption of a substantial percentage of the filtered sodium. For example, even with GFRs as low as 2 mL/min, 50 percent or more of the filtered sodium is resorbed (40). Thus there appears to be a limit to the degree to which resorption per nephron can be inhibited physiologically, and it is this limit plus the reduction in the number of nephrons that determines the ceiling for sodium excretion.

THE FLOOR FOR SODIUM EXCRETION

Because natriuretic forces presumably become increasingly marked as chronic renal disease advances, when salt intake is suddenly curtailed, these forces may not be immediately suppressible. The retention of anions in the blood such as sulfate and phosphate, which are only partially resorbed in the tubule and thus require the excretion of a cation, may also contribute to the sodium-losing state of chronic uremia. However, the possibility that functional defects in nephrons produced by anatomic abnormalities are responsible for the inability to conserve sodium maximally, once a commonly held explanation, now seems unlikely. Thus if the total nephron population is not markedly reduced (owing to the presence of the normal kidney), the diseased kidney does not manifest a sodium-losing tendency (52). Moreover, in patients with the nephrotic syndrome, the urine may be excreted virtually free of sodium despite far-advanced renal disease and uremia (9). Finally, it has recently been shown that if uremic patients are weaned slowly from dietary salt, the salt-losing state can be reversed totally (53).

In the latter studies, the sodium content of the diet of patients with GFRs varying from 5 to 16 mL/min was reduced very slowly over periods ranging from 4 to 14 weeks, under extremely close observation. Despite the development of a salt-losing tendency early in the study, each patient ultimately was able to establish sodium balance on a sodium intake of less than 10 meq/day (mean 5 meq/day). In none of the patients were there any adverse effects. Thus, the salt-losing tendency of chronic renal failure does appear to be a manifestation of the long-term adaptation for sodium excretion, rather than the result of intrinsic structural damage to the kidney or obligatory solute diuresis and can be shown to be reversible under appropriate dietary conditions.

CONCENTRATION AND DILUTION: THE EXCRETION OF WATER

A review of the normal concentrating and diluting mechanisms is presented in Chap. 12 and reference already has been made to alterations in these mechanisms that ensue in advancing renal disease. An abnormality in concentrating ability develops which ultimately limits the maximal achievable urinary osmolality to values only slightly in excess of those of the plasma; hence, if plasma osmolality is 300 mosm/kg water, 1 L water must be excreted for every 300 mosm of solute excreted. Dilution is better preserved than concentration in progressive renal disease, but the maximum increment in using volume during water diuresis depends upon how low the GFR is. Even if the patient with uremia were able to elaborate 10 mL "free water" per dL filtrate, this amounts to only 0.1 mL extra water per milliliter of glomerular filtrate. Hence, a patient with a GFR of 4 mL/min who excretes 600 mosm solute per day will have an obligatory urine volume of approximately 2 L/day (this assumes that the urine cannot be concentrated above the osmolality of plasma) and will be able to increase urine volume during maximal diluting ability only to approximately 2.6 L/day.

The restriction in the range of water excretion, therefore, is similar to that for sodium. There is an upper and lower limit, and for water the two tend to approach each other as the disease advances. In contrast to sodium, the average rate of water excretion (i.e., urine volume) in the uremic patient is higher than that in the normal individual, who will concentrate urine during part of the 24-h period. The uremic patient thus must maintain a larger intake of water than the average normal person. The uremic patient also tends to lose the diurnal pattern of water excretion and may excrete more water at night than during the day. With the formation of over 500 mL urine during the night and with a normal bladder capacity, nocturia is an inevitable consequence.

The obligatory loss of water imposed by the daily excretion of solute and a concentrating defect means that the urine volume does not diminish appreciably with water restriction or in the face of extrarenal losses of fluid (e.g., from sweating, vomiting, or diarrhea). Thus fluid losses must be replaced promptly, and the practice of placing patients with far-advanced uremia on water restriction for lengthy periods in order to perform tests such as intravenous pyelograms, gallbladder x-rays, or measurements of urinary concentrating ability is not without its risks. Hydropenia comparable to that produced in normal individuals subjected to complete water deprivation for 12 h or longer may be induced in the uremic patient by less severe water restriction for shorter periods of time.

The upper limit of water excretion may also lead to difficulties if an inappropriately large volume of fluid is ingested. Too often chronic water loading is prescribed in patients with advanced renal disease to "wash out" urea. Although the procedure will do very little to the blood urea levels, and nothing favorable for the uremic syndrome, it can result in water retention, hyponatremia, and water intoxication. An interesting social implication of the progressive limitation in the maximum volume of water that may be excreted during maximal dilution is that the increment in urine volume following alcohol ingestion (which is largely a function of inhibition of ADH release) will become smaller and smaller with time.

The fact that the urinary osmolality tends not to exceed that of the plasma appreciably in uremia conveys a certain amount of physiologic significance to a sudden fall in the volume of urine. If urine output diminishes substantially in a patient with chronic uremia, one may conclude that solute excretion has diminished in proportion to the decrement in volume. The two most likely causes of such a fall are (1) sudden reduction of GFR and (2) acute urinary retention. Thus an abrupt decrease in urine volume may be an indication that some acute, potentially catastrophic, but possibly reversible disorder has complicated the course of chronic progressive renal disease.

Despite its recognition for many years as an inherent feature of the uremic state, the mechanism of the concentrating defect has remained poorly understood. A number of possible explanations have been advanced which include (1) high rates of solute flow per nephron, (2) anatomic alterations distorting the medullary architecture, (3) an increase in blood flow through the medulla which dissipates the high interstitial: collecting tubule concentration gradient, (4) resistance of the collecting tubule to vasopressin, and (5) a defect in sodium chloride transport out of the ascending limb of the loop of Henle. None of these mechanisms is mutually exclusive and in view of the widely disparate forms of glomerular, tubular, and interstitial diseases which lead to a urinary concentrating defect, no single mechanism can explain the universality of the phenomenon.

Recently an abnormality of intrarenal recycling of urea has been demonstrated in the pyelonephritic animal (54). Failure to recycle urea and to sustain a high medullary interstitial solute concentration will, according to currently accepted theories of the countercurrent mechanism, lead to a concentrating defect. It is also possible that an acquired, impaired responsiveness to vasopressin occurs in the uremic state, and very recent observations on isolated cortical collecting tubules of the uremic rabbit have revealed a blunted water permeability response to vasopressin which appears to be linked to a decreased responsiveness of the adenylate cyclase system in this nephron segment (55).

CALCIUM AND PHOSPHORUS REGULATION (See also Chap. 8)

The control system serves admirably to maintain phosphate excretion equal to phosphate accession without phosphate retention in body fluids until GFR decreases to approximately 25 mL/min. Below a GFR of 25 mL/min, regulation persists, but serum phosphate concentrations rise because even in the face of high-grade phosphaturia per nephron, total excretion will decrease to less than intake with a normal rate of acquisition. As serum phosphate values increase, serum ionized calcium values will decrease reciprocally. An additional factor favoring a reduction in serum calcium concentration is the abnormality in vitamin D metabolism and the attendant impairment of calcium absorption from the gut that occurs in advancing renal disease.

Considerable evidence has been brought to bear on the nature of the calcium and phosphate control system in advancing renal disease (12, 56, 57). Certain of the basic facts have been established, and from these data a working hypothesis which is in general agreement with the data was proposed in 1969 (56). The general features of this hypothesis are depicted in Fig. 16-5.

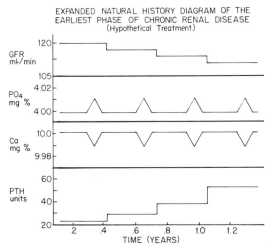

Figure 16-5. The reduction in GFR is intended to correspond to the decrease in nephron population and is shown occurring in sequential individual steps rather than as a continuum. With each decrement in GFR a transient period of phosphate retention ensues; this is followed by a reciprocal decrease in ionized calcium concentration, and the ionized calcium concentration effects an increase in PTH (parathyroid hormone) release. The increase in PTH results in a greater rate of phosphate excretion per residual nephron, and the plasma phosphate concentration returns to normal. The calcium concentration thereafter rises to normal, *but the PTH level must remain permanently elevated in order to prevent a recurrence of the hyperphosphatemia and hypocalcemia.* With each wave of nephron destruction the same cycle repeats itself; the detailed hypothetical sequence is described in the text.

On an average diet in the United States, phosphorus intake approximates 1 g/day, of which about 700 mg is absorbed and enters the extracellular fluid. Seven hundred milligrams of phosphorus, therefore, must be excreted daily for external balance to be maintained. If the GFR is 120 mL/min and the serum phosphate concentration is 4 mg/dL, approximately 7000 mg of phosphate will be filtered per 24 h. If there are 2 million nephrons contributing to phosphate excretion, the average rate of excretion per nephron will be 0.35 μg per 24 h. If renal disease then begins and the initial impact results in the loss of 20,000 nephrons, phosphate excretion will fall by 20,000 times 0.35 μg, or 7 mg/day. This unexcreted 7 mg will be distributed in the ECF and must lead to a finite increment in the serum phosphate concentration. For example, if the volume of distribution of the retained phosphate is 20 L, there will be an increase in serum phosphate concentration averaged over the 24-h period of 0.035 mg/dL. This rise in turn will lead to a reciprocal fall in ionized calcium of approximately 0.0035 mg/dL (57). The blood perfusing the parathyroid glands will reflect the decrease in calcium activity, and PTH secretion will be augmented. The blood perfusing the renal tubules will contain an increased concentration of PTH, and one of the key biologic effects of PTH is the reduction in tubular resorption of phosphate.

As PTH activity at the level of the nephron rises, phosphate excretion per residual nephron will increase, and not only will phosphate excretion by all the remaining nephrons return to the previous level, but the retained phosphate will be excreted. The serum phosphate concentration will thus return toward normal, and the serum calcium concentration will rise toward normal. Consequently, the stimulus to hypersecretion of PTH will abate. But as PTH levels start to fall, phosphate excretion per nephron will begin to fall, and the tendency to phosphate retention and hypocalcemia will recur. Thus, PTH levels must remain elevated, oscillating about a new normal level. The destruction of even 1 percent of the nephron population, according to this formulation, will lead to a persisting increase in the level of PTH activity.

With the next wave of nephron reduction the

same sequence will recur, and PTH levels will increase to a new steady-state range. Theoretically, this full cycle will repeat itself every time GFR diminishes. Thus PTH activity should increase throughout the natural history of chronic renal disease as long as phosphate intake and absorption are not reduced.

The role of vitamin D in the pathogenesis of hyperparathyroidism is not yet clearly established. Vitamin D_3 (cholecalciferol) is synthesized in the skin; it is converted to 25-OHD$_3$ in the liver and the latter is hydroxylated in the kidney to 1,25-(OH)$_2$D$_3$ (58). Both metabolites stimulate the enteric absorption of calcium, and although 1,25-(OH)$_2$D$_3$ is far more active mole for mole, it is present in the blood in far lower concentration. It thus is not clear which of the two metabolites plays the more important role in regulating intestinal calcium absorption in health. In relatively far advanced renal disease, 1,25-(OH)$_2$D$_3$ levels are low (17), presumably due to the loss of renal mass and despite the fact that PTH stimulates the l-hydroxylation of 25-OHD$_3$ in the kidney. The fall in 1,25-(OH)$_2$D$_3$ levels without a compensatory rise in 25-OHD$_3$ leads to the classic "vitamin D resistance" of advanced renal disease; and the latter will contribute to the forces favoring the production of secondary hyperparathyroidism; it will also favor the development of osteomalacia (58).

The possibility also exists, as was noted earlier, that chronic metabolic acidosis contributes to uremic osteodystrophy by virtue of buffering of hydrogen ions by skeletal carbonate and the release of calcium from bone as hydrogen ions are taken up (58).

According to the trade-off hypothesis expounded earlier, it should be possible to obviate the rise in parathyroid hormone levels by reducing phosphate intake in proportion to the reduction in nephron mass. This has been accomplished in experimental animals in which GFR was reduced in a stepwise fashion and dietary phosphorus reduced in proportion to the reduction in GFR. In contrast to uremic animals on a constant, normal phosphorus intake and in which parathyroid hormone levels were markedly elevated, the animals subjected to proportional reduction of phosphorus intake had normal parathyroid hormone levels (11).

In very recent studies (12), dogs subjected to "proportional reduction" of phosphorus intake were followed for up to 2 years in order to establish whether persistently normal parathyroid hormone levels would prevent the bone disease typical of prolonged secondary hyperparathyroidism. No evidence of osteitis fibrosa was found and bone histology revealed only osteomalacic change. In comparable animals supplemented with 25-OHD$_3$, the bones revealed no significant pathology. It appears, therefore, that the "tradeoff" skeletal complications of persistently elevated parathyroid levels are amenable to therapy and preventable by judicious dietary manipulation. This exciting approach remains to be fully evaluated in patients with chronic uremia.

ACID-BASE REGULATION

A primary charge to the acid-base control system is to effect the disposition of the hydrogen ions produced during metabolism without permitting the dislocation of the hydrogen ion concentration of body fluids from normal.[4] The influx of hydrogen ions into body fluids in a person on an average protein intake approximates 40 to 60 meq per 24 h. As was outlined in Chap. 6, these protons are buffered by extracellular fluid bicarbonate, converting the latter into carbonic acid, and the carbonic acid, which is in equilibrium with carbon dioxide, is maintained at a constant level by virtue of the excretion of carbon dioxide by the lungs. The kidneys must regenerate the bicarbonate that is lost in the buffering and simultaneously excrete the acquired hydrogen ions back into the environment. The regeneration of the bicarbonate and the excretion of the hydrogen ions is accomplished by a singular mechanism in the nephrons. This same mechanism effects the reclamation of all the filtered bicarbonate from the tubular fluid, a factor of great importance to acid-base homeostasis, for approximately 4800 meq bi-

---

[4] Drs. Schwartz and Cohen have recently presented a carefully reasoned argument against the existence of such a control system (60).

carbonate are filtered each day in a person with a normal nephron population.

The manner in which (1) bicarbonate is reclaimed from the glomerular filtrate, (2) new bicarbonate is formed, and (3) hydrogen ions are excreted is discussed in detail in Chap. 6.

The two main buffers present in the tubular fluid other than bicarbonate are phosphate and ammonia. Both have pK values sufficiently high so that when the urine pH is below 5.5, they are virtually maximally titrated with hydrogen ions. Hence, the total amount of hydrogen ions that may be excreted from the body in the urine and the total amount of new bicarbonate ions synthesized to reenter extracellular fluid will depend upon the absolute rate of excretion of phosphate plus ammonia. The rate of excretion of phosphate, however, is determined primarily by the need to maintain phosphate balance rather than by the state of acid-base balance, so that the contribution of phosphate to hydrogen excretion (and bicarbonate synthesis) may be considered as supportive but not sensitively attuned to the need for acid-base equilibrium. Precise regulation, therefore, must come from control of the rate of synthesis of ammonia.

The alterations in the acid-base control system that take place in renal disease may be described within the framework of the normal control system. The initial period of nephron reduction will lead to a transient decrease in hydrogen ion excretion and bicarbonate synthesis. Thus hydrogen ion retention and a decrease in plasma bicarbonate concentration will occur. Transient phosphate retention also occurs, as was noted in the discussion of the phosphate control system, and this is attended by an increase in PTH activity and a subsequent increase in phosphate excretion per residual nephron such that total phosphate excretion by the composite group of surviving nephrons will return to the previous level. Consequently, the hydrogen ions excreted as titratable acid (i.e., phosphate-buffered hydrogen ions) also will increase to the original level. But this alone will only partially restore hydrogen ion excretion and bicarbonate synthesis to the original level; ammonia excretion also must increase. The transient acidosis presumably induces adaptation of the ammonia synthetic system, and ammonia excretion per residual nephron increases, thereby allowing for hydrogen ion excretion per nephron to increase further and bicarbonate synthesis per nephron to increase in parallel. After compensation is complete, hydrogen ion balance may once again be maintained by the diminished population of nephrons, if the sum of phosphate excretion and ammonia excretion per nephron remain increased.

With each additional period of nephron destruction, the cycle should repeat itself. But as the nephron population diminishes progressively, the ability to compensate becomes less and less complete (see Fig. 16-6). Titratable acid remains nor-

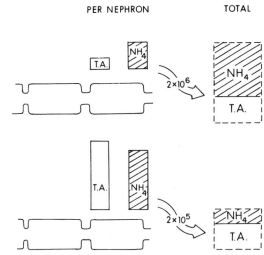

Figure 16-6. Response of a representative nephron to an average metabolic hydrogen ion load in health and in advanced renal disease. In the normal state, the total amount of acid excreted as titratable acid (i.e., phosphate-buffered hydrogen ions) and as ammonium is equal to the amount ingested, so that hydrogen ion balance is maintained. In advancing renal disease phosphate excretion per nephron increases sufficiently so that the total excretion rate of titratable acid tends to remain the same as that in health; ammonium excretion rates per nephron also increase markedly. However, the increment is limited by the metabolic pathways through which the ammonia is produced, and the *total* excretion rate of ammonia in uremia is lower than that in health. Consequently total hydrogen ion excretion is less than in health, and it is presumed that the difference between the rate of entry of hydrogen ions into body fluids and the rate of urinary excretion is accounted for by buffering by bone carbonate stores.

mal as long as phosphate intake is not diminished; however, the capacity to raise the rate of ammonia synthesis per nephron is limited and not sufficient to adjust quantitatively for the reduction of nephrons in the later stages of chronic renal disease.

In progressive renal disease, unless protein intake is restricted, hydrogen ion production from metabolism will remain comparable to that in the normal person. Titratable acid excretion may remain normal despite a marked reduction in nephron population if phosphate intake or enteric absorption is not reduced and external phosphate balance is preserved. However, total ammonia excretion diminishes despite an adaptive increase in ammonia production per nephron, and total hydrogen ion excretion and bicarbonate synthesis will fall below the rate of hydrogen ion production. This imbalance should lead to a progressive fall in arterial pH and a corresponding fall in plasma bicarbonate concentration, and death from metabolic acidosis should occur commonly and relatively early in chronic renal disease. However, this is not the case. Indeed, in patients with advancing renal disease, only moderately severe metabolic acidosis (which typically is well compensated) characteristically develops; once plasma bicarbonate concentrations fall to approximately 15 to 18 meq/L values tend to stay constant, in the absence of extenuating circumstances, until end-stage renal disease is approached. The fact that serum bicarbonate concentrations rarely fall below 15 meq/L in the face of a continuously positive hydrogen ion balance implies that continuous removal of hydrogen ions must be achieved by non-ECF buffers. As noted above, the present consensus is that the enormous bone stores of carbonate provide this buffering capacity, and it is probable that the "trade-off" is progressive loss of skeletal calcium and abnormalities of bone matrix (59), both of which contribute to the evolution of uremic osteodystrophy.

Most characteristically, the urine pH remains below 5.0 to 5.5 throughout the course of chronic renal disease. Thus, bicarbonate loss into the urine does not ordinarily contribute to the genesis of the metabolic acidosis. This in part is fortuitous, for plasma bicarbonate concentrations are low in uremia; hence, the concentration of bicarbonate in the glomerular filtrate is also low. When plasma bicarbonate concentrations are raised to the normal range in uremic patients, by feeding bicarbonate, reclamation may be less than complete, and a leak of bicarbonate into the urine may occur. The basis for this leak has been examined experimentally. The cumulative evidence indicates that the diminished ability to reabsorb bicarbonate represents a form of proximal renal tubular acidosis, which is due to a combination of an increase in parathyroid hormone activity and any other factor(s) that interfere with proximal sodium reabsorption (and proximal hydrogen secretion). In humans, the bicarbonate "leak" which follows the elevation of plasma bicarbonate toward normal levels makes it difficult to maintain a normal serum bicarbonate concentration by exogenous base administration. When bicarbonate is administered, the latter should not be the therapeutic goal.

POTASSIUM REGULATION

Because of the narrow limits of plasma potassium concentrations compatible with continuing life, adaptation of the potassium control system is critically important in patients with advancing renal disease. Potassium intake averages 60 to 80 meq/day on a normal diet, and until late in the course of renal disease, when protein may be restricted, potassium intake does not characteristically fall below this level. Thus, as with other solutes, the fewer the number of surviving nephrons, the higher must be the potassium excretion rate per nephron.

The definitive modulator of potassium excretion in uremia, as in health, continues to escape detection. Aldosterone must play a role, as evidenced clinically by the severe hyperkalemia which often develops in uremic patients receiving spironolactone. Nevertheless, aldosterone is probably not the fine modulator because renal potassium excretion can increase or decrease in accordance with dietary intake even in the presence of fixed levels of aldosterone activity (61). Hydrogen ion concentration can influence potassium secretion but cannot, on a priori grounds, modulate potassium secretion on a continuing basis.

The rate of sodium delivery to the distal tubule also is important as a conditioner of potassium excretion; but again cannot serve as a fine control mechanism, for patients maintain potassium balance in the face of changing sodium intake. Finally, the concentration of potassium in the plasma perfusing the kidney is important in influencing secretory rates (62), but exactly how important it is in fine modulation remains to be established. The adaptive increase in potassium excretion rate per nephron appears to be associated with a nonaldosterone-mediated increase in Na^+–K^+–ATPase (sodium–potassium-activated ATPase) activity similar to that which occurs in the kidneys of normal animals subjected to a chronic potassium load (63, 64). This change fails to occur if the adaptive kaliuresis per nephron is prevented by proportional reduction of potassium intake (63); nevertheless, the increased enzyme activity more likely supports rather than modulates the adaptive kaliuresis per nephron. It seems possible, therefore, that one or more additional and still unrecognized factors (such as a "kaliuretic hormone") could be involved in the defense of potassium homeostasis in uremia.

The adaptive potential of the nephron for potassium secretion is very great, and potassium excretion rates per nephron at low GFRs may be very large indeed. Furthermore, as in the case of other ions including sodium, the change in excretion rate per nephron in response to a small change in intake must become increasingly large as the number of nephrons diminishes. Because of the increased excretory contribution per nephron, however, it is not difficult to understand how the capacity to adapt further may be limited and how relatively modest acute increments in potassium intake in a uremic patient can initiate potentially serious degrees of hyperkalemia.

PRINCIPLES OF CONSERVATIVE MANAGEMENT

Many of the basic principles of conservative management of chronic progressive renal disease arise as direct and logical extensions of the concepts of pathophysiology described in this chapter. Part of the approach requires an understanding of the upper, and if relevant, the lower limit of excretory ability for key solutes and water. We believe that the trade-off hypothesis provides the basis for an additional part of the approach to conservative management. A further component relates to the loss of nonexcretory functions of the kidney. Finally, there still remains an element of conservative management that is empiric in nature.

Conservative management also involves the treatment of specific organ system abnormalities when they occur. For example, congestive heart failure, pericardial effusion, and gastrointestinal bleeding all require directed therapeutic efforts, and when drugs such as digoxin, aminoglycoside antibiotics, etc., are administered, the dose may have to be prorated on the basis of the level of renal function if the agent is excreted by the kidney or by the degree of uremia if the agent is metabolized, and the efficiency of metabolism is altered in uremia.

From the previous discussion of the control systems concerned with the excretion of individual solutes, a number of the key points in conservative management have emerged. At the risk of some repetition, it may be useful to summarize briefly in consecutive fashion the principles for each of the major functional systems.

It is the exception rather than the rule for abnormalities of sodium balance to evolve until relatively late in the course of chronic progressive renal disease in a patient maintained on an average salt intake (i.e., 5 to 7 g/day) unless the patient is nephrotic or has some other profound edema-forming stimulus. When abnormalities do evolve, they are more likely to relate to sodium loss from body fluids than to sodium retention.

Most patients will continue to maintain sodium balance with facility on an ad libitum salt intake until GFR is reduced to levels as low as 2 to 3 mL/min. However, as GFR falls below 20 to 30 mL/min, the obligatory loss of sodium in the urine becomes of practical importance, for if the dietary intake of salt falls below the "floor," negative sodium balance will ensue, and the sodium lost from the body must be replaced. Alternatively, if a patient exhibits sodium retention at any given level of salt intake, the intake obviously is too high and must be reduced. The use of furosemide to increase the rate of sodium excretion is an alternative for reducing the salt intake.

It often may be useful to establish the range of sodium excretion (i.e., both the floor and the ceiling) with some precision in order to set the dietary intake of sodium (as NaCl plus all other sodium-containing compounds). The patient thus will have freedom to vary salt intake in either direction about the prescribed level by as much as several grams a day.

The technique for determining the range of excretion of sodium is as follows: The patient is given a diet containing 1 g of salt/day or less and is instructed to maintain this diet for 8 days. On the fourth day, a 24-h urine sample is collected, and the excretion rate of sodium is determined. The value represents the obligatory rate of loss (i.e., the floor). The cumulative losses are replaced and for the next 4 days a total of 8 g of salt/day is provided either in the form of salt packets or a weighed salt shaker. The patient is instructed to add all the salt to his or her food each day and to eat all the food to which salt is added. (If some of the basic diet to which no salt is added is not eaten, the error in computation of sodium intake is negligible.) On the fourth day of the high-salt regimen, 24-h urinary sodium excretion again is determined, and an estimate of the upper limit or "ceiling" is provided. We have performed the semiquantitative balance studies on a large number of uremic patients and have found that the great majority of patients will maintain sodium balance on a diet containing from 2 to 8 g of salt/day. Thus a regular diet without added salt, which contains approximately 5 g of salt/day, will suffice for all but a small percentage of uremic patients.

A less quantitative technique for determining the range of sodium excretion consists of prescribing a diet of approximately 5 g of salt/day and instructing the patient to maintain an accurate chart of daily weights. Short-term increments or decrements in weight are very likely to reflect changes in salt (and water) balance.

TREATMENT OF SALT DEPLETION

The most challenging aspect of treating salt depletion in the uremic patient is the recognition of its existence. If the patient with advanced renal disease and uremia has been maintained on a dietary intake of salt below the "floor," he or she is very likely to have sustained a cumulative loss of sodium, chloride, and water. The advent of anorexia and nausea can contribute to negative sodium balance by decreasing the intake of salt, and any extra fluid lost through vomiting, diarrhea, or profuse sweating will add to the contraction of ECF volume. Negative sodium balance constitutes one of the most common causes of an acute exacerbation of the uremic state. The mechanism presumably relates to a functional decrease in GFR per nephron induced by ECF volume contraction. When salt depletion is suspected, supplementary sodium chloride may be administered either by mouth or parenterally. The latter route is often more satisfactory, for the clinical response may be assessed quickly and accurately. A solution containing sodium chloride and sodium bicarbonate (120 meq/L sodium and chloride and 22 meq/L sodium and bicarbonate) may be administered intravenously. As long as appropriate precautions are taken to avoid overexpansion of extracellular fluid volume, the infusion of 1 L to 2 L of this solution is safe and often results in a rise in GFR and in striking clinical improvement.

TREATMENT OF SALT RETENTION

As already indicated, an occasional uremic patient will have a low ceiling for sodium (i.e., less than 5 g of salt/day) without obvious explanation, but in most instances a low ceiling is explicable on the basis of some complicating process such as hypoalbuminemia, congestive heart failure, pericardial effusion, acute glomerulitis, or urinary retention.

Net loss of NaCl may be effected in an edematous uremic patient by prescribing a 1-g-salt diet and thereby reducing the level of intake below the floor for excretion. Diuretics also may be used to increase sodium excretion, but high-dosage levels tend to be required at low GFRs and the potential for toxicity is increased.

Once the extra fluid is excreted, it is essential to reestablish the proper range of sodium excretion and thereafter to maintain the intake within this range. If excessive salt restriction is continued, it ultimately will lead to sodium depletion even in a uremic patient who has been an edema former. However, one indication for continued salt restriction in uremia is severe hypertension; even here, however, caution must be exercised to avoid an unphysiologic degree of volume depletion, particularly if diuretics are also employed as antihypertensive agents.

CONCENTRATING AND DILUTING MECHANISMS

Most of the clinical principles relating to water requirements in uremia have already been considered. To reiterate, there is an obligatory minimal rate of water excretion. If 600 mosm solute is excreted per day and the urinary osmolality is fixed at approximately 300 mosm/kg water, 2 L of water will be excreted daily, even if the intake of water falls below this level. But the physician rarely has to be concerned with the water floor, for in the alert and responsive uremic patient the thirst mechanism will assure adequate replacement of water losses. Only if gastrointestinal complications develop (including severe stomatitis and glossitis as well as nausea, vomiting, and bleeding) which interfere either with the thirst mechanism or with the ingestion of water or if the patient's level of awareness decreases must fluid be given parenterally. Obviously, if water is restricted for any reason other than oliguria, negative water balance will develop.

There is also an upper limit of water excretion, but this rarely poses a problem clinically except when a patient becomes oliguric due to acute deterioration of renal function. However, if forced hydration is maintained and is excessive in degree, water retention and hyponatremia may occur in advanced disease. Because the rationale for forcing fluids is elusive at best, fluid intake should usually be conditioned by the patient's desires.

When the uremic patient presents with hyponatremia, the analysis of the abnormality requires a separate consideration of the preceding balance of sodium *and* the preceding balance of water (see Chaps. 12 and 13). In most cases it will be found that negative sodium balance rather than positive water balance has ensued, and an increase in so-

dium intake without water restriction will serve to correct the hyponatremia. If, on the other hand, the patient has received excessive amounts of hypotonic fluid, temporary water restriction below the obligatory rate of excretion with continued intake of sodium will correct the abnormality.

CALCIUM AND PHOSPHORUS

The most visible abnormality in calcium and phosphorus regulation (see also Chap. 20) is the occurrence of hyperphosphatemia and the reciprocal development of hypocalcemia at GFRs below 25 to 30 mL/min. It is at this state of chronic renal disease that phosphate-binding gels are traditionally prescribed. These antacids serve to bind phosphorus in the intestine and thereby to decrease the entry of phosphate into the extracellular fluid. Hyperphosphatemia is thus minimized, and its contribution to a decrease in ionized calcium concentration is reduced. Dietary restriction of phosphate will also facilitate the control of hyperphosphatemia.

On the basis of the information already presented in this chapter, there is a growing reason to believe that restriction of phosphate intake or absorption may be of value earlier in the course of chronic renal disease (before frank phosphate retention is evident). If phosphate absorption from the diet were decreased in exact proportion to the decrements in GFR, there would then be no temporary periods of phosphate retention, no reciprocal falls in calcium level, and no stimulus to the development of progressive hyperparathyroidism, at least prior to the development of vitamin D "resistance."

The early reduction of phosphate absorption could greatly retard the development of and the ultimate severity of secondary hyperparathyroidism; it would, thereby, prevent or reduce all of the symptoms and signs of uremia that are truly caused by high levels of PTH. It might also influence favorably the natural history of the underlying renal lesion, if recent studies on uremic rats have any relevance to uremic individuals.

Symptomatic hypocalcemia is uncommon even in the late stages of chronic uremia, especially if marked hyperphosphatemia is prevented. Rarely, however, tetany and even grand mal seizures may be precipitated in a hypocalemic, uremic patient by rapid correction (or overcorrection) of metabolic acidosis with bicarbonate infusion. If the manifestations of hypocalcemia are severe, short-term improvement can be obtained by the intravenous administration of calcium gluconate or calcium chloride, but caution should be exercised if the patient is receiving a digitalis preparation.

A detailed consideration of the treatment of uremic osteodystrophy is presented in Chap. 20 and is beyond the scope of this discussion, but a few general comments will be made. If the dominant skeletal lesion is osteitis fibrosa, an attempt to suppress PTH release medically may be made by the administration of phosphate-binding gels and oral calcium (2 to 4 g calcium gluconate or calcium lactate/day) for a period of at least 3 to 4 weeks. If this is unsuccessful, 25-OHD$_3$ or 1,25-(OH)$_2$D$_3$ may be added, but extreme caution is necessary to avoid hypercalcemia. If bone pain regresses, the regimen may be continued on a chronic basis, but close and continuing observation is mandatory to avoid the occurrence of an insidious rise in serum calcium levels because of the risk of widespread metastatic calcification. The administration of vitamin D (or a metabolite) and calcium also is of value in the correction of the osteomalacic component of uremic osteodystrophy. If uremic bone disease does not respond to the medical regimen and if osteitis fibrosa is the major lesion, subtotal parathyroidectomy may be indicated.

ACID-BASE REGULATION

Although the acidosis of chronic uremia usually is not progressive and plasma bicarbonate levels do tend to stabilize at approximately 16 to 18 meq/L, the decrease in bicarbonate concentration means that the total ECF base supply available to buffer any new incursion of hydrogen ions is diminished. Hence the uremic patient is more prone to develop sudden deviations in pH than is a normal individual. Care must be taken not to administer hydrogen ion donors over and above those derived from the diet. If acidosis does progress in a uremic patient or the plasma bicarbonate concentration stabilizes but at a level below 15 meq/L, decreasing the rate of formation of acid from metabolism (by means of protein restriction) or the administration of extra base (generally as orally administered sodium bicarbonate) is indicated.

A severe catabolic state, the intervention of a second form of acidosis (e.g., lactic acidosis, ketoacidosis, etc.), or an acute exacerbation of uremia, such as may occur following extracellular fluid volume depletion, acute pyelonephritis, or acute glomerulitis, can lead to a life-threatening intensification of the metabolic acidosis. The patient may enter the hospital with plasma bicarbonate concentrations of 5 meq/L or lower and arterial pH values below 7.0. Acidosis of this degree of severity constitutes a medical emergency and requires the intravenous administration of sodium bicarbonate in amounts which will restore the plasma bicarbonate to its previous steady-state level. If the administration of sodium poses a hazard, it may be necessary to initiate peritoneal or hemodialysis together with base administration.

Because the tendency toward metabolic acidosis probably begins early in the course of chronic renal disease, the buffering of a portion of the metabolic hydrogen ions by bone carbonate stores could take place over a period of many years. If extension of present information ultimately reveals that the long-term development of acidosis in uremia does in fact contribute importantly to the pathogenesis of uremic osteodystrophy by effecting slow but continuing dissolution of the mineral structure of the skeleton, a change in present therapeutic formulations may be indicated. Although alkali therapy is generally not prescribed before plasma bicarbonate concentrations fall to less than approximately 20 meq/L (and many authorities choose not to prescribe exogenous base at all), the alternative approach would be to administer approximately 20 meq of bicarbonate daily starting when the GFR is only modestly reduced (e.g., 40 to 50 mL/min).

POTASSIUM

Most patients with advancing chronic renal disease will maintain plasma potassium concentrations at a normal or only slightly elevated level on an average intake of potassium until virtually the end of the disease. This ability to preserve external potassium balance differentiates the patient with chronic renal disease from the one with acute tubular necrosis. However, in a rare patient who otherwise has typical chronic uremia, plasma potassium concentrations may stabilize at a level in excess of 6 to 7 meq/L. The majority of these patients appear to have diabetic nephropathy; many have been found to have both hyporeninemia and hypoaldosteronism. Moreover, they respond to the administration of mineralocorticoid hormone in large doses with a reduction of plasma potassium concentration. In some instances, dietary restriction of potassium (through the vehicle of protein restriction) may also be required and rarely both a low potassium intake and potassium-binding resins may be necessary.

Hyperkalemia may occur in any patient with advanced chronic renal disease who sustains an acute decrease in renal function and it must be treated as intensively and conscientiously as in the patient with acute renal failure (see Chap. 15). The infusion of glucose and insulin, sodium bicarbonate, or a calcium salt, the administration of potassium-exchange resins, and finally the extracorporeal removal of the potassium by dialysis may all be necessary.

When hyperkalemia occurs in a uremic patient treated (usually inappropriately) with spironolactone or a "potassium-sparing" diuretic (e.g., triamterene), it is usually necessary only to withdraw the offending drug. Hypokalemia, rather than hyperkalemia, may also be seen in an occasional patient with chronic renal disease and uremia. This finding generally relates to a combination of inadequate intake of potassium and extrarenal losses, and the treatment involves the judicious administration of supplementary potassium.

DIETARY CONSIDERATIONS

Unless there are special problems such as persistent hyperkalemia, hypertension, early and severe acidosis, etc., it seems advisable at the present time to maintain patients on an unrestricted diet as long as GFR is above 15 to 20 mL/min. We would advocate the use of phosphate-binding gels, however, earlier than this, probably when the GFR falls to the 30- to 40-mL/min range. Although protein restriction has been employed for many years, and specific regimens have been popularized by Giordano and Giovanetti (65, 66), the utility of marked protein restriction in patients with advancing chronic renal disease still remains to be established. Once GFR falls below approximately 10 mL/min, and before hemodialysis is instituted, some decrease in protein intake seems indicated in order to reduce the rate of acquisition of phosphorus and potassium and the rate of metabolic production of hydrogen ions. Recent observations suggest that the substitution of essential amino acids or their keto acid analogues may have the positive effects of protein restriction without the disadvantages of a very low protein diet (67).

Once dialysis is initiated, the diet may ordinarily be liberalized as long as precautions are taken to prevent either phosphorus retention or phosphorus depletion, hyperkalemia, and excessive interdialysis weight gain from volume expansion.

WHEN TO START DIALYSIS

To begin hemodialysis prematurely is to commit patients to a regimen to which they must adhere for the remainder of their lives, unless a successful renal transplant is performed. To wait too long, on the other hand, means that the patient will be subjected to unnecessary suffering and to a less than optimal chance for rehabilitation after dialysis is begun. It is common practice today to prepare patients with an AV (atrioventricular) fistula when GFR is approximately 5 to 7 mL/min and to institute dialysis within a month or two after creation of the fistula. But this must be individualized.

MISCELLANEOUS ASPECTS OF THERAPY

Treatment of anemia

Although anemia is a regular concomitant of advancing uremia, there are rarely any obvious physiologic abnormalities unless it is very severe.

Thus, if the hematocrit stabilizes above 20 percent, transfusion is rarely indicated. However, if there are abnormalities which appear to relate to diminished oxygen-carrying capacity of the blood (e.g., if congestive heart failure appears to be complicated by or caused by the anemia) elevation of the hematocrit is indicated. If bleeding contributes to the anemia, it is obviously important to control the bleeding diathesis, particularly if it is due to a discrete lesion in the gastrointestinal tract. When transfusion is employed, packed red blood cells should generally be used. If the patient is hyperkalemic, washed fresh cells should be used. In any event transfusions should be held to a minimum because of the risk of hepatitis.

Other forms of therapy for the anemia have been employed with variable results. These include androgenic steroids and cobalt salts. Although the latter may in some instances produce an increase in hemoglobin concentration, the side effects have been severe enough to preclude their routine use.

Treatment of hypertension

Hypertension occurs in patients with renal disease more often than it does in the general population. Its severity, however, varies considerably, and the intensity and urgency of treatment must be based upon the clinical status of the patient and the degree of advancement of the renal disease. In early or moderately advanced renal disease, the principles of treatment are not dissimilar from those employed in patients without renal disease. However, when renal failure is advanced, the approach to lowering the blood pressure is quite different. In general the pressure should be lowered gradually and titrated against the GFR, unless there is a life-threatening complication of hypertension, and great care should be taken not to render a patient hypotensive, even transiently. The choice of drugs depends in large part on the experience and preference of the therapist; however, α-methyldopa (Aldomet), in doses varying from 250 mg three times a day to levels as high as 2.5 g daily, has been used extensively, often in combination with propanolol (Inderal) or hydralazine (Apresoline). Moderate salt restriction with or without the addition of a diuretic may also facilitate the control of high blood pressure, but as emphasized previously precautions must be taken to avoid excessive volume depletion and the attendant risk of hypotension.

SUMMARY

We are born with approximately 1 million nephrons in each kidney. But many different disease entities have the capacity to destroy these nephrons over periods ranging from months to many years. Although there is an enormous reserve capacity and life may be sustained with as little as 5 percent (or perhaps even less) of the original nephron population, changes in the economy of the patients evolve with advancing nephron destruction in an inexorable fashion; such changes ultimately lead to the uremic syndrome, which without intervention culminates in death. Throughout the entire course of chronic renal disease, the response of the surviving nephrons is remarkable and is geared to ensure the maximal degree of preservation of homeostasis possible. It is because of the adaptations that take place in these residual units that serious abnormalities in the body fluids may not appear until more than 75 percent of the nephron population has been destroyed and that over 95 percent of the nephron population can be destroyed without completely disabling the patient. It has become increasingly apparent in recent years that the approach to the conservative treatment of chronic renal disease must be based to an increasing degree on an in-depth understanding of contemporary pathophysiologic concepts. Understanding the sequential changes in the biology of the uremic patient is greatly enhanced when the changes in renal function at each stage of chronic renal disease are clarified. Through such information it becomes possible to derive principles of therapy that are accurate, effective, and generally simple to execute. Ultimately, it should become possible to pinpoint the specific events that are responsible for the individual abnormalities of the uremic state, and from this type of exposition techniques may well evolve for preventing the occurrence, or at least diminishing the severity of, major abnormalities of the uremic state. The overall effect of a physiologic approach to chronic renal disease, therefore, should be translatable into ever-improved modalities of conservative therapy.

REFERENCES

1. Bricker, N. S.: On the pathogenesis of the uremic state: An exposition of the "trade-off hypothesis," *N. Engl. J. Med.*, **286**:1093, 1972.

2. Guisado, R., A. I. Arieff, and S. G. Massry: Changes in the electroencephalogram in acute uremia, *J. Clin. Invest.*, **55**:738, 1975.

3. Massry, S. G., J. W. Coburn, D. L. Hartenbower, J. H. Shinaberger, J. R. Depalma, E. Chapman, and C. R. Kleeman: Mineral contents of human skin in uremia: Effect of secondary hyperparathyroidism and hemodialysis, *Proc. Eur. Dialysis Transplant Assoc.*, **7**:146, 1970.

4. Perkow, J. W., B. S. Fine, and L. E. Zimmerman: Unusual ocular calcification in hyperparathyroidism, *Am. J. Ophthalmol.*, **66**:814, 1964.

5. Slatopolsky, E., S. Caglar, J. P. Pennell, D. D. Taggart, J. M. Canterbury, E. Reiss, and N. S. Bricker: On the pathogenesis of hyperparathyroidism in chronic experimental renal insufficiency in the dog, *J. Clin. Invest.*, **50**:492, 1971.

6. Bourgoignie, J. J., S. Klahr, and N. S. Bricker: Inhibition of transepithelial sodium transport in the frog skin by a low molecular weight fraction of uremic serum, *J. Clin. Invest.*, **50**:303, 1971.

7. Bourgoignie, J. J., K. H. Hwang, C. Espinel, S. Klahr, and N. S. Bricker: A natriuretic factor in the serum of patients with chronic uremia, *J. Clin. Invest.*, **51**:1514, 1972.

8. Kaplan, M. A., J. J. Bourgoignie, J. Rosecan, and N. S. Bricker: The effects of the natriuretic factor from uremic urine on sodium transport, water and electrolyte content, and pyruvate oxidation by the isolated toad bladder, *J. Clin. Invest.*, **53**:1568, 1974.

9. Bourgoignie, J. J., K. H. Hwang, E. Ipakchi, and N. S. Bricker: The presence of a natriuretic factor in urine of patients with chronic uremia. The absence of the factor in nephrotic uremic patients, *J. Clin. Invest.*, **53**:1559, 1974.

10. Fine, L. G., J. J. Bourgoignie, K. H. Hwang, and N. S. Bricker: On the influence of natriuretic factor from patients with chronic uremia on the bioelectric properties and sodium transport of the isolated mammalian collecting tubule, *J. Clin. Invest.*, **58**:590, 1976.

11. Slatopolsky, E., S. Caglar, Z. Gradowsky, J. M. Canterbury, E. Reiss, and N. S. Bricker: On the prevention of secondary hyperparathyroidism in experimental chronic renal disease using "proportional reduction" of dietary phosphorus intake, *Kidney Int.*, **2**:147, 1972.

12. Rutherford, W. E., P. Bordier, P. Marie, K. Hruska, H. Harter, A. Greenwalt, J. Blondin, J. Haddad, N. Bricker, and E. Slatopolsky: Phosphate control and 25-hydroxycholecalciferal administration in preventing experimental renal osteodystrophy in the dog, *J. Clin. Invest.*, **60**:332, 1977.

13. Naets, J. P., M. Wittek, C. Tanssant, and J. VanGeertruyden: Erythroporesis in renal insufficiency and in anephric man, *Ann. N.Y. Acad. Sci.*, **149**:143, 1968.

14. Davies, D. L., M. A. Schalekamp, D. G. Beevers, J. J. Brown, J. D. Briggs, A. F. Lever, A. M. Medina, J. J. Norton, J. I. S. Robertson, and M. Tree: Abnormal relation between exchangeable sodium and the renin angiotensin system in malignant hypertension and in hypertension with chronic renal failure, *Lancet*, **1**:683, 1973.

15. Tobian, L.: A viewpoint concerning the enigma of hypertension, *Am. J. Med.*, **52**:595, 1972.

16. Avioli, L. V., and J. G. Haddad: Vitamin D: Current concepts, *Metabolism*, **22**:507, 1973.

17. Haussler, M. R., M. R. Hyplies, J. W. Pike, and T. A. McCain: Radioligaud and receptor assay for 1,25-dehydroxy vitamin D: Biochemical, histologic and clinical applications, in A. W. Norman, K. Schaefer, J. W. Cobsrn, H. F. DeLuca, D. Fraser, H. Grigoleit, and D. V. Herrath (eds.), *Vitamin D: Biochemical, Chemical and Clinical Aspects Related to Calcium Metabolism*, Walter de Grüyter, Berlin, 1977, p. 473.

18. Hill, L. F., E. B. Mawer, and C. M. Taylor: Determination of plasma levels of 1,25-dehydroxycholecalciferol in man, in A. W. Norman, K. Schaefer, H. G. Grigoleit, D. V. Herrath, and E. Ritz (eds.), *Vitamin D and Problems Related to*

Uremic Bone Disease, Walter de Grüyter, Berlin, 1975, p. 755.

19. Bricker, N. S., S. Klahr, H. Lubowitz, and R. E. Rieselbach: Renal function in chronic renal disease, *Medicine (Baltimore),* **44:**263, 1965.

20. Bricker, N. S., L. G. Fine, M. A. Kaplan, M. Epstein, J. J. Bourgoignie, and A. Licht: "Magnification phenomenon" in chronic renal disease, *N. Engl. J. Med.,* **299:**1287, 1978.

21. Bank, N., and H. S. Aynedjian: Individual nephron function in experimental bilateral pyelonephritis. I. Glomerular filtration rate and proximal tubular sodium, potassium, and water reabsorption, *J. Lab. Clin. Med.,* **68:**713, 1966.

22. Lubowitz, H., M. L. Purkerson, M. Sugita, and N. S. Bricker: GFR per nephron and per kidney in the chronically diseased (pyelonephritic) kidney of the rat, *Am. J. Physiol.,* **217:**853, 1969.

23. Weber, H., K. Lin, and N. S. Bricker: Effect of sodium intake on single nephron glomerular filtration rate and sodium reabsorption in experimental uremia, *Kidney Int.,* **8:**14, 1975.

24. Rocha, A., M. Marcondes, and G. Malnic: Micropuncture study in rats with experimental glomerulonephritis, *Kidney Int.,* **3:**14, 1973.

25. Lubowitz, H., D. C. Mazundar, J. Kawamura, J. T. Grosson, F. Weisser, D. Rolf, and N. S. Bricker: Experimental glomerulonephritis in the rat: Structural and functional observations, *Kidney Int.,* **5:**356, 1974.

26. Allison, M. E. M., C. B. Wilson, and C. W. Gottschalk: Pathophysiology of experimental glomerulonephritis in rats, *J. Clin. Invest.,* **53:**1402, 1974.

27. Hayslett, J. P., M. Kashgarian, and F. H. Epstein: Functional correlation of compensatory renal hypertrophy, *J. Clin. Invest.,* **47:**774, 1968.

28. Fine, L. G., W. Trizna, J. J. Bourgoignie, and N. S. Bricker: Functional profile of the isolated uremic nephron. I: Control of fluid reabsorption by the proximal straight tubule, *J. Clin. Invest.,* **61:**1508, 1978.

29. Kleeman, C. R., D. A. Adams, and M. H. Maxwell: An evaluation of maximal water diuresis in chronic renal disease. I. Normal solute intake, *J. Lab. Clin. Med.,* **58:**169, 1961.

30. Tannen, R. L., E. M. Regal, M. J. Dunn, and R. W. Schrier: Vasopressin-resistant hyposthenu-ria in advanced chronic renal disease, *Am. J. Med.,* **42:**378, 1969.

31. Gonick, H. C., C. Goldberg, M. E. Rubin, and L. B. Guze: Functional abnormalities in experimental pyelonephritis. I. Studies of concentrating ability, *Nephron,* **2:**193, 1965.

32. Bricker, N. S., R. R. Dewey, H. Lubowitz, J. Stokes, and T. Kirgensgaard: Observations on the concentrating and diluting mechanisms of the diseased kidney, *J. Clin. Invest.,* **38:**516, 1959.

33. Thorn, G. W., G. F. Koepf, and M. Clinton, Jr.: Renal failure simulating adrenocortical insufficiency, *N. Engl. J. Med.,* **231:**76, 1944.

34. Lathem, W.: Hyperchloremic acidosis in chronic pyelonephritis, *N. Engl. J. Med.,* **258:**1031, 1958.

35. Scribner, B. H., and A. L. Babb: Evidence of toxins of "middle" molecular weight, *Kidney Int.,* **7:**s-349, 1975.

36. Furst, P., J. Bergstrom, A. Cordon, E. Johnsson, and L. Zimmerman: Separation of peptides of middle molecular weight from biologic fluids of patients with uremia, *Kidney Int.,* **7:**s-272, 1975.

37. Smith, H. W.: Salt and water volume receptors, *Am. J. Med.,* **23:**623, 1957.

38. Bricker, N. S.: Extracellular fluid volume regulation. On the evidence for a biologic control system, in M. Epstein (ed.), *The Kidney in Renal Disease,* Elsevier North-Holland Inc., New York, 1978, p. 19.

39. Schultze, R. G., H. Shapiro, and N. S. Bricker: Studies on the control of sodium excretion in experimental uremia, *J. Clin. Invest.,* **48:**869, 1969.

40. Slatopolsky, E., I. Elkan, C. Weerts, and N. S. Bricker: Studies on the characteristics of the control system governing sodium excretion in uremic man, *J. Clin. Invest.,* **47:**521, 1968.

41. Cope, C. L., and J. Pearson: Aldosterone secretion in severe renal failure, *Clin. Sci.,* **25:**331, 1963.

42. Weidman, P., M. H. Maxwell, and A. N. Lupu: Plasma aldosterone in terminal renal failure, *Am. Int. Med.,* **78:**13, 1973.

43. Berl, T., F. H. Katz, W. L. Henrich, A. de Torrente, and R. W. Schrier: Role of aldosterone in the control of sodium excretion in patients with advanced chronic renal failure, *Kidney Int.,* **14:**228, 1978.

44. Early, L. E.: Influence of hemodynamic factors on

sodium reabsorption, *Ann. N.Y. Acad. Sci.*, **139**:312, 1966.

45. Brenner, B. M., K. H. Falchuk, R. I. Keimowitz, and R. W. Berliner: The relationship between peritubular capillary protein concentration and fluid reabsorption by the renal proximal tubule, *J. Clin. Invest.*, **48**:1519, 1969.

46. Bricker, N. S., R. W. Schmidt, H. Favre, L. G. Fine, and J. J. Bourgoignie: On the biology of sodium excretion: The search for a natriuretic hormone, *Yale J. Biol. Med.*, **48**:293, 1975.

47. Schmidt, R. W., J. J. Bourgoignie, and N. S. Bricker: On the adaptation in sodium excretion in chronic uremia: The effects of "proportional reduction" of sodium intake, *J. Clin. Invest.*, **53**:1302, 1975.

48. Favre, H., K. H. Hwang, R. W. Schmidt, N. S. Bricker, and J. J. Bourgoignie: An inhibitor of sodium transport in the urine of dogs with normal renal function, *J. Clin. Invest.*, **56**:1302, 1975.

49. Epstein, M., N. S. Bricker, and J. J. Bourgoignie: Presence of natriuretic factor in urine of men undergoing water immersion, *Kidney Int.*, **13**:153, 1978.

50. Licht, A., S. Stein, and N. S. Bricker: Hormonal changes and transport adaptation in chronic renal failure: The possible role of a natriuretic hormone, *Biochem. Soc. Trans. (London)*, in press.

51. Fine, L. G., J. J. Bourgoignie, H. Weber, and N. S. Bricker: Enhanced end-organ responsiveness of the uremic kidney to the natriuretic factor, *Kidney Int.*, **10**:364, 1976.

52. Bricker, N. S., P. A. F. Morrin, and S. W. Kime, Jr.: The pathologic physiology of chronic Bright's disease, *Am. J. Med.*, **28**:77, 1960.

53. Danovitch, G. M., J. J. Bourgoignie, and N. S. Bricker: Reversibility of the "salt losing" tendency of chronic renal failure, *N. Engl. J. Med.*, **296**:14, 1977.

54. Gilbert, R. M., H. Weber, L. Turchin, L. G. Fine, J. J. Bourgoignie, and N. S. Bricker: A study of the intrarenal recycling of urea in the rat with chronic experimental pyelonephritis, *J. Clin. Invest.*, **58**:1348, 1976.

55. Fine, L. G., D. Schlondorff, W. Trizna, R. M. Gilbert, and N. S. Bricker: Functional profile of the isolated uremic nephron. II: Impaired water permeability and adenylate cyclase responsiveness of the cortical collecting tubule to vasopressin, *J. Clin. Invest.*, **61**:1508, 1978.

56. Bricker, N. S., E. Slatopolsky, E. Reiss, and L. V. Avioli: Calcium phosphorus and bone in renal disease and transplantation, *Arch. Int. Med.*, **123**:543, 1969.

57. Kaplan, M., J. M. Canterbury, G. Gavellas, D. Jaffe, J. J. Bourgoignie, E. Reis, and N. S. Bricker: Interrelations between phosphorus, calcium, parathyroid hormone, and renal phosphate excretion in response to an oral phosphorus load in normal and uremic dogs, *Kidney Int.*, **14**:207, 1978.

58. Haussler, M. R., and T. A. McCain: Basic and clinical concepts related to vitamin D metabolism and action, *N. Engl. J. Med.*, **297**:974, 1977.

59. Litzow, J. R., J. Lemman, and E. J. Lennon: The effect of treatment of acidosis on calcium balance in patients with chronic azotemic renal failure, *J. Clin. Invest.*, **46**:280, 1967.

60. Schwartz, W. B., and J. J. Cohen: The nature of the renal response to chronic disorders of acid-base equilibrium, *Am. J. Med.*, **64**:417, 1978.

61. Schultze, R. G., D. D. Taggart, H. Shapiro, J. P. Pennell, S. Caglar, and N. S. Bricker: On the adaptation in potassium excretion associated with nephron reduction in the dog, *J. Clin. Invest.*, **50**:1061, 1971.

62. Silva, P., B. D. Ross, A. N. Charney, A. Besarab, and F. H. Epstein: Potassium transport by the isolated perfused kidney, *J. Clin. Invest.*, **56**:862, 1975.

63. Schon, D. A., P. Silva, and J. P. Hayslett: The mechanism of renal potassium excretion in uremia, *Am. J. Physiol.*, **227**:1323, 1974.

64. Silva, P., J. P. Hayslett, and F. H. Epstein: The role of Na-K-activated adenosine triphosphatase in potassium adaptation stimulation of enzymatic activity by potassium loading, *J. Clin. Invest.*, **52**:2665, 1973.

65. Giordano, C.: Use of exogenous and endogenous urea for protein synthesis in normal and uremic subjects, *J. Lab. Clin. Med.*, **62**:231, 1963.

66. Giovanetti, S., and Q. Maggiore: A low nitrogen diet with proteins of high biological value for severe chronic uremia, *Lancet*, **1**:1000, 1964.

67. Mitch, W. E., and M. Walser: Effect of nutritional therapy of chronic renal failure: Quantitative assessment, *Clin. Res.*, **24**:407A, 1976.

17

Water, electrolyte, and acid-base disorders associated with acute and chronic dialysis

ARTHUR GORDON / MORTON H. MAXWELL

In 1960, Quinton, Dillard, and Scribner (1) described a technique permitting successful chronic cannulation of peripheral blood vessels, thereby facilitating simple, nontraumatic access to the circulation for the purpose of repetitively circulating blood extracorporeally through an artificial kidney. This single development has had far-reaching implications. Previously, the use of dialysis techniques for the treatment of uremia had been almost solely restricted to those patients who incurred an acute but potentially reversible deterioration of renal excretory function. The Quinton-Scribner "arteriovenous shunt" made repetitive, maintenance "chronic hemodialysis" feasible and the long-term treatment of patients with irreversible renal insufficiency a reality. Almost 20 years of experience, coupled with improvements in dialyzer and equipment design, have brought us presently to a point where more than 20,000 patients in the United States and 50,000 in the world who would otherwise have died from terminal renal failure are being maintained by chronic dialysis with mortality rates generally less than 10 percent per year (2).

Chronic dialysis has not been without complications. Indeed, dialysis patients can be considered to demonstrate a new syndrome with manifestations affecting virtually every organ system. Despite the vast amount of progress in the field in the past two decades, the full description of the dialysis syndrome, elucidation of its altered physiology, and determination of its optimal management are still to come. However, investigation of this syndrome has stimulated an extensive research program which has yielded valuable information in the understanding of the neurologic, bone, parathyroid, hypertensive, red blood cell, platelet, electrolyte, and nutritional complications of chronic uremia. Interest in the search for uremic toxic factors has been renewed.

Successful replacement of renal function by dialytic therapy requires not only substitution for impaired renal capacity to excrete metabolic waste products but also must provide for the maintenance of body fluid, electrolyte, and acid-base balance within viable and comfortable limits. It is these homeostatic functions of dialysis therapy which will be given major emphasis in this chapter.

GENERAL PRINCIPLES OF DIALYSIS

The principles of diffusion, osmosis, ultrafiltration, and passive and active transport are described in detail in Chap. 1, but will be reviewed briefly here as they relate to hemodialysis and peritoneal dialysis.

Dialysis may be defined as the differential diffusion of solutes and water through a passive porous membrane placed as a barrier between two solutions. The rate of diffusion for any given solute is largely determined by its relative concentration in each solution. When these concentrations are equal, dialyzable solutes will pass through the pores of the dialyzing membrane in both directions at equal rates, and there will be no *net transfer* of the solute between the two solutions. If, however, the concentration of the solute is higher in one solution than it is in the other, a *concentration gradient* is established, and net transfer of the solute (*diffusion*) will occur from the solution of higher concentration to the one of lower concentration at a rate dependent upon the magnitude of the gradient. Diffusion is also influenced by the molecular radius of each solute in relation to the cross-sectional size of the pores in the membrane. In clinical dialyzing techniques in which one of the solutions is the patient's plasma or blood, the dialyzing membrane must be selectively *semipermeable*; i.e., it must have a pore size large enough to transmit potentially toxic crystalloid solutes but small enough to be impermeable to serum proteins and other colloidal solutes, formed elements of the blood (blood cells, platelets), bacteria, and viruses. The movement of water is effected between solutions separated by a semipermeable dialyzing membrane by establishing either a hydrostatic pressure gradient or an osmotic pressure gradient, with water moving from the high hydrostatic pressure side to the low (i.e., by ultrafiltration—see below) or from the solution with the lower osmotic pressure to that with the higher (i.e., by osmosis).

These concepts of the dialysis principle are illustrated in Fig. 17-1, which diagrammatically depicts two solutions separated by a porous semipermeable membrane into two compartments. The black dots represent solutes whose molecular size and shape will permit them to pass through the pores of the membrane. By brownian movement, these solute particles in the solution "bombard" the membrane. Those particles which

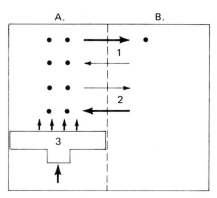

Figure 17-1. Diagrammatic representation of the processes of (1) diffusion, (2) osmosis, and (3) ultrafiltration (see text).

encounter a pore in the membrane will pass from one compartment to the other. Such brownian movement is directly related to temperature, but given equal temperatures the concentration, or number of particles in each solution, will determine the rate at which they contact and pass through the pores of the membrane. Thus, although solute particles will move across the membrane in both directions, the rate of movement is greater from the solution with the higher concentration. This net movement of solute from the solution of higher concentration (compartment A) to the one of lower concentration (compartment B) is the process of diffusion and is depicted in Fig. 17-1 by the upper arrows (1). The thickness of the arrow denotes the rate of movement in each direction.

The transmembrane movement of water as depicted by the lower arrows (2) occurs in a similar manner. Water moves from the compartment (B) with the higher "water concentration," i.e., lower solute concentration, or osmolality (see Chap. 1), to the compartment (A) with the lower "water concentration," i.e., higher solute concentration, or osmolality. This is the process of *osmosis*. Ultimately, the concentration of the solute and water in each compartment will equalize, at which time, although particles continue to move across the pores, the rate of movement is equal in each direction and there will be no further *net movement* of particles. Thus, at equilibrium, the compartments will contain equal quantities of solute and water.

If an external force, represented in Fig. 17-1 by

the piston (3), is applied to one compartment (A), it will literally "squeeze" both solute and solvent through the available pores of the membrane into compartment B at a rate proportional to the amount of force per unit area (pressure) applied. This movement of solute and water induced by a hydrostatic pressure differential can occur either with or against the existing chemical or osmotic concentration gradients and is referred to as the process of *ultrafiltration.* Similarly, a hydrostatic pressure gradient can be created by the application of a negative pressure (vacuum effect) to one compartment.

The movement of solute across the semipermeable membrane along concentration gradients is termed *diffusive transport. Convective transport* designates the movement of solute which accompanies the transmembrane transport of a solution along hydrostatic or osmotic pressure gradients (solvent drag).

The applicability of the principles of dialysis to the treatment of uremia is readily apparent. If uremic blood represents one of the solutions, the other solution, known as the *dialysate,* can be specifically designed to correct abnormalities in the concentration and the total body content of diffusible molecules in the uremic patient. Urea, phosphate, uric acid, creatinine, and other potentially toxic uremic solutes diffuse from the uremic plasma, where they are present in high concentrations, across the dialyzing membrane into the dialysate, which is prepared free of these solutes, thereby providing a maximal blood dialysate concentration gradient. The electrolyte composition of dialysate is designed to approximate normal serum concentrations, and thereby the process of diffusion will serve to correct toward normal any marked abnormalities in the electrolyte concentrations of the blood. Water flux can be controlled in regard to individual patient needs by the elective establishment of either hydrostatic pressure or osmotic pressure gradients. Such ultrafiltration also augments solute removal by the phenomenon of solvent drag, and indeed, in certain newly developed techniques (see *hemofiltration* and *diafiltration,* below), convective transport of uremic solutes largely or completely replaces diffusive transport.

Fortunately, both synthetic and natural membranes are readily available which function as appropriate semipermeable dialyzing membranes and permit the clinical application of dialysis principles, the specific details of which will be considered throughout this chapter.

COMPARATIVE ASSESSMENT OF HEMODIALYSIS AND PERITONEAL DIALYSIS

Hemodialysis and peritoneal dialysis represent the two major clinically effective dialysis techniques. In hemodialysis, blood is circulated extracorporeally through a hemodialyzer (artificial kidney) in which the process of dialysis occurs between the blood and the dialyzing solution separated by a membrane generally composed of cellophane or one of its derivatives. In peritoneal dialysis, dialysate is introduced into the peritoneal cavity where dialysis takes place between the capillary circulation within the peritoneal cavity and the instilled dialysate across a natural dialyzing membrane presumed to be the peritoneum.

Each of these techniques is capable of achieving essentially the same therapeutic end result, and in many instances, especially in the treatment of acute renal failure, the choice of dialysis method is based solely upon such logistic considerations as available facilities and experienced personnel, and the preference of the individual physician. As measured by relative urea clearances, peritoneal dialysis has only a fraction of the efficiency of hemodialysis. Urea clearances with peritoneal dialyses approximate 15 to 20 mL/min compared to urea clearances with hemodialyzers of 80 to 160 mL/min. However, essentially identical quantitative removal of solute and biochemical improvement can be effected by continuing peritoneal dialysis for time periods approximately three to six times longer than required for hemodialysis. This is demonstrated in Table 17-1, which compares the average change in blood urea nitrogen (BUN), serum creatinine, serum uric acid, and serum phosphorus obtained during 50 consecutive hemodialyses and peritoneal dialyses in patients with acute renal failure. The duration of the hemodialyses was 6 h, and the duration of the peritoneal dialyses averaged 30 h. Von Hartitzsch et al. (3) have compared predi-

Table 17-1. Average changes in serum chemistries with peritoneal dialysis and hemodialysis

| | PERCENT REDUCTION OF PREDIALYSIS SERUM CONCENTRATION | |
SOLUTE	PERITONEAL DIALYSIS	HEMODIALYSIS*
BUN	46	54
Creatinine	38	42
Uric acid	42	48
Phosphate	42	50

* High-efficiency, large-surface-area hemodialyzers are capable of achieving greater reductions.

alysis chemistries in a group of patients treated with chronic peritoneal dialysis and chronic hemodialysis, each modality being used for periods of 3 months or more, and have found no significant differences (Table 17-2).

Progress in membrane and dialyzer design in recent years has resulted in the development of even more efficient hemodialyzer function. Indeed dialyzers are now available which approach maximal attainable efficiency for clearance of low-molecular-weight solutes such as urea and creatinine, i.e., clearance approaches blood flow rate. Peritoneal dialysis appears, however, to be more efficient in its capacity to clear solutes of middle-molecular-weight configuration (4). Since the precise nature of uremic solutes of toxic consequence remains undefined, it is impossible at the present time to define the optimal level of dialysis efficiency. Experience to date would suggest however that despite differences in relative efficiency, clinical results, both with respect to acute and chronic dialysis, are comparable for peritoneal dialysis and hemodialysis.

The relative simplicity of acute peritoneal dialysis techniques permits this type of dialysis to be readily available at virtually any medical facility and to be performed by personnel with even minimal or no prior experience. It requires no special equipment other than commercially available dialysis solutions and catheters. In contradistinction, hemodialysis requires expensive equipment and facilities generally found only at the larger medical centers as well as an experienced, active professional team of physicians, nurses, and technicians. A word of caution is felt to be warranted here: The management of renal failure, whether acute or chronic,

often requires skills that extend far beyond the technical capacity to perform dialysis, and, accordingly, the mere availability of dialysis without the attendant nephrologic expertise does not necessarily offer the patient optimal care.

Although there are very few absolute contraindications to either method of dialysis, under certain clinical circumstances one dialysis technique may offer distinct advantages or lack certain disadvantages as compared to the other. In addition to selection based upon technical simplicity and ready availability, peritoneal dialysis might preferentially be used under the following conditions:

1. In acute, life-threatening emergency situations such as severe hyperkalemia or acidosis, the ability to institute peritoneal dialysis within minutes is of great value. Even if special dialysis solutions and equipment are not immediately available, one can readily introduce 2 L of 6/M sodium lactate, or, less desirably, isotonic saline solution or 5% dextrose in saline solution (generally immediately available on any ward), into the peritoneal cavity through any available long needle. Thereafter, the necessary equipment may be obtained to continue dialysis either with standard peritoneal dialysis techniques or, if desired, with hemodialysis. Even under emergency circumstances, it generally takes a minimum of 45 min and more often 1 to 3 h to institute hemodialysis, this time being required to place special catheters or cannulas into an artery and/or veins and to prepare the artificial kidney.

2. In the presence of active hemorrhage or bleeding diathesis, peritoneal dialysis has the ad-

Table 17-2. Predialysis chemistries with peritoneal dialysis and hemodialysis for 3 months or more

| | PERITONEAL DIALYSIS | HEMODIALYSIS |
SOLUTE	(9 H, 3 TIMES WEEKLY)	(5 H, 3 TIMES WEEKLY)
BUN	69 ± 12	69 ± 15
Creatinine	10.0 ± 3.9	10.3 ± 2.7
Uric acid	8.4 ± 1.6	8.0 ± 1.2
Phosphate	6.1 ± 2.1	5.9 ± 1.6

Source: Taken from Von Hartitzsch, et al. (3).

vantage of not requiring systemic anticoagulation. The extracorporeal circulation of blood during hemodialysis requires that anticoagulation with heparin be achieved to prevent clotting in the artificial kidney. This presents an appreciable risk to the patient with a hemorrhagic diathesis. The risk can be minimized by using the technique of regional heparinization (5) or constant slow infusion of heparin (6). With regional heparinization, heparin is infused into the blood as it enters the hemodialyzer and is neutralized by the infusion of protamine sulfate into the blood as it exits from the kidney and returns to the patient, thereby effectively anticoagulating the artificial kidney without inducing systemic anticoagulation. Constant slow heparin infusion techniques produce minimal levels of anticoagulation, barely adequate to prevent clotting in the artifical kidney. With experience and careful determination of periodic clotting times, the risk of systemic anticoagulation and hemorrhage can be minimized but not avoided. Methods for quantitating heparin requirements for repetitive dialysis have been reported (7).

3. The lesser efficiency of peritoneal dialysis minimizes the risk of inducing the dialysis disequilibrium syndrome, a phenomenon which seems to relate at least partially to the efficiency and rapidity of dialysis and/or of reduction in BUN concentration (8–13). Accordingly, in patients to be dialyzed who have a BUN concentration significantly in excess of 100 mg/dL, peritoneal dialysis might be favored to produce a more gradual reduction over a 24- to 48-h period of time as opposed to the similar biochemical change obtained more rapidly with hemodialysis. The disequilibrium syndrome has, however, occurred during peritoneal dialysis. Hemodialysis techniques can be modified, when indicated, to reduce efficiency and minimize this risk. Reduction in dialysis time, dialyzer surface area, dialysate and/or blood flow rates can be used individually or in combination to reduce hemodialysis efficiency (14).

4. The risk to the hypotensive patient is lower with peritoneal dialysis, since alterations in plasma volume are generally less abrupt and more predictable than they are with hemodialysis. Hemodialysis requires the extracorporeal circulation of a blood volume of at least 200 to 300 mL, and multiple factors including dialyzer dynamics, the nature of the dialyzing membrane, and the adequacy of the cannulas may result in variable and rapid ultrafiltration of plasma with worsening of hypotension. Although it is possible to replace such losses by the administration of volume expanders such as albumin, saline solution, or blood during hemodialysis or to attempt to quantitate these losses by using devices which permit either continuous or frequent weighing of the patient, these methods are not precise and may lead to inadequate or excessive fluid replacement. If peritoneal dialysis is conducted with 1.5% dextrose dialysate solutions, which are generally approximately isosmolar with the plasma of the average uremic patient, there will be little if any loss of plasma volume. Utilizing the dilution of instilled radioiodinated human serum albumin (RISA) concentration as a measure of intraperitoneal volume (15), we have found plasma volume losses of 0 to 100 mL/h. The underlying cause of existing hypotension should be ascertained and treated prior to or during the dialysis.

5. Although not as efficient as hemodialysis in removal of solutes, peritoneal dialysis is at least equally efficient in removal of water and correction of clinical states of overhydration. With the use of hyperosmolar dialyzing solutions (4.25% dextrose concentrations) we have achieved fluid losses as great as 1000 mL/h. Although such rapid depletion of extracellular fluid is rarely warranted or advisable, peritoneal dialysis can produce effective negative fluid balance and may be preferred when the principal purpose of dialysis is the correction of marked overhydration. For reasons as yet not clearly defined (see below), attempts to remove large quantities of fluid by ultrafiltration during hemodialysis are often frustrated by the development of hypotension, whereas equivalent volumes can be removed by peritoneal di-

alysis without attendant marked change in blood pressure. It may therefore require multiple hemodialyses to achieve safely the degree of negative fluid balance that is possible with one or two peritoneal dialyses. Recent modifications of hemodialysis techniques—sequential ultrafiltration and dialysis, diafiltration, hemofiltration and substitution of bicarbonate for acetate in dialysate (see below)—seem to provide successful methods for augmenting tolerable fluid removal capacity.

6. On very rare occasions a patient is encountered whose catabolic state is so marked that virtually continuous dialysis is required to prevent the development of severe uremia or life-threatening hyperkalemia. We have treated a patient in whom acute tubular necrosis developed following extensive muscle and bone trauma, and whose endogenous potassium source from the traumatized tissues and resultant hematomas was so massive that within 4 h of the completion of hemodialysis his serum potassium concentration had risen to 8 meq/L with associated electrocardiographic changes of hyperkalemia. He required continuous peritoneal dialysis for a period of 14 days as well as frequent enemas with cation exchange resins which were barely able to maintain his serum potassium concentration at 6.0 to 6.5 meq/L. Similar control of hyperkalemia would probably have required daily hemodialysis for prolonged periods of time. An increased risk of peritonitis has been reported with such prolonged peritoneal dialysis (16, 17). However, it is only in such unusual circumstances as the case cited that we ever feel continuation of dialysis beyond 24 to 48 h is indicated.

When hemodialysis is available or the patient's condition permits transfer to a hemodialysis center, it is the preferred technique under the following clinical conditions:

1. When the most rapid removal of dialyzable toxic solutes is indicated, the greater efficiency of hemodialysis becomes a highly desirable asset. This assumes its major clinical importance when one elects to use dialysis in the treatment of exogenous poisonings. The therapeutic goal is to augment maximally the usual excretory pathways for excretion or detoxification of the drug and thereby shorten the duration of drug-induced coma or minimize any direct organ-specific toxicity (e.g., nephrotoxicity, hepatotoxicity, cardiotoxicity). The clearance of virtually all dialyzable drugs is far greater with hemodialysis than with peritoneal dialysis (18). Certain additives such as albumin (19), lipids (20), and THAM (21) enhance peritoneal clearance of certain drugs by protein binding (barbiturates, salicylates), lipid binding (glutethimide), or ionization of weak acids (barbiturates, salicylates). However, clinical experience with these additives is minimal, and the limited increase in efficiency which they produce may not warrant the marked increase in expense and complexity of the procedure which their use entails. When part of the clinical syndrome induced by the drug intoxication includes severe acidosis, such as is seen with salicylates, ethylene glycol, and paraldehyde, prompt treatment with peritoneal dialysis can reverse the acidosis and should be used in those centers where hemodialysis is not available. The recent development of apparently safe and commercially available hemoperfusion devices provides the most efficient method for rapid and effective removal of exogenous toxins (22). There is little doubt that as increasing clinical experience with hemoperfusion devices confirms their safety and efficacy, they will become the treatment of choice for all poisonings with adsorbable toxins. Variable results have been obtained with these hemoperfusion devices in endogenous states of intoxication such as uremia and hepatic coma.

2. Although hemodialysis at present remains the modality of choice for chronic dialysis, improvements in automated equipment for peritoneal dialysis and increasing clinical experience with chronic maintenance peritoneal dialysis (23, 24) have apparently proven it to be a competitive therapeutic choice, no longer limited primarily to those patients unsuited for hemodialysis (25).

3. Hemodialysis may be required when perito-

neal dialysis is technically impossible. Dense intra-abdominal adhesions, inadvertent introduction of peritoneal dialysis solutions into the anterior abdominal wall, or extensive retroperitoneal hemorrhage may distort the anatomic integrity of the peritoneal cavity to such an extent that the satisfactory introduction of a peritoneal dialysis catheter becomes a virtual impossibility. After abdominal surgical treatment, external leakage of dialysis solutions from drains or leakage into the retroperitoneal space through surgically or traumatically created rents in the posterior peritoneum may make it impossible to maintain accurate fluid balance and/or achieve satisfactory drainage of dialysate. However, peritoneal dialysis has been (26) and often can be satisfactorily accomplished shortly after an abdominal operation if the surgeon has carefully reconstituted the anatomic continuity of the peritoneum.

4. Hemodialysis is generally preferable in patients with a localized intraperitoneal infection or abscess in whom the introduction of a catheter into the peritoneal cavity carries the risk of dissemination of the infection. Generalized peritonitis, either chemical or bacterial, does not per se contraindicate peritoneal dialysis, and indeed the procedure may have a therapeutic effect by virtue of the dilution and removal of bacteria or chemical irritants (26) and the introduction of antibiotics into the peritoneal cavity (27).

Other potential complications of both peritoneal and hemodialysis exist but generally do not affect the choice technique to be employed in the treatment of a given patient. These complications will be considered in the sections of this chapter dealing with the specific details of each dialysis technique.

INDICATIONS FOR DIALYSIS

Although renal failure constitutes the principal indication, dialysis has successfully been employed in a variety of disorders, as outlined in Table 17-3. Any clinical condition which has symptoms or signs that can be attributed to the effects

Table 17-3. Indications for dialysis*

Common
  Acute renal failure
  Chronic renal failure
  Exogenous poisonings
  Hyperkalemia
Infrequent
  Congestive heart failure (49)
  Refractory edematous states (50)
  Hypercalcemia (43, 44)
  Hypermagnesemia
  Hypernatremia (45)
  Metabolic acidosis (47, 48)
Rare
  Endogenous "poisonings"
    Hyperuricemia (35)
    Tophaceous gout (34)
    Hyperammonemia (30–32)
    Hyperbilirubinemia (33)
    Porphyria (42)
    Schizophrenia (51, 54)
    Myasthenia gravis (51)
    Endotoxin shock (53)
    Psoriasis (55)
Special
  Permit transfusion (57)
  Hypothermia (56)
  Parenteral fluid administration (58)

* Clinical experience is limited or based upon individual reports in all but those listed as common indications.

of dialyzable toxic solutes or to abnormalities in electrolyte, acid-base, or fluid balance can potentially be benefited by dialytic therapy. It is important, however, to be aware of the fact that the commercially available dialysate solutions for both hemodialysis and peritoneal dialysis are prepared primarily for the treatment of renal failure and may not be ideally suited for the treatment of other disease states. The overwhelming dominance of renal failure as an indication for dialysis seems to have deterred systematic evaluation of other potential applications of dialysis techniques. It is entirely possible that the future will see the development of several new dialysate compositions optimally designed for specific use in an increasing number of clinical conditions.

Acute renal failure can be managed medically without the use of dialysis (see Chap. 15), and it has yet to be convincingly demonstrated that dialysis improves the prognosis of all patients with this disorder. Nevertheless, dialysis greatly simplifies the management of these patients, generally improves patient comfort, facilitates the maintenance of better nutritional and clinical status, reduces the risk of infection, and unequivocally permits the survival of selected patients who because of prolonged oliguria, marked catabolic stimuli, or complicating systemic disorders would rarely recover without dialysis. Mortality in patients with acute renal failure treated by dialysis is generally due to complications of the precipitating disorder rather than to uremic complications.

There are varying criteria used to determine when in the patient's course dialysis should be instituted. Some elect to dialyze only for the control of uremic symptomatolgy; others choose an arbitrary BUN concentration, generally in the range of 100 mg/dL. Teschan et al. (28) have advocated a program of "prophylactic" daily hemodialysis for the purpose of permitting suitable patients liberal food and fluid intake and, if their condition permits, full ambulation. This regimen is designed to maintain optimal patient comfort and nutrition and to minimize the risks of uremia, such as infection and bleeding. It is our present practice to perform frequent dialyses in patients with acute renal failure, usually every 1 to 3 days, as determined by individual need and clinical circumstances.

The management of *chronic renal failure* has been revolutionized by the advent of dialysis techniques. The foremost indication for dialysis in this group is to sustain life and provide functional rehabilitation to the patient with terminal renal failure. This has been successfully achieved by the application of chronic maintenance hemodialysis techniques. Theoretically, such therapy is of potential benefit to any patient with terminal renal failure. In the past, the high cost of treatment and limitations in available facilities and trained personnel restricted its use to only a fraction of those patients in need. Various dialysis centers attempted to establish criteria for selection of patients. Statistically it was apparent that factors such as advanced age, the coexistence of complicating systemic diseases (such as sympto-

matic atherosclerosis, diabetes mellitus, malignant tumors, and systemic lupus erythematosus), psychologic instability and poor motivation, malnutrition, chronic active hepatitis (especially with ascites), and advanced uremic polyneuropathy were poor prognostic signs for either prolonged survival or successful rehabilitation. However, individual exceptions in each of these poor prognostic categories were not uncommon, and since the alternative to therapy is certain death from uremia, it often became morally and ethically difficult to refuse treatment to such patients. With financial restraints minimized by private and governmental insurance program support and with increasing availability of dialysis therapy, the majority of patients in need are now receiving treatment. The resulting increased experience with patients in these poorer prognostic categories has revealed that significant percentages of such patients are capable of doing well and currently there are few valid contraindications to chronic dialysis other than advanced malignant disease.

A variety of criteria have been suggested to ascertain the ideal time to begin chronic dialysis therapy. These include a serum creatinine concentration in excess of 10 mg/dL, creatinine clearance of less than 2 to 10 mL/min, and urine volume of less than 1000 to 1500 mL/day. It seems more reasonable, however, to utilize functional criteria and to begin chronic hemodialysis when, after maximal medical management has been accomplished and all potential reversible aspects of uremia have been considered and corrected, the patient's clinical condition and functional capacity remain worse than those which an experienced physician can anticipate achieving with dialysis therapy. Certain complications of uremia, particularly neuropathy and pericarditis, warrant prompt institution of dialysis. Symptomatic peripheral neuropathy can sometimes be avoided by serially following nerve conduction times and instituting adequate dialysis therapy when early evidence of progressive impairment occurs (29). Optimally, chronic therapy should be instituted before the ravages of symptomatic uremia have resulted in nutritional deficiency or organ damage. Dialysis may also be indicated in patients with compensated chronic renal insufficiency who develop transient deterioration of renal function due to superimposition of reversible processes, such as acute infection, congestive heart failure, or plasma volume depletion. In certain patients presenting with life-threatening uremia, it is impossible to determine from immediately available clinical data whether a potential for reversibility of the underlying parenchymal renal disease exists. In such patients dialysis is indicated to sustain and improve the patient while necessary diagnostic studies are obtained and a definitive therapeutic program established.

Dialysis is of great value in the support of patients undergoing *renal transplantation,* permitting maintenance of the patient during the stage of preparing for the transplant, achieving an optimal preoperative clinical state, sustaining the patient through periods of postoperative oliguria, and providing an alternative form of long-term therapy if the transplant should ultimately fail.

In addition to its proved value in the treatment of renal failure, dialysis is of potential value in the treatment of other clinical conditions, the manifestations of which relate to the presence of a dialyzable toxin of either endogenous or exogenous origin. Maher and Schreiner (18) have cited the following criteria for determining the applicability of dialysis for the treatment of exogenous poisonings: (1) the toxin should diffuse through a dialysis membrane at a reasonable rate, (2) a significant quantity of the poison should be in plasma water or rapidly equilibrate with it, (3) the intoxication should be directly related to the blood concentration, and (4) the amount of poison dialyzed must significantly add to the normal mechanisms for disposal of the toxin. It is apparent that the same or similar criteria relate to endogenous toxins. Accordingly, dialysis therapy has been utilized in the treatment of acute hepatic failure with ammonia intoxication and treatment of hyperuricemia. Clinical experience has been limited, however, and inadequate for making definitive recommendations regarding the ultimate role of dialysis in the management of these conditions. *Hepatic coma* and *ammonia intoxication* have been reported to exhibit at least transient improvement following either hemodialysis (30) or peritoneal dialysis (31). Ammonia

dialysance as high as 50 to 80 mL/min can be achieved with hemodialysis (32) and reduction in blood ammonia concentration obtained. However, both direct and indirect bilirubin are poorly dialyzed with dialysances during hemodialysis of 6.4 and 9.5 mL/min, respectively (18). Clearance of bilirubin with peritoneal dialysis is a mere 0.5 mL/min, with an increase to 1.0 mL/min obtained by the addition of albumin to the dialysate (33). The syndromes of acute hepatic failure and hepatic coma are complex and multifactorial and may in some patients have significant components which are not amenable to dialytic therapy.

Uric acid is dialyzable, and in a few reported cases dialysis has been successfully utilized for the treatment of chronic *tophaceous gout* (34) and of acute *hyperuricemia* following therapy of leukemia or lymphoma (35).

With the exception of renal failure, *exogenous poisonings* constitute the most common indication for dialysis. Table 17-4 presents a list of known dialyzable poisons, as compiled by Maher and Schreiner (18). It should be noted, however, that although the use of dialysis in the treatment of severe poisonings is advocated by some, others have demonstrated very high recovery rates with meticulous medical management without dialysis, at least in patients with barbiturate poisoning (36). Dialysis is unequivocally indicated in those poisonings in which there is a direct tissue toxicity which can be reduced by augmenting the rate and quantity of drug removal. It may also be of value in the treatment of poisonings which are associated with reversible biochemical abnormalities, such as the severe acidosis associated with salicylate, methanol, ethylene glycol, and paraldehyde poisoning.

Many toxins can be effectively and rapidly removed by hemoperfusion directly through a column of ion-exchange resin (37) or other adsorbents, particularly charcoal (38). These early attempts at application of hemoperfusion techniques were complicated by adverse effects upon the formed elements and proteins of blood. These side effects, however, have been minimized by currently commercially available hemoperfusion systems which utilize Amberlite compounds (39), coated activated carbon (40, 41) or fixed beds of

Table 17-4. Currently known dialyzable poisons

Barbiturates*	Alcohols	Metals	Miscellaneous substances
Barbital	Ethanol*	Arsenic	Thiocyanate*
Phenobarbital	Methanol*	Copper	Aniline
Amobarbitol	Isopropanol	Calcium	Sodium chlorate
Pentobarbital	Ethylene glycol	Iron	Potassium chlorate
Butabarbital	Analgesics	Lead	Eucalyptus oil
Secobarbital	Acetylsalicylic acid*	Lithium	Boric acid
Cyclobarbital	Methylsalicylate*	Magnesium	Potassium dichromate
Glutethimide*	Acetophenetidin	Mercury	Chromic acid
Depressants, sedatives, and	Dextropropoxyphene	Potassium	Digoxin
tranquilizers	Paracetamol	Sodium	Sodium citrate
Diphenylhydantoin	Antibiotics	Strontium	Dinitroorthocresol
Primidone	Streptomycin	Halides	*Amanita phalloides*
Meprobamate	Kanamycin	Bromide*	Carbon tetrachloride
Ethchlorvynol*	Neomycin	Chloride*	Ergotamine
Ethinamate	Vancomycin	Iodide	Cyclophosphamide
Methyprylon	Penicillin	Fluoride	5-Fluorouracil
Diphenhydramine	Ampicillin	Endogenous toxins	Methotrexate
Methaqualone	Sulfonamides	Ammonia	Camphor
Heroin	Cephalin	Uric acid*	Trichlorethylene
Gallamine triethiodide	Cephaloridine	Tritium*	Carbon monoxide
Paraldehyde	Chloramphenicol	Bilirubin	Chlorpropamide
Chloral hydrate	Tetracycline	Lactic acid	
Chlordiazepoxide	Nitrofurantoin	Schizophrenia	
Antidepressants	Polymyxin	Myasthenia gravis	
Amphetamine	Isoniazid	Porphyria	
Methamphetamine	Cycloserine	Cystine	
Tricyclic secondary amines	Quinine	Endotoxin	
Tricyclic tertiary amines		Hyperosmolar state*	
Monamine oxidase inhibitors		Water intoxication	
Tranylcypromine			
Pargyline			
Phenelzine			
Isocarboxazid			

* Kinetics of dialysis thoroughly studied and/or clinical experience extensive.
Source: Taken from Maher and Schreiner (18)

activated carbon (42). Experience with these devices is still limited, but it seems clear that hemoperfusion is destined to become the treatment of choice in poisonings with agents amenable to adsorption. Table 17-5 lists those toxins currently known to be adsorbable.

Since the electrolyte composition of dialysate is designed to approximate idealized potassium-free extracellular fluid, it is potentially capable of correcting a variety of fluid and electrolyte abnormalities. *Hyperkalemia* and *hypermagnesemia* occur almost solely in conjunction with oliguria and renal insufficiency and are effectively and ef-

ficiently corrected by dialysis (see Chaps. 4 and 19). *Hypercalcemia* of any cause can at least temporarily be corrected by dialysis (43, 44) but will recur unless the underlying cause of hypercalcemia is corrected or other forms of therapy are instituted (see Chaps. 10 and 11). Dialysis is also indicated in the treatment of the rare case of *hypernatremia* due to accidental salt poisoning (45). In rare instances of severe, symptomatic *hyponatremia* in diuretic-resistant patients with sodium and water excess, dialysis may be required as emergency therapy. Hypernatremia due to water depletion and hyponatremia associated with so-

Table 17-5. Currently known adsorbable poisons

Hypnotic drugs	Endogenous toxins
Barbiturates	Ammonia
Ethchlorvynol	"Middle molecules"
Glutethemide	Analgesics
Methyprylon	Acetylsalicylic acid
Methaqualone	Methyl salicylate
Meprobamate	Acetaminophen (paracetamol)
Others	
Amanita phalloides	
Atropine	
Demeton-S-methyl sulfoxide	
Dimethoate	
Paraquat	
Digoxin	
Morphine	
Benzodiazepines	

Source: After Winchester, Gelfand, Knepshield, and Schreiner.

dium depletion can generally be satisfactorily managed by intravenous fluid therapy and rarely if ever require consideration of dialysis therapy (see Chaps. 3 and 11). Dialytic correction of such abnormalities of serum electrolyte concentrations may at times require preparation of special dialysate solutions tailored specifically to enhance such correction. The low dialysate volume and electrolyte adsorption capacity of the REDY sorbent-based dialysate regeneration system (see below) makes it uniquely suited for modification of dialysate electrolyte composition (46).

Metabolic acidosis due to renal insufficiency and/or the ingestion of acidifying salts or drugs responds well to dialysis. Most dialyzing solutions contain bicarbonate precursor, in the form of either acetate or lactate in concentrations of 30 to 35 meq/L in hemodialysis solutions and 45 meq/L in peritoneal dialysis solutions, and therefore have an alkalinizing effect. Rarely, impaired peripheral or hepatic metabolic function fails to convert the precursor to bicarbonate, and acidosis may therefore not improve. Improvement in *lactic acidosis* has been reported with dialysis (47, 48) but may require the addition of supplemental sodium bicarbonate to the dialyzing solutions.

Surprisingly, although ultrafiltration during hemodialysis and the use of hyperosmolar dialysate in peritoneal dialysis have the capacity to induce rapid and marked negative fluid balance, dialysis has only rarely been used in the treatment of *congestive heart failure* and other edematous states (49, 50) such as *nephrosis* and *cirrhosis*. The ability to treat congestive heart failure and overhydration effectively has been repeatedly demonstrated in patients undergoing dialysis for renal failure. Presently available potent diuretics such as ethacrynic acid and furosemide have reduced the incidence of refractory heart failure and edema. Nevertheless, dialysis should be considered in the management of the rare cases of acute pulmonary edema, heart failure and edema, unresponsive to medical management, or in those cases where impending surgical treatment requires rapid, predictable negative fluid balance. An increased responsiveness to oral diuretic therapy has been noted after dialysis (50).

Individual reports have cited improvement with dialysis in *schizophrenia* and *myasthenia gravis* (51), *porphyria* (52), and *endotoxic shock* (53). Recent reports have confirmed the potential value of dialysis in the treatment of schizophrenia (54) and presented preliminary evidence of efficacy in psoriasis (55). Thus, a variety of diseases, the manifestations of which are known to relate to circulating dialyzable metabolites or toxins or suspected of doing so, may be potentially benefited by dialysis. The value of dialysis, perhaps using specially prepared dialyzing solutions, in the treatment of diabetic ketoacidosis, cystinosis, oxalosis, and other similar metabolic disorders has yet to be evaluated.

Peritoneal dialysis has been used to achieve rewarming in severe *hypothermia* (56). In those instances where intravenous therapy is not feasible due to such factors as poor veins or extensive burns of the extremities or in small infants, it is possible to administer *blood* (57) and certain *hypotonic solutions* (58) via the peritoneal cavity.

In the treatment of nonuremic patients with peritoneal dialysis it is important to be cognizant of the fact that the commercial dialysis solutions designed for use in renal failure may have undesirable side effects which must be compensated for by ancillary therapy. The minimal available osmolality is 372 mosm/L (1.5% dextrose solution), which is essentially isotonic in the uremic patient but is hypertonic in the nonuremic patient. This will result in negative salt and water balance, and if this is not desirable, salt and water must be replaced by appropriate fluids given orally or intravenously. It would be preferable to have isotonic or minimally hypertonic dialyzing solutions for the treatment of such patients. The calcium concentration of 3.5 to 4.0 meq/L is higher than the normal serum ionized calcium concentration and results in dialysis of calcium into the patient. This may be desirable for the acute treatment of the uremic patient who generally has hypocalcemia but may be hazardous if dialysis is performed for the treatment of congestive heart failure in a digitalized patient. Adequate potassium must also be added to prevent producing hypokalemia and precipitating or worsening digitalis intoxication. The high lactate or acetate concentration of 45 meq/L designed to correct the acidosis of renal failure may cause metabolic alkalosis in the nonuremic patient. It would seem desirable to have a variety of peritoneal dialyzing solutions, much as there are a variety of solutions for intravenous administration, each designed for the treatment of specific disorders. Presumably this will have to await the more widespread use of peritoneal dialysis in the treatment of nonuremic diseases.

Hemodialysis solutions are usually isosmolar or minimally hypoosmolar (negative fluid balance is achieved by ultrafiltration rather than by osmosis), have lower calcium and acetate concentrations, and generally do not require modification for the treatment of nonuremic states other than the selection of desirable potassium concentrations.

CONTRAINDICATIONS TO DIALYSIS

There are no true absolute contraindications to dialysis. Relative contraindications to hemodialysis are bleeding and hypotension. Localized intraperitoneal infection, loss of integrity of the peritoneum (especially the posterior peritoneum), abdominal drains, fistulae, or incompletely sutured wounds and extensive intra-abdominal adhesions constitute relative contraindications to peritoneal dialysis. Recent digitalis administration and/or digitalis intoxication are relative contraindications to either type of dialysis. The hypocal-

cemia and/or hyperkalemia which may be present in the uremic patient may mask evidence of digitalis intoxication; as these abnormalities, as well as hyponatremia and acidosis, are corrected by dialysis, digitalis effect may be enhanced and digitalis intoxication precipitated (59) or worsened with resultant severe arrhythmias which may prove fatal. Administration of digitalis to patients likely to require dialysis should be avoided unless absolutely indicated.

Perhaps the major contraindication to dialysis is lack of adequate experience on the part of the treatment team. The actual techniques of hemodialysis or peritoneal dialysis are relatively simple, but the nuances of therapy and the anticipation and management of complications of either dialysis or the underlying disease often require appreciable experience and expertise.

In the remainder of this chapter hemodialysis and peritoneal dialysis will be considered separately, with special emphasis on fluid and electrolyte aspects of each technique.

HEMODIALYSIS

Hemodialysis as a therapeutic modality has proved to be a successful means of maintaining life in patients with otherwise terminal renal failure. However, complications such as disequilibrium states, anemia, bleeding diatheses, neuropathy, pericarditis, hypertension, pseudogout, pruritus, metabolic bone disease, and metastatic calcification attest to the fact that artificial kidney treatment is at best an imperfect substitute for normal kidney function.

GENERAL PRINCIPLES

It is generally understood but rarely expressed that the term "artificial kidney," when applied to currently available hemodialyzers, is actually a misnomer. The normal kidney functions continuously and combines the process of glomerular filtration with tubular resorption and secretion to maintain the constancy of the composition of body fluids. In addition, the normal kidney has endocrine functions, secreting the hormones renin, erythropoietin, prostaglandin, and possibly others. Both renal excretory and endocrine functions are responsive to a variety of feedback systems (renin-angiotensin-aldosterone; parathyroid hormone-calcium-phosphorus-bone; third factor; antidiuretic hormone, etc.). Metabolic conversions of certain hormones including insulin, glucagon, gastrin, and vitamin D occur in the normal kidney. In contrast, the artificial kidney functions intermittently and is limited to the processes of diffusion, osmosis, and ultrafiltration. Obviously endocrine and metabolic function is lacking, and physiologic feedback systems do not exist. Furthermore, the available dialysis membranes used in artificial kidneys are not ideal and limit both the efficiency of hemodialysis and the nature of the solutes which can be dialyzed (see below).

The term *hemodialyzer* is therefore more precise than artificial kidney and denotes a dialysis system in which one of the solutions is whole blood; the other solution is specifically designed to approximate the composition of idealized extracellular fluid, modified slightly to enhance correction of the common fluid and electrolyte abnormalities of uremia (see below). Utilizing a suitable semipermeable synthetic dialyzing membrane (cellophane or its derivatives, polyacrylonitriles, or polycarbonates) and appropriate operational parameters (dialysate and blood flow rates and hydrostatic pressure gradients), the dialysis processes of differential diffusion along chemical and osmolar concentration gradients and ultrafiltration are capable of effecting (1) the removal of dialyzable solutes from serum, (2) the correction of electrolyte and acid-base abnormalities, and (3) the removal of significant volumes of body water. These functions, although limited when compared to normal kidney function, are capable in most instances of preventing death and disability from uremia and its complications.

The mathematical complexities of hemodialyzer kinetics (60, 61) are beyond the scope of this chapter. Basically, a hemodialyzer is a device in which solutes and water exchange between one moving solution (blood) and another (dialysate) across a semipermeable dialyzing membrane, the chemical concentration gradient between the so-

lutions providing the driving force for the movement of solutes, and osmotic or hydrostatic pressure gradients determining water movement, with additional significant effects upon solute movement (convective transport) by solvent drag effect (see Chap. 1). Hemodialyzer performance can be expressed by the dialysance formula (62)

$$\text{Dialysance} = \frac{Q_B(A - V)}{A - D}$$

where Q_B = blood flow rate through the hemodialyzer
A = concentration of solute in blood entering dialyzer
V = concentration of solute in blood leaving dialyzer
D = concentration of solute in dialysate

The term $Q_B(A - V)$ is a measure of the *mass transfer rate* for the solute, i.e., the amount removed from the blood in a given period of time. The term $A - D$ expresses the concentration gradient for the solute between blood and dialysate. If D can be kept at or near zero as it is in single-pass dialysate flow systems, then it can be eliminated from the formula, and the expression for dialysance becomes

$$\text{Dialysance} = \frac{Q_B(A - V)}{A}$$

The similarity to the clearance formula used to express the functional capacity of the human kidney for excretion of any given solute is apparent.

$$\text{Clearance} = \frac{UV}{P}$$

where UV = total amount of solute excreted, i.e., removed from the blood, in a given period of time = mass transfer rate
P = serum concentration of solute = A

Clearance thus serves as a measure of the capacity of a kidney, human or artificial, to transfer a given quantity of solute from the blood. Dialysance is a term used to express the same function in a system where a significant concentration of the solute exists in the dialysate. This lowers the chemical concentration gradient and thereby reduces the mass transfer rate, but the dialysance formula, by correcting for the concentration of the solute in the dialysate, permits assessment of the actual functional capacity of the hemodialyzer.

Dialysance and/or clearance formulas are clinically simple and useful means of assessing dialyzer performance but consider only the factors of blood flow rate, mass transfer rates, and concentration gradients. They fail to take into consideration a variety of factors which modify dialyzer performance and determine dialyzer efficiency. These include membrane properties, functional surface area of the hemodialyzer, and blood and dialysate flow characteristics. These characteristics become important considerations in optimization of dialyzer design and functional parameters (60, 61).

THE DIALYZING MEMBRANE

Abel et al. (63) used collodion tubes as the dialyzing membrane in the first artificial kidney. Biologic tissues, including intestinal and peritoneal membranes, were used by Love (64) and Necheles (65) in early artificial kidneys. In 1937, Thalheimer (66) was the first to use cellophane, and Kolff (67) selected this as the dialyzing membrane in the first clinically effective hemodialyzers. Despite extensive research subsequently in the development of improved membranes, including evaluation of collagen (68) and synthetic polymers (69), cellulosic membranes remain the membranes of choice in most presently used hemodialysis systems. Recent theoretic and probably practical considerations relative to potential benefits to be derived from the use of membranes with enhanced hydraulic permeability and transport characteristics for solutes of middle-molecular-weight configuration (70, 71) has led to the development and clinical use of thinner (and thereby more permeable) cuprophan membranes, "high-flux" polyacrylonitrile membranes (72, 73), and polycarbonate membranes (74). Clinically suitable dialysis membranes must be nontoxic, easily manufactured and readily available, inexpensive, sterilizable, resistant to tearing when handled or subjected to the pressures required for ultrafiltration, and must permit the effective movement of uremic solutes and water by differential diffusion and ultrafiltration.

Theoretically, the maximal achievable dialysance in a hemodialysis system is equal to the blood flow rate. For any given blood flow rate in a system which maintains optimal solute concentration gradients, the major resistance to mass transfer of solute is offered by the dialyzing membrane and its interfaces with both dialysate and with blood. Presently available clinical hemodialysis systems approach the attainment of maximal blood/dialysate concentration gradients by the use of single-pass dialysate flow systems, by combinations of single-pass and recirculation dialysate flow or by adsorption of dialyzed uremic solutes from a low-volume recirculating dialysate system. Therefore, the failure to attain optimal dialysance relates primarily to the dialyzing membrane and related features of dialyzer design.

The total membrane area of various clinical hemodialyzers varies from approximately 7600 to 25,000 cm², comparing favorably to the estimated 7600 cm² filtering area of the human kidney. Not all of this, however, is effective dialyzing area. In a coil-type hemodialyzer in which the blood passes through tubular channels or in a parallel-flow hemodialyzer in which blood flows through a rectangular "envelope," there are areas of "dead space" where there is poor blood and/or dialysate flow. By proper design of channel geometry and membrane-supporting structures, such dead space can be minimized, and optimal blood film thickness can be approached. Nevertheless, effective dialyzing area remains less than the actual physical area of the dialyzing membrane. This partially accounts for the fact that dialyzer function as quantitated by the actual mass transfer of solutes is less than one would anticipate from calculations based upon theoretical dialyzer kinetic data. In addition, during the course of dialysis, plasma proteins, particularly fibrinogen, and formed elements of blood may coat the membrane and gradually and progressively impair mass transfer by reducing effective dialyzing area.

More important, however, in preventing the attainment of maximal dialysance are the properties of the membrane itself, which offers a certain resistance to the passage of solute and water across it. This membrane resistance is dependent upon its permeability and relates primarily to the thickness of the membrane and its pore size. In addition to membrane resistance, both dialysate and blood offer resistance to solute transfer at their respective interfaces with the membrane. Thus, at any given blood flow rate, the mass transfer rate $[Q_B(A - V)]$ will be dependent upon the sum of the resistances to solute transport offered by the membrane and its dialysate and blood interfaces. By optimizing dialyzer design and geometry and maximizing dialysate and blood flow rates, blood and dialysate resistances to transfer of low-molecular-weight solutes can be minimized, and in modern dialyzers urea clearances can be achieved which approximate the blood flow rate through the dialyzer.

However, the membrane resistance remains a significant limiting factor to the transfer of less permeable solutes and particularly to those with molecular weights in excess of 200 daltons. For cuprophan, clinically the most commonly used cellulosic membrane, diffusive permeability decreases as solute molecular weight increases (75).

The thickness of the cellulosic membranes in clinical hemodialyzers is greater than optimal for maximal mass transfer, but a compromise is required to permit the membranes to maintain adequate tensile strength for the purpose of tolerating the pressure gradients necessary to permit required ultrafiltration rates. The pore size of these membranes is appreciably less than the apparent functional pore size of the glomerular membrane. The glomerular membrane permits filtration of solutes with molecular weights of at least 5200 (inulin) and possibly as high as 55,000. Although most known uremic metabolites and potential toxins have molecular weights below 200 daltons, it is possible that certain unidentified "middle molecules" with higher molecular weights are poorly dialyzed and may contribute to certain of the defects which complicate the course of patients on maintenance hemodialysis, e.g., neuropathy, anemia, and bleeding diathesis (76). There is some evidence that these middle molecules are dialyzed more effectively by peritoneal dialysis techniques than they are by hemodialysis

(25, 77). This membrane resistance to the mass transfer of solutes of middle-molecular-weight configuration has been reduced by the development of thinner cuprophan membranes or membranes with enhanced hydraulic and/or diffusive permeability. With polycarbonate (74) and polymethylmethacrylate (78) membranes, clearances for solutes in the molecular weight range of vitamin B_{12} (1355 daltons) and inulin (5200 daltons) are attainable which are twofold to fivefold greater than achieved with cuprophan membranes. Utilizing high-flux membranes with very high hydraulic permeability for the technique of hemodiafiltration (see below), transport characteristics for these higher-molecular-weight species approach those of urea (70, 71, 73). Augmentation of middle-molecular-weight solute transfer has also been achieved by the use of hemodialyzers with surface areas as large as 2.5 m².

THE DIALYSATE

The composition of commercially available dialysate is indicated in Table 17-6. Variations in hemodialysate composition are generally minor and basically the solution is designed to approximate the ionic composition of normal extracellular fluid, modified slightly to provide optimal correction of the common fluid and electrolyte disorders which accompany acute and chronic uremia. It is primarily an electrolyte solution; the only nonelectrolyte solute is glucose. In peritoneal dialysis solutions (see below), a high glucose concentration of the dialysate is used to create an osmotic concentration gradient, thereby providing a means of obtaining negative fluid balance. In hemodialysis, negative fluid balance is achieved pri-

Table 17-6. Hemodialysate composition

Na⁺	132 meq/L
K⁺	0–1 meq/L
Mg²⁺	1.5 meq/L
Ca²⁺	3.25 meq/L
Acetate	33 meq/L
Cl⁻	103–104 meq/L
Dextrose (glucose)	0–200 mg/dL
Osmolality	272–284 mosm/L

marily by ultrafiltration induced by hydrostatic pressure gradients. The absence of other solutes provides for the maximal removal of uremic metabolic waste metabolites such as urea, creatinine, uric acid, and phosphate. A relatively high concentration of bicarbonate precursor is provided to correct the metabolic acidosis which usually attends the uremic state.

Initially, when the use of dialysis was largely restricted to patients with acute renal failure, the sodium, chloride, calcium, and magnesium concentrations of dialysate were designed to approximate those of normal plasma. Diffusion along concentration gradients would tend to bring the patient's serum concentration of these electrolytes to normal. Hyperkalemia was a common problem in patients undergoing acute dialysis; potassium was eliminated from the dialyzing solutions, but could be added in desired concentrations, thereby permitting individualization according to the patient's needs. Since hypocalcemia was also common in these patients, a dialysate calcium concentration of 4 meq/L was chosen. This concentration is slightly higher than the normal *ionized* serum calcium concentration, and accordingly calcium would be dialyzed into the patient. Gross abnormalities in serum magnesium concentration are not common in the uremic patient, but the dialysate concentration of 1.5 meq/L assured correction of any abnormalities which might exist.

As experience in dialysis increased, and particularly when repetitive dialysis became feasible and widely used, it became apparent that these idealized electrolyte concentrations, although physiologically sound in concept for the treatment of acute renal decompensation, required modification when applied to patients undergoing regular, repetitive maintenance therapy.

SODIUM, CHLORIDE, AND OSMOLALITY

The *sodium concentration* of most hemodialysis solutions is slightly low in sodium (130 to 135 meq/L) when compared to the normal serum sodium concentration. The dialysate chloride concentration averages 103 meq/L, equivalent to a normal serum chloride concentration but relatively high compared to the dialysate sodium concentration. This *chloride* concentration is required to achieve electroneutrality of the hemodialysate. The only anions present are acetate and chloride. The concentration of acetate used is limited; therefore a chloride concentration which may be slightly higher than desirable is used. Fortunately, this does not appear to result in any significant clinical disturbances. It should be recognized however that little is known regarding the clinical significance of abnormalities in serum or total body chloride stores. The *osmolality* of hemodialysate is 265 to 280 mosm/L, equivalent to a level distinctly hypoosmolar to the osmolality of the serum of the uremic subject. The relatively low dialysate osmolality tends to result in the movement of water along osmolar gradients from the dialysate into the patient. In addition, the presence of plasma proteins in blood but not in dialysate results in an oncotic pressure gradient which also tends to move water from dialysate into the patient. These factors, however, are counterbalanced by the hydrostatic pressure required to propel blood through the hemodialyzer. These opposing forces for water movement tend to nullify one another. When desired, movement of water from the patient to the hemodialysate is effected by creating a hydrostatic pressure gradient from blood to dialysate.

Most commonly, the patient with oliguric renal failure, whether acute or chronic, presents with hyponatremia. Depending upon the appropriateness of the patient's medical management, his cooperation in adhering to required sodium and water restriction, and the presence or absence of significant extrarenal salt and water losses, the hyponatremia may result from a variety of combinations of salt and water excesses or deficits (see Chaps. 3 and 11), but usually is due to water excess with or without accompanying lesser degrees of sodium excess. Since hemodialysis therapy is intermittent rather than continuous, all sodium and water ingested in the interdialytic period in excess of the small amounts lost in residual urine volumes and by insensible losses will be retained. Therefore, total body sodium and water content is largely dependent upon the patient's ability to restrict intake between dialyses. Adherence to these restrictions is difficult and variable. Water excess will manifest itself as hyponatremia and weight gain; sodium excess will generally result in hypertension and/or edema. These clinical findings, i.e., weight gain, edema, hypertension, and hyponatremia, serve as indices of the total body water and sodium stores and the degree of patient cooperation in conforming with imposed restrictions. It becomes a requisite of intermittent dialysis therapy that these abnormalities be corrected during each dialysis.

The use of a dialysate sodium concentration lower than normal serum sodium concentration dates to the early days of dialysis when knowledge of dialysis kinetics, mechanisms of hypertension, and hypertension control was limited. The presumptive purpose was to create a concentration gradient for sodium, thereby enhancing diffusive transport of sodium out of the patient. Currently, necessary sodium removal is achieved primarily and probably adequately by the convective transport which attends ultrafiltration, and the need for and desirability of a hyponatric dialysate has been appropriately questioned. Stewart et al. (79, 80), using a dialysate sodium concentration of 145 meq/L, have demonstrated a lessening of intradialytic symptoms such as leg cramps and nausea without a sacrifice in the ability to achieve blood pressure control by appropriate ultrafiltration and maintenance of dry weight. It is very likely inertia rather than scientific and clinical proof or merit which perpetuates the use of low sodium concentration dialysate. The successful treatment of leg cramps with hypertonic saline (81) perhaps lends further credence to these concepts. Choice of dialysate sodium concentration must be made with due consideration given to the sodium content of local water supplies and the effects of various water treatment techniques on sodium content.

Ultrafiltration is produced by exerting a blood-to-dialysate hydrostatic pressure gradient, either by increasing the pressure within the blood compartment (positive pressure, used in coil or high-resistance artificial kidneys) or by exerting a vacuum effect in the dialysate compartment (nega-

tive pressure used in passive-flow, low-resistance artificial kidneys). Except in rare patients with residual urine volumes in excess of 500 mL/day who adhere strictly to the imposed restrictions in the intake of sodium and water, some degree of ultrafiltration is uniformly required to remove excesses of body sodium and water accumulated in the interdialytic period.

The attainable rate of ultrafiltration varies with the type of hemodialyzer employed and is dependent upon such factors as hydrostatic pressure gradient, effective dialyzing surface area, and membrane permeability (82). Ultrafiltration requirements are determined by the individual patient's need as assessed by interdialytic weight gain and the presence or absence of edema and hypertension. The goal is to maintain total-body sodium and water composition as near normal as possible. Although it is possible to reasonably predict the ultrafiltration for a given dialyzer (83, 84), the limiting factor in ultrafiltration is more often the patient rather than the dialyzer ultrafiltration capacity. For reasons as yet not clearly defined, certain patients seem extraordinarily intolerant to ultrafiltration, whereas others respond with remarkable ease.

Certain patients, even in the presence of objective evidence of gross sodium and water excess (edema and hypertension), respond to attempts at ultrafiltration by the development of significant and symptomatic hypotension requiring the discontinuation of ultrafiltration and the infusion of volume expanders. Hypoalbuminemic patients seem particularly prone to the development of ultrafiltration-induced hypotension, which, however, can often be counteracted by the infusion of salt-poor albumin. Infusions of significant volumes of saline solution counteract the intended purposes of ultrafiltration. In addition to hypovolemia, ultrafiltration seems capable of inducing symptoms such as leg cramps (81), headache, paresthesias, and other symptoms suggestive of dialysis disequilibrium (see below), which when severe can also limit the capacity to achieve adequate ultrafiltration. More important is the ability of any given patient to tolerate the acute loss of plasma volume induced by ultrafiltration. The ultrafiltrate has been shown to have an electrolyte composition similar or identical to that of plasma water, although at high ultrafiltration rates water removal rate slightly exceeds that of any solute movement (85, 86). The effects of ultrafiltration can therefore be considered as an acute depletion of plasma volume. The ability of any given patient to withstand such acute plasma volume depletion will depend upon such factors as the effective plasma volume at the start of dialysis, the capacity of fluid to move from the interstitial and intracellular fluid compartment into the plasma compartments, and the ability of the patient's cardiovascular system to respond with appropriate physiologic responses to the stimulus of acute volume depletion.

Recently various investigators have made the observations that, even in patients ordinarily intolerant to ultrafiltration during dialysis, large ultrafiltration volumes could be removed without inducing hypotension, leg cramps or other symptoms, by performing ultrafiltration and dialysis sequentially rather than concurrently (87, 88). With such techniques, the desired degree of ultrafiltration is accomplished before or after the actual dialysis procedure, with no ultrafiltration required during the dialysis phase itself. Using standard dialyzers, as much as 4 L of ultrafiltration can be accomplished in 90 min without inducing untoward symptomatology despite the previously demonstrated inability of a given patient to tolerate even lesser degrees of ultrafiltration during dialysis (89). Bergström et al. (88) and Shinaberger (89) attribute this phenomenon to the fact that ultrafiltration does not alter serum osmolality significantly or, if it has any effect, slightly raises it. Accordingly, as plasma volume falls with ultrafiltration, intracellular fluid can readily move to the extracellular space to support plasma volume. In contrast, when ultrafiltration is carried out during dialysis, the dialysis procedure lowers the serum osmolality by virtue of a fall in the BUN and water movement into the patient from the hyponatric, hypoosmolar dialysate. This fall in serum osmolality not only eliminates the capacity of the intracellular fluid to support the plasma volume but rather results in the movement of plasma and extracellular water into the cells, further augmenting plasma volume deple-

tion with resultant hypotension. Stewart et al. (90) utilize similar reasoning relative to osmotic dynamics between dialysate and serum in their recommendations for the use of higher dialysate sodium concentrations. Similar observations relative to minimizing hypotension and intradialytic symptomatology have been made by those using ultrafiltration (70, 71, 73) rather than dialysis techniques for end-stage renal disease therapy (see below). Others have suggested that dialysis-induced hypotension might relate to the effects of acetate dialyzed into the patient as a buffer precursor (91, 92). All buffers have the capacity to decrease myocardial contractility and vascular reactivity, but these effects are less pronounced with bicarbonate, and the suggestion has been put forth that substitution of bicarbonate for acetate in dialysate might be advantageous for acutely ill patients and those subject to dialysis-induced hypotension (92).

Although effective ultrafiltration can control hypertension in the majority of patients, those with renin-excess-related hypertension may not respond and, additionally, are very susceptible to development of hypotension during dialysis (see below).

It is possible to augment the effects of ultrafiltration by the creation of an osmotic gradient by the addition of high concentrations of glucose to the dialysate (cf. peritoneal dialysis). The *glucose concentration* in most dialysate solutions is 100 to 200 mg/dL. This approximates the usual blood glucose concentration and thereby eliminates any significant diffusion of glucose either into or out of the patient. It also increases the osmolality of dialysate sufficiently to obviate or minimize water movement from dialysate to uremic serum. The presence of glucose in the dialysate has certain disadvantages, notably its support of bacterial growth and its making the simple testing for formalin more difficult. DePalma et al. (93) have demonstrated that glucose can safely be eliminated from dialysate without inducing significant hypoglycemia or osmotic disequilibrium. There is some suggestion that the use of glucose-free dialysate might ameliorate the hypercholesterolemia and, to a lesser degree, the hypertriglyceridemia which attend uremia and dialysis (94).

Others have used high dialysate glucose concentrations (1500 mg/dL or higher) to create an osmotic concentration gradient and augment water and sodium removal during hemodialysis. Figure 17-2 is redrawn from the data of Mendelssohn et al. (95) and demonstrates a linear correlation between ultrafiltrate volumes (negative fluid balance) in milliliters per hour and the dialysate glucose concentration. If the plot is continued to zero glucose concentration in the bath, some 135 mL of ultrafiltrate per hour is still produced which can be explained by the 80 mmHg or more pressure gradient across the Kiil dialyzer used in these studies. Therefore, the ultrafiltration rate is graphed as the rate induced by the hypertonic glucose, corrected for that due to the pressure gradient. Increasing dialysate glucose concentration to 5200 mg/dL increased fluid removal a mere 365 mL/h, a rate readily achieved by hydrostatic pressure gradients alone.

When high dialysate glucose concentrations are employed, glucose dialyzes into the patient and may result in significant hyperglycemia. Although this increases serum osmolality and may offer some protection against cerebral edema (see discussion of delayed urea shift, below, under Dialysis Disequilibrium Syndromes), it has also been implicated in the causation of extreme hyperglycemia, partially due to the impaired glucose tolerance of the uremic patient. Fatal hyperglycemic nonketotic coma (96) as well as postdialysis hypoglycemic convulsions induced by sustained release of insulin with insulin overshoot postdialysis (97) has complicated the use of high glucose concentrations in dialysate. Hypertonic glucose solutions as a method of fluid removal probably have no place in modern hemodialysis techniques, and their use has been virtually abandoned.

Despite the increasing number of diabetics being treated with dialysis now, there are virtually no data about glucose transport phenomena in the diabetic during dialysis. Theoretically, a poorly controlled diabetic is subject to large glucose losses into the dialysate during the course of dialysis, and rapid falls in blood glucose levels are possible. We have seen instances of symptoms of hypoglycemia occurring at times when blood sugars were within normal range, apparently due to rapid falls from marked hyperglycemic levels. It would seem advisable to avoid glucose-free dialysate in diabetics to minimize glucose losses during dialysis and to avoid hypoglycemia. The usual standard glucose concentrations of 100 to 200 mg/dL are probably optimal.

An additional factor affecting extracellular fluid volume and blood pressure is that the hemodialyzer and its blood lines obligate the extracorporeal circulation of a significant quantity of blood in order to conduct effective dialysis. The earliest hemodialyzers had volume capacities ranging from 500 to 1000 mL, and in order to prevent hypotension due to *dialyzer phlebotomy* it was necessary to "prime" the dialyzers with whole blood, i.e., fill most or all of the dialyzer and blood lines with donor blood before instituting dialysis. This required the use of 1 or more units of blood with each dialysis and created a high risk of serum hepatitis, transfusion reaction, and hemosiderosis. Subsequent improvements in design have resulted in reduction of dialyzer volume, and most presently used dialyzers have extracorporeal volumes of less than 250 mL. These permit substitution of water or saline prime or self-prime for the previously required blood prime and obviate the need for the administration of blood except

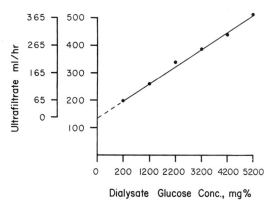

Figure 17-2. Augmentation of the rate of ultrafiltration by increasing the dialysate glucose concentration. The ultrafiltration rate is determined by a combination of hydrostatic and osmotic pressure gradients. The scale on the left represents the ultrafiltration rate produces by the osmotic pressure gradient created by the glucose concentration of the dialysate. (*After Mendelssohn et al.*)

when required for the treatment of symptomatic anemia.

With a water or saline prime, the dialyzer is filled with either 5% dextrose in water or with saline solution which is allowed to infuse into the patient as it is displaced by the patient's blood entering the hemodialyzer. These provide temporary support of plasma volume to counteract the hypotensive effect of dialyzer phlebotomy. With self-priming techniques the priming solutions are discarded as they are displaced by the patient's blood; i.e., there is no replacement of the blood as it moves from the patient to fill the dialyzer. The self-priming technique can be used only in those patients with stable cardiovascular responsiveness to hemodialysis who do not readily develop hypotension with plasma or circulating blood volume depletion. Saline prime offers greater support of the blood pressure than does water but does require additional ultrafiltration to remove the sodium contained in it. In addition to the volume lost in filling the dialyzer, there is an additional volume loss into the dialyzer when ultrafiltration is employed. The pressures required to induce effective ultrafiltration stretch the cellophane compartments and increase their capacity by as much as 400 mL. Thus, the blood compartment has an increase in its volume of whole blood (*dialyzer expansion phlebotomy*). These dialyzer phlebotomy effects tend to reduce whole-blood volume and either themselves induce hypotension or make the patient more susceptible to hypotension during attempts at ultrafiltration. This phenomenon is most pronounced in the coil-type dialyzers and least in the hollow fiber-type dialyzers.

Hypertension is present in the majority of patients presenting for dialysis and most often can be controlled effectively by restoring increased total body sodium stores to normal (98, 99) by means of dietary restriction and ultrafiltration. Both clinical and experimental evidence (100, 102) have suggested that sodium excess may affect arteriolar resistance in a manner which is not immediately reversible by returning total body sodium stores to normal, and it may require weeks at normal levels to achieve normotension. Vertes et al. (103) have described these patients as hav-

ing "saltwater-dependent" hypertension as characterized by the return to normotensive levels with adequate restoration of normal sodium stores over a period of time. The presumptive mechanism for such hypertension suggests that salt and water excess initially evokes hypertension due to a resultant increase in cardiac output. Subsequently, autoregulatory generalized vasoconstriction occurs in response to increased blood flow, restoring tissue perfusion towards normal, decreasing venous return, and thereby reducing cardiac output back towards normal. The hypertension, however, is perpetuated by this adaptive increase in peripheral resistance (104, 105). Correction of the primary salt and water excess state restores peripheral resistance and arterial blood pressure to normal (Fig. 17-3).

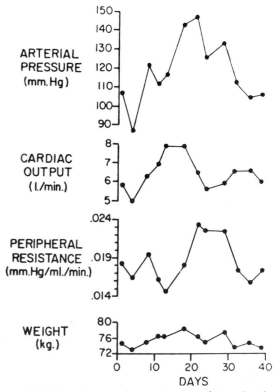

Figure 17-3. Hemodynamic changes in an anephric patient in response to body sodium and water fluctuations (as manifested by changes in body weight). (*From Coleman et al.*)

A second group of hypertensive patients, have been defined (103) comprising 10 to 15 percent of the dialysis population and generally characterized by markedly elevated predialysis peripheral plasma renin levels and resistance to blood pressure control despite frequent dialysis, vigorous ultrafiltration, negative sodium balance, and rigid dietary restriction. Such patients often respond to ultrafiltration by the development of hypotension during dialysis, only to manifest severe hypertension in the interdialytic period, often associated with intractable congestive heart failure, weight loss, progressive neuropathy, marked weakness, and malaise. This syndrome is generally seen in patients with glomerular disease or nephrosclerosis. Bilateral nephrectomy seems invariably to ameliorate the hypertension in these patients and to reverse many of the associated clinical symptoms. We have seen at least seven patients, apparently moribund, make dramatic symptomatic and clinical improvement virtually immediately after bilateral nephrectomy with marked lean body weight gain, improved strength, disappearance of neuropathy and rehabilitation (106). Resolution of intractable ascites has also been described following bilateral nephrectomy (107). Onesti et al. (108) indicated that the improvement in hypertension following nephrectomy resulted from reduction in peripheral resistance, and although they indicated that these patients seemed to be resistant to hypertension after bilateral nephrectomy, we have found them to be sensitive to sodium and volume overload and to manifest hypertension when exhibiting sodium excess.

We prefer to use predialysis blood pressure measurements as the critical index of blood pressure control. Postdialysis blood pressure not only is subject to the effect of pressure-lowering phenomena including dialyzer phlebotomy and ultrafiltration, but may, on occasion, present a paradoxical hypovolemic hypertension. This phenomenon has been described both in nonuremic patients (109) and with dialysis (110), but the mechanisms responsible for it are not clear. Exaggerated renin secretion in response to hypovolemia has been postulated as a possible cause (111).

In summary, most patients who present for di-

alysis with mild to marked hypertension can be controlled by sodium-restricted diet and progressive extracellular fluid volume reduction by ultrafiltration. Persistent hypertension may necessitate the temporary use of antihypertensive drugs. The use of antihypertensives may result in marked hypotension during dialysis and should be avoided unless required by the clinical effects of hypertension. Minimal doses should be used, and the effect of the blood pressure on end organs should be the major criterion for more vigorous treatment in the early months of hemodialysis. If after a suitable period of time severe hypertension persists or if the patient manifests rapid clinical deterioration due to the effects of hypertension, a peripheral renin assay should be obtained, and if it is markedly elevated, bilateral nephrectomy should be considered. Although bilateral nephrectomy almost invariably results in rapid cure or marked amelioration of hypertension and attendant symptomatology, the availability of effective antihypertensive agents permits a therapeutic alternative. Bilateral nephrectomy commits a patient to a marked anemia (hematocrit generally in the range of 15 to 23 volume percent) unresponsive to any currently available hematinic therapy other than transfusion, to anuria which imposes even stricter demands on salt and fluid restriction and eliminates renal excretion of middle molecules and, perhaps, makes a patient more subject to dialysis-induced hypotension (112). Furthermore, resistant high-renin hypertension has been described to ameliorate with time on continuation of maintenance dialysis (113) and, on rare occasions, patients with high-renin hypertension due to arteriolonephrosclerosis recover renal function after periods of 6 months or more on dialysis. The capacity of propranolol to suppress renin activity makes it an effective antihypertensive agent in dialysis patients with high renin levels, and alone, or when used in conjunction with minoxidil, it permits blood pressure control in virtually all such patients (114). Bilateral nephrectomy is probably best reserved for those patients unresponsive to drug therapy. Most patients with renin excess demonstrate a syndrome with manifestations suggestive of impaired perfusion of virtually all organs. The goal of drug therapy should be not only to control blood pressure but to control all evidence of tissue ischemia resulting from high renin activity. If drug therapy controls hypertension but not these other manifestations of the high-renin syndrome, nephrectomy may still be warranted.

The optimal *potassium concentration* of dialysate is variable and dependent on a variety of clinical factors. Generally, dialysate potassium concentrations of 2 meq/L or less are being used for both acute and chronic hemodialysis. Depending upon the predialysis serum potassium concentration, the duration of dialysis, and the efficiency of the hemodialyzer, the amount of potassium removed will vary from 70 to more than 200 meq per dialysis, reflecting loss from both extracellular and intracellular sites. Potassium dialyzes as well as or better than urea, and in the presence of hyperkalemia reductions in the serum potassium concentration of as much as 4.0 meq/L may occur.

Since, in the absence of significant gastrointestinal fluid losses, the excretion of potassium occurs only in the urine, total body potassium excess and/or hyperkalemia is a common accompaniment of acute or chronic oliguric renal failure. Hyperkalemia is a life-threatening abnormality (see Chap. 4), and potassium loads presented in the form of ingested potassium or derived from endogenous sources due to catabolic stimuli, tissue necrosis, or lysis of red blood cells must be removed during dialysis to prevent cardiotoxicity and death from hyperkalemia. Generally it is necessary to restrict rigidly the dietary intake of potassium, limiting it to 1.5 to 2.0 g daily (about 40 to 50 meq). Particular attention must be given to the complete avoidance of foods high in potassium content. Since potassium is ubiquitous, it is virtually impossible to achieve a diet with a content of less than 1.5 to 2 g daily. Assuming satisfactory patient compliance with dietary restrictions, there is an ingestion of a minimum of 280 to 350 meq potassium weekly which must be removed by dialysis in order to prevent hyperkalemia.

We have successfully used potassium-free dialysate (93) in our home dialysis patients for more than 7 years. This permits the patients to have a more liberal dietary potassium intake (60 to 80 meq daily). The average predialysis and postdialysis serum potassium concentrations have been 4.6 and 3.0 meq/L respectively. Johnson et al. (115) using potassium-free dialysate, noted a decrease in the serum potassium concentration postdialysis to as little as 2.7 meq/L but noted a rapid rebound within 3 h to 4 meq/L. We have not noted this rebound effect but rather a gradual increase to predialysis levels.

The possibility of the induction of hypokalemia and/or total body potassium depletion by a combination of dietary potassium restriction and frequent dialysis with low potassium concentration in the dialysate must be considered. Hypokalemia is a risk particularly in those patients with renal failure being treated with hyperalimentation regimens where high caloric intake and other anabolic stimuli result in the movement of potassium into glycogen depots and the intracellular space. Hypotension, fatigue, muscular weakness, myocardial necrosis, and cardiac arrhythmias may occur with potassium depletion. Also, hypokalemia can ultimately limit protein anabolic capacity and obviate the potential beneficial effects of hyperalimentation regimens.

Fine (116) has noted fatigue and hypotension attributed to hypokalemia occurring postdialysis in small children. Postmortem studies in five patients maintained on long-term home hemodialysis with potassium-free dialysate have failed to reveal any evidence of the single-fiber myocardial necrosis seen with experimental hypokalemia (117).

The potential induction of hypokalemia carries a special risk in patients receiving digitalis because of the danger of inducing digitalis intoxication and serious, potentially fatal arrhythmias (14). Similar risks of arrhythmias exist in patients who, although not receiving digitalis, have intrinsic heart or coronary artery disease. It seems best advised to use higher dialysate potassium concentrations in these patients (3 to 5 meq/L, depending upon the individual circumstances). This generally requires the use of individual dialysis systems, since we have found the use of oral potassium supplements or potassium infusions in such patients while they are dialyzed against a low potassium dialysate concentration from a central dialysate supply system to be unsatisfactory.

The reduction in serum potassium concentration may also relate to the glucose concentration of dialysate. If adequate glucose is dialyzed into the patient, glycogen deposition will occur; potassium is incorporated intracellularly during such glycogen deposition in the liver. This results in a lowering of the serum potassium concentration and thereby actually results in a decrease in the amount of extracellular potassium available for removal during the dialysis. Postdialysis glycogenolysis may occur and release the stored potassium back into the extracellular fluid causing rapid rises in serum potassium concentrations. Our studies would suggest that this phenomenon does not occur with the usual dialysate glucose concentrations of 200 mg/dL. It may, however, occur if high glucose concentrations are used in the hemodialysate or during peritoneal dialysis where dialysate glucose concentrations of 1500 to 4500 mg/dL are standard.

Dialysis may also induce respiratory alkalosis and at times metabolic alkalosis (118, 119), which could result in the movement of potassium from extracellular to intracellular sites, thereby also reducing the serum potassium concentrations but not total body potassium content.

The optimal *calcium* and *magnesium concentrations* of hemodialysate remain undefined. Various dialysis centers indicate a preference for calcium concentrations as disparate as 2.5 and 4.0 meq/L. The transfer of calcium and magnesium between dialysate and blood is related primarily to their respective ionic concentrations in each fluid (120, 121). A dialysate calcium concentration of 3 meq/L approximates the normal serum *ionized* calcium concentration (see Chap. 8) and generally will result in no net flux of calcium between dialysate and blood during dialysis in normocalcemic patients (120) and a movement of small quantities of calcium into the blood of hypocalcemic patients. Therefore this represents a satisfactory dialysate calcium concentration for patients undergoing acute hemodialysis. However, patients undergoing maintenance hemodialysis are exposed to the chronic effects of altered para-

thyroid physiology (secondary hyperparathyroidism) and the abnormalities of the calcium and phosphorus metabolism which attend chronic renal failure (see Chaps 9 and 11). The role which repetitive hemodialysis and specifically the dialysate calcium and magnesium concentrations plays in the amelioration or potentiation of these abnormalities remains unclear. The recent availability of parathyroid hormone assay and the intensive research directed at divalent cation metabolism in uremia and chronic dialysis offer hope that the question of optimal dialysate concentrations will soon be resolved. With the use of dialysate calcium concentrations in excess of 3.25 meq/L and simultaneous control of serum phosphate concentration with phosphate-binding antacids, the elevated parathormone levels present in uremia can be markedly reduced and renal osteodystrophy possibly ameliorated (122). Recently, Johnson (123) has recommended a dialysate calcium concentration of 3.5 meq/L, indicating that in chronic dialysis patients this results in normalization of the serum calcium concentration, transfer into the patient of sufficient calcium to balance fecal losses, prevention of loss of calcium from bone, and improvement in renal osteodystrophy.

The precise concentration of *magnesium* in dialysate seems less critical. Stewart et al. (124) have reported that not only is the use of magnesium-free dialysate well tolerated (most uremic subjects have mild degrees of hypermagnesemia) but it may improve neuropathy. The safety of magnesium-free dialysate has recently been confirmed and potential beneficial effects on renal osteodystrophy demonstrated (125). Most centers, however, use dialysate magnesium concentrations approximating 1.5 meq/L, which sustains a mild degree of hypermagnesemia in the patient and has at least the theoretical potential of minimizing the effect of parathyroid hormone on bone and decreasing parathyroid-hormone secretion. Posen and Kaye (126) have indicated that a dialysate magnesium concentration of 1.5 meq/L is without known untoward side effects and possibly is protective against metastatic calcification and neuropathy.

The risk of using significantly higher dialysate

calcium or magnesium concentrations seems clear. Earle et al. (127) indicated that acute hypercalcemia may result in the development of hypertension, and our group has noted that calcium infusions of 15 mg/kg body weight in uremic subjects commonly produce headache, nausea, vomiting, and an acute rise in blood pressure (128). The induction of hypermagnesemia by means of magnesium infusion has been noted to produce flushing, nausea, and hypotension. When dialysate calcium or magnesium concentrations significantly exceed their respective ionized fractions in the serum, then dialysis in effect results in the infusion of these cations into the patient. Drukker (129) described a syndrome manifested by rising blood pressure, nausea, vomiting, malaise, sweating, headache, somnolence, and intense burning of the skin which he termed the *hard water syndrome.* This syndrome has been primarily related to the use of dialysate in which the calcium concentration exceeds 5 meq/L. Although this occasionally may result from improperly prepared dialysate or dialysate concentrate, it most often occurs as the result of the presence of high calcium concentration (hard water) in the local water supply which is used in the preparation of dialysate. Accordingly, in areas where the local water supply is high in calcium or magnesium concentration, it becomes necessary to "treat" the water, either by deionization, water-softening techniques, reverse osmosis, or a combination of these methods. It is also possible to lower the calcium and/or magnesium concentrations in the dry chemicals or chemical concentrates used to mix with water for the preparation of dialysate and thereby allow the water containing these cations to bring the dialysate to desired levels, but this is not preferable to water treatment, since in many areas the divalent cation content of water is highly variable and in certain areas even exceeds the desired dialysate concentrations.

The accidental use of dialysate with a magnesium concentration of 15 meq/L has been reported to have resulted in flushing, muscular weakness, hyperreflexia, ataxia, and blurring of vision (130). Only one of the six exposed patients, however, developed hypotension. Hard water is usually characterized by excessive but variable calcium concentrations. Only modest amounts of magnesium are usually present. However, both calcium and magnesium may contribute to the hard water syndrome (131). The occurrence of hypertension, nausea, and vomiting favors calcium as the causative agent, whereas the development of central nervous system disturbances associated with hypotension would tend to implicate magnesium. Presently, when the risk and methods for prevention of the hard water syndrome are well known, it generally occurs as a result of malfunction of water treatment equipment.

In rare patients, hypercalcemia may result from the effect of severe secondary hyperparathyroidism. We have seen this result in a chronic syndrome manifested by hypertension, weakness, lethargy, and malaise, all of which symptoms disappeared following parathyroidectomy (132). The similarity of the symptoms resulting from hypercalcemia to those attributed to the dialysis disequilibrium syndrome should be noted and will be commented upon further (see below). The possible synergism between the deleterious effects of hypercalcemia and hypokalemia, especially those affecting cardiac function and/or sensitivity to digitalis, must be given special consideration in patients using potassium-free dialysis solutions. These real and potentially fatal risks of hypercalcemia demand that water treatment be employed in all areas where any significant concentrations of calcium and/or magnesium are present in local water supplies. Water used in dialysate preparation should preferably be free of calcium and magnesium. This can generally be achieved by the use of standard home water-softening units, generally composed of polystyrene resins which act as cation exchangers, exchanging sodium for divalent cations as well as iron, manganese, and aluminum. There may be, however, other contaminants of potential toxic significance present in any given water supply which are not removed by water-softening devices. No single water treatment technique removes all contaminants, and multiple water purification techniques may be required (133). Table 17-7 lists significant water contaminants other than calcium and magne-

Table 17-7. Water contaminants

CONTAMINANT	MAXIMAL* ACCEPTABLE WATER CONCENTRATION	MAJOR TOXIC POTENTIAL
Fluoride	0.2 mg/L	Bone disease (135)
Copper	0.0	Hemolysis (136, 137)
Lead	0.0	Neurologic complications
Aluminum	0.0	Neurologic complications
Arsenic	0.0	Neurologic complications
Tin	0.0	Neurologic complications
Other metals	0.0	Neurologic complications
Chloramines	0.1 mg/L	Hemolysis (138)
Nitrates	2 mg/L	Methemoglobinemia (139)
Pyrogens	0.0	Fever
Sulfate	100 mg/L	Nausea, vomiting, acidosis (133)
Iron	0.0	Iron storage disease (140), equipment damage (133)

*mg/L = parts per million

sium, their maximal recommended concentrations and their toxic potential. The minimal system recommended (133) consists of 5-μm and 1-μm sediment filters for removal of suspended particulate matter, a carbon filter for removal of free chlorine, chloramine, organic material and pyrogens, and a water softener. Iron concentrations greater than two parts per million require an oxidizing filter. If the resultant water contains fluorides, nitrates, or sulfates in excess of maximal acceptable levels, or significant concentrations of sodium (either derived from the water or the exchange for calcium by the water softener) or potassium, an auxiliary water treatment system utilizing reverse osmosis is warranted (134). Reverse osmosis is only 90 percent efficient in the removal of dissolved solids, so in those instances where high water content of nitrates (>10 mg/L) or flouride (>1.7 mg/L) exists, it becomes necessary to supplement these combined methods with a deionizer. It is readily apparent that decisions regarding optimal water treatment methodology require careful analyses of local water supplies.

A variety of other syndromes are seen in chronic dialysis patients which appear to relate to altered parathyroid function and abnormalities in calcium and phosphorus metabolism. Caner and Decker (141) called attention to an acute clinical syndrome occurring in chronic hemodialysis pa-

tients which resembled gouty arthritis and responded to therapy with colchicine. They attributed this, however, to the deposition of calcium phosphate in or around joints and termed the syndrome *pseudogout*. We have seen only a few instances of acute arthritis or peritendonitis in our dialysis patients. Of the seven patients who have had acute arthritis involving shoulder, wrist, finger, great toe, and ankle regions, four had a prior history of primary gout or hyperuricemia disproportionate to their renal failure. The remaining patients had no comparable history. The deposition of calcium pyrophosphate in knee cartilage and intervertebral disks described in pseudogout has never been observed in our patients. Colchicine usually effectively aborted the attack but was so often associated with nausea, vomiting, and debilitating diarrhea that we now preferentially treat with phenylbutazone, ACTH injections, or various analgesics once septic arthritis has been excluded.

We have observed no clear correlation between arthritis and the calcium-phosphorus product (serum calcium concentration × serum phosphorus concentration) or the predialysis serum uric acid. However, it is our impression that both uric acid and calcium are important factors in this syndrome. Some acute arthritic episodes have occurred in areas where there was evidence of metastatic calcification (see below). These metastatic calcifications usually are small, less than 1 cm in diameter, and may exist for many months prior to the onset of pain, swelling, and tenderness in this area. It seems probable, therefore, that this syndrome may be a disorder in which inflammation occurs in an area made susceptible by the presence of preexisting metastatic calcification.

Metastatic calcification, previously considered to be a relatively rare complication of chronic renal failure, has been seen more commonly in patients on chronic hemodialysis programs. Kaye et al. (142) indicated a correlation between the occurrence of soft-tissue calcification and the serum calcium-phosphorus product. Other factors, such as parathyroid hormone excess, postdialysis alkalosis, and local tissue changes, have also been implicated as possibly contributory to calcium deposition. Therapeutically, however, it appears that this complication can be minimized if not entirely eliminated by achieving satisfactory control of the serum phosphorus concentration. Dialysate contains no phosphorus, so that a maximal concentration gradient is achieved to assure optimal removal during dialysis. This, however, is inadequate for maintaining serum phosphorus concentrations at satisfactory levels. Phosphorus is a ubiquitous substance present in almost all foodstuffs. Between dialyses, the serum phosphorus concentration invariably rises due to dietary phosphorus loads, as well as endogenous phosphorus loads resulting from catabolic processes which liberate intracellular phosphorus stores. Satisfactory control of the serum phosphorus concentration, therefore, depends not only upon adequate dialysis but also upon limiting exogenous and endogenous phosphate loads. Rigid restriction of dietary phosphate intake results in a barely palatable diet and rarely meets with patient acceptance.

It is possible, however, to restrict the intake of foods which have particularly high phosphorus content such as milk and most dairy products. Antacids have the capacity to bind phosphorus within the gastrointestinal tract and can not only minimize the amount of ingested phosphorus available for absorption but can also deplete body phosphorus stores. Quantitatively, Basaljel is the antacid with the greatest phosphorus-binding capacity, but it, as well as many other antacids, seems to be poorly tolerated by most patients due to nausea, constipation, and aversion to the taste of the medication. Compliance with antacid therapy is often poor. Magnesium-containing antacids are contraindicated because absorption of even small amounts of magnesium coupled with impaired renal excretion can result in somnolence and life-threatening hypermagnesemia. Accordingly, aluminum-containing antacids are used preferentially. Recently, however, there has been a suggestion that the aluminum-containing antacids might also carry a risk. A syndrome, termed dialysis dementia, has been reported, generally manifesting itself after several years of dialysis and characterized by progressive speech disorders (dyspraxia), intellectual impairment, mutism, myoclonus, grand mal seizures, cerebel-

lar signs, electroencephalographic abnormalities, and ultimately death (143). A combination of presumptive evidence and the finding of elevated levels of aluminum in muscle, bone, and cerebral gray matter in these patients has led to the supposition that it may be a manifestation of aluminum toxicity arising from the use of antacids (144, 145, 146). Aluminum contamination of water supplies has also been suggested as a possible source for the increased body burden of aluminum in these patients (147). The relationship between this syndrome and aluminum intoxication is not yet so well documented as to permit recommendations regarding cessation of aluminum-containing antacid use, but certainly aluminum contamination of water when present should be eliminated by water treatment. At present there is little alternative to the use of these antacids and development of non-aluminum-containing phosphate binders seems a worthy research goal.

Endogenous phosphorus loads can be minimized by maintaining normal or positive nitrogen balance by the provision of adequate protein and caloric intake (see Chap. 10) and elimination of catabolic stimuli. Utilizing a combination of adequate dialysis, antacids, and dietary therapy, it is often possible to keep the serum phosphorus concentration constantly at 6 mg/dL or lower, thereby preventing marked elevation of the calcium-phosphorus product and reducing the risk of developing metastatic calcification. A combination of efficient dialysis, antacid administration, and poor dietary intake can result in phosphate depletion and a hypophosphatemic syndrome with weakness, anorexia, possibly worsening of anemia, and osteomalacia (148, 149). A high incidence of osteomalacia, hypophosphatemia, and an inappropriately low alkaline phosphatase has been reported in association with the dialysis dementia syndrome, though the etiologic role of phosphate in this syndrome could not be established (150).

Myocardial calcification is a particularly dangerous form of metastatic calcification characterized by microscopic myocardial calcification and fibrosis (151, 152) and clinically manifested by potentially fatal arrhythmias (153) electrocardiographic abnormalities, cardiomegaly, and congestive heart failure. These cardiac manifestations may occur in the absence of other evidence of soft-tissue calcification or metabolic bone disease (154). Unfortunately, the manifestations of myocardial calcification are nonspecific, and a diagnosis can be established antemortem only by excluding other causes of myocardial dysfunction. The cause of the myocardial localization of the calcification in these patients is unknown, but there does seem to be a relationship to elevated calcium-phosphorus product and the presence of secondary hyperparathyroidism. The serious nature of the complication demands a vigorous therapeutic approach with attempts to lower the serum phosphorus concentration as rapidly as possible and consideration of parathyroidectomy.

Pruritus is known to occur in uremia and has been attributed to the retention of undefined uremic toxins (155). It occurs, however, more frequently in chronic hemodialysis patients and appears, at least in part, to relate to abnormalities of calcium and phosphorus metabolism. Pruritus may occur acutely as a symptom of the hard water syndrome or may be a persistent, chronic, and distressing symptom. Although a definite correlation between the presence of pruritus and the serum concentration or skin content of calcium or the calcium-phosphate product has not been established, Massry et al. (156) have indicated complete or partial relief of pruritus following parathyroidectomy. It has been interesting to note that such relief may occur immediately following parathyroidectomy, often within 24 h of the operation, even before significant reductions have occurred in parathyroid hormone levels or skin content of calcium or phosphorus. Despite the fact that the precise biochemical abnormalities responsible for pruritus have not been defined, we have been so impressed with improvement following parathyroidectomy that we have undertaken such surgical treatment in patients who have no other manifestations of secondary hyperparathyroidism but have demonstrated elevated blood levels of immunoreactive parathormone in association with persistent intractable pruritus.

The osteodystrophy of uremia and other cutaneous, vascular, ocular, and visceral lesions occurring in association with abnormalities of para-

thyroid function and divalent ion metabolism in dialysis patients are fully discussed in Chap. 19.

In early dialysis systems, bicarbonate was added to dialysate to effect the correction of the metabolic acidosis present in most uremic patients. Since bicarbonate made the dialysate alkaline and tended to cause precipitation of calcium it was necessary to lower the dialysate pH by constantly bubbling 5% carbon dioxide through it. Dialysate *bicarbonate concentrations* approximated 35 meq/L, and bicarbonate diffused into the blood at a rate dependent upon the dialysate/blood concentration gradient and the efficiency of the hemodialyzer. These dialysis systems used chemicals which could be stored in a dry state and mixed with a given quantity of water in a reservoir to produce the desired dialysate solution (batch-type dialysate preparation system).

With the advent of single-pass dialysate flow systems, larger volumes of dialysate were required than for recirculating dialysate flow systems; the batch-type preparation of dialysate became impractical and was generally replaced by techniques providing for the continuous production of dialysate achieved by the mixing of fixed proportions of water and a specially prepared liquid chemical concentrate (proportioning dialysate preparation system). Sodium acetate is used in this system in place of sodium bicarbonate, since even in the liquid chemical concentrate it does not cause precipitation of calcium. Mion et al. (157) demonstrated that when dialysate containing acetate rather than bicarbonate was used, there occurred a slight reduction in the serum bicarbonate in the first half hour of dialysis as bicarbonate diffused from the patient into the bicarbonate-free dialysate at a rate approximating 90 meq/h. Subsequently, however, the serum bicarbonate concentration rose over the remainder of the dialysis as acetate was metabolized to bicarbonate.

With *acetate concentrations* of approximately 35 mg/L in the dialysate, acetate is dialyzed into the patient. It is readily metabolized by all tissues in the body, each mol of sodium acetate being metabolized to 1 mol of sodium bicarbonate. That Earnest et al. (118) and Rosenbaum et al. (119) were unable to measure detectable concentrations of acetate in the serum suggests rapid metabolic conversion to bicarbonate, but the latter group did describe a continuing rise in serum bicarbonate level in certain patients in the 12- to 18-h period postdialysis. This would indicate that under certain circumstances there may be a slow metabolic conversion of acetate to bicarbonate. These studies were conducted with relatively inefficient dialyzers characterized by bicarbonate and acetate dialysances of 55 to 70 ml/min and dialysis duration as long as 17 h. Less than 100 mmol/h of acetate dialyzed into the patient. With the development and clinical use of more efficient dialyzers, the acetate load during dialysis approached 300 mmol/h, the maximal rate at which acetate can be utilized by the normal adult (158). At such levels, blood acetate levels generally remain below 5 meq/L and are well tolerated (159). Even more efficient dialyzers currently available have the capacity to achieve bicarbonate and acetate dialysances in excess of 150 ml/min and deliver acetate loads as high as 400 mmol/h. A net result may be achieved whereby bicarbonate is dialyzed out of the patient at rates in excess of 100 meq/h and acetate is dialyzed into the patient at rates exceeding metabolic conversion capacity. The bicarbonate losses and the nonmetabolized acetate potentially causing a significant rise in blood acetate concentration can result in a worsening of acidosis during dialysis, especially in individual patients who might exhibit impaired capacity to metabolize acetate (159, 160). There is also the possibility that rapid infusion of acetate may result in the shunting of acetate metabolism into alternate pathways which culminate in the production of triglycerides and lipids and possibly contribute to the hyperlipidemia commonly seen in dialysis patients (161). Animal studies indicate that if this shunting does occur it does so to a minor, questionably significant, degree (162).

With some variation dependent upon diet and metabolic status, the average patient generates approximately 70 to 100 meq of acid daily. Approximately half of this is buffered intracellularly and by bone (see also Chap. 6). The remaining half in the extracellular fluid results in a fall in the serum bicarbonate concentration of about 2 or 3 meq/L daily. Predialysis serum bicarbonate concentrations of 19 to 20 meq/L were noted in chronic dialysis patients with a rise to normal or slightly elevated levels postdialysis (119, 163). However in more recent studies, utilizing more efficient dialyzers and shorter dialysis times, predialysis bicarbonate concentrations of 9 to 23 meq/L were found, and most patients showed postdialysis bicarbonate concentrations of 20 meq/L or less (89). It seems clear, therefore, that newer dialysis techniques and schedules have resulted in altered acid-base metabolic dynamics when compared to earlier methodologies. Only rarely have untoward effects been reported (160), but further experience and observations are required before optimal goals for acid-base aspects of dialysis therapy can be established.

Hypocapnia and respiratory alkalosis ordinarily compensate moderate degrees of uremic metabolic acidosis and result in essentially normal predialysis pH (119, 163) (see also Chap. 6). This hypocapnia persists even when the metabolic acidosis is corrected by dialysis and can thereby result in postdialysis alkalemia. The mechanisms resulting in the perpetuation of the respiratory alkalosis are uncertain but may result from uremic alteration in the respiratory threshold to P_{CO_2} (118, 164), persisting intracellular or cerebrospinal fluid acidosis, dialysis disequilibrium phenomena, or loss of CO_2 across the dailyzer (165–168). The clinical effects of this respiratory alkalosis are not clear, but physiologically it is associated with impaired release of oxygen from red blood cells and deposition of calcium and phosphorus in soft tissue. Alkalosis is poorly tolerated by uremic patients and may be responsible for symptoms such as headache, lethargy, nausea, and malaise.

Acetate has also been described as having a myocardial depressant effect (169) and a vasodilatory effect. Substitution of bicarbonate for acetate in dialysate has been recommended, at least in critically ill patients with an unstable cardiovascular status who tend to develop hypotension during dialysis, possibly as a consequence of acetate effects (91, 92, 171).

DIALYSIS DISEQUILIBRIUM SYNDROMES

The intermittent nature of hemodialysis therapy as presently applied requires that during the treatment period large quantities of uremic solute be removed and electrolyte and fluid abnormalities be corrected. Between dialyses, these abnormalities recur. Accordingly, the patient is repeatedly subjected to rapid wide swings in body biochemistry which, when graphed, assume a "sawtooth" pattern (Fig. 17-4). These abrupt biochemical changes have been implicated in the explanation of the mechanisms of a variety of signs and symptoms seen during dialysis and immediately post-dialysis. These have in the past been related to the phenomenon of a delayed or *reverse urea shift*, but it is more likely that in reality they relate to a variety of disequilibrium states brought about by the acute biochemical changes produced by dialysis and relating not only to urea but to other solutes as well.

Table 17-8 lists a variety of symptoms which have been attributed to the dialysis disequilibrium syndrome. The nonspecificity of these signs and symptoms is apparent. Neurologic

Table 17-8. Signs and symptoms associated with dialysis disequilibrium

Nausea and/or vomiting
Headache
Hypertension or hypotension
Visual blurring
Leg cramps
Peripheral parathesias
Mental clouding
Anxiety and/or agitation of unknown cause
Hyperventilation
Chest pain
Weakness, "washed-out feelings," or fatigue

symptoms such as twitching, confusion, convulsions, and coma have been noted with hemodialysis especially when the predialysis BUN exceeds 150 mg/100 ml. These neurologic complications, occurring during or shortly after completion of dialysis have been attributed to cerebral edema resulting from a slow transport of

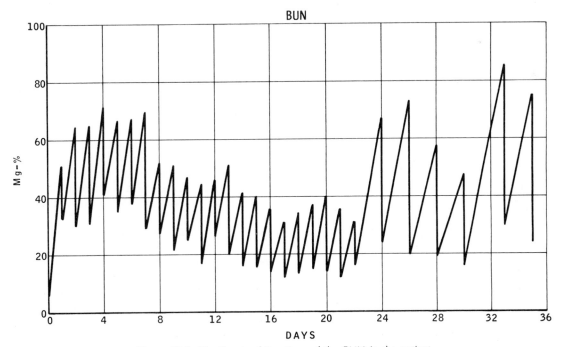

Figure 17-4. The "sawtooth" pattern of the BUN in the patient undergoing intermittent repetitive hemodialysis. The fluctuations are more pronounced as the frequency of dialysis is decreased.

urea across the blood-brain barrier (171). As dialysis lowers the blood urea concentration, the blood-brain barrier for urea impairs a correspondingly rapid reduction in the urea concentration in the brain and brain water. This urea disequilibrium creates an osmotic disequilibrium, and accordingly water moves into the hyperosmolar central nervous system causing cerebral edema and the accompanying clinical neurologic symptoms. Dossetor et al. (172) dialyzed uremic dogs and analyzed their cerebral cortices and white matter for water content, urea, sodium, and potassium. They demonstrated the development of cerebral edema without a change in the tissue sodium/potassium ratios and concluded that the cerebral edema resulted solely from osmotic changes induced by urea disequilibrium. Sitprija and Holmes (173) observed increases in intraocular pressure during hemodialysis which were independent of any associated changes in systemic blood pressure. Gilliland and Hegstrom (174) noted marked increases in cerebrospinal fluid pressure during dialysis which could be minimized by using dialysate solutions containing urea concentrations approaching that of uremic subjects, thereby preventing the dialysis of urea and avoiding reducing the BUN. Kennedy et al. (175) were able to prevent the electroencephalographic abnormalities associated with dialysis by increasing the serum osmolality either by infusing hypertonic fructose or by using high concentrations of glucose in dialysate (176).

The term *reverse urea effect*, or *shift*, derives from contrasting the dialysis phenomenon responsible for cerebral edema to the use of urea infusions, particularly by neurosurgeons, to reduce cerebral edema. Such reduction in cerebral edema is likewise based upon the blood-brain barrier for urea. The infused urea fails to diffuse rapidly into the central nervous system, an osmotic disequilibrium is created, and water, which readily crosses the blood-brain barrier, moves from the central nervous system and reduces cerebral edema. Carbon 14 urea studies have shown a 3- to 6-h delay in diffusion of urea into the brain (177). The term *delayed urea shift* is probably preferable to, and more precise than, reverse urea shift to describe this hemodialysis phenomenon.

Hampers and Schupak (178) have indicated, however, that they were unable to establish a definite correlation between dialysis-induced electroencephalographic abnormalities and urea shifts. Experimental studies in uremic dogs treated with dialysis have failed to demonstrate significant differences between urea concentration in blood and brain (179, 180). Arieff et al. have demonstrated in dogs that the induction of dialysis disequilibrium relates to the rapidity of dialysis (179). Rapid dialysis in acutely uremic dogs induced seizures, EEG changes, and cerebral edema. A significant osmotic gradient between blood and brain was found but could not be related to changes in the concentration of urea or the usually measured electrolytes. The osmotic gradient and resultant cerebral edema was attributed to the derivation of idiogenic osmols (181). An associated fall in cerebrospinal fluid and brain intracellular pH was found, despite a simultaneously rising arterial pH (182) (see Chap. 26). Several other acute biochemical changes occurring during hemodialysis have the capacity to induce neurologic disorders and other symptoms of the dialysis disequilibrium syndrome, and it seems most likely that this syndrome, much like the uremic syndrome itself, can be induced by a variety of factors acting singly or in combination with one another.

Postdialysis hypocapnia, either by virtue of its effect upon impairing oxygen dissociation from hemoglobin or the effect of respiratory alkalosis in reducing cerebral blood flow, may contribute to the central nervous system symptomatology. *Ultrafiltration* may result in plasma volume depletion and hypotension with resultant reduction in cerebral blood flow. Postdialysis fatigue seems to be a more prominent symptom in those dialyses where ultrafiltration is used to induce marked negative fluid balance. *Hyperosmolality*, generally induced by hyperglycemia resulting from the use of high dialysate glucose concentration (183, 184) (but rarely resulting from the accidental use of dialysate containing excess sodium or from the administration of excessive quantities of mannitol during attempts to produce diuresis in patients with acute renal failure), may result in hyperosmolar coma and related symptomatology resulting from cerebral dehydration.

When hyperglycemia does result from absorption of large quantities of glucose from dialysate high in glucose concentration, there may be an "overshoot" in insulin production with resultant reactive hypoglycemia (185) generally occurring 1 to 2 h after completion of dialysis. The symptoms of hypoglycemia may mimic those ascribed to dialysis disequilibrium. *Hypovolemic hypertension* (see above) may occur during dialysis and result in headaches, nausea, and vomiting or, if severe, in hypertensive encephalopathy.

Hypokalemia may result from dialysis with potassium-free or low potassium concentration dialysate and produce cardiotoxicity, hypotension, and/or fatigue. The *hard water syndrome* due to excess of calcium or magnesium in dialysate may result in a clinical picture compatible with the disequilibrium syndrome. The symptoms of acute copper intoxication may mimic those of dialysis disequilibrium. *Hyponatremia* resulting from low sodium concentration in the dialysate due either to an intentional reduction in an effort to enhance sodium removal or to an accidental preparation of low sodium dialysate may produce water intoxication with headache, nausea, convulsions, and cerebral edema. Erroneous production of dialysate with an excessively high sodium concentration may also produce neurologic symptoms.

Thus, although in most instances dialysis-induced cerebral edema is probably the major reason for many of the neurologic and nonspecific signs and symptoms of the dialysis disequilibrium syndrome, it must be considered a multifactorial condition with potential contributions by a variety of solute, hormonal, cardiovascular, and ionic abnormalities. When the symptoms are severe or life-threatening, all possible causes should be considered and appropriate diagnostic studies and therapeutic measures promptly instituted.

The patient undergoing hemodialysis may be exposed to a variety of potentially toxic substances which have the capacity of producing symptoms which may mimic those of the dialysis disequilibrium syndrome. *Heparin* is routinely administered during dialysis to prevent clotting of blood in the extracorporeal circuit. Although heparin is probably not directly toxic, it may potentiate bleeding with resultant hemorrhagic

shock or hemorrhagic cerebrovascular accidents. Both *formalin* and *sodium hypochlorite* are used in the cleaning and sterilization of dialysis systems and may produce toxic effects if accidentally infused into the patient. Although the infusion of several hundred milliliters of dilute formalin solution (2 to 6% formalin in water) from an artificial kidney has not resulted in any reported fatalities, the morbidity from such a misadventure may be alarming. With formalin infusion, the initial symptom of pain at the venous cannula site has shortly been followed by shortness of breath, chest pain, weakness, and hypotension. If sodium hypochlorite accidentally contaminates dialysis solutions, it is dialyzed into the patient and produces an acute and severe hemolysis.

Since clinically the more severe manifestations of the dialysis disequilibrium syndrome occur in those patients with high predialysis BUN levels, and since experimentally the syndrome relates to rapidity of dialysis, it becomes readily apparent that its occurrence can be minimized by modifying treatment in susceptible subjects in a manner designed to reduce dialysis efficiency. Thus, in patients with a high BUN (usually greater than 150 mg/dL), the duration of dialysis can be shortened, the surface area of the dialyzer used minimized, and the dialysate or blood flow rate reduced in order to effect a dialysis of limited efficiency. The use of anticonvulsants can be considered as well. The administration of osmotically active substances such as urea, glucose, mannitol, sodium salts, and glycerol has been suggested to avert or treat cerebral edema (181), but we have generally found no need to utilize these agents since limiting dialysis efficiency has been so effective as a preventive.

The less serious intradialytic symptoms such as headache, muscle cramps, nausea and vomiting probably result from different mechanisms unrelated to BUN levels and occur even during therapy in stabilized chronic dialysis patients. As noted above, these symptoms seem to be minimized or eliminated by increasing dialysate sodium concentration, substituting ultrafiltration techniques for dialysis, and minimizing osmotic gradients between blood and dialysate. When muscle cramps do occur, we have found the most effective therapy to be the intravenous administration of a bolus of 10 to 20 mL of hypertonic (22.5%) saline (185).

NEW TECHNOLOGIES

Recent developments have provided alternative methods for the extracorporeal treatment of uremic blood which have their own specific characteristics with reference to water and electrolytes. The standard hemodialysis techniques discussed above require the use of a minimum of 30 L and, more often, in excess of 100 L of dialysate per treatment. By the application of sorbent regeneration techniques, it has been possible to reduce total dialysate volumes to as low as 1 to 2 L (188), although in its currently clinically applicable form (REDY system) 5.5 L of dialysate are used. Regeneration of "spent" dialysate (dialysate containing dialyzed uremic solutes after it has passed through the hemodialyzer) is accomplished in a cartridge consisting of the five layers listed in Table 17-9. Conversion of urea to ammonium by urease is necessitated by the fact that essentially no known sorbents have the capacity to absorb significant quantities of urea at the temperature, pH, and electrolyte composition of dialysate. The first layer of the cartridge is termed a water decontaminant layer. It removes the majority of water contaminants and is placed proximal to the urease layer primarily to remove heavy and trace metal contaminants of tap water which, if present in significant concentrations, might inactivate the urease. The second layer contains the urease where urea is hydrolyzed to ammonium and carbonate. The third layer consists of zirconium phosphate, which essentially functions as a cation exchanger. When prepared in the sodium-hydrogen form it exchanges sodium and hydrogen for ammonium, calcium, magnesium, and potassium which are completely absorbed and removed from the dialysate (Fig. 17-5). The hydrogen ion combines with the carbonate derived from the urea to produce bicarbonate, water, and carbon dioxide. Although the precise reactions are uncertain, the ultimate reactions approximate the following:

Table 17-9. Component layers of REDY sorbent cartridge

1. Water decontaminant layer
2. Urease layer
3. Zirconium phosphate layer
4. Hydrous zirconium oxide layer
5. Activated carbon layer

$$C=O{<}{\begin{matrix} NH_2 \\ NH_2 \end{matrix}} + H_2O \rightarrow 2NH_4^+ + CO_3^{2-}$$
$$\text{urea}$$

$$CO_3^{2-} + H^+ \rightleftharpoons HCO_3^- + H^+ \rightleftharpoons H_2O + CO_2$$

Zirconium Phosphate Adsorption (Sodium—Hydrogen Form)

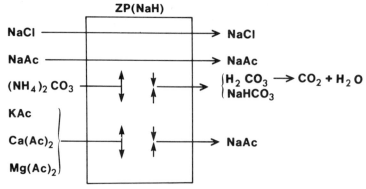

Figure 17-5. Functions of zirconium phosphate layer of sorbent cartridge. K^+, Ca^{2+}, and Mg^{2+} are absorbed in exchange for sodium. NH_4^+ is exchanged for H^+ and Na^+, thereby generating the addition of H_2CO_3 and $NaHCO_3$ to the dialysate.

Hydrous Zirconium Oxide Adsorption (Chloride Form)

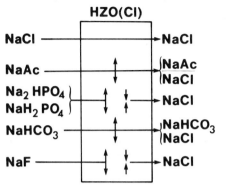

Figure 17-6. Functions of chloride form of hydrous zirconium oxide layer of sorbent cartridge. This functions primarily as an anion exchanger, adding chloride to the dialysate.

The next layer is an anion-exchange layer, hydrous zirconium oxide. When prepared in the chloride form, this layer adsorbs phosphate, fluoride, and, to a limited extent, bicarbonate, in exchange for chloride (Fig. 17-6). In the acetate form (Fig. 17-7) the exchange is for acetate rather than chloride. The final layer is composed of activated carbon which absorbs the nonurea nitrogenous uremic metabolites as well as a variety of water contaminants (Fig. 17-8). The ion exchangers also

Hydrous Zirconium Oxide Adsorption (Acetate Form)

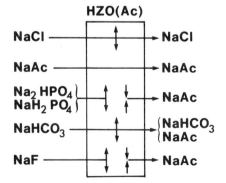

Figure 17-7. Functions of acetate form of hydrous zirconium oxide layer of sorbent cartridge. Acetate rather than chloride is added to the dialysate in exchange for adsorbed anions.

Carbon Adsorption

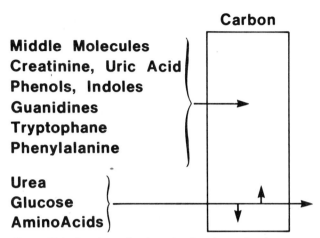

Figure 17-8. Functions of activated carbon layer of sorbent cartridge. Most organic solutes are adsorbed but urea-glucose and amino acids are only partially adsorbed.

function in essence as a deionizer water decontamination system. The dialysate flow system of the REDY is diagrammatically compared to the other available dialysate supply systems in Fig. 17-9. Sorbent regeneration of dialysate permits a low-volume recirculating dialysate system to maintain the maximal blood to dialysate concentration gradients for uremic solutes characteristic of single-pass, high-volume, dialysate delivery systems. In single-pass systems, a constant dialysate electrolyte composition is maintained by proportioning the admixture of fixed ratios of water and dialysate concentrate. In recirculating or combined recirculating single-pass dialysate flow systems, a given batch quantity of dialysate of fixed electrolyte composition is prepared by the mixing of appropriate portions of water and dry salts or dialysate concentrate. In contrast, in the sorbent regeneration system, the dialysate electrolyte composition is in an active state of flux as exchange occurs between the sorbents and the dialysate. Calcium, magnesium, and potassium are completely removed by the sorbents, necessitating reconstitution of prescribed concentrations by an infusion system located between the sorbent cartridge and the dialyzer. The composition of this infusate can be varied according to individual pa-

Dialysate supply systems

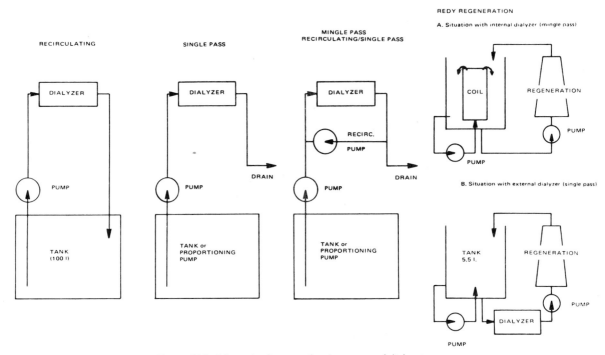

Figure 17-9. Schematic diagram of various types of dialysate supply systems.

tient needs to provide the desired dialysate concentrations of calcium, magnesium, and potassium. The cation exchange process by the zirconium phosphate adds significant quantities of sodium to the dialysate approximating 200 to 250 meq for a 6-h dialysis. To adapt for this, the sodium concentration of the dialysate with which dialysis is begun is appropriately lowered (110 to 115 meq/L). This is possible to do since the low total volume of the dialysate (5.5 L) in comparison to a given patient's extracellular and total body sodium and water volumes and the addition of sodium from the sorbents prevents any unusual major sodium or osmotic exchanges between blood and dialysate. Serum sodium concentration and other indicators of salt and water metabolism such as body weight and blood pressure are not significantly different in patients treated with the REDY

as compared to those treated with standard systems (189, 190, 191).

The sorbent system also differs from standard systems in that bicarbonate is generated by the cartridge. Bicarbonate concentrations of 15 to 20 meq/L are achieved so that bicarbonate losses from blood to dialysate are minimized. In contrast, less acetate is available with the sorbent system (191). Early studies with the REDY system indicated incomplete correction of acidosis in certain patients (190, 192, 193). This led to the substitution of the acetated form of zirconium oxide for the chloride form, thereby providing more acetate which was further augmented by changing the infused salts of calcium, magnesium, and potassium to acetate rather than chloride salts. These modifications have improved the correction of acidosis to a level comparable to that achieved with standard dialyses (89, 190, 191).

The ability to regenerate dialysate provides a low-volume system which is portable and independent of fixed water supply and water treatment systems. The system permits constant monitoring of ultrafiltration volumes and is readily modified to permit treatment of unusual clinical conditions occasionally occurring in conjunction with uremia such as hypernatremia, hyponatremia, hypercalcemia, and alkalosis (194). Most significantly, perhaps, it provides evidence that requisite dialysate volumes can be reduced to levels consistent with the potential ultimate development of a wearable ambulatory dialysis system.

Stimulated by the concepts of the middle-molecule hypothesis, membrane research has resulted in the development of dialyzer membranes with hydraulic permeability appreciably greater than that of Cuprophan and other cellulosic membranes used in standard dialysis systems. These "high-flux" water permeable membranes also have greater permeability for solutes, up to molecular weight ranges of 5000 to 40,000 daltons (195, 196). Such membranes have formed the basis for the development of ultrafiltration devices which utilize convective rather than diffusive transport (see above) for the purification of uremic blood (197, 198). No dialysate is required for these ultrafiltration techniques, but rather a large volume of sterile pyrogen-free solution is added to the blood as it enters (197) or leaves (198) the filtration device. This solution quantitatively replaces the volume removed by ultrafiltration, less that amount necessary to remove to correct the interdialytic salt and water gain. The composition of these fluids as used by the investigators reporting the initial clinical results with these systems is shown in Table 17-10.

Biochemical and clinical results with these ultrafiltration methods have generally been comparable to those obtained with hemodialysis with the added theoretic advantage of augmented middle-molecule removal and the observation by both groups of an unexplained improvement in hypertension (198, 199). No untoward effects were noted from amino acid and protein losses of 6.5 and 10 g respectively, and there was no evidence of a depletion syndrome. Much as was noted with

Table 17-10. Solutions used to replace ultrafiltrate in convective transport systems

	HEMODIAFILTRATION (197), meq/L	ULTRAFILTRATION KIDNEY (198), meq/L
Na^+	140	135
K^+	5.0	2.0
Cl^-	98	108.5
Lactate	—	33.75
Acetate	27	—
Gluconate	23	—
Ca^{2+}	2.5	3.75
Mg^+	3.0	1.5
Volume	70–80 L	18 L
Ultrafiltration rate	200–225 mL/min	70–75 mL/min

the sequential ultrafiltration-dialysis techniques previously discussed, intradialytic symptomatology and postdialysis fatigue were minimized when compared to their occurrence during standard dialysis. In their present form, these systems are somewhat complex, and the need for large volumes of sterile replacement fluids makes them costly. As more experience with these techniques accrues one can anticipate they will be simplified, but it should be readily apparent that a major simplification could result if the ultrafiltrate could be regenerated by appropriate sorbent agents and then returned directly to the patient. Such a system would require that the sorbents be sterile and that sorbent particles be prevented from infusing into the bloodstream. These same requirements exist for the application of sorbent methods to peritoneal dialyses and will be discussed below. Preliminary assessment of sorbent regeneration of ultrafiltrate is now being conducted (200).

PERITONEAL DIALYSIS

The concept that certain body tissues might clinically function as dialyzing membranes dates to 1922 and 1923, when, virtually simultaneously, Putnam (201) characterized "the living peritoneum as a dializing membrane," Ganter (202) reported on the biochemical and clinical effectiveness of pleural and peritoneal dialysis in the uremic dog and human, and Necheles (65) described successful extracorporeal hemodialysis utilizing excised peritoneum as the dialyzing membrane in dogs. Sporadic reports (203–209) subsequently confirmed the potential value of peritoneal dialysis in the treatment of uremia, but technical difficulties and frequent complications limited acceptance of the technique. In 1959, Maxwell et al. (210) and Doolan et al. (211) by virtue of technical improvements consisting of the design of a semirigid nylon catheter, standard commercially available dialyzing solutions, and a closed system of dialysate flow, established peritoneal dialysis as an effective, simple, and relatively safe therapeutic procedure. The simplicity of the technique gained it ready acceptance, even in those centers where hemodialysis was available (212). Although the dramatic advances in the field of chronic maintenance hemodialysis have commanded the major attention in the dialysis field, peritoneal dialysis remains an important therapeutic modality in the management of acute uremic states and has been gaining increasing acceptance as a satisfactory alternative to hemodialysis in the management of chronic uremia (213–215).

GENERAL PRINCIPLES

Much of our knowledge of the mechanisms and dynamics of peritoneal dialysis is empirically derived. Clinical experience and available kinetic data (216) have verified that the peritoneum acts as a passive dialyzing membrane (see below). Dialyzable solutes move between blood and the dialysate solution along their individual concentration gradients, and water moves along osmotic gradients, these movements occurring across a functionally semipermeable membrane which effectively retards any significant transmembrane passage of the formed elements of blood and high-molecular-weight blood components, such as serum proteins and other colloidal substances.

In hemodialysis, the extracorporeal circuit permits the accurate measurement of functional parameters and membrane characteristics. However, peritoneal dialysis is an in vivo process, and similar data can often be calculated only indirectly and with limited accuracy; the precise nature of the dialyzing membrane, factors affecting its permeability, the optimal composition, volumes and flow rates of dialysate, and the dynamics of peritoneal dialysis are poorly defined, often presumptive, and at best semiquantitatively determined.

THE DIALYZING MEMBRANE

The ability to conduct dialysis effectively within the peritoneal cavity has led to the conclusion that the peritoneum has the characteristics of a dialyzing membrane. The peritoneum has a large anatomic surface area (22,000 cm^2) approximating that of the glomerular capillaries and larger hemodialyzers (217, 218). The functional area involved in dialytic transport however is significantly less, probably less than 1000 cm^2 (60, 219). The larger surface area and richer vascular supply of the visceral peritoneum would suggest that it predominates over the parietal peritoneum. Although similar epithelial membranes such as frog skin and toad bladder have been demonstrated to have the capacity to transport ions actively, the peritoneum has been assumed to be inert and diffusion across it to be passive (220).

The actual pore size of the peritoneal membrane remains undetermined. There has been recent conjecture, however, based upon the observation that at equivalent levels of azotemia some patients undergoing maintenance peritoneal dialysis seem to manifest less evidence of uremic complications (25) than do patients on maintenance hemodialysis, that the peritoneal pore size is more compatible with the effective removal of certain uremic toxic factors than is the pore size of the artificial cellulosic membranes utilized in hemodialysis systems. The peritoneum appears to be significantly more soluble to solutes of middle-molecular-weight range (500 to 5000 daltons) than are hemodialyzer membranes (60, 221, 222).

The permeability of the membrane and diffusion coefficients vary for different solutes and accordingly affect their rates of diffusion and clearances. Maxwell et al. (210) and Boen (216) have shown clearances to be highest for urea and potassium; the clearance of other solutes decreases sequentially in the following order: chloride, sodium, creatinine, phosphate, uric acid, bicarbonate, calcium, and magnesium. A variety of factors may alter the permeability of the membrane and enhance solute clearance. The warming of dialysate to body temperature increases urea clearance by as much as 35 percent (223, 224). Pappenheimer (225), however, has ascribed this effect to changes in viscosity rather than to altered membrane permeability. Henderson and Nolph (222) have described increased peritoneal permeability with the use of hyperosmolar dialyzing solutions. Experimentally, alterations in solute transfer and/or membrane permeability have been demonstrated following the intraperitoneal or parenteral administration of drugs, such as vasopressin, streptokinase, serotonin, calcium chloride, epinephrine, dioctyl sodium sulfosuccinate, histamine, insulin, and dopamine. Calcium, vasopressin, and dopamine decrease transperitoneal diffusive transport, whereas the other agents appear to produce an increase (226–235). In human studies, isoproterenol, diazoxide, dipyridamole, and especially sodium nitroprusside have been found to augment diffusive transport, with such effects more marked for larger-molecular-weight solutes, suggestive evidence that these drugs enhance permeability or augment dialyzing surface area by opening new intraperitoneal capillary channels (236–238). As yet no clinical applications have resulted from these latter studies.

A question must be raised, however, as to whether the peritoneum is indeed the actual dialyzing membrane of the peritoneal cavity. Large particulate matter (such as india ink and red blood cells) introduced into the peritoneal cavity rapidly and completely enters the circulation (239–240). The intraperitoneal route has even been used for the administration of transfusions to infants and children (241, 242). Access to the circulation from the peritoneal cavity is gained via the lymphatics of the peritoneum and the diaphragm (240). When ^{131}ISA (radioiodinated serum albumin), a substance with a molecular weight considered to be higher than that which can readily pass the dialyzing membrane, is introduced into the peritoneal cavity, only small amounts (0.1 to 8 percent of the administered

dose) pass into the circulation within 2 to 6 h (243, 244). However, the ^{131}ISA which does enter the circulation also leaves the peritoneal cavity by way of the lymphatic circulation (245). Anatomically, the peritoneum is a thin membrane with a subperitoneal stratum containing a well-developed network of blood and lymph capillaries. Therefore, in order for ^{131}ISA or particulate matter to enter the lymphatics from the peritoneal cavity, the substance must pass across the peritoneum, suggestive evidence that the peritoneum may indeed be a permeable rather than a semipermeable membrane. Allen (246, 247) has suggested that these substances pass transperitoneally only at the diaphragm, where respiratory movements alter the anatomic relationships between pores of the peritoneum and the lymphatics to create directly communicating functional stomata of 2 to 20 μm diameter. Others, however, have demonstrated uptake of ^{131}ISA and red blood cells throughout the peritoneum (240, 245). If indeed the peritoneum itself is permeable to particulate and high-molecular-weight substances (248), then the true semipermeable dialyzing membrane of the peritoneal cavity must be some subperitoneal structure, most likely the capillary wall itself. These considerations in no way alter the clinical usefulness of peritoneal dialysis. However, they direct attention to the capillary network rather than the peritoneum in any experimental studies designed to elucidate or to change the permeability characteristics of the dialyzing "membrane."

THE DIALYSATE

The composition of commercially available dialysis solutions is essentially the same as that originally described by Maxwell and associates (210). Minor variations from this composition are present in the dialysate produced by an automated peritoneal dialysis proportioning system (249) (Table 17-11). They are designed to permit maximal removal of waste products and endogenous or exogenous toxins, to correct electrolyte or acid-base imbalance, to prevent significant absorption of the administered fluid from the peri-

Table 17-11. Peritoneal dialysis solutions

	BOTTLED SOLUTIONS	PROPORTIONING SYSTEM (249)
Na^+	140 meq/L	129–137 meq/L
K^+	0 meq/L	0
Ca^{2+}	3.5–4.0 meq/L	3.4–3.6 meq/L
Mg^{2+}	1.5 meq/L	0.5 meq/L
Sodium acetate	45 meq/L	37–39 meq/L
Cl^-	101 meq/L	96–102 meq/L
Dextrose	1500-4250 mg/dL	500-3500 mg/dL
Osmolality	372–525 mosm/L	300-450 mosm/L

toneal cavity, and, when indicated, to remove excess fluids. The solutions are prepared free of any nonelectrolyte solutes except glucose, thereby providing a maximal concentration gradient for the effective removal of uremic and other toxic solutes. The electrolyte concentrations are chosen to approximate idealized potassium-free extracellular fluid. Thus, any abnormalities in the serum concentrations of these electrolytes will tend to be corrected toward normal by movement along concentration gradients either into or out of the serum. Potassium is omitted, because hyperkalemia is often present in clinical situations where dialysis is required. If hyperkalemia is not present, potassium chloride may be added to adjust the concentration to any desired level. Dextrose is present to increase the osmolality. The minimal osmolality of 372 mosm (1.5% dextrose concentration) is somewhat higher than the usual serum osmolality of uremic patients. This prevents absorption of the administered fluid from the abdomen and the overhydration frequently reported with earlier techniques of peritoneal dialysis. When fluid removal is desired, an osmotic gradient is created by using solutions containing 4.25% dextrose (525 mosm/L). 7% dextrose solutions have been discontinued since their use is rarely indicated and the risks of severe hyperglycemia or dehydration are appreciable.

The *sodium* and *chloride* concentrations of 140 and 101 meq/L (Table 17-11) respectively, in dialysate are generally acceptable and result in normal serum concentrations of these ions at the end of dialysis in most cases (Tables 17-12 and 17-13). However, hypernatremia was noted after dialysis in 13 percent of this series of 50 patients

Table 17-12. Serum sodium concentration before and after peritoneal dialysis*

SERUM SODIUM CONCENTRATION, meq/L	PERITONEAL DIALYSIS	
	BEFORE	AFTER
< 126	7 (15%)	0
126–135	23 (50%)	7 (15%)
136–148	13 (28%)	33 (72%)
> 148	3 (7%)	6 (13%)

* Average duration of peritoneal dialysis, 30 h. Data are from a series of 50 consecutive patients with acute renal failure. Data were not available on all patients. The number of patients falling into each group is recorded in both absolute numbers and percentages, e.g., after peritoneal dialysis 33 patients or 72% of the group had a serum sodium concentration of 136–148 meq/L.

(sodium data available in 46 of these patients) with acute renal failure treated with peritoneal dialysis. In contradistinction, hypernatremia developed in only 1 percent of a similar group of patients treated with hemodialysis. Hypernatremia has been noted to occur when hyperosmolar ("hypertonic") dialyzing solutions are utilized for the purpose of removing excess fluid or edema (see below). Boyer et al. (250) attributed this phenomenon to the fact that the glucose present in high concentrations in hyperosmolar dialysate (4.25 to 7% dextrose) enters the blood faster than it can be metabolized, thereby causing hypergly-

Table 17-13. Serum chloride concentration before and after peritoneal dialysis*

SERUM CHLORIDE CONCENTRATION, meq/L	PERITONEAL DIALYSIS	
	BEFORE	AFTER
< 81	7 (16%)	0
81–95	19 (43%)	14 (32%)
96–108	17 (39%)	27 (61%)
> 108	1 (2%)	3 (7%)

* See footnote to Table 17-11.

cemia and a resultant rise in serum and extracellular fluid osmolality. Intracellular water then moves in response to this osmotic gradient into the extracellular space, and the intracellular osmolality rises to equate with the extracellular osmolality (see Chap. 1). When the excess glucose is metabolized after the completion of dialysis, serum osmolality falls, and water now moves from the extracellular space back into the cell; serum sodium concentration, which during dialysis has been maintained at a normal level by equilibration with the dialysate sodium concentration of 140 meq/L, rises to hypernatremic levels. Nolph et al. (251) observed that the "ultrafiltrate" induced by hyperosmolar dialyzing solutions has a low sodium concentration and they explained the hypernatremia on the basis that water was removed in excess of sodium relative to their concentrations in serum. They recommend prevention of this hypernatremia by partial replacement of the water losses intravenously when fluid losses induced by peritoneal dialysis exceed 3 or 4 L.

Our own studies with experimental peritoneal dialysis in dogs confirm the observation that the ultrafiltrate is low in sodium, but this mechanism alone is inadequate to explain our observation that hypernatremia is maximal several hours *after* completion of dialysis. This implies that the hypernatremia results from the postdialysis movement of water from the extracellular to the intracellular space as suggested by Boyer et al. (250). We have not, however, been able consistently to relate this to resolving hyperglycemia and feel that the exact mechanism must still be considered undetermined. If the dialysate is prepared with a sodium concentration of 120 to 130 meq/L, the ultrafiltrate is not as low in sodium, since sodium movement into the dialysate is enhanced by the concentration gradient. This increases the negative sodium balance achieved with hypertonic dialysis and seems to reduce the risk of hypernatremia (252). Reduction of the sodium concentration of peritoneal dialysate has been used to enhance negative sodium balance, especially in patients with severe hypertension or those undergoing chronic peritoneal dialysis (23).

Potassium is omitted from commercial peritoneal dialysis solutions to permit individualization for each patient. Potassium chloride may be added to the dialysate to produce any desired potassium concentration. Potassium-free solutions are used to treat hyperkalemia. The peritoneal clearance of potassium approximates that of urea, and as much as 200 meq of potassium may be removed during a single dialysis. In emergency situations, when hyperkalemia has progressed to the stage of cardiotoxicity, the electrocardiographic abnormalities may be improved in a matter of minutes, even before any detectable decrease in the serum potassium concentration can be measured. In patients in whom continued oliguria is anticipated and especially in those in whom catabolic stimuli (fever, tissue necrosis, infection, steroid hormones) or large endogenous sources of potassium (blood in the gastrointestinal tract, hematomas) predispose to rapid recurrence of hyperkalemia, the entire dialysis may be performed with potassium-free dialyzing solutions. Boen (216, 253) has reported that when potassium-free dialysate solutions were used for periods of 28 to 59 h, the lowest final serum potassium concentration observed was 3.4 meq/L. Although a negative potassium balance is usually induced by this technique, severe hypokalemia is prevented by the movement of intracellular potassium into the extracellular space. This state of total body potassium depletion serves to minimize any subsequent postdialysis rise in serum potassium concentration, presumably because newly formed potassium is initially incorporated into the depleted intracellular reservoir.

If dialysis is performed in patients without hyperkalemia, the dialysate potassium concentration is generally selected to reflect the final serum potassium concentration the physician wishes to achieve, generally about 4 meq/L. It must be remembered, however, that other factors may affect the serum potassium concentration (see Chap. 4). Correction of acidosis, the intracellular incorporation of potassium in the conversion of absorbed glucose to glycogen, and the enhanced loss of potassium with ultrafiltration all may serve to lower the serum potassium concentration to a level below that in the dialysate. Extreme caution is indicated in the selection of dialysate potassium concentration in patients who have received digitalis. Lowering of the serum potassium concentration may induce digitalis intoxication, especially in those cases where evidence of such intoxication may have been obscured by hyperkalemia. The simultaneous correction of hypocalcemia, acidosis, and hyponatremia may also enhance digitalis effects. Maher and Schreiner (14) have reported a high incidence of arrhythmias, several of which were fatal, in digitalized patients undergoing dialysis. Whenever possible, digitalis should be avoided in patients who may require dialysis. When dialysis is indicated in a digitalized patient, a dialysate potassium concentration of 4 to 5.5 meq/L should be employed, and the electrocardiogram should be monitored continuously (see also Chap. 4).

The *calcium* concentration of available solutions is 4.0 meq/L although in some solutions it has been reduced to 3.5 meq/L. These concentrations are higher than the normal physiologically significant ionized serum calcium concentration, and *calcium is generally dialyzed into the patients.* This tends to correct the hypocalcemia which frequently accompanies renal insufficiency. However, it may contribute to the precipitation of digitalis intoxication (see above), and if dialysis is performed repetitively or on a chronic basis, it may, if hyperphosphatemia coexists, pose a risk of metabolic calcification and perhaps several other syndromes related to abnormal calcium and phosphorus metabolism in dialysis (see above). Although Boen (253) has demonstrated the safety of using magnesium-free dialysate in acute cases, the *magnesium concentration* of the dialysate is 1.5 meq/L. The uremic patient, unless he has been exposed to large exogenous loads of magnesium, such as may be present in certain antacids and laxatives usually has a normal or mildly elevated ionized serum magnesium level, and the dialysate concentration of 1.5 meq/L serves to correct any existing significant abnormalities. The choice of these dialysate calcium and magnesium concentrations has in many respects been arbitrary, and as knowledge accrues regarding the intricacies of divalent ion metabolism in uremia and dialysis, they may well be subject to change (see also Chap. 20). The findings by Burnell (125) suggest-

ing that metabolic bone disease might be improved with the use of low-magnesium dialysate has led Tenckhoff to lower the magnesium concentration of peritoneal dialysate used for chronic dialysis to 0.5 meq/L.

Bicarbonate cannot be added to peritoneal dialysis solutions, since the simultaneous presence of calcium will cause the precipitation of calcium carbonate. Therefore, a bicarbonate precursor, either sodium *lactate* or sodium *acetate,* is added in concentrations of 45 meq/L. Lactate must be metabolized by the liver to provide available bicarbonate. In certain cases of severe hepatic insufficiency, circulatory insufficiency, or lactic acidosis, the inability to metabolize lactate effectively may impair bicarbonate production and the capacity to counteract acidosis (212). Acetate, which is largely metabolized by peripheral tissues and requires less oxygen for its metabolism, may be a more effective bicarbonate source and has largely replaced lactate in most dialysis solutions. It has also been suggested that acetate may have a bacteriostatic effect (249). Our own experience with peritoneal dialysis has shown uniform effectiveness in the improvement of acidosis as determined by clinical response and the correction of pH and carbon dioxide combining power toward normal (Table 17-14). In patients treated chronically with repetitive peritoneal dialysis, an acetate concentration of approximately 38 meq/L is required to prevent significant acidosis (249). As has been observed with hemodialysis, respiratory alkalosis may be present after peritoneal dialysis

Table 17-14. Serum carbon dioxide combining power before and after peritoneal dialysis*

SERUM CARBON DIOXIDE COMBINING POWER, meq/L	PERITONEAL DIALYSIS	
	BEFORE	AFTER
< 12	16 (35%)	0
13–19	15 (33%)	6 (13%)
20–30	14 (30%)	38 (83%)
> 31	1 (2%)	2 (4%)

* See footnote to Table 17-11.

due to a persistence of predialysis hyperventilation which may have existed as a respiratory compensatory response to the acidosis of the uremic patient. On occasion, especially with prolonged peritoneal dialysis, the absorption of large quantities of bicarbonate precursor may result in mild to moderate metabolic alkalosis. Postdialysis metabolic alkalosis is seen more often when the technique is utilized for the treatment of nonuremic, nonacidotic disorders, such as intoxications and congestive heart failure. The potential deleterious effects of using acetate as a buffer in hemodialysate (see above) have not been assessed as yet in either acute or chronic peritoneal dialysis, but it would seem likely that the significantly lesser efficiency of peritoneal dialysis would probably obviate any complications resulting from excessive rates of acetate diffusion into the patient.

Dextrose is added to augment the osmolality of the dialyzing solutions. The electrolyte composition of dialysate imparts an osmolality of approximately 290 mosm/L. The serum osmolality of most uremic patients is significantly higher than this, generally ranging from 310 to 350 mosm/L. An osmotic gradient of this magnitude could result in the absorption of significant quantities of water from the dialysate into the serum, creating a risk of overhydration of the patient (208). The addition of 15 g of dextrose to each liter (1.5% solutions) increases the dialysate osmolality to 365 or 372 mosm/L, thereby obviating the risk. Although the term is not precisely correct in this context, these 1.5% solutions are referred to as "isotonic" and generally in the uremic subject will not result in any major water shift between extracellular fluid and dialysate. In nonuremic patients (serum osmolality 280 to 300 mosm/L), however, these solutions are actually hyperosmolar ("hypertonic") and will produce negative fluid balance which, if marked, may result in significant depletion of the plasma volume and hypotension unless these losses are replaced. When such negative fluid balance is desirable for correction of states of overhydration, hypertonic dialyzing solutions are used. The osmolality of these solutions is increased by the addition of higher concentrations of dextrose. Hypertonic solutions are available with 4.25% dextrose concentrations

which have an osmolality approximating 525 mosm/L. 7% dextrose concentrations provide an osmolality of 678 mosm/L, but these solutions have been discontinued.

When repeated exchanges of 4.25% dextrose solutions are utilized, large quantities of dextrose may be absorbed, and hyperglycemia may result (see above). Although the uremic patient often manifests an impairment of glucose tolerance, we have rarely observed the blood glucose concentration to exceed 350 mg/dL except in the patients with diabetes mellitus, where concentrations in excess of 1000 mg/dL may occur. In diabetic patients, therefore, it is mandatory to follow serial blood glucose concentrations during dialysis and, when necessary, to administer insulin to counteract significant hyperglycemia. If a deterioration of the patient's state of consciousness occurs, one must be alert to the possibility that a hyperglycemic, hyperosmolar state may exist which, if unrecognized or uncorrected, may result in intracellular and cerebral dehydration and death (255).

It is rarely necessary to remove large quantities of extracellular fluid rapidly by hypertonic dialysis, and therefore it is our practice to achieve negative fluid balance by alternating the use of 4.25% dextrose and 1.5% solutions. With this technique, marked hyperglycemia or hyperosmolality rarely occurs, and a negative fluid balance of as much as 10 L can be achieved in a 24- to 36-h period. In those rare instances where greater fluid losses are desirable, we prefer to achieve it with a second peritoneal dialysis performed about 48 to 72 h after completion of the first.

When 2 L of hypertonic dialysis solutions is used, as much as 1000 mL of extracellular fluid may move into the peritoneal cavity within 30 to 45 min. In patients with cardiopulmonary disease, this large intraperitoneal volume may impair diaphragmatic movement and significantly increase dyspnea. Accordingly, in such patients, it may be advisable to use only 1 L of dialysate for each exchange.

The hypernatremia which may result from hypertonic peritoneal dialysis has already been discussed, as has been the fact that the "ultrafiltrate" is low in sodium, with a greater negative balance for water than for sodium. The composition of the ultrafiltrate with respect to other serum electrolytes has not yet been defined, but presumably the use of hypertonic solutions may enhance the negative balance for any dialyzable plasma solute, not only by virtue of the losses consistent with the ultrafiltrate volume, but by the additional effects of solute drag (256) and possibly by alteration of membrane permeability (222). This phenomenon, however, does not appear to be of major clinical importance for any other electrolyte except for potassium, where it may result in a final serum potassium concentration less than that of the dialysate potassium concentration. Also contributing to a lowering of the final serum potassium concentration is the fact that glucose absorbed from the dialysate is deposited as glycogen, and potassium is incorporated intracellularly in this metabolic process.

Occasionally, when dialysis is completed and the absorbed glucose is metabolized, reactive hypoglycemia may result (257) partially contributed to perhaps by the improvement in glucose metabolism resulting from the amelioration of uremia by the dialysis. For this reason, it is advisable, if insulin has been required during the dialysis, that doses be reduced or eliminated if possible toward the end of dialysis. Any postdialysis symptoms suggestive of hypoglycemia should be treated with orally or intravenously administered glucose.

There are several additives other than potassium chloride which may be added to the commercial dialysis solutions. *Aqueous heparin* in a dose of 1000 units per each 2-L exchange is added to prevent the clotting of any blood (from the puncture site or from the peritoneal surface) which may enter the peritoneal cavity, with possible occlusion of the dialysis catheter and interference with satisfactory drainage. When there is no intraperitoneal bleeding, as evidenced by the drainage of clear fluid from the patient, it is possible to discontinue the heparin.

The addition of antibiotics to the dialysis solutions is a matter of controversy. Maxwell et al. (210) originally recommended the addition of 25 mg of a tetracycline to each 2-L exchange. Subsequently, the demonstration of a prolonged half-life for tetracycline in renal failure and potential toxicity due to the antianabolic effect of tetracycline led to the suggestion that its use be abandoned (258). Even if all the tetracycline added to dialysate were absorbed in a 20-to-40 exchange dialysis, the maximal administered dose would be 500 to 1000 mg. We have never seen any postdialysis clinical complications attributable to tetracycline. Although we no longer routinely add antibiotics to dialysate, we strongly recommend their use where there is any indication that the procedure has not been conducted with the most scrupulous sterile technique by physician and nursing personnel thoroughly familiar with the necessary techniques. When antibiotics are needed, we continue to use tetracycline. There is some evidence that chloramphenicol may be preferable, since it is not significantly absorbed (258), but clinical experience is virtually totally lacking. Penicillin and its analogs are contraindicated because of the risk of sensitization, and kanamycin and neomycin because of the risk of nephrotoxicity and/or ototoxicity. There are no data referable to the use of other antibiotics as prophylactic additives to dialysate.

Antibiotics are not routinely used by those groups treating patients with chronic maintenance peritoneal dialysis. With the use of specially designed indwelling peritoneal catheters (259), a closed system for instilling and draining fluid, sterile solutions, reverse osmosis for treatment of water in those systems utilizing proportioning systems for dialysate preparation (260), and scrupulous sterile technique by patients and personnel, the incidence of bacterial peritonitis can be kept to as low as 0.12 percent (261). Sterile, cryptogenic peritonitis has been noted to occur, often clustered in "epidemic"-like outbreaks and possibly due to endotoxin (261, 262).

If significant pain occurs with the dialysis (usually while the fluid is being instilled or drained) 2 to 5 mL 1% *procaine hydrochloride* may be instilled via the dialysis tubing. If this is required more than two or three times, we prefer to attempt to reposition the catheter.

The use of other additives such as *albumin, alkali,* and *lipids* in an attempt to enhance the removal of certain solutes (principally toxins) has already been discussed.

Generally, 2 L of dialysate is introduced into the peritoneal cavity, although, as previously discussed, under special circumstances one might elect to infuse only 1 rather than 2 L for each exchange, specifically in those patients with cardiopulmonary disease in whom abdominal distention and limitation in diaphragmatic excursions are to be avoided. The rate of urea removal with 1-L exchanges can approximate that of 2-L exchanges if the time for a complete exchange (inflow, intraperitoneal dwell, and outflow) is halved (263). With 2-L exchanges and intermittent dialysate flow techniques, clinical (216) and theoretical (264) studies have suggested optimal dialysate exchange rates of 3.5 L/h. With the use of automated equipment, exchange times can be optimized and dialysate exchange rates as high as 12 L/h can be achieved with an increase of urea clearance from the usual 15 to 20 mL/min to as high as 40 mL/min (265). Ideally one would like to achieve a continuous flow of dialysate similar to that used in single-pass hemodialysis systems. Techniques to accomplish this, including the use of pumps and two dialysis catheters, have been reported (206, 223, 266–268). Shinaberger et al. (269) attempted to enhance dialysis efficiency and reduce total dialysate volume by continuously recirculating dialysate from the peritoneal cavity extracorporeally through an artificial kidney. Stephens et al. have utilized a similar recirculation technique also incorporating dialysate regeneration by activated charcoal (268). Gordon et al. (270) and Raja et al. (271) have performed continuous flow recirculating peritoneal dialyses utilizing the sorbent cartridge of the REDY system in dogs and have demonstrated the capacity to double the clearances achievable for low-molecular-weight solutes. Urea clearances as high as 60 mL/min have been achieved with such techniques (269, 270). None of these techniques, however, have as yet proved to be clinically satisfactory.

It is important to remember that *all* dialysis solutions are hyperosmolar to the usual patient undergoing dialysis and, except in the very rare case where the serum osmolality of the patient exceeds 370 mosm/L, dialysate will *never* be absorbed into the circulation over short periods of time. If all the instilled fluid is not returned (positive fluid balance), it means that the retained fluid is not draining for mechanical reasons or because it is filling intraperitoneal dead space. Some have suggested using 4.25% dextrose solutions when such positive balance occurs, in an attempt to restore fluid balance. Such an approach, however, can be potentially hazardous and should be undertaken only with full knowledge of the mechanisms involved. The 4.25% solution will move plasma water along osmolar concentration gradients into the peritoneal cavity, thereby increasing intraperitoneal volume. If the positive balance is due to incomplete filling of dead space, then this may result in improved drainage. Otherwise, it will merely deplete plasma volume, increased intraperitoneal volume, and fail to improve impaired drainage caused by an occluded catheter or dialysate leakage into extraperitoneal tissues. If resorted to repetitively in vain attempts to correct a positive fluid balance, it can result in plasma volume depletion and increasing distention of the abdomen. It may be attempted for one or possibly two exchanges in patients who are overhydrated and can tolerate depletion of the plasma volume. Otherwise, it is preferable to attempt to improve drainage by instilling an additional 500 or 1000 mL of dialysate. If these procedures fail to improve drainage, one is generally advised to remove the catheter, check it to see if it has become occluded, consider the possible causes of the poor drainage, and then introduce a new catheter.

When fluid has been inadvertently introduced into the abdominal wall or along fascial planes, it often becomes impossible to insert a catheter successfully thereafter. One should wait for this fluid to be absorbed into the circulation (generally about 24 h) before repeating attempts at peritoneal dialysis. This carries the risks of delay in starting dialysis, of overhydration when this fluid is absorbed, and, if hypertonic fluid has been used, of its functioning as a hyperosmolar clysis and drawing plasma into it. If the patient's condition does not permit acceptance of these risks, then hemodialysis will be required.

RESULTS OF PERITONEAL DIALYSIS

Peritoneal dialysis is a relatively inefficient technique when compared to hemodialysis. Boen

(120) has shown optimal clearances obtained with peritoneal dialysis to be as follows: urea 26 mL/min, potassium 21 mL/min, phosphate 16 mL/min, creatinine 15 mL/min, and uric acid 14 mL/min. Clearances for these solutes with hemodialysis are usually 300 to 600 percent higher. Therefore, it will take three to six times longer for peritoneal dialysis to achieve the solute removal obtained with hemodialysis, and accordingly peritoneal dialysis is usually conducted for 18 to 48 h in the treatment of the uremic patient. However, given this time, peritoneal dialysis accomplishes amelioration of the biochemical abnormalities of uremia which compares quite favorably to that achieved by hemodialysis.

Despite this relative inefficiency of peritoneal dialysis for the mass transfer of low-molecular-weight solutes, the clearance of middle-molecular-weight solutes such as inulin appears to be essentially identical (approximately 6 mL/min) to their clearance by hemodialyzers with similar functional dialysis areas (222). This is attributed presumptively to a peritoneal pore size and/or permeability (compared to hemodialysis membranes) more conducive to transport of middle-molecular-weight solutes. Removal of middle-molecular-weight solutes is almost certainly enhanced by the removal with each repetitive dialysis of the intraperitoneal reservoir accumulated in the interdialytic interval. Most chronic uremic patients have at least a small volume of peritoneal fluid and quantitatively the amount of middle-molecular-weight solute in this fluid is potentially a significant fraction of that removed with a dialysis. It is perhaps this relatively efficient mass transfer of middle-molecular-weight solutes which accounts for the low incidence of complications such as neuropathy seen in patients treated by chronic maintenance peritoneal dialysis despite lesser efficiency for mass transport of low-molecular-weight solutes such as urea and creatinine. Removal of these solutes can be augmented to approximate that of hemodialysis by prolonging treatment time for peritoneal dialysis. With the development of suitable implantable peritoneal catheters (259) and automated systems for the preparation and administration of large volumes of sterile peritoneal dialysate (272)

the capacity to perform repetitive maintenance peritoneal dialyses became a reality. Initially this therapy was reserved for patients not ideally suited for hemodialysis such as children, elderly patients with cardiovascular instability, those with no suitable vessels for vascular access, diabetics, and those incapable of successfully conducting home hemodialysis. Success in the treatment of these less than ideal patients has resulted in expansion of the indications for maintenance peritoneal dialysis, and it is perhaps not an exaggeration to state that it now represents a competitive technique to chronic hemodialysis in all patients with end-stage renal disease. The safety and simplicity of the technique makes it particularly suited to home dialysis and overnight use (273, 274).

Generally chronic peritoneal dialysis is conducted for 9 to 12 h, three or four times weekly. This generally results in a predialysis BUN below 100 mg/dL and creatinine below 15 mg/dL (273). The 10 to 20 g of protein lost with each dialysis is readily replaced by dietary protein intake of 1 g/kg per day. Table 17-15 shows comparative predialysis chemistries obtained in the same patients treated alternately with hemodialysis and peritoneal dialysis for periods in excess of 3 months with each technique (275).

In an attempt to simplify further the techniques of peritoneal dialysis, reduce required dialysate volumes, and possibly ultimately develop an am-

Table 17-15. Comparison of hemodialysis with peritoneal dialysis in 9 patients treated both ways for 3 months or more

	HEMODIALYSIS	PERITONEAL DIALYSIS
Na$^+$, meq/L	139 ± 4.0	139.0 ± 2.0
K$^+$, meq/L	4.7 ± 0.7	4.6 ± 0.7
CO$_2$, meq/L	21.0 ± 3.0	25.0 ± 2.0
BUN, mg/dL	64.0 ± 13.0	70.0 ± 12.0
Creatinine, mg/dL	9.9 ± 2.6	10.1 ± 3.7
Uric acid, mg/dL	7.9 ± 1.1	8.3 ± 1.6
Phosphorus, mg/dL	5.4 ± 1.6	5.9 ± 1.8
Protein, g/dL	6.8 ± 0.5	5.9 ± 0.7
Albumin, g/dL	3.7 ± 0.5	3.1 ± 0.5
Calcium, mg/dL	9.1 ± 0.4	8.4 ± 0.6
Hct, vol %	24.0 ± 4.0	27.0 ± 6.0
WBC	7.0 ± 1.4	7.8 ± 1.8

Source: From von Hartitzsch and Medlock. (275)

bulatory, wearable dialysis system, Lewin et al. have attempted to apply sorbent regeneration techniques to peritoneal dialysis, using the sorbents developed for the REDY system (276, 277). Sterilization of the sorbents has been achieved by gamma radiation and a system of filters adds further sterilization and renders the dialysate free of particles (276). Biochemically successful clinical functional dialyses have been achieved with total dialysate volumes of 6 L or less, but the full clinical application of the technique has been hampered by the occurrence of bacterial and aseptic, presumably chemical, peritonitis (277, 278). If this problem of peritonitis can be overcome, it is our opinion that the ultimate development of an ambulatory dialysis system is much more likely with peritoneal dialysis technology than with hemodialysis techniques.

REFERENCES

1. Quinton, W., D. Dillard, and B. H. Scribner: Cannulation of blood vessels for prolonged hemodialysis, *Trans. Am. Soc. Artif. Intern. Organs,* **6:**104, 1960.
2. Gurland, H. J., F. P. Brunner, C. Chantler, C. Jacobs, K. Schärer, N. H. Selwood, G. Spies, and A. J. Wing: Combined report on regular dialysis and transplantation in Europe, *Proc. Eur. Dial. Transplant Assoc.,* **3:**3, 1976.
3. von Hartitzsch, B., A. V. L. Hill, and T. R. Medlock: Nine hour peritoneal dialysis three times weekly—an alternative to conventional hemodialysis, *Proc. Eur. Dial. Transplant Assoc.,* **13:**306, 1976.
4. Babb, A. L., P. J. Johansen, M. J. Strand, H. Tenckhoff, and B. H. Scribner: Bidirectional permeability of the human peritoneum to middle molecules, *Proc. Eur. Dial. Transplant Assoc.,* **10:**247, 1973.
5. Maher, J. F., L. Lapierre, G. E. Schreiner, M. Geiger, and F. B. Westervelt, Jr.: Regional heparinization for hemodialysis: Technic and clinical experiences, *N. Engl. J. Med.,* **268:**451, 1963.
6. Kjellstrand, C. M.: Simple method for regional heparinization during dialysis avoiding rebound

7. Congdon, J. E., C. G. Kardenal, and J. D. Wallin: Monitoring heparin therapy in hemodialysis, *JAMA,* **226:**1529, 1973.
8. Kennedy, A. C., A. L. Linton, and J. C. Eaton: Urea levels in cerebrospinal fluid after hemodialysis, *Lancet,* **1:**410: 1962.
9. Hampers, C. L., P. B. Doak, M. N. Callaghan, H. R. Tyler, and J. P. Merrill: The electroencephalogram and spine fluid during hemodialysis, *Arch. Intern. Med.,* **118:**340, 1966.
10. Rosen, S. M., K. O'Connor, and S. Shaldon: Hemodialysis disequilibrium, *Br. Med. J.,* **2:**672, 1964.
11. Kennedy, A. C., A. I. Linton, S. Renfrew, R. G. Luke, and A. Dinwoodie: The pathogenesis and prevention of cerebral dysfunction during dialysis, *Lancet,* **1:**790, 1964.
12. Arieff, A. I., S. G. Massry, A. Barrientos, and C. R. Kleeman: Brain water and electrolyte metabolism in uremia: Effects of slow and rapid hemodialysis, *Kidney Int.,* **4:**177, 1973.
13. Arieff, A. I., R. Guisado, S. G. Massry, and V. C. Lazarowitz: Central nervous system pH in uremia and the effects of hemodialysis, *J. Clin. Invest.,* **58:**306, 1976.
14. Maher, J. F., and G. E. Schreiner: Hazards and complications of dialysis, *N. Engl. J. Med.,* **273:**370, 1965.
15. Gordon, A., and J. Astor: *Proc. III Int. Congr. Nephrol.,* 1966.
16. Le Grain, M., and J. P. Merrill: Short-term continuous transperitoneal dialysis, *N. Engl. J. Med.,* **248:**125, 1953.
17. Sarles, H. E., J. C. Lindley, and J. A. Fish: Peritoneal dialysis utilizing a millipore filter, *Kidney Int.,* **9:**54, 1976.
18. Maher, J. F., and G. E. Schreiner: Current status of dialysis of poisons and drugs, *Trans. Am. Soc. Artif. Intern. Organs,* **15:**461, 1969.
19. Berman, L. B., and P. Vogelsang: Removal rates for barbiturates using two types of peritoneal dialysis, *N. Engl. J. Med.,* **270:**77, 1964.
20. Shinaberger, J. H., L. Shear, L. E. Clayton, K. G. Barry, M. Knowlton, and L. R. Goldbaum: Dialysis for intoxication with lipid soluble drugs: Enhancement of glutethimide extraction with

phenomenon (abstract) *Trans. Amer. Soc. Nephrol.,* **3:**34, 1969.

lipid dialysate, *Trans. Am. Soc. Artif. Intern. Organs*, **11**:173, 1965.

21. Nahas, G. G., J. J. Giroux, J. Gjessing, M. Verosky, and L. C. Mark: The use of THAM in peritoneal dialysis, *Trans. Am. Soc. Artif. Intern. Organs*, **10**:345, 1964.

22. Winchester, J. F., M. C. Gelfand, J. H. Knepshield, and G. E. Schreiner: Dialysis and hemoperfusion of poisons and drugs, *Trans. Am. Soc. Artif. Int. Organs.*, **23**:762, 1977.

23. Boen, S. T., A. S. Mulinari, D. H. Dillard, and B. H. Scribner: Periodic dialysis in the management of chronic uremia, *Trans. Am. Soc. Artif. Intern Organs*, **8**:256, 1962.

24. von Hartitzsch, B., and T. R. Medloch: Chronic peritoneal dialysis—a regime comparable to conventional hemodialysis, *Trans. Am. Soc. Artif. Int. Organs*, **22**:595, 1976.

25. Tenckhoff, H., and F. K. Curtis: Experience with maintenance peritoneal dialysis in the home, *Trans. Am. Soc. Artif. Intern. Organs*, **16**:90, 1970.

26. Burns, R. O., L. W. Henderson, E. B. Hager, and J. P. Merrill: Peritoneal dialysis; clinical experience, *N. Engl. J. Med.*, **267**:1060, 1962.

27. Burnett, W. E., G. R. Brown, Jr., G. P. Rosemond, and H. T. Caswell: Treatment of peritonitis using peritoneal lavage, *Ann. Surg.*, **145**:675, 1957.

28. Teschan, P. E., C. R. Baxter, T. F. O'Brien, J. N. Freyhof, and W. H. Hall: Prophylactic hemodialysis in the treatment of acute renal failure, *Ann. Intern. Med.*, **53**:992, 1960.

29. Tenckhoff, H., R. H. Jebsen, and J. C. Honet: The effect of long-term dialysis treatment on the course of uremic neuropathy, *Trans. Am. Soc. Artif. Intern. Organs*, **13**:58, 1967.

30. Kiley, J. E., J. C. Pender, H. F. Welch, and C. S. Welch: Ammonia intoxication treated by hemodialysis, *N. Engl. J. Med.*, **259**:1156, 1958.

31. Nienhuis, L. I., E. I. Mulmed, and J. W. Kelley: Hepatic coma: Treatment emphasizing merit of peritoneal dialysis, *Am. J. Surg.*, **106**:980, 1963.

32. Kiley, J. E., H. F. Welch, J. C. Pender, and C. S. Welch: Removal of blood ammonia by hemodialysis, *Proc. Soc. Exp. Biol. Med.*, **91**:489, 1956.

33. Shoshkes, M., L. J. Kampel, J. Moss, B. Levinstone, and S. Ribot: The use of artificial renal dialysis techniques for the removal of bilirubin in the dog, *J. Newark Beth Israel Hosp.*, **14**:95, 1963.

34. Goldberg, M., L. Castelman, I. S. Friedman, and S. L. Wallace: The artificial kidney in the treatment of chronic tophaceous gout. Report of a case, *JAMA*, **182**:870, 1962.

35. Firmat, J., P. Vanamee, L. Klauber, I. Krakoff, and H. T. Randall: The artifical kidney in the treatment of renal failure and hyperuricemia in patients with lymphoma and leukemia, *Cancer*, **13**:276, 1960.

36. Clemmesen, C., and E. Nilsson: Therapeutic trends in the treatment of barbiturate poisoning, *Clin. Pharmacol. Ther.*, **2**:220, 1961.

37. Nealon, T. F., Jr., H. Surgerman, W. Shea, and E. Fleegler: An extracorporeal device to treat barbiturate poisoning: Use of anion-exchange resins in dogs, *JAMA*, **197**:118, 1966.

38. Yatzidis, H., D. Oreopoulos, D. Triantaphyllidis, S. Voudiclari, N. Tsaparas, C. Gavras, and A. Stravroulaki: Treatment of severe barbiturate poisoning, *Lancet*, **2**:216, 1965.

39. Rosenbaum, J. L., N. S. Kramer, and R. Raja: Resin hemoperfusion for acute drug intoxication, *Arch. Int. Med.*, **136**:263, 1976.

40. Chang, T. M. S., J. F. Coffey, P. Barre, A. Gonda, J. H. Dirks, M. Levy, and C. Lister: Microcapsule artificial kidney—treatment of patients with acute drug intoxication, *Can. Med., Assoc. J.*, **108**:429, 1973.

41. Gelfand, M. C., J. F. Winchester, J. H. Knepshield, K. M. Hanson, S. L. Cohan, B. S. Strauch, K. L. Geoly, A. C. Kennedy, and G. E. Schreiner: Treatment of severe drug overdosage with charcoal hemoperfusion, *Trans. Am. Soc. Artif. Intern Organs*, **23**:599, 1977.

42. Barbour, B. J., A. M. LaSette, and A. Koffler: Fixed-bed charcoal hemoperfusion for the treatment of drug overdose, *Kidney Int.*, **7**:S-333, 1976.

43. Rosenbaum, J. L., and O. P. Schumacher: Hemodialysis in the treatment of hypercalcemia, *Ohio State Med. J.*, **59**:1208, 1963.

44. Eisenberg, E., and F. A. Gotch: Normocalcemic hyperparathyroidism culminating in hypercalcemic crisis: Treatment with hemodialysis, *Arch. Intern. Med.*, **122**:258, 1968.

45. Finberg, L., J. Kiley, and C. N. Luttrell: Mass

accidental salt poisoning in infancy: A study of a hospital disaster, *JAMA*, **184**:187, 1963.

46. Richards, C. J., D. E. Gentile, C. R. P. George, W. J. Johnson, W. A. Lapkin, L. Lewin, W. B. Shapiro, L. J. Segal, T. I. Stainman, and F. B. Westervelt: Advantages of sorbent regeneration hemodialysis for acute renal failure. In press.

47. Westervelt, F. B., Jr., J. A. Owen, Jr., J. H. Hornbaker, Jr., and T. L. Gorsuch: Lactic-acidosis: A case treated with THAM and hemodialysis, *V. Med. Mon.*, **93**:251, 1966.

48. Jurgesen, J. C.: Dialysis for lactic acidosis, *N. Engl. J. Med.*, **278**:1350, 1968.

49. Maillou, L. U., C. D. Swartz, G. Onesti, C. Heider, O. Ramirez, and A. N. Brest: Peritoneal dialysis for refractory congestive heart failure, *JAMA*, **199**:873, 1967.

50. Rae, A. I., and J. Hopper, Jr.: Removal of refractory edema fluid by peritoneal dialysis, *Br. J. Urol.*, **40**:336, 1968.

51. Thölen, H., E. Stricker, H. Feer, M. A. Massini, and H. Staub: Über die Anwendung der Künstlichen Niere bei Schizophrenie und Myasthenia Gravis, *Dtsch. Med., Wochenschr*, **85**:1012, 1960.

52. Jutzler, G. A., S. Neuheisel, and P. Schmid: Experimental treatment of acute intermittent porphyria by extracorporeal hemodialysis, *Ger. Med. Mon.*, **9**:402, 1964.

53. Moyo, C. T. B., J. B. Dosseter, and L. D. MacLeau: Hemodialysis in the treatment of shock, *J. Surg. Res.*, **4**:380, 1964.

54. Wagemaker, H., Jr., and R. Cade: The use of hemodialysis in chronic schizophrenia, *Am. J. Psychiatry*, **134**:684, 1977.

55. Twardowski, Z. J.: Abatement of psoriasis and repeated dialysis, *Ann. Int. Med.*, **86**:509, 1977.

56. Lash, R. F., J. A. Burdette, and T. Ozdil: Accidental profound hypothermia and barbiturate intoxication: A report of rapid core rewarming by peritoneal dialysis, *JAMA*, **201**:269, 1967.

57. Cole, W. C. C., and J. C. Montgomery: Intraperitoneal blood transfusion: Report of 237 transfusions in 117 patients in private practice, *Am. J. Dis. Child.*, **37**:497, 1929.

58. Shear, L., C. Schwartz, J. A. Shinaberger, and K. G. Barry: Kinetics of peritoneal fluid absorption in adult man, *N. Engl. J. Med.*, **272**:123, 1965.

59. Maher, J. F., and G. E. Schreiner: Cause of death in acute renal failure, *Arch. Intern. Med.*, **110**:493, 1962.

60. Henderson, L. W.: Hemodialysis: Rationale and physical principles, in B. M. Brenner and F. C. Rector, Jr. (eds.), *The Kidney*, W. B. Saunders Company, Philadelphia, 1976, pp. 1643–1671.

61. Gotch, F. A.: Hemodialysis: Technical and kinetic considerations, in B. M. Brenner and F. C. Rector, Jr. (eds.), *The Kidney*, W. B. Saunders Company, Philadelphia, 1976, pp. 1672–1704.

62. Wolf, A. V., D. G. Remp, J. E. Kiley, and G. D. Currie: Artificial kidney function: Kinetics of hemodialysis, *J. Clin. Invest.*, **30**:1062, 1951.

63. Abel, J. J., L. G. Rowntree, and B. B. Turner: The removal of diffusible substances from the circulating blood by means of dialysis, *Trans. Assoc. Am. Physicians*, **28**:51, 1913.

64. Love, G. R.: Vividiffusion with intestinal membranes, *Med. Rec.*, **98**:649, 1920.

65. Necheles, H.: Über Dialysieren des stromenden Blutes am Lebenden, *Klin. Wochenschr.*, **2**:1257, 1923.

66. Thalheimer, W.: Experimental exchange transfusions for reducing azotemia: Use of artificial kidney for this purpose, *Proc. Soc. Exp. Biol. Med.*, **37**:641, 1937

67. Kloff, W. J.: *New Ways of Treating Uremia*, J. and A. Churchill, London, 1947.

68. Rubin, A. L., R. R. Riggio, R. L. Nachman, G. H. Schwartz, T. Miyata, and K. H. Stenzel: Collagen materials in dialysis and implantation, *Trans. Am. Soc. Artif. Intern. Organs*, **14**:169, 1968.

69. Markle, R., R. Falb, and R. Leininger: Development of improved membranes for artificial kidney dialysis, *Trans. Am. Soc. Artif. Intern. Organs*, **10**:22, 1964.

70. Henderson, L. W., L. Livoti, C. Ford, A. Kelly, and M. Lysaght: Clinical experience with intermittent hemodiafiltration, *Trans. Am. Soc. Artif. Intern. Organs*, **19**:119, 1973.

71. Silverstein, M. D., C. A. Ford, M. J. Lysaght, and L. W. Henderson: Response to rapid removal of intermediate molecular weight solutes in uremic man, *Trans. Am. Soc. Artif. Intern. Organs*, **20**:614, 1974.

72. Funck-Brentano, J. L., A. Sausse, N. K. Man, A. Granger, M. Rondon-Nucette, J. Zingraff, and P. Jungers: Une nouvelle methode d'hemodialyse

associant une membrane a haute permeabilite pour les moyennes molecules et un bain de dialyse en circuit ferme, *Proc. Eur. Dial. Transplant Assoc.*, **9**:55, 1972.

73. Quellhorst, E., J. Rieger, B. Doht, H. Beckmann, I. Jacob, B. Kraft, G. Mietzsch, and F. Scheler: Treatment of chronic uremia by an ultrafiltration kidney—first clinical experience, *Proc. Eur. Dial. Transplant Assoc.*, **13**:314, 1976.

74. Barbour, B. H., M. Bernstein, P. A. Cantor, B. S. Fisher, and W. Stone, Jr.: Clinical use of NISR polycarbonate membrane for hemodialysis, *Trans. Am. Soc. Artif. Intern. Organs*, **21**:144, 1975.

75. Farrell, P. G., and A. L. Babb: Estimation of the permeability of cellulosic membranes from solute dimensions and diffusivities, *J. Biomed. Mater. Res.*, **7**:275, 1973.

76. Babb, A. L., R. P. Popovich, T. G. Christopher, and B. H. Scribner: The genesis of the square meter-hour hypothesis, *Trans. Am. Soc. Artif. Intern. Organs*, **17**:81, 1971.

77. Babb, A. L., P. J. Johansen, M. J. Strand, H. Tenckhoff, and B. H. Scribner: Bi-directional permeability of the human peritoneum to middle molecules, *Proc. Eur. Dial. Transplant Assoc.*, **10**:247, 1973.

78. Ota, K., T. Okazawa, E. Kumagaya, T. Agishi, N. Sugino, N. Mitani, Y. Fujii, M. Kinura, Y. Nagao, H. Tsukamoto, H. Tanzawa, and Y. Sakai: Polymethylmethacrylate capillary kidney highly permeable to middle molecules, *Proc. Eur. Dial. Transplant Assoc.*, **12**:559, 1975.

79. Stewart, W. K., and L. W. Fleming: Blood pressure control during maintenance haemodialysis with isonatric (high sodium) dialysate, *Postgrad. Med. J.*, **50**:260, 1974.

80. Stewart, W. K., L. W. Fleming, and M. A. Manuel: Benefits obtained by the use of high sodium dialysate during maintenance haemodialysis, *Proc. Eur. Dial. Transplant Assoc.*, **9**:111, 1972.

81. Jenkins, P. G., and W. H. Dreher: Dialysis-induced muscle cramps: Treatment with hypertonic saline and theory as to etiology, *Trans. Am. Soc. Artif. Intern. Organs*, **21**:479, 1975.

82. Gotch, F. A., J. Autian, C. Colton, H. E. Ginn, B. J. Lipps, and E. Lowrie: The evaluation of hemodialyzers, Department of Health, Education, and Welfare Publication NIH 73-103.

83. Gotch, F. A.: Solute transport and ultrafiltration in hemodialysis, in S. G. Massry and A. L. Sellers (eds.), *Clinical Aspects of Uremia and Dialysis*, Charles C Thomas, Publisher, Springfield, Ill., 1976, pp. 639–658.

84. Nolph, K. D., T. D. Groshong, and J. F. Maher: Estimation of weight loss during coil dialysis, *Kidney Int.*, **1**:182, 1972.

85. Maher, J. F.: Discussion, *Trans. Am. Soc. Artif. Intern. Organs*, **7**:20, 1961.

86. Nolph, K. D., C. A. Hopkins, D. New, G. D. Antwiler, and R. P. Popovich: Differences in solute sieving with osmotic vs. hydrostatic ultrafiltration, *Trans. Am. Soc. Artif. Intern. Organs*, **22**:618, 1976.

87. Ing. T. S., D. L. Ashbach, and A. Kanter: Fluid removal with negative-pressure hydrostatic ultrafiltration using a partial vacuum, *Nephron*, **14**:451, 1975.

88. Bergström, J., H. Asaba, P. Fürst, and R. Oules: Dialysis, ultrafiltration and blood pressure, *Proc. Eur. Dial. Transplant Assoc.*, **13**:293, 1976

89. Shinaberger, J. A.: Dialysis, *Current Nephrology*, **1**:314, 1977.

90. Stewart, W. K., L. W. Fleming, and S. McLean: Is hyponatric dialysis appropriate, *Dialysis and Transplantation*, **6**:9, 1977.

91. Novello, A., R. C. Kelsch, and R. E. Easterling: Acetate intolerance during hemodialysis, *Clin. Nephrol.*, **5**:29, 1976.

92. Scribner, B. H.: Substitution of bicarbonate for acetate in the dialysate for care of a critically ill patient, *Dialysis and Transplantation*, **6**:26, 1977.

93. DePalma, J. R., A. Gordon, and M. H. Maxwell: Home hemodialysis using glucose and potassium free dialysate, *Proc. Int. Congr. Nephrol.*, **4**:55, 1969.

94. Swamy, A. P., R. V. M. Cestero, R. G. Campbell, and R. B. Freeman: Long term effect of dialysate glucose on the lipid levels of maintenance dialysis, *Trans. Am. Soc. Artif. Intern. Organs*, **22**:54, 1976.

95. Mendelssohn, S., C. D. Swartz, M. Yudis, G. Onesti, O. Ramirez, and A. N. Brest: High glucose concentration dialysate in chronic hemodialysis, *Trans. Amer. Soc. Artif. Intern. Organs*, **13**:249, 1967.

96. Potter, D. J.: Death as a result of hyperglycemia

without ketosis—a complication of hemodialysis *Ann. Intern. Med.*, **64**:399, 1965.

97. Gutman, R. A., R. O. Hickman, G. E. Chatrian, and B. H. Scribner: Failure of high dialysis-fluid glucose to prevent the disequilibrium syndrome, *Lancet*, **1**:295, 1967.

98. Blumberg, A., R. M. Hegstrom, W. B. Nelp, and B. H. Scribner: Extracellular volume in patients with chronic renal disease treated for hypertension by sodium restriction, *Lancet*, **2**:69, 1967.

99. Compty, C., H. Rottka, and S. Shaldon: Blood pressure control in patients with end-stage renal failure treated by intermittent hemodialysis, *Proc. Eur. Dial. Transplant. Assoc.*, **1**:209, 1964.

100. Hampers, C. L., J. J. Skillman, J. H. Lyons, J. E. Olson, and J. P. Merrill: A hemodynamic evaluation of bilateral nephrectomy and hemodialysis in hypertensive man, *Circulation*, **35**:272, 1967.

101. Merrill, J. P.: Discussion, *Trans. Am. Soc. Artif. Intern Organs*, **14**:365, 1968.

102. Douglas, B. H., A. C. Cuyton, J. B. Langston, and U. S. Bishop: Hypertension caused by salt loading. II. Fluid volume and tissue pressure changes, *Am. J. Physiol.*, **207**:669, 1964.

103. Vertes, V., J. L. Cangiano, L. B. Berman, and A. Gould: Hypertension in end-stage renal disease, *N. Engl. J. Med.*, **280**:978 1969.

104. Guyton, A. C., T. G. Coleman, A. W. Cowley, Jr., K. W. Schell, R. D. Manning, Jr., and R. A. Norma, Jr.: Arterial pressure regulation. Overriding dominance of the kidneys in long-term regulation of hypertension, *Am. J. Med.*, **52**:584, 1972.

105. Coleman, T. G., J. D. Bower, H. G. Langford, and A. C. Guyton: Regulation of arterial pressure in the anephric state, *Circulation*, **42**:509, 1970.

106. Popovtzer, M. M., B. J. Rosenbaum, A. Gordon, and M. H. Maxwell: Relief of uremic neuropathy after bilateral nephrectomy, *N. Engl. J. Med.*, **281**:949, 1969.

107. Feingold, L. N., F. X. Walsh, R. A. Gutman, J. C. Gunnells, and R. R. Robinson: Control of cachexia and ascites during chronic hemodialysis by bilateral nephrectomy, *Ann. Intern. Med.*, **78**:829, 1973.

108. Onesti, G., C. Swartz, O. Remirez, and A. N. Brest: Bilateral nephrectomy for control of hypertension in uremia, *Trans. Am. Soc. Artif. Intern. Organs,* **14**:361, 1968.

109. Cohn, J. N.: Paroxysmal hypertension and hypovolemia, *N. Engl. J. Med.*, **275**:643, 1966.

110. Brown, C. W.: Management of hypertension in chronic dialysis, *Proc. Third Annual S. E. Dialysis Conf.*, **3**:163, 1968.

111. Gleadle, R. I., J. J. Brown, J. R. Curtis, R. Fraser, D. H. Lawson, A. F. Lever, A. L. Linton, S. McVeigh, J. I. S. Robertson, H. E. DeWardener, and A. J. Wing: Plasma renin concentration and the control of blood pressure in patients with chronic renal failure. The effect of hemodialysis. *Proc. Eur. Dial. Transplant Assoc.*, **6**:131, 1969.

112. Rao, T. K. S., T. Manis, B. G. Delano, and E. A. Friedman: Continuing high morbidity during maintenance hemodialysis consequent to bilateral nephrectomy, *Trans. Am. Soc. Artif. Intern. Organs*, **19**:340, 1973.

113. Craswell, P. W., V. M. Hird, R. A. Baillod, Z. Varghese, and J. F. Moorhead: Significance of high plasma renin activity in patients on maintenance hemodialysis therapy, *Br. Med. J.*, **2**:741, 1973.

114. Hull, A. R., D. L. Long, R. C. Prati, W. A. Pettinger, and T. F. Parker: The control of hypertension in patients undergoing regular maintenance hemodialysis, *Kidney Int.*, **7**(suppl. 11):184, 1975.

115. Johnson, W. J., P. P. Frohnert, and N. P. Ladislaw: Potassium balance in patients maintained by long-term hemodialysis against potassium-free dialysate (abstract 1), *Proc. IV Int. Congr. Nephrol.*, **4**:303, 1969.

116. Fine, R. N.: Personal communication.

117. Rosen, V.: Personal communication.

118. Earnest, D. L., J. H. Sadler, R. H. Ingram, and E. J. Macon: Acid-base balance in chronic hemodialysis, *Trans. Am. Soc. Artif. Intern. Organs*, **14**:434, 1968.

119. Rosenbaum, B. J., J. W. Coburn, J. H. Shinaberger, and S. G. Massry: Acid-base status during the interdialytic period in patients maintained with chronic hemodialysis, *Ann. Intern. Med.*, **71**:1105, 1969.

120. Kaye, M., R. Mangel, and E. Neubauer: Studies in calcium metabolism in patients on chronic hemodialysis, *Proc, Eur. Dial. Transplant. Assoc.*, **3**:17, 1966.

121. Ogden, D. A., and J. H. Holmes: Changes in total and ultrafilterable plasma calcium and magne-

sium during hemodialysis, *Trans. Am. Soc. Artif. Intern. Organs*, **12**:200, 1966.

122. Goldsmith, R. S., and W. J. Johnson: Role of phosphate depletion and high dialysate calcium in controlling dialytic renal osteodystrophy, *Kidney Int.*, **4**:154, 1973.

123. Johnson, W. J.: Optimum dialysate calcium concentration during maintenance hemodialysis, *Nephron*, **17**:241, 1976.

124. Stewart, W. K., L. W. Fleming, D. C. Anderson, J. A. R. Lenman, and D. G. Hamieson: Changes in plasma electrolytes and nerve conduction velocities during chronic hemodialysis without magnesium, *Proc. Eur. Dial. Transplant. Assoc.*, **4**:285, 1967.

125. Burnell, J. M., and E. Teubner: Improvement of renal osteodystrophy by removal of magnesium from dialysate (abstract), Clin. Dial. and Transpl. Forum (1976).

126. Posen, G. A., and M. Kaye: Magnesium metabolism in patients on chronic dialysis, *Proc. Eur. Dial. Transplant. Assoc.*, **4**:224, 1967.

127. Earle, J. M., N. A. Kurtzman, and R. H. Moser: Hypercalcemia and hypertension, *Ann. Intern. Med.*, **64**:378, 1966.

128. Weidmann, P., S. G. Massry, J. W. Cobrun, M. H. Maxwell, J. Atleson, and C. R. Kleeman: Blood pressure effects of acute hypercalcemia. Studies in patients with chronic renal failure, *Ann. Intern. Med.*, **76**:741, 1972.

129. Drukker, W.: The hard water syndrome: A potential hazard during regular dialysis treatment, *Proc. Eur. Dial. Transplant. Assoc.*, **5**:284, 1968.

130. Govan, J. R., C. A. Porter, J. G. H. Cook, B. Dixon, and J. A. P. Trafford: Acute magnesium poisoning as a complication of chronic intermittent hemodialysis, *Br. Med. J.*, **2**:279, 1968.

131. Freeman, R. M., R. L. Lawton, and M. A. Chamberlain: Hard water syndrome, *N. Engl. J. Med.*, **276**:1113, 1967.

132. Cobrun, J. W., S. G. Massry, J. R. DePalma, and J. H. Shinaberger: Rapid appearance of hypercalemia with initiation of hemodialysis, *JAMA*, **210**:2276, 1969.

133. Comty, C. M., D. Luehmann, R. Wathen, and F. Shapiro: Water treatment for hemodialysis, *Dialysis and Transplantation*, **3**:26, 1974.

134. Madsen, R. F., B. Nielsen, O. J. Olsen, and F. Raaschou: Reverse osmosis as a method of preparing dialysis water, *Nephron*, **7**:545, 1970.

135. Nielsen, E., N. Solomon, N. J. Goodwin, N. Siddhivarn, R. Galonsky, D. Taves, and E. A. Friedman: Fluoride metabolism in uremia, *Trans. Am. Soc. Artif. Intern. Organs*, **19**:450, 1973.

136. Ivanovich, P., A. Manzler, and R. Drake: Acute hemolysis following hemodialysis, *Trans. Am. Soc. Artif. Intern. Organs*, **15**:316, 1969.

137. Matter, B. J., J. Pederson, G. Psimenos, and R. D. Lindemann: Lethal copper intoxication in hemodialysis, *Trans. Am. Soc. Artif. Intern. Organs*, **15**:309, 1969.

138. Yawata, Y., R. Howe, and H. S. Jacob: Abnormal red cell metabolism causing hemolysis in uremia, *Ann. Int. Med.*, **79**:362, 1973.

139. Carlson, D. J., and F. L. Shapiro: Methemoglobinemia from well water nitrates: A complication of home dialysis, *Ann. Int. Med.*, **73**:757, 1970.

140. Lawson, D. H., K. Boddy, P. C. King, A. L. Linton, and G. Will: Iron metabolism in patients with chronic renal failure on regular dialysis treatment, *Clin. Sci.*, **41**:345, 1971.

141. Caner, J. E. Z., and J. L. Decker: Recurrent acute (? gouty) arthritis in chronic renal failure treated by periodic hemodialysis, *Am. J. Med.*, **36**:571, 1964.

142. Kaye, M., R. Mangel, and E. Neubauer: Studies in calcium metabolism in patients on chronic hemodialysis, *Proc. Eur. Dial. Transplant. Assoc.*, **3**:17, 1966.

143. Alfrey, A. C., J. M. Mishell, J. Burks, S. R. Contiguglia, H. Rudolph, E. Lewin, and J. H. Holmes: Syndrome of dyspraxia and multifocal seizures associated with chronic hemodialysis, *Trans. Am. Soc. Artif. Intern. Organs*, **18**:257, 1972.

144. Berlyne, G. M.: Aluminum toxicity, *Lancet*, **1**:589, 1976.

145. Alfrey, A. C., G. R. LeGendre, and W. D. Kachney: *N. Engl. J. Med.*, **294**:184, 1976.

146. Ulner, D. M.: Toxicity from aluminum toxicity. *N. Engl. J. Med.*, **294**:184, 1976.

147. Flendrig, J. A., H. Kruis, and H. A. Das: Aluminum intoxication: The cause of dialysis dementia, *Proc. Eur. Dial. Transpl. Assoc.*, **13**:355, 1976.

148. Pieredes, A. M., H. A. Ellis, M. K. Ward, P. Aljama, J. Dewar, and D. N. S. Kerr: The need and

use of a phosphate-enriched dialysate during regular hemodialysis, *Trans. Am. Soc. Artif. Intern. Organs*, **23**:376, 1977.

149. Pierides, A. M., W. Simpson, H. A. Ellis, M. K. Ward, J. H. Dewar, and D. N. S. Kerr: Variable response to long-term 1, α-hydroxycholecalceferol in hemodialysis osteodystrophy, *Lancet*, **1**:1092, 1976.

150. Ward, M. K., A. M. Pieredes, P. Fawcett, D. A. Shaw, R. H. Perry; B. E. Tomlinson, and D. N. S. Kerr: Dialysis encephalopathy syndrome, Proc. *Eur. Dial. Transpl. Assoc.*, **13**:348, 1976.

151. Davidson, R. C., and J. P. Pendras: Calcium related cardio-respiratory death in chronic hemodialysis, *Trans. Am. Soc. Artif. Intern. Organs*, **13**:36, 1967.

152. Sokol, A., T. Gral, D. N. Edelbaum, V. Rosen, and M. E. Rubini: Correlation of autopsy findings and clinical experience in chronically dialyzed patients, *Trans. Am. Soc. Artif. Intern. Organs*, **13**:51, 1967.

153. Maher, J. F., R. B. Freeman, and G. E. Schreiner: Hemodialysis for chronic renal failure. II. Biochemical and clinical aspects, *Ann. Intern. Med.*, **62**:535, 1965.

154. Terman, D. S., A. C. Alfrey, W. C. Hammond, D. A. Ogden, and J. H. Homes: Metastatic calcification of the myocardium in uremia, *Proc. Am. Soc. Nephrol.*, **3**:67, 1969.

155. Schreiner, G. E., and J. F. Maher: *Uremia: Biochemistry, Pathogenesis and Treatment*, Charles C Thomas, Publisher, Springfield, Ill., 1962, p. 291.

156. Massry, S. G., M. M. Popovtzer, J. W. Coburn, D. L. Makoff, M. H. Maxwell, and C. R. Kleeman: Intractable pruritus as a manifestation of secondary hyperparathyroidism in uremia: Disappearance of itching after subtotal parathyroidectomy, *N. Engl. J. Med.*, **279**:697, 1968.

157. Mion, C. M., R. M. Hegstrom, S. T. Boen, and B. H. Scribner: Substitution of sodium acetate for sodium bicarbonate in the bath fluid for hemodialysis, *Trans. Am. Soc. Artif. Intern. Organs*, **10**:110, 1964.

158. Mudge, G. H., J. A. Manning, and A. Gilman: Sodium acetate as a source of fixed base, *Proc. Soc. Exp. Biol. Med.*, **71**:136, 1949.

159. Gonzales, F. M., J. E. Pearson, S. B. Gardus, and R. P. Nolbert: On the effects of acetate during hemodialysis. *Trans. Am. Soc. Artif. Intern. Organs*, **20**:169, 1974.

160. Novello, A., R. C. Kelsca, and R. E. Easterling: Acetate intolerance during hemodialysis, *Clin. Nephrol.*, **5**:29, 1976.

161. Bagdade, J. D., D. Porte, Jr., and E. L. Bierman: Hypertriglyceridemia: A metabolic consequence of chronic renal failure, *N. Engl. J. Med.*, **279**:181, 1968.

162. Rorke, S. J., W. D. Davidson, S. S. Guo, and R. J. Morin: Metabolic fate of ^{14}C-acetate during dialysis, *Proc. Eur. Dial. Transpl. Assoc.*, **13**:394, 1976.

163. Morgan, A. G., L. Burkinshaw, P. J. A. Robinson, and S. M. Rosen: Potassium balance and acid-base changes in patients undergoing regular hemodialysis, *Respiration*, **30**:889, 1973.

164. Gibson, G. J., and J. A. Streeton: Ventilatory response and acute acid-base changes in response to inhaled carbon dioxide in patients with chronic renal failure on long-term haemodialysis, *Respiration*, **30**:889, 1973.

165. Blumberg, A., and H. R. Marti: Mechanism of post-dialysis hyperventilation in patients with chronic renal insufficiency, *Clin. Nephrol.*, **5**:119, 1976.

166. Cowie, J., A. T. Lambie, and J. S. Robson: The influence of extracorporeal dialysis on the acid-base composition of blood and cerebrospinal fluid, *Clin. Sci.*, **23**:397, 1962.

167. Graziani, G., C. Ponticecchi, G. DiFilippo, and B. Radaelli: Acid-base changes in hemodialysis, *Br. Med. J.*, **2**:163, 1970.

168. Sherlock, J. E., J. W. Ledwith, and J. M. Letteri: Hemodialysis induced hypoxemia, *Dialysis and Transplantation*, **6**:34, 1977

169. Kirkendol, P. L., J. D. Bower, J. E. Pearson, and R. D. Holbert: The myocardial depressent effect of the hemodialysis buffer salt, sodium acetate, Abstr. Am. Soc. Nephrol, 1975, p. 31.

170. Graefe, U., W. Follette, J. Vizzo, and B. H. Scribner: Reduction in dialysis induced morbidity and vascular instability with the use of bicarbonate in dialysate. In preparation.

171. Peterson, H. deC., and A. G. Swanson: Acute encephalopathy occurring during hemodialysis, *Arch. Intern. Med.*, **113**:877, 1964.

172. Dosseter, J. B., J. Oh, L. Dayes, and H. M.

Pappins: Brain urea and water changes with rapid hemodialysis of uremic dogs, *Trans. Am. Soc. Artif. Intern. Organs,* **10**:323, 1964.

173. Sitprija, U., and J. H. Holmes: Preliminary observations on the change in intracranial pressure and intraocular pressure during hemodialysis, *Trans. Am. Soc. Artif. Intern. Organs,* **10**:323, 1962.

174. Gilliland, K. G., and R. M. Hegstrom: The effect of hemodialysis on cerebrospinal-fluid pressure in uremic dogs, *Trans. Am. Soc. Artif. Intern. Organs,* **9**:44, 1963.

175. Kennedy, A. C., A. L. Linton, R. G. Luke, and G. Renfrew: Electroencephalographic changes during hemodialysis, *Lancet,* **1**:408, 1963.

176. Kennedy, A. C., A. L. Linton, S. Renfrew, R. G. Luke, and A. Dinwoodie: The pathogenesis and prevention of cerebral dysfunction during dialysis, *Lancet,* **1**:790, 1964.

177. Schooler, J. C., C. F. Barlow, and L. J. Roth: The penetration of carbon-14 urea into cerebrospinal fluid and various areas of the cat brain, *J. Neuropathol. Exp. Neurol.,* **19**:216, 1960.

178. Hampers, C. L., and E. Schupak: *Long-Term Hemodialysis,* Grune & Stratton, Inc., New York, 1967, pp. 119-133.

179. Arieff, A. I., S. G. Massry, A. Barrientos, and C. R. Kleeman: Brain water and electrolyte metabolism in uremia. Effects of slow and rapid hemodialysis, *Kidney Int.,* **4**:177, 1973.

180. Wakim, K. G.: Predominance of hyponatremia over hypo-osmolality in simulation of the dialysis disequilibrium syndrome, *Mayo Clin. Proc.,* **44**:433, 1969.

181. Arieff, A. I., and S. G. Massry: Dialysis disequilibrium syndrome, in S. G. Massry and A. L. Selbers (eds.), *Clinical Aspects of Uremia and Dialysis,* Charles C Thomas, Publisher, Springfield, Ill., 1976, pp. 34-38.

182. Arieff, A. I., R. Gusado, S. G. Massry, and V. C. Lazarowtiz: Central nervous system pH in uremia and the effects of hemodialysis, *J. Clin. Invest.,* **58**:306, 1976.

183. Potter, D. J.: Death as a result of hyperglycemia without ketosis: A complication of hemodialysis, *Ann. Intern. Med.,* **64**:399, 1966.

184. Boyer, J., G. N. Gill, and F. H. Epstein: Hyperglycemia and hyperosmolality complicating peritoneal dialysis, *Ann. Intern. Med.,* **67**:568, 1967.

185. Rigg, G. A., and B. A. Bercu: Hypoglycemia—a complication of hemodialysis, *N. Engl. J. Med.,* **277**:1139, 1967.

186. Wakim, K. G., W. J. Johnson, and D. W. Klass: Role of blood urea and serum sodium concentrations in the pathogenesis of the dialysis dysequilibrium syndrome, *Trans. Am. Soc. Artif. Intern. Organs,* **14**:394, 1968.

187. Jenkins, P. G., and W. H. Dveher: Dialysis induced muscle cramps: Treatment with hypertonic saline and theory as to etiology, *Trans. Am. Soc. Artif. Intern. Organs,* **21**:479, 1975.

188. Gordon, A., T. Gral, J. R. DePalma, M. A. Greenbaum, L. B. Marantz, M. J. McArthur, and M. H. Maxwell: A sorbent-based low volume dialysate system: Preliminary studies in human subjects, *Proc. Eur. Dial. Transplant Assoc.,* **7**:63, 1970.

189. Gordon, A., O. S. Better, M. A. Greenbaum, L. B. Marantz, and M. H. Maxwell: Clinical maintenance hemodialysis with a sorbent-based, low volume dialysate regeneration system, *Trans. Am. Soc. Artif. Intern. Organs,* **17**:253, 1971.

190. Roberts, M., E. A. Pecker, A. J. Lewin, A. Gordon, and M. H. Maxwell: Clinical experience with absorptive recirculation dialysis, *Dialysis and Transplantation,* **6**:15, 1977.

191. Gordon, A., F. Parsons, and W. Drukker: Practical application of dialysate regeneration. In press.

192. Farrell, P. C., J. Mahony, J. Dawborn, A. Disney, B. Jones, and T. Mathew: Clinical evaluation of a dialysate regeneration system for maintenance dialysis, *Aust. N. Z. J. Med.,* **6**:292, 1976.

193. Hampl, M., M. Kessel, and G. Horn: Short duration dialysis employing the REDY (R) system with special consideration of buffer capacity, *Nieren U. Hochdruckkrankheiten* **5**(suppl. 1):34, 1976.

194. Richards, C. J., D. E. Gentile, C. R. P. George, W. J. Johnson, W. A. Lapkin, L. Lewin, W. B. Shapiro, L. J. Segal, T. I. Steinman, and F. B. Westervelt: Advantages of sorbent regeneration hemodialysis for acute renal failure. In press.

195. Henderson, L. W., C. Ford, C. K. Colton, L. W. Bluemle, Jr., and H. J. Bixler: Uremic blood cleansing by diafiltration using a hollow fiber ultrafilter, *Trans. Am. Soc. Artif. Intern. Organs,* **16**:107, 1970.

196. Man, N. K., A. Granger, M. Rondon-Nucete, J. Zingraff, P. Jungers, A. Sausse, and J. L. Funck-Brentano: One year follow-up of short dialysis with a membrane highly permeable to middle molecular, *Proc. Eur. Dial. and Transplant Assoc.*, **10:**236, 1973.

197. Henderson, L. W., L. Livoti, C. Ford, A. Kelly, and M. Lysaght: Clinical experience with intermittent hemodiafiltration, *Trans. Am. Soc. Artif. Intern. Organs*, **19:**1119, 1973.

198. Quellhorst, E., J. Roeger, B. Doht, H. Beckmann, I. Jacob, B. Kraft, G. Mietzsch, and F. Scheler: Treatment of chronic uraemia by an untrafiltration kidney—first clinical experience, *Proc. Eur. Dial. and Transpl. Assoc.*, **13:**314, 1976.

199. Henderson, L. W., C. A. Ford, M. J. Lysaght, R. A. Grossman, and M. E. Silverstein, Preliminary observations on blood pressure response with maintenance diafiltration, *Kidney Int.*, **7**(suppl. 3):S-413, 1975.

200. Shapiro, W., and M. Roberts: Personal communications.

201. Putnam, T. J.: The living peritoneum as a dialyzing membrane, *Am. J. Physiol.*, **63:**547, 1922–1923.

202. Ganter, G.: Über die Beseitigung giftiger Stoffe aus dem Blute durch Dialyse, *Münch Med. Wachenschr*, **70:**1478, 1923.

203. Heusser, H., and Werder, H.: Untersuchungen über Peritonealdialyse, *Bruns. Beitr. Klin. Chir.*, **141:**38, 1927.

204. Abbot, W. E., and P. Shea: Treatment of temporary renal insufficiency (uremia) by peritoneal lavage, *Am. J. Med. Sci.*, **211:**312, 1946.

205. Fine, J. H., H. A. Frank, and A. M. Seligman: The treatment of acute renal failure by peritoneal irrigation, *Ann. Surg.*, **124:**857, 1946.

206. Frank, H. A., A. M. Seligman, and J. H. Fine: Treatment of uremia after acute renal failure by peritoneal irrigation, *JAMA*, **103:**703, 1946.

207. Dérot, M.: Le dialyse péritonéale: Sa place dans le traitement de l'urémie aiguë, *Sem. Hôp. Paris*, **25:**3508, 1949.

208. Odel, H. M., D. O. Ferris, and H. Power: Peritoneal lavage as an effective means of extrarenal excretion, *Am. J. Med.*, **9:**63, 1950.

209. Grollman, A., L. B. Turner, and J. A. McLean: Intermittent peritoneal lavage in nephrectomized dogs and its application to the human being, *Arch. Intern. Med.*, **87:**379, 1951.

210. Maxwell, M. H., R. E. Rockney, and C. R. Kleeman: Peritoneal dialysis. 1. Technique and application, *JAMA*, **176:**917, 1959.

211. Doolan, P. D., W. P. Murphy, Jr., R. A. Wiggins, N. W. Carter, W. D. Cooper, R. H. Watten, and E. I. Alpern: An evaluation of intermittent peritoneal lavage, *Am. J. Med.*, **26:**831, 1959.

212. Burns, R. O., L. W. Henderson, E. B. Hager, and J. P. Merrill: Peritoneal dialysis: Clinical experience, *N. Engl. J. Med.*, **267:**1060, 1962.

213. von Hartitzsch, B., and T. R. Medloch: Chronic peritoneal dialysis—a regime comparable to conventional hemodialysis, *Trans. Am. Soc. Artif. Intern. Organs*, **22:**595, 1976.

214. Tenckhoff, H., C. R. Blagg, K. F. Curtis, and R. H. Hickman: Chronic peritoneal dialysis, *Proc. Eur. Dial. Transplant Assoc.*, **10:**363, 1973.

215. Scribner, B. H., C. Giordano, D. G. Oreopoulos, C. Mion, U. Buoncristiani, S. G. Davids, G. M. Gahl, and K. M. Jones: Long term peritoneal dialysis, *Proc. Eur. Dial. Transplant Assoc.*, **12:**131, 1975.

216. Boen, S. T.: *Peritoneal Dialysis in Clinical Medicine*, Charles C Thomas, Publisher, Springfield, Ill., 1964.

217. Dunea, G.: Peritoneal dialysis and hemodialysis, *Med. Clin. North Am.*, **55:**155, 1971.

218. Miller, R. B., and C. R.: Peritoneal dialysis, *N. Engl. J. Med.*, **281:**945, 1969.

219. Henderson, L. W.: The problem of peritoneal membrane area and permeability, *Kidney Int.*, **3:**409, 1973.

220. Berndt, W. O., and R. E. Gosselin: Physiologic factors influencing radiorubidium flux across isolated rabbit mesentery, *Am. J. Physiol.*, **200:**454, 1961.

221. Babb, A. L., P. J. Johansen, M. J. Strand, H. Tenckhoff, and B. H. Scribner: Bidirectional permeability of the human peritoneum to middle molecules, *Proc. Eur. Dial Transplant Assoc.*, **10:**247, 1973.

222. Henderson, L. W., and K. D. Nolph: Altered permeability of the peritoneal membrane after using hypertonic peritoneal dialysis fluid, *J. Clin. Invest.*, **48:**992, 1969.

223. Gross, M., and H. P. McDonald: Effect of dialy-

sate temperature and flow rate on peritoneal clearance, *JAMA*, **202**:363, 1967.

224. Gross, M., and H. P. McDonald, Jr.: Effects of dialysate temperature and flow rate on peritoneal clearance, *JAMA*, **202**:215, 1967.

225. Pappenheimer, J. R.: Passage of molecules through capillary walls, *Physiol. Rev.*, **38**:387, 1953.

226. Clark, A. L.: Absorption from the peritoneal cavity, *J. Pharmacol. Exp. Ther.*, **16**:415, 1921.

227. Fleisher, M. S., and L. Loeb: Studies in edema. VI. The influence of adrenalin on absorption from peritoneal cavity with some remarks on the influence of calcium chloride on absorption, *J. Exp. Med.*, **12**:288, 1910.

228. Berndt, W. O., and R. E. Gosselin: Action of vasopressin on the permeability of mesentery, *Science*, **134**:1987, 1961.

229. Wasserman, K., and H. W. Mayerson: Dynamics of lymph and plasma protein exchange, *Cardiology*, **21**:296, 1952.

230. Hare, H. G., H. Valtin., and R. E. Gosselin: Effects of drugs on peritoneal dialysis in the dog, *J. Pharmacol. Exp. Ther.*, **145**:122, 1964.

231. Shear, L., J. D. Harvey, and K. G. Barry: Peritoneal sodium transport: Enhancement by pharmacologic and physical agents, *J. Lab. Clin. Med.*, **67**:181, 1966.

232. Rasio, E. A.: Metabolic control of permeability in isolated mesentry, *Am. J. Physiol.*, **276**:1974.

233. Mattocks, A. M., and S. C. Penzotti: Acceleration of peritoneal dialysis with minimum amounts of dioctyl sodium sulfosuccinate, *J. Pharm. Sci.*, **61**:475, 1972.

234. Henderson, L. W., and J. E. Kintzel: Influence of antidiuretic hormone on peritoneal membrane area and permeability, *J. Clin. Invest.*, **50**:2437, 1971.

235. Gutman, R. A., W. P. Nixon, R. L. McRae, and H. W. Spencer: Effect of intraperitoneal and intravenous vasoactive amines on peritoneal dialysis: Study in anephric dogs, *Trans. Am. Soc. Artif. Intern. Organs*, **22**:570, 1976.

236. Nolph, K. D., A. J. Ghods, J. Van Stone, and P. A. Brown: The effects of intraperitoneal vasodilators on peritoneal clearances, *Trans. Am. Artif. Intern. Organs*, **22**:586, 1976.

237. Maher, J. F., and D. C. Hohnadel: Peritoneal

permeability and enhancement in uremia. Proc. 9th Annual Contractors' Conference. Artificial Kidney Chronic Uremia Program NIH NIAMDD, **9**:116, 1976.

238. Nolph, K. D., A. J. Ghods, P. Brown, J. Van Stone, F. N. Miller, D. L. Wiegmann, and P. D. Harris: Factor affecting peritoneal dialyses efficiency, *Dialysis and Transplantation*, **6**:52, 1977.

239. Cunningham, R. S.: The physiology of the serous membranes, *Physiol. Rev.*, **6**:242, 1926.

240. Hahn, P. F., L. L. Miller, F. S. Robscheit-Robbins, W. F. Bale, and G. H. Whipple: Peritoneal absorption: Red cells labeled by radio-iron hemoglobin move promptly from peritoneal cavity into the circulation, *J. Exp. Med.*, **80**:77, 1944.

241. Cole, W. C. C., and J. C. Montgomery: Intraperitoneal blood transfusion: Report of 237 transfusions on 117 patients in private practice, *Am. J. Dis. Child.*, **37**:497, 1929.

242. Mellish, P., and I. J. Wolman: Intraperitoneal blood transfusions, *Am. J. Med. Sci.*, **235**:717, 1958.

243. Shear, L., C. Swartz, J. A. Shinaberger, and K. G. Barry: Kinetics of peritoneal fluid absorption in adult man, *N. Engl. J. Med.*, **272**:123, 1965.

244. Gordon, A., and M. H. Maxwell: Kinetics of peritoneal dialysis: Transperitoneal movement of water, *Clin. Res.*, **13**:307, 1965.

245. Personal observations.

246. Allen, L.: The peritoneal stomata, *Anat. Rec.*, **67**:89, 1936.

247. Allen, L., and E. Vogt: A mechanism of lymphatic absorption from serous cavities, *Am. J. Physiol.*, **119**:776, 1937.

248. Nagel, W., and W. Kachinsky: Study of the permeability of the isolated dog mesentery, *Eur. J. Clin. Invest.*, **1**:149, 1970.

249. Tenckhoff, H.: Solutions and equipment, *Dialysis and Transplantation*, **6**:24, 1977.

250. Boyer, J., G. N. Gill, and F. H. Epstein: Hyperglycemia and hyperosmolality complicating peritoneal dialysis, *Ann. Intern. Med.*, **67**:568, 1967.

251. Nolph, K. D., J. E. Hano, and P. E. Teschan: Peritoneal sodium transport during hypertonic peritoneal dialysis: Physiologic mechanisms and clinical implications, *Ann. Intern. Med.*, **70**:931, 1969.

252. Ahearn, D. J., and K. D. Ahearn: Controlled so-

dium removal with peritoneal dialysis, *Trans. Am. Soc. Artif. Intern. Organs*, **18**:423, 1972.

253. Boen, S. T.: Kinetics of peritoneal dialysis: A comparison with the artificial kidney, *Medicine (Baltimore)*, **40**:243, 1961.

254. Borchardt, K. A., and J. A. Richardson: Adverse effect on bacteria of peritoneal dialysis solution containing acetate, *Clin. Res.*, **17**:425, 1969.

255. Whang, R.: Hyperglycemic non-ketotic coma induced by peritoneal dialysis, *Lancet*, **87**:453, 1967.

256. Henderson, L. W.: Peritoneal ultrafiltration dialysis: Enhanced urea transfer using hypertonic peritoneal dialysis fluid, *J. Clin. Invest.*, **45**:950, 1966.

257. Greenblatt, D. J.: Fatal hypoglycemia occurring after peritoneal dialysis, *Br. Med. J.*, **2**:270, 1972.

258. Bulger, R. J., J. V. Bennett, and S. T. Boen: Intraperitoneal administration of broad-spectrum antibiotics in paitnets with renal failure, *JAMA*, **194**:1198, 1965.

259. Tenckhoff, H.: A bacteriologically safe peritoneal access device, *Trans. Am. Soc. Artif. Intern. Organs*, **14**:181, 1968.

260. Petersen, N. J., L. A. Carson, and M. S. Favero: Microbiological quality of water in an automatic peritoneal dialysis system, *Dialysis and Transplantation*, **6**:38, 1977.

261. Sherrard, D. J., F. K. Curtis, P. Hanson, S. Terao, H. Harris, L. Laris, M. Klahn, and B. Thompson: Infection and other complications of peritoneal dialysis, *Dialysis and Transplantation*, **6**:28, 1977.

262. Gutman, R. A., and J. D. Shelburne: An outbreak of cryptogenic peritonitis, *Dialysis and Transplantation*, **6**:35, 1977.

263. Goldschmidt, Z. H., H. H. Pote, M. A. Katz, and L. Shear; Effect of dialysate volume on peritoneal dialysis kinetics, *Kidney Int.*, **5**:240, 1974.

264. Penzotti, S. C., and A. M. Mattocks: Effects of dwell time, volume of dialyses fluid and added accelerators on peritoneal dialysis of urea, *J. Pharm. Sci.*, **60**:1520, 1971.

265. Tenckhoff, H., G. Ward, and S. T. Boen: The influence of dialysate volume and flow rate on peritoneal clearance, *Proc. Eur. Dial. Transplant Assoc.*, **2**:113, 1965.

266. Lange, K., and G. Treser: Automatic continuous

high flow rate peritoneal dialysis, *Trans. Am. Soc. Artif. Intern. Organs*, **13**:164, 1967.

267. Peabody, A. M., and B. L. Martz: A method for continuous flow, single pass peritoneal dialysis: Preliminary communicaton, *J. Chronic Dis.*, **20**:163, 1967.

268. Stephen, R. L., E. Atkin-Thor, and W. J. Kolff: Recirculating peritoneal dialysis with subcutaneouscatheter, *Trans. Am. Soc. Artif. Intern. Organs*, **22**:575, 1976.

269. Shinaberger, J. H., L. Shear, and K. G. Barry: Increasing efficiency of peritoneal dialysis: Experience with peritoneal-extracorporeal recirculation dialysis, *Trans. Am. Soc. Artif. Intern. Organs*, **11**:78, 1965.

270. Gordon, A., A. J. Lewin, M. H. Maxwell, and N. D. Morales: Augmentation of efficiency by continuous flow sorbent regeneration peritoneal dialysis, *Trans. Am. Soc. Artif. Intern. Organs*, **22**:575, 1976.

271. Raja, R. M., M. S. Kramer, and J. L. Rosenbaum: Recirculation peritoneal dialysis with sorbent REDY cartridge, *Nephron*, **16**:134, 1976.

272. Tenckhoff, H., B. Meston, and G. Shilipetar: A simplified automatic peritoneal dialysis system, *Trans. Am. Soc. Artif. Intern. Organs*, **18**:436, 1972.

273. Tenckhoff, H.: Home peritoneal dialysis in S. G. Massry and A. L. Sellers (eds.), *Clinical Aspects of Uremia and Dialysis*, Charles C Thomas, Publisher, Springfield, Ill., 1976.

274. Oreopoulos, D. G., S. Karanicolas, and S. S. A. Fenton: Home peritoneal dialysis, *Dialysis and Transplantation*, **6**:70, 1977.

275. Hartitzsch, B. V., and T. R. Medlock: Chronic peritoneal dialysis—a regime comparable to conventional hemodialysis, *Trans. Am. Soc. Artif. Intern. Organs*, **22**:595, 1976.

276. Lewin, A. J., A. Gordon, M. Greenbaum, and M. H. Maxwell, Sorbent regeneration of peritoneal dialysate, *Trans. Am. Soc. Artif. Intern. Organs*, **20A**:130, 1974.

277. Lewin, A. J., A. Gordon, M. Blumenkrantz, J. Coburn, and M. H. Maxwell: Sorbent peritoneal dialysis—initial clinical trials, *Proc. Eur. Dial. Transplant Assoc.*, in press

278. Personal observations.

18

Disorders of the renal tubule that cause disorders of fluid, acid-base, and electrolyte metabolism*

R. Curtis Morris, Jr. / Anthony Sebastian

INTRODUCTION

In patients afflicted with what is now termed Type 1 RTA (renal tubular acidosis), Albright and his associates demonstrated that an unchanging dose of alkali therapy could sustain correction of metabolic acidosis caused by a persisting, non-azotemic disorder of renal acidification (1). With continued alkali therapy, hypercalciuria disappeared, gut absorption of calcium increased, the severity of hypocalcemia decreased, and the associated metabolic bone disease healed (1). Because of the great deficits of body calcium that can accrue in untreated patients with Type 1 RTA, Albright advised administration of vitamin D as well as of alkali to maximize the positive balance of calcium and thereby speed the healing of the metabolic bone disease. Albright and his colleagues had earlier demonstrated that administration of vitamin D could correct the hypocalcemia of non-

acidotic patients with pseudohypoparathyroidism (2) and heal the rickets of a patient with renal hypophosphatemic rickets (3), apparently without altering the presumably causal renal dysfunction of either disease.

Largely because of the scope and success of Albright's clinical investigations, and the logical appeal of the unilinear schemes of pathogenesis he formulated, three tacit assumptions have shaped most therapeutic approaches to renal tubular disorders that are causally associated with systemic metabolic derangements. These assumptions are: (1) Disorders of the renal tubule cause systemic metabolic derangements exclusively by causing disturbances of fluid and electrolyte homeostasis. (2) These disturbances derive exclusively and directly from the primary physiologic expression of the renal tubular disorders. (3) The kind and severity of the primary physiologic expression is determined only by the inherent and largely fixed character of the disease process affecting the renal tubule. Specifically, therapy aimed at directly correcting either the physiologic or metabolic consequences of a renal tubular disorder will not induce substantial changes in either the kind or severity of its primary physiologic expression. When made ex-

* Many of the research studies cited in this chapter were carried out in the General Clinical Research Center, University of California, San Francisco, with funds provided by the Division of Research Resources, RR-79, U.S. Public Health Service. This work was also supported by the following grants from the National Institutes of Health: AM 16764 and AM 21354.

plicit, these tacit assumptions are heuristically valuable and all may be valid in certain renal tubular disorders, e.g., Type 1 RTA in some adults (4–6). But in the very recent past, it has become clear that in most disorders of the renal tubule that are causally associated with systemic metabolic derangements, one or more of these assumptions is invalid in a way that has important therapeutic implications. For example, in patients with vitamin D dependency (7), administration of near "physiologic amounts of 1,25-$(OH)_2$ vitamin D_3 will within days not only initiate healing of the metabolic bone disease (8, 9) and correct hypocalcemia, but also will correct the complex dysfunction of the renal tubule. 1,25-$(OH)_2$ vitamin D_3, a hormone made uniquely in renal cortical tubules

Table 18-1. Physiologic characteristics of clinical disorders of renal acidification

| | RTA (RENAL TUBULAR ACIDOSIS) | | | | | | | |
| | TYPE 1 ("CLASSIC," "DISTAL") | | | TYPE 2 ("PROXIMAL") | | | | |
	NON-HCO_3^- WASTING	HCO_3^- WASTING	INCOMPLETE	TYPE 2 RTA	TYPE 1,2 HYBRID	INCOMPLETE	TYPE 4	UREMIC ACIDOSIS
Frank acidosis	Present	Present	Absent	Present	Present	Absent	Present	Present
Net renal H^+ secretion at normal $[HCO_3^-]_p$	Minimally reduced	Moderately reduced	Not reduced	Greatly reduced	Greatly reduced	Not reduced	Moderately reduced	Nearly normal to greatly reduced
Bicarbonaturia (percent of filtered HCO_3^- excreted) at normal $[HCO_3^-]_p$	<3–5%	5–10%	<1%	>15%	>15%	<2%	<2–15%	<3–>30%
TA+NH_4^+ excretion at normal $[HCO_3^-]_p$	Reduced	Reduced	Not reduced	Reduced	Reduced	Not reduced	Reduced	Reduced
Therapeutic alkali requirement (meq of HCO_3^-/kg body weight per day	1–3	5–10	None	2–>10	3–>10	None	1–2	1–3
Urinary acidification during acidosis	Impaired	Impaired	Impaired	Intact	Impaired	Intact	Intact	Intact
Bicarbonaturia (percent of filtered HCO_3^- excreted)	<3%	5–10%	<1%	None	<3%	None	None	None
TA+NH_4^+ excretion during acidosis	Reduced	Reduced	Not reduced or reduced	Not reduced	Reduced	Not reduced	Not reduced or reduced	Reduced
Carbon dioxide tension in HCO_3^--rich urine (UpH >BpH)								
$U_{P_{CO_2}}$ minus $B_{P_{CO_2}}$	<20	<20	<20	>20	<20	>20		
Serum potassium concentration	Normal or reduced	Usually reduced	Normal or reduced	Normal or reduced	Usually reduced	Low-normal	Increased	Normal or increased
Glomerular filtration rate	Normal or slightly reduced	Normal	Normal or slightly reduced	Normal or reduced	Usually reduced	Reduced	Normal to greatly reduced	Greatly reduced

ABBREVIATIONS: $[HCO_3^-]_p$, plasma bicarbonate concentration; TA, titratable acid; NH_4^+, ammonium; UpH, urine pH; BpH, blood pH; P_{CO_2}, carbon dioxide tension.

(10–12), is the most biologically active metabolite of vitamin D_3 known with respect to bone resorption (13), gut absorption of calcium (14), and healing of vitamin D-deficient rickets (15). In patients with pseudohypoparathyroidism it seems likely that both the metabolic derangements and the disturbances in electrolyte homeostasis are in part a consequence of reduced concentrations of circulating $1,25$-$(OH)_2$ vitamin D_3 (16–19). In most adult patients with Type 4 RTA the severity of the renal acidification defect is importantly determined by hypoaldosteronism (6, 20) and substantially mitigated by mineralocorticoid therapy (21). In previously untreated infants and children with Type 1 RTA, an increased severity of renal acidification defect predictably attends corrective alkali therapy and eventually dictates that its amount be increased, an increase in amount of alkali apparently being required to prevent or correct impaired growth (22).

RENAL TUBULAR ACIDOSIS

In the usual clinical instance in which impaired renal acidification causes acidosis, functioning renal mass is greatly reduced, as reflected by a large reduction in the GFR (glomerular filtration rate) and the syndrome of "uremic acidosis." RTA is a clinical syndrome of disordered renal acidification characterized by minimal or no azotemia, hyperchloremic acidosis, inappropriately high urinary pH, bicarbonaturia, and reduced urinary excretion of titratable acid and ammonium (1, 4–6, 22–35). The syndrome reflects a disorder of renal acidification that can cause acidosis with little or no reduction in renal mass. In recent years it has become apparent that several physiologically distinct disorders of renal acidification can give rise to RTA (Table 18-1).

TYPE 1 RTA ("CLASSIC," "DISTAL")

Physiologic character

In Type 1 RTA, urinary pH is inappropriately high during severe as well as mild degrees of acidosis (Fig. 18-1) (usually greater than 6), persisting urinary excretion of bicarbonate is characteristic (1, 4–6, 22–36), and the complex dysfunction

Table 18-2. Clinical spectrum of (classic Type 1, distal) RTA

Primary (no obvious systemic disease)
Sporadic (1, 22, 23, 26, 27, 31, 36)
Genetically transmitted (4, 22, 37)

Autoimmune disorders (30, 38–41)
Dysgammaglobulinemia
Hyperglobulinemic purpura (42)
Cryoglobulinemia (43)
Sjögren's syndrome (39, 40, 44, 45)
Chronic active hepatitis (46–51)
Primary biliary cirrhosis (48, 50–51)
Thyroiditis (52)
Fibrosing alveolitis (53)

Disorders causing nephrocalcinosis
Idiopathic hypercalciuria
Sporadic (54, 55)
Hereditary (56)
Primary hyperparathyroidism (57, 58)
Hyperthyroidism (59, 60)
Vitamin D intoxication (61)
Medullary sponge kidney (62, 63)
Hereditary fructose intolerance (64)
(after chronic fructose ingestion)
Wilson's disease (65)
Fabry's disease (66)

Drug- or toxin-induced nephropathy
Amphotericin B (67, 68)
Toluene (69)
Analgesics (69, 70)
Lithium (71)
Cyclamate (72)

Other renal diseases
Pyelonephritis (73)
Obtructive uropathy (74–77)
Renal transplantation (78–79)
Leprosy (80)

Genetically transmitted systemic diseases
Ehlers-Danlos syndrome (81)
Hereditary elliptocytosis (82)
Sickle-cell anemia (83, 84)
Marfan's syndrome (85)
Carbonic anhydrase B deficiency (86)

Hepatic cirrhosis (87–89)

of the proximal tubule characteristic of the Fanconi syndrome (impaired renal reabsorption of glucose, phosphate, and amino acids) is absent. Type 1 RTA can be the expression of a number of disease processes (Table 18-2) (4, 22, 37–89).

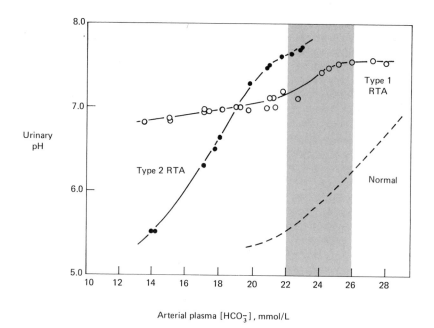

Figure 18-1. Relationship between urinary pH and plasma bicarbonate concentration in patients with prototypic Type 1 (classic) and Type 2 (proximal) RTA (renal tubular acidosis). In patients with Type 2 RTA, the urinary pH may be inappropriately high or appropriately low, depending on the degree of systemic acidosis. (Shaded area represents range of normal plasma bicarbonate concentrations.) [*From Sebastian et al. (6).*]

Adults. In adult patients with Type 1 RTA, the amount of bicarbonate excreted at both normal and reduced plasma bicarbonate concentrations is a near-trivial fraction of that filtered (Fig. 18-2). This finding, that the fractional excretion of filtered bicarbonate ($C_{HCO_3^-}/C_{in}$) is less than 5 percent over a broad range of normal and subnormal plasma bicarbonate concentrations, permits the inference that reabsorption of bicarbonate in the proximal renal tubule (and the distal tubule) is not substantially reduced, and indicates that impaired renal acid excretion need not be associated with renal "bicarbonate wasting" (5, 6, 25, 26, 30–36). In adult patients with Type 1 RTA, acidosis results principally from reduced urinary excretion of net acid (titratable acid + ammonium − HCO_3^-). Hence, correction of acidosis is characteristically sustained by an amount of alkali only a fraction more than the normal endogenous pro-

duction of nonvolatile acid, i.e., a fraction more than 1 meq/kg per day in adults (4–6, 90). In effect the endogenously produced nonvolatile acid is titrated with exogenously administered alkali.

Children. Until quite recently it was tacitly assumed that the physiologic character of Type 1 RTA in children was not significantly different from the prototypic dysfunction described in affected adults. It is now clear, however, that renal bicarbonate wasting will predictably occur in all short prepubertal children with idiopathic or familial Type 1 RTA who are given alkali therapy in amounts sufficient to sustain correction of acidosis (22, 36). RBW ("renal bicarbonate wasting") can be said to occur when the urinary excretion of net base (HCO_3^- − titratable acid + ammonium) exceeds the rate at which nonvolatile acid is endogenously produced (22, 36). Since endogenous production of nonvolatile acid may be as high as 3 meq/kg per day in rapidly growing children (91), RBW can be arbitrarily defined as net base excretion of greater than 3 meq/kg per day at normal (or reduced) plasma bicarbonate concentrations (36). So defined, RBW is quantitatively more important in the causation of acidosis than reduced excretion of acid per se (which predictably attends bicarbonate wasting because of the inappropriately high urinary pH at which bicarbonate wasting occurs). Reduced excretion of acid per se leads to acidosis only to the extent that the endogenously produced, nonvolatile acid titrates body buffers, including plasma bicarbonate. Such a loss of base is relatively minor and slowly developing compared to the loss of base which can result from a substantial fractional excretion of filtered bicarbonate. (This statement assumes that endogenous production of nonvolatile acid is not greatly supernormal, i.e., substantially greater than

3 meq/kg per day, as it can be in such conditions as lactic acidosis and diabetic ketoacidosis.) (See Chaps. 6 and 12.)

In affected infants RBW can be present from the outset (36) (Fig. 18-3), but usually occurs a few weeks after alkali therapy has been initiated. In older children RBW characteristically does not occur until several months after beginning alkali therapy, when growth velocity has greatly increased (Fig. 18-4). The occurrence of RBW in infants and children with Type 1 RTA does not appear to reflect a qualitative change in the character of the renal acidification defect: Over a broad range of normal and subnormal values of plasma bicarbonate concentration, $C_{\text{HCO}_3^-}/C_{\text{in}}$ remains relatively fixed, but ranges in value from 6 to 14 percent (Figs. 18-3 and 18-4). When RBW occurs in children with Type 1 RTA, the magnitude of RBW at normal plasma bicarbonate concentra-

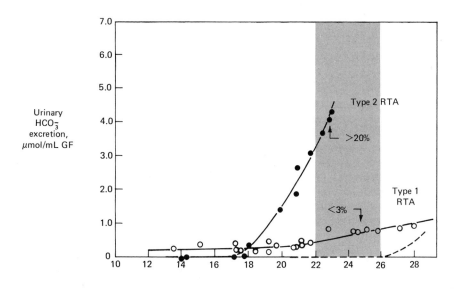

Figure 18-2. The relationship between urinary bicarbonate excretion and plasma bicarbonate concentration in patients with prototypic Type 1 (classic) and Type 2 (proximal) RTA. In patients with Type 1 RTA, the urine may contain bicarbonate even during severe degrees of acidosis, but at normal plasma bicarbonate concentrations the magnitude of bicarbonaturia is small, usually less than 5 percent of the filtered bicarbonate load. In patients with Type 2 RTA, the urine may be bicarbonate free during severe acidosis, but at normal plasma bicarbonate concentrations the magnitude of bicarbonaturia is large, often greater than 15 percent of the filtered bicarbonate load. (Shaded area represents range of normal plasma bicarbonate concentrations.) [*From Sebastian et al. (6).*]

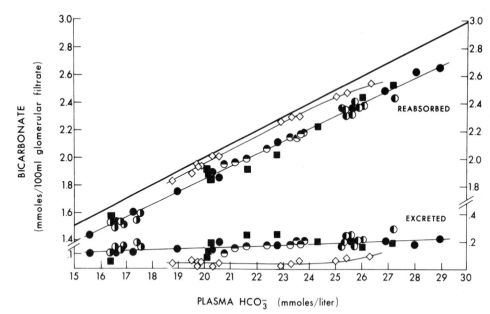

Figure 18-3. Relationship between plasma concentration, renal tubular reabsorption, and urinary excretion of bicarbonate (arterial plasma [HCO$_3^-$], THCO$_3^-$, and U$_{HCO_3}$V, respectively) during the first year of life in three infants with apparently Type 1 RTA, two with renal bicarbonate wasting (circles and squares), one without (diamonds).

tions is the major determinant of the amount of alkali required to sustain correction of their acidosis. This amount may range from 5 to 14 meq/kg per day, as opposed to an amount of 1 to 3 meq/kg per day, which is sufficient to correct acidosis in the absence of RBW. The persistence of RBW at reduced plasma bicarbonate concentrations accounts for the occurrence of strikingly severe acidosis, both before beginning, and soon after diminishing, corrective alkali therapy.

"Incomplete" Type 1 RTA. In patients with so-called "incomplete" Type 1 RTA, systemic acidosis is not present and net acid excretion does not appear to be frankly subnormal, although the pH of the urine is inappropriately high during NH$_4$Cl-induced acidosis (27). In these patients, urinary ammonium characteristically constitutes a greater-than-normal fraction of urinary net acid, both before and during induced acidosis; in some patients, ammonium excretion increases to frankly supernormal rates during NH$_4$Cl-induced aci-

dosis. In some patients with incomplete RTA, full-blown Type 1 RTA has occurred in association with a further reduction in renal function as reflected by a reduction in GFR (although not so much as to cause uremia) (92).

Mechanism and pathogenesis

The physiologic characteristics of Type 1 RTA (see also Chap. 6) can be explained as the consequence of an inability of the distal segments of the nephron to generate or maintain normally steep lumen-peritubular hydrogen ion gradients (4–6). At the minimal urinary pH attainable during acidosis, such a "gradient" defect would restrict the rate at which the distal nephron could secrete H$^+$ (given a normal content of the urinary buffers, Na$_2$HPO$_4$ and NH$_3$). Such a defect is not incompatible with the observation that C_{HCO_3}/C_{in} can exceed 5 percent at normal plasma bicarbonate concentrations in patients with bicarbonate-wasting Type 1 RTA (5). Yet, the net rate at which H^+ is secreted by the distal nephron might be greatly reduced in Type 1 RTA, even in the absence of a lumen-peritubular H^+ gradient (93): When patients with Type 1 RTA are loaded with sodium bicarbonate so that the pH of the urine exceeds that of the blood, the P_{CO_2} of urine does not greatly exceed that of the blood (93, 94) (as it does in normal subjects who are similarly loaded with sodium bicarbonate). If, in patients with Type 1 RTA, this phenomenon reflects a reduced amount of H_2CO_3 in the lumen of the distal nephron (93–96), the reduction could occur either because H_2CO_3 is generated at a reduced rate by the distal secretion of H^+ (93), or because H_2CO_3 is dissipated at an increased rate from the distal nephron (96). In Type 1 RTA, a single permeability defect of the distal nephron could permit both excessive back-diffusion of H_2CO_3, when the pH of the urine equals or exceeds that of the blood (during bicarbonate loading), and excessive back-diffusion of H^+ when the pH of the urine is less than that of blood (during acidosis) (96).

That an abnormality in permeability of the distal nephron to H^+ could underlie the impairment

of urinary acidification in patients with Type 1 RTA is suggested by the occurrence of apparently typical Type 1 RTA in patients with the nephropathy induced by amphotericin B (67). This antifungal antibiotic can alter cell membrane permeability (97, 98) and apparently increase passive H^+ permeability in certain H^+-secreting epithelia (43). Type 1 RTA occurs as an autosomal dominant genetic trait in patients without other apparent renal disease (4, 22), in patients with medullary sponge kidney (associated with Ehlers-Danlos syndrome) (81), and in patients with nephrocalcinosis in whom the primary expressed trait is not impaired renal acidification but apparently impaired proximal tubular reabsorption of calcium (in apparent association with impaired reabsorption of α-amino acids and lysozyme) (61). In adults, Type 1 RTA occurs predominantly in women, usually in association with disorders characterized by hypergammaglobulinemia (38–53), most commonly Sjögren's syndrome and less commonly "chronic active hepatitis" ("lupoid hepatitis"). The association of RTA and hypergammaglobulinemia appears to be more than coincidental, but RTA seems not to be caused by

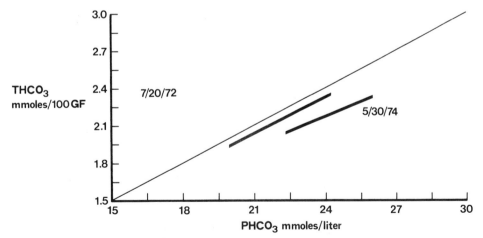

Figure 18-4. The change in the relationship between renal reabsorption of bicarbonate and plasma bicarbonate concentration in a young child with Type 1 RTA continuously treated with corrective alkali therapy. The downward displacement of the later "titration" curve translates to the occurrence of renal bicarbonate wasting. (*From McSherry et al., unpublished data.*)

hypergammaglobulinemia per se (41, 42). Rather, Type 1 RTA could appear to be the functional renal expression of a more general autoimmune disorder (e.g., Sjögren's syndrome) (4, 41) that can give rise to hypergammaglobulinemia. From evidence derived from both experimental models and human disease, a persuasive case can be made that lesions of the renal tubule (and interstitium) can result from immune complexes or autoantibodies directed against constituents of the basement membrane of the renal tubule (99, 100). Although these kinds of observations and considerations

might suggest that in most patients with Type 1 RTA the underlying abnormality is "structural" rather than "metabolic," the functional integrity of certain membranes involved in the renal acidification process might require a complete complement and specific arrangement of certain proteins which might have, or influence, enzymatic or metabolic activity.

Pathophysiology, metabolic derangement, and the effect of alkali therapy

Potassium and sodium. Hypokalemia, renal potassium wasting, renal sodium wasting, and secondary hyperaldosteronism are common complications of both Type 1 and Type 2 RTA (5, 6, 26–29, 33–36, 60, 101–103). Renal wasting of potassium can be said to occur when urinary excretion of potassium exceeds 40 meq/day despite hypokalemia (and in the absence of more than moderate metabolic alkalosis) (101) (Fig. 18-5). In patients with Type 1 RTA, but not in patients with Type 2 RTA, correction of acidosis with alkali therapy is predictably attended by a reduction in the urinary excretion rate of potassium, sodium, and aldosterone (Figs. 18-6 and 18-7); with sustained correction of acidosis, the external balances of potassium and sodium may become sufficiently positive to correct hypokalemia and sodium depletion (102). In most patients with Type 1 RTA, potassium supplements are not required to maintain normokalemia when correction of acidosis is sustained with alkali therapy.

These observations provide the basis for the inference that renal wasting of potassium and sodium in Type 1 RTA is a consequence of the renal acidification defect and not the consequence of independent abnormalities in renal conservation of sodium and potassium (4, 102). According to the conventional formulation of the pathogenetic mechanism, the gradient restriction of renal H^+ secretion reduces the rate of renal H^+–Na^+ exchange which in turn results in a "reciprocal" increase in renal K^+–Na^+ exchange and urinary sodium loss; sodium depletion leads to secondary hyperaldosteronism (102). With correction of acidosis, the attendant increase in intraluminal pH (reflected by the increase in uri-

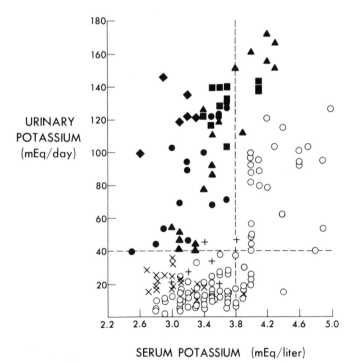

Figure 18-5. Relationship between urinary potassium excretion and serum potassium concentration in patients with RTA in whom correction of acidosis was sustained (●, ▲, ■, ◆) and in normal subjects experimentally depleted of potassium by dietary restriction (O, +, X). Some of the subjects represented by O were mildly alkalotic and were excreting significant amounts of urinary bicarbonate; the subjects represented by + were moderately alkalotic and were excreting more than 50 meq of urinary bicarbonate daily; the subjects represented by × were given large amounts of desoxycorticosterone after hypokalemia supervened. [*From A. Sebastian et al. (101).*]

nary pH) is presumed to remove the inferred gradient restriction on renal H^+ secretion. As a consequence, the rate of H^+–Na^+ exchange increases, the rate of K^+–Na^+ exchange decreases "reciprocally" and the urinary excretion rates of sodium and potassium decrease; correction of sodium depletion would lessen the stimulus to hyperaldosteronism (4, 102).

But the observation in patients with Type 1 RTA that urinary sodium and potassium excretion decreases when acidosis is corrected (59, 60, 101, 102) does not necessarily mean that renal wasting of these cations is a correctable consequence of the acidification defect only. In five of nine patients with Type 1 RTA studied during sustained correction of acidosis with potassium bicarbonate, a persisting impairment in renal conservation of sodium was observed when dietary intake of sodium was restricted (103) despite values of urinary pH near or greater than those of arterial blood, i.e., no apparent gradient restriction on H^+ secretion. Moreover, in some patients with Type 1 RTA, frank renal potassium wasting persists, in association with persisting hyperaldosteronism, despite sustained correction of acidosis with alkali therapy and the provision of a normal or even supernormal amount of dietary sodium (101). To what extent such impairment in the renal conservation of sodium and potassium might result from primary abnormalities of renal sodium and potassium transport, or from secondary functional or structural abnormalities of the kidney (e.g., juxtaglomerular cell hyperplasis, nephrocalcinosis), remains to be elucidated.

Calcium and phosphorus. Hypercalciuria and increased renal clearance of phosphate predictably occur during metabolic acidosis (1, 104, 105) (see also Chap. 19). It is not clear whether the magnitude of either phenomenon is abnormally great in untreated patients with Type 1 RTA. Medullary nephrocalcinosis (Fig. 18-8) and recurrent nephrolithiasis are characteristic and presumably a consequence of prolonged hypercalciuria (1, 4), and perhaps of diminished urinary excretion of citrate as well (106, 107). Urinary calcium chelated with citrate is soluble; calcium oxalate, the major constituent of urinary stones in Type 1 RTA, is relatively insoluble. Hypocal-

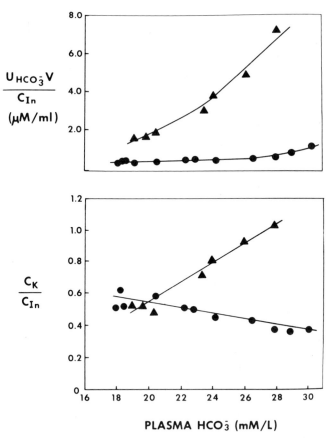

Figure 18-6. Effect of experimentally increasing plasma bicarbonate concentration (intravenous administration of sodium bicarbonate) on the fraction of the filtered load of potassium excreted in the urine (C_K/C_{in}) and urinary bicarbonate excretion $(U_{HCO_3}\text{-}V/C_{in})$ in a patient with Type 1 RTA (circles) and in a patient with Type 2 RTA (triangles). [*From R. C. Morris, Jr., et al. (5).*]

cemia, which may be a consequence of both hypercalciuria and impaired gut absorption of calcium (1, 4, 109), and hypophosphatemia are presumably causally related to the rickets and osteomalacia that can occur (1, 4) (Fig. 18-9). Chronic metabolic acidosis promotes mobilization of skeletal calcium (105) and may inhibit the uniquely renal conversion of 25-OH vitamin D_3 to 1,25-$(OH)_2$ vitamin D_3 (110), the biologically most active metabolite of vitamin D_3 known with respect to intestinal absorption of calcium, bone resorption, and the healing of rickets (13–15).The combination of nephrocalcinosis and rickets or osteomalacia is nearly specific for Type 1 RTA when hypervitaminosis D is excluded by the patient's history (111). In untreated patients with Type 1 RTA the plasma concentration of parathyroid hormone may be increased, a phenomenon that might be causally related to hypercalciuria as well as to hypocalcemia (112, 113).

With sustained correction of acidosis, hypercalciuria disappears (1, 22), citrate excretion increases (106–108), gut absorption of calcium in-

creases (1, 109), the renal clearance of phosphate decreases, and the serum concentrations of both phosphate and calcium become normal (1). Nephrocalcinosis and nephrolithiasis persist, but stones may be passed less frequently. Rickets and osteomalacia can heal with alkali therapy alone (114, 115). The administration of both alkali and vitamin D would, however, seem prudent in patients with Type 1 RTA in whom osteomalacia is severe.

In those patients in whom Type 1 RTA appears to be a late consequence of renal damage

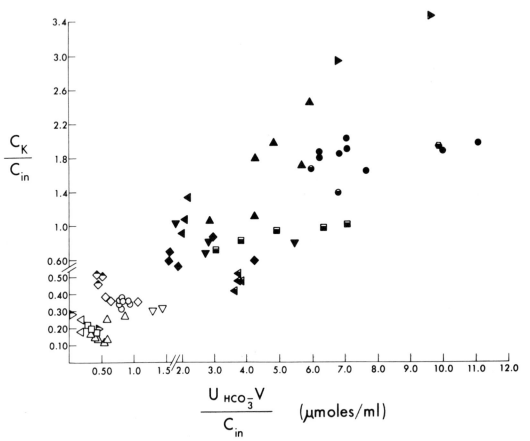

Figure 18-7. Relationship between fractional potassium excretion (C_K/C_{in}) and urinary bicarbonate excretion ($U_{HCO_3^-}\cdot V/C_{in}$) in patients with Type 2 RTA associated with Fanconi syndrome (closed and three-quarter-closed symbols) in whom plasma bicarbonate concentration was maintained at normal levels (22 to 26 μmol/L) for more than 2 months (closed and open symbols) or was rapidly increased to normal levels (intravenous administration of sodium bicarbonate) (three-quarter-open symbols). Each geometric symbol represents measurements made in a single patient. [*From A. Sebastian et al. (35).*]

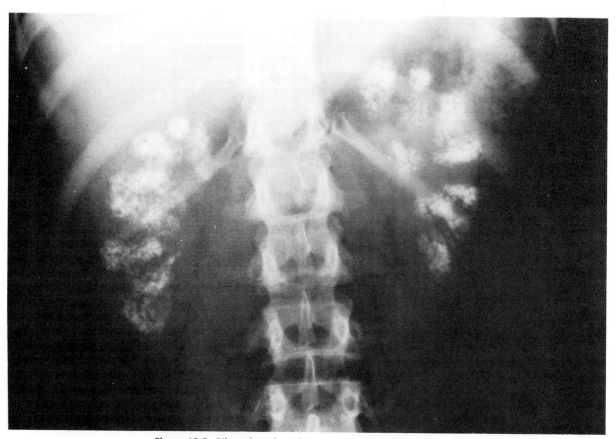

Figure 18-8. Bilateral nephrocalcinosis in a patient with Type 1 RTA.

caused by hypercalciuria and nephrocalcinosis (61), it is not known whether corrective alkali therapy affects the magnitude of hypercalciuria, urinary excretion of citrate, or the frequency of stone passage (61). In at least one genetically affected boy (hypercalciuria without RTA), bilateral nephrocalcinosis became radiographically demonstrable within months of starting alkali therapy.

Growth and nephrocalcinosis of children. In infants and young children with untreated Type 1 RTA, impaired growth is characteristic (see also Chap. 30), but normal growth is predictably attained and maintained when correction of acidosis is sustained with alkali therapy, even if frank stunting has occurred (22) (Fig. 18-10). In stunted infants with Type 1 RTA, the velocity of growth predictably increases strikingly within weeks of initiating alkali therapy and within 3 to 6 months, normal stature is predictably attained (22) (Fig. 18-11). Older children may require several years to attain normal height. Renal bicarbonate wasting tends to occur or increase in severity when growth velocity increases sharply. When greatly increased rates of somatic growth are sustained, the external balances of calcium and phosphorus, as well as of sodium and potassium, must perforce become strongly positive. In short children with renal osteodystrophy, a condition characterized by reduced circulating amounts of 1, 25-OH vitamin D_3, therapeutic administration of 1,25-$(OH)_2$ vitamin D_3 can induce increased rates of growth (as well as healing of rickets) (116). In short children with RTA, alkali-induced normalization of

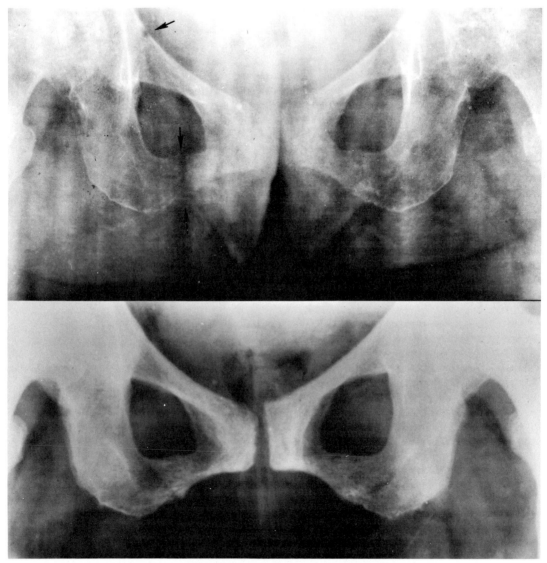

Figure 18-9. Osteomalacia with pseudofractures of the pubic ramus (arrows) with subsequent healing (lower picture).

growth might depend on a normalization in the metabolism of vitamin D. When initiated before the age of 3 years, continuously corrective alkali therapy appears to prevent nephrocalcinosis, possibly by preventing the hypercalciuria and hypo-citraturia that is otherwise predictable without alkali therapy (117). Accordingly, in children with Type 1 RTA both impaired growth and nephrocalcinosis can be regarded as preventable complications.

PATIENTS

BEFORE   AFTER

Standard   Tanner

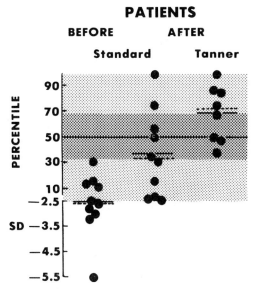

Figure 18-10. The effect of alkali therapy on height in 10 children with classic RTA. Height is expressed in percentiles relative to age- and sex-matched populations. "Tanner" values for patients' height potential (predicted from mean parental height) ("after") are derived as described by Tanner. (J. M. Tanner, *Growth at Adolescence*, Blockwell Scientific Publications, Ltd., Oxford, pp. 1–10.) Limits of the lightly shaded area indicate a ±2.5 S.D. (standard deviation) from the mean; the darker area, ±0.5 S.D. Solid horizontal lines indicate the mean for the group; dashed horizontal lines, the median. [*From E. McSherry and R. C. Morris, Jr.* (22).]

Clinical management (see also Chaps. 4, 6, and 30)

Emergencies. In patients with previously undiagnosed RTA, hypokalemia, severe acidosis, and hypocalcemia often coexist, and may require immediate therapeutic response (118). Hypokalemia-mediated respiratory depression and muscle weakness may be life threatening and necessitate hospitalization and careful monitoring of ventilatory rate and depth, as well as facilities for airway maintenance and assisted ventilation.

Hypokalemia should be corrected rapidly with intravenously administered potassium, and before correction of acidosis. The goal of emergency therapy is to maintain the serum potassium between 4.5 and 5.5 meq/L. It is better to err on the high than on the low side. Alkali should not be given until the serum concentration of potassium has been increased to normal values. With even partial correction of acidosis with alkali therapy, the severity of hypokalemia may increase because the ratio of extracellular/intracellular potassium decreases when blood pH–plasma bicarbonate concentration increases (119, 120). In practice, 40 meq of KCl in 500 mL of 5% glucose in water can be safely administered intravenously over 4 h. If the serum concentration of potassium is less than 2.0 meq/L, 20 meq of potassium can be administered during the first hour. Substantial correction of hypokalemia and dramatic clinical improvement may occur with as little as 20 meq of KCl, because the ratio of extracellular/intracellular potassium is increased during metabolic acidosis even when respiratory compensation normalizes arterial pH (119, 120). Hypokalemia in the presence of acidosis indicates a total body deficit of potassium in the range of 6 to 10 meq/kg. When normokalemia occurs, additional potassium should be administered only with alkali, otherwise frank hyperkalemia may result.

Acidosis should be corrected with $NaHCO_3$ (121). Rapid correction is unnecessary and even dangerous if the deficit of HCO_3^- is large, e.g., if the arterial HCO_3^- is less than 13 meq/L. Rapid replacement of a large HCO_3^- deficit may convert "compensated" metabolic acidosis to respiratory alkalosis, because the reduction of arterial P_{CO_2} that "compensates" the metabolic acidosis may persist for more than 24 h after correction of the HCO_3^- deficit. In the first 12 h, one-third to one-half of the approximate HCO_3^- deficit can be replaced; the remainder can be replaced over the next 36 h. The approximate deficit may be calculated as follows:

50% of patient's weight in kilograms
$$\times (25 - \text{venous serum } CO_2)$$

or

50% of patient's weight in kilograms
$$\times (22 - \text{arterial plasma } HCO_3^-)$$

In other words, the apparent HCO_3^- deficit or "CO_2 deficit" is multiplied by the apparent volume of the distribution of HCO_3^- or "HCO_3^--space."

During the first 4 to 6 h, the serum potassium

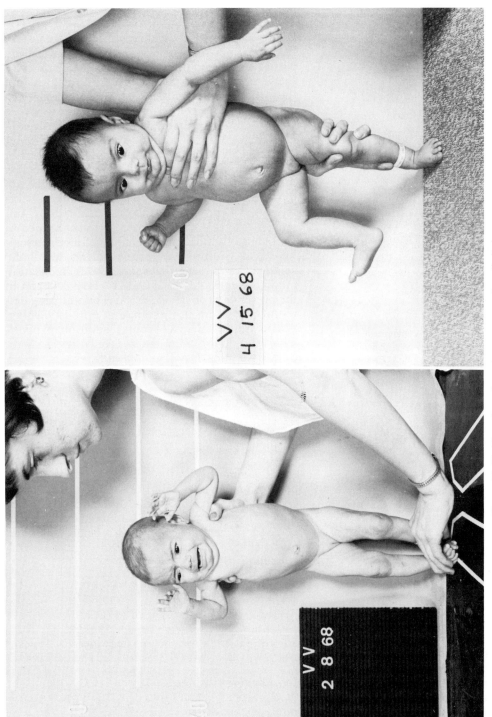

Figure 18-11. The effect of continuous, corrective alkali therapy on growth and development in an initially stunted infant girl with idiopathic Type 1 RTA. *Left.* Recorded February 8, 1968. *Right.* Recorded April 15, 1968. The limits of the lightly and darkly shaded enclosed areas on the growth "grid" (p. 897) indicate ±2.5 and ±1 S.D., respectively, of the mean stature for normal infant girls. [*From E. McSherry and R. C. Morris, Jr. (22).*]

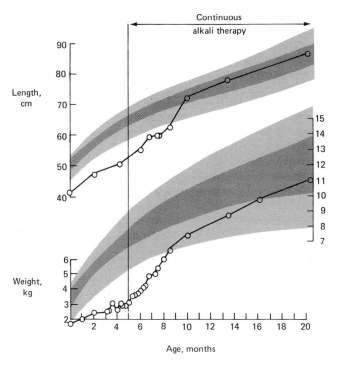

and CO_2 content should be measured every hour if possible, and for the following 12 h, every 4 h. If, during correction of the acidosis, potassium decreases to less than 4.0 meq/L, alkali therapy should be stopped until the serum potassium concentration increases. The rate of administration of KCl should be doubled to 20 meq/h if the serum potassium concentration decreases to less than 3.0 meq/L. If the serum potassium increases to greater than 5.5 meq/L, the infusion of potassium should be stopped until the serum potassium has decreased. If the serum potassium increases to greater than 6.5 meq/L, the rate of administration of alkali should be doubled as well.

Hypocalcemia is common in patients with untreated Type 1 RTA, and tetany prevented by acidosis and hypokalemia may occur with either alkali or potassium therapy. Accordingly, 10 mL of 10% calcium gluconate given intravenously over 10 min may be required every 2 to 4 h during initial correction of the acidosis and hypokalemia. With sustained correction of acidosis and hypokalemia, the tendency for tetany to occur de-

creases greatly even though the severity of hypocalcemia persists unchanged.

Chronic management

If belching and abdominal bloating is a serious problem in patients given $NaHCO_3$, alkali therapy can be given as Shohl's solution: 140 g of citric acid and 98 g of hydrated crystalline salt of sodium citrate are dissolved in water to a final volume of 1 L. Since 1 mL of Shohl's solution contains 1 meq of potential HCO_3^-, the dosage in adult patients is 50 to 100 mL/day in three divided doses. A range of serum CO_2 content of 23 to 28 meq/L indicates the probable adequacy of correction of acidosis.

Almost all children and infants are able to take $NaHCO_3$ in the amounts necessary to sustain correction of acidosis, even when these amounts are as great as 14 meq/kg per day. In young infants (less than 6 months), total alkali dosage is divided into equal portions and administered every 4 h with each feeding. In older infants and children, if their requirement is 10 meq/kg per day or less, alkali is administered four times per day in equal amounts. If their daily requirement exceeds 10 meq/kg per day, alkali therapy is administered five times per day, the first morning dose and the last evening dose being 125 to 150 percent of the other three equal doses (22).

It is important to remember that in most children with Type 1 RTA the dose of corrective alkali therapy will increase (meq/kg per day), usually when the rate of growth increases sharply (22). Hence, during rapid growth the adequacy of alkali therapy should be monitored with frequent measurements of venous CO_2 content: in young infants, weekly; in older infants, biweekly; in children every 2 to 3 months.

Prolonged administration of large amounts of pharmacy-prepared alkali can amount to a considerable financial expense. A glass bottle filled to the mark with 2.88 L of distilled water and the contents of an 8-oz box of Arm & Hammer baking soda (241.8 mg ± 2% of U.S.P. $NaHCO_3$) yields a solution with a bicarbonate concentration of 1 meq/mL. In our experience the solution is accurately and happily prepared by the affected child's parents; if the solution is kept refrigerated and capped between pourings, it is good for at least 2 months. Most of the children with Type 1 RTA followed in our clinic are treated with the home-prepared solution of $NaHCO_3$.

If dietary NaCl is restricted because of a sodium-retaining state, the amount of alkali necessary to correct acidosis is decreased. Indeed, the combination of NaCl restriction and 1 meq/kg per day of $NaHCO_3$ may give rise to frank metabolic alkalosis. Any portion of the alkali therapy usually can be given as potassium bicarbonate (or potassium citrate, potassium gluconate, or potassium acetate, the organic anion being converted to bicarbonate), but the possible complication of hyperkalemia should be kept in mind. In some patients, particularly those with "autoimmune" RTA, potassium supplements of 50 to 100 meq/day may be required to maintain normokalemia even after acidosis has been corrected.

The bone pain of osteomalacia usually disappears within 2 to 4 weeks of correcting acidosis. With recurrence of acidosis and continuing osteomalacia, bone pain may recur within a week. Thus, recurrence of bilateral bone pain suggests that correction of acidosis is not being sustained. Recurrence of unilateral pain, especially in the foot or toe, suggests that a frank bone fracture has occurred and appropriate x-rays should be taken. With correction of acidosis, hypokalemia, and hypocalcemia, bone pain may disappear and muscular strength may increase strikingly before much bone repair has occurred. Accordingly, the exercise program of patients with RTA and osteomalacia should be pointedly moderated and graduated, for overexercise may lead to bone fracture.

One of the frequent complications (and conceivably a cause) of Type 1 RTA is pyelonephritis, the optimal treatment of which has yet to be determined. Attempted eradication of the causal organism is rarely, if ever, successful and may be unrealistic, particularly in patients with nephrocalcinosis. The urine of patients with RTA is a good culture medium for *Escherichia coli* since urinary pH ranges from 6 to 7.5 and osmolality is often less than 500 μosm/kg (122). Moreover, with attempted eradication, a fairly innocuous *E. coli* may be replaced by a more destructive *Pseudomonas* or *Proteus*. Systematic studies of the renal handling of antibiotics have not been reported in patients with any kind of RTA. Some antibiotics are excreted in part by way of renal tubular secretion, a process which might be impaired in patients with RTA. We have had good experience with tetracycline in managing acute clinical episodes of pyelonephritis in patients with Type 1 RTA.

Prognosis

The prognosis of most well-managed adult patients with Type 1 RTA is determined more by the usually accompanying autoimmune disease, Sjögren's syndrome, or chronic liver disorder than by either the functional consequences of the renal disease or its complications, pyelonephritis, nephrocalcinosis, and nephrolithiasis. Morbidity generally considered causally related to the autoimmune state per se, such as Raynaud's phenomenon, recurrent purpura, and even the dry mouth of Sjögren's syndrome, may disappear with alkali therapy (123). In the great majority of well-managed adult patients with Type 1 RTA, the GFR and the severity of the acidification defect remain unchanged even when the GFR is substantially reduced when alkali therapy is started, and despite continuing bacteriologic evidence of chronic pyelonephritis (123) (Fig. 18-12). For many patients in whom Type 1 RTA occurs as part of Sjögren's syndrome, life is long and vigorous. In patients in whom Type 1 RTA occurs as an autosomal dominant trait, the prognosis is good with continued corrective alkali therapy.

TYPE 2 RTA ("PROXIMAL")

Physiologic character

In patients with Type 2 RTA (see also Tables 18-1 and 18-3, Fig. 18-2, and Chap. 6), the identifying observation that $THCO_3^-$ is reduced by at least 15 percent, at normal plasma bicarbonate concentrations, and under normal physiologic conditions, implicates the acidification process of the proximal tubule (4–6, 31–36) (Fig. 18-2). In prototypic Type 2 RTA, the urine pH is inappropriately high and bicarbonaturia occurs only dur-

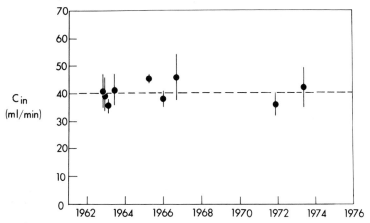

Figure 18-12. Values of inulin clearance (C_{in}) obtained over a 12-year period in a woman with Sjögren's syndrome, Type 1 RTA, nephrocalcinosis, and chronic bacteriuria. The patient was maintained in a nonacidotic and normokalemic state throughout by administration of alkali and supplemental potassium. [*From A. Sebastian et al. (6).*]

ing moderate or mild degrees of acidosis; during more severe degrees of acidosis, bicarbonaturia disappears, urinary pH decreases to normal minima, and acid excretion is not reduced, suggesting that the acidification process of the distal-most nephron is intact (4–6, 31–36) (Figs. 18-1 and 18-13). The physiologic characteristics of Type 2 RTA are those predicted by the formulation of Worthen and Good (124) (Figs. 18-2 and 18-13) and were first demonstrated by Lamy et al. in a child with Fanconi's syndrome as part of Lowe's syndrome (125). Type 2 RTA almost always occurs as part of a more complex dysfunction of the proximal tubule and is apparently always that type of RTA associated with the Fanconi syndrome (31, 32, 34, 126–154) (Table 18-3).

In some patients with a greater than 15 percent reduction in $THCO_3^-$ at normal plasma bicarbonate concentrations, the acidification process of the distal nephron also appears to be impaired; over a broad range of reduced plasma bicarbonate concentrations, $THCO_3^-$ is just less than complete and urinary pH remains inappopriately high. Such findings would appear to reflect a hybrid of Types 1 and 2 RTA (5, 6, 34).

As in children with bicarbonate-wasting Type 1 RTA (22), in patients with Type 2 RTA, the amount of alkali required to sustain the correc-

tion of acidosis is determined principally by the magnitude of bicarbonate wasting at normal plasma bicarbonate concentrations (5, 6, 31–34).

Mechanism and pathogenesis

The subcellular mechanisms of the transport impairment of Type 2 RTA have not been defined, with the exception of the state of carbonic anhydrase inhibition, in which Type 2 RTA occurs unassociated with Fanconi's syndrome (159, 160). The occurrence of Type 2 RTA and the Fanconi syndrome in genetically transmitted disorders of metabolism raises the possibility that in some cases the metabolic production or transduction of energy required for active transport may be impaired.

In adult patients, Type 2 RTA occurs most commonly in the clinical setting of intestinal malabsorption that gives rise to vitamin D deficiency, hypocalcemia, secondary hyperparathyroidism, and hypophosphatemia (5, 135, 137). Type 2 RTA also occurs in children with dietary deficiency of vitamin D (134, 136). In both circumstances, vitamin D therapy corrects the acidification dysfunction, and the usually accompanying complex renal tubular dysfunction like that of the Fanconi syndrome (Fig. 18-14). Although circulating parathyroid hormone can dampen the normal renal acidification process in humans (164), and primary hyperparathyroidism can *lead to* Type 2 RTA that persists after surgical correction of hyperparathyroidism (165), it seems unlikely that Type 2 RTA is caused by the physiologic effect of increased levels of circulating parathyroid hormone alone (5, 166). In the rat studied at normal plasma bicarbonate concentrations, systemically administered PTH (parathyroid hormone) in-

duces a substantial reduction of bicarbonate reabsorption in the proximal tubule, but bicarbonaturia does not occur, and net acid excretion is not decreased (167). In the dog and in humans studied at normal plasma bicarbonate concentrations (164, 168–170), experimentally administered PTH induces a reduction in net acid excretion and the occurrence of bicarbonaturia, but the amount of bicarbonate excreted is a trivial fraction of that filtered by the glomerulus. And, when plasma bi-

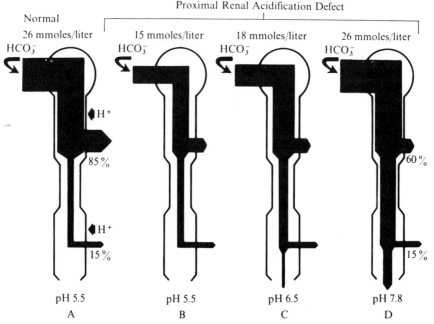

Figure 18-13. Schematic representation of the proximal renal acidification defect in Type 2 RTA. Effect of changes in plasma bicarbonate concentration on bicarbonate delivery to the distal nephron and, as a consequence, on urinary pH and bicarbonate excretion. (*A*) In normal subjects, at normal plasma bicarbonate concentrations, approximately 15 percent of the filtered HCO_3^- load escapes reabsorption proximally and is reabsorbed in the distal nephron; urinary bicarbonate excretion is nil, urinary pH is appropriately low, and net acid excretion is normal. (*B*) In patients with Type 2 RTA, at reduced plasma bicarbonate concentrations, bicarbonate excretion may also be nil, urinary pH may be appropriately low, and net acid excretion may not be reduced despite a reduction in the rate at which bicarbonate can be reabsorbed in the proximal tubule. This is because the amount of HCO_3^- escaping reabsorption proximally and delivered to the distal nephron may not be supernormal when the amount of bicarbonate presented to the proximal

tubule for reabsorption is also markedly reduced. (*C*) When, however, the plasma bicarbonate concentration is modestly increased (by administration of $NaHCO_3$), supernormal amounts of bicarbonate are delivered distally because the modest increase in filtered load of bicarbonate cannot be reabsorbed by the defective proximal tubule. As a consequence, some bicarbonate escapes reabsorption in the distal nephron, urinary pH becomes inappropriately high, and net acid excretion becomes reduced. (*D*) If the plasma bicarbonate concentration and filtered bicarbonate load are increased to normal levels, the amount of bicarbonate escaping reabsorption proximally greatly exceeds the reabsorptive capacity of the normal distal nephron and massive bicarbonaturia occurs. In the illustration of Type 2 RTA, renal tubular reabsorption of bicarbonate ($T_{HCO_3^-}$) at normal plasma bicarbonate concentration (26 mmol/L) is reduced by 25 percent.

Table 18-3. Clinical spectrum of Type 2 (proximal) RTA

Associated with multiple dysfunction of proximal tubule
(Fanconi syndrome)

Primary (no obvious systemic disease)
Sporadic (126, 127)
Genetically transmitted (128, 129)

Genetically transmitted systemic diseases
Cystinosis (31, 32, 124)
Lowe's syndrome (125)
Wilson's disease (130, 131)
Tyrosinemia (132)
Hereditary fructose intolerance (32)
(during fructose administration
or ingestion)
Pyruvate carboxylase deficiency (133)

Disorders associated with chronic hypocalcemia and second-
ary hyperparathyroidism
Vitamin D deficiency (5, 134–137)
Vitamin D dependency (138)

Drug- or toxin-induced nephropathy
Outdated tetracycline (139)
Methyl-5-chromon (diacramone) (140)
Streptozotocin (141)
Lead (142)

Other renal diseases
Amyloidosis (143)
Nephrotic syndrome (143–145)
Renal transplantation (146)
Sjögren's syndrome (34)
Medullary cystic disease (147)
Paroxysmal nocturnal hemoglobinuria (148)
Renal vein thrombosis (149)

Multiple myeloma (with monoclonal immunoglobulin-L-chain-
uria)
Fully expressed (35, 150, 151)
Harrison-Blainey syndrome (152–154)

Unassociated with multiple dysfunction of proximal tubule
Primary
Sporadic
Transient (155)
Persisting (156)
Genetically transmitted (157)
Osteopetrosis (158)
Carbonic anhydrase deficiency
Acetazolamide (159, 160)
Sulfanilamide (161)
York-Yendt syndrome (162)
Cyanotic congenital heart disease (163)

carbonate concentration is only minimally decreased (with ammonium chloride), experimentally administered PTH does not induce either bicarbonaturia or a reduction in net acid excretion (164, 170). Accordingly, one would expect that a disorder of renal acidification caused by PTH alone would not give rise to frank metabolic acidosis, but rather a slight decrease in plasma bicarbonate concentration. Indeed, a reversible impairment in renal acidification severe enough to cause frank acidosis has been demonstrated in nonazotemic patients with hyperparathyroidism only when the hyperparathyroidism was secondary to hypocalcemia and associated with both vitamin D deficiency and hypophosphatemia. In a recent study in thyroparathyroidectomized dogs, hypocalcemia induced by ethyleneglycol tetraacetic acid (EGTA) was attended by a decrease in the reabsorption of bicarbonate (171). In the otherwise intact dog, prolonged severe hypophosphatemia may be attended by a modest reduction in $THCO_3^-$, at normal plasma bicarbonate concentrations, and a slight decrease in plasma bicarbonate concentration (172). Emmett and his coworkers reported that in rats rendered chronically hypophosphatemic, a reduction in $THCO_3^-$ gave rise to frank metabolic acidosis only when an otherwise countervailing release of bone buffers was prevented by the administration of colchicine (173). Thus, in patients with hyperparathyroidism, vitamin D deficiency, and hypophosphatemia, the occurrence of frank metabolic acidosis might depend in part on the extent to which bones fail to release buffer salts. To the extent that vitamin D-deficient bones are unable to release buffer salts either because of their depletion of these salts, or because of the extant reduction in the circulating amount of 1,25-$(OH)_2D_3$, the potential for a modest reduction of $THCO_3^-$ to cause acidosis presumably would be enhanced.

Pathophysiology

Potassium, sodium, and water. In contrast to patients with Type 1 RTA, in patients with Type 2 RTA, renal potassium wasting and polyuria either occur (see also Chaps. 6 and 16), or become more severe, when correction of acidosis is

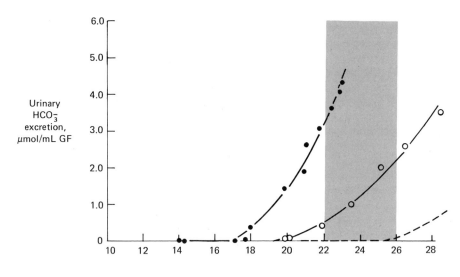

Figure 18-14. Relationship between urinary bicarbonate excretion and plasma bicarbonate concentration during intravenous administration of NaHCO₃ in a patient with Type 2 RTA and Fanconi syndrome associated with intestinal malabsorption. Before administration of vitamin D therapy (solid dots) serum Ca^{2+} = 7.5 mg/dL and $100 \cdot C_{HCO_3}/C_{in}$ = 18% at arterial plasma [HCO₃⁻] of 23 mmol/L; during administration of vitamin D therapy (open dots) Ca^{2+} = 8.5 mg/dL and $100 \cdot C_{HCO_3}/C_{in}$ = 3% at arterial plasma [HCO₃⁻] of 23 mmol/L. Normal subjects are represented by the broken line. The shaded area represents the normal range of arterial plasma bicarbonate concentration. [*From R. C. Morris, Jr., et al. (5).*]

sustained with alkali therapy alone (35, 174, 175) (Figs. 18-6 and 18-7). Because the capacity of the proximal tubule to reabsorb bicarbonate is greatly reduced, the distal nephron is swamped with bicarbonate when the plasma bicarbonate concentration is increased from subnormal to normal levels with alkali therapy (35) (Fig. 18-13). Furthermore, expanding an otherwise contracted ECF (extracellular fluid) volume has the effect of further reducing proximal reabsorption of Na⁺, HCO₃⁻, and Cl⁻ (174, 175). In the presence of a continued stimulus for sodium reabsorption in the distal nephron (e.g., hyperaldosteronism), the delivery of greatly supernormal amounts of sodium, bicarbonate, and chloride out of the proximal nephron would be expected to augment net potassium secretion in the distal nephron (35, 176), and thereby promote renal potassium wasting. During sustained correction of acidosis with alkali therapy the fraction of the filtered load of potassium excreted frequently exceeds 1.0 (which indicates

net renal secretion of potassium) and varies directly with the fractional excretion of filtered bicarbonate (35) (Fig. 18-7). In at least some patients with Type 2 RTA, as in some patients with Type 1 RTA, hyperaldosteronism (and hyperreninemia) persists despite sustained correction of acidosis and the provision of normal or supernormal amounts of dietary sodium (35). Potassium depletion causes not only an impairment in the renal concentrating function (177, 178) but also thirst and polydipsia as a primary phenomenon (179). These phenomena, combined with the greatly increased delivery of solute and water out of the proximal tubule, account for what is often strikingly severe polyuria. It is an important clinical point that in patients with Type 2 RTA (usually as part of the Fanconi syndrome) the urine can be dilute (i.e., hypoosmolar) despite dehydration.

Calcium and phosphorus. In patients diagnosed as having Type 2 RTA, transient (155) and persisting (156), in whom the renal dysfunction of the Fanconi syndrome was absent, hypocalcemia/hypercalciuria and hypophosphatemia/hyperphosphaturia did not occur (see also Chap. 19), despite metabolic acidosis; rickets also did not occur. Furthermore, hypokalemia did not occur either before or during alkali therapy, and potassium supplements were not required. In ways other than the absence of impaired renal reabsorption of glucose, phosphate, and α-amino acids, the renal dysfunction of these patients is clearly different from that of most patients in whom Type 2 RTA occurs in association with the Fanconi syndrome. (See the phosphorus and calcium section in the pathophysiology of Fanconi's syndrome.)

Treatment

The treatment of patients with Type 2 RTA is directed toward amelioration of their fluid, electrolyte, and acid-base disturbance, and when possible, correction of the underlying disease process. (Specific treatment of frequently accompanying vitamin D-resistant metabolic bone disease is considered under the section on the Fanconi syndrome.) Sustained correction of acidosis with alkali therapy requires the administration of alkali sufficient to balance the urinary excretion of net base plus the estimated endogenous production of nonvolatile acid. In these patients, net base excretion is essentially equal to bicarbonate excretion. The magnitude of renal bicarbonate excretion at normal plasma bicarbonate concentrations can vary from as little as 2 to 3 meq/kg body weight per day in patients with minimal impairment of proximal bicarbonate reabsorption, or marked reductions in GFR to values greater than 15 meq/kg body weight per day in patients with more marked dysfunction and/or more nearly normal GFR. The alkali and potassium requirements must then be determined empirically for each patient. When the amount of alkali required to correct acidosis is prohibitively large, hydrochlorothiazide can be a useful therapeutic adjunct (180–182). This agent is believed to increase proximal bicarbonate reabsorption by inducing

contraction of extracellular volume (157, 180–182). With hydrochlorothiazide, the severity of hypokalemia frequently increases. Restriction of dietary NaCl and water may also be useful in reducing the amount of alkali therapy required to correct acidosis, and in reducing the severity of renal potassium wasting and polyuria (175, 183).

TYPE 4 RTA

Physiologic character

In patients with Type 4 RTA, persisting hyperkalemia reflects a reduction in the renal clearance of potassium greater than that expected for the usually accompanying, often mild renal insufficiency (5, 6, 20, 21, 185, 191, 193–196, 208, 210, 211, 216, 222). At normal plasma bicarbonate concentrations, the C_{HCO_3}/C_{in} ranges from 2 to 14 percent; the magnitude of bicarbonaturia is greater than that expected for the degree of renal insufficiency, insufficient to implicate the acidification process of the proximal tubule and evident in the absence of hyperkalemia (20, 21, 185, 195, 210, 211, 222). During moderately severe acidosis, the urine is appropriately acidic (and hence bicarbonate-free) (20, 21). The urinary excretion of ammonium is, however, greatly reduced, even when the urine is very acidic. Hyperaminoaciduria, glucosuria, and increased renal clearance of phosphate are absent (5, 6, 20, 21). The physiologic characteristics are those predicted for an abnormality that disorders the "cation-exchange" segment of the distal nephron, and thereby causes a reduction in secretion rate of both hydrogen ion and potassium ion (230).

Pathogenesis (see also Chaps. 4 and 6)

In many if not most adults with Type 4 RTA, the severity of the impairment would appear to be critically determined by the usually accompany hyporeninemic hypoaldosteronism (20, 21, 193–196).

When administration of replacement mineralo-

Table 18-4. Clinical spectrum of Type 4 RTA

Aldosterone deficiency
  Combined deficiency of aldosterone and adrenal glucocorticoid
  hormones
    Addison's disease
    Bilateral adrenalectomy
    Inherited impairment of steroidogenesis 21-hydroxylase defi-
    ciency ("congenital adrenal hyperplasia") (184, 185)
  Selective deficiency of aldosterone
    Inherited impairment of aldosterone biosynthesis—corticos-
    terone methyl oxidase deficiency (186–189)
    Secondary to deficient renin secretion (190–196)
    Chronic idiopathic hypoaldosteronism in adults and children
    (197–200)

*Attenuated renal response to aldosterone (with secondary hyper-
reninemia and hyperaldosteronism)*
  Selective tubule dysfunction (186, 201–206)—"pseudohypoaldosteronism"
  Chronic tubulointerstitial disease with glomerular insufficiency
  (207)—"salt-wasting nephritis"

Attenuated renal response to aldosterone + aldosterone deficiency
  Selective tubule dysfunction with impaired renin secretion (208–
  213)
  Chronic tubulointerstitial disease with glomerular insufficiency
    Associated deficient renin secretion (191, 193, 214)
    Renin status uncertain (215–219)
  Renal transplantation with deficient renin secretion (220)
  Lupus nephritis with deficient renin secretion (221)

Uncertain pathophysiology (222–229)
  Chronic pyelonephritis (222, 223)
  Lupus nephritis (224)
  Renal transplantation (225)
  Acute glomerulonephritis (226)

corticoid hormone is discontinued in the adrenalectomized dog, net acid excretion decreases, and
hyperkalemic, hyperchloremic acidosis occurs and
persists (231). The reduction in net acid excretion is due largely to a reduction in urinary ammonium excretion, which in turn appears to be
due to diminished renal production of ammonia:
the reduction occurs despite a persistently reduced urinary pH (to values as low as 5.2) and no
decrease in urine flow. The reduction in ammonia production appears to be due in part to hyperkalemia, since the excretion rate of ammonium
correlates inversely with the plasma potassium
concentration and does not decrease when miner-

alocorticoid hormone is discontinued if hyperkalemia is prevented from occurring by restricting
intake of potassium. Although the ability to generate normally steep lumen-to-blood hydrogen ion
concentration gradients remains intact in the al-
dosterone-deficient dog, the ability of the distal
nephron to secrete hydrogen ion at normal rates
appears to be impaired (231). The impairment may
reflect a reduction in proton conductance at the
luminal membrane (232).

Renal ammonia production appears to be reduced also in patients with Type 4 RTA associated with hyporeninemic hypoaldosteronism; the
urinary excretion rates of ammonium in these patients are inappropriately low with respect to urinary pH and the degree of acidosis (21). In part,
this finding may reflect a reduction in the amount
of ammonia-producing parenchyma (4). In patients with Type 4 RTA and hyporeninemic hypoaldosteronism, urinary ammonium excretion
varies directly with urinary pH, and inversely with
serum concentration of potassium when the latter
is progressively reduced by administration of a
cation-exchange resin (214), restriction of dietary
potassium intake, or administration of exogenous
mineralocorticoid hormone (21) (Figs. 18-15, 18-
16, and 18-17).

In adult humans, it would appear that metabolic acidosis results from aldosterone deficiency
only when the deficiency is combined with nephron loss or some degree of renal tubular damage
(21, 196). Renal disease might contribute to the
pathogenesis of acidosis in aldosterone deficiency
in two ways: (1) by limiting renal ammoniagenesis, as previously discussed above, and (2) by
increasing distal delivery of bicarbonate to the al-
dosterone-deficient hydrogen ion secretory mechanism of the distal nephron. Reduced resorption
of bicarbonate in the proximal nephron is a predictable consequence of progressive nephron loss
(233).

In acidotic adult patients with Type 4 RTA,
continued administration of superphysiologic
amounts of 9α-fluorohydrocortisone (a synthetic
mineralocorticoid) can induce an increase in excretion of both titratable acid and ammonium
(when GFR is not reduced to values less than 20
mL/min) (21). Over a period of days or weeks, the

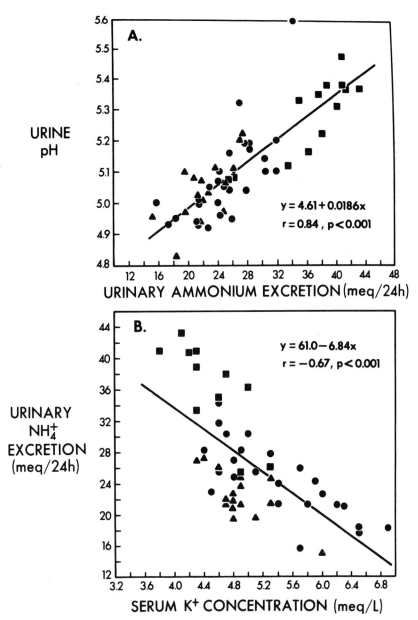

Figure 18-15. Relationship between urine pH and urinary ammonium excretion (A) and between the rate of urinary ammonium excretion and serum potassium concentration (B) during oral administration of 9α-fluorohydrocortisone therapy in three patients with hyporeninemic hypoaldosteronism without far-advanced chronic renal insufficiency (creatinine clearances: 35 mL/min per 1.73 m²; 31 mL/min per 1.73 m²; 44 mL/min per 1.73 m²). [*From A. Sebastian et al. (21).*]

increase in excretion of net acid is enough to sub-stantially ameliorate the acidosis (Fig. 18-16). The augmentation of ammonia production appears to be due to the correction of hyperkalemia. When

fluorohydrocortisone is discontinued and hyper-kalemia is prevented from reoccurring by dietary restriction of potassium, ammonium excretion does not decrease; titratable acid excretion does

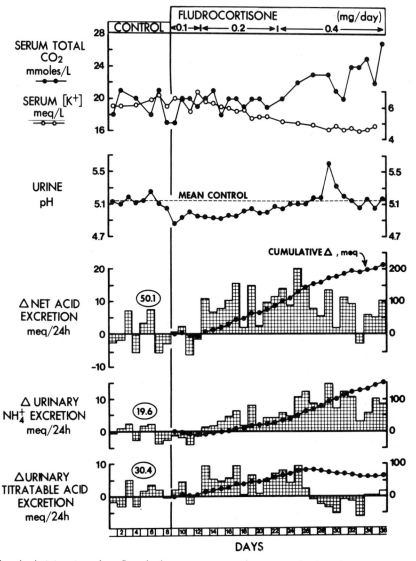

Figure 18-16. Effect of oral administration of 9α-fluorohydrocor-tisone on serum carbon dioxide and potassium concentration, urine pH, urinary titratable acid, ammonium, and net acid excre-tion in a patient with hyporeninemic hypoaldosteronism and chronic renal insufficiency (creatinine clearance 35 mL/min per 1.73 m²). Systemic acidosis had not previously been treated. In the three bottom panels the hatched bars represent the difference be-

tween the measured value of acid excretion and the mean pre-9α-fluorohydrocortisone value; the magnitude of these differences is indicated by the scale on the left-hand side of the panel. For ref-erence, the mean control value is designated by the numerals within the ellipses. The accumulated values of the daily differences are depicted by the solid circles and are indicated by the scale on the right-hand side of the panel. [*From A. Sebastian et al. (21).*]

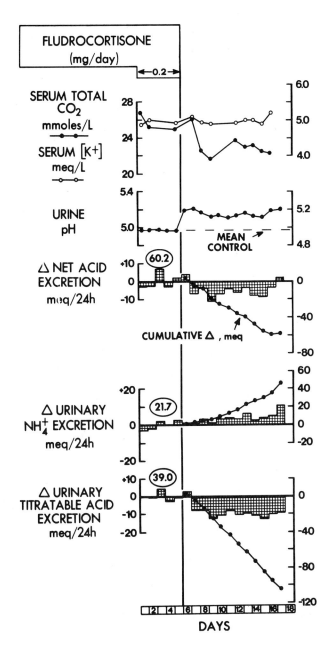

decrease and, as a consequence, acidosis reoccurs (Fig. 18-17). The requirement for superphysiologic amounts of exogenous mineralocorticoid hormone raises the possibility of renal hyporesponsiveness to the action of aldosterone.

Type 4 RTA in "pseudohypoaldosteronism" of infants and children constitutes an important example of a disorder of the renal tubule whose physiologic expression can change over time: Type 4 RTA can disappear in early childhood (206), even though the characteristic hyperreninemic hyperaldosteronism persists. The physiologic basis of the disappearance of the acidification dysfunction is not known. The disappearance might reflect the normal functional maturation of a nephron segment distal to that primarily affected. For example, the bicarbonate reabsorptive capacity of the cortical collecting duct may become great enough to "compensate" for a dysfunction in the distal convoluted tubule. In infants and children with Type 4 RTA, as in those with either Type 1 or Type 2 RTA, corrective alkali therapy can be attended by the rapid attainment of normal height and weight, even after frank stunting has occurred (206).

Treatment

In adult patients with hyporeninemic hypoaldosteronism, correction of systemic acidosis and hyperkalemia may be sustained by administration of 9α-fluorohydrocortisone in daily doses of 0.1 to 0.3 mg (231). Such therapy, however, may not always be indicated, since mineralocorticoid hormone may further increase ECF volume, and induce or increase the severity of hypertension. Restriction of dietary potassium, potassium-binding resins, and "loop" diuretics, e.g., furosemide, may be useful therapeutic adjuncts (234). Despite impairment in renal reabsorption of bicarbonate, administration of 1.5 to 2.0 meq sodium bicarbonate per

Figure 18-17. Effect of discontinuation of fluorohydrocortisone on serum carbon dioxide content and potassium concentration, urine pH and urinary titratable acid, ammonium, and net acid excretion in a patient with hyporeninemic hypoaldosteronism and chronic renal insufficiency (creatinine clearance, 35 mL/min per 1.73 m²). In this study dietary intake of potassium was reduced when therapy was discontinued; the serum potassium was reduced when therapy was discontinued; the serum potassium concentration remained constant. The rate of urinary ammonium excretion did not decrease when therapy was discontinued, despite a sustained increase in urine pH. [*From A. Sebastian et al. (21).*]

day may be sufficient to sustain correction of acidosis. Correction of acidosis usually mitigates the severity of hyperkalemia. The serum concentration of potassium can often be maintained at less than 5.0 meq/L with combined alkali therapy and modest dietary potassium restriction. The severity of hyperkalemia and acidosis can be predictably mitigated by oral administration of potassium-binding resins, but most patients find the medication distasteful.

In some children with Type 4 RTA correction of systemic acidosis and hyperkalemia can be sustained with administration of chlorothiazide alone (210, 211). In one patient this therapy was attended by a "growth spurt" (210).

CLINICAL EXPRESSIONS AND THERAPEUTIC PROBLEMS THAT INVOLVE MORE THAN ONE TYPE OF RTA

"Autoimmune" RTA

Of 14 patients with "autoimmune" RTA we have seen, all have been women; all but one have had Sjögren's syndrome (123). Twelve of the fourteen patients have had prototypic Type 1 RTA and one had a hybrid of Types 1 and 2. One patient had prototypic Type 2 RTA in association with the renal dysfunction of the Fanconi syndrome; in this patient evidence of impaired "distal" acidification was demonstrably absent. Joint disease has not been apparent clinically or radiographically, and eye findings are usually minimal. Not all of these patients complained of dry mouth, but histologic changes in salivary ducts diagnostic of Sjögren's syndrome have been invariable in buccal mucosa (except in the patient with "lupoid" hepatitis). Hypergammaglobulinemia (broad based) has been present in all patients with autoimmune RTA and in none of 15 patients with familial, genetically transmitted Type 1 RTA. In three patients, autoimmune Type 1 RTA first became apparent in the immediate postpartum period, when severe proximal muscle weakness occurred acutely in association with striking hypokalemia and renal potassium wasting (123). Persisting renal potassium wasting (despite alkali

therapy) and acute hypokalemic syndromes appear to be much more common in autoimmune Type 1 RTA than in familial or "idiopathic" Type 1 RTA.

Muscle weakness and metabolic bone disease

In patients with either Type 1 or 2 RTA, the rapidly occurring, severe muscle weakness of severe hypokalemia is the most dramatic and acutely life-threatening abnormality (118), and in patients with autoimmune Type 1 RTA the all-too-common initial clinical expression (see also Chaps. 19 and 20). But in patients with Type 2 RTA, muscle weakness is more commonly insidious in onset, less severe, and a consequence of the proximal myopathy that attends metabolic bone disease (235). In adult patients in whom Type 2 RTA occurs in the setting of intestinal malabsorption, hypocalcemia, secondary hyperparathyroidism, and hypophosphatemia, chronic weakness (of the proximal muscles) is often the major complaint (1, 235–237). Those affected typically have difficulty rising unassisted from a seated position. The weakness is usually associated with bone pain, symmetrical, often severe bone tenderness, and sometimes radiographic evidence of osteomalacia, most characteristically pseudofractures (1, 111). The metabolic bone disease may be of such striking clinical severity that even modest pretibial pressure elicits excruciating pain. The gait is characteristically slow and waddling (like a duck). All muscular effort may be attended by great discomfort. Deep tendon reflexes remain active (235). Electromyographic and histologic examination usually reveal little if any, objective evidence of muscle disease. Accordingly, and because the weakness is characteristically insidious in onset, the weakness is often mistaken as a psychoneurotic symptom. Although its pathogenetic mechanism is undefined, the myopathic disorder is predictably responsive to therapy that heals the associated metabolic bone disease. The myopathy is rare in children with Type 1 RTA. In affected adults with Type 1 RTA normal muscle strength returns with alkali therapy alone, but often only after several weeks. In affected patients with Type 2 RTA as part of the malabsorption syndrome, the myopathy responds dramatically and usually rapidly to therapy with alkali and vitamin D. By disturbing the metabolism of calcium and phosphate in muscles, a deficiency or disordered metabolism of vitamin D (238, 239) might be a pathogenetic factor in the myopathy that attends metabolic bone disease. Hyperparathyroidism and phosphate depletion might also be pathogenetic factors. In patients with renal osteodystrophy, striking and rapid amelioration of muscle weakness has been reported with the administration of 1,25-dihydroxy vitamin D_3 (240). The "metabolic" myopathy that attends metabolic bone disease also occurs in patients with idiopathic or tumor-caused "renal hypophosphatemic rickets" and in patients with Fanconi syndrome (as discussed in the specific sections dealing with these renal disorders).

pH-dependent urinary excretion of drugs

In patients with any type of RTA, corrective alkali therapy is invariably attended by intense alkalinity of the urine; the urinary pH is frequently greater than 8. This has important implications with respect to the clinical pharmacology of certain drugs whose urinary excretion is pH-dependent, and an important mode of their disposition (241, 242). As a group, the phenylalkylamines, including pseudoephedrine, have a high pK (greater than 8), and intense alkalinity of the urine greatly retards their excretion and acts to increase their blood level (243, 244). The cinchona alkaloids, quinidine and quinine, which also have a pK greater than 8, and salicylate are affected similarly (245, 246). Accordingly, in patients with any type of RTA, corrective alkali therapy predisposes them to certain kinds of drug toxicities. Frank psychosis has occurred in children with RTA who have received both a corrective dose of alkali therapy and the usual dose of pseudoephedrine for otitis media.

RENAL HYPOPHOSPHATEMIC RICKETS (AND OSTEOMALACIA) (TABLE 18-5)

This term refers to a group of disorders (see also Chap. 19) that have in common: (1) persisting hypophosphatemia caused by a reduction in renal tubular reabsorption of phosphate, expressed as an increased fractional excretion of filtered phosphate ($FEPO_4$) (or an increased renal clearance of phosphate); (2) a metabolic bone disease, usually rickets in childhood or osteomalacia in adulthood, that is "resistant" to treatment with vitamin D_2 in amounts many times that predictably curative of rickets or osteomalacia caused by simple deficiency of vitamin D (2, 247–274). The term implies the absence of impaired renal acidification and the complex renal dysfunction of the Fanconi syndrome. Modest renal glucosuria can occur. Neither the physiologic basis of the renal disorder nor a causal mechanism for the metabolic bone disease has been defined for any of these disorders, although in a very small number of patients the entire disorder can disappear with surgical removal of tumors of mesenchymal origin (253, 256, 257, 266–270), fibrous dysplasia of bone (271), or epidermal nevii (272, 273).

X-LINKED HYPOPHOSPHATEMIC RICKETS

The best-characterized and apparently most common kind of RHR (renal hypophosphatemic rickets) is that genetically transmitted as an X-linked dominant trait and first expressed clinically in early childhood (250, 255, 275). The severity of metabolic bone disease and of hypophosphatemia is greater in the affected male (hemizygote) than in the affected female, in whom expression of the disease can be quite mild (250). Growth impairment, which occurs in early childhood, appears to be of greater severity than can be accounted for by the characteristic leg bowing (250, 276, 277). In the rachitic bone disease of XLHR (X-linked hypophosphatemic rickets), in distinction from that of simple vitamin D deficiency, the long bones (on x-ray) have coarse trabeculations, thickened cortices, evidence of periosteal new bone formation, and boney overgrowth at muscle attachments (275). The serum concentrations of calcium are normal (250, 275) or modestly reduced (275, 278). Circulating concentrations of immunoreactive PTH are only modestly increased if at all (279–284). Alkaline phosphatase can be either normal or increased. Net gut absorption of calcium is reduced (285, 286); gut absorption of phosphate has been reported to be reduced (287), not reduced (288), or variably reduced (289). Plasma concentrations of 25-OH vitamin D_3 (290) and 1,25-$(OH)_2$ vitamin D_3 (291) are within the reported range of normal values (291).

Physiologic and metabolic character of the renal dysfunction

Glorieux, Scriver, and their coworkers have proposed that in XLHR the PTH-responsive component of renal phosphate transport is genetically disordered in a way that renders it physiologically unresponsive to circulating PTH (292). In affected hemizygotes, they observed that the $FEPO_4$ remained unchanged over a ten-fold increase in plasma concentration of endogenous PTH (3), and despite the intravenous administration of a large amount of PTH (7). They confirmed previous observations that experimental hypercalcemia is attended by a decrease in $FEPO_4$ (293–296), and interpreted this as evidence that the hypercalcemia per se increased renal phosphate reabsorption via a transport system independent of that normally responsive to PTH. Noting that phosphate, like

Table 18-5. Clinical spectrum of renal hypophosphatemic metabolic bone disease

Sporadic
　Childhood onset (254)
　Adulthood onset (260)

Genetically transmitted
　X-linked dominant
　　Childhood onset (250, 255)
　　Adulthood onset (262)
　Autosomal recessive (263)
　Autosomal dominant (264)
　Apparently autosomal dominant (258, 265)
　"Hypophosphatemic nonrachitic bone disease" (265)

Acquired (and often surgically reversible)
　Tumors of bone and soft tissue (253, 256, 257, 266–270)
　Fibrous dysplasia of bone (271)
　Epidermal nevus (271, 273)

Neurofibromatosis associated (247,274)

calcium, may equilibrate with a mitochondrial compartment during transepithelial absorption and that "negative reabsorption" of P_i can occur in patients with XLHR during acute phosphate loading, Scriver and his colleagues have suggested that "the (genetic) lesion in XLHR could be a defect permitting back-flux of P_i from cytosol at the luminal membrane by altering the normal Michaelis equilibrium [Scriver and Bergeron, 297], that permits net reclamation at that surface of the epithelium before equilibration with mitochondria" (261).

Most, if not all, of the patients with XLHR studied by Scriver and his colleagues appear to have been treated with large amounts of sodium phosphate, as well as with vitamin D. When PTE (parathyroid extract) was administered, the $FEPO_4$ was already quite high, although phosphate therapy had presumably been discontinued 12 to 18 h beforehand (265). In each of 16 patients with XLHR (from seven unrelated kindreds) who had not been treated with either phosphate or vitamin D and in whom $FEPO_4$ was relatively low (278) or negligible (experimental posthypercalcemia) (284), experimentally administered PTE induced an increase in $FEPO_4$ that was at least normal (278) or frankly exaggerated (284) (Fig. 18-18). In both the intact and parathyroidectomized dog and rat, renal handling of phosphate is greatly influenced by the prior intake of phosphate (298–302): At comparable plasma concentrations and filtered loads of phosphate, the $FEPO_4$ can be either greatly increased or reduced, depending on whether prior intake of phosphate has been high or low, respectively (300–302). A similar kind of phenomenon has been described in normal humans (303, 304) and in two adult patients with renal hypophosphatemic osteomalacia (258). In the patients with XLHR reported on by Scriver and his colleagues, the phenomena of a very greatly increased "basal" $FEPO_4$, a blunted phosphaturic response to administered PTH, and "negative" (renal) reabsorption of P_i during phosphate loading (292) all may reflect the capacity of prolonged administration of large amounts of phosphate to greatly alter the physiologic expression of the causal genetic defect.

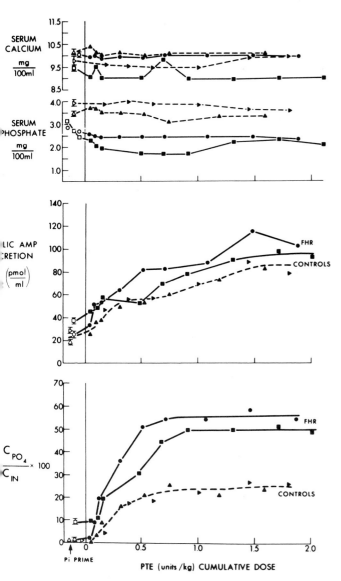

The metabolic derangement

XLHR has been considered by some to be a prototype of "phosphopenic refractory rickets" (261, 305). Normal renal reabsorption of filtered phosphate is of course critical to the "maintenance of the normal endogenous phosphate pool" (261), and the renal lesion of XLHR dictates a hypophosphatemic state. But, in patients with XLHR it seems unlikely that rickets results only from the hypophosphatemic state per se or that the hypophosphatemia reflects a generalized cellular depletion of phosphate. In patients with XLHR, rickets is predictably healed with massive amounts of vitamin D administered alone (2, 275, 306), and with little measured increase in the plasma concentration of phosphate (275, 307); phosphate therapy can "promote" or "initiate" healing of rickets (308–313), but apparently cannot induce or maintain complete healing unless administered in combination with vitamin D (258, 275, 311, 312). By contrast, phosphate therapy alone can heal the metabolic bone disease of patients with either Fanconi syndrome (314, 315) or renal hypophosphatemic rickets (259) that is not genetically transmitted. Thus, in patients with XLHR receiving high-dose phosphate, it seems likely that vitamin D therapy is not just an adjunct that limits or prevents the occurrence of secondary hyperparathyroidism (261, 305, 312), but a requirement for the complete healing of the metabolic bone disease.

Muscle weakness and other evidences of myopathy are conspicuously absent not only in both children and adults with XLHR (250, 255, 275), but in patients with other forms of genetically transmitted renal hypophosphatemic rickets as well (262–265). By contrast, striking muscle

Figure 18-18. Physiologic response to continuous intravenous administration of parathyroid extract (PTE) initiated almost immediately after termination of prolonged, experimentally induced hypercalcemia in two untreated adult hemizygotes with X-linked hypophosphatemic rickets (XLHR) (unbroken lines), who received an intravenously administered prime of neutral sodium phosphate ([●], 6.6 mmol; [■], 10.4 mmol) before clearance periods were begun, and in two normal control subjects (▲ and ▶, connected by broken lines.) Depicted are mean (±1 S.D.) of values from three successive clearance periods obtained immediately before PTE was initiated (open symbols) and individual values thereafter (closed symbols). Cyclic AMP (adenosine monophosphate) = 3′,5′-cyclic AMP in pmol/mL glomerular filtrate, a unit derived from urinary excretion rate (UV) divided by GFR (glomerular filtration rate) as measured by the renal clearance of inulin. C_{PO_4}/C_{in} = renal clearance of phosphate/renal clearance of inulin: fractional urinary excretion of filtered inorganic phosphate. [From E. Short et al. (284).]

weakness and general debility attend the hypophosphatemia and osteomalacia caused by the phosphate depletion induced in otherwise normal subjects by sustained restriction of phosphate absorption from the gut (orally administered aluminum hydroxide) (316–319). Furthermore, in children and adults with renal hypophosphatemic rickets that is *not* genetically transmitted, proximal muscle weakness is predictable (253, 256, 257, 259, 266–273, 320, 321), often striking, and can be responsive to phosphate therapy alone (259, 320), even though the hypophosphatemia of these patients is often no more severe than that of patients with XLHR. In patients with Fanconi syndrome, proximal muscle weakness occurs frequently and can be strikingly responsive to phosphate therapy alone (314, 315). In recently described children with a genetically transmitted "hypophosphatemic nonrachitic bone disease," and no evidence of myopathy, Scriver and his coworkers note that the bone disease is more benign than that of XLHR despite "the same low concentration of phosphate anion in the extracellular fluid" (265). They suggest that this disease and XLHR are "experiments of nature which may reveal a process regulating the distribution of inorganic phosphate between extracellular fluid and the bone compartment." Indeed, in XLHR, and possibly in other genetically transmitted forms of hypophosphatemic metabolic bone disease as well, the rachitogenic derangement in phosphate metabolism may be more one of cellular distribution than depletion of phosphate.

Mounting evidence indicates that vitamin D and its metabolites normally modulate not only the extracellular concentration and transcellular movement of phosphate and calcium but also the concentration of these ions within, and their movement between, cytoplasm and mitochondria (322–324). A genetic defect in either the cellular response to, or the kinds or amounts of species synthesized of, vitamin D metabolites (263, 268) could disorder the intracellular distribution and transport of phosphate and calcium in tissues normally acted upon by metabolites of vitamin D, including the bone. There is, however, no convincing evidence that either the metabolism of vitamin D or the cellular response to its metabolites is abnormal in any of the genetically transmitted diseases expressed as renal hypophosphatemic (vitamin D-resistant) metabolic bone disease.

Treatment

Healing of rickets in patients with XLHR and other forms of RHR requires large amounts of vitamin D_2. The starting dose should be 10,000 to 25,000 I.U. per day (275, 306). The amount is increased as needed to achieve evidence of healing, as judged by a falling serum level of alkaline phosphatase and radiographic improvement. Oral phosphate may be added as a neutral phosphate solution in amounts of 1 to 4 g of phosphorus per day (311–313). Although such phosphate therapy is not universally recommended for patients with XLHR (306, 325, 326), its use reduces the amount of vitamin D required to heal rickets (311–313) and may promote growth (312). We use phosphate therapy routinely in children with XLHR. Stamp (326) cites three disadvantages of phosphate therapy: (1) "the need to juggle two lots of pills instead of one; (2) the still-present danger of vitamin D intoxication if a patient should stop the phosphate supplement for any reason; (3) the increased secondary hyperparathyroidism which phosphate produces and to which these patients (XLHR) may be particularly liable." All seem agreed that phosphate therapy is useful in patients with adult-onset RHR that is not genetically transmitted.

Healing of rickets in patients with XLHR has been reported with long-term administration of 25-OH-cholecalciferol (327). Over the rather limited range of dosages investigated, $1,25\text{-}(OH)_2D_3$ has not been found to be a useful therapeutic agent in patients with XLHR (328, 329). Impressive claims have recently been made for the therapeutic use of $1\alpha\text{-}OHD_3$ (1α-hydroxyvitamin D_3), a synthetic analogue of $1,25\text{-}(OH)_2D_3$ (330): In 10 patients diagnosed only as having "vitamin D-resistant hypophosphatemic osteomalacia," Peacock and his associates reported that treatment with $1\alpha\text{-}OHD_3$ in high dose (3 to 6 μg/day) cured myopathy, increased calcium and phosphorus absorption (gut) and retention, and healed the osteomalacia. Phosphate supplements were not administered. In the four patients in whom the substance was measured, the circulating levels of $1,25\text{-}(OH)_2D_3$ attained with the high dose of 1α-OHD_3 were very much less than those induced with a lower dose of 1α-OHD_3 in patients with renal failure. These findings suggest the possibility that the metabolism of vitamin D could be abnormal in patients with some kinds of RHR.

ACQUIRED RENAL HYPOPHOSPHATEMIC RICKETS

These disorders are very rare and there are few published investigations of the character of either their renal dysfunction or metabolic derangement. Certain findings in several affected patients however, are of unusual interest and potential importance. In a 27-year-old man with apparently idiopathic, adult-onset renal hypophosphatemic osteomalacia, parathyroidectomy was attended by a striking clinical and radiographic improvement in the bone disease and a reduction in the requirement for vitamin D (331). In a 12-year-old boy with renal hypophosphatemic rickets, surgical excision of several fibroangiomas on the face and leg was attended by disappearance of all biochemical abnormalities and radiologic evidence of rickets (273). An extract of the excised tissue induced phosphaturia in a puppy. In a recently described 41-year-old woman with RHR and a giant cell tumor of the bone, the plasma concentration of $1,25\text{-}(OH)_2D_3$ was abnormally low; the plasma concentration of $25\text{-}OHD_3$ was normal (270). With short-term administration of $1,25\text{-}(OH)_2D_3$ in "replacement" amounts, hypophosphatemia disappeared, renal reabsorption of phosphate became normal, and healing of the metabolic bone disease began, as judged from histologic changes. Surgical removal of the tumor was attended by apparently complete remission of the RHR. These findings provide evidence that the tumor caused the RHR and that an abnormality in the metabolism of vitamin D was a necessary pathogenetic event. Unfortunately, measurements of plasma concentration of $1,25\text{-}(OH)_2D_3$ were not reported during the period in which administration of this metabolite was attended by reversal of the physiologic and metabolic abnormalities or during the

period after the tumor had been removed. If an abnormally high plasma concentration of $1,25\text{-}(OH)_2D_3$ were induced, it would be difficult to assign a precise pathogenetic role to the measured reduction in plasma concentration of $1,25\text{-}(OH)_2D_3$ per se.

FANCONI SYNDROME

PHYSIOLOGIC CHARACTER

Fanconi's syndrome (FS) consists of two components: (1) a complex dysfunction of the proximal renal tubule characterized by reduced net reabsorption of phosphate, glucose, amino acids, usually bicarbonate, and sometimes uric acid, expressed clinically as glucosuria, generalized hyperaminoaciduria, hyperphosphaturia (relative to concomitant hypophosphatemia), Type 2 (proximal) RTA, and sometimes hypouricemia; (2) a metabolic bone disease, characteristically rickets in children, osteomalacia in adults (332, 333). Although the clinical picture of FS is characteristically dominated by metabolic bone disease, and, in affected children, impaired growth and often frank stunting, disturbances in fluid and electrolyte homeostasis are usually continuously apparent. Thirst or polydipsia, polyuria, and the signs and symptoms of hypokalemia, acidosis, and depletion of ECF volume stem principally from impaired reabsorption of Na^+, HCO_3^-, Cl^-, and water in the proximal renal tubule (as detailed in the sections on the pathophysiology of Type 2 RTA). Such disturbances of fluid and electrolyte homeostasis may be explosive in onset and extreme in severity when the renal dysfunction occurs acutely, as with drug toxicity (139, 140), or in association with a systemic disturbance of metabolism, particularly one that also gives rise to lactic acidosis (334, 335).

PATHOGENESIS OF THE RENAL DISORDER

Metabolic

FS is a characteristic feature of several genetically transmitted metabolic diseases: cystinosis (332, 333), Lowe's syndrome (125, 336, 337), a certain kind of tyrosinemia (Type 1) (131, 338–340) when tyrosine or phenylalanine is not restricted (339), and HFI (hereditary fructose intolerance) when fructose is not restricted (341–343). In these diseases, FS invariably occurs in association with Type 2 RTA. FS also occurs in other genetically transmitted metabolic diseases, including Wilson's disease (129, 130, 344–346), galactosemia (347, 348), and a glycogen storage disorder (349, 350) characterized by galactose intolerance but not by a demonstrable enzyme deficiency. In these diseases, the occurrence of FS might represent a unit response to a disorder of some component of renal metabolism that is critical to the operation of all affected transport processes, for example, a component critical to the production on transduction of the energy required for the transport process. FS disappears in patients with galactosemia, tyrosinemia, Wilson's disease, and HFI when their systemic disorders of metabolism are corrected or attenuated by maneuvers that act to remove galactose (347), tyrosine (339, 340), copper (346), or fructose (32, 341–343), respectively. The abnormal gene products of these diseases do not then act directly to impair the operation of transport processes in the renal tubule. Rather, the expression of FS is pathogenetically linked to the abnormal gene product by way of a reversible abnormality of renal metabolism.

The reversible renal disorder of HFI constitutes a model of the renal dysfunction of FS that is uniquely susceptible to systematic analysis and uncomplicated by whatever secondary phenomena that attend the persisting renal disorders (32). Minutes after the experimental administration of fructose is initiated in patients with HFI, the multiple renal dysfunctions of FS occur simultaneously, persist for as long as fructose is continued, and disappear shortly after its discontinuance. The dysfunctions are dose-dependent and predictable in severity (32). As judged from clearance studies, net reabsorption of Na^+, HCO_3^-, Cl^-, and water are greatly reduced in the proximal renal tubule, and it seems likely that the dose-dependent aminoaciduria, glucosuria, and phosphaturia also result from disordered function of the proximal renal tubule (5, 32, 34). The renal disorder is caused by an abnormality of renal metabolism that is a direct consequence of an abnormal gene product, a kinetically deficient cytoplasmic, "soluble" enzyme, aldolase "B" (351, 352). In consequence of diminished renal cortical aldolase activity toward fructose 1-phosphate (F-1-P) and intact activity of fructokinase (which catalyzes the phophorylation of fructose of F-1-P), administration of fructose to patients with HFI evokes this sequence of biochemical events in the cytoplasm of cells of the proximal renal tubule (353): $\uparrow$F-1-P$\rightarrow$ $\downarrow$inorganic phosphate (P_i) (5). In these cells it seems likely that a reduction of cytoplasmic P_i causes a profound reduction in both the cellular concentration and rate of mitochondrial regeneration of ATP (354). Of perhaps greatest potential clinical significance is the observation that the experimental renal dysfunction induced by fructose can be greatly attenuated by prior loading with sodium phosphate (5). Presumably, by near prevention of the fructose-induced depletion of cellular P_i, this maneuver partially interrupts a sequence of biochemical events critical to the metabolic pathogenesis of the experimental renal disorder. It seems entirely possible that a number of renal diseases expressed clinically as FS, and possibly some that are not, may require a common pathogenetic sequence of biochemical events, and that more than one event in such a sequence may be susceptible to interdictive therapeutic attack.

Lysosomal

Lysosomes are cytoplasmic organelles which are bounded by a single membrane, and which contain hydrolases and other enzymes required for a variety of normal degradative processes, including the degrading of proteins and peptides. In the normal proximal convoluted tubule, pinocytotic vacuoles formed at the luminal border migrate inward and fuse with lysosomes, thereby completing a phagolysosomal continuum. Lysozyme is a small-molecular-weight protein (MW 15,000) that is readily filterable by the normal glomerulus, usually completely reabsorbed by the pinocytotic process of the renal tubule, and catabolized principally, if not entirely, by lysosomes in the proximal tubule (355–357). Lysozyme is then a normal constituent of renal lysosomes (358), but is not synthesized in the kidney (359). Lysozymuria is generally considered to reflect proximal tubule cell damage (360, 361). Other circulating small-molecular-weight proteins, including insulin (362), β_2-microglobulin (363–365), and immunoglobulin L chain (366), appear to be handled by the renal tubule in much the same way as lysozyme, and are characteristically excreted in the urine in greatly increased amounts in patients with nephropathic cystinosis and other genetically transmitted diseases causal of FS (362, 365, 367).

Lysozyme and light-chain nephropathy. Increased urinary excretion of substantial amounts of lysozyme and immunoglobulin L chain can also reflect their increased production (152–154, 368–371). When immunoglobulin L chain or lysozyme are filtered by the glomerulae at rates that overload the phagolysosomal system of the proximal tubule, structural damage (372) and dysfunction of the renal tubule can occur (150–154, 368–371). In patients with monocytic leukemia the not uncommon syndrome of renal potassium wasting appears to be a consequence of lysozyme-induced renal dysfunction (368–371). In patients ultimately diagnosed as having multiple myeloma, the occurrence of FS may precede by years other evidences of the disease and reflect an immunoglobulin-L-chain-induced nephropathy (152, 153). In this instance the immunoglobulin detected in the urine is presumably produced in excess by a single clone of myeloma cells, and hence is of but a single subtype, κ (152, 153), although one patient is described as having had only the λ subtype (373). Thus, when patients with FS excrete but one type of immunoglobulin L chains, monoclonal plasma cell dyscrasia, i.e., multiple myeloma, can be inferred to be causal (153). When increased urinary excretion of immunoglobulin L chain reflects a renal tubular dysfunction that is unassociated with increased production of L chain, both κ and λ subtypes are characteristically excreted (374, 375).

Some patients with FS excrete increased

amounts of lysosomal enzymes: N-acetylglucosaminidase is a "marker" lysosomal enzyme in hepatocytes (376), and in the renal cortex, the enzyme occurs predominantly in lysosomes (377, 378). Since the molecular weight of N-acetylglucosaminidase is approximately 250,000, increased excretion of this enzyme in patients with FS, in the absence of more than minimal albuminuria or a reduction in glomerular filtration, probably reflects a lysosomal abnormality (379, 380).

Cystinosis. In patients with cystinosis, the most common disease causally associated with FS in children, "storage" of cystine in lysosomes of the proximal renal tubule might be a primary pathogenetic event in the renal disorder (333). In so-called nephropathic or "infantile" cystinosis, FS is expressed within the first 12 months of life, progressive reduction in GFR leads to terminal uremia by midchildhood, and the free-cystine content of leukocytes is 80 times normal (381). In so-called benign cystinosis of adulthood, renal disease is absent (382), and the free-cystine content of leukocytes is 30 times normal (381). So-called adolescent or "intermediate" cystinosis is intermediate in severity with respect to the renal lesion and cystine content of leukocytes (383).

Whatever the pathogenicity of intracellular "storage" of cystine in nephropathic cystinosis is, the invariability and magnitude of the "storage" of cystine in certain cell types permits a biochemical diagnosis of the disease (384, 385). This is particularly important in those clinical situations in which the storage phenomenon does not give rise to observable crystals, as in the case of many infants homozygous for the trait, and in the special case of amniotic cells and affected fetal cells. Utilizing a pulse-labeling technique (386, 387) in which cultured amniotic cells accumulate abnormally large amounts of free ^{35}S-cystine, Schneider and his coworkers (388) have recently diagnosed nephropathic cystinosis in utero in an 18-week-old fetus homozygous for the trait. Excessive accumulation of free ^{35}S-cystine by either amniotic cells or white blood cells (as for the biochemical diagnosis of cystinosis in infants) (389) is easily detected in autoradiographs of thin-layer chromatograms (388, 389). The capability of diagnosing nephropathic cystinosis in utero has obvious therapeutic implications (388).

PATHOPHYSIOLOGY AND METABOLIC DERANGEMENT

Potassium and sodium

See the discussion of pathophysiology in Type 2 RTA for a description of the potassium and sodium metabolic derangement.

Phosphate and calcium

In FS sustained hypophosphatemia is a predictable consequence of the persisting impairment in renal reabsorption of phosphate and has generally been assumed to be the principal, if not sole, pathogenetic determinant of the metabolic bone disease (322–333). Phosphate therapy alone can heal the metabolic bone disease (314, 315). This therapeutic phenomenon would appear to have occurred most frequently in patients with adult-onset FS, but has been described in children with nephropathic cystinosis (333, 390). Metabolic bone disease, however, can antedate the occurrence of hypophosphatemia in patients with FS (391, 392), and can heal without measured change either in the severity of hypophosphatemia, or in the plasma calcium × phosphorus product, when large amounts of vitamin D are administered alone (393, 394). Furthermore, Dent and Harris found evidence of metabolic bone disease (and debility) in but one of four adult siblings with the renal dysfunction characteristic of FS, although hypophosphatemia (and mild metabolic acidosis) occurred in all and was severe in three (<2.0 mg/dL); hypocalcemia occurred in none (395). The apparent nonoccurrence of metabolic bone disease despite persisting, severe hypophosphatemia (1.7 mg/dL) and mild acidosis has recently been described in an adult woman with FS as part of "light-chain nephropathy" (154). It is clear that in some patients with the renal dysfunction of FS, rickets or osteomalacia is not a predictable consequence of plasma calcium × phosphorus product that is less than 30, as pointed out by Stanbury (393, 394).

Hypophosphatemia or phosphate depletion has been implicated in the pathogenesis of the proximal myopathy that frequently occurs in FS (259, 314, 315, 396). The myopathy can be reversed with phosphate therapy alone (259, 314, 315). Myopathy is, however, by no means predictable in FS, even when hypophosphatemia is severe (154, 395).

The renal dysfunction of FS usually does not give rise to hypocalcemia even after prolonged acidosis. Although hypercalciuria occurs (126, 150, 314, 380) and can disappear with alkali therapy (126, 345), its occurrence is not predictably related to that of acidosis (397). Hypercalciuria is characteristic of patients with Wilson's disease, irrespective of FS, and may reflect increased absorption of calcium from the gut (129, 345). In our experience hypercalciuria is usual in patients with cystinosis and its severity is unaffected by alkali therapy.

Nephrocalcinosis (and nephrolithiasis) occurs in FS (130, 314, 345, 380), but is quite uncommon, perhaps because urinary excretion of citrate is not reduced and is often increased (398, 399).

Vitamin D (See Chaps. 19 and 20)

Metabolic bone disease (including vitamin D dependency). FS occurs as part of vitamin D dependency, a rare disorder genetically transmitted as an autosomal recessive trait and characterized by hypocalcemia and secondary hyperparathyroidism but modest (or no) hypophosphatemia (7–9, 138, 400). When pharmacologic amounts of vitamin D_2 are administered to those affected, the rickets heal and the hypocalcemia (and hypophosphatemia) and renal dysfunction disappear (7, 138). Having found that in those affected "replacement" amounts of either $1,25\text{-}(OH)_2D_3$ or $1\alpha\text{-}OHD_3$ can, within days, correct the hypocalcemia and renal dysfunction, and initiate healing of rickets (8, 9, 401), Fraser and his colleagues have proposed that vitamin D dependency is caused by a genetic deficienty of $25\text{-}OHD_3$ 1-hydroxylase and consequent deficiency of circulating $1,25\text{-}(OH)_2D_3$ (8, 261, 305). Fraser and Scriver regard vitamin D dependency as a prototype of "calciopenic hereditary rickets" (305); the associated renal dysfunction is a consequence of secondary hyperparathyroidism.

Although plasma concentrations of $1,25\text{-}(OH)_2D_3$ have not been reported in patients with vitamin D dependency, and complete healing of rickets in those affected may require amounts of $1,25\text{-}(OH)_2D_3$ slightly greater than those required to heal vitamin D-deficient rickets (8, 9, 401), the phenomenon of vitamin D "dependency" compels an important question: Can disordered renal metabolism of vitamin D contribute to the phenomenon of vitamin D-resistant metabolic bone disease in patients with FS who are not hypocalcemic and in whom the renal dysfunction of FS is not reversed with vitamin D therapy? $1,25\text{-}(OH)_2D_3$ is synthesized exclusively in mitochondria of the renal cortex (10–12, 15), by the 1-hydroxylation of $25\text{-}OHD_3$, which is synthesized principally in the liver (402). By impairing either the 1-hydroxylation reaction per se or the accession of $25\text{-}OHD_3$ to the mitochondrial site of the reaction, abnormalities of the renal cortical tubule capable of causing persisting FS might greatly reduce the renal synthesis of $1,25\text{-}(OH)_2D_3$—and possibly other metabolites of $25\text{-}OHD_3$—and thereby contribute to the pathogenesis of the bone disease of FS (403). In animals, the experimental administration of maleic acid induces a reversible renal tubule dysfunction like that of FS (404, 405) and metabolic and structural changes in the renal cortical tubules, particularly in the mitochondria (406–409). In the vitamin D-deficient rat and chick, maleic acid induces a substantial reduction in the conversion of $25\text{-}OHD_3$ to $1,25\text{-}(OH)_2D_3$, and this reduction occurs without a significant decrease in GFR, where measured in the rat (403). Measurements of plasma concentrations of $25\text{-}OHD_3$ and $1,25\text{-}(OH)_2D_3$ have not been reported in patients with FS, but in one young girl with nephropathic cystinosis, treatment with a "physiologic" amount of $1,25\text{-}(OH)_2D_3$ (1 μg/day) was attended by rapid healing of rickets and an increase in linear growth

rate (410). Gertner et al. have also reported healing of rickets in three boys with cystinosis given $1\alpha\text{-}OHD_3$ (1α-hydroxycholecalciferol), a synthetic analogue of $1,25\text{-}(OH)_2D_3$ (411).

Renal dysfunction. The finding that vitamin D can reverse the complex renal tubular dysfunction of patients with either vitamin D "dependency" or deficiency suggests the possibility that an abnormality in the renal metabolism of $25\text{-}OHD_3$ or $1,25\text{-}(OH)_2D_3$ can contribute to the pathogenesis of the renal dysfunction of FS, and may be required for its expression in some cases. The renal dysfunction of vitamin D dependency and of vitamin D deficiency, of which hypophosphatemia has been considered to be an expression (400, 401), has usually been attributed to hyperparathyroidism secondary to hypocalcemia (261, 305, 400). But the demonstration in patients with these disorders that the renal dysfunction can be greatly attenuated by experimental correction of the hypocalcemia (5, 6, 400) and presumed suppression of secondary hyperparathyroidism need only mean that circulating PTH, possibly in increased amounts (and perhaps hypocalcemia), is required for the expression of FS. It would appear that hyperparathyroidism is causally associated with reversible FS (including Type 2 RTA) only when secondary to a deficiency, or disturbed metabolism, of vitamin D (see discussion in section on Type 2 RTA). In this regard it should be noted that when either vitamin D_2 or $1\alpha\text{-}OHD_3$ was experimentally discontinued in patients with vitamin D dependency, both the occurrence of hypophosphatemia and aminoaciduria antedated that of hypocalcemia (401). Conversely, hypophosphatemia and aminoaciduria appeared to persist for several days after hypocalcemia had been corrected with $1\alpha\text{-}OHD_3$ (401). Furthermore, in several patients with idiopathic FS unassociated with hypocalcemia (412–414), large-dose vitamin D therapy has been attended by correction of FS; and, in the one patient in whom the measurement was made, the plasma concentration of immunoreactive PTH was not increased (414). $25\text{-}OHD_3$ and, to a lesser extent, $1,25\text{-}(OH)_2D_3$ can act to increase renal reabsorption of phosphate, sodium, and calcium (415, 416). It is not known whether these actions depend on conversion of this metabolite to some metabolite of 25-OHD$_3$, or whether the normal operation of any renal tubular function depends on an effect of, or the renal metabolism of, 25-OHD$_3$ or 1,25-(OH)$_2$D$_3$.

THERAPY

The therapy of Fanconi's syndrome can be dramatically successful when substances critical to its causation can be removed, as in the case of HFI, galactosemia, Wilson's disease, and tyrosinemia (Type 1). But, in each of these diseases, morbidity and mortality may be determined more by extrarenal disorders, particularly liver disease (341, 343, 417, 418) and brain damage (341, 348, 419–422), which can persist despite removal of the specific toxic substances. In cystinosis, in which the renal disease is the principal determinant of morbidity and mortality, no therapy is known to attenuate the severity of FS or to prevent the inexorably progressive reduction in renal mass. Renal transplantation, however, has been lifesaving in a number of patients with cystinosis and otherwise fatal uremia (423–427). In some patients, growth spurts have occurred after renal transplantation (425, 427), but most children remain stunted. In the transplanted kidney, cystine crystals appear in the interstitial cells, but not in the tubule epithelial cells, and in only one instance in the glomerular cells (423). Recurrence of FS has not been reported. According to the recent report of the Advisory Committee to the Renal Transplant Registry (426), 24 patients with nephropathic cystinosis have received 27 transplanted kidneys. Of the 13 patients alive with functional transplanted kidneys in January 1974, 9 were well more than 3 years after transplantation.

The therapeutic approach to acidosis and hypokalemia is discussed under Type 2 RTA.

The approach to vitamin D therapy is much like that already considered in the section on RHR. Massive amounts of vitamin D$_2$, 100,000 to 300,000 U/day, may be required to heal rickets. It can be anticipated that the synthetic analogue of 1,25-(OH)$_2$D$_3$, 1α-OHD$_3$, will be widely used in the treatment of FS; both compounds have already been successfully used in "replacement" doses of 1 μg/day (410, 411). The very short biologic half-life of 1α-OHD$_3$ should minimize the danger of vitamin D intoxication, a common and serious problem with the use of vitamin D$_2$. Oral phosphate therapy would appear to be a useful therapeutic adjunct to vitamin D therapy, particularly in adult patients with idiopathic FS (257, 314, 315, 396).

PSEUDOHYPOPARATHYROIDISM

In 1942 Albright and his coworkers applied the term PHP (pseudohypoparathyroidism) (see also Chap. 19) to an inherited disorder characterized by hyperphosphatemia and hypocalcemia and the apparent cause of this combination, diminished renal and skeletal responsiveness to circulating PTH (2). Experimentally administered PTE failed to induce increases in either the urinary excretion of phosphate or the serum concentration of calcium as great as those occurring in normal subjects or patients with true HP (hypoparathyroidism).

TYPE 1 PHP

In the classic form of PHP, as originally described by Albright, and hereafter referred to as PHP-1, the metabolic derangements are commonly associated with dysmorphic syndrome that characteristically includes short stature, round face, short neck, thick, stocky habitus, and discrete abnormalities in individual bones of the skeleton; the metacarpal and metatarsal bones, and sometimes the phalanges, are shortened, apparently because of premature closure of the epiphyses (428).

Physiologic and metabolic character

Experimental administration of PTH or PTE to patients with PHP-1 fails to induce the 10- to 20-fold increase in urinary excretion of cAMP (3',5'-cyclic adenosine monophosphate) observed in subjects and patients with HP (429). This observation constitutes the most certain identifying metabolic characteristic of PHP-1 and provides insight into its pathogenesis. The normal phosphaturic response to administered PTH stems in large part from a reduction in phosphate reabsorption in the proximal tubule that requires the sequence of activation of adenyl cyclase at the contraluminal membrane, elevation of intracellular cAMP, and cAMP-dependent stimulation of a protein kinase located in the luminal membrane and presumably phosphorylation of this membrane (430–436). The PTH-induced increase in urinary excretion of cAMP is predominantly a consequence of increased production of cAMP by the renal tubule (437). PTH activated adenyl cyclase normally (in vitro) in the only renal cortical tissue so studied from a patient with PHP-1 (438). The log-linear dose response to PTH suggested that the genetic defect of PHP-1 ". . . is not a deletion either of the hormonal receptor or the enzyme adenyl cyclase" (438). In patients with PHP-1, the failure of administered PTH to induce a normal increase in the urinary excretion of cAMP and phosphate might reflect a failure to induce a normal increase in the concentration of cAMP at some locus of the renal tubule normally involved in mediating the phosphaturic effect of PTH.

Circulating immunoreactive PTH is increased to concentrations two to five times normal in patients with PHP-1 in apparent consequence of their hypocalcemia (428, 439). Osteitis fibrosa cystica can occur, yet bone density is usually normal or increased (428). The characteristic findings of diminished hypercalcemic response to administered PTE and reduced gut absorption of calcium can both be explained as consequences of a reduced concentration of circulating 1,25-$(OH)_2D_3$ (16–19). Vitamin D, presumably in the form of 1,25-$(OH)_2D_3$, is apparently required for PTH to induce both a normal hypercalcemic response and an increased gut absorption of calcium (440–443). Administration of vitamin D in pharmacologic amounts can restore hypercalcemic responsiveness to administered PTE in patients with PHP-1 (444, 445). Oral administration of 1,25-$(OH)_2D_3$ in apparently near "replacement"

amounts can both restore hypercalcemic responsiveness to PTH and increase gut absorption of calcium (17–19). Although correction of hypocalcemia might contribute to the restoration of hypercalcemic and phosphaturic responsiveness, in a recently reported patient with osseous hyporesponsiveness (but not renal hyporesponsiveness) to PTH, administration of 1,25-$(OH)_2D_3$ restored the hypercalcemic response to PTH even when the severity of hypocalcemia persisted undiminished (446).

In patients with PHP-1, long-term administration of pharmacologic amounts of vitamin D is characteristically attended not only by correction of hypocalcemia, but also by correction of hyperphosphatemia and increased renal phosphate clearance (428); in some patients the phosphaturic responsiveness to acutely administered PTH is restored (444, 445). In two patients with PHP-1, long-term administration of 1,25-$(OH)_2D_3$ or its synthetic analogue 1α-OHD_3 resulted in sustained normal serum concentrations of calcium and phosphorus (447). It has been proposed that the renal conversion of 25-OHD_3 to 1,25-$(OH)_2D_3$ is impaired in patients with PHP-1 (17–19). The PTH-induced stimulation of the uniquely renal cortical synthesis of 1,25-$(OH)_2D_3$ appears to require activation of renal cortical adenyl cyclase, and the consequent formation of cAMP (448). A genetic defect that disorders either PTH-dependent renal adenyl cyclase, or the normal metabolic disposition of PTH-dependent renal cortical cAMP, might then give rise to diminished synthesis of 1,25-$(OH)_2D_3$ and as a consequence skeletal, intestinal, and renal hyporesponsiveness to circulating PTH.

When the dysmorphic syndrome of PHP-1 occurs without the biochemical characteristics of HP, the disorder is termed PPHP (pseudopseudohypoparathyroidism) (449). In these patients, the phosphaturic response to administered PTH can be normal (429). PHP-1 and PPHP occur in siblings and in members of successive generations of a family (448, 450, 451). In the same person, PHP-1 may be expressed as PPHP at one time and as the fully expressed metabolic disorder at another (450, 452–454). In patients with PPHP, the PTH-induced increase in the urinary excretion of cAMP tends to be intermediate between that of patients with HP and those with fully expressed PHP (429). The increased concentration of calcitonin in the thyroid gland of patients with PHP-1 is not causally related to their hypocalcemia, and is almost certainly its consequence (455).

Treatment

In patients with PHP-1 or PHP-2, hypocalcemia and hyperphosphatemia are usually corrected with vitamin D, ergocalciferol (vitamin D_2), administered in doses of 25,000 to 200,000 U/day, and with dihydrotachysterol, in doses ranging from 0.25 to 1.0 mg/day. Vitamin D intoxication is less common in PHP-1 than in other types of hypoparathyroidism. Extensive long-term therapeutic experience with $1,25\text{-}(OH)_2D_3$ and $1\alpha\text{-}OHD_3$ has not yet been reported, but a dose of 0.5 μg/day is reported to have corrective metabolic effects qualitatively and quantitatively like those obtained with much larger amounts of vitamin D_2 (447). It seems likely that $1\alpha\text{-}OHD_3$ will become the therapeutic agent of choice.

TYPE 2 PSEUDOHYPOPARATHYROIDISM

Pseudohypoparathyroidism Type 2 (PHP-2) was first described by Drezner et al. (456) in a 22-month-old hypocalcemic infant boy in whom experimentally administered PTE induced only a trivial decrease in the Tm for phosphate reabsorption (normalized to GFR), but a striking increase in the urinary excretion rate of cAMP. These findings were interpreted as reflecting "... failure of intracellular reception of the cAMP message. . . ." These findings clearly indicate that PTH-induced activation of renal adenyl cyclase can occur in vivo without induction of the phosphaturic response. In a patient with PHP-2 in whom the phosphaturic response to administered PTE was restored to normal when hypocalcemia was corrected by calcium infusion, Rodriguez et al. (457) speculated that the metabolic defect in PHP-2 is "an inability of the cell membrane to respond to PTH with an increase in the permeability to calcium." Measurements of plasma con-

centrations of $1,25\text{-}(OH)_2D_3$ have not been reported in patients with PHP-2.

BARTTER'S SYNDROME

BS (Bartter's syndrome) (see also Chap. 23) consists of (1) renal potassium wasting (as defined in Pathophysiology of Type 1 RTA); (2) hypokalemic metabolic alkalosis; (3) hyperaldosteronism (without hypertension); (4) hyperreninemia; and (5) hyperplasia of the renin-producing juxtaglomerular cells in the afferent arteriole of the glomerulus (458). Increased urinary excretion of prostaglandin (and kallikrein) would appear to be usual and, in affected children, invariable (459–463). Glomerular filtration is usually normal (458, 464–469). The complex renal dysfunction of Fanconi syndrome is absent. Because experimentally administered angiotensin failed to induce a normal increase in blood pressure in those patients affected, Bartter and his associates proposed that their arteriolar smooth muscle was intrinsically hyporesponsive to endogenous angiotensin, and that as a consequence of the resultant circulatory insufficiency, chronic stimulation of renin secretion sustained circulating angiotensin at supernormal concentration (458). Hyperaldosteronism would be a predictable consequence of hyperangiotensinemia; juxtaglomerular cell hyperplasia could be attributed to chronic stimulation of the renin secretory process (458). It is at present unclear, however, what primary abnormality underlies BS or whether the syndrome can be the expression of more than one kind of primary abnormality.

The occurrence of BS in sibships (470–472) raises the possibility that it can reflect a genetically transmitted trait. The syndrome commonly occurs in early childhood and does not undergo remission. Salt craving, polydipsia, polyuria, impaired growth, and delayed puberty are characteristic; mental retardation may occur.

METABOLIC CHARACTER OF HYPERALDOSTERONISM

In some patients with BS the secretion rate of aldosterone may not be frankly supernormal, relative to the dietary intake of sodium, until the plasma concentration of potassium is increased toward normal by administration of potassium salts (465, 467, 468). But, in fact, the prior "normal" secretion rate is abnormally high relative to the prior severity of hypokalemia. The serum potassium concentration directly affects the adrenal secretion of aldosterone: In normal subjects, an increase in plasma potassium concentration almost immediately increases aldosterone secretion; a reduction in plasma potassium concentration decreases it (473–476). The striking increases in aldosterone secretion that can occur with only a lessened severity of hypokalemia (465, 468) may reflect the hyperplastic state of the chronically angiotensin-stimulated adrenal zona glomerulosa (458).

PATHOGENESIS OF RENAL POTASSIUM WASTING

Aldosterone

Renal potassium wasting occurs in patients with BS even when the secretion rate of aldosterone is not frankly supernormal (459, 465, 467–469, 477). Renal potassium wasting persists even when the secretion rate of aldosterone is reduced to normal values by maneuvers that suppress renin secretion [administration of albumin (477), propranolol (469), indomethacin (459)], or suppress aldosterone production (administration of aminoglutethimide) (477). Renal potassium wasting can persist even when secretion of aldosterone is abolished by adrenalectomy (471, 478). These findings indicate that in at least some patients with Bartter's syndrome hyperaldosteronism is not critical to the causation of renal potassium wasting, although its magnitude could well determine the severity of renal potassium wasting.

Impaired reabsorption of sodium

By causing the delivery of an abnormally large fraction of the filtered load of sodium to the potassium-secreting segments of the distal nephron, an impairment in the reabsorption of sodium in the proximal segments of the nephron (proximal tubule, loope of Henle) could give rise to renal potassium wasting (464). This possibility is sug-

gested by the finding that renal potassium wasting persists in patients with BS when dietary intake of sodium is restricted. By contrast, in patients with primary hyperaldosteronism, restriction of dietary sodium corrects renal potassium wasting. An abnormally large delivery of sodium to the potassium-secreting segments of the distal nephron might account for the persistence of renal potassium wasting in patients with Bartter's syndrome in whom the secretion rate of aldosterone is not greatly increased. In some patients with BS, renal conservation of sodium appears to be impaired (458, 464, 472). In two patients with BS in whom the volume of the extracellular compartment was rapidly expanded by intravenous administration of an isotonic solution of sodium chloride, the resultant diuresis of sodium occurred earlier and was of a greater magnitude than that in a control group of normal subjects in whom extracellular volume had been similarly expanded (472). It seems unlikely, however, that impairment in renal reabsorption of sodium per se could be the cause of renal potassium wasting, either by the mechanism of increased delivery of sodium to the (aldosterone-modulated) sodium-potassium exchange site or by causing sodium depletion, secondary hyperreninemia, and hyperaldosteronism. With the operation of either or both mechanisms, one would not expect renal potassium wasting to persist despite adrenalectomy or to be so resistant to either spironolactone which blocks the renal action of aldosterone, or agents which block synthesis of prostaglandin and secondarily dampen the synthesis of renin and aldosterone (vide infra).

Impaired reabsorption of chloride

The thick ascending limb is quantitatively the most important part of the "diluting segment" of the kidney. During water loading and suppression of release of antidiuretic hormone, the renal clearance of "solute-free water" (C_{H_2O}) provides a reliable estimate of the rate at which solute is reabsorbed in the thick ascending limb. In several studies of patients with BS undergoing water diuresis, C_{H_2O} has been abnormally and substantially reduced as a function of each of the various terms of solute delivery to the "diluting segment," including urine flow $(C_{H_2O} + C_{Na})$ and $(C_{H_2O} + C_{Cl})$ (466, 479, 480). This finding provides evidence that the rate at which solute is reabsorbed in the thick ascending limb is substantially reduced. The reduction appears not to be ascribable to chronic hypokalemia, metabolic alkalosis, hyperreninemia, hyperaldosteronism, or increased production of prostaglandin (480). An intrinsic impairment in the capacity of the thick ascending limb to reabsorb solute (the great bulk of which is NaCl) would imply an impairment in active reabsorption of chloride (481), the transport process that appears to provide the major if not exclusive driving force for sodium (chloride) reabsorption in the thick ascending limb (482, 483). Such an impairment might also reduce the rate of reabsorption of potassium in the thick ascending limb (481). As much as 30 to 40 percent of the filtered load of potassium may normally be reabsorbed in the ascending limb (484). By making the lumen of this segment electronegative, active reabsorption of chloride promotes the passive reabsorption of potassium. Diuretic agents that inhibit active chloride reabsorption in the thick ascending limb (485, 486) greatly increase the amount of potassium, as well as of sodium, entering the distal convoluted tubule (487). Administration of chloruretic agents (ethacrynic acid, furosemide) in humans and experimental animals also evokes an increase in renin secretion, in part, but apparently not entirely, as a consequence of contraction of ECF volume (488). An impairment of chloride transport in the loop of Henle could therefore account for the hyperreninemia (488, 489) as well as cause renal potassium wasting in Bartter's syndrome.

Primary impairment in renal reabsorption of potassium

Renal potassium wasting in patients with Bartter's syndrome might be the consequence of a primary impairment in potassium transport in segments of the nephron distal to the thick ascending limb (471, 490–493). In the rat the concentrations of potassium in the lumen of the distal convoluted tubule are lower than those predicted from the estimated electrochemical forces determining passive potassium movement; in response to deprivation of potassium, the tubule is capable of effecting net reabsorption of potassium against an electrochemical gradient. It has been postulated that the luminal membrane possesses an active potassium pump oriented toward the cell interior (176). Evidence suggests that a similar mechanism may be present in the medullary collecting duct (494). An impairment in the function of such a potassium reabsorptive mechanism might lead directly to renal potassium wasting in patients with BS.

METABOLIC DERANGEMENTS OF POTASSIUM DEPLETION AND ENHANCED SYNTHESIS OF PROSTAGLANDIN

Potassium depletion might account for the occurrence of hyperreninemia in Bartter's syndrome. Experimentally induced potassium depletion both in humans and dogs results in an increase in plasma renin activity not accounted for by changes in sodium balance (495, 496). Recent evidence suggests that potassium depletion might lead to the stimulation of renin secretion by stimulating renal production of prostaglandins (497–503). Experimentally induced potassium depletion in dogs results in parallel increases in plasma renin activity and urinary prostaglandin excretion; subsequent administration of chemical inhibitors of prostaglandin synthesis results in parallel decreases in plasma renin activity and prostaglandin excretion, despite persistence of potassium depletion (497). Administration of inhibitors of prostaglandin synthesis has also been found to inhibit the stimulation of renin secretion that normally results from sodium depletion or administration of furosemide (502).

Recent studies indicate that overproduction of prostaglandins by the kidney occurs in patients with Bartter's syndrome and contributes at least in part to the hypersecretion of renin (459–463, 504). Supernormal amounts of prostaglandins of renal origin are excreted in the urine of patients with the syndrome (459–463). Administration of inhibitors of prostaglandin synthesis (indomethacin, aspirin) results in a reduction in both prostaglandin excretion and plasma renin activity in the patients (459–462, 504). Plasma and urinary aldosterone concentration also decrease, as does urinary potassium excretion (459–462, 504). Prolonged administration of these inhibitors can greatly mitigate the severity of hyperreninemia, hyperaldosteronism, renal potassium wasting, and hypokalemia, but does not fully correct these disturbances. Thus, overproduction of prostaglandin can amplify renal potassium wasting in patients with BS, but is probably not the primary abnormality. By leading to stimulation of prostaglandin production, renal potassium wasting might be a self-amplifying disturbance, despite the suppres-

sive effect of potassium depletion on aldosterone production.

Prostaglandins have physiologic effects other than stimulation of renin secretion that may contribute to the pathophysiology of Bartter's syndrome. Prostaglandins have vasodilatory properties and are produced locally in the walls of arterial blood vessels (505). Increased production of prostaglandins therefore might limit the vasoconstrictor response of the blood vessels to angiotensin, thereby accounting for the subnormal blood pressure response to exogenously administered angiotensin (460). Administration of inhib-

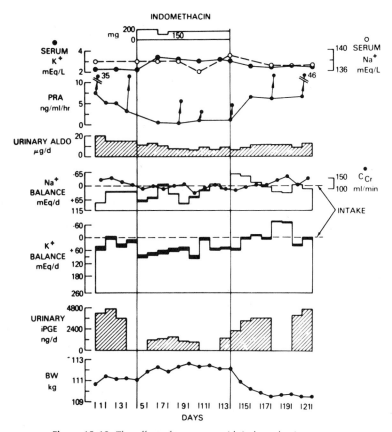

Figure 18-19. The effect of treatment with indomethacin on serum potassium (K+) and sodium (Na+), PRA (plasma renin activity), aldo (urinary aldosterone), C_{cr} (creatinine clearance), sodium and potassium balances, IPGE (urinary immunoreactive prostaglandin E-like material), and BW (body weight) on a 46-year-old woman with Bartter's syndrome. [*From Gill et al. (459).*]

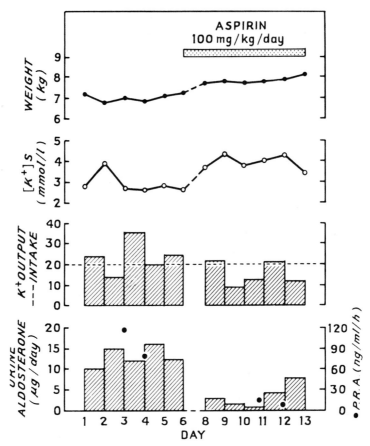

Figure 18-20. Effect of aspirin on plasma renin activity, aldosterone excretion, and potassium balance in a 22-month-old girl with Bartter's syndrome. [*From Norby et al. (461)*.]

itors of prostaglandin synthesis ameliorate the pressor hyporesponsiveness to infused angiotensin in patients with Bartter's syndrome (460, 504). Reninlike activity also is present in arterial walls, in amounts that vary inversely with sodium balance (506, 507). Angiotensin can apparently be generated locally in the blood vessel wall (508, 509). The intra-arterial overproduction of prostaglandin therefore may also limit the vasoconstrictor effect of angiotensin produced in situ. Similarly, intrarenal overproduction of prostaglandins may limit the intrarenal effects of locally produced angiotensin (510), which ordinarily may be suppressive of renin secretion (511, 512). The

juxtaglomerular apparatus is directly exposed to prostaglandins at the luminal surface of the macular densa, since prostaglandins produced in the kidney enter the tubular lumen in the loop of Henle and are excreted in the urine (513).

Prostaglandin has been shown to inhibit sodium reabsorption in the cortical segments of the renal collecting tubules (and possibly also the outer medullary segments) (514). Overproduction of intrarenal prostaglandins may account for the renal concentrating defect in Bartter's syndrome, since prostaglandin appears to antagonize the effect of antidiuretic hormone to promote water reabsorption in the distal nephron (515, 516).

TREATMENT

The treatment of patients with Bartter's syndrome is directed toward correcting hypokalemia. The commonly administered combination of spironolactone, an inhibitor of the renal action of the aldosterone, and potassium chloride will usually maintain serum concentration of potassium at values just below the normal range. Combined therapy with spironolactone and an agent that inhibits renin release, such as propranolol, would seem to be a rational therapeutic approach; administration of an inhibitor of renin secretion might be expected to blunt the increase in aldosterone secretion that would otherwise occur with the use of spironolactone alone. Combined administration of spironolactone, 100 to 200 mg/day, and propranolol, 100 to 200 mg/day, an inhibitor of renin secretion, can result in a sustained increase in the serum concentration of potassium, although usually not to normal values (468, 469). Unfortunately, gynecomastia can be a complication of spironolactone therapy.

Continuing administration of pharmacologic agents that inhibit renal prostaglandin synthesis, indomethacin, ibuprofen, and aspirin (459–461, 504), can also ameliorate hypokalemia and renal potassium wasting, hyperreninemia, and hyperaldosteronism in patients with Bartter's syndrome. Indomethacin has been employed at doses ranging from 1 to 2 mg/kg per day or 100 to 200 mg/day. In at least two patients, the use of indomethacin (504) (Fig. 18-19), or aspirin (461) (Fig. 18-20) alone has resulted in near correction of hypokalemia. Indomethacin has also been administered in combination with spironolactone, 200 mg/day (460). Although long-term experience with indomethacin has not yet been reported, the preliminary results appear encouraging.

REFERENCES

1. Albright, F., C. H. Burnett, W. Parson, E. C. Reifenstein, Jr., and A. Roos: Osteomalacia and late rickets: The various etiologies met in the United States with emphasis on that resulting from a specific form of renal acidosis, the therapeutic indications for each etiological sub-group, and the relationship between osteomalacia and Milkman's syndrome, *Medicine*, **25**:399–479, 1946.

2. Albright, F., C. H. Burnett, P. H. Smith, and W. Parson: Pseudohypoparathyroidism—an example of the "Seabright-Bantam" syndrome, *Endocrinology*, **30**:922, 1942.

3. Albright, F., A. H. Butler, and E. Bloomberg: Rickets resistant to vitamin D therapy, *Am. J. Dis. Child.*, **54**:529, 1937.

4. Seldin, D. W., and J. D. Wilson: Renal tubular acidosis, in J. B. Stanbury, J. B. Wyngaarden, and D. S. Fredrickson (eds.), *The Metabolic Basis of Inherited Disease*, 2d ed., McGraw-Hill Book Company, New York, 1966.

5. Morris, R. C., Jr., A. Sebastian, and E. McSherry: Renal acidosis, *Kidney Int.*, **1**:322–340, 1972.

6. Sebastian, A., E. McSherry, and R. C. Morris, Jr.: Metabolic acidosis with special reference to the renal acidoses, in B. M. Brenner and F. C. Rector, Jr. (eds.), *The Kidney*, W. B. Saunders Company, Philadelphia, 1976, chap. 16.

7. Prader, Von A., R. Illig, and E. Heierli: Eine besondere form der primaren vitamin-D resistenten rachitis mit hypocalcamie und autosomaldominanten erbgang: Die hereditare pseudo-mangelrachitis, *Helv. Paediatr. Acta*, **16**: 452, 1961.

8. Fraser, D., S. W. Kooh, H. P. Kind, M. F. Holick, Y. Tanaka, and H. F. DeLuca: Pathogenesis of hereditary vitamin D-dependent rickets. An inborn error of vitamin D metabolism involving defective conversion of 25-hydroxy-vitamin D to 1α,25-dihydroxyvitamin D, *N. Engl. J. Med.*, **289**: 817, 1973.

9. Balsan, S., M. Garabedian, R. Sorgniard, M. F. Holick, and H. F. DeLuca: 1,25-Dihydroxyvitamin D_3 and 1α-hydroxyvitamin D_3 in children: Biologic and therapeutic effects in nutritional rickets and different types of vitamin D resistance, *Pediatr. Res.*, **9**:586, 1975.

10. Fraser, D. R., and E. Kodicek: Unique biosynthesis by kidney of a biologically active vitamin D metabolite, *Nature*, **228**:764–766, 1970.

11. Gray, R. W., I. Boyle, and H. F. DeLuca: Vitamin D metabolism. The role of kidney tissue, *Science*, **172**:1232–1234, 1971.

12. Midgett, R. J., A. M. Speilvogel, J. W. Coburn, and A. W. Norman: Studies on calciferol metabolism.

VI. The renal production of the biologically active form of vitamin D, 1,25-dihydroxycholecalciferol; species, tissue and subcellular distribution, *J. Clin. Endocrinol. Metab.*, **36**:1153–1161, 1973.

13. Raisz, L. G., C. L. Trummel, M. F. Holick, and H. F. DeLuca: 1,25-Dihydroxycholecalciferol: A potent stimulator of bone resorption in tissue culture, *Science*, **175**:768–769, 1972.

14. Boyle, I. T., L. Miravet, R. W. Gray, M. F. Holick, and H. F. DeLuca: The response of intestinal calcium transport to 25-hydroxy and 1,25-dihydroxy vitamin D in nephrectomized rats, *Endocrinology*, **90**:605–608, 1972.

15. Norman, H. W., and H. Henry: 1,25-Dihydroxycholecalciferol—a hormonally active form of vitamin D₃, *Rec. Prog. Horm. Res.*, **30**:431–430, 1974.

16. Drezner, M. D., F. A. Neelon, M. Haussler, and H. McPherson: 1,25-Dihydroxycholecalciferol deficiency: The probable cause of hypocalcemia and metabolic bone disease in pseudohypoparathyroidism, *J. Clin. Endocrinol. Metab.*, **42**:621–628, 1976.

17. Kooh, S. W., D. Fraser, H. F. DeLuca, M. F. Holick, R. F. Belsey, M. B. Clark, and T. M. Murray: Treatment of hypoparathyroidism and pseudohypoparathyroidism with metabolites of vitamin D: Evidence for impaired conversion of 25-hydroxyvitamin D to 1α,25-dihydroxyvitamin D, *N. Engl. J. Med.*, **293**:840–914, 1975.

18. Sinha, T. K., and N. H. Bell: Letter: 1,25-Dihydroxyvitamin D₃ and pseudohypoparathyroidism, *N. Engl. J. Med.*, **294**:612, 1976.

19. Sinha, T. K., H. F. DeLuca, and N. H. Bell: Evidence for a defect in the formation of 1α,25-dihydroxyvitamin D in pseudohypoparathyroidism, *Metabolism*, **26**:731–738, 1977.

20. Sebastian, A., E. McSherry, M. Schambelan, D. Connor, E. Biglieri, and R. C. Morris, Jr.: Renal tubular acidosis (RTA) in patients with hypoaldosteronism caused by renin deficiency, *Clin. Res.*, **21**:706, 1973.

21. Sebastian, A., M. Schambelan, S. Lindenfeld, and R. C. Morris, Jr.: Amelioration of metabolic acidosis with 9α fluorohydrocortisone therapy in patients with hyporeninemic hypoaldosteronism, *N. Engl. J. Med.*, **297**:576–583, 1977.

22. McSherry, E., and R. C. Morris, Jr.: Attainment and maintenance of normal stature with alkali therapy in infants and children with classic renal tubular acidosis, *J. Clin. Invest.*, **61**:509–527, 1978.

23. Lightwood, R., W. W. Payne, and J. A. Black: Infantile renal acidosis, *Pediatrics*, **12**:628–644, 1953.

24. Pines, K. L., and G. H. Mudge: Renal tubular acidosis with osteomalacia: Report of three cases, *Am. J. Med.*, **11**:302–311, 1951.

25. Smith, L. H., Jr., and G. E. Schreiner: Studies on renal hyperchloremic acidosis, *J. Lab. Clin. Med.*, **43**:347–358, 1954.

26. Reynolds, T. B.: Observations on the pathogenesis of renal tubular acidosis, *Am. J. Med.*, **25**:503–515, 1958.

27. Wrong, O., and H. E. F. Davies: The excretion of acid in renal disease, *Q. J. Med.*, **28**:259–313, 1959.

28. Relman, A. S.: Renal acidosis and renal excretion of acid in health and disease, *Adv. Intern. Med.*, **12**:295, 1964.

29. Elkinton, J. R., D. K. McCurdy, and V. M. Bucklew, Jr.: Hydrogen ion and the kidney, in D. A. K. Black (ed.), *Renal Disease*, 2d ed., F. A. Davis Company, Philadelphia, 1967, pp. 110–135.

30. Morris, R. C., Jr., and H. H. Fundenberg: Impaired renal acidification in patients with hypergammaglobulinemia, *Medicine*, **46**:57–69, 1967.

31. Soriano, J. R., H. Biochis, and C. M. Edelmann, Jr.: Bicarbonate reabsorption and hydrogen ion excretion in children with renal tubular acidosis, *J. Pediatr.*, **71**:802–813, 1967.

32. Morris, R. C., Jr.: An experimental renal acidification defect in patients with hereditary fructose intolerance. II. Its distinction from classic renal acidification defect associated with the Fanconi syndrome of children with cystinosis, *J. Clin. Invest.*, **47**:1648–1663, 1968.

33. Soriano, J. R., and C. M. Edelmann, Jr.: Renal tubular acidosis, *Ann. Rev. Med.*, **20**:363–382, 1969.

34. Morris, R. C., Jr.: Renal tubular acidosis: Mechanisms, classification and implications, *N. Engl. J. Med.*, **281**:1405–1413, 1969.

35. Sebastian, A., E. McSherry, and R. C. Morris, Jr.: On the mechanism of renal potassium wasting in renal tubular acidosis associated with Fanconi syndrome (Type 2 RTA), *J. Clin. Invest.*, **50**:231–243, 1971.

36. McSherry, E., A. Sebastian, and R. C. Morris, Jr.:

Renal tubular acidosis in infants: The several kinds, including bicarbonate-wasting, classic renal tubular acidosis, *J. Clin. Invest.*, **51**:499, 1972.

37. Donckerwolcke, R. A., J. P. Van Biervliet, G. Koorevaar, R. H. Kuijten, and G. J. Van Stekelenburg: The syndrome of renal tubular acidosis with nerve deafness, *Acta Paediatr. Scand.*, **65**:100, 1976.

38. McCurdy, D. K., G. G. Cornwell, III, and V. J. De Pratti: Hyperglobulinemic renal tubular acidosis. Report of the two cases, *Ann. Intern. Med.*, **67**:110, 1967.

39. Talal, N., E. Zisman, and P. H. Schur: Renal tubular acidosis, glomerulonephritis and immunologic factors in Sjögren's syndrome, *Arthritis Rheum.*, **2**:774, 1968.

40. Mason, A. M. S., and P. L. Golding: Hyperglobulinaemic renal tubular acidosis: A report of nine cases, *Br. Med. J.*, **3**:143, 1970.

41. Pasternack, A., and E. Linder: Renal tubular acidosis: An immunopathological study on four patients, *Clin. Exp. Immunol.*, **7**:115, 1970.

42. Cohen, A., and B. J. Way: The association of renal tubular acidosis with hyperglobulinaemic purpura, *Aust. Ann. Med.*, **11**:189, 1962.

43. LoSpalluto, J., B. Dorward, W. Miller, and M. Ziff: Cryoglobulinemia based on interaction between a gamma macroglobulin and 7S gamma globulin, *Am. J. Med.*, **32**:142, 1962.

44. Shioji, R., T. Furuyama, S. Onodera, H. Saito, H. Ito, and Y. Sasaki: Sjögren's syndrome and renal tubular acidosis, *Am. J. Med.*, **48**:456, 1970.

45. Talal, N.: Sjögren's syndrome, lymphoproliferation, and renal tubular acidosis (editorial), *Ann. Intern. Med.*, **74**:633–634, 1971.

46. Read, A. E., S. Sherlock, and C. F. Harrison: Active "juvenile" cirrhosis considered as part of a systemic disease, *Gut*, **4**:378, 1963.

47. Seedat, Y. K., and E. R. Rain: Active chronic hepatitis associated with renal tubular acidosis and successful pregnancy, *S. Afr. Med. J.*, **39**:595, 1965.

48. Golding, P. L.: Renal tubular acidosis in chronic liver disease, *Postgrad. Med. J.*, **51**:550, 1975.

49. Bridi, G. S., P. W. Falcon, N. C. Brackett, Jr., W. J. S. Still, and I. N. Sporn: Glomerulonephritis and renal tubular acidosis in a case of chronic active hepatitis with hyperimmunoglobulinemia, *Am. J. Med.*, **52**:267, 1972.

50. Tsantoulas, D. C., I. G. McFarlane, B. Portman, A. L. W. F. Eddleston, and R. Williams: Cell-mediated immunity to human Tamm-Horsfall glycoprotein in autoimmune liver disease with renal tubular acidosis, *Br. Med. J.*, **4**:491, 1974.

51. Cochrane, A. M. G., D. C. Tsantoulos, A. Moussouros, I. G. McFarlane, A. L. W. Eddleston, and R. Williams: Lymphocyte cytotoxicity for kidney cells in renal tubular acidosis of autoimmune liver disease, *Br. Med. J.*, **2**:276, 1976.

52. Mason, A. M. S., and P. L. Golding: Renal tubular acidosis and autoimmune thyroid disease, *Lancet*, **2**:1104, 1970.

53. Mason, A. M. S., M. B. McIllmurray, P. L. Golding, and D. T. B. Hughes: Fibrosing alveolitis associated with renal tubular acidosis, *Br. Med. J.*, **4**:596, 1970.

54. Dent, C. E., C. M. Harper, and A. M. Parfitt: The effect of cellulose phosphate on calcium metabolism in patients with hypercalciuria, *Clin. Sci.*, **27**:463, 1964.

55. Parfitt, A. M., B. A. Higgins, J. R. Nassim, J. A. Collins, and A. Hilb: Metabolic studies in patients with hypercalciuria, *Clin. Sci.*, **27**:463, 1964.

56. Buckalew, V. M., M. L. Pruvis, M. G. Shulman, C. N. Herndon, and D. Rudman: Hereditary renal tubular acidosis, *Medicine (Baltimore)*, **53**:229, 1974.

57. Cohen, S. I., M. G. Fitzgerald, P. Fourman, W. J. Griffiths, and H. E. DeWardener: Polyuria in hyperparathyroidism, *Q. J. Med.*, **26**:423, 1957.

58. Reynolds, T. B., and J. E. Bethune: Renal tubular acidosis secondary to hyperparathyroidism, *Clin. Res.*, **17**:169, 1969.

59. Huth, E. J., R. L. Mayock, and R. M. Kerr: Hyperthyroidism associated with renal tubular acidosis, *Am. J. Med.*, **26**:818, 1959.

60. Zisman, E., R. A. Buccino, P. Gorden, and F. C. Bartter: Hyperthyroidism and renal tubular acidosis, *Arch. Intern. Med.*, **121**:118, 1968.

61. Ferris, T., M. Kashgarian, H. Levitin, I. Brant, and F. H. Epstein: Renal tubular acidosis and renal potassium wasting required as a result of hypercalcemic nephropathy, *N. Engl. J. Med.*, **265**:924, 1961.

62. Deck, M. D. F.: Medullary sponge kidney with renal tubular acidosis: A report of 3 cases, *J. Urol.*, **94**:330, 1965.

63. Morris, R. C., Jr., H. Yamauchi, A. J. Palubin-

skas, and J. Howenstine: Medullary sponge kidney, *Am. J. Med.,* **38:**883, 1965.

64. Mass, R. F., W. R. Smith, and J. R. Walsh: The association of hereditary fructose intolerance and renal tubular acidosis, *Am. J. Med. Sci.,* **251:**516, 1966.

65. Fulop, M., I. Sternlieb, and H. I. Scheinberg: Defective urinary acidification in Wilson's disease, *Ann. Intern. Med.,* **68:**770, 1968.

66. Yeoh, S. A.: Fabry's disease with renal tubular acidosis, *Singapore Med. J.,* **8:**275, 1967.

67. McCurdy, D. K., M. Frederic, and J. R. Elkington: Renal tubular acidosis due to amphotericin, *N. Engl. J. Med.,* **278:**124, 1968.

68. Patterson, R. M., and G. L. Ackerman: Renal tubular acidosis due to amphotericine B nephrotoxicity, *Arch. Intern. Med.,* **127:**241, 1971.

69. Taher, S. M., R. J. Anderson, R. McCartney, M. M. Popovitzer, and R. W. Schrier: Renal tubular acidosis associated with toluene "sniffing," *N. Engl. J. Med.,* **290:**765, 1974.

70. Steel, T. W., A. Z. Gyory, and K. D. G. Edwards: Renal function in analgesic nephropathy, *Br. Med. J.,* **2:**213, 1969.

71. Perez, G. O., J. R. Oster, and C. A. Vaamonde: Incomplete syndrome of renal tubular acidosis induced by lithium carbonate, *J. Lab. Clin. Med.,* **86:**386, 1975.

72. Yong, J. M., and K. V. Sanderson: Photosensitive dermatitis and renal tubular acidosis after ingestion of calcium cyclamate, *Lancet,* **2:**1273, 1969.

73. Cochran, M., M. Peacock, P. A. Smith, and B. E. C. Nordin: Renal tubular acidosis of pyelonephritis with renal stone disease, *Br. Med. J.,* **2:**721, 1968.

74. Berlyne, G. M.: Distal tubular function in chronic hydronephrosis, *Q. J. Med.,* **30:**339, 1961.

75. Better, O. S., A. I. Arieff, S. G. Massry, C. R. Kleeman, and M. H. Maxwell: Studies on renal function after relief of complete unilateral ureteral obstruction of three months' duration in man, *Am. J. Med.,* **54:**234, 1973.

76. Hutcheon, R. A., B. S. Kaplan, and K. N. Drummond: Distal renal tubular acidosis in children with chronic hydronephrosis, *J. Pediatr.,* **89:**372–376, 1976.

77. Wilson, D. R.: Renal function during and following obstruction, *Ann. Rev. Med.,* **28:**329–339, 1977.

78. Gyory, A. Z., J. G. Steward, C. R. O. George, D. J. Miller, and K. D. G. Edward: Renal tubular acidosis, acidosis due to hyperkalemia, hypercalcemia, disordered citrate metabolism and other tubular dysfunctions following human renal transplantation, *Q. J. Med.,* **38:**231, 1969.

79. Wilson, D. R., and A. A. Siddigui: Renal tubular acidosis after kidney transplantation, *Ann. Intern. Med.,* **79:**352, 1973.

80. Drutz, D. J., and R. A. Gutman: Renal tubular acidosis in leprosy, *Ann. Intern. Med.,* **75:**475, 1971.

81. Levine, A. A., and A. F. Michael, Jr.: Ehlers-Danlos syndrome with renal tubular acidosis and medullary sponge kidneys, *J. Pediatr.,* **71:**107, 1967.

82. Baehner, R. L., G. S. Gilchrist, and E. J. Anderson: Hereditary elliptocytosis and primary renal tubular acidosis in a single family, *Am. J. Dis. Child.,* **115:**414, 1968.

83. Goossens, J. P., L. W. S. Van Eps, H. Schouten, and A. L. Giterson: Incomplete renal tubular acidosis in sickle cell disease, *Clin. Chim. Acta,* **41:**149, 1972.

84. Ho Ping Kong, H., and G. A. O. Alleyne: Defect in urinary acidification in adults with sickle-cell anaemia, *Lancet,* **2:**954, 1968.

85. Takeda, R., S. Morimoto, M. Kuroda, and M. Murakami: Renal tubular acidosis, presenting as a syndrome resembling Bartter's syndrome, in a patient with arachnodatcyly, *Acta Endocrinol. (Kbh.),* **73:**531, 1973.

86. Shapira, E., Y. Ben-Yoseph, F. G. Eyal, and A. Russell: Enzymatically inactive red cell carbonic anhydrase B in a family with renal tubular acidosis, *J. Clin. Invest.,* **53:**59, 1974.

87. Better, O. S., Z. Goldschmid, C. Chaimowitz, and G. G. Alroy: Defect in urinary acidification in cirrhosis, *Arch. Intern. Med.,* **130:**77, 1972.

88. Oster, J. R., J. L. Hotchkiss, M. Carbon, and C. A. Vaamonde: Abnormal renal acidification in alcoholic liver disease, *J. Lab. Clin. Med.,* **85:**987, 1975.

89. Shear, L., H. L. Bonkowsky, and G. L. Gabuzda: Renal tubular acidosis in cirrhosis, *N. Engl. J. Med.,* **280:**1, 1969.

90. Relman, A. S., E. J. Lennon, and J. Lemann, Jr.: Endogenous production of fixed acid and the

measurement of the net balance of acid in normal subjects, *J. Clin. Invest.*, **40**:1621–1630, 1961.

91. Albert, M. S., and R. W. Winters: Acid-base equilibrium of blood in normal infants, *Pediatrics*, **37**:728–732, 1966.

92. Buckalew, V. M., Jr., K. D. McCurdy, G. D. Ludwig, L. B. Chaykin, and E. Elkinson, Jr.: The syndrome of incomplete renal tubular acidosis, *Am. J. Med.*, **45**:32, 1968.

93. Halperin, M. L., M. B. Godstein, A. Haig, M. D. Johnson, and B. J. Stienbaugh: Studies on the pathogenesis of type 1 (distal) renal tubular acidosis as revealed by the urinary P_{CO_2} tensions, *J. Clin. Invest.*, **53**:669, 1974.

94. Poy, R. K. P., and O. Wrong: The urinary P_{CO_2} in renal disease, *Clin. Sci.*, **19**:361, 1960.

95. Ochwadt, B. K., and R. F. Pitts: Effect of intravenous infusion of carbonic anhydrase on carbon dioxide tension of alkaline urine, *Am. J. Physiol.*, **195**:426, 1956.

96. Sebastian, A., E. McSherry, and R. C. Morris, Jr.: On the mechanism of the inappropriately low urinary carbon dioxide tension ($U_{P_{CO_2}}$) in classic (type 1) renal tubular acidosis (cRTA), *Clin. Res.*, **22**:544A, 1974.

97. Steinmetz, P. R., and L. R. Lawson: Defect in urinary acidification induced in vitro by amphotericin B, *J. Clin. Invest.*, **49**:596, 1970.

98. Finn, J. T., L. H. Cohen, and P. R. Steinmetz: Acidifying defect induced by amphotericin B: Comparison of bicarbonate and hydrogen ion permeabilities, *Kidney Int.*, **11**:261–266, 1977.

99. Steblay, R. W., and U. H. Rudofsky: Transfer of experimental autoimmune renal cortical tubular and interstitial disease in guinea pigs by serum, *Science*, **180**:166–168, 1973.

100. Andres, G. A., and R. T. McCluskey: Tubular and interstitial renal disease due to immunologic mechanisms, *Kidney Int.*, **7**:271–289, 1975.

101. Sebastian, A., E. McSherry, and R. C. Morris, Jr.: Renal potassium wasting in renal tubular acidosis (RTA); its occurrence in types 1 and 2 RTA despite sustained correction of systemic acidosis, *J. Clin. Invest.*, **50**:667, 1971.

102. Gill, J. R., Jr. N. H. Bell, and F. C. Bartter: Impaired conservation of sodium and potassium in renal acidosis and its correction by buffer anions, *Clin. Sci.*, **33**:577, 1967.

103. Sebastian, A., E. McSherry, and R. C. Morris, Jr.: Impaired renal conservation of sodium and chloride during sustained correction of systemic acidosis in patients with type 1, classic renal tubular acidosis, *J. Clin. Invest.*, **58**:454, 1976.

104. Farquharson, R. F., W. T. Salter, and D. M. Tibetts, et al.: Studies of calcium and phosphorus metabolism: XII. The effect of the ingestion of acid-producing substances, *J. Clin. Invest.*, **10**:221–249, 1931.

105. Lemann, J., Jr., J. R. Litzow, and E. J. Lennon: The effects of chronic acid loads in normal man: Further evidence for participation of bone mineral in the defense against chronic metabolic acidosis, *J. Clin. Invest.*, **45**:1608–1614, 1975.

106. Dedmon, R. E., and O. Wrong: The excretion of organic anion in renal tubular acidosis with particular reference to citrate, *Clin. Sci.*, **22**:19, 1962.

107. Morrisey, J. F., J. Ochoa, Jr., and W. D. Lotspeich, et al.: Citrate excretion in renal tubular acidosis, *Ann. Intern. Med.*, **58**:159, 1963.

108. Norman, M. E., R. M. Cohn, and D. K. McCurdy: Urinary citrate excretion in the diagnosis of distal renal tubular acidosis, *J. Pediatr.*, **92**:394–400, 1978.

109. Greenberg, A. J., H. McNamara, and W. W. McCrory: Metabolic balance studies in primary renal tubular acidosis: Effects of acidosis on external calcium and phosphorus balances, *J. Pediatr.*, **69**:610–618, 1966.

110. Lee, S. W., J. E. Russell, and L. V. Avioli: 25-OHD_3 to $1,25\text{-}(OH)_2D_3$ conversion impaired by systemic acidosis, *Science*, **195**:944–996, 1977.

111. Courey, R. W., and R. C. Pfister: The radiographic findings in renal tubular acidosis, *Diag. Radiol.*, **105**:497–504, 1972.

112. Coe, F. L.: Evidence for mild reversible hyperparathyroidism in distal renal tubular acidosis, *Arch. Intern. Med.*, **135**:1485, 1975.

113. Coe, F. L., J. J. Firpo, D. L. Hollandsworth, L. Segil, J. M. Canterbury, and E. Reiss: Effect of acute and chronic metabolic acidosis on serum immunoreactive parathyroid hormone in man, *Kidney Int.*, **8**:262, 1975.

114. Foss, G. L., C. B. Perry, and F. J. Y. Wood: Renal tubular acidosis, *Q. J. Med.*, **98**:185–199, 1956.

115. Richard, P., O. M. Wrong, and M. J. Chamberlain: Treatment of osteomalacia of renal tubular

acidosis by sodium bicarbonate alone, *Lancet*, **2:**994, 1972.

116. Chesney, R. W., A. V. Moorthy, J. A. Eisman, D. K. Jax, R. B. Mazess, and H. F. DeLuca: Increased growth after long term oral 1α,25-vitamin D_3 in childhood renal osteodystrophy, *N. Engl. J. Med.*, **298:**236–242, 1978.

117. McSherry, E., M. Pokroy, and R. C. Morris, Jr.: Prevention of nephrocalcinosis in infants and children with classic renal tubular acidosis with high dose alkali therapy. In press.

118. Owen, E. E., and J. V. Verner, Jr.: Renal tubular diseases with muscle paralysis and hypokalemia, *Am. J. Med.*, **28:**8, 1960.

119. Scribner, B. H., and J. M. Burnell: Interpretation of the serum potassium concentration, *Metabolism*, **5:**468, 1956.

120. Fraley, D. S., and S. Adler: Isohydric regulation of plasma potassium by bicarbonate in rat, *Kidney Int.*, **9:**333–345, 1976.

121. Schwartz, W. B., and W. C. Water, III: Lactate versus bicarbonate, *Am. J. Med.*, **32:**831, 1962.

122. Asscher, A. W., M. Sussman, W. E. Water, R. H. David, and S. Schick: Urine as a medium for bacterial growth, *Lancet*, **2:**1037, 1966.

123. Morris, R. C., Jr., A. Sebastian, and E. McSherry: Therapeutic experience in patients with classic renal tubular acidosis, *Proceedings VII International Congress of Nephrology*, S. Karger, Basel, 1978, p. 345.

124. Worthen, H. G., and R. A. Good: The de Toni-Fanconi syndrome with cystinosis, *Am. J. Dis. Child.*, **95:**653, 1958.

125. Lamy, M., J. Freza, J. Rey, and C. Larsen: Etude metabolique due syndrome de Lowe, *Rev. Eur. Etud. Clin. Biol.*, **7:**271, 1962.

126. Saville, P. D., J. R. Nassim, H. Stevenson, L. Mulligan, and N. Carey: The effect of A.T.10 on calcium and phosphorus metabolism in resistant rickets, *Clin. Sci.*, **14:**489, 1955.

127. Lee, D. B. N., J. P. Drinkard, V. J. Rosen, and H. C. Gonick: The adult Fanconi syndrome, *Medicine (Baltimore)*, **51:**107, 1972.

128. Hunt, D. D., G. Stearns, J. B. McKinely, E. Froning, P. Hicks, and M. Bonfiglio: Long-term study of a family with Fanconi syndrome without cystinosis (DeToni-Debre-Fanconi syndrome), *Am. J. Med.*, **40:**492, 1966.

129. Smith, R., R. H. Lindenbaum, and R. J. Walton: Hypophosphateamic osteomalacia and Fanconi syndrome of adult onset with dominant inheritance, *Q. J. Med.*, **179:**387–400, 1976.

130. Litin, R. B., R. V. Randall, N. P. Goldstein, N. H. Power, and G. R. Diessner: Hypercalciuria in hepatolenticular degeneration (Wilson's disease), *Am. J. Med. Sci.*, **238:**614, 1959.

131. Wilson, D. M., and N. P. Goldstein: Bicarbonate excretion in Wilson's disease (hepatolenticular degeneration), *Mayo Clin. Proc.*, **49:**394, 1974.

132. Gentz, J., R. Jagenburg, and R. Zetterstron: Tyrosinemia, *J. Pediatr.*, **66:**670, 1965.

133. Gruskin, A. B., M. S. Patel, M. Lindshaw, R. Ettenger, D. Huff, and W. Grover: Renal function studies and kidney pyruvate carboxylase in subacute necrotizing encephalomyelopathy (Leight's syndrome), *Pediatr. Res.*, **7:**932, 1973.

134. Guignard, J. P., and A. Torrado: Proximal tubular acidosis in vitamin D deficient rickets, *Acta Paediatr. Scand.*, **62:**543, 1973.

135. Muldowney, F. P., J. F. Donohoe, R. Freaney, C. Kampff, and M. Swan: Parathormone-induced renal bicarbonate wastage in intestinal malabsorption and in chronic renal failure, *Ir. J. Med. Sci.*, **3:**221, 1970.

136. Vainsel, M., Th. Manderlier, and H. L. Viss: Proximal renal tubular acidosis in vitamin D deficiency rickets, *Biomedicine*, **22:**35, 1974.

137. Scott, J., E. Elias, P. J. A. Moult, S. Barnes, and M. R. Wills: Rickets in adult cystic fibrosis with myopathy, pancreatic insufficiency and proximal renal tubular dysfunction, *Am. J. Med.*, **63:**488–492, 1977.

138. Stoop, J. W., M. J. C. Schraagen, and H. A. W. M. Tiddens: Pseudo-vitamin D deficiency rickets, *Acta Paediatr. Scand.*, **56:**607, 1967.

139. Wegienka, L. C., and J. M. Weller: Renal tubular acidosis caused by degraded tetracycline, *Arch. Intern. Med.*, **114:**232, 1964.

140. Otten, J., and H. L. Vis: Acute reversible renal tubular dysfunction following intoxication with methyl-3-chromone, *J. Pediatr.*, **73:**422, 1968.

141. Sadoff, L.: Neprotoxicity of streptozotocin, *Cancer Chemother. Rep.*, **54:**457, 1970.

142. Chisolm, J. J., H. C. Harrison, W. R. Eberlein, and H. E. Harrison: Amino-aciduria, hypophosphatemia, and rickets in lead poisoning, *Am. J. Dis. Child.*, **89:**159, 1955.

143. Sebastian, A., E. McSherry, I. Ueki, and R. C.

Morris, Jr.: Renal amyloidosis, nephrotic syndrome, and impaired renal tubular reabsorption of bicarbonate, *Ann. Intern. Med.*, **69**:541, 1968.

144. Stickler, G. B., J. W. Rosevear, and J. A. Ulrich: Renal tubular dysfunction complicating the nephrotic syndrome: The disturbance in calcium and phosphorus metabolism, *Mayo Clin. Proc.*, **37**:376, 1962.

145. Tegelaers, W. H. H., and H. W. Tiddens: Nephrotic-glucosuric-aminoaciduric dwarfism and electrolyte metabolism, *Helv. Paediatr. Acta,* **10**:269, 1955.

146. Massry, S. G., H. G. Preuss, J. F. Maher, and G. E. Schreiner: Renal tubular acidosis after cadaver kidney homotransplantation, *Am. J. Med.*, **42**:284, 1967.

147. Morris, R. C., Jr.: The clinical spectrum of Fanconi's syndrome, *Calif. Med.*, **108**:225, 1968.

148. Riley, A. L., L. M. Ryan, and D. A. Roth: Renal proximal tubular dysfunction and paroxysmal nocturnal hemoglobinurea, *Am. J. Med.*, **62**:125–129, 1977.

149. Cade, R., G. Spooner, L. Juncos, T. Fuller, D. Tarrant, D. Raulerson, J. Mahoney, M. Pckering, W. Grubb, and T. Marbury: Chronic renal vein thrombosis, *Am. J. Med.*, **63**:387–397, 1977.

150. Sirota, J. H., and D. Hamerman: Renal function studies in an adult subject with the Fanconi syndrome, *Am. J. Med.*, **16**:138, 1954.

151. Engle, R. L., and L. A. Wallis: Multiple myeloma and the adult Fanconi syndrome. I. Report of a case with crystal-like deposits in the tumor cells and in the epithelial cells of the kidney, *Am. J. Med.*, **22**:5, 1957.

152. Harrison, J. F., and J. D. Blainey: Adult Fanconi syndrome with monoclonal abnormality of immunoglobulin light chains, *J. Clin. Pathol.*, **20**:42, 1967.

153. Maldonado, J. E., et al.: Fanconi syndrome in adults: A manifestation of a latent form of myeloma, *Am. J. Med.*, **58**:354, 1975.

154. Smithline, N., J. P. Kassirer, and J. J. Cohen: Light-chain nephropathy: Renal tubular dysfunction associated with light-chain proteinuria, *N. Engl. J. Med.*, 294–271, 1976.

155. Nash, M. A., A. D. Torrado, I. Greifer, A. Spitzer, and C. M. Edelmann, Jr.: Renal tubular acidosis in infants and children, *J. Pediatr.*, **80**:738, 1972.

156. Donckerwolcke, R. A., G. J. Van Stekelenburg,

and H. A. Tiddens: A case of bicarbonate-losing renal tubular acidosis with defective carbonanhydrase activity, *Arch. Dis. Child.*, **45**:769, 1970.

157. Brenes, L. G., J. N. Brenes, and M. M. Hernandez: Familial proximal tubular acidosis, *Am. J. Med.*, **63**:244–252, 1977.

158. Vainsel, M., P. Fondu, S. Cadranel, C. L. Rocmans, and W. Gepts: Osteopetrosis associated with proximal and distal tubular acidosis, *Acta Paediatr.*, **61**:429–434, 1972.

159. Leaf, A., W. B. Schwartz, and A. S. Relman: Oral administration of a potent carbonic anhydrase inhibitor ("Diamox"), *N. Engl. J. Med.*, **250**:759, 1954.

160. Seldin, D. W., R. M. Portwood, F. C. Rector, Jr., and R. Cade: Characteristics of renal bicarbonate reabsorption in man, *J. Clin. Invest.*, **38**:1663, 1959.

161. Beckman, W. W., E. C. Rossmeisl, R. B. Pettingill, and W. Bauer: Study of effect of sulfanilamide on acid-base metabolism, *J. Clin. Invest.*, **19**:635, 1940.

162. York, S. E., and E. R. Yendt: Osteomalacia associated with renal bicarbonate loss, *Can. Med. Assoc. J.*, **94**:1329, 1966.

163. Rodriguez-Soriano, J., A. Vallo, M. Chouza, and G. Casstillo: Proximal renal tubular acidosis in tetralogy of fallot, *Acta Paediatr. Scand.*, **64**:671–674, 1975.

164. Hellman, D. E., W. Y. W. Au, and F. C. Bartter: Evidence for a direct effect of parathyroid hormone on urinary acidification, *Am. J. Physiol.*, **209**:643–650, 1965.

165. Siddiqui, A. A., and D. R. Wilson: Primary hyperparathyroidism and proximal renal tubular acidosis: Report of two cases, *Can. Med. Assoc. J.*, **106**:654–659, 1972.

166. Coe, F. L.: Magnitude of metabolic acidosis in primary hyperparathyroidism, *Arch. Intern. Med.*, **134**:262, 1974.

167. Bank, N., and H. S. Aynedjian: A micropuncture study of the effect of parathyroid hormone on renal bicarbonate reabsorption, *J. Clin. Invest.*, **58**:336–344, 1976.

168. Crumb, C. K., M. Martinez-Maldonado, G. Eknoyan, and W. N. Suki: Effects of volume expansion purified parathyroid extract and calcium on renal bicarbonate absorption in the dog, *J. Clin. Invest.*, **54**:1287–1294, 1974.

169. Karlinsky, M. L., D. S. Sager, and N. A. Kurtz-man: Effect of parathormone and cyclic adeno-sine monophosphate on renal bicarbonate reab-sorption, *Am. J. Physiol.*, **277**:1226–1231, 1974.

170. Hermkens, H., T. Nawar, C. Caron, and G. E. Plante: Effect of parathyroid hormone on renal excretion of sodium and hydrogen ions, *Can. J. Physiol. Pharmacol.*, **55**:628–638, 1977.

171. Farrow, S. L., D. R. Stienbaugh, and W. N. Suki: Effects of hypocalcemia on renal bicarbonate ab-sorption in the dog, *Kidney Int.*, **10**:489, 1976.

172. Farquharson, R. F., W. T. Salter, and D. M. Ti-betts, et al.: Studies of calcium and phosphorus metabolism: XII. The effect of the ingestion of acid-producing substances, *J. Clin. Invest.*, **10**:221–249, 1931.

173. Emmett, M., S. Goldfarb, Z. S. Agus, and R. G. Narins: The pathophysiology of acid-base changes in chronically phosphate-depleted rats, *J. Clin. Invest.*, **59**:291–298, 1977.

174. Edelmann, C. M., Jr., I. B. Houston, J. Rodri-guez-Soriano, H. Biochis, and H. Stark: Renal excretion of hydrogen ion in children with idio-pathic growth retardation, *J. Pediatr.*, **72**:443, 1968.

175. Arant, B. S., I. Greifer, C. M. Edelmann, Jr., and A. Spitzer: Effect of chronic salt and water load-ing on the tubular defects of a child with Fanconi syndrome (cystinosis), *Pediatrics*, **58**:3, 1976.

176. Giebisch, G.: Some reflections on the mecha-nism of renal tubular potassium transport, *Yale J. Biol. Med.*, **48**:315–335, 1975.

177. Rubini, M. E.: Water excretion in potassium de-ficient man, *J. Clin. Invest.*, **40**:2215–2224, 1961.

178. Mannitius, A., H. Levitin, D. Beck, and F. H. Ep-stein: On the mechanism of renal concentrating ability in potassium deficiencies, *J. Clin. Invest.*, **39**:684–692, 1960.

179. Berl, T., S. L. Linas, G. A. Aisenbrey, and R. J. Anderson: On the mechanism of polyuria in po-tassium depletion, *J. Clin. Invest.*, **60**:620–625, 1977

180. Rampini, S., A. Fanconi, R. Illig, and A. Prader: Effect of a hydrochloronthiazide on proximal renal tubular acidosis in a patient with idiopathic "de Toni-Debré-Fanconi syndrome," *Helv. Paediatr. Acta*, **23**:13, 1967.

181. Oetliker, O., and E. Rossi: The influence of ex-tracellular fluid volume on the renal bicarbonate threshold; a study in two children with Lowe's syndrome, *Pediatr. Res.*, **3**:140, 1969.

182. Donckerwolcke, R. A., G. J. Van Stekelenburg, and H. A. Tiddens: Therapy of bicarbonate-los-ing renal tubular acidosis, *Arch. Dis. Child.*, **45**:774, 1970.

183. VanBiervliet, J. P. G. M., R. A. M. G. Doncker-wolcke, G. L. VanStekelenburg, and S. K. Wad-man: Sodium chloride restriction and extracellu-lar fluid volume contraction in hyperphosphaturic vitamin D resistant rickets in the Lowe syn-drome, *Helv. Paediatr. Acta*, **30**:365–375, 1975.

184. Imai, M., Y. Igarashi, and H. Sokabe: Plasma renin activity in congenital virilizing adrenal hy-perplasia, *Pediatrics*, **41**:897, 1968.

185. Oetliker, O., and R. P. Zurbrugg: Renal tubular acidosis in salt-losing syndrome of congenital ad-renal hyperplasia (CAH), *J. Clin. Endocrinol. Me-tab.*, **31**:447, 1970.

186. Rosler, A., R. Theodor, H. Boichis, R. Gerty, S. Ulick, M. Alagem, E. Tabachnik, B. Cohen, and D. Rabinowitz: Metabolic responses to the administration of angiotensin II, K and ACTH in two salt-wasting syndromes, *J. Clin. Endocrinol. Metab.*, **44**:292–301, 1977.

187. Rosler, A., D. Rabinowitz, R. Theodor, L. C. Ra-mirez, and S. Ulick: The nature of the defect in a salt wasting disorder in Jews of Iran, *J. Clin. Endocrinol. Metab.*, **44**:297–291, 1977.

188. Ulick, S.: Diagnosis and nomenclature of the dis-orders of the terminal portion of the aldosterone biosynthetic pathway, *J. Clin. Endocrinol. Metab.*, **43**:92–96, 1976.

189. David, R., S. Golan, and W. Drucker: Familial aldosterone deficiency: Enzyme defect, diagnosis, and clinical course, *Pediatrics*, **41**:403–412, 1968

190. Schambelan, M., J. R. Stockgit, and E. G. Bigli-eri: Isolated hypoaldosteronism in adults, a renin deficiency syndrome, *N. Engl. J. Med.*, **287**:573–578, 1972.

191. Perez, G., L. Siegel, and G. E. Schreiner: Selec-tive hypoaldosteronism with hyperkalemia, *Ann. Intern. Med.*, **76**:757–763, 1972.

192. Brown, J. J., R. H. Chinn, R. Fraser, A. F. Lever, J. J. Morton, J. I. S. Robertson, M. Tree, M. A. Waite, and D. M. Park: Recurrent hyperkalaemia due to selective aldosterone deficiency: Correc-

tion by angiotensin infusion, *Br. Med. J.*, **1**:650–654, 1973.

193. Weidmann, P., R. Reinhart, M. H. Maxwell, P. Rowe, J. W. Coburn, and S. G. Massry: Syndrome of hyporeninemic hypoaldosteronism, *J. Clin. Endocrinol. Metab.*, **36**:965, 1973.

194. Oh, M. S., J. H. Carroll, J. E. Clemmons, A. H. Vagnucci, S. P. Levison, and E. S. M. Whang: A mechanism for hyporeninemic hypoaldosteronism in chronic renal disease, *Metabolism*, **23**:1157–1165, 1974.

195. Perez, G. O. J. R. Oster, and C. A. Vaamonde: Renal acidosis and renal potassium handling in selective hypoaldosteronism, *Am. J Med.*, **57**:809–816, 1974.

196. Perez, G. O., J. R. Oster, and C. A. Vaamonde: Renal acidification in patients with mineralocorticoid deficiency, *Nephron*, **17**:461–473, 1976.

197. Marieb, M. J., J. C. Melby, and S. S. Lyall: Isolated hypoaldosteronism associated with idiopathic hypoparathyroidism, *Arch Intern. Med.*, **134**:424–429, 1974.

198. Mellinger, R. C., F. L. Petermann, and J. C. Jurgenson: Hyponatremia with low urinary aldosterone occurring in an old woman, *J. Clin. Endocrinol. Metab.*, **34**:85–91, 1972.

199. McGiff, J. C., R. E. Muzzarelli, P. A. Duffy, Y. Gonzalez, C. E. Pierce, and T. F. Fawley: Interrelationships of renin and aldosterone in a patient with hypoaldosteronism, *Am. J. Med.*, **48**:247–253, 1970.

200. Russell, A., B. Levin, L. Sinclair, and V. G. Oberholzer: A reversible salt-wasting syndrome of the newborn and infant, *Arch. Dis. Child.*, **38**:313–325, 1963.

201. Postel-Vinay, M., G. M. Alberti, C. Ricour, J. Limal, R. Rappaport, and P. Royer: Pseudohypoaldosteronism: Persistence of hyperaldosteronism and evidence for renal tubular and intestinal responsiveness to endogenous aldosterone, *J. Clin. Endocrinol. Metab.*, **39**:1038–1044, 1974.

202. Rosler, A., E. Gazit, R. Theodor, H. Biochis, and D. Rabinowitz: Salt wastage, raised plasma-renin activity, and normal or high plasma-aldosterone: A form of pseudohypoaldosteronism, *Lancet*, 959–962, May 5, 1973.

203. Raine, D. N., and J. Roy: A salt-losing syndrome in infancy: Pseudohypoadrenocorticalism, *Arch. Dis. Child.*, **37**:548–556, 1962.

204. Lelong, M., D. Alagille, A. Phillippe, C. Gentil, and J. C. Gabilan: Diabete salin par insensibilite congenitale du tubule a l'aldosterone: "Pseudo-hypo-adrenocorticisme," *Rev. Fr. Etudes Clin. Biol.*, **5**:558–565, 1960.

205. Donnell, G. N., N. Litman, and M. Roldan: Pseudohypo-adrenalcorticism, *Am. J. Dis. Child.*, **97**:813–828, 1959.

206. Cheek, D. B., and J. W. Perry: A salt wasting syndrome in infancy, *Arch. Dis. Child.*, **33**:252–256, 1958.

207. Cogan, M. G., and A. I. Arieff: Sodium wasting, acidosis, and hyperkalemia induced by methicillin interstitial nephritis: Evidence for selective distal tubular dysfunction, *Am. J. Med.*, **64**:500, 1978.

208. Arnold, J. E., and J. K. Healy: Hyperkalemia, hypertension and systemic acidosis without renal failure associated with tubular defect in potassium excretion, *Am. J. Med.*, **47**:461–472, 1969.

209. Gordon, R. D., R. A. Geddes, C. G. K. Pawsey, and M. W. O'Halloran: Hypertension and severe hyperkalaemia associated with suppression of renin and aldosterone and completely reversed by dietary sodium restriction, *Aust. Ann. Med.*, **19**:288–294, 1970.

210. Spitzer, A., C. M. Edelmann, Jr., L. D. Goldberg, and P. F. H. Henneman: Short stature, hyperkalemia and acidosis: A defect in renal transport of potassium, *Kidney Int.*, **3**:251–257, 1973.

211. Weinstein, S. F., D. M. E. Allan, and S. A. Mendoza: Hyperkalemia, acidosis, and short stature associated with a defect in renal potassium excretion, *J. Pediatr.*, **85**:355, 1974.

212. Brautbar, N., J. Levi, A. Rosler, E. Leitesdorf, M. Djaldeti, M. Epstein, and C. R. Kleeman: Familial hyperkalemia, hypertension and hyporeninemia with normal aldosterone levels: A tubular defect in potassium handling, *Arch. Intern. Med.*, **138**:607, 1978.

213. Schambelan, M., A. Sebastian, and F. C. Rector, Jr.: Mineralocorticoid (MC) resistant renal potassium (K^+) secretory defect: Proposed distal tubule chloride shunt, *Clin. Res.*, **26**:545A, 1978.

214. Szylman, P., O. Better, C. Chaimowitz, and A. Rosler: Role of hyperkalemia in the metabolic

acidosis of isolated hypoaldosteronism, *N. Engl. J. Med.*, **294**:361, 1976.

215. Daughaday, W. H., and D. Rendleman: Severe symptomatic hyperkalemia in an adrenalectomized woman due to enhanced mineralocorticoid requirement, *Ann. Intern. Med.*, **66**:1197–1203, 1967.

216. Gerstein, A. R., C. R. Kleeman, E. M. Godl, S. S. Franklin, M. H. Maxwell, H. C. Gonick, M. L. Feffer, and T. I. Steinman: Aldosterone deficiency in chronic renal failure, *Nephron*, **5**:90–105, 1968.

217. Luke, R. G., M. E. M. Allison, J. F. Davidson, and W. P. Duquid: Hyperkalemia and renal tubular acidosis due to renal amyloidosis, *Ann. Intern. Med.*, **70**:1211–1217, 1969.

218. Vagnucci, A. H.: Selective aldosterone deficiency in chronic pyelonephritis, *Nephron*, **7**:524–537, 1970.

219. Rado, J. P., L. Szende, and L. Szucs: Hyperkalemia unresponsive to massive doses of aldosterone in a patient with renal tubular acidosis, *Endocrinology*, **68**:183–188, 1976.

220. DeFronzo, R. A., M. Goldberg, C. R. Cooke, C. Barker, R. A. Grossman, and Z. S. Agus: Investigation into the mechanisms of hyperkalemia following renal transplantation, *Kidney Int.*, **11**:357–365, 1977.

221. DeFronzo, R. A., R. Cooke, M. Goldberg, M. Cox, A. R. Myers, and Z. S. Agus: Impaired renal tubular potassium secretion in systemic lupus erythematosus, *Ann. Intern. Med.*, **86**:268–271, 1977.

222. Carroll, H. J., and S. J. Farber: Hyperkalemia and hyperchloremic acidosis in chronic pyelonephritis, *Metabolism*, **13**:808–817, 1964.

223. Lathem, W.: Hyperchloremic acidosis in chronic pyelonephritis, *N. Engl. J. Med.*, **258**:1031–1036, 1958.

224. Handler, N. M., J. R. Gill, Jr., and J. D. Gardner: Impaired renal tubular secretion of potassium, elevated sweat sodium chloride concentration and plasma inhibition of erythrocyte sodium outflux as complications of systemic lupus erythematosus, *Arthritis Rheum*, **15**:515–523, 1972.

225. Gyory, A. Z., J. H. Stewart, C. R. P. George, D. J. Tiller, and K. D. G. Edwards: Renal tubular acidosis, acidosis due to hyperkalemia, hypercalcaemia, disordered citrate metabolism and other tubular dysfunctions following human renal transplantation, *Q. J. Med.*, **38**:231–253, 1969.

226. Rubini, M. E., J. P. Sanford, and W. H. Meroney: Studies of potassium secretion in glomerulonephritis, *Am. J. Med.*, 790–797, Nov. 1977.

227. Posner, J. B., and D. R. Jacobs: Isolated analdosteronism: I. Clinical entity, with manifestations of persistent hyperkalemia, periodical paralysis, salt-losing tendency and acidosis, *Metabolism*, **13**:513–521, 1964.

228. Jacobs, D. R., and J. B. Posner: Isolated analdosteronism: II. The nature of the adrenal cortical enzymatic defect, and the influence of diet and various agents on electrolyte balance, *Metabolism*, **13**:522–531, 1964.

229. Hill, S. R., J. F. Nickerson, S. B. Chenault, J. H. McNeil, W. R. Starnes, and M. C. Gautney: Studies in man on hyper- and hypoaldosteronism, *Arch. Intern. Med.*, **104**:156–168, 1959.

230. Lemann, J., W. F. Pierling, and E. J. Lennon: Studies of the acute effects of aldosterone and cortisol on the interrelationship between renal sodium, calcium and magnesium excretion in normal man, *Nephron*, **7**:117, 1970.

231. Hulter, H., L. Ilnicki, J. Harbottle, and A. Sebastian: Impaired renal H^+ secretion and NH_3 production in mineralocorticoid-deficient glucocorticoid-replete dogs, *Am. J. Physiol.*, **232**:F136–F146, 1977.

232. Al-Awqati, Q., L. H. Norby, A. Mueller, and P. R. Steinmentz: Characteristics of stimulation of H^+ transport by aldosterone in turtle urinary bladder, *J. Clin. Invest.*, **58**:351, 1976.

233. Lubowitz, H., M. L. Purkerson, D. B. Rolg, F. Weisser, and N. S. Bricker: Effect of nephron loss on proximal tubular bicarbonate reabsorption in the rat, *Am. J. Physiol.*, **220**:457–461, 1971.

234. Sebastian, A., and M. Schambelan: Amelioration of type IV RTA in chronic renal failure with furosemide, *Kidney Int.*, **12**:534, 1977.

235. Vicale, C. T.: The diagnostic features of a muscular syndrome resulting from hyperparathyroidism, osteomalacia owing to renal tubular acidosis, and perhaps to related disorders of calcium metabolism, *Trans. Am. Neurol. Assoc.*, **74**:143–147, 1949.

236. Smith, R., and G. Stern: Muscular weakness in osteomalacia and hyperparathyroidism, *J. Neurol. Sci.*, **8**:511–520, 1969.

237. Mallette, L. E., B. M. Patten, and W. K. Engel: Neuromuscular disease in secondary hyperpara-

thyroidism, *Ann. Intern. Med.,* **82**:474–483, 1975.

238. Curry, O. B., J. F. Basten, M. J. O. Francis, and R. Smith: Calcium uptake by sarcoplasmic reticulum of muscle from vitamin D-deficient rabbits, *Nature,* **249**:83–84, 1974.

239. Birge, S. J., and J. G. Haddad, Jr.: 25-Hydroxycholecalciferol stimulation of muscle metabolism, *J. Clin. Invest.,* **56**:1100, 1975.

240. Henderson, R. G., J. G. G. Ledingham, and D. P. Oliver, et al.: Effects of 1,25-dihydroxycholecalciferol on calcium absorption, muscle weakness, and bone disease in chronic renal failure, *Lancet,* **1**:379, 1974.

241. Prescott, L. F.: Mechanisms of renal excretion of drugs, *Br. J. Anaesth.,* **44**:246, 1972.

242. Mudge, G. H., P. Silva, and G. R. Stibitz: Renal excretion by nonionic diffusion. The nature of disequilibrium, *Med. Clin. N. Am.,* **59**:681, 1975.

243. Beckett, A. H., and M. Rowland: Urinary excretion kinetics of amphetamine in man, *J. Pharm. Pharmacol.,* **17**:628, 1965.

244. Kuntzman, R. G., I. Tsai, L. Brand, and L. C. Mark: The influence of urinary pH on the plasma half-life of pseudoephedrine in man and dog and a sensitive assay for its determination in human plasma, *Clin. Pharmacol. Ther.,* **12**:62, 1971.

245. MacPherson, C. R., M. D. Milne, and B. M. Evans: The secretion of salicylate, *Br. J. Pharmacol.,* **10**:484, 1955.

246. Gerhardt, R. E., R. F. Knouss, P. T. Thyrum, R. J. Luchi, and J. J. Morris: Quinidine excretion in aciduria and alkaluria, *Ann. Intern. Med.,* **71**:927, 1969.

247. Dent, C. E.: Metabolic forms of rickets (and osteomalacia), in H. Bikel and J. Stern (eds.), *Inborn Errors of Calcium and Bone Metabolism,* University Park Press, Baltimore, 1976, pp. 124–149.

248. Dent, C. E.: Rickets and osteomalacia from renal tubule defects, *J. Bone Joint Surg.,* **34B**:266, 1952.

249. Dent, C. E., and H. Harris: Hereditary forms of rickets and osteomalacia, *J. Bone Joint Surg.,* **38B**:204, 1956.

250. Winters, R. W., J. B. Graham, T. F. Williams, V. W. McFalls, and C. H. Burnett: A genetic study of familial hypophosphatemia and vitamin D resistant rickets with a review of the literature, *Medicine,* **37**:97, 1958.

251. Stanbury, S. W.: Aspects of disordered renal tubular function, *Adv. Intern. Med.,* **9**:231, 1958.

252. Falkson, G., and B. Frame: Phosphate diabetes: A review, *Henry Ford Hosp, Med. Bull.,* **6**:244, 1958.

253. Prader, A., R. Illig, E. Uehlinger, and G. Stalder: Rachitis in folge knochentumors, *Helv. Paediatr. Acta,* **14**:544, 1959.

254. Winters, R. W., V. W. McFalls, and J. B. Graham: Sporadic hypophosphatemia in vitamin D resistant rickets, *Paediatrics,* **25**:959, 1960.

255. Greenberg, B. C., R. W. Winters, and J. B. Graham: The normal range of serum inorganic phosphorus and its utility as a discriminant in the diagnosis of congenital hypophosphatemia, *J. Clin. Endocrinol. Metab.,* **20**:364, 1960.

256. Dent, C. E., and M. Friedman: Hypophosphatemic osteomalacia with complete recovery, *Br. Med. J.,* **1**:1976, 1964.

257. Howard, J. E.: Case records of the Massachusetts General Hospital (B. Castleman), *N. Engl. J. Med.,* **273**:494, 1965.

258. Wilson, D. R., S. E. York, Z. F. Jaworski, and E. R. Yendt: Studies in hypophosphatemic vitamin D-refractory osteomalacia in adults, *Medicine,* **44**:99–134, 1965.

259. De Deuxchaisnes, C. N., and S. M. Crane: The treatment of adult phosphate diabetes and Fanconi syndrome with neutral sodium phosphate, *Am. J. Med.,* **43**:508–543, 1967.

260. Dent, C. E., and T. C. B. Stamp: Hypophosphatemic osteomalacia presenting in adults, *Q. J. Med.,* **40**:303–329, 1971.

261. Scriver, C. R., F. H. Glorieux, T. M. Reade, and H. S. Tenehouse: X-Linked hypophosphataemia and autosomal recessive vitamin D dependency: Models for the resolution of vitamin D refractory rickets, in H. Bikel and J. Stern (eds.), *Inborn Errors of Calcium and Bone Metabolism,* University Park Press, Baltimore, 1976, pp. 150–173.

262. Fryomyer, J. W., and W. Hodgkin: Adult-onset vitamin D-resistant hypophosphatemic osteomalacia, *J. Bone Joint Surg.,* **59A**:101–106, 1977.

263. Stamp, T. C. B., and L. R. I. Baker: Recessive hypophosphataemic rickets, and possible aetiology of the "vitamin D-resistant" syndrome, *Arch. Dis. Child.,* **51**:360–365, 1976.

264. Bianchine, J. W., A. A. Stambler, and H. E. Harrison: Familial hypophosphatemic rickets show-

ing autosomal dominant inheritance, *Birth Defects: The Endocrine System,* **7**:287–293, 1971.

265. Scriver, C. R., W. MacDonald, T. Reade, F. H. Glorieux, and B. Nogrady: Hypophosphatemic nonrachitic bone disease: An entity distinct from X-linked hypophosphatemia in the renal defect, bone involvement, and inheritance, *Am. J. Med. Genet.,* **1**:101–107, 1977.

266. McCance, R. A.: Osteomalacia with Looser's zones due to raised resistance to vitamin D acquired about the age of 15 years, *Q. J. Med.,* **16**:33, 1947.

267. Olefsky, J., R. Kempson, H. Jones, and G. Reaven: "Tertiary" hyperparathyroidism and apparent "cure" of vitamin D-resistant rickets after removal of an ossifying mesenchymal tumor of the pharynx, *N. Engl. J. Med.,* **286**:739–745, 1972.

268. Harrison, H. E.: Oncogenous rickets: Possible elaboration by a tumor of a humoral substance inhibiting tubular reabsorption of phosphate, *Pediatrics,* **52**:432, 1973.

269. Linovitz, R. J., D. Resnick, P. Keissling, J. J. Kondon, B. Sehler, R. J. Nejdl, J. H. Rowe, and L. J. Deftos: Tumor-induced osteomalacia and rickets: A surgically curable syndrome, *J. Bone Joint Surg.,* **58-A**:419, 1976.

270. Drezner, M. K., and M. N. Feinglos: Osteomalacia due to 1α,25-dihydroxycholecalciferol deficiency, *J. Clin. Invest.,* **60**:1046–1053, 1977.

271. Dent, C. E., and J. M. Gertner: Hypophosphataemic osteomalacia in fibrous dysplasia, *Q. J. Med.,* **179**:411–420, 1976.

272. Sugarman, G. I., and W. B. Reeds: Two unusual neurocutaneous disorders with facial cutaneous signs, *Arch. Neurol.,* **21**:242, 1969.

273. Aschinberg, L. C., L. M. Solomon, P. M. Zeis, P. Justice, and I. M. Rosenthal: Vitamin D-resistant rickets associated with epidermal nevus syndrome: Demonstation of a phosphaturic substance in the dermal lesions, *J. Pediatr.,* **91**:56–60, 1977.

274. Albright, F., and E. C. Reifenstein: *The Parathyroid Glands and Metabolic Bone Disease,* The Williams & Wilkins Company, Baltimore, 1948.

275. Williams, T. F., and R. W. Winters: in J. B. Stanbury, J. B. Wyngaarden, and D. S. Frederickson (eds.), *The Metabolic Basis of Inherited Disease,* McGraw-Hill Book Company, New York, 1972.

276. Harrison, H. E., H. C. Harrison, F. Lifshitz, and A. D. Johnson: Growth disturbance in hereditary hypoposphatemia, *Am. J. Dis. Child.,* **112**:290–297, 1966.

277. McNair, S. I., and G. B. Sticker: Growth in familial hypophosphatemic vitamin D-resistant rickets, *N. Engl. J. Med.,* **281**:511–516, 1969.

278. Hahn, T. J., C. R. Scharp, L. R. Halstead, J. G. Haddan, D. M. Karl, and L. V. Avioli: Parathyroid hormone status and renal responsiveness in familial hypophosphatemic rickets, *J. Clin. Endocrinol. Metab.,* **41**:926–937, 1975.

279. Arnaud, C., F. Glorieux, and C. R. Scriver: Serum parathyroid hormone in x-linked hypophosphatemia, *Science,* **173**:845–847, 1971.

280. Roof, B. S., C. F. Piel, and G. S. Gordan: Nature of defect responsible for familial vitamin D-resistant rickets (VDRR) based on radioimmunoassay for parathyroid hormone (PTH), *Trans. Assoc. Am. Physicians,* **85**:172–180, 1972.

281. Lewy, J. E., E. C. Cabana, H. A. Repetto, J. M. Canterbury, and E. Reiss: Serum parathyroid hormone in hypophosphatemic vitamin D-resistant rickets, *J. Pediatr.,* **81**:294–300, 1972.

282. Reitz, R. E., and R. L. Weinstein: Parathyroid hormone secretion in familial vitamin-D-resistant rickets, *N. Engl. J. Med.,* **289**:941–945, 1973.

283. Fanconi, A., J. A. Fischer, and A. Prader: Serum parathyroid hormone concentrations in hypophosphataemic vitamin D resistant rickets, *Helv. Paediatr. Acta,* **29**:187, 1974.

284. Short, E., R. C. Morris, Jr., A. Sebastian, and M. Spencer: Exaggerated phosphaturic response to circulating parathyroid hormone in patients with familial x-linked hypophosphatemic rickets, *J. Clin. Invest.,* **58**:152–163, 1976.

285. Stickler, G. B.: External calcium and phosphorus balances in vitamin D-resistant rickets, *J. Pediatr.,* **63**:942–948, 1963.

286. Soergel, K. H., K. H. Mueller, R. F. Gustke, and J. E. Geenen: Jejunal calcium transport in health and metabolic bone disease: Effects of vitamin D, *Gastroenterology,* **67**:28, 1974.

287. Short, E. M., H. J. Binder, and L. E. Rosenberg: Familial hypophosphatemic rickets: Defective transport of inorganic phosphate by intestinal mucosa, *Science,* **179**:700, 1973.

288. Glorieux, F. H., C. L. Morin, R. Travers, E. E.

Delvin, and R. Poirier: Intestinal phosphate transport in familial hypophosphatemic rickets, *Pediatr. Res.*, **10**:691–696, 1976.

289. Walton, J., M. E. Williams, D. Pool, and T. K. Gray: Jejunal transport of inorganic phosphate in familial hypophosphatemic rickets, *Clin. Res.*, **25**:34A, 1977.

290. Haddad, J. G., J. K. Chyu, T. J. Hahn, and T. C. B. Stamp: Serum concentrations of 25-hydroxy-vitamin D in sex-linked hypophosphataemic vitamin D-resistant rickets, *J. Lab. Clin. Med.*, **81**:22, 1973.

291. Haussler, M. R., D. J. Baylink, M. R. Hughes, P. F. Brumbaugh, J. E. Wergedal, F. H. Shen, R. L. Nielsen, S. J. Counts, K. M. Bursac, and T. A. McCain: The assay of 1α,25-dihydroxyvitamin D_3: Physiologic and pathologic modulation of circulating hormone levels, *Clin. Endocrinol.*, **5**:151s–165s, 1976.

292. Glorieux, F., and C. R. Scriver: Loss of a parathyroid hormone-sensitive component of phosphate transport in x-linked hypophosphatemia, *Science*, **175**:997–1000, 1972.

293. Lestradet, H., P. Royer, and D. Jacob: Resultats fournes par l'epreuve de perfusion calcique dans le rachitisme vitamine-resistant hypophosphate-mique idiopathique, *Rev. Fr. Etud. Clin. Biol.*, **3**:884–886, 1958.

294. Lamy, M., P. Royer, J. Frezal, and H. Lestradet: Le rachitisme vitamino-resistant familial hypophosphatemique primitif, *Arch. Fr. Pediatr.*, **15**:1–24, 1958.

295. Field, M. H., and E. Reiss: Vitamin D-resistant rickets: The effect of calcium infusion on phosphate reabsorption, *J. Clin. Invest.*, **39**:1807–1812, 1960.

296. Falls, W. F., Jr., N. W. Carter, F. C. Rector, Jr., and D. W. Seldin: Familial vitamin D-resistant rickets. Study of six cases with evaluation of the pathogenetic role of secondary hyperparathyroidism, *Ann. Intern. Med.*, **68**:533–560, 1968.

297. Scriver, C. R., and M. Bergeron: Aminoacid transport in kidney. The use of mutation to dissect membrane and transepithelial transport, in W. L. Nyhan (ed.), *Hereditable Disorders of Amino Acid Metabolism,* John Wiley and Sons, Inc., New York, 1974.

298. Foulks, J. G.: Homeostatic adjustment in the renal tubular transport of inorganic phosphate in the dog, *Can. J. Biochem. Physiol.*, **33**:638, 1955.

299. Foulks, J. G., and F. A. Perry: Renal excretion of phosphate following parathyroidectomy in the dog, *Am. J. Physiol.*, **195**:554, 1959.

300. Trohler, U., J-P. Bonjour, and H. Fleisch: Inorganic phosphate homeostasis. Renal adaption to the dietary intake in intact and thyroparathyroidectomized rats, *J. Clin. Invest.*, **57**:264–273, 1976.

301. Steele, T. H., and H. F. DeLuca: Influence of dietary phosphorus on renal phosphate reabsorption in the parathyroidectomized rat, *J. Clin. Invest.*, **57**:867–874, 1976.

302. Trohler, U., J-P. Bonjour, and H. Fleisch: Renal tubular adaptation to dietary phosphorus, *Nature*, **261**:145–146, 1976.

303. Thompson, D. D., and H. H. Hiatt: Effects of phosphate loading and depletion on the renal excretion and reabsorption of inorganic phosphate, *J. Clin. Invest.*, **36**:566–572, 1957.

304. Yendt, E. R., and Z. F. Jaworski: The relationship of urinary phosphate changes to parathyroid acivity, in R. O. Greep and R. V. Talmadge (eds.), *The Parathyroids*, Charles C Thomas, Publisher, Springfield Ill., 1961.

305. Fraser, D., and C. R. Scriver: Familial forms of vitamin D-resistant rickets revisited. X-linked hypophosphatemia and autosomal recessive vitamin D dependency, *Am. J. Clin. Nutr.*, **29**:1315–1329, 1976.

306. Dent, C. E., J. M. Round, and T. C. B. Stamp: Treatment of sex-linked hypophosphataemic rickets (SLHR), in B. Frame, A. M. Parfitt, and H. Duncan (eds.), *Clinical Aspects of Metabolic Bone Disease,* International Congress Series No. 270, Excerpta Medica, Amsterdam, 1973, p. 427.

307. Stanbury, S. W.: Osteomalacia, *Schweiz, Med. Wochenschr.*, **92**:883, 1962.

308. Fraser, D., N. T. Jaco, E. R. Yendt, J. D. Milne, and E. Lin: The induction of in vitro and in vivo calcification in bones of children suffering from vitamin D-resistant rickets without recourse to large doses of vitamin D, *Am. J. Dis. Child.*, **93**:84, 1957.

309. Fraser, D., D. W. Geiger, J. D. Munn, P. E. Slater, R. Jahn, and E. Lin: Calcification studies in clinical vitamin D deficiency and in hypophos-

phatemic vitamin D refractory rickets. The induction of calcium deposition in rachitic cartilage without administration of vitamin D, *Am. J. Dis. Child.,* **96**:460, 1958.

310. Frame, B., R. W. Smith, Jr., J. L. Fleming, and G. Manson: Oral phosphates in vitamin D-refractory rickets and osteomalacia, *Am. J. Dis. Child.,* **106**:147, 1963.

311. West, C. D., J. C. Blanton, F. N. Silverman, and N. H. Holland: Use of phosphate salt as an adjunct to vitamin D in the treatment of hypophosphatemic vitamin D refractory rickets, *J. Pediatr.,* **64**:469, 1964.

312. Glorieux, F. H., C. R. Scriver, T. M. Reade, H. Goldman, and A. Roseborough: Use of phosphate and vitamin D to prevent dwarfism and rickets in X-linked hypophosphatemia, *N. Engl. J. Med.,* **287**:481, 1972.

313. McEnery, P. T., F. N. Silverman, and C. D. West: Acceleration of growth with combined vitamin D-phosphate therapy of hypophosphatemic resistant rickets, *J. Pediatr.,* **80**:763, 1972.

314. Wilson, D. R., and E. R. Yendt: Treatment of the adult Fanconi syndrome with oral phosphate supplements and alkali, *Am. J. Med.,* **35**:487–511, 1963.

315. Smith, R., R. H. Lindenbaum, and R. J. Walton: Hypophosphataemic osteomalacia and Fanconi syndrome of adult onset with dominant inheritance, *Q. J. Med.,* **179**:387–400, 1976.

316. Lotz, M., E. Zisman, and F. C. Bartter: Evidence for a phosphorus-depletion syndrome in man, *N. Engl. J. Med.,* **278**:409–415, 1968.

317. Lotz, M., R. Ney, and F. C. Bartter: Osteomalacia and debility resulting from phosphorus depletion, *Trans. Assoc. Am. Physicians,* **77**:281–395, 1964.

318. Dent, C. E., and C. S. Winter: Osteomalacia due to phosphate depletion from excessive aluminum hydroxide ingestion, *Br. Med. J.,* **1**:551–552, 1974.

319. Baker, L. R. I., R. Ackrill, and W. R. Cattell, et al.: Iatrogenic osteomalacia and myopathy due to phosphate depletion, *Br. Med. J.,* **3**:150–152, 1974.

320. Schoot, G. D., and M. R. Wills: Myopathy in hypophosphataemic osteomalacia presenting in adult life, *J. Neurol. Neurosurg. Psychiatry,* **38**:297–304, 1975.

321. Teitelbaum, S. L., E. M. Rosenberg, M. Bates, and L. V. Avioli: The effects of phosphate and vitamin D therapy on osteopenic, hypophosphatemic osteomalacia of childhood, *Clin. Orthop. Related Res.,* **116**:38–47, 1976.

322. Borle, A. B.: Calcium and phosphate metabolism, *Ann. Rev. Physiol.,* **36**:361–390, 1974.

323. Borle, A. B.: Regulation of the mitochondrial control of cellular calcium homeostasis and calcium transport by phosphate, parathyroid hormone, calcitonin, vitamin D and cyclic AMP, in R. V. Talmage, M. Owen, and J. A. Parsons (eds.), *Calcium Regulating Hormones,* Fifth Parathyroid Hormone Conference, Oxford, 1974, American Elsevier Publishing Co., Inc., New York, 1974, chap. 8, p. 217.

324. Rasmussen, H., and P. Bordier: *The Physiological and Cellular Basis of Metabolic Bone Disease,* The Williams & Wilkins Company, Baltimore, 1974.

325. Stickler, G. B.: Comment on Ref. 313, *J. Pediatr.,* **80**:774, 1972.

326. Stamp, T. C. B.: Treatment of hereditary hypophosphataemic rickets (correspondence), *Arch. Dis. Child.,* **51**:988, 1976.

327. Puschett, J. B., M. Genel, A. Rastegar, C. Anast, H. F. DeLuca, and A. Friedman: Long-term therapy of vitamin D-resistant rickets with 25-hydroxycholecalciferol, *Clin. Pharmacol. Ther.,* **17**:202, 1975.

328. Brickman, A. S., J. W. Coburn, K. Kurokawa, J. E. Bethune, H. E. Harrison, and A. W. Norman: Actions of 1,25-dihydroxycholecalciferol in patients with hypophosphatemic, vitamin D-resistant rickets, *N. Engl. J. Med.,* **289**:495, 1973.

329. Russell, R. G. G., R. Smith, C. Preston, R. J. Walton, C. G. Woods, R. G. Henderson, and A. W. Norman: The effect of 1,25-dihydroxycholecalciferol on renal tubular reabsorption of phosphate, intestinal absorption of calcium and bone histology in hypophosphaaemic renal tubular rickets, *Clin. Sci. Molec. Med.,* **48**:177–186, 1975.

330. Peacock, M., P. J. Heyburn, and J. E. Aaron: Vitamin D resistant hypophosphataemic osteomalacia: Treatment with lα-hydroxyvitamin D_3, *Clin. Endocrinol.,* **7**:231S–237S, 1977.

331. Riggs, B. L., R. G. Sprague, J. Jowsey, and F. T. Maher: Adult-onset vitamin-D-resistant hypophosphatemic osteomalacia. Effect of total parathyroidectomy, *N. Engl. J. Med.,* **281**:762, 1969.

332. Leaf, A.: The syndrome of osteomalacia, renal

glycosuria, aminoaciduria, and increased phosphorus clearance (the Fanconi syndrome), in J. B. Stanbury, J. B. Wyngaarden, and D. S. Fredrickson (eds.), *The Metabolic Basis of Inherited Disease,* 2d ed., McGraw-Hill Book Company, New York, 1966, p. 1205.

333. Schneider, J. A., and J. E. Seegmiller: Cystinosis and the Fanconi syndrome, in J. B. Stanbury, J. B. Wyngaarden, and D. S. Fredrickson, (eds.), *The Metabolic Basis of Inherited Disease,* 3d ed., McGraw-Hill Book Company, New York, 1972, p. 1581.

334. Van Biervliet, J. P. G. M., L. Bruinvis, D. Ketting, P. K. De Bree, C. Van Der Heiden, S. K. Wadman, J. L. Willems, H. Bookelman, U. Van Haelst, and L. A. H. Monnens: Hereditary mitochondrial myopathy with lactic acidemia, a DeToni-Fanconi-Debré syndrome, and a defective respiratory chain in voluntary striated muscles, *Pediatr. Res.,* **11:**1088, 1977.

335. Bonnici, F., S. Smith, and H. De V. Heese: Letter to the editor, *Lancet,* **1:**1304, 1977.

336. Lowe, C. U., M. Terrey, and E. A. MacLachlan: Organoaciduria, decreased renal ammonia production, hydrophthalmos, and mental retardation: A clinical entity, *Am. J. Dis. Child.,* **83:**164, 1952.

337. Abbassi, V., C. U. Lowe, and P. L. Calcagno: Oculocerebrorenal syndrome, *Am. J. Dis. Child.,* **115:**145, 1968.

338. Fritzell, S., O. R. Jagenburg, and L. B. Schnurer: Familial cirrhosis of the liver, renal tubular defects with rickets and impaired tyrosine metabolism, *Acta Pediatr.,* **53:**18, 1964.

339. Halvorsen, S., and L. R. Gjessing: Studied on tyrosinosis. I. Effect of low-tyrosine and low-phenylalanine diet, *Br. Med. J.,* **2:**1171, 1964.

340. La Du, B. N., and L. R. Gjessing: Tyrosinosis and tyrosinemia, in J. B. Stanbury, J. B. Wyngaarden, and D. S. Fredrickson (eds.), *The Metabolic Basis of Inherited Disease,* 3d ed., McGraw-Hill Book Company, New York, 1972, p. 296.

341. Levin, B., G. J. A. I. Snodgrass, V. G. Oberholzer, E. A. Burgess, and R. H. Dobbs: Fructosaemia: Observations on seven cases, *Am. J. Med.,* **45:**826, 1968.

342. Wilson, D., G. Steiner, and M. Vranic: Studies of glucose turnover and renal function in an un-

usual case of hereditary fructose intolerance, *Am. J. Med.,* **62:**150, 1977.

343. Lameire, N., M. Mussche, and S. Ringoir: Une acidose tubulaire proximale chez une adulte, *J. Urol. Nephrol. (Paris),* **83:**911–915, 1977.

344. Bearn, A. G., T. F. Yu, and A. B. Gutman: Renal function in Wilson's disease, *J. Clin. Invest.,* **36:**1107, 1957.

345. Morgan, H. G., W. K. Stewart, K. G. Lowe, J. M. Stowers, and J. H. Johnstone: Wilsons disease and the Fanconi syndrome, *Q. J. Med.,* **31:**361, 1962.

346. Elsas, L. J., J. P. Hayslett, B. H. Spargo, J. L. Durant, and L. E. Rosenberg:Wilson's disease with reversible renal tubular dysfunction: Correlation with proximal tubular ultrastructure, *Ann. Intern. Med.,* **75:**427, 1971.

347. Cusworth, D. G., C. E. Dent, and F. V. Flynn: The aminoaciduria in galactosemia, *Arch. Dis. Child.,* **30:**150, 1955.

348. Komrower, G. M., V. Schwartz, A. Holzel, and L. Golberg: A clinical and biochemical study of galactosemia, *Arch. Dis. Child.,* **31:**254, 1956.

349. Fanconi, G., and H. Bickel: Die chronische aminosaurediabetes oder nephrotisch-glukosurischer zwergwuchs) bein der glykogenose und der cystinkrankheit, *Helv. Paediatr. Acta,* **4:**359, 1949.

350. Lampert, F., and G. Mayer: Glykogenose der leber mit galaktose-verwertungsstorung und schwerem Fanconi-syndrom, *Arch. Kinderheilkd.,* **98:**133, 1967.

351. Morris, R. C., Jr., I. Ueki, D. Loh, R. Z. Eases, and P. McLin: Absence of renal fructose-1-phosphate aldolase activity in hereditary fructose intolerance, *Nature (Lond.),* **214:**920, 1967.

352. Kranhold, J. F., D. Loh, and R. C. Morris, Jr.: Renal fructose-metabolizing enzymes: Significance in hereditary fructose intolerance, *Science,* **165:**402, 1969.

353. Wachsmuth, E. D., M. Thöner, and G. Pfleiderer: The cellular distribution of aldolase isozymes in rat kidney and brain determined in tissue sections by the immuno-histochemical method, *Histochemistry,* **45:**143–161, 1975.

354. Morris, R. C., Jr., K. Nigon, and E. B. Reed: Evidence that the severity of depletion of inorganic phosphate determines the severity of the disturbance of adenine nucleotide metabolism in the liver

and renal cortex of the fructose-loaded rat, *J. Clin. Invest.,* **61:**209–220, 1978.

355. Maunsbach, A. B.: Ultrastructure of the proximal tubule, in J. Orloff and R. W. Berliner (eds.), *Handbook of Physiology,* American Physiology Society, Washington, D.C., 1973, sect. 8, p. 31.

356. Christensen, E. I., and A. B. Maunsbach: Intralysosomal digestion of lysozyme in renal proximal tubule cells, *Kidney Int.,* **6:**396, 1974.

357. Maack, T., and D. Sigulem: Renal handling of lysozyme, in E. F. Osserman, R. E. Canfield, and S. Beychok (eds.), *Lysozyme,* Academic Press, Inc., New York, 1974, p. 321.

358. Shibko, S., and A. L. Tappel: Rat kidney lysosomes: Isolation and properties, *Biochem. J.,* **95:**731, 1965.

359. Osserman, E. F.: Lysozymuria in renal and nonrenal diseases, in Y. Manuel, J. P. Revillard, and H. Betuel (eds.), *Proteins in Normal and Pathological Urine,* Darger, New York, 1970, p. 260.

360. Hayslett, J. P., P. E. Perille, and S. C. Finch: Urinary muramidase and renal disease, *N. Engl. J. Med.,* **279:**506, 1968.

361. Barratt, T. M., and R. Crawford: Lysozyme excretion as a measure of renal tubular dysfunction in children, *Clin. Sci.,* **39:**457, 1970.

362. Chamberlain, M. J., and L. Stimmler: The renal handling of insulin, *J. Clin. Invest.,* **46:**911, 1967.

363. Berggård, I., and A. G. Bearn: Isolation and properties of a low molecular weight β_2-globulin occurring in human biological fluids, *J. Biol. Chem.,* **243:**4095, 1968.

364. Bernier, G. M., and M. E. Conrad: Catabolism of human β_2-microglobulin by the rat kidney, *Am. J. Physiol.,* **217:**1359, 1969.

365. Peterson, P. A., P.-E. Evrin, and I. Berggård: Differentiation of glomerular, tubular, and normal proteinuria: Determinations of urinary excretion of β_2-microglobulin, albumin, and total protein, *J. Clin. Invest.,* **48:**1189, 1969.

366. Mogielnicki, R. P., T. A. Waldmann, and W. Strober: The renal handling of low molecular weight proteins. I. L-chain metabolism in experimental renal disease, *J. Clin. Invest.,* **50:**901, 1971.

367. Waldmann, T. A., W. Strober, and R. P. Mogielnicki: The renal handling of low molecular weight proteins. II. Disorders of serum protein catabolism in patients with tubular proteinuria, the nephrotic syndrome, or uremia, *J. Clin. Invest.,* **51:**2162, 1972.

368. Osserman, E. F., and D. P. Lawlor: Serum and urinary lysozyme (muramidase) in monocytic and monomyelocytic leukemia, *J. Exp. Med.,* **124:**921–951, 1966.

369. Muggia, F. M., H. O. Heinemann, M. Farhangi, and E. F. Osserman: Lysozymuria and renal tubular dysfunction in monocytic and myelomonocytic leukemia, *Am. J. Med.,* **47:**351, 1969.

370. Pruzanski, W., and M. E. Platts: Serum and urinary proteins, lysozyme (muramidase), and renal dysfunction in mono- and myelomonocytic leukemia, *J. Clin. Invest.,* **49:**1694–1708, 1970.

371. Rudders, R. A., and K. J. Block: Myeloma renal disease: Evaluation of the role of muramidase (lysozyme), *Am. J. Med. Sci.,* **262:**79–85, 1971.

372. Clyne, D. H., L. Brendstrup, and M. R. First, et al.: Renal effects of intraperitoneal kappa chain injection: Induction of crystals in renal tubular cells, *Lab. Invest.,* **31:**131, 1974.

373. Rawlings, W., Jr., J. Griffin, T. Duffy, and R. Humphrey: Fanconi syndrome with lambda light chains in urine (correspondence), *N. Engl. J. Med.,* **299:**1351, 1976.

374. Walker, B. R., F. Alexander, and P. J. Tannenbaum: Fanconi syndrome with renal tubular acidosis and light chain proteinuria, *Nephron,* **8:**103, 1971.

375. Kamm, D. E., and M. S. Fischer: Proximal renal tubular acidosis and the Fanconi syndrome in a patient with hypergammaglobulinemia, *Nephron,* **9:**208, 1972.

376. Sellinger, O. Z., H. Beaufay, P. Jacques, A. Doyen, and C. de Duve: Tissue fractionation studies. 15. Beta-n-acetylglucosaminidase and beta-galactosidase in rat liver, *Biochem. J.,* **74:**450, 1960.

377. Price, R. G., and N. Dance: The cellular distribution of some rat-kidney glycosidases, *Biochem. J.,* **105:**877, 1967.

378. Dance, N., R. G. Price, D. Robinson, and J. L. Stirling: Beta-galactosidase, beta-glucosidase and N-acetyl-beta-glucosaminidase in human kidney, *Clin. Chim. Acta,* **24:**189, 1969.

379. Dance, N., R. G. Price, W. R. Cattell, J. Lansdell, and B. Richards: The excretion of beta-glucosaminidase and beta-galactosidase by patients

with renal disease, *Clin. Chim. Acta,* **27**:87, 1970.

380. Morris, R. C., Jr.: The clinical spectrum of Fanconi's syndrome, *Calif. Med.,* **108**:225, 1968.

381. Schneider, J. A., V. Wong, K. H. Bradley, and J. E. Seegmiller: Biochemical comparisons of the adult and childhood forms of cystinosis, *N. Engl. J. Med.,* **279**:1253, 1968.

382. Lietman, P. S., P. D. Frazier, V. G. Wong, D. Shotton, and J. E. Seegmiller: Adult cystinosis—a benign disorder, *Am. J. Med.,* **40**:511, 1966.

383. Scriver, C. R., and D. T. Whelan: Cystinuria: Concepts and new observations, in N. A. J. Carson and D. N. Raine (eds.), *Inherited Disorders of Sulphur Metabolism,* Churchill Livingston, Edinburgh, 1971, p. 70.

384. Schneider, J. A., K. Bradley, and J. E. Seegmiller: Increased cystine in leukocytes from individuals homozygous and heterozygous for cystinosis, *Science,* **157**:1321, 1967.

385. Schneider, J. A., F. M. Rosenbloom, K. H. Bradley, and J. E. Seegmiller: Increased free-cystine content of fibroblasts cultured from patients with cystinosis, *Biochem. Biophys. Res. Commun.,* **29**:527, 1967.

386. Schneider, J. A., K. H. Bradley, and J. E. Seegmiller: Transport and intracellular fate of cysteine-^{35}S in leukocytes from normal subjects and patients with cystinosis, *Pediatr. Res.,* **2**:441, 1968.

387. Schulman, J. D., W. Y. Fujimoto, and K. H. Bradley, et al.: Identification of heterozygous genotype for cystinosis in utero by a new pulse-labeling technique: Preliminary report, *J. Pediatr.,* **77**:468, 1970.

388. Schneider, J. A., F. M. Verroust, and W. A. Kroll, et al.: Prenatal diagnosis of cystinosis, *N. Engl. J. Med.,* **290**:878, 1974.

389. Willcox, P., and A. D. Patrick: Biochemical diagnosis of cystinosis using leucocytes, *Acta Paediatr. Scand.,* **64**:132, 1975.

390. Steendijk, R.: The effect of a continuous intravenous infusion of inorganic phosphate on the rachitic lesions in cystinosis, *Arch. Dis. Child.,* **36**:321, 1961.

391. Linder, C. C., C. M. Bull, and I. Grayce: Hypophosphatemic glycosuric rickets (Fanconi syndrome), *Clin. Proc. Child. Hosp.,* **8**:1, 1949.

392. Dent, C. E.: Commentary, *Clin. Proc. Child. Hosp.,* **8**:21, 1949.

393. Stanbury, S. W., and G. A. Lumb: Metabolic studies of renal osteodystrophy. I. Calcium, phosphorus and nitrogen metabolism in rickets, osteomalacia and hyperparathyroidism complicating chronic uremia and in the osteomalacia of the adult Fanconi syndrome, *Medicine,* **41**:1–31, 1962.

394. Stanbury, S. W.: in D. A. K. Black (ed.), *Bony Complications of Renal Disease,* Blackwell Scientific Publications, Oxford, 1962, p. 508.

395. Dent, C. E., and H. Harris: The genetics of "cystinuria," *Ann. Eugen.,* **16**:60, 1951.

396. Mallette, L. E., and B. M. Patten: Neurogenic muscle atrophy and osteomalacia in adult Fanconi syndrome, *Ann. Neurol.,* **1**:131–137, 1977.

397. Soriano, J. R., I. B. Houston, H. Boichis, and C. M. Edelmann, Jr.: Calcium and phosphorus metabolism in the Fanconi syndrome, *J. Clin. Endocrinol. Metab.,* **28**:1555–1563, 1968.

398. Milne, M. D., S. W. Stanbury, and A. E. Thomson: Observations on the Fanconi syndrome and renal hyperchloremic acidosis in the adult, *Q. J. Med.,* **21**:61, 1952.

399. De Toni, E., Jr., and S. Nordio: The relationship between calcium-phosphorus in metabolism, the "Krebs cycle" and steroid metabolism, *Arch. Dis. Child.,* **34**:371, 1959.

400. Arnaud, C., R. Maijer, T. Reade, C. R. Scriver, and D. T. Whelan: Vitamin D dependency: An inherited postnatal syndrome with secondary hyperparathyroidism, *Pediatrics,* **46**:871, 1970.

401. Reade, T. M., C. R. Scriver, F. H. Glorieux, B. Nogrady, E. Delvin, R. Poirier, M. F. Holick, and H. F. DeLuca: Response to crystalline 1α-hydroxyvitamin D_3 in vitamin D dependency, *Pediatr. Res.,* **9**:593, 1975.

402. Olson, E. B., J. C. Knutson, M. H. Bhattacharyya, and H. F. DeLuca: The effect of hepatectomy on the synthesis of 25-hydroxyvitamin D_3, *J. Clin. Invest.,* **57**:1213–1220, 1976.

403. Brewer, E. D., H. C. Tsai, K.-S. Szeto, and R. C. Morris, Jr.: Maleic acid-induced impaired conversion of $25(OH)D_3$ to $1,25(OH)_2D_3$: Implications for Fanconi's syndrome, *Kidney Int.,* **12**:244–252, 1977.

404. Berliner, R. W., R. J. Kennedy, and J. G. Hilton: Effect of maleic acid on renal function, *Proc. Soc. Exp. Biol. Med.,* **75**:791–794, 1950.

405. Harrison, H. E., and H. C. Harrison: Experimen-

tal production of renal glycosuria, phosphaturia, and aminoaciduria by injection of maleic acid, *Science,* **120:**606–608, 1954.

406. Gmaj, P., A. Hoppe, S. Angielski, and J. Rogulski: Effects of maleate and arsenite on renal absorption of sodium and bicarbonate, *Am. J. Physiol.,* **225:**90–94, 1973.

407. Rogulski, J., A. Pancanis, W. Adamowicz, and S. Angielski: On the mechanism of maleate action on rat kidney mitochondria: Effect on oxidative metabolism, *Acta Biochim. Pol.,* **21:**403–413, 1974.

408. Rosen, V. J., H. J. Kramer, and H. C. Gonick: Experimental Fanconi syndrome: II. Effect of maleic acid on renal tubular ultrastructure, *Lab. Invest.,* **28:**446–455, 1973.

409. Bergeron, M., L. Dubord, and C. Hausser: Membrane permeability as a cause of transport defects in experimental Fanconi syndrome, *J. Clin. Invest.,* **57:**1181–1189, 1976.

410. Etches, P., D. Pickering, and R. Smith: Cystinotic rickets treated with vitamin D metabolites, *Arch. Dis. Child.,* **52:**661, 1977.

411. Gertner, J. M., D. P. Brenton, C. E. Dent, and M. Demenech: Treatment of the rickets of cystinosis with lα-hydroxy vitamin D₃ (1976), XII European Symposium on Calcified Tissues, *Calcified Tissue Research,* **521:** 63–67, 1977.

412. Salassa, R. M., M. H. Power, J. A. Ulrick, and A. B. Hayles: Observations on the metabolic effects of vitamin D in Fanconi's syndrome, *Proc. Mayo Clin.,* **29:**214, 1954.

413. Bergstrom, W. H.: The response of multiple renal tubular dysfunction to calciferol, *Pediatr. Res.,* **2:**408, 1968.

414. Huguenin, M., R. Schacht, and R. David: Infantile rickets with severe proximal renal tubular acidosis, responsive to vitamin D, *Arch. Dis. Child.,* **49:**955, 1974.

415. Puschett, J. B., J. Moranz, and W. S. Kurnick: Evidence for a direct action of cholecalciferol and 25-hydroxycholecalciferol on the renal transport of phosphate, sodium, and calcium, *J. Clin. Invest.,* **51:**373, 1972.

416. Puschett, J. B., P. C. Fernandez, I. T. Boyle, R. W. Gray, J. L. Omdahl, and H. F. DeLuca: The acute renal tubular effects of 1,25-dihydroxycholecalciferol (36781), *Proc. Soc. Exp. Biol. Med.,* **141:**379, 1972.

417. Froesch, E. R.: Essential fructosuria and hereditary fructose intolerance, in J. B. Stanbury, J. B. Wyngaarden, and D. S. Fredrickson (eds.), *The Metabolic Basis of Inherited Disease,* 2d ed., McGraw-Hill Book Company, New York, 1966, p. 124.

418. Townsend, E. J., Jr., H. H. Mason, and P. S. Strong: Galactosemia and its relation to Laennec's cirrhosis: Review of the literature and presentation of six additional cases, *Pediatrics,* **7:**760, 1951.

419. Isselbacher, K. J.: Galactosemia, in J. B. Stanbury, J. B. Wyngaarden, and D. S. Fredrickson (eds.), *The Metabolic Basis of Inherited Disease,* 2d ed., McGraw-Hill Book Company, New York, 1966, p. 178.

420. Lindemann, R., L. R. Gjessing, B. Merton, A. C. Liken, and S. Halvorsen: Amino acid metabolism in hereditary fructosemia, *Acta Paediatr. Scand.,* **59:**141, 1970.

421. Walshe, J. M.: The biochemistry of copper in man and its role in the pathogenesis of Wilson's disease (hepatolenticular degeneration), in J. N. Cummings (ed.), *Biochemical Aspects of Nervous Diseases,* Plenum Press, Plenum Publishing Corporation, New York, 1972, p. 111.

422. Bearn, A. G.: Wilson's disease, in J. B. Stanbury, J. B. Wyngaarden, and D. S. Fredrickson (eds.), *The Metabolic Basis of Inherited Disease,* 3d ed., McGraw-Hill Book Company, New York, 1972, p. 1033.

423. Lucas, Z. J., R. L. Kempson, J. Palmer, D. Korn, and R. B. Cohn: Renal allotransplantation in man. II. Transplantation in cystinosis, a metabolic disease, *Am. J. Surg.,* **118:**158, 1969.

424. Hambidge, K. N., S. I. Goodman, P. A. Walravens, S. M. Mauer, L. Brettschneider, I. Penn, and T. E. Starzl: Accumulation of cystine following renal homotransplantation for cystinosis, *Pediatr. Res.,* **3:**364, 1969.

425. Mahoney, C. P., G. E. Striker, R. O. Hickman, G. B. Manning, and T. L. Marchioro: Renal transplantation for childhood cystinosis, *N. Engl. J. Med.,* **283:**397, 1970.

426. Advisory Committee to the Renal Transplant Registry: Renal transplantation in congenital and metabolic diseases. A report from the ASC/NIH Renal Transplant Registry, *J. Am. Med. Assoc.,* **232:**148, 1975.

427. Malekzadeh, M. H., H. B. Neustein, J. A. Schneider, A. J. Pennisi, R. B. Ettenger, C. H. Uittenbogaart, M. D. Kogut, and R. N. Fine: Cadaver renal transplantation in children with cystinosis, *Am. J. Med.*, **63:**525–533, 1977.

428. Potts, J. T., Jr.: Pseudohypoparathyroidism, in J. B. Stanbury, J. B. Wyngaarden, and D. S. Fredrickson (eds.), *The Metabolic Basis of Inherited Disease*, 3d ed., McGraw-Hill Book Company, New York, 1972, p. 1305.

429. Chase, L. R., G. L. Melson, and G. D. Aurbach: Pseudohypoparathyroidism: Defective excretion of 3′,5′-AMP in response to parathyroid hormone, *J. Clin. Invest.*, **48:**1832, 1969.

430. Agus, Z. S., J. B. Puschett, D. Senesky, and M. Goldberg: Mode of action of parathyroid hormone and cyclic adenosine 3′,5′-monophosphate on renal tubular phosphate reabsorption in the dog, *J. Clin. Invest.*, **50:**617–626, 1971.

431. Augus, Z. S., L. B. Gardener, L. H. Beck, and M. Goldberg: Effects of parathyroid hormone on renal tubular reabsorption of calcium, sodium and phosphate, *Am. J. Physiol.*, **224:**1143–1148, 1973.

432. Brunette, M. G., L. Taleb, and S. Carriere: Effect of parathyroid hormone on phosphate reabsorption along the nephron of the rat, *Am. J. Physiol.*, **225:**1076–1081, 1973.

433. Kinne, R., L. Schlatz, E. Kinne-Saffran, and I. Schwartz: Distribution of membrane-bound cyclic AMP-dependent protein kinase in plasma membranes of cells of the kidney cortex, *J. Membr. Biol.*, **24:**145–159, 1975.

434. Shlatz, L., I. Schwartz, E. Kinne-Saffran, and R. Kinne: Distribution of parathyroid hormone-stimulated adenylate cyclase in plasma membranes of cells of the kidney cortex, *J. Membr. Biol.*, **24:**131–144, 1975.

435. Hoffmann, N., M. Thees, and R. Kinne: Phosphate transport by isolated renal brush border vesicles, *Pflügers Arch.*, **362:**147–156, 1976.

436. Ullrich, K. J., G. Rumrich, and S. Klöss: Phosphate transport in the proximal convolution of the rat kidney. I. Tubular heterogeneity, effect of parathyroid hormone in acute and chronic parathyroidectomized animals and effect of phosphate diet, *Pflügers Arch.*, **372:**269–274, 1977.

437. Broadus, A. E., J. E. Mahaffey, F. C. Bartter, and R. M. Neer: Nephrogenous cyclic adenosine monophosphate as a parathyroid function test, *J. Clin. Invest.*, **60:**771, 1977.

438. Marcus, R., J. F. Wilbur, and G. D. Aurbach: Parathyroid hormone-sensitive adenyl cyclase from the renal cortex of a patient with pseudohypoparathyroidism, *J. Clin. Endocrinol. Metab.*, **33:**537, 1971.

439. Sinha, T. K., S. Miller, J. Fleming, R. Khairi, J. Edmondson, C. C. Johnston, Jr., and N. H. Bell: Demonstration of a diurnal variation in serum parathyroid hormone in primary and secondary hyperparathyroidism, *J. Clin. Endocrinol. Metab.*, **41:**1009–1013, 1975.

440. Rasmussen, H., H. DeLuca, and C. Arnaud, et al.: The relationship between vitamin D and parathyroid hormone, *J. Clin. Invest.*, **42:**1940–1946, 1963.

441. Gonnerman, W. A., W. K. Ramp, and S. U. Toverud: Vitamin D, dietary calcium and parathyroid hormone interactions in chicks, *Endocrinology*, **96:**275–281, 1975.

442. Au, W. Y. W., and L. G. Raisz: Restoration of parathyroid responsiveness in vitamin D-deficient rats by parenteral calcium or dietary lactose, *J. Clin. Invest.*, **46:**1572–1578, 1967.

443. Jonxis, J. H. P.: Some investigations on rickets, *J. Pediatr.*, **59:**607–615, 1961.

444. Stögmann, W., and J. A. Fischer: Pseudohypoparathyroidism: Disappearance of the resistance to parathyroid extract during treatment with vitamin D, *Am. J. Med.*, **59:**140–144, 1975.

445. Suh, S. M., D. Fraser, and S. W. Kooh: Pseudohypoparathyroidism: Responsiveness to parathyroid extract induced by vitamin D_2 therapy, *J. Clin. Endocrinol. Metab.*, **30:**609–614, 1970.

446. Metz, S. A., D. J. Baylink, M. R. Hughes, M. R. Haussler, and R. P. Robertson: Selective deficiency of 1,25-dihydroxycholecalciferol—a cause of isolated skeletal resistance to parathyroid hormone, *N. Engl. J. Med.*, **297:**1084–1090, 1977.

447. Werder, E. A., H. P. Kind, F. Egert, J. A. Fischer, and A. Prader: Effective long-term treatment of pseudohypoparathyroidism with oral 1α-hydroxy- and 1,25-dihydroxycholecalciferol, *J. Pediatr.*, **89:**266–268, 1976.

448. Horiuchi, N., T. Suda, H. Takahashi, E. Shimazawa, and E. Ogata: In vivo evidence for the intermediary role of 3′,5′-cyclic AMP in parathyroid hormone-induced stimulation of 1α,25-

dihydroxyvitamin D_3 synthesis in rats, *Endocrinology,* **101:**969–974, 1977.

449. Albright, F., A. P. Forbes, and P. H. Henneman: Pseudopseudohypoparathyroidism, *Trans. Assoc. Am. Physicians,* **65:**337, 1952.

450. Bartter, F. C.: Pseudohypoparathyroidism and pseudopseudohypoparathyroidism, in J. B. Stanbury, J. B. Wyngaarden, and D. S. Fredrickson (eds.), *The Metabolic Basis of Inherited Disease,* 2d ed., McGraw-Hill Book Company, New York, 1966, p. 1024.

451. Mann, J. B., S. Altermann, and A. G. Hills: Albright's hereditary osteodystrophy comprising pseudohypoparathyroidism and pseudopseudohypoparathyroidism: With a report of two cases representing the complete syndrome occurring in two successive generations, *Ann. Intern. Med.,* **56:**315, 1962.

452. Palubinskas, A. J., and H. Davies: Calcification of the basal ganglia of the brain, *Am. J. Roentgenol. Radium Ther. Nucl. Med.,* **82:**806, 1959.

453. Mautalen, C.A., J. F. Dymling, and M. Horwith: Pseudohypoparathyroidism 1942–1966. A negative progress report, *Am. J. Med.,* **42:**977, 1967.

454. Werder, E. A., R. Illig, S. Bernasconi, H. Kind, A. Prader, J. A. Fischer, and A. Fanconi: Excessive thyrotropin response to thyrotropin releasing hormone in pseudohypoparathyroidism, *Pediatr. Res.,* **9:**12, 1975.

455. Deftos, L. J., D. Powell, J. G. Parthemore, and J. T. Potts, Jr.: Secretion of calcitonin in hypocalcemic states in man, *J. Clin. Invest.,* **52:**3109, 1973.

456. Drezner, M., F. A. Neelson, and H. E. Lebovitz: Pseudohypoparathyroidism Type II: A possible defect in the reception of the cyclic AMP signal, *N. Engl. J. Med.,* **289:**1056, 1973.

457. Rodriguez, H. J., H. Villarreal, S. Klahr, and E. Slatopolsky: Pseudohypoparathyroidism Type II: Restoration of normal renal responsiveness to parathyroid hormone by calcium administration, *J. Clin. Endocrinol. Metab.,* **39:**693, 1974.

458. Bartter, F. C., P. Pronove, J. R. Gill, Jr., and R. C. MacCardle: Hyperplasia of the juxtaglomerular complex with hyperaldosteronism and hypokalemic alkalosis, *Am. J. Med.,* **33:**811, 1962.

459. Gill, J. R., Jr., J. C. Frolich, R. E. Bowden, A. A. Taylor, H. P. Keiser, H. W. Seyberth, J. A. Oates, and F. C. Bartter: Bartter's syndrome: A disorder characterized by high urinary prostaglandins and a dependence of hyperreninemia on prostaglandin synthesis, *Am. J. Med.,* **61:**43, 1976.

460. Fichman, M. P., N. Telfer, P. Zia, P. Speckart, M. Golub, and R. Rude: Role of prostaglandins in the pathogenesis of Bartter's syndrome, *Am. J. Med.,* **60:**785, 1976.

461. Norby, L., W. Flamenbaum, R. Lentz, and P. Ramwell: Prostaglandins and aspirin therapy in Bartter's syndrome, *Lancet,* **2:**604, 1976.

462. Lechi, A., G. Covi, C. Lechi, F. Mantero, and L. A. Scuro: Urinary kallikrein excretion in Bartter's syndrome, *Lancet,* **2:**604, 1976.

463. Dray, F.: Bartter's syndrome: Contrasting patterns of prostaglandin excretion in children and adults, *Clin. Sci. Molec. Med.,* **54:**115–118, 1978.

464. Cannon, P. J., J. M. Leeming, S. C. Sommer, R. W. Winter, and J. H. Laragh: Juxtaglomerular cell hyperplasia and secondary hyperaldosteronism (Bartter's syndrome): A re-evaluation of the pathophysiology, *Medicine,* **47:**107, 1968.

465. Brackett, N. C., Jr., M. Koppel, R. E. Randall, Jr., and W. P. Nixon: Hyperplasia of the juxtaglomerular complex with secondary aldosteronism without hypertension (Bartter's syndrome), *Am. J. Med.,* **44:**803, 1968.

466. Chaimovitz, C., J. Levi, O. S. Better, L. Oslander, and A. Benderli: Studies on the site of renal salt loss in a patient with Bartter's syndrome, *Pediatr. Res.,* **7:**89, 1973.

467. Erkelens, D. W., and L. W. Statius Van Eps: Bartter's syndrome and erythrocytosis, *Am. J. Med.,* **55:**711, 1973.

468. Solomon, R. J., and R. S. Brown: Bartter's syndrome: New insights into pathogenesis and treatment, *Am. J. Med.,* **59:**575, 1975.

469. Modlinger, R. S., G. L. Nicolis, L. R. Krakoff, and J. L. Gabrilove: Some observations on the pathogenesis of Bartter's syndrome, *N. Engl. J. Med.,* **289:**1022, 1973.

470. Greenberg, A. J., J. M. Arboit, M. I. New, and H. G. Worthen: Normotensive secondary hyperaldosteronism, *J. Pediatr.,* **69:**719, 1966.

471. Trygstad, C. W., J. A. Mangos, M. B. Bloodworth, Jr., and C. C. Lobeck: A sibship with Bartter's syndrome: Failure of total adrenalectomy to correct the potassium wasting, *Pediatrics,* **44:**234, 1969.

472. White, M. G.: Bartter's syndrome: A manifesta-

tion of renal tubular defects, *Arch. Intern. Med.,* **129:**41, 1972.

473. Cannon, P. J., R. P. Ames, and J. H. Laragh: Relation between potassium balance and aldosterone secretion in normal subjects and in patients with hypertensive or renal tubular disease, *J. Clin. Invest.,* **45:**865, 1966.

474. Brunner, J. R., L. Baer, J. E. Sealey, J. G. G. Ledingham, and J. H. Laragh: The influence of potassium loading and potassium deprivation on plasma renin in normal and hypertensive subjects, *J. Clin. Invest.,* **49:**2128, 1970.

475. Dluhy, R. G., L. Axelrod, R. H. Underwood, and G. H. Williams: Studies of the control of plasma aldosterone concentration in normal man. II. Effect of dietary potassium and acute potassium infusion, *J. Clin. Invest.,* **51:**1950, 1972.

476. Gann, D. S., C. S. Delea, J. R. Gill, Jr., J. P. Thomas, and F. C. Bartter: Control of aldosterone secretion by change of body potassium in normal man, *Am. J. Physiol.,* **207:**104, 1964.

477. Goodman, A. D., A. J. Vagnucci, and P. M. Hartroft: Pathogenesis of Bartter's syndrome, *N. Engl. J. Med.,* **281:**1435, 1969.

478. Louis, W. J., and A. E. Doyle: The effects of varying doses of angiotensin on renal function and blood pressure in man and dogs, *Clin. Sci.,* **29:**489, 1965.

479. Bartter, F. C.: The syndrome of juxtaglomerular hyperplasia with aldosteronism, hypokalemic alkalosis and normal blood pressure, *Birth Defects,* **X:**104, 1974.

480. Gill, J. R., Jr., and F. C. Bartter: Evidence for a prostaglandin-independent defect in chloride reabsorption in the loop of Henle as a proximal cause of Bartter's syndrome, *Am. J. Med.,* **65:**766–772, 1978.

481. Kurtzman, N. A., and L. F. Gutierrez: The pathophysiology of Bartter's syndrome, *JAMA,* **234:**758, 1975.

482. Burg, M., and N. Green: Function of the thick ascending limb of Henle's loop, *Am. J. Physiol.,* **224:**659, 1973.

483. Rocha, A. S., and J. P. Kokko: Sodium chloride and water transport in the medullary thick ascending limb of Henle. Evidence for active chloride transport, *J. Clin. Invest.,* **52:**612, 1973.

484. Wright, F.: Sites and mechanisms of potassium transport along the renal tubule, *Kidney Int.,* **11:**415, 1977.

485. Burg, M., and N. Green: Effect of ethacrynic acid on the thick ascending limb of Henle's loop, *Kidney Int.,* **4:**301, 1973.

486. Burg, M., L. Stoner, J. Cardinal, and N. Green: Furosemide effect on isolated perfused tubules, *Am. J. Physiol.,* **225:**119, 1973.

487. Durate, C. G., F. Chomety, and G. Giebisch: Effect of amiloride, ouabain, and furosemide on distal tubular function in the rat, *Am. J. Physiol.,* **221:**632, 1971.

488. Vander, A. J., and J. Carlson: Mechanism of the effects of furosemide on renin secretion in anesthetized dogs, *Circ. Res.,* **XXV:**145, 1969.

489. Cooke, R. C., T. C. Brown, B. J. Zacherle, and W. G. Walker: The effect of altered sodium concentration in the distal nephron segments on renin release, *J. Clin. Invest.,* **49:**1630, 1970.

490. Norby, L. H., G. J. Kaloyanides, and A. L. Mark: On the pathogenesis of Bartter's syndrome, *Clin. Res.,* **XXII:**540A, 1974.

491. Chonko, A. M., J. H. Stein, and T. F. Ferris: Renin and the kidney, *Nephron,* **15:**279, 1975.

492. Morris, R. C., Jr., R. R. McInnes, C. J. Epstein, A. Sebastian, and C. R. Scriver: Genetic and metabolic injury of the kidney, in B. M. Brenner and F. C. Rector (eds.), *The Kidney,* vol. II, W. B. Saunders Company, Philadelphia, 1976.

493. Kunau, R. T., and J. H. Stein: Disorders of hypo- and hyperkalemia, *Clin. Nephrol.,* **7:**173, 1977.

494. Diezi, J., P. Michoud, J. Aceves, and G. Giebisch: Micropuncture study of electrolyte transport across papillary collecting duct of the rat, *Am. J. Physiol.,* **224:**623, 1973.

495. Abbrecht, P. H., and A. J. Vander: Effects of chronic potassium deficiency on plasma renin activity, *J. Clin. Invest.,* **49:**1510, 1970.

496. Brunner, H. R., L. Baer, J. E. Sealey, J. G. G. Ledingham, and J. H. Laragh: The influence of potassium administration and of potassium deprivation on plasma renin in normal and hypertensive subjects, *J. Clin. Invest.,* **49:**2128, 1970.

497. Galvez, O. G., W. H. Bay, B. W. Roberts, and T. F. Ferris: The hemodynamic effects of potassium deficiency in the dog, *Circ. Res.,* **49** (suppl. 1):1–11, 1977.

498. Zusman, R. M., and H. R. Keiser: Prostaglandin biosynthesis by rabbit renomedullary interstitial

cells in tissue culture, *J. Clin. Invest.*, **60**:215, 1977.

499. Anderson, R. J., T. Berl, K. M. McDonald, and R. W. Schrier: Prostaglandins: Effects on blood pressure, renal blood flow, sodium and water excretion, *Kidney Int.*, **10**:205, 1976.

500. Larrson, C., P. Weber, and E. Anggard: Arachidonic acid increases and indomethacin decreases plasma renin activity in the rabbit, *Eur. J. Pharmacol.*, **28**:391, 1974.

501. Vander, A. J.: Direct effects of prostaglandin on renal function and renin release in anesthetized dog, *Am. J. Physiol.*, **214**:218, 1968.

502. Romero, J. C., C. L. Dunlap, and C. G. Strong: The effect of indomethacin and other anti-inflammatory drugs on the renin-angiotensin system, *J. Clin. Invest.*, **58**:282, 1976.

503. Werning, C., W. Vetter, P. Weidmann, U. Schwiekert, D. Stiel, and W. Siegenthaler: Effect of prostaglandin E_1 on renin in the dog, *Am. J. Physiol.*, **220**:852, 1971.

504. Verberckmoes, R., B. van Damme, J. Clement, A. Amery, and P. Michielsen: Bartter's syndrome with hyperplasia of renomedullary cells: Successful treatment with indomethacin, *Kidney Int.*, **9**:302, 1976.

505. Vane, J. R., and J. C. McGiff: Possible contributions of endogenous prostaglandins to the control of blood pressure, *Circ. Res.*, **36, 37** (suppl. 1):68, 1975.

506. Gould, A. B., L. T. Skeggs, and J. R. Kahn: Presence of renin activity in blood vessel walls, *J. Exp. Med.*, **119**:389, 1964.

507. Roschthal, J., R. Boucher, J. M. Rojo-Ortega, and J. Genest: Renin activity in aortic tissues of the rat, *Can. J. Physiol. Pharmacol.*, **47**:53, 1969.

508. Swales, J. D., and H. Thurston: Generation of angiotensin II at peripheral vascular level: Studies using angiotensin II antisera, *Clin. Sci. Molec. Med.*, **45**:691, 1973.

509. Thurston, H., and J. D. Swales: Action of angiotensin antagonists and antiserum upon the pressor responses to renin: Further evidence for the local generation of angiotensin II, *Clin. Sci. Molec. Med.*, **46**:273, 1974.

510. Aiken, J. W., and J. R. Vane: Intrarenal prostaglandin release attenuates the renal vasoconstrictor activity of angiotensin, *J. Pharmacol. Exp. Ther.*, **184**:678, 1973.

511. Blair-West, J. R., J. P. Coghland, D. A. Denton, J. W. Funder, B. A. Scoggins, and R. D. Wright: Inhibition of renin secretion by systemic and intrarenal angiotensin infusion, *Am. J. Phsyiol.*, **220**:1039, 1971.

512. Shade, R. E., J. O. Davis, J. A. Johnson, R. W. Gotshall, and W. S. Spielman: Mechanism of action of angiotensin II and antidiuretic hormone on renin secretion, *Am. J. Physiol.*, **224**:926, 1973.

513. Williams, W. M., J. C. Frolich, A. S. Nies, and J. A. Oates: Urinary prostaglandins: Site of entry into renal tubular fluid, *Kidney Int.*, **11**:256, 1977.

514. Stokes, J. B., and J. P. Kokko: Inhibition of sodium transport by prostaglandin E_2 across the isolated, perfused rabbit collecting tubule, *J. Clin. Invest.*, **59**:1099, 1977.

515. Grantham, J. J., and J. Orloff: Effect of prostaglandin E_1 on the permeability response of the isolated collecting tubule to vasopressin, adenosine 3′,5′-monophosphate, and theophylline, *J. Clin. Invest.*, **47**:1154, 1968.

516. Anderson, R. J., T. Berl, K. M. McDonald, and R. W. Schrier with tech. assist. of A. McCool and L. Gilbert: Evidence for an in vivo antagonism between vasopressin and prostaglandin in the mammalian kidney, *J. Clin. Invest.*, **56**:420, 1975.

19

Clinical disorders of calcium, phosphorus, and magnesium metabolism

A. M. PARFITT / M. KLEEREKOPER

INTRODUCTION AND SCOPE

This chapter presents the clinical phenomena which result from disturbances in the divalent-ion homeostatic system described in Chap. 8, and their investigation, diagnosis, and treatment. Three unifying principles underlie the discussion of pathogenesis: first, the remodeling cell system in bone regulates bone mass but not plasma calcium; second, a separate homeostatic system in bone controls plasma calcium; third, tubular reabsorption expressed as Tm/GFR (glomerular filtration rate) is the major mechanism determining the plasma levels of phosphate and magnesium and enables plasma calcium to be controlled with minimal changes in bone mass.

As with other electrolytes, clinical effects can result either from changes in the plasma concentration of a substance or from changes in the amount of the substance present in the body or in some body compartments. Just as hyponatremia and increased total body sodium can coexist, so can hypocalcemia and increased total body calcium, since the concentration and content of calcium, as of sodium, are regulated independently. The content of the soft tissues is more closely related to plasma concentrations than the content of bone, so that this dichotomy is less evident for phosphate and magnesium than for calcium, al-

though in the short term the intracellular and extracellular levels may change in opposite directions. The concentrations and amounts of substances in the urine are not homeostatically regulated, so that abnormalities in urinary excretion are of interest mainly for the light they shed on the recognition or understanding of abnormalities in body content or concentration.

LABORATORY INVESTIGATION OF THE DIVALENT-ION HOMEOSTATIC SYSTEM

The rationale of commonly used tests will be described. Some specialized procedures are covered in relation to specific diagnostic situations, and detailed protocols are given as an appendix.

PLASMA LEVELS OF CALCIUM, PHOSPHATE, AND MAGNESIUM

Plasma calcium[1] and its fractions

The determination of calcium in the laboratory is subject to many errors. In addition to the usual

---

[1] Plasma is the fluid phase of blood which circulates in vivo. Use of this term does not imply a choice of any particular fluid for analysis.

instrumental, technical, and human problems which can be detected by an adequate quality control system, there are several sources of contamination which may produce false elevation in individual samples even though overall quality control is undisturbed (1, 2). Falsely low results are less common so that in general when several results are discrepant the lowest is most likely to be correct. The overall precision of calcium determination with automated multichannel instruments such as the SMAC is in most laboratories as good as or better than manual methods, but erroneous high or low values are more common especially in patients with liver or renal failure or in lipemic or hemolyzed specimens. Any abnormal result should therefore be checked by a different method before any further action is taken. The blood for this should be drawn in the early morning after an overnight fast because dietary calcium produces an increase in plasma calcium of up to 0.15 mmol/L in some persons (3).

The total plasma calcium (Table 8-5) comprises three components—free ionized, complexed, and protein bound—of which only the first is subject to homeostatic control. These three components can vary independently, so that total calcium, like total leukocyte count, is an artifact of measurement convenience, not a real biologic quantity. If plasma proteins or the various complexing anions are diluted by an increase, or concentrated by a decrease, in plasma water, the ionized calcium changes in the same direction. Conversely if there is a gain or loss of protein or complexing anions by the plasma, ionized calcium changes in the opposite direction. But these changes are transient. If the homeostatic control system is functioning normally, ionized calcium will soon be restored to its previous level, so that chronic changes in the concentration of binding proteins or of complexing anions, however produced, lead to changes in protein-bound or in complexed calcium and consequently changes in total calcium but not in ionized calcium. Ideally, free ionized calcium would be measured routinely but this is not yet practicable. The available methods for this will be described first, and then various ways of estimating ionized calcium indirectly by simultaneous measurements of total calcium and total protein or albumin.

Direct measurement of plasma ionized calcium. At present, only the electrometric methods are likely to become routinely available. These depend on measuring the potential difference generated by contact of the unknown solution with an ion-specific electrode, and are therefore analogous to the measurement of pH. In the United States two suitable instruments are available—the Orion SS-20[2] using a flowthrough electrode system which is an automated version of the 99-20 (2) and the Schwartz System (4) which uses a solid-state dip electrode.[3] Both are designed for use with whole blood, serum, or plasma. The Orion instrument requires specimens to be handled anaerobically, while with the AMT instrument the pH of all specimens is adjusted to 7.4, so that specimens which have been allowed contact with air can be used. No direct comparison of these instruments has been reported, so that any advantage claimed for one system over the other remains unsubstantiated. The normal range for plasma ionized calcium measured on serum in our laboratory using the Orion system is 1.00 to 1.15 mmol/L. Values using plasma are approximately 5 percent lower than values using serum due to complexing of a small fraction of the ionized calcium by heparin. Normal ranges from different laboratories using the same equipment rarely differ by more than 5 to 10 percent.

Indirect estimation of plasma ionized calcium (5). Changes in plasma protein, particularly albumin, whether due to changes in hydration, posture, or nutrition, are responsible for about half the biologic variation in total calcium between different individuals (6), and for most of the variation on different occasions in the same individual (7). In persons with a normal ionized calcium the fraction of total calcium which is diffusible is not constant (as is frequently stated) but varies with the protein level (Table 19-1). At a constant level of protein, variations in ionized calcium do not affect percent diffusibility.

Some way of discounting the variation in total calcium due to changes in protein is clearly essential. Measurement of ultrafiltrable or diffusi-

[2] Orion Research Inc., Cambridge, Massachusetts 02139.

[3] Applied Medical Technology (AMT), Menlo Park, California 94025.

Table 19-1. Some effects of protein binding of calcium in normal subjects and patients with high or low plasma calcium

| | FREE IONIC CALCIUM | |
	NORMAL	ABNORMAL
Major source of variation in total calcium	Protein	Calcium
Diffusible calcium as percent of total	Variable	Stable
Correlation between total and ionic calcium	No	Yes

ble calcium will approximate ionized calcium but require meticulous care to avoid gross errors. It is desirable to standardize the conditions under which the blood is drawn. Increased venous pressure due to venous occlusion concentrates the plasma proteins by in vivo ultrafiltration across the wall of the vein into the interstitial space. Ideally, use of a tourniquet should be omitted, but this may make it difficult to get enough blood. Standing increases the venous pressure in the legs so that ideally the patients should be recumbent for 30 min before blood is drawn but this is not usually feasible for outpatients. Even if these precautions could be universally applied, they would not eliminate changes in plasma protein due to variation in sodium and water balance or to disease. The most accurate indirect method is by means of the McClean-Hasting nomogram based on the frog heart method (Fig. 8-1) (5). A formula which agrees well with the nomogram for total calcium values between 1.5 and 3.5 mmol/L is

$$Ca_c = \frac{Ca_m}{(0.55 + /\frac{TP}{16})}$$

where Ca_c = corrected total calcium (mmol/L)
$\quad Ca_m$ = measured total calcium
$\quad TP$ = measured total protein (g/dL)

Although objections can be raised against these and other methods (8, 9), they are all more accurate than making no correction at all. Hypoproteinemia should no longer be regarded as a cause of hypocalcemia, but as a compounding variable the effect of which must be eliminated. Routine protein correction largely eliminates variation due to posture or to the technique of venipuncture, and greatly reduces the likelihood of misclassifying a result as normal or abnormal (10).

Indirect estimates of ionized calcium are still necessary for routine use, but direct measure is especially important in the neonatal period (11),

whenever the complexed calcium is likely to be raised, as in chronic renal failure (8), when values for total protein or albumin are very high or very low, and in the presence of some abnormal globulins with unexpectedly high calcium-binding capacity (12). Finally, borderline hypercalcemia may be identified with greater certainty with the ionized than the corrected total calcium.

Statistical considerations. The variation among a set of single measurements has three components (13)—analytical variation, circadian and day-to-day variation in the same person (intraindividual variation), and true biologic variation between persons (interindividual variation). In the most careful hands and with replicate determinations almost complete elimination of analytical variation may be possible (1) with normal ranges for plasma calcium such as 2.40 ± 0.08 mmol/L, equivalent to a ±2 S.D. (standard deviation) range of 2.24 to 2.56 mmol/L and a CV[4] (coefficient of variation) of 3.3 percent. This is only marginally more than the CV due to biologic variation alone, but few laboratories can attain this degree of precision. More commonly the S.D. is greater, e.g., 2.40 ± 0.12 with a ±2 S.D. range of 2.16 to 2.64 mmol/L and a CV of 5 percent.

With any continuous variable it is necessary to think in quantitative rather than in categorical terms. For example, if the so-called upper limit of normal is 2.64 mmol/L, a "normal" value of 2.60 obviously has much more in common with an "abnormal" value of 2.68 than it does with another "normal" value of 2.20. The means of a number of sets of successive measurements in different normal subjects will vary over a narrower range than will the individual measurements. Such a set of results in a patient should be considered as a whole, by comparing the mean

---

[4] Coefficient of variation is the standard deviation expressed as a percentage of the mean.

and its standard error with the reference range appropriate to the number of tests. The difference between the quantitative and categorical approaches is shown in Fig. 19-1.

Plasma phosphate and magnesium

For all normal purposes only the total plasma inorganic phosphate need be determined. Measurement in the fasting state is more important than for calcium because the plasma phosphate is raised significantly by ingestion of phosphate-containing foods and lowered significantly by ingestion of carbohydrate. The relative proportions of monovalent and divalent ions can be calculated from the pH, but measurement of the other ionic species (Table 8-7) is neither practicable nor necessary. In an occasional patient with extreme

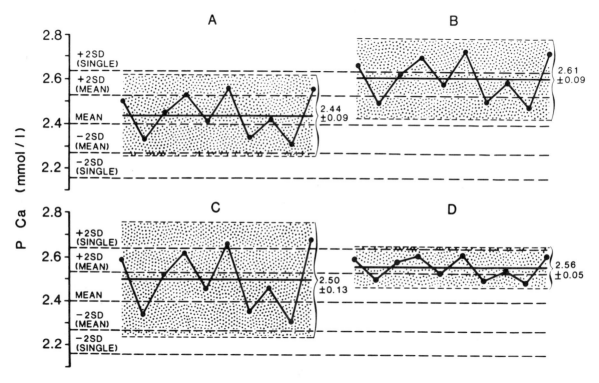

Figure 19-1. Four hypothetical sets of values for plasma calcium obtained on 10 consecutive days. In *A*, the mean of the set is within the normal [±2 S.D. (standard deviation)] range of means and the ±2 S.D. range of the set is within the normal range for a single measurement. The set would be described as normal by both the quantitative and categorical approaches. In *B*, the mean of the set is outside the normal range of means but is inside the normal range for a single measurement. The upper boundary of the ±2 S.D. range of the set is outside the normal range for a single measurement. By the quantitative approach the set would be described as having an upward shift of the mean of 0.21 mmol/L with normal variability about the mean. By the categorical approach the set would be described as oscillating between hypercalcemia and normocalcemia. In *C*, the mean of the set is within the normal range of means but the S.D. is higher than normal. The upper boundary of the ±2 S.D. range of the set is above the normal range for a single estimation. By the quantitative approach, the set would be described as having a normal mean with increased variability and by the categorical approach as intermittent hypercalcemia. In *D*, the mean of the set is above the normal range of means, but the S.D. is low so that the upper boundary of the ±2 S.D. range of the set is close to the upper boundary of the normal range for a single estimation, and each individual measurement is within that range. By the quantitative approach, the set would be described as having an upward shift of 0.16 mmol/L in mean value, with decreased variability, and by the categorical approach as normal. The difference in means between set *C* and set *D* is significant ($P < 0.02$).

hypercalcemia or hyperphosphatemia, or in studying the pathogenesis of soft tissue calcification, measurement of ultrafiltrable phosphate may be helpful.

There is significant protein binding of magnesium, and the free ionic magnesium would be the ideal quantity to measure, but no practicable method is yet available. Total magnesium can be corrected for total protein on the same lines as for calcium:

$$Mg_c = \frac{Mg_m}{0.76 + TP/30}$$

but the magnitude of the correction is usually so small that it could only rarely be of clinical importance.

PARATHYROID HORMONE

The only components of the major feedback loop which regulates plasma calcium are plasma calcium itself and PTH (parathyroid hormone). Both components must be known to understand the causes of either hyper- or hypocalcemia, but there are several problems in the usual measurement of PTH by radioimmunoassay. Some of these result from the lack of pure human hormone; this ideally should be used to generate antibodies and in the assay, both as a labeled reagent and as a standard (6). Many commercial PTH assays do not routinely include serial dilutions, so that no assurance can be given that displacement curves for standard and unknown are parallel. Other problems result from immunochemical heterogeneity such that native hormone, active and inactive fragments, and possibly precursor molecules may all contribute to the total immunoassayable material. For all these reasons adequate quality control is both more difficult and more important than when measuring a single substance of defined chemical composition (14). Although results may be expressed in terms of weight of bovine standard, they are only expressions of immunologic reactivity, and should be interpreted to mean that the unknown serum has displaced labeled hormone from antibody to the same extent as the stated quantity of the standard. The symbol iPTH is often used to reinforce this caution.

Characteristics of different PTH radioimmunoassays

Most clinically useful assays use antisera directed predominantly against immunogenic site(s) which are within the carboxy-terminal region of the PTH molecule (6). These react both with secreted hormone and with biologically inactive C-terminal fragments which have a much longer half-life. In the steady state, the plasma concentration of the C-terminal fragment will depend on the secretion rate of PTH, the fractional rate constant for cleavage of secreted hormone to fragment, and the metabolic clearance rate of the fragment (15). Not only the rate, but the site of cleavage may be important. Some biologically inactive fragments may be generated within the gland (16), thus contributing to the level of iPTH but not to the secretion of hormone. However, if cleavage and clearance are held constant, the level of C-terminal fragment will be proportional to the secretion rate of biologically active hormone. This is so even though the fragment itself is biologically inactive, and the concentration of the fragment may be 10 to 50 times the concentration of secreted hormone (15). Despite this the sensitivity of many assays is poor, a significant number of normal persons having no detectable iPTH (14).

Any change in the rate of metabolic clearance or in the rate of cleavage will alter the relationship between PTH secretion rate and level of iPTH, but so far this has been shown to occur only in chronic renal failure (17). The hormone is metabolized by the kidney, so that loss of functioning renal tissue will decrease its metabolic clearance rate (18). But since the hormone is part of a feedback loop, this alone will not raise the plasma level significantly, because the normal control mechanism would ensure that secretion rate were reduced in parallel. For example, hypothyroidism reduces the metabolic clearance rate of cortisol, but the secretion rate falls also, and only if exogenous hormone is provided at a constant rate does impaired clearance lead to clinical evidence of cortisol excess (19). But the C-terminal fragment is also metabolized by the kidney

(18), and decreased metabolic clearance of a biologically inactive substance will inevitably cause an increase in its plasma concentration. Consequently iPTH using a C-terminal assay will increase hyperbolically as GFR declines, irrespective of any change in PTH secretion rate, just like the concentration of creatinine. In renal failure a C-terminal PTH assay is mainly an expensive and indirect renal function test, and a high value may coexist with subnormal PTH secretion as judged by every other criterion. But if renal clearance does not change with time (as in most patients on chronic hemodialysis) serial changes in C-terminal iPTH will correctly identify the direction, although not the magnitude, of change in secretion rate.

Some assays are directed predominantly against immunogenic site(s) within the amino-terminal region of the molecule. These react both with secreted hormone and with any biologically active fragments which might be present, although none has so far been detected with certainty (15). Such N-terminal assays are much better suited to detect acute changes in hormone secretion rate, but in general are even less sensitive than C-terminal assays. Although assays are usually classified for convenience as predominantly C terminal or N terminal, there are at least three immunogenic sites in the PTH molecule, and every antiserum has a unique pattern of reactivity with the various molecular species present in the circulation.

Despite these problems clinically useful assays for PTH have been established, because the diagnostic value of a test depends solely on its predictive and correlative properties. C-terminal assays are useful in the diagnosis of primary hyperparathyroidism, and significant correlations have been demonstrated with plasma calcium level (6), size of gland at parathyroid surgery (14), Tm_p/ GFR, nephrogenous AMP (cyclic adenosine monophosphate), and degree of renal failure (14). The validity of these correlations and the diagnostic value of the test are not affected by the uncertainty about precisely what is measured, but this uncertainty imposes some limitations on the use of the assay to understand normal physiology or the pathogenesis of disease (15). It is evident that a C-terminal iPTH result is only an indirect estimate of hormone secretion rate, and conclu-

sions drawn should be supported wherever possible by some in vivo assessment of biologic activity. Many of these problems may disappear when cytochemical assays of greatly increased sensitivity and specificity become more widely available (20).

Relationship of PTH level to plasma calcium

The interactions between calcium and PTH in a feedback loop depend on two separate functional relationships (6). First, primary changes in plasma ionized calcium produce secondary changes in

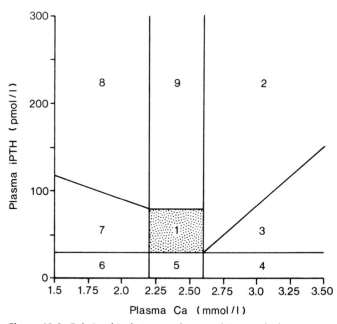

Figure 19-2. Relationship between plasma calcium and plasma iPTH (parathyroid hormone) showing diagnostic significance of various zones; in reality, the boundaries are much less clearly defined than are depicted. (1) Normal range, (2) primary hyperparathyroidism, (3) ectopic hyperparathyroidism, (4) nonparathyroid hypercalcemia, (5) increased dietary intake of calcium (depending on sensitivity of assay may also include normal range), (6) primary hypoparathyroidism, (7) partial hypoparathyroidism with increased proportion of biologically inactive metabolites; also magnesium depletion with reduced biologic effectiveness of hormone, (8) hypocalcemic (uncompensated) secondary hyperparathyroidism, (9) normocalcemic (compensated) secondary hyperparathyroidism.

Table 19-2. Diagnostic categories corresponding to various combinations of plasma calcium and iPTH results

iPTH	PLASMA CALCIUM		
	LOW	NORMAL	HIGH
Low	PTH-deficient hypoparathyroidism, magnesium intoxication	High net absorption of calcium	Nonparathyroid hypercalcemia
Normal	Magnesium depletion	Normality	Ectopic hyper-parathyroidism
High	1,25-DHCC deficiency, pseudohypoparathyroidism	Calcium depletion, increased PTH requirement	Hyperparathyroidism (primary or tertiary)

PTH in the opposite direction, so that calcium is the independent and PTH the dependent variable. Second, primary changes in PTH produce secondary changes in ionized calcium in the same direction, so that PTH is the independent and calcium the dependent variable. The interpretation of a PTH level depends on which of these relationships is dominant. Some assays show an inverse correlation between PTH and plasma calcium in normal subjects (6), suggesting that plasma calcium is driving PTH, but many assays show no correlation (14, 21), suggesting that neither relationship is dominant. But if primary changes in plasma calcium are experimentally imposed, for example by altering diet, the expected reciprocal changes in PTH will occur. By contrast, in patients with primary hyperparathyroidism all assays show a significant *direct* relationship between PTH and calcium. This is because differences in plasma calcium level between one patient and another depend mainly on differences in the secretion rate of PTH, which in turn depend on differences in tumor size and secretory activity. Using any assay which reflects steady-state PTH secretion and simultaneous plasma calcium measurement, it is possible to construct probability diagrams in which the likelihood of different clinical diagnoses varies between different diagnostic zones (Fig. 19-2 and Table 19-2).

The intermediate zones may require a dynamic rather than a static approach. The effect of an acute rise or fall in plasma calcium on PTH secretion can be determined using an N-terminal assay. For the duration of such an acute study, calcium is the independent and PTH the dependent variable (Fig. 19-3). The slope of the line relating the control and experimental points de-

pends partly on the number of functioning cells and partly on the ability of each cell to alter its rate of hormone secretion in response to a change

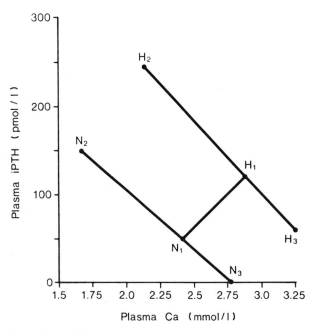

Figure 19-3. Different functional relationships between plasma Ca and PTH. N_1 marks the baseline values in a normal subject and N_2 and N_3 show the results of experimental manipulation of plasma calcium and corresponding changes in iPTH as the dependent variable. H_1 marks the baseline values in a patient with primary hyperparathyroidism, or a normal subject given excess PTH. The difference between N_1 and H_1 reflects the influence of PTH as the independent variable and calcium as the dependent variable. H_2 and H_3 show the effect of experimental manipulation of plasma calcium in the patient with hyperparathyroidism, with PTH again as the dependent variable. The slope of H_2-H_3 is greater than the slope of N_2-N_3, because of increased parathyroid cell mass.

in plasma calcium (22, 23). With a stimulation test [EDTA (ethylene diamine tetraacetic acid) infusion] an exaggerated increase in PTH level suggests an increase in the number of functioning cells (24), and a failure to increase PTH secretion suggests a reduced number of cells which are already maximally stimulated. With a suppression test (calcium infusion), a prompt fall in PTH suggests normal parathyroid function (25), and lack of suppression suggests parathyroid cell overactivity. There are several pitfalls in the interpretation of such tests (23), which are discussed further in the section on primary hyperparathyroidism.

URINARY EXCRETION AND TUBULAR REABSORPTION

The rate of urinary excretion of a divalent ion may be of interest for several reasons, each requiring a different method of data expression. When studying the pathogenesis of kidney stones, the appropriate expression is U_X (urinary concentration). The ratio of U_X to the total solute concentration (U_X/U_{osm}) of the highest mineral concentration which can occur when the urine is maximally concentrated; it has only been used for calcium (26). From the pH and the concentrations of all major cations and anions can be determined the activity products and degree of saturation with respect to various crystalline components of stones (27).

As a component of external balance, urinary excretion is a guide to intake, net absorption, or net loss from soft tissues or bone. For all these uses the appropriate expression is excretion per unit time (U_XV/t) either absolute or per kilogram of body weight. To circumvent the need for urinary collections to be both complete and accurately timed it is common practice to use creatinine as a referent. Creatinine excretion is correlated with height, weight, and muscle bulk (28) and is approximately 0.20 μmol/kg body weight per 24 h in man and 0.15 μmol/body weight per 24 h in women. Although subject to considerable day-to-day and month-to-month variation, both with a CV of about 10 to 15 percent (28), even larger errors may occur in urine collections outside a metabolic ward. Use of creatinine ratios (U_X/U_{Cr}) is reasonable for fasting or putative 24-h urine collections, but cannot be used for random specimens obtained at different times of day because of circadian variation in mineral excretion.

For assessment of tubular reabsorption the appropriate expression is excretion per unit of creatinine clearance [$U_XV/C_{Cr} = U_X/U_{Cr}(P_{Cr})$]. C_{Cr} (creatinine clearance) is the most convenient estimate of GFR glomerular filtration rate), an approximate index of the number of functioning nephrons. As explained in Chap. 8, tubular reabsorption per unit of creatinine clearance (TR_X/C_{Cr}) is given by

$$\frac{TR_X}{C_{Cr}} = P_X - \frac{U_XV}{C_{Cr}}$$

For phosphate this quantity is numerically equal to Tm_P/GFR above the saturation threshold, which occurs when TR_P is 80 percent or less. Below the saturation threshold, Tm_P/GFR can be calculated from the mathematical representation of the splay portion of the titration curve using either a programmable calculator (6) or a nomogram (29). Tm_P/GFR can also be calculated from published data using the relationship $TR_P/C_{Cr} = \%TR_P \cdot P_{Pi}$. For magnesium there is so little splay that Tm_{Mg}/GFR can be assumed equal to TR_{Mg}/C_{Cr} with minimal error when reabsorption is normal or low. When reabsorption is increased, no formula has been devised but the observed values for $U_{Mg}V/C_{Cr}$ and P_{Mg} can be compared with the normal relationship between these quantities (Chap. 8). For calcium, tubular reabsorption cannot be expressed as a single number because of uncertainty about the correct physiologic model and the relationship between $U_{Ca}V/C_{Cr}$ and P_{Ca} must be determined graphically (Fig. 19-4). Representative values in appropriate units for each of the three methods of data expression for each divalent ion are shown in Table 19-3. Further details will be given in individual sections.

NcAMP (NEPHROGENOUS CYCLIC ADENOSINE MONOPHOSPHATE)

Urinary excretion of cAMP occurs by both glomerular filtration and tubular secretion. The filtered load of cAMP ($P_{cAMP} \cdot C_{Cr}$) is derived mainly

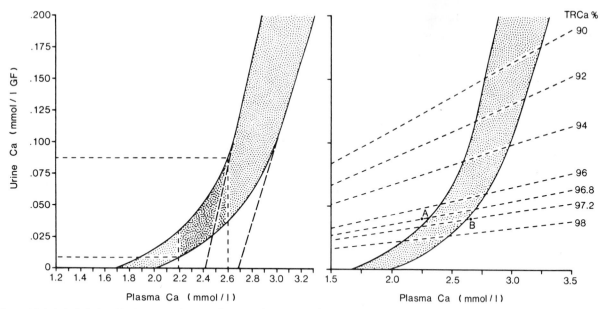

Figure 19-4. *Left.* Relationship between plasma calcium and urine calcium excretion per unit of GF. Light shaded area is the normal range; the slopes of the linear portion of the titration curves above the saturation threshold, and the shapes of the curvilinear portions below the saturation threshold, were determined by calcium infusion in normal subjects and patients with osteomalacia (Chap. 8). Heavy shaded area corresponds to normal ranges for plasma calcium of 2.2 to 2.6 mmol/L and for urine calcium of 1.25 to 12.5 mmol per 24 h, assuming a GFR of 1 dL/min. Because of these contraints the limits are closer together than usually depicted. *Right.* Correspondence between normal plasma/urine relationship depicted at left and percent tubular reabsorption, assuming that plasma calcium is 55 percent diffusible. Between point A (tubular reabsorption decreased) and point B (tubular reabsorption increased) there is a difference of only 0.5 in percent calcium reabsorption. It is evident that differences in percent reabsorption are influenced much more by change in load/GFR than by changes in reabsorption.

from the actions of catecholamines on liver, muscle, and other tissues and so is increased by exercise, emotion, sympathomimetic drugs, hyperthyroidism, and pheochromocytoma. To this is added cAMP formed within renal tubule cells as a result of activation of PTH or vasopressin, referred to as NcAMP, which is normally about one-quarter to one-half of total urinary cAMP (TcAMP) excretion (30). With impaired renal function P_{cAMP} rises as GFR falls so that the filtered load and the extrarenal contribution to TcAMP remain unchanged, but NcAMP falls in parallel with GFR (30). Although some PTH-generated cAMP enters the circulation, this is only a small fraction of the filtered load.

Like other urinary constituents either TcAMP or NcAMP can be expressed as excretion per unit time, per unit of creatinine excretion, or per unit of GFR. Of these, NcAMP/GFR is the best index

of parathyroid function (30, 31). This expression can be calculated as $TcAMP/C_{Cr} - P_{cAMP}$, analogous to similar calculations for tubular reabsorption. It eliminates variations due to the extrarenal contributions to TcAMP, correlates well with iPTH and with Tm_P/GFR, provides the best absolute separation between diagnostic groups, and can be used to compare patients with different degrees of renal failure. When related to plasma calcium NcAMP/GFR has the same diagnostic significance as iPTH, and is more accurate if renal

Table 19-3. Representative values for urinary excretion of divalent ions expressed in various ways

	CALCIUM	PHOSPHATE	MAGNESIUM
Concentration (mmol/L)	2–8	20–40	2–4
Amount (mmol/24 h)	2.5–10	25–50	2.5–5
Amount (mmol/mmol Cr)	0.2–0.8	2–4	0.2–0.4
Amount (μmol/LC$_{Cr}$)	15–60	150–300	15–30

function is impaired. The test should be conducted in the early morning fasting state during a water diuresis, which eliminates the small contribution of vasopressin as well as improving the accuracy of the urine collection. It can conveniently be combined with assessment of tubular reabsorption of phosphate, calcium, or magnesium in the same plasma and urine samples. In patients without renal failure or other causes of P_{cAMP} elevation, TcAMP/C_{Cr} provides almost as good diagnostic separation and eliminates the need for the less-precise measurement of plasma cAMP (30) but it correlates less well with iPTH and Tm_P/GFR. TcAMP/Cr gives poor absolute separation between diagnostic groups (32) but when related to plasma calcium gives almost as good discrimination as NcAMP/GFR (25). TcAMP/Cr accurately reflects rapid changes in PTH secretion in response to acute changes in plasma ionized calcium (25, 33) and so is superior to C-terminal iPTH for use in stimulation or suppression tests. Representative values for the different methods of expression with appropriate units are given in Table 19-4.

VITAMIN D

Vitamin D can be measured in blood only by inaccurate and insensitive chemical methods or by laborious bioassay, but 25-HCC (25-hydroxycholecalciferol) can be measured in plasma by either competitive protein-binding assay (34) or high-pressure liquid chromatography (35). Most assays do not separate 25-HCC from 25-HEC (25-hydroxyergocalciferol), but inclusion of both metabolites in a single result is satisfactory for most clinical purposes. 25-HEC is derived from EC (ergocalciferol) in the diet or taken as a nutritional supplement or as a medication (34). Unless

the contrary is stated, plasma 25-HCC includes both 25-HCC and 25-HEC. The plasma level of 25-HCC is the best index of total body stores of vitamin D and its metabolites. Intestinal absorption of vitamin D can be tested by measuring the plasma 25-HCC level before and 8 h after a single dose of 25 nmol/kg body weight of 25-HCC; the level should rise by at least 200 nmol/L (36). Several methods for assay of 1,25-DHCC have been developed but none is yet suitable for routine use.

CALCITONIN

Calcitonin assays using various provocative tests are essential in the diagnosis of medullary carcinoma of the thyroid and may be useful in studying the pathogenesis of osteoporosis, renal osteodystrophy, and other bone diseases, but are rarely helpful in patients with disordered mineral metabolism (37).

ASSESSMENT OF BONE TURNOVER

Measurement of bone turnover is most useful in the investigation and treatment of metabolic bone disease; it is only rarely needed in the differential diagnosis of disordered mineral metabolism but will frequently be referred to in discussions of pathogenesis. Three approaches are possible—histologic, biochemical, and radiokinetic.

Histologic methods

Turnover, defined as the fractional rate of bone volume replacement, can be measured by the in vivo double tetracycline-labeling technique which permits the bone formation rate to be related to the volume of bone in the biopsy sample. The fraction of surface engaged in resorption and formation depends on the time taken for bone cells to complete their work as well as on the rate of turnover, but such measurements can be used as indices of turnover provided that bone cell function is not greatly disturbed (38). Despite the serious sampling problems of bone biopsy, histologic indices of bone turnover correlate significantly with both biochemical and radiokinetic measurements (39).

Table 19-4. Representative values for either TcAMP (total cAMP) or NcAMP (nephrogenous cAMP) expressed in various ways

	NORMAL	HYPERPARATHYROIDISM
TcAMP nmol/min	1.5–5.0	2.0–10.0
nmol/μmol Cr	0.15–0.50	0.2–1.0
nmol/L C_{Cr}	15–50	20–100
NcAMP nmol/min	0.2–3.0	1.5–8
nmol/μmol Cr	0.02–0.30	0.15–0.80
nmol/L C_{Cr}	2–30	15–80

Biochemical methods

In general, urinary hydroxyproline excretion is an index of bone resorption and plasma alkaline phosphatase level is an index of bone formation (1). Hydroxyproline is an imino acid found only in collagen, and is formed by hydroxylation of proline after it has been incorporated into the collagen molecule (38). Hydroxyproline released by breakdown of bone is not recognized by any transfer RNA (ribonucleic acid) and so cannot be reutilized for collagen synthesis. Urinary hydroxyproline excretion can be used as an index of bone turnover subject to certain qualifications (40). First, the patient should be on a low dietary intake of gelatine (denatured collagen), beginning at least 12 h before and continuing during the urine collection. Second, the skin contains a substantial amount of collagen, and skin collagen turnover may be increased in various skin diseases and in adrenocortical overactivity, so that urinary total hydroxyproline excretion may be increased in the absence of bone disease. Third, of the hydroxyproline formed by the breakdown of collagen only between 10 and 20 percent appears in the urine. The remainder is oxidized within the liver to carbon dioxide and water, but little is known of the factors which regulate this process. Finally, only a very small fraction of total urinary hydroxyproline is normally excreted as the free imino acid; the bulk is in the form of hydroxyproline-containing peptides. A large number of such compounds have been identified, but separation into dialyzable and nondialyzable fractions is sufficient for practical purposes. The nondialyzable fraction is made up of high-molecular-weight peptides derived from the breakdown of recently formed immature soluble collagen and so reflects bone matrix formation. The dialyzable fraction comprises the small amount of free imino acid together with low-molecular-weight peptides derived from the breakdown of mature, insoluble collagen, and so reflects bone matrix resorption. Normally the dialyzable fraction is about 80 percent of the total; changes in total hydroxyproline mostly reflect changes in bone resorption but do not discriminate between normal and pathologic resorption. In healing osteitis fibrosa and in chronic renal failure, the nondialyzable fraction is relatively much larger, and values for total hydroxyproline excretion may then be misleading.

AP (alkaline phosphatase) is a family of enzymes which can release inorganic phosphate from a variety of organic phosphate substrates (40, 41). The optimum pH is much higher than ever occurs in vivo, and it is not certain that the activity measured has any physiologic function. Structurally and immunologically different AP are produced by the placenta, the biliary tract, the intestinal mucosa, and bone. The total AP level falls somewhat during early childhood, increases modestly during the adolescent growth spurt, falls substantially with the completion of growth (42), and increases slightly after 50 years (1). Below 50, the levels are 10 to 20 percent higher in males than in females. The values do not conform to a gaussian distribution and occasional high values are found in otherwise healthy persons. If the clinical context does not indicate which organ is the source of a raised AP, several techniques permit approximate estimates of whether bone or biliary phosphatase predominates, but precise numerical separation is not possible. Although skeletal AP is made by osteoblasts, there is little correlation between AP and the extent of lamellar bone formation. High levels are more often associated with increased woven bone formation as in fracture healing, Paget's disease, osteitis fibrosa, and osteoblastic metastases. A substantial increase in lamellar bone turnover in hyperthyroidism is associated with only a modest increase in AP. The AP may be normal in osteomalacia, and the reason for the more frequent increase is unknown; osteoblast function in this disease is impaired although total bone turnover may be increased. A further rise in AP is an early sign of healing, both in thyrotoxic osteopathy and in osteomalacia. The return of AP to normal is a warning sign that the dose of vitamin D may soon need to be reduced to prevent hypercalcemia.

Calcium isotope kinetics

These are mainly research tools rather than clinical methods. With serial observation of plasma, urinary, and fecal radioactivity after administration of radiocalcium, two quantities can be calculated—the size of the exchangeable pool and the accretion rate (38). Pool size reflects the level of plasma calcium, the amount of soft tissue calcium, and the amount of recently formed low-density bone, which is a function of bone turnover. The accretion rate represents the irreversible incorporation of calcium into the nonexchangeable fraction of bone calcium and includes primary mineralization, secondary mineralization, and periosteocytic mineral deposition. This corresponds approximately to organ-level bone formation determined morphologically. In osteomalacia, kinetic turnover may be increased when histologic turnover is normal or decreased. This is probably because of difficulty in separating accretion from short-term exchange in the presence of an excess of incompletely mineralized and abnormally permeable bone.

DISORDERS OF CALCIUM METABOLISM

THE CLINICAL PHYSIOLOGY OF CALCIUM

Background information is given in Chap. 8.

The regulation of total body calcium and of bone mass (38, 40)

Because almost all calcium in the body is in bone, total body calcium is determined almost entirely by bone mass. Accumulation of bone during growth occurs by enchondral ossification, which permits increase in length and creates new trabecular bone, and by net periosteal apposition and endosteal resorption, which together determine the thickness of the diaphyseal cortex. These processes, which increase the amount of bone (which is a tissue) and determine the shape of the bones (which are organs), are collectively referred to as modeling. Bone also turns over by the replacement mechanism of resorption followed by formation, referred to as remodeling; this is the only mechanism of turnover after cessation of growth. Turnover represents replacement, and so is equal to either whole body resorption or whole body formation, whichever is the smaller. Turnover as defined may be supplemented by an excess of resorption (negative bone balance) or by

an excess of formation (positive balance) or by neither (zero balance) but the deviation in balance is rarely more than 20 percent of turnover. Because of the discrete nature of bone turnover, changes in the amount of bone depend on two quantities which vary independently—the birth rate of new BRU (bone remodeling units) and the extent of remodeling imbalance, i.e., the mean net difference between total bone resorption and total bone formation within a single BRU. Remodeling imbalance is normally slightly positive on the periosteal surface, zero or slightly negative on the haversian surface, and from 10 to 30 percent negative on the endosteal surface after age 40 to 45 years. This leads to progressive thinning of trabeculae and of cortical bone from the inside, with a reduction in total bone mass of about 2 percent per annum in females for the first 5 to 10 years after the menopause, and about 1 percent per annum in females in later years and in males. Remodeling imbalance may or may not be associated with temporal uncoupling, or prolongation of the interval between completion of resorption and beginning of formation within a single BRU. There are two opposing views concerning the nature of involutional bone loss: either the bone is responding in an appropriate manner to some externally imposed constraint (such as dietary calcium deficiency), or the bone is imposing an additional load of mineral on the ECF (extracellular fluid) because of a primary defect in bone cell function. Probably both occur at different times and in different individuals. For example, the recommended dietary intake of calcium for adults in the United States is 20 mmol/day, but normal perimenopausal women need at least 30 mmol/day to remain in zero calcium balance (43). The usual response to removal of calcium to the body by any means is acceleration of bone loss in the interests of maintaining normocalcemia, rather than allowing the plasma calcium to fall in the interests of more efficient calcium conservation. On the other hand a high calcium intake may retard but certainly does not prevent involutional bone loss.

Remodeling imbalance within a single BRU can be increased either because more bone is removed (osteoclasts resorbing faster or for a longer time) or because less bone is replaced (osteoblasts forming more slowly or for a shorter time). The amount of bone removed and replaced in a BRU in cortical bone can be directly measured as the cement-line diameter and wall thickness of completed osteons, or their corresponding cross-sectional areas. The mean values of these quantities in an individual rarely depart by more than 5 to 10 percent from the population mean. Consequently, for both osteoclasts and osteoblasts the duration and rates of activity tend to vary inversely; the same probably holds true also on the cortical endosteal and trabecular surface. Within this framework, it is likely that several types of altered bone cell function contribute at different times and in different skeletal locations to both normal and abnormal bone loss. The most common response to increased demand for calcium from the skeleton is an increase in bone turnover with or without a decrease in bone formation within a single BRU. It must be emphasized that measurements of whole body bone turnover, whether by radiocalcium kinetics combined with balance studies or by urinary hydroxyproline excretion and AP, cannot provide any information about the disturbances in bone cell function which underlie remodeling imbalance within a single BRU. Whole body bone turnover is almost entirely determined by the birth rate of new BRU (activation frequency) and is quite independent of the function of individual osteoclasts and osteoblasts (38).

For a given extent of remodeling imbalance/BRU at a particular surface, the rate of loss (or gain) of bone is directly proportional to the rate of turnover, but the direction of change is not altered. However, if the extent of remodeling imbalance is sufficiently great, bone loss can be accelerated even if the rate of bone turnover is depressed. For example, an existing bone loss of 1 percent per annum will increase to 3 percent per annum if turnover increases from 10 to 30 percent per annum with no change in remodeling imbalance/BRU, or if bone turnover were halved to 5 percent per annum and remodeling imbalance increased from 10 to 60 percent, so that the osteoblasts put back only 40 percent of the bone removed instead of 90 percent in each BRU. As well as changing the rate of irreversible bone loss

in this way, turnover also influences the extent of reversible bone loss consequent on the remodeling process itself. Each BRU represents a temporary hole in the bone which will be refilled as the remodeling sequence is carried to completion. Each level of bone turnover is associated with a corresponding amount of temporarily missing bone, representing the sum total of all BRU throughout the skeleton. When bone turnover changes, the extent of temporarily missing bone changes over 3 to 6 months to the level appropriate to the new rate of bone turnover, and stays at that level for as long as the new rate of bone turnover persists. In summary, changes in bone mass which occur through the normal remodeling system depend on two independent variables—the birth rate of BRU and the extent of remodeling imbalance within a single BRU. The former reflects the rate of proliferation of precursor cells and determines the total number of osteoclasts and osteoblasts; the latter is the difference between the amount of bone removed and replaced in a single BRU, and depends on the function of individual osteoclasts and osteoblasts.

The regulation of plasma calcium

The relative importance of bone, kidney, and gut. It is a truism that for the plasma calcium to remain constant, the sum of all inputs into the ECF must balance exactly the sum of all outputs from the ECF, so that deviations in plasma calcium from normal must depend on imbalance between these various fluxes. This approach is appropriate when analyzing short-term transient changes. For example, if the plasma calcium falls, it is useful to consider where the calcium has gone, and if the plasma calcium rises, it is useful to consider where the calcium has come from. But these questions may be misleading with respect to long-term steady-state changes, since with persistent hypercalcemia or hypocalcemia, just as in the normal state, the total amount of calcium in the ECF is not changing with time.

By far the largest calcium fluxes in and out of the ECF occur at quiescent bone surfaces (about 100 mmol/day), and in the kidney by glomerular filtration and tubular reabsorption (about 200 mmol/day). The plasma calcium level is primarily determined by the level at which equilibration occurs at quiescent bone surfaces such that the total influx from ECF to bone fluid and total efflux from bone fluid to ECF are equal. This level will be increased or decreased either by an increase (or decrease) in the apparent solubility of bone mineral or by an increase (or decrease) in the outwardly directed surface calcium pump, mechanisms which are controlled principally by the synergistic effects of PTH and metabolites of CC (cholecalciferol), mainly 1,25-DHCC. The calcium homeostatic system is quite independent of bone turnover, and does not involve the activity of either osteoclasts or osteoblasts.

Although the kidney does not play the dominant regulatory role for plasma calcium that it does for plasma phosphate and magnesium, the interrelationships between plasma calcium and flow, GFR, and tubular reabsorption are nevertheless important. These can be expressed as

Filtered load or
$$P_{Ca(UF)} \times GFR = TR_{Ca} + L_{Ca} \quad (19\text{-}1)$$

Dividing through by GFR
$$P_{Ca(UF)} = \frac{TR_{Ca}}{GFR} + \frac{L_{Ca}}{GFR} \quad (19\text{-}1a)$$

For a representative value of 6 mmol/day for net absorption and urinary excretion of calcium, in the early morning fasting state TR_{Ca}/GFR would be about 1.28 mmol/L and L_{Ca}/GFR about 0.02 mmol/L, corresponding to a total excretion of 1 mmol during an 8-h period of overnight fasting. This nocturnal urinary excretion is widely believed to represent net bone resorption (44) but could easily be derived from the bone surface–perilacunar compartment, or from the interstitial fluid and connective tissue components of the exchangeable calcium pool. In the nonfasting state during the day, TR_{Ca}/GFR would be about 1.35 mmol/L and L_{Ca}/GFR about 0.05 mmol/L; during a 16-h period net absorption of 6 mmol would provide 5 mmol for urinary excretion and 1 mmol to replenish the soft tissue or bone compartments from which will be drawn the amount excreted during the subsequent 8-h nocturnal fast. Thus with normal renal function and a normal dietary

intake and absorption, the calcium load contributes only about 4 percent of the plasma ultrafiltrable calcium level during the day and about 2 percent during the night. However, it is clear from Eq. (19-1a) that this contribution will increase progressively as the GFR falls, and a combination of a modest increase in load derived either from gut or bone and a modest decrease in renal function could lead to significant hypercalcemia.

If tubular reabsorption of calcium is partitioned into the gradient-limited and capacity-limited components according to the Mioni model, the effect of load on plasma calcium is increased. According to this concept,

$$P_{Ca(UF)} = 0.4\, P_{Ca(UF)} + \frac{Tm_{Ca}}{GFR} + \frac{L_{Ca}}{GFR}$$

which on rearrangement yields

$$P_{Ca(UF)} = 1.7\left(\frac{Tm_{Ca}}{GFR} + \frac{L_{Ca}}{GFR} \right) \quad (19\text{-}2)$$

With this model the previous estimates of load would contribute about 7 percent of the plasma ultrafiltrable calcium during the day and about 3.5 percent at night.

Although short-term changes in the urinary excretion of calcium can reflect changes either in the bone surface–perilacunar compartments or in the soft tissue component of the exchangeable pool, in a steady state urinary calcium must be derived either from the diet or from stable bone mineral. It is therefore possible to resolve the total load into two components and rewrite Eq. (19-1) as

$$P_{Ca(UF)} = \frac{TR_{Ca}}{GFR} + \frac{NA}{GFR} + \frac{BR - BF}{GFR} \quad (19\text{-}3)$$

It is therefore evident that a primary change in the blood-bone equilibrium leading to a change in plasma calcium must be accompanied by a corresponding change in one or more of these three components. If the level of equilibration changes as a result of a change in PTH secretion, then TR_{Ca}/GFR will generally change in the same direction to about the same extent, because it also is controlled by PTH. If the level of equilibration should change for reasons other than a change in PTH secretion, as for example in mild hypervitaminosis D, then all three components may be involved. As far as possible the body attempts to keep net bone resorption constant in order to preserve bone mass, and adjustments are accomplished primarily in the other components. But if this is not possible, then bone mass will be sacrificed in the interests of maintaining a normal plasma calcium level.

The normal plasma calcium in relation to age, sex, and other variables. Except in the neonatal period described later the changes with age are small (1, 45–47). They are probably related to accelerated postmenopausal bone loss and to deterioration in renal function and vitamin D status in both sexes in the elderly. They should therefore be regarded as manifestations of disease rather than as reference values associated with ideal health. Provided that total calcium is routinely corrected for albumin or protein, the same normal range should be used for both sexes at all ages.

There is no significant seasonal change in plasma calcium (48). Changes in protein account entirely for the changes in total calcium which occur during the normal menstrual cycle, and largely for the fall in total calcium during late pregnancy (49), although there is a small fall in ionized calcium and increased secretion of PTH (50). The mean circadian changes in total calcium during normal eating and activity do not depart from fasting values by more than 0.05 mmol in either direction, but individual changes may be as high as 0.2 mmol/L (3). Total calcium values are higher in the erect posture than when recumbent because of increased transudation of water into the interstitial tissue of the dependent extremities, but there is no change in corrected calcium.

With serial indirect estimates of ionized calcium from total calcium and total protein in the fasting state, about half of the variation within the reference range is analytical, and about half interindividual, the latter corresponding to a CV of 2.7 percent. There is very little intraindividual variation on fasting measurements (7, 8). Because of this true biologic variation between persons, the means of sets of successive values are distributed approximately within the range of 2.27 to 2.53

mmol/L. Whether these small but significant interindividual differences are associated with similar differences in related measurements such as plasma phosphate or urinary calcium or are due to differences in diet, in PTH secretion, or in bone or renal responsiveness to PTH has not been determined.

HYPOCALCEMIA

Mechanisms and causes

There are several mechanisms which can lead to hypocalcemia and many clinical states in which hypocalcemia can occur. Nevertheless, since the maintenance of normocalcemia is almost entirely a function of PTH, persistent hypocalcemia can only occur as a result of either lack of PTH or of some impediment to its action. Such impediments are normally overcome by increased PTH secretion; if hypocalcemia persists despite an increased plasma PTH level, the calcium homeostatic system in bone is failing to respond to PTH in a normal manner.

The concept of bone cell resistance to PTH requires careful analysis, for it is of little value unless the particular cell function that exhibits such resistance can be specified. Such specificity is lacking in the usual methods of demonstrating PTH resistance in bone. Each of the three cell systems in bone—the remodeling system, the steady-state homeostatic system, and the error-correcting system—can contribute to the acute hypercalcemic response to exogenous PTH, but the presence or absence of such a response is not relevant to the pathogenesis of hypocalcemia (51). The acute release of calcium from bone, by whatever means, is unrelated to steady-state plasma calcium regulation. In fact, impairment of this process is more likely the result than the cause of sustained hypocalcemia, since it can be corrected in many instances by restoring normocalcemia by intravenous or oral calcium administration (52). It is the steady-state relationships between plasma ionized calcium and plasma PTH which defines the responsiveness to the hormone.

Resistance of the calcium homeostatic system to PTH defined in this way occurs either because of deficiency of cholecalciferol metabolites (mainly 1,25-DHCC) which act on the system, or because of primary resistance of the relevant bone cells (surface lining cells and osteocytes) to PTH as in pseudohypoparathyroidism, a disease in which, as explained later, there is also a partial deficiency of 1,25-DHCC. It follows that in all forms of sustained chronic hypocalcemia there is deficiency of either PTH or 1,25-DHCC (or other CC metabolites) or both. Hypocalcemia which occurs for reasons unrelated to PTH or CC metabolites can only be transient. Deficiency of PTH will affect the kidney and the bone remodeling system as well as the calcium homeostatic system, so that plasma phosphate will be raised and bone turnover will be depressed. By contrast, deficiency of CC metabolites leads to increased secretion of PTH and a fall in plasma phosphate unless there is target cell resistance to PTH in the kidney as well as in bone (as in pseudohypoparathyroidism) or an increase in phosphate load per nephron (as in chronic renal failure). Although the effects of PTH on the remodeling system may be blunted, bone turnover is often increased and PTH levels may be high enough to cause osteitis fibrosa; the coincidence of this with hypocalcemia is only explicable if they represent disturbances in different cell systems in bone (51).

It is necessary to distinguish between the pathogenesis of hypocalcemia and the pathogenesis of secondary hyperparathyroidism. The slight decrease in plasma calcium within the normal range which is needed to stimulate increased secretion of PTH is a signal which initiates a homeostatic defense mechanism, whereas persistent hypocalcemia indicates that the defense mechanisms have broken down (51). A raised PTH level acting on a normal calcium homeostatic system in bone is able to maintain normocalcemia in the face of dietary deficiency of calcium, intestinal malabsorption of calcium, decreased renal tubular reabsorption of calcium, or persistent hyperphosphatemia. These conditions may all cause transient hypocalcemia and secondary hyperparathyroidism, and may further worsen hypocalcemia if either PTH or CC metabolites are deficient, but do not by themselves cause sustained hypocalcemia. Transient hypocalcemia can also occur for many other

reasons. This analysis suggests a primary subdivision into five groups of conditions: first, PTH deficiency with hypocalcemia, hyperphosphatemia, and reduced bone turnover; second, deficiency of CC metabolites with hypocalcemic secondary hyperparathyroidism and usually hypophosphatemia; third, pseudohypoparathyroidism with hypocalcemic secondary hyperparathyroidism and usually hyperphosphatemia; fourth, chronic calcium depletion and other mechanisms leading to normocalcemic secondary hyperparathyroidism; and finally, a wide variety of causes of transient hypocalcemia.

PTH deficiency (53). HP (hypoparathyroidism) is associated with impaired renal 1-hydroxylation of 25-HCC (54) so that lack of PTH produces hypocalcemia both directly and via deficiency of 1,25-DHCC. Depending on the degree of PTH deficiency, plasma calcium can vary from about 1.2 mmol/L to low normal levels (55). The lowest values, which occur with complete absence of PTH, reflect the level of equilibration corresponding to the solubility of bone mineral in body fluids (56). Even with mild degrees of PTH deficiency the plasma calcium is less stable than normal. For example, hypocalcemia and tetany may be precipitated by corticosteroid-induced malabsorption of calcium (57), by mercurial-diuretic-induced hypercalciuria (57), or by estrogen-induced inhibition of bone resorption (58), processes which normally have only a trivial effect on plasma calcium. Plasma calcium also varies more with changes in calcium intake, and shows much greater reciprocal fluctuation with plasma phosphate than in normal subjects, because the plasma composition reflects more directly that of the bone ECF. Consequently, when PTH is only moderately deficient, hypocalcemia may occur only when the intake of calcium is deficient or the intake of phosphate is excessive.

As well as determining the steady-state level of plasma calcium, PTH also participates in the correction of deviations from the steady-state level; optimal recovery from induced hypocalcemia is dependent on a rapid increase in PTH secretion. By analogy with the early stages of Addison's disease, as parathyroid cell mass is reduced a point may be reached where maximally stimulated cells

Table 19-5. Metabolic data in surgical hypoparathyroidism classified according to severity*

	GRADE				
	1	2	3	4	5
Number of cases	10	10	9	8	5
Plasma Ca (mmol/L)	2.38 ± 0.03	2.30 ± 0.04	2.03 ± 0.02	1.71 ± 0.02	1.45 ± 0.03
Urine Ca (mmol/24 h)	3.17 ± 0.55	3.05 ± 0.56	1.60 ± 0.27	1.17 ± 0.22	1.15 ± 0.25
Urine Ca (μmol/L C_{Cr})	24.7 ± 2.2	21.7 ± 3.0	12.5 ± 2.0	9.0 ± 1.7	9.0 ± 2.0
Plasma P (mmol/L)	1.22 ± 0.04	1.33 ± 0.11	1.34 ± 0.07	1.63 ± 0.07	1.82 ± 0.10
Tm_P/GFR (mmol/L)	1.06 ± 0.06	1.05 ± 0.10	1.39 ± 0.09	1.80 ± 0.12	2.01 ± 0.16
Urine P (mmol/24 h)	21.7 ± 2.3	21.1 ± 1.2	14.7 ± 2.0	15.1 ± 2.2	16.7 ± 3.6
Urine P (μmol/L C_{Cr})	154.8 ± 13.1	182.6 ± 19.2	129.4 ± 18.8	115.8 ± 18.4	128 ± 29.5

	1 + 2	3 + 4 + 5	DIFFERENCE	P
Number of cases	20	22		
Urine P (mmol/24 h)	21.4 ± 1.3	15.6 ± 1.3	5.8 ± 1.9	<0.005
Urine P (μmol/L C_{Cr})	168.7 ± 13.4	124.2 ± 11.3	44.5 ± 17.5	<0.02

* Upper panel shows mean ± S.E. in each grade. Lower panel compares phosphate excretion between grades 1 and 2 (normocalcemic) and grades 3 to 5 (hypocalcemic).

are able to maintain a nearly normal basal level of hormone secretion but are unable to further augment secretion in response to increased physiologic demand. The recovery from induced hypocalcemia will then be retarded and incomplete. Based on these considerations five grades of severity of PTH-deficient HP have been defined (55) (Table 19-5). These divisions are arbitrary but are useful for descriptive and prognostic purposes.

NcAMP/GFR is decreased and TM$_P$/GFR increased in HP, but successive decrements in PTH and NcAMP/GFR have a progressively greater effect on TM$_P$/GFR because of operation on the splay portion of the titration curve at normal loads (Chap. 8). The rise in plasma phosphate is further offset by a reduction in L/GFR because of reduced gastrointestinal absorption (Table 19-5). Because less PTH is needed to inhibit phosphate reabsorption than to raise plasma calcium, hyperphosphatemia is a less constant finding than hypocalcemia, and with HP of moderate severity (grade 3) the plasma phosphate is usually normal (Table 19-5). However, plasma calcium and phosphate show a significant inverse correlation throughout the spectrum of PTH deficiency (55).

Although Tm$_P$/GFR is inversely related to NcAMP/GFR over a wide range, there are several factors which may disturb this relationship (Table 19-6). In normal subjects chlorpropamide

markedly reduces the cAMP response to small but not to large doses of exogenous PTH, but has no effect on the phosphaturic response (59). This suggests that much more cAMP is normally produced than is needed to activate the intracellular mechanisms which lead to reduced phosphate transport, and that the surplus is excreted in the urine. A similar disturbance in the normal relationship is produced by administration of acetazolamide, which increases phosphate excretion in PHP (pseudohypoparathyroidism) affecting cAMP excretion (60), and by certain synthetic analogues of PTH which increase excretion of phosphate in the rat but do not activate adenylate cyclase in isolated kidney membrane preparations (15).

Tm$_P$/GFR is affected by plasma calcium as well as by NcAMP/GFR. In a group of patients with nondetectable PTH and low values for NcAMP/GFR for a variety of reasons, Tm$_P$/GFR varied

Table 19-6. Some factors which alter the normal relationship between the NcAMP and phosphaturic response to exogenous PTH

NcAMP RESPONSE REDUCED, PHOSPHATURIC RESPONSE NORMAL	NcAMP RESPONSE NORMAL, PHOSPHATURIC RESPONSE REDUCED
Desamino b PTH 1-34	Hypocalcemia
Chlorpropamide	PHP Type 2
Acetazolamide	? Magnesium depletion
PHP Type 1 + calcium	

inversely with plasma calcium (Kleerekoper, unpublished data). Increased cell membrane permeability to calcium and consequent increased uptake of calcium by the renal tubule cell is probably an independent effect of PTH binding to receptor at the basal pole of the cell. The metabolic consequences of cell activation by PTH are mediated by the additive effects of increased intracellular cAMP and increased intracellular calcium (61); consequently, if calcium influx into the cell under the influence of PTH is reduced because of hypocalcemia, Tm_P/GFR will tend to be higher for the same level of NcAMP (Table 19-6). Because of the location of phosphate transport at the luminal pole of the tubule cell, increased tubular reabsorption of phosphate is associated with increased intracellular phosphate, and this together with reduced entry of cAMP and calcium inhibits l,α-hydroxylation of 25-HCC. Hypocalcemia may be a contributory factor in the low plasma levels of 1,25-DHCC in HP, and improved 1,25-DHCC synthesis may mediate part of the therapeutic response to calcium administration.

Most patients with surgical HP have a small amount of residual PTH secretion which may result in low but measurable levels of NcAMP/GFR, but this cannot accomplish normal tubular phosphate reabsorption because of the hypocalcemia. Sustained elevation of plasma calcium to normal, whether by intravenous calcium (62) or oral calcium (63), vitamin D, or 1,25-DHCC (63) reduces Tm_P/GFR and plasma phosphate toward normal; presumably there is no change in NcAMP but this has not been determined. Absence of any PTH, as in most cases of idiopathic HP, is associated with a small further decrement in plasma calcium, undetectable NcAMP excretion, and a substantially higher Tm_P/GFR and plasma phosphate which respond less readily to treatment.

When considered in isolation, the urinary excretion of calcium is low in HP, whether expressed as mmol/day or as mmol/L GFR (Table 19-5), but when related to plasma calcium, mean urinary calcium is higher in HP than in osteomalacia for the same degree of hypocalcemia because of impaired tubular reabsorption. However, there are many exceptions and tubular reabsorption of calcium is often normal (63). In the steady state the reduction in urinary calcium is a consequence of decreased net absorption of calcium due to 1,25-DHCC deficiency.

Because of lack of action of PTH on progenitor cell proliferation, the birth rate of BRU and bone turnover are reduced, whether measured by kinetic or morphologic techniques or by urinary hydroxyproline (51, 53), but this is unrelated to the hypocalcemia. The AP level is not consistently altered. Calcium balance is usually close to zero but may be significantly positive or negative (64); total body calcium tends to be slightly increased (65). The bones are usually radiographically normal although occasionally either osteopenia or osteosclerosis may occur. These differences have no effect on the plasma calcium.

PTH reduces the tubular reabsorption of bicarbonate as well as phosphate and in HP both the renal threshold and plasma level of bicarbonate are frequently raised. Although the CSF (cerebrospinal fluid) calcium does not fall as much as the plasma calcium, the sensitivity of the respiratory center to CO_2 is increased so that respiratory compensation for the raised plasma bicarbonate is incomplete and the plasma pH may be elevated (53).

The causes of PTH deficiency (53, 57, 66, 67) are classified in Table 19-7 as genetic, acquired, and transient.

Isolated Genetic HP. Congenital absence of the parathyroid gland causes tetany manifested at or soon after birth. As an isolated abnormality this is usually sporadic but both x-linked recessive and autosomal recessive inheritance may occur. More commonly it is associated with congenital absence of the thymus leading to profoundly depressed cell-mediated immunity and repeated severe infections (Di George syndrome), and multiple abnormalities due to maldevelopment of the 1st and 5th branchial clefts (branchial dysembryogenesis). Most patients die in infancy or early childhood but occasional survival into adolescence or adult life is possible, with partial improvement of both thymic and parathyroid function. Several other rare genetic entities cause HP in late childhood.

The MEDAC Syndrome (Multiple Endocrine Deficiency-Autoimmune-Candidiasis). This is a ge-

Table 19-7. The causes of PTH deficiency

Genetic HP
  Isolated
    Congenital absence of parathyroid glands
    Branchial dysembryogenesis
    Late onset
  Multiple endocrine deficiency-autoimmune-candidiasis
Acquired HP
  Surgical
  Other
    Irradiation
    Iron overload
    Neoplastic infiltration
    Idiopathic
    Miscellaneous
Transient and reversible HP
  Neonatal
  Transient dysplasia
  Suppression by hypercalcemia
  Maternal hyperparathyroidism
  Hypomagnesemia

netic disorder transmitted as an autosomal recessive trait comprising hypofunction of several endocrine glands often associated with organ-specific autoantibodies, variable involvement of other organs, and recurrent candida infections. The major independent components are chronic mucocutaneous candidiasis, HP, and Addison's disease, usually appearing in that order. When adrenal insufficiency becomes established, the plasma calcium may rise either from low to near-normal levels in untreated patients or from normal to high levels in patients on vitamin D (68). Other components of this syndrome include phlyctenular keratoconjunctivitis, alopecia, dental dysplasia, adult-type pernicious anemia, active chronic hepatitis, premature ovarian failure, and autoimmune thyroiditis. Steatorrhea may be produced by any of the three major components of the syndrome and also occurs as an independent component due to pancreatic fibrosis.

In some cases antiparathyroid antibodies have been found, although the prevalence varies considerably in different laboratories. Detection of these and other organ-specific antibodies may precede clinical manifestations and identify the syndrome in apparently normal family members. However, there is no evidence that the antibodies are directly involved in the destruction of parathyroid tissue.

SHP (Surgical Hypoparathyroidism). This is by far the commonest variety of HP. Thyroid surgery is less often performed in major medical centers than in the past, but the frequency in the total population remains high. With decreasing surgical experience, the incidence of parathyroid injury increases, so that the number of new cases may remain the same or even rise. Also, there has been a large increase in the number of parathyroid operations for mild hyperparathyroidism. The risk is higher in younger patients and with more extensive resections. With radical neck surgery for cancer, the incidence is markedly reduced by routine parathyroid autotransplantation (69).

It is important to distinguish between hypocalcemia and tetany, because the therapeutic and prognostic implications are quite different. Mild asymptomatic hypocalcemia occurs during and after surgery for several reasons unrelated to the parathyroid gland. After major cardiopulmonary operations there is a fall of 0.3 mmol/L in corrected total and calculated ionized calcium (70), which results from simultaneous increases in phosphate and lactate (because of impaired tissue oxygenation) and in citrate (because of transfusion of citrated blood). After operations on the thyroid gland there is a fall of about 0.2 mmol/L in corrected total calcium with a fall of 0.3 mmol/L in phosphate. These changes are unrelated either to the type of thyroid disease or the level of AP (71). Similar changes lasting from 1 to 2 h during operation are related to manipulation of the thyroid and so probably result from release of calcitonin (72). Larger postoperative falls occur in some patients with inadequate preoperative control of hyperthyroidism, due to reversal of negative bone and calcium balance (73), and delayed recovery from parathyroid suppression. However, although a disparity between total bone formation and resorption would begin immediately, it would not reach a maximum until about 4 weeks after operation, the duration of the resorptive phase of the normal remodeling cycle (74). Postthyroidectomy hypocalcemia from any of these causes is usually maximal on the first postoperative day and does not cause tetany. After operations on the parathyroid gland tetany may not occur until the third postoperative day or later, but there are many exceptions. In patients destined to develop permanent hypoparathyroidism after thyroid surgery, significant hypocalcemia and tetany may occur within 24 h, although the lowest level of plasma calcium may not be reached until the fourth day (53, 75). The occurrence of overt tetany after thyroid surgery is usually due to parathyroid gland injury whatever the time of onset, and the majority of such patients will never recover normal parathyroid function (53). The parathyroid injury is mainly the result of ischemia and reflects the extent of dissection and hemostasis necessary to achieve a dry operative field.

About half the patients who develop postthyroidectomy tetany will eventually recover sufficiently for treatment to be withdrawn. The chance of this is greater the earlier the onset and the lesser the severity of the tetany; it usually occurs within 6 months but may occasionally be delayed for up to 36 months. Apparent recovery is always associated with impaired parathyroid reserve, and may occasionally be followed many years later by the delayed recurrence of persistent hypocalcemia. Because of the tendency to recovery grades 1 to 3 are much commoner in SHP than in other forms of HP. In the remaining cases of postsurgical tetany, hypocalcemia persists indefinitely because of permanent chronic HP. Even so, most patients retain a small amount of residual PTH secretion; the PTH remnant probably fails to regenerate because of ischemia resulting from the operative trauma. Occasionally, hypocalcemia develops between 1 and 30 years after operation in the absence of tetany in the early postoperative period. The explanation for this is unknown but the practical lesson is clear—HP should be suspected in every patient with a scar in the neck however long ago the operation and whether or not the plasma calcium has previously been normal.

Other Forms of Acquired HP (53, 57, 66, 67). Permanent HP may very occasionally follow irradiation damage due to ^{131}I administration for hyperthyroidism or thyroid cancer, fibrosis, and atrophy due to iron deposition in hemochromatosis, thalassemia, and other causes of siderosis, and extensive destruction by metastatic disease. In rabbits, parathyroid necrosis can be produced by asparaginase; the use of this substance in the treatment of leukemia has been associated with hypocalcemia but the mechanism has not been established.

HP may first produce symptoms in adult life in the absence of any known cause. This is usually classified as idiopathic but it is invariably sporadic and without antiparathyroid antibodies. The onset may be at any age up to the eighth decade. Atrophy, fibrosis, and fatty infiltration and replacement have been found in the few reported autopsies. The mean interval between onset of symptoms and institution of treatment is about 8 years, but this may be reduced by multichannel biochemical screening; two cases have been diagnosed at Henry Ford Hospital in the last 2 years by this means.

Transient and Reversible HP. This can be due to delayed maturation of parathyroid function in the neonatal period, suppression of normal glands by hypercalcemia, or impaired hormone synthesis because of magnesium depletion.

During pregnancy calcium is transferred from the mother to the fetus by an active transport system in the placenta (76). After birth, plasma total and ionized calcium usually fall from the high levels found in cord blood by 0.2 to 0.3 mmol/L, the lowest point occurring within 24 to 72 h. Between 4 and 7 days of age both levels increase by about 0.08 mmol/L to reach the stable values of early infancy (77, 78). The early fall is accompanied by a parallel depression of PTH; both plasma calcium and PTH return to normal after 48 h (76, 78). Early neonatal tetany represents an exaggeration of this normal phenomenon which occurs especially in association with maternal diabetes, vitamin D deficiency, narcotic drug usage, and magnesium sulfate treatment for eclampsia, and with prematurity, low birth weight, and respiratory distress in the baby (76). Compared to infants without tetany the PTH level is lower and slower to rise to normal (78). Calcitonin levels are higher in premature than in full-term infants which may contribute to the increased incidence of tetany. Late neonatal tetany occurring after about 1 week usually follows cow's milk feeding and is associated with hyperphosphatemia and more severe symptoms. Occasionally persistent severe hypocalcemia is delayed for several weeks after birth, and associated with raised plasma phosphate and need for vitamin D to restore normocalcemia, a situation referred to as transient congenital dysplasia (53). After 3 to 6 months parathyroid function returns to normal and treatment can be withdrawn.

Normal parathyroid glands secrete less hormone in the face of hypercalcemia because of prolongation of the quiescent period so that a smaller fraction of cells is secreting PTH at one time, but this fraction cannot fall to zero. There is no evidence that even long continued suppression of hormone secretion produces parathyroid atrophy, so that recovery of normal function when hypercalcemia is corrected depends on quiescent cells reentering a secretory phase of the cell cycle, and not on regeneration of new tissue (53). Such temporary suppression may contribute to symptomatic hypocalcemia after thyroid or parathyroid surgery. A rare but interesting variant is the occurrence of hypocalcemic tetany as the presenting manifestation of primary hyperparathyroidism with bone disease, due to spontaneous infarction of an adenoma (79).

Infants born to mothers with primary hyperparathyroidism not uncommonly develop severe hypocalcemia (53). The symptoms usually begin within the first 2 weeks and complete recovery occurs after about 3 months, although one case of permanent HP has occurred. The mother's disease may otherwise be asymptomatic so that neonatal tetany may be the first clue to the diagnosis. PTH does not cross the placenta (80), and the cause is presumed to be depression of fetal parathyroid function because of transmission of maternal hypercalcemia via the placenta. In one case the level of PTH in the infant was raised and the hypocalcemia was attributed to hypomagnesemia. This causes hypocalcemia by multiple mechanisms (this is discussed in a later section). PTH levels have been undetectable in about half the cases, inappropriately low for the degree of hypocalcemia in about 40 percent, and modestly increased in about 10 percent (81). In some cases the plasma phosphate has been raised as in PTH deficiency from other causes (82).

Diagnosis of HP. The level of iPTH is usually lower than expected for the level of plasma calcium but may be as high as in normal persons because of an increased proportion of biologically inactive metabolites. Some assays can measure subnormal levels of iPTH (21) but most are insensitive. NcAMP/GFR may also be normal, but when related to plasma calcium gives better discrimination than iPTH. Although inconstant, hyperphosphatemia or other evidence of impaired phosphate reabsorption is present in most patients, but the combination of hypocalcemia and hyperphosphatemia can also occur in chronic renal failure, CC-metabolite deficiency, hypomagnesemia, intestinal malabsorption, endogenous or exogenous phosphate loads, and in PHP with or without the short metacarpal syndrome (53).

The recognition of latent or normocalcemic HP would be accomplished most reliably by demonstrating a subnormal increment in plasma iPTH in response to a hypocalcemic challenge, but a diagnostic test based on this principle has not yet been standardized. Although not yet validated by PTH measurements, delayed recovery from hypocalcemia induced by infusion of a chelating agent such as EDTA is analogous to impaired glucose tolerance in that it is a direct reflection of homeostatic control which can be used to assess parathyroid function provided the patient is euthyroid. Normally, the baseline level of plasma nonchelated calcium is restored within 10 h of the end of the infusion (6). The occurrence of hypocalcemia in response to cellulose phosphate and a low-calcium diet has a similar significance, and the two tests correlate well (83). In contrast to normal subjects, patients with an abnormal response to either test are unable to increase urinary hydroxyproline excretion or to increase tubular reabsorption of calcium in response to calcium deprivation. These tests have been used mainly in studying the natural history of HP; contrary to initial impression they have no value in identifying a need for treatment, but are useful in defining prognosis. The tests cannot be used to examine the possibility of recovery in patients on vitamin D unless combined with iPTH or NcAMP measurements. In this regard metabolic alkalosis may be a useful clue to persistence of HP.

Bone cell resistance to PTH: CC-metabolite deficiency with hypocalcemic secondary hyper-

parathyroidism. Increased secretion of PTH in CC-metabolite deficiency is initiated by intestinal malabsorption of calcium, and may be intensified by a direct effect on the parathyroid gland, but hypocalcemia does not occur until the calcium homeostatic system in bone begins to fail. Hypophosphatemia usually occurs much earlier because Tm_P/GFR is reduced both by increased PTH and directly as a result of CC-metabolite (probably 25-HCC) deficiency (84).

When hypocalcemia occurs it may disturb the relationship between NcAMP/GFR and Tm_P/GFR and so blunt the phosphaturic response to PTH. Occasionally, either because this effect of hypocalcemia is much more profound than usual or because of relative failure of PTH secretion, plasma phosphate may be normal or even increased (85, 86), producing a close biochemical resemblance to PHP. This is especially likely in patients with intestinal malabsorption and steatorrhea, in which there is also deficiency of magnesium and possibly of amino acid precursors required for PTH synthesis (87). Vitamin D deficiency does not directly alter the renal response to PTH (52). The lack of effect of endogenous PTH on phosphate reabsorption in severe rickets (88) is probably due to competition for receptors by endogenous PTH (89) as well as to hypocalcemia.

All three of the PTH-responsive cell systems in bone—the homeostatic system, the error-correcting system, and the remodeling system—require one or more metabolites of CC in order to function normally (51). Although 1,25-DHCC is probably the major metabolite of vitamin D which acts in concert with PTH, in some conditions lack of 25-HCC with a normal level of 1,25-DHCC may have similar effects. If CC metabolites are deficient, then despite an increase in PTH secretion the level of blood-bone equilibration may be reduced, recovery from induced hypocalcemia may be impaired, and the birth rate of BRU and bone turnover may be depressed. However, a sufficiently great increase in PTH secretion may overcome the effects of metabolite deficiency and restore both plasma calcium and bone turnover to normal or even supernormal levels, but still below those expected for the prevailing level of

PTH. The remodeling system is less dependent on CC metabolites than the homeostatic system, so that osteitis fibrosa, the most severe osseous effect of hyperparathyroidism, may develop despite persistent hypocalcemia. So long as this remains uncorrected, the stimulus to further parathyroid gland hyperplasia and PTH hypersecretion persists, so that parathyroid cell mass will tend to increase progressively.

The mechanisms of metabolite deficiency can be predicted from the normal metabolism of CC (90, 90a) (Table 19-8) and are associated with characteristic concentration profiles of the various compounds (Table 19-9). The time of onset of clinical effects will depend on the magnitude of body stores of both CC and 25-HCC. Since most 25-HCC normally escapes 1-hydroxylation,

Table 19-8. Causes of deficiency of vitamin D and/or its metabolites classified according to level of primary defect*

CC deficiency
  Atmospheric and other causes of ultraviolet light deprivation
  Dietary deficiency
  Intestinal malabsorption
    Hepatobiliary disease with lack of bile salts
    Severe pancreatic insufficiency
    Gastrointestinal disease
25-HCC deficiency
  Loss in enterohepatic circulation
  Impaired hepatic 25-hydroxylation
    Immaturity (neonatal)
    Hepatobiliary disease
  Increased renal excretion
    Biliary cirrhosis (loss of inactive metabolites)
    Nephrotic syndrome (loss of DBP + 25-HCC)
  Increased catabolism
    Anticonvulsant therapy
    Other causes of microsomal enzyme induction
1,25-DHCC deficiency
  Chronic renal failure
  Cystinosis
  Vitamin D dependency
  Tumor induced
  Hyperphosphatemia
  ? PTH deficiency†
  ?Pseudohypoparathyroidism†

* CC, cholecalciferol; 25-HCC, 25-hydroxycholecalciferol; DBP, vitamin D binding protein.
† 1,25-DHCC deficiency occurs in both, but it is not certain whether a mechanism other than hyperphosphatemia is involved.

Table 19-9. Plasma vitamin D metabolite profiles, according to cause of primary defect

PRIMARY DEFECT	CC	25-HCC	24,25-DHCC	1,25-DHCC
CC deficiency	↓	↓	↓	↓(or N*)
25-HCC deficiency	N	↓	↓	↓ (or N*)
1,25-DHCC deficiency (renal failure)	N	N (or ↓†)	↓‡	↓
1,25-DHCC deficiency (D dependent)	N	N	N (or ?↑)	↓
D "resistance"	N	N	N	N (or ?↑)

* Mild deficiency with secondary HP.

† Due to diet- or drug-induced enzyme induction.

‡ Not reduced as much as 1,25-DHCC because of extrarenal site(s) of 24-hydroxylation.

and this process is stimulated by PTH, the onset of 1,25-DHCC deficiency resulting from lack of its precursor will be further delayed by secondary hyperparathyroidism. The effects on mineral and bone metabolism of either 25-HCC or 1,25-DHCC deficiency will be modified by the presence or absence of deficiency of the other metabolite and of 24,25-DHCC. Although deficiency of 1,25-DHCC alone may cause both rickets and osteomalacia, this occurs more readily if 25-HCC or 24,25-DHCC are also deficient, in which case 1,25-DHCC alone is less able to restore bone mineralization to normal (84). Rickets and osteomalacia are discussed in more detail in the section on phosphate depletion. Many agents antagonize one or more of the effects of CC metabolites (90a), but true target cell resistance, implying a defect at or subsequent to the binding of hormone to receptor, has not been shown to occur. In one possible case (90b) there was hypocalcemia despite normal 25-HCC and high 1,25-DHCC and PTH levels, but 24,25-DHCC was not measured.

CC Deficiency. This can result either from reduced intake or intestinal malabsorption. The level of 25-HCC is normally higher in infants and children than in adults, and CC deficiency may lead to hypocalcemia and rickets at a 25-HCC level which in an adult would be entirely normal (91). Hypocalcemia may occur early while the plasma phosphate is still normal, thus reversing the more usual order in adults. At a later stage increased PTH secretion corrects the hypocalcemia and the plasma phosphate falls, but with even more severe deficiency hypocalcemia recurs despite a further increase in PTH secretion. The early hypocalcemic effect of CC deficiency is dependent on age, since hypocalcemia is the rule in young infants and normocalcemia is more common in older children (92). In adults, hypophosphatemia usually precedes hypocalcemia, which is often of only moderate severity. The mean plasma calcium was 2.1 mmol/L with 95 percent confidence limits of 1.6 to 2.6 mmol/L, in 29 patients assembled from the literature (93).

Any disease complicated by steatorrhea may be accompanied by malabsorption of both dietary CC and of the 25-HCC participating in the enterohepatic circulation (92), but this occurs more commonly with mucosal disease (as in gluten enteropathy) or loss of absorptive surface (as after bypass operations for obesity) than with maldigestion alone (as in pancreatic exocrine deficiency). The adverse effects may be intensified by malabsorption of calcium, phosphate, and magnesium also. The severity of absorptive defects for different substances varies considerably from patient to patient; in gluten enteropathy, osteomalacia may rarely occur in the absence of steatorrhea and steatorrhea may occur in the presence of constipation. In adults with osteomalacia due to gluten enteropathy the severity and variability of hypocalcemia are much the same as in dietary vitamin D deficiency (93). Hypocalcemia is less severe in postgastrectomy osteomalacia—mean value 2.2 mmol/L, with a 95 percent range of 1.8 to 2.6 mmol/L in 59 patients (93). In England, most patients with hypocalcemia or osteomalacia following gastrectomy have normal absorption of both radioactive CC and stable 25-HCC (92, 94), and can be cured by very small doses of vitamin D (93). This reflects the prevalence of subclinical vitamin D deficiency, which becomes overt with only a modest further reduction in intake. In the United States, patients with postgastrectomy hypocalcemia or osteomalacia more commonly have impaired CC absorption, but the mechanism of this is not clear.

25-HCC Deficiency. A contributory factor to neonatal hypocalcemia is a low 25-HCC level, either from maternal CC deficiency or from delayed maturation of the hepatic 25-hydroxylase (54). Low 25-HCC levels are commonly found in patients with alcoholic cirrhosis and other types of chronic liver disease, but they result more often from poor intake and intestinal malabsorption than from impaired 25-hydroxylation (95). In most such patients the formation of 25-HCC after administration of radioactively labeled precursor is normal for the prevailing body stores, as shown by the plasma level of 25-HCC (96). The 25-hydroxylase has a large reserve capacity, and extensive destruction of liver tissue is needed to impair 25-HCC formation. In biliary cirrhosis increased urinary excretion of biologically inactive polar metabolites contributes further to the low plasma 25-HCC level (97). In the nephrotic syndrome, because of the increased permeability of the glomerular basement membrane, the 25-HCC binding protein, in common with other plasma proteins of similar molecular weight, escapes into the urine carrying a significant amount of 25-HCC with it (98). Consequently, hypocalciuria, hypocalcemia, and secondary hyperparathyroidism are more severe than would be expected for the degree of renal insufficiency (99).

Low blood levels of 25-HCC, hypocalcemia, and occasionally osteomalacia occur in patients taking long-term anticonvulsant therapy, particularly phenytoin and phenobarbitone (90, 90a). The mean plasma calcium is reduced by 0.1 to 0.2 mmol/L, and the prevalence of hypocalcemia is about 10 to 20 percent with occasional values as low as 1.6 mmol/L. This may initiate a vicious circle of more frequent seizures, increased dosage of anticonvulsants, further worsening of hypocalcemia, and still further increase in number of seizures (100). Altered calcium metabolism is commoner in (but is not restricted to) institutionalized epileptics, and in most studies has been related to the number of drugs taken and to the dosage or duration of treatment. The plasma 25-HCC levels are reduced by 50 to 70 percent, showing the same

age and geographic differences as in normal subjects, and about 50 nmol of CC daily is needed to maintain normal vitamin D status, or 5 to 10 times the normal requirement. The conversion of labeled CC to 25-HCC is normal or even increased (101), but a much higher proportion of both CC and 25-HCC is converted to biologically inactive polar metabolites which are excreted in the bile. Accelerated catabolism of vitamin D by microsomes at the expense of mitochondria has been found in the rat liver (90, 90a), and most anticonvulsant-treated patients have increased urinary excretion of D-glucaric acid, an index of hepatic microsomal enzyme induction. This cannot be the whole explanation, since phenytoin is a less potent enzyme inducer than phenobarbitone, but more commonly leads to disordered calcium metabolism. Phenytoin impairs intestinal calcium absorption directly (90a), inhibits both PTH- and 25-HCC-induced bone resorption in mouse calvaria (102), and conceivably could also render the calcium homeostatic system in bone less responsive to PTH. This would account for disproportionate secondary hyperparathyroidism, and for histologic evidence of increased bone turnover without impaired bone mineralization in some anticonvulsant-treated patients (103). The plasma level of 1,25-DHCC is normal or even increased in both phenytoin- and phenobarbitone-treated patients (104), and conversion of 25-HCC to 1,25-DHCC in the rat is normal (90) so that the calcium and bone disturbances are presumably due to deficiency of both 25-HCC and 24,25-DHCC, which usually varies reciprocally with 1,25-DHCC.

1,25-DHCC Deficiency. By far the commonest cause of impaired 1-hydroxylation of 25-HCC is chronic renal failure, discussed in Chap. 16. As with deficiency of CC or 25-HCC, this is initially associated with impaired intestinal calcium absorption, hypocalciuria, secondary hyperparathyroidism, normocalcemia, and hypophosphatemia (105); only much later do the more characteristic plasma changes of hyperphosphatemia and hypocalcemia develop. In cystinosis, defective 1-hydroxylation and secondary hyperparathyroidism occur several years before the onset of chronic renal failure (p. 1076). Impaired 1-hydroxylation may also result from an unknown humoral agent secreted by certain tumors associated with rickets and osteomalacia (p. 1075).

In vitamin D dependency hypocalcemia and rickets begin in early infancy, and the clinical, biochemical, and radiographic features are identical with vitamin D deficiency, but the vitamin D nutritional status is normal and pharmacologic doses of CC or EC are needed for treatment (106). The condition is genetically transmitted as an autosomal recessive trait, and has frequently been confused with other forms of vitamin D refractory rickets associated with hypophosphatemia in which hypocalcemia and tetany do not occur (p. 1075). In vitamin D dependency, hypophosphatemia, aminoaciduria, and bicarbonate wasting are all due entirely to secondary hyperparathyroidism and are completely reversed by adequate treatment, which also restores normal growth, sometimes with a spectacular catch-up spurt (90). The patients are equally refractory to DHT (dihydrotachysterol) and 25-HCC. The plasma level of 1,25-DHCC is low despite normal levels of 25-HCC, and doses of 1,25-DHCC close to physiologic correct all manifestations of the disease (107), consistent with a genetic defect in 1-hydroxylation. More 1,25-DHCC may be required than in vitamin D deficiency, probably because of a greater degree of parathyroid hyperplasia due to the much longer delay in establishing effective treatment. The plasma phosphate levels are sometimes normal or even elevated, but similar variability occurs in vitamin D deficiency. A final difference from the usual form of vitamin D refractory rickets is that the need for treatment is life-long, hypocalcemia invariably recurring if it is withdrawn.

Bone cell resistance to PTH: PHP with hypocalcemic secondary hyperparathyroidism (66, 67, 105, 108). The term PHP (pseudohypoparathyroidism) has traditionally denoted the combination of target cell resistance to PTH with a cluster of osseous and other defects, of which short metacarpals is the most characteristic; when the osseous defects are present alone, the term PPHP (pseudopseudohypoparathyroidism) is commonly applied. Apart from its clumsiness, this term confuses two different situations which need to be distinguished. In PHP the biochemical changes in blood vary in severity with time and the plasma calcium and phosphate levels may sometimes be normal. Consequently the term PPHP may be applied to patients who have no metabolic disorder, and also to patients who are at risk of recurrence of hypocalcemia in the future. Since target cell resistance to PTH can also exist alone, it is essential for clarity of thought and exposition to have different terms for these two clinical syndromes which can occur either separately or together. In the ensuing discussion PHP will refer to primary target cell resistance to PTH, irrespective of the presence or absence of any other features; in this view there are no physical or radiographic features of PHP. The term SMS ("short metacarpal syndrome") will be used for the osseous and other defects, rather than Albright's hereditary osteodystrophy, which was originally defined to include both PHP and PPHP (109).

PHP with Short Metacarpal Syndrome. The age of onset of symptoms varies considerably between about 1 and 20 or more years, with a mean of about 8 years (108). The characteristic hypocalcemia and hyperphosphatemia may persist throughout life, but all cases adequately followed over long periods of time show considerable fluctuation, and spontaneous improvement may occur to the extent that treatment can be withdrawn for some years. Hypocalcemia usually recurs in time either because of the stress of pregnancy or intercurrent illness, or in later years for no apparent reason (110). The plasma calcium therefore overlaps the normal range, although less than in SHP, and the mean plasma calcium is significantly higher than in IHP. In contrast to IHP, the plasma phosphate shows less tendency to fall with age during childhood, and is higher for the same level of plasma calcium than in SHP or IHP. In mild cases the plasma calcium may be normal but plasma phosphate raised, a combination never seen either in SHP or IHP (55).

The SMS includes several components. There is shortening of metacarpals, especially the first, fourth, and fifth and occasionally all five. Affected metacarpals show retarded growth for several years before epiphyseal fusion; this is the result, not the cause, of the cessation of growth. As in any syndrome the most characteristic feature may sometimes be absent. There are also many other causes of short metacarpals which are genetically distinct from the SMS. Other skeletal abnormalities are short or deformed distal phalanges, multiple exostoses, abnormally thick calvarium, and Madelung and other deformities. Ectopic ossification and osteoma cutis are unrelated to the biochemical abnormalities in blood, and occur in SMS alone without PHP. They are quite distinct from the soft tissue calcium deposits in and around joints which are commoner in PHP than either SHP or IHP because of the higher plasma phosphate. A third form of ectopic calcium deposition is intracranial calcification, which occurs in all forms of HP of sufficient duration without treatment. Abnormal dermatoglyphic patterns and impairment of smell or taste are present in most cases and there is often a characteristic rounding of the face. Other obvious features are retarded growth and short stature, moderate obesity, and slight mental retardation. Although these are probably independent components of the SMS, they may be due in part to the frequently associated hypothyroidism (111). This is characteristically incomplete and nonprogressive, and the subject of frequent diagnostic equivocation. The defect may be hypothalamic, pituitary, or thyroid or at multiple levels; it is not clear whether it should be regarded as another independent component of the SMS or as another manifestation of endocrine target cell resistance. Similar comments apply to the frequently occurring deficiency of prolactin (90).

The mode of genetic transmission of PHP plus SMS is generally believed to be x-linked dominant, but there are equally good arguments for autosomal dominant (112). Although the two components can occur independently, there is evidently some form of genetic linkage between them. Within the same family there may be individuals with SMS alone and with SMS + PHP, but not with PHP alone. PTH-deficient IHP has occurred in association with SMS, so that the type of HP cannot be predicted with certainty from the patients' physical features (53).

There is general consensus concerning the pathogenesis of hyperphosphatemia in PHP, but considerable debate concerning the pathogenesis of hypocalcemia. The renal tubular generation of cAMP in response to PTH is defective; the baseline levels of NcAMP/GFR are low, as with deficiency of PTH but neither plasma cAMP nor NcAMP excretion increases normally in response to exogenous PTH. In both normal subjects and patients with SHP or IHP, after 200 units of bovine PTH plasma cAMP rises from a baseline of 10 to 30 nmol/L to 80 to 200 nmol/L, the peak value occurring within 5 to 10 min and returning to baseline levels by 60 min (113). In PHP, the baseline plasma cAMP is normal, and there is either no change or a small rise to less than 40 nmol/L in both normal subjects and patients with IHP or SHP. Total urinary cAMP excretion usually increases to greater than 40 nmol/min or 25 mmol/mg creatinine, in either the first or second half hour after intravenous administration of 300 units of PTH, but does not rise above 10 mmol/min or 8 mmol/mg creatinine in PHP (108). The 10- to 20-min delay between the peak increments in plasma and urinary cAMP represents the time between hormone-receptor interaction at the basal pole of the tubule cell, and transcellular migration of cAMP within the cell and subsequent transit in the urine to the bladder. The failure of normal hormone-receptor interaction in PHP is not due either to secretion of a biologically ineffective hormone or to blocking by the abnormally high plasma PTH (108). In one case studied postmortem, PTH-responsive adenylate cyclase activity in homogenized renal cortex was normal (114). This suggests that in vivo either the spatial relationship between receptor and enzyme is abnormal, some inhibitor is present, or cAMP is destroyed with unusual rapidity. The defect adequately accounts for the impaired phosphaturic response to endogenous and exogenous PTH and for the high Tm_P/GFR and plasma phosphate. However, as mentioned earlier, renal phosphate transport is influenced by plasma calcium as well as by cAMP. In some but not all patients with PHP, restoration of a normal plasma calcium by either EC or 1,25-DHCC lowers plasma phosphate to normal and partly restores the phosphaturic response to exogenous PTH (51, 108), even though urinary cAMP excretion is unaffected. Whether 1,25-DHCC increases tubule cell calcium uptake simply by restoring normocalcemia or whether it has an independent effect on membrane permeability to calcium is unclear. If only a small amount of cAMP is necessary for the intracellular changes which lead to decreased phosphate reabsorption, potentiation of this by increased entry of calcium could permit normal phosphate transport at the luminal pole of the cell, even though insufficient cAMP is generated to provide the large surplus in the urine which is usually found.

Patients with PHP uniformly have subnormal plasma levels of 1,25-DHCC as in PTH deficiency, and for the same reasons, namely, high intracellular phosphate associated with reduced entry of NcAMP and calcium. It has been proposed that this is the only reason for unresponsiveness of the calcium homeostatic system in bone to PTH and consequent hypocalcemia, and that there is no need to postulate defective cAMP generation by cells in bone as well as in the kidney, a unitary concept of the disease in which all features can be traced to a single defect (90, 115). Because of the secondary hyperparathyroidism, bone turnover and urinary THP excretion are higher than in PTH-deficient HP but are still usually lower than would be expected for the level of PTH, ranging from moderately below to substantially above normal (51). The variation in the calcemic response to prolonged administration of PTH probably reflects a comparable variation in the response of the remodeling system in bone. In some cases there is histologic or even radiographic evidence of osteitis fibrosa, indicating that the remodeling system is responding as expected (51, 67). A defect in bone mineralization has been found in a few cases as in PTH deficiency, but this has never produced any clinical or radiographic manifestations of rickets or osteomalacia. The spectrum of changes is similar to that found in chronic renal failure, and is consistent with varying degrees and durations of 1,25-DHCC deficiency. The rise of plasma calcium to normal, which occasionally follows the lowering of plasma phosphate by means of phosphate-restricted diets, aluminum-containing antacids, and probenecid (67, 108), could be due to increased

synthesis of 1,25-DHCC consequent on removing one of the inhibitory factors, although there are no direct measurements of plasma 1,25-DHCC levels before and after phosphate restriction in patients with PHP. The spontaneous variation in the degree of hypocalcemia with time is also more consistent with an indirect rather than a direct consequence of the abnormal genotype.

Nevertheless, it is premature to conclude that there is no primary target cell resistance to PTH of the calcium homeostatic system in bone. This belief rests heavily on the assumption (115) that the small doses of 1,25-DHCC needed to restore normocalcemia (0.5 to 1.5 μg daily) (105) are within the range of physiologic replacement, but the normal range of daily secretion rates of 1,25-DHCC is not yet known with sufficient precision to justify this assumption. The doses of 1,25-DHCC required to heal nutritional rickets, in which there is also deficiency of 25-HCC, are almost certainly higher than the normal secretion rate of 1,25-DHCC. In several instances, patients with PHP and hypocalcemia responsive to small doses of 1,25-DHCC have had high 25-HCC levels, due to previous or even concurrent treatment with vitamin D (115).

As well as these doubts concerning the major evidence for the unitary concept, there are additional arguments against it. The differences between PHP and vitamin D dependency, in which there is invariably florid clinical and radiographic rickets with minimal osteitis fibrosa, seem much too profound to attribute solely to the difference in plasma phosphate levels. If 1,25-DHCC deficiency and hyperphosphatemia were the only causes of hypocalcemia in PHP, the metabolic state should be indistinguishable from chronic renal failure, in which parathyroid hyperplasia is more massive, hypersecretion of PTH is greater, osteitis fibrosa more prevalent, and the plasma calcium more commonly normal or even elevated for the same degree of hyperphosphatemia.

Another physiologic action of PTH of uncertain status in PHP is tubular reabsorption of calcium. The occurrence of hypercalciuria at normal or subnormal plasma calcium levels during vitamin D treatment is less common in PHP than in PTH deficiency (108). In six unrelated patients the relationship between calcium excretion/GFR and plasma calcium during infusion showed normal or even increased tubular reabsorption, suggesting an appropriate or only slightly blunted response to elevated PTH (116). This is consistent with the unitary concept of the disease, and provides further evidence against the view that the kidney is the sole regulator of plasma calcium. However, in five patients from three families exogenous PTH failed to produce a normal increase in tubular reabsorption of calcium in relation to sodium (117). In three of these patients, calcium reabsorption showed a normal increase in response to bicarbonate infusion and a greater than normal increase in response to chlorothiazide, suggesting that defective reabsorption of calcium was secondary to defective reabsorption of bicarbonate (118).

Although the unitary concept of the disease is attractive, and may be applicable to some patients, the data as a whole are more consistent with multiple target cell involvement, each target cell manifesting a spectrum of responsiveness to PTH, the severity of which varies independently between one patient and another (108).

PHP without SMS. This is a heterogeneous group, which includes at least three distinct entities and possibly more. There are many theoretically possible mechanisms of target cell resistance to PTH (67, 105), but so far only a few have been shown to exist. In some patients the metabolic abnormality is similar to that associated with SMS, although the condition is genetically distinct. However, as a group patients without SMS have a much higher prevalence of severe osteitis fibrosa, with metaphyseal lesions resembling rickets, slipping of femoral capital epiphyses, and localized cystic changes. In a few cases in this group the response to exogenous PTH with respect to cAMP as well as phosphate excretion has been partly restored by treatment. In a very small number of other cases, the pathogenesis appears to be fundamentally different.

In three cases of PTH-resistant hypocalcemia with increased plasma PTH there was a normal increase in cAMP excretion in response to exogenous PTH (119–121). In one case the baseline NcAMP excretion was markedly increased and in the others it was normal. None of the three had short metacarpals although in one case there was short stature and a round face. In all three the plasma phosphate was normal or only slightly raised for the patient's age, but the phosphaturic response to exogenous PTH was slightly to severely blunted. The marked variation in age of onset (2, 26, and 79 years) and a variety of other differences suggest that they do not all have the same disease. Plasma 1,25-DHCC was measured in only one case and was very low although 25-HCC was normal (121); a bone biopsy in the same case showed a slight increase in surface extent of osteoid, but no increase in resorption. In no case was there radiographic evidence of osteitis fibrosa. In all three cases there was absence of a significant calcemic response to PTH given for 2 to 4 days; in one case this response was restored to normal by 1,25-DHCC 1.0 μg daily with attainment of a normal plasma level of 1,25-DHCC (121). In a further case, a subnormal phosphaturic response with a normal cAMP response to exogenous PTH was associated with chronic hyperphosphatemia, normocalcemia, and osteomalacia (122). In one of the three cases a normal phosphaturic response to exogenous PTH was restored by calcium infusion (120); as mentioned earlier, there may be an abnormal relationship between cAMP production and Tm_P/GFR in SHP simply because of hypocalcemia. The pathogenesis of the hypocalcemia is obscure; it cannot be due only to a primary defect in 1-hydroxylation of 25-HCC, otherwise the condition would be identical with vitamin D dependency.

Secretion of a structurally abnormal hormone was one of the early theories to account for PHP; it was discarded with cumulative evidence for Albright's original concept of target cell resistance and with the demonstration that PTH extracted from resected glands was biologically active (108). The concept has recently been revived to account for some unusual observations in a few patients, but conclusive proof is still lacking. In one such case, normal responsiveness to exogenous PTH with respect to phosphate excretion, cAMP excretion, and plasma calcium elevation was demonstrated. PTH was consistently raised with several assay systems, although normal with another. It was hypothesized that a structural defect in the molecule destroyed both biologic activity and immunogenic reactivity to one antiserum but not to others (123). We have encountered the same paradoxical combination of immunoassay findings in a patient with unequivocal SHP, in whom absence of hormone was confirmed by two additional assay systems. Accordingly, the single case of so-called pseudoidiopathic HP could represent an artifact of PTH assay in a patient with otherwise straightforward IHP. More recently, much stronger evidence for this concept was obtained in a patient with hypocalcemia, radiographic osteitis fibrosa, and markedly elevated iPTH by two different assays (124). After suppression of the iPTH level to normal with EC, endogenous PTH secretion was stimulated by induced hypocalcemia, but there was no significant change in phosphate or cAMP excretion. Exogenous PTH produced a normal increase in urinary cAMP and decrease in Tm_P/GFR, and 800 units of PTH daily for 2½ days raised plasma calcium from 1.4 to 2.4 mmol/L. In this patient the remodeling system was responsive both to exogenous and endogenous PTH, but the kidney (and presumably also the calcium homeostatic system in bone) was responsive to exogenous but not to endogenous PTH. This combination of findings indicates either an abnormal PTH molecule or abnormal receptors which recognize bovine but not human PTH.

Calcium deficiency and other causes of normocalcemic secondary hyperparathyroidism. A fall in plasma ionized calcium of as little as 0.01 mmol/L leads to a prompt increase in PTH secretion within a few minutes (Chap. 8). If the abnormal conditions leading to the fall persist, and the calcium homeostatic system in bone remains intact, a new equilibrium is reached in which plasma ionized calcium is slightly reduced and plasma PTH persistently raised. Ionized or corrected total calcium remains within normal limits, and the extent of the fall may be below the detection limits of current methodology. However, if only the ionic calcium-PTH feedback loop is involved, and the stimulus-response relationship of each component of the loop is unchanged, the original disturbance cannot be completely corrected; there has to be a continued stimulus to increased PTH secretion. Complete correction may be possible either if there is some stimulus to PTH secretion other than a fall in ionized calcium, or if the stimulus-response relationship of the gland changes in such a way that more PTH is secreted at the same plasma ionized calcium.

A sustained demand for increased PTH secretion usually leads to increased parathyroid cell mass because of hyperplasia (22). The stimulus for increased cell division and proliferation is not known, but may be related to a fall in the intracellular concentration of hormone (125). If maintenance of increased cell mass required a continuing increase in the fraction of cells undergoing cell division, then continuing stimulus to increased cell division would be needed. But once an increase in parathyroid cell mass has occurred, it could be maintained indefinitely if the birth rate and death rate of parathyroid cells (expressed as fractions of total cell mass) are the same as before, provided that the mean life span of the cell did not change. If each parathyroid cell retained the same stimulus-response relationship as before, the stimulus-response relationship of the whole gland would be changed such that more hormone would be secreted at the same level of plasma calcium (23). Consequently, the development of a sufficient degree of hyperplasia permits complete correction of the initial hypocalcemic stimulus, provided that the calcium homeostatic system in bone is intact. The hyperplasia will therefore be stable and nonprogressive. If the homeostatic system is not intact, then hypocalcemia may occur, existing hypocalcemia will be intensified, and parathyroid hyperplasia will tend to progress.

All of the causes of CC-metabolite deficiency initially bring about just such a sequence of events; the tendency to parathyroid hyperplasia may be augmented by loss of the hypothetical direct effect of 24,25-DHCC or 1,25-DHCC on the gland, which serves to delay the onset of 1,25-DHCC deficiency as explained earlier. Only with more severe deficiency does the calcium homeostatic system in bone begin to fail and hypocalcemia ensue. Apart from CC-metabolite deficiency, normocalcemic secondary hyperparathyroidism is produced by any process which tends to deplete the ECF of calcium, and by any process which increases the requirement for PTH of the calcium homeostatic system in bone (Table 19-10).

Reduced Net Intestinal Calcium Absorption. From a global viewpoint, this most commonly results from a simple reduction in intake. When this affects an entire community throughout life, as in the Bantu, little harm seems to result, possibly because of genetic adaptation (40). But if intake is reduced below the customary level for any reason, physiologic adaptation is necessary to minimize the extent of negative balance; the more abrupt the change the longer the time required to achieve maximum adaptation.

Net intestinal absorption may also be reduced because of increased fecal calcium excretion. Calcium absorption is relatively inefficient, and may be impaired because of defects in the intestinal mucosa as in sprue or gluten enteropathy,

Table 19-10. Causes of secondary hyperparathyroidism*

Hypocalcemic
  Resistance of homeostatic system to PTH
  Deficiency of vitamin D and/or its metabolites
  PHP ± SMS
Normocalcemic
  ECF calcium depletion
    Low dietary intake
    Intestinal malabsorption
    Decreased tubular reabsorption
    Pregnancy and lactation
    Increased net deposition in bone
    Dystrophic soft tissue calcification
    Hemodialysis
  Increased PTH requirement of calcium homeostatic system
    Hyperphosphatemia
    Fluorosis†
    Magnesium depletion‡
    Hypothyroidism
    Osteomalacia
    Corticosteroid excess

* The distinction between hypocalcemic and normocalcemic forms is useful but not absolute. Mild instances of the former may be normocalcemic, and severe instances of the latter may be transiently hypocalcemic.
† Fluorosis is the only normocalcemic cause which may become severe enough to cause osteitis fibrosa; this occurs much more commonly in the hypocalcemic group.
‡ PTH secretion is usually reduced by an independent effect.

trapping of calcium as soaps because of severe steatorrhea from any cause, impaired active transport due to CC-metabolite deficiency, or direct interference with the transport mechanism by corticosteroid excess (126). There may also be increased endogenous secretion of calcium, as in exudative enteropathy or in various diseases of the large bowel (127). Fecal calcium is usually increased in diseases such as hyperthyroidism or hypophosphatemic osteomalacia in which there is accelerated loss of bone or loss of bone mineral due to a primary disturbance in bone cell function. Throughout life, calcium absorption is regulated in some way by the need of the skeleton for calcium, independent of vitamin D status (128), although the mechanism is unknown. Occasionally fecal calcium may be so high that it exceeds intake and net absorption is negative. This precludes adaptation, but is rare unless dietary intake is also reduced. For example, fecal calcium exceeded intake in only one of nine patients with osteomalacia due to gluten enteropathy (129). In nutritional vitamin D deficiency, fecal calcium only rarely exceeds intake by more than 5 mmol/day and more commonly is approximately equal to intake.

The immediate response to decreased net absorption is increased tubular reabsorption of calcium probably due to secondary hyperparathyroidism. Urinary calcium excretion falls promptly but rarely below 1 mmol/day (83), so that a negative balance may still occur. This leads to accelerated loss of bone because of a combination of increased turnover (increased birth rate of BRU) and increased remodeling imbalance in each BRU. These changes are probably also due to secondary hyperparathyroidism, since kinetically determined bone turnover does not increase in response to a low-calcium diet in patients with HP (130). Severe calcium deficiency during rapid skeletal growth in infancy may lead to hypocalcemia, secondary hyperparathyroidism, hypophosphatemia, and rickets (131), but in adults hypocalcemia occurs only if calcium malabsorption is due to lack of CC metabolites, or is accompanied by PTH deficiency. In patients with normocalcemic HP (grades 1 and 2) simultaneous depletion of calcium and magnesium by means of cellulose phosphate leads to hypocalcemia, with failure to increase tubular reabsorption of calcium or urinary hydroxyproline excretion (83).

Decreased Renal-Tubular Reabsorption. If plasma calcium were regulated in the same way as plasma phosphate or magnesium, TR_{Ca}/GFR would be the major determinant of the plasma level, but there is no known instance of sustained hypocalcemia due to decreased tubular reabsorption of calcium alone. For calcium, as for glucose, the extrarenal mechanisms which maintain the plasma level ensure that decreased tubular reabsorption leads to increased urinary excretion, not to a fall in plasma level. For calcium, this only occurs if the homeostatic system in bone is defective. Decreased tubular reabsorption of calcium makes hypocalcemia more difficult to treat in HP and probably contributes to the hypocalcemia in chronic renal failure and the secondary HP of chronic corticosteroid therapy.

Although short-term increases in urinary calcium could be met by the bone surface–perilacunar compartment or by the interstitial fluid and soft tissue components of the exchangeable pool, sustained primary hypercalciuria must ultimately lead either to increased net intestinal absorption or to increased net bone resorption or both. The former response is clearly more desirable, and is mediated at least in part by secondary hyperparathyroidism and consequent increased synthesis of 1,25-DHCC. The mechanisms, causes, and effects of hypercalciuria are considered later in greater detail.

Other Mechanisms of Calcium Depletion. Increased net loss of calcium from the ECF occurs in the last trimester of pregnancy, with storage of approximately 600 mmol of calcium in the fetus, or about 7 mmol/day. This is associated with increases in PTH secretion (50), intestinal calcium absorption, and bone turnover (132). 1,25-DHCC synthesis may be stimulated not only by PTH, but independently by the hormonal changes of pregnancy, but the adaptive changes cannot be reproduced by ovarian hormones alone. Calcium absorption increases even in the second trimester before the onset of significant mineral accumulation by the fetus (132). All these changes continue and are intensified during lactation, which

removes as much as 12 mmol of calcium daily, but revert to normal within 3 months if lactation is terminated. The possible adverse effects of the calcium drain of pregnancy and lactation on bone are usually more than offset by the other endocrine changes of pregnancy, and bone mass measured by photon absorptiometry increases with parity (40). But when superimposed on nutritional vitamin D deficiency, the calcium drain of pregnancy and lactation intensifies both hypocalcemia and osteomalacia (93).

If osteosclerosis develops for any reason, there must for a period of time be increased net storage of calcium in bone and increased net intestinal absorption of calcium. Bone metastases from carcinoma of the prostate stimulate osteoblastic proliferation, and formation of new woven bone occurs much faster than bone destruction, leading to radiographic osteosclerosis. The same occasionally occurs with metastases from carcinoma of the lung or the breast (133, 134). Net storage of calcium, as shown by external calcium balance, may be in the range of 5 to 10 mmol/day with net intestinal calcium absorption greater than 50 percent and urine calcium excretion less than 1.5 mmol/day (133, 134). There is also comparable retention of phosphate with reduced urinary excretion. It is unclear whether these changes in mineral balance are mediated by increased secretion of PTH and 1,25-DHCC or by other homeostatic links between bone and gut. The same comment applies to the adaptive increase in calcium absorption which occurs during normal growth. The much more pronounced secondary hyperparathyroidism of fluorosis occurs by a different mechanism.

Too low a calcium concentration in the dialysate was a common cause of negative calcium balance and intensified secondary hyperparathyroidism and osteodystrophy during the early years of maintenance hemodialysis. A final route of loss of calcium from the ECF is into the soft tissues, and normocalcemic secondary hyperparathyroidism may occur in various types of calcinosis as described later. With both low-calcium dialysis and soft tissue deposition, loss of calcium from the ECF may be so rapid that it causes hypocalcemia. The same may occur with osteoblastic metastases but there are usually additional factors at work as described in the next section.

Increased Requirement for PTH of the Calcium Homeostatic System in Bone. The most important factor increasing PTH requirement is increased dietary intake of phosphate, or any other process tending to raise the plasma phosphate level. An increased phosphate concentration in the bone ECF must be associated with either decreased calcium concentration and an increased calcium gradient between systemic ECF and bone ECF, or no change in calcium with an increase in apparent solubility of bone mineral. In either case the necessary adjustments require an increased secretion of PTH. The kidney can excrete a moderately increased phosphate load by decreasing phosphate reabsorption by a mechanism which does not require an increase in PTH secretion, but a large increase in phosphate intake leads to persistent secondary hyperparathyroidism. Significant hypocalcemia occurs only if the calcium homeostatic system is defective, as in the neonatal period, in chronic renal failure, and in PTH deficiency or resistance. The subject is discussed further on p. 1090.

In chronic fluorosis the solubility of bone mineral is decreased by incorporation of fluoride, which would tend to lower the calcium concentration in the bone ECF and so in the plasma (51). This can be readily overcome by increased PTH secretion. Excluding CC-metabolite deficiency, fluorosis is the only cause of normocalcemic secondary hyperparathyroidism which may be associated with radiographic osteitis fibrosa. Loss of magnesium from the crystal surface and hydration shell impairs the release of calcium into the ambient fluid, so that chronic magnesium depletion may increase PTH requirement, but the inhibitory effect of hypomagnesemia on PTH synthesis may prevent an appropriate response (135).

Mild secondary hyperparathyroidism also occurs in hypothyroidism (136). Although reduced bone turnover modestly increases net calcium storage in bone, this is unlikely to be the sole explanation. More likely, thyroid hormone is necessary for normal functioning of the bone lining cell–osteocyte system, as it is for many other cells in the body. In normocalcemic HP (grades 1 and 2), hypothyroidism may lead to sustained hypocalcemia, correctable by thyroid administration alone (A. M. Parfitt, unpublished data). Both endogenous and exogenous cortisol excess reduce calcium absorption to an extent requiring 0.4 μg of 1,25-DHCC daily to overcome (90a) and modestly decrease the tubular reabsorption of calcium. In addition large doses of corticosteroids probably antagonize the effect of PTH on bone cells, by blocking inward transport and uptake of calcium (64).

A final cause of increased PTH requirement is osteomalacia, which occludes the quiescent bone surface required for operation of the homeostatic system, and increases the distance between the cells on the surface and the mineralized bone beneath. This is discussed further on p. 1081.

Miscellaneous causes of transient hypocalcemia. Many of the processes which cause normocalcemic secondary hyperparathyroidism may cause acute hypocalcemia if the loss of calcium from the ECF is sufficiently rapid. In addition a transient fall in ionized calcium may result from alteration of the normal relationships between calcium, protein, and complexing ions for a variety of reasons (Table 19-11), but this is quickly corrected if the PTH-homeostatic system is normal. Many agents including histamine, gastrin, ethanol, protamine, and imidazole cause acute hypocalcemia in experimental animals by various means (137) but have not yet been shown to have clinical relevance.

Fall in Ionized Calcium due to Intravascular Redistribution or Replacement. Exchange transfusion for neonatal hyperbilirubinemia is often carried out with stored blood preserved with ACD (acid-citrate-dextrose). The plasma ionized calcium may fall below 0.5 mmol/L during the exchange despite a rise in total calcium concentration (138). This occurs partly because of dilution by ACD and partly because of complexing by citrate; no significant change in ionized calcium occurs with heparinized blood. There is only a transient response to calcium gluconate. A fall in ionized calcium also occurs during plasma exchange as treatment for hyperglobulinemia or hypercholesterolemia, and can be prevented by the addition of calcium gluconate (139).

Table 19-11. Causes of transient hypocalcemia

Intravascular redistribution or replacement
  Exchange transfusion in neonates with ACD* blood
  Massive transfusion at any age with ACD blood
  Plasma exchange
  Rapid infusion of saline or hyperoncotic albumin
  Sudden increase in compexed calcium
   (phosphate, citrate, lactate, free fatty acids, bicarbonate,
   sulfate, EDTA)
Sudden increase in net deposition in bone
  Decrease in bone resorption
   (calcitonin, glucagon, mithramycin, actinomycin,
   diphosphonate, colchicine)
  Increase in mineralization of bone
    Early treatment of rickets
    Sudden hyperphosphatemia
  Increase in bone formation
    Osteoblastic metastases
    Healing osteitis fibrosa cystica
    Healing thyrotoxic osteopathy
Failure to increase bone resorption in response to calcium
 depletion
  Osteopetrosis
  Medullary carcinoma of the thyroid
  Normocalcemic HP
Sudden increase in net deposition in soft tissues
  Traumatic rhabdomyolysis
  Acute pancreatitis
  Rapid hyperphosphatemia
Multiple mechanisms and miscellaneous causes
  Magnesium infusion (also suppression of PTH)
  Hypernatremic dehydration in infants
  Aminoglycoside antibiotics
  Acute leukemia
  Hyperkalemic periodic paralysis (during attack) (200)
  Kenny syndrome (dwarfism plus medullary stenosis) (201)

* ACD, acid-citrate-dextrose; EDTA, ethylene diamine tetraacetic
acid.

Rapid administration of isotonic saline dilutes the ionized calcium faster than it can be mobilized from bone leading to an acute increase in PTH secretion and urinary cAMP excretion (140). Intravenous hyperoncotic albumin increases the protein-bound calcium at the expense of the ionized fraction with similar consequences (Chap. 8). The same mechanisms probably operate during infusion of all nonblood plasma expanders.

Complexing by citrate lowers ionized calcium during massive blood transfusion at any age (141), but the clinical importance of this and the need for treatment have been questioned (142). Citrate is metabolized rapidly by the normal liver; with impairment of hepatic function by anesthetic agents or hypoxia, the reduction in ionized calcium produced by citrate may persist for much longer than normal (141). A fall in ionized calcium due to an increase in complexed calcium may also result from lactate accumulation (143) due to exercise or ischemia, from a rise in plasma-free fatty acids (144) produced by epinephrine or ACTH (adrenocorticotrophic hormone) or occurring after pancreatitis or fat embolism, or from infusion of phosphate, bicarbonate, sulfate, or EDTA. In all these situations the immediate fall in ionized calcium is unrelated to the subsequent fate of the calcium complex which is formed. A rise in free fatty acids may also lower ionized calcium by increasing the affinity of albumin for calcium (144).

Many of these mechanisms operate in critically ill patients with sepsis, trauma, or shock (145). The changes during cardiopulmonary surgery were mentioned earlier. In patients undergoing extracorporeal perfusion, ionized calcium routinely falls to around 0.5 mmol/L in the absence of preventive measures (146). The effects resulting from accumulation of complexing anions in sick patients are sometimes compounded by impaired renal conservation of calcium. In addition, hypocalcemia may be a direct consequence of low cardiac output and impaired tissue perfusion since both improve with isoproterenol (147); whether this effect is on bone or on the parathyroid gland is not clear.

Increased Net Deposition in Bone. A decrease in activity of existing osteoclasts may lead to a transient fall in bone resorption and lower the plasma calcium, but hypocalcemia does not usually occur unless bone turnover is initially very high. Complete suppression of normal bone resorption for 3 h would remove approximately 1 mmol of calcium from the ECF and lower plasma calcium by about 0.05 mmol/L. However, if bone turnover were increased ten-fold, the number of osteoclasts would be similarly increased and complete suppression of resorption for the same time would lower plasma calcium by about 0.5 mmol/L. After 100 units of salmon calcitonin the plasma calcium fell by 0.05 mmol/L at 6 h in normal subjects and by 0.25 mmol/L in subjects with Paget's disease; there was a significant correlation between the fall in plasma calcium and the extent of trabecular bone surface covered by osteoblasts (148). Similar comments apply to the inhibition of bone resorption by other agents. For example, glucagon lowers plasma calcium by 0.1 mmol/L in normal subjects, by 0.17 mmol/L in primary hyperparathyroidism (149), and by 0.2 to 0.3 mmol/L in Paget's disease. Similar observations have been made with mithramycin, actinomycin, and various diphosphonates, compounds which will be discussed further in relation to the treatment of hypercalcemia. The hypocalcemia of colchicine poisoning (150) is due to inhibition of microtubular function both in the parathyroid gland leading to decreased PTH secretion and in osteoclasts leading to an acute decrease in bone resorption (151).

Prolonged treatment of Paget's disease with calcitonin reduces bone turnover and the number of osteoclasts, and leads to a progressive reduction in the acute hypocalcemic response, but does not lead to hypocalcemia or to any sustained increase either in basal PTH or the PTH increment in response to hypocalcemia (152). Similarly, in patients with medullary carcinoma of the thyroid and continued hypersecretion of calcitonin the mean plasma calcium is slightly decreased (37) and transient hypocalcemia may occur in response to intercurrent illness such as gastroenteritis, but sustained hypocalcemia unequivocally due to calcitonin excess has not been documented. Of four cases in which this has been suggested (153) two had steatorrhea, one had very slight hypocalcemia (mean 2.14 mmol/L) with no protein correction, and one had tetany after thyroid surgery with only a single high value for iPTH to rule out the obvious diagnosis of SHP. In two patients with chronic hypocalcemia total thyroidectomy was followed by a rise in plasma calcium, but this was short lived (37).

Although inhibition of resorption does not reduce steady-state plasma calcium levels (64), it may impair the response to dietary calcium depletion. This may account for the mild hypocalcemia which occurs in normocalcemic HP in response to a low-calcium diet combined with cellulose phosphate (83), and the more severe hypocalcemia with tetany which occurs with the same regimen in osteopetrosis (51). The same probably also applies to intermittent hypocalcemia in patients with medullary carcinoma of the thyroid.

Transient hypocalcemia may result from accelerated primary mineralization early in the treatment of rickets or osteomalacia or from accelerated secondary mineralization after administration of phosphate, but sustained deposition of calcium requires a substantial increase in formation of new bone, either woven bone as in fracture healing or osteoblastic metastases or lamellar bone as in healing thyrotoxic osteopathy or osteitis fibrosa. Several other mechanisms of increased net bone deposition were discussed in Chap. 8.

In osteoblastic metastases in bone, despite rapid net deposition of calcium, corrected plasma calcium usually remains normal; in one recent series (154) it was low in only 4 of 23 supposed cases of hypocalcemia, the remainder having a low total calcium due to hypoalbuminemia. But occasionally there may be significant hypocalcemia (1.5 to 2 mmol/L) with tetany, and the plasma phosphate may also be reduced (154, 155). Compared to patients without hypocalcemia the positive balance is even larger (in the range of 10 to 25 mmol/day) and fecal and urinary calcium excretion even lower (155). The total deposition of calcium in new bone must be even greater than the degree of net calcium retention, and may exceed the capacity of the normal homeostatic defenses, but this is unlikely to be the only factor. Bone formation may be accelerated still further by estrogen treatment in carcinoma of the prostate and by oophorectomy in carcinoma of the breast, but any fall in plasma calcium is usually small, transient, and asymptomatic. In some patients the plasma phosphate is raised, and in one case the metabolic data during life were indicative of HP and no parathyroid glands could be found at autopsy (156); metastatic disease is known to destroy the parathyroid glands in some cases (53). Another possible mechanism is the occurrence of bone formation over almost all free bone surfaces, such that the extent of quiescent surface available for the blood-bone equilibrium might be too small to sustain a normal plasma calcium. Unexplained hypocalcemia has been noted in cancer even without bone involvement. In one patient with myeloma, hypocalcemia was associated with low levels of cholesterol and fibrinogen, and all three rose to normal during remission induced by melphalan (157).

The most potent cause of hypocalcemia due to increased net bone formation is the so-called hungry bone syndrome which occurs during healing of osteitis fibrosa following either surgical resection or spontaneous infarction of an adenoma in primary hyperparathyroidism (79). Severe bone hunger develops more quickly and is much more severe than during healing of hyperthyroid bone disease (74) and the plasma calcium may fall so quickly that the patient gets convulsive seizures leading to multiple fractures. Tetany is refractory to treatment and occurs despite persistent elevation of plasma PTH. This is because conversion of resorptive to formative surfaces occurs within a few days rather than over several weeks as after correction of hypothyroidism. On all surfaces where resorption was previously in progress, osteoclasts rapidly disappear and new appositional bone formation begins. The hypocalcemia is usually accompanied by a substantial fall in both plasma phosphate and magnesium, and all three ions may practically disappear from the urine.

Pancreatitis and Other Causes of Abnormal Calcium Deposition in Soft Tissues. Extensive deposition of calcium salts may occur in necrotic muscle in traumatic rhabdomyolysis with acute renal failure (158). A similar mechanism operates in acute pancreatitis with retroperitoneal fat necrosis. One reason for the hypocalcemic effect of phosphate administration is the formation of colloidal calcium phosphate which is taken up by the macrophages and Kupffer cells in the liver (Chap. 8); whether calcium phosphate is deposited in other soft tissues is not known. The effects of hyperphosphatemia on plasma calcium are discussed further in relation to the treatment of hypercalcemia (p. 1035), and in the section on phosphate.

The frequency of hypocalcemia in acute pancreatitis has been overestimated because of failure to correct total calcium values for the usual fall in plasma albumin. In one large unselected series (159) the incidence of apparent hypocalcemia was 64 percent, but true hypocalcemia occurred only in 11 percent. In mild cases ionized calcium values often remain normal (160), but in severe cases the ionized calcium usually falls below 0.9 mmol/L, with occasional values as low as 0.3 mmol/L, the nadir occurring 48 to 72 h after the onset of the disease (161). The ionized calcium may be lower than expected from total calcium and albumin levels because of an increase in plasma free fatty acids.

The initial fall in plasma calcium is due to deposition of calcium as soaps in areas of lipolysis and fat necrosis, of which the calcium content is more than 200 mmol/kg (162). As much as 50 mmol of calcium has been recovered at autopsy, and disseminated fat necrosis may occur in the bone marrow and other areas because of circulating lipase, so that the total amount of calcium deposited is probably higher. In the pig, thyroidectomy abolishes the hypocalcemia of experimental pancreatitis, but calcitonin is a more important calcium-regulating hormone in this species than in humans (163). In patients, although calcitonin levels are sometimes markedly raised (probably in response to increased glucagon secretion), they do not correlate with the degree of hypocalcemia (161, 164). Calcitonin may contribute to delayed recovery, but it is probably not an important initiating factor. The same comment applies also to glucagon and to gastrin. The pancreas of the dog contains a hypocalcemic factor distinct from glucagon (165) but its role in human disease is unknown.

The plasma phosphate also usually falls in acute pancreatitis, following about 24 h after the fall in plasma calcium. In one series the mean was 0.8 mmol/L, with some values as low as 0.3 mmol/L (159). When measured Tm_P/GFR had been reduced (0.3 to 0.6 mmol/L, mean 0.5) and urinary cAMP excretion increased (164), most likely because of increased PTH secretion. Plasma iPTH levels have usually been increased (161) except in one study using a C-terminal assay (164). In some patients iPTH has been undetectable (166), and even when raised it is not clear whether the increase is appropriate for the degree of hypocalcemia. A suboptimal PTH response might result from hypomagnesemia or from proteolytic destruction of PTH within the circulation (166). The response to exogenous PTH is normal with respect both to plasma ionized calcium and urinary cAMP (164).

There are no data concerning urinary calcium excretion in acute pancreatitis prior to treatment. In some cases infused calcium has been promptly excreted with minimal increase in plasma level (167) and in other cases the plasma calcium has returned to normal (161). Possible causes for defective renal conservation of calcium include lack of PTH, the metabolic acidosis of tissue destruction, and the calciuretic effect of glucagon.

Multiple Mechanisms and Miscellaneous Conditions. Increased renal excretion rarely causes significant hypocalcemia alone, but probably contributes to several of the hypocalcemic states already discussed. Massive short-term losses (up to 40 mmol per 24 h) in various states of increased diuresis such as the recovery phase of acute renal failure may lead to transient hypocalcemia but this is more likely in patients with HP, in whom tetany may be precipitated by furosemide; this may lower ionized calcium by 0.15 mmol/L even in patients rendered normocalcemic with vitamin D (168). Hypermagnesemia resulting from treatment of eclampsia with magnesium salts has caused hypocalcemia (169), probably due to a combination of increased renal excretion of calcium resulting from competition between calcium and magnesium for the same reabsorptive mechanism, and depression of PTH secretion.

In infants during the first year of life, hypernatremia arising during the course of acute gastroenteritis, either present initially (hypertonic dehydration) (170) or after correction of metabolic acidosis (171), may be accompanied by moderate to severe hypocalcemia (1.4 to 2.0 mmol/L). The total plasma calcium is not correlated with phosphate, BUN (blood urea nitrogen), or protein but is inversely correlated with plasma sodium. Hypocalcemic infants are usually hypokalemic, and hypertonic saline lowers plasma calcium in potassium-depleted rats but not in normal rats (172). Conceivably some of the excess potassium in bone fluid may exchange for calcium, but no comparable phenomenon has been demonstrated in older children or adults.

Antibiotics of the aminoglycoside group occasionally induce a complex metabolic disorder comprising low blood levels of calcium, magnesium, potassium, and frequently phosphate. This has occurred with gentamycin, sisomicin, amikacin, tobramycin, viomycin, and capreomycin (173). The incidence is higher in patients with cancer, possibly because of an additive effect with adriamycin, an aminoglycoside antitumor agent. Streptomycin causes hypocalcemia in rats and has been successfully used to treat hypercalcemia in humans (174) but has not been reported to cause the complete syndrome. The plasma calcium corrected for albumin has ranged from 1.3 to 2.0 mmol/L. Hypokalemia and hypomagnesemia are due to impaired tubular reabsorption and consequent renal wasting. The PTH level is reduced to about half normal, and may be undetectable. The hypocalcemia does not respond to magnesium administration; this may be because sustained correction of magnesium depletion is not possible in the presence of a severe renal leak, or because PTH hyposecretion is due not only to magnesium depletion but to some additional effect of the drug. Plasma calcitonin levels are also normal or low. Whether renal wasting of calcium contributes to the hypocalcemia has not been determined. Complete recovery is usual within 2 to 8 weeks after cessation of the offending drug, but a few patients develop permanent and progressive renal failure.

Aminoglycoside antibiotics also cause muscle paralysis and respiratory depression because of blockade of neuromuscular transmission, particularly during and after anesthesia. This may be relieved by the administration of calcium, but is due to competition with calcium for receptors, not to a fall in plasma ionized calcium (175).

Many of the mechanisms already mentioned operate in patients with acute leukemia, with the additional effects of gram-negative septicemia, aminoglycoside and other antitumor agents, and both acute and chronic renal failure (176, 177). Severe hypocalcemia occurs in about one-third of adults and about 10 percent of children with acute leukemia; it is frequently terminal, occurring often within the last week of life.

Effects of hypocalcemia

HP is the major cause of symptomatic hypocalcemia (see Chap. 16) but it is not always clear whether the clinical features of HP are due to hypocalcemia alone, to other complications of HP such as hyperphosphatemia, or to other manifestations of the cause of the HP. There are interesting species differences in the response to hypocalcemia. In the cow this causes blockade of neuromuscular transmission and consequent paralysis (178) but in humans muscle weakness is very rare, except possibly in patients who have myasthenia gravis (179) or are receiving aminoglycoside antibiotics (175). The most frequent symptoms of hypocalcemia result from increased irritability of the nervous system, both peripheral and central (53, 180). This is related to the severity and rapidity of onset of hypocalcemia, not to its duration, but many of the other complications require a certain period of time to develop.

Tetany (53, 137, 180). It is convenient to use this term to denote the entire symptom complex due to increased neural excitability. A typical attack begins with sensations of tingling in the tips of the fingers, around the mouth, and less commonly in the feet. These gradually increase in severity and spread proximally along the limbs and over the face, and may be followed by numbness. The muscles of the extremities and sometimes the face then begin to feel tense and later go into spasm, progressing in the same pattern as the preceding sensory symptoms. Pain depends on the degree of tension developed in the muscle and may be very severe. Carpal spasm progresses to the classic "main d'accoucheur" posture, and less commonly similar changes occur in the lower limbs. Tetany is rarely dangerous but it is frequently alarming and the patient may be hyperventilating, both as a result of anxiety and as a reflex component of the syndrome. Both hypocapnia and increased adrenalin secretion worsen the tetany and produce their own effects, such as peripheral and circumoral pallor, sweating, and tachycardia.

Experimentally, a nerve exposed to a low concentration of calcium exhibits a reduced threshold of excitation, repetitive responses to a single stimulus, impairment of accommodation, and fi-nally, spontaneous activity. The manifestations of tetany are due to spontaneous discharges of both sensory and motor fibers in peripheral nerves which originate in the proximal part of the nerve even though the symptoms are felt earliest in the extremities.

Lesser degrees of neural excitability may be recognized by various signs for latent tetany. Chvostek's sign is elicited by tapping the facial nerve about 2 cm anterior to the earlobe just below the zygomatic process or between the zygomatic arch and the corner of the mouth. The responses consist of varying degrees of twitching of muscles supplied by the facial nerve. Trousseau's sign is elicited by inflating a sphygomanometer cuff on the upper arm to above the systolic blood pressure. The sensory and motor manifestations of tetany occur in sequence within 2 min, culminating in a typical attack of carpal spasm. The response depends on the induction of ischemia of the ulnar nerve immediately subjacent to the cuff. When the cuff is released, the muscles take about 5 to 10 s to relax; spasm which disappears immediately is unlikely to be genuine.

If a typical attack is witnessed or well described, the diagnosis of tetany will be obvious, but many variations are possible (53, 57, 180). The patient may describe the muscle spasm as a cramp, or as stiffness or clumsiness. Attacks are frequently precipitated by hyperventilation, whether due to emotional distress or to exercise. Spasm of the muscles of the larynx (laryngismus stridulus) fixes the vocal cords in the midline, but in adults laryngeal stridor is usually a result of hypocalcemia combined with vocal cord paralysis. In infants, carpopedal spasm is rare but tremors, twitches, and convulsive seizures are more common than in adults.

The effects of a rapidly falling calcium are more outspoken than those of a stable calcium at a lower level, and tetany may rarely be absent in long-standing hypocalcemia. Tetany may be masked by hypokalemia, hypermagnesemia, metabolic acidosis, uremia, or hypophosphatemia and worsened by withdrawal of thyroid medication, infection, diuretic administration, menstruation, and pregnancy, all with no change in plasma calcium level. Other causes of tetany include hyperkalemia, hypokalemia, hypomagnesemia, and both metabolic and respiratory alkalosis. As well as lowering ionized calcium, alkalosis has an independent and synergistic effect of increasing neural excitability. Patients with unrecognized hypocalcemia who are anxious and overbreathing may be dismissed from emergency rooms as hysterical.

Convulsive seizures (53, 180). Hypocalcemia increases neuronal irritability in the central as well as in the peripheral system and fits resembling those of epilepsy may occur. After parathyroid surgery these are very liable to cause fractures (181). There are two distinct types of seizure, although some patients may get both kinds. First, hypocalcemia lowers the excitation threshold for preexisting subclinical epilepsy. The attacks are indistinguishable from those occurring in the absence of hypocalcemia and may be of any form—focal, Jacksonian, petit mal, or grand mal. The EEG (electroencephalogram) shows the same range of findings as in epilepsy with normocalcemia, and remains abnormal with successful treatment even though the number of seizures is reduced (53). Second, generalized tetany may be followed by prolonged tonic spasms, more aptly referred to as cerebral tetany rather than epilepsy. There may be either an aura of the sensory symptoms of tetany or no aura at all, and tongue biting, loss of consciousness, incontinence, and postictal confusion may not occur. The EEG shows characteristic changes which gradually improve with treatment. Both types of seizure are usually refractory to anticonvulsant therapy (100); phenytoin masks the peripheral manifestations of tetany (182) and may initiate the vicious circle previously described.

Cardiovascular effects (see Chap. 14). Hypocalcemia delays ventricular repolarization and increases the Q-T interval and ST segment, which vary inversely with plasma calcium over the range 4 to 1 mmol/L. In neonates both total and ionized calcium correlate better with the $Q-T_c$ interval (i.e., the corrected Q-T interval) than the Q-T interval (183). The characteristic ECG (electrocardiogram) changes may lead to the recognition of hypocalcemia when other signs are lacking (184). With prolongation of electrical systole, the ventricles may fail to respond to the next atrial impulse, producing 2:1 heart block, and ventricular

arrhythmias (185) and refractoriness to digoxin in atrial fibrillation (186) may persist until hypocalcemia is corrected. These effects of hypocalcemia have been made use of in the treatment of digitalis-induced arrhythmias by EDTA infusion (187).

Calcium ion has a positive inotropic effect on the myocardium and is essential for coupling of excitation and contraction, but clinical effects of hypocalcemia on heart muscle function are rare. In the older literature, cardiac tetany was often reported in infants with rickets who developed dyspnea, tachycardia, and sudden death due to cardiac arrest in diastole. More recently a fall in ionized calcium due to excess citrate has been implicated in the fall in cardiac output and blood pressure induced by multiple blood transfusions (141). Routine monitoring of plasma ionized calcium in acutely sick patients has been advocated, but low values seem to be more the result than the cause of low cardiac output and impaired tissue perfusion (147). Severe hypotension and even shock may rarely be caused by acute hypocalcemia in various settings (184, 188), but the postural hypotension which occurs after EDTA infusion (189) is not due to a fall in ionized calcium because it is as common after calcium EDTA as after sodium EDTA.

In chronic hypocalcemia calcium infusion may increase both cardiac output and blood pressure, suggesting that cardiac function was suboptimal. There are also several well-documented instances in both children and adults of chronic hypocalcemia leading to congestive cardiac failure requiring digitalization and diuretic therapy, the need for which is abolished after restoration of normocalcemia for a few weeks or months (53).

Psychiatric effects. An acute toxic confusional psychosis may occur within 2 weeks of neck surgery, the patient being delirious, hallucinated, paranoid, or suicidal. This is commoner after parathyroid than after thyroid surgery and probably is related to hypomagnesemia as well as hypocalcemia. After recovery this acute psychosis does not recur even if hypocalcemia returns. In long-standing hypocalcemia many kinds of psychoneurosis, psychosis, and organic brain syndrome have been described. Subnormal intelligence occurs in about one-fifth of children with HP; it correlates with prolonged untreated hypocalcemia irrespective of its cause. Intelligence may increase with treatment or remain unchanged, despite improvement in personality. The wide variety of other syndromes suggests that, as with seizures, hypocalcemia has triggered a disorder to which the patient was already predisposed.

Ectodermal effects (53). The acute hypocalcemia after thyroidectomy may rarely be followed by a temporary arrest of growth of the hair and fingernails. The affected hair loses its luster and with resumption of growth (which may occur spontaneously even in the absence of treatment) it falls out extensively. In chronic hypocalcemia the skin may be dry and scaling, the nails brittle and fissured longitudinally, and the hair coarse, dry, fractured, and easily shed. Any existing dermatosis may be made worse.

Hypocalcemia affects a tooth only when it begins during the development of that tooth; teeth already formed are not affected. Hypoplasia of the enamel, with pitting, staining, superficial fractures, and increased liability to caries is the most characteristic finding. In HP, prolonged hypocalcemia is necessary to induce enamel hypoplasia, although this may follow transient neonatal hypocalcemia if there was maternal vitamin D deficiency.

Lenticular cataracts are the most common complication of chronic hypocalcemia (53). They begin as discrete punctuate or lamellar opacities in the cortex of the lens but separated from the capsule by a clear zone. These may occur in several distinct layers and are more evident in the posterior pole than in the anterior, but radially they are of even distribution. Eventually they may become confluent and produce total opacity of the lens. Cataracts occur in vitamin D deficiency with low plasma phosphate and high PTH, and in chronic renal failure with high plasma phosphate and high PTH, so that the hypocalcemia which occurs in all three conditions is the most likely immediate cause. This impairs the activity of an outwardly directed sodium pump, leading to increased entry of water into the lens and swelling, rupture, and degeneration of the lens fibers. The high calcium content of the affected lens is due

to dystrophic calcification; it is common to cataracts of all types and does not result from lack of a PTH effect on a calcium transport system.

Miscellaneous effects (53). In chronic hypocalcemia the function of many different organs may be disturbed, but the kinds of organ dysfunction which produce clinical effects are not always those which would be predicted from current knowledge of calcium at the molecular level. For example, the participation of ionic calcium in blood coagulation is known in considerable detail, but spontaneous bleeding is never caused by hypocalcemia. Calcium is important in the control of mitosis, but apart from one case of transient T cell deficiency in an infant (190) no clinical consequences of this have been reported.

Intestinal malabsorption and steatorrhea not only cause hypocalcemia but may be caused by hypocalcemia and disappear with its correction. Whichever comes first, a vicious circle may be established. In hypocalcemic steatorrhea jejunal villous atrophy does not respond to a gluten-free diet but is reversible by vitamin D.

Hypocalcemia per se probably has no direct effects on bone, although it may contribute to impaired mineralization in patients who also have CC metabolite deficiency (191). If bone changes occur they are more likely due either to deficiency or to excess of PTH. Untreated hypocalcemia in the mother during pregnancy may lead to neonatal secondary hyperparathyroidism and osteitis fibrosa; the bones spontaneously return to normal within a few months (53).

Mild papilledema is an occasional complication of hypocalcemia; it does not impair vision but if the patient also has seizures may lead to a mistaken diagnosis of cerebral tumor. It is due to increased secretion and hydrostatic pressure of the CSF and subsides quickly with treatment.

Basal ganglion calcification occurs in both HP and PHP of long-enough duration; in SHP the mean interval between operation and radiographic detection was 17 years (53). Other hypocalcemic states probably never remain untreated for so long, but hyperphosphatemia may also be important in pathogenesis. Often there is no neurologic disability, but a variety of extrapyramidal syndromes may occur; these usually improve with treatment but occasionally get worse.

Any differences noted in clinical features between idiopathic HP and SHP reflect differences in the severity of PTH deficiency and in the length of delay before diagnosis. In SHP which is not diagnosed for 10 years or more, the incidence of long-term complications such as cataracts and basal ganglion calcification is the same as in idiopathic HP (53).

Treatment of hypocalcemia

It is useful to distinguish between acute hypocalcemia, in which correction of symptoms is the main object and calcium salts the main agent used, and chronic hypocalcemia, in which attainment of normocalcemia is important even in the absence of symptoms and some form of vitamin D will usually be needed (53).

Table 19-12. Approximate values for increase in net flux of calcium (expressed as increase in urinary calcium excretion) required to produce successive increases in plasma calcium at normal or low values for tubular reabsorption, assuming a GFR of 1 dL/min*

| RISE IN PLASMA Ca, mmol/L | | RISE IN URINE Ca, mmol PER 24 H | |
FROM	TO	TR_{Ca} NORMAL	TR_{Ca} LOW
1.50	1.75	0.3	1.2
1.75	2.00	0.5	2.0
2.00	2.25	0.9	3.6
2.25	2.50	1.5	6.0
1.50	2.50	3.2	12.8

* At lower values for GFR correspondingly smaller increases in flux will be needed for the same rise in plasma calcium.

The response to treatment depends on the rate of obligatory incorporation of calcium into new bone and the extent to which the exchangeable pool in interstitial fluid, soft tissue, and bone is depleted. When these needs are satisfied, any net additional calcium entering the ECF will be excreted in the urine. The effect on plasma calcium of this increased flux of calcium through the body depends on GFR and on the characteristics of tubular reabsorption of calcium. At subnormal levels of plasma calcium the relationship between urine calcium excretion/L C_{Cr} and plasma calcium is approximately logarithmic (63), so that the increase in flux required to produce the same increase in plasma level gets progressively greater as the plasma calcium rises (Fig. 19-5 and Table 19-12). The diminishing effect of increasing load is especially evident when tubular reabsorption of calcium is depressed, as it is in some but not all patients with HP. Also, as GFR declines, so does the increase in flux required to achieve the same rise in plasma level.

Calcium preparations. Supplemental oral calcium increases the flux of calcium through the body, but in many patients with hypocalcemia the efficiency of calcium absorption is low because of 1,25-DHCC deficiency, so that only 5 to 10 percent of the amount given is absorbed. Frequent small doses are better than fewer large ones (192). The commonest mistake is to think in terms of weight of salt, rather than quantity of elemental calcium. There are large differences in calcium content between one salt and another (Table 19-

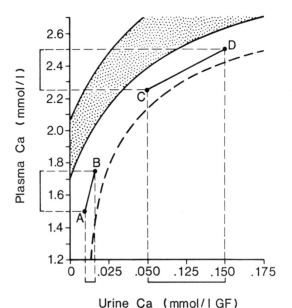

Figure 19-5. Relationship between calcium load requiring excretion (per unit of GF) and plasma calcium at subnormal levels. The shaded area is the normal range; the dotted line encloses the approximate range of decreased tubular reabsorption in hypoparathyroidism. Note that the increase in load required to produce the same rise in plasma calcium (0.25 mmol/L) is five times greater starting at 2.25 mmol/L (C to D) than starting at 1.5 mmol/L (A to B).

Table 19-13. Calcium content of different calcium salts used in treatment, and amounts of each salt needed to provide 25 mmol of calcium

ANION OF CALCIUM SALT	Ca CONTENT, mmol/g	AMOUNT, g PER 25 mmol
Carbonate	10	2.5
Chloride	9	2.8
Citrate	5.2	4.7
Lactate	3.2	7.7
Gluconate	2.2	11.0

13) but little difference in effect when prescribed in equimolar amounts. The most palatable preparation is an effervescent tablet made by Sandoz which is available everywhere in the world except in the United States. The widely used liquid preparation Neocalglucon is not recommended since in adequate amounts it frequently causes diarrhea; this effect may be sufficiently severe to *lower* the plasma calcium.

Intravenous calcium is usually given as the gluconate, available in ampuls of 10% solution. The nominal content is 2.25 mmol Ca per 10 mL, but the measured content may be as high as 3.25 mmol per 10 mL (146). The effect of a single injection may only last a few hours, and continuous intravenous infusion may be needed. This is safer than repeated injections, especially in infants in whom extravasation may lead to extensive subcutaneous calcification (193). The gluconate ion complexes calcium and is removed from the circulation by hepatic metabolism and renal excre-

tion at a variable rate; consequently there is little correlation between the increase in total plasma calcium and the increase in ionized calcium after calcium gluconate (146). Calcium chloride (10% solution; 9 mmol Ca/10 mL) produces a significantly higher ionized calcium than an equimolar amount of calcium gluconate, with a significant correlation between the increase in ionized calcium and increase in total calcium (146). For these reasons the chloride is the preferable salt when an immediate effect is urgently needed, but it is unsatisfactory for more general use because it is even more irritating than the gluconate and liable to cause sloughing if it escapes into the tissues.

Vitamin D and its metabolites. Because of the historical accident that they were synthesized first, EC (ergocalciferol) and DHT (dihydrotachysterol) have been mainly used in treatment, but both 25-HCC and 1,25-DHCC are likely to be available soon. Some clinical pharmacologic characteristics of these agents are compared in Table 19-14. They all raise plasma calcium by increasing intestinal absorption, and by raising the level of the blood-bone equilibrium in much the same way as PTH (53). In patients without osteomalacia the external balance is usually unchanged, the urinary excretion of calcium increasing by the same amount as net absorption, as with a pharmacologic dose in a normal person (194); in patients with osteomalacia urinary calcium remains low until the bones are repleted

Table 19-14. Clinical pharmacologic characteristics of substances with vitamin D action used in treatment

CHARACTERISTIC	CC OR EC	DHT	25-HCC	1,25-DHCC
Daily dose to prevent rickets (μg)*	2–10	20–100	1–5	?0.1–0.5†
Relative potency	1	$1/10$‡	2	20
Daily dose in HP (μg)	750–3000	250–1000	50–200	0.5–2
Relative potency	1	3‡	15	1500
Time to restore normocalcemia (weeks)§	4–8	1–2	2–4	½–1
Time to reach maximum effect (weeks)§	4–12	2–4	4–20	½–1
Persistence after cessation (weeks)	6–18¶	1–3	4–12	½–1

* All available preparations are presented and dispensed in mass, not molar units; 1 μmol is approximately 400 μg.
† Higher if 25-HCC is also deficient.
‡ Note that DHT is less potent than vitamin D in the treatment of rickets but more potent in the treatment of HP.
§ For constant daily dose; shorter if a loading dose is given.
¶ Up to 18 months after severe intoxication.

(92). A high dose of any form of vitamin D can increase bone turnover, but this usually does not occur in HP, and urinary total hydroxyproline excretion remains unchanged. This has led to the erroneous conclusion that the therapeutic effect of vitamin D does not involve the bones. But calcium fluxes between bone and blood increase before there is any change in calcium absorption or in plasma calcium. When used as a substitute for PTH, vitamin D largely restores the ability to recover from EDTA-induced hypocalcemia (196), and the fall in plasma calcium in response to a low-calcium diet is only about one-third of the rise with vitamin D.

Many of the difficulties encountered with vitamin D treatment are the result of defects in commercially available preparations (92). Even the products of reputable manufacturers may contain substantially more than the stated dose when new, and show significant loss of strength with storage. Enteric coated generic tablets are often very poorly absorbed. Preparations containing calcium or other vitamins as well as vitamin D are especially liable to oxidation or photochemical decomposition. Geltabs[5] calciferol U.S.P. is the only product with a capsule which is opaque to light and for which long-term stability of response has been documented (92). The 50,000 IU capsules should be assumed to contain 60,000 IU or 1.5 mg. DHT is available either as a capsule containing 0.125 mg (Hytakerol[6]) or tablets containing 0.125, 0.2, and 0.4 mg;[7] either is satisfactory. The nonencapsulated solution of DHT loses potency quickly because of repeated exposure to air and light.

Management of acute hypocalcemia with tetany. The objects of treatment are to relieve symptoms and forestall laryngeal obstruction or convulsive seizures. These are unlikely if the vocal cords are mobile and the plasma calcium is 1.8 mmol/L or higher. In adults, depending on the severity, 10 to 20 mL of 10% calcium gluconate

[5] The Upjohn Company, Kalamazoo, Michigan 49001.

[6] Winthrop Laboratories, 90 Park Avenue, New York, New York 10016.

[7] Phillips-Roxane Laboratories Inc., 330 Oak Street, Columbus, Ohio 43216.

is given by slow intravenous push allowing not less than 1 min per 10 mL. In patients who are digitalized sudden death from cardiac arrest has occurred with too rapid administration, and ECG control may be advisable. If the patient can swallow, oral calcium should be started immediately, giving 5 mmol Ca every 2 h of wakefulness, increasing each dose progressively to 10 mmol if required. If intravenous calcium is needed again within 6 h, continuous intravenous administration is advisable, beginning with 10 mL of 10% calcium gluconate added to 500 mL of intravenous fluid every 6 h. If the patient is an alcoholic or the response is poor, magnesium depletion is likely. Much higher doses (0.5 to 1 mmol/min of calcium chloride) may be needed to correct the low ionized calcium of critically ill patients (147). This can only be done safely with continuous monitoring of plasma ionized calcium, but the need to treat such transient hypocalcemia at all has not been convincingly established.

Based on the clinical response and plasma calcium levels during the first 24 to 48 h of treatment, and the likely duration of the underlying condition, DHT may be needed as well as calcium. A reliable regimen is 4 mg daily for 2 days, then 2 mg daily for 2 days, and then 1 mg daily until further dose adjustments are indicated. This should increase the plasma calcium to normal within a week or less. Intravenous calcium can be stopped within 48 h, but oral calcium should be continued until the plasma calcium returns to normal. If it rises too high it will quickly fall when the oral calcium is ceased. DHT is noncumulative so that its effect abates quickly when it is withdrawn; hypocalcemia will recur within 2 weeks or less if the underlying disease has failed to improve. 1,25-DHCC acts even more quickly than DHT and may become the drug of choice when a rapid effect is needed. It has been successfully used in neonatal hypocalcemia. 25-HCC acts no more quickly than DHT and is cumulative.

Management of chronic hypocalcemia. This is equivalent to the long-term management of HP, which is the most common cause of chronic hypocalcemia (53). If hypocalcemia is due to CC-metabolite deficiency, the patient probably also

Table 19-15. Effect of 25 to 50 mmol supplemental oral calcium in eight paients with grade 3 SHP*

	PRE	POST	CHANGE	GRADE 2
Plasma Ca (mmol/L)	2.01 ± 0.02	2.33 ± 0.02	+ 0.32	2.30 ± 0.04
Plasma P (mmol/L)	1.35 ± 0.05	1.29 ± 0.04	− 0.06	1.33 ± 0.11
Urine Ca (mmol/24 h)	1.42 ± 0.24	3.73 ± 0.50	+ 2.31	3.05 ± 0.36
Urine Ca (μmol/L GF)	11.2 ± 1.7	30.0 ± 3.6	+18.8	21.7 ± 3.0

* The relationship between the increases in plasma calcium and in urine calcium is within the limits given in Table 19-12. Note that urine calcium is higher in treated grade 3 than in grade 2 (data from Table 19-5) despite no difference in plasma calcium or phosphate.

has osteomalacia; the treatment of this is described elsewhere (92). The principles of treatment are the same in PHP, but the dose requirement may fall significantly after a few months (90, 90a). Most likely normocalcemia partly restores bone and renal responsiveness to PTH, but there may also be healing of subclinical osteomalacia.

The object of treatment is to keep the plasma calcium in the lower half of the normal range. If there is secondary hyperparathyroidism, optimum treatment should also lower iPTH to normal. Symptoms may improve or even disappear despite persistence of hypocalcemia and so symptoms cannot be used as a guide, but it is probably safe to leave mild asymptomatic hypocalcemia untreated for 3 months. If the plasma calcium is 1.9 mmol/L or higher (grade 3) it can usually be restored to normal by 25 to 50 mmol/day of oral calcium alone (Table 19-15) or by a combination of dietary salt restriction and chlorthalidone (197); urinary calcium increases with the former but decreases with the latter regimen. If the plasma calcium is below 1.9 mmol/L some form of vitamin D will usually be needed. It is safest to begin with a small dose which is cautiously increased at intervals no shorter than the time required for a maximum response (Table 19-14). This process is repeated until the plasma calcium is stabilized at the desired level.

Contrary to frequently expressed opinions, if a satisfactory preparation of vitamin D is used, the response is reasonably predictable. Once the correct dose is found it rarely needs to be changed, and in most patients the plasma calcium need only be measured at three monthly intervals. The doses required for maintenance fall within a fairly narrow range, unexplained or unpredictable changes

in plasma calcium almost never occur, and resistance to treatment is very uncommon; when it happens it involves all forms of vitamin D, including 1,25-DHCC (198). This is effective in much smaller doses (0.25 to 1.5 μg/day) (63, 199), but no long-term superiority over DHT has yet been demonstrated and the plasma calcium must be measured much more frequently to avoid dangerous hypercalcemia. Some causes of inadequate or excessive response are listed in Tables 19-16 and 19-17 and long-term results are summarized in Table 19-18.

If the patient's self-chosen intake of calcium is less than 25 mmol daily it should be made up to this figure with a calcium supplement. Restriction of milk and other dairy products is not necessary to control the plasma calcium level, but Tm_P/GFR usually does not fall to normal and

Table 19-16. Some causes of inadequate response to vitamin D or increase in dose requirement

Dose too small and/or duration too short
Noncompliance by patient
Manufacturing or dispensing error
Deteriorated preparation, especially unencapsulated liquid
Unabsorbed preparation, especially enteric coated tablet
Dietary calcium intake too low (optimum 20 to 30 mmol/day)
Magnesium depletion (202)
Hypothyroidism (except in children)
Any cause of ECF calcium depletion (Tables 19-10 and 19-11)
Severe impairment of calcium reabsorption (see Table 19-12)
Any defect in CC metabolism, especially anticonvulsant therapy (Table 19-8)
Infection, especially sinusitis
Treatment with corticosteroids (57)
Calcitonin excess (203)
True resistance (very rare); ? impaired vitamin D metabolism of unknown cause; ? impaired target cell responsiveness

Table 19-17. Some causes of excessive response to vitamin D or decrease in dose requirement

Use of long-acting preparation to treat acute hypocalcemia
Erratic patient compliance
Impatience—dose increased too frequently or by too large
  increments
Negligence—plasma calcium not measured frequently enough
Unsuspected change to stronger preparation due to manufacturing
  or dispensing error
Large increase in dietary calcium
Sudden breakdown of defense mechanism after prolonged
  subclinical overdosage
Thiazide diuretic administration (53)
Postpartum (mechanism unknown) (57)
After recovery from vitamin D intoxication (204)
Recurrence of hyperthyroidism
Immobilization (especially in children)
Coincidental development of sarcoidosis
Rapid mobilization of adipose tissue
Development of Addison's disease
Partial restoration of target cell responsiveness by normocalcemia
  in PHP

persistent mild hyperphosphatemia (Table 19-18) probably increases the risk of soft tissue calcification, nephrocalcinosis, and impaired renal function, all of which can occur without hypercalcemia. Wide fluctuation in dairy-product usage should be discouraged; an unrecognized increase in the consumption of milk or ice cream is a common reason for hypercalcemia. If symptoms of tetany persist despite correction of hypocalcemia, they may respond to phenytoin (53) which enhances the binding of calcium by phospholipids at the cell membrane (182); the required dose of vitamin D is likely to increase.

HYPERCALCEMIA

Mechanisms and causes: Equilibrium versus disequilibrium

There are many causes of hypercalcemia (Table 19-19) but only two fundamental mechanisms—in equilibrium hypercalcemia the level of equilibration between blood and bone (by whatever means this is accomplished) is raised, and in disequilibrium hypercalcemia the load of calcium cannot be excreted by the kidney at a normal plasma level

(64). Equilibrium hypercalcemia can be maintained indefinitely without continued loss of calcium from bone provided there are appropriate adjustments in the extraskeletal components of external balance. It is convenient to repeat the steady-state relationship previously described [Eq. (19-3), p. 962]:

$$P_{Ca(UF)} = \frac{NA}{GFR} + \frac{BR - BF}{GFR} + \frac{TR_{Ca}}{GFR} \quad (19\text{-}3)$$

The interrelationships between these variables are clearer if tubular reabsorption is partitioned into fractional and absolute components (Chap. 8), the former varying directly with plasma ultrafiltrable calcium:

$$P_{Ca(UF)} = P_{Ca(UF)_f} + \frac{TR_{Ca_{dist}}}{GFR} + \frac{NA}{GFR} + \frac{BR - BF}{GFR} \quad (19\text{-}4)$$

where f = the fraction of filtered calcium which undergoes gradient-limited reabsorption in the proximal tubule and loop of Henle

$TR_{Ca_{dist}}$ = the absolute capacity-limited reabsorption in the distal tubule and collecting duct which reaches a Tm_{Ca}/GFR as plasma calcium rises

On rearrangement this gives:

$$P_{Ca(UF)} = \frac{TR_{Ca_{dist}}}{(1 - f)GFR} + \frac{NA}{(1 - f)GFR} + \frac{BR - BF}{(1 - f)GFR} \quad (19\text{-}5)$$

Tubular reabsorption may change because of alteration either in f or in Tm_{Ca}/GFR; a change in total reabsorption due only to a change in plasma

Table 19-18. Effect of treatment with either EC or DHT (mean dose 0.70 ± 0.24 mg DHT equivalent daily) in 27 patients with chronic SHP for mean duration of 8 years (range 3 to 33 years)*

	UNTREATED	TREATED	DIFFERENCE
Plasma Ca (mmol/L)	1.59 ± 0.23	2.34 ± 0.09	$+0.75$
Plasma P (mmol/L)	1.65 ± 0.28	1.33 ± 0.14	-0.32

* Values are mean ± S.D. Note that the rise in calcium is greater than the fall in phosphate, and that variability is less for both.

Table 19-19. Causes of hypercalcemia

Parathyroid hormone excess	Sarcoidosis
Primary	Idiopathic
Secondary	Causes peculiar to children
Nonparathyroid neoplasia	Idiopathic infantile hypercalcemia
Local osteolysis	Hypothyroidism
Metastatic disease of bone	Blue-diaper syndrome
Myelomatosis	Hypophosphatasia
Humoral mechanisms	Miscellaneous causes
Ectopic hyperparathyroidism	Familial hypocalciuric hypercalcemia
Prostaglandin mediated	Pheochromocytoma
WDHA syndrome	Acromegaly
Lympho- and myeloproliferative disorders	Tuberculosis
Lymphoma	Berylliosis
Reticulosarcoma	Idiopathic periostitis
Acute or chronic leukemia	Metaphyseal chondrodysplasia
Other types of disequilibrium hypercalcemia	Adrenal cortical insufficiency
Immobilization after trauma	Rhabdomyolysis with acute renal failure
Hyperthyroidism	Iatrogenic hypercalcemia
Thiazide diuretics	Overdosage of parathyroid extract
Vitamin A intoxication	Ionic exchange resin in calcium phase
Hyperabsorption hypercalcemia	Total parenteral nutrition, especially if phosphate poor
Milk-alkali syndrome	Hard-water syndrome
Vitamin D intoxication	

calcium does not indicate a change in tubular transport activity.

Equilibrium hypercalcemia must be accompanied by some combination of increased net absorption, increased net bone resorption, or increased tubular reabsorption of calcium (due either to f or to Tm_{Ca}/GFR). Depending on how this is accomplished, external calcium balance may be zero, positive, or negative, but negative balance can only be avoided if tubular reabsorption or net absorption of calcium increases in parallel with the increase in level of blood-bone equilibrium. Because of the relative magnitude of these processes, the main task of protecting the bone must fall to the kidney. PTH increases tubular reabsorption directly and calcium absorption indirectly by increased 1,25-DHCC synthesis, but there may be other signals between bone, kidney, and gut which help to conserve bone mass. Provided the level of whatever agent is acting on the calcium homeostatic system does not change, hypercalcemia due to resetting of the blood-bone equilibrium is intrinsically stable. The plasma calcium will show the same degree of random fluctuation about the mean as normal, and will show no tendency to change with time. Equilib-

rium hypercalcemia is most commonly due to primary hyperparathyroidism.

The other fundamental mechanism of hypercalcemia is a need for a higher plasma level to enable the kidney to excrete the load entering the ECF from gut and bone. This load may increase either because of increased net absorption or increased net bone resorption. Net absorption of calcium only rarely exceeds 15 mmol/day, even when absorption is maximally stimulated by CC metabolites, unless the intake of calcium is enormous. Net bone resorption may increase transiently during the first few months after an increase in bone turnover, as explained in Chap. 8, and the magnitude of negative calcium balance may be as high as 10 mmol/day. Acceleration of any preexisting remodeling imbalance may add a further 5 mmol/day but the total negative calcium balance due to accelerated turnover is usually well below 20 mmol/day. A substantial negative bone balance is more easily produced by pathologic bone resorption, because the normal coupling between resorption and formation is in abeyance (Table 19-20), but even so the magnitude of negative calcium balance is almost always below 20 mmol/day. The extreme upper limit of increase in

Table 19-20. Comparison of normal bone resorption occurring during the process of normal turnover and abnormal bone resorption occurring in response to metastatic disease or myelomatosis

	NORMAL	RESORPTION
Purpose	Structural needs of body	"Lebensraum" for abnormal cells
Bone removed	Fatigued or dead	Indiscriminate
Depth and extent	Controlled	Uncontrolled
Subsequent formation	Coupled	Noncoupled
	Lamellar	Woven

load is probably 25 mmol/day, except in patients receiving calcium by intravenous infusion.

Calcium is excreted mainly by the kidneys, but if the calcium load is derived from bone the gut may also take part (205). If net bone resorption increases, net intestinal absorption usually decreases (possibly because 1,25-DHCC synthesis is depressed) and endogenous secretion may increase to the extent that net absorption is negative. Nevertheless, the prevention of hypercalcemia is primarily the function of the kidney, and the capacity of the normal kidney to excrete sur-

plus calcium is very large. From Fig. 19-6 it can be seen that a threefold increase in load could be excreted with a rise in plasma calcium from 2.4 to 2.8 mmol/L, even if tubular reabsorption of calcium were unchanged. If tubular reabsorption fell because of the expected suppression of PTH secretion, a threefold increase in load could be excreted with a rise in plasma calcium of only 0.1 mmol/L, and a fivefold increase in load excreted with a rise of less than 0.3 mmol/L. Consequently it is impossible for the steady-state plasma calcium level to remain above 3 mmol/L unless

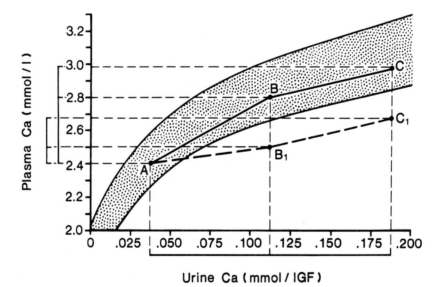

Figure 19-6. Relationship between calcium load requiring excretion and plasma calcium. Shaded areas indicate normal range from Fig. 19-4. A-B-C shows increase in plasma calcium produced by three- and fivefold increases in load with no change in tubular reabsorption. A-B_1-C_1 shows effect of the same increases in load with reduced tubular reabsorption.

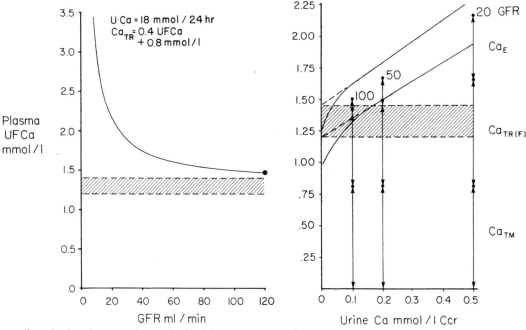

Figure 19-7. Effect of reduced GFR on plasma ultrafiltrable calcium (UFCa) in disequilibrium hypercalcemia. *Left.* Hyperbolic relationship between plasma UFCa and GFR at constant values for total urinary calcium and absolute component of tubular reabsorption of calcium. *Right.* Partition of plasma UFCa into load and tubular reabsorption at different levels of GFR. Horizontal shaded areas denote normal range for plasma UFCa. $Ca_{TR(F)}$, fractional tubular reabsorption of calcium/L C_{Cr}; Ca_{Tm}, absolute tubular reabsorption of calcium; CA_E, urinary excretion of calcium/L C_{Cr}. [*Reproduced from A. M. Parfitt (64) with permission.*]

either a decrease in GFR or an increase in tubular reabsorption of calcium. Mild hypercalcemia may result from this mechanism alone—in a geriatric population, no explanation other than mild renal insufficiency and dehydration could be found in three-quarters of the patients with a high corrected total calcium (206).

If GFR falls and both the calcium load to be excreted and tubular reabsorption are unchanged, calcium excretion by each nephron or each unit of GFR must increase, which is only possible with a rise in plasma level. The relationship between plasma calcium and GFR is hyperbolic (Fig. 19-7) so that the rise in plasma calcium is accelerated when GFR falls below 30 mL/min. This phenomenon is the opposite of the long-term effect of chronic renal failure to lower plasma calthere is some limitation in the ability of the kidneys to excrete calcium. This may result from

cium, which involves quite different mechanisms (Chap. 20). Hypercalcemia diminishes renal function (p. 1032) so that a vicious circle may be established whereby a rise in plasma calcium causes a fall in GFR, which limits the excretion of calcium, which causes a further rise in plasma calcium and a further fall in GFR (Fig. 19-8). Similarly, if tubular reabsorption increases and both load and GFR remain constant, the filtered load in each nephron must increase, which is only possible with a rise in plasma level. Tubular reabsorption of calcium may increase either in company with sodium as a result of ECF volume contraction (increase in f) or because of some humoral influence on calcium reabsorption in the distal nephron (increase in Tm_{Ca}/GFR). The effect on plasma calcium of increased tubular reabsorption by either means is shown in Fig. 19-9; a small change in tubular reabsorption has a more

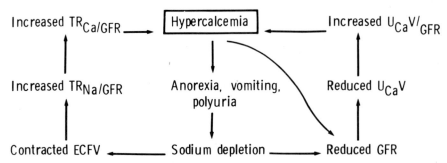

Figure 19-8. Vicious circles tending to instability and worsening of hypercalcemia. GFR, glomerular filtration rate; ECFV, extracellular fluid volume; TR, tubular reabsorption (Ca or Na). [*Reproduced from A. M. Parfitt (64) with permission.*]

immediate effect than a small change in GFR. Patients with hypercalcemia are subject to nausea, vomiting, and dehydration (p. 1034) so that another vicious circle may be set up whereby a rise in plasma calcium causes anorexia and vomiting, and the resulting sodium depletion and ECF volume contraction lead in turn both to a fall in GFR and to increased reabsorption of sodium and calcium (Fig. 19-8). Because of these vicious circles, hypercalcemia dependent only on a combination

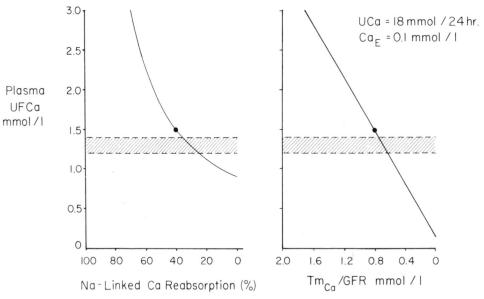

Figure 19-9. Effect of increase in tubular reabsorption of calcium on plasma ultrafiltrable calcium (UFCa) in disequilibrium hypercalcemia at constant values for total urinary calcium, GFR, and Ca_E (mmol/L GF). *Left panel*, effect of variation in sodium-linked fractional reabsorption; *right panel*, effect of variation in Tm-limited absolute reabsorption. [*Reproduced from A. M. Parfitt (64) with permission.*]

Table 19-21. Comparison of three types of hypercalcemia*

CHARACTERISTIC	VARIETY OF HYPERCALCEMIA		
	EQUILIBRIUM	DISEQUILIBRIUM	HYPERABSORPTION
Liability to change	Stable	Unstable	Usually stable
Rate of rise	Slow	Rapid	Usually slow
Calcium balance	Small negative	Large negative	Often positive
Increase in urinary calcium	Small	Large	Large
TR_{Ca}	Usually increased	Often increased	Often increased
Chronic renal failure—			
incidence	Low	High	High
Effect on plasma Ca	Fall	Rise	Fall
Effect of glucocorticoids	No change	Variable	Fall
Type of primary HP	Slow growth (Type 2)	Rapid growth (Type 1)	Type 2 + peptic ulcer

* Equilibrium hypercalcemia due to simultaneous resetting of the blood-bone equilibrium and of renal calcium threshold; disequilibrium hypercalcemia due to increased net bone resorption and decreased renal capacity to excrete calcium; and hyperabsorption hypercalcemia due to increased gastrointestinal absorption of calcium and either increased vitamin D action or increased tubular reabsorption of calcium.

SOURCE: Reproduced from A. M. Parfitt (64) with permission.

of increased load and decreased renal capacity to excrete calcium is intrinsically unstable. The plasma calcium is likely to show greater than normal fluctuation about the mean initially and progresses with time, sometimes very rapidly.

Disequilibrium hypercalcemia is most commonly due to metastatic disease of bone or other causes of greatly increased net bone resorption. An increase in load due to net absorption is usually smaller and not apt to change so rapidly because of the limitations imposed by suppression of PTH secretion and 1,25-DHCC synthesis. Hypercalcemia from excess vitamin D frequently includes an equilibrium component, and is therefore intermediate in its characteristics. Equilibrium, disequilibrium, and hyperabsorption are compared in Table 19-21. Many of the differences (64) will be described more fully in subsequent sections.

It is evident that various combinations of increased load to be excreted, increased tubular reabsorption, and decreased GFR occur in almost all patients with hypercalcemia regardless of the etiology. The magnitude of each of these disturbances can be determined by simultaneous measurements of plasma and urinary calcium and creatinine, and assessment of tubular reabsorption as described earlier. The relative contribu-

tions of the three mechanisms to the observed increase in plasma calcium can then be calculated provided the situation is not rapidly changing (207); a hypothetical example is shown in Fig. 19-10. Such calculations are useful in understanding pathogenesis, but do not differentiate between primary changes giving rise to disequilibrium hypercalcemia and changes which occur secondary to or in conjunction with resetting of the blood-bone equilibrium.

Accurate subdivision of the load component into net absorption and net bone resorption is only possible if a complete metabolic balance is performed, although an estimate can be made if absorption and bone turnover are separately determined by means of radiocalcium. Comparison of fasting with nonfasting urinary calcium is not valid in hypercalcemic patients because the soft tissue and interstitial components of the exchangeable pool take much longer than 12 h to equilibrate with the plasma. In patients with chronic hyperabsorption of calcium, even in the absence of radiographically detectable calcium deposits, mobilization of soft tissue calcium may sustain an increased urinary calcium excretion on a low-calcium diet for many weeks (208). Urinary total hydroxyproline excretion is an index of total

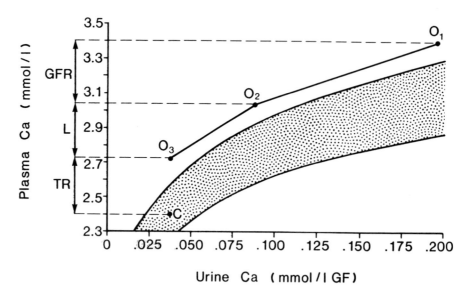

Figure 19-10. Method of partitioning hypercalcemia into different components. C, normal relationship between urine calcium per unit of glomerular filtrate and plasma calcium; O_1, observed relationship in a patient with hypercalcemia (3.4 mmol/L) and GFR of 45 mL/min. O_2 shows the effect of the same total load at a GFR of 1 dL/min; the vertical difference O_1-O_2 represents the contribution of reduced GFR to hypercalcemia. O_3 shows the effect of a normal load at a GFR of 1 dL/min; vertical difference O_2-O_3 represents the contribution of increased load to hypercalcemia. Residual vertical difference O_3-C represents the contribution of increased tubular reabsorption to hypercalcemia. Calculations assume 55 percent diffusibility of total plasma calcium.

bone resorption, and so of bone turnover, which varies independently of net bone resorption (the difference between total resorption and total formation). Most statements in the literature concerning the relative importance of increased net absorption and increased net resorption can only be regarded as approximations.

PTH excess

Classification and Pathogenesis. Increased secretion of PTH is the most common reason for the blood-bone equilibrium to be reset at a higher level with consequent hypercalcemia. This is usually referred to as primary hyperparathyroidism to distinguish it from various forms of secondary hyperparathyroidism described earlier. For many years the traditional distinction based on etiology was assumed without evidence to correspond to equally clear differences with respect to structure, function, biochemical effects, and treatment (Table 19-22). In reality a patient's status with respect to one of these characteristics gives no certain information about any of the oth-

ers, and separate assessment of all five is required for a complete description. Because of the confusion which exists it has been recommended that the traditional modifiers "primary" and "secondary" be abandoned, and hyperparathyroidism classified only on the basis of the level of plasma calcium (209). These terms are certainly in need of redefinition, and will be used here to refer solely to the origin of the hyperparathyroid state, not its behavior at the time it is recognized. On this basis it is proposed that hypercalcemic hyperparathyroidism be classified as primary, secondary, or ectopic (210) (Table 19-23). In the latter condition a substance identical to or closely resembling PTH is synthesized and released by nonparathyroid neoplasm; it will be described later in relation to other causes of humoral hypercalcemia in malignant disease.

Much confusion has arisen because the control of hormone secretion and the control of active cell mass have not been clearly separated (23). Most investigators have assumed that the former is the

Table 19-22. Traditional method of classifying hyperparathyroidism*

1. Etiologic	Primary	Secondary
2. Structural	Adenoma	Hyperplasia
3. Functional	Autonomous	Normally responsive
4. Biochemical	Hypercalcemia	Hypo- or normocalcemia
5. Therapeutic	Surgical	Medical

* It is often assumed that all five categories usually correspond, whereas in fact they usually vary independently.

most important and that hypercalcemic hyperparathyroidism is primarily a disorder in the control of hormone secretion. In fact it is always associated with an excess of active parathyroid tissue, and hormonal secretion by individual cells is abnormal only in a minority of cases. A sustained increase in demand for PTH secretion for any reason may lead to hyperplasia (p. 977), but cell proliferation and organ growth also occur for reasons unrelated to functional demand. This is the essence of the distinction between secondary and primary hyperparathyroidism, difficult as it may be to decide the correct classification in individual cases. For reasons which will be discussed later, a process which begins as hypocalcemic or normocalcemic secondary hyperparathyroidism may progress to hypercalcemia, a situation sometimes referred to as tertiary hyperparathyroidism.

Primary hypercalcemic hyperparathyroidism as defined may result from environmental agents or from an abnormal genotype. Of the former, only irradiation of the neck during childhood (211, D. S. Rao, unpublished data) and possibly administration of thiazide diuretics (212) or lithium salts (213) have been identified. In Sweden, hypercalcemic hyperparathyroidism is four to five times more prevalent in patients taking thiazide diuretics than in control subjects, but it is not known whether this preceded and contributed to the hypertension for which the thiazide was given, or was induced by the thiazide (212). In dogs, chronic thiazide administration leads to parathyroid hyperplasia (214) and the incidence of hyperparathyroidism seems to have increased substantially since thiazide diuretics were introduced in the early 1950s, but convincing epidemiologic evidence of a causal relationship is still lacking. There are at least five types of hereditary hyperparathyroidism (Table 19-24) (215–217), but collectively they account for no more than 10 to 20 percent of the total. The existence of the isolated adult form distinct from the MEN (multiple endocrine neoplasia) syndromes is disputed (215) because of the difficulty of excluding subclinical involvement of other glands in all affected individuals, but the indicated characteristics tend to be consistent within families (214). Familial hypocalciuric hypercalcemia (215) is considered separately, because although there is parathyroid hyperplasia it is by no means certain that the hypercalcemia is due to PTH excess. It must be emphasized that in the great majority of cases the cause is still unknown.

Secondary hypercalcemic hyperparathyroidism is rare, but occurs most commonly in chronic renal failure (218), intestinal malabsorption (219), and nonfamilial hypophosphatemic osteomalacia (220), but it may occasionally happen even in simple nutritional vitamin D deficiency (221). The reason for the transition from hypo- or normocalcemia to hypercalcemia is not known but three possible mechanisms can be suggested. First, deficiency of one or more CC metabolites may initiate parathyroid hyperplasia independent of any change in the plasma calcium (221). This could occur even in the absence of any effect of CC metabolites on hormone secretion, about which the evidence is inconclusive. Second, in normocal-

Table 19-23. Classification of hypercalcemic hyperparathyroidism*

1. Primary (genetic and/or environmental stimulus)
   a. Neoplastic (probably unicellular origin; carcinoma or adenoma)
   b. Hyperplastic (multicellular origin; "adenoma" or hyperplasia)
2. Secondary (initial secretory stimulus)
   a. Failure of involution after initial stimulus removed
   b. Continued growth due to acquired mitotic autonomy
3. Ectopic (secretion of PTH by nonparathyroid neoplasm)

* Categories 1a (+ possibly 2b) correspond to Lloyd Type 1, and 1b + 2a to Lloyd Type 2 (227). Acquired mitotic autonomy (2b) is sometimes referred to as tertiary hyperparathyroidism. See text and Fig. 19-11 for further details. In the majority of cases the stimulus (genetic, environmental, or secretory) cannot be identified.

Table 19-24. Five types of genetic hyperparathyroidism*

	NEONATAL	ADULT	MEN (1)	MEN (2)	FHH
Clinical points	Hypotonia, resp. distress, failure to thrive	Similar to nongenetic disease	PT, pituitary pancreatic islets (ZE or hyperinsulinemia)	PT, medullary Ca of thyroid, pheochromocytoma	Onset in childhood; hypermagnesemia, hypocalciuria
Severity	Always fatal	Variable	Mild	Very mild	Mild
Bone disease	Invariable	Common	Rare	Unknown	Unknown
Ulcer disease	Never	Rare	Common	Rare	Rare
Stone disease	Never	Common	Common	Rare	Rare
Transmission	Autosomal recessive	?Autosomal dominant	Autosomal dominant	Autosomal dominant	Autosomal dominant
No. of glands	Always multiple	Usually single	Usually multiple	Usually multiple	Always multiple

* MEN, multiple endocrine neoplasia; FHH, familial hypocalciuric hypercalcemia; ZE, Zollinger-Ellison syndrome.

cemic secondary hyperparathyroidism removal of the factor which increased the requirement for PTH would lead to mild hypercalcemia until the increased active cell mass returned to normal. The capacity of parathyroid tissue to undergo anatomic involution (which requires the individual parathyroid cell to have a finite life span) has been shown in the rat but has never been demonstrated in humans. The normal rate of cell turnover in the parathyroid gland is very low so that even with complete suppression of mitosis involution could only occur slowly. Failure of parathyroid involution accounts for the occurrence of hypercalcemia soon after the institution of chronic hemodialysis (Chap. 16) and for the occasional persistence of mild hypercalcemia for many years after renal transplantation (222). This mechanism would also explain the lack of progression of hypercalcemia with time which characterizes many patients with hypercalcemic hyperparathyroidism. A similar sequence of events after pregnancy has been invoked to explain the increased prevalence of hypercalcemic hyperparathyroidism in women, but whether the increased PTH secretion of pregnancy is accompanied by hyperplasia is not known. Third, the progressive parathyroid hyperplasia induced by persistent hypocalcemia (which only occurs in CC-metabolite deficiency) leads to mitotic autonomy in occasional patients with chronic renal failure and severe intestinal malabsorption, such that increased cell division

and tissue growth continue after the original stimulus is removed (218, 219). In renal failure, progression to hypercalcemia must be documented by measurement of ionized calcium, since an increase in total calcium may result simply from accumulation of organic acids which complex calcium. It is this process which most justifies the term tertiary hyperparathyroidism.

The anatomic basis of hypercalcemic hyperparathyroidism is variable and often difficult to categorize. Nodules of hyperplasia may produce mechanical compression of adjacent tissue, and adenomas may fail to show encapsulation; it is rarely possible to differentiate between adenoma and hyperplasia in a single gland (223). Single-gland and multiple-gland involvement must be distinguished, but the most important difference between an abnormal and a normal gland is in the total mass of active tissue, not in its histologic appearance (224). Although mean normal parathyroid weight is 30 to 40 mg, single glands as large as 70 to 80 mg may be found in normal persons. A gland of normal size may have more active tissue than normal because the fat has been replaced, but the great majority of glands causing disease are visibly enlarged (225). Recognition of single-gland disease is important because removal of only one gland will effect a cure, but most often the nature of the abnormal tissue is the same as in multiple-gland disease. Most so-called adenomas are multicellular in origin (226) and arise in the same settings as so-called hyperplasia (223). The occurrence of different anatomic responses to the same stimulus depends on differences in the degree of mitotic instability between different cells (Fig. 19-11). If the mitotic threshold is similar in all cells, hyperplasia affecting all glands will result, whereas foci of cells of low mitotic threshold lead to single or occasionally double adenomas (223, 227). There may initially be a stage of asymmetric hyperplasia which regresses when the "adenoma" secretes enough PTH to cause hypercalcemia. Alternatively, only the most mitotically unstable cells may respond to the stimulus (genetic, environmental, or secretory), with no change in the other glands. In patients with hypercalcemic hyperparathyroidism complicating intestinal malabsorption, the latter seems more probable (219). To indicate the fun-

Table 19-25. Comparison of two types of primary hyperparathyroidism based on a series analyzed by Lloyd (227)*

	TYPE 1	TYPE 2
Number of cases	44	88
Mean tumor weight (g)	5.90	1.05
Range	0.70–26.0	0.15–3.5
Length of history (years)	3.56 ± 4.8	6.66 ± 7.2
Doublings (from 50 mg)	6.9	4.3
Doubling time (months)	6.2	18.6
Linear growth rate (g/year)	1.64	0.15
Plasma Ca (mmol/L)	3.34 ± 0.60	2.91 ± 0.2
Plasma P (mmol/L), BUN 7.5	0.70 ± 0.13 (32)	0.76 ± 0.15 (86)
Plasma P (mmol/L), BUN 7.5	1.43 ± 0.43 (12)	1.05 ± 0.02 (2)
BUN (mmol/L)	9.3	5.5
Urinary Ca (mmol per 24 h)	8.42	10.20
Nephrolithiasis	5%	100%
Nephrocalcinosis	30%	25%
AP (K.A.U.)†	40.1 ± 23.2	8.1 ± 3.0
Bone disease	Osteitis fibrosa	Osteoporosis

* Numerical values are means ± 2 S.D. where appropriate. The number of doublings is calculated on the assumption of constant exponential growth. The nature of the bone disease and the presence of nephrocalcinosis was determined radiographically.
† K.A.U., King-Armstrong units.
SOURCE: Reproduced by permission from A. M. Parfitt (74).

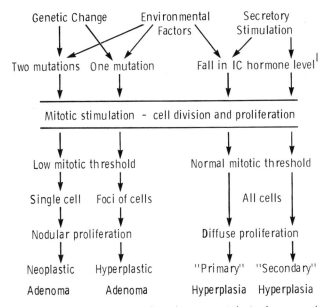

Figure 19-11. Interrelationships between etiologic factors and structural responses in the genesis of hyperparathyroidism. The link between increased demand for hormone and increased mitosis is unknown, but in other endocrine glands the intracellular concentration of hormone is an important factor (125). Neoplastic adenomas correspond to Lloyd Type 1 and hyperplastic adenomas to Lloyd Type 2 (227).

damental kinship in etiology, such tumors will be referred to as hyperplastic adenomas; they correspond to the Type 2 tumors of Lloyd (227).

It is reasonably certain that true tumors also occur in the parathyroid gland, although their unicellular origin has not yet been demonstrated. Such tumors (Lloyd Type 1) grow more rapidly and attain a larger size than Type 2 tumors and are occasionally malignant. They are associated with higher rates of DNA synthesis (H. M. Lloyd, personal communication), higher levels of iPTH and calcium in plasma, a higher prevalence of osteitis fibrosa and renal failure, and a lower incidence of renal stones (Table 19-25). Such tumors probably require at least two mutations (228), either two somatic mutations due to random concurrence of unknown environmental stimuli or one genetic and one somatic mutation, as when parathyroid carcinoma is found in the MEN Type 1 syndrome (229). Apart from malignant change, no histologic differences between Type 1 and 2 tumors have been described, but they have never

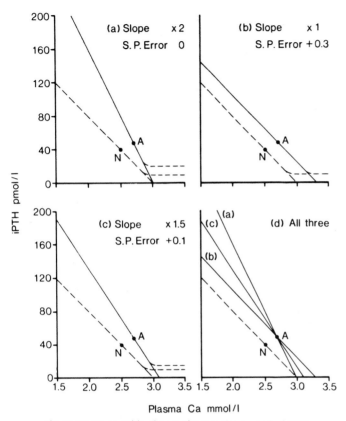

Figure 19-12. Possible abnormalities in the control of PTH secretion in hyperparathyroidism. In each panel point N identifies the mean normal value for PTH and plasma Ca, and the dotted line indicates the normal relationship between these variables; point A identifies the abnormal level of PTH and plasma Ca, and the solid line indicates the relationship between these variables. The horizontal dotted lines represent a possible nonsuppressible component of PTH secretion. In a the number of functioning cells is doubled, but each cell responds normally to changes in plasma calcium, so that the slope is increased but there is no set-point error. In b the number of cells is normal and each cell requires a higher level of plasma calcium to reduce PTH secretion by the same amount; the slope is normal but there is a set-point error. In c there is a combination of both abnormalities. In d the three hypothetical abnormal relationships are superimposed; the values were chosen so that the abnormal levels of PTH and plasma calcium were the same in each case. Current methods of assessing PTH secretion are not sensitive or precise enough to discriminate between these possibilities in an individual case. [*Modified after J. T. Potts and L. J. Deftos (56).*] If the nonsuppressible component is one-quarter of the basal secretion, it will not influence the relationship until the number of cells is increased more than sixfold.

been looked for with sophisticated cytochemical and quantitative methods. There are probably considerable differences in secretory activity, since tumors as small as 0.7 g may be associated with osteitis fibrosa and glands five times larger may lead only to Type 2 disease (227).

If the cells in the rim of normal tissue around an adenoma and in the other three glands are examined by electron microscopy, they are usually seen to be in the quiescent phase of the normal cell cycle (230). But with the light microscope the cells appear normal and atrophy of nonadenomatous tissue does not occur. This may be a residual effect of the original stimulus (genetic, environmental, or secretory) to all cells, but absence of atrophy occurs with neoplastic as well as hyperplastic adenomas so that more likely it is another instance of the extreme slowness and possible lack of any normal mechanism for producing parathyroid involution.

The study of the secretory response of abnormal parathyroid tissue in vivo is complicated by the uncertain relationship between plasma iPTH and PTH secretion (p. 954). Also, an increase in active parathyroid cell mass will increase the slope of the relationship between iPTH and calcium (23). In most patients with hypercalcemic hyperparathyroidism plasma iPTH and NcAMP increase in response to hypocalcemia induced by EDTA and decrease in response to hypercalcemia induced by calcium infusion (23–25, 33). But iPTH is still higher at all levels of plasma calcium than in normal persons. This could result from a set-point error at the level of the individual parathyroid cell, but the methods are probably too insensitive to distinguish between this abnormality and a simple increase in slope due to an increased number of cells (Fig. 19-12). Better evidence for a set-point error is that secretion may be increased by a fall in plasma calcium even though the level is still above normal (232). There is no consistent difference in secretory response between adenoma and hyperplasia, but a comparison between neoplastic adenomas and hyperplastic adenomas and hyperplasia combined would be more informative. It must be emphasized that no abnormality in the control of hormone secretion is needed to account for hypercalcemia. The normal parathyroid gland is unable to reduce hormone secretion to zero (Chap. 8); in the short term this can be demonstrated in individual cells, but in the long term continued hormone secretion despite hypercalcemia depends on an upper limit to the length of the quiescent period between successive cycles of secretory activity. Even if complete suppression of PTH secretion were possible, hypercalcemia would still occur if the number of functioning cells were sufficiently increased, although the plasma calcium would not rise above the level corresponding to zero hormone secretion (23).

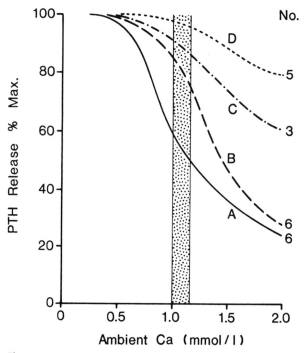

Figure 19-13. Four types of response of dispersed cells from abnormal human parathyroid glands to elevation of ambient calcium concentration (233). A, response of cells from hyperplastic glands (similar to response of normal bovine parathyroid cells); B, response of cells from adenomas; C and D, varying degree of autonomy of hormone secretion. Vertical shaded area encloses the normal range for plasma ionized calcium; the difference between hyperplastic and adenomatous cells is maximal in this region. At the highest calcium concentration most glands showed either normal suppression or virtual absence of suppression, with few in between. See text for further details.

More precise definition of the secretory behavior of abnormal parathyroid tissue can be accomplished in vitro. The maximum rate of hormone release by dispersed parathyroid cells varies over a ten-fold range; this is consistent with the range of secretory activity suggested previously, but there was no consistent relationship to histologic classification (233). In most cases of adenoma and hyperplasia hormone secretion could be reduced to 50 percent of maximum (or less) at an ambient calcium concentration of 2 mmol/L, but between 1 and 1.5 mmol/L cells from adenomas secrete significantly more hormone than cells from hyperplastic glands, which responded very much like cells from normal bovine glands (Fig. 19-13). This is direct evidence for a set-point error in the critical range of plasma calcium from normal to slightly above normal, such that a smaller increase in active cell mass is necessary to produce mild hypercalcemia and slight hypercalcemia could occur with no increase in cell mass at all. In a minority of cases PTH release could not be reduced below 80 percent of maximum; this occurred in 2 of 3 probable neoplastic adenomas and in 4 of 17 other cases. This partial autonomy of hormone secretion must be clearly distinguished from the autonomy of cell division mentioned previously. Similar observations have been made on incubated parathyroid tissue, with which a wide spectrum of secretory responses are found (234). Only tissue from a carcinoma failed to increase PTH release in response to low ambient calcium, but the response tended to decline after the first hour, possibly because of limited storage of hormone (235).

In summary, abnormalities in the control of hormone secretion (set-point error or less commonly true secretory autonomy) are present only in a minority of patients with hypercalcemic hyperparathyroidism. In the majority, hypersecretion of PTH is due mainly to an increase in the number of functioning cells because of some abnormality in the control of cell division and proliferation. This may be initiated by either genetic or environmental stimuli or occur as an inappropriate response to an increased demand for PTH secretion.

Effects, Diagnosis, and Treatment. In all cases

the level of plasma calcium correlates modestly but significantly both with plasma iPTH and with the weight of abnormal parathyroid tissue (205). The effects of hypercalcemia are similar whatever the cause and are described later, but there are important differences in the behavior of the hypercalcemia with time between different patients.

Differences in Clinical Course. Most patients with hyperparathyroidism have equilibrium hypercalcemia which is mild, of normal variability, and nonprogressive (Fig. 19-14). There is often no significant change with time even for many months, years, or even decades (205). This corresponds to Lloyd Type 2 disease (Table 19-25), identified in Table 19-23 with hyperplastic primary or noninvoluting secondary hyperparathyroidism. In a few patients the plasma calcium rises progressively with time; such patients usually have larger tumors and a high incidence of ostei-

tis fibrosa but a shorter duration of symptoms, indicating a more rapid growth of the tumor (Table 19-25). This corresponds with Lloyd Type 1 disease identified in Table 19-23 with neoplastic primary or tertiary hyperparathyroidism. Very rarely there may be rapid deterioration leading to a hypercalcemic crisis either due to unusually rapid tumor growth, or initiation of one of several kinds of vicious-circles, which produce disequilibrium hypercalcemia.

Biochemical Aspects. In most patients with Type 2 disease the short-term precision of plasma calcium control is as good as normal (Fig. 19-14) but in some patients there may be a short-term variation of 0.2 to 0.4 mmol/L presumably because of a greater degree of secretory autonomy (236). If renal function is normal, large changes in dietary calcium intake produce significant changes in net absorption (237), and if renal function is de-

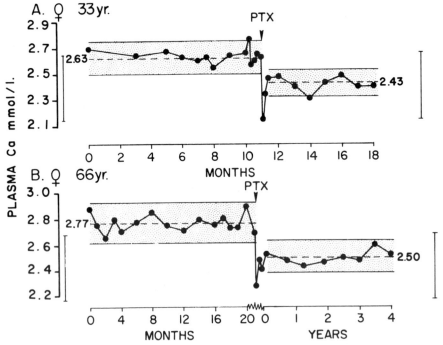

Figure 19-14. Serial plasma calcium measurements in two patients with primary hyperparathyroidism before and after parathyroidectomy (PTX). Shaded areas encompass mean ±2 S.D. ranges, vertical bars denote normal range. Note change in time scale in lower panel.

pressed large changes in dietary phosphate may produce significant changes in plasma phosphate and reciprocal changes in plasma calcium. Other causes of abnormal variability probably exist but have not been identified.

Hypercalcemia is the result of upward resetting of the blood-bone equilibrium and increased tubular reabsorption of calcium, but hypercalciuria is the result of increased net bone resorption and increased net intestinal absorption of calcium and so is an independent consequence of PTH excess. In most patients with Type 2 disease external calcium balance is close to zero or negative by no more than 2 mmol/day, with similar increases both in net absorption and urinary excretion of calcium (205). This is partly due to increased synthesis of 1,25-DHCC (54) but may reflect other adaptive mechanisms also (238), since it cont'nues after operation while bone mineral is being restored. If assessed solely on the basis of fasting urinary calcium excretion (239, 240) the degree of increased net bone resorption and negative balance is greatly overestimated. A substantial negative balance only occurs in patients with renal failure, presumably because of inability to increase 1,25-DHCC synthesis. This occurs most commonly in Type 1 disease and is frequently accompanied by osteitis fibrosa.

The mean value for Tm_{Ca}/GFR, whether calculated according to the Marshall or Mioni models, is significantly increased, but at least one-third of individual values are normal. Like other indices the results are most equivocal in patients with the mildest disease. When expressed as TR_{Ca}, tubular reabsorption of calcium is depressed in patients with nonparathyroid hypercalcemia (241), but this is due to an increase in L/GFR (Fig. 19-9), either because of increased net absorption, increased net bone resorption, or decreased GFR.

NcAMP is increased in almost all and Tm_P/GFR reduced in most patients, and both measurements correlate well with iPTH. Provided the data are expressed as Tm_P/GFR and not as $\%TR_P$, the discrimination between normality and hyperparathyroidism is not much improved by phosphate loading (Fig. 19-15) nor is there any evidence that this procedure leads to a greater increase in PTH secretion than in healthy per-

sons. If renal function is normal, the plasma phosphate is usually below or in the lower half of the normal range. The levels appear to be lower in England (Table 19-24) than in the United States, where as many as half the patients have a

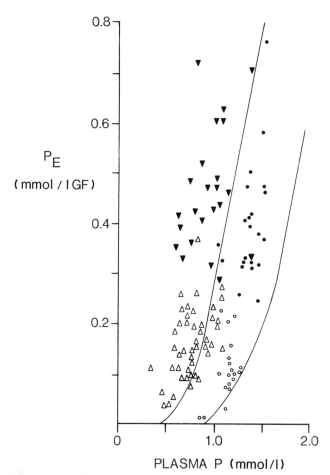

Figure 19-15. Effect of varying phosphate intake on relationship between phosphate excretion (mmol/L GF) and plasma phosphate, in normal subjects (open circles, normal or low phosphate intake; closed circles, high phosphate intake) and patients with primary hyperparathyroidism (open triangles, normal or low phosphate intake; closed triangles, high phosphate intake). The straight lines enclose the normal range for Tm_P/GFR. Although more of the hyperparathyroid points fall outside the normal range on the high phosphate intake, separation between the two groups has not been improved. [*Redrawn from Ref. 750 which gives the original sources of the data.*]

normal plasma phosphate; this is probably because of differences in dietary phosphate intake. However, even in England the plasma phosphate is usually above 0.6 mmol/L and is below 0.5 mmol/L in less than 5 percent of patients. Absence or reduction in amplitude of the normal circadian rhythm of phosphate excretion has been reported even though the normal nocturnal increase in plasma iPTH is usually preserved (242).

Absolute urinary phosphate excretion is either normal or moderately increased because of increased net absorption of phosphate in company with calcium (128), but a few patients are in greater negative balance for phosphate than would be predicted from the calcium balance. This is associated with negative nitrogen balance and results from a catabolic effect of excess PTH on muscle and other soft tissues (243), but loss of tissue phosphate may be even greater than in proportion to the loss of tissue nitrogen. The relationship between Tm_P/GFR, plasma phosphate, and intracellular phosphate depletion is discussed on p. 1059.

Plasma magnesium is usually normal but occasionally may be either low or high (244). These differences result from the opposing effects of hypercalcemia and PTH on tubular reabsorption of magnesium, which is decreased by the former (probably because of competition between calcium and magnesium for a common reabsorptive pathway), and increased by the latter (Chap. 8). Both intestinal absorption and urinary excretion of magnesium are often increased, but magnesium balance may be negative; this is due partly to the catabolic effect of PTH mentioned earlier and partly to disproportionate loss of magnesium from both soft tissues and bone.

Because of the effect of PTH on bicarbonate reabsorption and also because of mild phosphate depletion, the mean plasma chloride is increased and mean plasma bicarbonate decreased in hyperparathyroidism, but there is considerable overlap and the values are often normal (245). In occasional patients this effect is severe enough to produce proximal renal tubular acidosis with a low Tm_{HCO_3}/GFR (246). The opposite changes are frequently found in patients with nonparathyroid hypercalcemia. The plasma uric acid is often raised more than would be expected for the degree of renal impairment; this effect is probably indirect since acutely PTH has no effect on renal handling of urate (247).

Clinical Aspects. The clinical effects of hypercalcemia are described on p. 1031, and of hypophosphatemia on p. 1076. Among persons attending a general medical clinic in the United States the prevalence of hypercalcemic hyperparathyroidism was between 1 in 1000 and 1 in 800 (248) but in routine health screening of a large defined population in Stockholm with a 75 percent response, the prevalence was 1 in 300 (212). Most patients discovered in this way are asymptomatic, but a mild organic brain syndrome and subtle proximal limb girdle muscle weakness are easily missed unless looked for specifically. Hypertension is more prevalent and the mean blood pressure significantly higher in hyperparathyroidism than in normal controls, and may be the only manifestation of the disease (212). This cannot be explained simply as a consequence of hypercalcemia, and is not due only to hypercalcemic nephropathy because it is found in patients whose renal function is quite normal; subtle abnormalities of the renin-angiotensin system have been found in some patients. In Type 2 disease the most important consequence is nephrolithiasis. In Type 1 disease, as well as more severe hypercalcemia and osteitis fibrosa, the patients frequently have extensive weight loss (249); muscle wasting results from the neuromuscular effects of phosphate depletion, but excess PTH also has a more generalized catabolic effect. There may also be otherwise unexplained fever and a raised ESR (249). Significant anemia is also common, probably due to the bone marrow fibrosis of osteitis fibrosa.

Some patients with Type 1 disease may present with a hypercalcemic crisis characterized by severe gastrointestinal, renal, and cerebral symptoms of hypercalcemia, cardiac arrhythmias, abdominal pain, fever, rapidly rising levels of calcium, phosphate, and creatinine, initial hypertension but subsequent circulatory failure with oliguria or anuria, and a high death rate (205, 250). Widespread necrosis and calcification are found in the heart, lungs, stomach, blood vessels, and kidney at autopsy. A crisis may occur with other causes of hypercalcemia, but the complete clinicopathologic syndrome described occurs only in hyperparathyroidism. Very high levels of PTH may promote depolymerization of the glycosaminoglycans of connective tissue ground substance, which facilitates necrosis and tissue calcification in the presence of severe hypercalcemia. Increased blood viscosity due to intravascular formation of colloidal calcium phosphate may be an additional factor contributing to circulatory and renal failure (250). A crisis may be precipitated by immobilization, especially after fractures, development of concurrent hyperthyroidism, hepatitis (possibly because of reduced catabolism of PTH), thiazide diuretic administration, vitamin D repletion, sodium depletion, and dehydration or water depletion due to acquired diabetes insipidus. In hypercalcemic crisis the plasma calcium is usually more than 4 mmol/L and often more than 5 mmol/L, the AP is raised in 75 percent, radiographic osteitis fibrosa is present in about one-quarter, and a tumor is palpable in the neck in about half of the cases.

Bone Changes (74). In Type 2 disease, the bones are usually normal clinically and radiographically but bone turnover determined histologically or by calcium kinetics is often increased. Indices of cortical bone status in the extremities using either radiographic morphometry or photon absorptiometry are reduced by about 5 to 10 percent due to acceleration of involutional bone loss. Trabecular bone mass is even more reduced in the distal radial metaphysis, but is normal in the ilium (64). A 10 percent reduction in total body bone mass occurring over 5 years corresponds to a negative calcium balance of 1.5 mmol/day or less, in good agreement with direct measurements. An increased prevalence of vertebral compression fractures has been reported, but whether other fractures occur more commonly is not known. Traumatic fractures sometimes fail to heal until the hyperparathyroidism is cured.

In Type 1 disease, osteitis fibrosa eventually occurs in all patients unless the course is so rapid that there is insufficient time for the bones to respond. The essential characteristic of osteitis fibrosa is a breakdown in the normal coupling between resorption and formation, an increase in the size of resorption cavities (but not necessarily in the speed at which they are made), and replacement of normal lamellar bone by abnormal woven bone and fibrous tissue. The rate at which this replacement occurs depends on the rate of bone turnover, but the fundamental disturbance in bone cell function is independent of bone turnover, which is quite commonly reduced. The AP may be increased modestly as a result of increased bone turnover alone but substantial increases in AP only occur in patients with osteitis fibrosa. The most sensitive radiographic sign of osteitis fibrosa is subperiosteal resorption, which usually begins on the proximal shoulder of the radial border of the middle phalanx of the index finger of the dominant hand. Early changes are best seen by magnification of x-rays taken on fine-grain industrial film (251).

"Normocalcemic" Hyperparathyroidism. It has often been stated that a patient may have primary or autonomous secondary hyperparathyroidism without hypercalcemia. Such cases fall into three groups (Table 19-26). First, hypercalcemia may not be recognized because of technical and other errors, such as inadequate methodology, poor quality control, or failure to apply a protein cor-

Table 19-26. Reasons for apparent normocalcemia instead of hypercalcemia in hyperparathyroidism*

Failure to detect hypercalcemia
  Poor quality control or other laboratory error
  Failure to correct total calcium for protein
  Failure to determine ionized calcium
  Inadequate statistical analysis of repeated measurements
Diagnosis of hyperparathyroidism in error
  Overinterpretation of minor histologic changes
  Misinterpretation of iPTH levels
  Failure to recognize a fall in urinary calcium as transient
  Too short a period of follow-up
Genuine absence of hypercalcemia
  Initial or coincidental vitamin D deficiency
  Acute or chronic renal failure
  Acute pancreatitis
  Infarction of parathyroid adenoma
  ? High dietary intake of salt
  ? Low dietary intake of calcium

* In most instances the patient either does not have normocalcemia or does not have hyperparathyroidism.

rection. In many laboratories calcium still has the worst precision of all commonly performed measurements (252). "Normocalcemic" hyperparathyroidism is almost nonexistent if a sufficiently precise measurement of ionized calcium is obtained in all borderline cases (253, 254). Repeated measurements must be considered in quantitative rather than categorical terms, and in relation to an appropriate statistical model of inter- and intraindividual variation (p. 952). Second, patients with idiopathic hypercalciuria are sometimes mistakenly diagnosed as having primary hyperparathyroidism. Some reports are based on evident lack of familiarity with the normal variation in size and microscopic appearance of the human parathyroid gland (224, 225); minor ultrastructural changes resulting from the administration of phosphate as a diagnostic test have been misinterpreted as evidence of disease (255). Apparent benefits of surgical intervention may be claimed because of inadequate follow-up. Urinary calcium excretion may fall transiently after operative trauma to normal parathyroid glands for several reasons; net intestinal absorption may fall because of a reduction in 1,25-DHCC synthesis, and a depression of bone turnover will cause net calcium retention in bone for up to 6 months (Chap. 8). The question is discussed further in the section on hypercalciuria and nephrolithiasis. Third, autonomous hyperparathyroidism may be genuinely normocalcemic or even hypocalcemic because of some interference with the action of PTH on the calcium homeostatic system in bone. The best-documented reason for this is CC-metabolite deficiency, whether due to poor nutrition, malabsorption, or anticonvulsant drugs (256). This may either be the initial event leading to secondary hyperparathyroidism and mitotic autonomy, or

coincidental with unrelated primary hyperparathyroidism. In either case correction of the deficiency will lead to unequivocal hypercalcemia (74). In patients with renal failure the same may occur as a result of hyperphosphatemia; phosphate deprivation (see appendix) will lead to hypercalcemia in primary hyperparathyroidism or secondary hyperparathyroidism complicated by mitotic or secretory autonomy, otherwise, the plasma calcium will rise only to normal. Although not documented as causes of normocalcemic hyperparathyroidism, the plasma calcium might conceivably be lower than expected for the level of PTH because of high dietary intake of sodium and consequent reduction in sodium-linked calcium reabsorption, low dietary intake of calcium, or magnesium depletion.

Genuine absence of hypercalcemia may also occur temporarily as a result of acute renal insufficiency for any reason, even without hyperphosphatemia and acute pancreatitis, to which patients with hyperparathyroidism are predisposed; the plasma calcium should be measured at least 1 month after recovery in all patients with this disease. Remission of hypercalcemia for a longer time may result from infarction of an adenoma. In patients with osteitis fibrosa this may produce hypocalcemia and tetany, but in patients with Type 2 disease plasma calcium falls to normal and hypercalcemia may not recur for 6 to 12 months (257).

Diagnosis. Mild hypercalcemia with normal short-term random variability and no long-term change with time is almost always caused by hyperparathyroidism even when the patient is known to have some other disease capable of causing hypercalcemia. In such cases the hypercalcemia is usually due entirely to the hyperparathyroidism,

Table 19-27. Overall usefulness of various diagnostic procedures in the diagnosis of hypercalcemic hyperparathyroidism, based on both frequency of use and accuracy

	iPTH*	NcAMP	Tm$_p$/ GFR	HAND X-RAYS	HC	PD	TZ	DF
Renal stones	+	+++	++	+	+	−	+−	−
Hypercalcemic nephropathy	−	+	+	++	++	++	−	+−
Bone disease	−	−	−	+++	−	++	−	−
Acute hypercalcemia	++	+++	−	++	−	−	−	+
Accidental discovery	++	+++	+	+	+	+	+−	+

* iPTH, C-terminal iPTH; HC, hydrocortisone; PD, phosphate depletion; TZ, thiazide; DF, discriminant functions.

the second disease only very rarely making an independent contribution. Equilibrium hypercalcemia is occasionally seen in other disorders. CC and its metabolites raise the level of blood-bone equilibration to normal, and with mild overdosage to above normal in HP (64). Hypercalcemia due to nonparathyroid humoral agents secreted by neoplasms is usually progressive, but if a tumor is slowly growing it may mimic hyperparathyroidism for a time.

Hyperparathyroidism must be considered in five main situations, each calling for a different diagnostic approach. The fundamental diagnostic criteria of hypercalcemia—high iPTH for the level of plasma calcium, increased NcAMP, and decreased Tm_P/GFR—apply in all cases, but the relative importance of these and other procedures varies with the situation (Table 19-27). Tubular reabsorption of calcium is often increased in hyperparathyroidism, but so it is also in many other causes of hypercalcemia, although for different reasons (Fig. 19-16).

Calcium-containing Renal Stones. These are always due to Type 2 disease and the diagnosis depends almost entirely on the interpretation of biochemical tests. If undoubted hypercalcemia is found in a patient seeking medical advice because of symptoms due to calcium-containing renal stones, hyperparathyroidism is by far the most likely cause. The qualifications are important, since stones discovered incidentally in patients presenting in other ways have much less diagnostic significance. Very few other hypercalcemic disorders present in this manner. Renal stones and hypercalcemia may both follow immobilization but this diagnosis should be obvious. In sarcoidosis and mild vitamin D intoxication the hypercalcemia is suppressible by hydrocortisone. False-positive results in hyperparathyroidism are due to failure to apply a protein correction or use of too high a dose (61, 64). With the correct protocol (see Appendix), the plasma calcium falls only in Type 1 disease with disequilibrium hypercalcemia due to loss of the normal coupling between resorption and formation (64). If there is equivocal hypercalcemia, mild hyperparathyroidism must be differentiated from normality of calcium metabolism and from idiopathic hypercalciuria; the latter problem is dis-

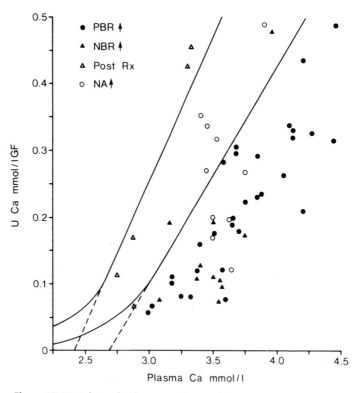

Figure 19-16. Relationship between urinary calcium excretion per unit of glomerular filtrate and plasma calcium in nonparathyroid hypercalcemia. Closed circles, 29 observations in 22 patients with increased PBR (pathologic resorption bone), 7 with bone metastases from breast cancer, 8 with bone metastases from other primary sources, 4 with myelomatosis, and 3 with lympho- or reticulosarcoma, comprising 18 personal cases and 4 reported by others. Closed triangles, 11 patients with greatly increased NBR (normal bone resorption), 5 with hyperthyroidism and 6 with immobilization. Open triangles, data in 5 patients after treatment including reexpansion of extracellular fluid volume. Open circles, 10 patients with hyperabsorption hypercalcemia (sarcoidosis, vitamin D poisoning, or milk-alkali syndrome), comprising 3 personal cases and 7 reported by others. Note that 31 of 33 patients with disequilibrium hypercalcemia due to increased net bone resorption have increased tubular reabsorption of calcium before treatment; this falls to normal with correction of volume depletion. Tubular reabsorption of calcium is also increased in half the patients with hyperabsorption hypercalcemia. The data attest to the importance of increased tubular reabsorption in the genesis of severe hypercalcemia of any etiology, but this measurement is of no value in differential diagnosis in a dehydrated patient. In hyperparathyroidism tubular reabsorption remains increased after correction of dehydration, whereas it falls to normal in nonparathyroid hypocalcemia.

cussed in the section on nephrolithiasis (p. 1048). The thiazide challenge test (see Appendix) may save time in the demonstration of definite hypercalcemia, but in most cases with a positive result there was already enough evidence to diagnose hyperparathyroidism before the test was performed. Some patients with unequivocal hypercalcemia show no greater rise in plasma calcium than normal (258); these different responses reflect different degrees of secretory versus mitotic autonomy.

Chronic Hypercalcemic Nephropathy (see p. 1032). The presence of nephrocalcinosis or other kinds of soft tissue calcification weights the diagnosis toward hyperabsorption hypercalcemia (p. 1022), but this may include hyperparathyroidism. C-terminal iPTH may be raised in chronic renal failure irrespective of PTH secretion (p. 954), and single estimations of both NcAMP/GFR and Tm$_p$/GFR become progressively less reliable as GFR declines. Even minor degrees of subperiosteal erosion of the phalanges are of great diagnostic importance (251). If there is undoubted hypercalcemia a hydrocortisone test should be performed (see Appendix) but if the plasma calcium is normal a phosphate deprivation test should be performed (Appendix); if hypercalcemia is unmasked its response to hydrocortisone can then be tested.

Bone Disease. The recognition of hyperparathyroidism depends almost entirely on the interpretation of bone x-rays (251), although occasionally a bone biopsy may be needed (74). Determination of the origin and current behavior of the hyperparathyroid state depends mainly on the history, the degree of renal failure, and the level of plasma calcium; the ionized calcium is of particular value in this context. Phosphate deprivation may be helpful and if a therapeutic trial of vitamin D is instituted, the possible emergence of hypercalcemia due to autonomous hyperparathyroidism must be kept in mind (256). The hydrocortisone test is of no value and may give false-positive results.

Acute Effects of Hypercalcemia. These will invariably be due to Type 1 disease. In a specialized center of referral the level of plasma calcium itself may be of no diagnostic value, but in less highly selected patients the higher the plasma calcium, the less likely is hyperparathyroidism (6). Subperiosteal resorption is of decisive importance if present, but may be absent if the history is very short. The iPTH gives clear-cut separation of hyperparathyroidism from other conditions but the blood must be drawn before any medical treatment is begun, otherwise the result may be uninterpretable. NcAMP is equally reliable and has the advantage that the result can usually be obtained much more quickly. Discriminant functions can be calculated using nomograms from simultaneous measurements of phosphate, bicarbonate, chloride, urea, and AP. These have no physiologic meaning but correctly identified the diagnosis in 90 percent of hypercalcemic patients (6). The hydrocortisone test may give false-positive results and should not be used.

Hypercalcemia Discovered by Accident. This may occur either as a result of investigation of an associated disease or of biochemical screening. Hyperparathyroidism is the most likely diagnosis because other hypercalcemic disorders are asymptomatic for a much shorter fraction of their total duration. However, the diagnostic problem may be more difficult because it encompasses all the known causes of hypercalcemia. The discriminant functions are also useful in this group because the necessary data will usually already be available.

Effects of Surgical Treatment. The need for operation in asymptomatic patients with minimal hypercalcemia, normal renal function, and normal bone mineral content is not established, but all criteria for Type 2 disease should be fulfilled before the decision is made to withhold treatment, since progressive disease cannot be excluded on the basis of a single plasma calcium determination. Such patients require life-long follow-up every 6 to 12 months. The best surgical approach represents a compromise between the sometimes conflicting objectives of precision of diagnosis, certainty of cure, and absence of permanent parathyroid injury. This raises issues beyond the scope of this chapter, but most patients have limited disease and can be cured by a limited operation (259). The early postoperative changes depend on the extent of removal of abnormal parathyroid tissue, the extent to which remaining normal parathyroid tissue is injured, the degree of so-called bone hunger, and the degree of renal failure.

In patients with good renal function an elevated iPTH usually returns to normal within 3 to 6 h, and plasma calcium within 24 h (249, 260). Hypocalcemia is rare in patients without bone disease in whom at least one gland is not subjected to operative trauma, but if all glands are biopsied the plasma calcium usually falls below normal, reaching its lowest value on the fourth or fifth day. A slower or incomplete fall may signify persistence of abnormal parathyroid tissue. NcAMP falls transiently below normal during the first 48 h, and the fall occurs earlier in patients who have sustained permanent parathyroid injury; hyperphosphatemia (greater than 1.8 mmol/L) is another indication of significant HP (249).

In patients with osteitis fibrosa the sudden switchover from resorption to formation throughout the skeleton leads to massive storage of bone mineral and intractable hypocalcemia (74). Positive calcium balances as high as 30 mmol/day can occur (261). There is also an abrupt fall in urinary hydroxyproline excretion and a temporary further increase in AP (262). Because bone mineral is alkaline, its rapid reconstitution leads to systemic metabolic acidosis. The plasma phosphate may fall even if the patient is hypoparathyroid as well and the invariable hypomagnesemia further worsens the hypocalcemia. Disturbed behavior, depression, and other psychiatric manifestations are more common than after thyroid surgery, but the most dangerous complication is convulsive seizures, which in a patient with osteitis fibrosa may cause simultaneous bilateral femoral neck fractures. The treatment is similar to hypocalcemia after thyroid surgery, except that magnesium must always be given and much larger doses of both vitamin D and calcium are needed (261). The severity of tetany is mitigated by preoperative administration of 25-HCC or DHT but this precaution is probably unnecessary if 1,25-DHCC is available.

The plasma magnesium can reach levels below 0.3 mmol/L (56, 57). This is usually explained as yet another consequence of bone hunger, but

storage of even 30 mmol of calcium a day would be accompanied by storage of only 1 mmol of magnesium, and urinary excretion could be reduced by this amount with only a trivial fall in plasma level. Consequently severe hyperparathyroidism must either be accompanied by preferential removal of magnesium from bone mineral or preferential loss of magnesium from within cells, so that restitution of normal bone or soft tissue composition requires a disproportionate amount of magnesium.

When studied 3 to 6 months later the patients usually have a normal plasma calcium, a plasma phosphate higher than before operation but often still slightly subnormal, significantly lower urinary calcium and urinary magnesium, and a modest increase in creatinine clearance (263). These changes occur irrespective of the presence or absence of symptoms at the time of surgery. In the majority of patients cured by removal of an adenoma, formation of new kidney stones is completely prevented (246), but stones present at the time of parathyroid surgery may continue to give symptoms and may even enlarge if the urine is infected.

If surgery is contraindicated or has failed, some form of medical treatment may be needed, but none is satisfactory. Deliberate induction of vitamin D deficiency would probably be effective but very difficult to accomplish. In postmenopausal women estrogen replacement produces a small but significant fall in plasma calcium sustained for at least several months (265), and very large doses of stilbestrol diphosphate have been temporarily effective in parathyroid carcinoma. A low-calcium diet with cellulose phosphate lowers plasma calcium by about 5 to 10 percent in some patients (237) but the duration of this effect is not known. Successful long-term control of hypercalcemia in hyperparathyroidism has been accomplished only by supplemental phosphate. This also unexpectedly healed subperiosteal erosion, but eventually led to widespread soft tissue calcification (266). The treatment of hypercalcemia in general is described later.

Nonparathyroid neoplasia. This is the most common cause of symptomatic hypercalcemia (Table 19-19), and several mechanisms have been described (56, 57, 267). Metastases in bone have been known for more than 200 years but correction of hypercalcemia by excision of a primary tumor indicates that metastases cannot be the whole explanation as was first thought. Neoplastic hypercalcemia probably always arises on the basis of secretion by the neoplastic cells of one or more substances which cause bone resorption. Most commonly these can only act locally, so that the secreting cells must be present within the bone, but if the potency or rate of secretion are high enough a systemic action from a distant site is possible. Although clinically useful, this distinction between local (primary or metastatic tumor) and systemic (humoral) causes of hypercalcemia is not absolute, since both mechanisms may be operative. Furthermore, other substances secreted by the tumor or other actions of the osteolytic agent may modify the clinical and biochemical findings. Consequently, a classification based on mechanisms does not correspond precisely with a classification based on the type of tumor.

There is a major unresolved disagreement concerning the frequency and significance of elevated iPTH in patients with neoplastic hypercalcemia. According to the traditional and still most widely held view, only a minority of neoplasms secrete a PTH-like substance (ectopic hyperparathyroidism), and iPTH levels are low or undetectable in the majority of patients with neoplastic hypercalcemia (267). By contrast, one group of investigators has reported raised iPTH levels in 103 of 108 unselected patients, including many with metastatic breast cancer and myelomatosis (268). They concluded that ectopic hyperparathyroidism was a major cause of hypercalcemia, irrespective of the type of tumor or the presence or absence of osseous metastases. There is much evidence against this conclusion. First, in both metastatic breast cancer (269) and myelomatosis (220) osteoclastic bone resorption is increased in proximity to the tumor cells but not elsewhere in the skeleton. Subperiosteal resorption in the phalanges is never seen except in a small minority of patients with authentic ectopic hyperparathyroidism, for which the best evidence is regression of the bone changes after excision of the tumor. Second, other mechanisms of hypercalcemia (such

as increased prostaglandin secretion) are being found in an increasing proportion of patients with low iPTH levels determined in other laboratories (271, 272). Third, in many patients with metastatic breast cancer and myelomatosis, tubular reabsorption of calcium and NcAMP excretion are consistent with normal or suppressed rather than raised iPTH levels. Tm_P/GFR is frequently reduced (273), but in most instances this is a nonspecific consequence of hypercalcemia.

The paradoxically high iPTH levels were obtained with a predominantly C-terminal assay (268). In patients with authentic ectopic hyperparathyroidism, gel filtration of the PTH-like material indicated that N-terminal iPTH (whole molecule or prohormone) was increased, and the relationship between N-iPTH and plasma calcium was the same in ectopic as in primary hyperparathyroidism (274). Unfortunately, this refinement was not carried out routinely in the later unselected series, so that increased biologically active PTH cannot be inferred with any certainty. Since most of the patients studied had a moderate degree of renal insufficiency, it is likely that the level of C-terminal fragment was raised as a nonspecific consequence of impaired renal function rather than because of increased PTH secretion.

Whatever the mechanism, patients with neoplastic hypercalcemia show certain features in common which set them apart from most patients with hypercalcemic hyperparathyroidism. They usually have disequilibrium rather than equilibrium hypercalcemia. The plasma calcium is higher and rises more rapidly, the history is shorter, weight loss more profound, and the patient sicker, but there are exceptions to each and sometimes all of these generalizations. The differences depend mainly on the rate of tumor growth; all the features just mentioned may be found in Type 1 hyperparathyroidism, and slowly growing nonparathyroid tumors may occasionally produce a clinical picture indistinguishable from Type 2 hyperparathyroidism.

Local Osteolysis. Bone destruction can be initiated by metastases from neoplasms arising elsewhere or by neoplasia of cells normally present in bone or bone marrow.

Metastatic Disease of Bone. The most common

cause is carcinoma of the female breast but the primary neoplasm may also be in the prostate, kidney, lung, thyroid, ovary, stomach or large bowel. Metastases are blood borne; they become established in the sinusoids of the red marrow (269), predominantly of the axial skeleton, and later invade the haversian canals of cortical bone. The effect on the bone includes both an increase in resorption and a reparative increase in woven bone formation. Bone scanning is much more sensitive than x-rays in the detection of metastases, the increased uptake depending entirely on the local increase in bone formation (275). Although resorption and formation are both increased they are not coupled as in normal bone remodeling units but can vary independently (Table 19-20). Depending on which predominates, the radiographic appearances can be classified as either osteoblastic or osteolytic. Predominantly osteoblastic metastases cause a net flux of calcium into bone and a tendency to hypocalciuria and hypocalcemia (p. 982). Predominantly osteolytic metastases cause a net loss of calcium from bone and a tendency to hypercalciuria and hypercalcemia (276). The ability to secrete chemical stimulators of bone resorption may be necessary for cancer cells to survive in bone. Both in breast cancer and in experimental metastases from VX_2 carcinoma, bone resorption is initiated by osteoclasts, which increase 10- to 20-fold in response to the secretion by the tumor cells of PGE_2 (prostaglandin-E_2) and of other unidentified substances. Later, resorption is continued directly by the tumor cells in the absence of osteoclasts (277).

In the early stages net loss of calcium from bone may be accommodated by decreased net absorption and increased endogenous secretion of calcium with no change in urinary calcium excretion (206), but as net bone resorption increases, first hypercalciuria and then hypercalcemia eventually occur. Progression of the disease (either spontaneous or hormonally induced) is usually associated with hypercalciuria, which occurs at some time in about 50 percent of patients (260). Conversely, regression (either spontaneous or in response to treatment) is associated with hypocalciuria, although this correlation was not found when only nocturnal calcium excretion was

measured (278). About 20 percent of patients have episodes of mild hypercalcemia (less than 3 mmol/L) which is asymptomatic and transient and does not need treatment, and about 15 percent develop severe symptomatic hypercalcemia (269). The plasma phosphate is often raised but in relation to the degree of renal failure may be low. Tubular reabsorption of phosphate is often normal in metastatic hypercalcemia in contrast to ectopic hyperparathyroidism, but may also be reduced despite suppression of PTH. This is most likely a nonspecific effect of hypercalcemia to reduce Tm_p/GFR.

Hypercalcemia is frequently preceded by worsening of bone pain and may occur spontaneously or be precipitated by hormonal therapy. Adrenalectomy, androgens, estrogens, progestogens, and the anti-estrogen tamoxifen (281) are all sometimes followed by hypercalcemia, presumably because of accelerated tumor growth, either transient or persistent. Estrogen dependence in breast cancer is usually manifest before the menopause, but fatal hypercalcemia may occasionally be precipitated by estrogen therapy in postmenopausal women, the plasma calcium rising by 2 to 2.5 mmol/L within 3 to 4 days (282). Hypercalcemia most often occurs as a complication of recognized disease, but may sometimes be the presenting feature. Florid radiographic evidence of osteolysis is usual, but rarely even the bone scan may be negative, the cause of the hypercalcemia being revealed by bone or bone marrow biopsy (283). Prolonged survival after recovery from hypercalcemia is possible, but most patients are dead within a year (269).

Net loss of calcium from bone is clearly the major cause of the hypercalcemia, but doubts have been expressed because of lack of correlation with the apparent extent of bone disease. Hypercalcemia is often preceded or accompanied by a fall in AP (279) and urinary total hydroxyproline may rise during recovery from hypercalcemia (284). Therefore, the imbalance leading to hypercalcemia may result from a suppression of bone formation, but radiocalcium kinetic studies usually do not show reduced accretion rate (279). Whatever the mechanism, the effect of net transfer of calcium from bone to blood depends on the relationships between the load of calcium requiring excretion, GFR, and tubular reabsorption of calcium. In a few cases in which all three variables have been measured, the degree of hypercalcemia has been consistent with the increase in load/GFR but in most cases tubular reabsorption of calcium is increased as well as load/GFR (Fig. 19-16), probably because of sodium depletion and ECF volume contraction.

Since tumor-induced osteolysis is chemically mediated, substances such as PGE_2 could conceivably have a systemic as well as a local effect. Plasma levels of PGE are high in many patients wtih bone metastases and hypercalcemia (272), but increased resorption has never been found in patients except in relation to tumor cells in bone. Furthermore, the production of hypercalcemia by net bone resorption depends on the magnitude of the calcium loss, not on its site of origin. It seems most likely that either a sudden increase in calcium release from bone (because of increased resorption or suppression of formation or both) or a reduction in GFR indicates the vicious circle characteristic of disequilibrium hypercalcemia.

As in other kinds of disequilibrium hypercalcemia there may be an excellent response to vigorous intravenous fluid therapy which simultaneously increases GFR and reduces the tubular reabsorption of calcium. Corticosteroids in adequate dose are usually effective but may need to be given parenterally rather than by mouth (285). Sustained correction of hypercalcemia may follow successful arrest of the underlying disease as with oophorectomy in a premenopausal patient. Other aspects of treatment are discussed in more detail on p. 1035.

Myelomatosis. In this disease hypercalcemia results from bone resorption initiated by neoplasia of plasma cells, which are a normal constituent of the bone marrow. Hypercalcemia occurs at some time in about 25 percent of patients (286) and its clinical and biochemical characteristics in general resemble those of metastatic hypercalcemia. In terms of the balance between increased resorption and increased formation, myeloma is at the opposite end of the scale from metastatic prostatic carcinoma (276, 279). Reparative woven bone formation is minimal, so that the AP is usu-

ally normal and the bone scan more often negative than in metastatic disease. However, a similar relationship exists between calcium balance and progression of the disease. A critical mass of tumor cells is a necessary but not a sufficient condition for the occurrence of hypercalcemia (287). Widespread disease is associated with increased bone resorption, a negative balance of up to 12 mmol daily, and a comparable degree of hypercalciuria (288).

As in metastatic disease, bone resorption in myeloma is mediated (at least initially) by osteoclasts (270). Cultured myeloma cells secrete a substance which stimulates bone resorption by increasing both the number and activity of osteoclasts, and which is similar to the OAF (osteoclast-activating factor) secreted by phytohemagglutinin-activated normal leukocytes. The chemical nature of OAF, either from normal leukocytes or myeloma cells, is unknown, although a larger molecule precursor has been found (288); it is not a prostaglandin, PTH, 1,25-DHCC, or any other chemically defined stimulator of bone resorption.

The hypercalcemia of myeloma has all the characteristics of a disequilibrium hypercalcemia; equilibrium hypercalcemia in a patient with a plasma protein dyscrasia is more likely due to primary hyperparathyroidism with benign monoclonal gammopathy (290). In some cases the relationship between calcium load/GFR and plasma calcium is normal (44) so that the factor limiting renal excretion is a fall in GFR, but in many patients there is increased tubular reabsorption of calcium (Fig. 19-16). As in all other varieties of hypercalcemia the tubular reabsorption of phosphate may be depressed; in one case the $Tm_P/$GFR was only 0.25 mmol/L, which led to a mistaken diagnosis of primary hyperparathyroidism (291). In different series the occurrence of hypercalcemia has been found to worsen (292) or to have no effect (293) on the long-term prognosis.

Very rarely in myeloma the total plasma calcium may increase because of a paraprotein with unusual calcium-binding capacity, the ionized calcium being normal (294). Subsequently, the calcium-binding activity was localized to the light chains of an IgGλ protein (12).

Humoral Mechanisms. If the plasma calcium falls to normal after removal of a tumor, it is reasonable to infer that some substance secreted by the tumor was the cause of the hypercalcemia, a conclusion which is strengthened if tumor extracts are able to resorb bone in vitro. If hypophosphatemia is also present and is similarly corrected, there is an obvious resemblance to hyperparathyroidism, but a reduction in Tm_p/GFR and hypophosphatemia is so commonly a nonspecific result of severe hypercalcemia that their presence is unhelpful in characterizing the nature of the humoral substance. There is no doubt that some tumors synthesize and secrete a substance closely resembling PTH, but other tumors secrete other hypercalcemic agents; in most published cases the humoral substance has not been identified with any certainty.

Ectopic Hyperparathyroidism. As currently used (295–298) this term identifies a clinical syndrome rather than a specific endocrinopathy. It usually resembles Type 1 primary hyperparathyroidism of the most rapidly progressive form. Renal calculi are rare (299); in the only personal case with a radiographic appearance resembling stone, it was due to calcification in the causative renal tumor. There may be histologic osteitis fibrosa (300), but in contrast to primary hyperparathyroidism, subperiosteal resorption is rarely seen in patients with acute hypercalcemia (299). In authentic cases the usual metabolic effects of PTH, including increased NcAMP excretion, reduced Tm_p/GFR, and increased tubular reabsorption of calcium, are invariably found when sought. An unexplained difference from primary hyperparathyroidism is that the plasma chloride tends to be reduced and plasma bicarbonate raised. A low plasma chloride is strong evidence against primary hyperparathyroidism but a normal or raised chloride does not rule out ectopic hyperparathyroidism (295). The difference has been attributed to a greater tendency to hypokalemia, possibly due to associated ectopic secretion of ACTH, but this is speculative. As in Type 1 primary hyperparathyroidism, the hypercalcemia responds to corticosteroids in a few patients but not in the majority. The plasma calcium and phosphate levels return to normal after excision of the primary tumor, as rapidly and completely as after parathyroidectomy in primary hyperparathyroidism.

The clinical syndrome of humoral hypercalcemia (absence of overt bone metastases and reversal by tumor excision) occurs most commonly in renal carcinoma and in epidermoid (squamous cell) carcinoma of the lung (301). The list of different tumors is very long and is still growing; the syndrome is very rare in carcinoma of the breast. Identification of PTH-like material in the blood or in the tumor has been accomplished in a much smaller number of patients, but the same two tumors predominate. Seen through immunofluorescence only some cells in any tumor appear to secrete PTH, the proportion varying from 15 to 90 percent, in contrast to the uniform secretory activity of all cells in parathyroid adenomas (302). Surviving tumor cells demonstrated biosynthesis of material similar to but probably not identical with PTH in one of seven cases tested (303).

The uncertainty concerning the frequency of ectopic hyperparathyroidism has already been mentioned. If only unequivocal instances are considered there is considerable evidence that the circulating iPTH is different from that in primary hyperparathyroidism (274). Some antisera do not react at all with ectopic PTH, whereas others react equally well with ectopic and with regular PTH. Using the GP1M antiserum, for the same level of plasma calcium there was considerably less total immunoreactive material in ectopic than in primary hyperparathyroidism. Conversely, for the same level of iPTH the plasma calcium was higher in ectopic than in primary hyperparathyroidism. Excellent discrimination between the two groups of patients was obtained if the plasma calcium was greater than 3.5 mmol/L (274). These differences are mainly due to a much smaller concentration of the biologically inert C-terminal fragment; there is also a larger amount of a higher-molecular-weight component, possibly pro-PTH. The data suggest that ectopic PTH is more resistant than regular PTH to enzymatic cleavage between residues 20 and 25. According to the repressor-deletion theory of ectopic hormone secretion, the primary structure of the initial polypeptide should be the same as in normal parathyroid glands, but lack of one or more cleavage enzymes might allow a larger precursor molecule to escape into the circulation. Alternatively, the primary structure of the polypeptide synthesized in ectopic hyperparathyroidism may differ from normal. Recent evidence suggests that in all ectopic hormone-producing tumors, the primary product of messenger RNA translation may be the same large-molecular-weight protein, from which different subunits can be cleaved by specific enzymes (304).

Nonparathyroid Humoral Hypercalcemia. In most patients with the clinical syndrome of pseudohyperparathyroidism, no PTH can be detected in the blood or in the tumor (305), although there are no clinical or biochemical differences between these cases and those with high iPTH levels. Failure of multiple assay systems to detect iPTH seems an unlikely explanation, but the humoral agents are still unknown in most cases. Humoral hypercalcemia may be due to benign lesions such as breast dysplasia (306), but most often the cause is a malignant neoplasm.

Prostaglandins in Neoplastic Hypercalcemia. As previously noted prostaglandins are probably involved in the localized osteolysis around metastases and may also have a systemic effect. Two kinds of transplantable tumor can induce experimental hypercalcemia—the $HDSM_1$ fibrosarcoma in the mouse and the VX_2 carcinoma in the rabbit (307); the latter also produces hypophosphatemia (308). In both cases the tumor secretes prostaglandins (particularly PGE_2), the plasma levels of PGE_2 in the transplanted animals are raised, increased resorption occurs in bones distant from the tumor, and both increased resorption (309) and hypercalcemia can be prevented by indomethacin, an inhibitor of prostaglandin synthetase (307). In some hypercalcemic patients without bone metastases and with suppressed PTH, increased urinary excretion of prostaglandin metabolites (310) and increased plasma levels of PGE_2 in the range associated with experimental hypercalcemia have been found (321); the hypercalcemia in such patients frequently responds to indomethacin (310, 311). Nevertheless, it is still uncertain whether humoral hypercalcemia is ever due to prostaglandins alone. Hypercalcemia is difficult to produce by prostaglandin administration in the rat unless

the rat is subjected to thyroparathyroidectomy (312) and has not been produced in the dog, a species whose calcium metabolism more closely resembles that of humans. Most patients with raised PGE_2 levels and hypercalcemia have had widespread metastases and such patients may have high PGE_2 levels without hypercalcemia (272). Finally, in no case has removal of a tumor been followed by correction of hypercalcemia, hypophosphatemia, and raised PGE_2 levels.

The WDHA Syndrome. The syndrome of WDHA (watery diarrhea, hypokalemia, and achlorhydria) or pancreatic cholera is associated with a non-β islet cell tumor of the pancreas. Of 62 cases recently reviewed 12 had hypercalcemia (313). This may be due to associated primary hyperparathyroidism but hypercalcemia may occur with suppressed iPTH (314); the tumor in such cases is usually benign. A variety of polypeptide hormones can be produced by these tumors; including secretin (313) and vasoactive intestinal polypeptide (314); both are possible causes of hypercalcemia in the WDHA syndrome. Nonparathyroid humoral hypercalcemia may also occur in islet cell carcinoma and respond to streptozotocin (315).

Other Suggested Mechanisms. The transplantable Leydig's cell tumor of the Fischer rat produces hypercalcemia by secreting an unidentified sterol (316). A variety of osteolytic plant sterols have been found in breast cancer tissue from hypercalcemic patients, but also from breast and other tumors unassociated with hypercalcemia; the blood levels of these sterols are no higher in patients with breast cancer than in control subjects (317). There is no evidence to support any role of vitamin D or its metabolites in tumor-induced hypercalcemia. Finally, many breast cancers are prolactin dependent; prolactin raises the plasma calcium in rats by about 0.5 mg/dL (318) but there is no evidence that prolactin can cause hypercalcemia in humans.

Lympho- and Myeloproliferative Disorders. Hypercalcemia may rarely occur in Hodgkin's disease and lymphosarcoma, reticulum cell sarcoma, and acute or chronic leukemia of any cytologic type (319). This group of disorders is considered separately because the reason for the hypercalcemia may be difficult to establish. In contrast to solid tumors definitive cure by surgery, which is the most convincing evidence for a humoral mechanism, is usually not possible, although hypercalcemia has remitted following excision of a solitary lymphoma of the spleen (320). The frequent response of the hypercalcemia to cytotoxic therapy is consistent with any mechanism. Ectopic secretion of PTH has been documented in Hodgkin's disease (299) and in myelogenous leukemia (321); the former patient had both subperiosteal resorption and renal stones. Hypercalcemia has occurred in reticulum cell sarcoma without bone involvement and with normal parathyroid glands and no PTH in the blood; an unidentified osteolytic agent could be extracted from the tumor (322). Some patients have been abnormally sensitive to vitamin D, as in sarcoidosis, and in other cases stimulation of bone resorption by tumor cells in bone probably contributes to the hypercalcemia.

In Hodgkin's disease less than 2 percent of the patients have hypercalcemia and only 6 percent of those with obvious bone lesions (323). This may be because the osseous response is more usually osteoblastic, or because of a humoral mechanism for hypercalcemia independent of net bone resorption. In one case lymphoma caused widespread diffuse bone resorption with multiple vertebral compression fractures resembling idiopathic osteoporosis, but there was only a trivial elevation of plasma calcium (324). The incidence of hypercalcemia is about the same in reticulum cell sarcoma and a similar uncertainty exists about the mechanisms. Absence of radiographic bone involvement is usual but diffuse infiltration may be found at autopsy (323). In both acute and chronic leukemia hypercalcemia occurs in 1 to 2 percent of cases (325). Although most patients have had abnormal bone x-rays, convincing evidence of bone resorption of sufficient severity to cause hypercalcemia is rare (326). The ages have ranged from 8 to 69 years and about one-third of the cases have been in children or adolescents.

In all three conditions the AP may be either normal or elevated, and the plasma phosphate normal or low, or high if, as commonly occurs, there is renal failure. None of the case reports have included sufficient data to characterize the relationship between calcium load, GFR, and tubular reabsorption.

Hyperparathyroidism in Neoplastic Hypercalcemia. In addition to ectopic hyperparathyroidism, various abnormalities of the parathyroid glands have been described in patients with neoplastic hypercalcemia. Apart from coexisting primary hyperparathyroidism the significance of the findings is questionable. A patient with cancer is not precluded from having other disease; in fact, various types of cancer may be associated with hyperparathyroidism more commonly than by chance, possible because of the mitogenic effect of hypercalcemia (327). Surgical cure of associated primary hyperparathyroidism is not only important in itself but may profoundly modify the prognosis and management of a patient mistakenly thought to have advanced or incurable disease on the basis of hypercalcemia (328). Very rarely hypercalcemia may be due both to primary and to ectopic hyperparathyroidism, two operations being needed to restore normocalcemia. In a personal case, a patient cured of primary hyperparathyroidism subsequently died of metastatic lung cancer with recurrence of hypercalcemia.

In most cases the parathyroid pathology has been a single adenoma but occasionally parathyroid hyperplasia is found. This has been attributed to renal failure and to phosphate administration, but also raises the possibility that the tumor was secreting a parathyrotropic substance, particularly when the clinical course suggests that hyperparathyroidism developed at the same time as the tumor (329). In some cases hyperplasia has been mistakenly diagnosed because of the absence of fat (a local manifestation of neoplastic cachexia) or of failure to recognize that an absence of parathyroid involution may be the normal response of parathyroid tissue to moderate hypercalcemia. In other cases the parathyroid parenchymal weight has been increased and hypercalcemia has regressed after subtotal parathyroidectomy (330). Coincidental primary chief cell hyperplasia seems the most likely explanation of this rare association. Finally, increased PTH secretion may rarely be produced by neoplastic infiltration of the parathyroid gland. Metastases to the parathyroid from a malignant melanoma have been associated with hypercalcemia and raised plasma iPTH (331), and a similar mechanism has been postulated with leukemic infiltration of the parathyroid glands.

Other causes of disequilibrium hypercalcemia. An abrupt and substantial increase in net bone resorption is a major cause of hypercalcemia in several other situations, but in many cases the data are insufficient to determine whether the necessary limitation in the capacity of the kidney to excrete calcium is due to increased tubular reabsorption or decreased glomerular filtration. The requirement for the simultaneous occurrence of two independent abnormalities is the reason why hypercalcemia occurs only in a small minority of patients with the disorders to be considered.

Immobilization after Trauma. Although slight elevation of total and especially ionized calcium is common in immobilized subjects (332), symptomatic hypercalcemia is rare, is virtually confined to adolescents, and is never produced by immobilization alone. Most cases occur after severe or multiple fractures (333), and a few after severe burns (334) or extensive traumatic paralysis (335). The ages have ranged from 9 to 22 years with a predominance of males, presumably because of increased liability to trauma. The symptoms usually begin rather abruptly a few weeks or months after the injury. The plasma calcium is often about 3.5 mmol/L, the plasma phosphate variable, and AP usually normal but occasionally raised. Urinary calcium usually ranges between 5 and 10 mmol per 24 h, and between 0.05 and 0.15 mmol/L GF. Tubular reabsorption of calcium is often increased (Fig. 19-16). iPTH in a few cases has been low, normal, or high (336); the latter values are probably the most reliable but are difficult to explain; whether they resulted from alterations in PTH secretion or in formation of catabolism of inactive metabolites is not known. Both hypercalcemia and high iPTH return to normal with remobilization. If this alone is ineffective or impractical, the hypercalcemia responds rapidly to corticosteroids (333) or calcitonin (337). Nephrolithiasis is a well-known complication of immobilization and together with hypercalcemia may suggest hyperparathyroidism, but few patients with immobilization hypercalcemia have had stones. Parathyroid exploration has been performed in a few cases but the correct diagnosis should be obvious. Immobilization may also precipitate or worsen hypercalcemia in patients on maintenance hemodialysis with secondary hyperparathyroidism, after fracture in primary hyperparathyroidism or Paget's disease, in hyperthyroidism (338), and after osteotomy in hypophosphatemic rickets treated with vitamin D (339). Hypercalcemia not precipitated by immobilization in Paget's disease is due to coexistent hyperparathyroidism.

The effects of immobilization on bone and bone mineral metabolism are complex and include separate components of recumbency, disuse, and trauma. Short-term bed rest (12 days) in healthy persons leads to an increase of about 10 percent in ionized calcium within a few days, urinary calcium rising more slowly (332). Prolonged bed rest (30 to 36 weeks) leads to a modest increase in urinary calcium, reaching a maximum in the seventh week and a more sustained increase in fecal calcium with negative calcium balances of about 5 mmol/day. The total plasma calcium usually remains normal, but urinary hydroxyproline increases by about 20 percent. Cumulative losses of about 1000 mmol of calcium can be sustained and the lost bone is restored at about the same rate after remobilization (340). These effects are consistent with a moderate increase in bone turnover with reversible bone loss (Chap. 8). The hypercalciuria of bed rest is reversed by quiet standing but not by exercise and so has been attributed to the gravitational effects of recumbency rather than to inactivity. The hypercalciuria is also reduced by oral phosphate supplements and by a low-sodium diet together with a thiazide diuretic.

Immobilization due to muscle paralysis after spinal cord injury or poliomyelitis leads to similar but much greater changes, with a two- to threefold increase in bone resorption determined by combined balance and kinetic studies, hydroxyproline excretion exceeding 100 mg per 24 h, mean urinary calcium in the 10- to 15-mmol per 24 h range, and negative calcium balances of about 12 mmol per 24 h (341). Bone histologic changes are best explained as consequences of a prolongation of the resorptive phase of the remodeling cycles, together with a severe depression of osteoblastic activity, causing a transient imbalance between resorption and formation. A new steady state is eventually established in which bone turnover is normal or depressed (341). Severe trauma produces in addition a very large local increase in bone turnover which augments the less-intense but more-generalized effects of recumbency and disuse. These effects are presumably greatest during the adolescent growth spur when bone turnover is already high. This accounts for the clinical setting in which hypercalcemia occurs but does not explain why only a small number of those at risk are affected. As in other situations, inappropriate renal retention of calcium may be a contributory factor (see Fig. 19-16).

Hyperthyroidism. Occasionally hyperthyroidism is complicated by severe symptomatic hypercalcemia. Eighteen cases were reviewed in 1970 (338) and about 12 have been reported since. This is not just an extreme form of the mild hypercalcemia due to increased bone turnover, because it is unrelated to the severity or duration of the hyperthyroidism, but like other forms of disequilibrium hypercalcemia, is probably due to a combination of increased net bone resorption and impaired renal excretion of calcium, either reduced GFR or increased tubular reabsorption (Fig. 19-16). Symptoms of hypercalcemia, especially anorexia, vomiting, thirst, and severe muscle weakness may dominate the clinical picture and mask those of hyperthyroidism, to the extent that the neck is explored for hyperparathyroidism. All degrees of hypercalcemic nephropathy may occur including nephrocalcinosis and acquired renal-tubular acidosis, but nephrolithiasis is unusual. The mean plasma calcium was 3.55 mmol/L, ranging from 2.95 to 4.80, with values exceeding 4.0 in about 20 percent of the cases. The mean plasma inorganic phosphate was 1.26 mmol/L ranging from 0.8 to 1.8, and mean 24-h urine calcium 13 mmol. The calcium balance is the same as in thyrotoxic patients without severe hypercalcemia (described later). PTH is usually undetectable, and NcAMP zero. The hypercalcemia invariably responds within a few weeks to correction of the hyperthyroidism, but normocalcemia may not be attained for as long as 8 weeks. Relapse of hyperthyroidism may occur both with or without recurrence of hypercalcemia. For very severe hypercalcemia additional treatment is needed and corticosteroids in adequate dose (equivalent to 40 to 80 mg of prednisone daily) have invariably reduced the plasma calcium to a safe level within 3 to 6 days (342). The β-adrenergic antagonist propanolol has been rapidly effective in three cases (343), which is paradoxical since it has no effect on urinary calcium or hydroxyproline excretion (344) or on the hypercalcemia of hyperparathyroidism. Phosphate and calcitonin have been successfully used in isolated cases. Renal function usually improves but not always to normal; indeed permanent renal insufficiency may progress to hypertension and death from renal failure.

Hypercalcemia in hyperthyroidism may also be due to concomitant hyperparathyroidism, the two diseases occurring in the same patient about 10 times more commonly than by chance and being present at the same time in about one-third of these patients (338). The development of hyperthyroidism may precipitate a hypercalcemic crisis. Hyperparathyroidism should be suspected if there is a history of kidney stones, a plasma phosphate below 0.8 mmol/L, subperiosteal resorption or lack of response of the hypercalcemia to antithyroid treatment and confirmed by NcAMP or iPTH assay.

Although severe hypercalcemia occurs only in a small minority of patients, bone and mineral metabolism are profoundly disturbed in almost all patients. Bone turnover is increased whether determined by calcium kinetics or bone morphologic or biochemical measures (64), presumably because of a direct effect of thyroxine on osteoclast precursor proliferation. This results in a transient negative skeletal balance (Chap. 8) of as much as 20 mmol of calcium daily (349), with a marked increase in both fecal and urinary calcium excretion. The negative balance persists only for about 8 months if skeletal balance were previously zero as in young adults, but in older persons an existing negative calcium balance of 1 mmol/day because of involutional bone loss will be amplified in proportion to the increase in turnover. As in other situations, the effect this has on the plasma calcium depends on how much of the calcium is lost in the stool and how much in the urine, and on the characteristics of renal-tubular reabsorption of calcium (Fig. 19-16). In several large series the total plasma calcium was increased by about 0.15 mmol/L but there was no correlation with plasma thyroxine (346). Albumin levels are often low in hyperthyroidism and a relatively greater increase in ionized calcium of about 0.1 mmol/L is found (344). There is an upward shift in the entire group, and about 20 to 30 percent of hyperthyroid patients have slight hypercalcemia, usually asymptomatic. Plasma calcium is raised much less than in hyperparathyroidism even though the increase in turnover and the degree of negative balance are much greater (Fig. 19-17). Because of increased net release of calcium from bone, PTH secretion is suppressed; this is

best shown by NcAMP which is uniformly low even though total cAMP excretion is high. This accounts for increased tubular reabsorption of phosphate and elevation of plasma phosphate (338), and for decreased tubular reabsorption of calcium. Although urinary calcium may be as high as 10 to 15 mmol per 24 h, this does not cause nephrolithiasis. The increased fecal calcium is not affected by vitamin D (345) but in one case was abolished by coincidental primary hyperparathyroidism (358). It is due to intestinal malabsorption rather than increased endogenous fecal calcium (348); malabsorption of other nutrients and abnormal mucosal histology are common in hyperthyroidism. After beginning antithyroid treatment the urinary calcium begins to fall within 1 to 2 weeks and the AP rises still further. The negative calcium balance is reversed in from 3 to 8 weeks; presumably this is followed by a

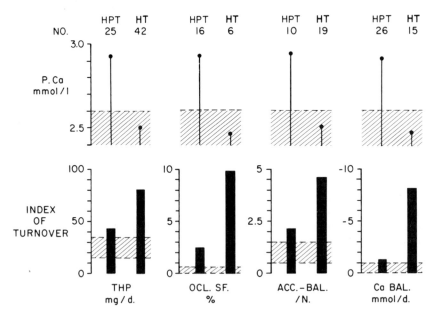

Figure 19-17. Comparison of mean values for plasma calcium (upper panel) and various indices of bone turnover (lower panel) in hyperparathyroidism (HPT—on left) and hyperthyroidism (HT—on right). The shaded areas denote normal ranges. THP, total urinary hydroxyproline in mg/24 h; OCL. SF, osteoclast-lined Howship's lacunar surface as a percentage of the total trabecular surface; ACC-BAL, net bone resorption (the difference between kinetic accretion and external balance) as a ratio to normal values; CaBal, external calcium balance; number of cases. [*Reproduced from A. M. Parfitt (64) with permission; sources given in original article.*]

positive balance for many months if the bone loss is repaired.

Thiazide Diuretics. The major effect of thiazide diuretics on bone mineral metabolism is a reduction in urinary calcium excretion which contrasts with the hypercalciuric effects of other agents causing hypercalcemia; this is considered on p. 1041. In the great majority of patients on long-term treatment with thiazides the plasma calcium remains normal, but very occasionally significant hypercalcemia occurs by one of several mechanisms. First, in patients with increased net bone resorption, hypercalciuria, and actual or incipient disequilibrium hypercalcemia, thiazides may induce or worsen hypercalcemia by limiting the capacity to excrete calcium. Second, in both primary and secondary hyperparathyroidism a rise in plasma calcium of 0.5 to 1 mmol/L may occur within a few days (349, 350). Chlorothiazide given intravenously produces a small increase in ionized calcium within 2 h which is absent in HP and exaggerated in hyperparathyroidism (351); this probably reflects a potentiation of some effect of PTH on bone. The use of thiazides in provocative tests for occult hyperparathyroidism was mentioned on p. 1010. Third, thiazides induce hypercalcemia in some patients receiving high doses of vitamin D (349, 352). In HP this is not due to reduced urinary calcium excretion and most likely results from augmented calcium release from bone. The hypercalcemia is usually self-limited, but may be sustained if there is also a fall in urinary calcium (352); the same may occur in some patients with sarcoidosis. Most rarely of all, thiazide diuretics may induce hypercalcemia in patients with no preexisting abnormality of calcium metabolism. In such cases the plasma calcium returns to normal within a few days or weeks of discontinuing the thiazide.

Although a substantial rise in plasma calcium is rare, minor changes are quite common. For a few days after beginning the administration of any diuretic there is a small and transient rise in total calcium due to concentration of plasma proteins resulting from volume depletion. In addition, with prolonged oral administration of thiazides there is a small rise in ionized calcium, the peak value occurring after about 2 weeks (353) but the level eventually returns to normal in most cases. When hypercalcemia is discovered in a patient taking a thiazide, it usually persists when the drug is stopped and is due to concomitant primary hyperparathyroidism.

Vitamin A Intoxication. This disorder is most common in children but can occur at any age (352). It is characterized by a dry, papular, seborrheic skin eruption with discoloration, pigmentation, and pruritus, fissuring of the mouth and tongue, alopecia, painful and tender bones with subcutaneous swellings and periosteal new bone on x-ray in children, and enlargement of the liver, often with prolonged prothrombin time and increased BSP retention. Hypercalcemia occurs most often in patients aged from 15 to 20 years, occasionally in children, and very rarely in older adults. The plasma calcium may exceed 2.5 mmol/L and the patient may have severe hypercalcemic symptoms and be quite ill, or there may be no symptoms other than those of the primary disease, for which there is always other evidence. Vitamin A has usually been taken for several years in a dose of 100,000 units daily or more, usually with small doses of vitamin D as well. The serum vitamin A level is two to four times the upper limit of normal, but in this respect there is no difference between patients with and without hypercalcemia, or even between patients with and without clinical intoxication. AP and urinary total hydroxyproline excretion may be raised and the calcium balance negative (353). Normocalcemia is usually restored in 1 to 3 weeks with intravenous fluids and withdrawal of vitamin A, and no permanent sequelae have occurred. As in other situations, hypercalciuria without hypercalcemia may occur. Case 3 of Frame et al. (354), reported as responsive to prednisone, can no longer be regarded as authentic since hypercalcemia has persisted despite cessation of vitamin A (B. Frame, personal communication). The cause of hypercalcemia in a small number of patients with vitamin A intoxication remains a mystery. Administration of 200,000 units daily to human subjects for 3 to 4 weeks *lowered* plasma and urinary calcium and led to increased retention of calcium and phosphate (356). Vitamin A causes increased bone resorption in tissue culture, but in one patient with intoxication there was increased surface extent of resorption by microradiography, but no hypercalcemia (357). Vitamin A stimulates PTH secretion in the rat, but the only reported PTH level in a patient was normal.

The syndrome of hyperabsorption hypercalcemia. This term includes a group of conditions which have in common an absolute increase in net calcium absorption, positive calcium balance, an increase in total body calcium, widespread soft tissue calcification, nephrocalcinosis with disproportionate renal failure, bones of normal or increased density, suppressed iPTH and NcAMP levels, and responsiveness of the hypercalcemia to hydrocortisone. This syndrome occurs in vitamin D poisoning, sarcoidosis, the milk-alkali syndrome, and in some cases of idiopathic infantile hypercalcemia. A closely similar clinical state may arise in primary hyperparathyroidism with peptic ulceration. In the early stages of vitamin D poisoning and sarcoidosis net bone resorption may be increased and calcium balance negative despite hyperabsorption, but once renal failure occurs the complete syndrome usually follows. It occurs in its most pure form in the milk-alkali syndrome, which will be described first. This is now much less common than in the past, although hyperabsorption hypercalcemia without the complete syndrome still occurs.

The Milk-Alkali Syndrome. This term originally denoted sustained hypercalcemia after prolonged ingestion of large quantities of mild and absorbable alkali for the treatment of peptic ulceration (358). The principal absorbable alkali is sodium bicarbonate. This is converted to sodium chloride in the stomach but if more is ingested than is needed to neutralize gastric HCl, both the sodium and bicarbonate ions are freely absorbed, leading to systemic alkalosis. The principal nonabsorbable antacid is aluminum hydroxide—$Al(OH)_3$. This is converted to $AlCl_3$ in the stomach, but all or most of this is reconverted to $Al(OH)_3$ by the sodium bicarbonate in pancreatic secretions, and there is normally no increase in fecal chloride excretion or systemic alkalosis (359). In chronic

renal failure very large amounts of $Al(OH)_3$ may lead to a modest increase in plasma bicarbonate, but the extent of this systemic effect is limited by the extent of gastric acid secretion. Calcium carbonate used to be considered a nonabsorbable antacid, but the doses used are so large that absorption of only 2 to 3 percent of the dose may represent a substantial calcium load. The great majority of patients with the milk-alkali syndrome have taken large quantities of calcium carbonate and many, perhaps all, of the features of the syndrome can be produced by calcium carbonate alone.

Calcium carbonate is converted to $CaCl_2$ in the stomach, and mostly reconverted by the alkaline pancreatic secretions to $CaCO_3$, in which form it is excreted in the stool (359), but very large doses may produce a significant rise in the plasma bicarbonate level. Single doses containing 100 mmol of elemental calcium will increase the plasma calcium by 0.25 to 0.5 mmol/L, with a peak at 2 h, persisting for 4 to 6 h (360); about 15 percent of the calcium is absorbed. With higher doses the peak increase lasts for several hours longer. Continued administration of calcium carbonate providing 200 to 400 mmol of elemental calcium daily produces a sustained increase in plasma calcium of 0.26 to 0.4 mmol/L and a 25 percent fall in creatinine clearance (361). About 10 to 15 percent of the extra calcium is absorbed and the urinary calcium increases by 5 to 8 mmol/day. The absorption of calcium from calcium carbonate has been reported to be related (362) or unrelated (363) to the presence or absence of gastric HCl secretion.

The acute milk-alkali syndrome (Cope-Wenger) occurred in about 1 percent of patients treated for peptic ulceration by the Sippy method with large quantities of milk and cream and 50 to 100 mmol of $CaCO_3$ each hour for a total of 500 to 1000 mmol of elemental calcium daily (368, 369). Symptoms of hypercalcemia, of which headache, dizziness, and mental confusion were especially prominent, began within a few days to a few weeks. The peak plasma calcium was 2.7 mmol/L on the sixth day of symptoms, with a BUN of 40 mmol/L, both falling to normal within 2 weeks of discontinuing calcium carbonate. Many cases had some predisposing condition such as renal disease or metabolic alkalosis due to loss of gastric acid. Calcium carbonate is a poor antacid and as a treatment for peptic ulcer it is now obsolete, but acute hypercalcemia due to calcium carbonate may occur in patients with chronic renal failure on maintenance hemodialysis (364).

Patients with chronic (irreversible) milk-alkali syndrome (Burnett) frequently have a long history of self-medication for dyspepsia. Small doses of calcium carbonate by mouth increase gastrin secretion and acid production by a local effect, without a significant rise in plasma calcium. Consequently, a vicious circle can be established with a progressive increase in the dose needed for symptomatic relief. The patients seek medical advice only when their own treatment is no longer effective, or because of symptoms of chronic hypercalcemia and renal failure. The distinctive characteristics of the syndrome result from a substantial increase in total body calcium. Almost all patients have ocular calcification, and many have periarticular lesions similar to tumoral calcinosis. Excess soft tissue calcium deposition can be demonstrated by kinetic studies even if not visible on x-rays (208). Nephrocalcinosis, radiographic or histologic, is universal and accounts for the disproportionate severity of the hypercalcemic nephropathy and renal failure in comparison with hyperparathyroidism. For example, the mean plasma calcium in 33 cases was 3.28 mmol/L but the mean BUN was about 70 mmol/L (358). Because of the renal failure, plasma phosphate is often raised and absolute urine calcium excretion low, but calcium excretion/L C_{Cr} may be high. Bone x-rays are either normal or show osteosclerosis.

The immediate cause of both acute and chronic syndromes is obvious, but why are only a few of those at risk affected? Excess intake of milk usually provides only a small part of the total calcium load and is not essential to the development of the syndrome. Persons with intrinsic hyperabsorption of calcium would presumably be more prone to the syndrome, but this has not been demonstrated. Metabolic alkalosis increases the tubular reabsorption of calcium (Chap. 8), so that excess absorbed calcium would be less readily excreted. Calcium excretion could also be impaired by preexisting renal disease and by sodium depletion from protracted vomiting. The limited data available (Fig. 19-16) suggest that tubular reabsorption of calcium at the time the diagnosis is made is sometimes increased and sometimes normal. Metabolic alkalosis also reduces bone turnover and reduces the capacity of bone to take up additional calcium; it has been claimed for this reason that calcium carbonate is more effective than other salts in raising the plasma calcium in HP (365). Finally, metabolic alkalosis may promote soft tissue calcium deposition (366). Although there is no evidence that excess milk and sodium bicarbonate alone can produce the syndrome, many patients have taken large quantities of sodium bicarbonate as well as calcium carbonate, both being freely available without prescription. Peptic ulcers are common in primary hyperparathyroidism and because of intestinal hyperabsorption and increased tubular reabsorption of calcium these patients are more than normally liable to increased total body calcium and soft tissue calcification in response to a high intake of milk and calcium carbonate. The question in such a patient is not whether the hypercalcemia is due to the milk-alkali syndrome *or* to primary hyperparathyroidism, but whether a patient who manifestly has the milk-alkali syndrome also has primary hyperparathyroidism. C-terminal iPTH may be raised in renal failure even if PTH secretion is reduced, but the hydrocortisone test is decisive.

Withdrawal of milk and alkali and institution of a low-calcium diet are the first steps in treatment but will be resisted by the patient, ostensibly because of intolerable dyspepsia. In the absence of hyperparathyroidism this will eventually restore a normal plasma calcium, but may take many months because the hypercalcemia is sustained by mobilization of the soft tissue calcium deposits. As in vitamin D poisoning, maintenance of normocalcemia may require corticosteroids as well as a low-calcium diet for several months. Although some improvement in renal function may take place, much of the impairment is permanent and terminal uremia may ensue despite removal of the underlying cause and correction of the hypercalcemia. The mechanism of action of corticosteroids in this context is not clear; the blood levels of the various vitamin D metabolites in the milk-alkali syndrome would be of great interest.

Vitamin D Intoxication. Forty years ago vitamin D in high dose was widely used in the treatment of arthritis and allergic disorders, and hypervitaminosis D was common (367). Today, hypercalcemia due to vitamin D is usually a complication of treatment in HP or refractory rickets and osteomalacia. It may also follow massive single-dose therapy for the treatment or prophylaxis of nutritional rickets, or simply from grossly excessive doses given through ignorance, for example, more than 2 mg daily for several months in small infants (368). A further outbreak of vitamin D intoxication may be expected to follow the current rush to use the newer metabolites and analogues of vitamin D in the treatment of osteoporosis; already several deaths have been reported with both vitamin D_2 and DHT. Since vitamin D is available without prescription, intoxication can also result from self-administration, which may be concealed (369). In a personal case, a patient given vitamin D for arthritis in 1942 continued to treat herself for 30 years before chronic hypercalcemic nephropathy was recognized. An unusual form of vitamin D intoxication occurs in grazing animals. For example, cattle in Argentina ingesting *Solanum malacoxylon* develop widespread calcinosis and renal failure. The plant contains a water-soluble ester, probably a glucuronide of 1,25-DHCC (54). A similar disease with a similar pathogenesis occurs in horses in Florida eating the shrub *Cestrum diurnum* (370). Human disease from the same cause has not yet been recognized.

In vitamin D intoxication the plasma level of 25-HCC is very high (1 to 4 μmol/L) (369, 371, 372). The level of 1,25-DHCC may be only slightly raised (10 to 15 pmol/L) or even undetectable (377) and intoxication can also occur in anephric subjects (371). Consequently both the therapeutic and toxic effects are probably mediated directly by 25-HCC. High doses of vitamin D simultaneously increase the intestinal absorption and urinary excretion of calcium and increase osteoclastic bone resorption and urinary excretion of calcium and increase osteoclastic bone resorption and turnover (Chap. 8); plasma calcium usually remains normal. Decreased tubular reabsorption of calcium is probably due to suppression of PTH secretion, but could also result from vitamin D-induced sodium retention and ECF volume expansion (373) or an increase in plasma level and urinary excretion of citrate (367).

In HP an exaggeration of the therapeutic effect of vitamin D on the blood-bone equilibrium may lead to mild equilibrium hypercalcemia (Fig. 19-18) but in severe hypercalcemia there is usually increased net bone resorption (371) and often increased tubular reabsorption of calcium (Fig. 19-16) (207). This may result from failure of one or more of the previously described mechanisms for decreasing calcium reabsorption or from a direct calcium-conserving effect of some metabolite of vitamin D. Other factors which may precipitate hypercalcemia in vitamin D-treated hyperparathyroidism are listed in Table 19-17. Immobilization is an important factor, particularly in children with vitamin D refractory rickets who are subjected to osteotomy (339). Several mechanisms help to postpone the onset of hypercalcemia in patients receiving too high a dose, but these eventually break down so that hypercalcemia may develop with explosive suddenness (53) (Fig. 19-18) even though in retrospect incipient intoxication has been present for many months.

In chronic vitamin D intoxication the clinical features are similar to those of the milk-alkali syndrome with a high incidence of ocular calcification and nephrocalcinosis. In patients given vitamin D for arthritis, soft tissue calcification occurred preferentially in and around the affected joints, the radiographic features sometimes resembling tumoral calcinosis (366); widespread arterial calcification is also common; these changes are due not only to hypercalcemia but to hyperphosphatemia, which results from increased intestinal phosphate absorption as well as from renal

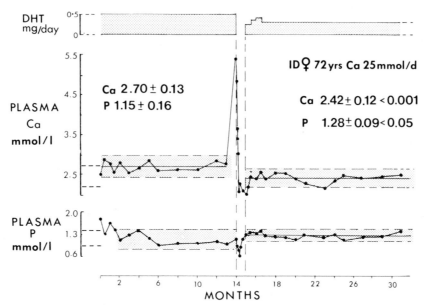

Figure 19-18. Serial values for plasma calcium and phosphate in a patient with SHP (surgical hypoparathyroidism) receiving DHT (dihydrotachysterol) and 25 mmol daily of calcium. Shaded areas denote means +2 S.D. ranges. Dotted lines at left denote normal ranges. Note initial mild equilibrium hypercalcemia, rapid onset of severe disequilibrium hypercalcemia, and restabilization on a lower dose of DHT. [*Reproduced from A. M. Parfitt (64) with permission.*]

failure. Anemia is often more severe than expected for the fall in GFR. In adults, bone biopsy may show increased surface extent of osteoclasts and decreased surface extent of osteoblasts; the AP is often low. In children there may be osteosclerosis resembling osteopetrosis, presumably because of suppression of the bone resorption necessary for normal modeling (367). The kidneys show basement membrane and interstitial calcification, especially in the medulla and around the distal tubules and collecting ducts. The changes resemble those due to hypercalcemia from other causes, but some differences between vitamin D- and PTH-induced nephrocalcinosis can be detected at the ultrastructural level (339).

There is a considerable body of experimental evidence suggesting that high doses of vitamin D may injure tissues directly and that the ensuing calcification is dystrophic as well as metastatic (366). In vitamin D refractory rickets, microscopic nephrocalcinosis is common and significant permanent impairment of renal function may occur after prolonged or repeated episodes of even mild hypercalcemia (374, 375). In HP, modest but significant impairment of renal function may occur after prolonged treatment in the absence of hypercalcemia (376). Hypercalciuria without hypercalcemia due to vitamin D may cause nephrolithiasis but whether it can impair renal function is unclear. The plasma calcium will eventually fall to normal if vitamin D is withheld and a low-calcium diet prescribed, but the plasma 25-HCC level may remain high for months and recovery is much more rapid if hydrocortisone is given (377). This probably does not directly antagonize vitamin D action, but produces independent effects on gut and bone in the opposite direction. Phosphate should never be used if the vitamin D was given for HP, but may be safe and effective if it was given for hypophosphatemic rickets.

Sarcoidosis. This disease is characterized by chronic noncaseating granulomas of multiple organs, but especially lung and liver. It is an important but still overlooked cause of hypercalcemia, usually of modest degree (3 to 3.5 mmol/L); rarely levels as high as 5.0 mmol/L may occur. It is manifested primarily by chronic hypercalcemic nephropathy and the other features of hyperabsorption hypercalcemia described earlier. Hypercalciuria is more common than hypercalcemia; as much as 25 mmol per 24 h may be excreted despite a normal plasma calcium (378). In one series 21 of 152 cases had nephrolithiasis (14 percent), about half of whom had hypercalcemia (379). However, others have found the incidence of nephrolithiasis to be no higher in sarcoidosis than in the general population (380).

Almost all patients have some other manifestation of the disease such as enlargement of the spleen, liver, or lymph nodes, excess keloid, iridocyclitis, erythema nodosum, abnormal serum protein electrophoretic pattern or abnormal chest x-ray with hilar adenopathy, diffuse infiltration, and pulmonary fibrosis, but none of these is particularly associated with hypercalcemia. The combination of hypercalcemia and splenomegaly usually indicates sarcoidosis or (less commonly) lymphoma. Occasionally hypercalcemia is the only sign of the disease; in several cases the diagnosis has been made by lymph node biopsy during neck exploration for suspected primary hyperparathyroidism (286). The incidence is about equal in blacks and whites and about 50 percent higher in males than in females. Most patients are between 20 and 45 years but extremes of 10 and 75 years have been reported.

The metabolic state in sarcoid hypercalcemia resembles vitamin D intoxication with increased intestinal absorption and decreased fecal excretion of calcium, suppressed or undetectable PTH, hypercalciuria, normal or raised but occasionally low plasma inorganic phosphate, increased bone turnover, and responsiveness to corticosteroids (381–384). Intestinal hyperabsorption and increased bone turnover are also found in normocalcemic patients with hypercalciuria (384). There is no relationship of the disturbed calcium metabolism to the presence of sarcoid granulomas in bone. In some patients hypercalcemia may be provoked by as little as 0.65 mmol of supplemental vitamin D, by ultraviolet irradiation of the skin

(381), by increased exposure to sunlight, or by small doses of 25-HCC or 1,25-DHCC, which do not induce hypercalcemia in normal persons (385). Blood levels of bioassayable vitamin D are normal, there is no increased formation of either 25-HCC or 1,25-DHCC after administration of labeled precursors, and the blood levels of these metabolites are usually normal (385). These data suggest that there is increased target cell responsiveness to physiologic amounts of active vitamin D metabolites, but the reason for this is quite unknown. There is also an exaggerated hypercalcemic response to exogenous PTH (385). In most patients gut, kidney, and bone are equally affected but differential sensitivity of these organs could explain occasional discrepancies such as the absence of hyperabsorption in patients with hypercalciuria or hypercalcemia (387, 388).

There is considerable geographic variation in the frequency of abnormal calcium metabolism in sarcoidosis. In North Carolina the mean plasma calcium in patients with sarcoidosis was significantly higher in the summer months than in the winter, and the incidence of hypercalcemia was 28 percent in the summer compared to 10 percent in the winter (389). However, in Philadelphia hypercalcemia is rare and confined to patients with long-standing and severe disease; hypercalciuria is no more common than in control subjects and there is no seasonal fluctuation (390). In subtropical Queensland, Australia, a compulsory annual chest x-ray leads to the diagnosis of sarcoidosis in many persons who are completely asymptomatic but who nevertheless manifest both hypercalciuria and hypercalcemia; the overall incidence of these abnormalities (including the subclinical cases) is about 45 and 30 percent, respectively. The rarity of abnormal calcium metabolism in some series has suggested that the metabolic disorder affects only a minority of patients. However, the high prevalence in asymptomatic patients in Queensland and the frequency of suppressed iPTH in patients without other calcium abnormalities (383) suggests that the metabolic defect affects the majority of, perhaps all, patients with sarcoidosis, but that its clinical expression depends on dietary, environmental, and other circumstances.

In addition to low or absent iPTH and NcAMP,

the standard hydrocortisone test is invariably positive in sarcoid hypercalcemia, although occasionally more than 10 days are needed to attain normocalcemia. If hypercalcemia persists it is likely due to concomitant primary hyperparathyroidism which seems to occur in sarcoidosis much more commonly than by chance (391). In such patients, as in other similar situations, the hypercalcemia is usually due entirely to the hyperparathyroidism, although occasionally corticosteroids may be needed to maintain normocalcemia after parathyroid surgery (392).

If the hypercalcemia responds to corticosteroids these are usually continued as treatment, since other manifestations of the disease may also benefit. During steroid treatment hyperabsorption of calcium is reversed (381) and low PTH levels return to normal (383); renal function improves to a varying extent, although in some cases permanent and occasionally progressive renal failure occurs. If the disordered calcium metabolism is the only manifestation of the disease alternative forms of treatment such as a low-calcium diet, sodium phytate, sodium phosphate, or cellulose phosphate may be preferable. Such measures are also best in patients with hypercalciuria alone, since any benefits from corticosteroids may be offset by their hypercalciuric effect. Thiazide diuretics effectively control hypercalciuria in sarcoidosis, although hypercalcemia may be induced in some patients. Chloroquin may correct the abnormal calcium metabolism (393) but it is uncertain whether this is due to reducing the effect of ultraviolet light on the skin or to a beneficial effect on the underlying disease process.

Idiopathic Hyperabsorption Hypercalcemia. Two siblings have been reported with recurrent nephrolithiasis, fluctuating hypercalcemia (2.7 to 3.6 mmol/L) and hypercalciuria (16 to 28 mmol per 24 h), intestinal hyperabsorption of calcium, normal bone turnover determined by calcium kinetics, indirect evidence of parathyroid suppression, and normal parathyroid glands on exploratory neck surgery (394). The metabolic state closely resembled sarcoidosis except that during a standard corticosteroid test there was no change in plasma calcium fractions or in urinary calcium excretion and a fall rather than a rise in fecal calcium excretion. The disorder is probably related to one form of idiopathic hypercalciuria with inadequate suppression of tubular reabsorption of calcium.

Hypercalcemia in children. Hyperparathyroidism and malignant neoplasia, the most common causes of hypercalcemia in adults, are much less common in children (395, 396). Although rare, hyperparathyroidism is usually much more severe than in adults—the plasma calcium exceeds 4 mmol/L in more than half the cases, osteitis fibrosa occurs in 75 percent, and renal stones only in 25 percent. This is because of the relative rarity of Type 2 disease, so that most children have Type 1 tumors. Primary neonatal hyperparathyroidism, due to a genetically distinct form of hereditary hyperplasia (Table 19-24), is uniformly fatal if surgical treatment is delayed. Hypercalcemic secondary hyperparathyroidism in neonates may be due to untreated maternal HP; neonatal hypercalcemia may also result from maternal vitamin D poisoning. Acute leukemia is the major neoplastic cause of hypercalcemia in children. Other adult causes to be considered are vitamin D intoxication, vitamin A intoxication, immobilization, Addison's disease, and familial hypocalciuric hypercalcemia (originally called benign familial hypercalcemia). There are also several causes of hypercalcemia which are peculiar to children.

Idiopathic Infantile Hypercalcemia. This disease usually begins between 3 and 7 months of age with failure to thrive and the fairly rapid onset of anorexia, vomiting, constipation, thirst, polyuria, dehydration, fever, hypotonia, and hyperreflexia (397). Two forms, mild and severe, have been described; the distinction refers to the presence or absence of associated abnormalities and to the prognosis, not to the severity of the hypercalcemia. In the "severe" form the birth weight is low and symptoms may begin soon after birth. There is an abnormal facies, strabismus, mental retardation, abnormal dentition, hypertension, and supravalvular aortic stenosis and other cardiovascular anomalies, collectively known as the Williams' syndrome (398). These features are absent in the "mild" form but all degrees of hypercalcemia can occur in either. Most patients with the Williams' syndrome do not have hypercalcemia even when looked for in the first year of life (398).

The level of plasma calcium may be between 3 and 4.5 mmol/L and may vary considerably from day to day. The plasma phosphate is normal and AP normal or reduced. There may be hypercalcemic nephropathy of varying severity. Plasma cholesterol and vitamin A levels are often raised. In the "severe" form, x-rays show hypertelorism and metaphyseal osteosclerosis. In both forms death may occur in the acute stage, but the plasma calcium eventually falls to normal even without treatment. In the "mild" form recovery is followed by normal health, but in the "severe" form 25 percent die within a few years and the mental retardation, physical stigmata, and cardiovascular anomalies are permanent and may permit retrospective diagnosis in normocalcemic patients with residual hypercalcemic nephropathy.

Whether the two forms represent different diseases or different degrees of severity of the same disease is not known. The metabolic state in both resembles vitamin D intoxication, with increased gastrointestinal absorption of calcium, exaggerated hypercalcemic response to a standard oral calcium load (399), and responsiveness to corticosteroids. Delayed restoration of normocalcemia after intravenous calcium was attributed to calcitonin deficiency (400) but could be a consequence of reduced turnover and hypermineralization of bone. In some cases hypercalcemia may be provoked by small doses of vitamin D, and in others bioassayable levels of vitamin D in blood have been raised (401). In England the incidence of the "mild" form declined substantially a few years after a reduction in the level of vitamin D fortification of dried milk powder used for infant feeding. The offspring of rabbits given vitamin D during pregnancy may have facial, dental, and cardiovascular anomalies similar to those of the human disease (402). Finally, skin fibroblasts from patients in the late normocalcemic stage of the "severe" form developed metachromasia in response to a small dose of vitamin D much more readily than control fibroblasts (403). The data suggest a disorder of vitamin D metabolism, possibly beginning in utero in the "severe" form, but not until late infancy in the "mild" form. In none of the published cases has vitamin D metabolism been studied by modern techniques.

Treatment consists of a low-calcium and vitamin D diet. If the plasma calcium is initially more than 3.5 mmol/L or if hypercalcemia persists, corticosteroids should be given as well.

Hypothyroidism. Children with hypothyroidism (especially cretins) may develop hypercalcemia and nephrocalcinosis. The plasma calcium may be raised initially and fall with treatment or may rise transiently after treatment has begun. Balance studies in affected children have shown both increased absorption and decreased urinary excretion of calcium (404) and as in idiopathic infantile hypercalcemia, various abnormalities in vitamin D metabolism have been postulated. Only one such case has been reported in adults (405); the plasma calcium fell from 3.15 mmol/L to normal after 3 weeks of treatment. Bone turnover is very low in hypothyroidism (338) and the sink capacity of the skeleton (Chap. 8) may be reduced, with increased susceptibility to hypercalcemia in response to increased calcium intake or absorption. This tendency may be augmented by calcitonin deficiency.

Blue-Diaper Syndrome. Hypercalcemia and nephrocalcinosis occurred in two siblings with a familial defect in tryptophane absorption (406). Bacterial degradation of unabsorbed tryptophane to indole metabolites led to indicanuria and blue discoloration of the diapers in infancy. Hypercalcemia was not noted until 1 year of age; it responded to a low-calcium diet and cortisone but could be reproduced by loading with tryptophane. Hypercalcemia also occurred from 8 to 36 h after tryptophane loading in about 50 percent of normal children (407), but not in adults (408). No similar case has been reported and the mechanism remains unknown.

Hypophosphatasia. In this rare disease there is virtual absence of skeletal AP, defective endochondral ossification, and radiographic appearances somewhat resembling rickets. Unexplained hypercalcemia occurs in most cases diagnosed before 6 months of age, the mean maximum level being about 3.5 mmol/L, with considerable fluctuation with time in the same patient (409). Hypercalcemia is less frequent with a later onset of symptoms, and does not occur at all in patients first diagnosed in adult life. The hypercalcemia is made worse if rickets is wrongly diagnosed and vitamin D is given. In some cases corticosteroids have produced apparent improvement in the x-ray appearances and a rapid fall in raised plasma calcium levels to normal.

Miscellaneous causes of hypercalcemia. Several rare causes of hypercalcemia have been too little studied to be placed in one of the preceding categories. Some persist indefinitely without treatment and others are self-limiting over a time scale varying from days to months. Many transient causes are complications of treatment.

Familial Hypocalciuric Hypercalcemia. Several kindreds have been reported in which many family members have hypercalcemia which is mild (2.7 to 3.2 mmol/L), nonprogressive, and asymptomatic (410). It has been detected as early as 12 months and as late as 76 years of age. About 1 patient in 10 gets kidney stones, but otherwise there are no ill effects and creatinine clearance is normal, although severe hypercalcemia has occurred in the neonatal period (217). The plasma phosphate is as low as in hyperparathyroidism, but plasma magnesium is significantly raised (0.85 to 1.2, mean 1.03 mmol/L). Urinary calcium excretion is below normal (mean 2.5 mmol per 24 h) and tubular reabsorption of calcium is more consistently increased than in hyperparathyroidism. Urinary magnesium is normal, but tubular reabsorption of magnesium is increased. The hypercalcemia shows no response to corticosteroids. Plasma iPTH is occasionally slightly raised, but is usually normal. Parathyroid histology may show mild hyperplasia, but subtotal parathyroidectomy does not correct the hypercalcemia so that making the correct diagnosis avoids unnecessary surgery. The disorder has been reported in the pediatric literature as benign familial hypercalcemia (411). The response of the parathyroid glands to changes in plasma calcium, although normal in direction and magnitude, was thought to be set at a higher level than normal with incomplete suppression of PTH. This abnormality could result from increased activity of the outwardly directed cell membrane pump which normally maintains very low intracellular calcium levels (23).

Pheochromocytoma. Hypercalcemia in a patient with pheochromocytoma is most commonly due to concomitant primary hyperparathyroidism (MEN Type 2) (412) but occasionally the plasma calcium may fall to normal a few days after adrenalectomy alone (413). In five reported cases the plasma calcium exceeded 3.3 mmol/L only once, and there were no symptoms of and no evident harmful effects from the hypercalcemia. Plasma phosphate and AP have not been consistently abnormal and urinary calcium has ranged from 6 to 20 mmol per 24 h; hypercalciuria without hypercalcemia has also been noted. Either epinephrine or norepinephrine may be the predominant hormone secreted and it has been suggested that α-adrenergic stimulation decreases tubular reabsorption of calcium, and β-adrenergic stimulation increases net bone resorption (414), possibly by stimulating bone adenylate cyclase. Catecholamines may stimulate PTH secretion (Chap. 8); PTH was raised in only one of the three cases tested, although an exaggerated rise in PTH in response to EDTA infusion was found in a normocalcemic patient (415). The tumor could also secrete other osteolytic substances such as prostaglandins.

Acromegaly. Hypercalcemia in a patient with acromegaly is usually due to concomitant primary hyperparathyroidism as a component of MEN Type 1, but occasionally mild hypercalcemia may be corrected by resection or irradiation of the pituitary tumor (416). More commonly, hypercalciuria without hypercalcemia is present and occasionally renal stones may result. Bone turnover is usually increased in acromegaly, and the presence or absence of hypercalcemia may reflect the relative preponderance of increased net absorption of calcium and decreased tubular reabsorption of calcium. Both changes have been ascribed to increased citrate production (417).

Tuberculosis. Hypercalcemia was found in about 1 percent of patients with tuberculosis needing hospital treatment (418). The plasma calcium was usually normal on admission, but rose 1 to 4 months later to 3 to 4 mmol/L. The plasma creatinine was moderately elevated (1.5 to 3.5 mg/dL) in about half, and AP, plasma phosphate, and tubular reabsorption of phosphate were normal. The hypercalcemia was fully responsive to prednisone and subsided permanently with discontinuation of calcium and vitamin D supplements and successful treatment of the tuberculosis. As in sarcoidosis, both increased sensitivity to vitamin D (418) and involvement of bone by the underlying disease (419) have been suggested as etiologic mechanisms. Hypercalcemia has also been observed in three cases of disseminated coccidioidomycosis, one of whom had bone destruction (420), and occasionally in histoplasmosis.

Berylliosis. Chronic industrial exposure to beryllium compounds may cause a granulomatous pneumonitis sometimes accompanied by enlargement of the liver, spleen, and lymph nodes. There is a radiographic and clinical resemblance to sarcoidosis but with less-marked hilar adenopathy. In a few patients mild transient hypercalcemia has occurred, usually with spontaneous resolution within a few months (421). Hypercalciuria on a low-calcium diet has been reported in about 25 percent of cases and recurrent renal stones in about 6 percent. The pulmonary complications are usually treated with corticosteroids but the effect of this treatment on the disordered calcium metabolism has not been carefully studied. In one case urinary calcium increased significantly during a short course of ACTH (422).

Idiopathic Periostitis. This is a rare and unusual disorder characterized by bone pain, fever, raised sedimentation rate, increased periosteal new bone in the absence of the usual causes, hypercalcemia with normal plasma phosphate and AP, and very high bone turnover. Some of the features resemble vitamin A poisoning, but in the one case reported in detail this was excluded and complete resolution occurred between 2 and 6 months after the onset (423). The hypercalcemia was unaffected by dietary calcium deprivation but in another case it responded to corticosteroids (424).

Metaphyseal Chondrodysplasia. This is a bizarre disorder of enchondral bone formation leading to gross dwarfism and deformity. In the only case diagnosed at Henry Ford Hospital, hypercalcemia (3.4 mmol/L) was found at the age of 5 (425). Fifteen years later mild hypercalcemia persists and has led to nephrolithiasis, nephrocalcinosis, and mild renal failure. All known causes of hypercalcemia have been excluded. Both plasma phosphate and Tm_P/GFR are low and tubular reabsorption of calcium increased, but iPTH is undetectable and NcAMP is normal. The hypercalcemia was unaffected by a standard hydrocortisone test. Most cases of this very rare disease have had hypercalcemia, which has tended to become less severe with time, with gradual improvement in the radiographic appearance of the bones (426).

Adrenocortical Insufficiency. An increase in plasma total calcium occasionally to as high as 4 mmol/L is about half as frequent as hyponatremia and may occur in as many as 25 percent of patients with acute symptomatic Addison's disease (427). In patients with MEDAC syndrome (p. 966) the addition of Addison's disease to previously well-controlled HP may precipitate hypercalcemia without change in the dose of vitamin D (68). In adrenalectomized dogs the increase in total calcium is due to increased concentration of plasma proteins due to volume contraction, increased calcium-binding affinity of plasma proteins due to hyponatremia, and an increase in calcium complexed to citrate and other organic anions, with a normal ionized calcium (428). By contrast, in the adrenalectomized rat, the ionized calcium is raised (429). Unfortunately, ionized calcium has not been reported in patients with Addison's disease, but in most patients the data are consistent with a normal value. Although hypercalcemia has led to investigation and even treatment for hyperparathyroidism, all the symptoms and laboratory data in most cases can be explained by Addison's disease alone. There are rare exceptions with genuine hypercalcemia, such as a 12-year-old child with nephrocalcinosis (430) and a unique case with neurologic symptoms probably due to hypercalcemia and phalangeal subperiosteal erosions; parathyroid exploration was negative and the bones healed after standard treatment of Addison's disease for 2 years (431). The urinary calcium may be normal, or may be increased to as high as 25 mmol per 24 h, but this is consistent with the increase in plasma complexed calcium.

Hypercalcemia and hypercalciuria also occur commonly during withdrawal of corticosteroid therapy, especially after adrenalectomy for Cushing's syndrome. The mechanism is presumably the same as in Addison's disease, although an increase in fecal as well as urinary calcium (432) is less easy to account for.

Rhabdomyolysis with Acute Renal Failure. Hypercalcemia may occur within a few weeks or months of acute renal failure associated with rhabdomyolysis, either traumatic, drug-induced, associated with malignant hyperthermia, or idiopathic (433). Most patients have been in the diuretic phase but hypercalcemia may occur despite persistent oliguria (434). At the onset of renal failure there is profound hyperphosphatemia and hypocalcemia but equally severe changes without muscle trauma are not followed by hypercalcemia, so that excessive parathyroid stimulation is not a factor; iPTH is not raised during the hypercalcemia. Massive muscular calcification occurs during the period of hypocalcemia, and absorption of this calcium may contribute to the hypercalcemia, but mobilization of stored 25-HCC as a result of muscle necrosis is probably more important. Resolution of soft tissue calcification may also contribute to hypercalcemia after renal transplantation (435) and in infants following neonatal subcutaneous fat necrosis; the latter responds rapidly to corticosteroid therapy (436).

Iatrogenic Hypercalcemia. Vitamin D intoxication, the milk-alkali syndrome, and thiazide diuretic effects are described separately. Simultaneous acute hypercalcemia and hypermagnesemia has followed the use of inadequately purified water for hemodialysis (hard-water syndrome) (437). Other mechanisms are overdosage of parathyroid hormone (438), oral administration of ion-exchange resins in the calcium phase, and excess intravenous or oral calcium (364), or of calcium salts in patients on vitamin D. Total parenteral nutrition, bypassing the regulatory influence of the gut, predisposes to a variety of electrolyte disorders and occasionally hypercalcemia may occur (439, 440). The kidney is unable to cope with the prescribed amount of calcium possibly because of phosphate depletion, immobilization, renal failure, or sodium depletion. In infants, phosphate depletion due to phosphate-free parenteral fluids may lead to hypercalcemia even without excess calcium in the solution (441).

Mild hypercalcemia may follow treatment with lithium for manic depressive psychosis (213) but

these patients usually have hyperparathyroidism, either uncovered or induced by the lithium treatment.

Effects of hypercalcemia

Many different effects on cell and organ function can be produced experimentally by hypercalcemia, but only those with clinical relevance will be described. Diseases causing hypercalcemia produce clinical consequences in several different ways. Those which can occur in any such disease are most likely due to hypercalcemia itself, but it is sometimes difficult to distinguish between the effects of hypercalcemia and those of other consequences of PTH excess. The effects depend on the rate of onset, the severity, and the duration of the hypercalcemia.

Soft tissue calcification. This is more commonly due to hyperphosphatemia than to hypercalcemia. Arterial and periarticular calcification are rare in hypercalcemic patients unless there is renal failure, but in three sites calcium deposits occur even if the plasma phosphate is low. The incidence of acute pyrophosphate arthropathy and chondrocalcinosis (366) is increased in hyperparathyroidism but not in other hypercalcemia disorders. Ocular calcification (corneal or conjunctival) occurs in chronic hypercalcemia of any etiology, but is more common in hyperabsorption hypercalcemia than in hyperparathyroidism. Renal calcification is the most important and is discussed separately in the next section.

The typical appearance of corneal calcification (Fig. 19-19a) is a crescent-shaped opacity close to but separated from the limbus at the nasal or temporal pole. With the naked eye it is best seen in relief when illuminated obliquely by reflection from the iris. It is easier to see with a slit lamp, but is often overlooked because it is erroneously described as "band keratopathy." This term refers to a horizontally disposed lesion spreading across the cornea (Fig. 19-19b), usually dystrophic calcification secondary to some disease of the eye. Band keratopathy also occurs in hypercalcemia (442), but is much less common than paralimbal calcification. Corneal calcification is usually asymptomatic and permanent, but conjunctival

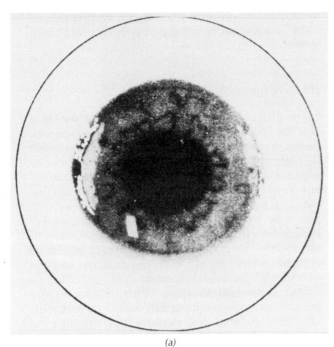

(a)

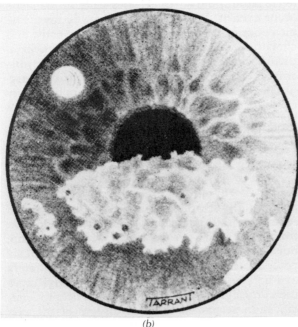

(b)

Figure 19-19. Two types of ocular calcification: a, typical para-limbal calcification of hypercalcemia; b, typical band keratopathy due to dystrophic calcification.

calcification may be associated with red and irritable eyes (366); the symptoms disappear promptly with correction of the hypercalcemia but the conjunctival lesions improve much more slowly. A similar relationship is found in the skin, where a combination of increased calcium deposition and high ionized calcium in the plasma leads to severe pruritus, which is relieved by a fall in plasma calcium before there has been time for any change in skin calcification (366).

Renal effects. Hypercalcemia is one of many causes of tubulointerstitial nephropathy, a group of conditions in which the pathologic process does not primarily involve the glomeruli so that there is a greater impairment of tubular than of glomerular function (443).

In acute experimental hypercalcemia (4 to 5 mmol/L) there is increased transit of calcium across the proximal tubular epithelium. In attempting to maintain a normal intracellular calcium concentration, the mitochondria swell, become overloaded with calcium, and eventually disintegrate, leading to necrosis of the cell (444, 445). Calcification of cellular debris causes obstruction within the tubular lumen, which may give rise to oliguria (339). The GFR is reduced because of vasoconstriction of afferent arterioles and decreased renal blood flow, redistribution of blood away from the cortex toward the medulla (444), and decreased permeability of the glomerular basement membrane (447), but there is a relatively greater impairment of Tm_{PAH}. With less-severe acute hypercalcemia there is polyuria due to impaired concentrating capacity and a smaller depression of GFR.

In chronic hypercalcemic nephropathy there is usually only a moderate reduction of creatinine clearance, impaired concentrating capacity with polyuria and nocturia, mild hypertension, few or no cells and casts in the urine, and only slight proteinuria (339, 448). Pathologic changes are seen around and between rather than within the tubules, and involve the distal tubules and collecting ducts rather than the proximal tubules. There is interstitial fibrosis and infiltration with chronic inflammatory cells, with collapse and atrophy of tubules, and hyalinization and fibrosis of the attached glomeruli. Calcification is located mainly in the interstitial tissue of the medulla and if sufficiently dense produces radiographic nephrocalcinosis of characteristic distribution.

Impaired ability to concentrate the urine is the most characteristic abnormality of function in hypercalcemic nephropathy; maximum urinary osmolality in response to pitressin shows all grades of impairment between normality and persistent isosthenuria, but in contrast to hypokalemic nephropathy, the latter is never seen with a normal GFR (448). The osmotic gradient within the medulla and papillae is reduced because of impaired sodium chloride transport in the ascending limb of the loop of Henle (449) and washout by the increase in medullary blood flow (446). Short-term hypercalcemia following calcium infusion reduces sodium reabsorption in the proximal tubule as well as in the loop; with chloride as the anion most of this additional sodium is reabsorbed in the distal nephron, but with gluconate most of the sodium is excreted in the urine (450). Very rarely, hypercalcemia caused acquired diabetes insipidus with urine which is persistently hypotonic to plasma (404). Hypercalcemia reduces the permeability to water of the collecting duct epithelium and impairs cAMP generation in response to ADH (antidiuretic hormone) (451); these experiments explain why hypotonicity occurs, but not why it is so rare. In some patients severe thirst and polyuria disappear within hours of removing a parathyroid tumor, suggesting that hypercalcemia may have a direct central effect on the thirst mechanism (404).

Many other disorders of tubular function occur in hypercalcemic patients. A decrease in Tm_P/GFR is a nonspecific consequence of the interaction between calcium and NcAMP (p. 966). Generalized aminoaciduria is probably due specifically to PTH excess rather than to hypercalcemia, but both tubular proteinuria and glycosuria are found in other hypercalcemic disorders. Reduction in proximal Tm_{HCO_3}/GFR in hyperparathyroidism is due to a combination of PTH excess and phosphate depletion, but a mild distal type of RTA (renal-tubular acidosis) may occur in any cause of hypercalcemia. This is usually obscured in diseases other than hyperparathyroidism by metabolic alkalosis due to a combination of PTH suppression, direct enhancement by hypercalcemia of hydrogen ion secretion (447), and

mobilization of alkaline bone salts (452). Defective reabsorption of potassium is common and probably contributes to the high prevalence of hypokalemia in hypercalcemic patients. This was found in 17 percent of patients with hyperparathyroidism but in 52 percent of patients with neoplastic hypercalcemia, because of its greater severity (453). Anorexia and vomiting also contribute to hypokalemia in these patients, which may be an additional reason for metabolic alkalosis.

With successful treatment of the hypercalcemia, hypercalcemic nephropathy may show complete recovery, partial recovery, no change, or progressive deterioration culminating in uremia (339). The prognosis depends on the extent of nephrocalcinosis and interstitial fibrosis, which reflects the duration rather than the severity of the hypercalcemia (339, 448, 454). The likelihood of improvement is also less if there is associated obstructive nephropathy due to stones, urinary tract infection, and hypertensive nephrosclerosis (339, 448). Although function may improve substantially, radiographic nephrocalcinosis is usually permanent. Other causes of nephrocalcinosis are listed in Table 19-28. Small concretions within the collecting ducts and minor calyces, more

Table 19-28. Causes of nephrocalcinosis*

Dystrophic (local factors predominant)
  Cortical
    Cortical necrosis
    Glomerulonephritis
  Medullary
    Tuberculosis
    Chronic pyelonephritis
  Papillary
    Analgesic nephropathy
    Sponge kidney
Metastatic (systemic factors predominant)
  Hypercalcemia of any cause
  Distal renal-tubular acidosis
  Oxalosis
  Chronic renal failure

* The distinction between dystrophic and metastatic calcification is not absolute because both local and systemic factors are often important. In sponge kidney, small concretions lie within cysts communicating with the terminal collecting ducts, and so represent nephrolithiasis rather than nephrocalcinosis, but radiographic differentiation may be difficult.

properly referred to as nephrolithiasis, may be difficult to distinguish from nephrocalcinosis.

Gastrointestinal effects. Anorexia and nausea are common in moderate hypercalcemia but the cause is more likely central than local. Constipation has been attributed to loss of smooth muscle tone, but may simply be a consequence of reduced food intake and dehydration. Repeated and intractable vomiting occurs in many patients with severe disequilibrium hypercalcemia, and the resultant depletion of salt and water is an important component of the vicious circle leading to further worsening of the hypercalcemia.

Peptic ulceration in hyperparathyroidism may be a manifestation of the Zollinger-Ellison syndrome in patients with MEN Type 1. Whether ulcers are more common than expected after these cases have been excluded is controversial (455, 456). In some patients ulcer-type dyspepsia may be relieved and ulcers heal more readily after parathyroidectomy. An acute rise in plasma calcium stimulates gastrin secretion (457), but plasma gastrin is not uniformly elevated in hyperparathyroidism. It falls in some but not all patients after surgical treatment, and is not clearly related either to gastric acid secretion or to peptic ulcer or dyspepsia. Neither gastrin levels nor the frequency and significance of dyspepsia has been systematically studied in other causes of hypercalcemia. Patients in hypercalcemic crisis frequently have abdominal pain, but the cause of this is unclear.

Acute pancreatitis is more common than expected by chance in hyperparathyroidism (458) but has also occurred in the hypercalcemia of vitamin D poisoning, metastatic breast cancer, myelomatosis, the hard-water syndrome, total parenteral nutrition, and calcium infusion as a diagnostic test (459). The apparently greater incidence in hyperparathyroidism may simply be due to a larger number of patient days of risk. Chronic pancreatitis with calcification also occurs in hyperparathyroidism but not in other hypercalcemic disorders. In some patients this association may represent hypercalcemic secondary hyperparathyroidism due to pancreatic steatorrhea (460), but more commonly the pancreatitis follows the hyperparathyroidism. Formation of pancreatic duct calculi, activation of trypsinogen by calcium, and occurrence of thromboarteritis due to intravascular coagulation have been suggested as etiologic factors for acute and chronic pancreatitis in hypercalcemic patients.

Cardiovascular effects. Despite the importance of calcium in myocardial function, mild chronic hypercalcemia usually has no detectable effect on the heart or circulation other than hypertension. With moderate to severe hypercalcemia there is shortening of the $Q-T_c$ interval (461), increased susceptibility to digitalis-induced arrhythmias, and occasionally varying degrees of heart block (462). In hypercalcemic crisis there is merging of the S and T waves and a variety of other electrocardiographic abnormalities (463); eventually there is central as well as peripheral circulatory failure and cardiac arrest. Acute hypercalcemia produced by calcium infusion leads to bradycardia and sinus arrhythmia due to vagal stimulation (464).

Hypertension is often found in patients with hypercalcemia. This is partly a result of hypercalcemic nephropathy but can occur when renal function is normal. Acute hypercalcemia, whether induced by calcium infusion or by disease, is usually accompanied by an acute rise in blood pressure; this effect is more evident in patients with impaired renal function (465). Possible mechanisms include a direct or indirect effect of calcium on peripheral resistance, increased cardiac output due to the positive inotropic effect of calcium, and changes in the renin-angiotensin system; the mechanisms in acute and chronic hypercalcemia are probably different (466).

Neurologic and psychiatric effects. Mild hypercalcemia in most cases has no discernible effect on the nervous system, although it may make existing disease worse. By contrast, most patients with severe hypercalcemia have an acute brain syndrome which may be the most obvious component of their illness. In chronic hypercalcemia some observers have detected apathy, lack of energy and spontaneity, anxiety, or depression in as many as 40 percent of patients (180), but it has not been demonstrated either that such symptoms are more common than in control subjects of the same age and sex, or that they are improved by restoring a normal plasma calcium level (467).

However, chronic recurrent headache and less commonly narcolepsy have been relieved by successful parathyroid surgery (180). A few patients have symptoms more likely to have a structural basis such as slowing of gait and movement, impairment of memory or slurred speech, and mild dementia. These symptoms are more often due to hypertensive cerebrovascular disease than to hypercalcemia alone, but the effects of existing cerebral ischemia are made worse by hypercalcemia. Signs of focal neurologic lesions may become manifest only when the plasma calcium is raised. In a personal case a hemiparetic recovered almost completely with resection of a lung cancer causing humoral hypercalcemia, but at autopsy a cerebral metastasis was found in the appropriate location. In alert patients without cerebral symptoms the EEG is invariably normal (468), although in a few cases hypercalcemia has led to convulsive seizures (469). A raised CSF protein without other cause has been reported. Some patients with hyperparathyroidism have weakness, especially of proximal limb girdle muscles, but it is unclear whether the lesion is in the muscle or in the peripheral nerve. There is no evidence in either case that hypercalcemia is responsible, and the matter is discussed in the section on phosphate depletion (p. 1077).

In severe hypercalcemia, especially with a hypercalcemic crisis, there are varying degrees of mental confusion and disorientation progressing to delirium, loss of contact with reality progressing to delusions and hallucinations, and depression of consciousness progressing to stupor and coma (180, 468). Many other neurologic syndromes have been described in individual cases including cerebellar ataxia, vertebrobasilar insufficiency, catatonia, a variety of parietal and frontal lobe syndromes, and convulsive seizures due to intravascular coagulation and microangiopathy (480, 489). The EEG frequently shows slowing of the postcentral rhythm below 8 Hz, and bilateral synchronous delta waves in the frontal leads suggestive of a midline lesion (470). These changes probably result from the combined effect of hypercalcemia, uremia, and acute hypertension and they may not return to normal for several weeks after the hypercalcemia has been corrected.

The EEG changes correlate with the severity of the clinical state, but may lead to an erroneous diagnosis of cerebral metastases in patients with hypercalcemia due to cancer (471).

Treatment of hypercalcemia

Too often, as soon as hypercalcemia is recognized, the regimen listed in some pocket guide to treatment is routinely ordered. In many cases the only effect is to confuse the interpretation of diagnostic tests and expose the patient to unnecessary inconvenience and risk. It must be emphasized that most patients with hypercalcemia need no treatment except for the underlying disease, as already described, and avoidance of inactivity, dietary calcium and vitamin D excess, thiazide diuretics, and fluid deprivation. But if severe or progressive, or causing distressing symptoms, the hypercalcemia itself must be treated in order to buy time to establish a diagnosis, get the patient well enough for parathyroid surgery, or allow other treatment to take effect. The degree of urgency is indicated by the severity of the symptoms, the level of plasma calcium, the state of the circulation, the adequacy of urinary output, the plasma levels of BUN and creatinine, and the ECG. The latter is particularly important in patients receiving or needing digitalis, which induces arrhythmias more readily in the presence of hypercalcemia (472).

Almost all patients needing treatment have disequilibrium hypercalcemia, and it is essential to interrupt the vicious circles described earlier and reverse the increase in net bone resorption. The ECF volume is contracted because of anorexia, vomiting, and polyuria. This worsens the hypercalcemia by limiting the capacity of the kidney to excrete calcium, both by further reducing GFR and by increasing tubular reabsorption of calcium, even in nonparathyroid hypercalcemia with suppression of PTH secretion (473) (Fig. 19-16). Intravenous 0.9% sodium chloride must be given with a judicious balance between the opposing needs for rapid reexpansion of ECF volume and for avoidance of circulatory overload. Hypokalemia is very frequent and should be corrected immediately, because it potentiates the harmful effects of hypercalcemia on the heart, but correction of hypomagnesemia should be postponed until the plasma calcium has begun to fall.

The preceding advice applies to all patients, and sometimes correction of fluid and electrolyte depletion alone may return the plasma calcium to a safe level, but most patients need also a more direct attack on the hypercalcemia. Many investigators have reported results of a single form of treatment applied to a miscellaneous group of patients but few have compared one form of treatment with another, and even fewer have developed criteria for selecting the combination of agents best suited to an individual patient. The physician must be guided by specific indications and contraindications, speed of action, efficacy, predictability, duration of action, liability to rebound, and safety (472) (Table 19-29). The individual agents will be described in relation to their probable mode of action, and an overall plan of management will then be given.

Intravascular sequestration of calcium. If the plasma calcium is 5 mmol/L or higher, particularly if the ECG is grossly abnormal, the patient is in imminent danger of death from cardiac arrest. The drug of choice in this rare situation is intravenous sodium EDTA, but this should not be used with a lesser degree of urgency. EDTA

forms a soluble but physiologically inert complex with calcium, and is the only agent which has an immediate effect of reducing the plasma ionized calcium (473a). Five grams of trisodium EDTA combines stoichiometrically with 14 mmol of calcium, and if given instantaneously would effectively lower the plasma calcium by about 4 mmol/L, but the fall would be about 2 mmol/L if given over 5 min and about 0.5 to 1 mmol/L if given over 2 h (473a). Between 3 and 5 g can be added to 500 mL of intravenous fluid and given over 20 to 60 min, the rate depending on the degree of urgency, with continuous ECG monitoring and frequent measurement of plasma ionized calcium. The calcium-EDTA complex is potentially nephrotoxic, but is normally subjected to tubular secretion and rapidly excreted in the urine. However, the therapeutic response does not depend at all on promotion of urinary calcium excretion, despite numerous statements to this effect. If renal function is poor, excretion is delayed, but the complex can readily be removed by hemodialysis. Removal can be monitored by the difference between total plasma calcium measured by atomic absorption (which includes the EDTA complex) and total plasma calcium measured by SMAC or autoanalyzer (which does not include the complex) (473a). The effect of EDTA does not last more than a few hours, but other measures should

Table 19-29. Comparison of various agents used in the treatment of hypercalcemia

	SPEED[a]	RELIABILITY, %[b]	PERSISTENCE[c]	SAFETY
EDTA	¼–1 h	100	1–2 h	+
Furosemide	4–8 h	75	4–6 h[d]	+++
Intravenous phosphate	4–8 h	90	3–6 days	++
Dialysis	4–8 h	75	4–6 h	+
Calcitonin	6–24 h[e]	75	12–24 h	++++
Mithramycin	12–36 h[e]	95–100	1–2 days	++
Oral phosphate	2–4 days[e]	60–80	3–6 days	++
Prednisone	3–6 days[e]	0–75[f]	4–8 days	+++

[a] Approximate time to useful therapeutic effect with usual dose; maximum effect may occur later.
[b] Approximate proportion of patients showing a worthwhile response.
[c] Approximate time after cessation before plasma calcium starts to rise again in the absence of other treatment.
[d] Much longer if vicious circles limiting renal excretion of calcium are interrupted.
[e] Plasma calcium may continue to fall for several days after the initial hypocalcemic effect.
[f] Depending on the type of tumor; 100 percent in hyperabsorption hypercalcemia.

by then have begun to take effect, and only under exceptional circumstances will a further dose of EDTA be needed. Intravenous sequestration may also be accomplished by intravenous sodium citrate, but this is rapidly metabolized and the effect on ionized calcium is unpredictable.

Increasing the loss of calcium from the body. Increasing fecal excretion of calcium is important only in hyperabsorption hypercalcemia, but increasing renal excretion is valuable in all patients. This will be accomplished by correction of ECF volume contraction, as already described, but intravenous fluids are often given unnecessarily to hypercalcemic patients without sodium depletion. The hypocalcemic effect of this procedure is commonly exaggerated by measuring only uncorrected plasma calcium, which falls because of dilution of plasma proteins even though corrected total calcium or ionized calcium does not change significantly. Sodium sulfate is more potent in promoting urinary calcium excretion than an equimolar amount of sodium chloride because of calcium-sulfate ion pair formation, but a greater hypocalcemic effect has not been convincingly demonstrated (474). Sodium sulfate may be safer because the sulfate ion is nonreabsorbable and cannot be retained in the circulation, so that pulmonary edema is less likely; severe hypernatremia may occur but is not necessarily indicative of hypertonicity in the presence of a multivalent anion (475).

A massive increase in urinary calcium excretion of up to 50 mmol per 24 h can be achieved by giving very high doses of potent nonthiazide diuretics such as furosemide or ethacrynic acid, with prompt and continuous replacement of urinary losses of water and all electrolytes other than calcium. The recommended regimen (476) calls for furosemide 100 to 200 mg to be given every 2 h; even the lower figure represents 30 times the usual therapeutic dose for a 24-h period. In addition to the amount of intravenous fluid and electrolytes needed to correct any existing deficit, 1.5 meq/min of sodium and 0.25 meq/min of potassium must be given, and urine must be collected in consecutive hourly periods. Ideally, replacement should be based on the volume and compo-

sition of each specimen, but in practice the concentrations of sodium, potassium, and magnesium measured on the first specimen can be combined with subsequent measurements of urinary volume alone to calculate the amounts needed for intravenous replacement. Circulatory and renal function should be monitored closely, and the procedure should not be continued for longer than 12 to 24 h. When given without other treatment this regimen produced a mean fall of plasma calcium of 0.8 mmol/L, mostly in the first 4 h, with considerable clinical improvement and a rise in creatinine clearance from 15 to 30 mL/min (476). Although evidently effective, the regimen is only rarely carried out as originally described. Patients with mild to moderate hypercalcemia are frequently given much smaller doses of furosemide (50 to 100 mg per 24 h), but there is no evidence that this is of the slightest benefit.

The rational use of intravenous fluids and diuretics in the treatment of hypercalcemia can be summarized as follows. First, it is of the utmost importance to correct existing deficits in all patients. Second, when this has been accomplished, either maintenance therapy related to the patient's tolerance for oral nourishment should be given without diuretics, or the combined high-dose regimen just outlined should be used. Any compromise between these alternatives merely complicates the patient's management to no useful purpose.

If renal function is too poor to permit a significant increase in urinary calcium excretion (plasma creatinine greater than 5.0 mg/dL), up to 60 mmol of calcium per 24 h can be removed by peritoneal dialysis using low-calcium or calcium-free dialysate and even more by hemodialysis, particularly in the ultrafiltration mode (476). This is especially useful in patients who need dialysis in any case because of oliguric renal failure, and in patients with renal failure which persists or appears after administration of EDTA. The fall in plasma calcium produced by dialysis is usually between 0.5 and 1.0 mmol/L (472), but the effect is inevitably transient. This form of treatment should never be used alone or continued beyond 12 to 24 h unless otherwise indicated. Calcium-free fluid for peritoneal dialysis must be specially prepared in the hospital pharmacy. Provision of dialysate fluid of individually specified composition for hemodialysis is even more difficult in most units, but a recirculating-adsorbent-based portable system (Redy) permits much greater flexibility.

Increasing net transfer of calcium into bone. Since a substantial disparity between total bone resorption and total bone formation is the main precipitating cause of disequilibrium hypercalcemia, a sustained fall in plasma calcium will not be achieved unless this imbalance is overcome.

Phosphate. Administration of phosphate reduces plasma calcium by several means, all imperfectly understood (Chap. 8). The $Ca \times P$ ion product in the bone fluid compartment is raised, with transient acceleration of primary mineralization, secondary mineralization, and bone crystal growth at quiescent bone surfaces. Bone resorption is reduced, probably by a direct effect on existing osteoclasts. A colloidal calcium-phosphate complex is formed within the ECF and is taken up by macrophages in the liver. Finally, calcium phosphate is deposited in many soft tissues, particularly if the plasma phosphate rises above 2 mmol/L or if soft tissue calcification has already been initiated. For the most rapid effect between 25 and 100 mmol of phosphate should be given intravenously over 6 or 8 h (472), using concentrated additive solutions containing 3 mmol/mL of either the sodium or potassium salts. The plasma calcium falls steadily during the infusion by an amount which is proportional both to the initial plasma calcium level and to the dose of phosphate; the mean fall is about 0.3 mmol/L with 25 mmol, 0.6 mmol/L with 50 mmol, 1.0 mmol/L with 75 mmol, and 1.5 mmol/L with 100 mmol (478). Only rarely should the initial dose exceed 50 mmol and the recommended rate of administration should never be exceeded. Intravenous phosphate should rarely be given if the initial plasma phosphate is above 1.5 mmol/L or plasma creatinine above 2.0 mg/dL after adequate rehydration. Plasma phosphate as well as calcium should be measured after 3 to 4 h, and the treatment should usually be terminated if the plasma phosphate rises above 2.0 mmol/L, or if the plasma calcium does not fall significantly. With these guidelines intravenous phosphate is an effective, safe, and predictable treatment for hypercalcemia, with the additional advantage that the plasma calcium may not begin to rise again for several days even if the underlying disease is not controlled (472). It is particularly suitable if the initial plasma phosphate is low because of either PTH excess or the nonspecific phosphaturic effect of hypercalcemia. But if the guidelines are not followed, several disastrous complications are possible. If given too rapidly or in too high a dose, hypocalcemia and severe hypotension may occur (189). If the plasma phosphate remains too high for too long, worsening of soft tissue calcification is inevitable. Either of these complications may lead to irreversible renal failure. Dangerous hyperphosphatemia is especially likely if the GFR remains low despite correction of volume depletion, because of significant structural damage to the kidney. Consequently, phosphate administration should normally be postponed for several hours while the response to 0.9% sodium chloride is observed. Hyperphosphatemia may persist even after phosphate administration is ceased, because an abnormally high $Ca \times P$ ion product is sustained by the calcium-phosphate deposits in the soft tissues, rather than by the bone (Fig. 19-20).

If the patient can tolerate oral nourishment and a rapid response is not required, phosphate can be given orally in doses of 30 to 60 mmol/day in divided doses, but it is unpleasant to take and often causes diarrhea. Although complications are less common than with intravenous phosphate, careful monitoring is still needed of both renal function and plasma phosphate, which should be kept below 1.5 to 1.8 mmol/L. If this precaution is not observed soft tissue calcification may be precipitated by oral as well as intravenous phosphate (479) (Fig. 19-20). Although oral phosphate may control hypercalcemia in some patients for prolonged periods, in others the plasma calcium begins to escape after about a week, and phosphate must then be withdrawn in favor of alternative measures.

Calcitonin. This decreases bone resorption both by reducing the activity of existing osteoclasts and by suppressing the recruitment of new osteoclasts from precursor cells. The acute effect depends more on the former mechanism, so that the hypocalcemic effect is proportional to the number of osteoclasts present and to the prevailing rate of bone resorption, whether normal or pathologic. The most commonly used doses have been in the range of 2 to 8 MRC units per kg body weight every 6 to 12 h, but in contrast to phosphate no consistent relationship between calcitonin dose and response has been established. Mean falls in plasma calcium between 0.4 and 0.6 mmol/L have been obtained with single doses ranging between 45 and 500 MRC units, and total daily doses up to 2500 units reduce plasma calcium by no more than 0.8 to 1 mmol/L (479, 482). A significant fall may occur within 4 h or not for 12 h or longer. The magnitude of the hypocalcemic effect is thus smaller than with phosphate and the response is usually slower and less predictable, occurring only in about 75 percent of cases. Nevertheless, calcitonin has a number of particular advantages. First, there are no known contraindications to its use and no significant adverse effects. Second, in contrast to phosphate, serious hypocalcemia cannot be produced by calcitonin. Third, there is essentially no upper limit to the dose which can be used. More commonly than with phosphate, some patients (particularly those with severe hyperparathyroidism) escape from the hypocalcemic effect of calcitonin after a few days to a week. This is presumably because calcitonin only affects the disequilibrium component of the hypercalcemia, and does not significantly reduce the level of blood-bone equilibration.

Mithramycin. This is a cytotoxic antibiotic originally introduced for the treatment of testicular tumors; its hypocalcemic effect was discovered accidentally. Its precise mode of action at the cellular level has not been determined in hypercalcemic patients, but it reduces both urinary hydroxyproline and kinetically determined bone turnover in Paget's disease and in patients with metastatic bone disease (56). It is given as a single intravenous dose of 25 μg/kg body weight, either as a bolus or as an intravenous infusion over 6 h. The plasma calcium falls by 0.4 to 0.8

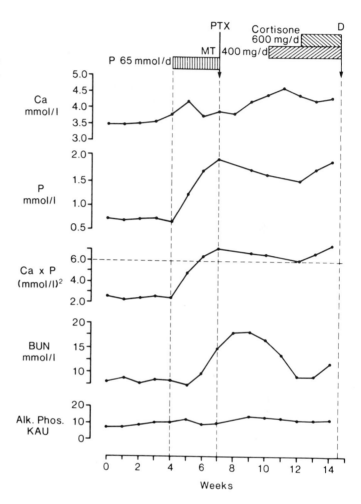

Figure 19-20. Effect of supplemental oral phosphate in a patient with parathyroid carcinoma (339). The plasma calcium was unaffected even though the plasma phosphate rose almost threefold; plasma phosphate remained abnormally high after the phosphate supplement was stopped, even when the BUN had fallen almost to the original level. Parathyroidectomy, MT (methylthiouracil) given in the hope of inducing hypothyroidism, and large doses of cortisone had no effect on the hypercalcemia. The plasma calcium and phosphate levels in the last 6 weeks of life suggest a equilibration with an extraosseous solid phase; the total Ca × P product was above the level (366) empirically related to secondary calcium-phosphate deposition (horizontal dotted line) for the last 8 weeks of life and at autopsy widespread massive soft tissue calcification was present.

mmol/L over 48 to 72 h, and the treatment should not be repeated unless the plasma calcium begins to rise again, which may not be for several more days (483, 484). The response is therefore less rapid than with calcitonin but it is more predictable. The time course is indicative of a slowly developing effect on existing osteoclasts, rather than suppression of osteoclast precursor proliferation. This is consistent with the action of mithramycin to inhibit synthesis of RNA, and therefore presumably protein, but not DNA (485). Mithramycin is potentially very toxic, and when given daily for 10 days as in antitumor treatment, there is a high incidence of bone marrow depression with leukopenia or thrombocytopenia, hepatotoxicity with elevation of liver enzymes and bilirubin, and renal toxicity with proteinuria and increased BUN and creatinine levels (484). In most cases these changes are reversible, and no permanent ill effects have occurred in the treatment of hypercalcemia when the same dose is given no more than every 3 to 4 days. Although in this dosage mithramycin acts on osteoclasts rather than on tumor cells, its use may make it more difficult to evaluate the patient's response to definitive antitumor therapy.

Corticosteroids. These are of major use in hyperabsorption hypercalcemia in which they are very effective in doses such as 20 to 40 mg daily of prednisone or equivalent dose of hydrocortisone, as described earlier. Somewhat larger doses in the range of 40 to 60 mg daily of prednisone have usually been effective in the hypercalcemia of hyperthyroidism, immobilization, idiopathic periostitis, tuberculosis, and Addison's disease. Corticosteroids have been widely used for many years in various forms of neoplastic hypercalcemia but in many cases they are ineffective, partly because the doses used are usually too small, partly because of oral rather than parenteral administration to a patient who is vomiting (285), but mainly because of large differences in responsiveness between one type of tumor and another. Doses in the range of 80 to 120 mg daily of prednisone are effective in about 75 percent of patients with hypercalcemia due to metastatic breast cancer (486) and in about 50 percent of patients with hypercalcemia due to myelomatosis (286), but other types of metastatic disease respond less well and often not at all. Even when effective, the maximum fall in plasma calcium may not occur for 7 to 10 days.

In neoplastic hypercalcemia corticosteroids act mainly by decreasing bone resorption (487), rather than decreasing net intestinal absorption as in hyperabsorption hypercalcemia. Possible mechanisms include suppression of osteoclast precursor proliferation as in many patients with corticosteroid-induced osteoporosis, inhibition of prostaglandin synthesis (488), and a cytotoxic effect on the tumor cells which is occasionally demonstrable as a diminution of lytic bone lesions on serial x-rays. If high-dose prednisone is to be included in the overall therapeutic regimen for a patient with either myelomatosis or metastatic breast cancer, it is sensible to use this agent in the treatment of hypercalcemia, but if corticosteroids are not otherwise indicated, more predictable methods for controlling the hypercalcemia should be sought.

Other agents and long-term treatment. Some patients with neoplastic hypercalcemia respond well to indomethacin, especially those who excrete increased amounts of prostaglandin metabolites in the urine (310), but the results of this test will not be rapidly available to most physicians. Demonstration of indomethacin responsiveness may be of diagnostic value in patients with chronic hypercalcemia, but in severely ill patients the response is too unpredictable to justify the withholding of other treatment.

Similar comments apply to the use of propranolol. This is effective in some patients with thyrotoxic hypercalcemia and ineffective in hyperparathyroidism, but urinary NcAMP is a much quicker and more reliable method of making this distinction. In severe thyrotoxic hypercalcemia propranolol may be a useful adjunct to corticosteroids or phosphate, but should not be relied upon alone.

It is much easier to lower the plasma calcium acutely than to maintain it at a satisfactory level in patients whose underlying disease is unresponsive to treatment, a dilemma which arises frequently in patients with neoplastic hypercalcemia. Daily oral phosphate, calcitonin every 1 to 2 days, or mithramycin every 3 to 4 days are worth a trial, but are rarely effective for more than a few weeks.

Overall plan of management. This is based on three principles (Table 19-30). First, the more sick the patient, the more important are both rapidity and certainty of action, even if the risk is greater. Second, a combination of agents is both safer and more effective than a single agent. Third, agents used together should be complementary with respect to both time course and mode of action. The validity of these principles is difficult to demonstrate rigorously, but they appear reasonable and apply in many other therapeutic situations. Most agents which inhibit bone resorption produce a modest fall in plasma phosphate which would partly offset the rise induced by phosphate treatment. In isolated patients, combinations such as phosphate with calcitonin (489) and calcitonin with prednisone (490) have been more effective than either agent used alone.

Every patient should have fluid and electrolyte deficits promptly corrected and should immediately be given one agent to reduce bone resorption, either calcitonin, mithramycin, or corticosteroids, the choice depending on the individual characteristics already described. If a more rapid effect is needed, either intravenous phosphate, high-dose furosemide, or dialysis should be started

after 2 h, the choice depending on the level of plasma phosphate, the degree of renal failure, and the response to volume expansion. This should be preceded by EDTA begun immediately if no time must be lost because of incipient cardiac arrest. When used in combination, the doses of EDTA and furosemide should be toward the lower end of previously suggested ranges, and the dose of phosphate should be chosen to produce one-third to one-half of the desired fall in plasma calcium. If maintenance treatment beyond the first few days is required, one of the agents which reduces bone resorption, either the same as used initially or another depending on the response, or oral phosphate, or some combination of these should be used. Definitive treatment for the underlying disease must be arranged with little or no delay.

DISORDERS OF URINARY CALCIUM EXCRETION

The urinary excretion of any divalent ion must be viewed from the perspectives of both overall mineral balance and of renal physiology. In terms of the simple model of the ECF developed in Chap. 8, control of the inlet tap is the concern of the former, and control of the outlet tap is the concern of the latter. For both phosphate and magnesium there is no extrarenal mechanism other than load for regulating the plasma level, which is governed primarily by tubular reabsorption. In the steady state a change in tubular reabsorption does not affect urinary excretion, since this is determined entirely by the load derived from net absorption, net bone resorption, and net loss from the soft tissues (Chap. 8). Consequently, there are no primary disorders of urinary excretion of either phosphate or magnesium. By contrast, the extrarenal mechanism for regulating plasma calcium ensures that primary changes in tubular reabsorption lead to steady-state changes in urinary excretion, not in plasma level. The regulation of calcium excretion is therefore much more complex than the regulation of phosphate or magnesium excretion and in different persons either renal (387) or extrarenal (491) factors may be of primary importance.

Table 19-30. Regimen for the treatment of moderate to severe hypercalcemia combining agents with different time course and mode of action

Essential
  Fluid and electrolyte replacement
  Reduction of bone resorption
    Either calcitonin, mithramycin, or corticosteroids
Options for more rapid effect
  Rapid
    Either intravenous phosphate, high-dose furosemide, or dialysis
  Very rapid
    Intravenous EDTA
Maintenance
  Either any agent reducing bone resorption, oral phosphate, or a combination

Mechanisms and causes of hypocalciuria

A fall in urinary calcium may be due to a primary reduction in calcium load and a secondary increase in tubular reabsorption, or a primary decrease in excretion and a secondary reduction in calcium load. There may also be a simultaneous decrease in load and increase in tubular reabsorption. The links between the primary and secondary events probably involve an increase in PTH secretion in the former case and a decrease in PTH secretion in the latter, but whether this is the only signal is not known.

A primary reduction in load may result from decreased net absorption or increased storage in bone or soft tissues. Decreased net absorption may result from decreased dietary intake, decreased intestinal absorption, or CC-metabolite deficiency. In contrast to sodium the maximum fall in urinary calcium excretion occurs on the first day after starting a low-calcium diet or cellulose phosphate (83). The long-term effects of dietary calcium restriction on urine calcium excretion are less well defined and can reflect differences in the efficiency of intestinal absorption and in the response of the bones as well as in renal conservation (492). Increased storage in bone occurs during growth, after reduction in bone turnover for any reason, during the development of osteosclerosis, and in chronic hypercapnia (493). Storage in fetal or infant bone drains calcium from the mother during pregnancy or lactation. Increased storage in soft tissues occurs during growth and during the development of soft tissue calcification. In all these situations there is decreased urinary excretion of calcium (Table 19-31). This is accomplished by an increase in tubular reabsorption with a minimal fall in plasma level if parathyroid function is normal, and by no change in tubular reabsorption and a substantial fall in plasma calcium level if parathyroid function is defective (83). If calcium is removed from the ECF quickly enough because of abrupt massive deposition in bone or soft tissues, both plasma and urinary calcium may fall transiently even if parathyroid function is normal. Similarly, intravenous infusion of a chelating agent such as EDTA decreases the urinary excretion of ionized cal-

Table 19-31. Causes of hypocalciuria classified according to mechanisms*

Primary reduction in load, secondary increase in reabsorption
  Reduced net absorption
    Decreased dietary intake
    Intestinal disease
    CC-metabolite deficiency
  Increased storage in bone
    Growth
    Fall in bone turnover (effect transient)
    Developing osteosclerosis
    Hypercapnia
  Miscellaneous
    Pregnancy
    Lactation
    Developing soft tissue calcification
Primary reduction in excretion, secondary reduction in load
  Fall in GFR, acute or chronic†
  Increased "proximal"‡ reabsorption
    CH_2O refeeding after starvation
    ECF volume contraction—postdiuretic; sodium intake ↓
    Developing edema
  Increased "distal" reabsorption
    Phosphate loading
    Magnesium depletion
    Metabolic alkalosis
    Thiazide diuretics

* Note that hypocalcemia is a cause of acute hypocalciuria, but not of chronic steady-state hypocalciuria.
† Depends on the balance between the decrease in TR_{Ca} and in NA_{Ca}.
‡ "Proximal" includes the proximal convoluted tubule and loop of Henle.

cium, even though total urinary calcium is increased (473a). But it is misleading to think of hypocalcemia as a cause of chronic steady-state hypocalciuria. The hypocalciuria associated with chronic hypocalcemia is due mainly to decreased intestinal calcium absorption resulting from 1,25-DHCC deficiency and to a lesser extent to decreased net bone resorption. This will lead to hypocalciuria whatever the level of plasma calcium, which will be determined by the interplay between the skeletal, hormonal, and renal mechanisms discussed earlier.

A primary reduction in renal excretion of calcium may result from a fall in GFR or an increase in tubular reabsorption. From Eq. (19-3)

(p. 962) it is evident that maintenance of normo-calcemia in the face of a decrease in GFR requires either a proportionate decrease in load or a decrease in tubular reabsorption. When the GFR falls abruptly due to circulatory changes (prerenal azotemia), the plasma calcium tends to rise; this is one of the vicious circles that leads to disequilibrium hypercalcemia as discussed on p. 995. By contrast, when the fall in GFR is associated with structural changes in the kidney, the plasma calcium tends to fall rather than to rise, due to a combination of 1,25-DHCC deficiency and hyperphosphatemia (54). In early chronic renal failure preservation of normocalcemia is achieved both by reduction in net absorption and in tubular reabsorption of calcium, but it is unclear to what extent these should be regarded as compensatory adjustments or as inevitable consequences of the primary renal disease. The reduction in GFR produced by unilateral nephrectomy is compensated entirely by decreased tubular reabsorption with no change in net absorption (494).

An increase in sodium-dependent calcium reabsorption in the proximal tubule and loop of Henle occurs whenever sodium excretion is decreased for a variety of reasons, but hypocalciuria so induced is not sustained. When carbohydrate is ingested after a period of starvation, there is retention of sodium, potassium, calcium, magnesium, and phosphate but this continues only for a few days (495). Calcium and sodium excretion also fall together as a result of ECF volume contraction. For example, after a single dose of any diuretic there is retention of sodium until the loss has been replaced, accompanied by a parallel retention of calcium (496). Transient hypocalciuria is uniformly observed in acute glomerulonephritis (497) and probably results from a combination of modest reduction in GFR, sodium retention, and decreased 1,25-DHCC synthesis. Urinary calcium also falls during the accumulation of edema for any reason. If dietary intake of sodium is reduced, there is a fall in urinary calcium as well as sodium excretion. However, after several weeks body weight is regained and although sodium excretion remains low, calcium excretion returns almost to the previous level (Fig. 19-21) (498). This escape is most likely due to a reduction in

reabsorption at the distal site where regulation of calcium absorption is independent of sodium.

A primary increase in sodium-dependent calcium reabsorption is offset by a compensatory decrease in homeostatic calcium reabsorption, so that whole kidney calcium reabsorption is unchanged. However, the converse is not true; with a primary increase in homeostatic reabsorption, the increase in whole kidney calcium reabsorption can be maintained indefinitely. The role of PTH in calcium conservation in a variety of circumstances has already been mentioned. PTH is also involved in at least the short-term hypocalciuric response to increased phosphate intake as described on p. 1090. Distal reabsorption of calcium is also increased in response to magnesium depletion and metabolic alkalosis (Chap. 8), but it is not known how long the fall in urine calcium excretion can be sustained. The only cause of sustained hypocalciuria due to a primary increase in tubular reabsorption of calcium is the long-term administration of thiazide diuretics.

Thiazide diuretics. Discovery of the hypocalciuric effect of thiazides is usually credited to Lamberg and Kuhlbach (499). They gave hydrochlorothiazide for 2 days to patients with cardiac failure and found postdiuretic hypocalciuria (Fig. 19-22), which occurs after all diuretics, as mentioned earlier. The sustained hypocalciuric effect of thiazides (Fig. 19-22) was first recognized by Lichtwitz and colleagues (500). They found that urinary calcium excretion fell to 40 to 60 percent of control values after 3 to 4 days of administration, remained at this level for as long as the thiazide was given, and could be produced by all thiazide diuretics.

Although the increase in tubular reabsorption of calcium is maintained indefinitely during thiazide administration, a sustained fall in urinary calcium must be accompanied by a corresponding fall in calcium load. There are no radiographic changes either in the bones or soft tissues even after 10 years of continued treatment with a cumulative reduction in urinary calcium of more than 50 percent of total body calcium. Consequently, long-term thiazide diuretic therapy must be accompanied by reduced net intestinal absorption of calcium. This has been shown by balance

SALT INTAKE

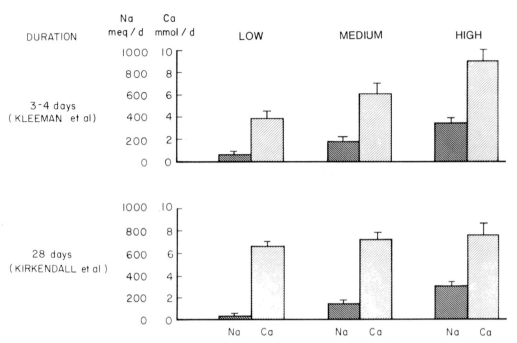

Figure 19-21. Comparison of short-term (3 to 4 days) and long-term (28 days) effects of varying dietary salt intake and consequent variation in urinary sodium excretion (heavy shading) on urinary calcium excretion (light shading). The scales are in proportion to plasma ultrafiltrable concentrations. Note that in the short term urinary calcium shows significant changes in the same direction as urinary sodium, but in the long term comparable changes in urinary sodium are not associated with significant change in urinary calcium. [*Data from C. Kleeman et al. (Chap. 8, Ref. 381) and W. M. Kirkendall, et al. (498).*]

studies performed after more than a few months of treatment (501), although in the first few weeks calcium absorption is temporarily increased. Failure to find decreased absorption uniformly after long-term treatment must be ascribed to limitations of the usual isotopic techniques which measure rapidity rather than completeness of absorption (502, 503). The obvious explanation for compensatory reduction in calcium absorption is that renal retention of calcium leads to a very slight rise in plasma calcium level, reduced PTH secretion, and reduced 1,25-DHCC synthesis. A fall in both PTH (504) and urinary hydroxyproline excretion (504, 505) has been found, but there are no measurements of 1,25-DHCC available. Diminished absorption could be an additional primary effect of the drug, a possibility which has not been tested in any in vitro system.

The acute effect of thiazides in humans is to increase urinary calcium excretion (496) but only by about half of the amount contained in the mobilized ECF, so that relative retention of calcium begins immediately. In the dog, micropuncture studies have shown that thiazides have no effect on calcium reabsorption at their site of action in the cortical diluting segment and early distal convoluted tubule (506). By contrast, with furosemide, ethacrynic acid, and mercurial diuretics (496), the increase in calcium excretion matches the lost ECF much more closely (Chap. 8). At the sites of action of these diuretics calcium and sodium are reabsorbed in about the same proportion as their concentrations in glomerular filtrate, but at the site of action of thiazides, calcium is reabsorbed proportionately less than sodium. With continued administration of any diuretic, urinary sodium excretion soon returns to the pretreatment level determined by dietary intake, because decreased reabsorption due to the diuretic is balanced by increased reabsorption elsewhere in the nephron. With both ethacrynic acid and furosemide this balance of sodium reabsorption at different sites is accompanied by a corresponding balance of calcium reabsorption, so that in the adapted state calcium excretion is unchanged. With thiazides, development of the same balance for sodium is accompanied by calcium retention, because the increase in calcium reabsortion at the site of compensatory increase in sodium reabsorption is greater than the decrease in calcium reabsorption at the site of diuretic action (373). This mechanism is undoubtedly important, but is unlikely to be the whole explanation for the hypocalciuric effect of thiazides for several reasons. First, in contrast to what happens after a few days, when thiazides are ceased after several weeks, urinary sodium excretion falls on the first day but calcium excretion rises (Fig. 19-22). Second, if the homeostatic calcium reabsorption mechanism can prevent long-term hypocalciuria in response to dietary sodium depletion, why does not the same effect occur with thiazide diuretic therapy? Subjects on a low-salt diet regain body weight presumably because they are able to maintain reduced sodium excretion by a mechanism which is not dependent on continued ECF volume contraction. However, this mechanism also operates in patients on long-term diuretics, in whom total body sodium and ECF volume usually return to baseline values after a few months. This suggests that thiazides have an additional effect of stimulating the homeostatic mechanism of calcium reabsorption. The acute renal responses to thiazides and to PTH are similar except for opposite effects on magnesium. The long-term hypocalciuric effect of thiazides in humans is markedly blunted in HP (490, 505, 507) despite a similar increase in sodium excretion. It has been suggested that patients with treated HP are in a state

of volume expansion because of vitamin D-induced sodium retention (373), but there are no data for or against such a possibility. The hypocalciuric effect is not augmented in hyperparathyroidism (508) but it is often enhanced by the temporary secondary hyperparathyroidism induced by cellulose phosphate. In both humans (509) and dog (510) the acute dissociation between sodium and calcium reabsorption is unaffected by the absence of PTH, indicating that the acute and chronic effects occur by different mechanisms. The concept of interaction between thiazide diuretics and PTH (507), although consistent with all available data, remains unexplained. Thiazides inhibit phosphodiesterase in vitro but less so than furosemide (506), do not potentiate the cAMP response to PTH, and have not been shown to affect NcAMP secretion in vivo.

Mechanisms and causes of hypercalciuria

This is due either to a primary increase in calcium load and secondary decreases in PTH secretion and tubular reabsorption, or a primary increase in excretion with secondary increases in PTH secretion and calcium load. There may also be a simultaneous increase in load and decrease in tubular reabsorption.

A primary increase in load may result from an increase either in net absorption or in net bone resorption, or mobilization of soft tissue calcium deposits. Increased net absorption may result from increased dietary intake, CC-metabolite excess, increased sensitivity to CC metabolites as in sarcoidosis, or primary hyperabsorption as discussed later. A rise in urinary calcium may follow within 10 days of increased exposure to sunlight (512), and variation in sun exposure and vitamin D synthesis probably contributes to seasonal fluctuations in urinary calcium excretion (513, 514). The hypercalciuria produced by a pharmacologic dose of vitamin D may persist for many months after its administration is discontinued (515). Net bone resorption is increased in the early phase of accelerated bone turnover for any reason, by metabolic acidosis, by phosphate depletion, during the development of osteoporosis, and from any cause

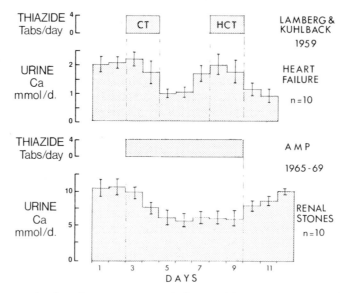

Figure 19-22. Comparison between 2- and 7-day administration of a thiazide diuretic. Upper panel, patients with congestive cardiac failure given a thiazide diuretic for 2 days on two separate occasions (499). Note that maximum fall in urinary calcium occurs on the first or second day, after cessation of the diuretic, during the period of postdiuretic sodium conservation; the same occurs with all types of diuretic. Lower panel, patients with nephrolithiasis and hypercalciuria given a thiazide diuretic for 7 days. Note that urinary calcium falls to a new stable level after 3 days, and after the diuretic is stopped increases progressively during the period of postdiuretic sodium retention, a response which does not occur with any other type of diuretic.

of pathologic bone resorption (Table 19-20). Most of the causes of disequilibrium of hyperabsorption hypercalcemia in their earlier stages or less severe forms may give rise to normocalcemic hypercalciuria (Table 19-19). Soft tissue calcium deposits can often be mobilized when the cause is removed, as when a low calcium intake is given in hyperabsorption hypercalcemia or the hyperphosphatemia of renal failure is corrected by renal transplantation (435). In all these situations there is an increased urinary excretion of calcium (Table 19-32). The rise in plasma calcium needed to accomplish this increase depends on the degree of suppression of PTH and on other factors influencing tubular reabsorption of calcium. It is misleading to think of hypercalcemia as a cause of steady-state hypercalciuria, since the urinary calcium excretion must equal the calcium load from gut or bone, whatever the level of plasma calcium. Similarly, the generally lower urinary calcium excretion of hyperparathyroidism than of

many other hypercalcemic states reflects a difference in load, not a difference in tubular reabsorption, which in this context determines not the size of the load but the level of plasma calcium needed to excrete it.

A primary increase in renal excretion of calcium may result from a rise in GFR or a fall in tubular reabsorption. A transient increase in GFR produced by renal vasodilators such acetylcholine or bradykinin leads to an equally transient increase in excretion of sodium and calcium (516). The possible contribution of a sustained increase in GFR to the increased urinary calcium excretion of hyperthyroidism (345) or increased dietary protein ingestion (512) is not known. A decrease in sodium-dependent calcium reabsorption occurs whenever sodium excretion is increased for a variety of reasons, but the hypercalciuria so induced is not always sustained. If dietary sodium intake is increased there is an increase in calcium as well as sodium excretion for a few days, but after several weeks the increased body weight returns to normal and calcium excretion returns almost to the previous level even though sodium excretion remains high (Fig. 19-21). This escape is most likely due to an increase in reabsorption at the distal site where regulation of calcium is independent of sodium. The natriuretic effect of continuous long-term administration of calcitonin (Chap. 8) (491) is also accompanied by hy-

Table 19-32. Causes of hypercalciuria classified according to mechanisms*

Primary increase in load, secondary decrease in reabsorption
  Increased net absorption
    Increased dietary intake
    CC-metabolite excess
    CC-metabolite hypersensitivity
  Decreased storage in bone
    Increase in bone turnover
    Developing osteoporosis
    Phosphate depletion
    Metabolic acidosis
    Pathologic bone resorption
  Miscellaneous
    Intravenous calcium, including TPN†
    Resolving soft tissue calcification
Primary increase in excretion, secondary increase in load
  Rise in GFR
    Acute—acetylcholine or bradykinin
    Chronic‡—high protein intake; hyperthyroidism
  Decreased "proximal"§ reabsorption
    ECF volume expansion
    Acute diuresis
    Bartter's syndrome
    Catecholamine excess
    Carbohydrate loading
    Calcitonin
    Proximal tubule damage
  Decreased "distal" reabsorption
    Phosphate depletion
    Magnesium excess
    Metabolic acidosis
    Medullary sponge kidney

* Note that hypercalcemia is a cause of acute hypercalciuria but not of chronic steady-state hypercalciuria.
† TPN, total parenteral nutrition.
‡ Depends on the balance between the increase in TR_{Ca} and in NA_{Ca}.
§ "Proximal" includes proximal convoluted tubule and loop of Henle.

percalciuria. This persists after sodium excretion returns to the baseline level because of volume depletion, indicating an effect of calcitonin of decreasing tubular reabsorption of calcium which is sustained for several weeks (491). In primary hyperaldosteronism with sustained ECF volume expansion there may be hypercalciuria, and even when baseline urinary calcium is normal, it shows an exaggerated increase in response to increased salt intake (518). Persistent hypercalciuria also occurs in some cases of Bartter's syndrome in which proximal tubular reabsorption is thought to be defective (519), and in several disorders in which there is structural damage to the proximal tubule such as idiopathic Fanconi syndrome (520), polyarteritis nodosa (521), Wilson's disease (522), and cadmium poisoning (523). However, in the latter two disorders urinary calcium excretion may fall substantially on a low-calcium diet (522, 526) so that the presumption of a primary renal-tubular defect may be incorrect.

Hypercalciuria may also result from a decrease in distal (homeostatic) calcium reabsorption. The role of suppression of PTH in permitting excretion of surplus calcium has already been mentioned. Distal reabsorption of calcium is also decreased in phosphate depletion, magnesium loading, and metabolic acidosis (Chap. 8). The transient increase in calcium excretion induced by carbohydrate ingestion is associated with a decrease in sodium excretion, but the mechanisms and site of action of carbohydrate are unknown. Hypercalciuria is common in medullary sponge kidney but whether this is a consequence or a cause of the structural defect is unclear (525).

In several conditions there is a simultaneous increase in load and decrease in tubular reabsorption. This occurs in metabolic acidosis, for example, in starvation ketosis (526) or ammonium chloride ingestion (527), in which bone resorption is increased, in phosphate depletion where decreased tubular reabsorption of calcium results in part from an unidentified humoral agent (p. 1064), in some cases of both exogenous and endogenous corticosteroid excess, in pheochromocytoma with simultaneous α- and β-adrenergic stimulation (414), and in some cases of acromegaly. If the increase in load and decrease in reabsorption were exactly balanced, there would be no need for an intermediary signal, but in metabolic acidosis the effect on the kidney is usually greater than the effect on bone, and PTH secretion is consequently increased (Chap. 8).

Idiopathic hypercalciuria and nephrolithiasis. A raised urinary calcium excretion is of interest mainly as a factor in the pathogenesis of calcium-containing kidney stones, of which a detailed account is beyond the scope of this chapter. About three-quarters of such stones are composed mostly of calcium oxalate and the remainder mostly of calcium phosphate or apatite. There is general agreement that an increase, either intermittent or continuous, in some ion activity product in the urine, a decrease in the excretion of some inhibitor of crystal formation, and an increase in urinary uric acid concentration are all important factors. But there is disagreement about which activity product is most relevant (528, 529), which inhibitor is most potent (530, 531), how uric acid promotes the precipitation of calcium salts (532), and how the degree of saturation of the urine is best determined (528, 529). The causes of hypercalciuria and stones (Table 19-33) are much fewer than the causes of hypercalciuria, partly because of differences in duration and partly because of many other factors which increase or decrease the risk of stones. There is no conclusive evidence that hypercalciuria has any other harmful effects (532). An acute increase in urinary calcium produced by diet may impair the ability to concentrate or acidify the urine, but these defects occur with the same frequency in chronic stone-formers with or without hypercalciuria (534). Nephrocalcinosis in patients with hypercalciuria is due either to hypercalcemia, to decreased tissue and urinary citrate as in RTA, to pyelonephritis, or to unrecognized medullary sponge kidney. A possible exception is a unique kindred in which nephrocalcinosis and distal RTA were preceded by hypercalciuria (535), but citrate metabolism was not examined.

Most patients with nephrolithiasis and hypercalciuria have none of the known causes (Table 19-33) and the hypercalciuria is consequently described as idiopathic. No precise definition of hypercalciuria can be given. Among normal persons the distribution of urinary calcium excretion is not gaussian but is skewed to the right; the values depend on the prevailing dietary habits and characteristics of intestinal absorption of the population studied and have probably increased in some countries in the last 20 years (536). Many normal persons excrete more than 10 mmol/day of calcium with no ill effects, but in a person forming calcium-containing stones, any calcium at all in the urine may be too much. To the extent that a high urinary calcium concentration is a risk factor for stone formation, the magnitude of risk is unrelated to the prevalence of particular levels of calcium excretion in the general population. The distribution of urinary calcium excretion among calcium stone-formers is similar to the distribution among healthy persons but in most (but not all) series is shifted upward by 1 to 2 mmol per 24 h (537). This suggests operation of the same factor(s) in the entire population of stone-formers, rather than a specific abnormality affecting one subgroup who thereby merit a separate designation. Further evidence for this viewpoint is that stone-formers as a group have an exaggerated increase in calcium excretion after carbohydrate ingestion, whatever their baseline level of calcium excretion (537). The most widely used "definition" of hypercalciuria is that originally proposed by Hodgkinson and Pyrah (539)—excretion on a free diet of more than 7.5 mmol per 24 h in men and more than 6 mmol per 24 h in women. The only purpose of this (or any other) definition is to identify groups of patients who have been investigated or treated in various ways, which will be described. It does not imply that

Table 19-33. Causes of hypercalciuria and nephrolithiasis*

Hyperparathyroidism	Acromegaly
Sarcoidosis	Large dietary calcium excess
Vitamin D excess	Prolonged intravenous calcium (TPN)
Immobilization	RTA
Cushing's syndrome	Medullary sponge kidney

* Note that these are many fewer than the causes of hypercalciuria. Most cases with this combination have none of these causes and are labeled "idiopathic" hypercalciuria.

stone-formers who meet this criterion have a disease that other stone-formers have escaped, or that urinary calcium values below this figure are not concerned in stone pathogenesis and so do not require treatment.

Idiopathic hypercalciuria denotes patients with nephrolithiasis in whom urinary calcium excretion is above the chosen level, but all the other conditions in Table 19-33 have been excluded. Such patients may be classified according to the source of the excess calcium or according to the supposed pathophysiologic mechanism. As already emphasized, all urinary calcium must ultimately be derived either from the diet (net absorption) or from the bone (net resorption). The relative contribution of these two sources can only be determined by measuring the external calcium balance. Several short cuts have been devised to circumvent the tedium and complexity of balance studies (540), but they cannot provide reliable answers to this question, however useful they may be in other ways. In individual patients the source may be entirely diet, entirely bone, or any combination in between, but mean values in groups of patients studied by the balance technique rather uniformly show that about two-thirds of the surplus urinary calcium is derived from net intestinal absorption and about one-third from net bone resorption (533, 541, 542).

But this does not permit the conclusion that idiopathic hypercalciuria is due in most cases to primary hyperabsorption of calcium and in the remainder to primary net bone resorption (536, 540). The data are equally consistent with a primary reduction in tubular reabsorption of calcium (387, 543) with varying degrees of intestinal compensation. Either increased absorption or decreased tubular reabsorption may be at fault in different groups of patients or both mechanisms may operate simultaneously in the same patients (532, 533, 544). More recently, a primary defect in tubular reabsorption of phosphate leading to hypophosphatemia has been proposed (532, 545). Some interrelationships between the various suggested mechanisms are shown in Fig. 19-23. They may represent simply the extremes of the normal distributions, which must apply to the various factors controlling the urinary excretion of calcium, rather than specific metabolic defects (536).

On the basis of combined measurements of TM_P/GFR and iPTH, hypercalciuric stone-formers can be classified into three groups—those with normal Tm_P/GFR and normal to low iPTH, those with low Tm_P/GFR and low iPTH, and those with low Tm_P/GFR and high iPTH (546). We have found a very similar grouping using NcAMP/GFR instead of iPTH (M. Kleerekoper, unpublished data). Unfortunately, tubular reabsorption of phosphate is an unsatisfactory basis for major pathophysiologic subdivision, because of the many nonspecific influences to which it is subject. For example, hypophosphatemia is common among stone-formers whatever their level of urinary calcium excretion (547), so that impaired phosphate reabsorption may be the result of the disease rather than a clue to its etiology. Another problem is that despite its crucial importance to the understanding of pathogenesis, no comparisons have been made of either ionized or corrected total calcium values between different patient groups. With these major reservations, the characteristics (Table 19-34) of the three main categories will now be described, but first an unnoticed paradox must be mentioned. Stone-formers as a group have high plasma levels of 1,25-DHCC (548), although probably for different rea-

Table 19-34. Three types of idiopathic hypercalciuria (552)*

TYPE	1	2	3
Primary defect (postulated)	Ca abs ↑	TR_P↓	TR_{Ca}↓
Fall in U_{Ca} on LCD† (mmol per 24 h)	4	1	1
Fasting Ca/Cr	N	↑	↑
Ca absorption	↑	↑	↑
Plasma 1,25-DHCC	↑	↑	↑
Plasma iPTH	N or ↓	↓	↑‡
NcAMP/GFR	N or ↓	↑	↑
Tm_P/GFR	N	↓	↓
U.THP	N or ↓	↑	↑
Bone mass	N	↓	N
Bone res. surface	N	↑	↑
Bone form. surface	N	↓	↓

* Numbers as in Fig. 19-23.
† LCD, low-calcium diet.
‡ Suppressible with thiazide diuretics or 25-HCC.

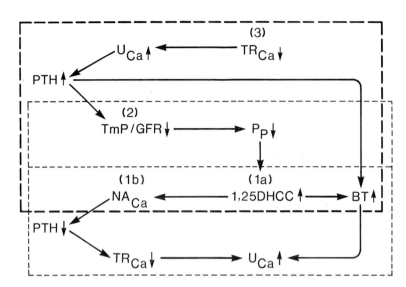

Figure 19-23. Interrelationships between different possible mechanisms for idiopathic hypercalciuria. In absorptive hypercalciuria (Type 1) increased net absorption of calcium (NA$_{Ca}$) causes a reduction in PTH secretion and tubular reabsorption of calcium, and an increase in urinary calcium. This may occur either with (1a) or without (1b) a primary increase in 1,25-DHCC synthesis causing a possible additional increase in BT (bone turnover). In Type 2 the same sequence of events is initiated by a primary reduction in tubular reabsorption of phosphate and consequent hypophosphatemia. In Type 3 a primary reduction of tubular reabsorption of calcium leads to increased urinary calcium and increased PTH secretion and eventually to a secondary increase in net absorption.

sons in different patients. This is currently regarded as the main cause of calcium hyperabsorption, whether primary or secondary. In all forms of idiopathic hypercalciuria, net intestinal absorption and urinary excretion of phosphate are also increased by about 10 to 15 mmol per 24 h (546), consistent with increased vitamin D action. But it has been shown several times that corticosteroids decrease fecal calcium and increase urinary calcium in patients with idiopathic hypercalciuria (532, 541, 542), which is the exact opposite of their effect in the two best-documented instances of vitamin D-dependent hyperabsorption of calcium, namely, sarcoidosis and vitamin D poisoning.

In primary hyperabsorption hypercalciuria, the slope relating changes in urinary calcium excretion to changes in dietary intake, normally between 5 and 10 percent, is increased to 20 percent or more (239, 240). Urinary calcium excretion falls substantially when a low-calcium diet is given for at least 4 days—for example, from 10.2 mmol per 24 h to 5.9 mmol per 24 h on an intake of 10 mmol/day (545) and from 11.2 mmol per 24 h to 4.7 mmol per 24 h on an intake of 3 to 4 mmol/day (547). These mean values are still significantly higher than are found in normal persons subjected to the same degree of dietary restriction, but there is considerable overlap between the two populations. In most patients an overnight fast will lower the urinary Ca/Cr ratio to the normal range, but in some an additional 10 to 12 h of fasting is needed (239). When extra calcium is given the rise in both plasma and urinary calcium is greater than normal (239, 536) but mean fasting plasma calcium is normal or even slightly reduced (550).

Intubation studies have demonstrated an increase in both the active and diffusional components of intestinal calcium transport (551). This results both from increased synthesis of 1,25-DHCC in the absence of either hypophosphatemia or increased PTH secretion, and increased responsiveness of intestinal calcium transport to 1,25-DHCC (550). iPTH and NcAMP may be moderately reduced or may be normal, presumably because of the relative insensitivity of these measurements to small decreases in PTH secretion within the normal range. Plasma phosphate and Tm_P/GFR are normal, probably because any effect of mild PTH deficiency is offset by the direct effect of calcium on phosphate transport. Urinary hydroxyproline excretion, bone turnover, and bone mass are usually normal but have not been studied in detail.

In primary hypophosphatemic hypercalciuria urinary calcium excretion falls only slightly on a low-calcium diet, for example, from 10.40 to 9.35 mmol per 24 h on an intake of 10 mmol/day (546), and the fasting urinary Ca/Cr is abnormally high. Tm_P/GFR and plasma phosphate are low by definition. The mean plasma calcium is usually normal, plasma 1,25-DHCC is increased by about 60 percent (545, 548), iPTH and NcAMP are low, and urinary hydroxyproline excretion is about 50 percent above normal. It is conceivable that this combination of abnormalities could result from primary hyperabsorption and secondary renal tubular damage either from obstruction, infection, or hypercalciuria itself, but there is a much higher incidence of bone disease than in other patients with hypercalcemia. Many have a generalized increase in radiolucency of bone on x-ray (546), radial bone mineral content measured by photon absorptiometry is low (545), AP is significantly raised, and bone biopsies show an increase in surface extent of osteoclasts and decrease in surface extent of osteoblasts, changes which become more normal with phosphate administration (545). It is possible that hypophosphatemia occurring for whatever reason provides the link, which has been suggested several times (552, 553) between some cases of idiopathic osteoporosis and idiopathic hypercalciuria, although there may also be a genetic link between these disorders (554). The reason for either osteoporosis or osteomalacia developing in different groups of patients with reduced tubular reabsorption of phosphate will be discussed in the section on phosphate metabolism.

In primary renal-tubular hypercalciuria, as in hypophosphatemic hypercalciuria, dietary calcium restriction has a minimal effect on urinary calcium excretion and fasting urinary Ca/Cr is raised (240). iPTH, NcAMP/GFR, and urinary hydroxyproline excretion are all increased by about 50 percent and Tm_P/GFR reduced to the same extent as in hypophosphatemic hypercalciuria (0.7 mmol/L), with a correspondingly low plasma phosphate (546, 548, 555). Plasma 1,25-DHCC is increased more than in primary hyperabsorption (547), and iliac bone biopsies show increased surface extent of both osteoclasts and osteoblasts (545). Both iPTH and urinary hydroxyproline excretion fall to normal with either thiazide diuretic or 25-HCC administration (504, 546); plasma phosphate rises significantly but not quite to normal.

All of these observations are consistent with secondary hyperparathyroidism, as is the increased bone turnover determined kinetically in unclassified patients with idiopathic hypercalciuria (541). But paradoxically the mean plasma calcium is often slightly raised (504, 543) rather than slightly reduced as would be expected. Apart from this the data conform to the original concept of Albright (542). The defect in calcium reabsorption is not due to staphylococcal pyelonephritis as he suggested, but its cause is still unknown. Some stone-formers have increased urinary excretion of sodium as well as calcium (555) but this is probably because dietary intake of both is increased. There is no evidence for chronic ECF volume expansion and detailed studies of sodium reabsorption have been normal (556). Tubular reabsorption of calcium during calcium infusion in hypercalciuric patients is normal (536), but this is consistent with impaired reabsorption in the basal state. Although the combination of decreased calcium reabsorption and increased iPTH suggests impaired renal-tubular responsiveness to endogenous PTH, the fall in urinary calcium in response to exogenous PTH is normal (557, 558). A structural defect in the PTH molecule with impaired binding to a calcium transport receptor in the renal tubule would account for many of the observations (558), but the PTH present in these patients appears to have normal biologic activity in every other respect.

The apparent frequency of these three mechanisms varies considerably in different parts of the world. Idiopathic hypercalciuria is predominantly absorptive in Leeds (536) and in Dallas (550) and predominantly hypophosphatemic in Seattle (545) and Milwaukee (547). In both Chicago and Houston thiazide-suppressible hyperparathyroidism is found in the majority of hypercalciuric stone-formers (504, 556) whereas at the Mayo Clinic stone-formers invariably have normal iPTH levels unless they have primary hyperparathyroidism (559). Whether there are genuine differences in epidemiology rather than simply in patient selection and data interpretation is an important but unanswered question.

The combination of secondary hyperparathyroidism and high normal plasma calcium in a hypercalciuric stone-former may be difficult to distinguish from mild primary hyperparathyroidism (253, 254, 560), particularly since some patients with the former condition may progress to autonomous secondary hyperparathyroidism with hypercalcemia (546). Although they are independent consequences of PTH excess, hypercalciuria and hypercalcemia would be expected to vary in the same direction in hyperparathyroidism. But, in fact, urinary calcium excretion is bimodally distributed with respect to plasma calcium, and is higher in patients with the smallest elevation of plasma calcium than in patients with more severe hypercalcemia, despite no difference in GFR (561). Thus, some patients with the mildest hypercalcemia have a substantial increase in load and a relative defect in tubular reabsorption of calcium, just as in idiopathic hypercalciuria. A compensatory increase in calcitonin secretion has been proposed as an explanation (562, 563), but the lack of long-term effects of endogenous calcitonin excess in humans (Chap. 8) makes this unlikely; the hypercalciuria of exogenous calcitonin has only been documented for a few weeks. Some of these patients may have phosphate depletion, which decreases tubular reabsorption of calcium by an unidentified humoral mechanism, and others may coincidentally have two unrelated disorders of calcium metabolism (564). But the most satisfactory explanation is that these patients have primary renal-tubular hypercalciuria with hypercalcemic secondary hyperparathyroidism (546). Parathyroid autonomy is indicated in such patients when a thiazide challenge (see Appendix) produces no change in plasma iPTH or urinary hydroxyproline excretion and a larger rise in plasma calcium than normal (546). As in hypercalcemic secondary hyperparathyroidism from other causes, the parathyroid pathology may be a single (hyperplastic) adenoma rather than hyperplasia of all glands. Hypercalciuria will persist or recur after operation, but the response to thiazide diuretic administration will now be normal (546). Thus, some patients with hypercalciuric nephrolithiasis and equivocal hypercalcemia need phosphate supplements, some need thiazide diuretic treatment alone, some need parathyroid surgery alone, and some need parathyroid surgery followed by thiazide diuretic treatment. Enthusiasm in the search for parathyroid pathology in such patients must be tempered by caution. Many physicians have forgotten that the original formulation of idiopatic hypercalciuria as a clinical entity was based on a completely negative parathyroid exploration in 17 cases (565). The worst therapeutic disaster which can befall a patient forming calcium stones is to be rendered hypoparathyroid by unnecessary and incompetent surgery, leaving a dismal choice between inadequate treatment of hypocalcemia and tetany, and further worsening of hypercalciuria and nephrolithiasis.

It would appear logical to match the treatment of hypercalciuria to its pathogenesis, and give a low-calcium diet and cellulose phosphate to patients with hyperabsorption hypercalciuria, phosphate supplements to patients with defective phosphate reabsorption and hypophosphatemia, and thiazide diuretics to patients with renal hypercalciuria. However, it is much easier to demonstrate a reduction in urinary calcium excretion than a reduction in stone formation. The risk of stone recurrence varies in a complex way with time since the first stone (566), so that depending on when it was begun, the apparent benefits of treatment may be over- or underestimated. Dietary calcium restriction leads to increased urinary oxalate excretion and so is unlikely to be effective unless combined with a low-oxalate diet. The long-term benefit of cellulose phosphate is not yet established (567) and different investigators have found conflicting results with sodium phosphate (560, 568, 569), probably because few patients will tolerate a dose high enough to be effective. The simplest and best-documented approach is to give thiazide diuretics to all normocalcemic calcium stone-formers, whatever the level of urinary calcium and whatever the supposed cause of hypercalciuria if present, and to give allopurinol as well to patients whose plasma and/or urinary uric acid levels are high, either initially or as a result of thiazide therapy (501, 570). In a few patients (less than 5 percent) the development of persistent hypercalcemia will indicate underlying hyperparathyroidism, either primary or secondary.

DISORDERS OF INORGANIC PHOSPHATE METABOLISM

Abnormalities of calcium and phosphate frequently go together, but hypophosphatemia and phosphate depletion may have wide-ranging effects on organic phosphate metabolism which are quite unrelated to calcium.

THE CLINICAL PHYSIOLOGY OF INORGANIC PHOSPHATE

Background information is given in Chap. 8.

The regulation of total body phosphate

Total body phosphate can fall substantially without causing any clinical effects of phosphate depletion. Conversely, serious phosphate depletion may occur even if total body phosphate is normal or only trivially reduced. A similar paradox exists for magnesium and much of the following analysis applies also to this ion. To resolve the paradox it is useful to consider the distinction between capacity, concentration, and content which was originally drawn for potassium by Scribner and Burnell (572). We may paraphrase their formulation and define the phosphate capacity as the sum total of all cations and other chemical groups outside the ECF which can associate in some way with phosphate. Phosphate depletion can then be defined on the basis of the content:capacity ratio rather than the absolute content. It is evident from the distribution of phosphate that substantial net loss from the body can only be met from bone or from within cells. The phosphate capacity of bone depends on the amount of mineralizable bone matrix. If the degree of mineralization and hence the phosphate "concentration" in bone is normal, loss of bone will be accompanied by loss of bone phosphate in the same proportion with a corresponding reduction in total body phosphate, but this will produce no clinical effects apart from those due to the bone loss itself. If the degree of mineralization is subnormal as in osteomalacia there is depletion of phosphate as well as of calcium. The regulation of bone mass was considered earlier and osteomalacia will be discussed later. Phosphate capacity will also increase if connective tissue protein matrices become mineralizable for any reason, as described later.

The phosphate capacity of the soft tissues depends upon the number of cells and on the amounts of intracellular protein, potassium, and water. For each tissue there are characteristic ratios of the major ions to cell protein and to each other (Table 19-35) which collectively determine its content:capacity ratio. For the body as a whole this ratio depends largely on muscle, which contains 75 to 80 percent of the total content of nitrogen, potassium, phosphate, and magnesium of the active cell mass (Chap. 8) (573). The acid-insoluble fraction of total intracellular phosphate includes phosphoglycerides and sphingolipids associated with the membranes of the cell and its organelles, and nucleic acids and nucleoproteins associated with the nucleus (574). In addition, phosphate is combined with, bound to, or otherwise sequestered by cell protein in some chemically undefined manner which ensures that gains or losses of protein by the cell are accompanied

Table 19-35. Ratios of intracellular ions to nitrogen and to each other in representative soft tissues

	K/N, mmol/g	P/N, mmol/g	P/K, mmol/mmol	Mg/N, mmol/g	Mg/K, mmol/mmol	Mg/P, mmol/mmol
Muscle	2.9	1.9	0.64	0.27	0.09	0.14
Liver	2.7	3.1	1.15	0.27	0.10	0.09
Brain	5.0	6.4	1.28	0.34	0.07	0.05
Lung	2.0	1.9	0.95	0.09	0.04	0.05
Red cells	2.7	0.5	0.19	0.11	0.04	0.20
Total ACM*	2.9	2.0	0.69	0.26	0.09	0.13

* ACM, active cell mass (573).

by corresponding gains or losses of phosphate. This relationship is expressed by the P/N ratio (Table 19-35), which varies over more than a 12-fold range between brain (6.4 mmol/g) and red cells (0.5 mmol/g). The acid-soluble fraction of total intracellular phosphate comprises nucleotides, glycolytic intermediates, phosphocreatine, and other miscellaneous organic phosphate compounds and a small amount of free P_i (inorganic phosphate). Together these form an important part of the total solute and total anion of cell water. The maintenance of electric neutrality ensures that gains or losses of potassium, the major intracellular cation, are accompanied by corresponding gains or losses of phosphate. This relationship is expressed by the P/K molar ratio, which varies over more than a sixfold range between brain (1.28) and red cells (0.19), much more than the K/N ratio (Table 19-35).

The regulation of plasma inorganic phosphate

Shifts between extra- and intracellular compartments. In a healthy person in nutritional equilibrium there can be no sustained net change in total IC (intracellular) phosphate, but several physiologic processes cause transient gains or losses by the cells (Tables 19-36 and 19-37); converse changes in plasma P_i levels occur which usually do not exceed 0.2 mmol/L (575). Since IC and EC (extracellular) P_i are in equilibrium, such shifts normally involve a change in IC acid-soluble organic phosphate, representing a transient change in soft tissue phosphate capacity. Inor-

ganic phosphate can enter the organic phosphate pool in only three ways. First, during glycolysis (Fig. 19-24) glyceraldehyde 3-phosphate combines with cytoplasmic P_i to form 1,3-diphosphoglycerate, which reacts with ADP (adenosine diphosphate) to form ATP (adenosine triphosphate) and 3-phosphoglycerate. In the red cell this reaction may take place at the cell membrane, the P_i coming directly from the ECF. However, P_i usually enters the cell as such, rather than by participating in a phosphorylation reaction. Second, during oxidative phosphorylation mitochondrial P_i is used directly to form ATP from ADP. Finally, during glycogenolysis P_i reacts directly with glycogen to form glucose 1-phosphate, which is

Table 19-36. Mechanisms of phosphate sequestration within cells

Short term
  Increase in glucose 6-phosphate
    Glycogenolysis (in muscle)
    Glucose uptake
  Increase in other phosphorylated glycolytic intermediates
    Stimulation of glycolysis
    Inhibition of glycolysis beyond 1,3-diphosphoglycerate
  Increase in ATP
    Stimulation of glycolysis
    Stimulation of oxidative phosphorylation
  Increase in P_i
    Hyperphosphatemia
    Glucose uptake
Long term
  Restoration of cell water and electrolytes
  Resynthesis of cell protein
  Resynthesis of glycogen
  Resynthesis of phosphocreatine (in muscle)

Table 19-37. Agents which produce a transient fall in plasma phosphate due to sequestration within cells by one or more of the mechanisms listed in Table 19-36

Epinephrine	Glucose	Lactate
Insulin	Fructose	Respiratory alkalosis
Glucagon	2-Deoxyglucose	Metabolic alkalosis

rapidly converted to glucose 6-phosphate. All other phosphorylations depend on the conversion of ATP to ADP with no net change in P_i, but regeneration of ATP by glycolysis or respiration may require a net influx of P_i into the cell. The normal content of glucose 6-phosphate and other phosphorylated intermediates (Fig. 19-24) in muscle is about 2.9 mmol/kg (576) for a total body content of about 90 mmol. If this were increased by only 5 percent, it would deplete the ECF by 4.5 mmol and reduce the plasma level by about 0.3 mmol/L, or a fall of 25 percent.

Glucose administration lowers plasma P_i within 1 to 2 h, usually by 0.05 to 0.15 mmol/L. This is mainly because hyperglycemia and consequent increase in insulin secretion increase muscle glucose 6-phosphate content (577), but red cell P_i rises initially (578), indicating that influx of P_i is an immediate consequence of hyperglycemia and is not mediated by glucose phosphorylation, which would lower IC P_i. The hypophosphatemic effect of the same amount of glucose is less when given by mouth than by vein because a higher proportion is taken up by the liver and converted to glycogen, so that a lesser proportion is available for phosphorylation in muscle. Hyperglycemia, however induced, also decreases the tubular reabsorption of phosphate for reasons described in Chap. 8, but urinary phosphate increases by too small an amount to contribute significantly to the fall in plasma P_i. The response to glucose is probably the major reason for the fall in plasma P_i which normally occurs after eating (579). There are cyclic changes in the glycogen content of both liver and muscle in relation to feeding and to short-term fasting (580) but these have only a small effect on plasma P_i.

A final cause of phosphate shifts between the EC and IC compartments is respiratory, and to a

lesser extent, metabolic alkalosis. Voluntary hyperventilation for only 3 to 5 min with a fall in P_{CO_2} to about 15 mmHg lowers plasma P_i by about 0.2 mmol/L. Compared with other causes of IC migration of phosphate, the hypophosphatemia of respiratory alkalosis lasts for much longer. When the same P_{CO_2} is maintained, the plasma P_i continues to fall to about 0.8 mmol below the baseline and stays at this level for up to 5 h, but returns to normal within an hour when normal ventilation is resumed (581). During such severe hypophosphatemia phosphate virtually disappears from the urine. Hyperventilation with a fall in P_{CO_2} has no effect on plasma P_i.

The relative importance of renal and extrarenal factors. The kidney plays no significant part in the acute and transient changes in plasma P_i just described, but it is the major determinant of the steady-state level. In accordance with the simple model described in Chap. 8 the plasma P_i concentration in the steady state automatically adjusts to ensure that the output of phosphate by the kidney balances exactly the net input of phosphate into the ECF from all sources. There is no extrarenal mechanism for regulating plasma P_i except this input, which constitutes the load of phosphate requiring excretion. The steady-state output must be equal to input (or load), so that the relative contributions of load, GFR, and tubular reabsorption to the plasma P_i level are defined by the relationship:

$$P_P \cdot GFR \text{ (filtered load)} = U_P V + TR_P \quad (19\text{-}6)$$

Dividing through by GFR

$$P_P = \frac{U_P V}{GFR} + \frac{TR_P}{GFR} \quad (19\text{-}6a)$$

where TR_P/GFR will usually be close to or equal to TM_P/GFR.

In the early-morning fasting state, with normal renal function, $U_P V/GFR$ is normally in the range of 0.05 to 0.2 mmol/L and tubular reabsorption accounts for about 90 percent of the plasma level (Chap. 8) (582). Since $U_{Ca}V/GFR$ in the early-morning fasting state is normally in the range of 0.01 to 0.04 mmol/L, and the molar Ca/P ratio in bone is 1.6, the contribution of net bone resorp-

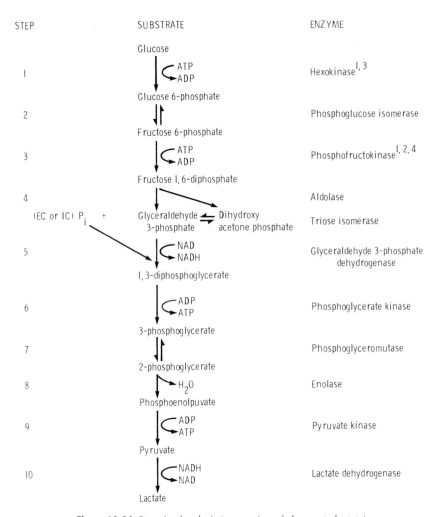

Figure 19-24. Steps in glycolysis (conversion of glucose to lactate). Note entry of P_i (inorganic phosphate) at step 5 (conversion of glyceraldehyde 3-phosphate to 1,3-diphosphoglycerate). In the red cell this comes directly from the EC (extracellular) pool; in other tissues it comes from the IC (intracellular) pool. 1, Stimulated by increase in P_i; 2, stimulated by decrease in [H$^+$]; 3, stimulated by increase in ATP; 4, inhibited by increase in ATP.

tion to fasting $U_P V/GFR$ can be no more than 0.006 to 0.025 mmol/L, which is less than 15 percent of the total (582). The remainder must be derived from the exchangeable pool in interstitial fluid, soft tissue, and bone, which during the course of an 8-h overnight fast becomes depleted to the extent of about 6 mmol.

In the nonfasting state, $U_P V/GFR$ is normally in the range of 0.1 to 0.4 mmol/L and tubular reabsorption accounts for about 80 percent of the plasma level. In an adult in zero external balance, despite the transient shifts between the IC and EC compartments just described, there can be no net contribution from bone or soft tissues, and $U_P V/$

GFR is derived entirely from NA (net absorption) and so from the diet. During the course of a 16-h period of food intake, net absorption of 30 mmol would provide about 24 mmol for urinary excretion and about 6 mmol to replenish the exchangeable pool in preparation for the next period of fasting and continued urinary excretion. In various disease states net bone resorption, net loss from within cells, and dissolution of soft tissue calcific deposits may contribute to the ECF input and hence to U_PV/GFR.

It is evident that with normal renal function TM_P/GFR is the dominant factor controlling the plasma P_i level. Large changes in load produce only small changes in plasma level and even these are partly offset by homeostatic adjustments in Tm_P/GFR in the opposite direction to the change in NA_P. Consequently, changes in plasma P_i in disease are mainly due to changes in Tm_P/GFR. There are two important exceptions to this generalization. The first concerns the effect of diminishing renal function. It is clear from Eq. (19-6a) that as GFR declines, the contribution of U_PV/GFR to plasma P_i must increase. Consequently, the lower the GFR, the greater is the effect on plasma P_i of a change in dietary phosphate intake or NA_P, or a change in net loss of phosphate from soft tissue or bone. The combination of a moderate reduction in GFR and a moderate increase in load may lead to severe hyperphosphatemia. The same principle operates in infants, in whom NA_P is high in relation to GFR. The second exception is that the kidney can only regulate plasma P_i if the net input of phosphate to the ECF is positive. If for any reason there is net extrarenal withdrawal of phosphate from the ECF into gut, soft tissue, or bone, the plasma P_i will progressively decline even though tubular reabsorption of phosphate is increased.

Three principles emerge from this discussion. First, the plasma P_i is normally regulated by Tm_P/GFR; changes in tubular reabsorption produce acute changes in urinary excretion, but the long-term effect is a change in plasma level and not a change in urinary excretion. Second, the contribution of load (U_PV/GFR) to plasma level is small with normal renal function, increases as GFR declines, and may become dominant when GFR falls

below 25 mL/min. Third, if net input of phosphate is negative, plasma P_i can no longer be regulated by the kidney and will continue to fall, either indefinitely or until a new equilibrium is attained.

The normal plasma phosphate in relation to age, sex, and other variables. The changes with age are depicted in Fig. 19-25. The accelerated pubertal fall occurs 1 to 2 years earlier in girls than in boys, but parallels the decline in total and osseous AP which begins in both sexes toward the

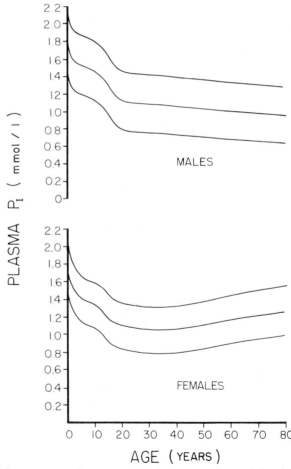

Figure 19-25. Changes in P_i with age in males and females [*Composite interpretation of data from several sources (42, 45, 367).*]

end of the adolescent growth spurt (42) (Fig. 19-26). It is due to a combination of fall in growth hormone secretion (582) and increased secretion of gonadal hormones (367) and PTH (45). The postmenopausal rise in women is due to estrogen deficiency. Tm_P/GFR is inversely related to plasma estradiol (585) and both the rise in Tm_P/GFR (584) and in plasma P_i (585) can be reversed by estrogen replacement. Whether this effect of estrogens on the renal tubule is direct or indirect is not known.

It appears from Fig. 19-25 that plasma P_i is not regulated as precisely as plasma Ca, with a CV of about 15 to 20 percent compared to 3 to 5 percent for calcium. This difference is biologic, not analytic, but it results mainly from a much greater variation *between* individuals for phosphate than for calcium (367). With serial measurements in normal subjects, the mean individual CV is about 6 to 8 percent (13), indicating homeostatic control which is about half as precise for P_i as for calcium. In contrast, some individuals consistently have values 50 to 60 percent higher than others with no overlap between them (367). These differences must reflect individual differences in

Tm_P/GFR, but it is not known whether this is due to genetic differences in transport capacity or differences in the levels of the many hormonal and other regulators of Tm_P/GFR.

SEVERE HYPOPHOSPHATEMIA AND PHOSPHATE DEPLETION

In accordance with the previous analysis, phosphate depletion is defined as a reduction in the content:capacity ratio, the P/N and P/K ratios of the active cell mass. This can arise either because of a primary loss of IC phosphate with a secondary negative external balance, or a primary negative balance with secondary loss of IC phosphate. It is convenient to classify hypophosphatemia on the basis of both severity and acuteness, because both the causes and effects may be different. Mild chronic hypophosphatemia (greater than or equal to 0.5 mmol/L) is usually due to a reduction in Tm_P/GFR, and is unaccompanied by phosphate depletion and is asymptomatic. Severe chronic hypophosphatemia (less than 0.5 mmol/L) is usually due to a primary negative balance, is

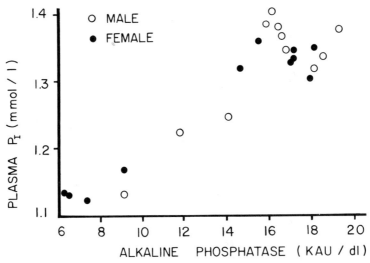

Figure 19-26. Relationship between plasma AP in KAU (King-Armstrong Units) and P_i during adolescence (42).

accompanied by phosphate depletion, and may cause muscle weakness and osteomalacia. However, there is only approximate correspondence between plasma P_i levels and the presence or absence of phosphate depletion or of symptoms. Acute hypophosphatemia is usually due to influx into cells, and if severe (less than 0.3 mmol/L) is usually preceded either by a reduction in IC phosphate or by chronic hypophosphatemia, and may cause a variety of severe disturbances in cell function.

Table 19-38. Causes of cell catabolism with loss of IC phosphate and magnesium either to the same degree as the loss of cell protein (proportional) or in excess of the loss of cell protein (disproportional)

PROPORTIONAL	DISPROPORTIONAL
Simple starvation	Protein-calorie malnutrition
Hyperthyroidism	Diabetic ketoacidosis
Infection	Alcoholic ketoacidosis
Trauma	Potassium depletion
Surgical operations	Hyperparathyroidism

Mechanisms and causes of phosphate depletion

Cell breakdown, proportional and disproportional. Simple starvation leads to catabolism of cell substance with loss of water, nitrogen, potassium, phosphate, and magnesium in the same proportion as in the tissues (Table 19-35). This process is shown diagrammatically in Fig. 19-27. The products of cell catabolism enter the ECF and are ultimately excreted in the urine. After the first month daily urinary losses stabilize at about 15 mmol of K, 10 mmol of P_i, and 1 mmol of Mg. By definition, this does not constitute phosphate depletion but it may set the stage for severe hypophosphatemia. Provision of carbohydrate after a prolonged fast leads to a prompt reduction in the excretion of K, P_i, and Mg (586, 587) as well as of Na and Ca. This is due partly to diversion into cells and partly to reduction of gluconeogenesis in the kidney and consequent greater availability of metabolic energy for other purposes (587). Complete simple starvation is uncommon, but a similar, albeit less severe, catabolic response occurs with partial starvation, hyperthyroidism, infection and other causes of fever, and trauma (Table 19-38). The combination of starvation and trauma underlies much of the normal catabolic response to surgical operations (588).

In several situations (Table 19-38) there is disproportionate cell breakdown with a relatively greater loss of K and P than of N. This occurs in states of chronic severe malnutrition in children such as kwashiorkor, as is shown by a fall in the K/N, and P/N ratios in muscle biopsies (590), and by a relatively greater whole body retention of K and P than of N during recovery (591). The deficit relative to N is greater for P than for K whereas in diabetic ketoacidosis and in other forms of severe metabolic acidosis associated with chronic alcoholism or ammonium chloride ingestion, the deficit relative to N is less for P than for K (591, 592). Nevertheless, increased net loss from cells and reduced GFR may combine to significantly raise the plasma P_i level in diabetic ketoacidosis. In alcoholic ketoacidosis the initial plasma P_i is often low because of the many other factors promoting phosphate depletion in these patients. In both experimental and clinical potassium depletion there is loss of about 10 percent of the N and about 20 percent of the P which would be proportional to the potassium loss (592), which cannot be repaired until the potassium depletion is corrected. Finally, in hyperparathyroidism the catabolic effect of excess PTH mentioned earlier is accompanied by relatively greater loss of P than of N from the soft tissues.

Primary negative phosphate balance—chronic hypophosphatemia. This may be due either to negative net intestinal absorption, enforced removal of P by dialysis (594), or reduction of Tm_P/GFR below the effective IC concentration. Primary negative balance leads to withdrawal of phosphate from within cells and (with calcium) from bone. These changes are thought to be mediated in some way by a fall in plasma P_i level. The effect of hypophosphatemia on bone is described later; a simple model of withdrawal of P_i from within cells is depicted in Fig. 19-27. EC and IC P_i are in equilibrium, but a modest fall in plasma P_i to 0.6 to 0.8 mmol/L (due, for example, to a low Tm_P/GFR) with or without a corresponding fall in free IC P_i does not lead to a loss of IC bound phosphate because a gradient can be maintained either between the EC and free IC compartments, or between the free IC and bound IC compartments, depending on the precise mechanism of phosphate sequestration. If for any reason the plasma level falls below 0.4 to 0.5

mmol/L, the maximum sustainable gradient is exceeded, P_i leaks out of the cells, and the organic-acid-soluble phosphate level declines. This is the likely explanation for the occurrence of phosphate depletion when plasma P_i is reduced to less than 0.5 mmol/L by a very low Tm_P/GFR, as in a few patients with primary hyperparathyroidism and in many patients with adult-onset non-

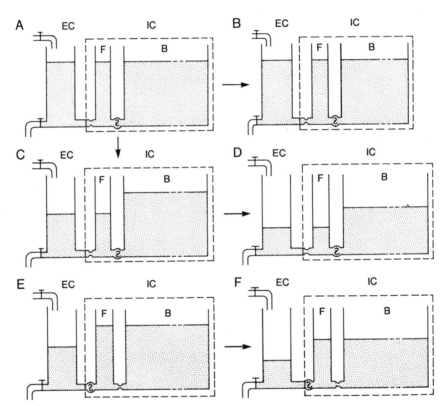

Figure 19-27. Model for relationship between EC and IC phosphate. IC phosphate comprises a free ionic component (F) which is in equilibrium with the ECF, and a much larger bound component (B). *A*, Normal state. In *B*, the capacity of B is reduced with a corresponding reduction in content, and no change in content:capacity ratio or concentration. While loss from B was occurring, the concentration in F and EC would be slightly increased; the diagram shows the steady state after these have returned to their previous level. *C* depicts the effect of a moderate reduction of concentration in EC; the concentration in F falls to the same extent but the mechanism of IC sequestration establishes

and maintains the gradient between the free and bound compartments. In *D* a further fall in concentration in EC has reduced the concentration in F to below the maximal substainable gradient, so that some phosphate is withdrawn from the bound compartment, a state of true IC depletion. *E* depicts an alternative method of restraining IC phosphate with the development of a gradient between EC and free IC compartments at the cell membrane. *F* shows the effect of a further fall in EC concentration below the maximum sustainable gradient, with corresponding removal of bound phosphate. It is likely that both of these mechanisms operate in different tissues.

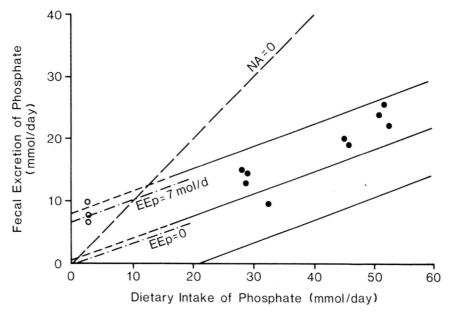

Figure 19-28. Relationship between fecal excretion of phosphate and dietary intake of phosphate; NA = O indicates that the two quantities are equal. The parallel solid lines indicate mean and 95 percent confidence limits of balance studies assembled by Stanbury (128). Dotted continuations are extrapolations below the lowest dietary intake at which measurements were made. The lower pair of dotted lines indicates fecal excretion = one-third of dietary intake + endogenous excretion of phosphate (EE$_P$) from 0 to 7 mmol/day. Closed circles, individual values obtained during balance studies in nine patients with idiopathic steatorrhea (129); open circles, mean values obtained during balance studies in normal subjects on very low dietary intake (596).

familial hypophosphatemia. This model fails to take into account the remarkable sex difference in the response to experimental P depletion of 2 to 3 weeks' duration (595). In men there is loss of minerals from soft tissues rather than from bone and plasma P$_i$ is maintained, whereas in women there is a loss of minerals from bone rather than from soft tissues and plasma P$_i$ falls. This is unlikely to be due simply to the difference in muscle mass.

For fecal phosphate excretion to exceed dietary intake (negative net absorption) either intake must be reduced, absorption impaired, or endogenous secretion increased. In contrast to calcium, adaptation of human subjects to a low intake of phosphate has been little studied. A model for the relationship between fecal and dietary phosphate is shown in Fig. 19-28; it is assumed that two-thirds of dietary intake is absorbed and that endogenous

excretion (unabsorbed endogenous secretion) varies from 0 to 7 mmol/day with a mean of 3.5 mmol/day. According to the model, the minimum intake required for an average person to avoid negative absorption varies from 0 to 10.5 mmol/day, with a mean of 5.25 mmol/day, a value of about 10 percent of the mean normal intake; this conclusion agrees with published balance studies (128). Consequently, reduced dietary intake can cause negative phosphate absorption only if associated with protracted vomiting or nasogastric suction (596) or as a component of generalized malnutrition.

Intestinal malabsorption of phosphate usually accompanies malabsorption of calcium and is frequently cited as a cause of hypophosphatemia (87), but fecal phosphate only rarely exceeds intake as a result of malabsorption alone. In gluten enteropathy, fecal phosphate is about 5 to 7 mmol higher than normal in relation to the intake (129) (Fig. 19-28) but net absorption exceeded 12 mmol/day in every case even during gluten-induced relapse with fecal fat excretion of more than 25 g/day. With normal renal function the observed degree of phosphate malabsorption would decrease plasma P_i by only 0.05 mmol/L. The passage of copious fluid stools in patients with ulcerative colitis, Crohn's disease, or recent intestinal-shunt surgery is probably associated with more severe malabsorption of phosphate, as of other ions.

Another possible cause of negative net absorption is ingestion of phosphate-binding antacids containing aluminum. These are converted to insoluble aluminum phosphate ($AlPO_4$) so that dietary phosphate is rendered unavailable for absorption. Calcium carbonate and magnesium-containing antacids also bind dietary phosphate but to a lesser extent than aluminum salts. Except in very high doses, antacids will only rarely cause negative phosphate balance unless combined with low intake, malabsorption, or chronic dialysis (597). Chronic alcoholism is a good example of the interplay of multiple mechanisms (575). These patients may have a poor food intake, frequent vomiting, intestinal malabsorption due to alcohol itself, to liver cirrhosis, or to pancreatitis, and they frequently use antacids for chronic gastritis.

Influx into cells or into bone—acute hypophosphatemia. The plasma P_i falls by 1 to 1.5 mmol/L within 4 to 6 h during hemodialysis and within 24 to 36 h after renal transplantation, but for the most part such rapid falls are due to increased influx into cells (Table 19-39). This normally causes only a modest fall in plasma P_i, but intravenous glucose was the cause in more than half of the patients with a plasma P_i of less than 0.7 mmol/L in one large series (596). In patients who already have a substantial loss of IC phosphate, whether from primary cell breakdown or from primary negative balance, profound hypophosphatemia can occur. Phosphate may enter cells because of restoration of cell water, reversal of preferential loss of IC phosphate, or resynthesis of glycogen and protein (Table 19-36). The more severe the IC deficit, the more profound the fall

in plasma P_i during recovery. Since the clinical effects of acute hypophosphatemia are all due to IC phosphate depletion, it is at first sight paradoxical that these effects should be precipitated by influx of phosphate into cells. The explanation is twofold. First, some low-bulk tissues may lose even more phosphate as high-bulk tissues such as muscle are gaining phosphate. This applies particularly to the cells of the blood; these show little change in composition during starvation and so have little tendency to sequester phosphate during recovery, but they combine direct exposure to hypophosphatemia with great susceptibility to its effects. Second, different phosphate pools within the same cell may change in opposite directions. For example, rapid resynthesis of cell protein may simultaneously increase the acid-insoluble phosphate and deplete the acid-soluble pool faster than it can be replenished by diffusion of P_i across the cell membrane. This applies particularly to muscle, which bears the main brunt of protein catabolism during starvation, and which because of its bulk is the main site of phosphate deposition during recovery. A further example is resumption of cell division in tissues which have suffered mitotic arrest during starvation, necessitating increased synthesis of DNA as well as protein in preparation for mitosis. This applies particularly to the gut, liver, and bone marrow.

Tale 19-39. Causes of acute hypophosphatemia due to increased influx into tissues

Severe
Diabetic ketoacidosis*
Acute alcoholism*
Total parenteral nutrition†
Resynthesis of bone
Mild
Surgical operations†
Heat stroke
Gram-negative septicemia†
Salicylate poisoning
Severe burns‡
Reyes' syndrome‡

* During recovery.
† Other mechanisms are also operative.
‡ Data are incomplete.

Clinically significant acute hypophosphatemia due to cell influx of phosphate occurs principally in diabetic ketoacidosis, acute alcoholism, and in total parenteral nutrition (Table 19-39). The latter condition is discussed separately because other mechanisms such as increased urinary loss are also involved. In diabetic ketoacidosis the initial plasma P_i may be as high as 2 to 2.5 mmol/L, associated with an increased rate of urinary phosphate excretion of 2.5 to 3.0 mmol/h (592, 600, 601). With effective correction of hyperglycemia and ketoacidosis by insulin and intravenous salt and water, with or without glucose or alkalies, phosphate moves rapidly into cells at a rate of 3 to 5 mmol/h. The plasma P_i may fall as much as 2 mmol/L in the first 4 h, but the lowest level usually occurs between 12 and 18 h after treatment was begun (575); urinary phosphate excretion also falls markedly in parallel with the plasma level.

In acutely ill patients with chronic alcoholism the initial plasma P_i is often below 0.8 mmol/L despite ketoacidosis (602, 603). As well as the multiple causes of phosphate depletion in these patients already mentioned, they may also have a low TM_P/GFR due to magnesium depletion (575). Withdrawal of ethanol and provision of calories is followed by a further fall which occurs more slowly than in diabetic ketoacidosis, the nadir usually being on the third or fourth day after admission (575). Phosphate influx into cells is probably promoted both by intravenous glucose and by hyperventilation, which is due to a combination of ammonium intoxication and the cerebral irritation of delirium tremens.

Hypophosphatemia commonly occurs in septicemia but values less than 0.2 mmol/L are rare (606). It is more prevalent in gram-negative than in gram-positive infections and is associated with hypotension, oliguric renal failure, and increased mortality. Hyperventilation is only part of the explanation but other etiologic factors have not been identified. A similar poor prognostic significance of unexplained hypophosphatemia has been observed in Reyes' syndrome (605) and in severe burns (575).

Multiple mechanisms: Negative balance com-bined with cell influx. Patients requiring TPN (total parenteral nutrition), often confusingly referred to as intravenous hyperalimentation, have usually suffered prolonged undernutrition or are in a catabolic state because of trauma. The solutions used vary in composition but all contain glucose, essential amino acids, sodium, and potassium (606). If no phosphate is included an initially normal plasma P_i falls by about 0.1 mmol/day, reaching the dangerous level of 0.2 mmol/L in about 10 days (607, 608). The usual explanation is that P_i is driven into cells by glucose uptake. The hypophosphatemic effect of glucose is enhanced by fasting and by intravenous administration, but when complete fasting in a previously healthy subject is interrupted by oral administration of carbohydrate alone, there is no change or even a slight rise in the plasma P_i level (495). The slow fall of P_i is consistent with the time scale of resynthesis of protein, but in the only published balance studies omission of phosphate during TPN prevented both nitrogen and phosphate retention (609). In rats there is increased phosphate turnover in muscle (610) but increased net deposition of phosphate has not been established. Urinary excretion of phosphate falls to less than 0.3 mmol/day during TPN, but such low levels are not attained for 8 to 10 days, during which 30 to 35 mmol of P_i are lost in the urine (607); this would deplete a normally sized exchangeable pool by 80 percent and lower plasma P_i to 0.25 mmol/L. Others have also found significant negative external balances for P_i during TPN (441). Despite frequent statements to the contrary (607, 610) and for whatever reason it occurs, urinary phosphate loss must contribute significantly to the hypophosphatemia of TPN, although it is not the whole explanation. There is a similar combination of increased cell influx (due to intravenous glucose) and increased urinary loss (due to intravenous sodium chloride) after uncomplicated surgical operations (611).

Effects of phosphate depletion

Patients with hypophosphatemia are often deficient in other substances such as potassium and magnesium but the clinical syndrome of phosphate depletion is reversed by phosphate administration alone. The syndrome occurs in its most pure form as a result of chronic antacid ingestion. Affected patients have a generalized malaise with tiredness and lack of energy, anorexia, severe muscle weakness, and bone pain due to osteomalacia. Patients with chronic renal failure who already have a defect in mineralization are especially liable to phosphate-depletion osteomalacia with the combination of antacids and hemodialysis (598). Chronic phosphate depletion also causes complex mineral and hormonal effects and sets the stage for acute phosphate depletion. Neither of these occurs in mild hypophosphatemia resulting from a low Tm_P/GFR which is frequently asymptomatic, but these patients may get both muscle weakness and osteomalacia just as in phosphate depletion if some additional factor is present, such as vitamin D depletion, increased PTH secretion, or phosphate transport defects in muscle or bone. The effects peculiar to phosphate depletion will be described here, and muscle weakness and osteomalacia will be described later.

Mineral and hormonal responses to negative phosphate balance. A moderate reduction in NA_P due to dietary restriction of $AlOH_3$ administration leads to a corresponding reduction in urinary phosphate excretion with unchanged or even more positive phosphate balance (599). The plasma P_i remains normal or even rises slightly in the early-morning fasting state when tubular reabsorption of phosphate is increased, but at other times of the day the plasma P_i is significantly reduced and accounts for the fall in urinary phosphate excretion without an increase in tubular reabsorption. Calcium absorption, urinary calcium excretion, and calcium balance do not change significantly. With more severe reduction in NA_P both in humans and in experimental animals, there is a rise in Tm_P/GFR which partly offsets the decrease in L/GFR and permits reduction in urinary phosphate excretion with minimal fall in plasma phosphate. This adjustment may be initiated by suppression of PTH secretion, but it is maintained by some other mechanism possibly dependent on IC de-

pletion of phosphate in the renal tubule. In phosphate-depleted rats the kidney is extremely resistant to the phosphaturic effect of PTH (612). Phosphate depletion also increases intestinal absorption and urinary excretion of calcium (by 7 to 15 mmol/day) and magnesium (by 2 to 4 mmol/day)(595), but urinary calcium does not usually increase unless urinary P_i excretion falls below about 4 to 5 mmol/day (613). During phosphate-free TPN, urine calcium may not increase above 5 mmol/day if calcium is also omitted from the solution.

The sex differences in the short-term responses to phosphate depletion, mentioned earlier, shed some light on the mechanism of these changes. In women, the plasma P_i falls and plasma 1,25-DHCC rises by about 40 percent whereas in men neither plasma P_i nor 1,25-DHCC changes (614). Intestinal absorption of both Ca and Mg increases to the same extent in both sexes, and so must occur by mechanisms which, as in the rat, are partly independent of increased 1,25-DHCC synthesis. Plasma iPTH also falls to the same extent in both sexes (595), so that phosphate depletion must inhibit PTH secretion by some means which is independent of the fall in plasma P_i. In men, urinary calcium increases only to the same extent as NA_{Ca} with no change in balance (unless the dietary calcium intake is low), whereas in women there is increased net bone resorption with a greater increase in urinary calcium and negative calcium balance. This is unlikely to be due solely to the modest increase in 1,25-DHCC level to 100 pm/L, because levels of 200 to 300 pm/L in idiopathic hypercalciuria (614) are associated with a much-smaller degree of negative calcium balance. Also phosphate depletion increases calcium release from bone even in the vitamin D-deficient rat (615).

Nothing is known of the histologic changes in bone remodeling or the precise skeletal sites from which calcium is released in humans, but in the rat phosphate depletion increases both osteoclastic and periosteocytic bone resorption despite the absence of PTH, and decreases the appositional bone-formation rate (615, 616). It is an interesting contrast that in response to phosphate depletion the growing rat sacrifices bone to permit normal soft tissue growth whereas adult men sacrifice soft tissue to protect bone, at least for a short time. The effects of phosphate depletion on bone formation and mineralization are further discussed on p. 1080. Whether in the long term phosphate depletion is a factor in bone loss and osteopenia is unknown.

Increased net bone resorption due to phosphate depletion may lead to hypercalcemia in both the dog (617) and the rat (615) after parathyroidectomy and vitamin D depletion, but in humans plasma calcium does not usually change significantly and may even fall slightly. However, TPN may lead to hypercalcemia (3 to 3.5 mmol/L) in premature neonates (441) and occasionally even in adults (607). The occurrence of severe hypercalciuria (often in excess of 10 mmol/day) with no rise in plasma calcium indicates that tubular reabsorption of calcium is depressed. This is partly due to PTH deficiency, but cross-circulation and kidney perfusion experiments strongly suggest an additional humoral factor, possibly released by bone, which reduces calcium reabsorption (618) in the distal tubule and collecting duct. Phosphate depletion also reduces the tubular reabsorption of bicarbonate (619) and of glucose (620), possibly because of a rise in intracellular pH.

Clinical and laboratory features of acute hypophosphatemia and phosphate depletion. The clinical features of acute hypophosphatemia are less well defined than of chronic hypophosphatemia (described later) because the patients are even more liable to other deficiencies and because of the wide variety of underlying diseases. Apart from nonspecific symptoms such as anorexia, nausea, and malaise, the major syndromes are a metabolic neuroencephalopathy sometimes progressing to coma, profound muscle weakness sometimes associated with rhabdomyolysis, hemolytic anemia, and impaired leukocyte and platelet function (575, 622).

Main Clinical Syndromes. The metabolic neuroencephalopathy can mimic a wide variety of primary neurologic diseases. A frequent early symptom is paraesthesiae beginning in the extremities and progressing centripetally associated with variable multimodal sensory impairment. Profound muscle weakness may develop rapidly; in contrast to the muscle weakness of chronic hypophosphatemia this is accompanied by depression or absence of deep tendon reflexes, is not predominantly proximal in distribution, and frequently involves muscles supplied by the cranial nerves, producing such signs as ptosis and difficulty in mastication. The available data for EMG, nerve-conduction velocity, and muscle biopsy are all consistent with a neurogenic rather than a myogenic cause of muscle weakness. Other features are tremor, ataxia, incoordination, ballismus, nystagmus, and unequal pupils. Dysarthria, dysphagia and shallow respiration may suggest bulbar involvement; in some patients ventilatory depression may be the major abnormality and may require tracheostomy and mechanically assisted respiration (622). A misdiagnosis of Guillain-Barré syndrome has initially been made in several patients. Cerebral symptoms include irritability, apprehension, disorientation, confusion, convulsive seizures, and coma, sometimes fatal. The EEG may be diffusely abnormal and the CSF protein level is usually increased. Hypophosphatemia may further worsen the cerebral depression and coma of diabetic ketoacidosis and hepatic encephalopathy. Phosphate depletion together with aluminum intoxication has also been incriminated in the pathogenesis of dialysis dementia (623). In experimental phosphate depletion with cerebral dysfunction the most striking abnormalities in the brain were diffuse hemorrhagic cerebral edema and intracerebral acidosis; inorganic phosphate (per kg dry weight) was paradoxically increased by about 15 percent (624).

Acute hypophosphatemia may also cause primary as well as neurogenic muscle weakness, similar to that of chronic hypophosphatemia but of more rapid onset. In alcoholic patients with prior phosphate depletion, hypophosphatemia induced by refeeding may be followed by clinical and laboratory evidence of rhabdomyolysis, with acute pain and tenderness as well as weakness of muscles, accompanied by a brisk rise in CPK (625). Soon after the plasma P_i may rise because of phosphate liberated from damaged cells. Lactate production in response to forearm exercise during ischemia may be subnormal, suggesting a defect in muscle glycogenolysis (626), or normal despite depletion of muscle glycogen (625). Even in the absence of skeletal muscle weakness, cardiac muscle function can be impaired, with reduced left ventricular stroke work and increased pulmonary artery wedge pressure (627); improvement in myocardial contractility occurred with phosphate repletion.

Many of these features can be explained as consequences of impaired tissue oxygenation because of deficiency of 2,3-DPG (2,3-diphosphoglycerate) in red cells combined with reduced availability of metabolic energy within affected tissues or organs because of ATP depletion (628).

Mechanisms and Consequences of Red Cell 2,3-DPG Deficiency. 2,3-DPG is the most abundant glycolytic intermediate in red cells, with a concentration of 4 to 5 mmol/L. It is formed by a diversion from the main sequence of glycolysis, the Rapoport-Luebering pathway (Fig. 19-29). A low plasma P_i (0.7 mmol/L) limits the formation of 1,3-DPG from glyceraldehyde 3-phosphate (Fig. 19-24). As a result triose phosphate and fructose diphosphate accumulate, glycolytic intermediates

formed subsequent to the block (especially 2,3-DPG) become depleted, and regeneration of ATP and ADP is impaired (629).

The most important effect of reduced red cell 2,3-DPG content is a shift to the left in the dissociation curve of oxyhemoglobin; this occurs because 2,3-DPG has a high binding affinity for hemoglobin and so displaces oxygen (630). Changes in the dissociation curve are usually expressed as values for P_{50}, which is the oxygen tension (P_{O_2}) corresponding to 50 percent dissociation. P_{50} values correlate both with red cell 2,3-DPG content and with plasma P_i during both diabetic ketoacidosis (531) and TPN (629). Even with extreme hypophosphatemia, red cell 2,3-DPG rarely falls below about 40 percent of normal, at which level oxygen release is decreased by about 15 percent when arterial P_{O_2} values are between 60 and 100 mmHg (632); this would be of little consequence in an otherwise healthy subject. However severe hypophosphatemia may prevent the normal adaptive increase in red cell 2,3-DPG which occurs in response to hypoxia, consequently it potentiates the harmful effects of anemia and may cause significant tissue hypoxia in sick patients in whom tissue perfusion is impaired. Severe hypophosphatemia therefore has the

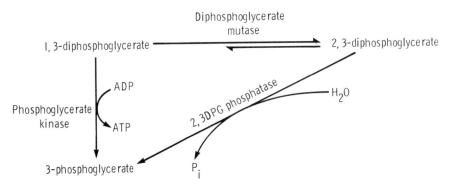

Figure 19-29. Formation of 2,3-DPG (2,3-diphosphoglycerate) as an additional intermediate in glycolysis in the red cell (Rapoport-Luebering pathway). Normally the concentration of 2,3-DPG is much higher than of 1,3-DPG. Formation of 1,3-DPG and hence 2,3-DPG is dependent on the availability of inorganic phosphate for step 5 of glycolysis (see Fig. 29-24).

potential for impairing the function of any organ in the body.

Mechanisms and Consequences of ATP Deficiency. In all cells the regeneration of ATP from ADP by either glycolysis or respiration is dependent on either EC or IC P_i (574). Consequently ATP deficiency is a predictable consequence of severe hypophosphatemia. The general consequences of ATP depletion include impaired control of energy production in mitochondria by oxidative phosphorylation, reduced activity of cell membrane $Na^+-K^+-ATPase$ (sodium–potassium–activated ATPase) leading to a loss of potassium by the cell and consequent influx of sodium, reduced RNA synthesis associated with fragmentation of the nucleus, reduced protein synthesis associated with disruption of the ribosomes in the rough endoplasmic reticulum, and hepatic accumulation of triglyceride (633). The magnitude of the ATP deficiency induced by hypophosphatemia and the extent to which this contributes to impaired cell function has been established only in the cells of the blood, probably because of their greater accessibility to study, but it is likely that the same mechanism operates in all tissues.

Red cells normally contain about 1 to 1.5 mmol/L ATP, and this may fall to 20 to 40 percent of normal with severe hypophosphatemia. The major consequence of red cell ATP depletion is hemolytic anemia, but this is uncommon and occurs only if the plasma P_i falls below 0.1 mmol/L and red cell ATP falls below 0.2 mmol/L. At this level the red cells become microspherocytic, abnormally rigid, and more quickly destroyed by the spleen (575, 621). This probably results from deficiency of ATP-dependent actomyosinlike contractile proteins which are responsible for the maintenance of cell shape (634). Apart from the adverse effects of anemia, increased red cell rigidity could reduce blood flow through the microcirculation and so further depress tissue oxygenation. In the dog, severe experimental hypophosphatemia (less than 0.3 mmol/L) causes ATP depletion in leukocytes with depression of cell motility and impairment of phagocytic and bactericidal activity; similar changes have occasionally been reported in patients (635). Similarly, re-

duced ATP content of platelets is associated with shortened life span, thrombocytopenia, poor clot retraction and increased liability to gastrointestinal hemorrhage, and bruising of the skin (621). Mild mucosal bleeding has been reported in some hypophosphatemic patients, but platelet dysfunction has not been documented in humans.

Possible Relationships with Clinical Syndromes. In principle, a combination of impaired tissue oxygenation and reduced availability of metabolic energy could adequately account for all the reported consequences of hypophosphatemia, but supporting evidence is still fragmentary. Early reports of reduced ATP levels in the brain of phosphate-depleted dogs were not confirmed (621), and in phosphate-depleted rats the level of ATP in the kidney does not fall for 6 weeks, although kidney P_i falls after 2 weeks (636). No other tissues have been examined directly, although the low resting E_M (transmembrane potential) of muscle in phosphate depletion (637) suggests impaired activity of the muscle-cell-membrane sodium pump, which is consistent with ATP deficiency. Impaired myocardial contractility in phosphate-depleted patients improve with no change in P_{50}, suggesting that ATP depletion rather than impaired oxygen transport was responsible (638). An adverse effect of reduced P_{50} on tissue oxygenation has been demonstrated only in the liver (639); with treatment, improved oxygen extraction correlated with a rise in P_{50}. This may account for the worsening of hepatocellular function which sometimes follows refeeding in alcoholic patients.

Prevention and treatment

Much remains to be learned about the pathogenesis of phosphate depletion and its complications, but prevention and treatment are usually simple. Careful monitoring of individual patients with respect to renal function as well as phosphate status should temper application of the following guidelines. As explained in Chap. 8 the meq is an unsatisfactory unit for phosphate and all doses should be prescribed and administered in mmol.

In patients taking high doses (80 mL/day or

more) of phosphate-binding antacids, plasma and urinary P_i should be measured every 3 to 6 months. Since the upper range of plasma P_i in phosphate-depleted patients overlaps the lower normal range, a 24-h urinary P_i excretion of more than 10 mmol provides the best assurance that the patient is not phosphate depleted. Lower values should lead to a reduction in dose or a change to aluminum phosphate or supplementary dietary or medicinal phosphate. Skim milk is an excellent source (containing 30 to 35 mmol/qt), and is useful in any disease predisposing to phosphate depletion.

Phosphate should be added to intravenous fluids much more frequently than has been customary in the past. Provided renal function is satisfactory, no harm can result and some patients assuredly will benefit. The dangers of hyperphosphatemia are real, but tolerance of surplus phosphate is much higher than is usually appreciated. If the plasma creatinine is normal (less than 1.2 mg/dL), the creatinine clearance will not be less than 50 mL/min even in a small-sized patient. At this level as much as 30 mmol of phosphate given in 24 h could not raise the plasma P_i by more than 0.5 mmol/L, a perfectly safe level, even if all the administered phosphate were to be excreted in the urine and none retained in the tissues. With muscle wasting the creatinine clearance could be overestimated, but tissue uptake of phosphate would be correspondingly increased. Except in patients with overt renal failure or other causes for hyperphosphatemia, any intravenous infusion which lasts for more than 24 h should provide at least 10 mmol of phosphate daily. This is easily accomplished by giving half the daily allotment of potassium as phosphate and half as chloride.

In diabetic ketoacidosis a minimum need of 50 mmol of phosphate in the first 24 h can be predicted. Even more phosphate is required in patients given bicarbonate because rapid correction of acidosis lowers P_{50} via the Bohr effect (640). Red cell 2,3-DPG is already low because of the acidosis and cannot be regenerated if the plasma P_i is allowed to fall. As with potassium, administration of phosphate should be delayed until the efflux of P_i from cells is reversed, but this usually occurs within a few hours of starting insulin. Many patients recover quickly without phosphate but it is difficult to predict those in whom it will be essential. Provision of phosphate enhances glucose utilization by stimulating glycolysis (575), returns P_{50} to normal, and accelerates recovery of consciousness (601, 631). The need for phosphate continues during cell restoration so that phosphate should be included as long as intravenous fluids are continued. Once normal feeding is resumed, supplemental phosphate is no longer needed.

In alcoholic patients requiring intravenous feeding some degree of phosphate depletion can be presumed and addition of phosphate should begin immediately. The amount required has not been established by balance measurements, but is unlikely to be less than the mean value for net intestinal absorption in normal subjects, or about 30 mmol/day. If intravenous feeding is not required, a normal plasma P_i will usually be restored without treatment (602).

In patients requiring TPN the need to include phosphate routinely is now generally appreciated and most commercially available amino acid solutions already contain phosphate. Amino acid solutions derived from hydrolysis of casein have always contained adequate phosphate, but those derived from hydrolysis of fibrins (such as Freamine) were initially phosphate-free (606). However, the Freamine II now available contains 10 mmol of phosphate/L. If this is mixed in equal parts with 50% dextrose, 3 L of the resultant solution contains only 15 mmol of phosphate so that some additional phosphate will almost always be needed. Provision of 10 to 15 mmol of phosphate per 100 kcal will maintain normal plasma P_i levels in most patients (608). The mean daily retention of phosphate was 27 mmol/day (or about 0.4 mmol/kg ideal body weight) in patients gaining 0.6 kg body weight daily, or about 43 mmol/kg weight gain (609). Allowing some surplus for urinary excretion, the daily requirement will usually be in the range of 30 to 50 mmol/day.

If phosphate depletion is already present on admission or if severe hypophosphatemia is allowed to develop because preventive measures are omitted, much larger amounts of phosphate are needed, in the range of 80 to 120 mmol/day. Also, some of the complications of phosphate depletion may become irreversible in extremely sick patients. If possible, phosphate supplements should be given by mouth; available preparations are discussed on p. 1083. Most often intravenous administration will be needed; both sodium and potassium phosphate are available in concentrated solutions of mixed monobasic and dibasic salts containing 3 mmol of P_i/mL which can be added to standard intravenous solutions.

The dangers of phosphate administration according to the preceding guidelines are negligible. However, if impaired renal function is not recognized, the recommended rates of administration may produce dangerous hyperphosphatemia, as described on p. 1086. As explained earlier, the rise in plasma P_i for a given increment in load increases hyperbolically as GFR declines. Occasionally, significant hypocalcemia and even tetany may result from administration of phosphate without calcium even though the plasma P_i does not rise above normal (607, 626). This only occurs in patients who are already phosphate depleted, probably because they have functional HP. Tetany has never been observed with the *prophylactic* administration of phosphate in the amounts recommended. Solutions for TPN routinely contain 2.5 mmol of Ca/L providing a daily intake of at least 5 mmol. Addition of calcium is not necessary if prophylactic phosphate is given for only a few days to diabetic or alcoholic patients. Other complications of phosphate administration may be due to the attendant cation, either sodium or potassium.

MILD TO MODERATE HYPOPHOSPHATEMIA WITHOUT PHOSPHATE DEPLETION

Primary hyperparathyroidism (p. 998) is the first cause of hypophosphatemia to be considered by most physicians, but this was present in only 1 of 100 instances accumulated in a 3-month period in a large general hospital (596). Most were due to one or more of the acute and transient causes already covered. Other causes of stable chronic hypophosphatemia are listed in Table 19-40.

Table 19-40. Causes of low Tm_P/GFR and consequent hypophosphatemia

Increased PTH secretion (see Tables 19-10, 19-19)
Other hormonal causes
Estrogens
Androgens and anabolic hormones
Oral contraceptives
Cushing's syndrome
Exogenous hypercortisonism
? Aldosterone excess
Metabolic causes
Hypercalcemia
Potassium depletion
Metabolic acidosis
Ammonium chloride
Renal-tubular acidosis
Ureterosigmoidostomy
? ECF volume expansion
Pharmacologic causes
Thiazide (? and other) diuretics
Probenecid
? Carbonic anhydrase inhibitors
Unclassifiable
Idiopathic hypercalciuria
Intrinsic or persistent renal-tubular defects (see Table 19-42)

Mechanisms and causes

It is convenient to repeat the fundamental relationship underlying the regulation of plasma phosphate:

$$P_P = \frac{L_P}{\text{GFR}} + \frac{TR_P}{\text{GFR}} \qquad (19\text{-}7)$$

When fractional phosphate reabsorption is less than 80 percent of the filtered load, which is almost always the case when the plasma phosphate is low for reasons other than phosphate depletion, the saturation threshold (Chap. 8) is exceeded and TR_P/GFR ($\%TR_P \cdot P_P/100$) is numerically equal to Tm_P/GFR. With a normal GFR and normal Tm_P/GFR, plasma P_i would remain within the normal range in most persons even if load were reduced to one-tenth of normal. Consequently, significant sustained hypophosphatemia is almost invariably due to a decrease in Tm_P/GFR. Such hypophosphatemia is usually stable, mild (0.6 to 0.9 mmol/L), refractory to treatment, and often asymptomatic. Because of the wide range of Tm_P/GFR between normal persons, a reduction of Tm_P/GFR of variable magnitude due to disease inevitably produces a wider range in both Tm_P/GFR and plasma P_i in the abnormal than in the normal population, with considerable overlap. A low Tm_P/GFR (Table 19-40) may be due to increased PTH secretion, primary or secondary, to a variety of other endocrine, metabolic, and pharmacologic causes, or to intrinsic defects (often genetic) of the renal tubule.

Increased PTH secretion. A low Tm_P/GFR due to an increase in PTH secretion for any reason is associated with a corresponding increase in nephrogenic cAMP/GFR (30, M. Kleerekoper, unpublished data). The low Tm_P/GFR of primary hyperparathyroidism and the causes of secondary hyperparathyroidism (Table 19-10) were discussed earlier. The plasma P_i is low and plasma calcium normal in most patients with vitamin D deficiency; in children this corresponds to Stage II (Table 19-41) but in adults Stage I is usually absent. The reduction in plasma P_i due to dietary deficiency or intestinal malabsorption of vitamin D is usually modest, with mean values in the range of 0.7 to 0.9 mmol/L (93). Nutritional vitamin D deficiency may be the most common cause of hypophosphatemia in geriatric practice in England, occurring in 40 percent of cases in one series (641), although this is a very rare cause in Australia and the United States. When measured, Tm_P/GFR has usually been low in vitamin D deficiency (93, 364). Whether the occasional exceptions are due to a subnormal PTH response (643) or to interference with PTH action on the kidney

(for example, by hypocalcemia) is not clear. In the rat, vitamin D depletion blunts both the NcAMP and phosphaturic response to exogenous PTH (644), so that the usual occurrence of hypophosphatemia in the human disease has been regarded as paradoxical. However, lack of vitamin D action on the renal tubule lowers Tm_P/GFR directly as well as by increased PTH secretion. This partly accounts for the paradox that PTH levels may be higher in Stage I vitamin D deficiency when the plasma P_i is normal than in Stage II when the plasma P_i is low but plasma 25-HCC is further reduced (Table 19-41). It also explains the prompt return of plasma P_i to normal within a few days or weeks of correcting vitamin D deficiency (645), even though increased PTH secretion persists for many months.

In hyperparathyroidism there is often impaired tubular reabsorption of bicarbonate and amino acids as well as phosphate. This is much more common in children than in adults and in secondary than in primary hyperparathyroidism (92). Although there is no doubt that increased PTH secretion is partly responsible, hypocalcemia and lack of vitamin D action on the renal tubule may also be important. All three defects in tubular reabsorption are reversed by vitamin D treatment. Although the Tm for glucose is usually high in primary hyperparathyroidism, secondary hyperparathyroidism may sometimes paradoxically be associated with glycosuria which, like the other renal-tubular abnormalities, disappears with vitamin D treatment (645).

Lack of vitamin D action on the intestine reduces the absorption of phosphate but this makes only a small contribution to the hypophosphatemia. Increasing the intake of calcium further reduces intestinal phosphate absorption in a vitamin D-deficient subject because of calcium phosphate precipitation; there is also a further depression in phosphate reabsorption (647), possibly due to the direct effect of calcium to potentiate the action of PTH. Despite an increase in net intestinal absorption of phosphate, urinary phosphate excretion may actually decline in the first few weeks of vitamin D repletion because of the rapidity with which phosphate is deposited with calcium in bone.

Table 19-41. Biochemical data in nine cases of nutritional rickets in infants classified according to increasing severity of radiographic changes and in six cases of rickets due to XLH* of comparable age (91)

PLASMA LEVEL	NORMAL	STAGE OF RICKETS			
		I	II	III	XLH
25-HCC (nmol/L)	85	47.5	40	20	90
Ca (mmol/L)	2.53	2.13	2.45	1.85	2.47
PTH (μL eq/L)	23	89	65	115	32
P (mmol/L)	1.94	1.77	0.87	0.81	0.84

* X-linked hypophosphatemic vitamin D refractory rickets.

The characteristic hyperphosphatemia of advanced chronic renal failure is so well known that the frequent fall in plasma P_i and occasional frank hypophosphatemia in early renal failure (648) is often overlooked. This early secondary hyperparathyroidism preceding phosphate retention is due to 1,25-DHCC deficiency. Chronic phosphate administration may cause secondary hyperparathyroidism if the dose is high enough; as explained later this may lower Tm_P/GFR so that plasma P_i in the fasting state may be subnormal. The secondary hyperparathyroidism of corticosteroid therapy reinforces the direct effect of corticosteroids on Tm_P/GFR (see below), but large doses of thyroid hormone have a direct phosphaturic effect so that the secondary hyperparathyroidism of hypothyroidism (649) is opposed by the direct action of thyroid hormone deficiency on renal phosphate transport; Tm_P/GFR is slightly reduced and occasional hypophosphatemia may result (650). Hypothyroidism also reduces the amplitude of the normal circadian variation in phosphate excretion (651).

Other endocrine, metabolic, and pharmacologic causes. The role of sex hormones in the physiologic regulation of plasma phosphate was discussed earlier. Estrogen administration to postmenopausal women can reduce the plasma P_i to below normal (585), particularly in patients with primary hyperparathyroidism (265). Oral contraceptives and anabolic steroids have a similar effect. Impaired phosphate reabsorption as a nonspecific consequence of hypercalcemia was mentioned on p. 1033. This is usually reversible but is occasionally a permanent consequence of hypercalcemic nephropathy (652), with other defects in proximal tubular reabsorption such as aminoaciduria and glycosuria.

Plasma phosphate is often low (0.8 to 1.0 mmol/L) in Cushing's syndrome and with chronic corticosteroid administration (655). This could be a direct renal-tubular effect or be due to secondary hyperparathyroidism or potassium depletion. ECF volume expansion is a less likely explanation because plasma P_i is usually normal in hyperaldosteronism (517), although there are occasional exceptions (655). The combination of hypophosphatemia and nephrolithiasis in Cushing's syndrome may suggest primary hyperparathyroidism. Somewhat paradoxically the normal rise in plasma and urinary phosphate between 8 A.M. and noon coincides with a *fall* in plasma hydrocortisone (656).

Plasma phosphate is often below 0.8 mmol/L and occasionally below 0.5 mmol/L in potassium depletion and hypokalemia, and returns to normal with potassium repletion (502, 657, 658). The metabolic acidosis of ammonium chloride administration (659), distal RTA, and ureterosigmoidostomy (93) is usually accompanied by mild persistent hypophosphatemia (0.7 to 0.8 mmol/L). In part this is the result of hypercalciuria and secondary hyperparathyroidism (Chap. 8) (660), but the rise in plasma P_i which follows alkali therapy is often accompanied or preceded by a rise in plasma potassium and may occur with no change in PTH secretion. Most likely metabolic acidosis impairs phosphate transport across the renal tubule independent of PTH or potassium depletion (661).

Most diuretics increase urinary phosphate excretion when the salt losses are replaced, but thiazide diuretics are unique in that phosphate excretion is increased despite ECF volume contraction. This effect begins immediately (496) and continues during chronic administration. Prolonged treatment of idiopathic hypercalciuria with a thiazide may lead to a persistent reduction in Tm_P/GFR and a fall in plasma P_i by 0.3 mmol/L. This is unaffected by potassium supplements, and may persist even after the drug is stopped (662). Probenecid decreases both tubular reabsorption and plasma level of P_i in some patients with HP, but usually has no detectable effect on phosphate metabolism in normal subjects (663).

Intrinsic or persistent defects of renal-tubular reabsorption. These are characteristically associated with rickets and osteomalacia, which do not occur in the disorders of the preceding section unless accompanied by abnormal vitamin D metabolism or metabolic acidosis. The difference is not simply one of degree of hypophosphatemia, but probably reflects the frequent and perhaps invariable association of similar transport defects in gut or bone. The clinical, radiographic, genetic, and biochemical aspects of the field are exceed-

Table 19-42. Intrinsic or persistent defects of renal-tubular reabsorption causing hypophosphatemia with rickets and/or osteomalacia

TYPE	ONSET
Phosphate alone ± glucose	
Familial hypocalcemic	Infancy
Familial normocalcemic	
Sex-linked dominant (XLH)	Infancy
Autosomal dominant	Infancy
Autosomal recessive	Infancy
Nonfamilial normocalcemic	
Permanent (NFH)	Adolescence or after
Transient	Adolescence
Oncogenic	Any age
Fibrous dysplasia	Any age
Neurofibromatosis	Any age
Postrenal transplantation	Any age
Multiple (Fanconi syndrome)*	
Primary: several genotypes	Variable
Secondary (genetic), e.g., cystinosis	Infancy
Secondary (acquired), e.g., heavy metal poisoning	Any age

* For further details of the Fanconi syndrome see Chap. 18.

ingly complex (56, 57, 90, 92) and only a brief summary is possible here. Further discussion is given in Chap. 18. The primary subdivision is into defects of phosphate transport alone with or without glucose and more global impairment of tubular function in the Fanconi syndrome (Table 19-42). The most important conditions in the first category are familial XLH (X-linked hypophosphatemic vitamin D refractory rickets) which usually presents in infancy, and NFH (nonfamilial hypophosphatemic vitamin D refractory osteomalacia), which usually presents in late adolescence or adulthood. These diseases differ markedly in many important respects (Table 19-43) and much of the confusion in the literature has arisen because conclusions drawn from the study of one disease have been uncritically and erroneously applied to the other.

XLH (X-linked Hypophosphatemia). XLH is characterized by five separate but interrelated abnormalities—hypophosphatemia, impaired mineralization of cartilage or bone leading to rickets and osteomalacia, retarded longitudinal growth, osteosclerosis, and ligamentous calcification (194). Bone pain and muscle weakness are either very mild or completely absent. Hypophosphatemia is a more sensitive genetic marker than bone disease and inheritance occurs as an X-linked dominant trait. Affected males are therefore hemizygous and affected females heterozygous for the abnormal gene. Most sporadic cases with onset in infancy are probably first-generation mutants for the XLH gene. Other modes of transmission such as autosomal dominant and autosomal recessive have been described in isolated families; these probably differ in phenotype as well as in genotype.

Hypophosphatemia can be detected soon after birth (provided normal values appropriate for the patient's age are used) and is lifelong. The plasma P_i varies with age in the same way as in normal subjects, and tends to remain throughout life at about the same level below the age-related mean. In adults, the plasma P_i is usually lower than in vitamin D deficiency (93) but in infants it is comparable to severe nutritional rickets (Table 19-41). Most estimates of Tm_P/GFR, whether by the traditional method of phosphate infusion or by the indirect method of Bijvoet, have been in the range of 0.4 to 0.8 mmol/L. The responses to phosphate loading and depletion are both qualitatively and quantitatively the same as in normal subjects, the points relating phosphate excretion per liter C_{Cr} and plasma P_i falling along a Tm_P/GFR line shifted to the left; as in primary hyperparathyroid-

Table 19-43. Differences between two forms of vitamin D refractory osteomalacia, XLH and NDH, excluding those dependent only on age of onset

	XLH	NFH
Muscle weakness	No	Yes
Bone pain	No	Yes
Increased glycinuria	No	Yes
Vertebral collapse	No	Yes
Loss of trunk height	No	Yes
Fractures*	No	Yes
Perilacunar low-density bone	Yes	No†
Osteosclerosis	Yes	No
Ligamentous ossification	Yes	No
Phosphate depletion†	No	Yes

* Looser zones (pseudofractures) occur in both.
† Evidence is inconclusive.
SOURCE: Modified from A. M. Parfitt (194).

ism (Fig. 19-15) the same automatic changes occur in phosphate clearance and fractional excretion. Calcium infusion increases phosphate reabsorption in XLH, and when calculated as $\%TR_P$ the data have frequently suggested a much greater increase in the patients than in the controls, which has been taken as evidence for secondary hyperparathyroidism (56). But when representative data were recalculated as Tm_P/GFR, the increase was found to be the same in both groups, in the range of 0.2 to 0.4 mmol/L (93). Values close to and sometimes within the normal range may be attained, but the difference between XLH and normal subjects remains the same throughout the infusion.

During childhood when rickets is active and growth retarded, there is net intestinal malabsorption and diminished urinary excretion of both calcium and phosphate. The malabsorption can be overcome by vitamin D, but in contrast to nutritional rickets tubular reabsorption of phosphate does not return to normal. Despite numerous statements to the contrary, the defect in phosphate absorption makes only a trivial contribution to the hypophosphatemia. For example, in the balance studies reviewed by Stickler (664) the mean urinary phosphate excretion was less than 3 mmol per 24 h below that of age-matched controls; assuming a GFR of 50 mL/min, this would have reduced plasma P_i by less than 0.05 mmol/L. Decreased net absorption of calcium when it occurs could be due to increased endogenous fecal calcium secretion rather than to decreased true absorption (665). Another unusual feature is that the rise in plasma calcium after an oral calcium load is normal (666) whereas in vitamin D deficiency the response is subnormal. In adults studied after attainment of skeletal maturity but with persistent hypophosphatemia, net intestinal absorption of both calcium and phosphate is normal in relation to intake over a wide range of intakes (128). This demonstrates that neither impaired intestinal absorption of calcium or phosphate can be the primary defect in the disease, but that both are the result of whatever mechanisms normally ensure that absorption is matched to skeletal need. In response to an oral phosphate load the rise in plasma P_i is subnormal (666); this is not due to differences in renal excretion but could be due to differences in net uptake by bone or soft tissues. Studies of phosphate transport in intestinal mucosal biopsies have given conflicting results (667, 668), but any defect present must affect the rate and not the completeness of phosphate absorption. A strain of mice with genetically determined hypophosphatemia has recently been discovered; as well as impaired proximal tubular phosphate reabsorption (669) the mice have a severe defect in intestinal transport of P_i which is refractory to 1,25-DHCC administration (670), an important difference from the human disease which should (but probably will not) engender caution in their use as an experimental model.

Despite the name given to the disease, there is no evidence for any abnormality of vitamin D metabolism. Early reports of increased formation of biologically inactive metabolites and decreased formation of 25-HCC probably resulted from an increase in the body pool of vitamin D due to previous treatment (90). Plasma 25-HCC levels are normal (Table 19-41) and the therapeutic response to 25-HCC is indistinguishable from that to EC except for the lower dose. This is simply because only 5 to 10 percent of a large pharmacologic dose of EC is 25-hydroxylated, so that only from one-tenth to one-twentieth of the dose of 25-HCC is needed for the same effect. Plasma levels of 1,25-DHCC have not been reported in detail, but long-term oral treatment produced no change in Tm_P/GFR despite a substantial increase in calcium absorption (671), which is quite different from the response in vitamin D dependency.

These patients do not (as Albright originally proposed and many still believe) have a primary defect in intestinal calcium absorption, but for reasons discussed later they do have mild secondary hyperparathyroidism; in the largest and most completely studied series both plasma PTH and urinary cAMP excretion were about twice normal (672). Plasma calcium levels were all within the normal range but were significantly lower than in normal controls by about 0.15 mmol/L. However, even the highest levels of PTH were too low to account for the observed reduction in Tm_P/GFR, which was 0.51 (versus 1.97 mmol/L) in males and 0.57 (versus 1.02 mmol/L) in females, with plasma phosphate levels about 0.15 mmol/L higher. In infants with severe nutritional rickets the PTH level is about four times higher than in XLH at equivalent plasma P_i levels (Table 19-41). There have been several reports of autonomous hyperparathyroidism in these patients, with hypercalcemia relieved by removal of a parathyroid adenoma or hyperplastic parathyroid tissue (673). Whether these are instances of hypercalcemic secondary hyperparathyroidism or represent the coincidence of two unrelated diseases is not known. Without exception, parathyroidectomy, whether performed for this or for any other reason, has had no significant effect on either Tm_P/GFR or plasma P_i.

All available data support the existence of an intrinsic and genetically determined defect in renal-tubular phosphate transport in XLH but there is still considerable controversy concerning its nature. It has been proposed that a PTH-sensitive component of renal phosphate transport is completely missing in hemizygotes and partially absent in heterozygotes, and that the response to calcium infusion represents a direct effect of calcium ion on a non-PTH-dependent component of renal phosphate transport (674). The data supporting this proposal are open to other interpretations (Chap. 18) and the phosphaturic response to exogenous PTH can be normal (672, 675) or even increased. Because of the insensitivity of most C-terminal assays to acute changes, whether PTH secretion changes sufficiently in response to calcium infusion to explain the observed change in Tm_P/GFR in both XLH and in normal subjects is still unknown, but this seems the most likely explanation.

NFH (Nonfamilial Hypophosphatemia). In NFH the onset may be at any age between 15 and 75 years but is most commonly between 20 and 40 years. The symptoms are typical of osteomalacia, with severe bone pain and generalized muscle weakness resembling a proximal limb girdle myopathy. There is often kyphosis and severe loss of trunk height due to vertebral compression and multiple fractures of long bones. A characteristic but unexplained feature is increased urinary excretion of glycine (194) (Table 19-43). The defect in phosphate reabsorption is usually worse than in XLH. For example, in six cases studied by

phosphate infusion the mean Tm_P/GFR was 0.31 mmol/L (676) and the mean plasma P_i in 27 cases tabulated by Fanconi (677) was 0.53 mmol/L, whereas in adults with XLH it is usually above 0.65 mmol/L. Despite this the rise in plasma P_i in response to an oral phosphate load is usually higher than in XLH and may be quite normal (678). In contrast to adults with XLH, patients with NFH have significant intestinal malabsorption of calcium. This is probably a reflection of the severity of the bone disease, since XLH adults with unusually severe bone disease also have calcium malabsorption. Intestinal calcium absorption increases significantly when the plasma phosphate is raised by either oral or intravenous administration of phosphate (57). As in XLH, absorption is controlled by the needs of the bone and the intestine is probably not the site of the primary defect. Urinary calcium excretion is high in relation to the severity of the bone disease, and may sometimes be high even in absolute terms (676). It may rise much more sharply with vitamin D treatment than in nutritional osteomalacia or XLH, long before the bones are healed, suggesting an additional defect in renal-tubular reabsorption of calcium.

Because of its greater rarity the nature of the phosphate transport defect has been less intensively studied than in XLH. Net tubular secretion of phosphate has been suggested (674) but this concept has not found general acceptance. There are several reports of PTH levels being up to six times normal (673), higher than is found in XLH, and there is a higher incidence of autonomous hyperparathyroidism—4 in a total of 44 published cases. This could result from a longer delay before diagnosis and treatment (mean greater than 6 years) or simply from a higher mean age of the patients. Apart from slight subperiosteal resorption in one case (676) there has been no radiographic evidence of hyperparathyroidism and the small number of bone biopsies have shown no evidence of increased resorption. Bone turnover determined by calcium kinetics or urinary THP is usually low. If endogenous PTH is suppressed by calcium infusion, the phosphaturic response to exogenous PTH is normal (678), but the response may be subnormal if this precaution is not taken. As in XLH surgical treatment of autonomous hyperparathyroidism has not restored the plasma P_i to normal, although in the only patient subjected to total parathyroidectomy the plasma P_i and tubular reabsorption of phosphate were in the HP range 20 years later with a normal or even exaggerated phosphaturic response to exogenous PTH (680). It is likely that PTH plays a permissive rather than a causal role since, as in XLH, treatment with vitamin D does not return the tubular reabsorption of phosphate or plasma P_i to normal despite a significant increase in intestinal calcium absorption or even the induction of hypercalcemia. In one patient who was initially indistinguishable from other cases of NFH of adolescent onset, the low plasma P_i unexpectedly returned to normal with DHT treatment alone and remained normal for 5 years after all treatment was stopped (681). Similar remissions have been observed by others (194).

In at least 15 cases of NFH, hypophosphatemia and osteomalacia have been abolished by excision of a tumor, permitting vitamin D treatment to be either withdrawn or withheld altogether; the time taken for the plasma P_i to rise to normal has varied from 1 to 8 weeks (194, 682). In three cases this rise was accompanied by chronic hypercalcemia which persisted after subtotal parathyroidectomy in one case but eventually subsided spontaneously in the other two. The tumors may arise in soft tissue or bone and are of mesenchymal or-igin but with very variable histology, often not typical of any existing category but most closely resembling a hemangiopericytoma. It is conceivable that such a tumor is present in all cases of NFH (194), since the tumors may be very small and slow growing, but in the first such patient diagnosed at Henry Ford Hospital (678), multiple contrast radiographic studies and bone and soft tissue scans are still quite normal more than 30 years after the onset of symptoms. A similar relationship has been observed in one of several cases of NFH associated with fibrous dysplasia, in which excision of most of the abnormal tissue was followed by healing of the rickets (683). The same might also apply to neurofibromatosis with NFH, in which widespread excision of the tumors is usually impractical.

It is likely that a humoral mechanism is operating but its nature is obscure. In one case the plasma 1,25-DHCC was low and both Tm_p/GFR and plasma phosphate returned to normal within 10 days on 3 μg of 1,25-DHCC daily (684). It is possible that the tumor was secreting some substance which inhibited the formation of 1,25-DHCC, but the PTH level was normal and did not change with treatment. After excision of the tumor with restoration of normal Tm_p/GFR and plasma P_i, a normal 1,25-DHCC level was not documented. The considerable differences between NFH and vitamin D dependency (Table 19-

Table 19-44. Differences between the main kinds of hypophosphatemic rickets and osteomalacia

	VITAMIN D DEFICIENT	VITAMIN D DEPENDENT	FANCONI SYNDROME[a]	RTA	XLH OR NFH
Plasma Ca (untreated)	N or ↓	↓	N[b]	N	N
PTH (untreated)	↑↑	↑↑	↑	↑	↑
Plasma P_i (treated)[c]	N	N	↓	N	↓
Plasma HCO_3^- (untreated)	↓	↓	↓	↓	N
Plasma HCO_3^- (treated)[d]	N	N	↓	↓	N
Urinary AA[e] (untreated)	↑	↑	↑	N	N[f]
Urinary AA (treated)	N	N	↑	N	N
Dose of vitamin D (mg/day)	0.025–0.25	1.5–5.0	1.0–10.0[g]	1.0–2.0	2.0–8.0

[a] Excluding cystinosis, which behaves like vitamin D dependency.
[b] May be low if renal failure is present.
[c] With vitamin D or alkali.
[d] With vitamin D alone.
[e] AA, amino acids.
[f] Except for glycine alone in NFH.
[g] Varies with degree of renal failure.
SOURCE: Modified from A. M. Parfitt (194).

44) indicate that some factor in addition to reduced synthesis of 1,25-DHCC must also be present in at least one of these diseases, probably in NFH. In a case of epidermal nevus syndrome with NFH, rickets was cured by excision of several fibrous tumors (685). An extract of the tumor increased phosphate excretion in a puppy whereas similar extracts from other tissues had no effect; no immunoassayable PTH or calcitonin was detectable. The same unknown inhibitor of phosphate reabsorption might also be secreted in neurofibromatosis, which resembles the epidermal nevus syndrome in several respects.

FS (Fanconi Syndrome). Despite its historical inaccuracy it is convenient to use this eponym to denote the association of multiple defects of proximal tubular reabsorption involving phosphate, glucose, amino acids, bicarbonate, and urate. Tubular proteinuria and defects in urinary concentration and acidification are frequently also present and renal wasting of sodium, potassium, or calcium less commonly. FS may be produced by a wide variety of morbid anatomic and biochemical insults to the proximal tubule (Chap. 18).

Several of the components of FS correspond to the renal-tubular actions of PTH and so may be produced by secondary hyperparathyroidism, and defective tubular reabsorption of phosphate could also be due to potassium depletion or metabolic acidosis (686). Only in very few cases have all three been adequately excluded; in many supposed instances a primary defect of phosphate transport has not been established, and FS as ordinarily understood and as defined earlier may not have been present. Ironically, this may even be so in cystinosis, the study of which led to the formulation of the FS concept, and which is still believed to be the most common cause of FS in children. Hypophosphatemic rickets, metabolic acidosis, and aminoaciduria are usually evident by the age of 6 to 12 months, while renal function is still normal or only very slightly impaired. Accordingly, these abnormalities are usually ascribed to primary defects in tubular transport even though cystine deposition in the proximal tubule cells is usually minimal or absent, and the shortening and swan neck deformity of the first third of the proximal convoluted tubule appears insufficient to account for the severity of the reabsorp-

tive defects (687). Recent observations have challenged this concept and suggested that deficiency of 1,25-DHCC and secondary hyperparathyroidism may occur very early in the course of the disease rather than being late and indirect consequences of destruction of renal tissue. In three cases hypophosphatemia was corrected (mean value 0.6 mmol/L rising to 1.2 mmol/L) and rickets healed with 1,σ-HCC 2 to 4 μg/day, doses only a little higher than have been found necessary in vitamin D dependency (688). PTH levels were high before treatment and fell significantly in two of the three cases. The hypophosphatemia of early cystinosis is therefore most likely due to secondary hyperparathyroidism; whether this is also responsible, at least in part, for the metabolic acidosis and aminoaciduria remains to be determined. It is conceivable that reduced activity of the 25-HCC 1-hydroxylase is a direct consequence of the structural changes in the proximal tubule, and more definitive localization of this enzyme would be of great interest. A rise in plasma P_i and Tm_P/GFR with vitamin D treatment occurs much more commonly in FS than in either XLH or NFH (687) even though the values usually remain below normal. Often there has also been lessening of aminoaciduria and a rise in plasma bicarbonate, and in isolated cases vitamin D has even reduced glucose excretion in FS (689), as has been observed in gluten enteropathy with secondary hyperparathyroidism (646).

Although the weight of evidence supports the existence of an irreversible defect of phosphate reabsorption in many patients with FS, particularly those with unequivocal structural damage to the proximal tubule, it will only be possible to examine the characteristics of this transport defect when the possible contributions of potassium depletion, metabolic acidosis, and secondary hyperparathyroidism have been eliminated. Consequently, no useful conclusions can be drawn from any of the previous studies which have attempted to elucidate these characteristics.

Effects

Mild hypophosphatemia, as in many of the conditions listed in Table 19-40, is usually completely asymptomatic. In less than 5 percent of the patients in Australia in whom hypophosphatemia was found by multichannel screening could any harmful effects be ascribed to it (596). In a large number of apparently healthy middle-aged men both systolic and diastolic blood pressures were found to correlate inversely with plasma P_i within the range of 0.5 to 1.2 mmol/L (690), but the significance and mechanism of this relationship are completely unknown. The effect of growth hormone on plasma P_i suggests that the higher plasma P_i of childhood may be necessary for normal growth. There is considerable evidence that hypophosphatemia contributes to the growth retardation and short stature in XLH, and that improved growth occurs if the plasma P_i is raised by whatever means (691). The same relationship was noted both before and after operation in a case of tumor-induced rickets (684) but changes in 1,25-DHCC synthesis might also have been responsible. The simplest explanation for the effect of hypophosphatemia on growth is that the proliferating chondroblasts in the growth plate require a particular level of plasma phosphate for optimum function. It has been suggested that growth in XLH is limited because red cell 2,3-DPG and P_{50} are low, and that restoration of normal oxygen transport is the reason for improved growth during supplemental phosphate treatment (692). This seems unlikely because the hyperphosphatemia of childhood is normally accompanied by a compensatory reduction in red cell 2,3-DPG (693). Several other groups have found red cell 2,3-DPG and P_{50} to be normal, and ATP to be normal or even increased in XLH (694, 695). None of the clinical effects which can be attributed to reduced red cell 2,3-DPG or reduced ATP content of any type of blood cell have been found in any of the conditions listed in Table 19-40. Some of the locomotor symptoms in adults with XLH are due to ligamentous ossification and are unrelated to the plasma phosphate, although the pain of osteomalacia may mimic a wide variety of rheumatologic disorders.

The occurrence of muscle weakness or osteomalacia in pure phosphate depletion probably reflects loss of phosphate from within the cells of muscle and bone; according to the model previously described (Fig. 19-27) this will occur if the plasma P_i falls below some critical value for any reason. The occurrence of the same complications in some patients whose plasma P_i does not fall below this value, but not in others with equivalent hypophosphatemia, requires some additional explanation.

Muscle weakness. The muscle weakness of pure phosphate depletion appears to be clinically indistinguishable from that occurring in vitamin D deficiency and in primary hyperparathyroidism but the latter conditions have been more fully studied (696). The distribution of weakness is similar to that of a proximal limb girdle myopathy, with difficulty in rising unaided from a chair or in climbing stairs. The affected muscles may be painful and tender, which can cause confusion with polymyositis (697). There is hypotonia but wasting is often less than expected. There is no fasciculation of myotonia and the tendon reflexes are normal or increased. Weakness of the pelvic girdle muscles can produce a characteristic ducklike, waddling gait and the most severely affected patients are unable to walk at all. The EMG shows motor unit potentials which are polyphasic and reduced in both duration and amplitude to an extent which correlates with plasma calcium but not with plasma P_i (616). Changes in muscle biopsies are either absent or mild and nonspecific, and plasma levels of muscle enzymes are always normal, except in the rhabdomyolysis of acute phosphate depletion. Most neurologists have concluded from these findings that the primary defect is in the muscle, and refer to the syndrome as a myopathy despite absence of the usual histologic and enzyme changes. A minority (698) believe that the weakness is neurogenic despite absence of the usual signs of denervation.

The prevalence of this syndrome approaches 100 percent in nutritional vitamin D deficiency (696) but is much less in patients with osteomalacia due to intestinal malabsorption (691). An identical syndrome, often very severe, occurs almost uniformly in osteomalacia associated with NFH, commonly in the adult Fanconi syndrome, and occasionally in renal-tubular acidosis; in all three conditions the weakness is often improved by phosphate treatment alone. By contrast, muscle weakness almost never occurs in XLH, with or without osteomalacia. In patients with primary hyperparathyroidism diagnosed because of symp-

Table 19-45. Comparison of six diseases associated with hypophosphatemia[a]

	PHOSPHATE DEPLETION	VITAMIN DEFICIENCY	PRIMARY HYPERPARA- THYROIDISM	NFH WITH OSTEO- MALACIA	XLH WITH OSTEO- MALACIA	RTA
Plasma calcium	N or ↑	↓	↑	N or ↓	N or ↓	N or ↓
Plasma 25-HCC	N	↓	N	N	N	N
Plasma PTH	↓[b]	↑	↑	N or ↑	N or ↑	N or ↑
Plasma P_i						
Direction	↓	↓	↓	↓	↓	↓
Magnitude[c]	0.4	0.8	0.9	0.5	0.7	0.8
Frequency of weakness (%)	100[d]	>90[e]	20[f]	>90	<5	10
Frequency of osteomalacia[g]	+	+++	+−	+++	++	+

[a] Note that proximal muscle weakness occurs without osteomalacia in hyperparathyroidism, osteomalacia without muscle weakness in XLH, and both osteomalacia and muscle weakness in the other four conditions.

[b] May be raised when osteomalacia occurs.

[c] Representative values in mmol/L.

[d] If experimentally induced; the frequency in spontaneous disease is unknown.

[e] Adequate testing may be precluded by pain.

[f] Excluding asymptomatic cases discovered by routine screening.

[g] Based on chemical and radiographic criteria, not on bone biopsy.

toms an identical syndrome occurs in about 20 percent. The prevalence is much less in patients diagnosed because of routine screening, although subtle changes may be found if looked for with great care (698).

The five main causes of the syndrome have in common only hypophosphatemia (Table 19-45) so that phosphate must somehow be involved in its pathogenesis. But differences in the level of plasma P_i alone cannot explain the complete absence of the syndrome in most patients in whom hypophosphatemia is due to a low Tm_P/GFR, or the variation in prevalence between the different disorders. Differences in IC P_i and in ATP and other organic phosphate compounds are likely to be much more critical. Loss of IC phosphate when the ECF P_i remains above the critical level of about 0.5 mmol/L requires some additional factor (Fig. 19-27); we are not concerned here with loss of phosphate as one component of general cell catabolism, although this also can cause muscle weakness. In RTA the degree of metabolic acidosis is not usually severe enough to be catabolic, but it could lead to preferential mobilization of muscle phosphate. Such a mechanism might also be activated by phosphate depletion itself, at least in males. In experimental phosphate depletion in male dogs, total muscle cell phosphate fell by 20 percent even though plasma P_i fell only to 0.54

mmol/L; there was a corresponding fall in resting E_M, consistent with loss of ATP (637). Whether female dogs would respond differently is not known. PTH also mobilizes muscle cell phosphate; in the parathyroidectomized rat this contributes about 60 percent of the increment in urinary phosphate excretion, only about 20 percent coming from bone and 20 percent from the ECF (700). This effect could give rise to a disproportionate loss of muscle cell phosphate in those patients with primary hyperparathyroidism who have severe muscle weakness (Table 19-46; Fig. 19-27).

The greater severity of muscle weakness in vitamin D deficiency than in XLH despite a lesser reduction in plasma P_i suggests that phosphate escapes more easily than normal from the muscle cell in response to hypophosphatemia (Table 19-46; Fig. 19-27). In the vitamin D-deficient rat, 25-HCC (but not 1,25-DHCC) increases P_i uptake

Table 19-46. Possible sites of impaired phosphate transport (intrinsic or extrinsic) in four diseases with hypophosphatemia

SITE OF DEFECTIVE TRANSPORT	VITAMIN D DEFICIENCY	PRIMARY HYPERPARA- THYROIDISM	NFH WITH OSTEOMALACIA	XLH WITH OSTEOMALACIA
Kidney	+	+	+	+
Bone	+	−	+	+
Muscle	+	+−	+	−
Gut	+	−	−	−

and ATP content of muscle, and vitamin D repletion restores muscle cell ATP more effectively than phosphate supplements alone, despite a lower plasma P_i level. These and other data suggest that one function of 25-HCC is to conserve tissue levels of phosphate in response to phosphate deprivation (701), an effect which is opposed to the acute mobilization of P_i by 1,25-DHCC. There is no direct evidence for this hypothesis in humans and 1,25-DHCC seems to be as effective as 25-HCC in improving muscle strength. The creatine phosphate and ATP in muscle were reported to be normal in one patient with postgastrectomy osteomalacia (702) but it is not clear that the appropriate referent was used. In nutritional rickets muscle cell actomyosin is reduced, a possible effect of ATP depletion (703). An alternative explanation for the additive effects of vitamin D depletion and hypophosphatemia on muscle weakness is that both vitamin D and phosphate are required for normal calcium transport in the sarcoplasmic reticulum (598).

Neither an effect of PTH nor of vitamin D can account for the severity of muscle weakness in NFH with osteomalacia and its absence in XLH. If the same general concept is valid, in NFH but not in XLH there must be an additional phosphate transport defect in the muscle cell membrane as well as in the renal tubule (Table 19-46; Fig. 19-27) such that phosphate leaks out of the cell more readily in response to hypophosphatemia. This is in keeping with the proposal of defective ion transport in multiple tissues as a unifying concept in the Fanconi syndrome (687).

Rickets and osteomalacia. These terms identify the state of the bones resulting from defective mineralization, before and after epiphyseal fusion; they are not used to denote the entire disease complex resulting from vitamin D deficiency which has been referred to as the osteomalacia syndrome (93). In rickets, mineralization of the cartilaginous growth plate and primary spongiosa is impaired, with accumulation of unmineralized cartilage and woven osteoid and eventual retardation or arrest of enchondral ossification. In osteomalacia, mineralization of lamellar bone is impaired, with accumulation of unmineralized lamellar osteoid and eventual retardation or arrest of appositional bone formation.

Although the mechanisms of mineralization in these tissues are not identical, they are sufficiently similar to be considered together for the purposes of this chapter. The clinical and radiographic features of rickets are the result of widening and broadening of the growth plate, swelling of the epiphyses, and skeletal deformities which are related to both age and activity. The clinical features of osteomalacia consist mainly of bone pain, especially of the spine, ribs, pelvis, and lower extremities, made worse by muscle strain, weight bearing, or pressure. The radiographic features consist of nonspecific demineralization with coarser trabeculation and occasional Looser zones or pseudofractures. There may also be thinning of cortices and subperiosteal resorption representing the osteoporosis and osteitis fibrosa of secondary hyperparathyroidism. More detailed accounts of various aspects of rickets and osteomalacia are given elsewhere (92, 93, 251); the remaining discussion will focus on the relationship between the state of the bones and the plasma P_i level.

The traditional histologic hallmark of osteomalacia is increased width of osteoid seams. Although the mineral appositional rate is reduced, the matrix appositional rate is reduced almost to the same extent so that osteoid seams grow in thickness quite slowly and persist for a long time. Osteoid covers a progressively increasing fraction of the bone surface and forms a progressively increasing fraction of the total volume of bone, but these changes are gradual. In most patients with osteomalacia of whatever etiology there is an increase in plasma AP and in kinetically determined calcium accretion rate, but these changes are not, as in other circumstances, indicative of increased osteoblastic activity. Total body bone formation and turnover may indeed be increased because of the frequently associated secondary hyperparathyroidism, but the function of individual osteoblasts is impaired (92). The rate of mineralization may be limited by the supply of calcium and phosphate ions, but in addition the maturation of matrix (which must occur prior to mineralization) is delayed and incomplete.

There is a generalized depression of osteoblast function in osteomalacia with respect to both matrix synthesis and mineralization and most likely a similar depression of chondroblast function in rickets. Both of these occur in phosphate depletion, vitamin D depletion, NFH, and XLH (Table 19-45), conditions which have in common only hypophosphatemia. The crucial importance of this in the pathogenesis of rickets and osteomalacia (Fig. 19-30) has been known for many years, and usually explained by failure of the ECF to attain some hypothetical solubility product, but there is no simple relationship between the plasma com-

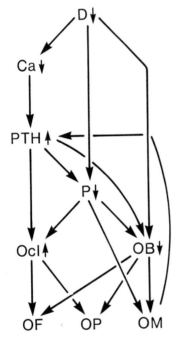

Figure 19-30. Interrelationships between disordered mineral metabolism and metabolic bone disease. Vitamin D deficiency (D↓) causes (a) hypocalcemia (Ca↓) directly and (b) hypophosphatemia (P↓) both directly and indirectly via secondary hyperparathyroidism (PTH↑) and (c) impaired osteoblast function (OB↓) directly and via hypophosphatemia. Secondary hyperparathyroidism increases osteoclast activity (Ocl↑) and contributes to further impairment of osteoblast function. Hypophosphatemia contributes to OM (osteomalacia) both directly and via impaired osteoblast function, and contributes further to increased osteoclast activity. Both increased osteoclast activity and decreased osteoblast function are concerned in the pathogenesis of both OF (osteitis fibrosa) and OP (osteoporosis), depending on the relative preponderance of different types of impaired cell function and the levels of plasma calcium and phosphate and other unknown factors.

position and the state of the bones (92). In chronic renal failure, what should be the protective effect of hyperphosphatemia might be offset by accumulation of mineralization inhibitors, but there are many other examples. Osteomalacia does not occur in most patients with hypophosphatemia due to a reduction in Tm_P/GFR (Table 19-40). In XLH, rickets may sometimes be delayed until adolescence (704) and many hypophosphatemic relatives have no clinical or radiographic evidence of bone disease throughout life (57). Such discordancies are to be expected in light of the impossibility of accounting for mineralization in purely physicochemical terms, and the crucial role of cells in the initiation and control of this process (Chap. 8).

In vitamin D deficiency the plasma P_i is usually not as low as in rickets and osteomalacia from other causes (93), and may be no lower than in many conditions not associated with rickets or osteomalacia such as Cushing's syndrome, estrogen treatment, or potassium depletion. This is partly due to the presence of hypocalcemia as well, but in addition to the experimental evidence presented in Chap. 8, there is much circumstantial clinical evidence for a role of vitamin D in mineralization, probably mediated by 24,25-HCC or 25-HCC or both. In rats, vitamin D is much more effective in preventing the histologic changes of rickets than $1,\alpha$-HCC, despite equivalent changes in plasma Ca and P_i levels (705). Similarly, in humans, a combination of 24,25-DHCC with 1,25-DHCC is more effective in correcting the abnormal bone mineralization of osteomalacia than 1,25-DHCC alone (84). The direct antirachitic effects of vitamin D metabolites are presumably mediated by actions on calcium and/or phosphate transport systems in bone cells, which are similar to those present in the gut and in the kidney (Table 19-46). Such ion transport systems might be concerned with uptake by the cell, transport within the cell, accumulation or release by mitochondria, extrusion from the cell, or the uptake and release of ions by membrane-bound matrix vesicles. A deficient supply or a fall in ionic activity of calcium or phosphate at the initial site of mineralization would therefore result from the additive effects of reduced ECF concentrations and defective membrane transport, or from either alone if sufficiently severe (Fig. 19-30).

This concept provides a satisfactory explanation for the variable effects of hypophosphatemia on bone, for the apparent resistance to vitamin D in phosphate depletion (706), and for the occurrence of rickets with the simultaneous hypocalcemia and hypophosphatemia of severe calcium deficiency in infancy (131), but the combination of a normal plasma Ca and low plasma P_i must still be reconciled with the blood-bone equilibrium at quiescent bone surfaces. Plasma is normally undersaturated with respect to secondary calcium phosphate, so that a fall in plasma P_i does not lead directly to any rise in plasma calcium. But if the bone fluid:P_i concentration fell to the same extent, dissolution of bone mineral would occur at the bone:fluid interface leading to a rise in bone fluid:calcium and eventually in plasma calcium; PTH secretion would fall, and the calcium homeostatic system would be inhibited (Table 19-47). According to either theory of the blood-bone equilibrium, a low plasma phosphate and normal plasma calcium can coexist in accordance with the physical chemistry of bone mineral, but only at the expense of a persistent decrease in PTH secretion.

The plasma iPTH does fall during phosphate depletion but how generally this occurs in asymptomatic hypophosphatemia due to a reduction in Tm_P/GFR is not known. Furthermore, when hypophosphatemia is accompanied by rickets or osteomalacia of whatever etiology, plasma iPTH is usually increased. Osteomalacia and secondary hyperparathyroidism are to be expected with de-

pletion of vitamin D or its metabolites, but both occur also in the absence either of abnormal vitamin D metabolism or of primary defects in intestinal absorption, as in XLH and NFH. Plasma iPTH is also raised in osteomalacia due to phosphate depletion alone (707) in which PTH secretion is initially reduced. The most likely explanation is that osteomalacia itself leads to mild hypocalcemia and secondary hyperparathyroidism because of increased surface extent of osteoid tissue. There is lack of available quiescent bone surface, not for osteoclastic resorption (a process which makes no contribution to steady-state plasma calcium regulation) but for operation of the calcium homeostatic system. Normally, osteoid seams are sites of net inward movement of calcium from blood to bone, but if mineralization becomes completely arrested, the cells on the surface of the osteoid become morphologically indistinguishable from the flat lining cells of normal bone. However, the ability of these cells to participate in the regulation of calcium homeostasis is likely to be impaired if they are separated from the mineralized bone by a thick layer of unmineralized osteoid tissue. The increasing and eventually complete envelopment of all bone surfaces by osteoid will inevitably increase the level of PTH required to maintain a normal plasma calcium (Fig. 19-30), but if the level of PTH is high enough even hypercalcemia may occur.

Any satisfactory theory of the pathogenesis of osteomalacia must account not only for the impairment of mineralization but for the defect in matrix synthesis, and there is considerable evidence that phosphate is concerned in this process

Table 19-47. Hypothetical adjustments to blood-bone equilibrium required to permit the plasma P_i to be changed without a change in plasma Ca, according to two different theories*

QUANTITY	PLASMA Pi DECREASED		PLASMA Pi INCREASED	
	NEUMAN	TALMAGE	NEUMAN	TALMAGE
Bone fluid: HPO_4^{2-}	↓	↓	↑	↑
Ca^{2+}	N	↑	N	↓
Activity product	↓	N	↑	N
H^+	↓	N	↑	N
Ca gradient—ECF:bone fluid	N	↓	N	↑
PTH secretion	↓	↓	↑	↑

* Both assume that HPO_4^{2-} is the same in both ECF and bone fluid (see Chap. 8).

also. In phosphate-depleted rats the rate of bone matrix synthesis is reduced by 60 percent (616). Furthermore, in rachitic rats deficient in vitamin D and phosphate, healing is associated with a substantial increase in total urinary hydroxyproline secretion which is due to increased collagen synthesis as well as to increased bone resorption (708). In patients with osteomalacia, vitamin D treatment frequently leads to similar changes in hydroxyproline excretion, probably for the same reasons, but in NFH this only occurs when phosphate is given as well (709). Bone formation determined by calcium kinetics increases significantly with vitamin D, and in NFH this occurs with phosphate treatment alone (710). The effects of phosphate on bone formation in tissue culture were described in Chap. 8.

These observations suggest a relationship between hypophosphatemia and impaired bone matrix synthesis in osteomalacia (Fig. 19-30). By analogy with muscle weakness, the most likely unifying principle is that impaired cell function (osteoblast or chondroblast) is due to IC depletion of P_i and consequently of ATP and other organic phosphate compounds. As in the muscle cell, IC depletion may be inevitable if the plasma P_i falls below 0.5 mmol/L but requires some additional factor if the plasma P_i remains above this level (Table 19-46 and Fig. 19-27). This factor is likely to be defective operation of a phosphate transport system in the osteoblast or chondroblast cell membrane such that IC P_i escapes more readily when the plasma P_i falls. This transport system could be the same as or distinct from that already postulated for the mineralization process, and this defect may be intrinsic and genetically determined in XLH and may be due to the unknown chemical mediator of hypophosphatemia in NFH, to metabolic acidosis in RTA, and to lack of 25-HCC or 24,25-DHCC in vitamin D depletion.

Treatment of hypophosphatemia

When this is due to a reduction in Tm_P/GFR it is difficult to correct except by removing the cause. Fortunately, in most of the conditions listed in Table 19-40 the hypophosphatemia requires no treatment. Both in NFH and XLH a modest increase in plasma P_i of 0.1 to 0.3 mmol/L may occur with vitamin D treatment for the rickets or osteomalacia, but whether this is due simply to suppression of PTH or to a direct effect of some vitamin D metabolite on the kidney is not known. The largest rise in plasma P_i and most favorable effect on growth occurred when renal failure was produced as a result of vitamin D intoxication (711). The diphosphonate EHDP raises the plasma P_i in normal subjects but in XLH the effect is small and the high doses needed would probably impair bone mineralization even further. None of the other known causes of increased Tm_P/GFR (p. 1083) could form the basis of an acceptable form of treatment, with the exception of ECF volume contraction. Although this does not produce chronic changes in plasma P_i in normal adults, dietary salt restriction in an infant with the oculocerebrorenal syndrome of Lowe reduced ECF volume and increased the tubular reabsorption of bicarbonate, amino acids, and phosphate, most likely in the proximal tubule. A significant increase in plasma P_i of 0.6 mmol/L was sustained for over 3 months and the rickets healed without any other treatment (712). In two cases of cystinosis similar results were achieved by a thiazide diuretic (713). The effect of ECF volume contraction in stimulating proximal reabsorption may have been reinforced by suppression of PTH as a result of renal retention of calcium. The opposite effect of thiazides on phosphate reabsorption and plasma P_i in idiopathic hypercalciuria indicates that the direct phosphaturic effect of the thiazides is predominant in adults, and the indirect antiphosphaturic effects are predominant in infants.

The only other way of raising the plasma P_i is by giving supplemental phosphate. Oral phosphate supplements may also be needed in the treatment of phosphate depletion, nephrolithiasis, and hypercalcemia. Several preparations are compared in Table 19-48. All are unpleasant to take and have a bitter, salty taste; they frequently cause abdominal pain and diarrhea. The most palatable is an effervescent tablet which is not available in

Table 19-48. Inorganic phosphate preparations for oral use*

NAME	FORM	CONTENT PER DOSAGE UNIT				
		P_i, mmol	Na, meq	K, meq	$\Delta H^+/P_i$,† meq/mmol	BUFFER,‡ meq/mmol
K Phos	Tablet	3.7	—	3.7	+0.80	0
K Phos Neutral	Tablet	8.0	12	2	+0.05	−0.74
Neutraphos	Capsule	8.0	7	7	+0.05	−0.74
Fleets phosphosoda	Solution (10 mL)	41.5	48	—	+0.63	−0.17

* Note difference in cation content and acid-base effect, calculated as: † Additional H^+ ions in relation to the HPO_4^{2-}:$H_2PO_4^-$ ratio in ECF; ‡ H^+ ions removed from the ECF, assuming complete excretion of the phosphate load at a urine pH of 5.0.

the United States. Unfortunately, the amounts required to increase the plasma P_i to normal are very large. In an adult with normal renal function an increase in plasma P_i of 0.5 mmol/L would require an increase in net input and output of 80 mmol per 24 h, corresponding to an increase in dietary intake of 120 mmol per 24 h; few patients can tolerate even as much as 60 mmol per 24 h for more than a short time. More success has been reported in children (692) but constant encouragement and close supervision of both mother and child were required. The effect on plasma P_i may be greater than predicted if metabolic acidosis is also present (714), since the commonly used preparations provide buffer as well as phosphate (Table 19-48). In XLH, phosphate supplements alone are ineffective (194) but they permit vitamin D to be given in smaller dosage and with greater safety. In NFH, phosphate supplements may be successful alone and are essential in all patients not only because of the greater phosphate depletion before treatment but because vitamin D alone may produce a large increase in urinary calcium excretion and little improvement in calcium balance (194, 676). Treatment of either XLH or NFH requires meticulous attention to detail continued over many years, and should be undertaken only by those with adequate knowledge and experience; further details are given elsewhere (645).

HYPERPHOSPHATEMIA

HP is the first cause of hyperphosphatemia to be considered by most physicians in the absence of renal failure, but this was present in only 1 of 84 cases accumulated in a 4-month period in a large general hospital (596). The many other causes are listed in Table 19-49; some of them are transient or asymptomatic and do not require extended discussion.

Table 19-49. Causes of hyperphosphatemia classified according to mechanism (see text for further details)

INCREASE IN Tm$_P$/GFR	INCREASE IN L/GFR	
HP	Decrease in GFR	Increase in L (endogenous)
PHP	Renal failure, acute or chronic	Respiratory acidosis
Hyperthyroidism	Increase in L (exogenous)	Diabetic ketoacidosis
Volume contraction	Too early weaning	Lactic acidosis
High temperature	Intragastric milk	Tissue ischemia
Juvenile hypogonadism	Increased absorption (vit. D)	Rhabdomyolysis
Postmenopausal state	Oral or intravenous phosphate	Malignant hyperpyrexia
Acromegaly	Laxatives or enemas	Cytotoxic therapy
Tumoral calcinosis	Transfusion of stored blood	Hemolysis
EHDP	White phosphorus burns	Familial

Mechanisms and causes

It is convenient to repeat the fundamental relationship underlying regulation of plasma phosphate:

$$P_p = \frac{L_p}{GFR} + \frac{TR_p}{GFR} \qquad (19\text{-}7)$$

With a normal GFR and normal Tm_p/GFR, plasma P_i would not rise above normal unless load were increased two- to threefold. Consequently, significant stable hyperphosphatemia with normal renal function is usually due to an increase in Tm_p/GFR. At normal loads persons with a high Tm_p/GFR are usually operating on the splay portion of the titration curve below the saturation threshold (Chap. 8), so that Tm_p/GFR may be appreciably greater than TR_p/GFR ($TR_p \times P_p/100$). Consequently an increase in Tm_p/GFR has a smaller effect on plasma P_i than a decrease in Tm_p/GFR by the same amount. For example, the increase in Tm_p/GFR of 0.95 mmol/L between grade 1 and grade 5 HP (Table 19-5) was accompanied by an increase in plasma P_i of only 0.60 mmol/L, although this was partly because L/GFR was reduced by 0.05 mmol/L. A high plasma P_i due only to a raised Tm_p/GFR rarely exceeds 2 mmol/L, and may not lead to any harmful effects. An increase in L/GFR is usually due to a fall in GFR alone; this is the most common single cause of hyperphosphatemia (596, 641) and is discussed in Chap. 20. An increase in load of sufficient magnitude can increase plasma P_i alone, but this occurs much more readily if GFR is also reduced. In this situation plasma P_i can rise rapidly and often causes serious harmful effects. Some hyperphosphatemic disorders have not been studied in sufficient detail to permit classification on this physiologic basis. For example, significant elevation of plasma P_i is found in muscular dystrophy (367) but the cause is unknown.

Increased Tm_p/GFR. An increase in the PTH-dependent component of whole kidney Tm_p/GFR is associated with a reduction in basel NcAMP excretion. This occurs with deficiency of PTH or resistance to its action; these disorders were discussed in relation to hypocalcemia. Temporary resistance to PTH occurs during infancy, and contributes to neonatal hyperphosphatemia (715). Resistance also occurs in magnesium depletion, but hyperphosphatemia (82) is due to reduced PTH secretion. Lithium, an inhibitor of adenylate cyclase activation in several tissues, has no effect on the renal-tubular response to PTH in humans (716). PTH is suppressed during calcium infusion, but the rise in plasma P_i occurs also in HP and is due more to an increase in load derived in some way from the soft tissues (367, 404). In nonparathyroid hypercalcemia, PTH is suppressed and NcAMP is low, but other factors (such as the phosphaturic effect of calcium) may work in the opposite direction, and plasma P_i is only rarely increased. A raised Tm_p/GFR ($+0.25$ to 0.3 mmol/L) and plasma P_i and suppressed NcAMP are regularly found in hyperthyroidism (707). About one-third of the patients have P_i values above the normal range, unless they have hyperparathyroidism as well; hyperthyroidism does not raise plasma P_i unless PTH secretion is suppressed. There is also an increase in load resulting from increased net bone resorption and progressive loss of muscle mass, but the negative balance rarely exceeds 6 to 8 mmol/day (345), which would raise the plasma P_i by only 0.05 mmol/L. The plasma P_i returns to normal in parallel with control of the disease. Tm_p/GFR is raised in phosphate depletion (612) and an immediate return to a normal phosphate intake conceivably could lead to transient hyperphosphatemia; this would be the converse of phosphate-induced hypophosphatemia but has not been reported in humans.

In the other causes of high Tm_p/GFR, normality of parathyroid function is usually presumed in the absence of data to the contrary, but detailed study is lacking and no measurements of NcAMP have been reported. ECF volume contraction after diuretic administration is associated with augmented phosphate reabsorption presumably in the proximal tubule. Together with a fall in GFR this may increase plasma P by 0.2 to 0.3 mmol/L, but this lasts only for a few hours (718). Chronic volume contraction as in Addison's disease is not accompanied by a rise in plasma P_i; correction of hypophosphatemia by volume contraction was mentioned earlier. A substantial rise in plasma P_i

from 1.3 mmol/L in winter to 2.0 mmol/L in summer with corresponding changes in Tm_P/GFR was noted in normal Japanese subjects (719); the mean plasma P_i correlated closely with atmospheric temperature throughout the year.

In juvenile hypogonadism in either sex there is a failure or delay in the normal fall in P_i which occurs during adolescence, so that the plasma P_i is high for the patients' age but not for their pubertal status (367); in adults with hypogonadism P_i is usually in the high normal range. The normal postmenopausal rise in Tm_P/GFR and P_i was mentioned earlier. In acromegaly both Tm_P/GFR and plasma P_i are increased by 0.2 to 0.4 mmol/L (17, 367) and about two-thirds of the patients have values above normal. The opposite effects of GH (growth hormone) and PTH on Tm_P/GFR are additive, but the effect of GH can be manifested in the absence of PTH (720). GH has no acute effect on phosphate reabsorption or excretion (721) so that its chronic effect may be indirect, mediated possibly by somatomedin.

A rare condition of considerable interest is familial tumoral calcinosis with hyperphosphatemia (366, 722). The plasma P_i is in the range of 2.5 to 3.5 mmol/L in children and 1.5 to 2.0 mmol/L in adults, with a corresponding elevation of Tm_P/GFR and normal GFR. Phosphate balance may be slightly positive but intestinal absorption and urinary excretion of phosphate are normal. In response to exogenous PTH both short-term changes in urinary phosphate excretion and long-term changes in plasma calcium have been normal. The high plasma P_i may precede the development of calcific lesions in some patients. Phosphate depletion by diet and aluminum hydroxide greatly reduces the size and number of the calcific deposits, whether the fall in plasma P_i is slight or substantial. Especially noteworthy is that the plasma calcium is normal or even slightly raised.

The last cause of raised Tm_P/GFR to be discussed is administration of EHDP (disodium etidronate; disodium-ethane-1-hydroxy-1,1-diphosphonate), a synthetic analogue of pyrophosphate which has found unexpected success in the treatment of Paget's disease. The effects on plasma P_i are dose dependent: with 20 mg/kg body weight per day plasma P_i rises slowly to a maximum of about 20 mmol/L after 3 weeks with a corresponding rise in Tm_P/GFR; with 5 mg/kg body weight per day there is no change in plasma P_i and with intermediate doses the rise is only transient despite continued administration (723, 724). EHDP has no effect on the plasma levels of PTH, growth hormone, cortisol, or thyroxine or on the response to exogenous PTH in terms of either cAMP or phosphate excretion (725). As in tumoral calcinosis the hyperphosphatemia of EHDP administration is unaccompanied by any change in plasma calcium.

Increased phosphate load. The phosphate load which has to be excreted by the kidney normally arises solely by absorption from the diet, but there are a variety of other exogenous and endogenous sources of surplus phosphate. With a continuous load arriving at a constant rate and a constant value for Tm_P/GFR the steady-state plasma P_i level varies both with load and with GFR (Fig. 19-31). Normally, as GFR falls Tm_P/GFR also falls because of secondary hyperparathyroidism, so that the plasma P_i does not rise as steeply as indicated. Load-dependent hyperphosphatemia much more commonly results from a large but transient excess, which produces an abrupt rise and fall in plasma P_i. If the load were to be delivered instantaneously, the maximum rise would be determined entirely by the volume of distribution and would be independent of GFR, but in practice the load is delivered over some period of time, usually between 6 and 18 h. The volume of distribution of a phosphate load must lie between the ECF volume (14 L) and the apparent volume of distribution corresponding to an exchangeable pool of 0.6 mmol/kg body weight, or 35 L for a 70-kg person. When 35 to 40 mmol of phosphate was infused over a 2-h period, the apparent volume of distribution was 22 L (724). The time course of the rise and fall of plasma P_i produced by a total load of 100 mmol arriving over either 6 or 24 h with a GFR of either 100 or 20 mL/min is shown in Fig. 19-32. With the slower delivery and normal GFR, a steady plasma level is attained after about 12 h. The lower GFR substantially increases the peak P_i level, but this effect is less with the shorter load; with both short and

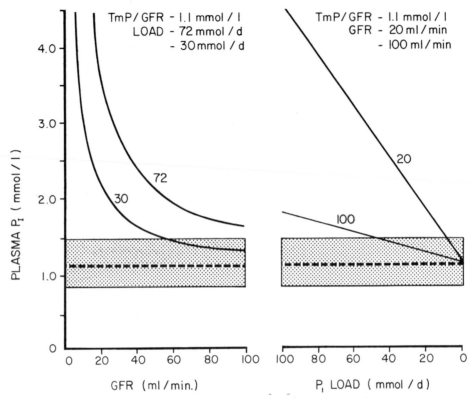

Figure 19-31. Steady-state P_i (plasma phosphate) concentrations at various levels of GFR and phosphate load, assuming a normal value for Tm_P/GFR. The shaded area encloses the normal range for plasma phosphate.

long loads the rate of decline is markedly reduced with the lower GFR. At these high blood levels, which are well above the saturation threshold, Tm_P/GFR has virtually no effect either on the peak level or on the rate of decline.

Exogenous Phosphate Loads. In infants the higher phosphate content of cow's milk than of human milk may contribute significantly to hyperphosphatemia, but in adults the dietary intake of phosphate is rarely high enough to raise the plasma P_i appreciably. However, continuous intragastric infusion of milk in the treatment of peptic ulceration may provide up to 60 to 100 mmol/day of phosphate and cause hyperphosphatemia (596) (Fig. 19-31). Vitamin D in large doses, either therapeutic or self-administered, increases phos-

phate absorption, which together with impaired renal function accounts for the frequent hyperphosphatemia in vitamin D poisoning and related disorders. Large amounts of oral phosphate are used in the treatment of osteomalacia, kidney stones, and hypercalcemia. Few patients can tolerate doses larger than 70 mmol/day; with net absorption of 60 percent the load would be 42 mmol/day. This would not produce hyperphosphatemia with normal renal function but only a modest decrease in GFR would be needed. Much larger loads can arise from ingestion of laxatives containing sodium phosphate such as Fleet's phosphosoda or sal hepatica. Fleet's phosphosoda contains 4.25 mmol of P_i/mL, appreciably more than the concentrated solution used as an intravenous additive. Not surprisingly, accidental poisoning sometimes occurs; as much as 1000 mmol of phosphate can be ingested in this way. With such enormous amounts much less than the usual 60 percent is absorbed, but even so the plasma P_i levels may rise as high as 10 to 20 mmol/L and

death may result (726). Less well known is that substantial absorption of P_i can occur from the large bowel when Fleet's phosphosoda is given as an enema, a procedure which has produced the highest plasma P_i levels (21 to 22 mmol/L) ever recorded (727, 728). One compulsive internal

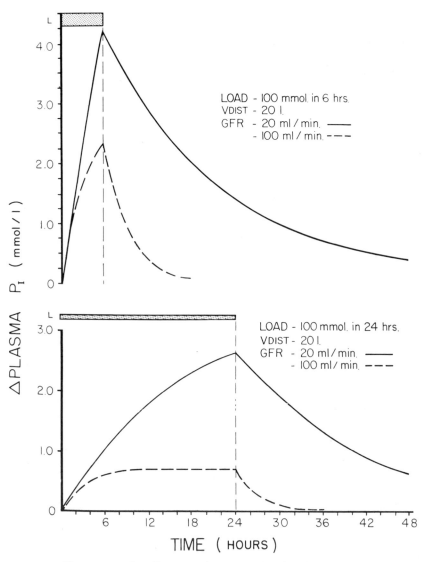

Figure 19-32. The effect on P_i of a sudden phosphate load of 100 mmol given over 6 h (upper panel) or 24 h (lower panel) at normal and at reduced GFR, assuming a volume of distribution of 20 L.

cleanser who lacked access to Fleet's phospho-soda used a phosphate-containing detergent for the same purpose (729). Most affected patients have been children, and many, but not all, have had either some disease of the bowel favoring prolonged retention of the enema or preexisting renal insufficiency. It is remarkable that no systematic study of plasma P_i levels in normal persons (adults or children) given sodium phosphate enemas has ever been carried out, and the widespread presumption of safety for this procedure is completely undocumented; several near fatalities have resulted. The abundance of sodium and the low pH (4.4 to 5.2) of the solution both favor absorption, and the massive influx of water produced by the hypertonicity could dissolve some of the precipitated phosphate already present in the stool.

Exogenous phosphate loads can also be given intravenously, either as an experimental procedure on in the treatment of phosphate depletion or hypercalcemia. The latter situation is much more dangerous, and the plasma P_i may rise precipitously if the guidelines given earlier are not followed. Phosphate can also be given unwittingly with blood transfusions. Even when stored under the most favorable conditions, the P_i concentration of blood rises steadily due to leakage from the cells and may reach 3 mmol/L by 3 weeks (141). However, the amount of phosphate given in this way will only rarely exceed 30 mmol, and the hyperphosphatemia reported during blood transfusion more likely results from the catabolic response to trauma, shock, or acidosis (741). Tetany during blood transfusion is related more to complexing of calcium by citrate than to the rise in plasma P_i. Phosphate may also be a contaminant in some preparations of heparin. A final route of entry of exogenous phosphate loads is via the skin, as a result of white phosphorus burns produced by incendiary bombs, a common occurrence during modern warfare (730). This substance ignites spontaneously on exposure to oxygen to form P_2O_5 (phosphorous pentoxide). On contact with water this forms pyrophosphoric acid ($P_2O_5 + 2H_2O \rightarrow H_2P_2O_7$) which in turn is converted to orthophosphoric acid ($H_2P_2O_7 + H_2O \rightarrow 2H_3PO_4$). Absorption of orthophosphate through the burned skin may raise the plasma P_i to 3 to 4 mmol/L in some patients with no change in others; a similar difference was noted with experimental white phosphorus burns in rabbits, much higher P_i (and lower Ca) levels occurring in the animals that died (730).

Endogenous Phosphate Loads. In contrast to exogenous phosphate loads in which external phosphate balance is positive, endogenous loads result from net loss of P_i from bone or soft tissues with negative external balance; the urinary excretion of phosphate is increased in both instances. Even with widespread osteolytic metastases net loss of P_i from bone rarely exceeds 5 to 10 mmol/day, which can cause no significant elevation of plasma P_i with normal renal function. The extent of resorption surface correlates with plasma P_i in osteoporosis (731), but this is because both are consequences of postmenopausal estrogen deficiency, not because increased bone resorption raises the plasma P_i. PTH-induced bone resorption is believed to contribute to hyperphosphatemia in chronic renal failure, but the fall in plasma P_i after parathyroidectomy is mainly a transient effect of greatly increased net bone formation, as occurs after parathyroidectomy in primary hyperparathyroidism with osteitis fibrosa. Bone marrow hyperplasia as in thalassemia or sickle cell anemia may lead to increased net bone resorption and account for a negative phosphate balance; a rise in plasma P_i is more likely due to hemolysis directly (596).

Experimental respiratory acidosis in the dog raises the plasma P_i to 5 to 6 mmol/L within a few hours (732), but whether the same rise occurs in patients with respiratory failure is not known. Hyperphosphatemia due to the catabolic effect of diabetic ketoacidosis was mentioned earlier. Lactic acidosis is even more prone to raise the plasma P_i; the mean value was 3.0 mmol/L in one series compared to 1.8 mmol/L in patients with diabetic ketoacidosis who had similar levels of blood pH and BUN (733). This most likely results from the tissue hypoxia which gives rise to lactic acidosis, with breakdown of ATP to AMP and P_i (734, 735). This mechanism probably contributes to the hyperphosphatemia which develops during major cardiopulmonary surgery (70).

Since muscle contains the bulk of soft tissue phosphate, necrosis of muscle tissue (rhabdomyolysis) is a potent cause of hyperphosphatemia. Rhabdomyolysis complicates a wide variety of diseases, including direct trauma, viral infections, envenomizations, heroin, ethanol and other toxic agents, heat stroke, and idiopathic paroxysmal myoglobinuria (736, 737). In heat stroke rhabdomyolysis leading to hyperphosphatemia may be preceded by hypophosphatemia due to hyperventilation (738). The situation is complicated by the frequent occurrence of acute renal failure due to myoglobin in patients with rhabdomyolysis, the original crush syndrome. The contribution of phosphate liberation from damaged muscle to the hyperphosphatemia is indicated by a higher phosphate/BUN ratio both in traumatic renal failure (239) and in nontraumatic rhabdomyolysis (737) than in nontraumatic renal failure. Individual values as high as 6 to 7 mmol/L may occur. A similar difference exists for potassium and presumably also for magnesium, although this is less well documented. The rise in plasma P_i may precede any rise in BUN or creatinine and occasionally may occur in the complete absence of renal failure (740).

A particularly interesting form of muscle injury leading to hyperphosphatemia occurs in malignant hyperpyrexia. Susceptible individuals usually have a mild but unusual subclinical myopathy, and soon after exposure to a wide variety of anesthetics their body temperature rises abruptly by 2 to 3°C/h due to excessive heat production by muscle. The underlying abnormality is thought to be inappropriate release or inadequate storage of calcium by the sarcoplasmic reticulum. Neither overt rhabdomyolysis with myoglobinuria nor acute renal failure occurs, but the muscles are often rigid, the CPK rises markedly within a few hours, and hyperkalemia is common. Histologic evidence of widespread muscle injury with focal necrosis is found at autopsy. Hyperphosphatemia has only rarely been sought, but levels as high as 4 to 5 mmol/L may occur within a few hours (741, 742).

Cytotoxic therapy is an important cause of massive cell destruction and liberation of IC constituents into the circulation. Particularly in acute lymphoblastic leukemia but also in various types of lymphoma and acute myeloproliferative syndromes, lysis of tumor cells beginning within 1 to 2 days of initiating treatment is soon followed by a rise in plasma P_i, usually accompanied also by a rise in plasma uric acid (743, 744). As judged by rates of urinary excretion, the increase in load begins within 12 h, persists for about 48 h, and may be as high as 100 to 200 mmol/day. This reflects the high total phosphate content of both lymphoblasts and myeloblasts, which is up to four times greater than the corresponding mature cells (743). Because of the slower rate of influx of phosphate than in rhabdomyolysis the plasma P_i usually does not rise above 2 to 3 mmol/L, although levels as high as 5 to 6 mmol/L can occur, particularly if the patient also gets acute urate nephropathy. Because of the age distribution of the underlying diseases, this phenomenon occurs most commonly in children and adolescents, but no age is immune. Hyperphosphatemia due to cell breakdown may also occur in hemolytic anemia, resolving hematomas, and in chronic myelogenous leukemia with massive leukocytosis even before treatment (596).

The rarest cause of an endogenous phosphate load is a bizarre disorder so far described only in three members of a single family (745). It is characterized by the onset in infancy of episodes of sudden, severe hyperphosphatemia (3 to 6 mmol/L) leading to tetany, with increased urinary phosphate excretion (50 mmol per 24 h), polyuria with hyposthenuria and minimal hypernatremia, fever, and convulsive seizures. In between attacks the patients were completely normal to extensive testing, and no functional abnormality of liver, brain, muscle, bone, or blood cells could be found during the attacks. The source of the excess phosphate could not be identified. A surreptitious exogenous source was ruled out by the occurrence of typical attacks in hospital under close scrutiny.

Effects

The most important long-term consequence of hyperphosphatemia is soft tissue calcification, which occurs mainly in patients with reduced GFR or high Tm_P/GFR. The most important short-term consequence is tetany, which occurs mainly in patients with an increase in phosphate load. The mild hyperphosphatemia of growth hormone excess or sex hormone deficiency has no known harmful effects.

In chronic renal failure hyperphosphatemia is accompanied by an increase in red cell 2,3-DPG with a corresponding increase in P_{50}; this partially protects against the adverse effects of anemia on tissue oxygenation. The hyperphosphatemia of normal growth is also accompanied by a high 2,3-DPG and P_{50} which may be the explanation for the so-called physiologic anemia of normal childhood (693); red cell glycolysis and ATP content are also increased by both normal and abnormal hyperphosphatemia. Similar changes in IC organic phosphate in other tissues may account for some of the effects of phosphate excess.

Mineral and hormonal effects of supplemental phosphate. In some ways these are the converse of the effects of phosphate depletion. In response to an increase in net absorption, plasma P_i rises at first, which leads to an increase in urinary phosphate excretion. In time the kidney adapts by decreasing Tm_P/GFR to partially offset the rise in L/GFR; this permits the surplus phosphate to be excreted with a minimal rise in the plasma P_i level (746, 747). For this reason the plasma P_i in the fasting state can be subnormal in a subject adapted to a high phosphate intake, even though the mean plasma P_i throughout the day is slightly increased.

The mechanism of this adaptive fall in Tm_P/GFR is not fully understood. As discussed later, the plasma calcium falls at first and PTH secretion increases, which initiates the fall in Tm_P/GFR. Later, some other mechanism, possibly a rise in IC phosphate within the renal tubule analogous to the changes in the red cells, maintains the reduction in Tm_P/GFR and PTH secretion returns to normal (559). The capacity of this intrinsic renal mechanism is limited; phosphate supplements in the range of 50 to 70 mmol/day corresponding to loads of 30 to 40 mmol/day can be accommodated in this way, but much larger loads lead to persistent secondary hyperparathyroidism and eventually to osteitis fibrosa in various animal species (748). Whether the long-term effect of moderate phosphate loads on bone is

good, bad, or indifferent is not known; support can be found for all three possibilities.

Although most of the surplus phosphate is excreted, phosphate administration consistently causes a small positive balance of phosphate and calcium in both normal subjects (749) and in patients with idiopathic hypercalciuria or primary hyperparathyroidism (553), presumably due to increased net storage in bone by one or more of the short-term mechanisms described in Chap. 8. The positive calcium balance is effected by a reduction in urinary calcium excretion, with no change in net absorption or fecal excretion of calcium. As with the decrease in tubular reabsorption of phosphate, the increase in tubular reabsorption of calcium may be initiated by increased PTH secretion, but it persists after the PTH level returns to normal and can occur in patients with HP (750). In normal subjects there is an inverse correlation between plasma P_i and plasma 1,25-DHCC (614), but the absence of a fall in calcium absorption with phosphate supplements in the range of 40 to 650 mmol/day makes it unlikely that there is any substantial fall in 1,25-DHCC production. Nevertheless, it is conceivable that much larger amounts of phosphate depress calcium absorption and lead to a sustained increase in PTH secretion, in part by reducing 1,25-DHCC synthesis.

A fall in plasma total and ionized calcium is a consistent effect of an abrupt rise in plasma P_i, which is discussed later in relation to phosphate-induced tetany, but in chronic hyperphosphatemia the plasma calcium remains normal unless there is deficiency of PTH, resistance to PTH, or deficiency of 1,25-DHCC as in HP, PHP, or chronic renal failure. The lack of hypocalcemia with EHDP-induced hyperphosphatemia is probably a result of binding of the EHDP to bone mineral at quiescent bone surfaces, thus insulating the bone from changes in the bone ECF. There is no tendency to hypocalcemia with the modest hyperphosphatemia of acromegaly or sex hormone deficiency or the severe hyperphosphatemia of tumoral calcinosis. The different responses to acute and chronic hyperphosphatemia indicate that phosphate retention cannot be the whole explanation for secondary hyperparathyroidism in chronic renal failure (Chap. 20).

The solubility of secondary calcium phosphate

at normal body pH is such that precipitation from the ECF would not occur unless the plasma P_i were raised above 2.5 mmol/L. Nevertheless, the combination of high plasma P_i and normal plasma calcium must require some adjustment in the blood-bone equilibrium. According to either the Talmage or the Neuman theories, by the converse of the changes postulated for a low plasma P_i (Table 19-47), a high plasma P_i and normal plasma calcium can coexist in accordance with the physical chemistry of bone mineral but at the expense of a persistent increase in PTH secretion. Data on plasma iPTH levels in chronic hyperphosphatemic states other than renal failure are meager, but indicate that PTH is not always raised.

Soft tissue calcification. This is an exceedingly complex subject, most of which is outside the scope of the present chapter (366). In dystrophic calcification the sequestered mineral withdrawn from the ECF would tend to lower the plasma calcium and P_i levels unless these are replaced. This could occur by increasing either net intestinal absorption or net bone resorption, or decreasing urinary excretion, or by a combination of these mechanisms. Limited data suggests that there is increased PTH secretion (751), increased tubular reabsorption of calcium, and increased bone turnover but no change in calcium absorption (752). Parathyroid hyperplasia has frequently been found at autopsy (753).

The relationship between prolonged hyperphosphatemia and metastatic soft tissue calcification is most clear in chronic renal failure (Chap. 20); the rate of decline of renal function may be influenced by the extent of soft tissue calcification in the kidney itself (754). Hyperphosphatemia also contributes to soft tissue calcification in the various forms of hyperabsorption hypercalcemia and in tumoral calcinosis, and soft tissue calcification may be worsened by phosphate treatment for hypercalcemia. Control of hyperphosphatemia by diet and aluminum hydroxide has led to improvement in soft tissue calcification in chronic renal failure (366) and in tumoral calcinosis (722). In calcinosis secondary to connective tissue disease, a small reduction in plasma P_i within the normal range produced by aluminum hydroxide and probenecid has improved soft tissue calcification even though hyperphosphatemia is not an etiologic factor (755). The milder hyperphosphatemia of vitamin D-treated HP may account for the not infrequent occurrence of calcific periarthritis in these patients, and probably contributes to their modest decline in renal function (376).

Hypocalcemia and tetany. An increased phosphate load from any source, exogenous or endogenous, frequently causes hypocalcemia and tetany (726–730, 740–744). There is a significant inverse relationship between plasma calcium and P_i, but the confidence limits are very wide so that for a plasma P_i of 4 mmol/L the total calcium could vary between 1.0 and 2.0 mmol/L; the relationship is the same in patients with rhabdomyolysis as in patients with an exogenous phosphate load or with lysis of tumor cells. Significant hypocalcemia and even tetany may occur with a plasma P_i of 2 mmol/L, a level which if reached slowly has little or no effect on plasma calcium. It is possible that after an initial rise of P_i to a higher level both calcium and phosphate fall together due to deposition in soft tissue or bone (Fig. 19-33).

In patients with either exogenous or endogenous phosphate loads, the plasma calcium falls by about 0.2 mmol/L for each 1.0-mmol/L rise in plasma P_i. In normal subjects given phosphate infusions the corresponding ratio has varied over a ten-fold range between 0.03 and 0.30 (756–758) (Table 19-50). Neither the amount infused, the duration or rate of infusion, the presence or absence of potassium in the infusate, nor whether or not total plasma calcium is corrected for dilution of plasma proteins accounts for this difference. When phosphate infusions are given to patients, the extent of the fall in plasma calcium varies directly with the initial plasma calcium level. This is in keeping with a purely physicochemical explanation in terms of exceeding the solubility product of secondary calcium phosphate (756). But the hypocalcemic effect is also greater in patients with metabolic bone disease of any kind than in those without (758), so that biologic factors, presumably involving differences in bone cell function, must also be important. For example, in untreated rickets a phosphate load may cause significant hypocalcemia, whereas after vitamin D treatment the same load produces no

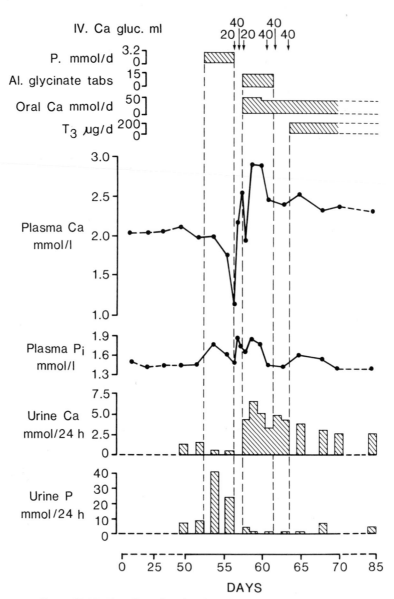

Figure 19-33. The effect of a phosphate load on a patient with partial HP (grade 3) (55) and mild hypothyroidism. After an initial rise in plasma phosphate both calcium and phosphate fell together, suggesting deposition of both in bone. This led to severe hypocalcemia and tetany. Normocalcemia was restored by correcting hypothyroidism and giving a calcium supplement. In patients receiving vitamin D the hypocalcemic effect of the same phosphate supplement is very much smaller (750).

Table 19-50. Effect of phosphate infusion on plasma calcium in normal subjects: Comparison of three different studies by Hebert (756), Better (757), and Stamp (758)

	HEBERT	BETTER	STAMP
Amount infused (mmol/kg)	1.81	1.5	1–1.2
Duration of infusion (h)	6	4	2½
Rate of infusion (mmol/kg per h)	0.3	0.4	0.4–0.6
Anion (Na/K)	8/1	8/1	All Na
Mean rise in P_i (mmol/L)	2.18	1.64	2.93
Mean fall in Ca (mmol/L)	0.18	0.51	0.08
$\Delta Ca/\Delta P$ (mmol/mmol)	0.08	0.31	0.03
Protein correction	No	No	Yes

change in plasma calcium despite the same or even greater rise in plasma P_i (759). The susceptibility to phosphate-induced hypocalcemia has been used as a diagnostic test for subclinical vitamin D deficiency in infants.

In acute traumatic renal failure with extensive muscle injury plasma calcium and P_i show a somewhat closer and more predictable relationship (760) (Fig. 19-34) than in acute hyperphosphatemia from other causes. The lesser fall in plasma calcium may result from a greater increase in PTH secretion but the hypocalcemia responds only transiently to calcium infusion. In dogs subjected to nephrectomy and muscle trauma, the damaged muscle increased its calcium content 10- to 15-fold with sufficient rapidity to be a major factor both in the genesis of hypocalcemia and its refractoriness to treatment (158). Once deposited, the calcium exchanges less freely and was presumed to be bound to denatured cell protein. In nontraumatic rhabdomyolysis, although phosphate is liberated from the injured muscle cell, the structure of the tissue is better preserved and denaturation of cell protein less evident, so that calcification is less extensive; the

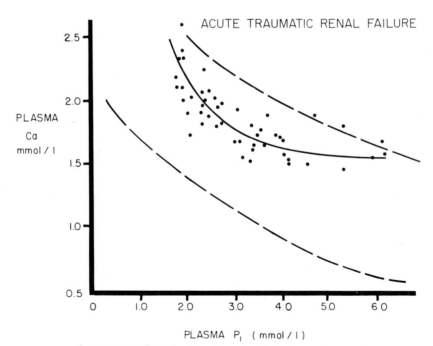

Figure 19-34. Effect of sudden hyperphosphatemia on plasma calcium in acute traumatic renal failure. Points and solid line taken from Meroney (760); dotted lines enclose a wide scatter of relationships observed with exogenous phosphate loads or endogenous loads with or without rhabdomyolysis.

lower plasma calcium levels of nontraumatic rhabdomyolysis cannot be attributed to increased soft tissue calcification. However, traumatic and nontraumatic rhabdomyolysis have in common the frequent occurrence of hypercalcemia during the diuretic recovery phase of myoglobinuric renal failure (736, 636). This has been ascribed to the severity of the hypocalcemia and consequent intensity of the stimulus to increased PTH secretion, but hypercalcemia has never followed the equally or even more severe hypocalcemia induced by hyperphosphatemia from other causes. Other mechanisms, such as increased mobilization of 25-HCC, must therefore contribute to the hypercalcemia (Chap. 20).

Treatment of hyperphosphatemia

Plasma P_i may be reduced by reducing Tm_P/GFR, increasing GFR, or decreasing L [Eq. (19-1)]. If none of these are possible, phosphate may be removed from the body by dialysis or temporarily sequestered in bone or soft tissues. If hyperphosphatemia is due to a high Tm_P/GFR, it will usually respond to treatment of the underlying disease. Apart from vitamin D or its metabolites given as a substitute for PTH, there is no satisfactory pharmacologic means of reducing Tm_P/GFR. Probenecid decreases tubular reabsorption of phosphate to a limited extent in patients with HP, but the response is unpredictable. Most diuretics increase urinary phosphate excretion acutely, and urinary phosphate may remain modestly increased during the first 1 to 2 weeks of thiazide administration, but long-term lowering of plasma P_i is unusual. In tumoral calcinosis and in chronic renal failure (excluding dialysis or transplantation) hyperphosphatemia can be controlled by restricting dietary intake and by giving aluminum hydroxide. The same measures with or without probenecid may be useful in load-dependent hyperphosphatemia, but more important are intravenous administration of calcium and urgent removal of phosphate by dialysis. If this is not available a small temporary fall in plasma P_i may follow administration of glucose and insulin, as in the emergency treatment of hyperkalemia. The

hyperphosphatemia of tumor cell lysis might be lessened by prior administration of allopurinol to prevent urate neuropathy.

DISORDERS OF MAGNESIUM METABOLISM

Because of its presence in bone, magnesium is closely related to calcium and phosphate, but because it is a major IC cation magnesium also resembles potassium in several respects, and is similarly influenced by the same agents and diseases.

THE CLINICAL PHYSIOLOGY OF MAGNESIUM

Background information is given in Chap. 8. In contrast to calcium and phosphate no known hormone has a dominant controlling effect on normal magnesium metabolism. For example, in high doses vitamin D increases intestinal absorption and PTH increases tubular reabsorption of magnesium, but changes in vitamin D status and PTH secretion within the normal range have no effect on magnesium metabolism.

The regulation of total body magnesium

As for phosphate, it is useful to distinguish between capacity, concentration, and content. The magnesium capacity and content of bone depend only on the total amount of bone mineral, but the concentration of magnesium in bone is so small that even large changes in bone mass or mineral content can have no detectable effects on plasma or urinary magnesium. Magnesium is not an integral component of bone mineral, but is confined to the hydration shell and crystal surface (Chap. 8), so that the concentration of magnesium in bone can vary much more readily than the concentration of calcium or phosphate. About 30 percent of bone magnesium is exchangeable in vitro, but in vivo only 1 percent is exchangeable within 24 h and 5 percent exchangeable within a week. As well as short-term gains or losses resulting from heteroionic exchange, the magnesium concentration of newly formed bone varies with the plasma magnesium level, so that long-term changes in bone magnesium can result from the normal process of bone turnover.

The magnesium capacity of soft tissues depends on the number of cells and the number of IC sites of magnesium binding or sequestration, which in turn depends on the amount of IC protein. The normal ratios of magnesium to nitrogen, potassium, and phosphate in some representative tissues are given in Table 19-35. Gains or losses of cell protein or cell potassium are accompanied by corresponding gains or losses of magnesium in accordance with these ratios; muscle is quantitatively the most important tissue, containing about 80 percent of the total magnesium of the active cell mass. Only about 10 percent of this is present as free ions in the cytosol (0.2 to 1.0 mmol/L), much less than predicted from the cell membrane potential by the Nernst equation, so that magnesium is probably pumped out of cells.

The regulation of plasma magnesium

In contrast to phosphate, there is no significant difference in plasma magnesium between the sexes, no significant effect of age in either sex, and much less intra- and interindividual variation (13, 42). Total plasma magnesium concentration measured by double-beam flame photometry or atomic absorption spectrophotometry varies little between different laboratories, with representative values of 0.85 ± 0.5 mmol/L with a ± 2 S.D. range of 0.75 to 0.95 mmol/L. Higher and more variable results were obtained with older chemical methods. The level of IC magnesium is usually stable, and net shifts between EC and IC compartments do not occur. For magnesium, as for phosphate, the kidney is the major determinant of the steady-state plasma level, which automatically adjusts so that output by the kidney balances net input to the ECF. The relative contributions of load, GFR, and tubular reabsorption to the plasma Mg level are defined by the relationship

$$P_{Mg} = \frac{U_{Mg}V}{GFR} + \frac{TR_{Mg}}{GFR} \qquad (19\text{-}8)$$

Normally TR_{Mg}/GFR is close to or equal to $Tm_{Mg} \cdot GFR$. In the early-morning fasting state with normal renal function U_{Mg}/GFR is normally in the range of 0.01 to 0.03 mmol/L, and tubular reabsorption accounts for about 97 percent of the plasma level (Chap. 8). Net bone resorption makes no detectable contribution to fasting $U_{Mg}V/GFR$, which is derived entirely from the exchangeable pool in interstitial fluid, soft tissue, and bone. During an 8-h overnight fast this becomes depleted to the extent of about 1 mmol. In the nonfasting state $U_{Mg}V/GFR$ is normally in the range of 0.02 to 0.04 mmol/L, and tubular reabsorption contributes about 95 percent to the plasma level. In an adult in zero external balance urinary magnesium is derived entirely from net absorption, and so from the diet. In normal subjects net absorption as judged by urinary excretion varies from 1.5 to 10 mmol/day with a mean value of around 4 to 5 mmol/day (761). During the course of a 16-h period of food intake, net absorption of 4 mmol would provide about 3 mmol for urinary excretion and about 1 mmol to replenish the exchangeable pool in preparation for the next period of fasting and continued urinary excretion.

The same three principles govern the regulation of plasma Mg in disease as of plasma phosphate. First, plasma Mg is normally regulated by TM_{Mg}/GFR. Second, the contribution of load ($U_{Mg}V/GFR$) to plasma level is small with normal renal function, increases as GFR declines, but does not become dominant until GFR falls below 10 mL/min. Third, if net input of magnesium into the ECF is negative, plasma Mg can no longer be regulated by the kidney and will continue to fall until mobilization from soft tissue and bone balances the external loss.

HYPOMAGNESEMIA AND MAGNESIUM DEPLETION (762–767)

Mechanisms and causes (Table 19-51)

In magnesium depletion there is a reduction in the Mg/N ratio in the active cell mass in the soft tissues and to a lesser extent a reduction in the Mg/Ca ratio in bone. A primary loss of IC mag-

Table 19-51. Causes of magnesium deficiency and hypomagnesemia

Internal redistribution[a]	Carbohydrate loading
Postparathyroidectomy	Osmotic diuresis
Acute pancreatitis	Saline diuresis
Treatment of diabetic ketoacidosis	Ammonium chloride
Correction of acidosis in renal failure	Post-urinary obstruction
Refeeding after starvation	Renal transplantation
Intravenous glucose and amino acids	Decreased Tm_{Mg}/GFR (extrinsic)
External losses	Primary hyperaldosteronism[e]
Nasogastric suction	Secondary hyperaldosteronism
Biliary fistula	Potassium depletion
Profuse sweating	ADH excess[e]
Massive lactation	Barrter's syndrome
Magnesium-free dialysis	Diuretic therapy
Extensive burns	Hyperthyroidism
Negative net absorption	Hypercalcemia[f]
Very low intake	HP
Excess fecal water	Decreased Tm_{Mg}/GFR (intrinsic)
Excess fecal fat[b]	Tubulointerstitial nephropathy
Malabsorption (generalized)[c]	Familial, with hypokalemia
Malabsorption (selective)	Aminoglycoside nephropathy
Increased renal excretion (transient)	Idiopathic—with other tubular disorders
Organic aciduria[d]	Idiopathic—without other tubular disorders
Ethanol loading	

[a] Particularly if preceded by cell catabolism (Table 19-38).

[b] Without mucosal disease, e.g., pancreatic deficiency or exudative enteropathy.

[c] Mucosal disease, with or without steatorrhea.

[d] For example, lactate or acetoacetate in poorly controlled diabetes.

[e] Due to ECF volume expansion.

[f] Including hyperparathyroidism.

nesium leads to a secondary negative external balance, and a primary negative balance causes secondary loss of IC and bone magnesium. In many disease states both processes occur with simultaneous losses from both IC and EC compartments. Chronic hypomagnesemia is usually due to a reduction in net intestinal absorption or in Tm_{Mg}/GFR, and in either case may occur with or without magnesium depletion and clinical effects, with only an approximate correspondence with the plasma magnesium level.

One source of confusion in the study of magnesium depletion is the use of inappropriate referents for the results of analysis of tissue composition. These are best referred to noncollagen nitrogen (768) or to IC protein nitrogen (769) but most published data use whole tissue wet weight or fat-free dry weight. In Table 19-52 various referents are compared for normal muscle, which

has been the tissue most frequently analyzed for diagnostic purposes. In catabolic states the amounts of connective tissue and of nuclear constituents change much less than the amount of tissue protoplasm. A 20 percent loss of cell substance without a change in composition will reduce all cell constituents expressed per kg dry weight by about 5 percent, and a 50 percent loss

Table 19-52. Composition of muscle by comparing various referents

REFERENT	N, g	Mg, mmol	K, mmol	P, mmol
kg fresh tissue (wet wt)*	31	8.3	92	59
kg fat-free dry wt*	148	39.5	438	281
g total tissue N	1	0.27	3.0	1.9
g intracellular N*	1.15	0.31	3.4	2.2
g noncollagen N†	1.15	0.31	3.5	2.1

* Data from Widdowson and Dickerson (769).

† Data from Baldwin et al. (68).

of cell substance will reduce the values by about 15 percent. These apparent changes will be larger in older persons who have a relatively greater amount of connective tissue.

The measurement of muscle Mg content is not invalidated by the usual close correlation between Mg and K in muscle (770). Loss of muscle K leads to a secondary depletion of muscle Mg, but the converse is also true: whichever is the primary deficit, its correction leads to restoration of both (771, 772). The general principle seems to be that because of the close relationship between K, P, and Mg within the cell, IC deficiency of any one element tends to cause loss of the others, although not necessarily in the same proportion as within the cell. K and Mg are also similarly affected by many diseases causing impaired absorption or increased renal loss. These varying causes of low muscle Mg will be associated with different values for the Mg/K ratio. Provided these pitfalls in interpretation are kept in mind, muscle Mg is a useful index of Mg depletion but K and noncollagen N should always be measured as well.

Magnesium depletion can be recognized without tissue analysis if there is a significant retention of magnesium when extra magnesium is given, but this requires measurement of external balance which is usually impractical. The same principle is made use of in the magnesium-load test, which requires only collection of urine (766, 773). In a normal subject 75 to 80 percent of an administered load is excreted in the urine within 24 h, but a magnesium-deficient subject will retain an abnormally high proportion of the load. The test is valid only if tubular reabsorption of magnesium is not impaired and if intestinal excretion of the load is insignificant; both of these assumptions can be in error in patients with chronic intestinal disease (765, 774). Red cell Mg reflects the ECF Mg at the time the cells were made, so that if red cell Mg is normal, a low plasma Mg is probably of recent onset. A similar comment applies to bone magnesium content, which varies with stable plasma magnesium level over a wide range and is the most accurate guide to total body magnesium (775).

Primary mobilization of IC Mg. Proportional cell breakdown occurs in partial starvation, hy-perthyroidism, infection, and trauma (Table 19-38); this will reduce total body magnesium but does not constitute magnesium depletion. Balance studies in obese subjects treated by prolonged total starvation showed loss of magnesium which was disproportionate to the loss of nitrogen with a fall in muscle Mg to around 30 mmol/kg fat-free weight (778); urinary magnesium is in the range of 1 to 3 mmol/day (775, 776), much higher than on a magnesium-free but otherwise adequate diet. This is probably due to the added effect of ketoacidosis, and the extra magnesium load is probably derived from bone as well as from soft tissues. (See also Chap. 27.) Disproportionate cell breakdown with relatively greater loss of Mg than of N also occurs in protein-calorie malnutrition in children, despite a relative increase in cell water. This was shown by a fall in the Mg/N ratio in muscle biopsies (589), and a relatively greater whole body retention of Mg than of N during recovery (590). The deficit relative to N is greater for Mg than for K in some cases (589), and greater for K than for Mg in others (777), presumably due to differences in the degree of dietary depletion. In diabetic ketoacidosis there is relatively greater loss of cell water and its attendant ions (Mg as well as K and P_i) than of cell substance (591, 592), with Mg deficits of 20 to 40 mmol. As for P_i and K, increased net loss from cells and reduced GFR may significantly raise the plasma Mg level in diabetic ketoacidosis. Chronic renal failure is another catabolic state sometimes associated with loss of muscle Mg (778).

As mentioned earlier, there is preferential loss of magnesium from both bone and soft tissue in hyperparathyroidism. In experimental hyperparathyroidism in the dog, diminished cell uptake of magnesium is a consequence of hypercalcemia, PTH itself having the opposite effect (779), but in human subjects PTH appears to have a generalized catabolic effect on soft tissues which is not found in other hypercalcemic states. Low values for muscle Mg were found in 12 of 18 patients with hyperparathyroidism, with a modest rise within 1 week of operation (780). There was a significant correlation between plasma and muscle Mg, but the plasma Mg was normal in most of the patients with low muscle Mg. Severe hypomagnesemia due to restoration of normal bone and soft tissue magnesium after parathyroidectomy (781) must be distinguished from mild asymptomatic hypomagnesemia which occurs frequently after all surgical operations (782).

With mobilization of IC Mg for whatever reason, plasma Mg is usually normal or raised, but severe acute hypomagnesemia may follow reversal of these shifts, as after successful parathyroid surgery, with effective treatment of diabetic ketoacidosis (783), provision of magnesium-free calories to a starved patient (784), or correction of metabolic acidosis in chronic renal failure (785). Plasma magnesium also falls after administration of amino acids and glucose in acute renal failure (786), and with deposition in necrotic tissue in acute pancreatitis (764, 766).

Primary negative magnesium balance. This is usually due either to negative net intestinal absorption or reduction of Tm_{Mg}/GFR below some critical level. Substantial losses of magnesium can occur with profuse sweating (762), in milk during excessive lactation (767), and during hemodialysis with a magnesium-free fluid (787), but clinically significant hypomagnesemia from any of these causes is rare. More important are losses of intestinal secretions, as with prolonged nasogastric suction, biliary fistula, or during the period of adaptation after an ileostomy (766). Loss from the body can also occur in severe burns; in one series a quarter of the patients had symptomatic hypomagnesemia, but this was probably due to secondary aldosteronism as well as to irrigation of the lesion (788). If the negative balance is transient, magnesium may be withdrawn only from the ECF with a fall in plasma level, but a sustained negative balance, however it occurs, must lead to net withdrawal of magnesium from within the cells and from bone. If this is a direct consequence of a fall in plasma level, the tissue losses are usually modest, but if there are additional effects of the primary disease, the losses can be much greater.

It is frequently assumed that much of the magnesium in bone and inside cells forms a reserve which can be drawn on to prevent a fall in plasma level. About 10 percent of total body magnesium (about 120 mmol) is exchangeable, but balance studies during the first week of a virtually magnesium-free diet indicated that only about 40 mmol was available to support the plasma level, which fell from 0.9 to 0.6 mmol/L (789). After about 3 months on the same diet the plasma level stabilized at about 0.2 mmol/L, with a calculated reserve of about 50 mmol, based on a mean negative balance of about 40 mmol and equivalent retention during recovery. In a patient on long-term cellulose phosphate treatment with a plasma magnesium of 0.4 mmol/L, the available reserve based on the measured retention during restoration of a normal plasma level was less than 20 mmol (790). In another study of experimental magnesium depletion in normal subjects, the plasma level fell no lower than 0.4 mmol/L, and there was no measurable fall in muscle magnesium content (791). Normal muscle magnesium content despite hypomagnesemia has also been found in some patients with steatorrhea (792).

A model of the relationship between EC and IC magnesium is shown in Fig. 19-35. If there is an inward electrochemical gradient for magnesium, the ECF concentration would have to fall low enough to abolish this gradient before there would be passive withdrawal of magnesium from the cell, unless in addition there was some process causing active mobilization of IC magnesium. This explains the usual stability of IC magnesium in normal subjects despite a significant fall in plasma level, and the small size of the magnesium reserve when depletion is induced by dietary means alone, in the absence of any process leading to cell catabolism.

Even less is known about the availability of bone magnesium. Although up to 30 percent is exchangeable in vitro, only about 1 percent or 5 to 10 mmol is rapidly exchangeable in vivo and the bulk of bone magnesium is accessible only through bone turnover. If bone of normal magnesium content were replaced by 50 percent magnesium-deficient bone at a rate of 10 percent per annum, between 25 and 50 mmol of magnesium could be released in a year. The distribution of magnesium in bone is not homogeneous, and trabecular and cortical bone must be analyzed separately (775). The range of normal values in a small sample is large, so that it is difficult to detect small

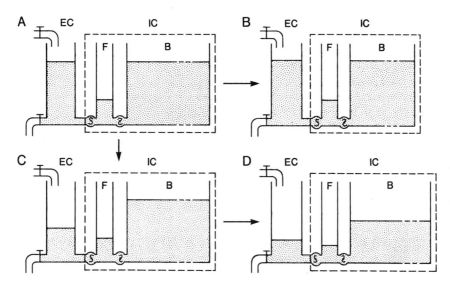

Figure 19-35. Model for relationship between EC (extracellular) and IC (intracellular) magnesium. In the normal state (*A*) the F (free) IC concentration is maintained at a low level by an outwardly directed pump at the cell membrane, and by the mechanisms of IC sequestration in the B (bound) compartment. *B* depicts the effect of cell catabolism with a reduction in magnesium capacity and content but not concentration. *C* shows the effect of a reduction in EC concentration; with a corresponding reduction in the activity of the cell membrane pump there would be no withdrawal of magnesium from inside the cell. *D* depicts the effect of a further reduction in EC concentration below the effective free IC concentration, leading to a fall in free IC and eventually in bound IC magnesium.

deficits in individual patients. Mean values which are normal for bone magnesium but low for muscle magnesium have been found in groups of patients with chronic diarrhea, cirrhosis of the liver, alcoholism, and chronic renal failure (778, 793–795). In none of these studies was muscle magnesium related to noncollagen nitrogen, and loss of muscle magnesium was at least partly a result of the catabolic state due to caloric deficiency rather than a response to hypomagnesemia. Nevertheless, the data indicate that although the magnesium stores in bone are larger than in muscle, they take much longer to be mobilized and provide no support for the suggestion that the ability to release magnesium from bone permits some persons to avoid hypomagnesemia in response to short-term magnesium deprivation (791). Low levels of bone magnesium have only been found in patients with chronic hypomagnesemia due to intestinal malabsorption (796), renal magnesium wasting, or chronic diarrhea (775), with

values between 10 and 30 percent below normal, corresponding to total deficits in the range of 50 to 200 mmol.

The ineffectiveness of soft tissue and bone magnesium in preventing a fall in plasma level also bears on the mechanism of renal conservation of magnesium. Early reports that this occurred by increased tubular reabsorption without a fall in plasma magnesium were based on inaccurate and insensitive methods. A reduction in dietary magnesium invariably causes a fall in plasma magnesium level when this is measured by atomic absorption spectrophotometry (Fig. 19-36) (244) and urinary magnesium falls exactly as predicted by the Tm_{Mg}/GFR model with no increase in tubular reabsorption, at least in the short term (Fig. 19-37). Even in the long term, it is uncertain that increased tubular reabsorption of magnesium ever occurs as a homeostatic response to magnesium depletion. During recovery from experimental magnesium deficiency of sev-

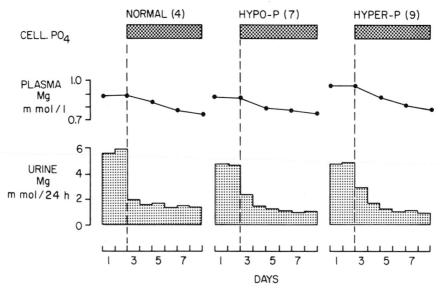

Figure 19-36. Effect of cellulose phosphate in normal subjects and in patients with latent (normocalcemic) HP and hypercalcemic hyperparathyroidism. Note prompt fall in both plasma and urinary magnesium in all three groups, with maximum urinary conservation occurring about 24 h earlier in the normal subjects than in those with impaired parathyroid function. [*Reproduced from A. M. Parfitt (244) with permission.*]

eral months' duration, urinary magnesium excretion rises in parallel with plasma magnesium (789), but in children recovering from protein-calorie malnutrition plasma magnesium returns to normal while urinary magnesium excretion is still low (784). Conceivably tubular reabsorption of magnesium, as of phosphate, could be increased as a result of IC depletion in the renal tubule.

According to the model, in the absence of negative balance the plasma magnesium should never fall below the appearance threshold, which seems to be about 0.5 mmol/L, but this assumes that below this level reabsorption is complete and urinary magnesium falls to zero. When measured by atomic absorption spectrophotometry, the urine has never been shown to become completely free of magnesium, so that some magnesium excretion probably continues at plasma levels much lower than the apparent threshold. There are also

many factors which impair renal magnesium conservation in disease. In patients convalescent from successful cancer surgery (789) the tubular reabsorption of magnesium on a magnesium-free diet was normal (Fig. 19-38), but in patients with inoperable cancer subjected to therapeutic magnesium depletion by dialysis (787), tubular reabsorption of magnesium was impaired (Fig. 19-38). This was most likely because of potassium depletion induced at the same time, although the patients were probably in a catabolic state as well. Tubular reabsorption of magnesium is also reduced by secondary hyperaldosteronism as will be discussed later. An important general principle is that clinically significant depletion usually requires more than one factor. For example, in previously healthy subjects complete exclusion of magnesium from the diet does not cause symptoms for several months, but in patients receiving magnesium-free parenteral fluids there is often impaired renal conservation of magnesium as well, and symptomatic hypomagnesemia occurs much sooner. Interaction of multiple causes is also characteristic in neonatal hypomagnesemia (798).

Negative or Reduced Net Intestinal Absorption. This occurs much more readily than with phosphate and is the most important single mechanism of magnesium depletion. For fecal magnesium excretion to exceed dietary intake either intake must be reduced, absorption impaired, or endogenous secretion increased. A model for the relationship between fecal and dietary magnesium is shown in Fig. 19-39. It assumes that 35 percent of ingested magnesium is absorbed and that endogenous excretion varies from 0 to 1.4 mmol/day. The model agrees with published balance data in normal subjects at very low (789) and very high intakes (799), and predicts that the minimum intake to avoid negative absorption varies

from 0 to 8 mmol/day with a mean of 4 mmol/day. This is about 30 to 40 percent of the mean normal intake, a much smaller margin of safety than for phosphate, so that reduced intake is more likely to cause depletion of magnesium than of phosphate. The dietary requirement to avoid negative balance has been variously estimated as between 9 and 12 mmol/day (800) or as high as 18 mmol/day (501), but if the latter figure is correct most apparently healthy persons are in a state of magnesium depletion. Other investigators have found no negative balances at intakes as low as 4 mmol/day (802). As much as 70 percent of dietary magnesium can be absorbed in severe magnesium depletion (803) or during growth (804).

Malabsorption is a more important cause of magnesium than of phosphate depletion; in 9 of 11 cases of intestinal disease with balance data fecal magnesium exceeded intake (Fig. 19-39) (774, 796, 805–807). Most of these patients had some form of short bowel syndrome (see also

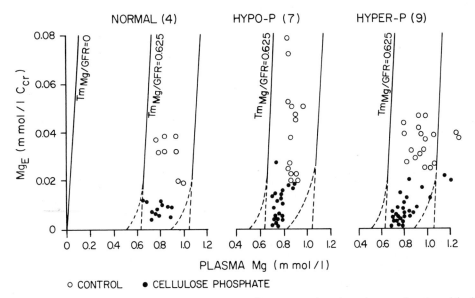

Figure 19-37. Relationship between plasma and urinary magnesium in the same subjects as in Fig. 19-36. Open circles, before cellulose phosphate; closed circles, during cellulose phosphate. Lower limit of Tm_{Mg}/GFR of 0.625 mmol is based on the assembled data for magnesium infusion in normal subjects. Dotted lines indicate uncertainty about the exact location of the lower end of the titration curve. Note the absence of any increase in tubular reabsorption of magnesium in any of the three groups. [*Reproduced from A. M. Parfitt (244) with permission.*]

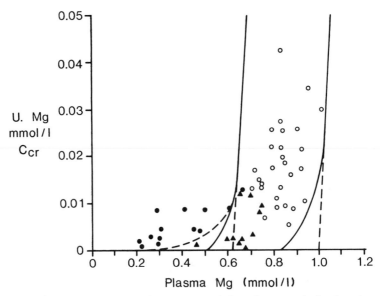

Figure 19-38. Renal conservation of magnesium in nonrenal magnesium depletion. Open circles, normal subjects; closed circles, patients with various forms of inoperable cancer subjected to therapeutic magnesium and potassium depletion by hemodialysis; both sets of data are redrawn from Nordin (797). Closed triangles, patients with oral cancer successfully treated by radical surgery and subjected to experimental magnesium depletion by dietary restriction; data are calculated on the assumption of a creatinine clearance of 80 mL/min. The normal range for Tm_{Mg}/GFR is as in Fig. 19-37. The curved dotted line represents the hypothetical lower segment of the magnesium titration curve permitting continuous leakage of magnesium at subnormal plasma levels. Note that patients with combined magnesium and potassium depletion have impaired tubular reabsorption of magnesium.

Chaps. 22 and 28), but four had nontropical sprue. As for potassium, fecal magnesium excretion is related to the total water content of the stool, so that patients with chronic diarrhea from any cause are liable to magnesium depletion and reduced muscle magnesium content (793). Fecal magnesium is also related to the fat content of the stool because of soap formation, and may be reduced by any measure (such as a low-fat diet or a gluten-free diet) which reduces the degree of steatorrhea (Fig. 19-39). Hypomagnesemia is common in all causes of intestinal malabsorption with steatorrhea, with an overall incidence of 20 to 40 percent (796) and values below 0.4 mmol in about 10 percent. Acute symptomatic hypomagnesemia can occur in the first few months after surgically induced malabsorption for the treatment of obesity (808). In the long term the mean plasma magnesium remains about 10 to 15 percent below normal indefinitely, but net absorption, although reduced, is still positive; most patients do not have IC depletion and are asymptomatic (809). In contrast to calcium and phosphate, malabsorption of magnesium does not usually occur in chronic renal failure (810).

Malabsorption of magnesium may also occur as an isolated abnormality without other evidence of intestinal disease (804, 811–814). Affected subjects have severe hypomagnesemia (0.2 to 0.4 mmol/L) and hypocalcemia, leading to tetany and convulsive seizures in early infancy which may be fatal without treatment. In some patients with a similar defect symptoms do not begin until adolescence (815). Fecal magnesium is much higher than in normal infants, who absorb about 65 to 75 percent of dietary magnesium (804), but in most cases it is in the normal range for adults (Fig. 19-40). This suggests a defect in whatever mechanism normally permits augmented magnesium absorption during growth.

Reduction of Tm_{Mg}/GFR. In one large series, uncontrolled diabetes mellitus and diuretic therapy were the most common causes of hypomagnesemia (816). The many other causes of impaired magnesium reabsorption are less common, but whatever the cause, most patients are asymptomatic if this is the only defect. Impaired reabsorption may also be a contributory or perpetuating factor in magnesium depletion due to some other cause, as mentioned earlier.

Plasma magnesium is reduced by about 0.1 mmol/L in primary hyperaldosteronism, most likely because sodium-linked magnesium reabsorption in the proximal convoluted tubule and the loop of Henle is reduced by chronic ECF volume expansion. These patients retain a substantial amount of magnesium when given spironolactone and after surgical cure (857) but aldosterone has no direct effect on magnesium reabsorption (Chap. 8). ECF volume expansion probably also accounts for the hypomagnesemia of inappropriate ADH secretion, as in porphyria (818); the

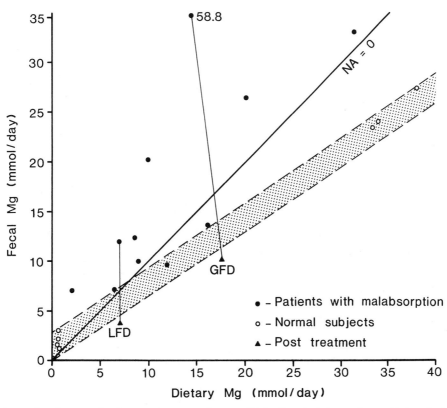

Figure 19-39. Relationships between fecal magnesium excretion and dietary magnesium intake. The solid line indicates equality with NA (net absorption) of zero. The dotted lines enclose a hypothetical normal range, assuming absorption of 35 percent of intake and intestinal excretion of 0 to 2.8 mmol/day. Open circles, normal subjects either on very low intake (789) or very high intake (799). Closed circles, patients with intestinal malabsorption (773, 796, 805–807); in 9 of 11 patients, fecal excretion exceeds dietary intake. The closed triangles show the effect of treatment, either a LFD (low-fat diet) in a patient with the short bowel syndrome (796), or a GFD (gluten-free diet) in an adolescent celiac disease (807).

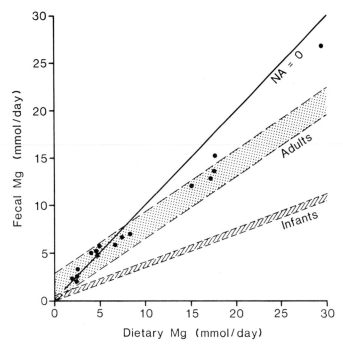

Figure 19-40. Relationship between fecal magnesium excretion and dietary magnesium intake in infantile primary hypomagnesemia. The solid and upper dotted lines are as in Fig. 19-39; lower dotted lines, hypothetical normal range in infants, assuming absorption of 65 percent of dietary intake and intestinal excretion of 0 to 0.6 mmol/day. Points represent individual balance periods in six patients studied at different intakes (811–815); most of them are in the normal range for adults, but absorption is much too low for normal growth.

apparent acute increase in magnesium excretion produced by ADH was probably a methodologic artifact (819). Whether a sustained increase in urinary magnesium can occur in response to a chronic increase in dietary sodium intake is not known; as mentioned earlier many persons can adapt to this without sustained volume expansion. Magnesium conservation is also impaired by potassium depletion, so that the effects of aldosterone excess could be due to this factor as well as to volume expansion. Hypomagnesemia is found in secondary hyperaldosteronism (820) in which plasma volume is usually reduced, even though total ECF volume is increased. Hypomagnesemia

also occurs in Bartter's syndrome (821), possibly because of impaired tubular reabsorption of magnesium as well as of calcium and sodium in the ascending limb of the loop of Henle. In chronic renal failure the reduced reabsorption of sodium due to the need to excrete more sodium per nephron is accompanied by reduced magnesium reabsorption, but usually this protects against hypermagnesemia rather than causes hypomagnesemia.

Magnesium excretion is increased acutely by all diuretics with the exception of acetazolamide (822), but cumulative losses only occur if the interval between successive doses is short in relation to the duration of action of the drug. This is most likely to occur with the thiazide diuretics, which can cause a sustained reduction in Tm_{Mg}/GFR and plasma magnesium, but in most patients the effect is small and the values remain within the normal range (507) (Fig. 19-41A). Transient severe hypomagnesemia (0.2 mmol) can occur during the massive diuresis which sometimes follows relief of urinary tract obstruction or renal transplantation (822), but acute osmotic diuresis due to mannitol infusion has relatively little effect on magnesium excretion (496). Increased urinary magnesium excretion at normal or subnormal plasma levels during uncontrolled diabetes mellitus (763) is probably due to complexing of magnesium by acetoacetate and other organic anions, as well as to the osmotic effect of glycosuria.

It is not known to what extent changes in the homeostatic reabsorption in the distal tubule can compensate for alterations in nonhomeostatic reabsorption, but abnormalities in the homeostatic reabsorption can also cause hypomagnesemia. Calcium infusion considerably increases urinary magnesium excretion because of competition of both ions for the same transport mechanism (823), and chronic hypercalcemia of many different causes may be associated with impaired magnesium reabsorption and low plasma magnesium for the same reason (824). In hypercalcemic hyperparathyroidism this effect is antagonized by the direct magnesium-conserving action of PTH (825), and in individual patients either may be predominant, accounting for the usual normality but greater variability of plasma magnesium (Fig. 19-37). Low values for Tm_{Mg}/GFR and plasma Mg occurred in 4 of 48 cases in one series (826) (Fig. 19-41B). The plasma magnesium is within the normal range in most patients with HP, but the mean level has been significantly reduced in several series (824, 827) and low values are found both before and during treatment with vitamin D. In 10 treated patients the values for plasma Mg and Tm_{Mg}/GFR were slightly low in 2 and slightly high in 2 (Fig. 19-41A), but low values in response to a thiazide diuretic occurred more commonly than in idiopathic hypercalciuria. The hypomagnesemia of HP is worsened by phosphate administration and improved by administration of parathyroid extract (826). In some patients there is increased retention of intravenously adminis-

tered magnesium, suggesting tissue depletion of magnesium as well (827), but in others retention has been normal (R. A. L. Sutton, personal communication).

In all the conditions mentioned so far the renal tubule has responded in an appropriate manner to some external stimulus, but intrinsic defects in magnesium reabsorption also occur. These normally produce more severe hypomagnesemia (Fig. 19-41C), with plasma magnesium levels often in the range of 0.2 to 0.4 mmol/L, but adverse effects due to magnesium depletion are rare. Impaired renal magnesium conservation occurs most often in chronic pyelonephritis or other causes of tubulointerstitial nephropathy (785); it is associated with reduced GFR and other evidence of impaired tubular function, and is an exaggeration of

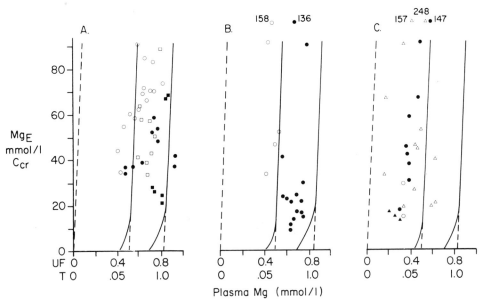

Figure 19-41. Relationship between urinary magnesium excretion (mmol/L C_{cr}) and plasma magnesium in three different situations, illustrating conformity to the Tm_{Mg}/GFR model of tubular reabsorption. *A.* Effect of thiazide diuretic for 6 days. Closed circles, patients with vitamin D-treated HP before thiazide; open circles, same patients after thiazide; closed squares, patients with hypercalciuria before thiazide; open squares, same patients after thiazide (507). *B,* Patients with primary hyperparathyroidism from two series. Closed circles (826); open circles (827). *C,* Patients reported to have renal wasting of magnesium. Closed circles, serial values in one patient (834); open triangles, single values of nine different patients (785); in three of these magnesium reabsorption is normal. Open circles, serial values in a single patient (832); closed triangles, single values in seven different patients (828–831, 833). Numbers indicate off-scale values for the ordinate.

the impaired magnesium reabsorption which normally occurs in chronic renal failure. In other cases there is also impaired tubular reabsorption of potassium and hypokalemia without other evidence of renal disease or of other renal-tubular dysfunction. This occurs in aminoglycoside nephropathy with severe hypomagnesemia (0.2 to 0.4 mmol/L) and hypocalcemia (173, 828), and in a rare familial disorder characterized by mild hypomagnesemia (0.4 to 0.6 mmol/L), an exaggerated fall in plasma magnesium in response to a magnesium-free diet, normal plasma calcium which paradoxically rises in response to magnesium deprivation, and a paradoxical increase in urinary magnesium excretion in response to spironolactone (829, 830). Impaired tubular reabsorption of magnesium has also occurred with a variety of other combinations of renal-tubular defects in isolated cases (831–833), and as an isolated defect without other detectable abnormalities (834).

Magnesium metabolism in specific clinical situations. Some disturbances of magnesium metabolism do not fit readily into the preceding simple classification or are sufficiently important to merit separate discussion.

Alcoholism, with or without Cirrhosis of the Liver (see also Chap. 21). This is currently the most common cause of symptomatic hypomagnesemia in the United States. In stable alcoholic subjects in good nutritional condition not requiring admission to hospital, the magnesium status is usually normal (835), but as a group patients requiring admission to hospital for treatment of alcoholism or its complications have chronic magnesium depletion with increased magnesium retention during parenteral administration, reduced exchangeable magnesium, and low muscle magnesium content (795, 835, 836). Plasma magnesium is often normal or only moderately reduced, except in patients with acute alcoholic poisoning or with the alcohol withdrawal syndrome. This is often accompanied by an abrupt fall in plasma magnesium and potassium (836, 837), particularly if calories from other sources are increased, but there is no correlation between the plasma magnesium level and the degree of IC deficit. In most patients the plasma magnesium

returns to normal within a week with the usual nutritional and supportive treatment, even without magnesium supplements (838). In more severely depleted patients, total retention during magnesium repletion is in the range of 50 to 200 mmol (795, 836). It is not clear whether the magnesium deficit is different between alcoholics with and without cirrhosis of the liver (794, 795). The plasma magnesium level may be reduced in patients with nonalcoholic liver disease but magnesium deficiency has not been demonstrated. The magnesium depletion of alcoholism is due to a combination of many factors, including reduced caloric intake and tissue wasting, reduced magnesium intake, intestinal malabsorption, due either to alcohol itself or to liver disease, episodic diarrhea, and impaired renal conservation due to secondary hyperaldosteronism, ketoacidosis, increased plasma and urinary lactate, and ethanol itself.

Acute administration of ethanol to normal subjects causes a significant, but transient, increase in urinary magnesium excretion (822), but the increase is much smaller when the plasma magnesium is low, and continued ethanol administration does not alter external magnesium balance (839).

Congestive Cardiac Failure. Patients under treatment for chronic heart failure as a group have a significant reduction in both plasma and red cell magnesium level and in muscle magnesium content, with values below normal in about 50 percent of the patients (840). Both urinary excretion and external balance of magnesium are closely correlated with potassium (841). As in alcoholism causes are multiple and include the catabolic effect of tissue hypoxia, reduced intake of both magnesium and total calories, the intestinal malabsorption of heart failure, and reduced tubular reabsorption of magnesium due to diuretic therapy reinforced by secondary hyperaldosteronism, potassium depletion, and possibly digoxin. The importance of magnesium deficiency in this group of patients is that it impairs renal conservation of potassium, encourages loss of potassium from heart muscle cells, and increases the risk of digitalis poisoning.

Surgical Operations. The special effects of gastrointestinal and parathyroid surgery on magnesium metabolism have already been described, but a fall of about 0.2 mmol/L in plasma magnesium often occurs in the first few days after any surgical operation (782, 842–844). It is due to a combination of reduced intake of magnesium, dilution of body fluids by hypotonic intravenous solutions, postoperative water retention, and impaired renal conservation of magnesium with rapid excretion of administered magnesium load. Often there is a corresponding fall in urinary magnesium excretion, but there may be no change or even a rise. The hypomagnesemia is usually of no clinical consequence, but has precipitated ventricular fibrillation after cardiac bypass (844). The level returns spontaneously to normal in about a week (843).

Magnesium Metabolism in Thyroid Disease. The plasma magnesium is reduced by 10 to 15 percent in hyperthyroidism, but total exchangeable magnesium determined by ^{28}Mg (most of which is IC soft tissue magnesium) is increased by 10 to 20 percent (845–847); in the rat the cell uptake of magnesium by the liver is increased by thyroxin (848). In addition there is increased net absorption and urinary excretion of magnesium with a positive magnesium balance. Increased magnesium excretion despite a reduced plasma level indicates reduced tubular reabsorption; the increase in GFR in hyperthyroidism is probably not great enough to account alone for the findings. In hypothyroidism the opposite changes of decreased exchangeable magnesium, increased plasma magnesium, decreased net absorption and urinary excretion with negative balance, and increased tubular reabsorption are found (845–847). The low plasma magnesium of hyperthyroidism correlates with indices of disease severity such as the degree of weight loss (843) and the plasma AP level (849). The lowest levels (0.3 to 0.4 mmol) were found in two patients with apathetic hyperthyroidism (849), the special features of which have been ascribed to hypomagnesemia. The positive magnesium balance continues for several weeks after onset of treatment but all abnormalities eventually return to normal, although this may take several months. Hyperthyroidism is associated with reduced PTH secretion but this could

account only for the decreased tubular reabsorption. Synthesis of 1,25-DHCC is presumably also impaired, but magnesium metabolism in hyperthyroidism more closely resembles the effects of vitamin D excess than vitamin D deficiency (850), and so most likely is a direct consequence of thyroid hormone action.

Clinical effects of magnesium depletion

There is a greater divergence of opinion concerning the clinical importance of magnesium deficiency than of deficiency of any other mineral or electrolyte (see also Chaps. 11 and 15). Some are reluctant to ascribe any symptoms to magnesium depletion even in the presence of substantial measurable deficits (851). At the other end of the spectrum, subclinical magnesium depletion is believed by some to be responsible for a wide variety of cardiovascular and hematologic complications (852), even in patients in whom all conventional tests of assessing magnesium status are normal.

A moderately skeptical view is justified, because the attribution of unexplained manifestations of disease to some measurable but irrelevant laboratory phenomenon is a common error of logic in medicine. Disappearance of symptoms after magnesium administration may result from its pharmacologic effects rather than from the correction of a deficiency (765), although the doses which produce clinical improvement often do not raise the plasma level above normal. Another contentious issue is the relative importance of IC and EC magnesium levels in the production of symptoms. In general, the EC level correlates better with the clinical state. For example, symptoms of magnesium intoxication occurred in a patient with acute renal failure and reduced muscle magnesium content (853). Substantial magnesium depletion can exist with a normal plasma magnesium level, but all clinical effects which are unequivocally due to magnesium deficiency are accompanied by significant hypomagnesemia and are relieved by restoration of the plasma magnesium level to normal. Nevertheless, equivalent degrees of hypomagnesemia may be associated with severe symptoms, or with no symptoms at all.

Hypomagnesemia is a necessary but not a sufficient condition for clinical effects and magnesium depletion at some critical IC location is probably also required. Most patients with symptomatic hypomagnesemia retain 50 to 150 mmol of magnesium during recovery (789, 795, 803, 836). There is a wealth of suggestive evidence that IC magnesium depletion can produce its own effects independent of the plasma level, but the precise nature of these effects and their frequency and importance are still undetermined.

It is convenient to consider separately those effects due to secondary changes in potassium metabolism, those due to secondary changes in calcium metabolism, and those due directly to hypomagnesemia.

Cardiac arrhythmias, muscle weakness, and potassium metabolism. The Na^+–K^+–ATPase which maintains the high concentration of potassium and low concentration of sodium within cells is activated by magnesium (765, 854). Consequently, in magnesium depletion there is increased loss of potassium as well as magnesium from the muscle cells as shown in clinical studies, and from the myocardium as shown in experimental animals. In the rat, loss of muscle potassium was associated with loss of nitrogen, reduction in cell size, and swelling and reduction in the number of mitochondria (855). Magnesium depletion also impairs the renal conservation of potassium so that despite increased loss from the cells, the plasma potassium level falls below normal. Both a negative potassium balance and a fall in plasma potassium have been observed in pure magnesium depletion in humans (789). The hypokalemia of magnesium depletion is refractory to conventional methods of potassium repletion, but clinical effects are related more to the loss of potassium from within the cell than to the plasma potassium level. The low level of muscle potassium is also resistant to administration of potassium, but is restored to normal when the magnesium depletion is corrected (771, 772).

The magnesium-dependent Na^+–K^+–ATPase is inhibited by digoxin and similar drugs and the effects of magnesium depletion and digoxin excess in promoting loss of potassium from the heart muscle cell are additive. Magnesium deficiency also increases the uptake of digoxin by the myocardium (856), so that there are several reasons for the enhanced sensitivity of magnesium-deficient patients to the toxic effect of digitalis. In experimental magnesium deficiency the dose of acetyl strophanthidin needed to induce arrhythmias is reduced. Arrhythmias are more prolonged and more often fatal, but are abolished by the administration of magnesium (857).

As a result of these interactions the precipitation of cardiac arrhythmias is an important effect of magnesium depletion; these occur particularly although not exclusively in patients who are digitalized (854, 858), and include ventricular tachycardia, often multifocal, ventricular fibrillation, and asystolic cardiac arrest; supraventricular arrhythmias are less common (283, 844, 854, 858). All are characterized by partial or complete refractoriness to the usual treatment until the hypomagnesemia is corrected. It is often difficult to separate the effects on the ECG of potassium and magnesium depletion, but in the absence of arrhythmias peaking of the T wave and prolongation of the QRS complex have been ascribed to magnesium depletion alone (859). Magnesium has sometimes been used in the treatment of arrhythmias without regard to their cause, but the response to magnesium is inconstant and short-lived unless the arrhythmia is associated with magnesium depletion. Most patients with magnesium-deficiency arrhythmias are normokalemic; such arrhythmias occur especially in circumstances favoring both potassium and magnesium depletion, when hypokalemia has been recognized and corrected but the equally (or sometimes more) important hypomagnesemia has been overlooked (783). The plasma magnesium is usually below 0.5 mmol/L. Mild hypomagnesemia is more likely a result than a cause of digitalis intoxication (860), because of anorexia and poor intake.

In alcoholics a reduction in muscle magnesium content both per kg FFW and Mg/K ratio was found in 10 patients with low plasma magnesium and was associated with reduction in the maximum force of voluntary isometric contraction of the quadriceps femoris muscle (861). There was also a significant reduction in phosphocreatinine and ADP but not ATP content. The plasma potassium was normal in all cases but muscle sodium and water content were increased. Magnesium depletion can impair the function of skeletal as well as cardiac muscle directly, and not just as a consequence of hypokalemia.

Hypocalcemic tetany in magnesium depletion. In experimental pure magnesium depletion in humans, the plasma calcium began to fall after 10 to 20 days, and eventually either stabilized at some level between 1.5 and 2 mmol/L or continued to fall until the experiment was terminated (789). Urinary calcium fell sooner and was usually below 0.25 mmol/day by the end of the first week. Fecal calcium excretion was also reduced, so that the subjects were in sustained positive balance for calcium, indicating that the release of calcium from bone by both the remodeling and homeostatic systems was impaired. Tetany due to hypocalcemia is a common complication of magnesium depletion in clinical practice; the development of tetany in an alcoholic patient is presumptive evidence of hypomagnesemia. The plasma phosphate is usually normal but is occasionally raised (82, 792), producing a biochemical resemblance to HP. There are unexplained differences in the incidence of this complication in different causes of hypomagnesemia. It is always present in children with primary intestinal malabsorption of magnesium, and is common but not universal in adults with reduced net intestinal absorption of magnesium for any reason. In hypomagnesemia due to primary reduction in tubular reabsorption, hypocalcemia is rare except in aminoglycoside nephropathy; in the familial disorder associated with hypokalemia, dietary depletion of magnesium and further depression of plasma magnesium produced a paradoxical *increase* in plasma calcium (829). The pathogenesis of the hypocalcemia is complex and at least three factors are involved—reduced secretion of PTH, impaired target cell responsiveness to PTH, and abnormal functioning of the blood-bone equilibrium independent of PTH.

The acute effect of a fall in plasma magnesium is to stimulate the release (and to a lesser extent the synthesis) of PTH (Chap. 8), but in severe chronic magnesium depletion PTH secretion is often reduced. Of 25 cases recently assembled (81), iPTH was high in 3, normal but inappropriately low for the plasma calcium in 12, and absolutely low or undetectable in 10. Thus, although impaired parathyroid function was demonstrated in the majority, this was sufficiently severe to explain the hypocalcemia in less than half the patients. What factors control the occurrence and timing of the transition from stimulant to suppressive effects of hypomagnesemia on PTH secretion are unknown.

Parathyroid function has been studied most intensively in patients with primary intestinal malabsorption of magnesium (812), but this disorder is almost certainly not representative of magnesium depletion in general. The low plasma magnesium is invariably accompanied by a low PTH, and when supplemental magnesium is withdrawn, iPTH falls immediately without even a transient increase as would normally occur (862). When magnesium administration is resumed, plasma iPTH rises within minutes (863), whereas in hypomagnesemic HP from other causes hours or days are required to restore normal iPTH levels and a week or longer to restore normocalcemia (81, 864). If the low plasma calcium is raised by calcium infusion above 2.0 mmol/L, PTH secretion is further suppressed in the magnesium-deficient state (863). These observations suggest a set-point error in the opposite direction to that found in some patients with hyperparathyroidism, such that a lower level of plasma calcium than normal is needed to suppress PTH release. The characteristics peculiar to this disorder are consistent with a defect in the transport of magnesium (and possibly calcium) in the parathyroid gland as well as in the intestinal mucosa.

Variable degrees of unresponsiveness to the effects of PTH on the kidney (phosphate and NcAMP excretion) and on bone (both short-term and long-term increase in plasma calcium) have often been found in patients with hypomagnesemia (865–867), but in others all tests of parathyroid responsiveness have been entirely normal (862, 868). In general, most subnormal responses have been obtained in patients with alcoholism or intestinal malabsorption who have been studied before treatment, and most normal responses have been obtained in infants and children in whom supplemental magnesium has only been recently discontinued (81). Although there are exceptions to this generalization (866, 868), the data as a whole suggest that target cell resistance to PTH is a function of the degree and/or duration of magnesium depletion, not of the plasma magnesium level at the time of the study (81, 866, 869). A subnormal calcemic response to PTH has been found more commonly than a subnormal phosphaturic or NcAMP response. Magnesium depletion has been also incriminated in the pathogenesis of hypophosphatemia, both in chronic alcoholism (575) and in intestinal malabsorption (774). A direct effect of reducing phosphate reabsorption independent of PTH could account for the rarity of hyperphosphatemia in magnesium depletion.

According to the concepts developed in an earlier section, the combination of a normal or raised iPTH and low plasma calcium is presumptive evidence for impaired action of PTH on the calcium homeostatic system in bone, irrespective of the response to exogenous PTH. Magnesium ions lost from the hydration shell and surface of the crystal lattice of bone mineral could be replaced by calcium ions by heteroionic exchange (868). As a result, the mineral would tend to be more stable and less soluble, so that the calcium concentration in bone fluid:ECF, and therefore in systemic ECF, would fall. Bone from magnesium-deficient rats behaves in this way in vitro (870) and such a defect would also impair the ability of both surface lining cells and osteocytes to mobilize calcium from bone in response to PTH. In addition there is a profound impairment of bone resorption in the magnesium-deficient dog (871), the severity of which is too great to attribute solely to PTH deficiency, indicating a defect in the remodeling system as well as in the homeostatic system. This concept is consistent with the positive calcium balances found in magnesium-deficient human subjects (789), and with correction of hypocalcemia despite continuing negative calcium

balance when magnesium-deficient patients with intestinal malabsorption were given supplemental magnesium (872). Plasma calcium may also increase before there has been a change in iPTH (864). It seems likely that impaired calcium release from bone initiates hypocalcemia in all cases, and that in different patients the hypocalcemia is sustained by varying combinations of reduced PTH secretion and impaired responsiveness of target cells to PTH (873).

Neuromuscular irritability. Classic overt tetany in a hypomagnesemic patient is almost always due to hypocalcemia. In a few cases the plasma total calcium has been normal (763), but overt tetany is the least-common direct complication of magnesium depletion. Neonatal tetany may be an exception, since this responds more quickly to magnesium than to calcium administration even if the plasma magnesium is normal (874). A syndrome comprising latent tetany, chronic anxiety with a variety of psychoneurotic symptoms, an abnormal EMG after hyperventilation, slight reduction of plasma and red cell magnesium, increased retention of an intravenous magnesium load, and clinical improvement with magnesium supplements has been extensively described in the French literature. There is considerable skepticism elsewhere about the reality of this syndrome, although one case has been diagnosed in the United States (875).

In experimental human magnesium depletion (789), anorexia and nausea were common early symptoms, followed by a coarse tremor in three of seven cases and muscle fibrillation in two cases, with a myopathic pattern on EMG. These phenomena were unrelated to the hypocalcemia, which was manifested chiefly by a positive Trousseau's sign; clinical improvement during magnesium repletion began before the plasma calcium rose. In spontaneous hypomagnesemia several types of spontaneous abnormal movements have been described, including both fine and coarse tremors, asterixis resembling hepatic failure, choreiform twitches, myoclonic jerks, and both focal and generalized convulsive seizures (469, 726–767). Quite often there is an alteration of mood with apathy, depression, apprehension, or extreme agitation, and sometimes an acute confusional state. Less commonly ataxia, vertigo, and muscle weakness have been described. Individually, many of these signs and symptoms can occur in hypocalcemia, but collectively the clinical picture is quite distinct from that of hypocalcemia due to reasons other than magnesium depletion. In many patients with the neuromuscular syndrome of magnesium deficiency the plasma calcium has been normal, and clinical improvement occurs in response to administration of magnesium but not calcium, whether the plasma calcium changes or not (767). Factors other than the plasma magnesium level determine the occurrence of the neuromuscular syndrome, since some patients with comparable degrees of hypomagnesemia are asymptomatic. The syndrome is common in the usual forms of neonatal hypomagnesemia, but not in primary intestinal malabsorption of magnesium. In adults, the syndrome is much more frequent in patients with intestinal malabsorption or alcoholism than in renal magnesium wasting. No consistent abnormalities have been found in the CSF magnesium concentration, which is normally about 20 percent higher than the plasma level (876).

The alcohol withdrawal syndrome is often associated with hypomagnesemia, and delirium tremens shows many resemblances to the neuromuscular syndrome of magnesium depletion, but there are many other electrolyte abnormalities in these patients (851). Delirium tremens often occurs with a normal plasma magnesium, and can recover spontaneously without magnesium supplements despite persistence of hypomagnesemia (469, 765). Alcohol withdrawal seizures are more likely to be related to hypomagnesemia (469). The risk of seizures is greater in patients with photomyoclonus (myoclonus induced by stroboscopic stimulation); this is related to the severity of hypomagnesemia and is improved by magnesium administration (877).

Other possible effects. In experimental magnesium deficiency in rapidly growing animals, abnormalities in almost every system have been described (762–765), but most of these have little or no relevance to clinical medicine. The relative magnitude of deficiency is much greater than ever occurs in humans, and the formation of new cells and tissues which are magnesium deficient from the outset is a fundamentally different process from the withdrawal of magnesium from tissue which has developed normally. A relationship suggested between the magnesium deficiency of growth and sudden unexpected infant death (878) remains unconfirmed. Magnesium supplementation in an uncontrolled study appeared to hasten recovery from protein-calorie malnutrition (879), but in a controlled study the outcome was unaffected (880). There are suggestive resemblances between the cardiovascular complications of experimental magnesium depletion and some neonatal cardiovascular disorders such as endomyocardial fibrosis (852), but no good evidence for an etiologic relationship.

The death rate from coronary artery disease is higher in areas where the natural water supply is soft rather than hard. It has been suggested that the low magnesium level in soft water is responsible, because the magnesium content of heart muscle was lower in patients who died from myocardial infarction than in patients who died from other causes (881). But the absolute concentration of myocardial magnesium was higher in the soft- than in the hard-water area, although the ratio of magnesium/potassium was lower (882). There was also no difference in the urinary excretion of magnesium, potassium, or calcium between persons living in hard- and soft-water areas (883). If there is a general relationship between occult magnesium depletion and cardiovascular and other degenerative diseases, it would be expected that the magnesium content of many tissues would decrease with age, but in fact there is no change apart from an increase in the aorta (884). An apparent atherogenic effect of low magnesium intake may reflect the low magnesium content of refined foods high in carbohydrate and fat (884).

Magnesium in urine may act as an inhibitor of mineralization, and urinary magnesium excretion is somewhat lower in patients with nephrolithiasis than in age- and sex-matched controls (761). Magnesium administration has been reported to be beneficial in the treatment of calcium oxalate nephrolithiasis, but there are no adequately controlled long-term studies.

The treatment of hypomagnesemia and magnesium depletion

There is no established method of raising the renal threshold of magnesium excretion by increasing Tm_{Mg}/GFR; whether induction of ECF volume depletion would have the same effect as on phosphate is not known. Apart from treatment of the underlying disease (Fig. 19-39), the only measure available is the administration of appropriate magnesium supplements (Table 19-53).

The most important aspect is prevention. As with phosphate, if oral intake is replaced by intravenous infusion for more than 1 to 2 days, it is sensible to give as much magnesium as would normally be absorbed. This is about 4 mmol per 24 h, provided by 2 mL of 50% magnesium sulfate. For no good reason it has become customary to use much larger amounts than this in patients receiving TPN (total parenteral nutrition), such as 0.25 mmol/kg body weight per 24 h, equivalent to 15 to 20 mmol per 24 h (606). In addition to a maintenance requirement, magnesium is needed

for repair of previous cell catabolism, but even so the amounts used are excessive. In the only comprehensive balance studies during TPN, magnesium was not measured, but based on the observed retentions of nitrogen, phosphate, potassium, and calcium, magnesium retention would have been no more than 2.9 mmol/day in patients gaining weight at an average rate of about 0.6 kg/day or a 4.6-mmol/kg weight gain (609). Even if this figure is doubled to allow for disproportionate loss of magnesium during cell catabolism, only 10 mmol per 24 h would be needed. As little as 0.04 mmol/kg body weight per 24 h has maintained a normal plasma magnesium level during TPN for as long as 6 months (885).

In the treatment of diabetic ketoacidosis, during the first few hours cell water is partially restored more rapidly than electrolytes as the blood glucose falls, but for the next 2 to 6 days there is restoration of K, P, and Mg without protein; if oral intake cannot be resumed, these elements should be added to the intravenous solution (591, 592). The total mean retention of magnesium is about 20 to 40 mmol, and an appropriate magnesium concentration for intravenous use is 2.5 mmol/L during this period (591, 592). Complete restoration of cell protein and its attendant ions may not occur for several weeks, but a normal diet without special supplements usually supplies a sufficient surplus. As with phosphate, it is important to monitor renal function and plasma magnesium levels periodically in patients receiving parenteral magnesium.

If significant magnesium depletion and hypomagnesemia has already developed, much larger amounts are needed (767). In a patient having convulsive seizures probably due to magnesium depletion, 4 mL of 50% magnesium sulfate solution (8 mmol) diluted to 1 dL should be given in 10 min. If the situation is less urgent 0.5 mmol/kg per 24 h should be given on the first day, preferably added to a continuous intravenous infusion. It can also be given by intramuscular injection of 2 mL of 50% magnesium sulfate (= 4 mmol) every 3 to 4 h, but the injections are quite painful. The amount recommended is about half the probable deficit estimated from balance stud-

Table 19-53. Magnesium preparations for oral and parenteral use[a]

ANION	FORM	Mg, mmol[b]
Chloride	Solution[c] (10 mL)	2.5
Citrate[d]	Solution (10 mL)	4.2
Gluconate	Tablet (500 mg)	1.2
Hydroxide[d]	Suspension (10 mL)	14.5
Hydroxide	Tablet (400 mg)[e]	3.5
Sulfate	Injection (2 mL)	4.0
Sulfate	Powder (15 g)[f]	61.2

[a] Magnesium glycerophosphate is often used in Europe but is not available in the United States.
[b] Content per dosage unit.
[c] Compounded with syrup.
[d] Marketed as a laxative (milk of magnesia) but sometimes prescribed for its magnesium content.
[e] A proprietary mixture of 200 mg each of magnesium and aluminum hydroxide (Maalox), widely used as an antacid.
[f] Usual cathartic dose (Epsom salts).

ies in symptomatic patients and is much smaller than the dose used in the treatment of eclampsia. Subsequently, 0.2 to 0.3 mmol/kg per day should be given for the next 3 to 5 days, depending on the clinical response.

Mild hypomagnesemia (less than or equal to 0.6 mmol/L) in an asymptomatic patient who has none of the clinical conditions associated with magnesium depletion needs no treatment, but many patients require long-term oral supplementation (Table 19-53). If the low plasma level is due to reduction in Tm_{Mg}/GFR, then, as for phosphate, the amount required to produce a significant rise in plasma level is very large, although, as for calcium, the splay at the lower end of the titration curve may decrease the amount needed to produce the same increase in plasma level. Above the saturation threshold with a GFR of 1 dL/min an increase in plasma magnesium of 0.1 mmol/L would require an increase in intake of 40 mmol per 24 h to provide the necessary increase in net absorption. Patients with intestinal malabsorption of magnesium, whether due to generalized mucosal disease or selective magnesium malabsorption, may also require 10 to 30 mmol per 24 h in infants and children, and 30 to 50 mmol per 24 h in adults. There is no good evidence for any difference in the availability of magnesium from different salts, but such large amounts can only be given with preparations of higher magnesium content. All magnesium salts tend to induce diarrhea in large doses, but this depends on the total osmotic load rather than on the chemical nature of the anion. Fortunately, the amount needed as a magnesium supplement is usually below the cathartic dose, which for magnesium sulfate is 15 g (60 mmol).

HYPERMAGNESEMIA

In the largest series of routine plasma magnesium measurements, high values occurred most commonly in patients with renal failure or taking magnesium-containing antacids, but less than 21 percent of more than 5000 determinations were

Table 19-54. Causes of hypermagnesemia

Decreased GFR*
Increased magnesium load*
  Endogenous
    Diabetic ketoacidosis
    Other cell catabolism
    Birth asphyxia
    Hibernation
  Exogenous
    Epsom salt poisoning
    Antacids and laxatives (Table 19-53)
    ?Vitamin D or metabolites
    Magnesium sulfate enema
    Treatment of eclampsia—mother
    Treatment of eclampsia—neonate
    Hemodialysis†
Increased Tm_{Mg}/GFR
  Hyperparathyroidism‡
  Familial hypocalciuric hypercalcemia
  Hypothyroidism
  Mineralocorticoid deficiency
  ?Aldosterone antagonists§

* Often both are present.
† Failure to soften hard water, or error in manufacture of concentrate.
‡ Effect is antagonized by hypercalcemia.
§ These raise low values to normal; hypermagnesemia is a theoretical but undocumented possibility.

above 1.04 mmol/L, mostly in patients sick enough to require admission to hospital (816). The frequency of different causes is quite different in the neonatal period (798).

Mechanisms and causes (Table 19-54)

Although the kidney is very efficient at excreting surplus magnesium, increased tubular reabsorption of magnesium is much less common than increased tubular reabsorption of calcium or phosphate. With a normal GFR and normal Tm_{Mg}/GFR, plasma magnesium would not rise above normal unless the load were increased fivefold, so that as with phosphate, an increased load is much more liable to cause hypermagnesemia if GFR is reduced. The general relationships between magnitude of load, rate of administration, volume of distribution, and GFR will be similar to those depicted for phosphate (Figs. 19-31 and 19-32) except that obligatory hypermagnesemia requires a more severe degree of renal failure.

Hypermagnesemia due to an increased endogenous magnesium load occurs as a result of cell catabolism in diabetic ketoacidosis, but the values rarely exceed 1.5 mmol/L. In birth asphyxia in neonates there is an inverse correlation between plasma magnesium and APGAR score (886); tissue anoxia probably causes release of IC cations as well as phosphate, but the plasma magnesium rarely exceeds 1.2 mmol/L from this cause alone. A similar mechanism may underlie the rise in plasma magnesium during hibernation.

Increased exogenous magnesium loads are most commonly due to magnesium-containing antacids or laxatives. Magnesium hydroxide or milk of magnesia has a very high magnesium content (Table 19-53); it is used by itself as a laxative and in combination with aluminum hydroxide as an antacid. As would be expected, patients with chronic renal failure are much more susceptible than normal subjects to hypermagnesemia as a result of antacid ingestion (887). The risk may be even greater in patients treated with potent vitamin D metabolites (888), but these do not always increase magnesium absorption (889). Combined high magnesium intake and impaired renal function can occur after renal transplantation, because antacids are routinely administered and the patient is at risk of abrupt reduction in renal function because of transplant rejection (890); this can precipitate symptomatic hypermagnesemia with values in the range of 3.5 to 6 mmol/L. Renal patients can also receive an exogenous magnesium load during hemodialysis, either because of an error in manufacture of the concentrate used for preparing the dialysate (891), or inadvertent use of excessively hard water (437).

In the past, many fatalities have resulted from poisoning with Epsom salts (magnesium sulfate), either accidental in children or deliberate in adults. In normal volunteers (892) 100 mmol of magnesium sulfate by mouth increased plasma magnesium only to about 1.7 mmol/L but the highest plasma magnesium ever recorded was 17.9 mmol/L in a patient estimated to have ingested more than 250 g of magnesium sulfate, or 1000 mmol of magnesium (893). Substantial absorption of magnesium can also occur from the large bowel. In normal subjects 400 to 800 mmol of magnesium sulfate per rectum increased the plasma magnesium roughly in proportion to the dose, with peak values between 3 and 8 mmol/L (892). Levels above 8 mmol/L have been produced by a therapeutic magnesium sulfate enema either as an evacuant or for the treatment of raised intracranial pressure, and at least one fatality has occurred (892). Perforation of the bowel and leakage of the solution into the peritoneum would further increase absorption.

Parenteral magnesium sulfate administration is still the treatment of choice for eclampsia. The optimum therapeutic blood level of magnesium is probably in the range of 3 to 4 mmol/L, but actual values at the time of delivery have varied from 1.2 to 7 mmol/L (894). Neonatal hypermagnesemia after maternal magnesium sulfate administration is common, with values in cord blood in the range of 1.5 to 6 mmol/L, correlating roughly with the maternal levels. This is especially likely if magnesium sulfate is given by continuous intravenous infusion to the mother for longer than 24 h. When intermittent intramuscular injections are given, the effect on the baby is much less (894).

Increased tubular reabsorption of magnesium occurs transiently during states of ECF volume contraction such as adrenal insufficiency or after diuretic administration. Aldosterone antagonists such as spironolactone (817) or potassium canrenoate (895) increase magnesium reabsorption when given to patients with hyperaldosteronism but have not been reported to cause hypermagnesemia. Increased Tm_{Mg}/GFR in familial hypocalciuric hypercalcemia, in some patients with primary hyperparathyroidism, and in hypothyroidism was mentioned earlier.

Effects of hypermagnesemia

The main pharmacologic actions of magnesium are blockade of neuromuscular transmission, depression of the conduction system of the heart, particularly at the sino-atrial and atrioventricular nodes, and depression of sympathetic ganglia (763, 764). The neuromuscular effect is qualitatively similar to that of curare, but results from presynaptic inhibition of acetylcholine release. All the actions of magnesium are antagonized by calcium. Contrary to earlier reports, there is no convincing evidence of any central depressive or anesthetic effect (767). Experimental hypermagnesemia in normal human subjects produced a transient sensation of warmth in the skin due to peripheral vasodilation, but no significant change in heart rate and only a slight fall in blood pressure. At plasma magnesium levels of 7 to 8 mmol/L there was complete paralysis of all skeletal muscles except the diaphragm, vocal cord adductors, and some facial muscles. There was no depression of consciousness or pain sensation, but lack of the normal means of communication gave a superficial appearance of CNS depression and coma (896). Symptomatic hypermagnesemia in patients is usually accompanied by nausea, vomiting, extreme lethargy, mental confusion, respiratory depression, dilated pupils, and absent deep tendon reflexes (887, 890, 893). In contrast to normal subjects significant hypotension and bradycardia are usual, and in isolated cases partial and complete heart block, junctional bradycardia, refractory hypotension (898), and cardiac arrest (887) have occurred. The adverse effects of magnesium may be worsened in uremic patients by hypocalcemia, hyperphosphatemia, and hyperkalemia (887), and attenuated by simultaneous hypercalcemia (437). There may also be smooth muscle paralysis leading to difficulty in micturition and defecation (887), and in neonates to inability to expel meconium (899). Transient hypocalcemia has occurred during the treatment of eclampsia (169, 900) due either to acute suppression of PTH secretion or to a substantial decrease in reabsorption and increase in urinary excretion of calcium because of competition of magnesium and calcium for the same transport mechanisms. An unexplained decrease in the anion gap may be a clue to unsuspected hypermagnesemia (901).

Chronic mild hypermagnesemia as in renal failure usually causes no symptoms, but may be associated with an increase in total body magnesium, both in bone and in soft tissue mineral deposits (902). Magnesium accumulation is probably a passive consequence of the higher plasma level, although the crystal structure of the mineral may be abnormal. In different experimental conditions magnesium may either inhibit or promote mineralization.

Treatment of hypermagnesemia

In most cases simple withdrawal of the exogenous source is all that is needed; there is no immediate danger if the deep tendon reflexes are still present. In the presence of severe respiratory depression or cardiac conduction defect, emergency treatment consists of support for ventilation and the intravenous administration of 2.5 to 5 mmol of calcium as a pharmacologic antagonist and of glucose and insulin to produce temporary influx into cells, as in the treatment of hyperkalemia. In the nephrectomized dog, uptake by soft tissue or bone may lower plasma magnesium by about 0.2 mmol/h (903). The most effective treatment is hemodialysis with a magnesium-free solution, which should produce a safe blood level within 4 to 6 h (890). This should be used in patients with impaired renal function with plasma levels greater than 5 mmol/L, or if there are any life-threatening complications. In neonatal hypermagnesemia, exchange transfusion has been effective (798).

APPENDIX: SPECIALIZED DIAGNOSTIC TESTS

HYDROCORTISONE TEST (424)

Hydrocortisone, 40 mg, should be given every 8 h and plasma corrected total or ionized calcium and phosphate measured 2 days and immediately before and then every 2 to 3 days for 10 to 14 days, or until the plasma calcium attains a stable level. The dietary calcium intake should be approximately constant. Other corticosteroids should not be used because they have been less-well standardized and occasionally produce different results. Higher doses should not be used because false-positive results in hyperparathyroidism are much more likely. The uncorrected total calcium may fall because of dilution of plasma proteins resulting from steroid-induced sodium retention, so that omission of a protein correction can lead to a false-positive result. Although rarely needed the test is exceedingly reliable and with the correct protocol false-positive results never occur in Type 2 hyperparathyroidism (647, 904). It must be emphasized that only negative inferences can be drawn; if the plasma calcium falls, the hypercalcemia is not due to hyperparathyroidism, whereas if the plasma calcium does not fall, the hypercalcemia is not due to sarcoidosis, vitamin D intoxication, or the milk-alkali syndrome. Urinary calcium excretion usually behaves like the plasma calcium but has been less-well standardized.

PHOSPHATE DEPRIVATION TEST (266)

This is useful in patients with equivocal hypercalcemia presenting with renal failure or osteitis fibrosa in whom hypercalcemia may be masked by a raised plasma phosphate, and in the investigation of patients with conditions thought to be associated with hyperparathyroidism in whom hypercalcemia may be masked by a high dietary intake of phosphate even without hyperphosphatemia. A low-phosphate diet (less than 15 mmol/day) and aluminum hydroxide gel 30 mL q.i.d. should be given for 6 days. Any other nonmagnesium aluminum-based antacid can be used provided the total dose of aluminum is approximately 2.5 g/day. Plasma corrected total or ionized calcium and phosphate should be measured 2 days and immediately before and then on alternate days (i.e., −2,0,2,4, and 6) and iPTH or NcAMP/GFR once before and on the sixth day after. If the plasma phosphate or iPTH falls and hypercalcemia does not occur, the patient probably has nonautonomous secondary hyperparathyroidism due to or complicated by renal failure or by excess dietary phosphate. If hypercalcemia occurs the patient probably has primary or autonomous secondary hyperparathyroidism, particularly if

iPTH remains high. The degree of phosphate depletion should be monitored by serial 24-h urine phosphate measurements; urine calcium excretion usually increases in all cases and is of much less discriminatory value than the change in plasma calcium.

THIAZIDE CHALLENGE TEST (349, 546)

This is useful in patients with equivocal hypercalcemia, hypercalciuria, and nephrolithiasis. A thiazide diuretic, one tablet every 6 or 12 h, should be given until unequivocal hypercalcemia occurs, but not for longer than 6 days unless continued as treatment. The minimum reliable dose has not been established. Plasma corrected total or ionized calcium and phosphate and 24-h urine calcium excretion should be measured 2 days and immediately before and then every 2 days (i.e., −2, 0, 2, 4, and 6), and plasma iPTH or NcAMP/GFR once before and on the sixth day or at the time of the highest plasma calcium. If urine calcium excretion and iPTH or NcAMP/GFR fall and hypercalcemia does not occur, the patient has renal-tubular hypercalciuria with secondary hyperparathyroidism. If hypercalcemia occurs and iPTH or NcAMP does not fall, the patient has either primary or autonomous secondary hyperparathyroidism. If neither urine nor plasma calcium changes, the test is uninterpretable. In patients with unequivocal hypercalcemic hyperparathyroidism, the response is variable (258), but the test is redundant.

REFERENCES

1. Goldsmith, R. S.: Laboratory aids in the diagnosis of metabolic bone disease, *Orthop. Clin. North Am.*, **3**:545–560, 1972.
2. Husdan, H., M. Leung, D. Oreopoulos, and A. Rapoport: Measurement of serum and plasma ionic calcium with the Space Stat 20 Ionized Calcium Analyzer, *Clin. Chem.*, **23**:1775–1777, 1977.
3. Wills, M. R.: The effect of diurnal variation on total plasma calcium concentration in normal subjects, *J. Clin. Pathol.*, **23**:772–777, 1970.

4. Schwartz, H. D.: New techniques for ion-selective measurements of ionized calcium in serum after pH adjustment of aerobically handled sera, *Clin. Chem.*, **22**:461–467, 1976.

5. Parfitt, A. M.: Investigation of disorders of the parathyroid glands, *J. Clin. Endocrinol. Metab.*, **3**:451–474, 1974.

6. Harris, E. K., and D. L. DeMets: Biological and analytic components of variation in long-term studies of serum constituents in normal subjects. V. Estimated biological variations in ionized calcium, *Clin. Chem.*, **17**:983–987, 1971.

7. Pedersen, K. O.: On the cause and degree of intraindividual serum calcium variability, *Scand. J. Clin. Lab. Invest.*, **30**:191–199, 1972.

8. Conceicao, S. C., D. Weightman, P. A. Smith, J. Luno, M. K. Ward, and D. S. Kerr: Serum ionised calcium concentration: Measurement versus calculation, *Br. Med. J.*, **1**:1103–1105, 1978.

9. Phillips, P. J., R. W. Pain, T. F. Hartley, and B. McL. Duncan: Current "corrected" calcium concept rechallenged, *Clin. Chem.*, **23**:1938–1939, 1977.

10. Aitken, R. E., P. C. Bartley, S. J. Bryant, and H. M. Lloyd: The effect of multiphasic biochemical screening on the diagnosis of primary hyperparathyroidism, *Aust. N.Z. J. Med.*, **5**:224–226, 1975.

11. Sorell, M., and J. F. Rosen: Ionized calcium: Serum levels during symptomatic hypocalcemia, *J. Pediatr.*, **87**:67–70, 1975.

12. Lindgärde, F., and O. Zettervall: Characterization of a calcium-binding IgG myeloma protein, *Scand. J. Immunol.*, **3**:277–285, 1974.

13. Young, D. S., E. K. Harris, and E. Cotlove: Biological and analytic components of variation in long-term studies of serum constituents in normal subjects. IV. Results of a study designed to eliminate long-term analytic deviations, *Clin. Chem.*, **17**:403–410, 1971.

14. Kleerekoper, M., J. P. Ingham, S. W. McCarthy, and S. Posen: Parathyroid hormone assay in primary hyperparathyroidism: Experiences with a radioimmunoassay based on commercially available reagents, *Clin. Chem.*, **20**:369–375, 1974.

15. Parsons, J. A.: Parathyroid physiology and the skeleton, in G. H. Bourne (ed.), *Biochemistry and Physiology of Bone*, vol. IV, Academic Press, Inc., New York, 1976.

16. Flueck, J. A., F. P. DiBella, A. J. Edis, J. M. Kehrwald, and C. D. Arnaud: Immuno-heterogeneity of parathyroid hormone in venous effluent serum from hyperfunctioning parathyroid glands, *J. Clin. Invest.*, **601**:1367–1375, 1977.

17. Freitag, J., K. J. Martin, K. A. Hruska, C. Anderson, M. Conrades, J. Landenson, S. Klahr, and E. Slatopolsky: Impaired parathyroid hormone metabolism in patients with chronic renal failure, *N. Engl. J. Med.*, **298**:29–32, 1978.

18. Hruska, K. A., K. Martin, P. Mennes, A. Greenwalt, C. Anderson, S. Klahr, and E. Slatopolsky: Degradation of parathyroid hormone and fragment production by the isolated perfused dog kidney: The effect of glomerular filtration rate and perfusate Ca^{++} concentrations, *J. Clin. Invest.*, **60**:501–510, 1977.

19. Parfitt, A. M.: Cushing's syndrome with normal replacement dose of cortisone in pituitary hypothyroidism, *J. Clin. Endocrinol.*, **25**:560–562, 1964.

20. Chambers, D. T., J. M. Zanelli, J. A. Parsons, L. Bitensky, and J. Chayen: A new ultra-structure cytochemical assay for measurement of biologically active parathyroid hormone in human plasma (abstract), *3rd International Workshop on Calcified Tissues*, Israel, 1978.

21. Christensen, M. S.: A sensitive radioimmunoassay of parathyroid hormone in human serum using a specific extraction procedure, *Scand. J. Clin. Lab. Invest.*, **36**:313–322, 1976.

22. Prien, E. L., E. B. Pyle, and S. M. Krane: Secondary hyperparathyroidism, in R. O. Greep, E. B. Astwood, and G. D. Aurbach (eds.), *Handbook of Physiology*, sec. 7, vol. VII, Am. Physiol. Soc., Washington, D.C., 1976, pp. 383–410.

23. Parfitt, A. M.: A theoretical model of the relationship between parathyroid cell mass and plasma calcium concentration in normal and uremic subjects: An analysis of the concept of autonomy and speculations on the mechanism of parathyroid hyperplasia, *Arch. Intern. Med.*, **124**:269–273, 1969.

24. Bouillon, R., and P. DeMoor: Parathyroid hormone secretion in primary hyperparathyroidism, *J. Clin. Endocrinol. Metab.*, **45**:261–269, 1977.

25. Shaw, J. W., S. B. Oldham, L. Rosoff, J. E. Bethune, and M. P. Fichman: Urinary cyclic AMP

analyzed as a function of the serum calcium and parathyroid hormone in the differential diagnosis of hypercalcemia, *J. Clin. Invest.*, **59:**14–21, 1977.

26. Chambers, R. McK., and T. L. Dormandy: Measurement and interpretation of hypercalciuria on twenty-four-hour urine series, *Lancet*, **4:**1378–1382, 1967.

27. Marshall, R. W., and W. G. Robertson: Nomograms for the estimation of the saturation of urine with calcium oxalate, calcium phosphate, magnesium ammonium phosphate, uric acid, sodium acid urate, ammonium acid urate and cystine, *Clin. Chim. Acta*, **72:**253–260, 1976.

28. Ransil, B. J., D. J. Greenblatt, and J. Koch-Weser: Evidence for systematic temporal variation in 24-hour urinary creatinine excretion, *J. Clin. Pharmacol.*, **17:**108–119, 1977.

29. Walton, R. J., and O. L. M. Bijvoet: Nomogram for derivation of renal threshold phosphate correlation, *Lancet*, **11:**309–310, 1975.

30. Broadus, A. E., J. E. Mahaffey, F. C. Bartter, and R. M. Neer: Nephrogenous cyclic adenosine monophosphate as a parathyroid function test, *J. Clin. Invest.*, **60:**771–783, 1977.

31. Babka, J. C., R. H. Bower, and J. Sode: Nephrogenous cyclic AMP levels in primary hyperparathyroidism, *Arch. Intern. Med.*, **136:**1140–1144, 1976.

32. Neelon, F. A.: cAMP and calcemia, *Ann. Intern. Med.*, **86:**821–822, 1977.

33. Broadus, A. E., L. J. Deftos, and F. C. Bartter: Effects of the intravenous administration of calcium on nephrogenous cyclic AMP: Use as a parathyroid suppression test, *J. Clin. Endocrinol. Metab.*, **46:**477–487, 1978.

34. Arnaud, S. B., M. Matthusen, J. B. Gilkinson, and R. S. Goldsmith: Components of 25-hydroxyvitamin D in serum of young children in upper midwestern United States, *Am. J. Clin. Nutr.*, **30:**1082–1086, 1977.

35. Schaefer, P. C., and R. S. Goldsmith: Quantitation of 25-hydroxycholecalciferol in human serum by high-pressure liquid chromatography, *J. Lab. Clin. Med.*, **91:**104–108, 1978.

36. Stamp, T. C. B.: Intestinal absorption of 25-hydroxycholecalciferol, *Lancet*, **3:**121–123, 1974.

37. Deftos, L. J.: Calcitonin in clinical medicine, *Adv. Intern. Med.*, **23:**159–193, 1978.

38. Parfitt, A. M.: The actions of parathyroid hormone on bone. Relation to bone remodelling and turnover, calcium homeostasis and metabolic bone disease. I. Mechanisms of calcium transfer between blood and bone and their cellular basis. Morphologic and kinetic approaches to bone turnover, *Metabolism*, **25:**809–844, 1976.

39. Lauffenburger, T., A. J. Olah, M. A. Dambacher, J. Guncaga, C. Lentner, and H. G. Haas: Bone remodeling and calcium metabolism: A correlated histomorphometric, calcium kinetic, and biochemical study in patients with osteoporosis and Paget's disease, *Metabolism*, **26:**589–606, 1977.

40. Parfitt, A. M., and H. Duncan: Metabolic bone disease affecting the spine, in R. Rothman and F. Simeone (eds.), *The Spine*, W.B. Saunders Company, Philadelphia, 1975, pp. 599–720.

41. Posen, S., C. Cornish, and M. Kleerekoper: Alkaline phosphatase and metabolic bone disorders, in L. V. Avioli and S. M. Krane (eds.), *Metabolic Bone Disease*, vol. 1, Academic Press, New York, 1977.

42. Round, J. M.: Plasma calcium, magnesium, phosphorus, and alkaline phosphatase levels in normal British schoolchildren, *Br. Med. J.*, **3:**137–140, 1973.

43. Heaney, R. P., R. R. Recker, and P. D. Saville: Calcium balance and calcium requirements in middle-aged women, *Am. J. Clin. Nutr.*, **30:**1603–1611, 1977.

44. Nordin, B. E. C.: Diagnostic procedures, in B. E. C. Nordin (ed.), *Calcium, Phosphate and Magnesium Metabolism*, Churchill-Livingstone, New York, 1976.

45. Arnaud, S. B., R. S. Goldsmith, G. B. Stickler, J. T. McCall, and C. D. Arnaud: Serum parathyroid hormone and blood minerals: Interrelationships in normal children, *Pediatr. Res.*, **7:**485–493, 1973.

46. Keating, F. R., J. D. Jones, and L. R. Elveback: Distribution of serum calcium and phosphorus values in unselected ambulatory patients, *J. Lab. Clin. Med.*, **74:**507–514, 1969.

47. Kelly, A., L. Munan, C. PetitClerc, K. P. Ho, and B. Billon: Use of values for calcium and protein in serum, and of a derived index obtained from a

probability population sample, *Clin. Chem.,* **22:**1723–1727, 1976.

48. Ljunghall, S., H. Hedstrand, K. Hellsing, and L. Wibell: Calcium, phosphate and albumin in serum: A population study with special reference to renal stone formers and the prevalence of hyperparathyroidism in middle-aged men, *Acta Med. Scand.,* **201:**23–30, 1977.

49. Graham, W. P., G. S. Gordan, H. F. Loken, A. Blum, and A. Halden: Effect of pregnancy and of the menstrual cycle on hypoparathyroidism, *J. Clin. Endocrinol.,* **24:**512–516, 1964.

50. Cushard, A., M. A. Crebtor, J. M. Canterbury, and E. Reiss: Physiologic hyperparathyroidism in pregnancy, *J. Clin. Endocrinol.,* **34:**767–771, 1972.

51. Parfitt, A. M.: The actions of parathyroid hormone on bone. Relation to bone remodelling and turnover, calcium homeostasis and metabolic bone disease. IV. The state of the bones in uremic hyperparathyroidism. The mechanisms of skeletal resistance to PTH in renal failure and pseudohypoparathyroidism and the role of PTH in osteoporosis, osteopetrosis and osteofluorosis, *Metabolism,* **25:**1157–1187, 1976.

52. Gerblich, A. A., S. M. Genuth, and J. G. Haddad: A case of idiopathic hypoparathyroidism and dietary vitamin D deficiency: The requirement for calcium and vitamin D for bone, but not renal responsiveness to PTH, *J. Clin. Endocrinol. Metab.,* **44:**507–513, 1977.

53. Parfitt, A. M.: Idiopathic, surgical and other varieties of parathyroid hormone deficient hypoparathyroidism, in L. DeGroot (ed.), *Metabolic Basis of Endocrinology,* Grune & Stratton Inc., New York. In press.

54. Haussler, M. R., and T. A. McCain: Basic and clinical concepts related to vitamin D metabolism and action, *N. Engl. J. Med.,* **297:**974–983 and 1041–1050, 1977.

55. Parfitt, A. M.: The spectrum of hypoparathyroidism, *J. Clin. Endocrinol. Metab.,* **34:**152–158, 1972.

56. Potts, J. T., and L. J. Deftos: Parathyroid hormone, calcitonin, vitamin D and bone mineral metabolism, in P. K. Bondy and L. E. Rosenberg (eds.), *Diseases of Metabolism,* 7th ed., vol. 2, W. B. Saunders Company, Philadelphia, 1974, pp. 1225–1430.

57. Yendt, E. R.: Disorders of calcium, phosphorus,

and magnesium metabolism, in M. H. Maxwell and C. R. Kleeman (eds.), *Clinical Disorders of Fluid and Electrolyte Metabolism,* 2d ed., McGraw-Hill Book Company, New York, 1972.

58. Burckhardt, P., B. Ruedi, and J. P. Felber: Estrogen-induced tetany in idiopathic hypoparathyroidism, *Hormone Res.,* **6:**321–328, 1975.

59. Coulson, R., and A. M. Moses: Effect of chlorpropamide on renal response to parathyroid hormone in normal subjects and in patients with hypoparathyroidism and pseudohypoparathyroidism, *J. Pharmacol. Exp. Ther.,* **194:**603–613, 1975.

60. Sinha, T. K., D. O. Allen,, S. F. Queener, and N. H. Bell: Effects of acetazolamide on the renal excretion of phosphate in hypoparathyroidism and pseudohypoparathyroidism, *J. Lab. Clin. Med.,* **89:**1188–1197, 1977.

61. Rasmussen, H., and P. J. Bordier: *The Physiological and Cellular Basis of Metabolic Bone Disease,* The Williams & Wilkins Company, Baltimore, 1974.

62. Eisenberg, E.: Effects of serum calcium level and parathyroid extracts on phosphate and calcium excretion in hypoparathyroid patients, *J. Clin. Invest.,* **44:**942–946, 1965.

63. Davies, M., C. M. Taylor, L. F. Hill, and S. W. Stanbury: 1,25-Dihydroxycholecalciferol in hypoparathyroidism, *Lancet,* **1:**55–58, 1977.

64. Parfitt, A. M.: Equilibrium and disequilibrium hypercalcemia—new light on an old concept, *Metab. Bone Dis. Rel. Res.* In press.

65. Cohn, S. H., M. S. Roginsky, J. F. Aloia, K. J. Ellis, and K. K. Shukla: Alterations in skeletal calcium and phosphorus in dysfunction of the parathyroids, *J. Clin. Endocrinol. Metab.,* **36:**750–755, 1973.

66. Schneider, A. B., and L. M. Sherwood: Pathogenesis and management of hypoparathyroidism and other hypocalcemic disorders, *Metabolism,* **24:**871–898, 1975.

67. Nusynowitz, M. L., B. Frame, and F. O. Kolb: The spectrum of the hypoparathyroid states: A classification based on physiologic principles, *Medicine,* **55:**105–119, 1976.

68. Farrell, P. M., H. Rikkers, and D. Moel: Cortisol-dihydrotachysterol metabolism in a patient with hypoparathyroidism and adrenal insufficiency:

Apparent inhibition of bone resorption, *J. Clin. Endocrinol.*, **42**:953–957, 1976.

69. Salander, H., and L.-E. Tisell: Incidence of hypoparathyroidism after radical surgery for thyroid carcinoma and autotransplantation of parathyroid glands, *Am. J. Surg.*, **134**:358–362, 1977.

70. Clowes, G. H. A., and F. A. Simeone: Acute hypocalcemia in surgical patients, *Ann. Surg.*, **146**:530–541, 1957.

71. Wilkin, T. J., T. E. Isles, C. R. Paterson, J. Crooks, and J. S. Beck: Postthyroidectomy hypocalcaemia: A feature of the operation or the thyroid disorder? *Lancet*, **1**:621–623, 1977.

72. Kaplan, E. L., R. Staroscik, G. W. Peskin, and C. D. Arnaud: Calcitonin-like responses in man during thyroid surgery, *J. Clin. Endocrinol.*, **28**:740–745, 1968.

73. Michie, W., J. M. Stowers, and S. C. Frazer: Postthyroidectomy hypocalcemia, *Lancet*, **1**:1051–1052, 1977.

74. Parfitt, A. M.: The actions of parathyroid hormone on bone. Relation to bone remodelling and turnover, calcium homeostasis and metabolic bone disease. III. PTH and osteoblasts, the relationship between bone turnover and bone loss, and the state of the bones in primary hyperparathyroidism, *Metabolism*, **25**:1033–1069, 1976.

75. Hans, S. S., and P. T. Lee: Post-thyroidectomy hypoparathyroidism, *Am. Surg.*, **42**:930–933, 1976.

76. Tsang, R. C., E. F. Donovan, and J. J. Steichen: Calcium physiology and pathology in the neonate, *Pediatr. Clin. North Am.*, **23**:611–626, 1976.

77. Bergman, L., and B. Isaksson: Plasma calcium fractions in normal subjects from birth to adult ages, *Acta Paediatr. Scand.*, **60**:630–636, 1971.

78. David, L., and C. S. Anast: Calcium metabolism in newborn infants: The interrelationship of parathyroid function and calcium, magnesium, and phosphorus metabolism in normal, "sick," and hypocalcemic newborns, *J. Clin. Invest.*, **54**:287–296, 1974.

79. Johnston, C. C., and R. B. Schnute: A case of primary hyperparathyroidism with spontaneous remission following infarction of the adenoma with development of hypocalcemic tetany, *J. Clin. Endocrinol. Metab.*, **21**:196–200, 1961.

80. Northrop, G., H. R. Misenhimer, and F. O. Becker: Failure of parathyroid hormone to cross the nonhuman primate placenta, *Am. J. Obstet. Gynecol.*, **129**:449–453, 1977.

81. Rude, R. K., S. B. Oldham, and E. R. Singer: Functional hypoparathyroidism and parathyroid hormone end organ resistance in human magnesium deficiency, *Clin. Endocrinol.*, **5**:209–244, 1976.

82. Medalle, R., and C. Waterhouse: A magnesium deficient patient presenting with hypocalcemia and hyperphosphatemia, *Ann. Intern. Med.*, **79**:76–79, 1973.

83. Parfitt, A. M.: The effect of cellulose phosphate on calcium and magnesium homeostasis, *Clin. Sci. Mol. Med.*, **49**:83–90, 1975.

84. Bordier, P., H. Rasmussen, P. Marie, L. Miravet, J. Gueris, and A. Ryckwaert: Vitamin D metabolites and bone mineralization in man, *J. Clin. Endocrinol. Metab.*, **46**:284–294, 1978.

85. Hosking, D. J., A. Williams, R. B. Godwin-Austen, and S. P. Allison: Osteomalacia presenting as chorea, *Br. Med. J.*, **3**:136–138, 1975.

86. Kanis, J. A., and R. J. Walton: Osteomalacia associated with increased renal tubular resorption of phosphate (hypohyperparathyroidism), *Postgrad. Med. J.*, **52**:295–297, 1976.

87. Muldowney, F. B., J. Donohoe, and C. Ryan: Bone disease in intestinal malabsorption, *Mod. Treat.*, **7**:686–702, 1971.

88. Steendijk, R.: The effect of parathyroid extract on the serum concentrations of calcium and inorganic phosphate in active and healing rickets, *Acta Paediatr.*, **53**:105–108, 1964.

89. Tomlinson, S., G. N. Hendy, D. M. Pemberton, and J. L. H. O'Riordan: Reversible resistance to the renal action of parathyroid hormone in man, *Clin. Sci. Mol. Med.*, **51**:59–69, 1976.

90. Coburn, J. W., and N. Brautbar: Disease states related to vitamin D, in A. W. Norman and M. Decker (eds.), *Vitamin D, Clinical and Nutritional Aspects*, New York. In press.

90a. Habener, J. L., and J. E. Mahaffey: Osteomalacia and disorders of vitamin D metabolism, *Ann. Rev. Med.*, **29**:327–342, 1978.

90b. Brooks, M. H., N. H. Bell, L. Love, P. H. Stern, E. Orfei, S. F. Queener, A. J. Hamstra, and H. F. DeLuca: Vitamin-D-dependent rickets type II: Resistance of target organs to 1,25-dihydroxyvitamin D, *N. Engl. J. Med.*, **298**:996–999, 1978.

91. Arnaud, S. B., G. B. Stickler, and J. C. Haworth: Serum 25-hydroxyvitamin D in infantile rickets, *Pediatrics*, **57**:221–225, 1976.

92. Frame, B., and A. M. Parfitt: Osteomalacia: Current concepts, *Ann. Intern. Med.*, **89**:966–982, 1978.

93. Morgan, B.: *Osteomalacia, Renal Osteodystrophy and Osteoporosis*, Charles C Thomas, Publisher, Springfield, Ill., 1973.

94. Gertner, J. M., M. Lilburn, and M. Domenech: 25-Hydroxycholecalciferol absorption in steatorrhoea and postgastrectomy osteomalacia, *Br. Med. J.*, **1**:1310–1312, 1977.

95. Lund, B., O. H. Sorensen, M. Hilden, and B. Lund: The hepatic conversion of vitamin D in alcoholics with varying degrees of liver affection, *Acta Med. Scand.*, **202**:221–224, 1977.

96. Mawer, E. B.: Aspects of the control of vitamin D metabolism in man, in A. W. Norman et al. (eds.), *Vitamin D: Biochemical, Chemical and Clinical Aspects Related to Calcium Metabolism*, Walter de Gruyter & Co., Berlin, 1977.

97. Krawitt, E. L., M. J. Grundman, and E. B. Mawer: Absorption, hydroxylation and excretion of vitamin D_3 in primary biliary cirrhosis, *Lancet*, **4**:1246–1249, 1977.

98. Barragry, J. M., M. W. France, N. D. Carter, J. A. Auton, M. Beer, B. J. Boucher, and R. D. Cohen: Vitamin D metabolism in nephrotic syndrome, *Lancet*, **3**:629–632, 1977.

99. Goldstein, D. A., Y. Oda, K. Kurokawa, and S. G. Massry: Blood levels of 25-hydroxyvitamin D in nephrotic syndrome, *Ann. Intern. Med.*, **87**:664–667, 1977.

100. Stamp, T. C. B.: Effects of long-term anticonvulsant therapy on calcium and vitamin D metabolism, *Proc. R. Soc. Med.*, **67**:64–68, 1974.

101. Silver, J., G. Neale, and G. R. Thompson: Effect of phenobarbitone treatment on vitamin D metabolism in mammals. *Clin. Sci. Mol. Med.*, **46**:433–448, 1974.

102. Jenkins, M. V., M. Harris, and M. R. Wills: The effect of phenytoin on parathyroid extract and 25-hydroxycholecalciferol-induced bone resorption: Adenosine 3′, 5′ cyclic monophosphate production, *Calcif. Tissue Res.*, **16**:163–167, 1974.

103. Mosekilde, L., F. Melsen, M. S. Christensen, B. Lund, and O. H. Sorensen: Effect of long-term vitamin D_2 treatment on bone morphometry and biochemical values in anticonvulsant osteomalacia, *Acta Med. Scand.*, **201**:303–307, 1977.

104. Jubiz, W., M. R. Haussler, T. A. McCain, and K. G. Tolman: Plasma 1,25-dihydroxyvitamin D levels in patients receiving anticonvulsant drugs, *J. Clin. Endocrinol. Metab.*, **44**:617–621, 1977.

105. Kleeman, K., and C. R. Kleeman: Parathyroid hormone and calcitonin, *The Year in Endocrinology*, 1977.

106. Prader, A., H. P. Kind, and H. F. DeLuca: Pseudovitamin D deficiency (vitamin D dependency), in H. Bickel and J. Stern (eds.), *Inborn Errors of Calcium and Bone Metabolism*, University Park Press, Baltimore, 1976.

107. Frame, B., and A. M. Parfitt: Vitamin D dependent bone disease: Long term response to vitamin D analogs and effect on tetracycline based bone dynamics, in A. W. Norman et al. (eds.), *Vitamin D: Biochemical, Chemical and Clinical Aspects Related to Calcium Metabolism*, Walter de Gruyter, Berlin, 1977.

108. Potts, J. T.: Pseudohypoparathyroidism, in J. B. Stanbury, J. B. Wyngaarden, and D. S. Fredrickson (eds.), *The Metabolic Basis of Inherited Disease*, 4th ed., McGraw-Hill Book Company, New York, 1978.

109. Mann, J. B., S. Alterman, and A. G. Hills: Albright's hereditary osteodystrophy comprising pseudohypoparathyroidism: With a report of two cases representing the complete syndrome occurring in successive generations, *Ann. Intern. Med.*, **56**:315–342, 1962.

110. Mautalen, C. A., J.-F. Dymling, and M. Horwith: Pseudohypoparathyroidism 1942–1966: A negative progress report, *Am. J. Med.*, **42**:977–985, 1967.

111. Marx, S. J., J. M. Hershman, and G. D. Aurbach: Thyroid dysfunction in pseudohypoparathyroidism, *J. Clin. Endocrinol. Metab.*, **33**:822–828, 1971.

112. Weinberg, A. G., and R. T. Stone: Autosomal dominant inheritance in Albright's hereditary osteodystrophy, *J. Pediatr.*, **79**:996–999, 1971.

113. Tomlinson, S., G. N. Hendy, and J. L. H. O'Riordan: A simplified assessment of response to parathyroid hormone in hypoparathyroid patients, *Lancet*, **1**:62–64, 1976.

114. Marcus, R., J. F. Wilber, and G. D. Aurbach:

Parathyroid hormone-sensitive adenyl cyclase from the renal cortex of a patient with pseudohypoparathyroidism, *J. Clin. Endocrinol.*, **33**:537–541, 1971.

115. Sinha, T. K., H. F. DeLuca, and N. H. Bell: Evidence for a defect in the formation of 1,25-dihydroxyvitamin D in pseudohypoparathyroidism, *Metabolism*, **26**:731–738, 1977.

116. Parfitt, A. M.: Tubular reabsorption of calcium in pseudohypoparathyroidism, in D. H. Copp and R. V. Talmadge (eds.), *Endocrinology of Calcium Metabolism*, Excerpta Medica, Amsterdam, 1978.

117. Moses, A. M., N. Breslau, and R. Coulson: Renal responses to PTH in patients with hormone-resistant (pseudo)hypoparathyroidism, *Am. J. Med.*, **61**:184–189, 1976.

118. Breslau, N., and A. M. Moses: Renal calcium reabsorption caused by bicarbonate and by chlorothiazide in patients with hormone resistant (pseudo) hypoparathyroidism, *J. Clin. Endocrinol. Metab.*, **46**:389–395, 1978.

119. Drezner, M., F. A. Neelon, and H. E. Lebovitz: Pseudohypoparathyroidism type II: A possible defect in the reception of the cyclic AMP signal, *N. Engl. J. Med.*, **289**:1056–1060, 1973.

120. Rodriguez, H. J., H. Villarreal, S. Klahr, and E. Slatopolsky: Pseudohypoparathyroidism type II: Restoration of normal renal responsiveness to parathyroid hormone by calcium administration, *J. Clin. Endocrinol. Metab.*, **39**:693–701, 1974.

121. Metz, S. A., D. J. Baylink, M. R. Hughes, M. R. Haussler, and R. P. Robertson: Selective deficiency of 1,25-dihydroxycholecalciferol—A cause of isolated skeletal resistance to parathyroid hormone, *N. Engl. J. Med.*, **297**:1084–1090, 1977.

122. Milgram, J. W., C. A. Engh, C. R. Haminton, and G. M. Kammer: Renal resistance to parathyroid hormone with hyperphosphatemic osteomalacia and osteitis fibrosa, *J. Bone Joint Surg.*, **56A**:1493–1500, 1974.

123. Nusynowitz, M. L., and M. H. Klein: Pseudoidiopathic hypoparathyroidism: Hypoparathyroidism with ineffective parathyroid hormone, *Am. J. Med.*, **55**:677–686, 1973.

124. Connors, M. H., J. J. Irias, and M. Golabi: Hypo-hyperparathyroidism: Evidence for a defective parathyroid hormone, *Pediatrics*, **60**:343–348, 1977.

125. Lloyd, H. M., J. D. Meares, and J. Jacobi: Effects of oestrogen and bromocryptine on *in vivo* secretion and mitosis in prolactin cells, *Nature*, **255**:497–498, 1975.

126. Wilkinson, R.: Absorption of calcium, phosphorus and magnesium, in B. E. C. Nordin (ed.), *Calcium, Phosphate and Magnesium Metabolism*, Churchill-Livingstone, New York, 1976.

127. Phillips, S. F., and J. Giller: The contribution of the colon to electrolyte and water conservation in man, *J. Lab. Clin. Med.*, **81**:733–746, 1973.

128. Stanbury, S. W.: Intestinal absorption of calcium and phosphorus in adult man in health and disease, in H. Bukel and J. Stern (eds.), *Inborn Errors of Calcium and Bone Metabolism*, University Park Press, Baltimore, 1976.

129. Nassim, J. R., P. D. Saville, P. B. Cook, and L. Mulligan: The effects of vitamin D and gluten-free diet in idiopathic steatorrhoea, *Q.J. Med.*, **28**:141–162, 1959.

130. Litvak, J., E. Oberhauser, J. Riesco, O. Lopez, R. Armendaris, I. Alliende, and F. Solis: Strontium-85 kinetics in hypoparathyroidism at different levels of calcium intake, *J. Nucl. Med.*, **8**:60–69, 1967.

131. Kooh, S. W., D. Fraser, B. J. Reilly, J. R. Hamilton, D. G. Gall, and L. Bell: Rickets due to calcium deficiency, *N. Engl. J. Med.*, **297**:1262–1266, 1977.

132. Heaney, R. P., and T. G. Skillman: Calcium metabolism in normal human pregnancy, *J. Clin. Endocrinol.*, **33**:661–670, 1971.

133. Schilling, A., D. Laszlo, J. Bellin, and E. D. Gottesman: The effect of diethylstilbestrol on the calcium, phosphorus and nitrogen metabolism of prostatic carcinoma, *J. Clin. Invest.*, **29**:918–924, 1950.

134. Spencer, H., R. Eisinger, and D. Laszlo: Metabolic and radioactive tracer studies in carcinoma of the prostate. Effect of diethylstibestrol and of orchiectomy, *Am. J. Med.*, **29**:282–296, 1960.

135. Chase, L. R., and E. Slatopolsky: Secretion and metabolic efficacy of parathyroid hormone in patients with severe hypomagnesemia, *J. Clin. Endocrinol. Metab.*, **38**:363–371, 1974.

136. Castro, J. H., S. M. Genuth, and L. Klein: Comparative response to parathyroid hormone in hyperthyroidism and hypothyroidism, *Metabolism*, **24**:839–848, 1975.

137. Isgreen, W. P.: Normocalcemic tetany: A problem of erethism, *Neurology*, **26:**825–834, 1976.

138. Maisels, M. J., T.-K. Li, J. T. Piechocki, and M. W. Werthman: The effect of exchange transfusion on serum ionized calcium, *Pediatrics*, **53:**683–686, 1974.

139. Buskard, N. A., Z. Varghese, and M. R. Wills: Correction of hypocalcaemic symptoms during plasma exchange, *Lancet*, **3:**344–346, 1976.

140. Shaw, J. W., S. B. Oldham, J. E. Bethune, and M. P. Fichman: Parathyroid hormone (PTH)-mediated rise in urinary cyclic AMP (UcAMP) during acute extracellular fluid (ECF) expansion natriuresis in man, *J. Clin. Endocrinol. Metab.*, **39:**311–315, 1974.

141. Bunker, J. P.: Metabolic effects of blood transfusion, *Anesthesiology*, **27:**446–453, 1966.

142. Howland, W. S., O. Schweizer, and C. P. Boyan: Massive blood replacement without calcium administration, *Surg. Gynecol. Obstet.*, **118:**814–818, 1964.

143. Schaer, H., and U. Bachmann: Ionized calcium in acidosis: Differential effect of hypercapnic and lactic acidosis, *Br. J. Anaesth.*, **46:**842–848, 1974.

144. Ladenson, J. H., and J. C. Shyong: Influence of fatty acids on the binding of calcium to human serum albumin, *Clin. Chim. Acta*, **75:**293–302, 1977.

145. Sibbald, W. J., V. Sardesai, and R. F. Wilson: Hypocalcemia and nephrogenous cyclic AMP production in critically ill or injured patients, *J. Trauma*, **17:**677–684, 1977.

146. White, R. D., R. S. Goldsmith, R. Rodriguez, E. A. Moffitt, and J. R. Pluth: Plasma ionic calcium levels following injection of chloride, gluconate, and gluceptate salts of calcium, *J. Thorac. Cardiovasc. Surg.*, **71:**609–613, 1976.

147. Drop, L. J., and M. B. Laver: Low plasma ionized calcium and response to calcium therapy in critically ill man, *Anesthesiology*, **43:**300–306, 1975.

148. Blanc, D., M.-C. Chapuy, and P. Meunier: Evaluation de l'activite osteoclastique par le test d'hypocalcemie provoquee par la calcitonine de saumon, *Nouv. Presse Med.*, **6:**2489–2494, 1977.

149. Birge, S. J., and L. V. Avioli: Glucagon-induced hypocalcemia in man, *J. Clin. Endocrinol.*, **29:**213–218, 1969.

150. Ellwood, M. G., and G. H. Robb: Self-poisoning with colchicine, *Postgrad. Med. J.*, **47:**129–138, 1971.

151. Heath, D. A., J. S. Palmer, and G. D. Aurbach: The hypocalcemic action of colchicine, *Endocrinology*, **90:**1589–1593, 1972.

152. Burkhardt, P. M., F. R. Singer, M. Peacock, and J. T. Potts: Parathyroid function in patients with Pagets disease treated with salmon calcitonin, in B. Frame, A. M. Parfitt, and H. Duncan (eds.), *Clinical Aspects of Metabolic Bone Disease*, Excerpta Medica, Amsterdam, 1973.

153. Keynes, W. M., and A. S. Till: Medullary carcinoma of the thyroid gland, *Q. J. Med.*, **40:**443–456, 1971.

154. Raskin, P., C. J. McClain, and T. A. Medsger: Hypocalcemia associated with metastatic bone disease: A retrospective study, *Arch. Intern. Med.*, **132:**539–543, 1973.

155. Randall, R. E., and D. S. Lirenman: Hypocalcemia and hypophosphatemia accompanying osteoblastic metastases, *J. Clin. Endocrinol.*, **24:**1331–1333, 1964.

156. Ehrlich, M., M. Goldstein, and H. O. Heinemann: Hypocalcemia, hypoparathyroidism, and osteoblastic metastases, *Metabolism*, **12:**516–526, 1963.

157. Coutant, G., J. Hamers, G. Baele, and W. Van Hove: Simultaneous occurrence of hypocholesterolemia, hypocalcemia and hypofibrinogenemia in a case of multiple myeloma, *Acta Haematol. (Basel)*, **54:**358–361, 1975.

158. Meroney, W. H., G. K. Arney, W. E. Segar, and H. H. Balch: The acute calcification of traumatized muscle, with particular reference to acute post-traumatic renal insufficiency, *J. Clin. Invest.*, **36:**825–832, 1957.

159. Imrie, C. W., B. F. Allam, and J. C. Ferguson: Hypocalcaemia of acute pancreatitis: The effect of hypoalbuminaemia, *Curr. Med. Res. Opin.*, **4:**101–116, 1976.

160. Allam, B. F., and C. W. Imrie: Serum ionized calcium in acute pancreatitis, *Br. J. Surg.*, **64:**665–668, 1977.

161. Weir, G. C., P. B. Lesser, L. J. Drop, J. E. Fischer, and A. L. Warshaw: The hypocalcemia of acute pancreatitis, *Ann. Intern. Med.*, **83:**185–189, 1975.

162. Turner-Warwick, R. T.: Hypocalcaemia in acute pancreatitis, *Lancet*, **3:**546–547, 1956.

163. Norberg, H. P., J. DeRoos, and E. L. Kaplan: Increased parathyroid hormone secretion and hypocalcemia in experimental pancreatitis: Necessity for an intact thyroid gland, *Surgery,* **77**:773–778, 1975.

164. Robertson, G. M., E. W. Moore, D. M. Switz, G. W. Sizemore, and H. L. Estep: Inadequate parathyroid response in acute pancreatitis, *N. Engl. J. Med.,* **294**:512–516, 1976.

165. Sowa, M., H. E. Appert, and J. M. Howard: The hypocalcemic activity of pancreatic tissue homogenate in the dog, *Surg. Gynecol. Obstet.,* **144**:365–370, 1977.

166. Condon, J. R., D. Ives, M. J. Knight, and J. Day: The aetiology of hypocalcaemia in acute pancreatitis, *Br. J. Surg.,* **62**:115–118, 1975.

167. Hayes, M. A.: A disturbance in calcium metabolism leading to tetany occurring early in acute pancreatitis, *Ann. Surg.,* **142**:346–350, 1955.

168. Gabow, P. A., T. J. Hanson, M. M. Popovtzer, and R. W. Schrier: Furosemide-induced reduction in ionized calcium in hypoparathyroid patients, *Ann. Intern. Med.,* **86**:579–581, 1977.

169. Eisenbud, E., and C. C. LoBue: Hypocalcemia after therapeutic use of magnesium sulfate, *Arch. Intern. Med.,* **136**:688–691, 1976.

170. Finberg, L., and H. E. Harrison: Hypernatremia in infants: An evaluation of the clinical and biochemical findings accompanying this state, *Pediatrics,* **16**:1–12, 1955.

171. Rapoport, W., K. Dodd, M. Clark, and I. Syllm: Postacidotic state of infantile diarrhea: Symptoms and chemical data, *Am. J. Dis. Child.,* **73**:391–000, 1947.

172. Finberg, L., and E. Fleishman: Experimental studies of the mechanisms producing hypocalcemia in hypernatremic states, *J. Clin. Invest.,* **36**:434–439, 1957.

173. Keating, M. J., M. R. Sethi, G. P. Bodey, and N. A. Samaan: Hypocalcemia with hypoparathyroidism and renal tubular dysfunction associated with aminoglycoside therapy, *Cancer,* **39**:1410–1414, 1977.

174. Roediger, W. E. W., D. Ludwin, and R. A. Hinder: Hypocalcaemic response to streptomycin in malignant hypercalcaemia, *Postgrad. Med. J.,* **51**:399–401, 1975.

175. Pittinger, C., and R. Adamson: Antibiotic blockade of neuromuscular function, *Ann. Rev. Pharmacol.,* **12**:169–184, 1972.

176. Alberts, D. S., A. A. Serpick, and W. L. Thompson: Hypocalcemia complicating acute leukemia, *Med. Pediatr. Oncol.,* **1**:289–295, 1975.

177. McKee, L. C.: Hypocalcemia in leukemia, *South. Med. J.,* **68**:828–832, 1975.

178. Bowen, J. M., D. M. Blackmon, and J. E. Heavner: Neuromuscular transmission and hypocalcemic paresis in the cow, *Am. J. Vet. Res.,* **31**:831–839, 1970.

179. Patten, B. M.: A hypothesis to account for the Mary Walker phenomenon, *Ann. Intern. Med.,* **82**:411–415, 1975.

180. Frame, B.: Neuromuscular manifestations of parathyroid disease, in H. L. Klawans (ed.), *Handbook of Clinical Neurology,* vol. 27, North-Holland Publishing Company, Amsterdam, 1976, pp. 283–320.

181. Sakai, S., D. David, H. Shoji, K. H. Stenzel, and A. L. Rubin: Bone injuries due to tetany or convulsions during hemodialysis, *Clin. Orthop.,* **118**:118–123, 1976.

182. Goldberg, M. A.: Phenytoin, phospholipids, and calcium, *Neurology,* **27**:827–833, 1977.

183. Colletti, R. B., M. W. Pan, E. W. P. Smith, and M. Genel: Detection of hypocalcemia in susceptible neonates: The Q-oTc interval, *N. Engl. J. Med.,* **290**:931–935, 1974.

184. Kriesler, B., A. Dinbar, and D. B. Tulcinsky: Postoperative atetanic hypocalcemic coma: Report of a case, *Surgery,* **65**:916–918, 1969.

185. Kambara, H., B. J. Iteld, and J. Phillips: Hypocalcemia and intractable ventricular fibrillation, *Ann. Intern. Med.,* **86**:583–584, 1977.

186. Chopra, D., P. Janson, and C. T. Sawin: Insensitivity to digoxin associated with hypocalcemia, *N. Engl. J. Med.,* **296**:917–918, 1977.

187. Soffer, A., T. Toribara, D. Moore-Jones, and D. Weber: Clinical applications and untoward reactions of chelation in cardiac arrhythmias, *Arch. Intern. Med.,* **106**:824–833, 1960.

188. Shackney, S., and J. Harson: Precipitous fall in serum calcium, hypotension and acute renal failure after intravenous phosphate therapy for hypercalcemia, *Ann. Intern. Med.,* **66**:906–916, 1967.

189. Llach, F., P. Weidmann, R. Reinhart, M. H. Maxwell, J. W. Coburn, and S. G. Massry: Effect

of acute and long-standing hypocalcemia on blood pressure and plasma renin activity in man, *J. Clin. Endocrinol. Metab.*, **38**:841–847, 1974.

190. Fossard, C., M. J. Tarlow, and R. A. Thompson: Transient hypocalcaemia and T-cell deficiency in an infant, *Br. Med. J.*, **2**:950, 1977.

191. Drezner, M. K., F. A. Neelon, J. Jowsey, and H. E. Lebovitz: Hypoparathyroidism: A possible cause of osteomalacia, *J. Clin. Endocrinol. Metab.*, **45**:114–122, 1977.

192. Kales, A. N., and J. M. Phang: Effect of divided calcium intake on calcium metabolism, *J. Clin. Endocrinol.*, **32**:83–87, 1971.

193. Harris, V., R. S. Ramamurthy, and R. S. Pildes: Late onset of subcutaneous calcifications after intravenous injections of calcium gluconate, *Am. J. Roentgenol. Radium Ther. Nucl. Med.*, **123**:845–849, 1975.

194. Parfitt, A. M.: Hypophosphatemic vitamin D refractory rickets and osteomalacia, *Orthop. Clin. North Am.*, **3**:653–680, 1972.

195. Neer, R. M., M. F. Holick, H. F. DeLuca, and J. T. Potts: Effects of 1α-hydroxyvitamin D_3 and 1,25-dihydroxy-vitamin D_3 on calcium and phosphorus metabolism in hypoparathyroidism, *Metabolism*, **24**:1403–1413, 1975.

196. Parfitt, A. M.: The actions of parathyroid hormone on bone. Relation to bone remodelling and turnover, calcium homeostasis and metabolic bone disease. II. PTH and bone cells: Bone turnover and plasma calcium regulation, *Metabolism*, **25**:909–955, 1976.

197. Porter, R. H., B. G. Cox, D. Heaney, T. H. Hostetter, B. J. Stinebaugh, and W. N. Suki: Treatment of hypoparathyroid patients with chlorthalidone. *N. Engl. J. Med.*, **298**:577–581, 1978.

198. Chesney, R. W., S. D. Horowitz, B. E. Kream, J. A. Eisman, R. Hong, and H. F. DeLuca: Failure of conventional doses of 1α,25-dihydroxycholecalciferol to correct hypocalcemia in a girl with idiopathic hypoparathyroidism, *N. Engl. J. Med.*, **297**:1272–1275, 1977.

199. Rosen, J. F., A. R. Fleischman, L. Finberg, J. Eisman, and H. F. DeLuca: 1,25-Dihydroxycholecalciferol: Its use in the long-term management of idiopathic hypoparathyroidism in children, *J. Clin. Endocrinol. Metab.*, **45**:457–468, 1977.

200. Dyken, M. L., and G. D. Timmons: Hyperka-lemic periodic paralysis with hypocalcemic episode, *Arch. Neurol.*, **9**:508–517, 1963.

201. Kenny, F. M., and L. Linarelli: Dwarfism and cortical thickening of tubular bones: Transient hypocalcemia in a mother and son, *Am. J. Dis. Child*, **111**:201–207, 1966.

202. Rosler, A., and D. Rabinowitz: Magnesium-induced reversal of vitamin-D resistance in hypoparathyroidism, *Lancet*, **2**:803–805, 1973.

203. Paterson, C. R.: Vitamin D resistance in hypoparathyroidism with medullary carcinoma of the thyroid, *Br. Med. J.*, **2**:952, 1977.

204. Chertow, B. S., S. R. Plymate, and F. O. Becker: Vitamin-D-resistant idiopathic hypoparathyroidism: Acute hypercalcemia during acute renal failure, *Arch. Intern. Med.*, **133**:838–840, 1974.

205. Coombes, R. C., M. K. Ward, P. B. Greenberg, C. J. Hillyard, B. R. Tulloch, R. Morrison, and G. F. Joplin: Calcium metabolism in cancer. Studies using calcium isotopes and immunoassays for parathyroid hormone and calcitonin, *Cancer*, **38**:2111–2120, 1976.

206. Hodkinson, H. M.: Serum calcium in a geriatric inpatient population, *Age and Aging*, **2**:157–162, 1973.

207. Nordin, B. E. C., M. Peacock, and R. Wilkinson: The relative importance of gut, bone and kidney in the regulation of serum calcium, in Calcium, parathyroid hormone and the calcitonins, *Proceedings of the IV Parathyroid Conference*, Chapel Hill, N.C., March 15-19, 1971, pp. 263-272.

208. Henneman, P. H., and W. H. Baker: Two mechanisms of sustained hypercalcemia following hypervitaminosis D and the milk-alkali syndrome, *J. Clin. Invest.*, **36**:889, 1957.

209. Reiss, E., and J. M. Canterbury: Spectrum of hyperparathyroidism, *Am. J. Med.*, **56**:794–799, 1974.

210. Potts, J. T., and W. T. St. Goar: Case records of the Massachusetts General Hospital (in discussion), *N. Engl. J. Med.*, **298**:271, 1978.

211. Tissell, L.-E., S. Carlsson, S. Lindberg, and I. Ragnhult: Autonomous hyperparathyroidism: A possible late complication of neck radiotherapy, *Acta Chir. Scand.*, **142**:367–373, 1976.

212. Christensson, T., K. Hellström, and B. Wengle: Hypercalcemia and primary hyperparathyroidism. Prevalence in patients receiving thiazides as de-

tected in a health screen, *Arch. Intern. Med.,*
137:1138–1142, 1977.

213. Christiansen, C., P. C. Baastoup, and I. Transbol: Lithium induced primary hyperparathyroidism, *Calcif. Tissue Res.* (suppl),**22:**341–343, 1977.

214. Pickleman, J. R., F. H. Straus, M. Forland, and E. Paloyan: Thiazide-induced parathyroid stimulation, *Metabolism,* **18:**867–873, 1969.

215. Marx, S. J., A. M. Spiegel, E. M. Brown, and G. D. Aurbach: Family studies in patients with primary parathyroid hyperplasia, *Am. J. Med.,* **62:**698–706, 1977.

216. Goldsmith, R. E., G. W. Sizemore, I.-W. Chen, E. Zalme, and W. A. Altemeier: Familial hyperparathyroidism: Description of a large kindred with physiologic observations and a review of the literature, *Ann. Intern. Med.,* **84:**36–43, 1976.

217. Spiegel, A. M., H. E. Harrison, S. J. Marx, E. M. Brown, and G. D. Aurbach: Neonatal primary hyperparathyroidism with autosomal dominant inheritance, *J. Pediatr.,* **90:**269–272, 1977.

218. Bergdahl, L., and L. Boquist: Secondary hypercalcemic hyperparathyroidism, *Virchows Arch [Pathol Anat],* **358:**225–239, 1973.

219. Smith, J. F.: Parathyroid adenomas associated with the malabsorption syndrome and chronic renal disease, *J. Clin. Pathol.,* **23:**362–369, 1970.

220. Kleerekoper, M., R. Coffey, T. Greco, S. Nichols, N. Cooke, W. Murphy, and L. V. Avioli: Hypercalcemic hyperparathyroidism in hypophosphatemic rickets, *J. Clin. Endocrinol. Metab.,* **45:**86–94, 1977.

221. Lumb, G. A., E. B. Mawer, and S. W. Stanbury: The apparent vitamin D resistance of chronic renal failure: A study of the physiology of vitamin D in man, *Am. J. Med.,* **50:**421–441, 1971.

222. Bigos, S. T., R. M. Neer, and W. T. St. Goar: Hypercalcemia of seven years' duration after kidney transplantation, *Am. J. Surg.,* **132:**83–88, 1976.

223. Black, W. C., and J. R. Utley: The differential diagnosis of parathyroid adenoma and chief cell hyperplasia, *Am. J. Clin. Pathol.,* **49:**761–775, 1968.

224. Bruining, H. A.: *Surgical Treatment of Hyperparathyroidism,* Charles C Thomas, Publisher, Springfield, Ill., 1971.

225. Edis, A. J., O. H. Beahrs, J. A. van Heerden, and O. E. Akwari: "Conservative" versus "liberal" approach to parathyroid neck exploration, *Surgery,* **82:**466–473, 1977.

226. Fialkow, P. J., C. E. Jackson, M. A. Block, and K. A. Greenawald: Multicellular origin of parathyroid "adenomas," *N. Engl. J. Med.,* **3:**696–698, 1977.

227. Lloyd, H. M.: Primary hyperparathyroidism: An analysis of the role of the parathyroid tumor, *Medicine,* **47:**53–71, 1968.

228. Jackson, C. E., and L. Weiss: Endocrine tumor genetics, in H. T. Lynch (ed.), *Cancer Genetics,* Charles C Thomas, Publisher, Springfield, Ill.

229. Mallette, L. E., J. P. Bilezikian, A. S. Ketcham, and G. D. Aurbach: Parathyroid carcinoma in familial hyperparathyroidism, *Am. J. Med.,* **57:**642–648, 1974.

230. Roth, S. I.: Recent advances in parathyroid gland pathology, *Am. J. Med.,* **50:**612–622, 1971.

231. Monchik, J. M., H. L. Wray, M. Schaaf, and J. M. Earll: Nonautonomy of parathyroid hormone and urinary cyclic AMP in primary hyperparathyroidism, *Am. J. Surg.,* **133:**498–505, 1977.

232. Lockefeer, J. H., W. H. L. Hackeng, and J. C. Birkenhäger: Parathyroid hormone secretion in disorders of calcium metabolism studied by means of EDTA, *Acta Endocrinol. (kbh),* **75:**286–296, 1974.

233. Brown, E. M., M. F. Brennan, S. Hurwitz, R. Windeck, S. J. Marx, A. M. Apiegel, J. O. Koehler, D. G. Gardner, and G. D. Aurbach: Dispersed cells prepared from human parathyroid glands: Distinct calcium sensitivity of adenomas vs. primary hyperplasia, *J. Clin. Endocrinol. Metab.,* **46:**267–276, 1978.

234. Birnbaumer, M. E., A. B. Schneider, D. Palmer, D. A. Hanley, and L. M. Sherwood: Secretion of parathyroid hormone by abnormal human parathyroid glands in vitro, *J. Clin. Endocrinol. Metab.,* **45:**105–113, 1977.

235. Chertow, B. S., D. J. Manke, G. A. Willisma, G. R. Baker, G. K. Hargis, and R. J. Buschmann: Secretory and ultrastructural responses of hyperfunctioning human parathyroid tissues to varying calcium concentration and vinblastine, *Lab. Invest.,* **36:**198–205, 1977.

236. Edmondson, J. W., and T.-K. Li: The relationship of serum ionized and total calcium in primary hyperparathyroidism, *J. Lab. Clin. Med.,* **87:**624–629, 1976.

237. Parfitt, A. M.: The effect of cellulose phosphate in primary hyperparathyroidism, *Clin. Sci. Mol. Med.*, **49:**91–98, 1975.

238. Stanbury, S. W.: Parathyroid hormone and the intestinal absorption of calcium in man, in *International Symposia on the Metabolism of Water and Electrolytes*, Siena, Italy, November 9–11, 1972, pp. 241–260.

239. Nordin, B. E. C., M. Peacock, and R. Wilkinson: Hypercalciuria and calcium stone disease, *Clin. Endocrinol. Metab.*, **1:**169–183, 1972.

240. Pak, C. Y. C., M. Ohata, E. C. Lawrence, and W. Snyder: The hypercalciurias: Causes, parathyroid functions, and diagnostic criteria, *J. Clin. Invest.*, **54:**387–400, 1974.

241. Transbøl, I., I. Hornum, S. Hahnemann, E. Hasner, H. Øhlenschlaeger, H. Diemer, and K. Lockwood: Tubular reabsorption of calcium in the differential diagnosis of hypercalcaemia: Further experience, *Acta Med. Scand.*, **188:**505–522, 1970.

242. Sinha, T. K., S. Miller, J. Fleming, R. Khairi, J. Edmondson, C. C. Johnston, and N. H. Bell: Demonstration of a diurnal variation in serum parathyroid hormone in primary and secondary hyperparathyroidism, *J. Clin. Endocrinol. Metab.*, **41:**1009–1013, 1975.

243. Landau, R. L., and A. Kappas: Anabolic hormones in hyperparathyroidism. With observations on the general catabolic influence of parathyroid hormone in man, *Ann. Intern. Med.*, **62:**1223–1233, 1965.

244. Parfitt, A. M.: The effect of cellulose phosphate on plasma and urinary magnesium at different levels of parathyroid function in man, *Clin. Sci. Mol. Med.*, **51:**161–168, 1976.

245. Coe, F. L.: Magnitude of metabolic acidosis in primary hyperparathyroidism, *Arch. Intern. Med.*, **134:**262–265, 1974.

256. Muldowney, F. P., D. V. Carroll, J. F. Donohoe, and R. Freaney: Correction of renal bicarbonate wastage by parathyroidectomy, *Q. J. Med.*, **40:**487–498, 1971.

247. Shelp, W. D., T. H. Steele, and R. E. Rieselbach: Comparison of urinary phosphate, urate and magnesium excretion following parathyroid hormone administration to normal man, *Metabolism*, **18:**63–70, 1969.

248. Boonstra, C. E., and C. E. Jackson: Hyperpara-

thyroidism detected by routine serum calcium analysis: Prevalence in a clinic population, *Ann. Intern. Med.*, **63:**468–474, 1965.

249. Mallette, L. E., J. P. Bilezikian, D. A. Heath, and G. D. Aurbach: Primary hyperparathyroidism: Clinical and biochemical features, *Medicine*, **53:**127–146, 1974.

250. Thomas, W. C., J. G. Wiswell, T. B. Connor, and J. B. Howard: Hypercalcemic crisis due to hyperparathyroidism, *Am. J. Med.*, **24:**229–239, 1958.

251. Parfitt, A. M.: The clinical and radiographic manifestations of renal osteodystrophy, in D. J. David and J. Wiley (eds.), *Perspectives in Hypertension and Nephrology: Calcium Metabolism in Renal Failure and Nephrolithiasis*, 1977.

252. Ross, J. W., and M. D. Fraser: Analytical clinical chemistry precision: State of the art for fourteen analytes, *Am. J. Clin. Pathol.*, **68:**130–141, 1977.

253. Muldowney, F. P., R. Freaney, J. P. McMullin, R. P. Towers, A. Spillane, P. O'Connor, P. O'Donohoe, and M. Moloney: Serum ionized calcium and parathyroid hormone in renal stone disease, *Q. J. Med.*, **65:**75–86, 1976.

254. Transbøl, I.: On the diagnosis of so-called normocalcaemic hyperparathyroidism, *Acta Med. Scand.*, **202:**481–487, 1977.

255. Shieber, W., S. J. Birge, L. V. Avioli, and S. L. Teitelbaum: Normocalcemic hyperparathyroidism with "normal" parathyroid glands, *Arch. Surg.*, **103:**299–302, 1971.

256. Broadus, A. E., T. A. S. Hanson, F. C. Bartter, and J. Walton: Primary hyperparathyroidism presenting as anticonvulsant-induced osteomalacia, *Am. J. Med.*, **63:**298–305, 1977.

257. Johnson, R. D., and J. W. Conn: Hyperparathyroidism with a prolonged period of normocalcemia, *JAMA*, **210:**2063–2066, 1969.

258. Jørgensen, F. S., I. Transbøl, and C. Binder: The effect of bendroflumethiazide on total, ultrafiltrable and ionized calcium in serum in normocalcaemic renal stone formers and in hyperparathyroidism, *Acta Med. Scand.*, **194:**323–326, 1973.

259. Purnell, D. C., D. A. Scholz, and O. H. Beahrs: Hyperparathyroidism due to single gland enlargement. Prospective postoperative study, *Arch. Surg.*, **112:**369–372, 1977.

260. Muls, E., R. Bouillon, and P. DeMoor: Hormonal and biochemical changes in patients successfully

operated for primary hyperparathyroidism, *Acta Endocrinol.*, **83:**549–555, 1976.

261. Jackson, W. P. U., and C. P. Dancaster: Hyperparathyroidism with bone disease. Use of calciferol and milk in postoperative management, *Metabolism*, **11:**123–135, 1962.

262. Smith, R.: Dissociation between changes in urinary total hydroxyproline and plasma alkaline phosphatase after removal of parathyroid tumor, *Clin. Chim. Acta*, **23:**421–426, 1969.

263. Kaplan, R. A., W. H. Snyder, A. Stewart, and C. Y. C. Pak: Metabolic effects of parathyroidectomy in asymptomatic primary hyperparathyroidism, *J. Clin. Endocrinol. Metab.*, **42:**415–426, 1976.

264. Harrison, A. R., and G. A. Rose: The late results of parathyroidectomy in patients with calculus or nephrocalcinosis, in *Urinary Calculi Int. Symp. Renal Stone Res., Madrid, 1972*, Karger, Basel, 1973, pp. 354–357.

265. Gallagher, J. C., and R. Wilkinson: The effect of ethinyloestradiol on calcium and phosphorus metabolism of post-menopausal women with primary hyperparathyroidism, *Clin. Sci. Mol. Med.*, **45:**785–802, 1973.

266. Dent, C. E.: Some problems of hyperparathyroidism, *Br. Med. J.*, **2:**1419–1425, 1495–1500, 1962.

267. Schneider, A. B., and L. M. Sherwood: Calcium homeostasis and the pathogenesis and management of hypercalcemic disorders, *Metabolism*, **23:**975–1007, 1974.

268. Benson, R. C., B. L. Riggs, B. M. Pickard, and C. D. Arnaud: Radioimmunoassay of parathyroid hormone in hypercalcemic patients with malignant disease, *Am. J. Med.*, **56:**821–826, 1974.

269. Galasko, C. S. B.: Skeletal metastases and mammary cancer, *Ann. R. Coll. Surg. Engl.*, **50:**3–28, 1972.

270. Mundy, G. R., L. G. Raisz, R. A. Cooper, G. P. Schechter, and S. E. Salmon: Evidence for the secretion of an osteoclast stimulating factor in myeloma, *N. Engl. J. Med.*, **291:**1041–1046, 1974.

271. Robertson, R. P., D. J. Baylink, S. A. Metz, and K. B. Cummings: Plasma prostaglandin E in patients with cancer with and without hypercalcemia, *J. Clin. Endocrinol. Metab.*, **43:**1330–1335, 1976.

272. Demers, L. M., J. C. Allegra, H. A. Harvey, A.

Lipton, J. R. Luderer, R. Mortel, and D. E. Brenner: Plasma prostaglandins in hypercalcemia patients with neoplastic disease, *Cancer*, **39:**1559–1562, 1977.

273. Zilva, J. F., and J. P. Nicholson: Plasma phosphate and potassium levels in the hypercalcemia of malignant disease, *J. Clin. Endocrinol. Metab.*, **36:**1019–1026, 1973.

274. Benson, R. C., B. L. Riggs, B. M. Pickard, and C. D. Arnaud: Immunoreactive forms of circulating parathyroid hormone in primary and ectopic hyperparathyroidism, *J. Clin. Invest.*, **54:**175–181, 1974.

275. Galasko, C. S. B.: The pathological basis for skeletal scintigrophy, *J. Bone Joint Surg. [Br.]*, **57:**353–359, 1975.

276. Spencer, H., and I. Lewin: Derangements of calcium metabolism in patients with neoplastic bone involvement, *J. Chronic Dis.*, **16:**713–726, 1963.

277. Powles, T. J.: Mechanisms for the development of bone metastases and hypercalcaemia in patients with breast cancer, *Proc. R. Soc. Med.*, **70:**199–201, 1977.

278. Gardner, B., and G. S. Gordan: Does urinary calcium excretion reflect growth or regression of disseminated breast cancer? *J. Clin. Endocrinol.*, **22:**627–630, 1962.

279. Myers, W. P. L.: Hypercalcemia associated with malignant diseases, in *Endocrinology Year Book, and Endocrinology Hormone Producing Tumors*, Med Publishers, Chicago, 1973.

280. Davis, H. L., A. N. Wiseley, and G. Ramirez: Hypercalcemia complicating breast cancer, *Oncology*, **28:**126–137, 1973.

281. Veldhuis, J. D.: Tamoxifen and hypercalcemia, *Ann. Intern. Med.*, **88:**574–575, 1978.

282. Cornbleet, M., P. K. Bondy, and T. J. Powles: Fatal irreversible hypercalcemia in breast cancer, *Br. Med. J.*, **1:**145, 1977.

283. Becker, F. O., and T. B. Schwartz: Normal fluoride 18 bone scans in metastatic bone disease, *JAMA*, **225:**628–629, 1973.

284. Lee, C. A., and H. M. Lloyd: Bone collagen and calcium metabolism in normocalcemic and hypercalcemic patients with breast cancer, *Cancer*, **27:**1099–1105, 1971.

285. Thalassinos, N. C., and G. F. Joplin: Failure of corticosteroid therapy to correct the hypercalcae-

mia of malignant disease, *Lancet,* **3:**537–538, 1970.

286. David, N. J., J. V. Verner, and F. L. Engel: The diagnostic spectrum of hypercalcemia: Case reports and discussion, *Am. J. Med.,* **33:**88–110, 1962.

287. Durie, B. G. M., G. R. Mundy, and S. E. Salmon: Multiple myeloma, clinical staging and role of osteoclast-activating factor in localized bone loss, in J. E. Horton, T. M. Tarpley, and W. F. Davis (eds.), *Mechanisms of Localized Bone Loss, Calc. Tiss. Abst.,* 1978(suppl.).

288. Lazor, M. Z., L. E. Rosenberg, and P. Carbone: Studies of calcium metabolism in multiple myeloma with calcium[47] and metabolic-balance techniques, *J. Clin. Invest.,* **42:**1238–1247, 1963.

289. Mundy, G. R., L. G. Riasz, J. L. Shapiro, J. G. Bandelin, and R. J. Turcotte: Big and little forms of osteoclast activating factor, *J. Clin. Invest.,* **60:**122–128, 1977.

290. Dexter, R. N., F. Mullinax, H. L. Estep, and R. C. Williams: Monoclonal IgG gammopathy and hyperparathyroidism, *Ann. Intern. Med.,* **77:**759–764, 1972.

291. McGeown, M. G., and D. A. D. Montgomery: Multiple myelomatosis simulating hyperparathyroidism, *Br. Med. J.,* **1:**86–88, 1956.

292. Kyle, R. A., and L. R. Elveback: Management and prognosis of multiple myeloma, *Mayo Clin. Proc.,* **51:**751–760, 1976.

293. Witts, L. J., et al.: Report on the first myelomatosis trial. Part I. Analysis of presenting features of prognostic importance. Report of the Medical Research Council's Working Party for Therapeutic Trials in Leukaemia, *Br. J. Haematol.,* **24:**123–139, 1973.

294. Lindgärd, F., and O. Zettervall: Characterization of a calcium-binding IgG myeloma protein, *Scand. J. Immunol.,* **3:**277–285, 1974.

295. Lafferty, F. W.: Pseudohyperparathyroidism, *Medicine,* **45:**247–260, 1966.

296. Omenn, G. S., S. I. Roth, and W. H. Baker: Hyperparathyroidism associated with malignant tumors of nonparathyroid origin, *Cancer,* **24:**1004–1012, 1969.

297. Buckle, R.: Ectopic PTH syndrome, pseudohyperparathyroidism; hypercalcaemia of malignancy, *J. Clin. Endocrinol. Metab.,* **3:**237–251, 1974.

298. Heath, D. A., and G. D. Aurbach: Ectopic production of parathyroid hormone: A prototype of nonendocrine hormone synthesis, in C. J. Kryston and R. A. Shaw (eds.), *Endocrinology and Diabetes,* Grune and Stratton, Inc., New York, 1975, pp. 215–225.

299. Scholz, D. A., B. L. Riggs, D. C. Purnell, R. S. Goldsmith, and C. D. Arnaud: Ectopic hyperparathyroidism with renal calculi and subperiosteal bone resorption: Report of a case, *Mayo Clin. Proc.,* **48:**124–126, 1973.

300. Azzopardi, J. G., and R. S. Whittaker: Bronchial carcinoma and hypercalcemia, *J. Clin. Pathol.,* **22:**718–724, 1969.

301. Bender, R. A., and H. Hansen: Hypercalcemia in bronchogenic carcinoma. A prospective study of 200 patients, *Ann. Intern. Med.,* **80:**205–208, 1974.

302. Palmieri, G. M. A., R. E. Nordquist, and G. S. Omenn: Immunochemical localization of parathyroid hormone in cancer tissue, *J. Clin. Invest.,* **53:**1726–1735, 1974.

303. Hamilton, J. W., C. R. Hartman, D. H. McGregor, and D. V. Cohn: Synthesis of parathyroid hormone-like peptides by a human squamous cell carcinoma. *J. Clin. Endocrinol. Metab.,* **45:**1023–1030, 1977.

304. Lips, C. J. M., J. van der Sluys Veer, J. A. van der Donk, R. H. van Dam, and W. H. L. Hackeng: Common precursor molecule as origin for the ectopic-hormone-producing-tumor syndrome, *Lancet,* **1:**16–18, 1978.

305. Powell, D., F. R. Singer, T. M. Murray, C. Minkin, and J. T. Potts: Nonparathyroid humoral hypercalcemia in patients with neoplastic diseases, *N. Engl. J. Med.,* **289:**176–181, 1973.

306. Marx, S. J., R. M. Zusman, and W. O. Umiker: Benign breast dysplasia causing hypercalcemia, *J. Clin. Endocrinol. Metab.,* **45:**1049–1052, 1977.

307. Tashjian, A. H., J. E. Tice, and K. Sides: Biological activities of prostaglandin analogues and metabolites on bone in organ culture, *Nature,* **266:**645–647, 1977.

308. Schtacher, G.: Selective renal involvement in the early development of hypercalcemia and hypophosphatemia in VX-2 carcinoma-bearing rabbits: Study on serum and tissues alkaline phos-

phatase and renal handling of phosphorus, *Cancer Res.*, **29:**1512–1518, 1969.

309. Hough, A., H. Seyberth, J. Oates, and W. Hartmann: Changes in bone and bone marrow of rabbits bearing the VX-2 carcinoma: A comparison of local and distant effects, *Am. J. Pathol.*, **87:**537–552, 1977.

310. Seyberth, H. W., G. V. Segre, P. Hamet, B. J. Sweetman, J. T. Potts, and J. A. Oates: Characterization of the group of patients with the hypercalcemia of cancer who respond to treatment with prostaglandin synthesis inhibitors, *Trans. Assoc. Am. Physicians*, **89:**92–104, 1976.

311. Robertson, R. P., D. J. Baylink, J. J. Marini, and H. W. Addison: Elevated prostaglandins and suppressed parathyroid hormone associated with hypercalcemia and renal cell carcinoma, *J. Clin. Endocrinol. Metab.*, **41:**164–167, 1975.

312. Robertson, R. P., and D. J. Baylink: Hypercalcemia induced by prostaglandin E_2 in thyroparathyroidectomized but not intact rats, *Prostaglandins*, **13:**1141–1145, 1977.

313. Hirose, S., K. Kobayashi, K. Kajikawa, and N. Sawabu: A case of watery diarrhea, hypokalemia and hypercalcemia associated with nonulcerogenic islet cell tumor, *Am. J. Gastroenterol.*, **64:**382–391, 1975.

314. Holdaway, I. M., M. C. Evans, and E. D. Clarke: Watery diarrhoea syndrome with episodic hypercalcaemia, *Aust. N.Z. J. Med.*, **7:**63–65, 1977.

315. Cryer, P. E., and G. J. Hill: Pancreatic islet cell carcinoma with hypercalcemia and hypergastrinemia. Response to streptozotocin, *Cancer*, **38:**2217–2221, 1976.

316. Rice, B. F., L. M. Roth, F. E. Cole, A. A. MacPhee, K. Davis, R. L. Ponthier, and W. H. Sternberg: Hypercalcemia and neoplasia: Biologic, biochemical and ultrastructural studies of a hypercalcemia-producing Leydig cell tumor of the rat, *Lab. Invest.*, **33:**428–439, 1975.

317. Haddad, J. G., S. J. Couranz, and L. V. Avioli: Circulating phytosterols in normal females, lactating mothers and breast cancer patients, *J. Clin. Endocrinol. Metab.*, **30:**174–180, 1970.

318. Mahajan, K. K., C. J. Robinson, and D. F. Horrobin: Prolactin and hypercalcaemia, *Lancet*, **1:**1237–1238, 1974.

319. Libnoch, J. A., K. Ajlouni, W. L. Millman, A. R. Guansing, and G. B. Theil: Acute myelofibrosis and malignant hypercalcemia, *Am. J. Med.*, **62:**432–438, 1977.

320. Kippen, D. A., and J. B. Freeman: Isolated histiocytic lymphoma of the spleen causing fever and hypercalcemia, *Arch. Surg.*, **112:**1233–1234, 1977.

321. Zidar, B. L., R. K. Shadduck, A. Winkelstein, Z. Ziegler, and C. C. Hawker: Acute myeloblastic leukemia and hypercalcemia: A case of probable ectopic parathyroid hormone production, *N. Engl. J. Med.*, **295:**692–694, 1976.

322. Singer, F. R., D. Powell, C. Minkin, J. E. Bethune, A. Brickman, and J. W. Coburn: Hypercalcemia in reticulum cell sarcoma without hyperparathyroidism or skeletal metastases, *Ann. Intern. Med.*, **78:**365–369, 1973.

323. Canellos, G. P.: Hypercalcemia in malignant lymphoma and leukemia, *Ann. N.Y. Acad. Sci.*, **230:**240–246, 1974.

324. Child, J. A., and I. E. Smith: Lymphoma presenting as "idiopathic" juvenile osteoporosis, *Br. Med. J.*, **1:**720–721, 1975.

325. McKee, L. C.: Hypercalcemia in leukemia, *South Med. J.*, **67:**1076–1079, 1974.

326. Joyner, M. V., P. Dujardin, J. P. Cassuto, and P. Audoly: Hypercalcaemia as complication of accelerated chronic granulocytic leukaemia, *Br. Med. J.*, **4:**1060, 1977.

327. Farr, H. W., T. J. Fahey, A. G. Nash, and C. M. Farr: Primary hyperparathyroidism and cancer, *Am. J. Surg.*, **126:**539, 1973.

328. Vichayanrat, A., A. Avramides, B. Gardner, S. Wallach, and A. C. Carter: Primary hyperparathyroidism and breast cancer, *Am. J. Med.*, **61:**136–139, 1976.

329. Jung, A., R. Millet, P. Schneider, and R. J. Walton: Hypercalcaemia and parathyroid hyperplasia associated with renal adenocarcinoma, *Postgrad. Med. J.*, **52:**106–108, 1976.

330. Kohout, E.: Serum calcium levels and parathyroid glands in malignant disorders, *Cancer*, **19:**925–939, 1966.

331. Borden, H., J. Hummer, C. W. Landon, and J. Paris: The use of procaine in acquired malignant melanoma metastatic to the parathyroid gland: A case report, *Can. Anaesth. Soc. J.*, **23:**616–623, 1976.

332. Heath, H. III, J. M. Earll, M. Schaaf, J. T. Piech-

ocki, and T.-K. Li: Serum ionized calcium during bed rest in fracture patients and normal men, *Metabolism*, 21:633–640, 1972.

333. Wolf, A. W., R. G. Chuinard, R. S. Riggins, R. M. Walter, and T. Depner: Immobilization hypercalcemia, *Clin. Orthop.*, **118**:124–129, 1976.

334. Berliner, B. C., I. R. Shenker, and M. S. Weinstock: Hypercalcemia associated with hypertension due to prolonged immobilization (an unusual complication of extensive burns), *Pediatrics*, **49**:92–96, 1972.

335. Claus-Walker, J., R. E. Carter, R. J. Campos, and W. A. Spencer: Hypercalcemia in early traumatic quadriplegia, *J. Chronic Dis.*, **28**:81–90, 1975.

336. Lerman, S., J. M. Canterbury, and E. Reiss: Parathyroid hormone and the hypercalcemia of immobilization, *J. Clin. Endocrinol. Metab.*, **45**:425–428, 1977.

337. Pezeshki, C., and A. F. Brooker: Immobilization hypercalcemia: Report of two cases treated with calcitonin, *J. Bone Joint Surg. [Am.]*, **59**:971–973, 1977.

338. Parfitt, A. M., and C. E. Dent: Hyperthyroidism and hypercalcaemia, *Q. J. Med.*, **39**:171–187, 1970.

339. Parfitt, A. M.: Hypercalcaemic nephropathy, *Med. J. Aust.*, **2**:127–134, 1964.

340. Donaldson, C. L., S. B. Hulley, J. M. Vogel, R. S. Hattner, J. H. Bayers, and D. E. McMillan: Effect of prolonged bed rest on bone mineral, *Metabolism*, **19**:1071–1084, 1970.

341. Minaire, P., P. Meunier, C. Edouard, J. Bernard, P. Courpron, and J. Bourret: Quantitative histological data on disuse osteoporosis, *Calcif. Tissue Res.*, **17**:57–73, 1974.

342. Meier, D. A., A. R. Arnstein, and J. I. Hamburger: Symptomatic thyrotoxic hypercalcemia, *Mich. Med.*, **73**:19–24, 1974.

343. Rude, R. K., S. B. Oldham, F. R. Singer, and J. T. Nicoloff: Treatment of thyrotoxic hypercalcemia with propranolol, *N. Engl. J. Med.*, **294**:431–433, 1976.

344. Georges, L. P., R. P. Santangelo, J. F. Mackin, and J. J. Canary: Metabolic effects of propranolol in thyrotoxicosis. I. Nitrogen, calcium, and hydroxyproline, *Metabolism,* **24**:11–21, 1975.

345. Cook, P. B., J. R. Nassim, and J. Collins: The effects of thyrotoxicosis upon the metabolism of calcium, phosphorus, and nitrogen, *Q. J. Med.*, **28**:505–529, 1959.

346. Gordon, D. L., S. Suvanich, V. Erviti, M. A. Schwartz, and C. J. Martinez: The serum calcium level and its significance in hyperthyroidism: A prospective study, *Am. J. Med. Sci.*, **268**:31–36, 1974.

347. Burman, K. D., J. M. Monchik, J. M. Earll, and L. Wartofsky: Ionized and total serum calcium and parathyroid hormone in hyperthyroidism, *Ann. Intern. Med.*, **84**:668–671, 1976.

348. Singhelakis, P., C. C. Alevizaki, and D. G. Ikkos: Intestinal calcium absorption in hyperthyroidism, *Metabolism*, **23**:311–321, 1974.

349. Parfitt, A. M.: Chlorothiazide induced hypercalcemia in juvenile osteoporosis and primary hyperparathyroidism, *N. Engl. J. Med.*, **281**:55–59, 1969.

350. Koppel, M. H., S. G. Massry, J. H. Shinaberger, D. L. Hartenbower, and J. W. Coburn: Thiazide-induced rise in serum calcium and magnesium in patients on maintenance hemodialysis, *Ann. Intern. Med.*, **72**:895–901, 1970.

351. Popovtzer, M. M., V. L. Subryan, A. C. Alfrey, E. B. Reeve, and R. W. Schrier: The acute effect of chlorothiazide on serum-ionized calcium: Evidence for a parathyroid hormone–dependent mechanism, *J. Clin. Invest.*, **55**:1295–1302, 1975.

352. Parfitt, A. M.: Thiazide-induced hypercalcemia in vitamin D–treated hypoparathyroidism, *Ann. Intern. Med.*, **77**:557–563, 1972.

353. Stote, R. M., L. H. Smith, D. M. Wilson, W. J. Dube, R. S. Goldsmith, and C. D. Arnaud: Hydrochlorothiazide effects on serum calcium and immunoreactive parathyroid hormone concentrations: Studies in normal subjects, *Ann. Intern. Med.*, **77**:587–591, 1972.

354. Frame, B., C. E. Jackson, W. A. Reynolds, and J. E. Umphrey: Hypercalcemia and skeletal effects in chronic hypervitaminosis A, *Ann. Intern. Med.*, **80**:44–48, 1974.

355. Katz, C. M., and M. Tzagournis: Chronic adult hypervitaminosis A with hypercalcemia, *Metabolism*, **21**:1171–1176, 1972.

356. Dull, T., P. F. Maurice, D. H. Henneman, and P. H. Henneman: Early effects of vitamin A on calcium, citrate and phosphorus metabolism in man, *J. Clin. Invest.*, **40**:1035, 1961.

357. Jowsey, J., and B. L. Riggs: Bone changes in a patient with hypervitaminosis A, *J. Clin. Endocrinol. Metab.*, **28:**1833–1835, 1968.

358. Punsar, S., and T. Somer: The milk-alkali syndrome, *Acta Med. Scand.*, **173:**435–449, 1963.

359. Hurst, P. E., R. B. I. Morrison, J. Timoner, A. Metcalfe-Gibson, and O. Wrong: The effect of oral anion exchange resins on faecal anions. Comparison with calcium salts and aluminum hydroxide, *Clin. Sci.*, **24:**187–200, 1963.

360. Epstein, S., W. Van Mieghem, J. Sagel, and W. P. U. Jackson: Effect of single large doses of oral calcium on serum calcium levels in the young and the elderly, *Metabolism*, **22:**1163–1173, 1973.

361. McMillan, D. E., and R. B. Freeman: The milk alkali syndrome: A study of the acute disorder with comments on the development of the chronic condition, *Medicine*, **44:**485–501, 1965.

362. Ivanovich, P., H. Fellows, and C. Rich: The absorption of calcium carbonate, *Ann. Intern. Med.*, **66:**917–923, 1967.

363. Vincent, P. C., and F. J. Radcliff: The effect of large doses of calcium carbonate on serum and urinary calcium, *Am. J. Dig. Dis.*, **11:**286–295, 1966.

364. Ginsburg, D. S., E. L. Kaplan, and A. I. Katz: Hypercalcaemia after oral calcium-carbonate therapy in patients on chronic haemodialysis, *Lancet*, **1:**1271–1274, 1973.

365. Thomas, W. C., A. M. Lewis, and E. D. Bird: Effect of alkali administration on calcium metabolism, *J. Clin. Endocrinol. Metab.*, **27:**1328–1336, 1967.

366. Parfitt, A. M.: Soft tissue calcification in uremia, *Arch. Intern. Med.*, **124:**544–556, 1969.

367. Danowski, T. S.: *Clinical Endocrinology*, vol III, *Calcium, Phosphorus, Parathyroids and Bone*, The Williams and Wilkins Company, Baltimore, 1962.

368. Najjar, S. S., S. F. Aftimos, and R. F. Kurani: Furosemide therapy for hypercalcemia in infants, *J. Pediatr.*, **81:**1171–1174, 1972.

369. Belchetz, P. E., R. D. Cohen, J. L. H. O'Riordan, and S. Tomlinson: Factitious hypercalcaemia, *Br. Med. J.*, **1:**690–691, 1976.

370. Krook, L., R. H. Wasserman, J. N. Shively, A. H. Tashjian, T. D. Brokken, and J. F. Morton: Hypercalcemia and calcinosis in Florida horses: Implication of the shrub, Cestrum Diurnum, as the causative agent, *Cornell Vet*, **65:**26–56, 1975.

371. Counts, S. J., D. J. Baylink, F.-H. Shen, D. J. Sherrard, and R. O. Hickman: Vitamin D intoxication in an anephric child, *Ann. Intern. Med.*, **82:**196–200, 1975.

372. Hughes, M. R., D. J. Baylink, P. G. Jones, and M. R. Haussler: Radioligand receptor assay for 25-hydroxyvitamin D_2/D_3 and 1,25-dihydroxyvitamin D_2/D_3, *J. Clin. Invest.*, **58:**61–70, 1976.

373. Martinez-Maldonado, M., G. Eknoyan, and W. N. Suki: Diuretics in non-edematous states, *Arch. Intern. Med.*, **131:**797–808, 1973.

374. Paunier, L., P. E. Conen, A. A. M. Gibson, and D. Fraser: Renal function and histology after long-term vitamin D therapy of vitamin D refractory rickets, *J. Pediatr.*, **73:**833–844, 1968.

375. Moncrieff, M. W., and G. W. Chance: Nephrotoxic effect of vitamin D therapy in refractory rickets, *Arch. Dis. Child.*, **44:**571–579, 1969.

376. Parfitt, A. M.: Renal function in vitamin D treated hypoparathyroidism, in S. G. Massry and E. Ritz (eds.), *Phosphate Metabolism*, Plenum Press, New York, 1977.

377. Shetty, K. R., K. Ajlouni, P. S. Rosenfeld, and T. C. Hagen: Protracted vitamin D intoxication, *Arch. Intern. Med.*, **135:**986–988, 1975.

378. Thomas, G. O.: Hypercalciuria in sarcoidosis treated with inorganic phosphates, *Br. Med. J.*, **2:**96–98, 1969.

379. Lebacq, E., H. Verhaegen, and V. Desmet: Renal involvement in sarcoidosis, *Postgrad. Med. J.*, **46:**526–529, 1970.

380. Murphy, G. P., and H. K. Schirmer: Nephrocalcinosis, urolithiasis and renal insufficiency in sarcoidosis, *J. Urol.*, **86:**702–706, 1961.

381. Dent, C. E.: Calcium metabolism in sarcoidosis, *Postgrad. Med. J.*, **46:**471–477, 1970.

382. Bell, N. H., and F. C. Bartter: Studies of ^{47}Ca metabolism in sarcoidosis: Evidence for increased sensitivity of bone to vitamin D, *Acta Endocrinol.*, **54:**173–180, 1967.

383. Cushard, W. G., A. B. Simon, J. M. Canterbury, and E. Reiss: Parathyroid function in sarcoidosis, *N. Engl. J. Med.*, **286:**395–398, 1972.

384. Reiner, M., G. Sigurdsson, V. Nunziata, M. A. Malik, G. W. Poole, and G. F. Joplin: Abnormal

calcium metabolism in normocalcaemic sarcoidosis, *Br. Med. J.*, **2**:1473–1476, 1976.

385. Bell, N. H., T. K. Sinba, P. H. Stern, and H. F. DeLuca: Sarcoidosis and its relationship to vitamin D, in *Vitamin D: Biochemical, Chemical and Clinical Aspects Related to Calcium Metabolism*, Walter de Gruyter & Co., Berlin, 1977.

386. Rhodes, J., E. H. Reynolds, J. D. Fitzgerald, and P. Fourman: Exaggerated response to parathyroid extract in sarcoidosis, *Lancet*, **2**:598–601, 1963.

387. Jackson, W. P. U., and C. Dancaster: A consideration of the hypercalciuria in sarcoidosis, idiopathic hypercalciuria, and that produced by vitamin D. A new suggestion regarding calcium metabolism, *J. Clin. Endocrinol.*, **19**:658–680, 1959.

388. Hendrix, J. Z.: Abnormal skeletal mineral metabolism in sarcoidosis, *Ann. Intern. Med.*, **64**:797–805, 1966.

389. Taylor, R. L., H. J. Lynch, and W. G. Wysor: Seasonal influence of sunlight on the hypercalcemia of sarcoidosis, *Am. J. Med.*, **34**:221–227, 1963.

390. Goldstein, R. A., H. L. Israel, K. L. Becker, and C. F. Moore: The infrequency of hypercalcemia in sarcoidosis, *Am. J. Med.*, **51**:21–30, 1971.

391. Aberg, H., H. Johansson, I. Werner, and L.-G. Wiman: Sarcoidosis, hypercalcemia and hyperparathyroidism, *Scand. J. Respir. Dis.*, **53**:259–264, 1972.

392. Dawidson, I., and S. Jameson: Sarcoidosis with hypercalcemia, reversible uremia and hyperparathyroidism, *Scand. J. Urol. Nephrol.*, **6**:308–311, 1972.

393. Hunt, B. J., and E. R. Yendt: The response of hypercalcemia in sarcoidosis to Chloroquine, *Ann. Intern. Med.*, **59**:554–564, 1963.

394. Hornum, I., I. Transbol, S. Hahnemann, and B. Halver: An endocrine and metabolic study of idiopathic hyperabsorption hypercalcemia in the adult, *Proc. Fifth Europ. Calc. Tiss. Symp.*, in *Tissus Calcifies*, pp. 307–312.

395. Bjernulf, A., K. Hall, I. Sjögren, and I. Werner: Primary hyperparathyroidism in children: Brief review of the literature and a case report, *Acta Paediatr. Scand.*, **59**:249–258, 1970.

396. Mannix, H.: Primary hyperparathyroidism in children, *Am. J. Surg.*, **129**:528–531, 1975.

397. Fraser, D., B. S. L. Kidd, S. W. Kooh, and L. Paunier: A new look at infantile hypercalcemia, *Pediatr. Clin. North. Am.*, **13**:503–525, 1966.

398. Jones, K. L., and D. W. Smith: The Williams elfin facies syndrome: A new perspective, *J. Pediatr.*, **86**:718–723, 1975.

399. Barr, D. G. D., and J. O. Forfar: Oral calcium-loading test in infancy, with particular reference to idiopathic hypercalcemia, *Br. Med. J.*, **1**:477–480, 1969.

400. Forbes, G. B., M. F. Bryson, J. Manning, G. H. Amirhakimi, and J. C. Reina: Impaired calcium homeostasis in the infantile hypercalcemic syndrome, *Acta Paediatr. Scand.*, **61**:305–309, 1972.

401. Seelig, M. S.: Vitamin D and cardiovascular, renal and brain damage in infancy and childhood, *Ann. N.Y. Acad. Sci.*, **147**:537–582, 1969.

402. Friedman, W. F., and L. F. Mills: The relationship between vitamin D and the craniofacial and dental anomalies of the supravalvular aortic stenosis syndrome, *Pediatrics*, **43**:12–18, 1969.

403. Becroft, S. M. O., and D. Chambers: Supravalvular aortic stenosis-infantile hypercalcemia syndrome: In vitro hypersensitivity to vitamin D_2 and calcium, *J. Med. Genet.*, **13**:223–228, 1976.

404. Fourman, P., and P. Royer: *Calcium Metabolism and the Bone*, 2d ed., Blackwell Scientific Publications, Ltd., Oxford, 1968.

405. Lowe, C. E., E. D. Bird, and W. C. Thomas: Hypercalcemia in myxedema, *J. Clin. Endocrinol.*, **22**:261–267, 1962.

406. Drummond, K. N., A. F. Michael, R. A. Ulstrom, and R. A. Good: The blue diaper syndrome: Familial hypercalcemia with nephrocalcinosis and indicanuria, *Am. J. Med.*, **37**:928–948, 1964.

407. Michael, A. F., K. N. Drummond, D. Doeden, J. A. Anderson, and R. A. Good: Tryptophan metabolism in man, *J. Clin. Invest.*, **43**:1730–1740, 1964.

408. McIlwaine, C. L. K.: Tryptophan loading and hypercalcaemia, *Lancet*, **2**:395, 1966.

409. Fraser, D.: Hypophosphatasia, *Am. J. Med.*, **22**:730–746, 1957.

410. Marx, S. J., A. S. Spiegel, E. M. Brown, J. O. Koehler, D. G. Gardner, M. F. Brennan, and G. D. Aurbach: Divalent cation metabolism in familial hypocalciuric hypercalcemia versus in typical primary hyperparathyroidism, *Am. J. Med.* In press.

411. Foley, T. P., H. C. Harrison, C. D. Arnaud, and H. E. Harrison: Familial benign hypercalcemia, *J. Pediatr.*, **81**:1060–1067, 1972.

412. Miller, S. S., G. W. Sizemore, S. G. Sheps, and G. M. Tyce: Parathyroid function in patients with pheochromocytoma, *Ann. Intern. Med.*, **82**:372–375, 1975.

413. DePlaen, J. F., F. Boemer, and C. Van Ypersele de Strihou: Hypercalcaemic phaeochromocytoma, *Br. Med. J.*, **3**:734, 1976.

414. Skrabanek, P.: Catecholamines cause the hypercalciuria and hypercalcaemia in phaeochromocytoma and in hyperthyroidism, *Med. Hypoth.*, **3**:59–62, 1977.

415. Bouillon, R., and P. De Moor: Pheochromocytoma and hyperparathyroidism, *Ann. Intern. Med.*, **81**:131, 1974.

416. Shai, F., R. K. Baker, J. R. Addrizzo, and S. Wallach: Hypercalcemia in mycobacterial infection, *J. Clin. Endocrinol.*, **34**:251–256, 1972.

417. Braman, S. S., A. L. Goldman, and M. I. Schwarz: Steroid-responsive hypercalcemia in disseminated bone tuberculosis, *Arch. Intern. Med.*, **132**:269–271, 1973.

418. Lee, J. C., A. Catanzaro, J. G. Parthemore, B. Roach, and L. J. Deftos: Hypercalcemia in disseminated coccidioidomycosis, *N. Engl. J. Med.*, **297**:431–433, 1977.

419. Nadarajah, A., M. Hartog, B. Redfern, N. Thalassinos, A. D. Wright, G. F. Joplin, and T. R. Fraser: Calcium metabolism in acromegaly, *Br. Med. J.*, **4**:797–801, 1968.

420. Hanna, S., M. T. Harrison, I. MacIntyre, and R. Fraser: Effects of growth hormone on calcium and magnesium metabolism, *Br. Med. J.*, **2**:12, 1961.

421. Stoeckle, J. D., H. L. Hardy, and A. L. Weber: Chronic beryllium disease: Long-term follow up of sixty cases and selective review of the literature, *Am. J. Med.*, **46**:545–561, 1969.

422. Hardy, H. L., F. C. Bartter, and A. E. Jaffin: Metabolic study of a case of chronic beryllium poisoning treated with ACTH, *Arch. Indust. Hyg. Occup. Med.*, **3**:579–582, 1951.

423. Dimich, A., S. Brown, S. Minkowitz, and S. Wallach: Idiopathic periostitis with hypercalcemia, *Am. J. Med.*, **42**:828–837, 1967.

424. Dent, C. E., and L. Watson: The hydrocortisone test in primary and tertiary hyperparathyroidism, *Lancet*, **3**:662–664, 1968.

425. Gram, P. B., J. L. Fleming, B. Frame, and G. Fine: Metaphyseal chrondrodysplasia of Jansen, *J. Bone Joint Surg.*, **41A**:951–959, 1959.

426. Frame, B.: Conditions which may be confused with rickets. Presented at Symposium on Pediatric Diseases Related to Calcium, New Orleans, La., May 1978.

427. Jorgensen, H.: Hypercalcemia in adrenocortical insufficiency, *Acta Med. Scand.*, **193**:175–179, 1973.

428. Walser, M., B. H. B. Robinson, and J. W. Duckett: The hypercalcemia of adrenal insufficiency, *J. Clin. Invest.*, **42**:456–465, 1963.

429. Raman, A.: Effect of adrenalectomy on ionic and total plasma calcium in rats, *Horm. Metab. Res.*, **2**:181–183, 1970.

430. Prader, V. A., E. Uehlinger, and R. Illig: Hypercalcämie bei morbus addison im kindesalter, *Helv. Paediatr. Acta*, **14**:607–617, 1959.

431. Downie, W. W., A. Gunn, C. R. Paterson, and G. F. A. Howie: Hypercalcaemic crisis as presentation of Addison's disease, *Br. Med. J.*, **1**:145–146, 1977.

432. Tuttle, S. G., and W. G. Figueroa: Hypercalciuria associated with reduction in corticoid therapy after prolonged administration of prednisone and after bilateral adrenalectomy for Cushing's syndrome, *J. Clin. Invest.*, **37**:937, 1958.

433. Koffler, A., R. M. Friedler, and S. G. Massry: Acute renal failure due to nontraumatic rhabdomyolysis, *Ann. Intern. Med.*, **85**:23–28, 1976.

434. de Torrente, A., T. Berl, P. D. Cohn, E. Kawamoto, P. Hertz, and R. W. Schrier: Hypercalcemia of acute renal failure, *Am. J. Med.*, **61**:119–123, 1976.

435. Hornum, I.: Post-transplant hypercalcemia due to mobilization of metastatic calcifications: An alternative to tertiary hyperparathyroidism, *Acta Med. Scand.*, **189**:199–205, 1971.

436. Michael, A. F., R. Hong, and C. D. West: Hypercalcemia in infancy, associated with subcutaneous fat necrosis and calcification, *Am. J. Dis. Child.*, **104**:235–244, 1962.

437. Freeman, R. M., R. L. Lawton, and M. A. Chamberlain: Hard-water syndrome, *N. Engl. J. Med.*, **276**:1113–1118, 1967.

438. Howenburg, H., and T. M. Ginsburg: Acute hypercalcemia: Report of a case, *JAMA*, **99**:1166, 1932.

439. Ulstrom, R. A., and D. M. Brown: Acute iatrogenic hypercalcemia in an infant on hyperalimentation, *J. Pediatr.*, **81**:419–420, 1972.

440. Manson, R. R.: Acute pancreatitis secondary to iatrogenic hypercalcemia, *Arch. Surg.*, **108**:213–215, 1974.

441. Heird, W. C.: Disorders of calcium and phosphorus metabolism, in R. G. Winters and E. G. Hasselmayer (eds.), *I.V. Nutrition in the High Risk Infant*, John Wiley & Sons, Inc., New York, 1975.

442. Porter, R., and A. L. Crombie: Corneal calcification as a presenting and diagnostic sign in hyperparathyroidism, *Br. J. Ophthal.*, **57**:665–668, 1973.

443. Suki, W. N., and G. Eknoyan: Tubulo-interstitial diseases, in B. M. Brenner and F. C. Rector (eds.), *The Kidney*, vol. II, W.B. Saunders Company, Philadelphia, 1976.

444. Duffy, J. L., Y. Suzuki, and J. Churg: Acute calcium nephropathy: Early proximal tubular changes in the rat kidney, *Arch. Pathol.*, **91**:340–350, 1971.

445. Ganote, C. E., D. S. Philipsborn, E. Chen, and F. A. Carone: Acute calcium nephrotoxicity: An electron microscopical and semiquantitative light microscopical study, *Arch. Pathol.*, **99**:650–657, 1975.

446. Brunette, M. G., J. Vary, and S. Carrière: Hyposthenuria in hypercalcemia: A possible role of intrarenal blood-flow (IRBF) redistribution, *Pfluegers Arch.*, **350**:9–23, 1974.

447. Benabe, J. E., and M. Martinez-Maldonado: Hypercalcemic nephropathy, *Arch. Intern. Med.*, **138**:777–779, 1978.

448. Epstein, F. H.: Calcium nephropathy, in M. B. C. Strauss and L. G. Welt (eds.), *Diseases of the Kidney*, 2d ed, Little, Brown and Company, Boston, 1971.

449. Guignard, J.-P., N. F. Jones, and M. A. Barraclough: Effect of brief hypercalcaemia on free water reabsorption during solute diuresis: Evidence for impairment of sodium transport in Henle's loop, *Clin. Sci.*, **39**:337–347, 1970.

450. DiBona, G.: Effect of hypercalcemia on renal tubular sodium handling in the rat, *Am. J. Physiol.*, **220**:49–53, 1971.

451. Beck, N., H. Singh, S. W. Reed, H. V. Murdaugh, and B. B. Davis: Pathogenic role of cyclic AMP in the impairment of urinary concentrating ability in acute hypercalcemia, *J. Clin. Invest.*, **54**:1049–1055, 1974.

452. Heinemann, H.O.: Metabolic alkalosis in patients. with hypercalcemia, *Metabolism*, **14**:1137–1152, 1965.

453. Aldinger, K. A., and N. A. Samaan: Hypokalemia with hypercalcemia, *Ann. Intern. Med.*, **87**:571–573, 1977.

454. Connor, T. B., and H. Lovice: Observations on renal function before and after correction of hypercalcemia, *Trans. Am. Clin. Climatol. Assoc.*, **74**:139–151, 1963.

455. Dent, R. I., J. H. James, C.-A. Wang, L. Deftos, R. Talamo, and J. E. Fischer: Hyperparathyroidism: Gastric acid secretion and gastrin, *Ann. Surg.*, **176**:360–369, 1972.

456. Stremple, J. F., and C. G. Watson: Serum calcium, serum gastrin and gastric acid secretion before and after parathyroidectomy for hyperparathyroidism, *Surgery*, **75**:841–852, 1974.

457. Trudeau, W. L., and J. E. McGuigan: Effects of calcium on serum gastrin levels in the Zollinger-Ellison syndrome, *N. Engl. J. Med.*, **281**:862–866, 1969.

458. Rosin, R. D.: Pancreatitis and hyperparathyroidism, *Postgrad. Med. J.*, **52**:95–101, 1976.

459. Gafter, U., E. M. Mandel, L. Har-Zahav, and S. Weiss: Acute pancreatitis secondary to hypercalcemia: Occurrence in a patient with breast carcinoma, *JAMA*, **235**:2004–2005, 1976.

460. Plough, J. C., and L. M. Kyle: Pancreatic insufficiency and hyperparathyroidism, *Ann. Intern. Med.*, **47**:590–598, 1957.

461. Bronsky, D., A. Dubin, S. S. Waldstein, and D. S. Kushner: Calcium and the electrocardiogram. II. The electrocardiographic manifestations of hyperparathyroidism and of marked hypercalcemia from various other etiologies, *Am. J. Cardiol.*, **I**:833–843, 1961.

462. Ginsberg, H., and K. V. Schwartz: Hypercalcemia and complete heart block, *Ann. Intern. Med.*, **79**:903, 1973.

463. Bradlow, B. A., and N. Segel: Acute hyperparathyroidism with electrocardiographic changes, *Br. Med. J.*, **2**:197–200, 1956.

464. Smallwood, R. A.: Some effects of the intravenous administration of calcium in man, *Aust. Ann. Med.,* **16**:126–131, 1967.

465. Weidmann, P., S. G. Massry, J. W. Coburn, M. H. Maxwell, J. Atleson, and C. R. Kleeman: Blood pressure effects of acute hypercalcemia: Studies in patients with chronic renal failure, *Ann. Intern. Med.,* **76**:741–745, 1972.

466. Kleerekoper, M., D. S. Rao, and B. Frame: *Hypercalcemia, Hyperparathyroidism and Hypertension, Cardiovasc. Med.,* **3**:1283–1295, 1978.

467. Pratley, S. K., S. Posen, and T. S. Reeve: Primary hyperparathyroidism: Experiences with 60 patients, *Med. J. Aust.,* **1**:421–426, 1973.

468. Cohn, R., and J. Sode: The EEG in hypercalcemia, *Neurology (Minneap.),* **21**:154–161, 1971.

469. Katzman, R., and H. M. Pappas: *Brain Electrolytes and Fluid Metabolism,* The Williams & Wilkins Company, Baltimore, 1971.

470. Allen, E. M., F. R. Singer, and D. Melamed: Electroencephalographic abnormalities in hypercalcemia, *Neurology,* **20**:15–22, 1970.

471. Strickland, N. J., A. M. Bold, and W. E. Medd: Bronchial carcinoma with hypercalcaemia simulating cerebral metastases, *Br. Med. J.,* **3**:590–592, 1967.

472. Goldsmith, R. S.: Treatment of hypercalcemia, *Med. Clin. North Am.,* **56**:951–960, 1972.

473. Jessiman, A. G., K. Emerson, R. C. Shah, and F. D. Moore: Hypercalcemia in carcinoma of the breast, *Ann. Surg.,* **157**:377–393, 1963.

473a. Parfitt, A. M.: The study of parathyroid function in man by EDTA infusion, *J. Clin. Endocrinol.,* **29**:569–580, 1969.

474. Lemann, J., and M. P. Mehr: Sodium sulfate infusions and hypercalcemia, *JAMA,* **194**:224–225, 1965.

475. Walser, M.: Treatment of hypercalcemias, *Mod. Treat.,* **7**:662–674, 1970.

476. Suki, W. N., J. J. Yium, M. Von Minden, C. Saller-Hebert, G. Eknoyan, and M. Martinez-Maldonado: Acute treatment of hypercalcemia with furosemide, *N. Engl. J. Med.,* **283**:836–840, 1970.

477. Canary, J. J.: Treatment of hypercalcemia, in S. Spitzer and D. W. W. Oaks (eds.), *Emergency Medical Management, The 21st Hahnemann Symposium,* Grune & Stratton, Inc., New York, 1971, pp. 104–112.

478. Fulmer, D. H., A. B. Dimich, E. O. Rothschild, and W. P. L. Myers: Treatment of hypercalcemia: Comparison of intravenously administered phosphate, sulfate and hydrocortisone, *Arch. Intern. Med.,* **129**:923–930, 1972.

479. Ayala, G., B. S. Chertow, J. H. Shah, G. A. Williams, and S. C. Kukreja: Acute hyperphosphatemia and acute persistent renal insufficiency induced by oral phosphate therapy, *Ann. Intern. Med.,* **83**:520–521, 1975.

480. Sørensen, O. H., T. Friis, I. Hindberg, and S. P. Nielsen: The effect of calcitonin injected into hypercalcaemic and normocalcaemic patients, *Acta Med. Scand.,* **187**:283–290, 1970.

481. Silva, O. L., and K. L. Becker: Salmon calcitonin in the treatment of hypercalcemia, *Arch. Intern. Med.,* **132**:337–339, 1973.

482. Vaughn, C. B., and V. K. Vaitkevicius: The effects of calcitonin in hypercalcemia in patients with malignancy, *Cancer,* **34**:1268–1271, 1974.

483. Elias, E. G., G. Reynoso, and A. Mittelman: Control of hypercalcemia with Mithramycin, *Ann. Surg.,* **175**:431–435, 1972.

484. Smith, I. E., and T. J. Powles: Mithramycin for hypercalcaemia associated with myeloma and other malignancies, *Br. Med. J.,* **1**:268–269, 1975.

485. Kennedy, B. J.: Metabolic and toxic effects of Mithramycin during tumor therapy, *Am. J. Med.,* **49**:494–503, 1970.

486. Manheimer, I. H.: Corticosteroids in hypercalcaemia, *Cancer,* **18**:679–691, 1965.

487. Bentzel, C. J., P. P. Carbone, and L. Rosenberg: The effect of prednisone on calcium metabolism and Ca^{47} kinetics in patients with multiple myeloma and hypercalcemia, *J. Clin. Invest.,* **43**:2132–2165, 1964.

488. Tashjian, A. H., E. F. Voelkel, and L. Levine: Effects of hydrocortisone on the hypercalcemia and plasma levels of 13,14-dihydro-15-keto-prostaglandin E_2 in mice bearing the $HSDM_1$ fibrosarcoma, *Biochem. Biophys. Res. Commun.,* **74**:199–207, 1977.

489. Brautbar, N., and R. Luboshitzky: Combined calcitonin and oral phosphate treatment for hypercalcemia in multiple myeloma, *Arch. Intern. Med.,* **137**:914–916, 1977.

490. Au, W. Y. W.: Calcitonin treatment of hypercalcemia due to parathyroid carcinoma, *Arch. Intern. Med.*, **135**:1594–1597, 1975.

491. Bijvoet, O. L. M.: Kidney function in calcium and phosphate metabolism, in L. V. Avioli and S. M. Krane (eds.), *Metabolic Bone Disease*, vol. 1, Academic Press, Inc., New York, 1977.

492. Malm, O. J.: Calcium requirement and adaptation in adult men. Oslo University Press, *Scand. J. Clin. Lab. Invest. suppl. 36*, 1958.

493. Davies, D. M.: Sixty days in a submarine: The pathophysiological and metabolic cost, *J. R. Coll. Physicians Lond.*, **7**:132–144, 1973.

494. Boner, G., M. Newton, and R. E. Rieselbach: Exaggerated carbohydrate-induced calciuria in the remaining kidney of transplant donors, *Kidney Int.*, **3**:24–29, 1973.

495. Brickman, A. S., E. J. Drenick, I. F. Hunt, and J. W. Coburn: Studies of water (H$_2$O) and electrolyte (E) retention (R) following carbohydrate administration (CH) to fasting (F) obese subjects, *Clin. Res.*, **17**:167, 1969.

496. Parfitt, A. M.: The acute effects of mersalyl, chlorothiazide and mannitol on the excretion of calcium and other electrolytes in man, *Clin. Sci.*, **36**:267–282, 1969.

497. Wilson, R. J.: Renal excretion of calcium and sodium in acute nephritis, *Br. Med. J.*, **4**:713–715, 1969.

498. Kirkendall, W. M., W. E. Connor, F. Abboud, S. P. Rastogi, T. A. Anderson, and M. Fry: The effect of dietary sodium chloride on blood pressure, body fluids, electrolytes, renal function and serum lipids of normotensive man, *J. Lab. Clin. Med.*, **87**:418–434, 1976.

499. Lamberg, B.-A., and B. Kuhlback: Effect of chlorothiazide and hydrochlorothiazide on the excretion of calcium in urine, *Scand. J. Clin. Lab. Invest.*, **11**:351–357, 1959.

500. Lichwitz, A., R. Parlier, S. deSèze, D. Hioco, and L. Miravet: L'effect hypocalciurique des sulfamides diurétiques, *Sem. Hop. Paris*, **37**:2351–2362, 1961.

501. Yendt, E. R., and M. Cohanim: Thiazides and calcium urolithiasis, *CMA J.*, **118**:755–758, 1978.

502. Ehrig, U., J. E. Harrison, and D. R. Wilson: Effect of long-term thiazide therapy on intestinal calcium absorption in patients with recurrent renal calculi, *Metabolism*, **23**:139–149, 1974.

503. Barilla, D. E., R. Tolentino, R. A. Kaplan, and C. Y. C. Pak: Selective effects of thiazide on intestinal absorption of calcium in absorptive and renal hypercalciurias, *Metabolism*, **27**:125–131, 1978.

504. Coe, F. L., J. M. Canterbury, J. J. Firpo, and E. Reiss: Evidence for secondary hyperparathyroidism in idiopathic hypercalciuria, *J. Clin. Invest.*, **52**:134–142, 1973.

505. Middler, S., C. Y. C. Pak, F. Murad, and F. C. Bartter: Thiazide diuretics and calcium metabolism, *Metabolism*, **22**:139–146, 1973.

506. Edwards, B. R., P. G. Baer, R. A. L. Sutton, and J. H. Dirks: Micropuncture study of diuretic effects on sodium and calcium reabsorption in the dog nephron, *J. Clin. Invest.*, **52**:2418–2427, 1973.

507. Parfitt, A. M.: Interactions of thiazide diuretics with parathyroid hormone and vitamin D. Studies in patients with hypoparathyroidism, *J. Clin. Invest.*, **51**:1879–1888, 1972.

508. Jørgensen, F. S., and I. Transbøl: The effect of bendroflumethiazide on the renal handling of calcium, magnesium and phosphate in normocalcaemic renal stone formers and in hyperparathyroidism, *Acta Med. Scand.*, **194**:327–334, 1973.

509. Costanzo, L. S., A. M. Moses, K. J. Rao, and I. M. Weiner: Dissociation of calcium and sodium clearances in patients with hypoparathyroidism by infusion of chlorothiazide, *Metabolism*, **24**:1367–1373, 1975.

510. Quamme, G. A., N. L. M. Wong, R. A. Sutton, and J. H. Dirks: Interrelationship of chlorothiazide and parathyroid hormone: A micropuncture study, *Am. J. Physiol.*, **229**:200–205, 1975.

511. Marcus, R., F. Orner, G. Arvesen, and C. Lundquist: Thiazide diuretics do not potentiate c'AMP response to parathyroid hormone, *Metabolism*, **27**:701–710, 1978.

512. Parry, E. S., and I. S. Lister: Sunlight and hypercalciuria, *Lancet*, **2**:1063–1065, 1975.

513. Transbøl, I., F. S. Jørgensen, B. Lund, and O. H. Sørensen: Importance of season and clearance correction in the definition of hypercalciuria, *Acta Med. Scand.*, **199**:127–128, 1976.

514. Robertson, W. G., A. Hodgkinson, and D. H. Marshall: Seasonal variations in the composition

of urine from normal subjects: A longitudinal study, *Clin. Chim. Acta*, **80**:347–353, 1977.

515. Freedman, P.: Renal colic and persistent hypercalciuria following self-administration of vitamin D, *Lancet*, **1**:668–669, 1957.

516. Gonda, A., N. Wong, J. F. Seely, and J. H. Dirks: The role of hemodynamic factors on urinary calcium and magnesium excretion, *Can. J. Physiol. Pharmacol.*, **47**:619–626, 1969.

517. Linkswiler, H. M., C. L. Joyce, and C. R. Anand: Calcium retention of young adult males as affected by level of protein and of calcium intake, *Trans. N.Y. Acad. Sci.*, **36**:333–340, 1974.

518. Rastegar, A., Z. Agus, T. B. Connor, and M. Goldberg: Renal handling of calcium and phosphate during mineralocorticoid "escape" in man, *Kidney Int.*, **2**:279–286, 1972.

519. Fanconi, A., G. Schachenmann, R. Nussli, and A. Prader: Chronic hypokalaemia with growth retardation, normotensive hyperrenin-hyperaldosteronism ("Bartter's syndrome"), and hypercalciuria: Report of two cases with emphasis on natural history and on catch-up growth during treatment, *Helv. Paediatr. Acta*, **26**:144–163, 1971.

520. Soriano, J. R., I. B. Houston, H. Boichis, and C. M. Edelmann: Calcium and phosphorus metabolism in the Fanconi syndrome, *J. Clin. Endocrinol.*, **28**:1555–1563, 1968.

521. Darmady, E. M., W. J. Griffiths, H. Spencer, D. Mattingly, F. Stranak, and H. E. de Wardener: Renal tubular failure associated with polyarteritis nodosa, *Lancet*, **1**:378–383, 1955.

522. Litin, R. B., R. V. Randall, N. P. Goldstein, M. H. Power, and G. R. Diessner: Hypercalciuria in hepatolenticular degeneration, *Am. J. Med. Sci.*, 614–620, 1959.

523. Kazantsis, G.: in G. E. W. Wolstenholme and J. Knight (eds.), *The Balkan Nephropathy. Ciba Foundation Study Group #30*, Little, Brown and Company, Boston, 1967.

524. Randall, R. V., N. P. Goldstein, J. B. Gross, J. W. Rosevear, and W. F. McGuckin: Urinary excretion of calcium in Wilson's disease (hepato-lenticular degeneration), *J. Clin. Invest.*, **40**:1074, 1961.

525. Rao, D. S., B. Frame, M. A. Block, and A. M. Parfitt: Hyperparathyroidism and medullary sponge kidney, *JAMA*, **238**:212, 1977.

526. Garnett, J., E. S. Garnett, R. J. Mardell, and D. L. Barnard: Urinary calcium excretion during ketoacidosis of prolonged total starvation, *Metabolism*, **19**:502–508, 1970.

527. Beck, N., and S. K. Webster: Effects of acute metabolic acidosis on parathyroid hormone action and calcium mobilization, *Am. J. Physiol.*, **230**:127–131, 1976.

528. Robertson, W. G., M. Peacock, R. W. Marshall, D. H. Marshall, and B. E. C. Nordin: Saturation-inhibition index as a measure of the risk of calcium oxalate stone formation in the urinary tract, *N. Engl. J. Med.*, **294**:249–252, 1976.

529. Pak, C. Y. C., Y. Hayashi, B. Finlayson, and S. Chu: Estimation of the state of saturation of brushite and calcium oxalate in urine: A comparison of three methods, *J. Lab. Clin. Med.*, **89**:891–901, 1977.

530. Howard, J. E.: Studies on urinary stone formation: A saga of clinical investigation, *Johns Hopkins Med. J.*, **139**:239–252, 1976.

531. Baumann, J. M., S. Bisaz, R. Felix, H. Fleisch, U. Ganz, and R. G. G. Russell: The role of inhibitors and other factors in the pathogenesis of recurrent calcium-containing renal stones, *Clin. Sci. Mol. Med.*, **53**:141–148, 1977.

532. Coe, F. L., and A. G. Kavalach: Hypercalciuria and hyperuricosuria in patients with calcium nephrolithiasis, *N. Engl. J. Med.*, **291**:1344–1350, 1974.

533. Parfitt, A. M., B. A. Higgins, J. R. Nassim, J. A. Collins, and A. Hilb: Metabolic studies in patients with hypercalciuria, *Clin. Sci.*, **27**:463–482, 1964.

534. Lavan, J. N., F. C. Neale, and S. Posen: Urinary calculi: Clinical, biochemical and radiological studies in 619 patients, *Med. J. Aust.*, **2**:1049–1061, 1971.

535. Buckalew, V. M, M. L. Purvis, M. G. Shulman, C. N. Herndon, and D. Rudman: Hereditary renal tubular acidosis: Report of a 64 member kindred with variable clinical expression including idiopathic hypercalciuria, *Medicine*, **53**:229–254, 1974.

536. Nordin, B. E. C.: Hypercalciuria, *Clin. Sci. Mol. Med.*, **52**:1–8, 1977.

537. Robertson, W. G., and D. B. Morgan: The distribution of urinary calcium excretions in normal

persons and stone-formers, *Clin. Chim. Acta,* **37**:503–508, 1972.

538. Lemann, J., W. F. Piering, and E. J. Lennon: Possible role of carbohydrate-induced calciuria in calcium oxalate kidney-stone formation, *N. Engl. J. Med.,* **280**:232–237, 1969.

539. Hodgkinson, A., and L. N. Pyrah: The urinary excretion of calcium and inorganic phosphate in 344 patients with calcium stone of renal origin, *Br. J. Surg.,* **46**:10–18, 1958.

540. Pak, C. Y. C., D. A. East, L. J. Sanzenbacher, C. S. Delea, and F. C. Bartter: Gastrointestinal calcium absorption in nephrolithiasis, *J. Clin. Endocrinol. Metab.,* **35**:261–270, 1972.

541. Edwards, N. A., and A. Hodgkinson: Metabolic studies in patients with idiopathic hypercalciuria, *Clin. Sci.,* **29**:143–157, 1965.

542. Liberman, U. A., O. Sperling, A. Atsmon, M. Frank, M. Modan, and A. De Vries: Metabolic and calcium kinetic studies in idiopathic hypercalciuria, *J. Clin. Invest.,* **47**:2580–2590, 1968.

543. Henneman, P. H., P. H. Benedict, A. P. Forbes, and H. R. Dudley: Idiopathic hypercalciuria, *N. Engl. J. Med.,* **259**:802–807, 1958.

544. Lichtwitz, A., S. de Séze, D. Hioco, R. Parlier, C. Lanham, and L. Miravet: Les formes rénales et entéro-rénales du diabéte calcique essai d'individualisation biochimique, *Sem. Hop. Paris,* **37**:663–681, 1961.

545. Shen, F. H., D. J. Baylink, R. L. Nielsen, D. J. Sherrard, J. L. Ivey, and M. R. Haussler: Increased serum 1,25-dihydroxyvitamin D in idiopathic hypercalciuria, *J. Lab. Clin. Med.,* **90**:955–962, 1977.

546. Bordier, P., A. Ryckewart, J. Gueris, and H. Rasmussen: On the pathogenesis of so-called idiopathic hypercalciuria, *Am. J. Med.,* **63**:398–409, 1977.

547. Edwards, N. A., and A. Hodgkinson: Phosphate metabolism in patients with renal calculus, *Clin. Sci.,* **29**:93–106, 1965.

548. Caldas, A. E., R. W. Gray, and J. Lemann: The simultaneous measurement of vitamin D metabolites in plasma: Studies in healthy adults and in patients with calcium nephrolithiasis, *J. Lab. Clin. Med.,* **91**:840–849, 1978.

549. Harrison, A. R.: Some results of metabolic investigations in cases of renal stone, *Br. J. Urol.,* **31**:398–403, 1959.

550. Kaplan, R. A., M. R. Haussler, L. J. Deftos, H. Bone, and C. Y. C. Pak: The role of 1,25-dihydroxyvitamin D in the mediation of intestinal hyperabsorption of calcium in primary hyperparathyroidism and absorptive hypercalciuria, *J. Clin. Invest.,* **59**:756–760, 1977.

551. Wilkinson, R.: Absorption of calcium, phosphorus and magnesium, in B. E. C. Nordin (ed.), *Calcium, Phosphate and Magnesium Metabolism,* Churchill-Livingstone, New York, 1976.

552. Jackson, W. P. U.: Osteoporosis of unknown cause in younger people: Idiopathic osteoporosis, *J. Bone Joint Surg. [Br.],* **40**:420–441, 1958.

553. Bordier, Ph. J., L. Miravet, and D. Hioco: Young adult osteoporosis, *J. Clin. Endocrinol. Metab.,* **2**:277–292, 1973.

554. Sperling, O., A. Weinberger, I. Oliver, U. A. Liberman, and A. De Vries: Hypouricemia, hypercalciuria and decreased bone density: A hereditary syndrome, *Ann. Intern. Med.,* **80**:482–487, 1974.

555. Phillips, M. J., and J. N. C. Cooke: Relation between urinary calcium and sodium in patients with idiopathic hypercalciuria, *Lancet,* **2**:1354–1357, 1967.

556. Suki, W. N., G. Eknoyan, N. Samaan, C. Dichoso, P. C. Johnson, and M. Martinez-Maldonado: Idiopathic hypercalciuria: Its diagnosis, pathogenesis and treatment, in E. L. Becker (ed.), *Cornell Seminars in Nephrology, Perspectives in Nephrology and Hypertension,* vol. 2, John Wiley and Sons, New York, 1973, pp. 229–246.

557. Edwards, N. A., and A. Hodgkinson: Studies of renal function in patients with idiopathic hypercalciuria, *Clin. Sci.,* **29**:327–338, 1965.

558. Birge, S. J.: In discussion of F. L. Coe, J. Canterbury, and E. Reiss: Hyperparathyroidism in idiopathic hypercalciuria: Primary or secondary? *Trans. Am. Assoc. Physicians,* **84**:159, 1971.

559. Smith, L. H., W. C. Thomas, and C. D. Arnaud: Orthophosphate therapy in calcium renal lithiasis, *Urinary Calculi Int. Symp. Renal Stone Res., Madrid 1972,* Karger, Basel, 1973, pp. 188–197.

560. Johansson, H., L. Thorén, I. Werner, and L. Grimelius: Normocalcemic hyperparathyroidism, kidney stones, and idiopathic hypercalciuria, *Surgery,* **77**:691–696, 1975.

561. Wibell, L., and I. Werner: Serum phosphate and calcium and phosphate excretion at different levels of serum calcium in hyperparathyroidism, *Acta Med. Scand.*, **193**:161–165, 1973.

562. Pak, C. Y. C.: Parathyroid hormone and thyrocalcitonin: Their mode of action and regulation, *Ann. N.Y. Acad. Sci.*, **179**:450–474, 1977.

563. Liberman, U. A., and A. De Vries: Idiopathic hypercalciuria: A state of compensated hyperparathyroidism? *Rev. Europ. Etudes Clin. et Biol.*, **16**:860–865, 1971.

564. Smith, L. H.: Medical evaluation of nephrolithiasis. Etiologic aspects and diagnostic evaluation, *Urol. Clin. N. Am.*, **1**:241–260, 1974.

565. Cope, O., B. A. Barnes, B. Castleman, G. C. E. Mueller, and S. I. Roth: Vicissitudes of parathyroid surgery: Trials of diagnosis and management in 51 patients with a variety of disorders, *Ann. Surg.*, **154**:491–508, 1961.

566. Coe, F. L., J. Keck, and E. R. Norton: The natural history of calcium urolithiasis, *JAMA*, **238**:1519–1523, 1977.

567. Pak, C. Y. C., C. S. Delea, and F. C. Bartter: Successful treatment of recurrent nephrolithiasis (calcium stones) with cellulose phosphate, *N. Engl. J. Med.*, **290**:175–225, 1974.

568. Thomas, W. C.: Medical aspects of renal calculous disease: Treatment and prophylaxis, *Urol. Clin. N. Am.*, **1**:261–278, 1974.

569. Ettinger, B.: Recurrent nephrolithiasis: Natural history and effect of phosphate therapy. A double-blind controlled study, *Am. J. Med.*, **61**:200–000, 1976.

570. Coe, F. L.: Treated and untreated recurrent calcium nephrolithiasis in patients with idiopathic hypercalciuria, hyperuricosuria or no metabolic disorder, *Ann. Intern. Med.*, **87**:404–410, 1977.

571. Adelman, R. D., S. B. Abern, D. Merten, and C. H. Halsted: Hypercalciuria with nephrolithiasis: A complication of total parenteral nutrition. *Pediatrics*, **59**:473–475, 1977.

572. Scribner, B. H., and J. M. Burnell: Interpretation of the serum potassium concentration, *Metabolism*, **5**:468–479, 1956.

573. Passmore, R., and M. H. Draper: The chemical anatomy of the human body, in R. H. S. Thompson and D. P. Wootten (eds.), *Biochemical Disorders in Human Disease*, 3d ed., Churchill, London, 1970.

574. Lehninger, A. L.: *Biochemistry*, 2d ed., White Publishers, Inc., New York.

575. Knochel, J. P.: The pathophysiology and clinical characteristics of severe hypophosphatemia, *Arch. Intern. Med.*, **137**:203–220, 1977.

576. Soskin, S., and R. Levine: *Carbohydrate Metabolism*, 2d ed., The University of Chicago Press, Chicago, 1952.

577. Danowski, T. S.: *Diabetes Mellitus*, The Williams & Wilkins Company, Baltimore, 1957.

578. Russell, R. G. G., S. Foden, J. Lorains, J. A. Kanis, J. Phillips, and S. Tomlinson: Method for measuring inorganic phosphate in red blood cells and its application to disturbances of phosphate metabolism in man (abstract), in *3rd International Workshop on Calcified Tissues*, Kiriat Anavim, Israel, March 1978.

579. Annino, J. S., and A. S. Pelman: The effect of eating on some of the clinically important constituents of the blood, *Am. J. Clin. Pathol.*, **31**:155–159, 1954.

580. Conlee, R. K., M. J. Rennie, and W. W. Winder: Skeletal muscle glycogen content: Diurnal variation and effects of fasting, *Am. J. Physiol.*, **231**:614–618, 1976.

581. Mostellar, M. E., and E. P. Tuttle: Effects of alkalosis on plasma concentration and urinary excretion of inorganic phosphate in man, *J. Clin. Invest.*, **43**:138–149, 1964.

582. Robertson, W. G.: Plasma phosphate homeostasis, in B. E. C. Nordin (ed.), *Calcium, Phosphate and Magnesium Metabolism*, Churchill-Livingstone, New York, 1976.

583. Lindsay, R., J. R. T. Coutts, and D. M. Hart: The effect of endogenous oestrogen on plasma and urinary calcium and phosphate in oophorectomized women, *Clin. Endocrinol. (Oxf.)*, **6**:87–93, 1977.

584. Nassim, J. R., P. D. Saville, and L. Mulligan: The effect of stilboestrol on urinary phosphate excretion, *Clin. Sci.*, **15**:367–371, 1956.

585. Aitken, J. M., D. M. Hart, and D. A. Smith: The effect of long-term mestranol administration on calcium and phosphorus homeostasis in oophorectomized women, *Clin. Sci.*, **41**:233–236, 1971.

586. Rapoport, A., G. L. A. From, and H. Husdan:

Metabolic studies in prolonged fasting. I. Inorganic metabolism and kidney function, *Metabolism*, **14**:31–46, 1965.

587. Fleming, L. W., and W. K. Stewart: Effect of carbohydrate intake on the urinary excretion of magnesium, calcium and sodium in fasting obese patients, *Nephron*, **16**:64–73, 1976.

588. Moore, F. D.: *Metabolic Care of the Surgical Patient*, W. B. Saunders Company, Philadelphia, 1959.

589. Metcoff, J., S. Frenk, I. Antonowicz, G. Gordillo, and E. Lopez: Relations of intracellular ions to metabolite sequences in muscle in Kwashiorkor. A new reference for assessing the significance of intracellular concentrations of ions, *Pediatrics*, **26**:960–972, 1960.

590. Linder, G. C., J. D. L. Handsen, and C. D. Karabus: The metabolism of magnesium and other inorganic cations and of nitrogen in acute Kwashiorkor, *Pediatrics*, **31**:552–568, 1963.

591. Butler, A. M.: Diabetic coma, *N. Engl. J. Med.*, **4**:648–659, 1950.

592. Nabarro, J. D. N., A. G. Spencer, and J. M. Stowers: Metabolic studies in severe diabetic ketosis, *Q. J. Med.*, **21**:225–248, 1952.

593. Mahler, R. F., and S. W. Stanbury: Potassium-losing renal disease. Renal and metabolic observations on a patient sustaining renal wastage of potassium, *Q. J. Med.*, **25**:21–52, 1956.

594. Bishop, M. C., J. G. G. Ledingham, and D. O. Oliver: Phosphate deficiency in haemodialysed patients, *Proc. Europ. Dial. and Transpl. Assoc.*, **8**:106–114, 1971.

595. Dominguez, J. H., R. W. Gray, and J. Lemann: Dietary phosphate deprivation in women and men: Effects on mineral and acid balances, parathyroid hormone and the metabolism of 25-OH-vitamin D, *J. Clin. Endocrinol. Metab.*, **43**:1056–1068, 1976.

596. Betro, M. G., and R. W. Pain: Hypophosphatemia and hyperphosphatemia in a hospital population, *Br. Med. J.*, **1**:273–276, 1972.

597. Lotz, M., E. Zisman, and F. C. Bartter: Evidence for a phosphorus-depletion syndrome in man, *N. Engl. J. Med.*, **278**:409–452, 1968.

598. Baker, L. R. I., P. Ackrill, W. R. Cattell, T. C. B. Stamp, and L. Watson: Iatrogenic osteomalacia and myopathy due to phosphate depletion, *Br. Med. J.*, **3**:150–152, 1974.

599. Cam, J. M., V. A. Luck, J. B. Eastwood, and H. E. de Wardener: The effect of aluminum hydroxide orally on calcium, phosphorus and aluminum metabolism in normal subjects, *Clin. Sci. Mol. Med.*, **51**:407–414, 1976.

600. Seldin, D. W., and R. Tarail: The metabolism of glucose and electrolytes in diabetic acidosis, *J. Clin. Invest.*, **29**:552–565, 1950.

601. Franks, M., R. F. Berris, N. O. Kaplan, and G. B. Myers: Metabolic studies in diabetic acidosis. II. The effect of the administration of sodium phosphate, *Arch Intern. Med.*, **81**:42–55, 1948.

602. Stein, J. H., W. O. Smith, and H. E. Ginn: Hypophosphatemia in acute alcoholism, *Am. J. Med. Sci.*, **252**:78–87, 1966.

603. Territo, M. C., and K. R. Tanaka: Hypophosphatemia in chronic alcoholism, *Arch. Intern. Med.*, **134**:445–447, 1974.

604. Riedler, G. F., and W. A. Scheitlin: Hypophosphataemia in septicaemia: Higher incidence in gram-negative than in gram-positive infections, *Br. Med. J.*, **1**:753–756, 1969.

605. Cooperstock, M. S., R. P. Tucker, and J. V. Baublis: Possible pathogenic role of endotoxin in Reye's syndrome, *Lancet*, **2**:1272–1274, 1975.

606. Shils, M. E.: *Minerals in Total Parenteral Nutrition*, P. C. White and M. E. Nagy (eds.), Publishing Sciences Group, American Medical Association, 1974.

607. Dudrick, S. J., B. V. Macfadyen, C. T. Van Buren, R. L. Ruberg, and A. T. Maynard: Parenteral hyperalimentation. Metabolic problems and solutions, *Ann. Surg.*, **176**:259–264, 1972.

608. Sheldon, G. F., and S. Grzyb: Phosphate depletion and repletion: Relation to parenteral nutrition and oxygen transport, *Ann. Surg.*, **182**:683–689, 1975.

609. Rudman, D., W. J. Millikan, T. J. Richardson, T. J. Bixler, W. J. Stackhouse, and W. C. McGarrity: Elemental balances during intravenous hyperalimentation of underweight adult subjects, *J. Clin. Invest.*, **55**:94–104, 1975.

610. Hill, G. L., E. J. Guinn, and S. J. Dudrick: Phosphorus distribution in hyperalimentation induced hypophosphatemia, *J. Surg. Res.*, **20**:527–531, 1976.

611. Guillou, P. J., D. G. Morgan, and G. L. Hill: Hy-

pophosphataemia: A complication of "innocuous dextrose-saline," *Lancet*, **4:**710–712, 1976.

612. Steele, T. H., J. L. Underwood, B. A. Stromberg, and C. A. Larmore: Renal resistance to parathyroid hormone during phosphorus deprivation, *J. Clin. Invest.*, **58:**1461–1464, 1976.

613. Shorr, E., and A. C. Carter: Aluminum gels in the management of renal phosphatic calculi, *JAMA*, **144:**1549–1556, 1950.

614. Gray, R. W., D. R. Wilz, A. E. Caldas, and J. Lemann: The importance of phosphate in regulating plasma 1,25(OH)$_2$-vitamin D levels in humans: Studies in healthy subjects, in calcium-stone formers and in patients with primary hyperparathyroidism, *J. Clin. Endocrinol. Metab.*, **45:**299, 1977.

615. Baylink, D., J. Wergedal, and M. Stauffer: Formation, mineralization and resorption of bone in hypophosphatemic rats, *J. Clin. Invest.*, **50:**2519–2530, 1971.

616. Cuisinier-Gleizes, P., M. Thomasset, F. Sainteny-Debove, and H. Mathieu: Phosphorus deficiency, parathyroid hormone and bone resorption in the growing rat, *Calcif. Tissue Res.*, **20:**235–249, 1976.

617. Coburn, J. W., and S. G. Massry: Changes in serum and urinary calcium during phosphate depletion: Studies on mechanisms, *J. Clin. Invest.*, **49:**1073–1087, 1970.

618. Massry, S. G.: Effect of phosphate depletion on renal tubular transport, in L. V. Avioli et al. (eds.), *Phosphate Metabolism, Kidney and Bone*, Armour Montague, Paris, 1976.

619. Emmett, M., S. Goldfarb, Z. S. Agus, and R. G. Narins: The pathophysiology of acid-base changes in chronically phosphate-depleted rats, *J. Clin. Invest.*, **59:**291–298, 1977.

620. Gold, L. W., S. G. Massry, and R. M. Friedler: Effect of phosphate depletion on renal tubular reabsorption of glucose, *J. Lab. Clin. Med.*, **89:**554–559, 1977.

621. Fitzgerald, F. T.: Hypophosphatemia, *Adv. Intern. Med.*, **23:**137–157, 1978.

622. Newman, J. H., T. A. Neff, and P. Ziporin: Acute respiratory failure associated with hypophosphatemia, *N. Engl. J. Med.*, **296:**1101–1103, 1977.

623. Dialysis dementia (editorial), *Br. Med. J.*, **4:**6046–6047, 1976.

624. Rosen, R., W. Leach, and A. Arieff: Central nervous system dysfunction and hypophosphatemia (HP), *Proc. Amer. Soc. Nephrol., Kidney Internatl.*, **12:**460, 1977.

625. Knochel, J. P., G. L. Bilbrey, T. J. Fuller, and N. W. Carter: The muscle cell in chronic alcoholism: The possible role of phosphate depletion in alcoholic myopathy, *Ann. N.Y. Acad. Sci.*, **252:**274–291, 1975.

626. Klock, J. C., H. E. Williams, and W. C. Mentzer: Hemolytic anemia and somatic cell dysfunction in severe hypophosphatemia, *Arch. Intern. Med.*, **134:**360–364, 1974.

627. O'Connor, L. R., W. S. Wheeler, and J. E. Bethune: Effect of hypophosphatemia on myocardial performance in man, *N. Engl. J. Med.*, **297:**901–903, 1977.

628. Kreisberg, R. A.: Phosphorus deficiency and hypophosphatemia, *Hosp. Prac.*, **1:**121–128, 1977.

629. Travis, S. F., H. J. Sugerman, R. L. Ruberg, S. J. Dudrick, M. Delivoria-Papadopoulos, L. D. Miller, and F. A. Oski: Alterations of red-cell glycolytic intermediates and oxygen transport as a consequence of hypophosphatemia in patients receiving intravenous hyperalimentation, *N. Engl. J. Med.*, **285:**763–767, 1971.

630. Thomas, H. M., S. S. Lefrak, R. S. Irwin, H. W. Fritts, and P. R. B. Caldwell: The oxyhemoglobin dissociation curve in health and disease, *Am. J. Med.*, **57:**331–335, 1974.

631. Ditzel, J.: Effect of plasma inorganic phosphate on tissue oxygenation during recovery from diabetic ketoacidosis, *Adv. Exp. Biol. Med.*, **37A:**163–172, 1971.

632. Duhm, J.: 2,3-DPG-induced displacements of the oxyhemoglobin dissociation curve of blood: Mechanisms and consequences, *Adv. Exp. Boil. Med.*, **37A:**179–186, 1971.

633. Farber, E.: ATP and cell integrity, *Fed. Proc.*, **32:**1534–1539, 1973.

634. Lichtman, M. A.: Hypoalimentation during hyperalimentation, *N. Engl. J. Med.*, **2:**1432–1433, 1974.

635. Craddock, P. R., Y. Yawata, L. VanSanten, S. Gilberstadt, S. Silvis, and H. S. Jacob: Acquired phagocyte dysfunction. A complication of the hypophosphatemia of parenteral hyperalimentation, *N. Engl. J. Med.*, **290:**1403–1407, 1974.

636. Kreusser, W. J., K. Kurokawa, E. Aznar, and S. G. Massry: Phosphate depletion. Effect of renal inorganic phosphorus and adenine nucleotides, urinary phosphate and calcium and calcium balance, *Min. Electrolyte Metab.*, **1**:30–42, 1978.

637. Fuller, T. J., N. W. Carter, C. Barcenas, and J. P. Knochel: Reversible changes of the muscle cell in experimental phosphorus deficiency, *J. Clin. Invest.*, **57**:1019–1024, 1976.

638. O'Connor, L. R., W. S. Wheeler, and J. E. Bethune: Letter to the editor, *N. Engl. J. Med.*, **298**:341, 1978.

639. Rajan, S., R. Levinson, and C. M. Leevy: Hepatic hypoxia secondary to hypophosphatemia, *Clin. Res.*, **21**:521, 1973.

640. Alberti, K. G. M. M., J. H. Darley, P. M. Emerson, and T. D. R. Hockaday: 2,3-Diphosphoglycerate and tissue oxygenation in uncontrolled diabetes mellitus, *Lancet*, **2**:391–395, 1972.

641. Hodkinson, H. M.: Serum inorganic phosphate in a geriatric in-patient population, *Gerontol. Clin. (Basel)*, **15**:45–49, 1973.

642. Dent, C. E., and T. C. B. Stamp: Theoretical renal phosphorus threshold in investigation and treatment of osteomalacia, *Lancet*, **2**:857–860, 1970.

643. Thalassinos, N. C., S. Wicht, and G. F. Joplin: Secondary hyperparathyroidism in osteomalacia, *Br. Med. J.*, **1**:76–79, 1970.

644. Forte, L. R., G. A. Nickols, and C. S. Anast: Renal adenylate cyclase and the interrelationship between parathyroid hormone and vitamin D in the regulation of urinary phosphate and adenosine cyclic 3′,5′-monophosphate excretion, *J. Clin. Invest.*, **57**:559–568, 1976.

645. Parfitt, A. M., and B. Frame: Drug treatment of rickets and osteomalacia, *Semin. Drug Treat.*, **2**:83–115, 1972.

646. MacCuish, A. C., J. F. Munro, and W. L. Lamb: Reversible renal tubular defects in gluten enteropathy with osteomalacia, *Br. Med. J.*, **2**:343–344, 1970.

647. Snapper, I., and A. Kahn: Tubular reabsorption of phosphorus in avitaminosis D, *Clin. Orthop.*, **17**:297–302, 1960.

648. Friis, T., S. Hahnemann, and E. Weeke: Serum calcium and serum phosphorus in uremia during administration of sodium phytate and aluminium hydroxide, *Acta Med. Scand.*, **183**:497–505, 1968.

649. Bouillan, R., and D. DeMoor: Parathyroid function in patients with hyper- or hypothyroidism, *J. Clin. Endocrinol. Metab.*, **38**:999–1004, 1974.

650. Adams, P., T. M. Chalmers, B. L. Riggs, and J. D. Jones: Parathyroid function in spontaneous primary hypothyroidism, *J. Endocrinol.*, **40**:467–475, 1968.

651. Mintz, D. H., D. E. Hellman, and J. J. Canary: Effect of altered thyroid function on calcium and phosphorus circadian rhythms, *J. Clin. Endocrinol.*, **28**:399–411, 1968.

652. Lordon, R. E., J. J. McPhaul, and D. A. McIntosh: Hypoparathyroidism with hypophosphatemia: A clinical paradox due to acquired renal hyperphosphaturia, *Ann. Intern. Med.*, **64**:1066–1070, 1966.

653. Ross, E. J., P. Marshall-Jones, and M. Friedman: Cushing's syndrome: Diagnostic criteria, *Q.J. Med.*, **35**:149–189, 1966.

654. Anderson, J., and J. B. Foster: The effect of cortisone on urinary phosphate excretion in man, *Clin. Sci.*, **18**:437–439, 1959.

655. Gordon, G. B., and A. Eichenholz: Unusual renal function associated with saluresis accompanying water loading in a case of primary aldosteronism, *J. Lab. Clin. Med.*, **57**:257–265, 1961.

656. Goldsmith, R. S., A. W. Siemsen, A. D. Madon, and M. Forland: Primary role of plasma hydrocortisone concentration in the regulation of the normal forenoon pattern of urinary phosphate excretion, *J. Clin. Endocrinol.*, **25**:1649–1659, 1965.

657. Anderson, D. C., T. J. Peters, and W. K. Stewart: Association of hypokalaemia and hypophosphataemia, *Br. Med. J.*, **4**:402–403, 1969.

658. Vianna, N. J.: Severe hypophosphatemia due to hypokalemia, *JAMA*, **215**:1497–1498, 1971.

659. Weber, H. P., R. W. Gray, J. H. Dominguez, and J. Lemann: The lack of effect of chronic metabolic acidosis on 25-OH-vitamin D metabolism and serum parathyroid hormone in humans, *J. Clin. Endocrinol. Metab.*, **43**:1047–1055, 1976.

660. Lee, D. B. N., J. P. Drinkard, H. C. Gonick, W. F. Coulson, and A. Cracchiolo: Pathogenesis of renal calculi in distal renal tubular acidosis, *Clin. Orthop.*, **121**:234–242, 1976.

661. Mautalen, C., R. Montoreano, and C. Labarrere: Early skeletal effect of alkali therapy upon the os-

teomalacia of renal tubular acidosis, *J. Clin. Endocrinol. Metab.*, **42**:875–881, 1976.

662. Condon, J. R., and R. Nassim: Hypophosphatemia and hypokalaemia, *Br. Med. J.*, **1**:110, 1970.

663. Spurr, C. L., R. V. Ford, and J. H. Moyer: The effect of probenecid (Benemid) on phosphate excretion and other metabolic processes, *Am. J. Med. Sci.*, **228**:256–261, 1954.

664. Stickler, G. B.: External calcium and phosphorus balances in vitamin D–resistant rickets, *J. Pediatr.*, **63**:942–948, 1963.

665. Hall, B. D., D. R. MacMillan, and F. Bronner: Vitamin D–resistant rickets and high fecal endogenous calcium output, *Am. J. Clin. Nutr.*, **22**:448–457, 1969.

666. Condon, J. R., J. R. Nassim, and A. Rutter: Pathogenesis and osteomalacia in familial hypophosphataemia, *Arch. Dis. Child.*, **46**:269–272, 1971.

667. Short, E. M., H. J. Binder, and L. E. Rosenberg: Familial hypophosphatemic rickets: Defective transport of inorganic phosphate by intestinal mucosa, *Science*, **179**:700–702, 1973.

668. Glorieux, F. H., C. L. Morni, R. Travers, E. E. Delvin, and R. Poirier: Intestinal phosphate transport in familial hypophosphatemic rickets, *Pediar. Res.*, **10**:691–696, 1976.

669. Giasson, S. D., M. G. Brunetti, G. Danan, N. Vigneault, and S. Carriere: Micropuncture study of renal phosphorus transport in hypophosphatemic vitamin D resistant rickets mice, *Pfluegers Arch.*, **371**:33–38, 1977.

670. O'Doherty, P. J. A., H. F. DeLuca, and E. M. Eicher: Lack of effect of vitamin D and its metabolites on intestinal phosphate transport in familial hypophosphatemia of mice. *Endocrinol.*, **101**:1325–1330, 1977.

671. Russell, R. G. G., R. Smith, C. Preston, R. J. Walton, C. G. Woods, R. G. Henderson, and A. W. Norman: The effect of 1,25-dihydroxycholecalciferol on renal tubular reabsorption of phosphate, intestinal absorption of calcium and bone histology in hypophosphataemic renal tubular rickets, *Clin. Sci. Mol. Med.*, **48**:177–186, 1975.

672. Hahn, T. J., C. R. Scharp, L. R. Halstead, J. G. Haddad, D. M. Karl, and L. V. Avioli: Parathyroid hormone status and renal responsiveness in familial hypophosphatemic rickets, *J. Clin. Endocrinol. Metab.*, **41**:926–937, 1975.

673. Kleerekoper, M., R. Coffey, T. Greco, S. Nichols, N. Cooke, W. Murphy, and L. V. Avioli: Hypercalcemic hyperparathyroidism in hypophosphatemic rickets, *J. Clin. Endocrinol. Metab.*, **45**:86–94, 1977.

674. Glorieux, F., and C. R. Scriver: Loss of a parathyroid hormone–sensitive component of phosphate transport in X-linked hypophosphatemia, *Science*, **175**:997–1000, 1972.

675. Magid, G. J., J. R. Maloney, J. H. Sirota, and E. A. Schwab: Familial hypophosphatemia. Studies on its pathogenesis in an effected mother and son, *Ann. Intern. Med.*, **64**:1009–1027, 1966.

676. Dent, C. E., and T. C. B. Stamp: Hypophosphataemic osteomalacia presenting in adults, *Q. J. Med.*, **40**:303–329, 1971.

677. Fanconi, G., E. Rossi, A. Prader, E. Gautier, G. Stalder, and P. E. Ferrier: Idiopathische hypophosphatamische osteomalazie mit beginn in der adoleszenz, *Helv. Paediatr. Acta*, **26**:535–549, 1971.

678. Frame, B., R. W. Smith, and G. M. Wilson: Acquired non-familial osteomalacia of vitamin-D-resistant type, *Henry Ford Hospital Med. Bull.*, **9**:548–558, 1961.

679. Scriver, C. R., R. B. Goldbloom, and C. C. Roy: Hypophosphatemic rickets with renal hyperglycinuria, renal glucosuria and glycyl-prolinuria, *Pediatrics*, **34**:357–371, 1964.

680. Riggs, B. L., R. G. Sprague, J. Jowsey, and F. T. Maher: Adult-onset vitamin-D-resistant hypophosphatemic osteomalacia: Effect of total parathyroidectomy, *N. Engl. J. Med.*, **281**:762–766, 1969.

681. Dent, C. E., and M. Friedman: Hypophosphataemic osteomalacia with complete recovery, *Br. Med. J.*, **1**:1676–1679, 1964.

682. Linovitz, R. J., D. Resnick, P. Keissling, J. J. Kondon, B. Sehler, R. Nejdl, J. H. Rowe, and L. J. Deftos: Tumor-induced osteomalacia and rickets: A surgically curable syndrome, Report of two cases, *J. Bone Joint Surg. [Am.]*, **58**:419–423, 1976.

683. Dent, C. E., and J. M. Gertner: Hypophosphataemic osteomalacia in fibrous dysplasia, *Q. J. Med.*, **65**:411–420, 1976.

684. Drezner, M. K., and M. N. Feinglos: Osteomalacia due to 1,25-dihydroxycholecalciferol defi-

ciency: Association with a giant cell tumor of bone, *J. Clin. Invest.*, **60**:1046–1053, 1977.

685. Aschinberg, L. C., L. M. Solomon, P. M. Zeis, P. Justice, and I. M. Rosenthal: Vitamin D–resistant rickets associated with epidermal nevus syndrome: Demonstration of a phosphaturic substance in the dermal lesions, *J. Pediatr.*, **91**:56–60, 1977.

686. Stanbury, S. W.: Aspects of disordered renal tubular function, *Adv. Intern. Med.*, **9**:22–31, 1958.

687. Lee, D. B. N., J. P. Drinkard, V. J. Rosen, and H. C. Gonick: The adult Fanconi syndrome: Observations on etiology, morphology, renal function and mineral metabolism in three patients, *Medicine*, **51**:107–138, 1972.

688. Gertner, J. M., D. P. Brenton, C. E. Dent, and M. Domeneds: Treatment of the rickets of cystinosis with lα hydroxycholecalciferol, *Calcif. Tissue Res.*, **22**(suppl.):63–67, 1977.

689. Salassa, R. M., M. H. Power, J. A. Ulrich, and A. B. Hayles: Observations on the metabolic effects of vitamin D in Fanconi's syndrome, *Mayo Clin. Proc.*, **29**:214–224, 1954.

690. Ljunghall, S., and H. Hedstrand: Serum phosphate inversely related to blood pressure, *Br. Med. J.*, **1**:553–554, 1977.

691. McEnery, P. T., F. N. Silverman, and C. D. West: Acceleration of growth with combined vitamin D-phosphate therapy of hypophosphatemic resistant rickets, *J. Pediatr.*, **80**:763–774, 1972.

692. Glorieux, F. H., C. R. Scriver, T. M. Reade, H. Goldman, and A. Roseborough: Use of phosphate and vitamin D to prevent dwarfism and rickets in X-linked hypophosphatemia, *N. Engl. J. Med.*, **287**:481–487, 1972.

693. Card, R. T., and M. C. Brain: The "anemia" of childhood: Evidence for a physiologic response to hyperphosphatemia, *N. Engl. J. Med.*, **288**:388–392, 1973.

694. Cartier, P., J. P. Leroux, S. Balsan, and P. Royer: Etude de la glycolyse et de la permeabilite des erythrocytes aux ions orthophosphates dans le rachitisme vitaminoresistant hypophosphatemique hereditaire, *Clin. Chim. Acta*, **29**:261–271, 1970.

695. Munk, P., M. H. Freedman, M. L. Greenberg, and H. Levison: Hemoglobin-oxygen affinity in hypophosphatemic rickets, *Acta Paediatr. Scand.*, **65**:97–99, 1976.

696. Skaria, J., B. C. Katiyar, T. P. Srivastava, and B. Dube: Myopathy and neuropathy associated with osteomalacia, *Acta Neurol. Scand.*, **51**:37–58, 1975.

697. Searles, R. P., A. D. Bankhurst, T. D. Ahlin, and R. P. Messner: Antacid-induced hypophosphatemia: An unusual cause of "pseudo-myopathy," *J. Rheumatol.*, **4**:176–178, 1977.

698. Patten, B. M., J. P. Bilezikian, L. E. Mallette, A. Prince, W. K. Engel, and G. D. Aurbach: Neuromuscular disease in primary hyperparathyroidism, *Ann. Intern. Med.*, **80**:182–193, 1974.

699. de Seze, S., A. Lichtwitz, D. Hioco, P. Bordier, and L. Miravet: Hypophosphataemic osteomalacia in the adult with defective renal tubular function, *Ann. Rheum. Dis.*, **23**:33–44, 1964.

700. Meyer, R. A., and M. H. Meyer: Soft tissue phosphate loss accompanying the hyperphosphaturic effect of parathyroid hormone in rats, *Endocrinology*, **94**:1331–1336, 1974.

701. Birge, S. J.: Vitamin D, muscle and phosphate homeostasis, *Min. Electrol. Metab.*, **1**:57–64, 1978.

702. Wortsman, J., C. Y. C. Pak, F. C. Bartter, L. Deftos, and C. S. Delea: Pathogenesis of osteomalacia in secondary hyperparathyroidism after gastrectomy, *Am. J. Med.*, **52**:556–564, 1972.

703. Stroder, J.: The content of actomyosin in the skeletal muscle of rats with experimentally induced rickets, *Helv. Paediat. Acta*, **21**:323–326, 1966.

704. Frymoyer, J. W., and W. Hodgkin: Adult-onset vitamin D-resistant hypophosphatemic osteomalacia. A possible variant of vitamin D-resistant rickets, *J. Bone Joint Surg. [Am.],* **59**:101–106, 1977.

705. Edelstein, S., D. Noff, A. Ornoy, E. Sekeles, S. Dekel, D. Goodwin, Y. Messer, and J. G. Ghazarian: Vitamin D and the bone (abstract), in *Third International Workshop on Calcified Tissues*, Kiriat Anavim, Israel, March 1978, p. 43.

706. Muldowney, F. P.: Metabolic bone disease secondary to renal and intestinal disorders, *Calif. Med.*, **110**:397–409, 1969.

707. Lee, D. B. N., B. G. Mills, A.-S. Brickman, and S. G. Teitelbaum: Osteomalacia. A comparative study of the separate effects of intravenous calcium (Ca) and phosphorus (P) on parathyroid function, intestinal Ca absorption and bone mor-

phology, in A. W. Norman et al. (eds.), *Vitamin D and Problems Related to Uremic Bone Disease*, Walter De Gruyter, Berlin, 1975.

708. Parsons, V., C. Davies, and M. Self: Total urinary hydroxyproline excreted in healing experimental rat rickets, studied with ¹⁴C proline, *Calcif. Tissue Res.*, **12**:47–58, 1973.

709. Smith, R., and M. Dick: The effect of vitamin D and phosphate on urinary total hydroxyproline excretion in adult-presenting "vitamin D resistant" type I renal tubular osteomalacia, *Clin. Sci.*, **35**:575–587, 1968.

710. de Deuxchaisnes, C. N., and S. M. Krane: The treatment of adult phosphate diabetes and Fanconi syndrome with neutral sodium phosphate, *Am. J. Med.*, **43**:508–543, 1967.

711. Harrison, H. E., H.-C. Harrison, F. Lifshitz, and A. D. Johnson: Growth disturbance in hereditary hypophosphatemia, *Am. J. Dis. Child.*, **112**:290–297, 1966.

712. Van Biervliet, J. P. G. M., R. A. M. G. Doncerwolcke, G. J. Van Stekelenburg, and S. K. Wadman: Sodium chloride restriction and extracellular fluid volume contraction in hyperphosphaturic vitamin D resistant rickets in the Lowe syndrome, *Helv. Paediatr. Acta*, **30**:365–375, 1975.

713. Callis, L., F. Castello, G. Fortuny, A. Vallo, and A. Ballabriga: Effect of hydrochlorothiazide on rickets and on renal tubular acidosis in two patients with cystinosis, *Helv. Paediatr. Acta*, **25**:602–619, 1970.

714. Rose, G. A.: Role of phosphate in treatment of renal tubular hypophosphataemic rickets and osteomalacias, *Br. Med. J.*, **2**:857–861, 1964.

715. Linarelli, L. G., J. Bobik, and C. Bobik: Newborn urinary cyclic AMP and developmental renal responsiveness to parathyroid hormone, *Pediatrics*, **50**:14–23, 1972.

716. Spiegel, A. M., R. H. Gerner, D. L. Murphy, and G. D. Aurbach: Lithium does not inhibit the parathyroid hormone–mediated rise in urinary cyclic AMP and phosphate in humans, *J. Clin. Endocrinol. Metab.*, **43**:1390–1393, 1976.

717. Malamos, B., P. Sfikakis, and P. Pandos: The renal handling of phosphate in thyroid disease, *J. Endocrinol.*, **45**:269–273, 1969.

718. Haug, T. O.: Time course of changes in concentration of some plasma components after frusemide. *Br. Med. J.*, **3**:622, 1976.

719. Iwanami, M., S. Osiba, T. Yamada, and H. Yoshimura: Seasonal variations in serum inorganic phosphate and calcium with special reference to parathyroid activity, *J. Physiol.*, **149**:23–33, 1959.

720. Corvilain, J., M. Abramow, and A. Bergans: Effect of growth hormone on tubular transport of phosphate in normal and parathyroidectomized dogs, *J. Clin. Invest.*, **43**:1608–1612, 1964.

721. Westby, G. R., S. Goldfarb, M. Goldberg, and Z. S. Agus: Acute effects of bovine growth hormone on renal calcium and phosphate excretion, *Metabolism*, **26**:525–530, 1977.

722. Mozaffarian, G., F. W. Lafferty, and O. H. Pearson: Treatment of tumoral calcinosis with phosphorus deprivation, *Ann. Intern. Med.*, **77**:741–745, 1972.

723. De Vries, H. R., and O. L. M. Bijvoet: Results of prolonged treatment of Paget's disease of bone with disodium ethane-1-hydroxy-1, 1-diphosphonate (EHDP), *Neth. J. Med.*, **17**:281–298, 1974.

724. Walton, R. J., R. G. G. Russell, and R. Smith: Changes in the renal and extrarenal handling of phosphate induced by disodium etidronate (EHDP) in man, *Clin. Sci., Mol. Med.*, **49**:45–56, 1975.

725. Recker, R. R., G. S. Hassing, J. R. Lau, and P. D. Saville: The hyperphosphatemic effect of disodium ethane-1-hydroxy-1, 1-diphosphonate (EHDP™): Renal handling of phosphorus and the renal response to parathyroid hormone, *J. Lab. Clin. Med.*, **81**:258–266, 1973.

726. McConnell, T. H.: Fatal hypocalcemia from phosphate absorption from laxative preparation, *JAMA*, **216**:147–148, 1971.

727. Honig, P. J., and P. G. Holtzapple: Hypocalcemic tetany following hypertonic phosphate enemas, *Clin. Pediatr.*, **14**:678–679, 1975.

728. Sotos, J. F., E. A. Cutler, M. A. Finkel, and D. Doody: Hypocalcemic coma following two pediatric phosphate enemas, *Pediatrics*, **60**:305–307, 1977.

729. Rao, K. J., M. Miller, and A. M. Moses: Hypocalcemic tetany. Result of high-phosphate enema, *N.Y. State J. Med.*, **76**:968–969, 1976.

730. Bowman, T. E., T. J. Whelan, and T. G. Nelson: Sudden death after phosphorus burns: Experimental observations of hypocalcemia, hyperphosphatemia and electrocardiographic abnormalities

following production of a standard white phosphorus burn, *Ann. Surg.,* **174**:779–784, 1971.

731. Kelly, P. J., J. Jowsey, B. L. Riggs, and L. R. Elveback: Relationship between serum phosphate concentration and bone resorption in osteoporosis, *J. Lab. Clin. Med.,* **69**:110, 1967.

732. Giebisch, G., L. Berger, and R. Pitts: The extrarenal response to acute acid-base disturbances of respiratory origin, *J. Clin. Invest.,* **34**:231–245, 1955.

733. O'Connor, L. R., K. L. Klein, and J. E. Bethune: Hyperphosphatemia in lactic acidosis, *N. Engl. J. Med.* **297**:707–709, 1977.

734. Hems, D. A., and J. T. Brosnan: Effects of ischaemia on content of metabolites in rat liver and kidney in vivo, *Biochem. J.,* **120**:105–111, 1970.

735. Opie, H., M. Thomas, P. Owen, and G. Shulman: Increased coronary venous inorganic phosphate concentrations during experimental myocardial ischemia, *Am. J. Cardiol.,* **30**:503–513, 1972.

736. Grossman, R. A., R. W. Hamilton, B. M. Morse, A. S. Penn, and M. Goldberg: Nontraumatic rhabdomyolysis and acute renal failure, *N. Engl. J. Med.,* **291**:807–811, 1974.

737. Koffler, A., R. M. Friedler, and S. G. Massry: Acute renal failure due to nontraumatic rhabdomyolysis, *Ann. Intern. Med.,* **85**:23–28, 1976.

738. Knochel, J. P., and J. H. Caskey: The mechanism of hypophosphatemia in acute heat stroke, *JAMA,* **238**:425–426, 1977.

739. Meroney, W. H.: The phosphorus to nonprotein nitrogen ratio in plasma as an index of muscle devitalization during oliguria, *Surg. Gynecol. Obstet.,* **100**:309–314, 1955.

740. Minow, R. A., S. Gorbach, B. L. Johnson, and L. Dornfeld: Myoglobinuria associated with influenza A infection, *Ann. Intern. Med.,* **80**:359–361, 1974.

741. Denborough, M. A., J. F. A. Forster, M. C. Hudson, N. G. Carter, and P. Zapf: Biochemical changes in malignant hyperpyrexia, *Lancet,* **2**:1137–1140, 1970.

742. Pollock, R. A., and R. L. Watson: Malignant hyperthermia associated with hypocalcemia, *Anesthesiology,* **34**:188–194, 1971.

743. Zusman, J., D. M. Brown, and M. E. Nesbit: Hyperphosphatemia, hyperphosphaturia and hypocalcemia in acute lymphoblastic leukemia, *N. Engl. J. Med.,* **289**:1335–1340, 1973.

744. Brereton, H. D., T. Anderson, R. E. Johnson, and P. S. Schein: Hyperphosphatemia and hypocalcemia in Burkitt lymphoma, *Arch. Intern. Med.,* **135**:307–309, 1975.

745. Miller, W. L., W. J. Meyer, and F. C. Bartter: Intermittent hyperphosphatemia, polyuria, and seizures—a new familial disorder, *J. Pediatr.,* **86**:233–235, 1975.

746. Edwards, N. A., R. G. G. Russell, and A. Hodgkinson: The effect of oral phosphate in patients with recurrent renal calculus, *Br. J. Urol.,* **37**:390–398, 1965.

747. Ettinger, B., and F. O. Kolb: Inorganic phosphate treatment of nephrolithiasis, *Am. J. Med.,* **55**:32–37, 1973.

748. Stanbury, S. W.: Bone disease in uremia, *Am. J. Med.,* **44**:714–724, 1968.

749. Spencer, H., J. Menczel, I. Lewin, and J. Samachson: Effect of high phosphorus intake on calcium and phosphorus metabolism in man, *J. Nutr.,* **86**:125–132, 1965.

750. Parfitt, A. M., and B. Frame: Phosphate loading and depletion in vitamin D treated hypoparathyroidism. Implications for different physiological models of phosphate reabsorption, in L. V. Avioli et al. (eds.), *Phosphate Metabolism, Kidney and Bone,* Armour Montague, Paris, 1976.

751. Phelps, P., and C. D. Hawker: Serum parathyroid hormone levels in patients with calcium pyrophosphate crystal deposition disease (chondrocalcinosis, pseudogout), *Arthritis Rheum.,* **16**:590–596, 1973.

752. Kales, A. N., and J. M. Phang: Dietary calcium perturbation in patients with abnormal calcium deposition, *J. Clin. Endocrinol. Metab.,* **31**:204–212, 1970.

753. Samuelsson, S.-M., and I. Werner: Systemic scleroderma, calcinosis cutis and parathyroid hyperplasia, *Acta Med. Scand.,* **177**:673–684, 1965.

754. Ibels, L. S., A. C. Alfrey, L. Haut, and W. E. Huffer: Preservation of function in experimental renal disease by dietary restriction of phosphate, *N. Engl. J. Med.,* **298**:122–126, 1978.

755. Dent, C. E., and T. C. B. Stamp: Treatment of calcinosis circumscripta with probenecid, *Br. Med. J.,* **1**:216–218, 1972.

756. Hebert, L. A., J. Lemann, J. R. Petersen, and E. J. Lennon: Studies of the mechanism by which phosphate infusion lowers serum calcium concentration, *J. Clin. Invest.*, **45:**1886–1894, 1966.

757. Better, O. S., G. K. Kyriakides, and D. Barzilai: Influence of age on the phosphaturic response to induced hypocalcemia in man, *J. Clin. Endocrinol. Metab.*, **31:**665–669, 1970.

758. Stamp, T. C. B.: The hypocalcaemic effect of intravenous phosphate administration, *Clin. Sci.*, **40:**55–65, 1971.

759. Jonxis, J. H. P.: Some investigations on rickets, *J. Pediatr.*, **59:**607–615, 1961.

760. Meroney, W. H., and R. F. Herndon: The management of acute renal insufficiency, *JAMA*, **155:**877–883, 1954.

761. Evans, R. A., M. A. Forbes, R. A. L. Sutton, and L. Watson: Urinary excretion of calcium and magnesium in patients with calcium-containing renal stones, *Lancet*, **4:**958–961, 1967.

762. MacIntyre, L.: An outline of magnesium metabolism in health and disease—A review, *J. Chronic Dis.*, **16:**201–215, 1963.

763. Wacker, W. E. C., and A. F. Parisi: Magnesium metabolism, *N. Engl. J. Med.*, **278:**658–663, 712–716, 772–776, 1968.

764. Foster, G. V.: Magnesium metabolism, in S. C. Dyke (ed.), *Recent Advances in Clinical Pathology*, 2d ed., Churchill-Livingstone, New York, 1969.

765. Gitelman, H. J., and L. G. Welt: Magnesium deficiency, *Adv. Intern. Med.*, **20:**233–241, 1969.

766. Thoren, L.: Magnesium metabolism, *Prog. Surg.*, **9:**131–156, 1971.

767. Flink, E. B.: Magnesium deficiency and magnesium toxicity in man, in A. S. Prasad (ed.), *Trace Elements in Human Health and Disease*, vol. II, Academic Press, Inc., New York, 1976.

768. Baldwin, D., P. K. Robinson, K. L. Zierler, and J. L. Lilienthal: Interrelations of magnesium, potassium, phosphorus, and creatinine in skeletal muscle of man, *J. Clin. Invest.*, **31:**850–858, 1952.

769. Widdowson, E. M., and J. W. T. Dickerson: Chemical composition of the body, in C. L. Comar and F. Bronner (eds.), *Mineral Metabolism*, vol. IIA, Academic Press, Inc., New York, 1964.

770. Alfrey, A. C., N. L. Miller, and D. Butkut: Evaluation of body magnesium stores, *J. Lab. Clin. Med.*, **84:**153–162, 1974.

771. Whang, R., and J. K. Aikawa: Magnesium deficiency and refractoriness to potassium repletion, *J. Chron. Dis.*, **30:**65–68, 1977.

772. Dyckner, T., and P. O. Wester: Intracellular potassium after magnesium infusion, *Br. Med. J.*, **2:**822–823, 1978.

773. Fourman, P., and D. B. Morgan: Chronic magnesium deficiency, *Proc. Nutr. Soc.*, **21:**34–41, 1962.

774. Petersen, V. P.: Metabolic studies in clinical magnesium deficiency, *Acta Med. Scand.*, **173:**285–298, 1963.

775. Alfrey, A. C., and N. L. Miller: Bone magnesium pools in uremia, *J. Clin. Invest.*, **52:**3019–3027, 1973.

776. Drenick, E. J., I. F. Hunt, and M. E. Swendseid: Magnesium depletion during prolonged fasting of obese males, *J. Clin. Endocrinol. Metab.*, **29:**1341–1348, 1969.

777. Alleyne, G. A. O., D. J. Millward, and G. H. Scullard: Total body potassium, muscle electrolytes, and glycogen in malnourished children, *J. Pediatr.*, **76:**75–81, 1970.

778. Lim, P., and E. Jacob: Magnesium status in chronic uraemic patients, *Nephron*, **9:**300–307, 1972.

779. Wallach, S., J. V. Bellavia, J. Schorr, and A. Schaffer: Tissue distribution of electrolytes, ^{47}Ca and ^{28}Mg in experimental hyper- and hypoparathyroidism, *Endocrinology*, **78:**16–28, 1966.

780. Hessman, Y., and L. Thoren: Extra- and intracellular magnesium in hyperparathyroidism, *Acta Chir. Scand.*, **139:**431–436, 1973.

781. Potts, J. T., and B. Roberts: Clinical significance of magnesium deficiency and its relation to parathyroid disease, *Am. J. Med. Sci.*, **235:**206–219, 1958.

782. Heaton, F. W.: Magnesium metabolism in surgical patients, *Clin. Chim. Acta*, **9:**327–333, 1964.

783. McMullen, J. K.: Asystole and hypomagnesaemia during recovery from diabetic ketoacidosis, *Br. Med. J.*, **1:**690, 1977.

784. Cadell, J. L., and R. E. Olson: An evaluation of the electrolyte status of malnourished Thai children, *J. Pediatr.*, **83:**124–128, 1973.

785. Randall, R. E.: Magnesium metabolism in chronic renal disease, *Ann. N.Y. Acad. Sci.*, **162:**831–846, 1969.

786. Abel, R. M., W. M. Abbott, and J. E. Fischer: In-

travenous essential L-amino acids and hypertonic dextrose in patients with acute renal failure, *Am. J. Surg.*, **123**:632–638, 1972.

787. Parsons, F. M., G. F. Edwards, C. K. Anderson, S. Ahmad, P. B. Clark, C. Hetherington, and G. A. Young: Regression of malignant tumours in magnesium and potassium depletion induced by diet and haemodialysis, *Lancet*, 1:243–244, 1974.

788. Broughton, A., I. R. M. Anderson, and C. H. Bowden: Magnesium-deficiency syndrome in burns, *Lancet*, 2:1156–1158, 1968.

789. Shils, M. E.: Experimental human magnesium depletion, *Medicine*, **48**:61–85, 1969.

790. Sutton, R. A. L.: Hypomagnesaemia and magnesium deficiency, *J. R. Coll. Physicians. Lond.*, **2**:358–370, 1968.

791. Dunn, M. J., and M. Walser: Magnesium depletion in normal man, *Metabolism*, **15**:884–895, 1966.

792. Muldowney, F. P., T. J. McKenna, L. H. Kyle, R. Freaney, and M. Swan: Parathormone-like effect of magnesium replenishment in steatorrhea, *N. Engl. J. Med.*, **282**:61–68, 1970.

793. Lim, P., and E. Jacob: Tissue magnesium level in chronic diarrhea, *J. Lab. Clin. Med.*, **80**:313–321, 1972.

794. Lim, P., and E. Jacob: Magnesium deficiency in liver cirrhosis, *Q. J. Med.*, **41**:291–300, 1972.

795. Lim, P., and E. Jacob: Magnesium status of alcoholic patients, *Metabolism*, **21**:1045–1051, 1972.

796. Booth, C. C., N. Barbouris, S. Hanna, and I. MacIntyre: Incidence of hypomagnesaemia in intestinal malabsorption, *Br. Med. J.*, **2**:141–144, 1963.

797. Nordin, B. E. C.: Plasma calcium and plasma magnesium homeostasis, in B. E. C. Nordin (ed.), *Calcium, Phosphate and Magnesium Metabolism*, Churchill-Livingstone, New York, 1976.

798. Tsang, R. C.: Neonatal magnesium disturbances, *Am. J. Dis. Child.*, **124**:282–293, 1972.

799. Heaton, F. W., and F. M. Parsons: The metabolic effect of high magnesium intake, *Clin. Sci.*, **21**:273–284, 1961.

800. Jones, J. E., R. Manaol, and E. B. Flink: Magnesium requirements in adults, *Am. J. Clin. Nutr.*, **20**:632–635, 1967.

801. Seelig, M. S.: The requirement of magnesium by the normal adult. Summary and analysis of published data, *Am. J. Clin. Nutr.*, **14**:342, 1964.

802. Marshall, D. H., B. E. C. Nordin, and R. Speed: Calcium, phosphorus and magnesium requirement, *Proc. Nutr. Soc.*, **35**:163–173, 1976.

803. Barnes, B. A., O. Cope, and E. B. Gordon: Magnesium requirements and deficits: An evaluation in two surgical patients, *Ann. Surg.*, **152**:518–532, 1960.

804. Nordio, S., A. Donath, F. Macagno, and R. Gatti: Chronic hypomagnesemia with magnesium-dependent hypocalcemia, *Acta Paediatr. Scand.*, **60**:441–448, 1971.

805. Fletcher, R. F., A. A. Henley, H. G. Sammons, and J. R. Squire: A case of magnesium deficiency following massive intestinal resection, *Lancet*, 1:522–525, 1960.

806. Opie, L. H., B. G. Hunt, and J. M. Finlay: Massive small bowel resection with malabsorption and negative magnesium balance, *Gastroenterology*, **47**:415–420, 1964.

807. Goldman, A. S., D. D. Van Fossan, and E. E. Baird: Magnesium deficiency in celiac disease, *Pediatrics*, **29**:948–952, 1962.

808. Lipner, A.: Symptomatic magnesium deficiency after small-intestinal bypass for obesity, *Br. Med. J.*, 1:148, 1977.

809. Parfitt, A. M., M. J. Miller, D. L. Thomson, A. R. Villanueva, D. S. Rao, I. Oliver, and B. Frame: Metabolic bone disease after intestinal bypass for treatment of obesity, *Ann. Intern. Med.*, **89**:193–199, 1978.

810. Clarkson, E. M., S. J. McDonald, H. E. de Wardener, and R. Warren: Magnesium metabolism in chronic renal failure, *Clin. Sci.*, **28**:107–115, 1965.

811. Friedman, M., G. Gatcher, and L. Watson: Primary hypomagnesaemia with secondary hypocalcaemia in an infant, *Lancet*, 1:703–705, 1967.

812. Paunier, L., I. C. Radde, S. W. Kooh, P. E. Conen, and D. Fraser: Primary hypomagnesemia with secondary hypocalcemia in an infant, *Pediatrics*, **41**:385–402, 1968.

813. Strømme, J. H.: Familial hypomagnesemia. Biochemical, histological and hereditary aspects studied in two brothers, *Acta Paediatr. Scand.*, **58**:433–444, 1969.

814. Smales, O. R. C.: Primary infantile hypomagnesaemia, *Proc R. Soc. Med.*, **67**:759–762, 1974.

815. Coenegracht, J. M., and H. G. J. Houben: Idiopathic hypomagnesemia with hypocalcemia in an adult, *Clin. Chim. Acta*, **50**:349–357, 1974.

816. Jackson, C. E., and D. W. Meier: Routine serum magnesium analysis. Correlation with clinical state in 5,100 patients, *Ann. Intern. Med.*, **69:**743–748, 1968.

817. Horton, R., and E. G. Biglieri: Effect of aldosterone on the metabolism of magnesium, *J. Clin. Endocrinol.*, **22:**1187–1192, 1962.

818. Nielsen, B., and N. A. Thorn: Transient excess urinary excretion of antidiuretic material in acute intermittent porphyria with hyponatremia and hypomagnesemia, *Am. J. Med.*, **38:**345–350, 1965.

819. Fisch, L., L. H. Miller, and C. R. Kleeman: Effect of vasopressin on calcium and sodium excretion in hydrated normal subjects, *Proc. Soc. Exp. Biol. Med.*, **119:**719–222, 1965.

820. Cohen, M. I., H. McNamara, and L. Finberg: Serum magnesium in children with cirrhosis, *J. Pediatr.*, **76:**453–455, 1970.

821. Sutherland, L. E., P. Hartroft, J. U. Balis, J. D. Bailey, and M. J. Lynch: Bartter's syndrome: A report of four cases, including three in one sibship, with comparative histologic evaluation of the juxtaglomerular apparatuses and glomeruli, *Acta Paediatr. Scand.* (Suppl.):201, 1970.

822. Massry, S. G.: Pharmacology of magnesium, *Ann. Rev. Pharmacol. Toxicol.*, **17:**67–82, 1977.

823. Davis, B. B., H. G. Preuss, and H. V. Murdaugh: Hypomagnesemia following the diuresis of post-renal obstruction and renal transplant, *Nephron*, **14:**275–280, 1975.

824. Eliel, L. P., W. O. Smith, R. Chanes, and J. Hawrylko: Magnesium metabolism in hyperparathyroidism and osteolytic disease, *Ann. N.Y. Acad. Sci.*, **162:**810–830, 1969.

825. Hornum, I., and I. Transbøl: Partial escape of magnesium from the renal action of parathyroid hormone in hyperparathyroidism, *Acta Med. Scand.*, **193:**325–330, 1973.

826. King, R. G., and S. W. Stanbury: Magnesium metabolism in primary hyperparathyroidism, *Clin. Sci.*, **39:**281–303, 1970.

827. Jones, K. H., and P. Fourman: Effects of infusions of magnesium and of calcium in parathyroid insufficiency, *Clin. Sci.*, **30:**139–150, 1966.

828. Bar, R. S., H. E. Wilson, and E. L. Mazzaferri: Hypomagnesemia hypocalcemia secondary to renal magnesium wasting, *Ann. Intern. Med.*, **82:**646–649, 1975.

829. Gitelman, H. J., J. B. Graham, and L. G. Welt: A familial disorder characterized by hypokalemia and hypomagnesemia, *Ann. N.Y. Acad. Sci.*, **162:**856–864, 1969.

830. Paunier, L., and P. C. Sizonenko: Asymptomatic chronic hypomagnesemia and hypokalemia in a child: Cell membrane disease? *J. Pediatr.*, **88:**51–55, 1976.

831. Michelis, M. F., A. L. Drash, L. G. Linarelli, F. R. De Rubertis, and B. B. Davis: Decreased bicarbonate threshold and renal magnesium wasting in a sibship with distal renal tubular acidosis (evaluation of the pathophysiologic role of parathyroid hormone), *Metabolism,* **21:**905–920, 1972.

832. Booth, B. E., and A. Johanson: Hypomagnesemia due to renal tubular defect in reabsorption of magnesium, *J. Pediatr.*, **85:**350–354, 1974.

833. Runeberg, L., Y. Collan, E. J. Jokinen, J. Lahdevirta, and A. Aro: Hypomagnesemia due to renal disease of unknown etiology, *Am. J. Med.*, **59:**873–881, 1975.

834. Freeman, R. M., and E. Pearson: Hypomagnesemia of unknown etiology, *Am. J. Med.*, **41:**645–656, 1966.

835. Mendelson, J. H., B. Barnes, C. Mayman, and M. Victor: The determination of exchangeable magnesium in alcoholic patients, *Metabolism*, **14:**88–98, 1965.

836. Jones, J. E., S. R. Shane, W. H. Jacobs, and E. B. Flink: Magnesium balance studies in chronic alcoholism, *Ann. N.Y. Acad. Sci.*, **162:**934–946, 1969.

837. Mendelson, J. H., M. Ogata, and N. K. Mello: Effects of alcohol ingestion and withdrawal on magnesium states of alcoholics: Clinical and experimental findings, *Ann. N.Y. Acad. Sci.*, **162:**918–933, 1969.

838. Jeaton, F. W., L. N. Pyrah, C. C. Beresford, R. W. Bryson, and D. F. Martin: Hypomagnesaemia in chronic alcoholism, *Lancet*, **2:**802–805, 1962.

839. Dick, M., R. A. Evans, and L. Watson: Effect of ethanol on magnesium excretion, *J. Clin. Pathol.*, **22:**152–153, 1969.

840. Lim, P., and E. Jacob: Magnesium deficiency in patients on long-term diuretic therapy for heart failure, *Br. Med. J.*, **3:**620–622, 1972.

841. Lazara, R. K., T. K. Yun, W. C. Balck, J. J. Walsh, and G. E. Burch: Magnesium and potassium metabolism in patients with idiopathic cardiomyop-

athy and chronic congestive heart failure, *Proc. Soc. Exp. Biol. Med.,* **120**:110–114, 1965.

842. Sawyer, R. B., M. A. Drew, M. H. Gesink, K. C. Jr. Sawyer, and K. C. Sawyer: Postoperative magnesium metabolism, *Arch. Surg.,* **100**:343–348, 1970.

843. Holden, M. P., M. I. Ionescu, and G. H. Wooler: Magnesium in patients undergoing open-heart surgery, *Thorax,* **27**:212, 1972.

844. Scheinman, M. M., R. W. Sullivan, and K. H. Hyatt: Magnesium metabolism in patients undergoing cardiopulmonary bypass, *Circulation,* **39, 40**(suppl. 1): 235–241, 1969.

845. Rizek, J. E., A. Dimich, and S. Wallach: Plasma and erythrocyte magnesium in thyroid disease, *J. Clin. Endocrinol.,* **25**:350–358, 1965.

846. Dimich, A., J. E. Rizek, S. Wallach, and W. Siler: Magnesium transport in patients with thyroid disease, *J. Clin. Endocrinol.,* **26**:1081–1092, 1966.

847. Jones, J. E., P. C. Desper, S. R. Shane, and E. B. Flink: Magnesium metabolism in hyperthyroidism and hypothyroidism, *J. Clin. Invest.,* **45**:891–900, 1966.

848. Wallach, S., J. V. Ballavia, P. J. Gamponia, and P. Bristrim: Thyroxine-induced stimulation of hepatic cell transport of calcium and magnesium, *J. Clin. Invest.,* **51**:1572–1577, 1972.

849. Marks, P., and H. Ashraf: Apathetic hyperthyroidism with hypomagnesaemia and raised alkaline phosphatase concentration, *Br. Med. J.,* **2**:821–822, 1978.

850. Wallach, S., J. V. Bellavia, J. Schorr, and P. J. Gamponia: Effect of vitamin D on tissue distribution and transport of electrolytes, ^{47}Ca and ^{28}Mg, *Endocrinology,* **79**:773–782, 1966.

851. Fankushen, D., D. Raskin, A. Dimich, and S. Wallach: The significance of hypomagnesemia in alcoholic patients, *Am. J. Med.,* **37**:802–812, 1964.

852. Seelig, M. S.: Magnesium deficiency with phosphate and vitamin D excesses: Role in pediatric cardiovascular disease? *Cardiovasc. Med.,* 637–650, June 1978.

853. Lim, P., and O. T. Khoo: Hypermagnesaemia in presence of magnesium depletion in acute-on-chronic renal failure, *Br. Med. J.,* **1**:414–416, 1969.

854. Iseri, L. T., J. Freed, and A. R. Bures: Magnesium deficiency and cardiac disorders, *Am. J. Med.,* **58**:837–846, 1975.

855. George, G. A., and F. W. Heaton: Changes in cellular composition during magnesium deficiency, *Biochem. J.,* **152**:609–615, 1975.

856. Goldman, R. H., R. E. Kleiger, E. Schweizer, and D. C. Harrison: The effect on myocardial ^{3}H-digoxin of magnesium deficiency, *Proc. Soc. Exp. Biol. Med.,* **136**:747–749, 1971.

857. Seller, R. H., J. Cangiano, K. E. Kim, S. Mendelssohn, A. N. Brest, and C. Swartz: Digitalis toxicity and hypomagnesemia, *Am. Heart J.,* **79**:57–68, 1970.

858. Chadda, K. D., E. Lichstein, and P. Gupta: Hypomagnesemia and refractory cardiac arrhythmia in a nondigitalized patient, *Am. J. Cardiol.,* **31**:98–100, 1973.

859. Seelig, M. S.: Electrocardiographic patterns of magnesium depletion appearing in alcoholic heart disease, *Ann. N.Y. Acad. Sci.,* **162**:906–917, 1969.

860. Kim, Y. W., C. E. Andrews, and W. E. Ruth: Serum magnesium and cardiac arrhythmias with special reference to digitalis intoxication, *Am. J. Med. Sci.,* **242**:127–132, 1961.

861. Stendig-Lindberg, G., J. Bergstrom, and E. Hultman: Hypomagnesaemia and muscle electrolytes and metabolites, *Acta Med. Scand.,* **201**:273–280, 1977.

862. Suh, S. M., A. J. Tashjian, N. Matsuo, D. K. Parkinson, and D. Fraser: Pathogenesis of hypocalcemia in primary hypomagnesemia: Normal end-organ responsiveness to parathyroid hormone, impaired parathyroid gland function, *J. Clin. Invest.,* **52**:153–160, 1973.

863. Anast, C. S., J. L. Winnacker, L. R. Forte, and T. W. Burns: Impaired release of parathyroid hormone in magnesium deficiency, *J. Clin. Endocrinol. Metab.,* **42**:707–717, 1976.

864. Wiegmann, T., and M. Kaye: Hypomagnesemic hypocalcemia. Early serum calcium and late parathyroid hormone increase with magnesium therapy, *Arch. Intern. Med.,* **137**:953–955, 1977.

865. Estep, H., W. A. Shaw, C. Watlington, R. Hobe, W. Holland, and S. G. Tubker: Hypocalcemia due to hypomagnesemia and reversible parathyroid hormone unresponsiveness, *J. Clin. Endocrinol.,* **29**:842–848, 1969.

866. Woodard, J. C., P. D. Webster, and A. A. Carr: Primary hypomagnesemia with secondary hypocalcemia, diarrhea and insensitivity to parathyroid hormone, *Am. J. Dig. Dis.,* **17**:612–618, 1972.

867. Connor, T. B., P. Toskes, J. Mahaffey, L. G. Martin, J. B. Williams, and M. Walser: Parathyroid function during chronic magnesium deficiency, *Johns Hopkins Med. J.*, **131**:100–117, 1972.

868. Chase, L. R., and E. Slatopolsky: Secretion and metabolic efficacy of parathyroid hormone in patients with severe hypomagnesemia, *J. Clin. Endocrinol. Metab.*, **38**:363–371, 1974.

869. Michelis, M. F., R. W. Bragdon, R. D. Fusco, A. Eichenholz, and B. B. Davis: Parathyroid hormone responsiveness in hypoparathyroidism with hypomagnesemia, *Am. J. Med. Sci.*, **270**:412–418, 1975.

870. MacManus, J., F. W. Heaton, and P. W. Lucas: A decreased response to parathyroid hormone in magnesium deficiency, *J. Endocrinol.*, **49**:253–258, 1971.

871. Levi, J., S. G. Massry, J. W. Coburn, F. Llach, and C. R. Kleeman: Hypocalcemia in magnesium-depleted dogs: Evidence for reduced responsiveness to parathyroid hormone and relative failure of parathyroid gland function, *Metabolism*, **23**:323–335, 1974.

872. Heaton, F. W., and P. Fourman: Magnesium deficiency and hypocalcaemia in intestinal malabsorption, *Lancet*, **2**:50–52, 1965.

873. Shils, M. E.: Magnesium deficiency and calcium and parathyroid hormone interrelations, in A. S. Prasad (ed.), *Trace Elements in Human Health and Disease*, vol. II, Academic Press, Inc., New York, 1976.

874. Turner, T. L., F. Cockburn, and J. O. Forfar: Magnesium therapy in neonatal tetany, *Lancet*, **1**:283–284, 1977.

875. Seelig, M. S., A. R. Berger, and N. Spielholz: Latent tetany and anxiety, marginal magnesium deficit and normocalcemia, *Dis. Nerv. Syst.*, **36**:461–465, 1975.

876. Pallis, C., I. Macintyre, and H. Anstall: Some observations on magnesium in cerebrospinal fluid, *J. Clin. Pathol.*, **18**:762–764, 1965.

877. Wolfe, S. M., and M. Victor: The relationship of hypomagnesemia and alkalosis to alcohol withdrawal symptoms, *Ann. N.Y. Acad. Sci.*, **162**:973–984, 1969.

878. Caddell, J. L.: Magnesium deprivation in sudden unexpected infant death, *Lancet*, **2**:258–261, 1972.

879. Caddell, J. L.: Magnesium deficiency in protein-calorie malnutrition: A follow-up study, *Ann. N.Y. Acad. Sci.*, **162**:874–890, 1969.

880. Rosen, E. U., P. G. Campbell, and G. M. Moosa: Hypomagnesemia and magnesium therapy in protein-calorie malnutrition, *J. Pediatr.*, **77**:709–714, 1970.

881. Chipperfield, B., and J. R. Chipperfield: Heart-muscle magnesium, potassium, and zinc concentrations after sudden death from heart-disease, *Lancet*, **2**:293–295, 1973.

882. Chipperfield, B., J. R. Chipperfield, G. Behr, and P. Burton: Magnesium and potassium content of normal heart muscle in areas of hard and soft water, *Lancet*, **1**:121–122, 1976.

883. Dauncey, M. J., and E. M. Widdowson: Urinary excretion of calcium, magnesium, sodium and potassium in hard and soft water areas, *Lancet*, **1**:711–715, 1972.

884. Schroeder, H. A., A. P. Nason, and I. H. Tipton: Essential metals in man: Magnesium, *J. Chronic Dis.*, **21**:815–841, 1969.

885. Jacobson, S.: Complete parenteral nutrition in man for seven months, in G. Berg and G. Thieme (eds.), *Advances in Parenteral Nutrition*, Verlag, Stuttgart, 1970.

886. Engel, R. R., and R. J. Elin: Hypermagnesemia from birth asphyxia, *J. Pediatr.*, **77**:631–637, 1970.

887. Randall, R. E., M. D. Cohen, C. C. Spray, and E. C. Rossmeisl: Hypermagnesemia in renal failure: Etiology and toxic manifestations, *Ann. Intern. Med.*, **61**:73–88, 1964.

888. Sorensen, E., L. Tougaard, and Brochner-Mortensen: Iatrogenic magnesium intoxication during 1-α-hydroxycholecalciferol treatment, *Br. Med. J.*, **3**:215, 1976.

889. Kanis, J. A., R. Smith, R. J. Walton, and M. Bartlett: Effect of 1-alpha-hydroxycholecalciferol on magnesium metabolism in chronic renal failure, *Br. Med. J.*, **1**:211, 1977.

890. Alfrey, A. C., D. S. Terman, L. Brettschneider, K. M. Simpson, and D. A. Ogden: Hypermagnesemia after renal homotransplantation, *Ann. Intern. Med.*, **73**:367–371, 1970.

891. Govan, J. R., C. A. Porter, J. G. H. Cook, B. Dixon, and J. A. P. Trafford: Acute magnesium poisoning as a complication of chronic intermittent haemodialysis, *Br. Med. J.*, **2**:278–279, 1968.

892. Stevens, A. R., and H. G. Wolff: Magnesium in-

toxication: Absorption from the intact gastrointestinal tract, *Arch. Neurol.,* **63:**749–759, 1950.

893. Ditzler, J. W.: Epsom-salts poisoning and a review of magnesium-ion physiology, *Anesthesiology,* **32:**378–380, 1970.

894. Lipsitz, P. J.: The clinical and biochemical effects of excess magnesium in the newborn, *Pediatrics,* **47:**501–509, 1971.

895. Lim, P., and E. Jacob: Magnesium-saving property of an aldosterone antagonist in the treatment of oedema of liver cirrhosis, *Br. Med. J.,* **1:**755–756, 1978.

896. Somjen, G., M. Hilmy, and C. R. Stephen: Failure to anesthetize human subjects by intravenous administration of magnesium sulfate, *J. Pharmacol. Exp Ther.,* **154:**652–659, 1966.

897. Berns, A. S., and K. R. Kollmeyer: Magnesium-induced bradycardia, *Ann. Int. Med.,* **85:**760–761, 1976.

898. Mordes, J. P., R. Swartz, and R. A. Arky: Extreme hypermagnesemia as a cause of refractory hypotension, *Ann. Intern. Med.,* **83:**657–658, 1975.

899. Sokal, M. M., M. R. Koenigsberger, J. S. Rose, W. E. Berdon, and T. V. Santulli: Neonatal hypermagnesemia and the meconium-plug syndrome, *N. Engl. J. Med.,* **286:**823–825, 1972.

900. Monif, G. R. G., and J. Savory: Iatrogenic maternal hypocalcemia following magnesium sulfate therapy, *JAMA,* **219:**1469–1470, 1972.

901. Emmett, M., and R. G. Narins: Letter to the editor, *Ann. Intern. Med.,* **84:**340–341, 1976.

902. Contiguglia, S. R., A. C. Alfrey, N. Miller, and D. Butkus: Total-body magnesium excess in chronic renal failure, *Lancet,* **1:**1300–1302, 1972.

903. Grantham, J. J., W. H. Tu, and P. R. Schloerb: Acute magnesium depletion and excess induced by hemodialysis, *Am. J. Physiol.,* **198:**1211–1216, 1960.

904. Evans, R. A., R. E. Benson, and N. Wyndham: Primary hyperparathyroidism, *Aust. N.Z. J. Surg.,* **40:**348–351, 1971.

20

Altered divalent ion metabolism in renal disease and renal osteodystrophy

JACK W. COBURN / KIYOSHI KUROKAWA /
FRANCISCO LLACH

INTRODUCTION

An association between renal disease, skeletal abnormalities, and hyperplasia of the parathyroid glands has been known for several decades (1–4). The studies of Stanbury and Lumb (5, 6) and of Dent et al. (7) opened an era of extensive investigation into the basic processes leading to abnormalities of divalent ion metabolism, parathyroid structure and function, vitamin D metabolism, and bone in patients with renal insufficiency.

The lives of patients with chronic renal failure are now prolonged by better conservative therapy, widespread maintenance dialysis, and successful renal transplantation; consequently, the morbidity associated with disordered divalent ion metabolism, soft tissue calcification, and osseous pathology has assumed greater clinical significance. The clinical features of renal osteodystrophy have been better defined, and more rational approaches to the prevention and treatment of renal osteodystrophy have been developed. In this discussion, the term *renal osteodystrophy* is used in a generic sense to include all the various skeletal diseases which have been reported in patients with renal

failure, i.e., retardation of growth, osteomalacia, osteitis fibrosa, osteosclerosis, and osteoporosis.

PATHOGENESIS

A large amount of information has accumulated in recent years (8–21) which has greatly furthered our knowledge of the mechanisms that underlie the development of altered divalent ion metabolism in renal insufficiency. Nonetheless, there is uncertainty about the initial steps in the pathogenesis of either secondary hyperparathyroidism or altered metabolism of vitamin D and the degree of interaction between various pathogenic factors. It is likely that processes which cause disordered divalent ion metabolism become operative in the early stages of renal insufficiency and then continue throughout the life of the patient. The initiation of maintenance dialysis leads to improvement of some of the clinical and biochemical manifestations of uremia; however, the patient is continually exposed to various pathogenic factors which may aggravate the skeletal disease. We suggest that this chapter be read in conjunction with Chaps. 8 and 19 by Parfitt and Kleerekoper; many of the concepts set forth here are presented in a more general manner.

SECONDARY HYPERPARATHYROIDISM

There is little doubt that parathyroid hyperplasia and high circulating levels of PTH (parathyroid hormone) are among the most consistent abnormalities of divalent ion metabolism present in patients with chronic renal failure. There is considerable evidence that the blood levels of PTH

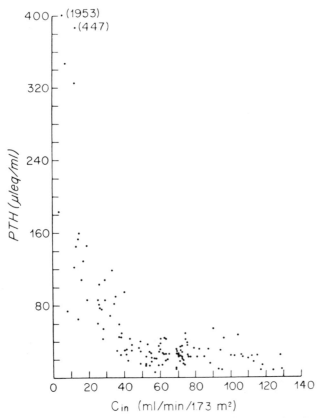

Figure 20-1. Relationship between the renal clearance of inulin and serum level of iPTH (immunoreactive parathyroid hormone) in patients with varying levels of renal function. Immunoassay of PTH was done utilizing an antiserum that recognizes the 1-84 PTH as well as its fragments. [*Arnaud et al. (23) by permission from Kidney Int.*]

become elevated early in the course of renal insufficiency; thus, increased levels of iPTH (serum immunoreactive parathyroid hormone) have been reported in patients with only mild elevations in serum creatinine or blood urea nitrogen (22) or with inulin clearances that are only slightly decreased, as is shown in Fig. 20-1 (23). Moreover, patients with mild renal insufficienty exhibits a greater than normal rise in serum iPTH in response to induced hypocalcemia (Fig. 20-2).

The main factor which leads to PTH secretion and causes hyperplasia of the parathyroid glands in uremic patients is perfusion of the glands with blood containing reduced ionized calcium. In recent years, considerable investigation has sought the causes of hypocalcemia and consequent secondary hyperparathyroidism in renal insufficiency. Factors which may lead to hypocalcemia include (1) phosphate retention with a rise in serum P_i and a reciprocal change in serum calcium, (2) altered vitamin D metabolism with intestinal malabsorption of calcium, (3) skeletal resistance to the calcemic action of PTH, (4) an altered feedback relationship between serum calcium and secretion of PTH, which may be related to abnormal vitamin D metabolism, and (5) impaired degradation of PTH secondary to reduced renal mass.

Phosphate retention

The role of of phosphate retention as a major factor in the pathogenesis of secondary hyperparathyroidism has been emphasized by Slatopolsky, Bricker, and their colleagues (25, 26). As the phosphate retention theory developed, it was postulated that a transient and possibly undetectable increase in serum phosphorus occurs in early renal failure in association with a small decrement in renal function (27). The transient hyperphosphatemia was believed to temporarily decrease the blood ionized calcium, which in turn stimulated PTH secretion. The higher levels of PTH would reduce tubular reabsorption of phosphorus, cause phosphaturia, and return both serum phosphorus and calcium toward normal but at the expense of a higher level of PTH.

Considerable evidence supports an important

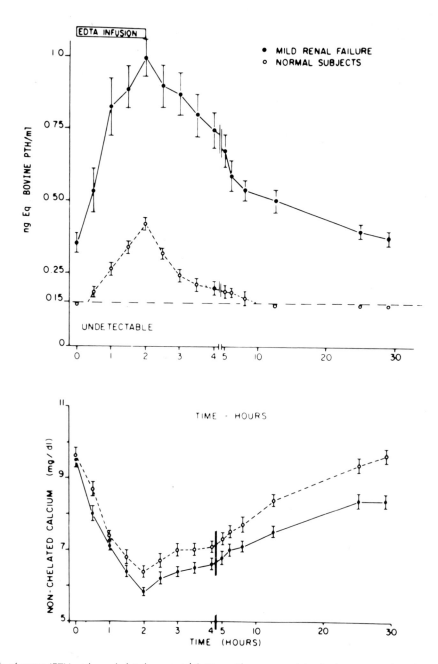

Figure 20-2. Levels of serum iPTH and nonchelated serum calcium [mean ± S.E. (the standard error)] in relationship to time during and after the infusion of EDTA (ethylenediaminetetraacetic acid). Concentrations of small iPTH below 0.15 mg/mL (the horizontal interrupted line) are generally not detected with high accuracy.

There was a delay in the recovery from hypocalcemia in patients with mild renal failure compared to observations in normal subjects. [Llach et al. (24) by permission from J. Clin. Endocrinol. Metab.]

role of phosphate retention in producing secondary hyperparathyroidism: Reiss et al. (28) demonstrated that an oral phosphorus load, which provides 0.5 g of elemental phosphorus, led to a modest increase in serum phosphorus, a fall in blood ionized calcium, and an increase in serum iPTH (Fig. 20-3). Others have shown that the long-term feeding of animals with a high-phosphate diet let to parathyroid hyperplasia, high levels of iPTH, and a mild reduction in serum calcium level (29, 30). Studies with experimentally

induced renal failure have shown that a reduction in dietary phosphate intake in proportion to the decrease in GFR (glomerular filtration rate) could prevent the development of secondary hyperparathyroidism in dogs with uremia of 2 months' duration (26) and substantially reduce the serum iPTH levels in animals with renal failure of 2 years' duration (31) (Fig. 20-4). Preliminary observations indicate that a reduction of dietary phosphate intake in proportion to the decrease in GFR for 2 months in patients with mild renal in-

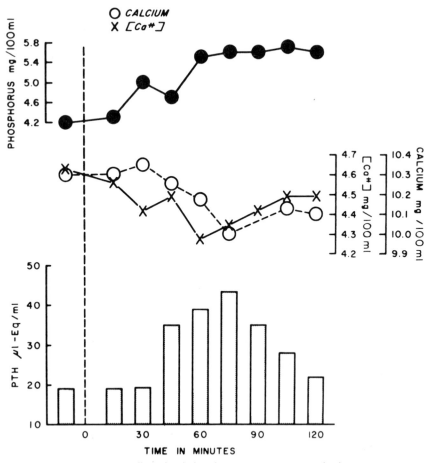

Figure 20-3. Effect of oral phosphate on serum iPTH, total calcium, ionized calcium, and phosphorus in a normal human being. The normal ranges of PTH are 10 to 60 μeq/mL; total calcium, 10.9 to 10.5 mg/dL; ionized calcium, 4.08 to 4.80 mg/dL; and phosphorus, 3.5 to 4.5 mg/dL. [*Reprinted from Reiss et al. (28) by permission from J. Clin. Invest.*]

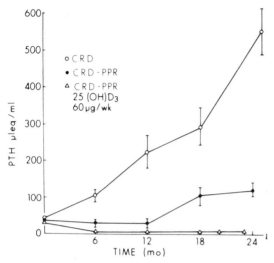

Figure 20-4. Serial values of iPTH in dogs with chronic renal insufficiency; values are mean ± S.E. Dogs received a normal constant phosphate intake (o), a phosphate intake reduced in proportion to the decrease in GFR (glomerular filtration rate) (●), or a proportional reduction in phosphate intake plus 24-hydroxyvitamin D_3 (25-HCC) 60 μg/week (Δ). [*Reprinted from Rutherford et al. (31) by permission from J. Clin. Invest.*]

sufficiency and creatinine clearances of 50 to 90 mL/min was followed by a decrease in serum iPTH to normal (24). When dietary P_i was reduced and aluminum hydroxide gel was given to patients with more advanced renal insufficiency (creatinine clearance of 22 to 63 mL/min), serum iPTH fell substantially, but the values remained above the normal range (32). Other studies have shown that serum iPTH levels correlate positively with the degree of hyperhphosphatemia in patients undergoing dialysis (33), observations providing support for a role of hyperphosphatemia in causing parathyroid hyperplasia, particularly in patients with advanced uremia.

In patients with mild renal insufficiency, slightly low serum phosphorus levels have been reported (24, 34, 35); these observations indicate that a slight decrease in serum calcium, which is sometimes noted as well in such patients (34), cannot arise as a direct consequence of hyperphosphatemia. Such phosphorus levels were from fasting morning blood samples, and it may be argued that they are not representative of the values that would be seen throughout the day; thus,

blood phosphorus levels could be higher in azotemic patients after a phosphate-containing meal than in normal subjects. In a preliminary study in patients with renal insufficiency, no differences were found in postabsorptive levels of serum phosphorus between normal subjects and mildly azotemic patients (36). However, serum phosphorus was elevated to a great extent, ionized blood calcium fell more, and serum iPTH rose higher over a 6-h period after an oral phosphate load in dogs with renal insufficiency compared to control animals (37). Chronic phosphate loading of normal animals produces mild fasting hypophosphatemia despite the existence of parathyroid hyperplasia (30). Thus, phosphate loading may augment PTH secretion through some effect other than a fall in blood ionized calcium. As discussed below, phosphate loading may decrease the renal production of 1,25-dihydroxyvitamin D_3 (1,25-DHCC) (38). Such an effect may allow greater secretion of PTH for any given level of serum calcium.

As renal disease advances and GFR falls below 25 mL/min, hyperphosphatemia usually develops (39, 40); under such circumstances hypocalcemia is more directly related to the level of serum phosphorus. Some of the factors which aggravate the degree of hyperphosphatemia in advanced renal failure and in patients treated with hemodialysis are noted in Table 20-1.

Table 20-1. Factors which influence serum phosphorus levels in patients with renal failure*

1. Dietary phosphorus intake
2. Residual renal function
3. Ingestion of phosphate-binding compounds
4. Secretion of PTH (parathyroid hormone) and responsiveness of the skeleton to the PTH
5. Balance between degradation and synthesis of protoplasm
6. Extent of vitamin D deficiency and treatment with active vitamin D compounds
7. Rate of skeletal accretion (i.e., healing of osteomalacia or osteitis fibrosa)
8. Hypomagnesemia
9. Parenteral alimentation
10. Intake of large amounts of supplemental Ca
11. Phosphate-containing enemas
12. Frequency duration and efficienty of dialysis

* See text; modified from Coburn and Llach (18).

Alterations in vitamin D metabolism

Abnormal conversion of vitamin D_3 to its active hormonal form probably contributes to the development of hypocalcemia in renal insufficiency. The evidence that vitamin D metabolism is altered in renal failure is strong: Intestinal absorption of calcium is diminished, and this defect is poorly responsive to vitamin D (41). In patients with advanced renal insufficiency, metabolic balance studies reveal that fecal calcium excretion is equal to or even greater than the amount ingested in the diet (5, 7, 42). Radioisotopic methods indicate that intestinal absorption of calcium is reduced in most patients with advanced uremia (34, 43–45). Liu and Chu (41) found no improvement of osteomalacia or calcium balance in uremic patients treated with usual oral doses of vitamin D and conceived the idea that uremia impairs the response to vitamin D. Subsequently, it was shown that intestinal malabsorption of calcium could be overcome by the administration of vitamin D in doses of 100,000 to 300,000 I.U./day (5–7). With such treatment, calcium absorption increased and rickets or osteomalacia was generally healed.

These observations led to the speculation that the intestinal absorptive mechanism for calcium was unresponsive unless total vitamin D "activity" present in serum was increased to very high levels (46). The discovery that the kidney is the only organ capable of converting 25-hydroxyvitamin D_3 (25-HCC) to 1,25-DHCC (47) provided the framework for the hypothesis that vitamin D metabolism is altered in uremia. Thus anephric rats are unable to produce 1,25-DHCC from its precursor (47), an observation which led to speculation that impaired renal production of 1,25-DHCC accounts for impaired calcium absorption and osteomalacia in uremia.

Several observations support this premise: The failure of nephrectomized rats to produce 1,25-DHCC has been verified in several laboratories (48, 49); Hartenbower et al. (50) found reduced intestinal calcium transport and diminished intestinal localization of radiolabeled 1,25-DHCC following the injection of radiolabeled vitamin D_3 to chicks with impaired renal function. Mawer et al. (51) and Schaefer et al. (52) observed considerably displacement or "loss" of tritium (^3H) compared to ^{14}C after giving vitamin D_3, which is labeled both with ^3H in the 1- and 25-positions and with ^{14}C in the 4-position, to patients with normal renal function and nutritional vitamin D deficiency. On the other hand, there was no loss of tritium in anephric or uremic individuals. Such data provide indirect evidence for the failure of the uremic patient to hydroxylate 25-HCC at the 1-position and produce 1,25-DHCC. Piel et al. (53) found a metabolite of radiolabeled-administered vitamin D_3 that was chromatographically identical to 1,25-DHCC in the plasma of two children with kidney transplants, whereas none could be identified in the same children studied prior to the successful renal transplantation. Gray et al. (54) could not regularly identify a chromatographic peak identical to 1,25-DHCC in the plasma of normal, vitamin D-replete humans given radiolabeled 25-HCC. Presumably this occurs because of the presence of a large pool of nonlabeled 25-HCC in normal subjects and because of the relatively low specific activity of the radiolabeled 25-HCC administered.

With the development of a receptor assay using nuclear chromatin from the intestine, Brumbaugh et al. (55) were able to measure plasma levels of 1,25-DHCC. The levels of 1,25-DHCC have been uniformly found to be decreased in patients with chronic renal failure (56–58).

The nature of the response to replacement with various vitamin D metabolites also supports the view that impaired conversion of 25-HCC to 1,25-DHCC is of importance in renal failure. Thus, minute amounts of 1,25-DHCC, but not 25-HCC, can improve calcium transport and mobilize bone mineral in acutely uremic rats (59). Moreover, 1,25-DHCC in doses of 0.6 to 1.0 μg/day can increase ^{47}Ca absorption to normal in uremic patients (60, 61), while the quantity of 25-HCC that augments calcium absorption in uremia is 100 to 500 μg (62, 63) and the amount of vitamin D_3 needed is even greater (34). The effects of these sterols on calcium absorption are shown in Fig. 20-5.

A suggestion that the conversion of vitamin D_3 to 25-HCC is abnormal in renal failure was proposed by Avioli et al. (65), who found an usually rapid turnover of radiolabeled D_3 with increased

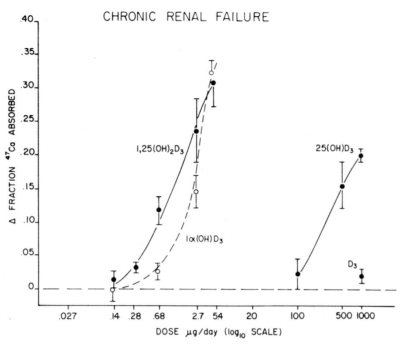

Figure 20-5. Changes (Δ) in the fraction of ^{47}Ca absorbed in patients studied before and 8 to 10 days after treatment with the various vitamin D sterols. Values are mean ± S.E. The data are adapted from Coburn et al. (34), Brickmen et al. (64), and Colodro et al. (63).

production of nonactive, more polar metabolites. Russell and Avioli (66) reported low plasma levels of 25-HCC in uremic rats compared to pair-fed, sham-operated controls. In contrast to such observations, Lumb et al. (67) and Mawer and co-workers (68) provided data indicating that the metabolism of radiolabeled vitamin D_3 to 25-HCC was normal in uremic patients. They concluded that previous results had been obtained because the dietary intake of nonradiolabeled vitamin D was lower in the uremic patients. In an estimate of the metabolism of 25-HCC, Gray et al. (54) concluded that its turnover rate was slower in anephric patients than in normal subjects. Plasma levels of 25-HCC have commonly been normal or close to normal in uremic patients, although low values may occur in response to decreased intake of foods containing vitamin D (69–71). Eastwood et al. (72, 73) have stressed the value of plasma 25-HCC levels in predicting the occurrence of osteomalacia in patients with renal insufficiency.

Thus, most data indicate that the conversion of vitamin D_3 to 25-HCC is unaltered in renal failure, while the production of 1,25-DHCC has been uniformly found to be reduced.

The consequences of reduced generation of 1,25-DHCC in renal failure deserve consideration: The problems that may arise from a deficiency of this active form of vitamin D include (1) decreased intestinal absorption of calcium and phosphorus, (2) decreased calcemic action of PTH on the skeleton, and (3) increased PTH secretion at any given level of serum calcium. The possibility that vitamin D or one of its metabolites may exert a direct action on the parathyroid glands and thereby inhibit PTH secretion has received considerable support: There are specific receptors for 1,25-DHCC in the parathyroid glands (74, 75); also, Chertow et al. (76) found PTH suppression 4 h after the administration of 1,25-DHCC in vivo; also, experiments in vitro indicate that 1,25-DHCC could reduce PTH release from parathyroid gland slices. Oldham et al. (77) found that iPTH fell more readily during calcium infusion in rachitic puppies given 1,25-DHCC 6 h earlier compared to those given vehicle alone. On the other hand, 1,25-DHCC had little or no effect on PTH secretion independent of its action on serum calcium when given to humans with intact vitamin D status (78) or in dogs with normal access to vitamin D (79).

The net effect of reduced calcium absortion and resistance to the skeletal action of PTH noted above would be to lower ionized calcium in the blood and thereby enhance PTH secretion and lead to secondary hyperparathyroidism. Moreover, lack of 1,25-DHCC might lead to decreased PTH suppression for any given level of ionized calcium in the blood. Although this fact is often unappreciated, severe secondary hyperparathyroidism with skeletal lesions showing some degree of fibroosteoclasia are common in patients with nutritional vitamin D deficiency (80). Thus, disordered vitamin D metabolism, which may cause both hypocalcemia and also directly alter feedback suppression of PTH secretion, is a major factor, perhaps of equal importance to phosphate retention, in the genesis of secondary hyperparathyroidism in renal failure (81).

When in the course of progressive renal insufficiency does the abnormality of vitamin D metabolism occur? The answer to this important question remains at present uncertain. Intestinal absorption of calcium has generally been normal in patients with serum creatinine levels below 2.5 mg/dL (34). Preliminary observations suggest that plasma levels of 1,25-DHCC may be normal in patients with this level of renal function (82). Such observations suggest that altered vitamin D metabolism may not occur in the early stage of renal insufficiency. On the other hand, the methods for measuring intestinal calcium absorption may be too insensitive to detect a minor abnormality since there is large intersubject variation in the comparison of the two population groups (34). Moreover, enhanced PTH secretion could restore the renal production of 1,25-DHCC toward normal, particularly during the early phases of renal insufficiency when renal mass is not greatly reduced; this could explain the maintenance of both normal intestinal calcium absorp-

tion and the level of 1,25-DHCC in early renal failure.

An inverse relationship between intestinal calcium absorption and serum urea nitrogen or serum creatinine levels has been noted in patients with advanced renal failure (34, 83). Observations that intestinal calcium absorption fell from subnormal to even lower values after bilateral nephrectomy in uremic patients who were undergoing dialysis suggest that the remnant kidney is capable of producing a small amount of 1,25-DHCC (84). Rutherford et al. (31) found that the additional treatment of uremic dogs with 25-HCC in addition to the reduction in dietary phosphorus intake in proportion to the decrease in GFR completely corrected secondary hyperparathyroidism and restored the skeleton to normal, providing support for a significant role of altered vitamin D metabolism in uremia. A reduced phosphorus intake may stimulate, while a high phosphorus intake can inhibit the generation of 1,25-DHCC (38); thus, phosphate retention in renal failure could be responsible for the altered vitamin D metabolism, thereby leading to secondary hyperparathyroidism.

Despite the finding of low plasma levels of 1,25-DHCC in uremic patients reported to date (56–58), intestinal absorption of calcium is not uniformly reduced in patients with renal failure, and certain uremic patients may actually exhibit increased absorption of calcium (83). Also, lesions of osteomalacia occur in only a fraction of patients with uremia. Thus, skeletal biopsies may reveal little or no evidence of vitamin D deficiency, even in anephric subjects (85). It is uncertain why signs and symptoms of vitamin D deficiency do not develop more frequently in uremic patients who have not received treatment with large doses of vitamin D or a similar sterol. The normal or elevated levels of serum phosphorus present in patients with advanced renal failure may protect the skeleton from the mineralizing defect that is so common in nutritional vitamin D deficiency.

Skeletal resistance to PTH

Skeletal resistance to the calcemic action of PTH is another important cause of hypocalcemia in patients with renal insufficiency. Evanson (86) noted that the calcemic response to an infusion of parathyroid extract was significantly lower in hypocalcemic patients with renal failure than was observed in normal subjects or patients with hypoparathyroidism. In the study of many more patients, Massry et al. (87) found that the calcemic response to a standardized infusion of PTH (parathyroid extract) was significantly lower than normal in patients with advanced renal failure, in those with moderate renal failure (creatinine clearance of 27 to 87 mL/min), and in those undergoing regular dialysis. This reduced calcemic response was unrelated to the initial serum calcium, phosphorus, or iPTH levels. In patients with mild renal insufficiency and creatinine clearances of 34 to 93 mL/min, Llach et al. (24) found a delayed recovery from induced hypocalcemia in the patients compared to normal subjects, despite a greater augmentation in serum iPTH levels (Fig. 20-2). These observations indicate that skeletal resistance to endogenous PTH appears early in the course of renal insufficiency. Such data suggest that a greater circulating PTH level may be required for the maintenance of a normal serum calcium level in patients with renal failure. Preliminary data in dogs with short-term renal failure indicate that a restriction in dietary phosphorus intake in proportion to the fall in GFR prevented a rise in serum iPTH, while the skeletal resistance to the calcemic action of PTH persisted (88); it was concluded that the blunted response to PTH is not a primary factor responsible for the secondary hyperparathyroidism of uremia. In contrast to these data, Llach et al. (35) found that dietary phosphate restriction in patients with mild renal insufficiency improved the calcemic response to a standardized infusion of PTE.

The factors responsible for skeletal resistance to the calcemic action of PTH are, at present, uncertain. In dogs with acute renal failure (89), and rats with chronic renal failure (90), which have a blunted calcemic response to PTE, the administration of 1,25-DHCC resulted in partial correction of the skeletal response. Such data support the possibility that altered vitamin D metabolism plays a role. Other preliminary observations in rats suggest that hyperphosphatemia is responsible for

the skeletal resistance to PTE (91). In studies carried out in an organ culture system of bone, the serum of uremic patients was found to inhibit PTH-stimulated release of calcium from the bone. The addition of several uremic metabolites caused a similar inhibition but only in concentrations substantially higher than those present in vivo (92). Thus, the factor in uremic serum responsible for impaired PTH action on bone could be some unidentified substance, or the resistance could arise through a synergistic action of several of the uremic "toxins" studied.

Altered degradation of PTH

It has been generally accepted that an increased rate of secretion of PTH is the major mechanism responsible for high plasma levels of iPTH in renal insufficiency. There is considerable evidence that the kidney plays an important role in the degradation of PTH and that the metabolic clearance of PTH is reduced in renal failure. A reduced renal degradation of PTH could contribute to the hyperparathyroid state in uremia. A brief review of PTH metalolism is necessary before one considers how it may be altered in renal failure.

Berson and Yalow (93) reported the finding of immunochemical heterogeneity of PTH in the plasma of uremic patients; they suggested that the presence of more than one peptide fragment of PTH and altered metabolism of the hormone could account for the observed heterogeneity. This initial discovery has been followed by extensive research into the biochemistry and metabolism of PTH (94, 95).

Intact PTH is secreted from the gland into the circulation as a MW9500, 84 amino acid peptide chain (1–84); its biologic activity resides in the amino terminal (N terminal) 1–34 amino acids. The 1–84 molecule is rapidly degraded, and several inactive fragments containing the carboxyl terminal (C terminal) of the peptide chain appear in the serum. Due to the shorter half-life of the intact (and N terminal) molecule, the C-terminal fragments are the predominant PTH peptides found in the circulation. There is still some controversy as to whether the parathyroid gland secretes the intact 1–84 amino acid polypeptide exclusively or whether some fragments are also directly secreted into the circulation (96–98).

The intact 1–84 molecule is rapidly degraded in the peripheral tissues, particularly the kidney and liver (99). The liver has a large capacity to degrade the intact molecule, but it may not play an important role in degradation of either the C- or N-terminal fragments (100). By contrast, the kidney can extract and degrade the intact 1–84 molecule and both the C- and N-terminal fragments (101–103). In the presence of chronic renal disease, the metabolism and degradation of PTH is altered, resulting in decreased degradation of PTH and its fragments (104–106). Such events could be additional mechanisms accounting for elevated iPTH levels in patients with renal failure.

There is clear evidence for a role of decreased renal degradation of PTH in leading to high levels of iPTH, particularly when the latter is measured with a C-terminal antiserum. Thus, plasma PTH levels are much higher in patients with secondary hyperparathyroidism due to chronic renal failure than in those with primary hyperparathyroidism (106). Second, the disappearance of iPTH from the circulation after parathyroidectomy is much slower in patients with chronic renal failure than in patients with primary hyperparathyroidism (93, 106). Third, renal transplantation results in the disappearance of iPTH from the circulation at a rate that is significantly faster than is observed when parathyroidectomy is done in dialysis patients (106). Studies of the turnover of intact 1–84 PTH have generally been obtained with the infusion of exogenous bovine PTH because of the very low levels of 1–84 PTH that are normally circulating. Nonetheless, Papapoulus et al. (107) studied the metabolic clearance rate of bovine 1–84 PTH and found a somewhat lower clearance of the hormone in patients with chronic renal failure than in normals. However, there was considerable variation, with some uremic patients having clearance rates that were within the normal range. The clearance of PTH containing the amino terminal region was much more rapid than was the case for the C-terminal fragment in patients with chronic renal failure.

Knowledge of the rates of degradation of various circulating forms of PTH is important both because there are differences in biologic activity of different PTH fragments and also because various antisera used to measure iPTH recognize different parts of the PTH molecule. Many immunoassays utilize antisera directed toward the C-terminal fragments, and the values obtained with this assay are often markedly elevated in uremia, as is noted above. Different specificities of antisera probably account for the variability of iPTH levels reported from various laboratories. Also, there will be apparent nonsuppressibility of the parathyroid glands during a calcium infusion in uremic patients when tested with antisera against the C terminus (108), while iPTH levels fall when measured with an N-terminal antiserum (Fig. 20-6).

The relative roles of phosphate retention, altered vitamin D metabolism, skeletal resistance to PTH, and altered degradation and metabolism of PTH in the pathogenesis of hypocalcemia and secondary hyperparathyroidism in renal failure are uncertain. In early renal failure, serum calcium levels and values for intestinal calcium absorption have generally been normal, while serum phosphorus levels are either normal or low. Serum iPTH levels are commonly increased (22, 23), although they may be normal when an amino terminal immunoassay is utilized (24). The likelihood that complex feedback loops exist between the synthesis of 1,25-DHCC and PTH secretion creates an added complexity. Observations that the restriction of dietary phosphate intake, carried out early in the course of failure, can greatly reduce the magnitude of secondary hyperparathyroidism and largely restore the responsiveness of the skeletons to PTH indicate that phosphate retention is an important pathogenic factor. However, the finding of normal or low serum levels of phosphorus in early renal failure suggests that phosphate retention may induce secondary hyperparathyroidism through a mechanism other than via a change in serum phosphorus level.

DEFECTIVE MINERALIZATION

Another feature of skeletal disease in patients with advanced renal failure is that of defective mineralization or osteomalacia. In contrast to the large

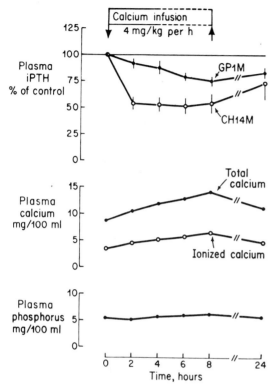

Figure 20-6. Changes in total and ionized calcium, phosphorus, and iPTH, expressed as mean ± S.E., before, during, and after an 8-h calcium infusion. The values for iPTH were measured utilizing antiserum GP1M which recognizes the C-terminal portion of circulating PTH as well as the intact molecule, and antiserum CH14M which more specifically recognizes only the intact PTH molecule; these are expressed as a percentage of control values. For total calcium, ionized calcium, and phosphorus, the S.E. was less than the height of the symbols showing the mean values. [*Reproduced from Goldsmith et al. (108) by permission from J. Clin. Invest.*]

amount of experimental and clinical data concerned with the causes of secondary hyperparathyroidism in renal failure, convincing data on the pathogenesis of impaired skeletal mineralization are quite limited. Although it may be convenient to attribute impaired mineralization to altered vitamin D metabolism, other pathogenic factors may also be implicated.

Role of vitamin D

Despite the observations that plasma levels of 1,25-DHCC are very low in all uremic patients

studied and that a marked abnormality of intestinal calcium transport is common in uremia (109), overt osteomalacia or even histologic evidence of impaired mineralization is found in only a small fraction of patients with end-stage uremia (8, 110, 111). Moreover, evidence of osteomalacia may be absent even in anephric patients (85). Several factors could contribute to the low frequency of osteomalacia in uremic patients. Thus, impaired mineralization could arise because of factors unrelated to the absence of 1,25-DHCC, because of the absence of another metabolite of vitamin D, or because some factor in uremia may "protect" most patients from the development of abnormal mineralization despite the absence of 1,25-DHCC. Some evidence can be gathered in support of each of these hypotheses.

In the United Kingdom, defective skeletal mineralization is more common in uremic patients than in North America. Eastwood et al. (76) have suggested that uremic osteomalacia correlates with decreased plasma levels of 25-HCC. Low plasma levels of 25-HCC probably reflect total vitamin D production and intake, and relative vitamin D deficiency is more common in Northern Europe than in the United States because of reduced sunlight exposure and lack of widespread fortification of foods with vitamin D. It is not surprising that vitamin D deficiency would lead to greater impairment of skeletal mineralization in patients with renal failure. Low plasma levels of 25-HCC are not infrequent in patients with uremia (70), and a good correlation was found between plasma levels of 25-HCC and the protein content of the diet. Under such conditions, low levels of 25-HCC probably reflect reduced dietary intake of the sterol. Enhanced renal losses of 25-HCC, as may occur with the marked proteinuria of the nephrotic syndrome (112, 113), may contribute to low levels of 25-HCC in azotemic patients who excrete a significant amount of protein in their urine.

The mechanism whereby the absence of vitamin D or a related sterol leads to impaired mineral deposition in bone is poorly understood (see Chaps. 8 and 19). Whether vitamin D (or 1,25-DHCC) directly stimulates bone mineralization or whether it produces bone mineralization by increasing the levels of calcium and phosphate in the ECF (extracellular fluid) surrounding bone is a matter of considerable controversy. Also, it is possible that a vitamin D sterol other than 1,25-DHCC, i.e., 24,25-DHCC (114) or 25-HCC (115), may have a major action to stimulate skeletal mineralization.

Plasma phosphorus levels

The level of plasma phosphorus may be an important determinant regarding the presence of impaired mineralization in uremic patients. Stanbury and Lumb (6) found an association between the presence of osteomalacia and a low plasma calcium × phosphorus product. Kanis et al. (116) found an inverse relationship between the number of osteoid lamellae, which provides an index

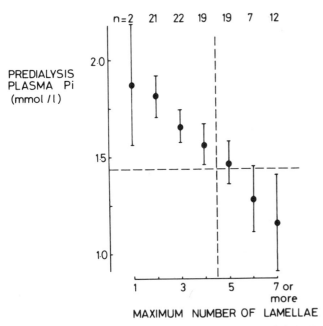

Figure 20-7. The relationship between mean predialysis P_i (plasma phosphorus) and the maximum number of lamellae seen on bone biopsy, as an index of osteomalacia in a large group of patients undergoing regular hemodialysis. Osteomalacia (five or more lamellae) was uncommon in patients with high levels of plasma phosphorus while there was evidence for a mineralization defect in many patients whose plasma phosphorus lay below the upper limits of normal (horizontal dashed line). [*Reprinted from Kanis et al. (116) by permission of W. de Gruyter.*]

of osteomalacia, and the predialysis plasma phosphorus levels in a large group of patients undergoing regular hemodialysis (Fig. 20-7). Evidence for a mineralization defect was common in patients whose mean plasma phosphorus lay below the lower limit of normal. The development of osteomalacia in humans may require both a lack of vitamin D and the presence of hypophosphatemia, although the latter may be a more important determinant.

Altered collagen synthesis and maturation

As reviewed in Chap. 8, the formation of bone requires both the generation and maturation of collagen. Without the maturation of collagen and the development of specific cross-linkages between collagen molecules, mineral deposition may not proceed normally. There is considerable evidence for an abnormality in collagen synthesis and maturation in uremia. Thus, rats with experimental uremia failed to develop mature, insoluble collagen and exhibit a preponderance of immature, soluble collagen that fails to mineralize normally (117). The mechanism underlying this abnormality in collagen synthesis is uncertain; however, similarities exist between the abnormalities of collagen maturation observed in uremia and those found in vitamin D deficiency (118, 119). Russell and Avioli (120) found that treatment of uremic animals with 25-HCC largely restored collagen maturation toward normal, providing additional evidence for a role of altered vitamin D metabolism in producing defective collagen maturation. Such abnormal collagen synthesis and maturation could be a factor that contributes to impaired mineralization of bone in uremic patients. However, it may not be warranted to extend to humans with end-stage uremia the observations made in experimental animals with short-term renal insufficiency.

Bone crystal maturation

The formation of mineralized bone normally involves the initial precipitation of amorphous calcium phosphate and its subsequent transformation into crystalline hydroxyapatite. This trans-

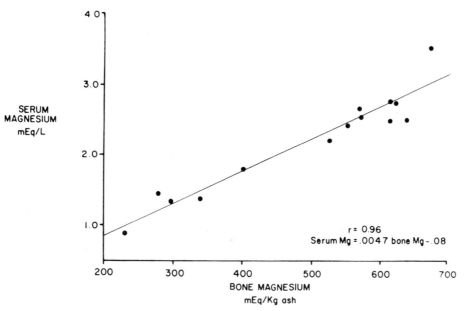

Figure 20-8. Relationship between serum magnesium and bone magnesium in samples obtained at postmortem examination from patients with renal insufficiency as well as other disorders. [*Reproduced from Alfrey et al. (123) by permission from J. Lab. Clin. Med.*]

formation occurs as part of the maturation of bone, and it is a necessary process in forming bone of high structural integrity. One characteristic of immature bone is the presence of large quantities of amorphous calcium phosphate, identifiable because of its low density. The evaluation of animals with chronic uremia has revealed a correlation between the skeletal content of amorphous calcium phosphate and the quantity of immature, soluble collagen (117). In the study of bone material obtained postmortem (121) or by biopsy (122) from uremic humans, the presence of more severe renal osteodystrophy was correlated with a decrease in bone density and a decrease in the carbonate content of the skeleton.

The reasons for the delay in the progressive maturation of bone mineral is uncertain, but several features known to exist in uremia may contribute. These include increased bone magnesium, elevated level of pyrophosphate content, and diminished carbonate. Alfrey et al. (123) and Burnell et al. (122) have found elevated magnesium

content in bone from uremic patients, and Alfrey et al. (123) found a close correlation between bone magnesium content and serum magnesium levels (Fig. 20-8). Alfrey and Solomon (124) noted a fourfold increase in bone pyrophosphate content in bone samples obtained from uremic patients compared to nonuremic controls. There was an associated increase in magnesium content, and they suggest that pyrophosphate may be present in a transphosphorylated form which is resistant to breakdown. This pyrophosphate may impair the normal conversion of amorphous calcium phosphate to crystalline apatite (125). Thus, an increase in bone pyrophosphate could contribute to altered crystal maturation (124). Alfrey et al. (126) also suggested that pryophosphate may exist as its magnesium salt, which is less susceptible to degradation by naturally occurring pyrophosphatases. In support of a role of magnesium, Kaye (127) found that the rate of bone crystal maturation could be modified by altering dietary magnesium intake.

Thus, several features of uremia, which include abnormal vitamin D metabolism, decreased bone carbonate, increased skeletal magnesium, and increased pyrophosphate, may play a role in leading to impaired collagen maturation and defective bone crystal development. Factors related to acidosis are discussed below. A possible role of some toxic factor related to uremia per se has not been excluded. The role of these factors in contributing to symptomatic bone disease in patients with chronic renal failure remains poorly understood. Initiating regular dialysis may introduce additional pathogenic mechanisms, which are discussed below.

THE ROLE OF ACIDOSIS

A role of acidosis in contributing to mineral abnormalities in patients with renal failure is a matter of controversy. A number of metabolic studies carried out in patients with uremia implicate a role of acidosis in leading to negative calcium balance and possibly contributing to the skeletal disease in renal failure. Thus, the observation that patients with stable chronic renal failure can maintain a stable level of serum bicarbonate despite a continued dietary acid load and a marked reduction in renal acid excretion (128) suggests the existence of continued buffering of $[H^+]$ by the body and, in particular, in bone. Also, Litzow et al. (129) found that alkali treatment of azotemic patients with chronic acidosis reduced both urinary and fecal losses of calcium, inducing a balance for calcium that was indistinguishable from zero. However, the correction of acidosis did not induce net calcium retention.

Observations on the role of bone in buffering the continued acid load in uremia have been derived from analysis of the mineral content of bone obtained either at postmortem or by bone biopsy. It has been suggested that hydrogen ion accumulates in bone in association with the quantitative loss of calcium carbonate from bone (121). However, the existence of crystalline calcium carbonate itself in bone is a matter of some controversy. During acute acid infusion the carbonate is lost from bone in association with sodium rather than calcium, and Burnell et al. (122) suggested that the carbonate and sodium exist in the hydration shell. Although bone may act to buffer an acid load through the release of carbonate (or bicarbonate), there is the acceptance of hydrogen ion in association with bone resorption and apatite dissolution, no matter what causes bone resorption. It has been shown that the buffering provided by bone during acidosis is more effective in animals with intact parathyroid glands, presumably because bone turnover is more rapid (130).

In a study of autopsy material, Pellegrino and Biltz (121) found that the reduction in carbonate and calcium from uremic bone was proportional to the duration of uremia; on the other hand, Burnell et al. (122) observed no correlation between the degree of acidosis and the quantity of bone carbonate in dialysis patients. Pellegrino and associates (131) found an increase in phosphate content of bone in patients treated with dialysis, while Burnell et al. (122) found no change in phosphate content, except in patients with marked osteitis fibrosa who exhibited a decrease in bone phosphorus. Kaye et al. (132) found an increase in bone phosphorus content in association with a decrease in carbonate in their study of postmortem material. On the basis of the reciprocal relationship between changes in phosphate and bicarbonate, Kaye et al. (132) suggested that there was formation of apatite which was deficient in carbonate in uremia, with phosphate substituted for carbonate; they suggested that this change may occur with only minimal alteration in crystal symmetry and size. The failure of Burnell et al. (122) to find an increase in phosphorus despite reduced carbonate suggests that the loss of carbonate does not require replacement with phosphate; the data could also reflect a different degree of renal failure and the use of dialysis treatment in the patients studied in Seattle by Burnell and coworkers.

On the other hand, other observations point to a minor role of acidosis in producing bone disease in uremia. Therapy of patients suffering from overt renal osteodystrophy with alkali (5, 7) failed to produce healing of the bone lesion. On the other hand, pharmacologic doses of vitamin D lead to healing even in the presence of acidosis (133). Moreover, long-term acid feeding of animals produces skeletal lesions more akin to osteoporosis, with a decrease in both bone mineral and bone matrix rather than evidence of secondary hyperparathyroidism (134). It was concluded that long-term acid feeding may produce an increase in bone resorption, although the major skeletal findings were those of osteoporosis.

A combination of renal failure and acidosis may have effects different from those of acidosis per se. Also, the matter may be even more complex in dialysis patients, because the restoration of body and bone buffer may be totally incomplete with the use of acetate-containing dialysate. Bone carbonate is generally reduced, and Burnell has suggested (135) that the carbonate in bone may affect crystal growth and maturation, thereby providing a mechanism whereby acidosis could indirectly affect the skeleton.

ROLE OF CALCITONIN

Plasma levels of calcitonin, as measured by radioimmunoassay, have generally been found to be increased in patients with both acute or chronic renal failure (136–138). There is evidence for immunoheterogeneity of circulating plasma calcitonin, which may account for wide differences in values reported from different laboratories. Lee et al. (138) suggested a different chromatographic pattern of iCT (immunoreactive calcitonin) in patients with chronic renal failure compared to medullary carcinoma of the thyroid. The uremic patients had a much greater fraction of iCT present in a high-molecular species that was different from intact calcitonin; the latter represented only a small fraction of immunoreactivity. Whether different forms of calcitonin found in chronic renal failure are biologically active remains unknown, and immunoassays used may detect inactive forms of the peptide hormone.

The biological significance of increased levels of calcitonin in uremia at this time remains uncertain, although recent reports by Heynen, Kanis, and coworkers (139, 140) suggest a different relation between serum iCT and iPTH levels in uremic patients having features of renal osteodystrophy than in those wihout: Dialysis patients were separated into two groups on the basis of a

bimodal distribution of plasma alkaline phosphatase. The patients with normal alkaline phosphatase levels had mean values of serum iPTH that were lower and serum iCT levels that were higher than values observed in dialysis patients with elevated alkaline phosphatase activities; serum levels of calcium and phosphorus did not differ between the two groups. A positive correlation between plasma iPTH and plasma iCT was noted in the uremic patients with normal alkaline phosphatase levels and also in normal subjects. On the other hand, the patients with elevated alkaline phosphatase levels demonstrated a negative correlation between serum iPTH and iCT, with higher serum iPTH levels and lower iCT values; the result was a higher ratio of iPTH to iCT (Fig. 20-9). They suggest that the high iCT levels in patients with normal alkaline phosphatase levels

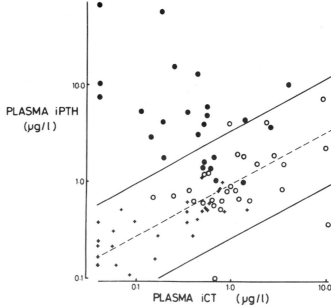

Figure 20-9. The relationships between iPTH (immunoreactive parathyroid hormone) and iCT (calcitonin) in normal subjects (+) and patients with chronic renal failure maintained on hemodialysis with either normal (o) or increased (●) activities of plasma alkaline phosphatase. The hormone concentrations are plotted on logarithmic scales; the interrupted line shows the regression slope with 95 percent confidence limits (——) for values from normal subjects and renal patients with normal levels of plasma alkaline phosphatase. [*Reproduced from Kanis et al. (140a) by permission from Calcif. Tissue Res.*]

may have inhibited or blocked the action of PTH on bone. Thus, a normal alkaline phosphatase activity may occur due to the action of calcitonin to block the rapid turnover of bone associated with high iPTH levels. Patients with elevated alkaline phosphatase activities and over renal osteodystrophy may have an excess of circulating PTH accompanied by a relative deficiency of calcitonin. The reason for such an apparent "deficiency" of the thyroid C cells to secrete calcitonin is unclear; these authors suggest it could represent either a lack of adequate stimulus for calcitonin secretion or be due to the failure of normal calcitonin synthesis and secretion in response to an appropriate stimulus. In another group of patients, under treatment with regular hemodialysis, Kanis et al. (141) noted a fall in plasma alkaline phosphatase, a decrease in the number of osteoblasts seen on bone biopsy, a decrease in plasma phosphorus, and a rise in plasma iCT in association with bilateral nephrectomy. Plasma calcium and iPTH were unchanged. They suggest that the rise in plasma calcitonin may be responsible for the transient decrease in bone turnover observed following bilateral nephrectomy. Such observations provide some additional support for their contention that low levels of calcitonin may contribute to increased bone turnover in uremic patients.

HISTOLOGIC FEATURES OF BONE

Interest in the study of bone itself as a means of understanding the pathophysiologic events and as a guide to appropriate management of renal osteodystrophy has increased substantially. Although the techniques for obtaining, preparing, and interpreting microscopic sections of bone have shown advancement, a paucity of specialized laboratories for the evaluation of bone limits the use of this technique to careful clinical investigation. The technique for obtaining, processing, and carrying out quantitative analysis of bone biopsies is described by Parfitt in Chap. 19. These techniques have been applied widely and with considerable safety in patients with renal osteodystrophy studied in various centers throughout the world (110, 142–147).

A major group of patients with uremic bone disease exhibits skeletal changes that are similar to those seen in primary hyperparathyroidism; these features include osteitis fibrosa, increased numbers of osteoclasts, increased woven osteoid, and the appearance of many Howslip's lacunae. It should be remembered that osteitis fibrosa or fibroosteoclasia may occur due to any factor that causes an increase in bone formation (111); thus, it is a nonspecific reaction of the skeleton to either local (i.e., fracture) or systemic (thyroxine, PTH) stimuli. Woven osteoid differs from the usual regular, lamellar osteoid pattern and shows a disordered, haphazard arrangement of the collagen fibers. Woven osteoid is capable of becoming mineralized in the absence of vitamin D (148); however, the calcium is often deposited as amorphous calcium phosphate rather than as hydroxyapatite. Such deposition in woven osteoid may explain the presence of osteosclerosis (111). Under normal circumstances, the lamellar structure of osteoid may permit osteocytes to sense mechanical stresses and strains on bone which are transformed in turn into electric potentials via piezoelectric properties. It has been suggested that the chaotic arrangement of collagen fibrils in woven bone may modify these stress-strain relationships, resulting in greater synthesis of inferior, woven bone for any particular degree of stress; this could lead to a tendency toward osteosclerosis (111). Thus, osteosclerosis is commonly associated with other evidence of fibroosteoclasia.

Another major abnormality of bone that may occur in uremia is defective mineralization. It must be stressed that the presence of increased unmineralized osteoid, by itself, does not imply the presence of a mineralization defect. Thus, increased quantities of unmineralized osteoid appear under any condition associated with high rates of skeletal turnover, as mineralization tends to lag behind bone resorption and synthesis of the matrix. Disagreement exists as to the most sensitive and accurate histologic method for identifying delayed mineralization; the methods utilized include (1) measurement of the width of the osteoid seams, (2) identification and counting of the number of unmineralized osteoid lamellae in the osteoid seams, (3) measurement of the extent of bone surface covered with osteoid, (4) calculation of the relative volume of osteoid from the fraction of total bone surface covered with unmineralized osteoid, and (5) evaluation of the osteoid surface covered with osteoblasts. In addition, tetracycline can be given, preferably in two separate doses, to label newly forming bone; then, the width between the two tetracycline lines is measured as the apposition rate. In addition to these methods, the "calcification front," identified with toluidine blue, has been utilized by Bordier and Tun-Chot (149). Of these methods, double tetracycline labeling in conjunction with quantitative histologic techniques probably provides the best means for identifying defective mineralization (150).

Patients with advanced renal failure commonly exhibit manifestations of fibroosteoclasia, defective mineralization, or both. It is important to consider when these abnormalities occur in the course of renal insufficiency.

MILD RENAL FAILURE

Malluche et al. (151) carried out bone biopsies in 22 patients with mild to moderate renal insufficiency, defined by having creatinine clearances between 40 and 117 mL/min per 1.73 m^2 body surface area. Among those patients having a creatinine clearance above 60 mL/min, 40 percent exhibited an increase in woven osteoid, a finding which probably indicates the previous existence of increased osteoclastic resorption and higher bone turnover. The fraction of surface showing active osteoclasts and the osteoid volume were normal in these patients. Evidence for a mineralization defect, although present in some patients with creatinine clearances above 40, was unusual; moreover, a severe mineralizing defect was seen only in patients with more advanced renal failure. Malluche et al. (151) interpreted their findings in early renal failure as consistent with changes induced by excess PTH acting on bone.

ADVANCED RENAL FAILURE

As renal failure advances, the incidence of overt skeletal disease is more common. There appears to be considerable variation in the incidence and severity of bone disease from one part of the world to another. Some of the factors that may contribute to such variation are discussed below. Although it is not certain whether histologic features of uremia are necessarily different in patients undergoing dialysis compared to those in patients with stable, advanced renal failure, certain investigators have suggested that differences do occur. Geographic and environmental factors may play a role in the occurrence of certain types of bone disease. Some investigators have found it convenient to divide patients with advanced renal failure into various groups depending on the subcategories of skeletal disease (6, 110, 145), while others favor the evaluation of patients in a single group (111, 142). As is pointed out later, there may be advantages in attempting to separate certain clinical syndromes based on the histologic features that are present. These specific syndromes are described below.

Stanbury and Lumb (6) recommended that uremic patients should be subgrouped according to the presence of divergent forms of skeletal disease. One group exhibits a preponderance of osteomalacia while others have features of secondary hyperparathyroidism. The latter patients generally exhibit a higher product of calcium × phosphorus product in serum. In these patients, active resorption surface, number of osteoclasts, and/or increased fibrosis each correlated either with parathyroid gland weight or serum levels of iPTH (143, 144, 152).

Other patients have shown a preponderance of a mineralizing defect. Most of these patients exhibit features characteristic of secondary hyperparathyroidism as well, with increased areas of fibrosis and resorptive surface (153). These patients usually have a tendency toward hypocalcemia and a low calcium × phosphorus product (6). Sherrard et al. (110) have found that bone turnover rate, as studied by double tetracycline labeling, is markedly increased in the patients with osteitis fibrosa, while it is slowed in the patients showing a mineralizing defect or osteomalacia.

The reasons why some patients show a preponderance of osteitis fibrosa while others show defective mineralization remain obscure. Stanbury and Lumb (6) suggested that abnormal vitamin D metabolism or resistance to vitamin D might lead to hypocalcemia and unresponsiveness to the cal-cemic action of PTH in patients with a mineral-izing defect, while other patients have a more re-sponsive skeleton and thereby elevate their serum calcium and phosphorus to normal, or even above, in response to increased secretion of PTH.

There is clearly great variation in the type of skeletal disease seen in different geographic lo-cations. In Israel, Italy, and in certain parts of the United Kingdom (46, 154, 155), the preponderant bone disease may be that of osteomalacia, while investigators in Germany (111), the Netherlands (142), and the United States (110) have found le-sions of secondary hyperparathyroidism to be more common. A lower incidence of osteitis fibrosa has been attributed to lower dietary phosphorus in-take in Israel (154) and in Italy (155), and intake of diets low in protein and phosphorus content may increase the frequency of osteomalacia (156). Differences in latitude and climate are known to have a major effect on vitamin D production, as measured by plasma levels of 25-HCC (157); also, there are differences in the foods that are fortified with vitamin D, varying from extensive in the United States, where milk, other dairy products, and bread have vitamin D added, to restricted, as in the United Kingdom, where only margarine has vitamin D added. Such factors may contribute to differences in the type of skeletal disease seen in various parts of the world. Dietary calcium intake is variable under different cultural circumstances, providing yet another possible factor. Data on dif-ferences in dietary intake that are obtained under comparable circumstances are not available for various places around the world; hence, it is dif-ficult to be conclusive. It seems likely that uremic patients who consume lower dietary phosphorus exhibit less fibroosteoclasia, observations that fit with those of Rutherford et al. (31) in experimen-tal animals. Moreover, isolated cases of patients showing osteomalacia secondary to phosphate de-pletion have also been clearly documented (158, 159).

PATIENTS UNDERGOING REGULAR DIALYSIS

There is disagreement about whether dialysis treatment can lead to specific qualitative differ-ences in the skeletal disease present or whether dialysis merely prolongs the lives of patients with end-stage uremia and thereby exposes them to the various pathogenic factors for a longer period of time. There are certain factors unique to dialysis patients: these include administration of heparin, the exposure to fluoridated water, exposure to high concentrations of acetate, the periodic removal of bicarbonate, the exposure to varying concentra-tions of calcium and magnesium in dialysate, and the presence of various trace elements or other substances in dialysate. Such factors make pa-tients undergoing dialysis unique and may mod-ify the appearance of osteodystrophy.

From their observations on patients studied in Heidelberg, Ritz et al. (111) concluded that there are no qualitative differences between the find-ings in bones of patients undergoing dialysis compared with those in patients with advanced chronic uremia. On the other hand, Ellis and co-workers in Newcastle (143, 153) concluded that a different pathologic pattern is seen in dialysis pa-tients compared to patients with stable advanced uremia. Thus, Newcastle patients with advanced renal failure but not treated with dialysis exhib-ited skeletal lesions which were predominantly those of osteitis fibrosa, with a small percentage showing osteomalacia. On the other hand, a pro-gressive increase in the incidence of osteomalacia was seen with the duration of dialysis. Many pa-tients showing osteomalacia also exhibit a com-ponent of fibroosteoclasia with increased resorp-tion surface and marrow fibrosis.

In addition to these patients, the group in New-castle (153, 160) and Coburn et al. (161) have identified a subgroup of dialysis patients who ex-hibit only osteomalacia or a mineralizing defect that is associated with little or no evidence of sec-ondary hyperparathyroidism. Such patients fail to show improvement following treatment with 1α-HCC or 1,25-DHCC, an observation suggesting little or no relationship between their bone dis-ease and altered vitamin D metabolism. This type of skeletal disease has not been clealy docu-mented in uremic patients not undergoing di-alysis. Whether this syndrome is related to a sin-gle pathogenic factor related to the dialysis procedure per se or is related to the prolonged pe-riod of exposure of such patients to the uremic milieu remains, at this time, uncertain. In reports that have appeared over the last several years, investigators from Newcastle have suggested that this condition may arise due to inadequate dialysis (162), fluoride in dialysate (163), concomitant treatment with phenytoin and anticonvulsants (164), phosphate depletion (165), or a failure to remove aluminum from dialysate with adequate water treatment (166).

Thus, the factors that lead to a high incidence of various types of skeletal disease in patients with advanced uremia and in those undergoing dialysis are not clearly defined. The finding of certain skeletal lesions by bone biopsy may depend on the selection of patients with specific symptoms or features for the biopsy procedure. Rarely are data provided to indicate that all uremic patients seen have had skeletal biopsies. Despite this constraint, certain observations suggest that some patients with advanced renal failure or undergoing long-term dialysis exhibit only minor abnormalities of calcium or parathyroid metabolism and may have skeletal features that are totally normal. Other patients with advanced renal failure of the same extent and duration or treated with the same dialysis procedure may become totally disabled with severe skeletal disease.

CLINICAL AND BIOCHEMICAL FEATURES OF ALTERED DIVALENT ION METABOLISM

Despite the evidence that the pathophysiologic alterations develop early in the course of renal insufficiency, signs and symptoms due to altered calcium homeostasis generally appear only in patients with advanced uremia. In part, this may occur because some symptoms, such as muscle weakness, are so insidious in their appearance that they are not even noticed by the patient. Moreover, many symptoms may be attributed to "uremia" per se by a physician caring for the patient. In contrast to this late appearance of symptoms, a number of biochemical alterations regularly appear early in the course of progressive renal insufficiency. Because the evaluation of altered calcium homeostasis and osteodystrophy is made commonly from biochemical measurements, the latter will be reviewed before specific clinical signs and symptoms are considered.

BIOCHEMICAL FEATURES

Serum phosphorus levels

Serum phosphorus levels are usually slightly lower than normal (24, 34) or normal (39, 167) in the early stages of renal failure. Studies of random, fasting levels of serum phosphorus, evaluated in relation to the GFR in a large number of patients with renal insufficiency, indicate that hyperphosphatemia is absent until renal function falls to 20 to 30 percent of normal (39, 40). Even in patients with creatinine clearance rates below 20 mL/min, serum phosphorus levels show wide variation, with values ranging from 2.5 to 15 mg/dL in individual patients.

Serum phosphorus is acutely affected by dietary intake of phosphorus, which causes an increase in serum level, and by the intake of carbohydrate-rich foods, which lowers serum phosphorus levels. Slatopolsky et al. (21) have suggested that postprandial levels of serum phosphorus may show a marked rise in uremic patients compared to normal subjects. However, other data suggest little differences in serum phosphorus after a phosphorus load in normal individuals and patients with renal failure (36).

Some of the factors that may affect the serum phosphorus level in patients with renal insufficiency are shown in Table 20-1. The dietary phosphorus intake and the fraction of phosphorus absorbed from the intestinal tract have an important effect on blood phosphorus levels, particularly those in advanced renal failure. In advanced renal failure, there is reduced net absorption of phosphorus, determined from metabolic balance studies (5, 41, 168, 169), and from studies using radiophosphate (170). The relationship between the daily fecal losses of phosphorus and dietary phosphorus intake for patients with advanced renal failure is shown in relationship to similar observations in normal subjects (Fig. 20-10). Many of the observations on fecal phosphorus excretion in the patients with renal failure lie either above the mean regression line for normal subjects or beyond the normal limits, indicating reduced net absorption of phosphorus. The factors responsible for this mildly impaired phosphorus absorption are unknown; increased endogenous

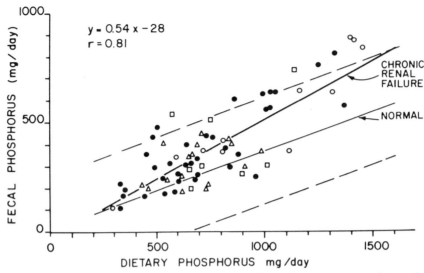

Figure 20-10. The relationship between daily fecal phosphorus excretion and dietary intake of phosphorus in patients with advanced renal failure. The regression line for normals has been adapted from Stanbury (168). Sources of other data collected from the literature are indicated by Coburn et al. (169). The interrupted lines indicate the 95 percent confidence limits for normal data while the solid heavy line indicates the regression slope for data in patients with chronic renal failure. [*Reproduced from Coburn et al. (169) by permission from Wiley Medical Publishers.*]

fecal phoshporus excretion secondary to hyperphosphatemia might play a role, although Kopple and Coburn (42) found no relationship between the fecal phosphorus and the level of serum phosphorus; such observations suggest that endogenous fecal losses of phosphorus were so small in relation to total fecal phosphorus that the total loss was not modified by serum phosphorus levels. It is well known that 1,25-DHCC can stimulate phosphorus absorption in the intestine (171), and it seems most likely that the hypoabsorption of phosphorus in uremia arises from the same abnormality in vitamin D metabolism that causes impaired calcium absorption.

The dietary content of phosphorus has a major effect on serum phosphorus levels; the intake of phosphorus varies considerably in various parts of the world depending on cultural habits. In the United States, dietary intake of phosphorus is often higher than in many other parts of the world, and it is not uncommon for normal individuals to have a dietary intake of 1500 to 2000 mg of phosphorus per day. In the usual patients treated with dialysis, this quantity may fall to 1000 to 1500 mg/day. A certain degree of rigid dietary restriction is needed to reduce dietary phosphorus intake below this level. With the use of very low protein diets, dietary phosphorus intake readily falls to 300 to 400 mg/day (42). Low-protein diets, as utilized for the management of uremia in Italy and Germany, with a substantial fraction of calories supplied as pasta in Italy (156) or as potatoes in Germany (172), contain low amounts of phosphorus.

Aluminum-containing gels, which bind phosphate in the intestine and render it nonabsorbable, are commonly employed to reduce the absorption of phosphorus in uremia. The two compounds utilized most frequently are aluminum hydroxide gel and aluminum carbonate gel. The liquid gels are generally more effective in binding phosphate than are dried powders of the same compounds (173). However, the liquid aluminum-containing gels are so unpalatable that patient compliance is very difficult to achieve; thus, patients may find it much easier to ingest larger quantities of the capsules containing dried aluminum hydroxide or aluminum carbonate gel. In general, the relationship between the dose of aluminum hydroxide ingested and the satisfactory control of serum phosphorus levels is derived by the empiric adjustment of the dosage.

There are some specific data on the effect of these compounds that are derived from metabolic balance studies (168, 174) which indicate that the intake of 75 to 200 mL/day of aluminum hydroxide gel can enhance the fecal losses of phosphorus by 30 to 144 percent. However, there was not a very strong relationship between the quantity of aluminum hydroxide gel taken and either the net or relative increases in fecal phosphorus. In studies carried out with dietary phosphorus intake below 1.0 g/day, fecal phosphorus exceeded the dietary intake when aluminum hydroxide was taken; however, when dietary phosphorus was increased to 2.0 g/day or above, fecal phosphorus was less than total dietary intake despite ingestion of aluminum hydroxide gel. Thus, intake of a diet high in phosphorus content can overcome the effect of ingesting substantial amounts of aluminum hydroxide or aluminum carbonate. A certain degree of dietary phosphorus restriction carried out in conjunction with regular ingestion of aluminum hydroxide or aluminum carbonate is usually needed to prevent hyperphosphatemia in patients with advanced renal failure and in those undergoing regular dialysis.

The effect of PTH on serum phosphorus levels is dependent on the degree of renal insufficiency. With mild or only moderate impairment of renal function, an increase in the secretion of PTH decreases renal-tubular phosphate reabsorption and leads to a reduction in serum phosphorus levels. However, as glomerular insufficiency progresses, there is a limited renal capacity to excrete phosphorus, even in the face of very high levels of PTH. The PTH may continue to act on the bone, causing osteoclastic reabsorption with the release of phosphorus and calcium into the ECF. Thus, PTH favors an increase in serum phosphorus levels in patients with advanced renal failure, and serum phosphorus levels are often higher in uremic patients with overt secondary hyperparathyroidism compared to patients with an equal degree of renal insufficiency but lacking overt secondary hyperparathyroidism (133, 175). Thus, the removal of the parathyroid glands in patients with advanced renal failure is almost invariably associated with a marked decrease in serum phosphorus levels as well as a decrease in serum calcium concentration (Fig. 20-11). It is evident that the serum phosphorus levels can be altered in patients with little or no residual renal function by events which lead to a change in the balance between bone formation and bone resorption. The initial healing of either osteomalacia or osteitis fibrosa is often associated with a fall in serum phosphorus concentration, presumably because bone formation and the deposition of calcium and phosphorus in the skeleton are increased out of proportion to the rate of bone resorption.

The administration of active forms of vitamin D and probably the status of body stores of vitamin D, i.e., vitamin D deficiency, may have a marked effect on levels of serum phosphorus. The effects of active forms of vitamin D on serum phosphorus levels can occur due to their direct effect on phosphorus homeostasis or indirectly via

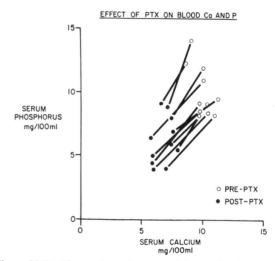

Figure 20-11. Changes in total serum calcium and P_i levels in 11 uremic patients before and following subtotal PTX (parathyroidectomy) for overt secondary hyperparathyroidism. [*From Massry et al. (175) by permission from Arch. Intern. Med.*]

an effect on PTH. Studies employing pharmacologic doses of vitamin D or dihydrotachysterol indicate that intestinal absorption of phosphorus is increased (5, 168, 170). Stanbury and Lumb (5) suggested that there were equimolar increments in the intestinal absorption of calcium and phosphorus in uremic patients with osteomalacia following treatment with vitamin D; it was initially suggested that vitamin D augments the absorption of phosphorus secondary to the effect on calcium. However, more recent studies in experimental animals clearly indicate that the active form of vitamin D, 1,25-DHCC, can augment intestinal transport of phosphorus, even in the absence of phosphate in the luminal surface (171, 176). Studies utilizing 1,25-DHCC in humans suggest that the stimulation of absorption of calcium and phosphorus is not equimolar (177) (Fig.

20-12). Moreover, studies carried out in animals indicate that phosphorus transport may be stimulated by 1,25-DHCC in segments of the intestine where its effect on calcium is far less marked (171). Since a major action of vitamin D on phosphorus homeostasis is to enhance phosphorus absorption in the gut, one might anticipate that serum phosphorus would be increased following the administration of 1,25-DHCC to uremic patients. However, the administration of either vitamin D in pharmacologic amounts or of 1,25-DHCC in small quantities may suppress secondary hyperparathyroidism in uremic patients; this may lead to reduced bone resorption with the deposition of calcium and phosphous in bone. The healing of vitamin D-deficiency osteomalacia is often associated with a transient decrease in serum phosphorus levels as well. Thus, in actual practice, one commonly observes a fall in serum phosphorus level and a decreased need for aluminum hydroxide or aluminum carbonate during the first 2 to 3 months of treatment of uremic patients with 1,25-DHCC (152); later, the serum phosphorus levels may increase. This may occur after a period of rapid skeletal remineralization is complete. With abrupt cessation of treatment with 1,25-DHCC, the serum phosphorus levels commonly fall quickly (Fig. 20-13).

Another mechanism whereby vitamin D may affect serum phosphorus levels is by enhancing the intracellular flux of inorganic phosphate; thus, in vitamin D-deficient animals the administration of either vitamin D_3 or 25-HCC leads to the movement of intracellular phosphate (178). Whether such an effect occurs in uremic humans is unknown.

The serum phosphorus level is also influenced by the balance between synthesis and degradation of body proteins. Thus, marked hyperphosphatemia can appear during a hypercatabolic state. Such an effect is magnified in a patient with markedly decreased renal function; even a mild infection may be associated with disproportionate increases in serum urea nitrogen and phosphorus levels compared to serum creatinine. In an opposite way, periods of increased protein anabolism may be associated with the development of hypophosphatemia due to the deposition of phospho-

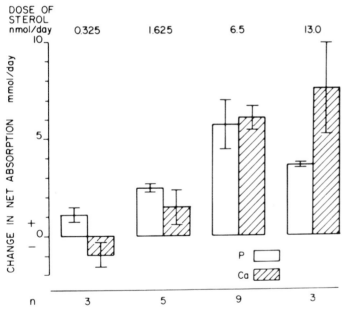

Figure 20-12. The effect of 1,25-DHCC or 1α-HCC on net absorption of calcium (Ca) and phosphorus (P) in patients with advanced renal failure who were studied on the metabolic balance ward. Values shown are mean ± S.E. and the number of observations (n) are show below. The daily doses of 1.25-DHCC of 0.325, 1.625, 6.5, and 13 nmol/day correspond to 0.13, 0.68, 2.7, and 5.4 μg/day, respectively. [*Reprinted from Coburn et al. (177a) by permission from Plenum Press.*]

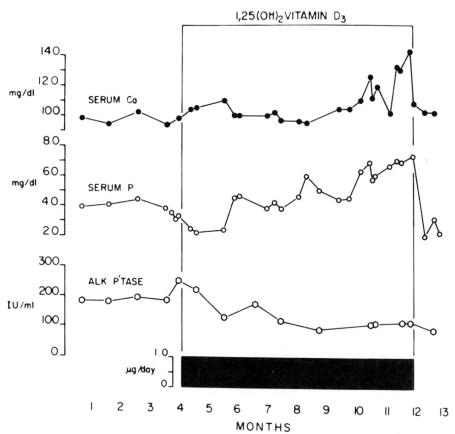

Figure 20-13. Changes in serum Ca, P, and alkaline phosphatase activity in a 56-year-old man treated with regular hemodialysis. During this time, serum iPTH fell from 1580 to 220 pg/mL (normal less than 400 pg/mL). Notable are the early fall and the late rise in serum phosphorus. The latter occurred after the alkaline phosphatase fell and coincident with the development of hypercalcemia. [*Reprinted from Coburn et al. (152) by permission from W. de Gruyter.*]

rus into tissues. Hypophosphatemia may be seen with refeeding following a period of starvation or protein depletion. The administration of diets markedly restricted in proteins and containing only small quantities of essential amino acids and reduced quantities of phosphate may be associated with the appearance of marked hypophosphatemia and hypercalcemia (179).

The treatment of uremic patients with protein restriction utilizing natural foods rarely leads to hypophosphatemia despite restriction of phosphorus intake to 300 to 400 mg/day (42). The administration of a diet comprising essential amino

acids may stimulate protein anabolism to a degree not seen with a low-protein diet composed of natural foods, thereby decreasing serum phosphorus even further. During the infusion of amino acids and hypertonic glucose for total parenteral nutrition, a substantial decrease in serum phosphorus is common unless phosphorus is added to the parenteral solution (Chap. 10). The oral administration of very large quantities of calcium salts, such as calcium carbonate, may lead to phosphate binding in the intestine and thereby reduce phosphorus absorption. The ingestion of calcium-containing compounds may suppress

PTH secretion, a factor which would also reduce serum phosphorus levels.

Although uremic patients generally exhibit an increase in net phosphorus absorption as dietary phosphorus is increased, occasional uremic or dialysis patients exhibit normal or even low levels of plasma phosphorus, despite the ingestion of a normal diet and little or no intake of phosphate-binding gels (159, 180). The reason for such hypophosphatemia is uncertain; some patients could have a greater degree of malabsorption of phosphorus than exists in the usual uremic patient, although no direct measurements of phosphorus absorption are available in such patients. The suggestion that the frequency of osteomalacia may rise in uremic patients fed either a low-phosphate diet (156) or given aluminum hydroxide (181) indicates that phosphate restriction must be used with some caution, and serum phosphorus levels should be monitored.

From this review, it is apparent that a variety of factors may have either long-term or short-lived effects on serum phosphorus levels in uremic patients. Other events that can affect the serum phosphorus levels in nonuremic patients, such as acute respiratory alkalosis or metabolic alkalosis, may have an effect in uremia, but they have not been studied extensively. Whether abrupt changes in acid-base status can affect the serum phosphorus level in uremic patients is also uncertain.

An important pathogenic role of hyperphosphatemia in either leading to or aggravating secondary hyperparathyroidism in renal insufficiency has been discussed. Hypophosphatemia may also occur and may predispose to impaired skeletal mineralization. Attention must be given to the prevention of hyperphosphatemia as well as a depression in serum phosphorus levels. Kanis et al. (116) have found that the number of osteoid lamellae, an index of osteomalacia, correlated inversely with the predialysis level of serum phosphorus in a large population of dialysis patients (Fig. 20-7).

There are no definite data to indicate that phosphate depletion can develop without a fall in serum phosphorus to below normal levels. Patients with stable chronic uremia (42) and those undergoing dialysis (182) can be in negative balance and yet persist in showing modest hyperphosphatemia. The lack of correlation of the negative phosphorus balance with those of either nitrogen or calcium (42) suggests that excess phosphorus is deposited in certain tissues. Indeed body composition data from neutron activation provide some support for this view (183).

A possible role of hyperphosphatemia and phosphate retention in either accelerating or aggravating the progression of renal failure itself is suggested from recent observations made in experimental animals (184). Treatments of subtotally nephrectomized rats with a diet markedly restricted in phosphorus content was associated with either stabilization or improvement of renal function, while animals receiving a normal phosphorus diet exhibited progressive renal failure. Tissue levels of calcium and phosphorus in the kidneys of patients with advanced uremia were increased compared to other tissues (185). A preliminary report raises the possibility that the induction of marked phosphate depletion may be associated with stabilization or even improvement of renal function in certain patients with advanced renal failure (186), while the administration of 1,25-DHCC, which may augment intestinal calcium and phosphorus absorption, led to a modest decrease in renal function when it was used without dietary phosphate restriction (187). Such observations are preliminary, but they raise the possibility that phosphate retention could play a role in the pathogenesis of progressive renal insufficiency. Studies in the dog with a reduced GFR revealed no differences in renal function in animals with normal or restricted dietary phosphorus intakes (31). If phosphate depletion and osteomalacia can be avoided, there may be some merit in restricting phosphate absorption in the early phases of renal insufficiency; however, careful clinical trials are needed before such an approach is applied with safety on a wide-scale basis.

Hypocalcemia

A fall in total serum calcium is a common but not invariable finding in patients with advanced renal failure. Although the mean serum calcium level in patients with advanced renal failure and clearance rates between 5 and 20 mL/min is significantly lower than that observed in normal subjects, only 40 percent of uremic patients were found to have total serum calcium levels below the 95 percent confidence limits of normal (40). Moreover, levels below 7.5 mg/dL were observed infrequently. An increase in the complexed fraction of calcium has been observed in patients with advanced uremia (40, 188); this presumably occurs because of an increased complexing of calcium to various anions. If the fraction of complexed calcium can increase substantially, the ionized blood calcium may be below normal, despite normal levels of total serum calcium. This may be observed after hemodialysis when hemoconcentration adds to the component that is protein bound (189). With greater availability of the specific ion electrode for measuring blood ionized calcium, it will be possible to identify true decreases in calcium levels with greater accuracy in uremic patients. There is generally some disagreement as to whether there is an alteration in the fraction of calcium-bound protein in uremia. Patients studied in our laboratory have generally shown a normal fraction of calcium bound to protein (40), while Weeke and Friis (167) noted a reduced fraction of calcium bound to protein. Acidosis can decrease the degree of protein binding, and marked acidosis, present in some uremic patients, could be sufficient to induce such an effect in vivo.

The value of measuring ionized calcium in patients with renal disease is exemplified by findings in patients with the nephrotic syndrome. Thus, a low total serum calcium level would be expected in such patients because of the decrease in serum albumin, although it may have been assumed that ionized calcium was normal in such patients. However, the measurement of ionized calcium with a specific ion electrode has revealed the prevalence of a decrease in ionized calcium in such patients (190). The pathogenesis of altered calcium homeostasis in the nephrotic syndrome is discussed in detail below.

A decrease in the level of total and ionized calcium has been observed in stable chronic uremia in relation to the level of serum creatinine; however, the range of individual values was wide. The initiation of regular hemodialysis is generally associated with an increase in total serum calcium

toward normal (179, 191). Moreover, this increase in serum calcium has been observed despite the use of low levels of dialysate calcium and despite the presence of marked hyperphosphatemia (179). Such an observation, made several years ago when the control of hyperphosphatemia was poor, points to the existence of some unknown factor related to dialysis per se, which tends to correct uremic hypocalcemia. When dialysis is carried out utilizing modern techniques, the incidence of hypocalcemia may be low; the frequency distribution of serum calcium levels in dialysis patients studied in Seattle in 1975 and 1976 is shown in Fig. 20-14. The causes of hypocalcemia in renal failure are reviewed under the section on Pathogenesis.

Hypercalcemia in chronic renal failure

Although uncommon, hypercalcemia also occurs in patients with renal failure, particularly in those undergoing long-standing hemodialysis. Some of the causes of hypercalcemia in patients with advanced renal failure are listed in Table 20-2. Hypercalcemia, when it develops in uremic patients, may be associated with greater symptomatology than is the situation in patients with normal renal function. Thus, the cause of such hypercalcemia should be delineated.

Transient hypercalcemia can be seen in uremic patients ingesting large quantities of calcium carbonate or other calcium salts, during treatment with vitamin D sterols, and in some but not all dialysis patients after the prolonged use of dialysate containing calcium in a concentration of 7 to 8 mg/dL (193). Hypercalcemia of a more persistent type can occur in patients with severe or "overt" secondary hyperparathyroidism; such hypercalcemia may appear within weeks to months after hemodialysis has been initiated. The explanation for the hypercalcemia is not particularly clear, but the initiation of dialysis may render these patients somewhat more responsive to the calcemic action of PTH; moreover, high rates of PTH secretion may continue due to massive parathyroid hyperplasia and despite an increase in serum calcium to elevated levels.

In the absence of high serum iPTH levels or radiographic evidence of bone resorption, one cannot assume that high levels of PTH are re-

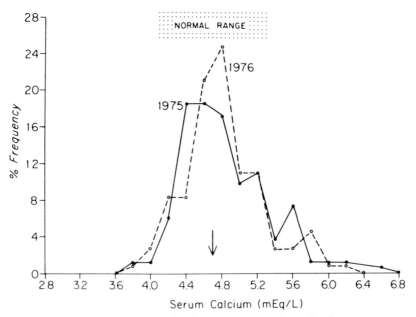

Figure 20-14. Frequency distribution of serum calcium levels in patients undergoing regular hemodialysis under the care of the Northwest Kidney Center, Seattle, Washington. Dialysate magnesium was 1.0 meq/L in 1975 and 0.5 meq/L in 1976. [*Reproduced from Burnell and Teubner (192) by permission from Proc. Clin. Dial. Transpl. Forum.*]

sponsible for an elevated serum calcium. Thus, persistent elevation of serum calcium levels has been found among dialysis patients who have a peculiar disorder of the skeleton, characterized by a marked defect in mineralization, the absence of osteitis fibrosa, and serum iPTH levels that are normal or even unmeasurable. X-rays show only "osteopenia." In these patients hypercalcemia may appear or be aggravated when they receive oral calcium supplements, small amounts of vitamin D, or are treated with dialysate containing a high calcium concentration (161). Hypercalcemia has been reported with the use of a calcium-containing exchange resin (194), in association with marked phosphate restriction and hypophosphatemia (179), in conjunction with immobilization, and during the ingestion of thiazide diuretics (195). Uremic patients may also develop hypercalcemia due to associated illnesses, i.e., multiple myeloma, sarcoidosis. Under certain circumstances, hypercalcemia may occur or be pro-

longed in uremic patients because the loss of renal function leads to absence of the ability of the body

Table 20-2. Conditions associated with hypercalcemia in patients with renal failure

1. Severe secondary hyperparathyroidism
2. High dietary calcium intake
3. Treatment with vitamin D sterols
4. Use of high dialysate calcium
5. Phosphate restriction and hypophosphatemia
6. Mineralization defect (osteomalacia without secondary hyperparathyroidism)
7. Immobilization (in association with no. 1)
8. Administration of thiazide diuretics
9. Use of calcium-cycle ion exchange resins
10. Use of low-protein, amino acid diets (usually low in phosphate)
11. Coexistence of diseases causing hypercalcemia, e.g., multiple myeloma, sarcoidosis, metastatic malignancy
12. Recovery phase of acute renal failure
13. Following successful renal transplantation

to excrete calcium mobilized from bone or absorbed through the intestine.

Hypermagnesemia

Serum magnesium levels are commonly elevated in patients with advanced renal insufficiency. Despite this finding, the homeostasis of body magnesium in renal failure has received less attention than has the study of calcium or phosphorus metabolism. Normally, the kidney provides for the regulation of body magnesium; hence, the loss of renal excretory capability leads to altered homeostasis for this major intracellular action. Studies of magnesium balance suggest that net magnesium absorption does not deviate markedly from normal in patients with advanced renal failure (169). With the presence of normal intestinal absorption and reduced renal excretion, a tendency to develop hypermagnesemia can be readily understood.

The levels of serum magnesium generally are normal unless the creatinine clearance rate is below 30 mL/min (40). With a further decrease in renal function, a larger number of uremic patients exhibit increased serum magnesium levels. As noted in Chap. 8, approximately 20 percent of magnesium is bound to albumin, a fraction that is unchanged in renal failure despite an increase in total serum magnesium level (40, 123). The increase in serum magnesium levels is associated with an increase in skeletal magnesium content (122, 123), a factor which may have an adverse effect on crystal formation in the skeletal tissues (126).

There is little evidence that intracellular stores of magnesium are particularly altered in uremia. If cellular magnesium is decreased, this is commonly associated with malnutrition and diminished intracellular potassium (123).

Whether intestinal handling of magnesium may be altered in uremia is open to question. On one hand, net absorption has been found to be normal; on the other hand, a reduction in intestinal transport of magnesium of the jejunum and ileum has been reported in uremic patients studied by means of perfusion of different intestinal segments. Moreover, treatment with 1α-HCC re-

stored magnesium transport to normal (196). The last observation contrasts to the absence of an effect of either 1,25-DHCC or 1α-DHCC when their effects on net absorption (169) were studied (Fig. 20-15). The reasons for discrepancies between observations utilizing intestinal perfusions and those derived from metabolic balance conditions remain uncertain. It is possible that the magnesium transport is markedly impaired in one portion of the intestine while it is normal or even increased in another, resulting in normal net magnesium absorption by the entire intestinal tract.

A small increase in magnesium intake in patients with advanced renal failure generally leads to an equal increase in urinary excretion of magnesium (42), an observation suggesting that patients accumulate magnesium slowly. In the usual patient with advanced renal failure who is not under treatment with dialysis, the major factor that affects the serum magnesium level and produces hypermagnesemia is an increase in dietary magnesium intake. With the intake of magnesium-containing antacids or magnesium-containing cathartics, abrupt and marked hypermagnesemia may occur. An increase in magnesium may also occur when enemas are given with magnesium-containing solutions. In uremic patients undergoing dialysis, the level of magnesium in the dialysate is a major factor influencing the serum magnesium level. Based largely on "tradition," many dialysis centers use dialysate which contains magnesium in a concentration of 1.5 meq/L, a value that is similar to the non-protein-bound or diffusible level in normal serum. The tap water used to prepare dialysate may contain magnesium, 0.5 to 5.1 meq/L. With the use of high magnesium concentrations in dialysate, blood levels of 2.5 to 4.0 meq/L are common (40). Using dialysate that contains magnesium in a concentration of 0.5 to 0.7 meq/L results in serum magnesium concentrations that are close to normal in most dialysis patients (192).

The clinical consequences of hypermagnesemia and increased skeletal content of this cation in uremia are not resolved. Most uremic patients exhibit no apparent sequelae due to steady-state moderate hypermagnesemia, although the hy-

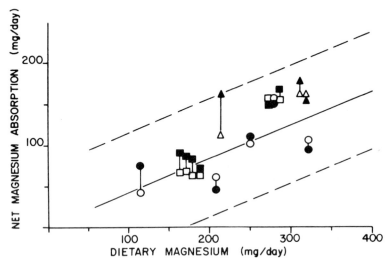

Figure 20-15. The effect of 1,25-DHCC and 1α-HCC on net intestinal magnesium absorption in normal individuals (Δ) and patients with stable advanced renal failure (o, □). Open symbols represent pretreatment values, while closed symbols are measurements during treatment. The patients with renal failure received either 1,25-DHCC (o) or 1α-HCC (□), while the normal subjects received 1,25-DHCC (Δ). The solid line and interrupted lines represent the regression slope and 95 percent confidence limits for net magnesium absorption in normal individuals. [*Reprinted from Coburn et al. (169) by permission of Wiley Medical Publishers.*]

pothermia of uremia has been attributed, in part, to magnesium retention (197). When serum magnesium is increased to very high levels (greater than 3.5 to 5.0 meq/L), flushing and burning of the skin may occur. Such symptoms have developed when the water purification system used for preparing dialysate has suddenly failed (198). An acute elevation of serum magnesium is known to suppress the secretion of PTH (199, 200), and it is possible that hypermagnesemia may reduce the degree of secondary hyperparathyroidism that occurs in uremia (200a). However, there are no convincing data to suggest that long-standing hypermagnesemia has any significant effect on PTH secretion; it is likely that an effect of hypermagnesemia to suppress PTH secretion is completely offset by the stimulation of the parathyroid glands produced by hypocalcemia, albeit mild.

When patients with renal insufficiency also have intestinal malabsorption, poor nutritional intake, or marked renal magnesium wasting, hypomagnesemia may develop (201). Such hypomagnesemia is associated with impaired secretion of PTH and marked hypocalcemia (202).

Plasma alkaline phosphatase, hydroxyproline, and AMP

Serum alkaline phosphatase is made up of isoenzymes that arise from the intestine, liver, kidney, and bone. Despite the heterogeneity of this enzyme, the measurement of alkaline phosphatase can provide a rough indication of increased osteoblastic activity; moreover, studies of isoenzymes have shown that the increased alkaline phosphatase in uremia arises primarily from bone (203, 204). We have found serum total enzyme levels to be commonly increased in association with osteitis fibrosa, osteomalacia, or mixed lesions, although markedly elevated levels are said to be more characteristic of fibroosteoclasia (205) which shows a high rate of bone turnover. Nonetheless, serial measurements of plasma alkaline phosphatase may provide a useful clinical guide for monitoring the therapy of skeletal disease with calcium compounds and/or vitamin D sterols, and these serial measurements can also record the slow progression in a uremic patient who is developing skeletal disease. It should be kept in mind that uremic patients can exhibit significant and overt skeletal disease and yet have normal plasma alkaline phosphatase activity. Since coexisting hepatic abnormalities are particularly common in patients undergoing regular dialysis, it is essential that liver disease is excluded as a cause of elevated alkaline phosphatase. Thus, its measurement is clinically useful in many patients with advanced uremia; however, a major pitfall to avoid is the assumption that normal alkaline phosphatase activities implies the absence of significant skeletal disease in any given individual patient. In studies of large numbers of patients, alkaline phosphatase activities correlate with skeletal histologic features, with positive correlations between alkaline phosphatase and percentage of osteoblastic surface and the percent of active resorption surface (206, 207).

Peptides containing hydroxyproline and free hydroxyproline itself are released in association with the degradation of bone collagen; normally, the free and peptide-bound hydroxyproline are excreted in the urine (208). In patients with impaired urinary excretion due to advanced renal failure, the plasma levels of both free and peptide-bound hydroxyproline are elevated. With any increase in bone resorption and collagen degradation, plasma levels of hydroxyproline may increase even further (209, 210). Varghese and colleagues (211) have reported that total plasma hydroxyproline may provide a valuable index for the assessment of the extent of bone resorption and further evaluation of the response to therapy. Thus, the plasma levels of hydroxyproline were noted to fall in association with improvement of the skeletal disease that can follow either subtotal parathyroidectomy or treatment with 1,25-DHCC. Hart et al. (212) have noted that the plasma concentrations of free but not peptide-bound hydroxyproline correlated with certain abnormalities of bone histology which suggest increased bone resorption. Despite these claims for the utility of its measurements, the hydroxyproline measurement has not gained wide popularity in the United States compared to its use in the United Kingdom.

Plasma levels of AMP (cyclic adenosine monophosphate) have been noted to be increased in uremic patients (213): normally, plasma levels of AMP may be expected to reflect activity of PTH. However, no correlation has been found between plasma cAMP levels and the degree of secondary hyperparathyroidism; moreover, the levels may remain elevated for some time after parathyroidectomy (213). The reasons for the elevated levels of cAMP in patients with renal failure remain obscure. They may be related to catecholamines or the action of other peptide hormones.

Serum iPTH

Serum iPTH levels, as noted earlier, are commonly elevated in patients with renal insufficiency; the degree of elevation may be striking. Serum levels are strikingly elevated when measured with an antisera directed primarily toward the C terminus of the PTH molecules, while the degree of elevation is far less when they are measured with an antisera directed toward the intact molecule or the N terminus. Despite these limitations, experience indicates that iPTH levels often correlate with the presence or extent of overt skeletal disease. Bordier et al. (144) found a good correlation between serum iPTH levels and histomorphometric features of fibroosteoclasia (Fig. 20-16). Glassford et al. (214) found higher iPTH levels in dialysis patients with roentgenographic evidence of bone disease. However, one cannot compare values of serum iPTH determined in different laboratories because of the use of different antisera and different standards. Thus, it is best that sequential observations in the same patient are obtained with the same antisera and in the same laboratory.

Although pathogenic mechanisms responsible for elevation of serum iPTH levels exist in all patients with reduced renal failure, serum iPTH levels are sometimes normal or undetectable. Such a finding may occur in uremic patients with concomitant hypomagnesemia (202); also, low or normal levels of serum iPTH have been found in dialysis patients who exhibit a mineralizing defect with no evidence of fibroosteoclasia. The mechanism for reduced serum iPTH levels in the latter group remains uncertain.

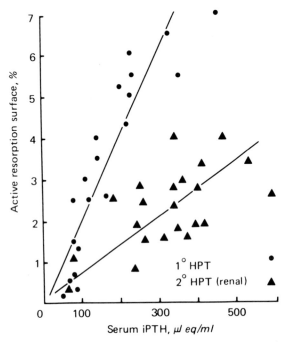

Figure 20-16. Relationship between "active" resorption surface (percent of total cancellous bone surface) and serum iPTH in patients with renal osteodystrophy (▲) or primary hyperparathyroidism (●). [*Reprinted from Bordier et al. (144) by permission of Kidney Int.*]

It has been popular to consider that certain uremic patients with marked hyperplasia may have "autonomous" secretion of PTH; however, most evidence suggests that serum iPTH levels do fall during either a calcium infusion or during dialysis using a high calcium level in dialysate. It may be necessary for the serum calcium to be raised to hypercalcemic levels before a fall in iPTH is seen. It is known that a certain amount of basal PTH secretion occurs despite marked elevation of serum Ca, as is shown in Fig. 20-17 (215). The presence of the massive hyperplasia of the parathyroid glands may be responsible for maintaining serum calcium in the moderately elevated range (i.e., 11 to 12 mg/dL) in association with elevated levels of serum iPTH. In such patients, subtotal parathyroidectomy may result in the return of more normal suppression of iPTH levels during induced hypercalcemia (216, 217).

CLINICAL SIGNS AND SYMPTOMS OF OSTEODYSTROPHY

A number of signs and symptoms in addition to bone pain and fractures in association with altered divalent ion metabolism and the secondary hyperparathyroidism that exists in end-stage uremia. Moreover, the symptoms that appear in association with osteodystrophy are quite subtle, insidious in their onset, and often difficult to separate from other features of uremia itself. Although fortunately not common, bone pain may develop and slowly progress to the point that the patient is totally disabled. This can occur independent of whether the pathology of the skeleton shows primarily fibroosteoclasia, osteomalacia, or a mixture of both. The pain is generally vague and deep seated, and it may be located in the low back, hips, knees, or legs. It often varies in intensity from time to time and is often aggravated by weight bearing or by sudden movement or pressure. Occasionally, pain is localized around the

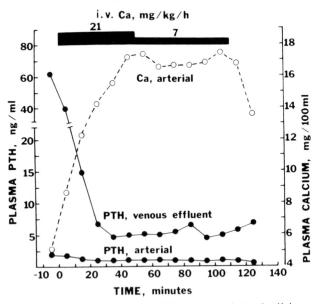

Figure 20-17. Changes in plasma PTH in an anesthetized calf during induced hypercalcemia. Effluent blood samples were collected via a surgically cannulated vein draining the superior parathyroid gland. These data demonstrate incomplete suppression of parathyroid secretion by hypercalcemia. [*Reprinted from Mayer et al. (215) by permission of J. Clin. Invest.*]

knee, ankle, or heel and may be of such sudden appearance as to suggest acute arthritis. Pain in the low back may arise from collapse of a vertebral body, and sharp chest pain may be the first indication of a rib fracture that has occurred during a cough, sneeze, or even normal breathing. A change in position, such as sitting up from the supine position or spontaneous rolling over during sleep, may evoke generalized pain throughout the back, hips, and chest. Pain is not relieved by massage or local heat, and the patient usually perceives the pain as being more deeply seated than in the joints or muscle.

The severity of symptoms often does not correlate closely with radiologic or histologic changes. Thus, patients may exhibit severe abnormal skeletal x-rays or bone biopsies and yet be totally asymptomatic. Uremic patients or patients undergoing regular hemodialysis, who are normally active and totally without symptoms, may develop, within several weeks to months, pain to a degree that they have difficulty walking across a room. Others experience such slow and gradual progression of symptoms that little notice is given until total debility has occurred.

Physical findings are frequently lacking; occasionally there may be localized tenderness. This may occur with pressure on the chest wall, lateral compression of the pelvis, or there may be localized tenderness over the vertebral spine or rib.

Myopathy and muscle weakness

Muscular weakness largely limited to the proximal musculature can be a serious and debilitating problem in patients with renal osteodystrophy. The afflicted patient may be confined to a wheelchair or may be unable to hold his arms above his head because of shoulder girdle weakness. This myopathy resembles in many ways the muscle weakness reported in vitamin D deficiency (218–220). In both forms of myopathy, plasma levels of muscle enzymes, such as creatine phosphokinase, are usually normal, and electromyographic abnormalities are either absent or nonspecific. The muscle weakness appears slowly, with the patient unable to climb stairs easily or rise from a sitting position without help. The gait may become abnormal so the patient waddles from side to side with the so-called "penguin" gait.

The pathogenesis of this muscle weakness is uncertain but (1) secondary hyperparathyroidism (221), (2) altered phosphate metabolism, and (3) abnormal metabolism of vitamin D have each been incriminated. Striking improvement in muscle weakness has been observed in uremic patients following the administration of either 1,25-DHCC, 1 to 5 μg/day (61, 210), or 25-HCC, 20 to 100 μg/day (222), and following successful renal transplantation (223). The prompt improvement in muscle weakness that follows treatment with vitamin D may imply a role of abnormal vitamin D metabolism in causing the abnormality. Moreover, altered muscle contraction and relaxation has occurred in vitamin D-deficient rats (224). Muscle biopsy, carried out in selected patients, has revealed mild, nonspecific myopathic alterations by light microscopy and severe degenerative changes by electron microscopic examination (223). In three patients with severe to mild muscle weakness, electron micrographs revealed localized areas of severe disorganization of the myofibrils, with dispersion of z-band material; the latter reverted to normal following treatment with 25-HCC (222). In an experimental animal model of uremia, Matthews et al. (225) found defective transport of calcium by sarcoplasmic reticulum isolated from skeletal muscle of uremic rabbits; this was reversed by treatment with 1,25-DHCC. On the other hand, the addition of 1,25-DHCC to vesicles of muscle sarcoplasm, in vitro, failed to correct the defective calcium transport. Calcium transport by the sarcoplasmic reticulum may be an important process regulating muscle retraction; these studies may provide insight into the functional nature of altered muscle function in uremia, supporting an interaction between myopathy and aberrant vitamin D metabolism.

All muscle abnormalities present in uremia should not be attributed to altered vitamin D metabolism, because features of protein-calorie malnutrition are common in uremia, and decreases in alkali-soluble protein, as described in muscle from uremic patients (226), may contribute to muscle dysfunction. It has been suggested that muscular weakness may arise in secondary hyperparathyroidism on a neuropathic basis (221), and uremic polymyopathy, whatever its pathogenesis, may contribute to muscular weakness (227). The prompt improvement of muscle weakness in uremic patients following treatment with 1,25-DHCC (210, 228) before serum iPTH levels fall or with doses that are too low to reduce serum iPTH points to a major role of altered vitamin D metabolism rather than secondary hyperparathyroidism.

Pruritus

Itching, a common symptom in patients with advanced renal failure, often improves and may disappear following initiation of regular hemodialysis. However, pruritus sometimes persists and is of such intensity that it prevents sleep and interferes with a patient's normal activities. This symptom is common in patients with clinically evident secondary hyperparathyroidism, and pruritus improves or may totally disappear within a few days after subtotal parathyroidectomy (229, 230). The mechanism whereby secondary hyperparathyroidism can lead to pruritus is uncertain. Elevated levels of calcium in the skin have been reported in such patients (229); however, the increased calcium content in the skin is probably not responsible for the itching because the latter improves in a few days following surgery while a longer time is required before the skin calcium content decreases. Moreover, reversible itching may develop in uremic patients with the administration of pharmacologic doses of vitamin D and during infusions of calcium; such observations suggest that an elevated concentration of ionic calcium in the ECF may be an important factor contributing to the pruritus. Recent observations which suggest that there may be relief of uremic pruritus following the intravenous injection of lidocaine (231) or following treatment with ultraviolet light (232) point to the fact that uremic pruritus is multifactorial. In the absence of specific evidence of secondary hyperparathyroidism, i.e., very high levels of iPTH and radiographic evidence of resorption, parathyroid surgery is not indicated. However, the presence of pruritus should direct a clinician to seek evidence of secondary hyperparathyroidism.

Calciphylaxis (tissue necrosis and cutaneous ulcerations)

The occurrence of an unusual clinical entity, typified by peripheral ischemic necrosis and vascular calcification, has been noted for many years in isolated patients with chronic renal failure (223–240). This syndrome usually appears in patients with end-stage uremia and a long-standing history of renal failure, although patients have developed the syndrome following successful renal transplantation. The syndrome has been observed in association with renal diseases of varying causes, and there has been no predilection for a specific age or sex.

The skin lesions make their appearance as superficial violacious discolorations, in a mottled, circumscribed pattern; the lesions may involve the tips of the toes or fingers or occur about the ankles, thighs, or buttocks. The lesions are often accompanied by pain. As the lesions progress they become hemorrhagic with ischemic, "dry" necrosis. Frequently, boring ulcerations and eschar formation occur; lesions of the terminal phalanges often exhibit clear demarcation and even self-amputation (Fig. 20-18) Such lesions resemble those which accompany a vasculitis; however, biopsy specimens fail to show fibrinoid necrosis or granulomatous inflammation. All patients with these lesions have demonstrated evidence of medial calcinosis of small- and medium-sized arteries; skin biopsies generally reveal the presence of medial calcification and intimal thickening. Ischemic myolysis, ischemic cardiac disease, and hemorrhagic panniculitis have been reported in individual cases.

The pathogenesis of this syndrome is uncertain; extensive medical calcinosis of arteries can occur in patients with renal failure and yet not lead to gangrene and ulceration; the possibility that there may be mechanical obstruction attributable to calcium deposition has been considered; however, the favorable response to some patients to parathyroidectomy within a few days

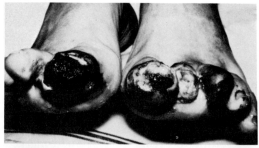
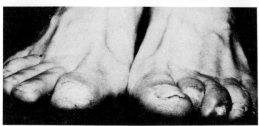

Figure 20-18. Ischemic and necrotic lesions of the toes which appeared after successful renal transplantation (top) in a patient with hypercalcemia due to secondary hyperparathyroidism. The lesions healed within 3 to 4 months following subtotal parathyroidectomy (bottom). [*Reprinted from Massry et al. (237) by permission from Arch. Intern. Med.*]

suggests that mechanical obstruction cannot totally explain the ischemia. Vascular spasms related either to serum calcium levels (241) or an effect of PTH itself (242) may be implicated. The occurrence of such lesions after renal transplantation in patients receiving glucocorticoids (240, 243) raises the possibility that steroids may play a role. Selye (244) showed that this syndrome was more likely in an animal model if the animals were given large doses of glucocorticoids.

Most uremic patients presenting with this syndrome have had previous or present evidence of overt secondary hyperparathyroidism, and a sizeable fraction of such patients (240) have shown substantial improvement following subtotal parathyroidectomy. Without treatment the lesions often progress with varying degrees of rapidity; a number of afflicted patients have died, usually from secondary infection (235, 140). Because of the unfavorable natural history and the poor prognosis, we have recommended subtotal parathyroidectomy when such lesions appear in con-

junction with any evidence of secondary hyperparathyroidism (high serum iPTH and bone erosions) (240).

Arthritis and periarthritis

The development of acute pain, redness, and swelling around one or more joints can occur due to altered metabolism of calcium and phosphorus in uremia. Rarely, pain in the ankle or foot which lacks local signs except for vague tenderness may be associated only with radiographic changes of subperiosteal resorption and/or periosteal new bone formation. Evidence that such symptoms are related to secondary hyperparathyroidism is provided by the observation that such discomfort can disappear completely within 1 to 2 weeks following subtotal parathyroidectomy. The syndrome, calcific periarthritis, is probably caused by the deposition of hydroxyapatite crystals, and it usually accompanies marked hyperphosphatemia (245). This syndrome must be differentiated from either pseudogout or gouty arthritis; the last two are characterized by a true monoarticular arthritis, and they can be differentiated by the identification of specific crystals of either urate or calcium pyrophosphate within the synovial fluid (246). Because of vague pain in bones and joints or because of muscle weakness, uremic patients with osteomalacia or osteitis fibrosa are often seen by rheumatologists or internists before the relationship between their symptoms and altered calcium and phosphorus homeostasis is recognized.

Spontaneous tendon rupture

Spontaneous tendon rupture also occurs with unusual frequency in patients with long-standing renal failure, and this complication is usually associated with evidence of marked secondary hyperparathyroidism (247, 248). The syndrome has been reported in association with primary hyperparathyroidism (249, 250) and other causes of secondary hyperparathyroidism (251), and it has been suggested that an abnormality of collagen metabolism, as exists in uremic bone (252), may occur in the tendon and cause weakening (240). An effect of systemic acidosis causing elastosis of the involved tendon has also been proposed as a causal factor (253).

Rupture has occurred most commonly in the quadriceps tendons, triceps tendons, or in extensor tendons of the fingers. Typically, the quadriceps tendon ruptures while the patient is walking, descending stairs, or after stumbling; the patient is unable to extend the leg, and a palpable gap and ecchymoses above the tendon are pathognomonic. Surgical treatment with slow rehabilitation has resulted in satisfactory results (250).

Skeletal deformities

True deformities of bone are quite common in uremic children, in whom the bone undergoes growth, modeling, and remodeling; on the other hand, skeletal deformities occasionally occur in adults; such deformities arise from abnormalities of skeletal remodeling and from recurrent fractures. The deformities commonly seen in children include bowing of the tibia and femur and those arising from slipped epiphyses (254). Slipped epiphyses occur more commonly in children with long-standing congenital renal disease than in children undergoing dialysis (254). Most commonly the problem becomes manifest in preadolescence; the hip is the most common site afflicted, followed by the radius and ulna, with lower humeral, lower femoral, and lower tibial sites more rarely involved (255). With hip involvement, a limp is the most common feature, and pain is absent in half of the cases. When the radius and ulna are involved, local swelling and ulnar deviation of the hands appear. The histologic abnormalities associated with slipped epiphyses are those of secondary hyperparathyroidism, and the radiolucent zone between the epiphyseal ossification and the metaphysis arises due to an accumulation of poorly mineralized woven bone and/or fibrous tissue (254) and not from an excess of cartilage and chondro-osteoid, as is typical of true vitamin D-deficient rickets.

Rarely, children with "renal rickets" exhibit the typical radiographic findings of vitamin D deficiency (81). Bowing of the long bones may occur in early childhood, but it is generally not severe until adolescence. Chronic renal insufficiency is a common cause of adolescent "knock-knee" or genu valgum (256). This can appear within a few months, with difficulty in walking and pain in the knees the common presenting symptom.

In adults with renal failure, particularly those with an isolated mineralizing defect, marked skeletal deformities may occur. Lumbar scoliosis, thoracic kyphosis, and deformities of the rib cage may lead to a marked loss of height and limitation of ventilation (Fig. 20-19). Such marked deformities may develop in uremic patients over a period of 1 to 2 years.

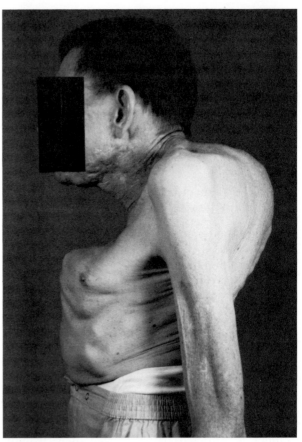

Figure 20-19. Marked kyphoscoliosis in a patient undergoing regular hemodialysis who developed a marked mineralizing defect of bone that was associated with normal levels of iPTH and was unresponsive to treatment with 1,25-DHCC. This deformity developed over a 2-year period following rejection of a renal homograft.

Retardation of growth

Growth failure is a common feature in children with renal insufficiency; this growth retardation exists both before and during treatment with maintenance hemodialysis. Clearly, growth retardation may occur when there is no evidence of renal osteodystrophy. A number of factors contribute to the retarded growth of uremic children; these include malnutrition (257), chronic acidosis, impaired intestinal absorption of calcium and phosphorus, renal osteodystrophy, and certain hormonal factors, such as low levels of somatamedin (258, 259). Before dialysis, one-third to one-half of children with a "predeterminal" stage of chronic renal failure had heights below the third percentile (260), and the growth velocity is below normal limits for age in two-thirds of children treated with dialysis (261). There is some delay in the appearance of puberty, but nonetheless growth potential is decreased. The addition of caloric supplements has been reported to improve growth (262), although this view is not universally accepted (263). Improved or even "catch-up" growth has also been reported during treatment with 1,25-DHCC (264). Studies showing that correction of acidosis can improve growth in children with renal-tubular acidosis suggest that long-standing acidosis in azotemic children could have a deleterious effect on growth (265). During treatment with 1,25-DHCC, catch-up growth did not occur during the early period of treatment when the serum iPTH levels were still elevated and renal osteodystrophy was still evident, but catch-up growth began after the apparent "healing" of the renal osteodystrophy. Such apparent improvement in growth during treatment with 1,25-DHCC suggests a possible role of altered vitamin D metabolism in causing retardation of growth.

Other uremic symptoms and secondary hyperparathyroidism

A number of nonskeletal symptoms that commonly coexist in uremic patients with overt renal osteodystrophy could arise as a consequence of a common pathogenic mechanism leading to both the skeletal disease and the other symptoms. The view that PTH, when present in great excess, may be a uremic toxin has been voiced (266). Indeed, the "trade-off" hypothesis of Bricker (267) suggests that the price that must be paid for the maintenance of calcium and phosphorus homeostasis in early renal failure leads to the skeletal abnormalities of secondary hyperparathyroidism; very high levels of PTH may also contribute to the uremic syndrome (268). A number of features of the uremic state which may be related to the marked secondary hyperparathyroidism are shown in Table 20-3.

There is evidence that the secondary hyperparathyroidism that occurs experimentally in acute renal failure can lead to increase in the calcium content of the brain in association with abnormal EEG (electroencephalogram) (269, 270). Probable relevance of these animal experiments to acute renal failure in humans has been provided by Cooper et al. (271), who found that EEG abnormalities, increased levels of iPTH, and an increase in brain calcium content all occur early in the course of acute renal failure in humans. During the diuretic and recovery phases, a decrease in serum iPTH to normal and normalization of the EEG were observed.

A role of high PTH levels in leading to alterations of the CNS (central nervous systm) in chronic renal failure and in dialysis patients is less well established. The EEG abnormalities of uremia may change toward normal with regular and

Table 20-3. Symptoms, signs, and other features of uremia associated with renal osteodystrophy and secondary hyperparathyroidism*

Bone pain	Hypertension
Muscular weakness	Ischemic skin ulcers (calciphylaxis)
Fractures	Central nervous system abnormalities—abnormal EEG
Skeletal deformities	Anemia and pancytopenia
Pseudogout	? Impotence
Acute periarthritis	? Peripheral neuropathy
Pruritus	? Dialysis dementia syndrome
Spontaneous tendon rupture	? Hyperlipidemia and arteriosclerosis

* See text; modified from Coburn and Llach (18).

adequate dialysis (272); however, brain calcium levels were normal in most patients with chronic renal failure (271). The anecdotal experience that there may be rather striking improvement of behavioral abnormalities following subtotal parathyroidectomy in some uremic patients with secondary hyperparathyroidism (273) may indicate a significant neurotoxic role of PTH in certain patients; preliminary observations provide support for such a role (274).

It has been suggested that peripheral neuropathy may occur with greater frequency in uremic patients with secondary hyperparathyroidism (275), although this premise has been challenged (276); Arieff and Schmidt found no association between motor nerve conduction velocity and iPTH levels. In an experimental study of acute uremia, increased nerve content of calcium and prolonged motor nerve conduction velocity were found and were related to increased activity of the parathyroid glands (277), but Arieff and coworkers have failed to find such an abnormality (278). Thus, present available information provides strong support for the view that PTH acts as a neurotoxin in the CNS; whether it plays a role in peripheral neuropathy remains unsettled.

The clinical syndrome of dialysis dementia, characterized by dyspraxia, dyslexia, myoclonus, altered behavior, and progressing to dementia with seizures, psychosis, and even death, is often associated with overt renal osteodystrophy (279). A possible link between dialysis dementia and secondary hyperparathyroidism may be strengthened by the finding of enhanced aluminum accumulation in the brain of patients with the syndrome (280) and the report that PTH may enhance the uptake of aluminum by the brain (281). Recent epidemiologic observations suggest that dialysate containing a high content of aluminum is associated with a higher incidence of skeletal disease (166). This association does not imply a cause-and-effect relationship. However, there have been isolated cases of dialysis dementia which showed improvement following parathyroidectomy (282) or after successful renal transplantation (283); further information is needed to clarify the relationship between dialysis dementia, altered calcium and phosphorus metabolism, overt bone disease, and aluminum exposure in uremic patients.

The possibility that secondary hyperparathyroidism could be a factor contributing to the impotence found in patients with end-stage renal failure has also been suggested (18, 284). This suggestion is supported by our anecdotal observation that libido and sexual function improve in uremic patients with secondary hyperparathyroidism following either subtotal parathyroidectomy or suppression of PTH during treatment with 1,25-DHCC. In a preliminary report of a prospective study, the administration of 1,25-DHCC was associated with an increase in potency in two of seven dialysis patients. There was a concomitant fall in plasma luteinizing hormone in one and a rise in plasma testosterone in the other (285). The impotence seen in chronic uremia is probably multifactorial, but it seems possible that excess PTH may play a role in its genesis in certain cases.

Extensive marrow fibrosis and sclerosis of bone can develop in uremic patients as a consequence of secondary hyperparathyroidism; such alterations could contribute to the hematologic abnormalities present in uremia. An association between renal osteodystrophy, myelofibrosis, and abnormal hematopoiesis has been reported by Weinberg et al. (286), who noted that patients with leukopenia, thrombocytopenia, and a more severe degree of anemia were more likely to have overt bone disease. They suggest that the splenomegaly present in certain uremic patients may arise as a hematologic compensatory mechanism due to replacement of normal erythroid tissue by osteitis fibrosa. An increased incidence of anemia is known in patients with primary hyperparathyroidism (287) and this correlates with the extent of marrow fibrosis (1). Preliminary reports suggest that the hematocrit may increase in uremic patients with secondary hyperparathyroidism following subtotal parathyroidectomy (288). It seems logical to assume that the suppressive effect of PTH on erythropoietic function is related to the local factors produced by marrow fibrosis; however, a direct effect of PTH on erythroid precursors has not been excluded.

There are other features of the uremic state that may also be related to secondary hyperparathyroidism. Elevated blood concentrations of triglycerides have been reported in a substantial fraction of patients with advanced uremia (289, 290). In experimental animals with acute nephrectomy, a condition known to produce the rapid appearance of secondary hyperparathyroidism, an increase in blood lipids has also been noted (291, 292). Cantin (293) reported that parathyroidectomy partially inhibited the increase in lipids observed after bilateral nephrectomy, while the administration of PTE restored the hyperlipidemia in parathyroidectomized uremic rats. Such data provide some support for the possibility that hyperlipidemia present in uremia may have some relationship to secondary hyperparathyroidism. Other observations suggest that resistance to insulin action and the hyperglycemia sometimes observed in uremia may be related to the presence of secondary hyperparathyroidism (294).

From the above discussion, it seems that it is necessary to revise one's view about target organs and actions of PTH; in chronic renal failure the tissues are subjected to continued increased concentrations of PTH, far beyond those seen in most other conditions; it is generally assumed on the basis of actions of PTH in slices of renal cortex that the N-terminal fragment of PTH is the only portion of PTH that is active; it remains equally possible that other PTH fragments, particularly when present in the level seen in chronic renal failure, might be responsible for some of these actions. Obviously, this is speculative, but further investigation about the role of high levels of PTH in uremia will undoubtedly clarify its precise role as a "uremic toxin."

X-RAY FEATURES OF RENAL OSTEODYSTROPHY

Both the type of radiographic abnormality seen and the incidence of various radiographic alterations of bone vary considerably in reports from different centers which have evaluated patients with advanced renal failure (10). Such differences probably reflect a true variation in the type of skeletal disease, which may be due to differences in the age of the patients, the management employed, and the duration of uremia and dialysis in the patients being reported. However, it is likely that differences in radiographic techniques employed including the type of film and the interest of the radiologist are of substantial importance. X-rays of bone that are obtained utilizing standard x-ray film and automatic film developing procedures result in films of much poorer quality than those that were available 20 years ago (256, 295). Techniques to increase the sensitivity of x-rays are particularly useful in views of the hands; these include the use of fine-grain film (i.e., Kodak M industrial film or mammography film), the use of manual rather than automatic film developing method, and the omission of grid or screen techniques. Magnification techniques can add further to the sensitivity. Meema et al. (296) found the phalanges to be normal in 67 percent of uremic patients from films obtained and viewed with conventional techniques, and only 8 percent showed subperiosteal resorption. With the introduction of better film and the use of magnification techniques, only 26 percent were normal while 29 percent exhibited substantial subperiosteal resorption. There is some danger in overreading films with the use of these magnification techniques, and familiarity with normal variation is required (297).

X-ray characeristics of secondary hyperparathyroidism

One of the principal radiographic features of secondary hyperparathyroidism is the presence of resorption, which may occur on the subperiosteal, intracortical, and endosteal surface of cortical bone (Fig. 20-20). Another radiographic feature of excess parathyroid activity seen in azotemic patients is new bone formation at the periosteal surface, a process termed periosteal neostasis by Meema et al. (298). Finally, alterations of the trabecule of spongy bone may lead to either osteosclerosis or osteopenia.

Erosions occurring in conjunction with new bone formation may take the form of cysts or osteoclastomas, although these are believed to be less common in uremic secondary hyperparathyroidism than in primary hyperparathyroidism (256, 299). Occasionally, cystic lesions or brown tu-

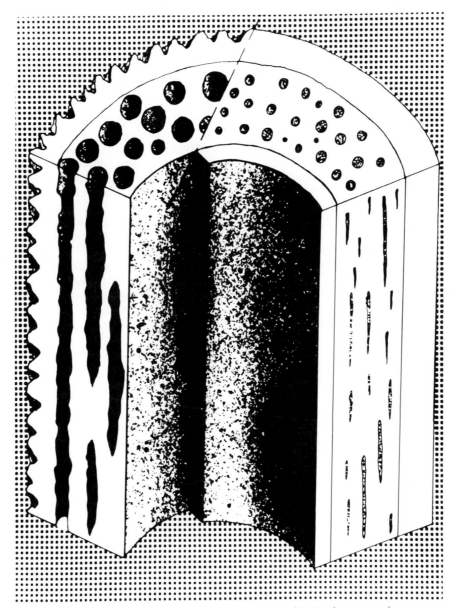

Figure 20-20. Diagrammatic representation showing three types of resorption: on the right is a normal cortical bone while that occurring with secondary hyperparathyroidism is shown on the left. Bone resorption is occurring at the endosteal, intracortical (haversian), and periosteal surfaces. [*Reprinted from Mehls et al. (297a) by permission from Pediatr. Radiol.*]

mors are associated with pain; they may alter the configuration of the teeth when they occur in the jaw; areas of subperiosteal erosions almost invariably accompany such lesions. With healing the cystic areas are replaced by areas of sclerosis.

Identification of subperiosteal resorption of the phalanges with the use of fine-grain radiographs of the hands is thought to be the most sensitive radiographic sign of secondary hyperparathyroid-ism (295, 300). Abnormalities have been found on x-ray in approximately half of the patients who show increased resorption surface on bone biopsy (296, 297, 300, 301): this frequency can be increased with magnification radiographs. The appearance of bone erosions has been shown to correlate reasonably well with the serum levels of iPTH (214, 297).

The earliest lesions usually appear on the ra-

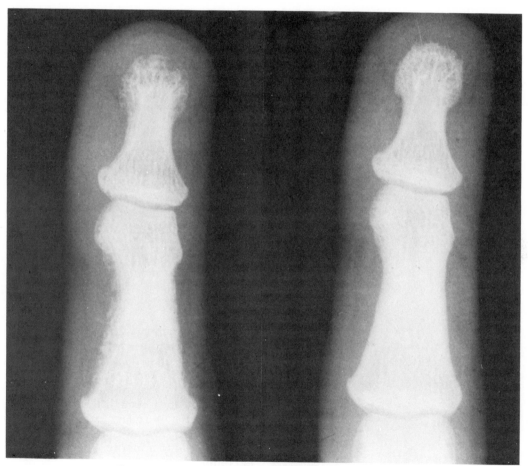

Figure 20-21. The middle and distal phalanx of the third digit of a patient with osteodystrophy are shown on the left, while the same digit, after treatment with 1,25-DHCC, is shown on the right. Subperiosteal erosions can be seen to be much more marked on the radial (left) surface of the middle phalanx although they are also present on the ulnar surface in this patient. The marked erosions in the distal phalanx are also evident.

dial surface of the middle phalanx of the second or third digit of the dominant hand; they first appear as a slight irregularity near either the proximal or distal shoulder formed by the metaphysis of the phalanx (256); as the lesions progress the erosions extend along a greater length of the shaft of the phalanx (Fig. 20-21), involve other digits, adjacent proximal and distal phalanges, and eventually appear on the ulnar border. The evolution of such lesions has been described in detail by Parfitt (256). Although such erosions are generally asymptomatic, they occasionally produce erosive synovitis which leads to soft tissue swelling, pain, and stiffness.

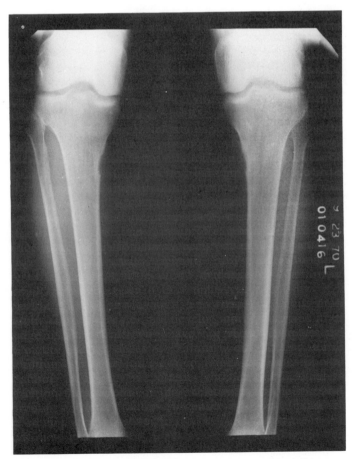

Figure 20-22. Subperiosteal erosions, occurring bilaterally, near the junction of the metaphysis with the shaft of the tibia, a common site involved with subperiosteal resorption (see text).

The tuft of the terminal phalanx, usually of the second or third digit, commonly shows resorption areas. Such tuft erosions (Fig. 20-21) are more easily identified in uremic secondary hyperparathyroidism than in primary hyperparathyroidism, perhaps because of the common coexistence of osteomalacia in the former (256, 302). Because of the natural occurrence of irregularities of the tuft, the recognition that the cortical margin is lost may be difficult. Nonetheless, it has been possible to quantitate and grade the extent of such erosions (297). When the terminal tuft erosion is severe, there may be marked loss of the terminal phalanx leading to collapse of the soft tissues; this may change the contour of the fingers to an extent that they apear to show "clubbing" (303). Healing of erosions of the tuft and phalanges is believed to occur initially with replacement of poorly mineralized fibrous tissue and woven bone. Despite successful treatment and healing, the shape of the bone may not be reversed to normal (304).

Other sites commonly showing bone erosions include the upper end of the tibia, the neck of the femur or humerus, the lower end of the radius and ulna and the lower surface of the medial end of the clavicle. The predilection for subperiosteal erosions to occur near the junction of the metaphysis with the shaft (Fig. 20-22) is believed to be because the modeling of bone during growth into a triangular shape with typical metaphyseal flaring requires that the surplus bone on the outer cortex be removed. Consequently, the precursor cells of mesenchymal origin at this site are more prone to differentiate into osteoclasts. Such areas are often the first site of subperiosteal resorption in uremic children (255). Although typical resorption of the phalanges is uncommon in young children, it does occur in older adolescents and young adults; it is less common in uremic patients over 40 (305). Resorption can be seen in the skull, leading to a mottled lucent appearance; this is commonly associated with areas of osteosclerosis, as is noted below.

One boney site that exhibits erosion in primary hyperparathyroidism but is rarely affected in uremic secondary hyperparathyroidism is the lamina dura (306). Another type of bone erosion that occurs with secondary hyperparathyroidism is intracortical or haversian erosion which is manifested by the presence of intracortical striations on x-ray films in a number of pathophysiologic processes associated with increased bone turnover, i.e., hyperthyroidism, acromegaly, and rapid growth spurt at adolescence (307). These cortical striations are not as specific for hyperparathyroidism as are subperiosteal erosions (297), 307–309). Increased endosteal resorption can also occur as a manifestation of secondary hyperparathyroidism; this may produce scalloping of the endosteal surface or it may produce widening of the central canal of the long bones.

Meema et al. (298) applied the term periosteal neostasis to the appearance of new woven bone within fibrous tissue underlying the periosteum. When such bone is newly formed, it is separated from the preexistent bone by radiolucent area which represents an interposed area of fibrous tissue. As the process progresses, the lucent zone may calcify and disappear, and the existence of such new bone formation may be recognized from an increase in the outer diameter of bone (Fig. 20-23).

Osteosclerosis represents another radiographic feature of osteitis fibrosa that arises due to an increase in the thickness and number of trabeculae present in spongy bone. It is generally apparent only in skeletal areas that are comprised largely of cancellous bone with very little contribution of compact bone; these areas include the vertebrae, pelvis, skull, clavicle, proximal humerus, and proximal and distal femur and tibia. In the spine, osteosclerosis may lead to a characteristic "rugger jersey" appearance.

Radiographic alterations of the skull have been classified into four types (310): (1) a diffuse "ground-glass" appearance, with loss of sharp margins at the vascular grooves and diploic venous channels; (2) a diffuse mottled or granular appearance, which is the most frequent abnormality type, and probably arises from a network of enlarged resorption spaces within the tables of the skull; (3) the presence of focal lucent defects, 1 to 3 cm in diameter, which may be present with or without a "ground-glass" or mottled appearance of surrounding areas; and (4) the presence of focal areas of sclerosis. The lesions may be confused with those of Paget's disease or multiple myeloma. These abnormalities of the skull

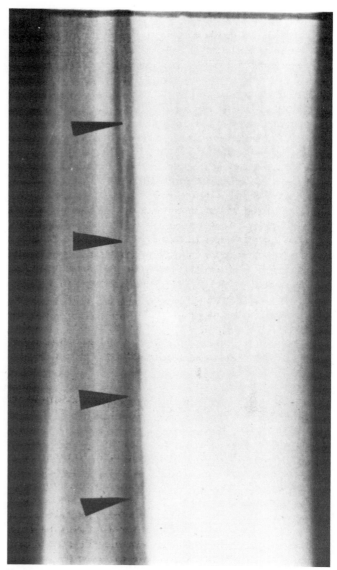

Figure 20-23. Area of periosteal new bone formation, termed periosteal neostasis (298), along the tibia in a patient undergoing regular hemodialysis.

may disappear completely after appropriate treatment (Fig. 20-24).

Although radiographic changes may correlate roughly with the degree of iliac crest histology, the correlation may not invariably be close in an individual patient. Such lack of correlation may be related, in part, to the fact that radiographic

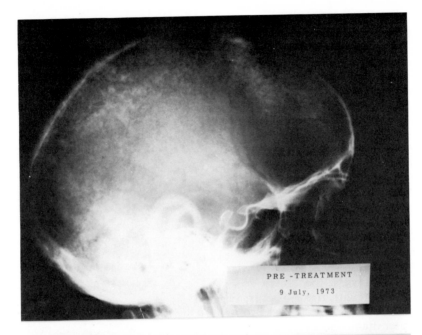

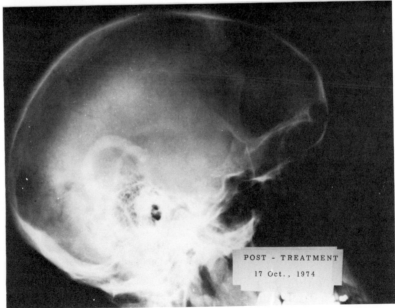

Figure 20-24. Radiographs of the skull in patients with overt renal osteodystrophy. The upper figure shows areas of modeling, granularity, and increased sclerosis, while the lower radiograph was obtained after 10 months of treatment with 1,25-DHCC. [*Reprinted from Coburn and Llach (18) by permission of N. Nijhoff.*]

abnormalities are most easily seen in cortical bone, while iliac crest bone biopsy involves the evaluation of trabecular bone.

Radiographic features of osteomalacia

The radiographic features of osteomalacia are far less distinctive than those arising from secondary hyperparathyroidism. Once the epiphyses have closed, the typical radiographic finding of rickets, with widening of the epiphyseal growth plate and other classic deformities, do not occur. The only pathognomonic finding of osteomalacia present in adults is the Looser zone or pseudofracture. The Looser zone, which has been well described by Parfitt (256), is a straight wide band of radiolucency which abuts onto the cortex and is usually perpendicular to the long axis of the bone; it is often symmetrical and may or may not be accompanied by a narrow area of sclerosis or a small, poorly mineralized callus (311–313). Healing or callus formation is usually minimal unless specific treatment is given. The means for distinguishing a Looser zone from a stress fracture have been outlined by Parfitt (256). One important difference is that the initial hairline break of a stress fracture does not enlarge but heals with normal callus formation. In uremic patients, spontaneous stress fractures commonly occur in the metatarsals or ribs with variable degrees of pain; these fractures tend to heal spontaneously, albeit more slowly than normal, with good callus formation. With mechanical stress or when vitamin D deficiency is very severe and prolonged, the Looser zone, like other stress fractures, may extend across the full width of bone to produce a true fracture with displacement of the fragments (311). The presence of Looser zones has been remarkably infrequent in our experience, and fewer than 2 percent of German dialysis patients exhibited this feature (314); however, Looser zones were reported in 20 percent of uremic Australian patients with symptomatic osteodystrophy (256). The reason for this different incidence is unknown.

Protusio acetabuli, identified because of a convex bulging into the pelvis over the acetabulum, may occur as a specific feature of osteomalacia (313). Skeletal demineralization is a feature of osteomalacia; however, this is a nonspecific finding. Features such as increased haziness or coarsening of the trabeculae, biconcavity of the vertebral bodies, particularly in association with normal bone density, and bending deformities of long bones have been said to be typical of osteomalacia (295); however, few radiologists can make such distinctions. Uremic patients with osteomalacia commonly have pronounced secondary hyperparathyroidism as well, and bone erosions commonly coexist. Thus, the findings of osteomalacia are predominantly microscopic, and one can only be certain of this diagnosis on the basis of bone histology.

Osteopenia or osteoporosis

A common radiographic feature present in patients with advanced renal failure is decreased density of bone: this can arise as a consequence of secondary hyperparathyroidism or osteomalacia and is thus nonspecific. Parfitt and coworkers (315) have used the term "dialysis osteopenia" to indicate a syndrome characterized by a substantial reduction in the amount of bone and an increased incidence of bone pain and fractures that are out of proportion to the radiographic and histologic evidence for osteomalacia or osteitis fibrosa. The radiographic findings have been likened to those seen in the idiopathic osteoporosis of young adults. There is loss of cortical bone from the endosteal surface, periarticular rarefaction, a loss of trabecular bone with honeycomb or fishnet pattern, and the occurrence of fractures that are somewhat intermediate in appearance between stress fractures and the typical Looser zones. Unfortunately, extensive histologic studies of patients with this syndrome are not available, and it is not altogether certain whether this syndrome is the same as that reported from Newcastle, as was suggested by Parfitt (256). In the latter patients, skeletal biopsies commonly show the presence of osteomalacia (309). The failure of "dialysis osteopenia" to respond adequately to subtotal parathyroidectomy or treatment with large doses of vitamin D has been one of the principal means for separating this lesion retrospectively from other bone diseases seen in uremia (315).

Quantitative measurements of bone mineral

Cortical thickness measurements: the metacarpal index. The metacarpal index can be obtained by measuring the dimensions of the cortex of a metacarpal bone on x-ray film utilizing magnification and a special caliper (316). Normal data are available for the second left metacarpal, and the metacarpal index is the ratio of cortical to total bone width. On the basis of the assumption that this bone is a perfect cylinder, the cross-sectional ratio of cortical area to total area can be calculated (317). The metacarpal index has been validated by direct comparison to measurement of bone ash (318). Observations in primary hyperparathyroidism have suggested that total bone area is increased, while the cortical area is reduced (319). In patients with chronic renal failure and not treated with dialysis, the metacarpal index was found to be reduced in 20 to 40 percent of patients (296, 307, 320). Several studies suggested that there may be a progressive decrease in the metacarpal index with duration of dialysis (321). This method is particularly useful for serial measurements in the same patient or for the evaluation of various modalities in large groups of patients.

Photon absorptiometry. Another noninvasive method for the serial evaluation of the skeleton is photon absorptiometry. With this technique, the absorption of photons emitted from an isotopic source is utilized to assess the mineral content of bone. The isotopes utilized, either ^{125}I or [241]Am, emit photons of specific, narrow wavelengths and low energy (322). Such measurements are taken over the phalanges, the radius and ulna, and the femur. Hahn et al. (323) have measured both the distal radius, which is primarily made up of trabecular bone, and the midshaft of the radius, which comprises cortical bone; this has enabled them to evaluate the ratio of these two forms of bone, which undergo turnover at different rates. Griffiths et al. (324) found the mineral content of the midradius and ulna to be significantly lower in uremic patients undergoing dialysis than in age-matched controls; they also observed a progressive loss of bone with an increasing duration of therapy with dialysis in a center using a dialy-sate calcium level of 5.2 mg/dL. In a subsequent study, they (325) reported that most women undergoing dialysis maintained stable bone mineral, whereas 44 percent of men lost bone mass. This method appears to be more accurate than are most methods which measure the density of bone from x-ray film; however, the equipment is expensive and measurements are limited to certain sites of the skeleton, primarily comprising cortical bone. Moreover, bone mineral content can be reduced for several reasons: (1) because there is a primary reduction in the volume of bone tissue; (2) due to an increase in intercortical porosity as a consequence of enlarged resorption spaces; or (3) because normally mineralized bone is replaced by unmineralized osteoid or poorly mineralized woven bone (256). The measurement of bone density by photon absorptiometry does not allow distinction between these causes of decreased bone density; this technique is best used when serial measurements are obtained for the quantitation of bone mineral and when results are evaluated in terms of observations obtained from fine-detail radiographs.

Neutron activation provides a more accurate method for measuring total calcium or bone mineral in either the entire body or in isolated parts of the skeleton. This technique requires the availability of a neutron source for the activation of calcium and other elements in the skeleton and immediate access to a whole body counter for quantitation of the short-lived radionuclides. This technique has proven useful in research studies (326, 327) of bone mineral content in uremic patients. This technique may be particularly useful when serial measurements can be obtained for evaluation of the effects of a specific modality of treatment. Some of the results obtained with these quantitative techniques are discussed below (see Management).

Scintiscan. Skeletal scintigraphy, which is done utilizing a [99]TcM pyrophosphate, provides a sensitive method for the detection of skeletal alterations in patients with renal failure. The technique allows for follow-up evaluation of the response to treatment. Although the mechanism responsible for the accumulation of pyrophosphates in bone is not entirely certain, there is evidence to indicate that these pyrophosphates accumulate in areas of increased bone turnover (328). Rosenthal and Kaye (329) suggested that pyrophosphate accumulates in areas with abnormal collagen metabolism, including both osteitis fibrosa and osteomalacia. By serially evaluating the uptake of the isotopes over the distal femur, Lien et al. (330) calculated the bone:soft tissue ratio of isotope uptake. An abnormal uptake was found in 78 percent of long-term dialysis patients

and a similar proportion of patients with chronic renal failure who were not undergoing regular dialysis. On the basis of correlation between bone uptake of ^{99}TcM pyrophosphate and urinary excretion of hydroxyproline, Weigmann et al. concluded that an increased skeletal uptake in uremia was related to the presence of immature collagen. Others (331) found abnormal scintiscans in 13 of 14 patients undergoing dialysis. Symmetrically increased activity was noted over

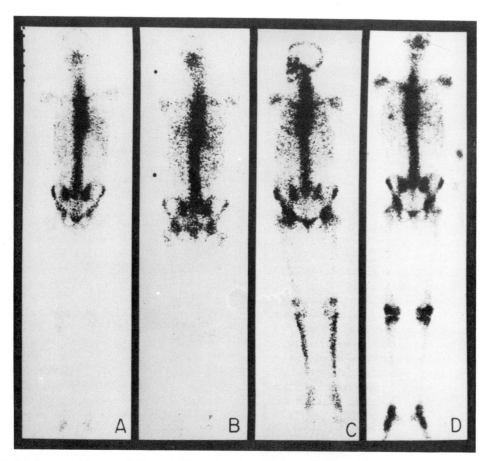

Figure 20-25. Scintigrams of bone utilizing technitium-labeled pyrophosphate in a normal subject and in patients with renal failure. The severity of the abnormality has been graded: A—grade 0, normal scintigram; B—grade 1, scintigram showing normal uptake in the femoral heads with an extension into the femoral neck and trochanteric region; C—grade 2, scintigram showing abnormal uptake in the femoral head and neck and in the proximal half of the tibial shaft; D—grade 3, scintigram showing extensive uptake in the femoral head and marked uptake in the femoral and tibial condyles, the tarsis, and the proximal part of the metatarsis. [*Reproduced from Olgaard et al. (332) by permission of Nephron.*]

the skull, mandible, sternum, shoulders, vertebrae, and distal aspects of the femur and tibia. Uptake of the labeled pyrophosphate over certain areas, such as the mandible, was pronounced and appeared earlier than did radiographic abnormalities. Ølgaard et al. (332) found that 90 percent of patients undergoing regular dialysis had pathologic accumulation on scintigrams, while x-ray abnormalities were seen in only one-third of the patients (Fig. 20-25). Abnormal scintigrams were more common in dialysis patients who had been previous recipients of renal homografts. They suggest that intensive glucocorticoid treatment may aggravate the abnormality reponsible for an abnormal scintiscan. The diphosphate scintiscan can be used to detect soft tissue calcification, particularly with regard to pulmonary calcifications (333, 334). This technique can detect abnormal uptake of calcium in muscles following acute muscle injury, a common precursor to acute renal failure (335).

Extraskeletal calcifications

Soft tissue calcifications, of several distinct types, occur commonly in patients with end-stage renal disease. The factors which predispose to their development include an increase in the calcium $\times$ phosphorus product in plasma, the degree of secondary hyperparathyroidism, the level of blood magnesium, alkalosis, and local tissue injury (336). Three major clinical varieties of extraskeletal calcification occur in uremia: (1) calcification of medium sized arteries, (2) periarticular or tumoral calcifications, and (3) visceral calcifications, which can involve the heart, lung, and kidney. Parfitt (336) has separated periarticular calcifications into three further types: (1) periarticular chondrocalcinosis, which occurs in primary hyperparathyroidism as well as in secondary hyperparathyroidism; (2) calcific periarthritis, which may have calcification very similar to that seen with typical dystrophic calcifications; and (3) tumoral calcinosis, quite common in the early years of hemodialysis (337) but which is now usual. Occasionally there may be pain, stiffness, and soft tissue swelling associated with calcific periarthritis. Calcification commonly involves the eye, when it may affect the sclerae (band keratopathy) or the conjunctiva, when it produces the whitish plaques (338), or can induce an acute inflammatory response due to crystal phagocytosis and lead to the "red eye" of uremia (339). A rise in local pH due to the loss of CO_2 into the air is believed to predispose to such ocular calcifications.

The appearance of arterial calcifications is usually distinct (Fig. 20-26); they are diffuse and continuous along the vessel, and such calcifications involve the media of the vessel; its appearance contrasts to the dense, irregular discrete appearance of calcified intimal plaques. Vascular

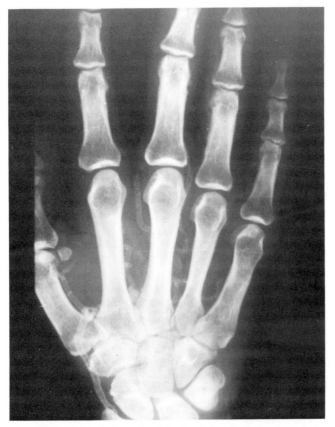

Figure 20-26. Radiograph of the hand showing extensive calcification of the radial artery and various digital vessels. These calcifications show features characteristic of calcification involving the media of the artery (see text).

calcifications may be first identified in the dorsalis pedis artery where it descends between the first and second metatarsals and where it is often seen as a ring or tube (305). Other common sites involved are the ankles, followed by abdominal aorta, feet, pelvis, hands, and wrists. Arterial calcifications often occur without any symptoms; however, rigidity and lack of compressibility may make it difficult to palpate pulses or hear the Kortkoff's sounds; also, vascular access for dialysis may be difficult to achieve. Occasionally, extensive vascular calcifications are associated with ischemic lesions and the syndrome of calciphylaxis (240).

An evaluation of the incidence of vascular calcification suggests that they are age related; thus, an incidence of 50 percent was found in dialysis patients aged 40 to 50, compared to 30 percent in the 15- to 30-year age group. Vascular calcifications are exceedingly uncommon in children with renal failure (340). Meema et al. (341) documented calcifications in 36 percent of uremic patients not treated with dialysis, 19 percent of those treated with peritoneal dialysis, 13 percent of those after receiving a renal transplant, and 8 percent of those undergoing hemodialysis.

The pathogenesis of these different types of extraskeletal calcification may vary; thus, visceral calcifications can occur in patients totally lacking arterial and periarticular calcification, and the converse also occurs. Most experience indicates that periarticular or tumoral calcifications can be reversed by phosphate restriction with a reduction of the calcium × phosphorous product in plasma (336, 342, 343). Such calcification is clearly related to the solubility product of calcium phosphate, but the possibility exists that PTH may enhance the accumulation of calcium into soft tissues (229).

Contiguglia et al. (344) separated two types of extraskeletal calcification on the basis of their chemical characteristics: (1) visceral calcification and (2) arterial and periarticular calcification. Visceral calcium existed as amorphous calcium phosphate. Usually, such amorphous calcium phosphate is rapidly converted to apatite at a physiologic pH; the lack of such conversion led to the evaluation of pyrophosphate content of bone

and serum in patients exhibiting visceral calcification (124, 126). Despite the suggestion that soft tissue calcification may be associated with secondary hyperparathyroidism, Contiguglia et al. (344) could find no relationship between evidence of secondary hyperparathyroidism, on the basis of parathyroid size, or the serum calcium × phosphorus product, and the extent of soft tissue calcifications found at autopsy in uremic patients.

Visceral calcification may give rise to serious symptoms depending on the organ involved. Thus, heart block has been reported due to deposition of calcium in the cardiac conduction system (345, 346), and cardiac failure has been associated with extensive replacement of myocardium with calcification (344). Extensive pulmonary calcification, which may be found in alveolar septal and vascular walls, may be associated with pulmonary fibrosis and septal thickening. Such calcification is only rarely extensive enough to provide radiographic evidence of calcification (347). Various alterations of pulmonary function, including reduced vital capacity, reduced carbon monoxide diffusion, and a low P_{O_2} have been found antemortum in patients subsequently found to have severe pulmonary calcification. Such pulmonary calcification (Fig. 20-27) may be detected with the technetium pyrophosphate scan (333, 334). Kuzela et al. (185) found morphologic evidence of visceral calcification in 6 of 56 patients dying with chronic renal failure. Such calcification was more common in patients who had undergone treatment with dialysis than in uremic patients who had not been treated with dialysis.

EFFECT OF DIALYSIS ON DIVALENT ION METABOLISM

Hemodialysis itself has many effects upon mineral metabolism in patients with advanced renal failure. Several of the dialysis-related factors that may affect divalent ion homeostasis include (1) the concentrations of calcium and magnesium in dialysate; (2) the efficiency of the dialyzer, which can affect the rate of movement of various ions across the membrane, and the duration and frequency of dialysis; (3) periodic fluctuations of blood phosphorus, calcium, and pH and the levels of various uremic "toxins" that fall with each

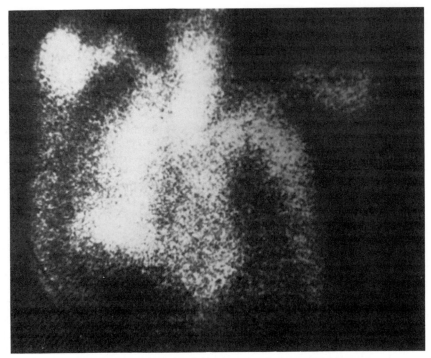

Figure 20-27. Scintiscan of the chest showing severe pulmonary calcification in a patient with advanced uremia. [*Reprinted from Devancaanthan et al. (333) by permission of Clin. Nephrol.*]

dialysis. Such effects may modify skeletal responsiveness to PTH, improve intestinal calcium absorption (348), and modify the flux rates of calcium and phosphorus from one body compartment to another; (4) the effect of glucose, which is often added in dialysate, on plasma levels of magnesium and phosphorus; (5) the levels of trace substances, such as fluoride or aluminum, in the water used to prepare dialysate and which may have an effect on the skeleton; (6) the effect of heparin which is given during each hemodialysis; and (7) the effect of a general and gradual improvement of uremia that occurs following the initiation of regular hemodialysis. There are no physiologic conditions that mimic the sawtooth pattern of certain biochemical parameters, such as phosphorus, magnesium, and [H$^+$] ion, due to the intermittency of hemodialysis. Whether or not such intermittent variations have an effect on divalent ion homeostasis is unknown.

Within a few months after initiation of regular hemodialysis, the predialysis concentrations of serum calcium generally reach levels between 9.0 and 10.0 mg/dL. Thus, an increase in the serum calcium level generally occurs in patients who were previously hypocalcemic, while little or no change occurs in patients with initial serum calcium levels near normal (179, 191, 194, 349). Such increments in serum calcium levels occur with the initiation of hemodialysis despite marked hyperphosphatemia or the use of dialysate with a calcium level lower than that in the blood. The mechanism responsible for this increase in serum calcium level is unknown; no improvement of the calcemic response to PTH has been detected with the initiation of dialysis (87). Initiation of regular hemodialysis has been found to produce no change in intestinal calcium absorption (34, 350, 351), although a transient increase immediately after dialysis was reported by Chanard et al. (348).

With regular dialysis using a dialysate having a calcium level of 6 to 7 mg/dL, the predialysis serum calcium levels are frequently normal; there may be an increased incidence of patients with normal or increased serum calcium when dialysate magnesium is reduced so that persistent hypermagnesemia is reversed (192). In a small number of patients, overt and persistent hypercalcemia appears some time after the initiation of hemodialysis (191, 349, 352).

There is almost invariably an increase in total serum calcium level during the dialysis procedure; this occurs due to an increase in albumin level secondary to the ultrafiltration and hemoconcentration that accompanies hemodialysis; there may be an increase in the affinity of plasma albumin for calcium as a result of a rise in blood pH. Studies carried out with calcium-specific electrodes indicate the ionized blood calcium can fall during hemodialysis even as total blood calcium *increases*; this occurs when dialysis is carried out with a dialysate calcium level of 2.5 meq/L (189). When the same evaluation is made during dialysis with a dialysate calcium level of 6.0 to 7.0 mg/dL, there is an increase in the ionized calcium level (189). Other studies show an acute decrease in the level of iPTH (353), but the decrease in iPTH produced may be transient and increase to predialysis levels before the next dialysis.

A number of investigators have measured the quantity of calcium moving across the dialyzer during dialysis (354–357), although most studies were carried out using dialyzers of lower efficiency than those commonly used at present. In a study utilizing a Kiil dialyzer, the dialysance of calcium, calculated from the ultrafiltrable fraction of plasma calcium, was 60 to 70 percent of the dialysance of urea (355). In this study influx and efflux of radiolabeled calcium were similar; however, others (357) have suggested that hyperphosphatemia had a mild effect to inhibit calcium transfer from dialysate into the patient. The total quantity of calcium transferred into a patient during over 10 h of dialysis utilizing such a Kiil dialyzer was 700 to 1100 mg when the dialysate calcium concentration exceeded the diffusible level of plasma by 1.5 to 2.0 mg/dL (356). The quan-

tities of calcium transferred with use of high-surface-area dialyzers and short (3.5 to 4.5 h) dialysis are likely to be lower than those measured with a Kiil dialyzer and 10 to 11 h of dialysis.

The level of magnesium in dialysate has a major influence on the serum magnesium levels in the dialysis patients; serum magnesium levels ranged from 1.5 to 2.4 meq/L in a center employing a dialysate magnesium concentration of 0.5 meq/L; on the other hand, serum levels of magnesium were 2.5 to 4.5 meq/L in patients using a dialysate magnesium level of 1.5 meq/L (40). Burnell et al. (192) reported that lowering the dialysate magnesium concentration from 1.0 to 0.5 meq/L resulted in the slow reduction of predialysis plasma magnesium from values that were persistently elevated to levels nearer to normal (Fig. 20-28).

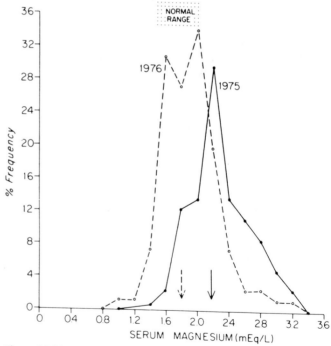

Figure 20-28. Frequency distribution of serum magnesium levels in patients undergoing regular dialysis under the care of the Northwest Kidney Center, Seattle, Washington. Dialysate magnesium concentration was 1.0 meq/L in 1975 (*n* = 109) and 0.5 meq/L in 1976 (*n* = 81). [*Reproduced from Burnell and Teubner (192) by permission of Proc. Clin. Dial. Transpl. Forum.*]

Serum phosphorus is acutely decreased by 50 to 60 percent during each dialysis procedure; the magnitude of decrease is usually less than that observed for creatinine and uric acid, and the dialysance of inorganic phoshorus is 25 to 35 percent of the rates of urea (358). Some patients exhibit a rapid rebound of the postdialysis serum phosphorus level so that it returns close to the predialysis value within 12 to 18 h after completion of dialysis (40). The total amount of phosphorus removed during dialysis is determined both by the concentration of plasma phosphorus and the efficiency of the dialyzer used. Thus the quantity removed may be 1000 to 1200 mg during a standard dialysis (182). A patient eating 1100 to 1300 mg/day of phosphorus with net absorption of 45 percent (169) can be in neutral or positive phosphorus balance unless intestinal absorption of phosphorus is curtailed.

The presence of significant fluoride in the tap water used for the preparation of dialysate results in the movement of significant quantities of fluoride into the patient (359, 360); the content of fluoride in blood, tissues, and bone increases to very high levels following repeated dialysis with fluoride-containing dialysate (360, 361) since such patients lack the normal mechanism for renal excretion of fluoride (362). Posen et al. (361) reported a high incidence of clinically significant osteodystrohy in patients undergoing hemodialysis in a community utilizing fluoridated water. These patients experienced bone pain, arthralgias, and muscle weakness; x-rays of bone revealed Looser zones, decreased density, and fractures. The histologic study of bone revealed osteomalacia. Other uncontrolled studies also suggested that there was a high incidence of overt bone disease in patients using fluoridated water for preparation of dialysate (163, 363, 364). The clinical findings in the dialysis patients exposed to fluoridated water differ significantly from clinical and experimental features of fluorosis in nonuremic patients; in the latter, the lesions are predominantly those of exostoses and osteosclerosis (365, 366). In a controlled study, Oreopolous et al. (367) failed to detect differences in the rate of progression of skeletal disease in patients treated with dialysate prepared from fluoridated water compared to other patients treated with dialysate lacking fluoride. There was a higher incidence of osteosclerosis in the former group, an effect believed to be due to fluoride. However, the control patients were drinking some amount of fluoridated water, a factor which may have contributed to a lack of difference between the two groups. Others have also expressed an opinion that use of fluoridated water does not hasten the development or progression of renal osteodystrophy (368); hence its role in causing bone disease remains uncertain.

It has been suggested that aluminum, sometimes present in a water supply, may accumulate in the patient during dialysis; the use of such water has been associated with a high incidence of bone disease (166). It is possible that the reported higher incidence of bone disease in association with the use of fluoridated water may have occurred because of the presence of aluminum rather than fluoride in the water. Appropriate water treatment could remove both trace elements from the water and lead to a reduced incidence of incapacitating skeletal disease. The present state of the art would seem to dictate that water treatment should be employed when there is a substantial incidence of overt skeletal disease in dialysis patients. This would be particularly true when the skeletal disease is osteomalacia and when the usual findings of secondary hyperparathyroidism are lacking.

Patients undergoing regular dialysis regularly receive injections of heparin, and clinical and experimental studies suggest that heparin, when given repeatedly, is associated with decreased skeletal mineralization and may predispose to fractures in patients without renal disease. Thus, osteoporosis has been reported in patients receiving 15,000 to 30,000 units of heparin/day over long periods of time (369); also, multiple fractures (370) and pseudoarthrosis (371) have been reported. Osteoporosis did not develop in patients receiving lower doses, i.e., 10,000 units/day (369), and dialsysis patients may not receive quantities of heparin large enough to cause difficulties. With the use of more efficient dialyzers and the reduction in time for each dialysis, the total quantity of heparin given is less, and any potential adverse effect of heparin on the skeleton may be less than existed in the past. Presently, it is not possible to carry out regular hemodialysis without using heparin; hence, it is not possible to test the theory that heparin administration plays a role in the pathogenesis of bone disease in dialysis patients.

ALTERED MINERAL METABOLISM IN ACUTE RENAL FAILURE

A number of abnormalities of calcium and phosphorus homeostasis occur in acute renal failure. These are of interest because the pathogenic factors are of recent onset and may be less complex than is the case for chronic renal failure; therefore, they can be more easily evaluated both in humans and in experimental animals.

In studies of patients with acute renal failure, hypocalcemia, hyperphosphatemia, and elevated levels of iPTH exist early in the oliguric phase (372, 373). The degree of hypocalcemia is variable, but it develops within the first few days of acute renal failure and often persists into the diuretic period when serum phosphorus levels often fall to or below normal (Fig. 20-29). There was no correlation between serum levels of phosphorus and calcium, suggesting that hypocalcemia was not caused by hyperphosphatemia per se. An inverse correlation between serum calcium and iPTH levels was observed, indicating an appropriate response of PTH secretion to the hypocalcemia. Nonetheless, the infusion of PTE to patients with acute renal failure has failed to raise plasma calcium levels appropriately both during the oliguric and diuretic periods. These observations are consistent with the development of skeletal resistance to the calcemic action of PTH early in the course of acute renal failure (372). Also, it has been shown that the administration of 1,25-DHCC to dogs made acutely uremic by bilateral nephrectomy partially restored the calcemic response to PTE (89). It was suggested that the renal production of 1,25-DHCC may cease with the development of acute renal failure, and the skeletal unresponsiveness to PTH could arise from such a dificiency of 1,25-DHCC. In rats with acute renal failure, treatment with 1,25-DHCC

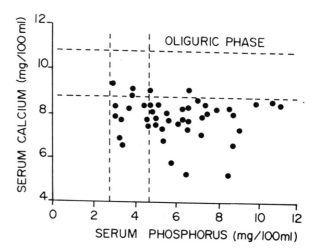

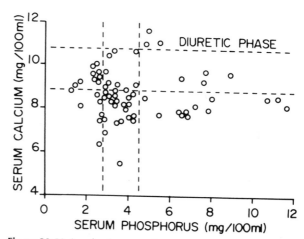

Figure 20-29. Levels of serum calcium and phosphorus in patients with acute renal failure studied during both the oliguric and diuretic phases. Hypocalcemia occurred under both circumstances, and serum calcium was independent of serum phosphorus level. [*Reprinted from Massrv et al. (372) by permission of Kidney Int.*]

failed to restore a normal calcemic response to PTH; thus, the mechanism for skeletal resistance remains controversial (90).

Pietrek et al. (374) reported a rapid fall in the plasma levels of 25-HCC during the course of acute renal failure (Fig. 20-30). Although the mechanisms responsible for the fall in plasma 25-HCC are unknown, their observations suggest that

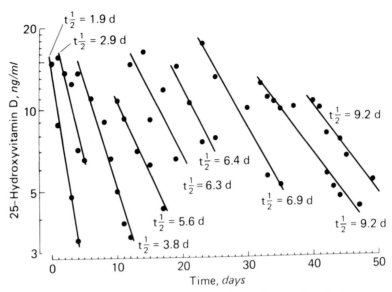

Figure 20-30. Plasma levels of 25-HCC obtained serially in patients with acute renal failure. The values are plotted on a logarithmic scale and the apparent half-time for decrease in plasma levels is shown for individual patients. [*Reprinted from Pietrek et al. (374) by permission of Kidney Int.*]

the turnover of this sterol is enhanced. A decrease in the level of 25-HCC may limit the substrate available for the generation of 1,25-DHCC by the damaged kidney.

Elevated plasma levels of iPTH may play a casual role for certain uremic symptoms noted in patients with acute renal failure. Thus, the brain calcium content increases in association with the appearance of an abnormal EEG pattern in an experimental animal with acute renal failure; this increase in brain calcium and the abnormal EEG can be prevented by parathyroidectomy (269). Observations in patients with acute renal failure support an etiologic role of PTH in the genesis of CNS dysfunction (271).

Although hypocalcemia is a common feature of acute renal failure, patients occasionally demonstrate hypercalcemia during the diuretic phase of acute renal failure. This may occur when there is still substantial impairment of GFR. Most patients who develop hypercalcemia have developed acute renal failure following rhabdomyolysis (375, 376). It has been suggested that large amounts of

calcium may be deposited in the damaged muscle tissue during the initial period of acute renal failure (377). The presence of large quantities of calcium and phosphate in damaged muscle has been demonstrated by x-ray (378) and by technetium diphosphonate scan (335), and in muscle specimens obtained at biopsy (379) or autopsy (380). During the diuretic phase, the sequestered calcium and phosphate may be released into the circulation. The capacity of the kidney to excrete the calcium released into the circulation from the devitalized muscle may not be sufficient to prevent the development of hypercalcemia.

During the diuretic phase, serum phosphorus often falls to normal or below. Serum phosphorus may fall as urinary phosphorus excretion increases due to an osmotic diuresis, from the extracellular volume expansion that often exists, and from high circulating levels of PTH. An improved nutritional status may lead to the intracellular movement of phosphate as well.

Although the hypercalcemia seen in acute renal failure may be transient and resolved within a few days, some patients may have serum calcium levels of 13 to 15 mg/dL for as long as 3 to 4 weeks (381). Treatment may include saline infusion and furosemide (382) or calcitonin, and these have been partially effective. It is probably unwise to administer phosphate salts, either by mouth or parenterally, unless the serum phosphorus level is low or normal; this would be particularly true if the renal function has not yet returned to normal. Glucocorticoids should also be given only with caution, as patients in the early recovery phase of acute renal failure may be particularly susceptible to the catabolic side effects of steroids.

CALCIUM HOMEOSTASIS IN THE NEPHROTIC SYNDROME

Certain alterations of calcium metabolism, including hypocalcemia, hypocalciuria, and intestinal malabsorption of calcium, are known to occur in patients with the nephrotic syndrome. The hypocalcemia is generally ascribed to a reduction in the protein-bound fraction of calcium due to the hypoalbuminemia, and it has been assumed that the levels of ultrafiltrable or ionized calcium are normal. However, Lim et al. (383) and Goldstein et al. (190) have shown that plasma ionized calcium is significantly reduced in patients with the nephrotic syndrome. Hypocalciuria is common in patients with the nephrotic syndrome (384, 385); such hypocalciuria could arise from the avid sodium retention that is usually present in nephrotic patients since the renal handling of calcium and sodium are so closely related. However, Jones et al. (385) failed to find a relationship between urinary calcium and sodium excretion in their study of 30 nephrotic patients. Metabolic balance studies have indicated the presence of reduced intestinal absorption of calcium in nephrotic patients (384, 386), although the levels of renal function were not reported in many of these patients with the nephrotic syndrome and others were receiving treatment with glucocorticoids, which are known to alter calcium metabolism.

Recent studies have revealed the existence of both abnormal calcium metabolism and altered vitamin D metabolism in nephrotic patients; indeed, abnormal vitamin D metabolism could be responsible for the former. Thus, plasma levels of 25-HCC have been found to be low in patients with the nephrotic syndrome and normal renal function (112, 113, 190). A positive correlation between plasma level of 25-HCC and serum albumin and an inverse correlation between plasma 25-HCC level and urinary protein excretion were found by Goldstein et al. (190), although Schmidt-Gayk et al. did not find such a correlation (112). The 25-HCC present in plasma is specifically bound to a vitamin D binding protein, which migrates with a globulin on cellulose acetate electrophoresis and has a molecular weight of approximately 59,000 daltons. In the nephrotic syndrome, the permeability of glomerular basement membrane is markedly increased for proteins with a molecular weight near that of albumin (approximately 69,000) and it is likely that the vitamin D binding protein is filtered through the glomerular basement membrane in large amounts and consequently lost in the urine.

Haddad and Walgate (387) have demonstrated a decrease in serum levels of vitamin D binding protein in hypoproteinemic disorders, including the nephrotic syndrome. The low plasma vitamin D binding protein in patients with the nephrotic syndrome was confirmed by other investigators (112, 113), who also demonstrated excess urinary loss of this protein, while no detectable vitamin D binding protein was found in the urine of normal subjects. A study of the appearance of radiolabeled vitamin D metabolites in the urine after oral ingestion of labeled vitamin D was carried out in nephrotic patients and in normal controls. During the first 24 h after ingestion of ^3H cholecalciferol a significant amount of ^3H cholecalciferol appeared in the urine of the nephrotic patient; ^3H 25-HCC excretion was maximal and constituted the major fraction of urinary radioactivity from 24 to 48 h after the dose, and it was the only radioactive vitamin D metabolite detectable after 48 h. The urinary excretion of ^3H vitamin D and its metabolites was negligible in the normal subjects. The radioactivity from vitamin D and the urinary vitamin D binding protein comigrated during the chromatographic separation of urine from the nephrotic patients. Other investigators have demonstrated the rapid urinary excretion of intravenously administered [3]H 25-HCC in rats with experimental nephrotic syndrome from glomerulonephritis (388). Such data provide support for the view that significant urinary losses of 25-HCC occur in the nephrotic syndrome.

The quantitative aspects of these urinary losses in the nephrotic syndrome were also evaluated: Barragry et al. (113) estimated the loss of vitamin D and its metabolites to be 2.5 μg/day, while Schmidt-Gayk et al. (112) found 3.2 μg/day of 25-HCC in the urine. These quantities are equivalent to 100 to 120 I.U. of vitamin D, an amount that may be equal to daily intake in parts of the world where foods are not regularly fortified with vitamin D; hence, such losses could lead to a significant deficiency of vitamin D.

The pathophysiologic role of a low serum 25-HCC level in the altered divalent ion metabolism observed in the nephrotic syndrome is not clear. Lim et al. (386) studied calcium balance in 13 nephrotic patients and 8 patients during clinical remission from the nephrotic syndrome. Mean values of creatinine clearance and the duration of the nephrotic syndrome in 13 patients were 91.6 mL/min (range, 81 to 122 mL/min) and 14 months (range, 2 to 24 months), respectively; creatinine clearance in 8 patients in remission was 96.9 mL/min (range, 85 to 126 mL/min). A marked decrease in net intestinal absorption of calcium was observed in the nephrotic patients, and stool calcium equaled or exceeded dietary calcium intake in 8 of the 13 patients. These data confirmed a previous observation of Emerson and Beckman (384). In contrast, a study of intestinal calcium absorption, measured by a double radioisotope method, demonstrated a significant reduction in intestinal calcium absorption in patients with the nephrotic syndrome *only* when significant renal failure was present; 10 patients with the nephrotic syndrome and normal serum creatinine levels did not exhibit any decrease in intestinal calcium absorption (389). These discrepant results may be due, at least in part, to the different methods employed.

Intestinal calcium malabsorption may be responsible for the hypocalciuria seen in patients with the nephrotic syndrome. A study of the relationship between C_{Ca}/GFR and C_{Na}/GFR in patients with the nephrotic syndrome revealed a slope lower than that seen in volume-expanded dogs, normal dogs given furosemide, or in patients with advanced renal failure but without the nephrotic syndrome (190). The slope was similar to that observed in calcium-deficient dogs undergoing extracellular volume expansion (390). These data suggest that there may be strong forces acting to retain calcium in the nephrotic syndrome; moreover, the hypocalciuria cannot be explained simply by the avid sodium reabsorption.

Although there is good evidence for the presence of altered vitamin D metabolism and even calcium deficiency in the nephrotic syndrome, their clinical consequences are not apparent at the present time. In association with a reduction in plasma ionized calcium, elevated plasma iPTH levels also have been found (190). Bone biopsy specimens obtained from seven patients with nephrotic syndromes revealed no evidence of osteomalacia or osteitis fibrosa from conventional histologic examination (186). On the other hand, another study indicates the presence of early osteomalacia in patients with the nephrotic syndrome (391). The presence of vitamin D deficiency in patients with the nephrotic syndrome even before renal insufficiency develops could contribute to the development of a pattern of renal osteodystrophy which may be different from that seen in other uremic patients without the nephrotic syndrome. Data are not available comparing the extent of skeletal disease in uremic patients with a past history of the nephrotic syndrome to other uremic patients lacking a history of the nephrotic syndrome.

RENAL TRANSPLANTATION AND DIVALENT ION METABOLISM

Many features of renal osteodystrophy and altered divalent ion metabolism are corrected after successful renal transplantation. With the introduction of normal functioning kidney, the production of 1,25-DHCC begins and iPTH may rapidly disappear from the circulation since the kidney is a major site for PTH degradation. Moreover, the kidney will begin to play an "excretory" role in homeostasis of phosphorus and calcium, and the renal handling of these ions will be influenced by several factors, including the level of function of the transplanted kidney, the circulating levels of iPTH, the degree of osmotic diuresis present, and the extent of extracellular volume expansion. Corticosteroids, which are employed to suppress the tissue rejection, may have significant modulating effects on divalent ion metabolism in transplant recipients.

Although the occurrence of autonomous parathyroid hyperfunction has been reported in patients with chronic renal failure (392), such hyperplastic parathyroid glands are, in general, thought to be responsive to the usual feedback mechanisms. With a return of the ability of the kidney to excrete phosphorus and produce 1,25-DHCC and improved responsiveness of the skeleton to the calcemic action of PTH, the serum calcium levels return to normal; the hyperplastic parathyroid glands begin the process of involution. The time required for these glands to return to normal size probably varies depending on their size and other factors which may regulate parathyroid gland function, including the levels of vitamin D sterols.

In a majority of transplant recipients, serum iPTH returns to normal within 1 to 4 months after successful transplantation (343, 393, 394). However, a state with relatively normal vitamin D metabolism combined with hyperfunction of the parathyroid glands may exist in some patients after renal transplantation, and hypercalcemia may ensue. David et al. (395) found elevated plasma iPTH levels in 11 of 15 transplant recipients with normocalcemia and each of 7 patients with hypercalcemia, 1 to 3 years after renal transplantation. The plasma iPTH levels were higher in the hypercalcemic patients than would be expected in the presence of hypercalcemia. Thus, PTH secretion may not be completely suppressed even in the presence of hypercalcemia, and the amount of PTH secreted from the glands may remain high in hypercalcemic transplant recipients. Secretion of a certain amount of hormone by normal parathyroid glands is known to be continued independent of an increase in calcium concentration (215). Thus, very large hyperplastic glands may secrete an amount of PTH that is sufficient to cause hy-

percalcemia. Evidence for such a theory is provided by an animal model of hypercalcemia due to a large mass of normal parathyroid tissue; Gittes and Radde produced persistent hypercalcemia by transplanting 40 normal parathyroid glands into a single rat (396).

While it is likely that persistent hyperparathyroidism plays a major role in the genesis of posttransplant hypercalcemia, other factors may contribute. Alfrey et al. (343) noted hypophosphatemia in the majority of transplant recipients and suggested that a reduction in body phosphate stores with phosphate depletion was responsible, at least in part, for the hypercalcemia. After renal transplantation body phosphate stores may be depleted because of lowered intestinal phosphate absorption as a consequence of intense antacid therapy, secondary to increased renal clearance of phosphate due to residual hyperparathyroidism and steroid treatment, or due to an acquired renal defect in renal-tubular transport of phosphate (397). Persistent parathyroid hyperplasia may be unmasked by coexistent phosphate depletion, and the appearance of hypercalcemia may be related to the interval required for a critical level of phosphate depletion to develop. In support of this contention is the finding of an inverse correlation between serum calcium and inorganic phosphate levels in transplant recipients (398), with most hypercalcemic patients exhibiting concomitant hypophosphatemia. Furthermore, the administration of supplemental phosphate may reduce plasma calcium levels to normal in many hypercalcemic transplant recipients, as is shown in Fig. 20-31 (343). Glucocorticoids have an effect to lower serum calcium levels, and they may modify the appearance of the hypercalcemia. Often, hypercalcemia appears only when the dose of prednisone is reduced (398).

Posttransplant hypercalcemia is more frequent in patients with x-ray evidence of severe bone disease and metastatic calcification during the course of renal failure than in patients lacking these findings. The mobilization of extraskeletal calcification may be another factor contributing to this hypercalcemia (395, 398).

The incidence of significant secondary hyperparathyroidism, defined by the presence of hypercalcemia, hypophosphatemia, and increased renal

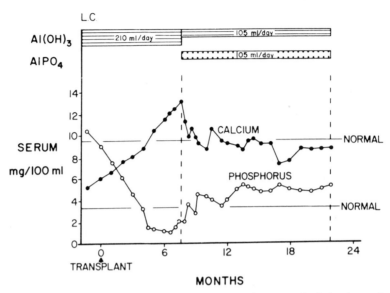

Figure 20-31. Levels of serum calcium and phosphorus in a renal transplant recipient. During the initial 7 months, as the patient received aluminum hydroxide [Al(OH)₃], there was a fall in serum phosphorus to below 2 mg/dL and hypercalcemia occurred; sub-sequently, the patient had aluminum phosphate gel (AlPO₄) sub-stituted: serum phosphorus rose into the normal range and hyper-calcemia was controlled. [*Reproduced from Alfrey et al. (343) by permission of N. Engl. J. Med.*]

clearance of phosphate, is 15 to 35 percent in transplant recipients (393, 395, 398–400). The hypercalcemia usually appears between a few days to several months after the transplant surgery, and in most cases it appears within the first 6 months (343, 395). However, the delayed appearance of hypercalcemia until 2 to 3 years after transplantation has been reported (399). The hypercalcemia may be persistent, and mild hypercalcemia lasting for more than 1 year is not infrequent. When the hypercalcemia is mild (less than 12 mg/dL), medical management with oral phosphate supplements is often sufficient. Surprisingly, most transplant patients have no clinical signs or symptoms which could be attributed to such hypercalcemia and the hypercalcemia may have no deleterious effects on renal function even over several years. We have observed a renal homograft recipient who has been totally without symptoms and with excellent graft function for 12 years with a serum calcium of 11 to 12 mg/dL.

There are a number of situations that suggest a need for parathyroidectomy in renal transplant recipients. Some patients may develop severe hypercalcemia, i.e., serum calcium greater than 13 mg/dL, and subtotal parathyroidectomy may be indicated. Subtotal parathyroidectomy should also be considered when there is deterioration of renal transplant function in association with hypercalcemia; such surgery has been reported to halt the progression of or even restore lost renal function (398). Thus, evidence for hyperparathyroidectomy (erosions and elevated serum iPTH) should be sought in renal transplant recipients with deterioration of graft function in conjunction with hypercalcemia, albeit mild. Parathyroidectomy may result in easier control of hypertension, and surgery should be strongly considered in transplant recipients who develop soft tissue ischemia and necrosis, i.e., calciphylaxis (240).

In most instances treated surgically, subtotal parathyroidectomy effectively corrects the hypercalcemia, and the surgically removed specimens reveal chief cell hyperplasia. However, the effects of the remnant parathyroid tissue on serum calcium levels cannot be easily predicted preoperatively, and hypercalcemia may persist or reappear in rare instances. In these instances a repeat neck operation may be required but only with certain technical difficulties and a high incidence of damage to the recurrent laryngeal nerve. Also, surgical hypoparathyroidism sometimes occurs. To obviate such technical problems, Wells et al. (401, 402) have recommended parathyroid autotransplantation in the management of parathyroid hyperplasia. In this procedure, the four parathyroid glands are identified and removed from the neck, and small pieces of parathyroid tissue are transplanted into the forearm muscle. These transplanted parathyroid gland fragments function normally and respond appropriately to hyper- and hypocalcemic stimuli (404). If graft-dependent hypercalcemia develops, the transplanted parathyroid tissue is accessible for partial removal under local anesthesia. Other surgeons feel that this procedure involves unnecessary surgery with an added risk of infection. An alternative is the quick freezing and storage of the parathyroid tissue, with subsequent transplantation if the patient develops persistent hypoparathyroidism.

Successful renal transplantation generally leads to gradual and steady improvement in renal osteodystrophy (405, 406). Serial bone biopsy specimens have shown complete resolution of osteomalacia in 81 percent of patients after 1 year. By contrast, osteitis fibrosa tends to resolve at a slower rate and may not resolve completely years after transplantation. This may not be too surprising, since the GFRs are mildly reduced in most successful renal transplant recipients, and they are similar to those observed in patients with early renal insufficiency in whom abnormal divalent ion metabolism and secondary hyperparathyroidism have been shown to exist. Thus, features of mild hyperparathyroidism, as exist in mild renal insufficiency, are not surprising in patients with a successfully functioning transplant.

Serum phosphorus levels may fall to very low levels after renal transplantation. Such severe hypophosphatemia may lead to osteomalacia (397). Furthermore, steroid-induced osteopenia may gravely complicate the metabolic bone disease that already existed prior to renal transplantation.

A distressing complication of an otherwise successful renal transplantation is the development of aseptic necrosis of bone, a problem occurring in 7 to 29 percent of transplant recipients (407). The most commonly affected site is the femoral head, but the femoral condyles, the head of the humerus, and the talus can also be involved. The factors contributing to the genesis of aseptic necrosis in transplant recipients are not fully understood; the administration of glucocorticoids, the presence or absence of osteoporosis, fat emboli, local hemodynamic factors induced by renal allograft, and/or severe secondary hyperparathyroidism have each been implicated (399, 408). Although infrequent, aseptic necrosis has been reported in patients treated with regular dialysis, even though they have never had a renal transplant or glucocorticoid treatment (409).

The severe pain and crippling that occur as a consequence of aseptic necrosis may restrict significantly the rehabilitation of these patients; surgical intervention, such as femoral head replacement or total hip replacement, is then indicated.

Growth of children may improve following renal transplantation, and catch-up growth has been observed in many instances (411, 412). However, considerable retardation of growth often occurs (259), and it seems likely that the degree of prednisone is a major factor causing poor growth after transplantation. The use of alternate-day therapy with prednisone has resulted in considerable improvement in the rate of growth in transplant recipients (412).

PREVENTION AND MANAGEMENT

The objectives of management of altered divalent ion metabolism and osteodystrophy in patients with renal failure should be (1) to keep the blood concentrations of calcium and phosphorus as near normal as possible, (2) to prevent the development of hyperplasia of the parathyroid glands, or, if this has already occurred, to suppress parathyroid secretion and hyperplasia, (3) to restore the skeleton to normal, and (4) to prevent and reverse extraskeletal calcification.

The intensity of treatment and the specific treatment modality will vary with the stage of renal insufficiency, whether or not there is evidence of overt osteodystrophy, and depending on whether regular dialysis has been initiated. Some of the specific methods used in the management of renal osteodystrophy are given in Table 20-4, with details provided in the text.

PREVENTION OF PHOSPHATE RETENTION AND HYPERPHOSPHATEMIA

The hyperphosphatemia of uremia is one of the major factors responsible for the development and maintenance of secondary hyperparathyroidism in renal failure. Slatopolsky, Bricker, and their associates have demonstrated that reducing dietary phosphorus intake in proportion to the decrease in GFR in uremic dogs could largely prevent the development of secondary hyperparathyroidism (25, 26, 31). Results from a preliminary study (35) suggest that the reduction in dietary phosphorus intake in proportion to the decrease in GFR in the patient with mild renal insufficiency can reduce the levels of plasma iPTH and improve the calcemic response of the skeleton to PTE. Also, in patients treated with regular dialysis, high plasma levels of phosphorus contribute to the development of soft tissue calcification. Thus, the restriction of dietary phosphorus intake and the prevention of development of hyperphosphatemia is of prime importance in the treatment of renal osteodystrophy.

The dietary intake of phosphorus depends primarily on the intake of meat and dairy products. The usual intake of phosphorus by normal adults in the United States varies between 1.0 and 1.8 g/day. One could reduce dietary intake of phosphate in proportion to the decrease in GFR in patients with mild chronic renal insufficiency. With elimination or restriction of dairy products and rigid adherence to 40 g of protein per day, the dietary intake of phosphorus can be reduced to 600 to 900 mg/day, a quantity that is approximately 60 percent of a normal dietary intake of phosphorus (42). Thus, one can envision great difficulty in

Table 20-4. Guidelines for management of renal osteodystrophy

1. Control of serum phosphorus
   a. Restrict dietary phosphorus intake to 0.8 to 1.0 g/day
   b. Phosphate-binding antacids: aluminum hydroxide or carbonate
   c. Avoid hypophosphatemia
2. Dietary calcium supplements
   a. Oral calcium to supply 1 g/day, but only if serum phosphorus is controlled
   b. Dialysate calcium, 6.0 to 6.5 mg/dL (3.0 to 3.25 meq/L)
3. Vitamin D sterols
   A. Indications
      a. Hypocalcemia
      b. Overt 2° hyperparathyroidism (high iPTH, bone erosions) with serum calcium less than 11.0 mg/dL
      c. Osteomalacia (with 2° hyperparathyroidism)
      d. Children with chronic renal failure
      e. Concomitant anticonvulsant therapy
      f. ? Prophylaxis
   B. Types and appropriate doses
      a. Vitamin D_2 or D_3, 10,000 to 200,000 I.U. (0.25 to 5 mg)
      b. Dihydrotachysterol, 0.25 to 2.0 mg/day
      c. 25-HCC (calcifediol), 25 to 100 μg/day
      d. 1,25-DHCC (calcitriol), 0.25 to 1.0 μg/day
      e. 1α-HCC, 0.5 to 2.0 μg/day
4. Parathyroidectomy: Indications and evidence of secondary hyperparathyroidism (erosions and increased iPTH)
   a. Persistent hypercalcemia (serum calcium greater than 11.5 to 12.0 mg/dL)
   b. Progressive extraskeletal calcification
   c. Persistently elevated serum calcium × phosphorus product
   d. Pruritus unresponsive to medical treatment
   e. Calciphylaxis (ischemic ulcers and necrosis)
   f. Symptomatic hypercalcemia after renal transplantation
5. Other factors in management
   a. Dialysate magnesium, 0.7 to 1.2 mg/dL (0.5 to 0.7 meq/L)
   b. Water treatment: ? remove aluminum, fluoride, excess calcium, and magnesium
   c. Avoid concomitant treatment with barbiturates, phenytoin, or gluthemide
   d. Normalize acid-base status

restricting phosphate intake in proportion to a fall in GFR in patients with more advanced renal failure by simply reducing the dietary phosphorus intake. In such patients, a proportional reduction of dietary phosphorus intake is impractical, as such a diet is unpalatable to North American tastes. Other measures are required to reduce the intestinal absorption of dietary phosphorus, and phosphate-binding antacids must be given to restrict intestinal absorption of phosphorus (33, 413). The aluminum-containing compounds used to bind phosphorus in the intestinal tract include the aluminum hydroxide and aluminum carbonate gels; these are available as liquid gels, tablets, and capsules. The capsules are less effective than liquid gels in binding phosphorus (173); however, patient compliance is usually much better with capsules than is the case for either liquids or tablets. The goals of such antacid therapy are to reduce the serum phosphorus levels to or near normal; in dialysis patients, predialysis serum phosphorus levels are ideally maintained between 3.5 and 5.0 mg/dL. In patients with advanced renal failure (creatinine clearance less than 10 mL/min) and in those treated with dialysis, dietary phosphorus should be restricted to 800 to 1000 mg/day, and aluminum hydroxide or aluminum carbonate capsules should be prescribed, 3 to 4 capsules with each meal. Serum phosphorus levels should be monitored at least once monthly in dialysis patients to permit appropriate adjustment of the phosphate-binding compounds. If serum phosphorus decreases too much or remains above the desired range, the number of capsules should be decreased or increased to 1 to 3 capsules/day. Antacids containing magnesium should be avoided.

The fall in serum phosphorus level during dietary phosphate restriction and therapy with phosphate-binding antacids is usually associated with a rise in serum calcium level (174, 175). If the magnitude of rise in serum calcium is adequate, a decrease in the blood levels of iPTH may occur (174); this, in turn, will contribute to the maintenance of the serum phosphorus level at a lower value, because a high PTH level contributes to the elevated serum phosphate levels in chronic renal failure.

It is equally important to avoid lowering serum phosphorus to levels lower than normal to prevent the development of phosphate depletion in uremic patients. Some patients require no phosphate-binding gels. Their overzealous use can produce severe hypophosphatemia and phosphate depletion in uremic patients. This problem can

aggravate the bone disease and cause overt osteomalacia (158, 414, 415).

It is generally assumed that aluminum hydroxide and aluminum carbonate are nonabsorbable and are safe. However, there is evidence both in humans and in experimental animals suggesting that orally administered aluminum may be absorbed to a significant extent and lead to an increase in plasma aluminum levels and increased aluminum content in various tissues (280, 416). Moreover, hyperparathyroidism may aggravate the tissue accumulation of aluminum (281). Several lines of evidence suggest that certain symptoms of uremia in hemodialysis patients, such as dialysis dementia and some forms of renal osteodystrophy (166), may be related to aluminum accumulation in tissues.

Epidemiologic data suggest that aluminum which is accumulated in the body of dialysis patients from water used to prepare dialysis is more important in leading to these syndromes than is the aluminum absorbed from the intestinal tract (166, 280). Nonetheless, Mayor et al. have shown that excess PTH may enhance the intestinal absorption of aluminum and its deposition in tissues of experimental animals (281). Thus, the relative roles of the "body burden" of aluminum arising from dialysate compared to that from orally administered phosphate-binding gels in leading to the deposition of aluminum in tissues are not settled. Presently, there are no means for controlling hyperphosphatemia other than by use of aluminum-containing compounds; weighing the known hazards of hyperphosphatemia with the theoretical risk of aluminum toxicity, the physician is left with little choice other than using these compounds as needed to control serum phosphorus levels appropriately. In the future we may know whether there is, indeed, significant toxicity of oral aluminum, and there is the possibility of the development of other agents that may effectively block phosphorus absorption.

DIETARY SUPPLEMENTS OF CALCIUM

Oral supplements of calcium should be considered in patients with advanced chronic renal failure and those undergoing dialysis for two reasons: first, impaired intestinal absorption of calcium exists in these patients, and second, the diets generally consumed by the uremic patients contain reduced amounts of dairy products and, consequently, a low quantity of calcium. The dietary calcium intake in a large population of patients with advanced renal failure was estimated to be 400 to 700 mg/day (42). The evaluation of net intestinal calcium absorption by metabolic balance procedures suggests that a neutral or positive balance for calcium can be achieved in uremic patients with the supplementation of the diet with calcium carbonate (417), calcium citrate (418), or calcium lactate (417) to increase the total intake of calcium to 1.5 g or more per day (42, 419). Calcium carbonate also acts to bind phosphorus in the intestine, which may aid in the reduction of serum phosphorus. The question of when in the course of renal failure calcium supplements should be given is uncertain; Coburn et al. (34) found normal intestinal calcium absorption in male patients with serum creatinine levels below 2.5 mg/dL while Werner et al. (420) found a decrease in intestinal calcium absorption in certain patients with GFRs of 20 to 50 mL/min. Patients with more advanced renal failure may be more prone to develop hypercalcemia with oral calcium supplementation since they lack the renal avenue for calcium excretion should net calcium absorption increase more than anticipated.

The long-term effects of oral supplements of calcium on the progression of bone disease have been reported from several laboratories. Meyrier et al. (421) compared two groups of patients undergoing maintenance hemodialysis, one receiving calcium carbonate, 5 to 20 g/day, and a control group receiving no calcium supplementation. Bone biopsies obtained after 8 months showed a significant difference between the two groups. There was a lower incidence of resorptive lesions in patients receiving calcium supplements. Moreover, fewer patients exhibited x-ray evidence of skeletal disease, spontaneous fractures, pseudogout, or extraskeletal calcifications in the group given calcium supplements. Hypercalcemia, which occurred in most of the patients, resolved following a reduction in intake of calcium. Curtis et al. (422) found plasma alkaline phosphatase levels and serum iPTH levels to be lower in uremic patients with overt secondary hyperparathyroidism given supplements of calcium carbonate or, in those with low blood phosphorus levels, calcium phosphate. Eastwood et al. (303, 423) compared the effect of vitamin D with that of calcium carbonate supplements by bone biopsy in uremic patients with renal osteodystrophy. In patients receiving only calcium supplements, they observed the diffuse patchy deposition of calcium in osteoid without the development of a distinct "calcification front" that was regularly seen in biopsies from the patients given vitamin D. This study provides important clinical evidence that vitamin D is more effective than calcium supplementation in reversing overt skeletal disease in uremia.

Treatment with oral calcium supplements is not without certain risk. It is unwise to administer large amounts of oral calcium compounds in a patient with hyperphosphatemia because of the risk of an elevation in the calcium × phosphorus product, thereby predisposing to extraskeletal calcification. Hypercalcemia may develop in uremic patients (421, 424, 425) as in patients with normal renal function (426) during therapy with large quantities of oral calcium salts. Hypercalcemia may be more likely to occur in patients who have had the concomitant rapid lowering of serum phosphorus values below 2 to 3 mg/dL (179). Some uremic patients who have mild hypercalcemia (11 to 12 mg/dL) are asymptomatic; other patients may exhibit symptoms despite only a modest elevation of serum calcium levels. In addition to nausea, anorexia, vomiting, mental confusion, and lethargy, patients with advanced renal failure may develop pruritus (229) or an acute elevation in blood pressure (241).

In patients with advanced renal failure and GFRs below 10 mL/min and in patients undergoing regular hemodialysis, it is reasonable to recommend calcium supplements to provide 1.0 g/day of elemental calcium; if the serum calcium level exceeds 10.5 mg/dL the quantity should be halved. In patients with serum calcium levels below 8.0 mg/dL, the quantity of calcium supplements should be increased. Calcium supplements should not be initiated until the serum phosphorus levels are below 5.5 to 6.0 mg/dL. Frequent monitoring of serum calcium and phosphorus levels is important because there is considerable variability in the response of individual patients to the same dosage of supplemental calcium (421). Calcium carbonate is the first choice as a source of supplemental calcium because it contains a higher fraction of calcium, is inexpensive, tasteless, and relatively well tolerated. Forty percent of calcium carbonate is elemental calcium compared to only 12 percent of calcium lactate and 18 percent of calcium gluconate. Calcium carbonate is available in several flavored proprietary preparations, including Titralac and Tums. To maximize the absorption of calcium, it is best that the quantity of calcium be divided into several doses taken throughout the day rather than administering it in one or two doses (427).

In patients undergoing regular hemodialysis, serum calcium levels, obtained just before dialysis, may spontaneously reach levels of 10.0 to 11.0 mg/dL (192). Under such conditions, calcium supplements should be used with caution, although Goldsmith (428, 429) reported the prevention and management of renal osteodystrophy with phosphate restriction and oral calcium supplements in dialysis patients.

CONCENTRATION OF CALCIUM IN DIALYSATE

When the use of dialysate concentrate was introduced for the preparation of dialysate, a concentrate was chosen that provided 2.6 to 2.7 meq/L (5.2 to 5.4 mg/dL) of calcium when diluted 35:1. This value was selected because it resulted in a final dialysate calcium concentration of 6.0 mg/dL when it was diluted with the tap water that was typically found to contain calcium in a level of 0.5 to 1.0 mg/dL. As dialysis became widespread, many communities found it necessary to purify their water supplies so that the water utilized had no added calcium, and the dialysate used in many areas contained only 5.2 to 5.6 mg/dL of calcium. The use of such dialysate, which lowers ionized calcium during each dialysis, probably aggravates secondary hyperparathyroidism in many patients. Thus, dialysis treatment using a dialysate cal-

cium of 5.0 to 5.5 mg/dL is associated with a progressive increase in iPTH levels over the first few months of hemodialysis (200a, 429).

Johnson et al. (394) found that predialysis iPTH levels were indirectly related to plasma calcium levels in patients treated with dialysis for more than 6 months with a dialysate calcium level below 6.0 mg/dL. Goldsmith et al. (108) found that plasma iPTH levels fell with use of dialysate calcium above 6.5 mg/mL and when serum phosphorus was maintained below 6.0 mg/dL. Atkinson et al. (430) reported progressive loss of bone mineral from the femur, as measured by photon absorptiometry, in dialysis patients utilizing a dialysate calcium of 6.0 mg/dL. Utilizing a whole body counter, Denney et al. (326) found that total body calcium decreased or was unchanged in patients treated with dialysate calcium of 6.0 mg/dL, while total body calcium either did not change or showed a slight increase in those utilizing a dialysate calcium of 8.0 mg/dL. Chamberlain and Robinson (431) reported a fall in total body calcium in most dialysis patients using a dialysate calcium of 6.0 mg/dL. Catto et al. (432) reported evidence for loss of bone, either by x-ray, neutron activation, or photon absorptiometry, in a substantial fraction of patients undergoing dialysis using a calcium level of 5.3 to 5.5 mg/dL. Bone et al. (321) assessed bone mineral content from the metacarpal index in patients using a dialysate calcium of either 5.0 mg/dL or 7.0 mg/dL. In the former group, there was a significant fall in the metacarpal index, while no change was seen in the latter group. Regan et al. (193) evaluated radiographs, bone morphometry, and plasma biochemical changes in dialysis patients using a dialysate calcium level that was progressively increased from 4.5 to 5.0 mg/dL and then to 7.0 mg/dL. Predialysis serum calcium concentrations increased from 9.4 to 9.7 mg/dL and then to 10.0 mg/dL. Plasma iPTH levels were increased in all patients, and they did not show a significant change for any group, although values decreased in individual patients. Two of six patients with radiologic signs of bone disease showed improvement, while three other patients developed bone disease during the study. Morphometric measurements of bone indicated that bone loss occurred primarily in male patients; soft tissue calcifications continued to appear during the study. It was concluded that dialysis using a calcium of 7.0 mg/dL offered little or no benefit; an occasional patient showed some benefit, but this was totally unpredictable. Mountokalakis et al. (433) confirmed this observation of a greater tendency for bone loss to occur in male rather than female dialysis patients. They suggested that bone loss occurred from factors other than treatment with hemodialysis per se. In an extensive study of the effect of dialysate calcium on serum iPTH levels, Bouillon et al. (353) reported an acute reduction of serum iPTH following dialysis using a dialysate calcium of 7.5 mg/dL. However, serum iPTH levels returned to the same predialysis levels within 1 to 2 days after dialysis, and predialysis iPTH levels were no different in patients using a dialysate calcium of 7.5 mg/dL compared to those using 6.0 mg/dL. They observed suppression of predialysis serum levels of iPTH only in patients given pharmacologic doses of vitamin D. Evans and Somerville (434) found no improvement in uremic patients with osteomalacia following use of a dialysate calcium of 8.6 mg/dL.

Others have reported that the slow appearance of bone disease occurs relentlessly and independent of changes in dialysate calcium levels (305). Thus, the incidence of vascular calcification, fractures, periarticular calcifications, and subperiosteal erosions was unchanged over the years despite introduction of changes in treatment modalities.

From available information, the use of dialysate containing a calcium level below 6.0 to 6.5 mg/dL may predispose to progressive bone loss and an increased frequency of bone erosions. Such a progressive development of bone disease may be modified if the dialysate calcium level is increased to 6.0 to 6.5 mg/dL. It is less certain that an increase in the dialysate calcium level above 7.0 mg/dL leads to any beneficial effect, and it may lead to persistent predialysis hypercalcemia. On the other hand, there is no evidence that the use of dialysate with a calcium above 6.5 to 7.0 mg/dL is effective in reversing secondary hyperparathyroidism. The appropriate use of phosphate restriction, dietary calcium supplements, and/or

vitamin D treatment may be more effective than is the use of a dialysate calcium above 7.0 mg/dL, perhaps because the former modalities exert a continuous effect compared to the intermittent effect of a high calcium dialysate.

USE OF VITAMIN D STEROLS

Despite adherence to therapy with appropriate dietary phosphate restriction, adequate intake of phosphate binders, the use of appropriate levels of calcium in dialysate, and an adequate dietary intake of calcium, a significant number of patients with advanced renal failure develop disabling bone disease. The clarification of the role of the kidney in generating 1,25-DHCC, the active hormonal form of vitamin D, has prompted a reevaluation of the use of vitamin D in treating such patients. A case can be raised in support of the theoretical use of vitamin D sterols early in the course of renal insufficiency (20). However, there are no data available regarding the efficacy or safety of the use of vitamin D sterols in a prophylactic manner in such patients. There are a number of reports of clinical trials employing one of the vitamin D analogues for the management of bone disease in uremic patients. In most clinical trials reported, each patient has served as his or her own control, and the studies usually involved the use of only one form of vitamin D. There are limited data available comparing the efficacy of different vitamin D sterols.

When uremic patients exhibit evidence of secondary hyperparathyroidism with bone erosions, high blood levels of iPTH, and elevated plasma alkaline phosphatase activity, treatment with an adequate quantity of one of the various forms of vitamin D often results in improvement. Pharmacologic doses of vitamin D_2 itself (5, 7), dihydrotachysterol (435, 436), 25-HCC or calcifidiol (146, 437, 438), 1α-HCC (439, 440), and 1,25-DHCC (61, 152, 441) have each been reported to lead to improvement of symptoms, improvement of x-rays toward normal, amelioration of bone pathology, and a fall in plasma levels of alkaline phosphatase and serum iPTH.

Although vitamin D_2 or D_3 and dihydrotachysterol have been available for a long period of time, there are only a few well-documented reports on their efficacy (5, 7, 41, 435). There is evidence that vitamin D induces bone mineralization that is more nearly normal than occurs following calcium supplementation alone (423). Stanbury and Lumb (5) and Dent et al. (7) have shown that vitamin D_2, 50,000 to 200,000 I.U./day, improves the overt skeletal disease in many patients with advanced renal failure. However, there is great variation in the responsiveness of individual patients, and Lumb et al. (67) found that 4000 to 18,000 I.U./day (0.10 to 0.45 mg/day) may be effective in certain uremic patients. Potter et al. (442) reported improvement of radiographic evidence of bone disease in five of six uremic children given vitamin D, 32,000 to 57,000 I.U./day, for 5 to 13 months. The only problem was mild hypercalcemia which resolved on reduction of dose.

The use of vitamin D or other active sterols is not without hazard. Hypercalcemia can occur even in the anephric patients (443), and the hypercalcemia may require several weeks for resolution. When hypercalcemia occurs, it arises as a consequence of high blood levels of 25-HCC, while the levels of 1,25-DHCC are not increased (444).

Vitamin D or other vitamin D sterols should not be used when serum phosphorus levels are elevated as an increase in the calcium × phosphorus product can occur with the appearance of extraskeletal calcification (445). On the other hand, treatment with vitamin D, when carried out in conjunction with adequate control of hyperphosphatemia, may be associated with regression of extraskeletal calcifications, including those in blood vessels (446).

During the last few years, several highly active naturally occurring forms of vitamin D, including 25-HCC, 1,25-DHCC, 24,25-DHCC, and 1,24,25-THCC (1,24,25-trihydroxyvitamin D_3) have been introduced for either brief or long-term clinical trials. Also, several synthetic analogues have been introduced which bypass the need for renal 1-hydroxylation. These include 1α-HCC, 5-6-trans-25-HCC, and 5-6-trans-vitamin D_3. Of these, 25-HCC, 1,25-DHCC, and 1α-HCC have had the widest use. Reports describing the use of

these sterols, the doses given, and the overall results obtained, are reviewed below.

25-HCC (calcifediol)

Despite the availability of 25-HCC for investigational use since 1969 (447), reports of its use in substantial numbers of patients with renal osteodystrophy have only recently appeared. Intestinal absorption of calcium can be increased with 25-HCC, 100 μg/day (62, 63), while the amount that augments calcium absorption in normal subjects is as low as 20 μg/day (63). Nonetheless, available data suggest that uremic patients do respond favorably to daily treatment doses below 100 μg/day. Teitlebaum et al. (146) treated five patients with 40 μg/day for 3 to 9 months; there was a decrease in serum iPTH and alkaline phosphatase, and serial bone biopsies showed a decrease in the number of osteoclasts, a decrease in osteoid surface covered with active osteoblasts, and a decrease in marrow fibrosis. Serum calcium levels rose to above 12.0 mg/dL in three of the five cases. Witmer and colleagues (437) treated nine uremic children with 25-HCC. Five had severe osteodystrophy that previously failed to respond to vitamin D, 350 to 700 μg/day (13,000 to 27,000 I.U./day) before 25-HCC treatment was initiated. There was a decrease in osteitis fibrosa, a reduction in the number of osteoblasts, and a decrease in marrow fibrosis with use of 25 to 200 μg/day. Other children, who had normal or near-normal skeletal x-rays at the initiation of hemodialysis, were given (1) either 25-HCC, 25 to 50 μg/day plus oral calcium supplement or (2) oral calcium alone. There was progressive worsening of bone lesions in the group receiving only oral calcium; however, skeletal biopsies showed improved mineralization and decreased fibrosis in the patients given 25-HCC. Two patients in the latter group developed severe hypercalcemia, an observation suggesting that less sterol may be tolerated in patients with mild skeletal disease. Fournier et al. (448) noted a rise in plasma alkaline phosphatase and an increase in active formation surface of trabecular bone in three patients given 25-HCC, 200 to 300 μg, three times per week for 4 to 8 weeks. These actions differed from those observed in other patients given 1α-HCC over the same period. Early results from a five-center study have been summarized by Recker and colleagues (438); these patients, all treated with hemodialysis, received 200 μg three times weekly for 29 weeks with the dose adjusted to avoid hypercalcemia and a final dose that averaged 46 μg/day. As a group, the patients noted a significant improvement in symptoms, with decreased bone pain and tenderness and a better overall clinical status. There was a small increase in serum calcium, a small but barely significant increase in serum phosphorus, and serum alkaline phosphatase fell. Plasma iPTH was not changed for the entire group, although many patients exhibited a significant decrease depending on the immunoassay utilized. Bone biopsies disclosed an increase in resorption surface in

conjunction with a decrease in the amount of fibrosis. Plasma levels of 25-HCC rose to 200 to 300 ng/mL concomitant with the maximum elevation of serum calcium (Fig. 20-32). In each of the series reported, several noted hypercalcemia.

Eastwood et al. (73) gave 25-HCC, 20 to 40 μg/day, intravenously to five patients for 4 weeks; there was improved bone mineralization, increased muscle strength, and a substantial rise in plasma 25-HCC level. The greatest improvement was noted in patients having low plasma levels of 25-HCC with an increase to normal with treatment.

Thus, 25-HCC appears to be effective in patients with renal osteodystrophy; it is available in parts of Europe and is under investigational use in the United States. A major unanswered ques-

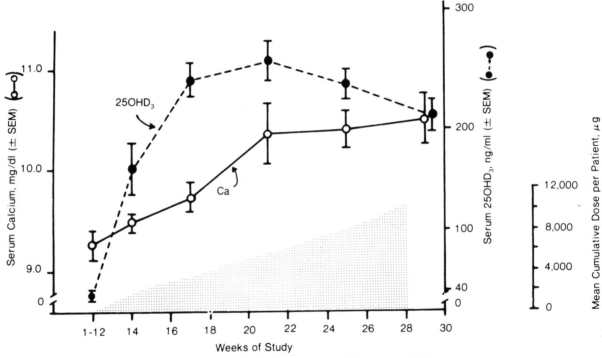

Figure 20-32. Levels of calcium and 25-HCC (mean ± S.E.) in 44 patients with renal osteodystrophy undergoing long-term hemodialysis and being treated with 25-HCC. Also, the cumulative dose of 25-HCC, calcifediol, is also shown in the stippled area. [Reprinted from Recker et al. (438) by permission of Arch. Intern. Med.]

tion is whether 25-HCC may be more effective than 1,25-DHCC or 1α-HCC in inducing mineralization of bone in uremic patients, as has been suggested by Bordier et al. (115) in patients with vitamin D deficiency.

1α,25-DHCC (calcitriol)

With the availability of 1,25-DHCC, initially prepared biosynthetically and then from efficient chemical synthesis, a number of clinical trials have been reported indicating its efficacy in treating patients with renal osteodystrophy. In an early study, Brickman et al. (449) reported observations in eight patients given 1,25-DHCC, 0.14 to 0.68 μg/day by mouth, for 2 to 4 months. Patients with secondary hyperparathyroidism and osteitis fibrosa showed a decrease in serum iPTH, a fall in marrow fibrosis, and an increase in resorption surface. Patients with muscle weakness observed an increase in muscle strength. There was some improvement in the mineralization front in those with osteomalacia. Similar observations were reported by Henderson et al. (210) in two patients and by Silverberg et al. (441) in one case, the last being treated intravenously. Striking improvement in muscle strength was noted (210, 441, 449), and there was increased bone mineralization in the patient with osteomalacia (441). Also, Eastwood et al. (450) gave 1,25-DHCC intravenously, 0.54 to 1.35 μg/day, to five patients for 4 weeks and noted better bone mineralization with an improved calcification front in three patients. Pierides et al. (451) reported five patients treated with 1,25-DHCC, 1.0 to 1.5 μg/day, for 6 to 8 months. They again noted improvement in secondary hyperparathyroidism as evidenced by changes in bone histology, skeletal x-ray, and serum iPTH and alkaline phosphatase. Bone mineralization was improved but this occurred more slowly. There was electromyographic improvement with an increase in the duration of the action potential. A series of 40 patients from Los Angeles, Seattle, and Hawaii was treated with 1,25-DHCC, with an average dose of 0.62 μg/day for 4 to 90 weeks (152); there was a striking improvement in symptoms of bone pain and muscle weakness in 71 and 85 percent, respectively. A

group of patients were identified who did not show a favorable clinical response; this group had a higher pretreatment mean serum calcium level (10.3±0.21 mg/dL) than did the patients who showed a favorable response (8.99 ± 0.26 mg/dL). Serum phosphorus levels did not differ in the two groups. Subsequently, the "treatment failure" patients were divided into two separate groups: (1) those with a bone biopsy showing a mineralizing defect or "pure" osteomalacia with little or no evidence of secondary hyperparathyroidism, and (2) those who had marked osteitis fibrosa, high plasma levels of iPTH, and pretreatment serum calcium levels above 10.8 mg/dL (452). In both groups, serum calcium levels rose promptly with treatment, and there was no subjective or objective evidence of improvement.

Many of the patients showing a favorable response had a decrease in serum phosphorus level within the first 1 to 3 months of treatment; subsequently, an increase in serum phosphorus often

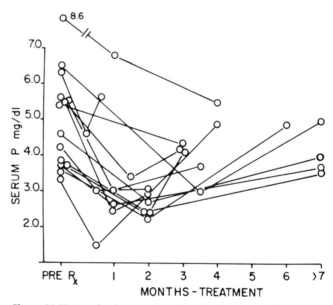

Figure 20-33. Levels of serum phosphorus before, at a nadir, and at the end of 5 to 7 months of treatment with 1,25-DHCC for overt renal osteodystrophy. This is shown in relationship to the duration of treatment, and the final value represents the last observation during treatment. [*Reprinted from Coburn and Brickman (452a) by permission of Plenum Press.*]

occurred in conjunction with the rise in serum calcium level (Fig. 20-33). Sherrard and colleagues (453) evaluated control and posttreatment bone biopsies in a group of uremic patients treated with 1,25-DHCC and two control groups of patients undergoing dialysis using either 6.0 or 8.0 mg/dL calcium in dialysate. The control groups both received vitamin D_3, 500 I.U./day. The pretreatment bone biopsies showed more extensive

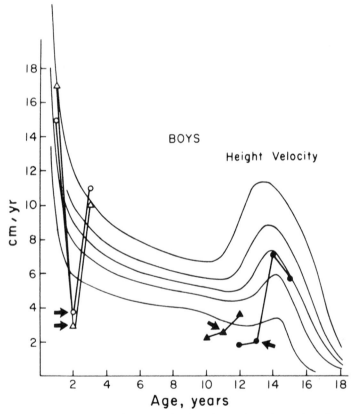

Figure 20-34. The Tanner height-velocity plots of growth in four children treated with 1,25-DHCC. Height-velocity is shown in cm/ year. The arrows denote the initiation of therapy. Height-velocity was normal during the first year of life for cases 1 and 2 (△, o) but fell below the third percentile during months 12 to 24. Height-velocity increased in each patient after therapy was begun. The percentile lines from top to bottom are 97th, 75th, 50th, 25th, and 3d. [*Reproduced from Chesney et al. (264) by permission of N. Engl. J. Med.*]

lesions in patients given 1,25-DHCC than the other groups; however, there was a marked decrease in fibrosis in 10 of 11 with osteitis fibrosa, and there was a striking increase in mineralization in 16 of 17 patients treated with 1,25-DHCC. On the other hand, patients treated with the two levels of calcium in dialysate showed little or no improvement. It was concluded that 1,25-DHCC was more effective than supplemental calcium added to the dialysate in both improving mineralization and in reversing secondary hyperparathyroidism.

There is recent experience in treating children with 1,25-DHCC. Six children ages 3 months to 14 years, with evidence of severe skeletal disease, received 1,25-DHCC, 0.014 to 0.041 µg/kg body weight per day, for 4 to 26 months (264). The patients had hypocalcemia initially and showed a slight increase in serum calcium with treatment. There was a decrease in serum iPTH and a fall in alkaline phosphatase; of great interest was a marked increase in growth velocity in four children (Fig. 20-34). This increase in growth occurred after serum iPTH and alkaline phosphatase had decreased toward normal, observations suggesting that healing of renal osteodystrophy was necessary prior to the onset of catch-up growth.

Ahmed and colleagues (228) reported five patients given a low dose of 1,25-DHCC, 0.5 µg/day, for 4 to 16 months. There was a return of plasma alkaline phosphatase, hydroxyproline, and iPTH to normal in four cases. Bone histology showed improved mineralizaton and remodeling of the trabecular architecture in all patients and a decrease in fibrosis in the patients with evidence of parathyroid overactivity before treatment. The use of 0.5 µg/day was associated with only mild hypercalcemia, which readily reversed upon temporarily discontinuing the sterol.

Improvement in muscle strength has been a constant observation in all series. This often was noted between 1 and 6 weeks after initiation of treatment. In several cases (152, 228), muscular strength improved with 1,25-DHCC, 0.25 µg/day, even though serum iPTH showed no change or actually rose. Such anecdotal experience suggests that the muscular weakness may be reversed with

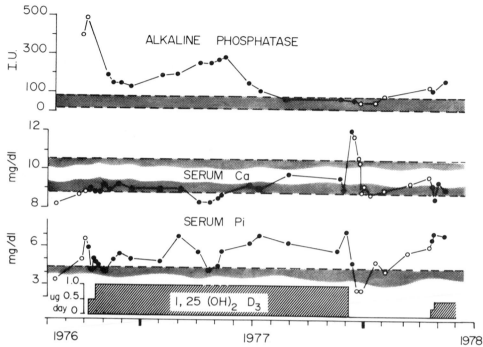

Figure 20-35. Course of a patient with overt renal osteodystrophy due to marked secondary hyperparathyroidism which shows serial values of serum alkaline phosphatase, calcium and phosphorus (P$_i$) in relationship to the daily dose of 1,25-DHCC. After a period of 14 months, during which the patient received 1.0 μg/day, abrupt hypercalcemia occurred. This dissipated following withdrawal of treatment, and the patient subsequently did not have hypercalcemia while receiving 0.5 μg/day. [*Courtesy of Winkler and Coburn, unpublished observations.*]

smaller quantities of 1,25-DHCC than are required to reverse the secondary hyperparathyroidism.

In general, the trials utilizing 1,25-DHCC and 1α-HCC suggest that these sterols are most effective in treating patients with secondary hyperparathyroidism, particularly when there is either normal or decreased serum calcium; when overt osteomalacia and secondary hyperparathyroidism coexist, a favorable response is usual. Whether or not long-term treatment can restore bone histology totally to normal remains unresolved. The very slow rate of bone remodeling may indicate that 1 to 2 years of treatment might be required to restore the skeleton to normal. Long-term studies indicate that the amount of 1,25-DHCC tolerated without hypercalcemia may be 1.0 to 2.0 μg/day during the period when bone is rapidly

remineralizing. Once healing has slowed or stopped, as evidenced by a fall in alkaline phosphatase, hypercalcamia may occur despite use of a dose that was well tolerated for many months (Fig. 20-35). The data of Ahmed et al. (228) suggest that doses above 1.0 μg/day may not be required at the outset, but further observations are necessary to answer this question. The administration of 1,25-DHCC may help to identify patients with an isolated defect in mineralization (452) and those with marked parathyroid hyperplasia where the large mass of the hyperplastic glands necessitates parathyroid surgery. Whether treatment with one of these sterols will be useful in prophylaxis of skeletal disease in patients with less severe or early bone lesions has not been established. Clearly, patients with mild skeletal disease are more prone to develop episodes of hypercalcemia (454). With 1,25-DHCC (calcitriol) now available in the United States and 1α-HCC now marketed in Europe, the United Kingdom, and Japan, further and wide experience with these sterols will soon be available.

1α-HCC

This synthetic analogue was successfully synthesized in substantial quantities before 1,25-DHCC became available. In vivo, it undergoes 25-hydroxylation in the liver to 1,25-DHCC prior to exerting an action. It is very active in patients with advanced uremia, and the dose required to increase intestinal calcium absorption is only 1.5 times to twice that needed for 1,25-DHCC (64); following promising short-term clinical studies (455, 456) numerous therapeutic trials with 1α-HCC have been reported in uremic patients with symptomatic skeletal disease. Chan et al. (439) administered 1α-HCC for 5 to 8 months and noted an improvement in radiographic manifestations of bone disease and a decrease in alkaline phosphatase in one patient; also, an increase in growth velocity was noted during treatment with 1α-HCC (457).

Total body calcium measured with neutron activation either increased or failed to decrease during treatment with 1α-HCC compared to the usual decrease observed in other dialysis patients given calcium supplements (458, 459). A favorable response has been reported by others (448, 460–462), with a decrease in alkaline phosphatase, a fall in iPTH, and/or improvement in the bone biopsy in patients exhibiting marked abnormalities. Naik and colleagues (463) found no change in body calcium or plasma alkaline phosphatase in patients without overt bone disease, observations which contrast with those noted in patients with significant skeletal disease at the outset. Although a decrease in serum iPTH was generally noted in conjunction with an increase in serum calcium, certain patients exhibited a fall in plasma iPTH without a change in serum calcium, particularly early in the course of treatment with 1α-HCC (462).

Pierides et al. (160) were the first to observe that responsiveness of the patients to 1α-HCC varied from patient to patient; thus, those with significant osteitis fibrosa, either with or without concomitant osteomalacia on bone biopsy, had a favorable response, while patients who showed osteomalacia alone had little or no improvement. In the histologic evaluation of a larger number of patients treated with 1α-HCC (153), improvement was noted in 12 of 16 cases with evidence of osteitis fibrosa present; however, when osteomalacia was present, there was improvement in only 8 of 22 cases, and most of the patients with osteomalacia who improved had concomitant osteitis fibrosa. Kanis et al. (464, 465) observed that relief of skeletal symptoms, improvement in x-rays, and a fall in plasma alkaline phosphatase occurred commonly, i.e., in 87, 76, and 75 percent, respectively, of patients treated with 1α-HCC, but there was improvement of bone biopsy in only 46 percent of treated patients. When patients showing improvement on skeletal biopsy were separated from those who failed to improve, those with a combination of osteitis fibrosa and osteomalacia generally improved, while patients showing either "pure" osteitis fibrosa or osteomalacia alone were less likely to improve. The best predictive factor separating the two groups was a low plasma calcium before treatment in the patients showing improvement. Such a separation of groups could not be made on the basis of response to treatment by Melsen et al. (466), who noted a decrease in osteoid surface, improved percent mineralization of osteoid, and augmented rate of mineralization after 6 months of treatment with 1α-HCC. Serum iPTH levels fell in 14 of 16 patients with treatment, and there was an inverse relationship between iPTH and serum calcium during the course of treatment in most patients (467). A reduction in serum iPTH levels often occurred in conjunction with a fall in serum calcium during treatment with a 1α-HCC as shown in Fig. 20-36 (440, 468); however, this change did not occur in all patients and patients with high levels of serum calcium before treatment failed to exhibit a change in iPTH. Similar observations were obtained in a larger group of patients by Peacock et al. (469), although changes in serum alkaline phosphatase, phosphorus, and calcium often occurred without a fall in serum iPTH; bone histology often im-

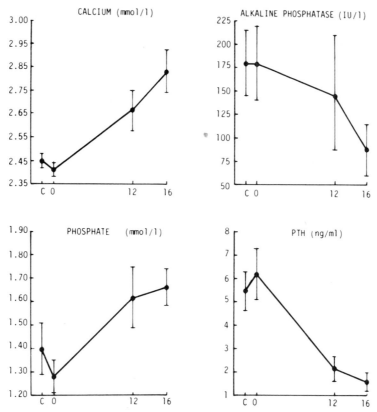

Figure 20-36. Mean values of plasma calcium, phosphorus, alkaline phosphatase, and serum iPTH in 10 dialysis patients according to the duration of treatment with 1α-HCC, indicated in months. The initial dose was 1.0 μg/day and the dosage was adjusted in each patient during the trial. [*Reproduced from Papapoulus et al. (440) by permission of W. de Gruyter.*]

proved with reduced features of secondary hyperparathyroidism, i.e., reduced resorption surface and/or improved osteomalacia, evidenced by reduced osteoid volume and osteoid surface and increased calcification front. Bone (470) observed that patients with skeletal erosions and high serum iPTH and alkaline phosphatase levels required a long period of treatment with 1α-HCC before serum calcium rose, while dialysis patients without erosions and normal or only slightly increased iPTH and alkaline phosphatase levels exhibited a more rapid rise in serum calcium during treatment. Patients in both groups showed improvement in bone pain and muscle strength.

The importance of concomitant use of aluminum hydroxide for intestinal phosphate binding was stressed by the results of Davison et al. (471); 20 patients receiving 1α-HCC and no aluminum hydroxide were compared with a group given aluminum hydroxide to reduce serum phosphorus below 5.0 mg/dL before treatment with 1α-HCC was initiated. In the former, the incidence of corneal calcifications, pruritus, and radiographic evidence of soft extraskeletal calcifications was higher. Bone erosions resolved in an equal number in both groups, but there was a higher incidence of periosteal new bone formation in the group not given phosphate-binding gels. It was shown that 1α-HCC caused a significant increase in phosphate absorption in these patients (471). These observations underscore the need for administration of phosphate binders during such treatment.

Children and adults not yet teated with dialysis and with only mild hyperparathyroidism had a favorable response to 1α-HCC, although two patients with evidence of "autonomous hyperparathyroidism" did not respond (472). Postlewaite and Houston (473) evaluated children, ages 5 to 17, treated with 1α-HCC, 0.04 to 0.08 μg/kg per day: there was improvement in 11 of 12 cases with a decrease in plasma alkaline phosphatase and an increase in serum calcium. Five of the twelve received prior treatment with vitamin D, in doses from 50 to 100 μg/day, without effect; such a favorable effect of 1α-HCC in a patient previously unresponsive to a large dose of vitamin D was reported by Hirooka et al. (474).

In a double-blind study, Tougaard et al. (475) gave either 1α-HCC, 1.0 μg/day, or a placebo for 11 weeks. They noted a rise in serum calcium and a fall in iPTH levels; however, plasma alkaline phosphatase, the degree of bone mineralization measured by phosphorus:hydroxyproline ratio in bone, and bone mineral content of the forearm measured by photon absorptiometry were no different in the 1α-HCC, or the placebo-treated groups. This study suggested little beneficial effect of 1α-HCC in preventing bone mineral loss, although the duration of treatment was very short. In another evaluation of the prophylactic use of 1α-HCC, Walker et al. (476) noted an increase in serum calcium and a fall in serum phosphorus in patients treated with 1α-HCC when dialysis was first initiated. Serum alkaline phosphatase and iPTH levels were not changed. However, there was development of ocular calcification and radiographic evidence of increased extraskeletal calcification during the treatment period; they had no control observations to indicate whether such extraskeletal calcifications may have occurred with the progression of renal failure alone or whether they were due to the treatment with 1α-HCC. Bone biopsies disclosed a decrease in resorption surfaces when they were abnormally high, and x-rays indicated reversal of erosions in approximately one-third of patients. Measurements of bone mass by neutron activation indicate that 1α-HCC either resulted in a reduced rate of fall in bone mineral content or increased the bone mineral content (463, 477). In another study, total body calcium was evaluated by neutron activation and forearm bone content was measured by photon absorptiometry; there was an increase in body calcium but there was no change in forearm calcium content during treatment with 1α-HCC. It was concluded that treatment with 1α-HCC may increase the spinal calcium content, which correlates with total body calcium, while the calcium content of the peripheral skeleton was unaltered. Such results could be due to the more rapid effect of 1α-HCC on trabecular bone that primarily makes up the axial skeleton, while an effect on cortical bone may occur much more slowly.

An evaluation of treatment with 1α-HCC was compared to results seen in patients treated using a dialysate calcium of either 5.5 or 7.0 mg/dL (478). The group receiving 1α-HCC utilized a dialysate calcium of 5.5 mg/dL. In the last group, serum calcium rose, plasma alkaline phosphatase and iPTH decreased, there was a reduced incidence of bone erosions, and bone calcium, measured by neutron activation, increased. However, the patients treated with dialysate calcium levels of either 5.5 or 7.0 mg/dL exhibited no change in any of these parameters. These observations are similar to those with 1,25-DHCC (453), which indicate that an active vitamin D compound is more effective in reducing the degree of secondary hyperparathyroidism than is an increase in the calcium content in dialysate alone.

Other vitamin D sterols and general considerations regarding vitamin D use

In addition to the 1α-hydroxylated sterols discussed above, several other synthetic sterols have been introduced for brief trials. Several of these sterols have the A ring rotated 180° about the 5,6-double bond, thereby converting the orientation from a cis to a trans configuration with the normal 3-hydroxyl group assuming a geometric position equivalent to that of the 1α-hydroxyl radial.

This may be referred to as a "pseudo 1α-hydroxyl" configuration. Studies in humans have shown that 5,6-trans-vitamin D_3 can enhance intestinal absorption of calcium in uremic patients when it is administered in doses of 0.25 to 5 mg/day (479, 480). Lower quantities of 5,6-trans-vitamin D_3 were effective in stimulating intestinal calcium absorption and elevating serum calcium levels in patients with chronic renal failure (481). Grigoleit et al. (482) noted improved intestinal calcium absorption and reversal of x-ray abnormalities in uremic patients given 5,6-trans-25-HCC, 50 to 125 μg/day for an average duration of 33 weeks. Some patients noted improvement in symptoms, and there was reversal of x-ray abnormalities and some improvement in histologic findings. Schulz et al. (483) reported experience with 14 patients who were treated with 5,6-trans-25-HCC, 100 to 250 μg/day. Serum calcium rose, and there was a reduction in unmineralized osteoid and a decrease in bone resorption. Such observations are of interest, but it is not clear whether these compounds will have advantage over the natural 1-hyroxylated sterols or dehydrotachysterol itself, which is also active by virtue of its "pseudo-1α-hydroxyl" characteristics.

One major feature of 1,25-DHCC and 1α-HCC is their relative rapid turnover compared to vitamin D itself. Brickman et al. (64) found the halftime of reversal of hypercalciuria to be approximately 50 to 75 percent greater for 1α-HCC than 1,25-DHCC. Kanis and Russell (484) evaluated the rate of reversal of hypercalcemia or hypercalciuria induced by vitamin D_3, dihydrotachysterol, 1α-HCC, and 1,25-DHCC. The half-time for reversal of the effects was shorter after discontinuing 1,25-DHCC than was the case for 1α-HCC, vitamin D_3, or dihydrotachysterol, and the differences were independent of the dose given or the length of treatment. Thus 1,25-DHCC shows a rapid dissipation of effect, a useful feature should toxicity occur. In addition, there are several well-documented cases who responded to 1,25-DHCC, 25-HCC, or 1-HCC after no response to vitamin D_3 or dihydrotachysterol (152, 437, 473, 474).

One consideration in the choice of either 1α-HCC or dihydrotachysterol is their lack of 25-hydroxyl group, and thus, hepatic 25-hydroxylation is necessary before they act. The concomitant treatment with a drug such as phenobarbital, phenytoin, or glutethemide, which impairs the hepatic 25-hydroxylation (17, 485, 486), may result in impaired action of the vitamin D sterol. Indeed Pierides et al. have reported that anticonvulsant therapy had an adverse effect on the response to 1α-HCC (487).

Another question raised is whether or not the active vitamin D compounds have a major effect on magnesium homeostasis in uremic patients. Sörenson et al. (488) suggested that these active sterols might induce magnesium intoxication; however, Kanis et al. (489, 490) and we (169, 491) have carried out metabolic balance studies in uremic patients treated with 1,25-DHCC or 1α-HCC and found little or no effect of these sterols on serum magnesium level or magnesium balance.

Only fragmentary data are available about the effect of 24,25-DHCC in uremia. Kanis et al. (114, 491) reported qualitative differences between the actions of 24,25-DHCC and 1,25-DHCC in normal humans. Llach et al. (492) found that 24,25-DHCC, in doses of 2.0 to 4.0 μg/day, produced a slight decrease in serum calcium level and a rise in alkaline phosphatase activity in dialysis patients. These latter effects are clearly different from those of 1,25-DHCC, but there are insufficient data available to suggest a known therapeutic role of 24,25-DHCC; further observations are needed to clarify its role.

SUBTOTAL PARATHYROIDECTOMY

The various medical modalities described above can often produce some degree of suppression of the parathyroid glands, with improvement of symptoms and altered divalent ion metabolism in uremic patients. However, these measures may not be successful in certain patients, and the appearance of certain manifestations of secondary hyperparathyroidism may necessitate subtotal parathyroidectomy. The clinical presentations which indicate the need for subtotal parathyroidectomy include (1) persistent hypercalcemia in conjunction with evidence of hyperparathyroidism particularly when the former produces symptoms; (2) severe and intractable pruritus that does not respond to dialysis and other medical treatment, and which occurs in association with evidence of secondary hyperparathyroidism (bone erosions and high serum iPTH); (3) a serum calcium × phosphorus product that consistently exceeds 75 to 80 and when there is progressive, severe extraskeletal calcifications; (4) severe or progressive skeletal and articular pain; and (5) the appearance of calciphylaxis, i.e., ischemic lesions and necrosis of soft tissues, and vascular calcifications (10, 493–495).

The appearance of persistent, significant hypercalcemia (greater than 11 mg/dL) is not common in patients with end-stage renal failure under treatment with regular dialysis. The appearance of persistent hypercalcemia, particularly with clinical signs and symptoms attributed to hypercalcemia (i.e., peptic ulcer disease, nausea, and vomiting), may indicate the need for subtotal parathyroidectomy. It should be remembered that hypercalcemia can occur in uremia without secondary hyperparathyroidism (161); thus, parathyroid surgery should not be done for hypercalcemia in the absence of bone erosions and elevated plasma levels of iPTH. Significant hypercalcemia also may appear in patients with successfully functioning renal transplants and may also necessitate parathyroid surgery as is noted above.

The occurrence of plasma calcium and phosphate levels that are increased to produce a calcium × phosphorus product that consistently exceeds 75 to 80 is often associated with severe and progressive extraskeletal calcifications and/or rapidly progressive skeletal disease. When there is a persistently elevated calcium × phosphorus product that does not respond to aggressive treatment with dialysis, dietary control, and treatment with phosphate-binding gels, a physician must consider the possible need for subtotal parathyroidectomy, particularly when serum iPTH levels are elevated and bone erosions are present. After successful surgery, both serum calcium and phosphorus levels generally fall, and extraskeletal calcifications may slowly resolve over a period of weeks to months.

Severe pruritus that is unresponsive to aggressive dialysis and medical treatment has been suggested to be an indication for subtotal parathyroidectomy (229, 493). In some patients, pruritus disappears or improves within 24 to 48 h after subtotal parathyroidectomy; however, other patients show no response. Lidocaine, 200 mg IV, may effectively suppress the pruritus present in some dialysis patients (231); this effect of lidocaine persists for 2 to 3 days, and it has few side effects. We have also been impressed by the effectiveness of intravenous lidocaine injections for dialysis patients suffering with severe pruritus that was previously unresponsive to other treatment. Other investigators have reported successful treatment of pruritus by phototherapy with ultraviolet light; eight exposures of the entire skin to long-wave ultraviolet light over a 4-week period was said to produce prolonged relief of pruritus in many dialysis patients (232). From available information, we do not recommend subtotal parathyroidectomy surgery for pruritus unless there are other features of hyperparathyroidism (bone erosions and high plasma iPTH); even then efforts should be made to suppress the parathyroid hyperplasia with the methods noted above.

Occasionally, severe skeletal and articular pain occur in association with an elevated plasma iPTH level and osteitis fibrosa may incapacitate the patient. These symptoms may disappear or improve within a matter of a few days to several weeks after subtotal parathyroidectomy.

The syndrome of calciphylaxis, with ischemic lesions of soft tissue leading to ulcerations and necrosis, is a serious complication in patients with end-stage chronic renal failure (Fig. 20-18); this may progress and lead to death from sepsis unless it is appropriately treated. Often, other medical treatment has been unsuccessful, and subtotal parathyroidectomy has been the only method effective in reversing this serious complication. The ulcerative lesions may slowly heal over a period of days to weeks in the majority of cases so far reported (240). In some patients serum iPTH levels are found to be low and marked phosphate restriction may be attempted in the hope of reversing this lesion (240).

A situation creating a difficult dilemma to the

physician is the occurrence of marked hyperphosphatemia and overt secondary hyperparathyroidism in a noncompliant patient. Such patients often have marked hyperphosphatemia, extraskeletal calcifications, bone erosions, and high plasma iPTH levels. The serum calcium level may be normal or slightly elevated. Under such conditions, parathyroid surgery may permit the reduction of blood phosphorus and the resolution, albeit temporarily, of the ectopic calcifications. However, unless the patient then follows the prescribed treatment with dietary phosphate restriction and aluminum hydroxide or carbonate, the problem is likely to recur.

At surgery for a subtotal parathyroidectomy, the four parathyroid glands should be identified first. Then the surgeon should choose a gland to be partially removed. Usually, the gland that appears less hyperplastic than the others but has an adequate blood supply is the best to partially resect; or one may choose the gland that shows more fat cells among the hyperplastic chief cells on microscopic sections. Part of this gland should be removed, leaving 100 to 200 mg of the tissue. After visually observing the preservation of satisfactory blood supply in the remnant parathyroid gland that is to remain in place, the surgeon can totally excise the three other glands. The residual parathyroid tissue sometimes undergoes hyperplasia necessitating a second surgical procedure; therefore, it is recommended that the remnant gland be marked by a metal clip and/or a long black silk suture (398, 496). Occasionally, only three parathyroid glands are found in the neck or in the upper anterior thorax that are accessible at the time of neck exploration. We usually recommend the removal of all three glands if only three are found under an assumption that the fourth gland is located elsewhere. However, such patients can develop hypoparathyroidism, indicating the existence of only three glands; more commonly, there is only partial correction of the overt hyperparathyroidism. In certain unusual cases, five and even six parathyroid glands may be present. Good judgment and, even more important, extensive experience of the parathyroid surgeon are clearly important for the identification and management of such atypical cases. Technical problems during the surgical procedure should be few, and blood loss should be minimal. The patient usually can leave the hospital within a week. A dialysis patient should be treated with dialysis 1 day prior to surgery.

The main problem encountered in the postoperative period is control of blood calcium concentration. Blood calcium levels do not invariably fall after removal of three or more parathyroid glands, and the magnitude and duration of hypocalcemia varies from patient to patient. Profound and persistent hypocalcemia often develops in certain patients, particularly those with x-ray evidence of skeletal erosions. The serum phosphate levels usually diminish postoperatively; however, hyperphosphatemia may persist and contribute to the decrease in serum calcium. With the use of dialysate containing calcium in a concentration of 6.0 to 7.0 mg/dL there is an increase in blood calcium during each dialysis, and this may alleviate hypocalcemia during the interdialytic interval. Uremic patients who are not yet treated with maintenance dialysis and who undergo subtotal parathyroidectomy may require frequent intravenous infusions of calcium gluconate and supplementation of oral calcium and vitamin D to combat postoperative hypocalcemia (493).

Tetany may occur in such patients during the postoperative period, and hemodialysis, perhaps from its alkalinizing effect, may predispose to tetany. When the serum calcium level falls below 7.5 mg/dL, oral calcium supplements should be given to prevent a further decrease of serum calcium level. The quantity of oral calcium needed is often quite large; initial treatment should provide at least 2.0 g of elemental calcium, and this amount can be increased by 0.5 to 1.0 g/day at intervals of 3 to 7 days until serum calcium begins to increase. If the concentration of serum calcium falls below 7 mg/dL and if tetany appears, intravenous calcium should be given as well. In patients with profound and sustained hypocalcemia, treatment with vitamin D or one of its active forms is indicated. With such therapy, careful monitoring of serum calcium is mandatory, and phosphate-binding compounds should be adjusted to maintain serum phosphorus in the range of 3.5 to 5.0 mg/dL. Tetany occurring in a uremic patient with severe bone disease may be catastrophic, and the simultaneous fracture of scapula, clavicle, and both femoral necks has been reported during a single short episode of tetany during dialysis (497); we have observed major fracture (i.e., a spiral fracture of the femur or femoral neck fracture) in three patients after parathyroid surgery; they occurred 1 to 3 weeks after surgery, and, of interest, each occurred late during the hemodialysis procedure. In postoperative patients with marked periarticular calcifications, it may be wise to maintain modest hypocalcemia, i.e., serum calcium of 8.0 and 9.0 mg/dL, until the ectopic calcifications have resolved.

In occasional patients with very marked skeletal disease, the hypocalcemia that appears after parathyroidectomy may persist for 2 to 3 months despite treatment with large amounts of oral calcium supplements and with vitamin D or a related sterol. Serum phosphorus and magnesium levels may also decrease during this time. If the serum magnesium falls below 1.5 mg/dL (1.2 meq/L), supplemental magnesium can be given by mouth. For the hypophosphatemia, there is a greater dilemma as the administration of phosphate salts can markedly aggravate the hypocalcemia. If the serum phosphorus falls below 2.5 mg/dL, aluminum-containing gels should be reduced or stopped, but no effort should be made to increase the phosphorus above 3.5 to 4.0 mg/dL. During the period of hypocalcemia, remineralization of the skeleton is usually occurring, and once the "hungry bones" have reached or neared saturation, the blood calcium will start to rise and the requirement for calcium and vitamin D will decrease markedly. If their dosages are not reduced, hypercalcemia may ensue. The fall of a markedly elevated plasma alkaline phosphatase level to near normal may indicate that the bone is reaching a stage when healing is largely completed; when this occurs, the calcium supplements and vitamin D dosage should be reduced.

Occasionally, the residual parathyroid tissue undergoes hyperplasia, and a second operation may be necessary. The second operation may have greater technical difficulties, and it is not without significant complications, such as damage to the recurrent laryngeal nerve. Wells et al. (401, 402) have suggested the use of autotransplantation of the parathyroid glands. This procedure involves the removal of *all* four parathyroid glands from the neck, with the implantation of multiple small fragments of parathyroid tissue in the forearm muscle of the patient. Most of the fragments of parathyroid tissue implanted do not undergo necrosis but may function normally and show an appropriate response to hypercalcemic and hypocalcemic stimuli (404). If the clinical manifestations of overt secondary hyperparathyroidism recur, some of the implanted parathyroid fragments can be easily identified and removed. Parathyroid glands can also be stored frozen, and some of the stored parathyroid tissue can be successfully implanted into forearm muscle if persistent hypocalcemia should continue (402).

New insight into the role of vitamin D and its active metabolites on the regulation of PTH secretion and the availability of these highly active forms of vitamin D for the management of uremic patients should make the management of secondary hyperparathyroidism easier to achieve in patients with end-stage renal failure; thus, there may be a reduced need for subtotal parathyroidectomy in these patients.

OTHER TREATMENT CONSIDERATIONS

Other management considerations, some of which have been alluded to earlier, will depend on special circumstances encountered. Excess quantities of trace substances, such as fluoride or aluminum, present in water used to prepare dialysate may have a pathogenic role in producing a high incidence of bone disease (166, 280, 364). Although the data supporting such a theory are largely epidemiologic, it would seem that a dialysis center which encounters a high incidence of serious skeletal disease should carefully evaluate the relative purity of the water supply and the water treatment in use. A dialysis center encountering a high incidence of osteomalacia should initiate the appropriate means for water purification. Loss of skeletal carbonate (or bicarbonate) may be another factor that has a deleterious effect on the skeleton; in totally refractory bone disease, a therapeutic trial with bicarbonate-containing dialysate may also be reasonable, although there is no evidence to suggest that it will be of value. Treatment with a β-adrenergic blocking drug, such as propanolol, may reduce the manifestations of secondary hyperparathyroidism (499), suggesting a possible role for such agents. On the other hand, it is likely that other side effects of such drugs may limit their use to patients requiring them for their antihypertensive value. Clearly, further exploration of the effects of these agents on bone disease is certainly warranted.

It is possible that calcitonin may be useful in certain cases when the secondary hyperparathyroidism is inoperable or when it cannot be managed with a vitamin D sterol because of hypercalcemia (139, 140). It may act to suppress certain effects of excess PTH; a single report of its short-term administration in uremic patients indicated very little overall effect (500).

An appropriate means for managing extraskeletal calcifications, when they do not respond to control of serum phosphorus level or parathyroidectomy, poses a serious dilemma. Zucchelli et al. (501) reported experience with treating nine dialysis patients with the diphosphonate EHDP (disodium-ethane-1-hydroxyl-1, 1-diphosphonate) 7.5 to 10 mg/kg body weight for 5 to 9 months. It was given to patients who had well-controlled serum phosphorus levels but persistent ectopic calcification. No change was seen in five, but two had complete regression of the ectopic calcification and another showed a reduction of arterial calcification. Bone biopsies showed that treatment with EHDP led to a significant increase in osteoid volume and osteoid surface without modifying the calcification front. There were slight increases in serum alkaline phosphatase levels in most of the patients. Thus, they note that the EHDP was well tolerated; however, a risk of developing osteomalacia with such treatment (328, 502) suggests that its use should be limited to cases with severe extraskeletal calcification that is posing a serious threat to the patient and when all other therapeutic modalties have failed.

MANAGEMENT OF FRACTURES

Rib fractures, which are probably the most frequent fractures seen in uremic patients, usually heal very slowly over a period of several months. They are usually asymptomatic and little specific treatment is required. Traumatic fractures of the long bones and of the femoral neck may have a poor union even after several months. When fractures occur in patients with marked secondary hyperparathyroidism, the appropriate surgical repair should be considered since prolonged immobilization can create even greater complications in such patients. The successful use of femoral head prosthesis has been reported in patients with end-stage uremia and those on dialysis (503). When secondary hyperparathyroidism exists in a patient with a fracture, it seems preferable to treat such a patient with an active form of vitamin D rather than with parathyroidectomy, because of the risk of tetany and seizures in such patients.

ACKNOWLEDGMENTS

This research was supported in part by Grant AM 14750 and Contract AM 7-2204 with the U.S.P.H.S. and by Research Funds from the Veterans Administration.

Outstanding secretarial assistance was provided by Patti Kentor and Harriet Goldware-Sorkin; Sally Shupien and Dr. Kornel Gerszi assisted in the bibliographic search and Dr. Jeffrey Kraut kindly reviewed the manuscript.

REFERENCES

1. Albright, F., T. G. Drake, and H. W. Sulkowitch: Renal osteitis fibrosa cystica: Report of case with discussion of metabolic aspects, *Johns Hopkins Med. J.*, **60**:377, 1937.
2. Follis, R. H., Jr., and D. A. Jackson: Renal osteomalacia and osteitis fibrosa in adults, *Johns Hopkins Med. J.*, **72**:232, 1943.
3. Pappenheimer, A. M.: Effect of an experimental reduction of kidney substance upon parathyroid glands and skeletal tissue, *J. Exp. Med.*, **64**:965, 1936.
4. Pappenheimer, A. M., and S. L. Wilens: Enlargement of the parathyroid glands in renal disease, *Am. J. Pathol.*, **11**:73, 1937.

5. Stanbury, S. W., and G. A. Lumb: Metabolic studies of renal osteodystrophy: I. Calcium, phosphorus and nitrogen metabolism in rickets, osteomalacia and hyperparathyroidism complicating chronic uremia and the osteomalacia of the adult Fanconi syndrome, *Medicine (Baltimore)*, **41**:1, 1962.

6. Stanbury, S. W., and G. A. Lumb: Parathyroid function in chronic renal failure: A statistical survey of the plasma biochemistry in azotaemic renal osteodystrophy, *Q. J. Med.*, **35**:1, 1966.

7. Dent, C. E., C. N. Harper, and G. R. Philpot: Treatment of renal-glomerular osteodystrophy, *Q. J. Med.*, **30**:1, 1961.

8. Avioli, L. W., and S. L. Titelbaum: The renal osteodystrophies, in B. M. Brenner and F. C. Rector, Jr. (eds.), *The Kidney*, W. B. Saunders Company, Philadelphia, 1976, pp. 1542–1591.

9. Bronner, F. (ed.): Symposium on recent advances in vitamin D: Clinical implications, *Am. J. Clin. Nutr.*, **29**:1257–1329, 1976.

10. Massry, S. G., and J. W. Coburn: Divalent ion metabolism and renal osteodystrophy, in S. G. Massry and A. L. Sellers (eds.), *Clinical Aspects of Uremia and Dialysis*, Charles C Thomas, Publisher, Springfield, Ill., 1976, p. 304.

11. Coburn, J. W., and D. L. Hartenbower: Physiology of calcium, phosphorus and magnesium and disorders affecting their metabolism, in H. C. Gonick (ed.), *Current Nephrology*, vol. I, Pinecliff Medical Publishing Co., Pacific Palisades, Calif., 1977, pp. 99–171.

12. David, D. S. (ed.): *Calcium Metabolism in Renal Failure and Nephrolithiasis*, John Wiley & Sons, Inc., New York, 1977, 402 pp.

13. DeLuca, H. F.: Vitamin D endocrine system, *Adv. Clin. Chem.*, **19**:125–174, 1977.

14. Haussler, M. R., and T. A. McCain: Basic and clinical concepts related to vitamin D metabolism and action, *N. Engl. J. Med.*, **297**:974–983 and 1041–1050, 1977.

15. Norman, A. W., K. Schaefer, J. W. Coburn, H. F. DeLuca, D. Fraser, H. G. Grigoleit, and D. V. Herrath (eds.): *Vitamin D: Biochemical, Chemical and Clinical Aspects Related to Calcium Metabolism*, Walter de Gruyter & Co., Berlin, 1977, 973 pp.

16. Peacock, M. (ed.): The clinical uses of 1α-hydroxyvitamin D_3, *Clin. Endocrinol.*, **7**(suppl.):1s–246s, 1977.

17. Coburn, J. W., D. L. Hartenbower, and C. R. Kleeman: Divalent ion metabolism, in N. Freinkel (ed.), *The Year in Metabolism*, Plenum Publishing Corporation, New York, 1978, pp. 327–377.

18. Coburn, J. W., and F. Llach: Renal osteodystrophy and maintenance dialysis, in W. Drukker, F. M. Parsons, and J. F. Mater (eds.), *Renal Osteodystrophy and Maintenance Dialysis*, M. Nijhoff, The Hague, Netherlands, 1978, pp. 571–600.

19. DeLuca, H. F.: Vitamin D metabolism and function, *Arch. Intern. Med.*, **138**:836, 1978.

20. Massry, S. G., and E. Ritz: The pathogenesis of secondary hyperthyroidism of renal failure, *Arch. Intern. Med.*, **138**:853, 1978.

21. Slatopolsky, E., W. E. Rutherford, K. Hruska, K. Martin, and S. Klahr: How important is phosphate in the pathogenesis of renal osteodystrophy? *Arch. Intern. Med.*, **138**:848, 1978.

22. Reiss, E., J. M. Canterbury, and R. T. Bilinsky: Measurement of serum parathyroid hormone in renal insufficiency, *Trans. Assoc. Am. Physicians*, **81**:104, 1968.

23. Arnaud, C. D.: Hyperparathyroidism and renal failure, *Kidney Int.*, **4**:89, 1973.

24. Llach, F., S. G. Massry, F. R. Singer, K. Kurokawa, J. H. Kaye, and J. W. Coburn: Skeletal resistance of endogenous parathyroid hormone in patients with early renal failure: A possible cause for secondary hyperparathyroidism, *J. Clin. Endocrinol. Metab.*, **41**:338, 1975.

25. Slatopolsky, E., S. Caglar, J. P. Pennell, D. B. Taggart, J. M. Canterbury, E. Reiss, and N. S. Bricker: On the pathogenesis of hyperparathyroidism in chronic experimental renal insufficienty in the dog. *J. Clin. Invest.*, **50**:492, 1971.

26. Slatopolsky, E., S. Caglar, L. Gradowska, J. Canterbury, E. Reiss, and N. S. Bricker: On the prevention of secondary hyperparathyroidism in experimental chronic renal disease using "proportional reduction" of dietary phosphorus intake, *Kidney Int.*, **2**:147, 1972.

27. Slatopolsky, E., and N. Bricker: The role of phosphorus restriction in the prevention of secondary hyperparathyroidism in chronic renal disease, *Kidney Int.*, **4**:141, 1973.

28. Reiss, E., J. M. Canterbury, M. A. Bercowitz, and E. L. Kaplan: The role of phosphate in the secretion of parathyroid hormone in man, *J. Clin. Invest.*, **49**:2146, 1970.

29. LaFlame, G. H., and J. Jowsey: Bone and soft tissue changes with oral phosphate supplements, *J. Clin. Invest.*, **51**:2834, 1972.

30. Jowsey, J., E. Reiss, and J. M. Canterbury: Long term effects of high phosphate intake on parathyroid hormone levels and bone metabolism, *Acta Orthop. Scand.*, **45**:801, 1974.

31. Rutherford, W. E., P. Bordier, P. Marie, K. Hruska, H. Harter, A. Greenwalt, J. Blondin, J. Haddad, N. Bricker, and E. Slatopolsky: Phosphate control and 25-hydroxycholecalciferol administration in preventing experimental renal osteodystrophy in the dog, *J. Clin. Invest.*, **60**:332, 1977.

32. Fotino, S.: Phosphate excretion in chronic renal failure: Evidence for a mechanism other than circulating parathyroid hormone, *Clin. Nephrol.*, **8**:499, 1977.

33. Fournier, A. E., C. D. Arnaud, W. J. Johnson, W. F. Taylor, and R. S. Goldsmith: Etiology of hyperparathyroidism and bone disease during chronic hemodialysis: II. Factors affecting serum immuno-reactive parathyroid hormone, *J. Clin. Invest.*, **50**:599, 1971.

34. Coburn J. W., M. H. Koppel, A. S. Brickman, and S. G. Massry: Study of intestinal absorption of calcium in patients with renal failure, *Kidney Int.*, **3**:264, 1973.

35. Llach, F., S. G. Massry, A. Koffler, H. H. Malluche, F. R. Singer, A. S. Brickman, and K. Kurokawa: Secondary hyperparathyroidism (2° HPTISM) in early renal failure (ERF): Role of phosphate (P) retention. Proc. 10th Annu. Meet., Am. Soc. Nephrol., *Kidney Int.*, **12**:459, 1977.

36. Massry, S. G., E. Ritz, and R. Verberckmoes: Role of phosphate in the genesis of secondary hyperparathyroidism of renal failure, *Nephron*, **18**:77, 1977.

37. Kaplan, M. A., J. M. Canterbury, G. Gavellas, D. Jaffe, J. Bourgoignie, E. Reiss, and N. S. Bricker: Interrelations between phosphorus, calcium, parathyroid hormone, and renal phosphate excretion in response to an oral phosphorus load in normal and uremic dogs, *Kidney Int.*, **14**:20, 1978.

38. Tanaka, Y., and H. F. DeLuca: The control of 25-hydroxy-vitamin D metabolism by inorganic phosphorus, *Arch. Biochem. Biophys.*, **154**:566, 1973.

39. Goldman, R., and S. H. Bassett: Phosphorus excretion in renal failure, *J. Clin. Invest.*, **33**:1623, 1954.

40. Coburn, J. W., M. Popovtzer, S. G. Massry, and C. R. Kleeman: The physicochemical state and renal handling of divalent ions in chronic renal failure, *Arch. Intern. Med.*, **124**:302, 1969.

41. Liu, S. H., and H. I. Chu: Studies of calcium and phosphorus metabolism with special reference to pathogenesis and effects of dihydrotachysterol (A.T.10) and iron, *Medicine (Baltimore)*, **22**:103, 1943.

42. Kopple, J. D., and J. W. Coburn: Metabolic studies of low protein diets in uremia: II. Calcium, phosphorus and magnesium, *Medicine*, **52**:597, 1973.

43. Kaye, M., and M. Silverman: Calcium metabolism in chronic renal failure, *J. Lab. Clin. Med.*, **66**:535, 1965.

44. Ogg, C. S.: The intestinal absorption of ^{47}Ca by patients in chronic renal failure, *Clin. Sci.*, **34**:467, 1968.

45. Parker, T. F., P. Vergne-Marini, A. R. Hull, C. Y. C. Pak, and J. S. Fordtran: Jejunal absorption and secretion of calcium in patients with chronic renal disease on hemodialysis, *J. Clin. Invest.*, **54**:358, 1974.

46. Stanbury, S. W., G. A. Lumb, and E. B. Mawer: Osteodystrophy developing spontaneously in the course of chronic renal failure, *Arch. Intern. Med.*, **124**:274, 1969.

47. Fraser, D. R., and E. Kodicek: Unique biosynthesis by kidney of a biologically active vitamin D metabolite, *Nature*, **228**:764, 1970.

48. Gray, R., I. Boyle, and H. F. DeLuca: Vitamin D metabolism: The role of kidney tissue, *Science*, **172**:1232, 1971.

49. Norman, A. W., R. J. Midgett, J. F. Myrtle, and H. G. Nowicki: Studies on calciferol metabolism: I. Production of vitamin D metabolite 4B from 25-OH-cholecalciferol by kidney homogenates, *Biochem. Biophys. Res. Commun.*, **42**:1082, 1971.

50. Hartenbower, D. L., J. W. Coburn, C. R. Reddy, and A. W. Norman: Calciferol metabolism and

intestinal calcium transport in the chick with reduced renal function, *J. Lab. Clin. Med.*, **83**:38, 1974.

51. Mawer, E. B., J. Backhouse, and C. M. Taylor: Failure of formation of 1,25-dihydroxy-cholecalciferol in chronic renal insufficiency, *Lancet*, **1**:626, 1973.

52. Schaefer, K., D. von Herrath, and R. Stratz: Metabolism of 1,2 H^3-4-C^{14}-cholecalciferol in normal, uremic and anephric subjects, *Isr. J. Med. Sci.*, **8**:80, 1972.

53. Piel, C. F., B. S. Roof, and L. V. Avioli: Metabolism of tritiated 25-hydroxycholecalciferol in chronically uremic children before and after successful renal homotransplantation, *J. Clin. Endocrinol. Metab.*, **37**:944, 1973.

54. Gray, R. W., H. P. Weber, J. H. Dominguez, and J. Lemann, Jr.: The metabolism of vitamin D_3 and 25-hydroxy-vitamin D_3 in normal and anephric human, *J. Clin. Endocrinol. Metab.*, **39**:1045, 1974.

55. Brumbaugh, P. F., D. H. Haussler, R. Bressler, and M. R. Haussler: Radio-receptor assay for 1α,25-dihydroxy-vitamin D_3, *Science*, **183**:1089, 1974.

56. Haussler, M. R., D. J. Baylink, M. R. Hughes, P. F. Brumbaugh, J. E. Wergedal, F. H. Shen, R. L. Nielsen, S. J. Counts, K. M. Bursac, and T. A. McCain: The assay of 1-alpha,25-dihydroxy-vitamin D_3: Physiologic and pathologic modulation of circulating hormone levels, *Clin. Endocrinol.*, **5**:151s, 1976.

57. Hill, L. F., and S. W. Stanbury: Vitamin D and the kidney, *Nephron*, **15**:369, 1975.

58. Eisman, J. A., A. J. Hamstra, B. E. Kream, and H. F. DeLuca: 1,25-Dihydroxyvitamin D in biological fluids: A simplified and sensitive assay, *Science*, **193**:1021, 1976.

59. Wong, R. G., A. W. Norman, C. R. Reddy, and J. W. Coburn: Biological effects of 1,25-dihydroxycholecalciferol (a highly active vitamin D metabolite in acutely uremic rats, *J. Clin. Invest.*, **51**:1287, 1972,

60. Brickman, A. S., J. W. Coburn, and A. W. Norman: Action of 1,25-dihydroxycholecalciferol, a potent, kidney-produced metabolite of vitamin D_3, in uremic man, *N. Engl. J. Med.*, **287**:891, 1972.

61. Brickman, A. S., J. W. Coburn, S. G. Massry, and A. W. Norman: 1,25-Dihydroxy-vitamin D_3 in normal man and patients with renal failure, *Ann. Intern. Med.*, **80**:161, 1974.

62. Rutherford, W. E., J. Blondin, K. Hurska, R. Kopelman, S. Klahr, and E. Slatopolsky: Effect of 25-hydroxy-cholecalciferol on calcium absorption in chronic renal disease, *Kidney Int.*, **8**:320, 1975.

63. Colodro, I. H., A. S. Brickman, J. W. Coburn, J. W. Osborn, and A. W. Norman: Effect of 25-hydroxy-vitamin D_3 on intestinal absorption of calcium in normal man and patients with renal failure, *Metabolism*, **27**:745, 1968.

64. Brickman, A. S., J. W. Coburn, G. R. Friedman, W. H. Okamura, S. G. Massry, and A. W. Norman: Comparison of effects of 1α-hydroxy-vitamin D_3 and 1,25-dihydroxy-vitamin D_3 in man, *J. Clin. Invest.*, **57**:1540, 1976.

65. Avioli, L. V., L. Birge, S. W. Lee, and E. Slatopolsky: The metabolic fate of vitamin D_3 ^{3}H in chronic renal failure, *J. Clin. Invest.*, **47**:2239, 1968.

66. Russell, J. E., and L. V. Avioli: Effect of experimental chronic renal insufficiency on bone mineral and collagen maturation, *J. Clin. Invest.*, **51**:3072, 1972.

67. Lumb, G. A., E. B. Mawer, and S. W. Stanbury: The apparent vitamin D resistance of chronic renal failure: A study of the physiology of vitamin D in man, *Am. J. Med.*, **50**:421, 1971.

68. Mawer, E. B., G. A. Lumb, K. Schaeffer, and S. W. Stanbury: The metabolism of isotopically labeled vitamin D_3 in man: The influence of the state of vitamin D nutrition, *Clin. Sci.*, **40**:39, 1971.

69. Bayard, F., P. Bec, H. Ton That, and J. P. Louvet: Plasma 25-hydroxycholecalciferol in chronic renal failure, *Eur. J. Clin. Invest.*, **3**:447, 1973.

70. Offerman, G., D. von Herrath, and K. Schaefer: Serum 25-hydroxycholecalciferol in uremia, *Nephron*, **13**:269, 1974.

71. Shen, F. U., D. J. Baylink, D. J. Sherrard, L. Shen, N. A. Maloney, and J. E. Wergedal: Serum immunoreactive parathyroid hormone and 25-hydroxy-vitamin D in patients with uremic bone disease, *J. Clin. Endocrinol. Metabol.*, **40**:1009, 1975.

72. Eastwood, J. B., E. Harris, T. C. B. Stamp, and H. E. DeWardener: Vitamin-D deficiency in the osteomalacia of chronic renal failure, *Lancet*, **2**:1209, 1976.

73. Eastwood, J. B., T. C. Stamp, H. E. DeWardener, P. J. Bordier, and C. D. Arnaud: The effect of 25-hydroxyvitamin D_3 in osteomalacia of chronic renal failure, *Clin. Sci. Mol. Med.*, 52:499, 1977.

74. Henry, H. L., and A. W. Norman: Studies on the mechanism of action of calciferol: VII. Localization of 1,25-dihydroxyvitamin D_3 in chick parathyroid glands, *Biochem. Biophys. Res. Commun.*, 62:781, 1975.

75. Brumbaugh, P. F., M. R. Hughes, and M. R. Haussler: Cytoplasmic and nuclear binding components for 1-alpha,25-dihydroxyvitamin D_3 in chick parathyroid glands, *Proc. Natl. Acad. Sci. U.S.A.*, 72:4871, 1975.

76. Chertow, B. S., D. J. Baylink, J. E. Wergedal, M. H. H. Su, and A. W. Norman: Decrease in serum immunoreactive parathyroid hormone in rats and parathyroid hormone secretion in vitro by 1,25-dihydroxycholecalciferol, *J. Clin. Invest.*, 56:668, 1975.

77. Oldham, S. B., R. Smith, D. L. Hartenbower, H. L. Henry, A. W. Norman, and J. W. Coburn: The acute effects of 1,25-dihydroxycholecalciferol on serum immunoreactive parathyroid hormone in the dog, *Endocrinol.*, (in press) 1978.

78. Llach, F., J. W. Coburn, A. S. Brickman, K. Kurokawa, A. W. Norman, and E. Reiss: Acute actions of 1,25-dihydroxy-vitamin D_3 in normal man: Effect on calcium and parathyroid status, *J. Clin. Endocrinol. Metab.*, 44:1054, 1977.

79. Canterbury, J. M., S. Lerman, A. J. Claflin, H. Henry, A. W. Norman, and E. Reiss: Inhibition of parathyroid hormone secretion by 25-hydroxycholecalciferol and 24,25-dihydroxycholecalciferol in the dog, *J. Clin. Invest.*, 61:1375, 1977.

80. Stanbury, S. W., and G. A. Lumb: Parathyroid function in chronic vitamin D deficiency in man: A model for comparison with chronic renal failure, *Calcif. Tissue Res.*, 21(suppl.):185, 1976.

81. Stanbury, S. W.: The role of vitamin D in renal bone disease, *Clin. Endocrinol.*, 7(suppl.):255, 1977.

82. Slatopolsky, E., R. Gray, N. D. Adams, J. Lewis, K. Hruska, K. Martin, S. Klahr, H. DeLuca, and J. Lemann: Low serum levels of 1,25(OH)$_2$D$_3$ are not responsible for the development of secondary hyperparathyroidism in early renal failure (abstract), *Kidney Int.*, 14:000, 1978.

83. Recker, R. R., and P. D. Saville: Calcium absorption in renal failure: Its relationship to blood urea nitrogen, dietary calcium intake, time on dialysis, and other variables, *J. Lab. Clin. Med.*, 78:380, 1971.

84. Oettinger, C. W., R. Merrill, T. Blanton, and W. Briggs: Reduced calcium absorption after nephrectomy in uremic patients, *N. Engl. J. Med.*, 291:458, 1975.

85. Bordier, P. J., S. Tun-Chot, J. B. Eastwood, A. Fournier, and H. E. De Wardener: Lack of histological evidence of vitamin D abnormality in the bones of anephric patients, *Clin. Sci.*, 44:33, 1973.

86. Evanson, J. M.: The response to the infusion of parathyroid extract in hypocalcemic states, *Clin. Sci.*, 31:63, 1966.

87. Massry, S. G., J. W. Coburn, D. B. N. Lee, J. Joswey, and C. R. Kleeman: Skeletal resistance to parathyroid hormone in renal failure: Study in 105 human subjects, *Ann. Intern. Med.*, 78:357, 1973.

88. Kaplan, M. A., J. M. Canterbury, D. Jaffe, G. Gavellas, J. Bourgoignie, E. Reiss, and N. S. Bricker: Effect of dietary phosphorus (P) on the phosphaturic and calciuric responses to parathyroid hormone (PTH) in the uremic dog (abstract), *Kidney Int.*, 12:457 1977.

89. Massry, S. G., R. Stein, J. Garty, A. I. Arieff, J. W. Coburn, A. W. Norman, and R. M. Friedler: Skeletal resistance to the calcemic action of parathyroid hormone in uremia: Role of 1,25(OH)$_2$D$_3$, *Kidney Int.*, 9:467–474, 1976.

90. Somerville, P. J., and M. Kaye: Resistance to parathyroid hormone in renal failure: Role of vitamin D metabolites, *Kidney Int.*, 14:245, 1978.

91. Somerville, P. J., and M. Kaye: Parathyroid resistance in acute renal failure is caused by phosphate retention, *Abstr. 7th Int. Congr. Nephrol.*, *Montreal*, June 18–23, 1978, p. E3.

92. Wills, M. R., and M. V. Jenkins: The effect of uremic metabolites on parathyroid extract-induced bone resorption in vitro, *Clin. Chim. Acta*, 73:121, 1976.

93. Berson, S. A., and R. S. Yalow: Immunochemical heterogeneity of parathyroid hormone in plasma, *J. Clin. Endocrinol.*, 28:1037, 1968.

94. Arnaud, C. D.: Parathyroid hormone: Coming of age in clinical medicine, *Am. J. Med.*, 55:577, 1973.

95. Habener, J. F., and J. T. Potts, Jr.: Biosynthesis of parathyroid hormone, *N. Engl. J. Med.,* **299:**580–585 and 635–644, 1978.

96. Silverman, R., and R. S. Yalow: Heterogeneity of parathyroid hormone: Clinical and physiologic implications, *J. Clin. Invest.,* **52:**1958, 1973.

97. Flueck, J. A., F. P. Di Bella, A. J. Edis, J. M. Kehrwald, and C. D. Arnaud: Immunoheterogeneity of parathyroid hormone in venous effluent serum from hyperfunctioning parathyroid glands, *J. Clin. Invest.,* **60:**1367, 1977.

98. Habener, J. F., D. Powell, T. M. Murray, G. P. Mayer, and J. T. Potts, Jr.: Parathyroid hormone: Secretion and metabolism, in vivo, *Proc. Natl. Acad. Sci. U.S.A.,* **68:**2986, 1971.

99. Catherwood, B. D., R. M. Friedler, and F. R. Singer: Sites of clearance of endogenous parathyroid hormone in the vitamin D-deficient dog, *Endocrinology,* **98:**228, 1976.

100. Martin, K., K. Hruska, A. Greenwalt, S. Klahr, and E. Slatopolsky: Selective uptake of intact parathyroid hormone by the liver: Differences between hepatic and renal uptake, *J. Clin. Invest.,* **58:**781, 1976.

101. Hruska, K. A., R. Kopelman, W. E. Rutherford, S. Klahr, and E. Slatopolsky: Metabolism of immunoreactive parathyroid hormone in the dog: The role of the kidney and the effects of chronic renal disease, *J. Clin. Invest.,* **56:**39, 1975.

102. Hruska, K. A., K. Martin, P. Mennes, A. Greenwalt, C. Anderson, S. Klahr, and E. Slatopolsky: Degradation of parathyroid hormone and fragment production by the isolated perfused dog kidney: The effect of glomerular filtration rate and perfusate Ca⁻⁻ concentrations, *J. Clin. Invest.,* **60:**501, 1977.

103. Martin, K. J., K. A. Hruska, J. Lewis, C. Anderson, and E. Slatopolsky: The renal handling of parathyroid hormone: Role of peritubular uptake and glomerular filtration, *J. Clin. Invest.,* **60:**808, 1977.

104. Melick, R. A., and T. J. Martin: Parathyroid hormone metabolism in man: Effect of nephrectomy, *Clin. Sci.,* **37:**667, 1969.

105. Massry, S. G., J. W. Coburn, M. Peacock, and C. R. Kleeman: Turnover of endogenous parathyroid hormone in uremic patients and those undergoing hemodialysis, *Trans. Am. Soc. Artif. Intern. Organs,* **18:**416, 1972.

106. Freitag, J., K. J. Martin, K. A. Hruska, C. Anderson, M. Conrades, J. Ladenson, S. Klahr, and E. Slatopolsky: Impaired parathyroid hormone metabolism in patients with chronic renal failure, *N. Engl. J. Med.,* **298:**29, 1978.

107. Papapoulos, S. E., G. N. Hendy. S. Tomlinson, I. G. Lewin, and J. L. H. O'Riordan: Clearance of exogenous parathyroid hormone in normal and uraemic man, *Clin. Endocrinol.,* **7:**211, 1977.

108. Goldsmith, R. S., J. Furszyfer, W. J. Johnson, A. E. Fournier, G. W. Sizemore, and C. D. Arnaud: Etiology of hyperparathyroidism and bone disease during chronic hemodialysis: III. Evaluation of parathyroid suppressibility, *J. Clin. Invest.,* **52:**173, 1973.

109. Vergne-Marini, P., T. F. Parker, C. Y. C. Pak, A. R. Hull, H. F. DeLuca, and J. S. Fordiran: Jejunal and ileal calcium absorption in patients with chronic renal disease: Effect of lα-hydroxycholecalciferol, *J. Clin. Invest.,* **57:**861, 1976.

110. Sherrard, D. J., D. J. Baylink, J. E. Wergedal, and N. Maloney: Quantitative histological studies on the pathogenesis of uremic bone disease, *J. Clin. Endocrinol.,* **39:**119, 1974.

111. Ritz, E., H. H. Malluche, B. Krempien, and O. Mehls: Bone histology in renal insufficiency, in David S. David (ed.), *Perspectives in Nephrology and Hypertension,* John Wiley & Sons, Inc., New York, 1977, pp. 197–233.

112. Schmidt-Gayk, H., W. Schmitt, C. Grawuner, E. Ritz, W. Tschöpe, V. Pietsch, K. Andrassy, and R. Bouillon: 25-Hydroxy-vitamin D in nephrotic syndrome, *Lancet,* **2:**105, 1977.

113. Barragry, J. M., M. W. France, N. D. Carter, J. A. Auton, M. Beer, B. J. Boucher, and R. D. Cohen: Vitamin-D metabolism in nephrotic syndrome, *Lancet,* **2:**629, 1977.

114. Kanis, J. A., T. Cundy, M. Bartlett, R. Smith, G. Heynen, G. T. Warner, and R. G. G. Russell: Is 24,25-dihydroxycholecalciferol a calcium regulating hormone in man? *Brit. Med. J.,* **1:**1382, 1978.

115. Bordier, P., H. Rasmussen, P. Marie, L. Miravet, J. Gueris, and A. Ryckwaert: Vitamin D metabolites and bone mineralization in man, *J. Clin. Endocrinol. Metab.,* **46:**284, 1978.

116. Kanis, J. A., N. D. Adams, M. Earnshaw, G.

Heynen, J. G. G. Ledingham, D. O. Oliver, R. G. G. Russell, and C. G. Woods: Vitamin D, osteomalacia and chronic renal failure, in A. W. Norman, K. Schaefer, J. W. Coburn, H. F. De-Luca, D. Fraser, H. G. Grigoleit, and D. von Herrath (eds.), *Vitamin D: Biochemical, Chemical and Clinical Aspects Related to Calcium Metabolism*, Walter de Gruyter & Co., Berlin, 1977, pp. 671–673.

117. Russell, J. E., J. D. Termine, and L. V. Avioli: Abnormal bone mineral maturation in the chronic uremic state, *J. Clin. Invest.*, **52**:2848, 1973.

118. Mechanic, G. L., S. U. Toverud, and W. K. Ramp: Quantitative changes of bone collagen cross-links and precursors in vitamin D deficiency, *Biochem. Biophys. Res. Commun.*, **47**:760, 1972.

119. Russell, J. E., L. V. Avioli, and G. Mechanic: The nature of the collagen cross-links in bone in the chronic uraemic state, *Biochem. J.*, **145**:119, k975.

120. Russell, J. E., and L. V. Avioli: Twenty-five hydroxycholecalciferol-enhanced bone maturation in the parathyroprivic state, *J. Clin. Invest.*, **56**:792, 1975.

121. Pellegrino, E. D., and R. M. Biltz: The composition of human bone in uremia, *Medicine,* **44**:397, 1965.

122. Burnell, J. M., E. Teubner, J. E. Wergedal, and D. J. Sherrard: Bone crystal maturation in renal osteodystrophy in humans, *J. Clin. Invest.*, **32**:52, 1974.

123. Alfrey, A. C., N. L. Miller, and D. Butkus: Evaluation of body magnesium stores, *J. Lab. Clin. Med.*, **84**:153, 1974.

124. Alfrey, A. C., and C. C. Solomons: Bone pyrophosphate in uremia and its association with extraosseous calcification, *J. Clin. Invest.*, **57**:700, 1976.

125. Termine, J. D., and A. S. Posner: Amorphous/crystalline interrelationships in bone mineral, *Calcif. Tissue Res.*, **1**:8, 1967.

126. Alfrey, A. C., C. C. Solomons, J. Ciricillo, and N. L. Miller: Extraosseous calcification: Evidence for abnormal pyrophosphate metabolism in uremia, *J. Clin. Invest.*, **57**:692, 1976.

127. Kaye, M.: Magnesium metabolism in the rat with chronic renal failure, *J. Lab. Clin. Med.*, **84**:536, 1974.

128. Goodman, A. D., J. Lemann, Jr., E. J. Lennon,

and A. S. Relman: Production, excretion and net balance of fixed acid in patients with renal acidosis, *J. Clin. Invest.*, **44**:495, 1965.

129. Litzow, J. R., J. Leann, Jr., and E. J. Lennon: The effect of treatment of acidosis on calcium balance in patients with chronic azotemic renal disease, *J. Clin. Invest.*, **46**:280, 1967.

130. Nichols, G., Jr., and N. Nichols: Effect of parathyroidectomy on content and availability of skeletal sodium in the rat, *Am. J. Physiol.*, **198**:749 1960.

131. Pellegrino, E. D., R. M. Biltz, and J. M. Letteri: Interrelationships of carbonate, phosphate, monohydrogen phosphate, calcium, magnesium and sodium in uraemic bone: Comparison of dialyzed and non-dialyzed patients, *Clin. Sci. Mol. Biol.*, **53**:307, 1977.

132. Kaye, M., A. J. Fruch, M. Silverman, J. Henderson, and T. Thibault: A study of vertebral bone powder from patients with chronic renal failure, *J. Clin. Invest.*, **49**:442, 1970.

133. Stanbury, S. W.: Bone disease in uremia, *Am. J. Med.*, **44**:714, 1968.

134. Barzel, U. S., and J. Jowsey: The effects of chronic acid and alkali administration on bone turnover in adult rats, *Clin. Sci.*, **36**:517, 1969.

135. Burnell, J. M., E. J. Teubner, and A. G. Miller: Acid-base chemistry and human bone, in *Proc. 10th Annu. Contractors' Conf. Artif. Kidney Program, Natl. Inst. Arthritis, Metab. Digest. Dis.*, U.S. Dept. HEW (NIH 77-1442), Bethesda, Md., 1977, pp. 35–37.

136. Heynen, G., and P. Franchimont: Human calcitonin radioimmunoassay in normal and pathologic conditions, *Eur. J. Clin. Invest.*, **4**:213, 1974.

137. Isaac, R., P. Nivez, G. Piamba, J. P. Fillastre, and R. Ardaillou: Influence of calcium infusion on calcitonin and parathyroid hormone concentration in normal and hemodialyzed patients, *Clin. Nephrol.*, **3**:14, 1975.

138. Lee, J. C., J. G. Parthemore, and L. J. Deftos: Immunochemical heterogeneity of calcitonin in renal failure, *J. Clin. Endocrinol. Metab.*, **45**:528, 1977.

139. Heynen, G., J. A. Kanis, D. Oliver, and M. Earnshaw: Evidence that endogenous calcitonin protects against renal bone disease, *Lancet,* **2**:1322, 1976.

140. Kanis, J. A., M. Earnshaw, G. Heynen, R. G. G. Russell, and C. G. Woods: The possible role of calcitonin deficiency in the development of bone disease due to chronic renal failure, *Calcif. Tissue Res.*, **22**(suppl.):147, 1977.

140a. Kanis, J. A., M. Earnshaw, G. Heynen, R. G. G. Russell, and C. G. Woods: The possible role of calcitonin deficiency in the development of bone disease due to chronic renal failure, *Calcif. Tissue Res.*, **22**(suppl.):147, 1977.

141. Kanis, J. A., M. Earnshaw, G. Heynen, J. G. G. Ledingham, D. O. Oliver, R. G. G. Russell, C. G. Woods, P. Franchmont, and S. Gaspar: Changes in histological and biochemical indexes of bone turnover after bilateral nephrectomy in patients on hemodialysis: Evidence for a possible role of endogenous calcitonin, *N. Eng. J. Med.*, **19**:1073, 1977.

142. Duursma, S. A., W. J. Visser, and L. Njio: A quantitative histological study of bone in 30 patients with renal insufficiency, *Calcif. Tissue Res.*, **9**:216, 1972.

143. Ellis, H. A., and K. M. Peart: Azotaemic renal osteodystrophy, a quantitative study on iliac bone, *J. Clin. Pathol.*, **26**:83, 1973.

144. Bordier, P. J., P. J. Marie, and C. D. Arnaud: Evolution of renal osteodystrophy: Correlation of bone histomorphometry and serum mineral and immunoreactive parathyroid hormone values before and after treatment with calcium carbonate or 25-hydroxycholecalciferol, *Kidney Int.*, **7**:S-102, 1975.

145. Delling, G., A. Schulz, and W. Schulz: Morphologische klassifikation der renden osteopathic, *Mels. Med. Met.*, **49**:133, 1975.

146. Teitelbaum, S. L., J. M. Bone, P. M. Stein, J. J. Gilden, M. Bates, V. C. Boisseau, and L. V. Avioli: Calcifediol in chronic renal insufficiency: Skeletal response, *JAMA*, **235**:164, 1976.

147. Malluche, H. H., E. Ritz, H. P. Lange, D. Arras, and W. Schoeppe: Bone mass in maintenance haemodialysis: Prospective study with sequential biopsies, *Eur. J. Clin. Invest.*, **6**:265, 1976.

148. Ball, J., and A. Garner: Mineralisation of woven bone in osteomalacia, *J. Pathol. Bacteriol.*, **91**:563, 1966.

149. Bordier, P. J., and S. Tun-Chot: Quantitative histology of metabolic bone disease, *Clin. Endocrinol. Metab.*, **1**:197, 1972.

150. Frost, H. M.: The dynamics of human osteoid tissue, in D. J. Hioco (ed.), *L'ostéomalacie*, Masson & Cie, Paris, 1967, pp. 3–18.

151. Malluche, H. H., E. Ritz, H. P. Lange, J. Kutschera, M. Hodgson, U. Seiffert, and W. Schoeppe: Bone histology in incipient and advanced renal failure, *Kidney Int.*, **9**:355, 1976.

152. Coburn, J. W., A. S. Brickman, D. J. Sherrard, F. R. Singer, D. J. Baylink, E. G. C. Wong, S. G. Massry, and A. W. Norman: Clinical efficacy of 1,25-di-hydroxy-vitamin D_3 in renal osteodystrophy, in A. W. Norman, K. Schaefer, J. W. Coburn, H. F. DeLuca, D. Fraser, H. G. Grigoleit, and D. von Herrath (eds.), *Vitamin D: Biochemical, Chemical and Clinical Aspects Related to Calcium Metabolism*, Walter de Gruyter & Co., Berlin, 1977, pp. 657–666.

153. Ellis, H. A., A. M. Pierides, T. G. Feest, M. K. Ward, and D. N. S. Kerr: Histopathology of renal osteodystrophy with particular reference to the effects of 1α-hydroxyvitamin D_3 in patients treated by long-term haemodialysis, *Clin. Endocrinol.*, **7**(suppl.):31S, 1977.

154. Berlyne, G. M., J. Ben-Arie, N. Epstein, E. M. Booth, and R. Yagil: Rarity of renal osteodystrophy in Israel due to low phosphorus intake: A natural experiment, *Nephron*, **10**:141, 1973.

155. Maschio, G., E. Bonucci, G. Mioni, A. D'Angelo, E. Ossi, E. Valvo, and A. Lupo: Biochemical and morphological aspects of bone tissue in chronic renal failure, *Nephron*, **12**:437, 1974.

156. Fiaschi, E., E. Maschio, A. D'Angelo, E. Bonucci, N. Tessitore, and P. Messa: Low-protein diets and bone disease in chronic renal failure, *Kidney Int.*, **12**(suppl. 8):S79, 1978.

157. Neer, R., M. Clark, V. Friedman, R. Belsey, M. Sweeney, J. Buonchristiani, and J. Potts, Jr.: Environmental and nutritional influences on plasma 25-hydroxy vitamin D concentration and calcium metabolism in man, in A. W. Norman, K. Schaefer, J. W. Coburn, H. F. DeLuca, D. Fraser, H. G. Grigoleit, and D. von Herrath (eds.), *Vitamin D: Biochemical, Chemical, and Clinical Aspects Related to Calcium Metabolism*, Walter de Gruyter & Co., Berlin, 1977, pp. 595–606.

158. Baker, L. R. N., P. Ackrill, W. R. Cattell, C. B.

Stamp, and L. Watson: Iatrogenic osteomalacia and myopathy due to phosphate depletion, *Br. Med. J.*, **3:**150, 1974.

159. Ahmed, K. Y., Z. Vargese, M. R. Wills, E. Meinhard, R. K. Skinner, R. A. Baillad, and J. F. Moorhead: Persistent hypophosphatemia and osteomalacia in dialysis patients not on oral phosphate binders: Response to dihydrotachysterol therapy, *Lancet*, **2:**439 1976.

160. Pierides, A. M., H. A. Ellis, W. Simpson, J. H. Dewar, M. K. Ward, and D. N. S. Kerr: Variable response to long-term 1α-hydroxycholecalciferol in haemodialysis osteodystrophy, *Lancet*, **1:**1092, 1976.

161. Coburn, J. W., A. S. Brickman, D. J. Sherrard, E. G. C. Wong, F. R. Singer, and A. W. Norman: Defective skeletal mineralization in uremia without relation to vitamin D, serum calcium or phosphorus (abstract), *Kidney Int.*, **12:**455, 1977.

162. Kerr, D. N. S., J. Walls, H. Ellis, W. Simpson, P. R. Uldall, and M. K. Ward: Bone disease in patients undergoing regular haemodialysis, *J. Bone J. Surg.*, **51B:**578, 1969.

163. Siddiqui, J. Y., W. Simpson, H. A. Ellis, and D. N. S. Kerr: Serum fluoride in chronic renal failure, *Proc. Eur. Dial. Transplant Assoc.*, **7:**110, 1970.

164. Pierides, A. M., H. A. Ellis, M. Ward, W. Simpson, K. M. Peart, F. Alvarez-Ude, P. R. Uldall, and D. N. S. Kerr: Barbiturate and anticonvulsant treatment in relation to osteomalacia with haemodialysis and renal transplantation, *Br. Med. J.*, **1:**190, 1976.

165. Pierides, A. M., H. A. Ellis, M. K. Ward, P. Aljama, J. Dewar, and D. N. S. Kerr: The need and use of a phosphate-enriched dialysate during regular hemodialysis, *Trans. Am. Soc. Artif. Intern. Organs*, **23:**376, 1977.

166. Ward, M. K., T. G. Feest, H. A. Ellis, I. S. Parkinson, D. N. S. Kerr, J. Herrington, and G. L. Goode: Osteomalacic dialysis osteodystrophy: Evidence for a water-borne aetiological agent, probably aluminum, *Lancet*, **1:**841, 1978.

167. Weeke, E., and T. H. Friis: Serum fractions of calcium and phosphorus in uremia, *Acta Med. Scand.*, **189:**79, 1971.

168. Stanbury, S. W.: The phosphate ion in chronic renal failure, in D. J. Hioco (ed.), *Phosphate In-organique, Biologie et Physiopathologie, Int. Symp.*, Sandoz, Paris, 1970, pp. 187–208.

169. Coburn, J. W., D. L. Hartenbower, A. S. Brinkman, S. G. Massry, and J. D. Kopple: Intestinal absorption of calcium, magnesium, and phosphorus in chronic renal insufficiency, in D. S. David (ed.), *Calcium Metabolism in Renal Failure and Nephrolithiasis*, John Wiley & Sons, Inc., New York, 1977, pp. 77–109.

170. Caniggia, A., and C. Gennari: Intestinal absorption of radiophosphate after physiologic doses of 25(OH)D$_3$ in normals, liver cirrhosis and chronic renal failure patients, in A. W. Norman, K. Schaefer, J. W. Coburn, H. F. DeLuca, D. Fraser, H. G. Grigoleit, and D. von Herrath (eds.), *Vitamin D: Biochemical, Chemical and Clinical Aspects Related to Calcium Metabolism*, Walter de Gruyter & Co., Berlin, 1977, pp. 755–757.

171. Walling, M. W.: Intestinal calcium and phosphate transport: Differential responses to vitamin D$_3$ metabolites, *Am. J. Physiol.*, **233:**E488, 1977.

172. Kluthe, R., D. Oechslen, H. Quirin, and H. J. Jesdinsky: Six years' experience with a special low-protein diet, in R. G. Kluthe, G. Berlyne, and B. Burton, *Uremia, An International Conference on Pathogenesis, Diagnosis and Therapy*, Georg Thieme Verlag, Stuttgart, 1972, p. 250.

173. Rutherford, E., A. Mercado, K. Hruska, H. Harter, N. Mason, R. Sparks, S. Klahr, and E. Slatopolsky: An evaluation of a new and effective phosphorus binding agent, *Trans. Am. Soc. Artif. Intern. Organs*, **19:**446, 1973.

174. Clarkson, E. M., V. A. Luch, W. V. Hynson, R. R. Bailey, J. B. Eastwood, J. S. Woodhead, V. R. Clements, J. L. H. Oriordan, and H. E. De Wardener: The effect of aluminum hydroxide on calcium, phosphorus and aluminum balances, the serum parathyroid hormone concentration and the aluminium content of bone in patients with chronic renal failure, *Clin. Sci.*, **43:**519, 1972.

175. Massry, S. G., J. W. Coburn, M. M. Popovtzer, J. H. Shinaberger, M. H. Maxwell, and C. R. Kleeman: Secondary hyperparathyroidism in chronic renal failure: The clinical spectrum in uremia, during hemodialysis and after renal transplantation, *Arch. Intern. Med. (Chicago)*, **124:**431, 1969.

176. Walling, M. W., and D. V. Kimberg: Effects of 1-alpha,25-dihydroxy-vitamin D$_3$ and solanum

glaucophyllum on intestinal calcium and phosphate transport and on plasma Ca, Mg, and P levels in the rat, *Endocrinology*, **97**:1567, 1975.

177. Brickman, A. S., D. L. Hartenbower, A. W. Norman, and J. W. Coburn: Actions of 1α-hydroxy-vitamin D₃ and 1,25-dihydroxy-vitamin D₃ on mineral metabolism in man. I. Effects on net absorption of phosphorus, *Am. J. Clin. Nutr.*, **30**:1064, 1977.

177a. Coburn, J. W., A. S. Brickman, D. L. Hartenbower, and A. W. Norman: Intestinal phosphate absorption in normal and uremic man: Effects of 1,25(OH)₂-vitamin D₃ and 1α(OH)-vitamin D₃, in S. G. Massry and E. Ritz (eds.), *Phosphate Metabolism*, Plenum Press, New York, 1977, pp. 549–557.

178. Birge, S. J., and J. G. Haddad: 25-Hydroxycholecalciferol stimulation of muscle metabolism, *J. Clin. Invest.*, **56**:1100, 1975.

179. Coburn, J. W., A. S. Brickman, and S. G. Massry: Medical treatment in primary and secondary hyperparathyroidism, *Semin. Drug Treat.*, **2**:117, 1972.

180. Shah, S., C. Cruz, and W. Castillo: Persistent hypophosphatemia in patients on chronic hemodialysis without phosphate binding gels (abstract), *Kidney Int.*, **10**:526, 1976.

181. Hill, A. V. L., F. Alvarez-Ude, A. M. Pierides, D. N. S. Kerr, H. A. Ellis, and K. M. Peart: The effects of calcium carbonate, aluminum hydroxide and dihydrotachysterol on haemodialysis bone disease, in A. W. Norman, K. Schaefer, H. V. Grigoleit, D. von Herrath, and E. Ritz (eds.), *Vitamin D and Problems Related to Uremic Bone Disease*, Walter de Gruyter & Co., Berlin, 1975, pp. 643–650.

182. Bishop, M. C., J. G. G. Ledingham, and D. O. Oliver: Phosphate deficiency in haemodialysed patients, *Proc. Eur. Dial. Transplant Assoc.*, **8**:106, 1971.

183. Letteri, J. M., K. J. Ellis, D. P. Orofino, S. Ruggieri, S. N. Asad, and S. H. Cohn: Altered calcium metabolism in chronic renal failure, *Kidney Int.*, **6**:45, 1974.

184. Ibels, L. S., A. C. Alfrey, L. Hand, and W. E. Huffer: Preservation of function in experimental renal disease by dietary restriction of phosphate, *N. Engl. J. Med.*, **298**:122, 1978.

185. Kuzela, D. C., W. E. Huffer, J. D. Conger, S. D. Winter, and W. S. Hammond: Soft tissue calcification in chronic dialysis patients, *Am. J. Pathol.*, **86**:403, 1977.

186. Collier, V. U., W. Mitch, and M. Walser: The effect of spontaneous or induced lowering of plasma Ca × P product on progression of chronic renal failure, *Clin. Res.*, **26**:564A, 1978.

187. Christiansen, C., P. Rødbro, M. S. Christensen, B. Hartnack, and I. Transbøl: Deterioration of renal function during treatment of chronic renal failure with 1,25-dihydroxycholecalciferol, *Lancet*, **2**:700, 1978.

188. Walser, M.: The separate effects of hyperparathyroidism, hypercalcemia of malignancy, renal failure and acidosis on the state of calcium, phosphate and other ions in plasma, *J. Clin. Invest.*, **41**:1454, 1962.

189. Raman, A., Y. K. Chong, and G. A. Sreenevasan: Effects of varying dialysate calcium concentration on the plasma calcium fractions in patients on dialysis, *Nephron*, **16**:181, 1976.

190. Goldstein, D. A., Y. Oda, K. Kurokawa, and S. G. Massry: Blood levels of 25-hydroxy-vitamin D in nephrotic syndrome: Studies in 26 patients, *Ann. Int. Med.*, **87**:664, 1977.

191. Wing, A. J., J. R. Curtis, J. B. Eastwood, E. K. M. Smith, and H. E. DeWardener: Transient and persistent hypercalcaemia in patients treated by maintenance haemodialysis, *Br. Med. J.*, **4**:150, 1968.

192. Burnell, J. M., and E. Teubner: Effects of decreasing magnesium in patients with chronic renal failure, *Proc. Clin. Dial. Transplant Forum*, **5**:191, 1976.

193. Regan, R. J., M. Peacock, S. M. Rosen, P. J. Robinson, and A. Horsman: Effect of dialysate calcium concentration on bone disease in patients on hemodialysis, *Kidney Int.*, **10**:246, 1976.

194. Papadimitriou, M., J. C. Gingell, and G. D. Chisholm: Hypercalcemia from calcium ion-exchange resins in patients on regular hemodialysis, *Lancet*, **2**:948, 1968.

195. Koppel, M. H., S. G. Massry, J. H. Shinaberger, D. L. Hartenbower, and J. W. Coburn: Thiazide induced rise in serum calcium and magnesium in patients on maintenance hemodialysis, *Ann. Intern. Med.*, **72**:895, 1970.

196. Brannan, P. G., P. Vergne-Marini, C. Y. C. Pak, A. R. Hull, and J. S. Fordiran: Magnesium absorption in the human small intestine: Results in patients with absorptive hypercalciuria, *J. Clin. Invest.*, **57**:1412, 1976.

197. Freeman, R. M.: The role of magnesium in the pathogenesis of azotemic hypothermia, *Proc. Soc. Exp. Biol. Med.*, **137**:1069, 1971.

198. Freeman, R. M., R. L. Lawton, and M. A. Chamberlain: Hard-water syndrome, *N. Engl. J. Med.*, **276**:1113, 1967.

199. Massry, S. G., J. W. Coburn, and C. R. Kleeman: Evidence for suppression of parathyroid gland by hypermagnesemia, *J. Clin. Invest.*, **49**:1619, 1970.

200. Habener, J. F., and J. T. Potts, Jr.: Relative effectiveness of magnesium and calcium on the secretion and biosynthesis of parathyroid hormone in vitro, *Endocrinology*, **98**:197, 1976.

200a. Pletka, P., D. S. Bernstein, C. L. Hampers, J. P. Merrill, and L. M. Sherwood: Effects of magnesium on parathyroid hormone secretion during chronic hemodialysis, *Lancet*, **2**:462, 1971.

201. Randall, R. E., Jr., M. D. Cohen, C. C. Spray, Jr., and E. C. Rassmeisl: Hypermagnesemia in renal failure: Etiology and toxic manifestations, *Ann. Intern. Med.*, **61**:73, 1964.

202. Mennes, P., R. Rosenbaum, K. Martin, and E. Slatopolsky: Hypomagnesemia and impaired parathyroid hormone secretion in chronic renal disease, *Ann. Intern. Med.*, **88**:206, 1978.

203. Naik, R. B., P. Gosling, and C. P. Price: Comparative study of alkaline phosphatase isoenzymes, bone histology, and skeletal radiography in dialysis bone disease, *Br. Med. J.*, **1**:1307, 1977.

204. Skillen, A. W., and A. M. Pierides: Serum alkaline phosphatase isoenzyme patterns in patients with chronic renal failure, *Clin. Chim. Acta*, **80**:339, 1977.

205. Alvarez-Ude, F., T. G. Feest, M. K. Ward, A. M. Pierides, H. A. Ellis, K. M. Peart, W. Simpson, D. Weightman, and D. N. S. Kerr: Hemodialysis bone disease: Correlation between chemical, histologic, and other findings, *Kidney Int.*, **14**:68, 1978.

206. Ritz, E., H. Malluche, J. Bommer, O. Mehls, and B. Krempien: Metabolic bone disease in patients on maintenance hemodialysis, *Nephron*, **12**:393, 1974.

207. Duursma, S. A., R. G. van Kesteren, W. J. Visser, J. M. M. Roelofs, and J. A. Raymakers: Serum alkaline phosphatase: Its relation to bone cells and its significance as an indicator for vitamin D treatment in patients with renal insufficiency, in A. W. Norman, K. Schaefer, H. G. Grigoleit, D. von Herrath, and E. Ritz, *Vitamin D and Problems Related to Uremic Bone Disease*, Walter de Gruyter & Co., Berlin, 1975, pp. 167–171.

208. Prockop, D. J., and K. I. Kivirikko: Relationship of hydroxyproline excretion in urine to collagen metabolism, *Ann. Intern. Med.*, **66**:1243, 1967.

209. Kowalewski, J., J. Tomaszewski, J. Hanzlik, H. Sawislak, and A. Zbikowska: The elimination of free, peptide-bound and protein-bound hydroxyproline into dialysate during peritoneal dialysis in patients with renal failure, *Clin. Chim. Acta*, **34**:123, 1971.

210. Henderson, R. G., R. G. G. Russell, J. G. G. Ledingham, R. Smith, D. O. Oliver, R. J. Walton, D. G. Small, C. Preston, G. T. Warner, and A. W. Norman: Effects of 1,25-dihydroxycholecalciferol on calcium absorption, muscle weakness, and bone disease in chronic renal failure, *Lancet*, **1**:379, 1974.

211. Varghese, Z., J. F. Moorhead, R. A. Baillod, and M. R. Wills: Plasma hydroxyproline in renal osteodystrophy, *Proc. Eur. Dial. Transplant Assoc.*, **10**:187, 1973.

212. Hart, W., S. A. Duursma, W. J. Visser, and L. K. F. Njio: The hydroxyproline content of plasma of patients with impaired renal function, *Clin. Nephrol.*, **4**:104, 1975.

213. Hamet, P., D. A. Stouder, H. Z. Ginn, J. G. Hardman, and G. W. Liddle: Studies of the elevated extracellular concentration of cyclic AMP in uremic man, *J. Clin. Invest.*, **56**:339, 1975.

214. Glassford, D. M., A. R. Remmers, Jr., H. E. Sarles, J. D. Lindley, M. T. Scurry, and J. C. Fish: Hyperparathyroidism in the maintenance dialysis patient, *Surg. Gynecol. Obstet.*, **142**:328, 1976.

215. Mayer, G. P., J. F. Habener, and J. T. Potts, Jr.: Parathyroid hormone secretion in vivo: Demonstration of a calcium-independent non-suppressible component of secretion, *J. Clin. Invest.*, **57**:678, 1976.

216. Popovtzer, M. M., S. G. Massry, D. L. Makoff, M. H. Maxwell, and C. R. Kleeman: Renal han-

dling of phosphate in patients with chronic renal failure: The role of variations in serum phosphorus and parathyroid activity, *Isr. J. Med. Sci.*, **5**:1018, 1969.

217. Slatopolsky, E., W. E. Rutherford, F. H. Hoffsten, I. O. Elkan, H. R. Butcher, and N. S. Bricker: Non-suppressible secondary hyperparathyroidism in chronic progressive renal disease, *Kidney Int.*, **1**:38, 1972.

218. Smith, R., and G. Stern: Myopathy, osteomalacia and hyperparathyroidism, *Brain*, **90**:593, 1967.

219. Schott, G. D., and M. R. Wills: Muscle weakness in osteomalacia, *Lancet*, **1**:626, 1976.

220. Birge, S. J.: Vitamin D, muscle and phosphate hoemostasis, *Miner. Electrolyte Metab.*, **1**:57, 1978.

221. Mallette, L. E., B. M. Patten, and W. K. Engel: Neuromuscular disease in secondary hyperparathyroidism, *Ann. Intern. Med.*, **82**:474–483, 1975.

222. Schoenfeld, P. J., J. A. Martin, B. Barnes, and S. L. Teitelbaum: Amelioration of myopathy with 25-hydroxyvitamin D_3 therapy ($25(OH)D_3$) in patients on chronic hemodialysis, *Third Workshop on Vitamin D, Book of Abstracts*, Asilomar, Calif., 1977, p. 160.

223. Floyd, M., D. R. Ayyar, D. D. Barwick, P. Hudgson, and D. Weightman: Myopathy in chronic renal failure, *Q. J. Med.*, **43**:509, 1974.

224. Rodman, J. S., and T. Baker: Changes in the kinetics of muscle contraction in vitamin D-depleted rats, *Kidney Int.*, **13**:189, 1978.

225. Matthews, C., K. W. Heimberg, E. Ritz, B. Agostini, J. Fritzsche, and W. Hasselbach: Effect of 1,25-dihydroxycholecalciferol on impaired calcium transport by the sarcoplasmic reticulum in experimental uremia, *Kidney Int.*, **11**:227, 1977.

226. Delaporte, C., J. Bergstrom, and M. Broyer: Variations in muscle cell protein of severely uremic children, *Kidney Int.*, **10**:239, 1976.

227. Jebsen, R. H., H. Tenckhoff, and J. C. Honet: Natural history of uremic polyneuropathy and effects of dialysis, *N. Engl. J. Med.*, **277**:327, 1967.

228. Ahmed, K. Y., M. R. Wills, Z. Varghese, E. A. Meinhard, and J. F. Moorhead: Long-term effects of small doses of 1,25-dihydroxycholecalciferol in renal osteodystrophy, *Lancet*, **1**:629, 1978.

229. Massry, S. G., M. M. Popovtzer, J. W. Coburn, D.L. Makoff, M. H. Maxwell, and C. R. Kleeman: Intractable pruritus as a manifestation of 2°

hyperparathyroidism in uremia: Disappearance of itching following subtotal parathyroidectomy, *N. Engl. J. Med.*, **279**:697, 1968.

230. Hampers, C. L., A. I. Katz, R. E. Wilson, and J. P. Merrill: Disappearance of "uremic" itching after subtotal parathyroidectomy, *N. Engl. J. Med.*, **279**:695, 1968.

231. Tapia, L., J. S. Cheigh, D. S. David, J. F. Sullivan, S. Seal, M. M. Reidenberg, K. H. Stenzel, and A. L. Rubin: Parenteral lidocaine in treatment of pruritus in dialysis patients, *N. Engl. J. Med.*, **296**:261, 1977.

232. Gilchrest, B. A., J. W. Rowe, R. S. Brown, T. I. Steinman, and K. A. Arndt: Relief of uremic pruritus with ultraviolet phototherapy, *N. Engl. J. Med.*, **297**:136, 1977.

233. Richard, D. G. B.: Chronic renal disease with secondary hyperparathyroidism, *Br. Med. J.*, **1**:67, 1951.

234. Anderson, D. C., W. K. Steward, and I. M. Piercy: Calcifying panniculitis with fat and skin necrosis in a case of uremia with autonomous hyperparathyroidism, *Lancet*, **2**:323, 1968.

235. Richardson, J. A., G. Herron, R. Reitz, and R. Layzer: Ischemic ulcerations of skin and necrosis of muscle in azotemic hyperparathyroidism, *Ann. Intern. Med.*, **71**:126, 1969.

236. Friedman, S. A., S. Novack, and G. E. Thomson: Arterial calcification and gangrene in uremia, *N. Engl. J. Med.*, **280**:1392, 1969.

237. Massry, S. G., A. Gordon, J. W. Coburn, L. Kaplan, S. S. Franklin, M. H. Maxwell, and C. R. Kleeman: Vascular calcification and peripheral necrosis in a renal transplant recipient: Reversal of lesions following subtotal parathyroidectomy, *Am. J. Med.*, **49**:416, 1970.

238. Rosen, H., S. A. Friedman, and A. E. Raizner: Azotemic arteriopathy, *Am. Heart J.*, **84**:250, 1972.

239. Conn, J., Jr., F. A. Krumbovsky, F. Del Greco, and N. M. Simon: Calciphylaxis: Etiology of progressive vascular calcification and gangrene, *Ann. Surg.*, **177**:206, 1973.

240. Gipstein, R. M., J. W. Coburn, D. A. Adams, D. B. M. Lee, K. P. Parsa, A. Sellers, W. N. Suki, and S. G. Massry: Calciphylaxia in man: A syndrome of tissue necrosis and vascular necrosis in patients with chronic renal disease, *Arch. Intern. Med.*, **136**:1273, 1976.

241. Weidmann, P., S. G. Massry, J. W. Coburn, J. Atleson, M. H. Maxwell, and C. R. Kleeman: Effect of acute hypercalcemia on blood pressure in patients with chronic renal failure, *Ann. Intern. Med.*, **76**:741, 1972.

242. Charbon, G. A.: Parathormone: A selective vasodilator, in R. V. Talmadge and L. F. Balander (eds.), *Parathyroid Hormone—Thyrocalcitonin (Calcitonin)*, Excerpta Med. Found., Amsterdam, 1969, pp. 475–484.

243. Karanda, F. C., E. M. Dehmel, and G. Kahn: Cutaneous complications of immunosuppressed renal homograft recipients, *JAMA*, **299**:419, 1974.

244. Selye, H.: *Calciphylaxis*, The University of Chicago Press, Chicago, 1962.

245. Mirahmadi, K. S., J. W. Coburn, and R. Bluestone: Calcific periarthritis and hemodialysis, *JAMA*, **223**:548, 1973.

246. Massry, S. G., R. Bluestone, J. R. Klinenberg, and J. W. Coburn: Abnormalities of the musculoskeletal system in hemodialysis patients, *Semin. Arthritis Rheum.*, **4**:321, 1975.

247. Lotem, M., M. D. Robson, and J. B. Rosenfeld: Spontaneous rupture of the quadriceps tendon in patients on chronic hemodialysis, *Ann. Rheum. Dis.*, **33**:428, 1974.

248. Lotem, M., J. Bernheim, and B. Conforty: Spontaneous rupture of tendons: A complication of hemodialyzed patients treated for renal failure, *Nephron*, **21**:201, 1978.

249. Preston, F. S., and A. Adicoff: Hyperparathyroidism with avulsion of three major tendons, *N. Engl. J. Med.*, **266**:968, 1962.

250. Preston, E. T.: Avulsion of both quadriceps tendons in hyperparathyroidism, *JAMA*, **221**:406, 1972.

251. Cirincione, R. J., and B. E. Baker: Tendon rupture with secondary hyperparathyroidism, *J. Bone J. Surg.*, **57**:852, 1975.

252. Avioli, L. V.: Collagen metabolism, uremia and bone, *Kidney Int.*, **4**:105, 1973.

253. Murphy, K. J., and I. Mc Phee: Tears of major tendons in chronic acidosis with elastosis, *J. Bone Jt. Surg.*, **53**:510, 1971.

254. Mehls, O., E. Ritz, K. Burkhard, G. Gilli, W. Link, E. Willich, and K. Scharer: Slipped epiphysis in renal osteodystrophy, *Arch. Dis. Child.*, **50**:545, 1975.

255. Mehls, O., E. Ritz, B. Krempien, E. Willich, J. Bommer, and K. Schärer: Roentgenological signs in the skeleton of uremic children, *Pediatr. Radiol.*, **1**:183, 1973.

256. Parfitt, A. M.: Clinical and radiographic manifestations of renal osteodystrophy, in D. S. David (ed.), *Calcium Metabolism in Renal Failure and Nephrolithiasis*, John Wiley & Sons, Inc., New York, 1977, p. 150.

257. Chantler, C., and M. A. Holliday: Growth in children with renal disease, with special reference to the effects of calorie malnutrition: A review, *Clin. Nephrol.*, **1**:230, 1973.

258. Saenger, P., E. Weidmann, E. Schwartz, S. Kenth-Schulz, J. E. Lewy, R. R. Reggio, A. L. Rubin, K. H. Stenzel, and M. I. New: Somatomedin and growth after renal transplantation, *Pediatr. Res.*, **8**:163, 1974.

259. Pennisi, A. J., G. Costin, L. S. Phillips, C. Vittenbogaart, R. B. Ettenger, M. H. Malekzadeh, and R. N. Fine: Linear growth in long-term renal allograft recipients, *Clin. Nephrol.*, **8**:415, 1977.

260. Schärer, K.: Growth in children with chronic renal failure, *Kidney Int.*, **13**(suppl. 8):S68, 1978.

261. Chantler, C., R. A. Donckerwolcke, F. P. Brunner, H. J. Gurland, R. A. Hathway, C. Jacobs, N. H. Selwood, and A. J. Wing: Combined report on regular dialysis and transplantation of children in Europe, 1976, *Proc. Eur. Dial. Transplant Assoc.*, **14**:70, 1977.

262. Simmons, J. M., C. J. Wilson, D. E. Porter, and M. A. Holliday: Relation of calorie deficiency to growth failure in children on hemodialysis and the growth response to calorie supplementation, *N. Engl. J. Med.*, **285**:653, 1971.

263. Betts, P. R., and G. Magrath: Growth pattern and dietary intake of children with chronic renal insufficiency, *Brit. Med. J.*, **2**:189, 1974.

264. Chesney, R. W., A. V. Moorthy, J. A. Eisman, D. K. Jax, R. B. Mazess, and H. F. DeLuca: Increased growth after long-term oral $1\alpha,25$-vitamin D_3 in childhood renal osteodystrophy, *N. Engl. J. Med.*, **298**:238, 1978.

265. McSherry, E., and R. C. Morris: Attainment and maintenance of normal stature with alkali therapy in infants and children with classic renal tubular acidosis (RTA), *J. Clin. Invest.*, **61**:509, 1978.

266. Massry, S. G., and D. A. Goldstein: Role of para-

thyroid hormone in uremic toxicity, *Kidney Int.*, **13**(suppl. 8):S39, 1978.

267. Bricker, N. S.: On the pathogenesis of the uremic state: An exposition of the "trade-off" hypothesis, *N. Engl. J. Med.*, **286**:1093, 1972.

268. Bricker, N. S., and L. G. Fine: The trade-off hypothesis: Current status, *Kidney Int.*, **13**(suppl. 8):S5, 1978.

269. Arieff, A. I., and S. G. Massry: Calcium metabolism of brain in acute renal failure: Effects of uremia, hemodialysis and parathyroid hormone, *J. Clin. Invest.*, **53**:387, 1974.

270. Guisado, R., A. I. Arieff, and S. G. Massry: Changes in the electroencephalogram in acute uremia: Effects of parathyroid hormone and brain electrolytes, *J. Clin. Invest.*, **55**:738, 1975.

271. Cooper, J. D., V. C. Lazarowitz, and A. I. Arieff: Neurodiagnostic abnormalities in patients with acute renal failure: Evidence for neurotoxicity of parathyroid hormone, *J. Clin. Invest.*, **61**:1448, 1978.

272. Kiley, J. E., N. W. Woodruff, and K. L. Pratt: Evaluation of encephalopathy by EEG frequency analysis in chronic dialysis patients, *Clin. Nephrol.*, **5**:245, 1976.

273. Ball, J. H., J. W. Johnson, C. L. Hampers, and J. P. Merrill: The many facets of secondary hyperparathyroidism, *Arch. Intern. Med.*, **131**:746, 1973.

274. Arieff, A. I., C. Covey, and V. Lazarowitz: Nervous system abnormalities in uremia. Program, 11th Annu. Contractors' Conf. *Artif. Kidney–Chronic Uremia program*, NIAMDD, Bethesda, Md., 1978, pp. 100–103.

275. Avram, M. M., D. A. Feinfeld, and A. H. Huatuco: Search for the uremic toxin: Decreased motor nerve conduction velocity and elevated parathyroid hormone in uremia, *N. Engl. J. Med.*, **298**:1000, 1978.

276. Arieff, A. I., and R. W. Schmidt: Parathyroid hormone as a uremic neurotoxin, *N. Engl. J. Med.*, **299**:362, 1978.

277. Goldstein, D. A., L. A. Chui, and S. G. Massry: Effect of parathyroid hormone and uremia on peripheral nerve calcium and motor nerve conduction velocity, *J. Clin. Invest.*, **62**:88, 1978.

278. Cooper, J. D., A. I. Arieff, V. C. Lazarowitz, and R. Guisado: Effects of chronic renal failure on central nervous system in dogs, *Clin. Res.*, **25**:428A, 1977.

279. Ward, M. K., A. M. Pierides, P. Fawcett, D. A. Shaw, R. H. Perry, B. E. Tomlinson, and D. N. S. Kerr: Dialysis encephalopathy syndrome, *Proc. Eur. Dial. Transplant Assoc.*, **13**:348, 1976.

280. Alfrey, A. C., G. R. LeGendre, and W. D. Kaehny: Dialysis encephalopathy syndrome: Possible aluminum intoxication, *N. Engl. J. Med.*, **294**:184, 1976.

281. Mayor, G. H., J. A. Keiser, and P. K. Ku: Aluminum absorption and distribution: Effect of parathyroid hormone, *Science*, **197**:1187, 1977.

282. Ball, J. H., D. E. Butkus, and D. S. Madison: Effect of subtotal parathyroidectomy on dialysis dementia, *Nephron*, **18**:151, 1977.

283. Sullivan, P. A., D. J. Murnaghan, and N. Callaghan: Dialysis dementia: Recovery after transplantation, *Br. Med. J.*, **2**:740, 1977.

284. Loew, H., H. Schultz, and G. Busch: Klinische aspekte der impotency mannlicher dauer-dialyse-patienten, *Med. Welt.*, **26**:1651, 1975.

285. Massry, S. G., D. A. Goldstein, W. R. Procci, and O. A. Kletzky: Impotence in patients with uremia: A possible role for parathyroid hormone, *Nephron*, **19**:305, 1977.

286. Weinberg, S. G., A. Lubin, S. N. Wiener, M. P. Deoras, M. K. Ghose, and R. C. Kopelman: Myelofibrosis and renal osteodystrophy, *Am. J. Med.*, **63**:755, 1977.

287. Boxer, M., L. Ellman, R. Geller, and C.-A. Wong: Anemia in primary hyperparathyroidism, *Arch. Intern. Med.*, **137**:588, 1977.

288. Bettor, O. S., S. M. Shasha, J. Windver, and C. Chaimovitz: Improvement in the anemia of hemodialysis patients following parathyroidectomy, *Proc. Am. Soc. Nephrol.*, **9**:1, 1976.

289. Bagdade, J. D., D. Porte, Jr., and E. L. Biermann: Hypertriglyceridemia: A metabolic consequence of chronic renal failure, *N. Engl. J. Med.*, **279**:181, 1968.

290. Losowsky, M., and D. H. Kenward: Lipid metabolism in acute and chronic renal failure, *J. Lab. Clin. Med.*, **71**:736, 1968.

291. Winkler, A. W., S. H. Durlacher, H. E. Hoff, and E. B. Man: Changes in lipid content of serum and of liver following bilateral renal ablation or ureteral ligation, *J. Exp. Med.*, **77**:473, 1943.

292. Svanborg, A.: Studies on renal hyperlipemia, *Acta Med. Scand.*, **141**(suppl. 264):1, 1951.

293. Cantin, M.: Kidney, parathyroid and lipemia, *Lab. Invest.*, **14**:1691, 1965.

294. Lindall, A., R. Carmena, S. Cohen, and C. Compty: Insulin hypersecretion in patients on chronic hemodialysis: Role of parathyroids, *J. Clin. Endocrinol.*, **32**:653, 1971.

295. Dent, C. E., and C. J. Hodson: Radiological changes associated with certain metabolic bone diseases, *Br. J. Radiol.*, **27**:605, 1954.

296. Meema, H. E., S. Rabinovich, S. Meema, G. J. Lloyd, and D. G. Oreopoulos: Improved radiological diagnosis of azotemic osteodystrophy, *Radiology*, **102**:1, 1972.

297. Ritz, E., P. Prager, B. Krempien, J. Bonner, H. H. Malluche, and H. Schmidt-Gayk: Skeletal x-ray findings and bone histology in patients on hemodialysis, *Kidney Int.*, **13**:316, 1978.

297a. Mehls, O., E. Ritz, B. Krempien, E. Willich, J. Bronner, and K. Schäfer: Roentgenological signs in the skeleton of uremic children: An analysis of the anatomical principles underlying the roentgenological changes, *Pediatr. Radiol.*, **1**:183, 1973.

298. Meema, H. E., D. G. Oreopoulos, S. Rabinovich, H. Husdan, and A. Rapaport: Periosteal new bone formation (periosteal neostasis) in renal osteodystrophy, *Radiology*, **110**:513, 1974.

299. Craven, J. D.: Renal glomerular osteodystrophy, *Clin. Radiol.*, **15**:210, 1964.

300. Doyle, F. H.: Radiological patterns of bone disease associated with renal glomerular failure in adults, *Br. Med. Bull.*, **28**:220, 1972.

301. Doyle, F. H., T. Aung, R. N. P. Carroll, E. D. Williams, and R. Shackman: Bone resorption in chronic renal failure: A comparison of radiological and histological assessments, *Br. Med. Bull.*, **28**:225, 1972.

302. Genant, H. K., L. L. Heck, L. H. Lanzl, K. Rossmann, J. Vander Horst, and E. Paloyan: Primary hyperparathyroidism, *Radiology*, **109**:513, 1973.

303. Eastwood, J. B., Ph. J. Bordier, and H. E. DeWardener: Some biochemical, histological, radiological and clinical features of renal osteodystrophy, *Kidney Int.*, **4**:128, 1973.

304. Webster, G. D., Jr.: Azotemic renal osteodystrophy, *Med. Clin. N. Am.*, **47**:985, 1963.

305. Tatler, G. L. V., R. A. Baillad, Z. Varghese, W. B. Young, S. Farrow, M. R. Wills, and J. F. Moorhead: Evolution of bone disease over 10 years in 135 patients with terminal renal failure, *Br. Med. J.*, **4**:315, 1973.

306. Prager, P., R. Singer, E. Ritz, and B. Krempien: Diagnostischer stellenwert der lamina dura dentium beim sekundären hyperparathyreoidismus, *Fortschr. Röntgenstr.*, **129**:237, 1978.

307. Meema, H. E., and S. Meema: Comparison of microradioscopic and morphometric findings in the hand bones with densitometric findings in the proximal radius in thyrotoxicosis and in renal osteodystrophy, *Invest. Radiol.*, **7**:88, 1972.

308. Meema, H. E., and D. L. Schatz: Simple radiologic demonstration of cortical bone loss in thyrotoxicosis, *Radiology*, **97**:9, 1970.

309. Simpson, W., H. A. Ellis, D. N. S. Kerr, M. McElroy, R. A. McNay, and K. N. Peart: Bone disease in long-term hemodialysis: The association of radiological with histologic abnormalities, *Br. J. Radiol.*, **49**:105, 1976.

310. Ellis, K., and R. J. Hochstim: The skull in hyperparathyroid bone disease, *Am. J. Roentgenol.*, **83**:732, 1960.

311. Chalmers, J., W. D. H. Conacher, D. L. Gardner, and P. J. Scott: Osteomalacia—a common disease in elderly women, *J. Bone Jt. Surg.*, **49-B**:403, 1967.

312. Simpson, W., J. R. Young, and F. Clark: Fractures resembling stress fractures in Punjabi immigrants with osteomalacia, *Clin. Radiol.*, **24**:83, 1973.

313. Norfray, J., L. Calenoff, F. Del Greco, and F. A. Krumlovsky: Renal osteodystrophy in patients on hemodialysis as reflected in the bony pelvis, *Am. J. Roentgenol., Radium Ther. Nucl. Med.*, **125**:352, 1975.

314. Ritz, E., B. Krempien, O. Mehls, and H. Malluche: Skeletal abnormalities in chronic renal insufficiency before and during maintenance hemodialysis, *Kidney Int.*, **4**:116, 1973.

315. Parfitt, A. M., S. G. Massry, and A. C. Winfield: Osteopenia and fractures occurring during maintenance hemodialysis: A "new" form of renal osteodystrophy, *Clin. Orthop.*, **87**:287, 1972.

316. Nordin, B. E. C., J. MacGregor, and D. A. Smith: The incidence of osteoporosis in normal women:

Its relation to age and menopause, *Q. J. Med.*, **35**:25, 1966.

317. Garn, S. M., A. K. Poznanski, and J. M. Nagy: Bone measurement in the differential diagnosis of osteopenia and osteoporosis, *Radiology*, **100**:509, 1971.

318. Gryfe, C. I., A. N. Exton-Smith, and R. J. C. Steward: Determination of the amount of bone in the metacarpal, *Age and Ageing*, **1**:213, 1972.

319. Parfitt, A. M.: The actions of parathyroid hormone on bone: Relation to bone remodeling and turnover, calcium homeostasis and metabolic bone disease. Part III of IV parts: PTH and osteoblasts, the relationship between bone turnover and bone loss, and the state of the bones in primary hyperparathyroidism, *Metabolism*, **25**:1033, 1976.

320. Cochran, M., L. Bulusu, A. Horsman, L. Stasiac, and B. E. C. Nordin: Hypocalcemia and bone disease in chronic renal failure, *Nephron*, **10**:113, 1973.

321. Bone, J. M., A. M. Davison, and J. S. Robson: Role of dialysate calcium concentration in osteoporosis in patients on hemodialysis, *Lancet*, **1**:1047, 1972.

322. Cameron, J. R., R. B. Mazess, and J. A. Sorensen: Precision and accuracy of bone mineral determination by direct photon absorptiometry, *Invest. Radiol.*, **3**:9, 1968.

323. Hahn, T. J., and B. H. Hahn: Osteopenia in patients with rheumatic diseases: Principles of diagnosis and therapy, *Semin. Arthritis Rheum.*, **6**:165, 1976.

324. Griffiths, H. J., R. E. Zimmerman, G. Bailey, and R. Snider: The use of photon absorptiometry in the diagnosis of renal osteodystrophy, *Radiology*, **109**:277, 1973.

325. Griffiths, H. J., R. E. Zimmerman, M. Lazarus, E. Lowrie, M. N. Gottlieb, E. Phillips, and K. Pomerantz: The long-term follow-up of 195 patients with renal failure: A preliminary report, *Radiology*, **122**:643, 1977.

326. Denney, J. D., D. J. Sherrard, W. R. Nelp, C. H. Chestnut, and D. J. Baylink: Total body calcium and long term calcium balance in chronic renal disease, *J. Lab. Clin. Med.*, **82**:226, 1973.

327. Letteri, J. M., and S. H. Cohn: Total body neutron activation: Analysis in the study of mineral homeostasis in chronic renal disease, in D. S. David (ed.), *Calcium Metabolism in Renal Failure and Nephrolithiasis*, John Wiley & Sons, Inc., New York, 1977, pp. 249–278.

328. Fleisch, H., and R. G. G. Russell: Experimental clinical studies with pyrophosphate and diphosphonates in D. S. David (ed.), *Calcium Metabolism in Renal Failure and Nephrolithiasis*, John Wiley & Sons, Inc., New York, 1977, pp. 293–336.

329. Rosenthall, L., and M. Kaye: Observations on the mechanism of ^{99m}Tc-labeled phosphate complex uptake in metabolic bone disease, *Nucl. Med.*, **5**:59, 1976.

330. Lien, J. W. K., T. Wiegmann, L. Rosenthall, and M. Kaye: Abnormal ^{99m}technetium-tin-pyrophosphate bone scans in chronic renal failure, *Clin. Nephrol.*, **6**:509, 1976.

331. Sy, W. M., and A. K. Mittal: Bone scan in chronic dialysis patients with evidence of secondary hyperparathyroidism and renal osteodystrophy, *Br. J. Radiol.*, **48**:878, 1975.

332. Olgaard, K., J. Heerfordt, and S. Madsen: Scintigraphic skeletal changes in uremic patients on regular hemodialysis, *Nephron*, **17**:325, 1976.

333. Devacaanthan, K., A. U. Yap, Z. Chayes, and R. M. Stein: Pulmonary calcification in chronic renal failure: Use of diphosphonate scintiscan as a diagnostic tool, *Clin. Nephrol.*, **6**:488, 1976.

334. Davis, B. A., K. P. Poulose, and R. C. Reba: Scanning for uremic pulmonary calcifications, *Ann. Intern. Med.*, **85**:132, 1976.

335. Siegel, B. A., W. K. Engel, and E. C. Derrer: Localization of technicium-99m diphosphonate in acutely injured muscle: Relationship to muscle calcium deposition, *Neurology*, **27**:230, 1977.

336. Parfitt, A. M.: Soft tissue calcification in uremia, *Arch. Intern. Med.*, **124**:544, 1969.

337. Johnson, C., C. B. Graham, and F. K. Curtis: Roentgenographic manifestations of chronic renal disease treated by periodic hemodialysis, *Am. J. Roentgenol.*, **101**:915, 1967.

338. Berlyne, G. M.: Microcrystalline conjunctival calcification in renal failure: A useful clinical sign, *Lancet*, **2**:366, 1968.

339. Berlyne, G. M., and A. G. Shaw: Red eyes in renal failure, *Lancet*, **1**:4, 1967.

340. Ritz, E., O. Mehls, J. Bommer, H. Schmidt-Gayk, P. Fiegel, and H. Reitinger: Vascular calcifica-

tions under maintenance hemodialysis, *Klin. Wochenschr.*, **55**:375, 1977.

341. Meema, H. E., D. G. Oreopoulos, and G. A. DeVeber: Arterial calcifications in severe chronic renal disease and their relationship to dialysis treatment, renal transplant, and parathyroidectomy, *Radiology*, **121**:315, 1976.

342. Caner, J. E., and J. L. Decker: Recurrent acute (gouty?) arthritis in chronic renal failure treated with periodic hemodialysis, *Am. J. Med.*, **36**:571, 1964.

343. Alfrey, A. C., D. Jenkins, C. G. Groth, W. S. Schorr, L. Gecelter, and D. A. Ogden: Resolution of hyperparathyroidism after renal transplantation, *N. Engl. J. Med.*, **279**:1349, 1968.

344. Contiguglia, S. R., A. C. Alfrey, N. L. Miller, D. E. Runnells, and R. Z. LeGeros: Nature of soft tissue calcification in uremia, *Kidney Int.*, **4**:229, 1973.

345. Dreher, W., and W. Shelp: Atrioventricular block in a long term dialysis patient: Reversal after parathyroidectomy, *JAMA*, **234**:954, 1975.

346. Schwartz, K. V.: Heart-block in renal failure and hypercalcemia, *JAMA*, **235**:1550, 1976.

347. Conger, J. D., W. S. Hammond, A. C. Alfrey, S. R. Contiguglia, R. E. Stanford, and W. E. Huffer: Pulmonary calcification in chronic dialysis patients: Clinical and pathologic studies, *Ann. Int. Med.*, **82**:330, 1975.

348. Chanard, J., J. Assailly, C. Bader, and J. Funck-Brentano: Rapid method for measurement of fractional intestinal absorption of calcium, *J. Nucl. Med.*, **15**:369, 1974.

349. Katz, A. I., C. L. Hampers, and J. P. Merrill: Secondary hyperparathyroidism and renal osteodystrophy in chronic renal failure, *Medicine (Baltimore)*, **48**:333, 1969.

350. Messner, R. P., H. T. Smith, F. L. Shapiro, and D. H. Gregory: The effect of hemodialysis, vitamin D, and renal homotransplantation on the calcium malabsorption of chronic renal failure, *J. Lab. Clin. Med.*, **74**:472, 1969.

351. Genuth, S. M., V. Vertes, and J. R. Leonard: Oral calcium absorption in patients with renal failure treated by chronic hemodialysis, *Metabolism*, **18**:124, 1969

352. Coburn, J. W., S. G. Massry, J. R. DePalma, and J. H. Shinaberger: Rapid appearance of hypercal-cemia with initiation of hemodialysis, *JAMA*, **210**:2276, 1969.

353. Bouillon, R., R. Verberckmoes, and P. D. Moor: Influence of dialysate calcium concentration and vitamin D on serum parathyroid hormone during repetitive dialysis, *Kidney Int.*, **7**:422, 1975.

354. Wing, A. J.: Optimum calcium concentration of dialysis fluid for maintenance haemodialysis, *Br. Med. J.*, **4**:145, 1968.

355. Strong, H. F., B. C. Schatz, J. H. Shinaberger, and J. W. Coburn: Measurement of dialysance and bidirectional fluxes of calcium in vivo using radiocalcium, *Trans. Am. Soc. Artif. Intern. Organs*, **17**:108, 1971.

356. Mirhamadi, K. S., B. S. Duffy, J. H. Shinaberger, J. Jowsey, Massry, and J. W. Coburn: A controlled evaluation of clinical and metabolic effects of dialysate calcium levels during regular dialysis, *Trans. Am. Soc. Artif. Intern. Organs*, **17**:118, 1971.

357. Goldsmith, R. S., J. Furszyter, W. J. Johnson, G. W. Beeler, Jr., and W. F. Taylor: Calcium flux during hemodialysis, *Nephron*, **20**:132, 1978.

358. Wolf, A. V., D. G. Remp, J. E. Kiley, and G. D. Currie: Artificial kidney function: Kinetics of hemodialysis, *J. Clin. Invest.*, **30**:1062, 1951.

359. Taves, D. R., R. Terry, F. A. Smith, and D. E. Gardner: Use of fluoridated water in long term hemodialysis, *Arch. Intern. Med.*, **115**:167, 1965.

360. Taves, D. R., R. B. Freeman, D. E. Kamm, L. P. Ramos, and B. H. Scribner: Hemodialysis with fluoridated water, *Trans. Am. Soc. Artif. Intern. Organs*, **14**:412, 1968.

361. Posen, G. A., J. R. Marier, and Z. F. Jaworski: Renal osteodystrophy in patients on long-term hemodialysis with fluoridated water, *Fluoride*, **4**:114, 1971.

362. Walser, M., and W. J. Rahill: Renal tubular transport of fluoride compared with chloride, *Am. J. Physiol.*, **210**:1290, 1966.

363. Nielsen, E., N. Solomon, N. J. Goodwin, N. Siddhwarn, R. Galonsky, D. Taves, and E. P. Friedman: Fluoride metabolism in uremia, *Trans. Am. Soc. Artif. Intern. Organs*, **19**:450, 1973.

364. Cordy, P., R. Gagnon, D. R. Taves, and M. Kaye: Fluoride and hemodialysis, *Trans. Am. Soc. Artif. Intern. Organs*, **20**:197, 1974.

365. Weatherell, J. A., and S. M. Weidmann: The

skeletal changes in chronic experimental fluorosis, *J. Pathol. Bacteriol.*, **78**:233, 1959.

366. Faccini, J. M.: Fluoride and bone, *Calcif. Tissue Res.*, **3**:1, 1969.

367. Oreopoulos, D. G., D. R. Taves, S. Rabinovich, H. E. Meema, T. Murray, S. S. Fenton, and G. A. de Veber: Fluoride and dialysis osteodystrophy: Results of a double blind study, *Trans. Am. Soc. Artif. Intern. Organs*, **20**:203, 1974.

368. Hampers, C. L., E. Schupak, E. G. Lowrie, and J. M. Lazarus: *Long-Term Hemodialysis*, 2d ed., Grune & Stratton, Inc., New York, 1973, p. 21.

369. Griffith, G. C., G. Nichols, Jr., J. D. Asher, and B. Flanagan: Heparin osteoporosis, *JAMA*, **195**:1089, 1966.

370. Jaffe, M. D., and P. W. Wellis, III: Multiple fractures associated with long-term sodium heparin therapy, *JAMA*, **193**:152, 1965.

371. Stinchfield, F. E., B. Sanlcaran, and R. Samilson: The effect of anticoagulant therapy on bone repair, *J. Bone Jt. Surg., Br. Vol.*, **35A**:270, 1956.

372. Massry, S. G., A. I. Arieff, J. W. Coburn, G. Palmieri, and C. R. Kleeman: Divalent ion metabolism in patients with acute renal failure: Studies on the mechanism of hypocalcemia, *Kidney Int.*, **5**:437, 1974.

373. Kokot, F., and J. Kuska: Der Einfluss der Hemodialyse auf die Parathormonkonzentration bei akuter Niereninsuffizienz, *Z. Gesamte Inn. Med. Ihre Grezgeb.*, **29**:916, 1974.

374. Pietrek, J., F. Kokot, and J. Kuska: Serum 25-hydroxyvitamin D and parathyroid hormone in patients with acute renal failure, *Kidney Int.*, **13**:178, 1978.

375. Grossman, R. A., R. W. Hamilton, B. M. Morse, A. S. Penn, and M. Goldberg: Nontraumatic rhabdomyolysis and acute renal failure, *N. Engl. J. Med.*, **291**:807, 1974.

376. Koffler, A., R. M. Friedler, and S. G. Massry: Acute renal failure due to nontraumatic rhabdomyolysis, *Ann. Intern. Med.*, **85**:23, 1976.

377. Meroney, W. H., G. K. Arney, W. E. Segar, and H. H. Balch: The acute calcification of traumatized muscle with particular reference to acute post-traumatic renal insufficiency, *J. Clin. Invest.*, **36**:825, 1957.

378. Clark, T. G., and M. D. Sumerling: Muscle necrosis and calcification in acute renal failure due to barbiturate intoxication, *Br. Med. J.*, **2**:214, 1966.

379. Mautner, L. S.: Muscle necrosis associated with carbon monoxide poisoning, *Arch. Pathol.*, **60**:136, 1955.

380. DeTorrente, A., T. Berl, P. D. Cohn, E. Kawamoto, D. Hertz, and R. W. Schrier: Hypercalcemia of acute renal failure, *Am. J. Med.*, **61**:119, 1976.

381. Miach, P. J., J. K. Dawborn, M. C. Douglas, G. Jerums, and J. M. Xipell: Prolonged hypercalcemia following acute renal failure, *Clin. Nephrol.*, **4**:32, 1975.

382. Suki, W. N., J. J. Yium, M. Van Minden, C. Saller-Hebert, G. Eknoyan, and M. Martinez-Maldonado: Acute treatment of hypercalcemia with furosemide, *N. Engl. J. Med.*, **283**:836, 1970.

383. Lim, P., E. Jacob, L. F. Chio, and H. S. Pwee: Serum ionized calcium in nephrotic syndrome, *Q. J. Med.*, **45**:421, 1976.

384. Emerson, K., Jr., and W. W. Beckman: Calcium metabolism in nephrosis: I. A description of an abnormality in calcium metabolism in children with nephrosis, *J. Clin. Invest.*, **24**:564, 1945.

385. Jones, J. H., D. K. Peters, D. B. Morgan, G. A. Coles, and N. P. Mallick: Observations on calcium metabolism in the nephrotic syndrome, *Q. J. Med.*, **36**:301, 1967.

386. Lim, P., E. Jacob, E. P. C. Tock, and H. W. Pwee: Calcium and phosphorus metabolism in nephrotic syndrome, *Q. J. Med.*, **46**:327, 1977.

387. Haddad, J. G., Jr., and T. Walgate: Radioimmunoassay of the binding protein for vitamin D and its metabolites in human serum: Concentrations in normal subjects and patients with disorders of mineral homeostasis, *J. Clin. Invest.*, **58**:1217, 1976.

388. Nishii, Y., K. Kumaki, M. Fukushima, T. Shimizu, M. Ono, H. Okawa, R. Niki, I. Matsunaga, K. Ochi, Y. Tohira, S. Sasaki, and T. Suda: Metabolism of 25-hydroxy-vitamin D_3 and 1α-hydroxy-vitamin D_3 in experimental rats with chronic renal failure, in A. W. Norman, K. Schaefer, J. W. Coburn, H. F. DeLuca, D. Fraser, H. G. Grigoleit, and D. von Herrath (eds.), *Vitamin D: Biochemical, Chemical and Clinical Aspects Related to Calcium Metabolism*, Walter de Gruyter & Co., Berlin, 1977, pp. 179–181.

389. Mountokalakis, T. H., C. Virvidakis, P. Singhellakis, C. Alevizaki, and D. Ikkos: Intestinal calcium absorption in the nephrotic syndrome, *Ann. Intern. Med.*, **86**:746, 1977.

390. Brickman, A. S., S. G. Massry, and J. W. Coburn: Effect of calcium deprivation on renal handling of calcium during repeated infusion of saline, *Am. J. Physiol.*, **220**:44, 1971.

391. Malluche, H. H., D. A. Goldstein, and S. G. Massry: Osteomalacia and hyperparathyroid bone disease in patients with nephrotic syndrome, *J. Clin. Invest.*, **63**:000, 1979.

392. McIntosh, D. A., E. W. Peterson, and J. J. McPhare: Autonomy of parathyroid function after renal homotransplantation, *Ann. Intern. Med.*, **65**:900, 1966.

393. Schwartz, G. H., D. S. David, R. R. Riggio, P. D. Saville, J. C. Whitsell, K. H. Stenzel, and A. L. Rubin: Hypercalcemia after renal transplantation, *Am. J. Med.*, **49**:42, 1970.

394. Johnson, W. J., R. S. Goldsmith, and C. D. Arnaud: Prevention and treatment of progressive secondary hyperparathyroidism in advanced renal failure, *Med. Clin. North Am.*, **56**:961, 1972.

395. David, D. S., S. Sakai, B. L. Brennen, R. A. Riggio, J. Cheigh, K. H. Stenzel, A. L. Rubin, and L. M. Sherwood: Hypercalcemia after renal transplantation: Long-term follow-up data, *N. Engl. J. Med.*, **289**:398, 1973.

396. Gittes, R. F., and I. C. Radde: Experimental model for hyperparathyroidism: Effect of excessive numbers of transplanted isologous parathyroid glands, *J. Urol.*, **95**:595, 1966.

397. Moorhead, J. F., M. R. Wills, K. Y. Ahmed, R. A. Baillod, Z. Varghese, G. L. V. Tatler, and A. Fairney: Hypophosphatemic osteomalacia after cadaveric renal transplantation, *Lancet*, **1**:694, 1974.

398. Geis, W. P., M. M. Popovtzer, J. L. Corman, C. G. Halgrimson, C. G. Groth, and T. E. Starzl: The diagnosis and treatment of hyperparathyroidism after renal homotransplantation, *Surg. Gynecol. Obstet.*, **137**:997, 1973.

399. Chattergee, S. N., R. M. Friedler, T. V. Berne, S. B. Oldham, F. R. Singer, and S. G. Massry: Persistent hypercalcemia after successful renal transplantation, *Nephron*, **17**:1, 1976.

400. Christensen, M. S., H. E. Nielsen, and S. Tør-ring: Hypercalciuria and parathyroid function after renal transplantation, *Acta Med. Scand.*, **201**:35, 1977.

401. Wells, S. A., J. C. Gunnell, J. D. Shelburne, A. B. Schneider, and L. M. Sherwood: Transplantation of the parathyroid glands in man: Clinical indications and results, *Surgery*, **78**:34, 1975.

402. Wells, S. A., G. J. Ellis, J. C. Gunnells, A. B. Schneider, and L. M. Sherwood: Parathyroid autotransplantation in primary hyperparathyroid hyperplasia, *N. Engl. J. Med.*, **295**:57, 1976.

403. Wells, S. A., Jr., J. A. Stirman, R. M. Bolman, and J. C. Gunnells: Transplantation of the parathyroid glands, *Surg. Clin. North Am.*, **58**:391, 1978.

404. Schneider, A. B., S. A. Wells, J. C. Gunnells, J. B. Leslie, and L. M. Sherwood: Regulation of function of transplanted parathyroid glands in man, *Am. J. Med.*, **63**:710, 1977.

405. Carroll, R. N. P., E. D. Williams, T. Aung, E. Yeboah, and R. Shackman: The effect of renal transplantation on renal osteodystrophy, *Proc. Eur. Dial. Transplant Assoc.*, **10**:446, 1973.

406. Pierides, A. M., H. A. Ellis, K. M. Peart, W. Simson, P. R. Uldall, and D. N. S. Kerr: Assessment of renal osteodystrophy following renal transplantation, *Proc. Eur. Dial. Transplant Assoc.*, **11**:481, 1974.

407. Gustafsson, L. A., M. H. Meyers, and T. V. Berne: Total hip replacement in renal transplant recipients with aseptic necrosis of the femoral head, *Lancet*, **2**:606, 1976.

408. Habermann, E. T., and R. L. Cirstofaro: Avascular necrosis of bone as complication of renal transplantation, *Semin. Arthritis Rheum.*, **6**:189, 1976.

409. Baily, G. L., H. J. L. Griffiths, A. J. Mocelin, D. H. Gundy, C. L. Hampers, and J. P. Merrill: Avascular necrosis of the femoral head in patients on chronic hemodialysis, *Am. Soc. Artif. Intern. Organs*, **18**:401, 1972.

410. Gottlieb, M. N., M. K. Stephens, E. G. Lowrie, J. M. Lazarus, H. J. Griffiths, J. E. Kenzora, T. B. Strom, E. Phillips, and J. P. Merrill: Bone disease following renal transplantation, in D. S. David (ed.), *Calcium Metabolism in Renal Failure and Nephrolithiasis*, John Wiley & Sons, Inc., New York, 1977, pp. 279–292.

411. Potter, D., F. O. Belzer, L. Rames, M. A. Holli-

day, S. L. Kovatz, and J. S. Najorian: The treatment of chronic uremia in childhood, *Pediatrics*, **45**:432, 1970.

412. McEnery, P. T., L. L. Gonzales, L. W. Martin, and C. D. West: Growth and development of children with renal transplants: Use of alternate day steroid therapy, *J. Pediatr.*, **83**:806, 1973.

413. Fournier, A. E., W. J. Johnson, D. R. Taves, J. W. Beabout, C. D. Arnaud, and R. S. Goldsmith: Etiology of hyperparathyroidism and bone disease during chronic hemodialysis: I. Association of bone disease with potentially etiologic factors, *J. Clin. Invest.*, **50**:592, 1971.

414. Abrams, D. E., R. B. Silcott, R. Terry, T. V. Berne, and B. H. Barbour: Antacid induction of phosphate depletion syndrome in renal failure, *West. J. Med.*, **120**:157, 1974.

415. Mahony, J. F., J. M. Hayes, J. P. Ingham, and S. Posen: Hypophosphataemic osteomalacia in patients receiving hemodialysis, *Br. Med. J.*, **2**:142, 1976.

416. Berlyne, G. M., J. Ben-Ari, D. Pest, J. Weinberger, M. Stern, G. R. Gilmore, and R. Levine: Hyperaluminaemia from aluminum resins in renal failure, *Lancet*, **2**:494, 1970.

417. Clarkson, E. M., S. J. McDonald, and H. E. De Wardener: The effect of a high intake of calcium carbonate in normal subjects and patients with chronic renal failure, *Clin. Sci.*, **30**:425, 1966.

418. McDonald, S. J., E. M. Clarkson, and H. E. De Wardener: The effect of a large intake of calcium citrate in normal subjects and patients with chronic renal failure, *Clin. Sci.*, **26**:27, 1964.

419. Clarkson, E. M., J. B. Eastwood, K. G. Koutsaimanis, and H. E. De Wardener: Net intestinal absorption of calcium in patients with chronic renal failure, *Kidney Int.*, **3**:258, 1973.

420. Malluche, H. H., E. Werner, and E. Ritz: Intestinal absorption of calcium and whole body calcium retention in incipient and advanced renal failure, *Miner. Electrolyte Metab.*, **1**:263, 1978.

421. Meyrier, A., J. Marsac, and G. Richet: The influence of a high calcium carbonate intake on bone disease in patients undergoing hemodialysis, *Kidney Int.*, **4**:146, 1973.

422. Curtis, J. R., H. E. De Wardener, P. E. Gower, and J. B. Eastwood: The use of calcium carbonate and calcium phosphate without vitamin D in the management of renal osteodystrophy, *Proc. Eur. Dial. Transplant Assoc.*, **7**:141, 1970.

423. Eastwood, J. B., P. J. Bordier, and H. E. De Wardener: Comparison of the effect of vitamin D and calcium carbonate in renal osteomalacia, *Q. J. Med.*, **40**:569, 1971.

424. Makoff, D. L., A. Gordon, S. S. Franklin, A. R. Gerstein, and M. H. Maxwell: Chronic calcium carbonate therapy in uremia, *Arch. Intern. Med.*, **123**:15, 1969.

425. Ginsberg, D. S., E. L. Kaplan, and A. I. Katz: Hypercalcemia after oral calcium carbonate therapy in patients on chronic hemodialysis, *Lancet*, **1**:1271, 1973.

426. McMillan, D. E., and R. B. Freeman: The milk alkali syndrome: A study of the acute disorder with comments on the development of the chronic condition, *Medicine*, **44**:485, 1965.

427. Phang, J. M., A. N. Kales, and T. J. Hahn: Effect of divided calcium intake on urinary calcium excretion, *Lancet*, **1**:84, 1968.

428. Goldsmith, R. S., and W. J. Johnson: Role of phosphate depletion and high dialysate calcium in controlling dialytic renal osteodystrophy, *Kidney Int.*, **4**:154, 1973.

429. Goldsmith, R. S.: The effects of calcium and phosphorus in hemodialysis, *Annu. Rev. Med.*, **27**:181, 1976.

430. Atkinson, P. J., D. A. Hancock, V. N. Acharya, F. M. Parsons, E. A. Proctor, and G. W. Reed: Changes in skeletal mineral in patients on prolonged maintenance dialysis, *Br. Med. J.*, **4**:519, 1973.

431. Chamberlain, M. J., and B. H. B. Robinson: Whole body calcium changes during long term dialysis, *Proc. Eur. Dial. Transplant Assoc.*, **8**:126, 1970.

432. Catto, G. R. D., J. A. R. McIntosh, A. F. MacDonald, and M. MacLeod: Haemodialysis therapy and changes in skeletal calcium, *Lancet*, **1**:1150, 1973.

433. Mountokalakis, Th., A. Symvoulidis, K. Ntalles, and D. Ikkos: Bone loss in chronic renal failure, *Lancet*, **1**:363, 1977.

434. Evans, R. A., and P. J. Somerville: The use of high calcium dialysate in the treatment of renal osteomalacia, *Aust. N. Z. J. Med.*, **6**:10, 1976.

435. Kaye, M., G. Chatterjee, G. F. Cohen, and S. Sagar: Arrest of hyperparathyroid bone disease with

dihydrotachysterol in patients undergoing chronic hemodialysis, *Ann. Intern. Med.*, **73**:225, 1970.

436. Kaye, M., and S. Sagar: Effect of dihydrotachysterol on calcium absorption in uremia, *Metabolism,* **21**:815, 1972.

437. Witmer, G., A. Margolis, O. Fontaine, J. Fritsch, G. Lenoir, M. Broyer, and S. Balsan: Effects of 25-hydroxycholecalciferol on bone lesions of children with terminal renal failure, *Kidney Int.*, **10**:395, 1976.

438. Recker, R., P. Schoenfeld, J. Letteri, E. Slatopolsky, R. Goldsmith, and A. Brickman: The efficacy of calcifediol in renal osteodystrophy, *Arch. Intern. Med.*, **138**:857, 1978.

439. Chan, J. C. M., S. B. Oldham, M. F. Holick, and H. F. DeLuca: 1α-hydroxyvitamin D_3 in chronic renal failure: A potent analogue of the kidney hormone, 1,25-hydroxycholecalciferol, *J. Am. Med. Assoc.*, **234**:47, 1975.

440. Papapoulos, S. E., A. M. Brownjohn, F. J. Goodwin, W. Hartey, I. D. Marsh, and J. L. H. O'Riordan: The effect of 1α-hydroxycholecalciferol on secondary hyperparathyroidism of chronic renal failure, in A. W. Norman, K. Schaefer, J. W. Coburn, H. F. DeLuca, D. Fraser, H. G. Grigoleit, and D. von Herrath (eds.), *Vitamin D: Biochemical, Chemical and Clinical Aspects Related to Calcium Metabolism,* Walter de Gruyter & Co., Berlin, 1977, pp. 693–695.

441. Silverberg, D. S., K. B. Bettcher, J. B. Dossetor, T. R. Overton, M. F. Holick, and H. F. DeLuca: Effect of 1,25-dihydroxycholecalciferol in renal osteodystrophy, *Can. Med. Assoc. J.*, **112**:190, 1975.

442. Potter, D. E., C. J. Wilson, and M. B. Ozonoff: Hyperparathyroid bone disease in children undergoing long-term hemodialysis: Treatment with vitamin D, *J. Pediatr.*, **85**:60, 1974.

443. Counts, S. G., D. J. Baylink, F. H. Shen, D. J. Sherrard, and R. O. Hickman: Vitamin D intoxication in an anephric child, *Ann. Intern. Med.*, **82**:196, 1975.

444. Hughes, M. R., D. J. Baylink, P. G. Jones, and M. R. Haussler: Radioligand receptor assay for 25-hydroxyvitamin D_2/D_3, *J. Clin. Invest.*, **58**:61, 1976.

445. Mallick, N. P., and G. M. Berlyne: Arterial calcification after vitamin-D therapy in hyperphosphatemic renal failure, *Lancet,* **2**:1316, 1968.

446. Verberckmoes, R., R. Bouillon, and B. Krempien: Disappearance of vascular calcifications during treatment of renal osteodystrophy, *Ann. Intern. Med.*, **82**:529, 1975.

447. DeLuca, H. F., and L. V. Avioli: Treatment of renal osteodystrophy with 25-hydroxycholecalciferol, *Arch. Intern. Med.*, **126**:896, 1970.

448. Fournier, A. E., P. J. Bordier, J. Gueris, J. Chanard, P. Marie, C. Ferriere, M. Osario, J. Bedrossian, and H. F. DeLuca: 1α-Hydroxycholecalciferol and 25-hydroxycholecalciferol in renal bone disease, *Proc. Eur. Dial. Transplant Assoc.*, **12**:227, 1976.

449. Brickman, A. S., D. J. Sherrard, J. Jowsey, F. R. Singer, D. J. Baylink, N. Maloney, S. G. Massry, A. W. Norman, and J. W. Coburn: 1,25-Dihydroxycholecalciferol: Effect on skeletal lesions and plasma parathyroid hormone in uremic osteodystrophy, *Arch. Intern. Med.*, **134**:883, 1974.

450. Eastwood, J. B., M. E. Phillips, H. E. De Wardener, P. J. Bordier, P. Marie, C. D. Arnaud, and A. W. Norman: Biochemical and histological effects of 1,25-dihydroxycholecalciferol in the osteomalacia of chronic renal failure, in A. W. Norman, K. Schaefer, H. G. Grigoleit, D. von Herrath, and E. Ritz (eds.), *Vitamin D and Problems Related to Uremic Bone Disease,* Walter de Gruyter & Co., Berlin, 1975, p. 595.

451. Pierides, A. M., M. K. Ward, F. Ude-Alvarez, H. A. Ellis, K. M. Peart, W. Simpson, D. N. S. Kerr, and A. W. Norman: Long term therapy with 1,25 $(OH)_2D_3$ in dialysis bone disease, in J. F. Moorhead (ed.), *Proceedings, European Dialysis and Transplant Assn.,* vol. 12, Putnam Med. and Scientific Publ., New York, 1975, p. 237.

452. Coburn, J. W., A. S. Brickman, D. J. Sherrard, F. R. Singer, E. G. C. Wong, D. J. Baylink, and A. W. Norman: Use of 1,25$(OH)_2$ vitamin D_3 to separate "types" of renal osteodystrophy, *Proc. Eur. Dial. Transplant Assoc.*, **14**:442, 1977.

452a. Coburn, J. W., and A. S. Brickman: Current status of the use of newer analogs of vitamin D in the management of renal osteodystrophy, in S. G. Massry, E. Ritz, and A. Rapado (eds.), *Homeostasis of Phosphate and Other Minerals,* Plenum Press, New York, 1978, pp. 473–486.

453. Sherrard, D. J., J. W. Coburn, A. S. Brickman, D. J. Baylink, A. W. Norman, and N. Maloney: A his-

tologic comparison of 1,25(OH)$_2$ vitamin D treatment with calcium supplementation in renal osteodystrophy, in A. W. Norman, K. Schaefer, J. W. Coburn, H. F. DeLuca, D. Fraser, H. G. Grigoleit, an D. von Herrath (eds.), *Vitamin D: Biochemical, Chemical and Clinical Aspects Related to Calcium Metabolism*, Walter de Gruyter & Co., Berlin, 1977, pp. 719–721.

454. Winkler, S., A. S. Brickman, E. G. C. Wong, D. J. Sherrard, R. B. Miller, C. M. Bennett, and J. W. Coburn: Hypercalcemia during treatment of uremic patients with 1,25(OH)$_2$D$_3$: Analysis of 30 cases (abstract), *Kidney Int.*, **14**:000, 1978.

455. Chalmers, T. M., M. W. Davie, J. O. Hunter, K. F. Szaz, B. Pelc, and E. Kodicek: 1α-Hydroxycholecalciferol as a substitute for the kidney hormone, 1,25-dihydroxycholecalciferol, in chronic renal failure, *Lancet*, **2**:696, 1973.

456. Peacock, M., J. J. Gallagher, and B. E. C. Nordin: Action of 1α-hydroxy-vitamin D$_3$ on calcium absorption and bone resorption in man, *Lancet*, **1**:385, 1974.

457. Chan, J. C. M., and H. F. DeLuca: Growth velocity in a child on prolonged hemodialysis: Beneficial effect of 1α-hydroxy-vitamin D$_3$, *J. Am. Med. Assoc.*, **238**:2053, 1977.

458. Catto, G. R. D., M. MacLeod, B. Pek, and E. Kodicek: 1α-Hydroxycholecalciferol: A treatment for renal bone disease, *Br. Med. J.*, **1**:12, 1975.

459. Catto, G. R., and M. MacLeod: The investigation and treatment of renal bone disease, *Am. J. Med.*, **61**:64, 1976.

460. Madsen, S., and K. Ølgaard: 1-Alpha-hydroxycholecalciferol treatment of adults with chronic renal failure, *Acta Med. Scand.*, **200**:1, 1976.

461. Nielsen, S. P., E. Binderup, W. O. Godtfredsen, H. Jensen, and J. Ladefaged: 1α-Hydroxycholecalciferol. Long-term treatment of patients with uraemic osteodystrophy, *Nephron*, **16**:359, 1976.

462. Davie, M. W. J., T. M. Chalmers, J. O. Hunter, B. Pelc, and E. Kodicek: 1-Alpha-hydroxycholecalciferol in chronic renal failure: Studies of the effect of oral doses, *Ann. Intern. Med.*, **84**:281, 1976.

463. Naik, R. B., J. T. Dabek, G. Heynen, H. M. James, J. A. Kanis, P. W. Robertson, B. H. B. Robinson, and C. G. Woods: Measurement of whole body calcium in chronic renal failure: Effects of 1α-hydroxyvitamin D$_3$ and parathyroidectomy, *Clin. Endocrinol.*, **7**(suppl.):139S, 1977.

464. Kanis, J. A., M. Earnshaw, R. G. Henderson, G. Heynen, J. G. G. Ledingham, R. B. Naik, D. O. Oliver, R. G. G. Russell, R. Smith, R. H. Wilkinson, and C. G. Woods: Correlation of clinical, biochemical and skeletal responses to 1α-hydroxyvitamin D$_3$ in renal bone disease, *Clin. Endocrinol.*, **7**(suppl.):45S, 1977.

465. Kanis, J. A., R. G. G. Russell, R. B. Naik, M. Earnshaw, R. Smith, G. Heynen, and C. G. Woods: Factors influencing the response to 1α-hydroxyvitamin D$_3$ in patients with renal bone disease, *Clin. Endocrinol.*, **7**(suppl.):51S, 1977.

466. Melsen, F., H. E. Nielsen, and M. S. Christensen: Bone histomorphometry in patients with chronic renal failure: Effect of 1α-hydroxyvitamin D$_3$, *Clin. Endocrinol.*, **7**(suppl.):39S, 1977.

467. Nielsen, H. E., M. S. Christensen, F. Melsen, F. K. Rømer, and H. E. Hansen: Effect of 1α-hydroxyvitamin D$_3$ on parathyroid function in patients with chronic renal failure, *Clin. Endocrinol.*, **7**(suppl.):67S, 1977.

468. Papapoulos, S. E., A. M. Brownjohn, B. J. R. Junor, F. P. Marsh, F. J. Goodwin, W. Hately, I. G. Lewin, S. Tomlinson, G. N. Hendy, and J. L. H. O'Riordan: Hyperparathyroidism in chronic renal failure, *Clin. Endocrinol.*, **7**(suppl.):59S, 1977.

469. Peacock, M., J. E. Aaron, G. S. Walker, and A. M. Davison: Bone disease and hyperparathyroidism in chronic renal failure: The effect of 1α-hydroxyvitamin D$_3$, *Clin. Endocrinol.*, **7**(suppl.):73S, 1977.

470. Bone, J. M.: Hyperparathyroidism and the predictability of response to 1α-hydroxyvitamin D$_3$, *Clin. Endocrinol.*, **7**(suppl.):83S, 1977.

471. Davison, A. M., M. Peacock, G. S. Walker, D. H. Marshall, M. S. F. McLaughlin, and P. J. A. Robinson: Phosphate and 1α-hydroxy-vitamin D$_3$ therapy in haemodialysis patients, *Clin. Endocrinol.*, **7**(suppl.):91S, 1977.

472. Pierides, A. M., H. A. Ellis, W. Simpson, D. Cook, and D. N. S. Kerr: The effect of 1α-hydroxyvitamin D$_3$ in predialysis renal bone disease, *Clin. Endocrinol.*, **7**(suppl.):109S, 1977.

473. Postlethwaite, R. J., and I. B. Houston: Bone disease in children with chronic renal failure: Therapy with 1α-hydroxyvitamin D$_3$, *Clin. Endocrinol.*, **7**(suppl.):117S, 1977.

474. Hirooka, M., H. Wako, C. Kaneko, M. Ishikawa, S. Sasaki, and T. Suda: Curative effects of 1-

alpha-hydroxycholecalciferol on calcium metabolism and bone disease in patients with chronic renal failure, *J. Nutr. Sci. Vitaminol. (Tokyo)*, **21**:277, 1975.

475. Tougaard, L., E. Sorensen, J. Brochner-Mortensen, M. S. Christiansen, P. Rodbro, and A. W. W. Sorensen: Controlled trial of 1α-hydroxy-cholecalciferol in chronic renal failure, *Lancet*, **1**:1044, 1976.

476. Walker, G. S., M. Peacock, J. Aaron, P. J. A. Robinson, and A. M. Davison: Prophylactic 1α-hydroxyvitamin D₃ therapy in haemodialysis patients, *Clin. Endocrinol.*, **7**(suppl.):125S, 1977.

477. Junor, B. J. R., and G. R. D. Catto: The effect of 1α-hydroxy-vitamin D₃ on calcium and mineral content of bone in renal osteodystrophy, *Clin. Endocrinol.*, **7**(suppl.):131S, 1977.

478. Winney, R. J., P. Tothill, J. S. Robson, S. R. Abbot, G. P. Lidgard, E. H. D. Cameron, M. A. Smith, J. N. MacPherson, and J. A. Strong: The effect of dialysate calcium concentration and 1α-hydroxyvitamin D₃ on skeletal calcium loss and hyperparathyroidism in haemodialysis patients, *Clin. Endocrinol.*, **7**(suppl.):151S, 1977.

479. Gagnon, R., G. W. Ogden, G. Just, and M. Kaye: Comparison of dihydrotachysterol and 5,6-trans vitamin D₃ on intestinal calcium absorption in patients with chronic renal failure, *Can. J. Physiol. Pharmacol.*, **52**:272, 1974.

480. Rutherford, W. E., K. Hruska, J. Blondin, M. Holick, H. F. DeLuca, S. Klahr, and E. Slatopolsky: The effect of 5,6-trans vitamin D₃ on calcium absorption in chronic renal disease, *J. Clin. Endocrinol. Metab.*, **40**:13, 1975.

481. Kraft, D., and G. Offermann: The effect of high doses of 5,6-trans-25-hydroxycholecalciferol on calcium metabolism in relative vitamin D resistancy (hypoparathyroidism and chronic renal failure), in A. W. Norman, K. Schaefer, J. W. Coburn, H. F. DeLuca, D. Fraser, H. G. Grigoleit, and D. von Herrath (eds.), *Vitamin D: Biochemical, Chemical and Clinical Aspects Related to Calcium Metabolism*, Walter de Gruyter & Co., Berlin, 1977, pp. 679–680.

482. Grigoleit, H. G., K. Schaefer, D. Kraft, G. Offerman, D. von Herrath, and D. G. Delling: Clinical efficacy of 5,6-trans-25-OHCC in chronic renal failure, in A. W. Norman, K. Schaefer, J. W. Coburn, H. F. DeLuca, D. Fraser, H. G. Grigo-

leit, and D. von Herrath (eds.), *Vitamin D: Biochemical, Chemical and Clinical Aspects Related to Calcium Metabolism*, Walter de Gruyter & Co., Berlin, 1977, pp. 701–713.

483. Schulz, W., R. Heidler, P. Spiegel, U. Gessler, A. Schulz, and G. Delling: The treatment of renal osteopathy with 5,6-trans-25-OHCC: A report of experiments made during 32 months therapy, in A. W. Norman, K. Schaefer, J. W. Coburn, H. F. DeLuca, D. Fraser, H. G. Grigoleit, and D. von Herrath (eds.), *Vitamin D: Biochemical, Chemical and Clinical Aspects Related to Calcium Metabolism*, Walter de Gruyter & Co., Berlin, 1977, pp. 715–718.

484. Kanis, J. A., and R. G. Russell: Rate of reversal of hypercalcaemia and hypercalciuria induced by vitamin D and its 1α-hydroxylated derivatives, *Brit. Med. J.*, **1**:78, 1977.

485. Silver, J.: Anticonvulsant osteomalacia. An overview, in A. W. Norman, K. Schaefer, J. W. Coburn, H. F. DeLuca, D. Fraser, H. G. Grigoleit, and D. von Herrath (eds.), *Vitamin D: Biochemical, Chemical and Clinical Aspects Related to Calcium Metabolism*, Walter de Gruyter & Co., Berlin, 1977, pp. 835–837.

486. Hahn, T. J., and L. V. Avioli: Anticonvulsant osteomalacia, *Arch. Intern. Med.*, **135**:997, 1975.

487. Pierides, A. M., D. N. Kerr, H. A. Ellis, J. L. H. O'Riordan, and H. F. DeLuca: 1α-Hydroxycholecalciferol in hemodialysis renal osteodystrophy: Adverse effects of anticonvulsant therapy, *Clin. Nephrol.*, **5**:189, 1976.

488. Sörensen, E., L. Tougaard, and J. Bröchner-Mortensen: Iatrogenic magnesium intoxication during 1α-hydroxycholecalciferol treatment, *Br. Med. J.*, **2**:215, 1976.

489. Kanis, J. A., R. Smith, R. J. Walton, and M. Bartlett: Magnesium intoxication during 1-alpha-hydroxycholecalciferol treatment, *Br. Med. J.*, **2**:878, 1976.

490. Kanis, J. A., R. Smith, R. J. Walton, and M. Bartlett: Effect of 1-alpha-hydroxycholecalciferol on magnesium metabolism in chronic renal failure, *Br. Med. J.*, **1**:211, 1977.

491. Kanis, J. A., G. Heynen, R. G. G. Russell, R. Smith, R. J. Walton, and G. T. Warner: Biological effects of 24,25-dihydroxycholecalciferol in man, in A. W. Norman, K. Schaefer, J. W. Coburn, H. F. DeLuca, D. Fraser, H. G. Grigoleit,

and D. von Herrath (eds.), *Vitamin D: Biochemical, Chemical and Clinical Aspects Related to Calcium Metabolism,* Walter de Gruyter & Co., Berlin, 1977, p. 793.

492. Llach, F., A. S. Brickman, K. E. Gerszi, A. W. Norman, and J. W. Coburn: Actions of 24,25-dihydroxy-vitamin D_3 in uremic patients (abstract), *Clin. Res.,* **26:**543A, 1978.

493. Wilson, R. E., C. L. Hampers, D. S. Bernstein, J. W. Johnson, and J. P. Merrill: Subtotal parathyroidectomy in chronic renal failure, *Ann. Surg.,* **174:**640, 1971.

494. David, D. S.: Calcium metabolism in renal failure, *Am. J. Med.,* **58:**48, 1975.

495. Katz, A. D., and L. Kaplan: Parathyroidectomy for hyperplasia in renal disease, *Arch. Surg.,* **107:**51, 1973.

496. Gordon, H. E., J. W. Coburn, and E. Passaro: Surgical management of secondary hyperparathyroidism, *Arch. Surg.,* **104:**520, 1972.

497. Sakai, S., D. David, H. Shoji, K. Stenzel, and A. Rubin: Bone injuries due to tetany or convulsion during hemodialysis, *Clin. Orthop.,* **118:**118, 1976.

498. Fischer, J. A., J. W. Blum, and U. Binswanger: Acute parathyroid hormone response to epinephrine *in vivo, J. Clin. Invest.,* **52:**2434, 1973.

499. Caro, J., A. Besarab, J. F. Burke, and J. A. Glennon: A possible role for propranolol in the treatment of renal osteodystrophy, *Lancet,* **2:**451 1978.

500. Delano, B. G., R. Baker, B. Gardner, and S. Wallach: A trial of calcitonin therapy in renal osteodystrophy, *Nephron,* **11:**287, 1973.

501. Zucchelli, P., M. Fusaroli, L. Fabbri, P. Pavlica, S. Casanova, G. Viglietta, and M. Sasdelli: Treatment of ectopic calcification in uremia, *Kidney Int.,* **13**(suppl. 8):S86, 1978.

502. Fleisch, H., and J. P. Bonjour: Diphosphonate treatment in bone disease, *N. Engl. J. Med.,* **289:**1419, 1973.

503. Zingroff, J., T. Drucke, J.-P. Roux, M. Rodon-Nucete, N. K. Man, and P. Jungers: Bilateral fracture of the femoral neck complicating uremic bone disease prior to chronic hemodialysis, *Clin. Nephrol.,* **2:**73, 1974.

21

Water, electrolyte, and acid-base disorders in liver disease

T. B. REYNOLDS

SODIUM RETENTION, ASCITES, AND EDEMA

Ascites caused by liver disease is always accompanied by portal hypertension, and this is the reason for localization of fluid in the peritoneal cavity. Portal hypertension is more important in the pathogenesis of ascites than is lowered serum oncotic pressure since ascites regularly disappears when portal hypertension is relieved by side-to-side portacaval shunt, even when serum protein levels are unchanged. There is evidence that the major site of fluid transudation from the vascular tree is the sinusoidal bed of the liver. In experimental portal hypertension, fluid has been seen to appear on the liver surface (1), and pleural effusion instead of ascites develops when the liver is transferred into the right pleural cavity (2). The hepatic lymphatics are distended in patients with ascites; this is suggestive of increased fluid transudation from the liver sinusoids (3). Probably some of the ascitic fluid comes from the mesenteric and intestinal capillaries which are also hypertensive (4,5). Ascites caused by liver disease is a transudate, though the protein content is often higher than usually seen in transudates—reaching 50 percent of the serum protein level in about 10 percent of patients (6).

During ascites formation, urinary sodium content is usually very low (less than 10 meq per 24 h) and the patient gains ascites in direct proportion to sodium intake. The concentration of sodium in ascites is 0.9 × serum sodium (Donnan effect), so there will be a weight gain of 1 kg for each 110 to 120 meq of sodium in the diet. During the very earliest stages of ascites formation or during early spontaneous regression of ascites, the urinary sodium content may be quite variable, occasionally low and occasionally high, and, in general, nearly in balance with the sodium intake.

The most widely accepted theory for the pathogenesis of sodium retention in ascites maintains that ascites formation occurs because of the elevated intrahepatic sinusoidal pressure and precedes sodium retention. The loss of sodium and water into the peritoneal space causes a reduction of plasma volume which is perceived by the vascular volume-sensing apparatus as a need for vascular expansion, to be achieved by renal sodium and water retention. The retained sodium and water fail to relieve the plasma contraction because most of the retained fluid is extruded into the peritoneal space. Whether or not the leakage of sodium and water would ever cease if pressure in the peritoneal cavity rose sufficiently has not, to my knowledge, been tested in animals or human beings.

Plasma volume has been measured by many different investigators in patients with liver disease and ascites. All have found increased rather than decreased values (7). However, increased total plasma volume could be due to dilatation of the hypertensive portal venous bed, with the nonportal or "effective" plasma volume actually low, as postulated in the above theory of pathogenesis of ascites. Lieberman and colleagues, impressed with the magnitude and consistency of plasma volume expansion found in patients with liver disease, have proposed the "overflow" theory of ascites formation (8). They propose that sodium retention and plasma volume expansion appear first, prior to ascites formation. Ascites develops when the combination of plasma expansion and portal hypertension causes overflow into the peritoneal cavity. Denison et al. provided some support for this theory when they showed that ascites could be initiated in patients with portal hypertension by administration of the sodium-retaining hormone deoxycorticosterone acetate (DOCA) (9). The frequent finding of increased plasma renin and aldosterone in patients with sodium retention and ascites appears to support the standard theory for sodium retention and ascites formation, since "effective" plasma volume contraction would provide a logical stimulus for increased renin secretion. However, as suggested by Rosoff et al. (10), and Wilkinson et al. (11), increased plasma renin might be caused by a shift in intrarenal blood flow from outer cortical toward juxtamedullary nephrons with longer loops of Henle. The primary event in sodium retention might then be disturbance in intrarenal blood flow caused by some still unknown abnormality.

Increased plasma renin activity and aldosterone content and increased urinary aldosterone frequently accompany cirrhosis with ascites. Though aldosterone metabolism by the liver is impaired in cirrhosis, the rise in plasma aldosterone is due primarily to increased adrenal output rather than to delayed degradation (12, 13). Proximal tubular sodium retention appears to be much more important than aldosterone-mediated distal tubular sodium reabsorption, however. In our experience, markedly elevated values for plasma renin and aldosterone are confined to patients with very tight sodium retention (urinary sodium less than 2 meq per 24 h). Some patients with ascites and urinary sodium levels of 2 to 15 meq per 24 h have normal or nearly normal plasma renin and aldosterone (14). Normalization of plasma aldosterone with aminoglutethimide did not cause a marked natriuresis in three patients reported by Rosoff et al. (12), and one of their patients had marked spontaneous natriuresis without change in plasma aldosterone.

Edema formation in patients with liver disease is somewhat difficult to explain. When it accompanies tense ascites, it can be a hydrostatic phenomenon due to pressure on the vena cava with impaired drainage from the leg vessels. However, edema sometimes precedes ascites formation in patients with chronic liver disease. When the serum albumin is quite low, edema could be due to decreased plasma oncotic pressure. Many patients who have dependent edema antedating ascites have plasma protein levels nearly in the normal range, however. Raised inferior vena caval pressure due to narrowing of the vena cava in its course past the posterior aspect of the liver has been reported in some patients (15). However, to my knowledge no one has measured inferior vena caval pressures in patients who have dependent edema without ascites. The overflow theory of Lieberman provides a better explanation for dependent edema in the absence of ascites then does the classical theory for sodium retention.

HYPONATREMIA AND WATER BALANCE (See also Chap. 12)

As is true in the other edematous states, it has become increasingly obvious that hyponatremia in patients with cirrhosis and ascites is a manifestation of water excess rather than of sodium depletion. Though hyponatremia has been attributed to diuretic therapy, many patients have hyponatremia in the untreated state. Hyponatremia is rare in the absence of sodium retention and ascites. Mild hyponatremia is quite common in ascitic patients, but levels of serum sodium below 125 meq/L tend to be seen only in sicker patients, particularly those with the hepatorenal syndrome. Hyponatremia of a marked degree is considered a serious prognostic sign.

Impaired free water clearance is demonstrable in many patients with liver disease (16, 17). The pathogenesis of this impaired water tolerance is still not entirely certain. Schedl and Bartter proposed that markedly increased proximal sodium and water reabsorption lead to impairment in water diuresis because of reduced delivery of filtrate distally (18). They showed increases in free water clearance after mannitol infusion. Vesin claims increased water tolerance in some patients given glucocorticoids (19), but cortisol deficiency seems an unlikely explanation for the impaired water clearance in liver disease. Currently, the most reasonable explanation for impaired water diuresis is increased vasopressin concentration either due to impaired hepatic inactivation, "inappropriate" increase in secretion, "appropriate" increase in secretion, or some combination of these phenomena (see Chap. 12). Data on plasma levels of immunoactive vasopressin in patients with cirrhosis and hyponatremia are limited at this time, though Skowsky et al. have reported moderately elevated levels and markedly decreased rates of hepatic inactivity in six patients with cirrhosis (20).

If, in fact, a strong tendency for water retention exists in many patients who have liver disease and sodium retention, then dietary factors may contribute to hyponatremia. We found that serum sodium fell significantly in ascitic patients treated with diuretics and a low-sodium diet whereas it was unchanged in comparable patients given diuretics with a normal salt intake (21). Water intake was not controlled during this study; probably water restriction would have protected similarly against hyponatremia.

Moderate water restriction is the usual therapy for hyponatremia with ascites. It is unusual to find central nervous system symptoms attributable to hyponatremia, and serum sodium levels below 110 meq/L are exceptional. However, extremely low serum sodium is most often found in the patient with severe liver disease who may well have some degree of hepatic encephalopathy. The neurological symptoms of encephalopathy may be difficult to differentiate from the somnolence and

confusion of hyponatremia. In such situations, we recommend administration of hypertonic saline in sufficient quantity to raise the serum sodium to approximately 120 meq/L. Most of the infused saline ends up in the peritoneal cavity, but this presents no immediate threat to life, and a 2- to 3-L therapeutic paracentesis can be performed with relative safety if the ascites is uncomfortably tense. Diuretic therapy is not contraindicated, in our view, in hyponatremic patients. Ring-Larsen et al. employed peritoneal dialysis for hyponatremia in cirrhotic patients with no noted improvement in mental state in spite of an increase in serum sodium (22).

ACID-BASE ABNORMALITIES (See also Chap. 6)

The major acid-base abnormalities occur as often in patients with chronic liver disease as in the general population. These include metabolic acidosis due to lactic acid accumulation or diabetic ketosis, metabolic alkalosis from vomiting, and respiratory acidosis from chronic pulmonary disease. Seen in increased freqency in liver disease are (1) disturbance related to diuretic therapy (see below), (2) renal tubular acidosis, and (3) respiratory alkalosis.

RENAL TUBULAR ACIDOSIS

Renal tubular acidosis (RTA) was reported in a patient with cirrhosis of the liver by Smith, Middleton, and Williams in 1967 (23). In 1969, Shear et al. reported an abnormal response to an acid load in 9 of 15 patients with cirrhosis—2 had overt hyperchloremic acidosis and the other 7 had a defect shown only by acid loading (24). There have been many subsequent publications pointing out a relationship between liver disease and RTA. When present, the metabolic acidosis is rarely severe or symptomatic; serum bicarbonate levels usually are in the 15 to 20 meq/L range and blood pH is nearly normal. The relative hyperchloremia may be overlooked if there is concomitant hyponatremia and the anion gap is not calculated. "Incomplete" RTA with hyperchloremic acidosis evident only after acid loading is more common than is overt RTA. The disorder is seen in alcoholic liver disease, cryptogenic cirrhosis, and chronic active hepatitis. It is particularly frequent in primary biliary cirrhosis (25). The RTA is of the "distal" or "gradient" type with the lower limit of urine pH in the 5.8 to 6.5 range, a reduced urinary titratable acidity, and a urinary ammonium content that is relatively high for the urine pH (25, 26). Hypokalemia is present in some patients. Shear et al. believed that hypokalemia could cause hepatic encephalopathy by stimulating renal ammonia production, with much of this ammonia ending up in the renal venous blood because of lack of urine acidity (24).

The reason for an association between distal RTA and liver disease is uncertain. Most such patients have some degree of hyperglobulinemia, as do many patients with primary, distal RTA, but there is no close correlation between the magnitude of globulin increase and urinary acidification (25). Better suggests that the defect in urine acidification is the result of increased proximal tubular sodium reabsorption which leaves no opportunity for distal tubular sodium-hydrogen exchange (27). However, many patients with RTA and liver disease have no evidence of ascites or sodium retention. An immunologic cause for the RTA is suggested by the relative frequency of mild acidification defect found in primary biliary cirrhosis and chronic active hepatitis (25), diseases with immunologic overtones. However, we have seen mild RTA relatively frequently in patients with alcoholic liver disease. At this time, the relationship between RTA and liver disease seems definite, but the basic reason for the relationship remains obscure. RTA with cirrhosis can be confused with mild hyperchloremic acidosis resulting from the inhibiting action of large doses of spironolactone on sodium-hydrogen exchange and with the chemical changes accompanying prolonged respiratory alkalosis.

RESPIRATORY ALKALOSIS

Hyperventilation with respiratory alkalosis was described in patients with chronic liver disease by Vanamee et al. in 1956 (28) and this association has been confirmed repeatedly since then both in chronic (29–34) and acute (35) liver disease. When the hyperventilation is prolonged, there may be compensatory renal lowering of serum bicarbonate to levels of 10 to 15 meq/L. Casey and coworkers noted a significant relationship between respiratory alkalosis and hyperammonemia in their patients, consistent with a direct effect of ammonia on the respiratory center (31). Roberts et al. showed that intravenous ammonium acetate in dogs caused both hyperammonemia and respiratory alkalosis (36). However, Dölle found no correlation between either arterial or venous ammonia levels and P_{CO_2} (33). Mild degrees of arterial hypoxemia are common in patients with chronic liver disease. Heinemann and colleagues found some correlation between hyperventilation and hypoxemia (29), but Snell and Luchsinger failed to find any correlation in 15 patients (30). The cause of the hyperventilation of liver disease remains uncertain, therefore. Its detection may alert the clinician to the presence of otherwise unsuspected hepatic encephalopathy.

It has been suggested that respiratory alkalosis may contribute to hepatic encephalopathy by impairing oxyhemoglobin dissociation and by raising the NH_3/NH_4^+ ratio with increased penetration of NH_3 into the brain. Posner and Plum treated patients with mild hepatic encephalopathy and respiratory alkalosis by inhalation of 5% carbon dioxide (37). Though arterial NH_3 declined and cerebral NH_3 uptake decreased, the patient's clinical status worsened and cerebral oxygen uptake fell. Clinical deterioration also ensued when the respiratory alkalosis was treated with intravenous acetazolamide. Attempts to treat hyperventilation by respiratory center sedation obviously would be risky in patients with severe liver disease. For all of these reasons, treatment of respiratory alkalosis in patients with liver disease is not advisable.

HYPOKALEMIA (See also Chap. 4)

Hypokalemia is sometimes found in patients with liver diseases in the absence of any exposure to diuretic drugs. Serum potassium levels below 2.0

meq/L may occur, sometimes with accompanying muscle weakness. In our experience such patients have usually had alcoholic liver disease. The relative importance of vomiting, diarrhea, and increased urinary loss from secondary hyperaldosteronism has never been satisfactorily assessed in this type of patient. The limited data available do not point to increased urinary loss as an important mechanism (37–39).

Total exchangeable potassium often is below normal in patients with chronic liver disease even in the absence of hypokalemia (38, 40, 41). This low body potassium seems resistant to administration of potassium supplements and may be due, in some degree, to the low muscle mass characteristic of chronic liver disease. Additionally, it has been postulated that some as yet unidentified cellular abnormality accounts for the lower than normal exchangeable intracellular potassium.

DIURETIC-INDUCED ELECTROLYTE ABNORMALITIES

HYPOKALEMIA

This is the most common diuretic-induced electrolyte abnormality in patients with liver disease and sodium retention. Most of today's potent diuretics (furosemide, ethacrynic acid, thiazides, bumetanide, metolazone) block sodium chloride reabsorption in the proximal nephron and/or the ascending limb of Henle's loop. This increases the concentration and amount of sodium reaching the distal tubular Na^+/K^+ exchange site and, if hyperaldosteronism is present, kaliuresis is increased. An additional factor promoting hypokalemia and kaliuresis is the metabolic alkalosis that accompanies the normal action of these diuretics. Metabolic alkalosis results in potassium entry to the intracellular space and favors potassium rather than hydrogen exchange for sodium in the distal tubule. The severity of hypokalemia seen with diuretics is related to the magnitude of the natriuresis, the degree of secondary hypoaldosteronism, and the dietary intake of potassium. Serum potassium levels less than 2 meq/L were seen frequently during the early days of use of these diuretics when no measures were taken to

prevent hypokalemia. Oral potassium supplements are now widely used and are quite effective in preventing hypokalemia. Though it tends to cause gastric irritation, potassium chloride is preferable to the alkaline salts of potassium since it helps prevent metabolic alkalosis. Several commercial preparations of varied palatability are available. An inexpensive method of administration is granular potassium chloride used as artificial salt. Most patients will accept at least 40 mmol daily in this form without gastric upset. Of all potassium chloride preparations, probably the most acceptable, from the patient's standpoint, is "Slow-K" a slow-release tablet in a wax base. However, serious small-bowel pathology lead to the abandonment of another form of slow-release potassium chloride in 1965 (42), and reports are now beginning to appear in Britain (43–45) and the United States (46) of esophageal and small-intestinal ulceration attributed to "Slow-K."

A very satisfactory method of avoiding hypokalemia in patients with ascites who are given diuretics is the concomitant administration of one of the distally acting diuretics (spironolactone, triamterene or amiloride). On our liver unit we rarely administer a proximally acting diuretic alone to a patient with ascites. If brief or intermittent diuresis is desired, we use triamterene, 100 or 200 mg once or twice daily, and if continuous diuresis is elected, we administer spironolactone, 100 to 400 mg daily, as required. Amiloride is an excellent antikaluretic drug, as potent as spironolactone in our experience (47) but not yet available in the United States. With these combinations, the need for potassium chloride supplements to prevent hypokalemia is greatly reduced. Occasional patients still require oral potassium chloride, but this should not be given routinely since dangerous hyperkalemia can occasionally result.

Effective diuresis can be induced in almost all patients with ascites and normal renal function using spironolactone alone (48). Daily doses of 200 to 400 mg are usually required, and the dose may have to be raised to as high as 800 mg per day. Hypokalemia and metabolic alkalosis do not occur when spironolactone is used alone; in fact, mild hyperchloremic acidosis is customary because of the inhibition of Na^+/H^+ exchange in the distal tubules. Disadvantages of large-dose spironolactone therapy that make it less suitable for nonhospital use include (1) gastric discomfort from a large number of 25-mg tablets, (2) slow onset and cessation of diuretic action, and (3) the danger of serious hyperkalemia if patients are inadvertently given potassium chloride supplements or if they develop renal insufficiency.

METABOLIC ALKALOSIS

Metabolic alkalosis is very common in ascitic patients treated with thiazides, ethacrynic acid, furosemide, metolazone or bumetanide. There are at least three mechanisms responsible for the alkalosis. First, if potassium deficiency occurs there is migration of hydrogen intracellularly with resultant extracellular alkalosis. Second, the movement of increased amounts of sodium into the distal tubule promotes increased Na^+/H^+ exchange over and above the amount needed to balance the metabolic production of hydrogen. Third, extracellular fluid volume is reduced by diuresis of urine that contains sodium, potassium, and chloride but little or no bicarbonate (because of the increased Na^+/H^+ exchange in the distal tubule). Substantial contraction of the extracellular fluid without concomitant loss of bicarbonate causes "contraction alkalosis."

Prevention of alkalosis with diuretics can be approached in three different ways:

1. Large potassium chloride supplements will reduce the Na^+/H^+ exchange in the distal tubule by providing more potassium for exchange with sodium. Some urinary excretion of bicarbonate may ensue. Less bicarbonate will be generated by urinary hydrogen secretion, and there will be less tendency for intracellular hydrogen shift because there will be less potassium deficiency.
2. Concomitant use of triamterene, spironolactone, or amiloride interferes with urinary Na^+/H^+ exchange, reduces renal bicarbonate regeneration, and promotes urinary bicarbonate loss.
3. Oral supplementation with lysine or arginine

hydrochloride provides hydrochloric acid which restores normal serum bicarbonate and chloride concentrations. These amino acids are palatable as 10% solutions and can be given in amounts of 50 to 100 mmol daily without gastric irritation.

HYPERCHLOREMIC ACIDOSIS

As indicated earlier, when either spironolactone or amiloride is used in effective doses alone, a mild degree of hyperchloremic acidosis frequently ensues (serum chloride 110 to 115 meq/L, serum bicarbonate 14 to 19 meq/L). This is due to interference by the diuretic with Na^+/H^+ exchange in the distal tubule. Urine pH tends to be somewhat higher (6.5–7.0) with these diuretics than with the proximally acting diuretics, and the urine contains appreciable amounts of bicarbonate.

RENAL IMPAIRMENT

Moderate elevations of serum creatinine and urea nitrogen are frequent accompaniments of diuretic administration in patients with liver disease and ascites. This is more common in patients whose ascites is refractory or moderately refractory to diuretics; approximately 15 percent of such patients will have a doubling of serum creatinine during diuresis. In our opinion, this impairment of renal function is not closely related to the hepatorenal syndrome (49). Diuretic-induced renal insufficiency disappears promptly if saline is administered to replace diuretic-induced losses, even if diuretic administration is continued. One explanation for diuretic-induced renal impairment is hypovolemia due to removal of sodium and water from the plasma at a faster rate than they can be repleted from the ascites. Shear and coworkers showed that the maximum rate of movement of ascites to plasma during diuresis was approximately 900 mL/day (50).

In a randomized, controlled trial of different regimens of diuresis we found statistically significant rises in serum urea nitrogen and creatinine in all groups of patients given diuretics to the

point of complete or near complete relief of ascites (21). On the other hand, we found no
changes in urea nitrogen or creatinine in groups
of patients given diuretics with the objective of
partial removal of ascites to the point of achieving patient comfort.

HEPATORENAL SYNDROME

DEFINITION

Hecker and Sherlock described patients with cirrhosis, ascites, hyponatremia, and terminal renal
failure in 1956 (51). Though hepatorenal syndrome (HRS) is the term most widely used for
this disorder, functional renal failure, suggested
by Vesin (52) is the more pathogenetic designation. It is a functional disturbance of the kidney
of unknown cause that is often seen in patients
with severe liver disease. Anatomically the kidneys are normal and their dysfunction has been
shown to be reversible when reunited with a normal liver either after renal (53) or liver (54) transplantation.

CHARACTERISTICS

There are no pathognomonic features that allow a
definite diagnosis of HRS. However, most other
causes of renal dysfunction in the setting of severe liver disease can be identified; in the absence
of any identifiable renal disease, then HRS is
likely. The liver disease with HRS always is severe. Most patients with fulminant acute hepatic
necrosis have some degree of renal failure, presumably due to HRS, just prior to death. In our
liver unit, about half of the patients who die from
chronic or subacute liver disease have evidence of
HRS (Table 21-1). Thomsen and Juhl found that
41 of 104 patients dying with cirrhosis of the liver
had a serum creatinine above 2.0 mg/dL during
the last week of life (55). Patients with severe
acute alcoholic hepatitis are particularly prone to
develop HRS, and almost all of such patients who
die do so with an elevated serum creatinine.
Renal dysfunction is seen occasionally in patients with bile duct obstruction, particularly after

Table 21-1. Prognostic value of various biochemical tests in 406 hospitalized patients with subacute or chronic liver disease*

	SURVIVED THE HOSPITALIZATION	DIED
Total patients	305	101
Serum albumin		
2.0 g/100 mL or less	104	53
Above 2.0 g/100 mL	199	45
Serum bilirubin		
Above 20 mg/100 mL	19	23
20 mg/100 mL or less	285	76
Prothrombin activity		
Less than 30% of control	50	40
30% or greater	250	56
Serum urea nitrogen		
Above 40 mg/100 mL	18	68
40 mg/100 ml or less	273	33
Serum creatinine		
Above 2.4 mg/100 mL	8	54
2.4 mg/100 mL or less	297	47

* The records of all patients hospitalized on the liver unit at John Wesley County Hospital with subacute or chronic liver disease during an 18-month period in 1968 and 1969 were surveyed and the most abnormal result for each of the laboratory tests was used to construct the table. For each test except serum creatinine, there were a few patients who had no measurement made.
Source: From F. Schaffner, S. Sherlock, and C. Leevy (eds.), *The Liver and Its Diseases,* Intercontinental Medical Book Corp., New York, 1974, p. 308.

surgery or sepsis; whether this renal lesion is
HRS or acute tubular necrosis remains unsettled,
though available evidence favors the latter (56,
57). Renal failure is often seen with severe toxic
hepatitis (acetaminophen, carbon tetrachloride,
allopurinol, *Amanita phalloides* ingestion, methoxyflurane, halothane). Probably there is direct
renal damage from most of these substances,
though this has not been proven for acetaminophen and halothane.

Many patients with HRS have oliguria early in
the course of the renal lesion, and nearly all develop oliguria before death. However, about half
of the patients will continue to have urine volumes over 500 mL per 24 h when the renal disorder is first detected (Table 21-2). The urine
contains little or no protein, and there are few
cells or casts in the sediment. Unlike the findings
in acute tubular necrosis, urine sodium concentration tends to be quite low and osmolality is

Table 21.2. Clinical and laboratory features in 15 patients who survived the hepatorenal syndrome, group A, and 15 who did not, group B*

	A	B
Age, mean and range	44 (31–56)	47 (29–60)
Sex	9M, 6F	9M, 6F
Type of liver disease		
Subacute	14	13
Chronic	1	2
Hospital day when renal dysfunction detected, mean and range	18 (1–90)	20 (1–79)
Days from detection of renal dysfunction to death or normal renal function, mean & range	54 (13–105)	21 (1–90)
Clinical features at detection of renal dysfunction		
Jaundice	14/15	13/15
Ascites	14/15	15/15
Encephalopathy	13/15	12/15
Preceding neomycin therapy	11/15	9/15
Preceding diuretic therapy	7/15	9/15
Laboratory test results at detection of renal dysfunction, mean and range		
Serum bilirubin, mg/dL	21 (0.9–47)	21 (0.9–38)
Serum albumin, gm/dL	2.2 (1.5–3.3)	1.9 (1.7–2.5)
Serum globulin, gm/dL	4.6 (3.0–5.8)	4.9 (3.8–6.3)
SGOT, Karmen U/mL	134 (45–366)	131 (70–280)
Prothrombin, % of normal	50 (25–88)	51 (10–90)
Serum urea nitrogen/creatinine, mg/dL	20 (8–44)	19 (9–37)
Serum Na^+, meq/L	128 (115–140)	128 (115–141)
At detection of renal dysfunction, number of patients with		
24-h urine volume >500 mL	11/15	3/14
Urine Na^+ >10 meq/L	1/14	1†/13

* All patients had serum creatinine levels of 2.5 mg/dL or above.
†Urine Na^+ 60 meq/L, while receiving diuretics.
Source: After F. Schaffner, S. Sherlock, and C. Leevy (eds.), *The Liver and Its Diseases*, Intercontinental Medical Book Corp., New York, 1974, p. 310.

usually moderately higher than that of plasma. Some insist that a low urine sodium concentration (less than 15 meq/L) must be present in order to allow a diagnosis of HRS. However, about 3 percent of the patients in whom we diagnose HRS do not have a low concentration of sodium in the urine and yet, otherwise, they seem typical in every respect (58). Ascites is very common in patients with HRS accompanying subacute or chronic liver disease but is not present in every case, in our material. Hypertension and severe acidosis are exceptional. In spite of the reputed inability of the damaged liver to manufacture urea normally, the serum urea nitrogen/creatinine ratio is somewhat increased in HRS, averaging 20 in the 30 patients described in Table 21-2.

The rate of progression of renal dysfunction in patients with HRS is extremely variable. Some have continuous, stable serum urea and creatinine elevations for months before recovery or death with progressive hepatic and renal failure (Fig. 21-1). Others have total loss of renal function over a relatively brief period of time.

DIFFERENTIAL DIAGNOSIS

A common dilemma in diagnosis is the patient with known liver disease who develops renal dysfunction after receiving diuretics or a potentially nephrotoxic antibiotic such as gentamicin. The urinary findings should resemble those of acute tubular necrosis in the second instance, though it is difficult to predict urine sodium concentration in a patient with ascites and marked sodium retention who develops superimposed gentamicin toxicity. The renal insufficiency caused by diuret-

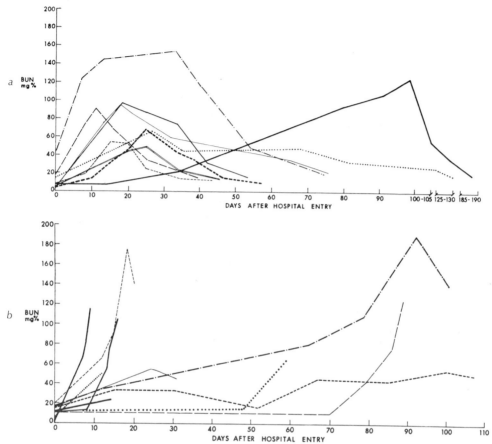

Figure 21-1. Variable course of the blood urea nitrogen in 10 patients who survived the hepatorenal syndrome (a) and 10 patients who expired (b).

ics rarely progresses beyond a serum creatinine of 2.5 mg/dL unless there is underlying chronic nephropathy, and it usually disappears rapidly when diuretic use is stopped or when saline is given. Patients with alcoholic liver disease may develop pyelonephritis with papillary necrosis, oliguria, and renal failure (59). The urine of these patients invariably contains bacteria and large numbers of leucocytes, and the kidneys are often increased in size on x-ray. Leptospirosis can cause both jaundice and renal insufficiency. Urinary findings resemble those of a nephritis, fever is usually prominent, and the serologic test for leptospirosis should become abnormal within two weeks after

onset of the illness. There are a number of medications and toxins that cause simultaneous liver and kidney damage including carbon tetrachloride, methoxyflurane, allopurinol, and *Amanita phalloides*. Acetaminophen and halothane sometimes are associated with both jaundice and renal failure; whether the renal failure is due to HRS or to tubular damage is unsettled.

PROGNOSIS

HRS was considered to be invariably fatal until the report of four survivors by Goldstein and Boyle in 1965 (60). A review of 18 months' experience in our liver unit in 1973 showed 8 survivors among 62 patients (13 percent) with HRS associated with chronic or subacute liver disease. HRS was defined as any otherwise unexplained elevation of serum creatinine above 2.4 mg/dL. In comparing 15 selected patients with HRS who survived (the 8 mentiond above together with 7 additional survivors) with 15 consecutive patients who did not (Table 21-2) we found no differences in clinical features, hepatic biochemical tests, or prior use of neomycin or diuretics. Only 24-h urine volume was different; it was greater than 500 mL at the time of detection of renal dysfunction in 11 of the survivors and in only 3 of the fatal cases.

The prognosis of HRS is so grim that, in patients with subacute or chronic liver disease, the serum creatinine and urea nitrogen are far more accurate predictors of survival than are any of the standard hepatic tests. Table 21-1 compares the prognostic accuracy of extreme abnormality in bilirubin (above 20 mg/dL), albumin (below 2.0 g/dL) and prothrombin activity (less than 30 percent of control) with that of serum urea nitrogen over 40 mg/dL and serum creatinine over 2.4 mg/dL. The case material consists of 406 consecutive patients hospitalized in our liver unit during an 18-month period with a diagnosis of subacute or chronic liver disease. Approximately 86 percent of the prognostications based on serum urea nitrogen or creatinine abnormality were correct as compared to 76 percent based on bilirubin, 63 percent on albumin, and 73 percent on prothrombin.

PATHOGENESIS

Patients with HRS consistently show a decrease in renal blood flow with an increase in renal vascular resistance (61–65) and a change in intrarenal blood flow distribution with decrease in outer cortical and relative increase in juxtamedullary blood flow (65, 66). It is unlikely that these alterations are a reflex renal response to low cardiac output or to extensive shunting of blood through superficial skin vessels. These same abnormalities are often present to a lesser degree in patients with ascites and marked sodium retention who have a normal creatinine clearance (67). Whether or not the abnormalities could be a reflex response to decreased "effective" plasma volume remains unsettled. Total plasma volume is consistently increased in patients with chronic liver disease, and we found no differences between patients with and without HRS (7). However, the increase in total plasma volume could be due to expansion of the portal venous bed from portal hypertension, and the "effective" plasma volume might still be decreased. Tristani and Cohn found short-term increases in renal blood flow after dextran infusion in 13 of 21 patients (62). We found temporary improvement in renal function in 9 of 16 patients with HRS given plasma expander (68). Improvement in HRS described after side-to-side portacaval shunt (69) could be due to effective plasma volume increase resulting from reduction in portal hypertension. Improvement in HRS described after LeVeen shunt placement (70) could be due to plasma volume expansion. On the other hand, 7 of our 16 patients showed no response at all to plasma expansion and 15 of the total of 16 patients died during the hospitalization. McCloy et al. (71) and Baldus (61) found no improvement in renal hemodynamics or renal function following either single or multiple infusions of albumin solution. The possible role of decreased effective plasma volume remains unsettled, therefore.

To us it seems quite unlikely that diuretics play any part in the pathogenesis of HRS (49). Many patients with the syndrome have never received diuretics. Diuretic-induced renal insufficiency rarely causes a creatinine increase of greater than 2.5 mg/dL, and it disappears rapidly when diuretics are discontinued or when saline is given. Since HRS patients usually have ascites, it is only natural that many will have received diuretics during the onset of the renal dysfunction and that there will be instances of progression from diuretic-induced renal insufficiency to HRS that could be purely coincidental.

Deficiency or accumulation of some vasoactive substance normally supplied by or removed by the liver could cause the renal hemodynamic changes of HRS. For example, Berkowitz suggested that a deficiency of renin substrate might cause renal vasoconstriction (72). Horisawa tested this general theory by performing exchange transfusions with fresh whole blood in 10 patients with HRS (73). There was no correlation between increase in renin substrate levels and improvement in renal function. Though renin substrate levels increased in most patients after exchange, only two showed improvement in renal function, and only one survived. Therefore, it is unlikely that slow accumulation of a toxic humoral agent or deficiency of any long-lived humoral substance is a cause of HRS.

Fischer and colleagues have proposed that accumulation of false neurotransmitters at sympathetic nerve endings might explain renal dysfunction as well as encephalopathy in liver disease (74). However, failure of dopamine therapy to correct the HRS (75) is against this concept.

An important role of prostaglandins in the hepatorenal syndrome is suggested by the recent findings of Boyer (76). Administration of indomethacin to patients with ascites and tight sodium retention consistently caused prompt fall in renal clearances of para-aminohippurate and creatinine and a rise in serum creatinine. These changes could be prevented by an intravenous infusion of prostaglandin $A_1(PGA_1)$. In following up these findings, Zipser and colleagues showed that plasma prostaglandin levels were markedly increased in similar patients and that the levels fell after indomethacin or ibuprofen, coincident with the decrease in creatinine clearance (14). Prostaglandin administration does not seem helpful in patients with HRS, however (77, 78). We postulate that the marked increase in plasma prostaglandin found in patients with ascites and sodium retention represents a compensatory response attempting to maintain normal renal vasodilatation and that this compensatory response has been overcome by some powerful vasoconstrictor stimulus in patients who develop HRS.

TREATMENT

There are a number of excellent reviews of HRS including those by Summerskill (79), Vesin (52), and Conn (80) that discuss therapy.

That treatment of HRS is unsatisfactory at this time is hardly surprising in view of the gravity of the underlying liver disease and the lack of understanding of the pathogenesis of the syndrome. Though it has frequently been stated that most patients with HRS die *with* rather than *from* uremia, it is tempting to think that mortality from the liver disease might be lowered if it were possible to treat the renal dysfunction effectively. Though many patients with HRS receive an occasional peritoneal or hemodialysis, there are limited published data on the effect of intensive dialysis on mortality rate (81). Many vasoactive drugs have been tried without clear-cut benefit. They include metaraminol (82), dopamine (75), phentolamine (65), and octapressin (83). We and others (65) have given vasodilator drugs directly into the renal artery without benefit. Conn mentioned possible benefit from corticosteroid therapy (80); we found no increase in survival from this treatment in a controlled trial involving 38 patients (84). In spite of the evidence that indomethacin administration can cause a renal circulatory dysfunction closely resembling HRS (76), administration of prostaglandin E_2 directly into the renal artery was not helpful in three patients with HRS (77), and intravenous PGA_1 did not consistently improve renal hemodynamics in patients with impaired renal function studied by Arieff and Chidsey (78). We have given prolonged PGA_1 infusions (0.3 $\mu g/kg$ per min) to two patients with HRS without benefit.

A major unresolved therapeutic question in HRS is the role of plasma expansion with albumin solution or ascitic fluid. Recently, encouraging results in a few patients of our own with daily albumin infusions or with placement of a LeVeen peritoneal-jugular shunt have prompted us to begin a controlled trial of these two modes of therapy. Until more data are available we advise at least a brief trial of plasma expansion therapy in most patients. If urinary creatinine shows a definite increase with expansion then it may be worthwhile continuing this treatment on a daily basis as long as benefit can be documented. Probably there is a risk of precipitating variceal hemorrhage with expansion of blood volume so that expansion therapy should not be continued for long if there is no definite improvement in renal function.

REFERENCES

1. Hyatt, R. E., G. H. Lawrence, and J. R. Smith: Observations on the origin of ascites from experimental hepatic congestion, *J. Lab. Clin. Med.*, **45**:274, 1955.

2. Freeman, S.: Recent progress in physiology and biochemistry of liver, *Med. Clin. North Am.*, **37**:109, 1953.

3. Baggenstoss, A. H., and J. C. Cain: The hepatic hilar lymphatics of man: their relation to ascites, *N. Engl. J. Med.*, **256**:531, 1957.

4. Losowsky, M. S., and C. S. Davidson: The source of ascitic fluid in cirrhosis of the liver, *Arch. Intern. Med.*, **110**:279, 1962.

5. Witte, M. H., C. L. Witte, and A. E. Dumont: Progress in liver disease: physiological factors involved in the causation of cirrhotic ascites, *Gastroenterology*, **61**:742, 1971.

6. Sampliner, R., and F. Iber: High protein ascites in patients with uncomplicated hepatic cirrhosis, *Am. J. Med. Sci.*, **267**:275, 1974.

7. Lieberman, F. L., and T. B. Reynolds: Plasma volume in cirrhosis of the liver: its relation to portal hypertension, ascites and renal failure, *J. Clin. Invest.*, **46**:1297, 1967.

8. Lieberman, F. L., E. K., Denison, and T. B. Reynolds: The relationship of plasma volume, portal hypertension, ascites formation and renal sodium retention in cirrhosis: the overflow theory of ascites, *Ann. N.Y. Acad. Sci.*, **170**:202, 1970.

9. Denison, E. K., F. L. Lieberman, and T. B. Reynolds: 9—fluorohydrocortisone induced ascites in alcoholic liver disease, *Gastroenterology*, **61**:497, 1971.

10. Rosoff, L., J. Williams, P. Moult, H. Williams, and S. Sherlock: Renal hemodynamics and the renin-angiotensin system in cirrhosis: their relationship to sodium retention, *Gastroenterology*, **70**:133A, 1976.

11. Wilkinson, S. P., A. Alam, H. Moodie, and R. Williams: Renal retention of sodium in cirrhosis and fulminant hepatic failure, *Postgrad. Med. J.*, **51**:527, 1975.

12. Rosoff, L., Jr., P. Zia, T. B. Reynolds, and R. Horton: Studies of renin and aldosterone in cirrhotic patients with ascites, *Gastroenterology*, **69**:698, 1975.

13. Coppage, W. S., Jr., D. P. Island, A. E. Cooner, and G. W. Liddle: The metabolism of aldosterone in normal subjects and in patients with hepatic cirrhosis, *J. Clin. Invest.*, **41**:1672, 1962.

14. Zipser, R. D., J. C. Hoefs, P. F. Speckart, P. K. Zia, and R. Horton: Prostaglandins: modulators of renal function and pressor resistance in chronic liver disease. Submitted for publication.

15. Mullane, J. F., and M. L. Gliedman: Elevation of the pressure in the abdominal inferior vena cava as a cause of a hepatorenal syndrome in cirrhosis, *Surgery*, **59**:1135, 1966.

16. Papper, S., and L. Saxon: The diuretic response to administered water in patients with liver disease. II. Laennec's cirrhosis of the liver, *Arch. Intern. Med.*, **103**:750, 1959.

17. Shear, L., P. W. Hall, III, and G. J. Gabuzda: Renal failure in patients with cirrhosis of the liver. II. Factors influencing maximal urinary flow rate, *Am. J. Med.*, **39**:198, 1965.

18. Schedl, H. P., and F. C. Bartter: An explanation for and experimental correction of the abnormal water diuresis in cirrhosis, *J. Clin. Invest.*, **39**:248, 1960.

19. Vesin, P.: Le traitement des cirrhoses ascitiques éthyliques par la delta-cortisone, *Arch. Fr. Mal. App. Dig.*, **48**:1497, 1959.

20. Skowsky, R., J. Riestra, I. Martinez, L. Swan, and T. Kikuchi: Arginine vasopressin kinetics in hepatic cirrhosis, *Clin. Res.*, **24**:101A, 1976.

21. Reynolds, T. B., A. Goodman, and E. Savage: Treatment of ascites without dietary sodium restriction, *Clin. Res.*, **24**:147A, 1976.

22. Ring-Larsen, H., E. Clausen, and L. Ranek: Peritoneal dialysis in hyponatremia due to liver failure, *Scand. J. Gastroenterol.*, **8**:33, 1972.

23. Smith, P. M., J. E. Middleton, and R. Williams: Renal tubular acidosis and cirrhosis, *Postgrad. Med. J.*, **43**:439, 1967.

24. Shear, L., H. L. Bonkowsky, and G. J. Gabuzda: Renal tubular acidosis in cirrhosis. A determinant of susceptibility to recurrent hepatic precoma, *N. Engl. J. Med.*, **280**:1, 1969.

25. Golding, P. L.: Renal tubular acidosis in chronic liver disease, *Postgrad. Med. J.*, **51**:550, 1975.

26. Vesin, P., J. Gouerou, M. Dervichian, D. Agar,

M. Azogui, and D. Cattan: Acidose tublaire rénale et hépatopathies alcooliques, *Arch. Fr. Mal. App. Dig.*, **65**:209, 1976.

27. Better, O. S., Z. Goldschmid, C. Chaimowitz, and G. G. Alroy: Defect in urinary acidification in cirrhosis, *Arch. Intern. Med.*, **130**:77, 1972.

28. Vanamee, P., J. W. Poppell, A. S. Glicksman, H. T. Randall, and K. E. Roberts: Respiratory alkalosis in hepatic coma, *Arch. Intern. Med.*, **97**:762, 1956.

29. Heinemann, H. O., C. Emirgil, and J. P. Mijnssen: Hyperventilation and arterial hypoxemia in cirrhosis of the liver, *Am. J. Med.*, **28**:239, 1960.

30. Snell, R. E., and P. C. Luchsinger: The relation of arterial hypoxemia to the hyperventilation of chronic liver disease, *Am. J. Med. Sco.*, **245**:289, 1963.

31. Casey, T. H., W. H. J. Summerskill, R. G. Dickford, and J. W. Rosewear: Body and serum potassium in liver disease. II. Relationships to arterial ammonia, blood pH and hepatic coma, *Gastroenterol.*, **48**:208, 1965.

32. Mulhausen, R., A. Eichenholz, and A. Blumentals: Acid-base disturbances in patients with cirrhosis of the liver, *Medicine (Baltimore)*, **46**:185, 1966.

33. Dölle, W.: Störungen des Säure-Basenstoffwechsels bei chronisch Leberkranken, in G. A. Martini (ed.), *Aktuelle Probleme der Hepatologie*, George Thieme Verlag, Stuttgart, 1962, p. 128.

34. Prytze, H. and A. C. Thomsen: Acid-base status in liver cirrhosis. Disturbances in stable, terminal and portacaval shunted patients, *Scand. J. Gastroenterol.*, **11**:249, 1976.

35. Record, C. O., R. A. Iles, R. D. Cohen, and R. Williams: Acid-base and metabolic disturbances in fulminant hepatic failure, *Gut*, **16**:144, 1975.

36. Roberts, K. E., F. G. Thompson, III, J. W. Poppell, and P. Vanamee: Respiratory alkalosis accompanying ammonium toxicity, *J. Appl. Physiol.*, **9**:367, 1956.

37. Posner, J. B. and F. Plum: The toxic effects of carbon dioxide and acetazolamide in hepatic encephalopahty, *J. Clin. Invest.*, **39**:1246, 1960.

38. Roberti, A., H. Traverso, P. Vesin, R. Viguié, and P. Blanchon: Etude du Na et du K échangeables et des liquides extracellulaires dans les cirrhosis éthyliques, *Sem. Hop. Paris*, **42**:1714, 1966.

39. Vesin, P.: Le métabolisme du potassium chez l'homme. II. Problèmes de physiopathologie digestive, *Presse Med.*, **77**:1853, 1969.

40. Casey, T. H., W. H. J. Summerskill, and A. L. Orvis: Body and serum potassium in liver disease. I. Relationship to hepatic function and associated factors, *Gastroenterology*, **48**:198, 1961.

41. Negant deDeuxchaisnes, C., R. A. Collet, R. Busset, and R. S. Mach,: Exchangeable potassium in wasting, amyotrophy, heart disease and cirrhosis of the liver, *Lancet*, **1**:681, 1961.

42. Baker, D. R., W. H. Schrader, and C. R. Hitchcock: Small-bowel ulceration apparently associated with thiazide and potassium therapy, *JAMA*, **290**:586, 1964.

43. Heffernan, S. J., and J. J. Murphy: Ulceration of small intestine and slow-release potassium tablets (correspondence), *Br. Med. J.*, **1**:746, 1975.

44. Farquharson-Roberts, M. A., A. E. B. Giddings, and A. S. Nunn: Perforation of small bowel due to slow release potassium chloride (Slow-K), *Br. Med. J.*, **2**:206, 1975.

45. McCall, A. J.: Slow-K ulceration of oesophagus with aneurysmal left atrium (correspondence) *Br. J. Med.*, **2**:230, 1975.

46. Weiss, S. M., H. L. Rutenberg, D. L. Paskin, and H. A. Zaren: Gut lesions due to slow-release KCl tablets (letters), *N. Engl. J. Med.*, **296**:111, 1976.

47. Yamada, S., and T. B. Reynolds: Amiloride (MK-870) a new antikaluretic diuretic: comparison to other antikaluretic drugs in patients with liver disease and ascites, *Gastroenterology*, **59**:833, 1970.

48. Eggert, R. C.: Spironolactone diuresis in patients with cirrhosis and ascites. *Br. Med. J.*, **4**:401, 1970.

49. Lieberman, F. L. and T. B. Reynolds: Renal failure with cirrhosis. Observations on the role of diuretics, *Ann. Intern. Med.*, **64**:1221, 1966.

50. Shear, L., Ching, S., and Gabuzda, G. J.: Compartmentalization of ascites and edema in patients with hepatic cirrhosis, *N. Engl. J. Med.*, **282**:1391, 1970.

51. Hecker, R., and S. Sherlock: Electrolyte and circulatory changes in terminal liver failure, *Lancet*, **2**:1121, 1956.

52. Vesin, P.: Late functional renal failure in cirrhosis with ascites: pathophysiology, diagnosis and treatment, in G. A. Martini and S. Sherlock (eds.),

Aktuelle Probleme der Hepatologie, George Thieme Verlag, Stuttgart, 1962, p. 118.

53. Koppel, M. H., J. W. Coburn, M. M. Mims, H. Goldstein, J. D. Boyle, and M. E. Rubini: Transplantation of cadaveric kidneys from patients with hepatorenal syndrome, *N. Engl. J. Med.,* **280:**1367, 1969.

54. Iwatsuki, S., M. M. Popovtzer, J. L. Corman, M. Ishikawa, C. W. Putnam, F. H. Katz, and T. E. Starzl: Recovery from "hepatorenal syndrome" after orthotopic liver transplantation, *N. Engl. J. Med.,* **289:**1155, 1973.

55. Thomsen, A. C., and E. Juhl: Renal failure in terminal cirrhosis of the liver, *Scand. J. Gastroenterol.,* **7:**117, 1970.

56. Dawson, J. L.: Renal failure in obstructive jaundice—clinical aspects, *Postgrad. Med. J.,* **51:**510, 1975.

57. Wardle, E. N.: Renal failure in obstructive jaundice—pathogenic factors, *Postgrad. Med. J.,* **51:**512, 1975.

58. Reynolds, T. B.: The hepatorenal syndrome, in F. Schaffner, S. Sherlock, and C. M. Leevy (eds.), *The Liver and Its Diseases,* Intercontinental Medical Book Corp., New York, 1974.

59. Edmondson, H. A., T. B. Reynolds, and H. G. Jacobsen: Renal papillary necrosis with special reference to chronic alcoholism: A report of 20 cases, *Arch. Intern. Med.,* **118:**255, 1966.

60. Goldstein, H., and J. D. Boyle: Spontaneous recovery from the hepatorenal syndrome: report of four cases, *N. Engl. J. Med.,* **272:**895, 1965.

61. Baldus, W. P.: Etiology and management of renal failure in cirrhosis and portal hypertension, *Ann. N.Y. Acad. Sci.,* **170:**267, 1970.

62. Tristani, F. E., and J. N. Cohn: Systemic and renal hemodynamics in oliguric hepatic failure: effect of volume expansion, *J. Clin. Invest.,* **46:**1894, 1967.

63. Schroeder, E. T., L. Shear, S. M. Sancetla, and G. J. Gabuzda: Renal failure in patients with cirrhosis of the liver. III. Evaluation of intrarenal blood flow by para-aminohippurate extraction and response to angiotensin, *Am. J. Med.,* **43:**887, 1967.

64. Tyler, J. M., J. L. Jeffries, and C. E. Wilder: A study of the renal blood flow by nitrous oxide technique in normal and oliguric patients with cirrhosis of the liver, *Clin. Res.,* **10:**194, 1962.

65. Epstein, M., D. P. Berk, N. K. Hollenberg, D. F. Adams, T. C. Chalmers, H. L. Abrams, and J. P. Merrill: Renal failure in the patient with cirrhosis: the role of active vasoconstriction, *Am. J. Med.,* **49:**175, 1970.

66. Kew, M. C., P. W. Brunt, R. R. Varma, K. J. Hourigan, H. S. Williams, and S. Sherlock: Renal and intrarenal blood flow in cirrhosis of the liver, *Lancet,* **2:**504, 1971.

67. Baldus, W. P., W. H. J. Summerskill, J. C. Hunt, and F. T. Maher: Renal circulation in cirrhosis: observations based on catheterization of the renal vein, *J. Clin. Invest.,* **43:**1090, 1964.

68. Reynolds, T. B., F. L. Lieberman, and A. G. Redeker: Functional renal failure with cirrhosis: the effect of plasma expansion therapy, *Medicine (Baltimore),* **46:**191, 1967.

69. Schroeder, E. T., P. J. Numann, and B. E. Chamberlain: Functional renal failure in cirrhosis: recovery after portacaval shunt, *Ann. Intern. Med.,* **72:**923, 1970.

70. LeVeen, H. H., G. Christoudias, I. P. Moon, R. Luft, G. Falk, and S. Grosberg: Peritoneo-venous shunting for ascites, *Ann. Surg.,* **180:**580, 1974.

71. McCloy, R. M., W. P. Baldus, F. T. Maher, and W. H. J. Summerskill: Effects of changing plasma volume, serum albumin concentration and plasma osmolality on renal function in cirrhosis, *Gastroenterology,* **53:**229, 1967.

72. Berkowitz, H. D., C. Galvin, and L. D. Miller: Significance of altered renin substrate in the hepatorenal syndrome, *Surg. Forum,* **23:**342, 1972.

73. Horisawa, M., and T. B. Reynolds: Exchange blood transfusion for hepatorenal syndrome in severe liver disease, *Arch. Intern. Med.,* **136:**1135, 1976.

74. Fischer, J. E., and J. H. James: Treatment of hepatic coma and hepatorenal syndrome: mechanism of action of L-Dopa and aramine. *Am. J. Surg.,* **123:**222, 1972.

75. Barnado, D. E., W. P. Baldus, and F. T. Maher: Effects of dopamine on renal function in patients with cirrhosis, *Gastroenterology,* **58:**524, 1970.

76. Boyer, T. D., and T. B. Reynolds: Prostaglandin insufficiency: a role in the hepatorenal syndrome? *Gastroenterology,* **71:**899, 1976.

77. Zusman, R. M., N. E. Tolkoff-Rubin, L. Axelrod, and A. Leaf: Treatment of the hepatorenal syn-

drome (HRS) with intrarenal prostaglandin E_1 (PGE), *Kidney Int.*, **8:**422, 1975.

78. Arieff, A. I., and C. A. Chidsey: Renal function in cirrhosis and the effect of prostaglandin A_1, *Am. J. Med.*, **56:**695, 1974.

79. Summerskill, W. H. J.: Hepatic failure and the kidney, *Gastroenterology*, **51:**94, 1966.

80. Conn, H. O.: A rational approach to the hepatorenal syndrome, *Gastroenterology*, **65:**321, 1973.

81. Parsons, V., S. P. Willkinson, and M. J. Weston: Use of dialysis in the treatment of renal failure in liver disease, *Postgrad. Med. J.*, **51:**515, 1975.

82. Lancestremere, R. G., E. L. Klingler, E. Frisch, and S. Papper: Simultaneous determination of cardiac output and renal function in patients with Laennec's cirrhosis during the administration of the pressor amine, metaraminol, *J. Lab. Clin. Med.*, **61:**820, 1963.

83. Cohn, J. N., F. E. Tristani, and I. M. Khatri: Systemic vasoconstriction and renal vasodilator effects of PLV-2 (Octapressin) in man, *Circulation*, **38:**151, 1964.

84. Denison, E. K., L. Goldstein, and T. B. Reynolds: Unpublished observations.

22

Water and electrolytes in gastrointestinal disease

SIDNEY F. PHILLIPS

The physiology of secretion and absorption of water and electrolytes is understood quite well since it is based on a considerable body of experimental work. Although information on the pathophysiology of these systems in disease is being accumulated, much of it has not yet been integrated. The subject of water and electrolyte metabolism in gastrointestinal disease is best approached by first comprehending normal mechanisms, and then outlining abnormal states.

NORMAL PHYSIOLOGY

The gastrointestinal tract is a large body compartment containing isotonic solutions of electrolytes. Gastrointestinal contents differ in composition from the extracellular fluid because the various mucosal membranes which are interposed actively modify the equilibrium between the two. Mucosal secretion and absorption can greatly influence body water and electrolyte content, since the magnitudes of the exchanges involved far exceed those of other systems; with normal fluid intake and normal endogenous secretion of fluids, some 9 L enters the upper intestine daily. During passage through the bowel the

mixture is selectively altered and then so efficiently conserved that 200 mL or less of water is excreted in the feces.

The major physiologic functions of the gastrointestinal tract are *motility,* for propulsion and mixing of foodstuffs; *secretion,* whereby fluids of widely differing electrolyte composition, containing enzymes and bile acids essential to digestion, are added to the intestinal contents; *digestion,* a sequence of physicochemical reactions which break down dietary components to simpler compounds which can be absorbed; and selective *absorption* of the products of digestion and of water, electrolytes, and bile acids secreted earlier.

Most of these functions are relatively quiescent under basal circumstances, variably stimulated by sensory (cephalic) stimuli, and evoked by the ingestion of food. The concept that different organs and functions are normally integrated by hormonal and neural mechanisms into a precisely coordinated whole is central to an understanding of how localized disease can derange water and electrolyte metabolism throughout the system. Nevertheless, each specialized region of the gastrointestinal tract must be studied separately to be understood as a part of the whole.

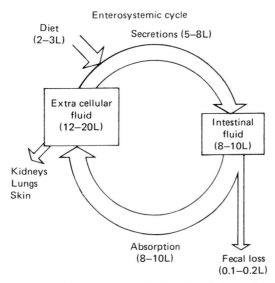

Figure 22-1. Cycling of water and electrolytes between the alimentary canal and ECF is represented by entry into the bowel (diet and secretions) and exit from the bowel (absorption and fecal loss).

ENTEROSYSTEMIC CYCLING OF WATER AND ELECTROLYTES (Fig. 22-1)

A large proportion of the extracellular fluid enters the alimentary canal daily. For example, in a 70-kg adult, about half the extracellular fluid volume is secreted into the upper gastrointestinal tract, far more fluid than is added through the diet. The average daily intake of sodium (150 meq), potassium (50 meq), and chloride (200 meq) is similarly trivial compared with the amounts secreted into the intestinal lumen during 24 h (Table 22-1) or present in the body.

Food entering the upper gastrointestinal tract promotes simultaneous or sequential secretions of saliva, gastric juice, bile, and pancreatic juice; these fluids contain widely varying concentrations of sodium, potassium, chloride, bicarbonate, and hydrogen ions (Table 22-1). Mixing, propulsion, digestion, and progressive equilibration toward the physiologic extracellular pH and osmolality occur in the stomach and duodenum. In the small intestine an uncertain volume of isotonic, neutral, small-bowel secretion (succus entericus) is added to the contents (Table 22-1). In the jejunum this fluid is rich in chloride; in the ileum, bicarbonate is the predominant anion.

Absorption of different nutrients begins in the small intestine and peaks for most in the proximal jejunum. The jejunum receives 8 to 10 L of isotonic electrolyte solution per 24 h; resorption preserves some 9 L of water, more than 500 meq each of sodium and chloride, 200 meq of bicarbonate, and 100 meq of potassium. Absorption of water and electrolytes continues in the ileum and is completed in the colon, where each day 1 to 2 L of semiliquid material is progressively desiccated to feces. Some 500 mL of water and 100 meq of cation per 24 h is simultaneously recycled through the enterohepatic circulation.

Some organs, such as the stomach, have a primarily secretory function, although they are capable of limited absorption (e.g. of some water and alcohol). Other organs, such as the small or large intestine, are primarily areas for absorption, although capable of secretion under abnormal circumstances. Since secretion is stimulated mainly by food intake and absorption is believed to be largely obligatory, homeostasis of the whole organism must be adjusted through changes in renal and not gastrointestinal function.

Table 22-1. Approximate composition of diet and gastrointestinal secretions per 24 h

	FLUID, L	SODIUM, meq	POTASSIUM, meq	CHLORIDE, meq	BICARBONATE, meq	CONCENTRATION, meq/L				
						Na	K	Cl	HCO$_3$	pH
Diet	2–3	150	50	200						
Saliva	1.0	50	20	40	50	20–80	10–20	20–40	20–60	7.0–8.0
Gastric juice	1–2	40–160	15	200	—	20–100	5–10	120–160	—	1.0–7.0
Bile	1.0	100	5	40	40	150–250	5–10	40–80	20–40	7.0–8.0
Pancreatic juice	1.0–2.0	150	5	40	120	120	5–10	10–60	80–120	7.0–8.0
Succus endericus	1.0–2.0	140–280	5–10	Variable	Variable	140	5	Variable	Variable	7.0–8.0

SECRETION

Principles of measurement

Secretion is a sequence of synthesis and active and passive transport to the lumen of fluids containing electrolytes, digestive compounds, and enzymes. It is executed by specialized glandular cells in or under the intestinal mucosa; these cells create very different physicochemical environments, adjusted for regional functions, in the bowel lumen. For example, the acid pH in the stomach is essential to peptic digestion but also precipitates certain bile acids and inactivates pancreatic enzymes if these reflux from the duodenum. The alkaline secretions in the duodenum neutralize gastric juice and inactivate pepsin but provide a milieu in which pancreatic enzymes can hydrolyze food and in which fatty acids and monoglycerides, by forming micelles with bile salts, become water-soluble and absorbable. The reason for specific intraluminal fluid composition in other areas is less evident, but the differences also presumably reflect regional specializations of mucosal transport. For example, ileal and colonic mucosa contain high levels of carbonic anhydrase, secrete bicarbonate, and maintain a relatively alkaline intraluminal pH. It has been suggested that the ileum and colon, by secreting bicarbonate ions in exchange for chloride, conserve the "fixed" anion (chloride) and excrete an ion that is readily available from local cellular metabolism.

Basal secretion of digestive juices is continuous; in response to the sight or smell of food (cephalic stimulation), vagal impulses initiate greater amounts of secretion. Increased output is maintained during eating and digestion by an interplay of neural and multihormonal mechanisms. The hormones are released from the mucosa by digestive products (amino acids or fats), chemical changes in the lumen (especially pH), or alterations in intraluminal pressure (1). Complex interactions may occur following the simultaneous release of several hormones which can produce different physiologic responses in more than one target organ. For example, cholecystokinin-pancreozymin (CCK-PZ) and gastrin may act synergistically or competitively at the same

receptor site in various organs by virtue of their common terminal amino acid sequence (2, 3). Secretin, which is chemically dissimilar, probably has a different receptor site (which may be shared with glucagon) in these organs and usually exerts an opposing effect.

Secretory function is conventionally measured first under basal or fasting circumstances and then in response to a stimulus. The stimuli are either test meals and food derivatives or compounds which mimic the hormones or neurotransmitters involved in secretion. Stimuli are customarily given in a maximum dose, so as to induce a peak response by activating all secretory cells. The responses probably parallel those which are evoked physiologically by foods. The results of secretory tests are best expressed as total output per unit time of the most relevant component (e.g. hydrochloric acid in the stomach; water, bicarbonate, or enzymes from the pancreas). These data can be refined by feeding nonabsorbable marker substances; this permits calculation of secretions lost in transit or gained in reflux between organs (4).

Salivary secretion

Saliva is mixed with food by chewing, thus preparing a bolus for propulsion, and initiates carbohydrate digestion with salivary amylase. Saliva is hypotonic, and when swallowed, it may modify the composition of gastrointestinal contents at lower levels. The parotid glands contribute most of the surprisingly large amount of water and electrolyte constituting salivary flow (Table 22-1). Basal secretion is approximately 0.5 mL/min. Peak flow of some 3 to 4 mL/min is evoked by chewing or by parasympathetic stimulation, and the fluid produced is modified (5): Osmolality is increased due to a higher sodium content, and pH changes from 5.5 to 7.8 as a result of increased secretion of bicarbonate. The major control of secretion is probably neural, but mineralocorticoids can increase the potassium/sodium ratio.

Gastric secretion

When food enters the stomach, onward passage is slowed to aid mixing of the contents and peptic digestion. An enormous increase in hydrogen ion concentration, produced by parietal cell secretion of hydrochloric acid, creates the optimum environment (pH 2 to 4) for the action of pepsin. Gastric acid secretion is controlled by two complementary mechanisms: vagal stimulation and gastrin secretion. Fasting and nocturnal (basal) secretion is usually less than 50 mL/h and is mainly controlled by vagal impulses. Immediately before, during, and after meals, secretion is augmented by release of gastrin from the antral mucosa in response to cephalic (vagal), mechanical (distention), and chemical (products of protein digestion or pH) stimuli in the antrum. Secretory volume increases some fivefold as a result of these stimuli, and acidity usually increases.

Secretion of hydrochloric acid raises the concentration of hydrogen ions in the gastric lumen more than a million times above that in the extracellular fluid. Carbon dioxide enters the parietal cell from the plasma and is hydrated in the reaction catalyzed by carbonic anhydrase (6):

$$CO_2 + H_2O \rightarrow H_2CO_2 \rightarrow H^+ + HCO_3^-$$

Hydrogen ions acidify gastric juice, whereas bicarbonate ions diffuse back into the plasma, producing the postcibal "alkaline tide." Simultaneously chloride ions are transported by the parietal cell from the plasma into gastric juice. Passage of sodium into gastric juice and back-diffusion of hydrogen ions into the circulation are restricted in health by a functional mucosal barrier.

Gastric juice also contains a nonparietal alkaline fluid with electrolytes and pepsin. The proportions of acid and alkaline secretion may vary greatly, but both are isotonic with plasma. The composition of gastric contents is modified by age, sex, disease, and admixture with salivary, pancreatic, or biliary secretion.

Biliary secretion

Bile contains water, electrolytes, and several other compounds, including bilirubin, neutral fat, cholesterol, lecithin, and bile salts. The last are of the greatest physiologic importance, since they are essential for micellar solubilization of fat prior to its efficient absorption. Secretion of bile involves several different active and passive mechanisms which transport the various constituents from liver cells into the biliary ductules. Nervous, humoral, and chemical mechanisms control secretion. Of these, the choleretic effects of secretin, released from the small-intestinal mucosa, and of bile salts, resorbed from the small intestine, are rated most important (7). Secretin increases the volume, and bicarbonate concentration of bile may increase to 60 meq/L (pH 8) and thus help neutralize acid gastric contents. During fasting, bile is stored in the gallbladder, since resting common bile duct pressure is low and does not overcome the resistance of the sphincter of Oddi. Active and passive absorption of sodium and water by the gallbladder concentrates the bile fivefold (8). Contraction and emptying of the gallbladder is induced mainly by CCK-PZ, which is secreted from the small-intestinal mucosa in response to the products of fat and protein digestion.

Pancreatic secretion

Pancreatic juice has two components with different functions and cellular origins (9). The components vary in proportion, depending upon the nature of the stimulus to secretion. One, an alkaline watery fluid containing a high concentration of bicarbonate, is derived from the ductular cells; these remove carbon dioxide from arterial blood and hydrate it to carbonic acid, which dissociates into hydrogen and bicarbonate. Cations in this secretion are in concentrations similar to those in the plasma. The second, a more viscous secretion of acinar cells, contains digestive enzymes including trypsin, amylase, and lipase. A small, continuous, basal secretion of pancreatic juice occurs during fasting, and a cephalic phase of secretion mediated through the vagus has been demonstrated. Hormones released from the mucosa of the upper small intestine are the major controls of pancreatic secretion. Secretin is released particularly through acidification of duodenal contents and promotes volume and bicarbonate secretion. CCK-PZ promotes simultaneous output of digestive enzymes and contraction of the gallbladder (10). Gastrin probably stimulates pancreatic enzyme output and may, to a lesser degree, increase volume and bicarbonate secretion, but the relative importance of the second mechanism in human beings is unknown.

Succus entericus

In health, the intestine continuously secretes small volumes (50 mL/h or less) of an isotonic, alkaline mixture of goblet-cell mucus, intestinal (Brunner's) gland secretions, desquamated epithelium containing intracellular enzymes, and an ultrafiltrate of plasma. The contribution of this secretion, succus entericus, to the normal enterosystemic cycle is uncertain, and accurate measurements of the volume and composition of succus entericus are not available for healthy human beings. Diseases are known, however, in which the volume increases to many liters per day (11), e.g., in pancreatic cholera or the Zollinger-Ellison syndrome, which are caused by hormone-secreting tumors, usually of pancreatic origin.

The integration of propulsion, secretion, digestion, and absorption in the duodenum is important to the subsequent metabolism of water and electrolytes in the remainder of the gastrointestinal tract. At least 1500 mL of fluid traverses the duodenum after each meal. The acid pH of gastric contents is neutralized by bicarbonate from pancreatic juice and bile, and additional absorption or secretion of water and electrolytes brings duodenal contents to isotonicity with extracellular fluid (12). Hydrolysis of proteins and polypeptides is completed by proteolytic enzymes from the pancreas; digestion of carbohydrate is completed by pancreatic amylase and the action of disaccharidases localized in the brush borders of intestinal mucosal cells; and simultaneously hydrolysis of fat is completed by pancreatic lipase. Fatty acids and monoglycerides then react with bile acids to produce water-soluble micelles, in which fats are dispersed and absorbed (13). Thus, by the formation of an isotonic mixture of monosaccharides, amino acids, micellar fat, and electrolytes, requirements for absorption are met.

Duodenal function is facilitated by the fine control of gastric emptying which is evoked by the entrance of food into the duodenum. Emptying of gastric contents into the duodenum is slow and intermittent; both propulsion and retropulsion occur. The hormones that coordinate the flow of gastric, pancreatic, and biliary secretions simultaneously influence motility: Gastrin and CCK-PZ increase gastric motility (14, 15), whereas secretin delays gastric emptying. Osmolality of the duodenal contents also controls gastric emptying through osmoreceptors in the duodenal wall (16). Neural impulses carried by the vagi probably mediate and integrate both the release of the hormones and the contractile response of the stomach.

Although clinical associations between disorders of motility and abnormal water and electrolyte metabolism are often striking, the normal relationships between motility, secretion, and absorption of electrolytes in the intestine are poorly understood. Intestinal motility studies have been performed, but their validity is uncertain. Simple measurements involve timing the passage of barium, radiopaque pellets, or dye markers as they travel through the intestine. More refined techniques record pressures at different sites by the use of balloons or open-tip tubes. The significance of the patterns of contraction thus derived is not always obvious in health and is incompletely documented in disease.

ABSORPTION

Absorption moves nutrients, ions, and water from the lumen of the bowel into portal venous blood and abdominal lymphatics. The different elements are carried by different active and passive transport systems. Absorption may be modified by "solvent drag," i.e., incorporation of solute into the bulk flow of water from the lumen into the circulation. Most nutrients are absorbed by active mechanisms, which probably require specific mucosal "carriers" (17, 18). Net movement of electrolytes and water is the sum of rapid, simultaneous, bidirectional fluxes (Fig. 22-2) by which as many as 5 to 10 ions or molecules traverse the mucosa in both directions for each net ion or

BIDIRECTIONAL FLUXES IN INTESTINE

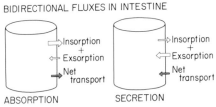

Figure 22-2. Simultaneous bidirectional fluxes of electrolytes and water across the intestinal mucosa determine the direction and magnitude of net transport (absorption or secretion). Fluxes are demonstrable by changes in the specific activities of water (labeled with deuterium or tritium) and radioactive electrolytes (see Ref. 19).

molecule "absorbed" or "secreted." Passive ion transport is determined by relative chemical (concentration) and electric (mucosal-serosal potential difference) forces on the mucosal and serosal (vascular) surfaces of the intestine. Active transport involves movement not explicable by, and sometimes against, electrochemical gradients. Solvent drag is related to the size of the particles contained in the solution relative to hypothetical, water-filled "pores" through which solvent moves

(Fig. 22-3). Diamond (19) has described the functional variability of "pores." It appears that epithelial surfaces vary greatly in their degree of "tightness" or "leakiness," reflecting the function of "pores." These watery channels are thought by some to be located in the junctions between epithelial cells.

Absorption of sodium is considered essential to absorption of water, other electrolytes, and certain nutrients throughout the intestines (17). Sodium transport is active throughout the small and large intestine, although there are regional variations in its efficiency (20). Failure of active sodium absorption leads to net secretion of sodium into the lumen, creating an osmotic gradient along which water flows. It has been proposed that an ATP-dependent "sodium pump," which normally transports sodium from lumen to blood (21), is sensitive to a variety of toxic, humoral, or mechanical insults, and that its inhibition reveals a simultaneous, but previously masked, mechanism for loss of sodium from extracellular fluid into the lumen.

Poorly understood additional factors influence the transport of water and electrolytes in the in-

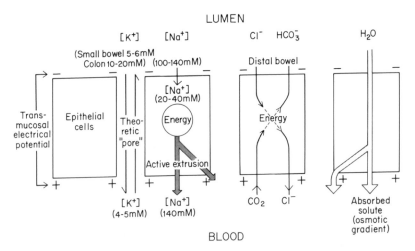

Figure 22-3. Mechanisms proposed for intestinal transport of electrolytes and water. Active sodium transport in the jejunum, ileum, and colon increases in efficiency distad. Potassium moves passively and is "secreted" into the colon due to a large negative mucosal potential. Chloride absorption and bicarbonate secretion predominate distad. Water transport is by diffusion along osmotic gradients.

testines; they are considered relatively unimportant. Aldosterone decreases potassium absorption and increases sodium absorption, especially in the colon (22). Some evidence exists that other hormones (antidiuretic hormone, gastrin, secretin, and CCK-PZ) may affect the absorption of water and certain electrolytes.

Intestinal absorption is conventionally measured by balance studies which record oral intake, urine loss, and fecal output. Until the 1960s, only net absorption or secretion by the entire gastrointestinal tract could be so studied. The use of transintestinal intubation, especially when combined with nonabsorbable marker substances and isotopic labeling, now allows absorption to be quantified regionally during steady-state perfusion of the human intestine in vivo (23).

Absorption in the jejunum

Sodium is absorbed actively against a small electrochemical gradient and also moves with bulk flow of water through large mucosal "pores." Glucose, other actively absorbed monosaccharides, certain amino acids, and bicarbonate enhance sodium absorption (20), possibly by direct stimulation of the sodium pump; sodium in turn augments glucose and amino acid transport (24, 25). Large osmotic gradients are created, along which water moves. Thus, the simultaneous presence of sodium, bicarbonate, digestive and products, and water permits maximum absorption of all.

Water transport is considered to be passive and osmotically dependent (17). Potassium also moves across the mucosa following its concentration gradient between the lumen and blood, modified by the small negative electric potential of jejunal mucosa. Chloride mostly follows sodium, to preserve electric neutrality in the lumen. Bicarbonate disappears rapidly from the lumen by a mechanism involving either active absorption or neutralization of bicarbonate by hydrogen ions secreted by the mucosa (26). Figure 22-4 shows the composition to which an isotonic fluid placed in the jejunum, ileum, or colon is adjusted by absorption and secretion of electrolytes and water.

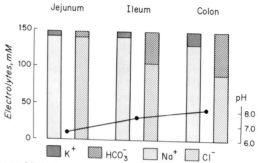

Composition of solutions at equilibrium in bowel

Figure 22-4. Composition of isotonic electrolyte solutions which develop and equilibrate in the small and large bowel. These compositions approximate those of chyme or fasting intestinal content at the same sites.

Intestinal contents at these sites have the same compositions.

Absorption in the ileum

Each day, 2 to 3 L of neutral, isotonic chyme enters the ileum. The ileal mucosa is less permeable than the jejunal to simple diffusion of ions; however, sodium is absorbed actively against larger electrochemical gradients, and water follows (20). Movement of potassium across the mucosa of the ileum can be explained by electrochemical gradients (27), but the mechanisms of anion movement are more complex. Absorption of chloride and secretion of bicarbonate are coupled by a process which may involve active transport of one or both ions (20, 28). It follow that pH and bicarbonate concentrations increase in the distal small bowel (Fig. 22-4).

Distally, the small bowel also has supplementary capacity for the absorption of nutrients and a specific capacity to absorb vitamin B_{12} and bile acids.

Absorption in the colon and rectum

Highly efficient mechanisms for absorption of water and electrolytes are present in the colon; 1 to 2 L of liquid ileal contents is converted to formed feces each 24 h, and more than 90 percent

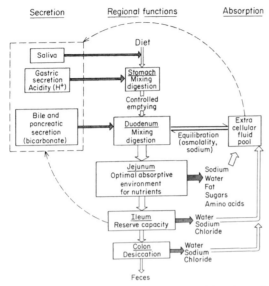

Figure 22-5. Summary of specialized, regional functions of the gastrointestinal tract by which the enterosystemic circulation of electrolytes and water is maintained.

of the sodium and chloride entering the cecum is subsequently absorbed (29). Sodium transport is active and occurs against very large concentration gradients; chloride is absorbed simultaneously by a passive process, thereby establishing osmotic gradients necessary for passive absorption of water. Active bicarbonate secretion occurs in the colon, and organic anions, arriving from the proximal intestine, may modify pH and ionic exchanges between the lumen and circulation (30). Though the colon absorbs potassium in health, small amounts of potassium may be secreted by the colon under certain circumstances. The process is predominantly passive, as potassium diffuses along the electric gradient created by the highly negative colonic mucosa (31). In addition, some potassium may be secreted in the mucus discharged by the abundant goblet cells of the colon. This loss may contribute to potassium depletion in disease states characterized by excess loss of intestinal mucus (32).

The function of the colon in conserving water and electrolytes (29) can be demonstrated by comparing the composition of normal feces (approximately 100 mL water and less than 5 meq sodium/day) with that of discharge from ileostomies

or the material estimated to enter the colon in health (1500 mL and more than 150 meq sodium/day). Conservation of sodium by the colon is particularly important, since the small intestine cannot absorb sodium sufficiently well to maintain sodium balance on diets greatly restricted in sodium (22). It is likely that some regional specialization exists in the colon for transport of water and electrolytes. Studies thus far indicate that the cecum and ascending colon absorb the major proportion of sodium and water and that the rectum plays only a small role (Fig. 22-5).

PATHOPHYSIOLOGY

Water and electrolyte metabolism can be deranged when gastrointestinal motility, digestion, or absorption is altered by disease. Mismanaged fluid is either lost to the outside or sequestered inside the body. Vomiting, diarrhea, and fistulas are routes of external loss, whereas internal loss by sequestration is characteristic of obstruction, ileus, and peritonitis (Fig. 22-6). The fluid lost is usually isotonic, and in most instances, the most important deficits are of water and sodium. In addition, potassium depletion can be expected in chronic conditions or with severe diarrhea, while alkalosis may be superimposed when vomiting

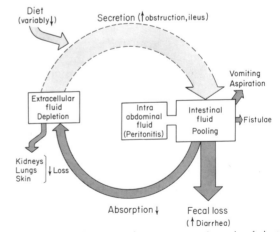

Figure 22-6. Disturbances of the enterosystemic cycle of electrolytes and water produced by disease and resulting in external loss or internal sequestration of fluid.

with loss of acid gastric secretion has been prominent. These characteristic patterns depend on the source and duration of fluid loss. However, variations are common, since more than one problem is often present. For example, obstruction of the small bowel may result in both intestinal sequestration of fluid and massive vomiting.

Loss of isotonic fluid diminishes the plasma volume and may precipitate hypovolemic shock. Usually plasma concentrations of electrolytes are initially preserved, but if the patient drinks large amounts of electrolyte-free water, the plasma will become progressively dilute and particularly hyponatremic (33). Compensatory or aggravating disorders of fluid, electrolyte, or acid-base balance may be superimposed on gastrointestinal disease when changes in renal, cardiac, or pulmonary function result from alterations in the extracellular fluid volume, its pH, or its electrolyte composition.

The effects of disease on the normal functions of the gastrointestinal tract and their integration remain mostly conjectural. For example, the effect of intestinal obstruction on secretion in the proximal intestine is largely unknown. The major reasons for our ignorance are the difficulties of applying more sophisticated investigative techniques to seriously ill patients and the questionable validity of the findings in the absence of steady-state conditions.

VOMITING

Definition and basic mechanisms

Vomiting involves forceful expulsion from the mouth of material from the upper gastrointestinal tract. The neuromuscular reflexes involved are controlled through the vomiting center, which is located in the lateral reticular formation of the medulla. Vomiting is activated by afferent nerves coming from the gastrointestinal tract or from chemoreceptors adjacent to the vomiting center.

Clinical causes

Vomiting commonly reflects one of a diverse variety of visceral causes originating within or ad-

jacent to the gastrointestinal tract; obstruction is the most important in terms of immediate severity and metabolic consequences. In addition, nonobstructive intra-abdominal diseases such as peptic ulcer, pancreatitis, peritonitis, and infections act through this mechanism. Central factors (certain drugs, infections, pregnancy, and irradiation), metabolic disorders (diabetic ketosis and uremia), and elevation of intracranial pressure (malignant hypertension or tumor) also play a role.

Metabolic consequences

Vomiting depletes gastric hydrochloric acid and leads to dehydration and alkalosis, with secondary hypokalemia (see below) and tetany. If the vomitus comes from the small intestine, especially from the duodenum, greater losses of sodium, potassium, and water can occur; however, the loss of alkaline duodenal secretions may balance acidic gastric loss and minimize the acid-base disturbance. The pattern may be modified by internal sequestration of fluid and electrolytes, ingestion of absorbable alkali, or achlorhydria (as when gastric outlet obstruction complicates carcinoma of the stomach). The composition of gastric contents is also extremely variable as a result of different ratios of basal/stimulated gastric juice, basal/swallowed saliva, and basal/fluid refluxing from the duodenum. Randall (34) reports enormous ranges for sodium (6 to 157 meq/L), potassium (1 to 65 meq/L), and chloride (13 to 167 meq/L) in the composition of gastric aspirates. Thus, the metabolic effects of vomiting are often unpredictable, and simple "gastric alkalosis" is the exception rather than the rule.

The development and consequences of gastric alkalosis due to depletion of hydrochloric acid have been described by Kassirer and Schwartz (35) (Fig. 22-7). They repeatedly aspirated the stomachs of healthy volunteers over a 2- to 6-day period and continued water and electrolyte balance observations for a further 4 to 8 days. Sodium, potassium, chloride, and volume lost in the gastric aspirates were replaced with dietary supplements. During the period of drainage, progressive alkalosis developed. Mean plasma bicarbonate concentration and blood pH increased from

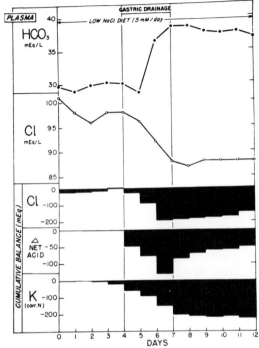

Figure 22-7. Plasma concentrations of anions and net balance of chloride, potassium, and hydrogen ions during the development of metabolic alkalosis induced by selective depletion of gastric hydrochloric acid. Note that alkalosis and negative potassium balance persisted during the postdrainage period (days 7 to 12) despite a dietary intake of 70 meq potassium per day. (*From J. P. Kassirer and W. B. Schwartz, Am. J. Med., 40:10–18, 1966. By permission of the Ruben H. Donnelley Corporation.*)

28.6 to 37.5 meq/L and 7.4 to 7.5, respectively. Urinary pH also increased from 6.4 to 7.5, reflecting loss of the sodium bicarbonate generated by gastric acid losses. Isotonic amounts of water accompanied the sodium bicarbonate into the urine, causing mild volume depletion.

During the period of nasogastric suction the alkalinization of extracellular fluid was testament to the prevailing negative acid balance, i.e., more hydrogen ions were lost from the body than were being produced through intermediary metabolism. The mean net balance between gastrointestinal (GI) bicarbonate generation and renal bicarbonate excretion was *positive*, resulting in net gain of 144 meq of alkali.

If the kidney were able to excrete all the so-dium bicarbonate generated by unreplaced hydrochloric acid losses, serum bicarbonate concentration would remain normal and acid-base balance would be maintained. A severe price, however, would be paid for the prevention of alkalosis. Progressive urinary loss of sodium bicarbonate and water would lead to progressive volume depletion, hypotension, and eventually to shock.

With continued GI losses the kidney, in fact, becomes progressively *less able* to excrete the increased load of bicarbonate delivered. The retention of this sodium bicarbonate, and the water it obligates, mitigates loss of extracellular and intravascular fluids, thereby helping to ensure circulatory competence.

Thus, when faced with the choice of maintaining acid-base stability or intravascular volume, the kidney responds in the host's best interest by sustaining circulatory competence, a function clearly more vital for survival.

The initial volume losses initiate a series of stimuli—fall in renal perfusion and glomerular filtration rate (GFR), increased aldosterone, and perhaps decreased humoral-salt-wasting factors—which cause avid renal sodium retention. As positively charged sodium cations are reabsorbed from the glomerular filtrate, negatively charged anions must accompany them to preserve electroneutrality. Chloride and bicarbonate are therefore reabsorbed along with sodium, the former most likely passively following the actively reabsorbed sodium, whereas hydrogen ions must be secreted to catalyze reabsorption of bicarbonate. These points are more fully discussed in Chap. 6.

DIARRHEA

Definition and basic mechanisms

Diarrhea is characterized by increased frequency and excess water content of the stools. Individual bowel habits vary, but more than four soft or watery bowel movements each 24 h is abnormal. Diarrheal fluid is isotonic with extracellular fluid, and sodium, chloride, and potassium are the predominant solutes. A good quantity of bicarbonate may also be present (36). Diarrhea always results from impaired absorption or excessive secretion of solute, usually sodium; the excess water simply follows solute along an osmotic gradient. Increased fecal losses of sodium occur when the intestinal mucosa is diseased or insufficient in area to resorb sodium, or when chemical toxic or exudative processes provoke excessive secretion of sodium (see below). In some cases, malabsorption of carbohydrates, long-chain fatty acids, or bile acids provides an environment in which colonic bacteria can produce compounds (short-chain organic acids, hydroxy-fatty acids, dihydroxy-bile acids) thought to inhibit sodium absorption in the colon. Malabsorption of chloride (chloridorrhea) or secretion of potassium (villous adenoma) can also produce the osmotic force that retains water in the bowel. Organic anions may contribute much of the solute in carbohydrate malabsorption.

Pathophysiology

Diarrhea can be caused by excessive intake, maldigestion, malabsorption, abnormal fluid secretion (including exudation), and changes in intestinal motility.

Excessive intake. This rarely causes diarrhea in health, since the capacity of the intestines for absorption of water and solute is great, and volumes which exceed it are usually rejected by vomiting. Occasionally, excessive intake of fat can cause steatorrhea. Certain laxatives (those containing polyvalent, slowly absorbed ions such as $MgSO_4$) act by osmotic effects, and in excessive amounts can produce diarrhea. Osmotic diarrhea can also follow the ingestion of poorly absorbed compounds such as mannitol or lactulose.

Maldigestive diarrhea. Many pathologic conditions impair normal digestion and hence prevent effective absorption of nutrients. Osmotic diarrhea results. The most common causes of steatorrhea are digestive defects: In pancreatic insufficiency, hydrolysis of fat is impaired because of inadequate pancreatic lipase secretion; in bile acid deficiency due to hepatobiliary diseases, micellar solubilization of fatty acids by bile acids is reduced; and after gastric surgery, mixing of digestive secretions and nutrients is poorly coordinated. Carbohydrate absorption is decreased when the brush border enzymes which hydrolyze disaccharides to monosaccharides are deficient. For example, lactase deficiency is extremely common in some races (Orientals, blacks), and diarrhea should be anticipated in such patients if they ingest lactose (milk sugar). Maldigestive diarrhea is closely related to malabsorptive diarrhea and resembles it.

Malabsorptive diarrhea. This results from mucosal or submucosal diseases which impair absorption by the small or large intestine. Loss of mucosal surface area, as with resection of the bowel or certain fistulas, has the same result. Mucosal disease may impair sodium transport mechanisms directly, or the presence of unabsorbed dietary or digestive components (such as fat, disaccharides, or bile acids) may inhibit sodium absorption in the colon (37). Rarely, deficiency of a mucosal cell active transport system (as for monosaccharides) may cause an osmotic diarrhea.

Secretory diarrhea. This results from changes in structure or function of the intestines. Structural changes usually result in generalized secretion (exudation). For example, in ulcerative colitis, diffuse mucosal ulceration permits blood, mucus, protein, and electrolytes to exude into the bowel. Increased secretion of water and electrolytes, without structural change in the intestine, is also a common cause of diarrhea (38). The ability of intestinal mucosa to secrete isotonic fluid has been known for many years but largely ignored. The stimuli known to increase intestinal secretion are diverse (Table 22-2). Certain bacterial enterotoxins, such as those of *Vibrio cholerae* and *Escherichia coli,* induce secretion by increasing cyclic adenosine monophosphate (cAMP) in

Table 22-2. Intestinal secretion and diarrhea

DISORDER	SECRETORY STIMULUS
Asiatic cholera, staphylococcal and clostridial food poisoning, *E. coli* diarrheas ("turista")	Bacterial enterotoxins (heat-stable and heat-labile forms have been described)
Islet-cell tumors (pancreatic cholera, WHDA)	Gastrointestinal hormones (vasoactive intestinal polypeptide [VIP], possibly others)
Medullary thyroid cancer	Calcitonin
Steatorrhea	Long-chain fatty acids
Ileal resection	Dihydroxy-bile acids
Laxative abuse	Anthraquinone cathartics
Intestinal obstruction	Stimulus unknown

mucosal cells. The cAMP system has been studied intensively and is conceived of as an "intracellular messenger" for the secretion process. "Traveler's diarrhea" is probably due to enterotoxigenic strains of *E. coli* in about a third of cases.

The experimental observation that glucose absorption continues despite marked secretion of electrolytes and fluid has led to the use of oral glucose-electrolyte solutions in the treatment of cholera and other secretory diarrheas. It is clear that such therapy can reduce the volume of intestinal fluid loss by promoting the absorption of fluid with glucose.

Partial or recently relieved intestinal obstruction is often associated with diarrhea. Obstruction may impair normal absorption and increase proximal secretion as well.

The diarrhea that accompanies steatorrhea appears to have a secretory as well as an osmotic component. Dietary oleic acid is chemically similar to ricinoleic acid (the active principle of castor oil) and shares with it the property of stimulating intestinal fluid secretion in the small and large bowel. Bile acid malabsorption is often associated with steatorrhea, usually when the underlying disease involves the ileum. Bile acids are mucosal secretagogues, and when excess bile acids enter the colon, they act as endogenous cathartics.

Hormones may also stimulate small-bowel secretion of fluids. Certain neoplasms (pancreatic islet-cell tumors, bronchogenic carcinomas, and ganglioneuromas) produce hormones such as vasoactive intestinal polypeptide (VIP) which dramatically increase small-intestinal secretion.

Zollinger-Ellison syndrome. The diarrhea of the Zollinger-Ellison syndrome probably involves several mechanisms, most of them dependent on hypersecretion of gastric fluid. Excessive acid in the small intestine damages the mucosa and also leads to steatorrhea, because lipase and bile acids are inactivated at a low pH. It has also been suggested that hypergastrinemia may directly stimulate bowel secretion.

Metabolic consequences

Severe diarrhea can lead to a daily loss of 5 to 10 L of fluid together with large amounts of sodium,

potassium, and bicarbonate. Dehydration, decrease in body sodium, hypokalemia, and acidosis result. Hyponatremia may secondarily be produced by ingestion of sodium-free liquids or parenteral replacement of water in excess of sodium. In some osmotic diarrheas, water may be lost in excess of sodium, as solutes other than sodium (disaccharides, organic acids) also trap water in the lumen. Disproportionate loss of water can lead to hypernatremic dehydration, which may be aggravated by the use of replacement fluids high in solutes, especially sodium. This "hypertonicity syndrome" is seen particularly in young children (under 2 years of age) and requires cautious and appropriate fluid replacement (see also Chap. 30).

Secretion of potassium appears to reach a maximum output (36) and is augmented little when the volumes of stool increase further (Fig. 22-8). Clinically significant depletion of total body potassium is to be expected only in severe or chronic diarrhea. Rarely, massive secretion of colonic mucus may occur, and hypokalemia characterizes some islet-cell tumors ("pancreatic cholera") or severe laxative abuse (37, 39). Prolonged hypokalemia may injure the renal medulla in such a way that urinary concentrating ability is lost (see also Chap. 4).

The anions in stools are bicarbonate and or-

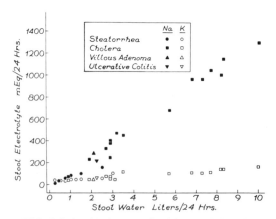

Figure 22-8. Relationship between fecal losses of electrolytes and water in certain diarrheal diseases. Note that sodium loss increases with greater loss of volume whereas potassium loss remains constant despite fecal volumes of 5 to 10 L/day. (*From J. S. Fordtran and J. M. Dietschy, Gastroenterology, 50:263–285, 1966. By permission of The Williams & Wilkins Company, Baltimore.*)

ganic radicals derived from the fermentative action of colonic bacteria. The relative excretion of acid or base in the stools can be estimated from fecal concentrations of sodium, potassium, and chloride. When the sum of sodium and potassium exceeds the fecal chloride plus the plasma bicarbonate concentration, bicarbonate (or its organic equivalent) is being excreted to excess, and acidosis may be predicted. However, great deviations from normal acid-base balance are unusual in diarrhea.

The metabolic consequences of diarrhea at their most acute and extreme develop in infantile diarrhea and Asiatic cholera (40); in the latter, 10 to 20 L of isotonic fluid may be lost per day. Each liter of stool contains 100 to 140 meq of sodium, 20 to 40 meq of potassium, 80 to 100 meq of chloride, and 30 to 50 meq of bicarbonate, with insignificant protein, fat, and sugar. Dehydration, acidosis, and hypokalemia develop rapidly, and acute renal failure may be an early complication. Adequate therapy often requires an initial 3 to 6 L of fluid given intravenously, followed by continuous replacement of subsequent losses. The huge quantity involved in one successful course of treatment is depicted in Fig. 22-9.

INTESTINAL FISTULAS AND RESECTION OF THE INTESTINES

Definition and basic mechanisms

Fistulas are abnormal communications between the bowel and the skin (external fistula) or another hollow viscus (internal fistula). Fistulas arise spontaneoulsy as a result of gastrointestinal disease or are surgically created as stomas; the same disturbances of absorption may develop with either form. Loss of absorptive surface, from either resection or short-circuiting, causes most of the problems. Contamination of the proximal bowel with fecal organisms may also occur (as in the blind-loop syndrome). Some of these bacteria

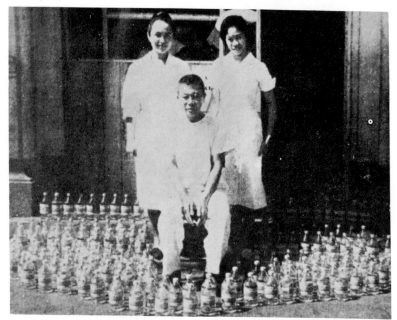

Figure 22-9. Patient after recovery from Asiatic cholera. This 53-kg man required 60 L intravenous fluid replacement during 5 days of acute symptoms. (*From R. A. Phillips, Fed. Proc., 23:705–712, 1964. By permission of the Federation of American Societies for Experimental Biology.*)

deconjugate and dehydroxylate bile acids, precipitating them in the lumen; the precipitated bile salts cannot form micelles with fat (41). Maldigestion of fat with steatorrhea and loss of sodium, water, and other ions, including calcium and magnesium, follows. Some bacteria also consume essential materials, such as vitamin B_{12}, and deprive the host of nutrients.

Bypass or resection of the terminal ileum causes unique problems. Absorption of bile acids at the normal site in the ileum is impossible, and bile acids are lost into the colon (42). Depletion of the bile acid pool may be severe, impairing digestion of fat in the proximal small intestine and leading to steatorrhea. The presence of excessive amounts of bile acids in the colon blocks sodium and water absorption there and adds a watery component to the steatorrhea.

After ileal resection or bypass, a syndrome of hyperoxaluria and renal calculi may develop (42). This syndrome is produced by increased absorption of dietary oxalate, due to increased passive permeability of colonic mucosa to oxalate and to binding of calcium ions in the bowel lumen by ionized fatty acids; the reduction of intraluminal free calcium increases oxalate solubility. When ileal bypass is performed for obesity, two specific complications occur: hepatic steatosis, which can lead to coma and death, and a migratory polyarthralgia.

Changes in intestinal transit may further compromise digestion and absorption, and increased gastric secretion sometimes occurs after extensive resection of the small intestine. Such abnormalities are poorly understood and may be due to insufficiency of the hormones normally secreted from the mucosa of the small intestine.

Clinical causes

Spontaneous fistulas are usually complications of peptic ulcer, neoplasia, inflammatory bowel disease, or pancreatitis. Fistulas may also result from trauma. Postoperative fistulas, which usually follow leakage from anastomoses, are numerically important. Intestinal resections are usually performed for inflammatory, vascular, or malignant disease of the bowel. Ileal bypass procedures are sometimes recommended in the treatment of morbid obesity or hyperlipidemia (see also Chap. 28).

Metabolic consequences

External gastric, duodenal, and jejunal fistulas. These can discharge up to 5 L of fluid daily (43). The fluid is isotonic and contains high concentrations of sodium; dehydration and sodium depletion are, therefore, common. The anions lost depend on the exact site of the fistula. Acidosis may develop if primarily duodenal secretion is lost; alkalosis may develop if loss is mostly gastric. Pancreatic enzymes may digest the abdominal wall. Fistulas of the jejunum are not common and rarely cause severe electrolyte disturbance; however, in about 15 percent of cases, enough fluid is lost to produce dehydration. Normal acid-base balance is usually preserved, since the effluent has an approximately neutral pH.

Biliary and pancreatic fistulas. Sodium and water are lost through a biliary fistula, but the loss is not usually a problem. Pancreatic fistulas are more serious: the loss of fluid can amount to a liter daily, acidosis may result from the loss of bicarbonate, and the condition is often complicated by severe autolysis of the abdominal wall due to pancreatic enzymes.

Fistulas of the ileum or colon. These seldom produce serious disorders of water and electrolyte metabolism unless the rest of the intestine is diseased, as, for example, with Crohn's disease. A patient with an ileostomy may constantly lose water and electrolytes and may be chronically water- and sodium-depleted (44). Sodium balance may be precarious even when stomal function appears normal, since the colon, which normally preserves sodium, is nonfunctional. Consequently, ileostomies may discharge up to 100 meq of sodium each day, regardless of the state of body sodium balance. The water content (up to 1 L daily) is also greater than that of feces. Since the patient tends toward a low body water and has an obligatory loss via the ileostomy, urine volume is usually low; this may contribute to the increased incidence of urinary calculi following such operations. Hypomagnesemia is common and may require therapy.

Internal fistulas. A fistula between the upper

and lower intestine reroutes intestinal contents past some of the mucosa available for absorption. Bacterial overgrowth in the upper intestine often contributes to symptomatology. Inadvertent gastroileostomy is most serious, since inadequately digested food is delivered from the stomach directly to the distal small bowel. In most other circumstances, relatively little food is short-circuited; gastrocolic fistulas, for example, cause malabsorption and diarrhea as consequences of contamination of the upper intestine by fecal bacteria.

Short-bowel syndrome. After massive intestinal resection, usually for mesenteric vascular disease or regional enteritis, a syndrome of chronic "intestinal insufficiency" may develop, with multiple disturbances of nutrition, hydration, and electrolyte metabolism (45). As little as 12 in of the duodenojejunal segment may barely support life, but a patient with less than 50 in of small intestine usually needs specific therapy to combat the malabsorptive effects of minimal absorptive surface, hypermotility, and rapid transit of nutrients, reduced bile acid pool, lack of gastrointestinal mucosal hormones, bacterial colonization of the small bowel, and poor digestion. Some of these unfortunate patients can now be managed with total parenteral nutrition (46) (see also Chap. 10).

Chronic malnutrition secondary to malabsorption leads to an increase in extracellular relative to intracellular volume, presumably due to hypoalbuminemia, dilutional hyponatremia, and loss of intracellular potassium. Although total body potassium may be markedly reduced, transfer of potassium to the extracellular compartment secondary to diarrheal acidosis may produce hyperkalemia unless additional potassium is lost, as with severe diarrhea.

INTESTINAL SEQUESTRATION: OBSTRUCTION AND ILEUS

Definition and basic mechanisms

Mechanical obstruction or atonic arrest of the intestine (ileus) has characteristic consequences.

In mechanical obstruction, distal progress of air, saliva, food, and secretions ceases. The prox-imal bowel distends and becomes compromised, further reducing absorption and propulsion. In experimental obstruction of the canine small intestine, absorption from distended bowel segments diminishes after 6 to 12 h and is replaced by secretion of sodium and water (47). Increased intraluminal pressure, elevation of portal venous and lymphatic pressures, ischemia, and the toxic effects of rapid bacterial multiplication in the involved segment are among the mechanisms proposed to account for these changes.

Once obstruction is established, edema, petechial hemorrhages, and finally necrosis and gangrene develop in the bowel wall. These changes are most pronounced when occlusion or strangulation of the vasculature occurs, or in closed-loop obstruction, which produces exceedingly high intramural pressure. Excessive permeability of the damaged intestinal mucosa allows loss of proteins from the blood to the intestinal lumen, while bacteria and their toxins move simultaneously in the opposite direction. Peritonitis, therefore, frequently complicates untreated obstruction. Additional injury to ischemic mucosa may be caused by compounds in the intestinal lumen, including pancreatic enzymes, bile acids, and their derivatives, and bacterial exotoxins. However, the sequence whereby untreated obstruction leads to irreversible shock and death is uncertain. Volume depletion, free perforation of the bowel, bacterial toxins, gram-negative septicemia, and splanchnic vasoconstriction have been implicated. The general role of bacteria is well established experimentally, since mortality from obstruction is reduced in newborn or germ-free animals, or when broad-spectrum antibiotics have been given previously (48).

Functional obstruction of the bowel (ileus) occurs most frequently in association with peritonitis. The pathogenesis of ileus is unknown, but the condition has conventionally been subdivided into two entities. In *spastic ileus*, a ring of muscle, constricted because of altered autonomic innervation through the celiac ganglion, is thought to occlude the bowel. *Adynamic ileus* is postulated to result from neural inhibition of coordinated motor activity, producing atony of the entire small and large bowel. Ileus may complicate spinal injuries and can be induced by ganglionic blocking agents. Hypokalemia is thought to produce adynamic ileus by decreasing the contractibility of smooth muscle. The metabolic consequences of ileus are the same whatever the source, and it is hard to justify the maintenance of two different classifications.

Pseudoobstruction is clinically similar to ileus. It is believed to be a manifestation of chronic neuromuscular disease of the gastrointestinal tract. Pathogenetic mechanisms are thought to include autonomic denervation (diabetic visceral neuropathy), replacement of smooth muscle by connective tissue (systemic sclerosis and other connective tissue disease), and incoordination of muscular contraction or relaxation (the aganglioneurosis of congenital megacolon).

Clinical causes

Mechanical obstruction of the bowel is caused either by lesions involving the entire circumference of the intestine (as with volvulus, certain congenital malformations, hernias, and adhesive bands) or by those which encroach upon the lumen (usually tumors or inflammatory disease). Less often, foreign bodies may occlude the bowel by impaction. Ileus (atonic obstruction) is often a temporary reaction to laparotomy. Several intra-abdominal diseases, especially pancreatitis, peritonitis, intra-abdominal hemorrhage, or occlusive vascular disease, constitute the majority of other instances. Ileus may also occur during the course of systemic disorders, including uremia and septicemia, and it may have a neurogenic basis (see earlier).

Metabolic consequences

Hypovolemia, hyponatremia, and hypochloremia are the major abnormalities observed in most cases (33). During the course of obstruction or ileus, several liters of extracellular fluid may become sequestered in the intestine. Within 24 h of experimental obstruction of the distal small bowel, 50 percent or more of the plasma volume has been thus lost (49). Additional amounts may accumulate in the peritoneal cavity. The degree of total fluid loss varies with the site, duration, and degree of obstruction, but may be sufficiently

acute and extensive to precipitate hypovolemic shock. Plasma concentrations of electrolytes are initially preserved since the fluid lost is isotonic, but the patient usually becomes thirsty and drinks sodium-poor fluid, so that he is often hyponatremic when first seen. Body chloride is depleted through vomiting. Loss of bicarbonate, impairment of renal function due to hypovolemia, and starvation with consequent ketosis may individually or collectively produce mild acidosis. *Alkalosis* may be prominent and early in obstruction of the upper intestine associated with severe vomiting, but when reflex vomiting is associated with distal obstruction, acidosis is to be expected.

The outcome of relieved obstruction is largely determined by the presence of complications: gram-negative sepsis, peritonitis, bowel perforation, acute renal failure (50). When vascular insufficiency is present in obstruction, bowel is more permeable and quickly becomes less viable, complications are common, and mortality is far greater than in simple obstruction.

In a volume-repleted patient, recovery from intestinal obstruction may be associated with a sudden diuresis as the sequestered intraluminal fluid is reabsorbed.

PERITONITIS

Definition and basic mechanisms

Peritonitis is an inflammation of the peritoneal membrane due to bacterial or chemical injury. When acute and generalized, it leads to major metabolic disorders and changes in intestinal function. Normally, the large surface area of the peritoneum mediates rapid transport of water and electrolytes between the peritoneal cavity and the circulation. In disease, impairment of these transport mechanisms leads to sequestration of fluid and electrolytes within the peritoneal cavity; the amount may be augmented by the osmotic effects of concomitant exudation of protein.

Clinical causes

Acute peritonitis is usually a complication of either intra-abdominal or pelvic disease. Perforation of the intestine or gallbladder, pancreatitis, penetrating wounds (including laparatomy), and pelvic infections account for most cases. Primary peritoneal infection with pyogenic organisms occurs rarely in children. Tuberculous peritonitis is now uncommon but may manifest as ascites.

Metabolic consequences

Peritonitis primarily causes loss of sodium and water into the peritoneal cavity, but the condition is often complicated by perforation of a viscus or by ileus. Reflex hypotension and shock may predominate immediately after perforation. As large volumes of fluid accumulate, hypovolemia, hyponatremia, acidosis, and renal failure may develop.

IATROGENIC DISORDERS

Iatrogenic disturbances of water and electrolyte metabolism are common in gastrointestinal disease, particularly after abdominal surgery (see also Chap. 31). *Excessive replacement of fluid and electrolytes,* especially as parenteral sodium chloride solutions but also as enemas containing absorbable sodium, represents the most common problem. The decreased ability of the kidneys to excrete sodium in the immediate postoperative period is often the precipitating factor. Fluid overload leading to water intoxication or sodium retention leading to pulmonary edema or cardiac failure may result, especially in patients with coexistent cardiopulmonary or renal disorders. Depletion of fluid and electrolytes may be produced by prolonged suction of the stomach or intestines if parenteral replacement is inadequate or inappropriate. Certain diets and medication may also produce characteristic syndromes affecting water and electrolyte metabolism. The *milk-alkali syndrome,* usually found when compulsive patients with peptic ulcer follow an overrigorous therapeutic program, develops from absorption of excessive calcium (prescribed as milk or as an antacid) and absorbable alkali. Alkalosis and hypercalcemia result, and later developments include nephrocalcinosis, metastatic calcification, and ultimate renal failure. Vomiting is common and may aggravate the alkalosis, dehydration, and im-

pairment of renal function. *Anticholinergic drugs,* if given to patients with incipient pyloric obstruction, may initiate or aggravate vomiting and cause "gastric alkalosis." Diarrhea, sometimes with dehydration and hypokalemic alkalosis, is a feature of *laxative abuse* or the prolonged use of enemas and may occur acutely or as a late chronic complication in patients receiving *radiotherapy.*

EVALUATION OF WATER AND ELECTROLYTE DISORDERS IN ABDOMINAL DISEASE

HISTORY

The *clinical history,* while primarily directed toward a specific diagnosis, should include questions designed to yield information about probable fluid and electrolyte losses, thirst, and urine volume. If vomiting has been prominent, the volume, duration, and character should be ascertained. Large amounts of vomitus, especially if projectile and "fecal" in character, suggest intestinal obstruction. The presence of bile implies patency of the pyloroduodenal canal, whereas identification of undigested food eaten more than 12 h previously is characteristic of pyloric obstruction. If blood is present, the nature (fresh or coffee-ground appearance) and amount should be assessed. With *diarrhea,* its duration and the frequency of the stools should be noted. The appearance of the stools is also important; for example, "rice-water" stools, typical of cholera, imply loss of large volumes of isotonic fluid; fatty stools indicate maldigestion or malabsorption, and a silver color connotes the admixture of blood with fat. Red blood usually originates from the colon but can occur with massive hemorrhage from gastric lesions. Melena usually originates from bleeding located above the ileocecal valve, most often in the stomach or upper small intestine. Large amounts of mucus suggest a colonic source and a relative increase in loss of potassium in relation to that of other cations.

Similar questions about the volume and character of discharges are relevant to *external fistulas.* The appearance of fistulous discharges often yields a clue to the visceral origin of the fistula and thus to the composition of the loss. Clear fluid or undigested food (stomach), bile (duodenum and upper small intestine), or fecal material (from the colon) are examples. The degree and composition of internal fluid loss (in ileus, obstruction, and peritonitis) cannot be evaluated by the history.

Age, sex, associated diseases, and body contour are important in evaluating potential imbalance of water and electrolytes. Children, women, and obese individuals have smaller total volumes of body water relative to weight than lean adult males and, therefore, withstand fluid loss less well. Evaluation of cardiopulmonary and renal function is important, especially if parenteral fluid therapy is under consideration.

PHYSICAL EXAMINATION

The degree of dehydration is first evaluated by standard, albeit relatively crude, clinical methods; about 60 mL fluid per kg body weight must be lost before dehydration is evident on examination. The rate, depth, and nature of respiratory movement may indicate the presence of acid-base imbalance. In addition, clinical evidence of depletion of specific substances (for example, latent tetany due to hypocalcemia, or the flaccidity of severe hypokalemia) is sought when the history is consistent with such possibilities (see also Chap. 11). *On inspection*, the abdominal contour may provide diagnostic assistance. A scaphoid abdominal wall, through which the outlines of hollow organs may be observed, is characteristic of advanced emaciation and dehydration. Distention, often accompanied by a tympanitic percussion note, is suggestive of obstruction or ileus, and the site may sometimes be predicted: Pyloric obstruction yields signs in the left upper quadrant, small-bowel obstruction causes central abdominal distention, and obstruction in the distal colon first results in bulging of the flanks.

Peristalsis may be visible proximal to the site of obstruction, and further clues may be gained by palpating an abdominal mass or examining the rectum and hernial orifices. Bowel sounds are often increased and changed in character with obstruction, whereas absent or grossly diminished bowel sounds suggest ileus. Abdominal wall tenderness, rebound, and rigidity indicate an inflammatory lesion and peritonitis; shifting dullness is the cardinal sign of free peritoneal fluid. The appearance of fistulas and their discharges are also examined; severe autodigestion of surrounding tissues suggests trypsin secretion and therefore a fistula originating in or near the duodenum.

INVESTIGATIONS

Standard tests are performed immediately to assess water and electrolyte depletion and renal function and to serve as a baseline against which future progress can be evaluated. Urinalysis, including determination of specific gravity, serum concentrations of sodium, potassium, chloride, and bicarbonate, should be obtained. It is often advisable to measure serum calcium and magnesium concentrations. Acid-base balance should be evaluated, the Astrup method being one convenient way. Blood urea nitrogen or, when intestinal bleeding is suspected, serum creatinine concentrations should be obtained. The hemoglobin and hematocrit will be important in evaluating blood loss and volume depletion.

A variety of routine diagnostic tests may be employed to determine the site and nature of the primary disease. Endoscopy, with or without biopsy of the stomach or distal large bowel, is easy to perform when indicated. Flat plates of the abdomen taken with the patient in the upright position as well as in supine or lateral positions are also standard procedures. From these, evidence of perforation (free air under the diaphragm), ileus, or obstruction (distended loops of bowel with or without fluid levels) may be obtained. A hazy "ground-glass" appearance, obscuring the usual structures, especially the psoas shadows, indicates intra-abdominal fluid.

More specific information may also be gained from these procedures. Thus, the approximate location of intestinal obstruction may be evident from the haustral markings of involved bowel, volvulus can often be identified, and characteristic patterns of mucosal abnormality (as in toxic megacolon) may be evident. Possible biliary disease may be signaled by air in the biliary system. And calcific shadows, such as gallstones or pancreatic or vascular calcification, can provide important clues to the diagnosis. A routine chest x-ray, viewed in conjunction with an abdominal flat plate, assists identification of abnormalities in the subdiaphragmatic area. More extensive radiologic investigations are feasible, even in acutely or severely ill patients. Contrast studies of the stomach and intestine, using media of the radiologists's choice and with his careful collaboration, can be made under special circumstances, even in the presence of obstruction, ileus, or perforation. Angiography, intravenous cholangiography, and excretory urography may also be feasible and occasionally indicated.

Laboratory tests of a less routine nature are sometimes helpful in evaluating loss of water and electrolytes, as well as the site and nature of the lesion responsible. Various specimens can be utilized for a variety of purposes, including measurements of pH, electrolyte, fat, and enzyme content; culture, microscopic investigation, and cytologic examination can be useful.

RECORDING OF DATA

Material aspirated from the stomach, intestines, or (by paracentesis) from the abdominal cavity, stool, vomitus, and fistulous discharge should all be inspected by the physician. Details of daily fluid balance must be tabulated meticulously for all patients with abdominal disease involving present or potential disorders of water and electrolyte metabolism. For reliable balance charts, the cooperation of an informed, motivated, and accurate nursing staff is vital, and repeated efforts to educate all paramedical personnel in this regard are essential. Records must include the volume and nature of *intake*, conventionally subdivided as *oral, intravenous,* or *other* (such as the volume given by enema less the volume returned). The volume and electrolyte content of *intravenously administered fluids*, including blood, are of particular importance. *Fluid output* is also charted by category as *urine, stool volume, vomitus, aspiration,* and *other* (such as fistulous discharges).

Daily *net fluid balance* must be calculated accurately. In addition, body weight should be recorded daily, whenever possible. Modifications due to excessive sweating and insensible loss are computed by the physician. In the majority of critically ill patients, frequent recording of blood pressure and pulse rate is indicated. Monitoring of central venous pressure may also be necessary and is particularly crucial when the balance between loss and requirements cannot be precisely determined and if cardiac or renal function is suspect.

TREATMENT

GENERAL PRINCIPLES

In most instances, the history and physical examination will, at best, yield only a rough approximation of the amount of fluid and the nature of the electrolytes required for managing any clinical problem. Usually it is possible to await the results of appropriate laboratory investigations before embarking upon a specific course of therapy. The questions immediately posed revolve around the *need to give fluids, the route* whereby fluids should be administered, and whether, in addition, *aspiration* of the gastrointestinal tract should be performed. At the same time, one prepares for rapid delivery of specific therapy for the causative lesion, if such is available. When early but not emergency *surgical treatment* of the condition is needed, effective intestinal intubation and preoperative correction of water, electrolyte, and acid-base disorders should be completed within 24 or, at the most, 48 h.

The *oral* route provides the simplest way of replacing fluid and electrolytes, but it is often contraindicated, most commonly by vomiting, suspicion of certain lesions (such as perforation or complete bowel obstruction), the possibility of early abdominal surgical treatment, or the presence of hypovolemic shock. In such instances, or if dehydration is clinically apparent and thus consistent with a volume deficit of 5 L or more in the adult, the *parenteral* route for fluid replacement is preferred. Under rare circumstances, fluid can be administered by other methods, including the *peritoneal, rectal,* and even *subcutaneous* routes. Alternatives to oral or intravenous fluid replacement are, in general, unsatisfactory, and secure placement of a needle in an adequate vein is a prime objective.

The decision to intubate the gastrointestinal tract should be made thoughtfully. Continued vomiting, abdominal distention (especially if fluid levels are visible in distended bowel on radiologic examination), obstruction, ileus, and suspected perforation of a viscus are common indications for intubation and aspiration. Both are often required as preoperative measures when obstruction, ileus, or perforation is suspected or proved. On the other hand, intubation with suction can aggravate disorders of water and electrolyte metabolism if it is not intelligently and carefully managed.

Once the decision to intubate the gastrointestinal tract beyond the stomach has been made, the tip of the tube should be advanced to a point just proximal to the site of the lesion, with the guidance of a radiologist and under fluoroscopic control. Much time and frustration can be saved by this approach, especially when the tube is traversing the gastroduodenal area. Once securely placed in the second part of the duodenum, the tube may be advanced at intervals from the bedside. Periodic fluoroscopic monitoring is essential. A wide variety of tubes and suction instruments is available. We prefer a sump-type tube for aspiration of the stomach or upper part of the small intestine, and employ the Miller-Abbot tube for distal lesions (Fig. 22-10); the Gomco apparatus is satisfactory for suction. But if these measures are to be truly effective, an alert and informed nursing staff to supervise their operation is essential.

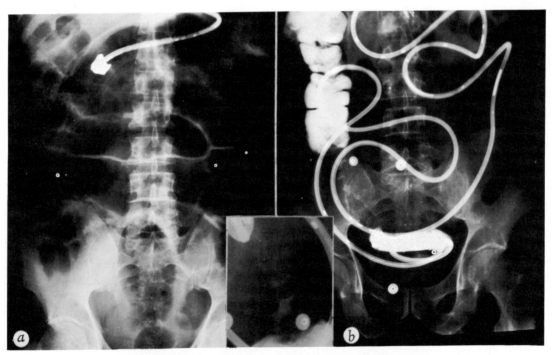

Figure 22-10. Plain x-ray films of the abdomen. *a.* During acute intestinal obstruction. *b.* After passage of Miller-Abbott tube into the small intestine and effective "decompression." Water-soluble radiopaque medium introduced through the tube shows (in inset) the obstructing lesion, acute regional enteritis.

If cardiac, pulmonary, and renal functions are satisfactory, normal saline is usually a good choice. If hypovolemia or shock predominate, colloidal solutions (blood, plasma, or dextran) are preferred. When laboratory and other data become available, therapy can be appropriately modified. After adequate replacement of the initial deficit is achieved, as judged by the clinical condition, vital signs, and urine flow, further replacement of losses is dictated by the fluid balance and the clinical findings.

The amount and nature of replacement therapy cannot be specified in advance. Each patient presents an individual problem, often involving a combination of disorders, and an approach based on an appreciation of the pathophysiology, evaluation of all information, and response to initial therapy is essential.

MANAGEMENT OF CHARACTERISTIC COMBINED DISORDERS

Hypokalemic, hypochloremic alkalosis (see also Chaps. 4 and 6)

This sequence results most often from prolonged vomiting or aspiration of gastric contents and reflects predominant loss of hydrochloric acid. Fluid replacement can be mainly sodium chloride, and provided the output of urine is adequate

(greater than 600 mL/day), potassium chloride (40 to 100 meq/day) can be added. The degree of alkalosis and its response to treatment determine whether acidifying agents (such as ammonium chloride, 1% solution), combination solutions (containing sodium, potassium, ammonium, and chloride), or lysine monohydrochloride should be used. During the administration of acidifying agents, blood pH or bicarbonate content should be monitored daily. Simultaneously, the serum potassium concentrations serve as a guide to the need for continuing potassium replacement. Since complete pyloric obstruction is unusual, and as continuous aspiration of gastric contents aggravates the loss of electrolytes and alkalosis, the stomach should be aspirated as infrequently as possible. Serial measurements of the volumes recovered reflect the degree of obstruction and its response to conservative treatment.

Hyponatremic, hypokalemic acidosis (see also Chaps. 4 and 6)

Loss of isotonic fluid into distended loops of obstructed bowel, from fistulas, or in diarrhea leads to progressive hyponatremia and, when diarrhea is prominent, may also produce acidosis and hypokalemia. Initially, replacement of plasma volume with isotonic sodium chloride may be urgent, and in adults 4 to 6 L can be required to restore the blood pressure and urine output. Aci-

Table 22-3. Precipitating factors and treatment of common metabolic disorders

METABOLIC DISORDER	COMMON PRECIPITATING FACTORS	TREATMENT
Volume depletion	Severe vomiting or diarrhea	Sodium chloride or colloids.
Sodium depletion with "dilutional hyponatremia"	Diarrhea, obstruction, peritonitis, ileostomy	Sodium chloride.
Potassium depletion	Diarrhea, vomiting	Potassium chloride.
Alkalosis	Vomiting	Ammonium chloride, lysine monohydrochloride.
Acidosis	Diarrhea, obstruction, ileus	Sodium lactate or bicarbonate.
Sodium excess	Sodium chloride overload	Stop fluids; give diuretics.
Water excess	Overload with sodium-poor fluids	Stop fluids; if severe, use hypertonic saline solution.
Calcium depletion	Malabsorption, acute pancreatitis	Parenteral or oral gluconate, calcium, vitamin D.
Magnesium depletion	Prolonged parenteral feeding, ileal disease, diarrhea	Parenteral magnesium sulfate.

dosis can be treated with one-sixth molar ($M/6$) sodium lactate, or solutions containing either bicarbonate (50 to 80 meq/L with sodium chloride) or acetate. In less severe examples, orally administered fluids may facilitate resorption of intestinal secretions, as shown in cholera or infantile gastroenteritis when glucose taken by mouth reduces the volume of stools (51).

Short-bowel syndrome; hyponatremia and malnutrition

Treatment should be based upon the oral intake of rapidly absorbed nutrients, including artificial dietary supplements. Steatorrhea can be lessened by replacement of dietary fat with medium-chain triglycerides; fat-soluble vitamins may be required; and partially or completely hydrolyzed carbohydrates and protein can be prescribed as peptides, oligosaccharides, glucose, or amino acid mixtures. Sodium, potassium, calcium, and anion supplements may also be needed and can be given in a form convenient for absorption as an oral supplement of isotonic electrolytes with glucose. Acute derangements, usually involving sodium and water balance, may necessitate treatment with intravenous solutions. Magnesium depletion, which may be recurrent and severe, requires therapy with regular parenteral magnesium sulfate.

When total parenteral nutrition is being considered, several well-known complications must be kept in mind before proceeding with this form of therapy. These include (1) mechanical complications of the catheter (pneumothorax, catheter emboli, etc.), (2) infections, (3) metabolic disturbances (46). Among the latter, hyperosmolar coma, azotemia, hyperammonemia, hypercalcemia, hypophosphatemia, trace-metal deficiency, vitamin deficiency, and vitamin toxicity have been described.

REFERENCES

1. Gregory, R. A.: *Secretory Mechanisms of the Gastro-Intestinal Tract*, Edward Arnold (Publishers) Ltd., London, 1962.
2. Mutt, V., and J. E. Jorpes: Isolation of aspartyl-phenylalanine amide from cholecystokinin-pancreozymin, *Biochem. Biophys. Res. Commun.*, **26**:392–397, 1967.
3. McGuigan, J. E.: Antibodies to the C-terminal tetrapeptide amide of gastrin: Assessment of antibody binding to cholecystokinin-pancreozymin, *Gastroenterology*, **54**:1012–1017, 1968.
4. Go, V. L. W., A. F. Hofmann, and W. H. J. Summerskill: Simultaneous measurements of total pancreatic, biliary, and gastric outputs in man using a perfusion technique, *Gastroenterology*, **58**:321–328, 1970.
5. Burgen, A. S. V., and N. G. Emmelin: *Physiology of the Salivary Glands*, The Williams & Wilkins Company, Baltimore, 1961.
6. Davenport, H. W.: *Physiology of the Digestive Tract: An Introductory Text*, 2d ed., Year Book Medical Publishers, Inc., Chicago, 1966.
7. Wheeler, H. O., E. D. Ross, and S. E. Bradley: Canalicular bile production in dogs, *Am. J. Physiol.*, **214**:866–874, 1968.
8. Diamond, J. M.: The reabsorptive function of the gall-bladder, *J. Physiol. (London)*, **161**:442–473, 1962.
9. Dreiling, D. A., H. D. Janowitz, and C. V. Perrier: *Pancreatic Inflammatory Disease: A Physiologic Approach*, Paul B. Hoeber, Inc., New York, 1964.
10. Go, V. L. W., A. F. Hofmann, and W. H. J. Summerskill: Pancreozymin bioassay in man based on pancreatic enzyme secretion: Potency of specific amino acids and other digestive products, *J. Clin. Invest.*, **49**:1558–1564, 1970.
11. Hendrix, T. R., and T. M. Bayless: Intestinal secretion, *Annu. Rev. Physiol.*, **32**:139–164, 1970.
12. Fordtran, J. S., and T. W. Locklear: Ionic constituents and osmolality of gastric and small-intestinal fluids after eating, *Am. F. Dig. Dis.*, **11**:503–521, 1966.
13. Hofmann, A. F.: Clinical implications of physicochemical studies on bile salts, *Gastroenterology*, **48**:484–494, 1965.
14. Gregory, R. A., and Hilda J. Tracy: The constitution and properties of two gastrins extracted from hog antral mucosa, *Gut*, **5**:103–114, 116–117, 1964.
15. Brown, J. C., and C. O. Parkes: Effect on fundic pouch motor activity of stimulatory and inhibitory fractions separated from pancreozymin, *Gastroenterology*, **53**:731–736, 1967.

16. Hunt, J. N.: The duodenal regulation of gastric emptying, *Gastroenterology*, **45**:149–156, 1963.

17. Schultz, S. G., and P. F. Curran: Intestinal absorption of sodium chloride and water, in C. F. Code and W. Heidel (eds.), *Handbook of Physiology: A Critical, Comprehensive Presentation of Physiological Knowledge and Concepts*, sec. 6, vol. III, *Intestinal Absorption*, American Physiological Society, Washington, D. C., 1968, pp. 1245–1275.

18. Fordtran, J. S., and F. J. Ingelfinger: Absorption of water, electrolytes, and sugars from the human gut, in C. F. Code and W. Heidel (eds.), *Handbook of Physiology: A Critical, Comprehensive Presentation of Physiological Knowledge and Concepts*, sec. 6, vol. III, *Intestinal Absorption*, American Physiological Society, Washington, D. C. 1968, pp. 1457–1490.

19. Diamond, J. M.: Tight and leaky junctions of epithelia: A perspective on kisses in the dark, *Fed. Proc.*, **33**:2220–2224, 1974.

20. Fordtran, J. S., F. C. Rector, Jr., and N. W. Carter: The mechanisms of sodium absorption in the human small intestine, *J. Clin. Invest.*, **47**:884–900, 1968.

21. Katz, A. I., and F. H. Epstein: Physiologic role of sodium-potassium-activated adenosine triphosphatase in the transport of cations across biologic membranes, *N. Engl. J. Med.*, **278**:253–261, 1968.

22. Phillips, S. F.: Absorption and secretion by the colon (editorial), *Gastroenterology*, **56**:966–971, 1969.

23. Cooper, H., R. Levitan, J. S. Fordtran, and F. J. Ingelfinger: A method for studying absorption of water and solute from the human small intestine, *Gastroenterology*, **50**:1–7, 1966.

24. Olsen, W. A., and F. J. Ingelfinger: The role of sodium in intestinal glucose absorption in man, *J. Clin. Invest.*, **47**:1133–1142, 1968.

25. Esposito, G., A. Faelli, and V. Capraro: Influence of the transport of amino acids on glucose and sodium transport across the small intestine of the albino rat incubated in vitro, *Experientia*, **20**:122–124, 1964.

26. Turnberg, L. A., J. S. Fordtran, N. W. Carter, et al.: Mechanism of bicarbonate absorption and its relationship to sodium transport in the human jejunum, *J. Clin. Invest.*, **49**:548–556, 1970.

27. Giller, J., and S. F. Phillips: Electrolyte absorption and secretion in the human colon, *Amer. J. Dig. Dis.*, **17**:1003–1011, 1972.

28. Turnberg, L. A., F. A. Bieberdorf, S. G. Morawski, et al.: Interrelationships of chloride, bicarbonate, sodium and hydrogen transport in the human ileum, *J. Clin. Invest.*, **49**:557–567, 1970.

29. Phillips, S. F., and J. Giller: The contribution of the colon to electrolyte and water conservation in man, *J. Lab. Clin. Med.*, **81**:733–746, 1973.

30. Devroede, G. J., and S. F. Phillips: Conservation of sodium, chloride and water by the human colon, *Gastroenterology*, **56**:101–109, 1969.

31. Geall, M. G., R. J. Spencer, and S. F. Phillips: Transmural electrical potential difference of the human colon, *Gut*, **10**:921–923, 1969.

32. Crane, C. W.: Observations on the sodium and potassium content of mucus from the large intestine, *Gut*, **6**:439–443, 1965.

33. Moore, F. D.: *Metabolic Care of the Surgical Patient*, W. B. Saunders Company, Philadelphia, 1959.

34. Randall, H. T.: Symposium on basic sciences in surgical practice: Water and electrolyte balance in surgery, *Surg. Clin. North Am.*, **32**:445–469, 1952.

35. Kassirer, J. P., and W. B. Schwartz: The response of normal man to selective depletion of hydrochloric acid: Factors in the genesis of persistent gastric alkalosis, *Am. J. Med.*, **40**:10–18, 1966.

36. Fordtran, J. S., and J. M. Dietschy: Water and electrolyte movement in the intestine, *Gastroenterology*, **50**:263–285, 1966.

37. Phillips, S. F.: Diarrhea: A current view of the pathophysiology, *Gastroenterology*, **63**:495–518, 1972.

38. Phillips, S. F., and T. S. Gaginella: Intestinal secretion as a mechanism in diarrheal disease, in G. B. J. Glass (ed.), *Progress in Gastroenterology*, vol. III, Grune and Stratton, Inc., New York, 1977. In press.

39. Verner, J. V., and A. B. Morrison: Endocrine pancreatic islet disease with diarrhea, *Arch. Int. Med.*, **133**:492–500, 1974.

40. Phillips, R. A.: Water and electrolyte losses in cholera, *Fed. Proc.*, **23**:705–712, 1964.

41. Krone, C. L., E. Theodor, M. H. Sleisenger, and G. H. Jeffries: Studies on the pathogenesis of malabsorption: Lipid hydrolysis and micelle for-

mation in the intestinal lumen, *Medicine (Baltimore),* **47:**89–106, 1968.

42. Hofmann, A. F.: The entero-hepatic circulation of bile acids in man, *Adv. Intern. Med.,* **21:**501–534, 1976.

43. Edmunds, L. H., Jr., G. M. Williams, and C. E. Welch: External fistulas arising from the gastrointestinal tract, *Ann. Surg.,* **152:**445–469, 1960.

44. Hill, G. L.: *Ileostomy: Surgery, Physiology, and Management,* Grune & Stratton, New York, 1976.

45. Winawer, S. J., S. A. Broitman, D. A. Wolochow, M. P. Osborne, and N. Zamcheck: Succesful management of massive small-bowel resection based on assessment of absorption defects and nutritional needs, *N. Engl. J. Med.,* **274:**72–78, 1966.

46. Fleming, C. R., D. B. McGill, and H. N. Hoffman: Total parenteral nutrition, *Mayo Clin. Proc.,* **51:**187–199, 1976.

47. Shields, R.: Surgical aspects of the absorption of water and electrolytes by the intestine, *Monogr. Surg. Sci.,* **1:**119–172, 1964.

48. Cohn, I., Jr.: *Strangulation Obstruction,* Charles C. Thomas, Publisher, Springfield, Ill., 1961.

49. Fine, J., F. Fuchs, and S. Gendel: Changes in plasma volume due to decompression of the distended small intestine, *Arch. Surg.,* **40:**710–716, 1940.

50. Ellis, H.: Acute intestinal obstruction: General considerations, in R. Maingot: *Abdominal Operations,* 5th ed., Appleton-Century-Crofts, Inc., New York, 1969, pp. 1497–1518.

51. Pierce, N. F., R. B. Sack, R. C. Mitra, J. G. Banwell, K. L. Brigham, D. S. Fedson, and A. Mondal: Replacement of water and electrolyte losses in cholera by an oral glucose-electrolyte solution. *Ann. Intern. Med.,* **70:**1173–1181, 1969.

23

Fluid and electrolyte disorders of endocrine diseases

JAMES T. HIGGINS, JR. / PATRICK J. MULROW

INTRODUCTION

In this chapter we shall discuss some of the electrolyte abnormalities which may be seen in endocrine diseases. Although the broadest definition of electrolytes could include all electrically charged solutes in body fluids, we shall confine ourselves for the most part to sodium and potassium and consider the clinical situations in which endocrine diseases result in abnormalities in the total body content or in the extracellular concentration of these minerals. Divalent cations are covered elsewhere, as are acid-base metabolism and bicarbonate ion. Although water metabolism is discussed in detail in another chapter, we will touch on water balance in this chapter as it influences the concentrations of the electrolytes sodium and potassium.

We shall orient the discussion around the endocrine diseases as the primary event and then explore the electrolyte abnormalities which might result from the hormonal imbalance. While acknowledging that virtually any hormone can affect electrolyte metabolism, especially when it is present in enormous amounts, we shall confine ourselves primarily to mechanisms of clinical importance in human beings.

BASIC ELECTROLYTE PHYSIOLOGY

As living organisms become more complex, evolving first into collections of connected and interdependent cells and then adapting to varied habitats, it became necessary for the organism to control for itself the environment of its cell. This process of preservation of the milieu intérieur is as important to the multicellular organism as is nutrition or reproduction, and it is not surprising that the mechanisms which control the content of the extracellular fluids evolved early and through the eons became extremely complex (1–5). See also Chaps. 1 to 6.

Ultimately there evolved organisms so large that circulation of tissue fluids became necessary, and consequently it was necessary to maintain the volume as well as the constituents of those fluids. Thus in the highly developed organisms such as the mammals we find an exceedingly complex array of mechanisms for maintenance of both the volume and the composition of the extracellular fluid (ECF). The survival value of ECF volume and composition is so important that each is regulated by a number of humoral, physical, and neural mechanisms, with extensive interplay among the control mechanisms. Moreover, such important hormones as aldosterone and vasopressin appear to participate in the regulation of both volume and composition of ECF.

GENERAL CONSIDERATIONS

Next let us consider some ways by which hormones can affect the concentration of electrolytes in the ECF. In describing a simple model cell it is pointed out that the cell must expend energy to maintain the high intracellular potassium concentration and low intracellular sodium concentration, referable to the concentration of these ions in the ECF (5, 6). The gradients of these ions across the cell membrane are maintained in part by this energy-consuming active transport and in part by the relative resistance of the cell membrane to passive diffusion of the ions down their chemical and/or electric gradients. Thus, hormones which (1) influence the supply of energy to the active transport site, (2) act on the components of the transport mechanism itself, or (3) change the passive permeability of the cell membrane can result in shifts in the distribution of

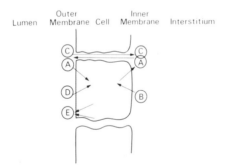

Figure 23-1. Model of epithelial cells separating luminal fluid and interstitial fluid. Solute A diffuses from luminal fluid down its electrochemical gradient and is actively transported up an electrochemical gradient to the interstitial fluid. Solutes B and D are transported up their electrochemical gradient into the cytoplasm through basal or luminal membranes which may have quite different transport characteristics. Solute C is shown moving across the epithelium through the intercellular space. Solute E is secreted into the luminal fluid, passively down an electrochemical gradient, or actively up a gradient.

sodium, potassium, other solutes, and water itself between intracellular fluid (ICF) and ECF (3, 7). Considering the differences in the concentrations of these ions which normally exist across the cell membranes, and the fact that the intracellular volume is about twice the volume of the extracellular space, it is apparent that shifts in the distribution of sodium and potassium across the cell membrane can result in marked abnormalities in the concentrations of these ions in the ECF (or, clinically speaking, in the serum).

Now, suppose we take a large number of the simple model cells and spread them out in a sheet, like the stones of a cobblestone street. Allow the top surface membranes (outward-facing) and the bottom surface membranes (inward-facing) to assume different physical and chemical properties which will affect how solutes move across these membranes, and finally we have an epithelium. The simple cell first described might be thought of as symmetrical, because the membrane all around the cell is homogenous. An epithelial cell, however, is asymmetrical or polar because the membranes making up the two faces of the epithelial sheet are dissimilar (8–11). Variations in the properties of the inward- and outward-facing membranes, and differing degrees of "leakiness" between the cells of the sheet (or between the "cobblestones") will allow the epithelia to achieve an almost infinite variety of transport characteristics (11). A model of an epithelial cell is shown in Fig. 23-1. Mechanisms by which hormones might influence transport through such a tissue are obvious. If solute A diffuses into the cell through the outer membrane and is pumped out across the inner membrane by an active transport process, then a hormone might affect the passive properties of the outer membrane, or the pump action on the inner membrane. Another hormone might control active uptake of a substance (B or D) across either membrane. Another might control extrusion of a solute E from the cell across the outer membrane ("secretion") either by actively transporting it across this membrane or by creating favorable electrochemical gradients for its diffusion from the cell. A characteristic of many epithelia is the ability to maintain a steep osmotic gradient between the two solutions it separates, so permeability to water is another important parameter which may be hormonally controlled. Examples of hormones which accomplish these effects are known and will be described later. Finally, it is tempting to speculate that hormonal control of the passive leak through the intercellular spaces of an epithelium might modulate the overall transport properties of the tissue. Solute C, for instance, might move in either direction between the cells of the epithelium under the effect of concentration gradients or electric potential gradients, or it might be washed along with bulk flow of water which is moving along an osmotic gradient ("solvent drag"). The transport processes of ions and other solutes which establish these chemical, electric, or osmotic gradients might also, of course, be under hormonal regulation. To date, however, there is no evidence for hormonal control of the passive leak properties of the intercellular communications, although striking structural and functional changes in epithelial intercellular spaces have been produced experimentally (12).

Hormones may, and frequently do, interact to affect electrolyte balance either competitively or cooperatively. They may act on the same tissue, or their sites of action may be far apart and interaction take place as the altered electrolyte solution circulates from one organ to another. In some cases, the interaction appears to be almost accidental, as when a homeostatic process for maintenance of blood volume produces an electrolyte concentration abnormality by changing sodium and water balance during correction of a volume disturbance. Finally, since secretion of a hormone by an endocrine cell is usually a membrane-mediated mechanism, another hormone with a cell membrane effect may affect the rate of secretion by the cell (13–16).

The hormones whose primary function is regulation of water and electrolyte metabolism act upon the kidney, and principal among these are aldosterone and antidiuretic hormone (ADH). These two hormones are the most important for net electrolyte and water balance and for control of electrolyte concentration in the ECF. Other hormones appear to affect electrolytes significantly only in abnormal circumstances when these hormones are present in abnormal amounts, or when a disturbance in aldosterone or ADH allows the effects of these hormones upon electrolytes and water to become physiologically significant.

Consideration must also be given to end-organ responsiveness. For instance, a small amount of aldosterone will cause marked renal sodium conservation in an individual with heart failure, whereas the same amount would cause little net sodium retention in a normal subject. Similarly, a small amount of ADH may be adequate for water conservation in a patient with adrenal insufficiency, but if cortisol replacement is given, water diuresis ensues despite the continued presence of the small amount of ADH. Further consideration of these important points will be given as each hormone and the pathological states are considered.

SPECIFIC INTERACTIONS OF HORMONES AND ELECTROLYTES

ADRENAL CORTICAL HORMONES

The adrenal cortical hormones play a role in salt and water homeostasis equalled only by the role of the antidiuretic hormone. All hormones of the adrenal cortex (and the gonads) are derivatives of cholesterol, and all have the basic cyclopentenophenanthrene structure with its four rings of carbon atoms (Figs. 23-2 and 23-3). The structural variations which account for the different physiological effects of the hormones occur through addition of carbon side chains at the 10, 13, and 17 positions of the cyclopentanophenanthrene ring, through unsaturation of the carbon-carbon bonds at several loci, and through hydroxylation of any of several carbon atoms (Fig. 23-3). The three major categories of steroid hormones are the corticoids, the androgens, and the estrogens. The corticoids or cortiscosteroids are synthesized in the adrenal cortex and are characterized by the addition of four carbon atoms (methyl groups at

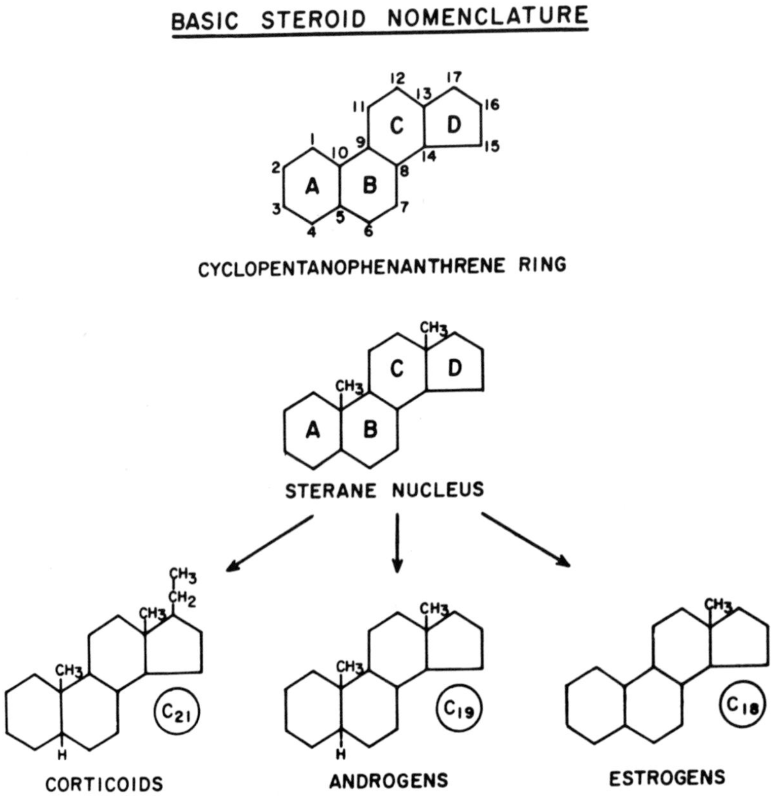

BASIC STEROID NOMENCLATURE

CYCLOPENTANOPHENANTHRENE RING

STERANE NUCLEUS

CORTICOIDS   ANDROGENS   ESTROGENS

Figure 23-2. Steroid structure, nomenclature, and numbering system.

positions 10 and 13 and an ethyl group at position 17) to the 17 carbon atoms of the cyclopentanophenanthrene ring, hence the name C-21 steroids for this group. Androgens have only the two methyl groups at positions 10 and 13 and hence are termed C-19 steroids. Finally, estrogens with their methyl group at position 13 are the C-18 steroids (Fig. 23-2). The corticosteroids are divided into two major groups, those with a dominant effect on intermediary metabolism (the glucocorticoids) and those whose principal effect is on mineral metabolism (the mineralocorticoids). Actually, all of these C-21 hormones have a combination of glucocorticoid (including anti-inflammatory) and mineralocorticoid effects, but the relative potency for these effects varies from compound to compound, and the arbitrary assignment of a compound to the glucocorticoid or mineralocorticoid category depends upon which of its physiological effects appears to be most important. The obvious consequence of this spectrum of actions is that, in sufficiently large amounts, any corticosteroid compound can have the same effect as any other. Cortisol, which in normal amounts has important effects on intermediary metabolism and water balance, in large amounts will mimic fully the mineralocorticoid effects of aldosterone. Aldosterone, although principally responsible for regulation of mineral metabolism, can be shown to affect intermediary metabolism and the inflammatory response when it is given in excessive amounts. The relative glucocorticoid and mineralocorticoid potencies of the most important natural and synthetic corticosteroids are shown in Table 23-1.

The laboratory technique of competitive binding assay has led to an understanding of why a corticosteroid can have both glucocorticoid and mineralocorticoid metabolic effects. It has been shown that the respective metabolic process is initiated when the hormone binds to a nuclear receptor in the target tissue's cells, and the specific-

ity resides in the receptor rather than in the hormone (17). There are two major classes of receptors which have different affinities for the various steroid molecules, and the affinity of a specific receptor for the corticosteroids corresponds to the relative biological potencies of the hor-

BIOSYNTHESIS OF ADRENAL STEROIDS

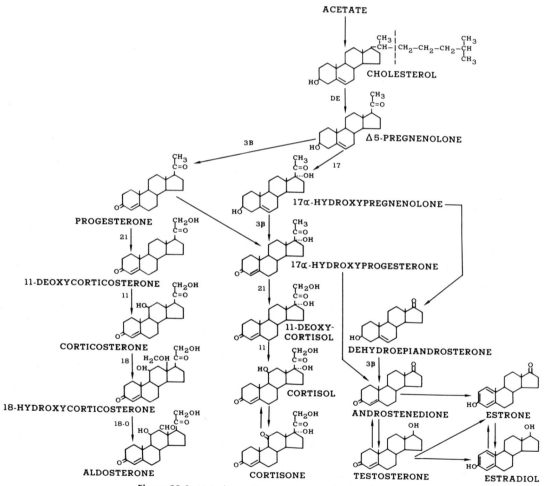

Figure 23-3. Main biosynthetic pathways of adrenal steroidogenesis. Letters and numbers at the arrows denote specific enzymes: DE = demolase, or debranching enzyme; 3β = 3β-ol-dehydrogenase with $\Delta 4,\Delta 5$-isomerase; 11 = C_{11}-hydroxylase; 17 = C_{17}-hydroxylase; 21 = C_{21}-hydroxylase; 18 = C_{18}-hydroxylase; 18-0 = 18-oxidase.

Table 23-1. Relative in vivo potency of some natural and synthetic corticoid preparations*

STEROID COMPOUND	ESTIMATED POTENCIES	
	GLUCOCORTICOID	MINERALOCORTICOID
Cortisol	1	1
Cortisone	0.8	0.8
Desoxycorticosterone	0	25
Aldosterone	?+	200–400
Prednisolone	5	0.5
Prednisone	4	0.5
Methylprednisolone	8–10	?±
Triamcinolone	6–8	?±
Dexamethasone	25–50	?±
Fludrocortisone	10–25	100

* Potencies of the various steroids are compared with cortisol, which is given a value of 1 for its glucocorticoid and mineralocorticoid effects

mones (18–21). For instance, one receptor isolated from renal cortex of adrenalectomized rats avidly binds aldosterone; it binds deoxycorticosterone to a lesser degree, and cortisol still less. A second renal cortical receptor shows much greater affinity for cortisol than for the mineralocorticoids. The ability of one hormone to displace another from the receptor is also a function of its biological potency, thus deoxycorticosterone will displace cortisol from the mineralocorticoid receptor, and aldosterone will displace deoxycorticosterone. Furthermore, the failure of a hormone to bind to a specific receptor provides strong evidence that the hormone does not mediate the in vivo biological effect of that receptor (21). The relative affinities of some corticosteroids for mineralocorticoid receptors, as revealed by competitive binding techniques, are shown in Table 23-2. It can be seen that the values compare quite well with the commonly accepted relative potencies obtained by biological response and shown in Table 23-1. Also illustrated by these data is the effect of plasma proteins to bind some corticoids more than others. In plasma, cortisol has only 1/250th the activity of aldosterone because of the greater protein-binding of cortisol, whereas in protein-free buffer the ratio is reduced to 45:1.

Cortisol and related glucocorticoids

Cortisol (hydrocortisone, compound F) is the principal glucocorticoid in man. Corticosterone (compound B) appears to assume this role in some other species such as the rat and bullfrog. Glucocorticoid secretion is primarily from the zona fasiculata, and the rates of synthesis and secretion are under control of adrenocorticotrophic hormone (ACTH) from the anterior pituitary.

The glucocorticoids exert an effect on electro-

Table 23-2. Relative in vitro potency of various corticoid compounds to compete for aldosterone-binding sites in kidney slices*

STEROID COMPOUND	ESTIMATED POTENCIES	
	IN PLASMA	IN BUFFER
Cortisol	1	1
Aldosterone	250	45
Desoxycorticosterone	40	18
Spironolactone	0.12	0.18

* Potencies of the various steroids are compared with cortisol as in Table 23-1.
Source: After Baxter et al. (21).

Table 23-3. Classification of hyponatremia

I. "APPARENT" HYPONATREMIA DUE TO DISPLACEMENT OF PLASMA WATER

A. Hyperlipidemia
B. Hyperproteinemia

II. HYPONATREMIA DUE TO REPLACEMENT OF ELECTROLYTES BY OSMOTICALLY ACTIVE SOLUTE SUCH AS GLUCOSE IN EXTRACELLULAR SPACE

III. TRUE HYPONATREMIA DUE TO ABNORMALITIES OF SODIUM AND/OR WATER BALANCE

A. Hyponatremia with overhydration due to increases in total body water content in excess of sodium
   1. Heart, liver, or renal failure
   2. Oral or intravenous water load
B. Hyponatremia with dehydration secondary to sodium depletion
   1. Natural loss due to mineralocorticoid insufficiency, gastrointestinal loss, sweating, renal salt wasting
   2. Iatrogenic due to diuretics, paracentesis, usually combined with severely limited intake
C. Hyponatremia with renal water retention, without heart, liver, or renal disease (excessive antidiuretic hormone)
   1. Secretion of vasopressinlike material from nonendocrine tumors
   2. Inappropriate secretion of vasopressin by normal neurohypophysis
      a. Intracranial lesion such as inflammation, trauma, metabolic disease (myxedema, porphyria)
      b. Intrathoracic lesion such as infection, surgery

lyte metabolism via their effects on the kidney. The effect on glomerular filtration rate (GFR) is evidenced by the low GFR in adrenally insufficient individuals, and by the increase in GFR in normal or adrenally insufficient subjects given exogenous glucocorticoid hormone in pharmacological amounts. Glucocorticoids also exert another important effect to augment renal water excretion (see also Chap. 12). Patients with adrenal insufficiency are unable to dilute urine sufficiently to excrete a water load normally, and consequently the ECF becomes diluted. Before the ready availability of steroid assays for clinical diagnosis, use was made of this phenomenon by challenging patients with suspected adrenal insufficiency with a water load (Fig. 23-4) (22). This inability to dilute the urine maximally is only partially explained by the low GFR and has been shown also to be due to abnormalities in renal tubular transport. Adrenal insufficiency is usually associated with some degree of sodium depletion and ECF volume contraction, and in this state fractional reabsorption of filtrate in the proximal tubule is augmented. The result is a decrease in delivery of fluid out of the proximal tubule to more distal sites where urine dilution takes place by reabsorption of sodium and chloride, and thus the patient is unable to produce a dilute urine. Excretion of a dilute urine also requires maintenance of impermeability to water in the collecting duct, so that water cannot readily diffuse from the dilute urine in the tubule back into the circulation. The impermeability to water depends upon the absence of ADH, and the glucocorticoids appear to inhibit secretion of ADH, especially that part of ADH secretion which is controlled by hypothalamic osmoreceptors. This is accomplished by raising the threshold for stimulation of the osmoreceptors, so that a higher serum osmolality is required to stimulate the secretion of ADH (23). The glucocorticoids also, especially in conjunction with the mineralocorticoids, help to restore the contracted plasma volume of the patient with adrenal cortical insufficiency and thus reduce the stimulation to ADH secretion which is mediated by the thoracic volume receptors. Finally, there is evidence that the glucocorticoids act directly upon the distal renal tubular cells, independent of the effects of ADH,

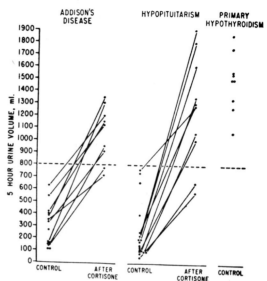

Figure 23-4. Results of water-loading tests in patients with Addison's disease, hypopituitarism, and primary hypothyroidism. 1500 mL tap water was given orally over a 15- to 45-min period after an overnight fast. Note the substantial increase in 5-h urine volume in patients with Addison's disease and hypopituitarism when tests were repeated 2 h after the oral administration of 50 mg cortisone. (*From A. M. Moses et al.*)

to decrease the water permeability in this segment (24–26).

As mentioned above, the glucocorticoids all have some mineralocorticoid effect, although of low potency (Table 23-1), and if present in sufficiently large amount can produce renal sodium retention and potassium and hydrogen ion excretion. The systemic effect of the glucocorticoid hormones is catabolic, and this causes loss of potassium from cells with an increase in extracellular potassium concentration and in urinary potassium excretion.

Aldosterone and other mineralocorticoid hormones (see also Chap. 14)

Of all the steroid hormones synthesized in the adrenal cortex, aldosterone has the strongest sodium-conserving actions in the intact animal. Although all of the hormones normally secreted by the adrenal cortex share this property (progesterone, a precursor of other adrenocortical hormones, causes sodium wasting as described subsequently but is not normally secreted in large amounts by the adrenal cortex), the mineralocorticoid effect of all except aldosterone becomes important only in pathological conditions of excessive secretion.

As with cortisol, the primary determinant of the effective circulatory level of aldosterone is its secretory rate. The secretory rate of aldosterone is controlled by ACTH, the renin-angiotensin system, and serum potassium concentration, but the most important of these is the renin-angiotensin system. Aldosterone secretion rate is determined by the circulating blood level of angiotensin II, which appears to be dependent primarily upon the secretion rate of renin (27, 28). Renin is a proteolytic enzyme secreted by specialized granular cells in the walls of the renal afferent arterioles. This enzyme acts upon a circulating globulin termed angiotensinogen or renin substrate, which is synthesized in the liver, to split off a decapeptide, angiotensin I. Angiotensin I is subsequently cleaved by a peptidase, the converting enzyme (29), to release the octapeptide angiotensin II, which is both an aldosterone stimulator and a potent vasoconstrictor substance. The converting enzyme also acts as a degrading enzyme or kininase for the vasodilator kinins such as bradykinin (29, 30). Even though the converting enzyme is found in plasma, in the kidney, and in other organs, its concentration appears to be greatest in the lung, where it acts on circulating angiotensin I (31, 32). Although renin substrate levels are found to be reduced in liver disease or elevated by estrogen administration, and converting enzyme activity is lower in lung disease such as sarcoidosis, nevertheless the final determinant of angiotensin II level in the blood appears to be the secretion rate of renin. A naturally occurring heptapeptide fragment of angiotensin II, desaspartyl¹-angiotensin II (or angiotensin III, as it has come to be known) has been found to be a potent stimulator of adrenal cortical secretion of aldosterone (33–35). In vitro, it appears to be more potent as an aldosterone stimulator than is angiotensin II. Whether the heptapeptide is formed in the blood and functions as a circulating hormone mediating the aldosterone-stimulating effects of the renin-angiotensin system, or whether it is formed at the target tissue to act as an intracellular mediator is currently unknown. However, it now appears likely that the heptapeptide desaspartyl¹-angiotensin II must be considered a physiologically important link in the renin-angiotensin-aldosterone system. To date, no clinical implications are known.

There are two major circulatory variables controlling renin secretion, renal arterial blood pressure, and ionic composition of the plasma and the tubular fluid (28, 36, 37). A reduction in arterial perfusion pressure, whether caused by hemorrhage, heart failure, dehydration, or stenosis of the renal artery, is a potent stimulus for renin secretion. Renin secretion is also influenced by changes in the ionic composition of the blood perfusing the kidney, perhaps because changes in the plasma electrolytes result in changes in the composition of the tubular fluid which reaches the macula densa. Potassium, for instance, plays a role with increased dietary intake (38, 39) or hyperkalemia (40, 41) suppressing renin secretion, and potassium depletion has been shown to stimulate renin secretion in human beings (39). The mechanism by which potassium influences renin release remains unidentified (37). Whether or not variations in plasma sodium concentration within the physiological range directly control renin secretion in unknown, but infusion of hypertonic saline directly into the renal artery suppresses renin secretion, probably by a macula densa mechanism (41, 42). Drugs which alter reabsorption in the more proximal portions of the renal tubule change the composition of the tubular fluid which is delivered to the macula densa, and this is undoubtedly one way by which pharmacological agents affect renin secretion (43). The relative roles of blood pressure receptors in the afferent arterioles and chemoreceptors in the macula densa remain to be proven, but an interplay between them is probable (37). Finally, the sympathetic nervous system appears to play an important role in control of renin secretion. Infusion of catecholamines into normal animals or human subjects results in stimulation of renin and aldosterone secretion (44–47), and studies with isolated renal slices (48, 49), as well as pharmacological studies in human beings (50, 51), re-

veal this to be mediated by beta-adrenergic receptors. In addition to an effect of circulating
catecholamines, a direct stimulatory effect on
renin secretion by renal sympathetic nerves has
been demonstrated (45, 47, 52). However, relative
roles of the adrenergic nervous system and direct
stimulation of the renal afferent arteriolar baroreceptors in mediation of the renin secretory response to ECF volume depletion remain to be
elucidated.

The role of ACTH in control of aldosterone secretion is probably a permissive one. Certainly
administration of exogenous ACTH is a potent
stimulus for aldosterone secretion, but the patient
with anterior pituitary insufficiency is frequently
found to regulate sodium and potassium balance
quite well with glucocorticoid replacement but no
exogenous mineralocorticoid. Eventually such a

patient usually acquires a need for mineralocorticoid replacement as the adrenal cortex undergoes atrophy in the absence of ACTH. In the normal individual, or in patients with low-renin
hypertension, an effect of ACTH upon aldosterone secretion can be inferred from the small cyclical fluctuations of plasma aldosterone levels
which occur in concert with the circadian rhythm
of ACTH secretion (53, 54).

Changes in ionic composition of the plasma
perfusing the adrenal cortex also act directly to
control aldosterone secretion. Hyponatremia in
the blood perfusing the isolated or in situ adrenal
gland of the dog (Fig. 23-5) or sheep directly
stimulates secretion of aldosterone (55, 56). It is
doubtful whether this is physiologically significant, however, for hyponatremia is frequently associated with disorders of water metabolism in

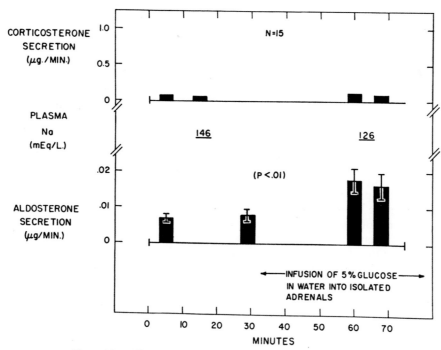

Figure 23-5. Effects of infusion of 5% glucose solution into arterial
supply of isolated adrenal glands of 15 hypophysectomized, nephrectomized dogs. (Mean values and standard errors are presented
for aldosterone secretion.) With the production of hyponatremia
there was a significant increase in aldosterone secretion but no
change in corticosterone secretion. (*From J O. Davis et al.*)

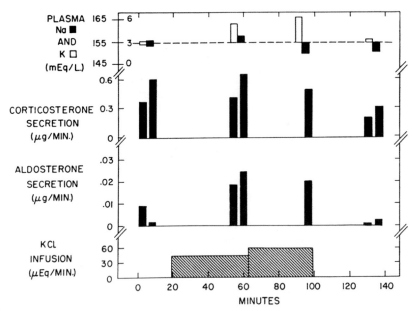

Figure 23-6. Typical changes in aldosterone and corticosterone secretion rates before and during infusion of potassium chloride into the arterial supply of isolated adrenals of a hypophysectomized, nephrectomized dog. (*From J. O. Davis et al.*)

which the volume of the ECF is changed, and secretion of aldosterone responds appropriately to changes in renin secretion which are mediated by the volume disturbance. For instance, hyponatremia associated with water overload due to hypotonic fluid administration or excessive secretion of vasopressin is accompanied by normal, not augmented, aldosterone secretion (57–59). Changes in the serum potassium concentration, on the other hand, can have profound effects on aldosterone secretion rate. Increased potassium concentration in the blood perfusing the animal adrenal (Fig. 23-6) or brought about by feeding potassium will stimulate aldosterone secretion rate (55, 56). In human beings increased dietary potassium intake (60) or intravenous potassium infusion (61) stimulates aldosterone secretion even when serum potassium concentration shows little or no change (Fig. 23-7). This effect occurs without change in plasma renin activity (61) and in anephric humans (62). Potassium depletion (39, 60) or an acute reduction in serum potassium concentration (62) suppresses aldosterone secretion (Fig. 23-8).

The net effect of aldosterone in the intact animal is urinary sodium conservation and potassium excretion, which are accomplished by the distal portions of the renal tubule (63). Aldosterone can also be shown to have effects on transport by epithelia in the colon (64, 65), sweat glands (66), and salivary glands (67, 68), but the magnitude of the responses of these tissues is so small that they probably play minor roles in electrolyte homeostasis. Determination of rectal transepithelial electric potential difference has been proposed as a diagnostic test for presence of primary aldosteronism (69), but the accuracy and specificity of this test have been questioned (70). The mineralocorticoid hormones also play an important role in sodium conservation in the lower vertebrates, and much of our knowledge of the effects of aldosterone at the cellular level has come from study of the response of the amphibian urinary bladder to aldosterone. It may be significant that all of the epithelia which display striking changes in ion transport under the influence of aldosterone would appear to be "tight" epithelia with low permeability for passive diffusion of solutes (11). The transport of sodium across the epithelia of renal distal tubule, mammalian colon, or amphibian bladder is thought to follow the route of solute A in the model epithelium depicted in Fig. 23-1. Aldosterone has been shown to increase the net active transport of sodium from the luminal side of these epithelia to the serosal side (71, 72), but whether it does this by increasing passive sodium permeability through the luminal membrane (73, 74) or by increasing the energy supply to the pump at the serosal membrane (75, 76) remains unknown. It has been convincingly shown that aldosterone must gain access to the interior of the cell, that it binds to the cell nucleus, and that mediation of its effect is dependent upon synthesis of new ribonucleic

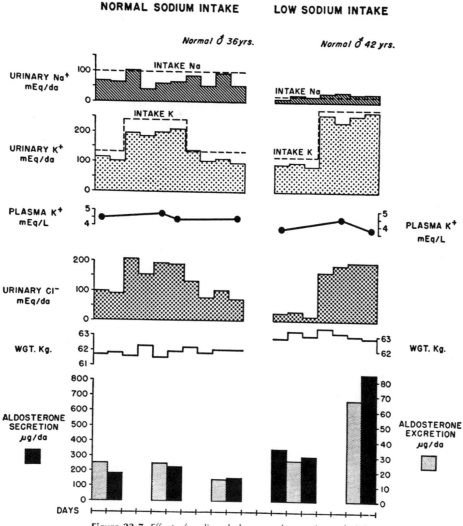

Figure 23-7. Effect of sodium balance and potassium administration upon aldosterone secretion in normal subjects. Note that potassium loading had little effect on aldosterone secretion when sodium intake was normal but significantly increased aldosterone secretion during sodium deprivation. (*From P. J. Cannon et al.*)

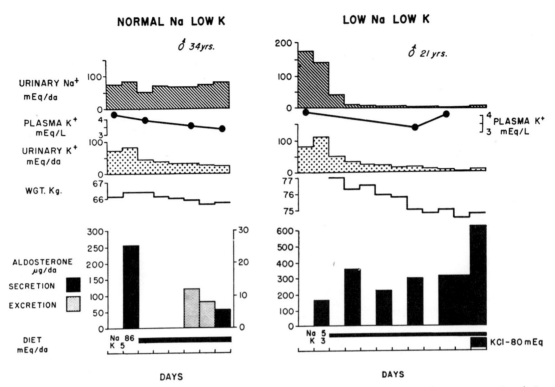

Figure 23-8. Effect of dietary potassium deprivation and sodium balance on aldosterone secretion in normal subjects. Note the striking fall in aldosterone secretion induced by potassium deprivation while subject was on a normal sodium intake (shown on left). In the study at the right, potassium deprivation blunted the usual rise which occurs in aldosterone secretion during sodium deprivation. On the final day potassium chloride administration markedly stimulated aldosterone secretion. (*From P. J. Cannon et al.*)

acid and protein (77, 78). This protein, of course, could theoretically be a carrier protein which augments the movement of the hydrophilic sodium ion through the lipids of the luminal membrane of the cell, it could be a protein component of the pump mechanism on the serosal face of the cell, or it could be an enzyme participating in provision of energy to the pump mechanism. Recent studies of amphibian urinary bladder have revealed profound spontaneous variations in the ionic conductivity of the epithelium which correlate directly with changes of net sodium transport (79). Microelectrode studies have localized the conductivity changes to the cell membrane (80), providing evidence for physiological control of sodium transport through changes in passive cell permeability to ions, and supporting the evidence that aldosterone affects luminal membrane transport (73, 74).

The effect of aldosterone on potassium secretion appears to be indirectly linked to sodium transport. In this case, the bulk of our knowledge comes from study of the distal renal tubule, where it has been shown that reabsorption of sodium leads to steep electric gradients across the entire epithelium, lumen negative to interstitium. The cell interior is negative to the lumen, but the potassium concentration in the cell is sufficiently higher than that of the tubular fluid that there is a net driving force for passive movement into the luminal fluid (24, 81, 82). Also in this portion of the renal tubule hydrogen ion is secreted, creating a pH gradient, and the movement of the positively charged hydrogen ion discharges some of the electric gradient established by sodium transport from the luminal fluid. Control of the net secretory rates of potassium and hydrogen ions, and the stoichiometric relationship to sodium reabsorption remain unknown but undoubtedly are related to the stores of potassium and hydrogen ion inside the cells (83–85).

There is also evidence that aldosterone may play a role in the uptake of potassium into non-epithelial cells. This is suggested by the protective effect which aldosterone gives to potassium-loaded rats (86). On the other hand, incubation of rat diaphragm with aldosterone in vitro is associated with a loss of potassium from the tissues (87). Patients with hyporeninemic hypoaldosteronism are usually hyperkalemic, and although this may be due primarily to lack of the kaliuretic action of aldosterone (88–90), a recent study of diabetic patients with hyporeninemic hypoaldosteronism showed that mineralocorticoid hormone administration partially blocked the efflux of potassium from cells in response to hyperglycemia (91). Thus it would appear likely that while aldosterone exerts its effects on potassium metabolism primarily by its actions on epithelia, there may be other actions influencing distribution of potassium between the intracellular and extracellular fluid spaces.

The response of the kidney to aldosterone is complicated and depends greatly upon the state of salt and water balance of the subject and upon the functional status of the cardiovascular system. Soon after the availability of synthetic mineralocorticoid hormones made such a study possible, it was observed that a normal human subject on a normal diet responded to exogenously administered aldosterone or deoxycorticosterone by reducing urinary sodium excretion, thus going into positive sodium balance. This positive sodium balance lasted only a few days, however, and then urinary sodium excretion increased to equal intake despite continued mineralocorticoid administration (Fig. 23-9). This phenomenon became known as renal escape from the sodium-retaining effect of the mineralocorticoid hormone (92–95). Escape is still incompletely understood, but it has

been shown that it is not dependent upon increased blood pressure, increased GFR, presence of the adrenal glands, or diminution of ADH secretion (96, 97). Because the subject is in a state of net positive sodium balance due to the retention of sodium before escape occurred, and because the various characteristics concerning GFR, blood pressure, other hormones, etc., are shared with the renal response to intravenous or oral salt loading, it is assumed that both take place by the same mechanisms (98). A full discussion of the natriuresis of escape and saline loading will not be attempted here, but it is important to note that existence of a natriuretic hormone has been proposed for more than a decade (99). Isolation of such a hormone and even conclusive proof of its existence remain elusive (100, 101). An important mechanism contributing to renal escape, perhaps the dominant mechanism, is decreased net and fractional reabsorption in the proximal renal tubule (102, 103). The most obvious result of decreased proximal tubular reabsorption is increased excretion of sodium and water, but other reabsorptive processes such as those of glucose and phosphorus are depressed as well (104–107). Fractional reabsorption rate of sodium in the proximal tubule has an important effect on excretion rate of potassium and hydrogen ions. Decreased proximal fractional reabsorption as occurs in escape causes increased delivery of sodium to distal sites where it is reabsorbed leading to increased secretion of potassium and hydrogen ions. In contrast, avid reabsorption in the proximal tubule, as occurs in heart failure, cirrhosis or the nephrotic syndrome, or after sodium depletion, results in decreased sodium delivery to distal reabsorption sites and thus to lower potassium and hydrogen ion secretion rates even though these pathological states are associated with high endogenous aldosterone secretion.

Other aldosterone-responsive tissues such as the salivary glands (67, 68), sweat glands (66), and colonic mucosa (64, 65, 69) do not participate in the escape phenomenon, and in the kidney potassium excretion remains elevated after escape from the renal sodium-retaining effect of excessive mineralocorticoid hormone. Thus there is an increase in the potassium/sodium concentration ra-

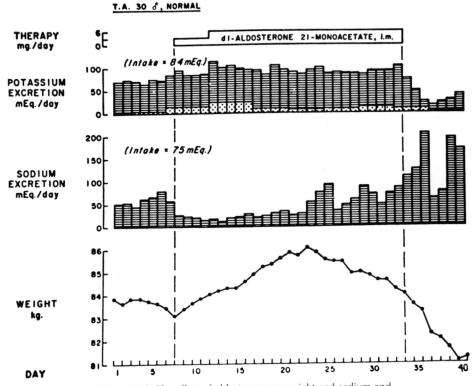

Figure 23-9. The effect of aldosterone on weight and sodium and potassium excretion in a normal subject. (*From J. T. August et al.*)

tios of the urine and the secretions of these glands and an elevated transepithelial electric potential in the colon of many of the individuals who show escape from the renal sodium-retaining effects of the mineralocorticoid hormones. This continued potassium wasting can lead to depletion of body stores of this mineral.

In contrast to the ease with which normal subjects escape from the renal sodium-retaining effects of mineralocorticoids, those with vascular lesions are unable to escape. A good example is the patient with heart failure and a high level of endogenous aldosterone who continues to retain sodium avidly. A similar response to exogenously administered mineralocorticoid hormone is seen in dogs with arteriovenous fistulas or inferior vena caval constriction who may retain sodium to the point of death (96). This striking sensitivity to the sodium-retaining effect of mineralocorti-

coids in cardiovascular disease is not due exclusively to high distal tubular reabsorption rates, for these subjects may be able to maintain sodium balance in the absence of external mineralocorticoid hormone. The defect may be a failure to decrease proximal reabsorption when extracellular fluid volume expansion results from the effect of the mineralocorticoid hormones on the distal tubule. Here also, the existence of an unidentified hormone has been proposed to explain this aspect of escape (96).

OTHER STEROID HORMONES

Progesterone

Progesterone is a precursor of the corticosteroids and is usually secreted only in small quantities by the adrenal cortex. It is secreted in rather large amounts by the corpus luteum of the ovary and by the placenta during pregnancy. It is bound to a significant extent by the cellular mineralocorticoid receptors, and thus if progesterone is present in large quantities it may compete with aldosterone for the binding sites, thus producing an inhibitory effect on the sodium-retaining response to the mineralocorticoid hormones (108–110). In pregnancy and to a lesser degree in the luteal phase of the menstrual cycle, the increased progesterone secretion interferes with the action of aldosterone. Use has been made of this fact by pharmaceutical chemists who have synthesized a progesteronelike steroid compound which has minimal intrinsic biological activity but which competes with aldosterone for cell binding and thus inhibits the mineralocorticoid effects of aldosterone (111, 112). This compound, spironolactone, has proved to be useful clinically to block the effects of aldosterone and related mineralocorticoid hormones in various states of sodium retention (see Chap. 13).

Estrogens

Estrogenic steroids secreted by the adrenal cortex, ovary, or placenta have no intrinsic effect on electrolyte metabolism. However, the high blood levels of estrogens found during pregnancy, or during administration of exogenous estrogens, can indirectly affect electrolytes by their effect on the liver to stimulate increased synthesis of the renin substrate. This results in a complex biological response discussed elsewhere (Chap. 25), and it suffices here simply to point out that increased renin substrate may force the renin reaction to the right, resulting in more angiotensin generation and thus in increased aldosterone secretion with all of its consequences (113–115).

Androgens, glucocorticoid and mineralocorticoid precursors

The androgens have no direct effect on electrolyte metabolism. However, their anabolic effects on the tissues necessitate the retention in the body of substances needed for cell growth, including water and minerals. Abnormalities in adrenal androgen secretion may occur simultaneously with electrolyte disturbances in a group of disorders of adrenal hormone synthesis known collectively as the adrenogenital syndromes or congenital adrenal hyperplasia. In these conditions, discussed more fully below, defects in the enzyme pathways for corticosteroid synthesis lead to decreased production of cortisol. Since the rate of ACTH secretion is determined by the feedback effect of serum cortisol concentration, ACTH secretion increases in order to stimulate adrenal cortisol synthesis. The enzymatic defect is usually not complete, so under the stimulus of continued high levels of ACTH, the output of cortisol rises toward normal levels. The problem, however, lies in the fact that the precursor steroids which are synthesized at steps prior to the step involving the defective enzyme accumulate in large amounts and ultimately spill over into the circulation. Although the glucocorticoid or mineralocorticoid potency of these steroids is weak relative to the potencies of cortisol or aldosterone, respectively, the large amounts which ultimately appear in the blood can have profound metabolic effects. For example, the increased progesterone and 17-hydroxyprogesterone production may contribute to sodium wasting by competing with aldosterone for the mineralocorticoid receptors.

ANTIDIURETIC HORMONE

Antidiuretic hormone and water metabolism are described in detail in Chap. 12. It will suffice here to reiterate that in humans ADH appears to be involved exclusively with water conservation by the kidney. Its secretory rate is responsive to changes in both extracellular solute concentration and volume. Because of this involvement of ADH and water metabolism with both volume and ionic composition, there is extensive interplay between this system and the volume and composition-regulating mechanisms of the adrenal cortex and the kidney. As already discussed, cortisol affects the responsiveness of the hypothalamic volume receptor to changes in plasma solute concentration and affects the renal tubular response to ADH. Excessive ADH secretion, by expanding the ECF volume, can both inhibit renin secretion and suppress renal tubular sodium reabsorption so that urinary sodium wasting occurs.

THYROID HORMONE

The thyroid hormones, principally thyroxin and triiodothyronine, produce the same cellular effects and differ only in potency. They are important for growth, for regulation of intermediary metabolism rate, and for thermogenesis in homeothermic animals. These hormones are not usually considered to be important in the normal physiological regulation of water and electrolyte metabolism, but at extremes of hypo- and hyperfunction of the thyroid gland there may be profound disturbances.

Many of the effects of thyroid disorders on water and electrolytes are indirect. In hypothyroidism, blood volume is reduced, the cardiac output is low, and blood flow to the kidneys and GFR are reduced (116–119). There is a decrease in the ability to excrete an acutely administered water load which is probably due to the diminished GFR (120–123). Studies in the hypothyroid rat have shown that sodium reabsorption in the diluting segment of the renal tubule is normal, and a more dilute urine can be elaborated if GFR is increased or if proximal tubular reabsorption is inhibited (124). When treated with thyroid hormone replacement, hypothyroid patients show an increase in GFR and restoration of ability to dilute the urine after a water load (117, 121). There is no evidence for abnormality in control of ADH secretion in most cases of hypothyroidism, but isolated cases of excessive secretion of ADH with concomitant dilutional hyponatremia (an example of the so-called syndrome of inappropriate ADH secretion) have been reported (125). Water excretion in hypothyroid patients is discussed more fully in the following section on clinical disorders.

In hyperthyroidism, on the other hand, there is peripheral vasodilatation and increased cardiac output. Total renal blood flow, as evidenced by clearance of hippuric acid derivatives, is increased (118, 119). An increase in the renal medullary blood flow probably results in a reduction of the medullary interstitial solute concentration so that the osmotic gradient from tubule to interstitium is reduced. This would explain the observation in hyperthyroid human beings and experimental animals that the urine cannot be maximally concentrated in response to dehydration or ADH administration (126–128).

There are also direct effects of the hypothyroid state on renal function. Thyroid hormone is a trophic hormone, required for normal growth, and the developing hypothyroid animal has been shown to have smaller than normal kidneys. Microdissection study has revealed the proximal convoluted tubule of the hypothyroid rat to be shortened (129), and it has been postulated that this may be one mechanism for the decreased fractional reabsorption of sodium observed in hypothyroidism (see below). Transport rates of organic compounds are reduced in hypothyroidism as evidenced by the subnormal transport maxima for para-aminohippurate, glucose, and Diodrast (117–119, 130). These defects are repaired by treatment with thyroid hormone.

Although sodium reabsorption in the diluting segment of the renal tubule appears to be normal, as described above, there may be some impairments of electrolyte transport in more distal segments of the tubule. When given an acute hypertonic saline load, the hypothyroid rat responds with an exaggerated natriuresis due to diminished tubular reabsorption (131). In hypothyroid humans given an isotonic saline load, the sodium excretion rate does not increase to a significantly greater degree than that of euthyroid subjects, but the fractional excretion is higher. Furthermore, in both rat (131) and humans (132), the kidney does not respond normally to administered aldosterone or 9-α-fluorocortisone, either with enhanced sodium reabsorption or an increase in potassium excretion. Probably related to this tubular abnormality is the failure to reabsorb filtered sodium normally in response to the upright posture (132). Despite these defects, however, day-to-day sodium balance and serum electrolyte concentrations are usually normal in hypothyroidism.

Myxedematous patients accumulate ECF which is rich in protein, and when treated with thyroid hormone they frequently respond with a diuresis and natriuresis. Despite this indirect evidence for sodium accumulation in the hypothyroid state, there is no evidence for extensive sodium retention, and in the hypothyroid rat measurement of inulin space actually shows significant reduction in the ECF volume.

The mechanisms by which thyroid hormone exerts its effects on cellular metabolism have remained elusive despite decades of research. A series of elegant studies published in the past several years provides strong evidence that a major part of thyroid thermogenesis in homeothermic animals occurs because of an effect of the thyroid hormone on cell plasma membrane ATPase mediated sodium and potassium transport (133–136). Although there is no evidence at present to suggest that this mechanism is important for electrolyte balance, concentration or distribution in the clinical sense, the fact that sodium and potassium transport is involved may ultimately prove to have important clinical implications and deserves mention here. It has been shown that a significant portion of the increase in oxygen consumption by thyroid hormone–stimulated tissue is sodium dependent and is accompanied by increased sodium-potassium-activated ATPase (Na^+–K^+–ATPase) activity. Triiodothyronine given to either euthyroid or hypothyroid rats was found to reduce the intracellular Na/K ratio of heart and diaphragm, but no significant change in serum electrolyte concentrations was seen. A similar effect on intracellular Na/Ka ratio of liver was seen in vitro. This effect of thyroid hormone on cell membrane Na^+–K^+–ATPase does not appear to be a universal one in all tissues, however, for it has been shown by other investigators that enzyme activity is low and intracellular sodium concentration high in red blood cells of hyperthyroid patients (137). It has been suggested that this effect of thyroid hormone on membrane ATPase activity may be mediated via new ribonucleic acid (RNA) and protein synthesis, analogous to the effect of mineralocorticoid hormones on epithelial cells, but this remains to be established. Such an effect on sodium and potassium transport across the cell membrane has obvious implications for cell volume regulation and electrochemical gradients of sodium and potassium, but no clinical or biological consequences are known beyond those of oxygen and substrate utilization and heat generation.

Finally, it should be acknowledged that iodide itself is an electrolyte, and its availability, uptake, and organification by the thyroid gland are essential for life in virtually all vertebrates.

PARATHYROID HORMONE

The major role of parathyroid hormone is in calcium metabolism as described in Chaps. 8 and 9. Parathyroid hormone does have an indirect effect on electrolyte metabolism, due to the renal effects of hypercalcemia (138–141). Hypercalcemia produces first functional and then structural changes in the kidney which impair the urinary concentrating response to ADH, a form of nephrogenic diabetes insipidus. In the early functional changes there are minimal morphological lesions, but later there develop an interstitial nephritis, nephrocalcinosis, and stone formation in the collecting system. These latter lesions can lead to obstruction and infection with varying degrees of renal excretory failure and its metabolic consequences.

The action of parathyroid hormone on the proximal renal tubule is adenylate cyclase–mediated (142–144), and in addition to promoting increased reabsorption of filtered calcium it inhibits reabsorption of phosphorus, sodium, and bicarbonate. Although increased sodium excretion can be shown after stimulation of parathyroid hormone secretion (145, 146), this natriuresis does not appear to be of sufficient degree to cause clinically significant sodium depletion. The bicarbonate diuresis which occurs in response to the action of parathyroid hormone on the renal proximal tubule may produce clinically apparent metabolic acidosis with low serum bicarbonate and high chloride concentrations in patients with hyperparathyroidism (147). In contrast, hypoparathyroidism may be associated with metabolic alkalosis.

Finally, the parathyroid hormone–mediated

changes in ECF calcium concentration may influence the function of other hormonal systems because of the effects of calcium on membrane stability and hormone secretion. For instance, calcium has been shown to be essential for the exocytotic process of catecholamine secretion by the adrenal medulla (13).

THYROCALCITONIN

Administration of thyrocalcitonin to human beings has been reported to cause increased urinary excretion of calcium and phosphorus (148, 149) by a mechanism independent of parathyroid hormone (148). One study also reported increased excretion of sodium and chloride in normal humans (150), but other investigators have found variable increases in urinary phosphorus excretion and no change in sodium excretion in response to thyrocalcitonin administration (151). The phosphaturic response to thyrocalcitonin seen in rats (152) and dogs (153–155) is abolished by parathyroidectomy (154, 155), indicating that the renal response is an indirect one induced by the increase in parathyroid hormone secretion which occurs in reaction to the fall in serum calcium caused by thyrocalcitonin. Patients with thyrocalcitonin-secreting medullary carcinoma of the thyroid show no electrolyte disturbance other than hypocalcemia, and thus it is felt that this hormone is not important for regulation of water and electrolyte homeostasis. Nevertheless, thyrocalcitonin-sensitive adenylate cyclase activity has been found in the medullary ascending limb, cortical ascending limb, and early distal convoluted tubule of the rabbit renal tubule, suggesting a specific biological action of this hormone on the kid-157).

INSULIN

Insulin has been thought to have no direct effect on water and electrolyte metabolism, but its universal effect on carbohydrate metabolism throughout the organism has indirect effects. For instance, the membrane effects of aldosterone and ADH on epithelial sodium transport, as seen in the amphibian skin or urinary bladder, are augmented by insulin (158). The hyperglycemia and metabolic acidosis associated with insulin deficiency can have profound indirect effects on water and electrolyte homeostasis. The hyperglycemia itself lowers extracellular sodium concentration and causes depletion of total body stores of sodium and water. The accumulated extracellular glucose serves as an osmotically active agent moving water out of cells, thus diluting extracellular solutes. As the maximum glucose reabsorptive capacity of the renal tubules is exceeded by the increasing amount of glucose in the glomerular filtrate, glucose is lost in the urine where it serves as an osmotic agent to increase excretion of sodium and water. Finally, the secretion rate of renin in response to volume changes may be impaired in long-standing diabetes, thus contributing an additional sodium-losing mechanism (159). In summary, then, insulinopenic hyperglycemia is associated with hyponatremia, sodium wasting, and dehydration (Table 23-3; see also Chap. 24).

Two further mechanisms may operate to cause hyponatremia in the diabetic. The first of these is not a true hyponatremia, for the concentration of sodium in plasma water is normal. It occurs in patients who have a severe elevation of serum lipids, principally very low density lipoproteins (VLDL). The VLDL may occupy a significant volume in the intravascular space and actually displace plasma. Since the clinical laboratory assays the electrolyte content of all of the noncellular supernatant of centrifuged blood, the apparent plasma or serum electrolyte concentration will be reduced to the extent that plasma water is displaced by lipid. Formulas for calculation of the effects of hyperglycemia (160, 161) and hyperlipidemia (162, 163) on plasma sodium concentration have been published.

True hyponatremia may be seen in some diabetics who are treated with chlorpropamide and respond by retaining water, excreting a relatively concentrated urine. Although it was originally proposed that chlorpropamide might have an intrinsic antidiuretic action (164), it is now commonly accepted that it acts on the renal collecting ducts to potentiate the effect of endogenous ADH.

The metabolic acidosis which may occur in insulinopenic diabetes may itself produce an abnormality in potassium homeostasis. As metabolic intermediates such as the keto acids accumulate, cells take up hydrogen ions and give up potassium to the ECF. This potassium load into the ECF is excreted by the kidneys, leaving the patient with a net potassium deficit. During insulin treatment, potassium is reaccumulated by cells as the acidosis is corrected and the ECF concentration of potassium falls, frequently to abnormally low levels. This phenomenon has been taken advantage of for emergency treatment of hyperkalemia in the nondiabetic patient, in whom infusion of insulin and glucose causes transport of potassium into cells, resulting in a redistribution of potassium between intracellular and extracellular water and a fall in extracellular potassium concentration.

Insulin has not been thought to play a role in potassium homeostasis in the absence of diabetic ketoacidosis. However, hyperkalemia has frequently been recognized in patients with hyporeninemia, hypoaldosteronism, and mild renal dysfunction (89, 90, 165, 166), and recently a group of patients has been described who had mild diabetes as well (92, 166). In these patients it was necessary to administer insulin as well as

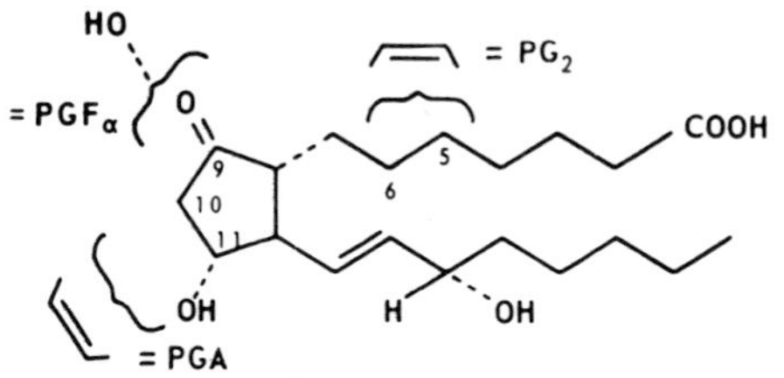

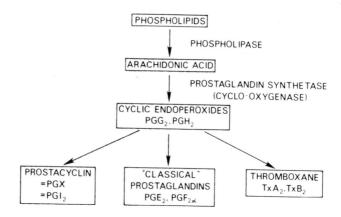

BIOSYNTHESIS OF PROSTAGLANDINS

Figure 23-11. Main biosynthetic pathways of prostaglandins. Note that the synthesis of the cyclic endoperoxides from arachidonic acid by prostaglandin synthesis is central to synthesis of all of the naturally occurring prostaglandins. Prostaglandin synthetase activity is inhibited by a number of drugs in clinical use.

mineralocorticoid hormone to restore serum potassium to normal levels (92). Since the fall in serum potassium concentration could not be fully accounted for by urinary excretion, it was assumed that the insulin and aldosterone both mediated cell uptake of potassium.

PROSTAGLANDINS

Prostaglandins are naturally occurring 20-carbon unsaturated fatty acids containing a five-membered ring (167, 168). The names and formulas are shown in Fig. 23-10. They are synthesized from polyunsaturated fatty acids and do not exist free in tissue in any significant amounts; rather, they are synthesized and released in response to stimuli.

A diagram of the biosynthesis of prostaglandins is shown in Fig. 23-11. The first step is the activation of a phospholipase A to hydrolyze arachidonic acid from the phospholipid. An enzyme formerly called prostaglandin synthetase but presently termed cyclooxygenase then converts

Figure 23-10. General chemical structure of the prostaglandins. Prostaglandins are naturally occurring 20-carbon unsaturated fatty acids containing a five-membered ring (1, 2). The basic chemical structure of the "classical" prostaglandins is shown here. In PG_2 the carbon-carbon bond at position 5-6 is unsaturated, in PGA the 10-11 bond is unsaturated, and the oxygen at position 9 is reduced to a hydroxy group in PGFα.

the arachidonic acid to the intermediate endoperoxides which may be converted to prostaglandin E (PGE), prostaglandin F (PGF), or prostacyclin (PGI), and under certain circumstances, to thromboxanes. This synthetase is present in a great variety of tissues.

The major synthesis of prostaglandins in the kidney occurs in the interstitial cells of the renal medulla and papilla, and also in the epithelial cells of the medullary collecting duct. These locations suggest a role for prostaglandins in control of water excretion. The main prostaglandins in the kidney are prostaglandins E and F. They are produced by both cortical and medullary tissue, but the medulla is the major site of prostaglandin synthesis, whereas the cortex is the major site of destruction (169). PGE_2 appears to be the major prostaglandin produced; however, more recent data indicate that endoperoxides and PGI are also produced. Small amounts of PGA are found, although the origin of PGA is a matter of dispute. Under ordinary circumstances, little if any thromboxanes are made by the kidney, but kidneys with experimentally produced obstruction appear to make large amounts of thromboxanes (170). Although much of the literature is concerned with renal PGE production, it should be recognized that such measurements may be merely an index of prostaglandin synthesis, and other prostaglandins may play important physiological roles.

Once formed, prostaglandins are rapidly metabolized, particularly by the lungs. This rapid metabolism makes it unlikely the prostaglandins made by the kidney are hormones in the classic sense, but they may act as local hormones either within the cell in which they are formed, or on nearby cells. The major prostaglandin metabolizing enzyme, the 15-hydroxydehydrogenase, has its highest activity in the cortex and has little activity in the renal medulla (170). This dissociation between synthesis and degradation may have important biological implications.

The prostaglandins are among the most active natural substances known. The actions of the different prostaglandins differ quantitatively and qualitatively, and it is by no means clear which actions are physiological and which are pharmacological. There are qualitative differences between biological actions of the prostaglandins of the F series and those of the E and A series. The prostaglandins E and A resemble each other in their biological action, but PGE_2 is more potent for the renovascular bed (171). $PGF_{2\alpha}$ does not affect renal blood flow and urine formation. PGE compounds oppose both neural and hormonal vasoconstrictor stimuli, whereas $PGF_{2\alpha}$ augments the vasoconstriction produced by adrenergic nervous activity and pressor hormones. As mentioned previously, both PGE and PGF compounds are rapidly cleared by the lungs, while PGA is not; thus, only the latter can behave as a systemic hormone. However, there is considerable debate as to whether PGA is a naturally occurring compound (172–175). No specific enzyme for the synthesis of PGA has been found in the renal medulla.

Several lines of evidence suggest that prostaglandins may regulate renal blood flow (176–180). Infusion of PGE or PGA into human beings or animals or directly into the renal artery causes renal vasodilatation. However, pharmacological doses of prostaglandins have been used in most of these studies and therefore the results may not imply that prostaglandins have a physiological control over renal blood flow. McGiff and coworkers (181, 182) have emphasized the possible intrarenal role of PGE_2 as a modulator of renal blood flow. Infusion of angiotensin II or norepinephrine into the renal artery caused an initial fall in renal blood flow, followed by an increase in prostaglandin synthesis and a reversal of the vascular effects of the vasoconstrictor hormone. These authors argue that PGE_2 regulates the renal circulation since release of PGE_2 is associated with recovery of renal blood flow and urine flow during the vasoconstrictor stimulus. When angiotensin II failed to release PGE_2 from the kidney, renal vasoconstrictor and antidiuretic responses were sustained. Furthermore, these investigators (181, 183) presented evidence that PGE acts locally on the renal medullary vasculature. Inhibition of PGE synthesis with indomethacin reduced inner cortical blood flow in the isolated perfused canine kidney. Aiken and Vane (184) demonstrated that indomethacin increased the renal vasoconstrictor action of angiotensin II and was associated with failure of release of prostaglandins. Furthermore, inhibition of renal prostaglandin synthesis by indomethacin abolished renal autoregulation in the anesthetized dog.

Another line of evidence has been presented by Tannenbaum et al. (185). These authors infused the prostaglandin precursor sodium arachidonate into the renal artery of a dog and demonstrated an increase in renal blood flow and renal venous prostaglandinlike substances. Infusion of an inhibitor of prostaglandin synthetase activity blocked this response. Acute renal ischemia may also increase prostaglandin release in both the ipsilateral and contralateral kidneys (186). This bilateral effect may be due to the release of renin from the constricted side. Presumably the released renin generates peripheral blood angiotensin II which, in turn, stimulates the contralateral kidney to release prostaglandins. Prostaglandins may also mediate other factors which cause renal vasodilatation. Increases in renal blood flow following bradykinin or furosemide infusion or ureteral obstruction have been found to be abolished or attenuated by indomethacin administration (187–190). The vasodilatation following ureteral obstruction may be due to the production of thromboxanes (170).

In spite of these results, there is considerable controversy over the role of prostaglandins in the regulation of renal blood flow, especially in the conscious animal. It had been suggested that renal autoregulation is controlled by prostaglandins (191). However autoregulation of renal blood flow and glomerular filtration rate in perfused dog kidneys was maintained when prostaglandin production was inhibited with indomethacin, and many subsequent experiments have confirmed these findings (192–194). These differences, noted particularly between conscious and anesthetized animals, may be explained by the increased vascular resistance that is present in the anesthetized animal. The increased renovascular resistance may be due to enhanced activity of the renin-angiotensin or adrenergic systems. Thus, when the baseline resistance is high, it appears

easier to demonstrate a role for prostaglandins in the regulation of renal blood flow. Furthermore, stimuli such as intrarenal infusion of vasoconstrictors and stimulation of renal nerves decrease renal blood flow while increasing production of renal prostaglandins.

In summary, a number of studies suggest that endogenous prostaglandins attenuate a variety of renal vasoconstrictor stimuli in the kidney. Whether or not prostaglandins regulate basal renal blood flow is unclear, but renal autoregulation is maintained even when prostaglandin synthesis is inhibited.

There is considerable controversy about the effect of prostaglandins on sodium excretion by the kidney. Prostaglandins may influence renal excretion of sodium by at least two mechanisms. One mechanism is by vasodilatation and another may be a direct action on the renal tubule. When prostaglandins of the PGE or PGA series are infused either systemically or into the renal artery, there is an increase in renal blood flow and renal sodium excretion in anesthetized dogs and in conscious humans (176–180, 187, 195). The demonstration of enhanced free water clearance associated with the natriuresis suggests that prostaglandins decrease sodium reabsorption in the proximal tubule (178–180). In micropuncture studies, a more distal site of action of prostaglandins has been suggested (196). There are problems with the interpretation of these investigations since pharmacological doses of prostaglandins were used, and the intrarenal infusion of these substances may not stimulate the naturally occurring intrarenal synthesis and action.

The most convincing evidence that endogenous prostaglandins are natriuretic is the work of Tannenbaum et al. (185). The intrarenal infusion of arachidonic acid to anesthetized dogs caused an ipsilateral increase in sodium excretion associated with an increase in PGE in the renal venous blood. This enhanced renal sodium excretion occurred with doses of arachidonic acid that did not change glomerular infiltration rate or renal blood flow. The natriuresis was prevented by administration of an inhibitor of prostaglandin synthesis.

In contrast, data of Kirchenbaum et al. (197)

suggest that prostaglandins decreased sodium excretion. They reported that arachidonic acid does not increase renal sodium excretion in the prostaglandin-depleted kidney and that prostaglandin inhibition causes a natriuresis in the conscious dog. Furthermore, in humans indomethacin can attenuate furosemide-induced natriuresis and diminish the renal sodium and potassium wasting in patients with Bartter's syndrome. In vitro PGE_1 can directly enhance transmembrane sodium transport in the toad bladder and frog skin (198, 199). It is possible, therefore, that prostaglandins can decrease renal sodium excretion by enhancing tubular sodium reabsorption, but this antinatriuretic effect may be obscured by prostaglandin-induced renal vasodilatation which, in turn, decreases tubular sodium reabsorption.

The response of prostaglandin levels in the kidney or peripheral blood levels to changes in sodium intake is still unclear. Although early data suggested that sodium loading decreased while sodium depletion increased PGA content of the rat kidney, or peripheral plasma levels of PGA in humans (200), there is serious doubt that PGA is a naturally occurring substance.

In summary, the role of endogenous prostaglandins on sodium balance is not clear, and further studies are necessary to resolve their action.

The high concentration of prostaglandin in the interstitial cells of the renal medulla suggests that prostaglandin may play a role in the control of renal water excretion (201). In vitro studies with prostaglandins support this contention. In the toad bladder, prostaglandins do not have an effect on basal water transport but do antagonize the action of vasopressin and theophyllin, but not of cAMP (202–207). Since vasopressin increases cAMP by stimulating adenylate cyclase activity, PGE most likely affects water transport at a step proximal to cAMP generation, possibly by altering vasopressin affinity for the adenylate cyclase receptor. Indeed PGE can inhibit vasopressin-stimulated adenylate cyclase activity in the medulla of the rat (208). In vivo experiments also suggest an effect of prostaglandins on renal water excretion. Intrarenal administration of PGE_1 increases urine flow and free water clearance, possibly as a result of increased renal blood flow. In anesthetized hy-

pophysectomized dogs undergoing a water diuresis, inhibitors of prostaglandin synthesis potentiated the effect of exogenous vasopressin (209). In humans undergoing a water diuresis, indomethacin enhanced the response of urinary osmolality to exogenous vasopressin (210). These data suggest that prostaglandins play a role in renal water excretion by antagonizing the action of ADH. Additional hemodynamic effects may also play a role.

Previously cited data indicated that angiotensin II infusion increases PGE release, and it was postulated that angiotensin II may control prostaglandin production by the kidney. Early studies by Vander (195) in dogs showed no effect of PGE on renin release. However the demonstration in patients with Bartter's syndrome (see below) that indomethacin treatment or aspirin administration inhibited prostaglandin production and lowered renin levels suggested that prostaglandins may control renin release. More recent data by Carlson et al. (211) showed that PGE or PGA infusions increased renin production. Furthermore, indomethacin administration reduces the basal levels of renin in human beings and blocks the increased renin secretion which follows furosemide stimulation (212). These data suggest that endogenous renal prostaglandins may play an important role in the control of renin release. Indeed, in the dog with a nonfiltering kidney, indomethacin can block the rise of renin secretion which follows a decrease in perfusion pressure to the kidney (213). Preliminary data by Franco (214) indicate that a number of prostaglandins can increase renin release in the superfused rat kidney.

The role of prostaglandins in regulating blood pressure in experimental hypertension has been studied in animals mainly by measuring prostaglandins in renal vein blood, renal content of prostaglandins, or prostaglandin production in vitro, or by observing blood pressure changes following treatment of an animal with inhibitors of prostaglandin synthesis. The results have been conflicting, but alterations of prostaglandin levels, particularly PGE, have been reported. Jaffe et al. (215) reported increased PGE levels in the ischemic kidney and elevated serum PGE levels in chronic renovascular hypertension. In vitro production of PGE by kidneys of rats with renal clip hypertension was reduced in reports of Pugsly et al. (216) and Sirois et al. (217). In fact, the latter group found reduced PGE production by genetically hypertensive rats and an inverse correlation between the height of the blood pressure and the production of PGE_2, while Dunn on the other hand found increased renal medullary prostaglandin synthesis in the Okamoto strain of spontaneously hypertensive rat (SHR) (218). In another type of genetic hypertensive rat, the New Zealand strain, Armstrong et al. (219) reported decreased prostaglandin inactivation by the 15-hydroxydehydrogenase in kidney homogenates. The authors suggest that in these rats, PGE augments noradrenaline vasoconstriction and the excess PGE, as a result of decreased destruction, may lead to changes in renal resistance and the development of hypertension.

In most reports, the inhibition of prostaglandin synthesis has increased blood pressure in experimental hypertension in rats and rabbits, particularly during acute phase of development of the hypertension. Romero and Strong (220) treated rabbits with severe hypertension and high plasma renin levels with indomethacin. This treatment resulted in renal failure, malignant hypertension, and death. Hornych et al. (221) reported increased peripheral PGA levels in renal hypertensive patients which they interpreted as an adaptive mechanism, whereas Patak et al. (222) found that giving indomethacin to hypertensive patients blocked the natriuretic and hypotensive effects of furosemide. PGA is an attractive candidate for a renal hormone since it escapes metabolism by the lung and could have a peripheral effect whereas PGE is rapidly cleared by the lung. Nevertheless, as mentioned previously, there is considerable doubt about the natural occurrence of PGA.

Prostaglandins may also control blood pressure by acting as a local vasodilator. Release of prostaglandins by perfused arteries and veins suggest that this may occur. Angiotensin II, bradykinin, or norepinephrine can release PGE from perfused vascular tissue. Both arteries and veins synthesize PGE, and more recently Moncada, Higgs, and Vane (223) showed that these vessels produced an important inhibitor of platelet aggregation, PGI, which is also vasocative in certain vascular beds. Arteries and veins from the SHR rat have been reported to produce increased amounts of PGE in vitro (224, 225). Possibly this is an adaptive mechanism to lower the blood pressure. Furthermore, inhibitors of prostaglandin synthesis increase peripheral resistance in several animal species.

In addition to prostaglandins, other lipids from the kidney may be vasodepressors. Investigations by Muirhead (226, 227) suggest the renal medulla contains a nonprostaglandin neutral lipid which serves a vasodepressor function. Although semipurified extracts of this material have no immediate vasodepressor action, chronic administration can lower the blood pressure of animals with experimental hypertension. Autotransplants of renal medulla into rats with malignant hypertension lowered the blood pressure, while transplants of renal cortex had no effect. Examination of the surviving renal medullary tissue showed the presence of renal medullary interstitial cells. Transplantation of interstitial cells from tissue culture lowers the blood pressure even when prostaglandin production is inhibited with indomethacin. Muirhead and his colleagues (226, 227) have evidence that the activity resides in the neutral lipid extract. This antihypertensive action of the renal medullary tissue appears to be effective in a wide variety of hypertensive models including renovascular hypertension, mineralocorticoid and salt-loading hypertension, and angiotensin-induced hypertension.

BRADYKININ

The renal kallikrein-bradykinin system is proposed as a local hormonal system which is involved in the regulation of renal blood flow and sodium excretion. Renal kallikrein is produced by the cortex of the kidney and is excreted in considerable amounts into the urine. It appears to act within the kidney on a substrate called kininogen to produce an active kinin, kallidin, which has a natriuretic effect on the kidney as well as a vasodilator action. Stop-flow studies suggest that an important site of kinin production may be in the distal tubule of the kidney (228). Margolius et al. (229) reported that a low sodium intake caused a progressive increase while a high sodium intake decreased kallikrein excretion. Administration of a mineralocorticoid hormone increased kallikrein excretion, while aldosterone antagonists such as spironolactone lowered kallikrein excretion. These workers proposed that kallikrein excretion is related to the level of mineralocorticoid hormone and have reported that, in vitro, aldosterone can stimulate kallikrein production by cultured renal tubular cells. There is some controversy over the effect of sodium intake upon kallikrein excretion. Some workers have proposed that kallikrein may be positively correlated with sodium excretion and may play a role in the natriuresis following salt loading.

In patients with essential hypertension, urinary kallikrein excretion is low, and it is also low in nonhypertensive members of their families (230). In primary aldosteronism kallikrein excretion is elevated and can be diminished by spironolactone administration (230). The excretion of subnormal amounts of kallikrein by hypertensive patients may represent a defect in the renal vasodilator system. Such a defect could play a role in increased renal vascular resistance seen in hypertensive patients.

The kallikrein-bradykinin system may interact with the prostaglandin system. Perfusion of the kidney with bradykinin can transiently increase PGE release. In transformed mouse fibroblasts, bradykinin appears to stimulate PGE production by activating a phospholipid deacylating enzyme (231), and in arterial smooth muscle cells in vitro, bradykinin can stimulate PGE production (232, 233). Although part of the renal vasodilatation produced by infusion of the bradykinin may be due to PGE release, there is another component as well since indomethacin treatment does not block the vasodilatation caused by infusions of bradykinin (234).

PROLACTIN

Prolactin is a hormone of major importance in the regulation of fluid and electrolyte balance in fishes, amphibians, and birds, but its role is still not clear in mammalian electrolyte metabolism. In the rat and in the perfused cat kidney, prolactin preparations from several animal species can stimulate renal retention of water, sodium, and potassium (235–237). When ovine prolactin is administered to humans, it produces renal retention of water, sodium, and potassium (238).

In teleost fish, removal of the pituitary gland leads to loss of ability to survive in fresh water. Survival requires that a fish be able to retain sodium within the body without having an accumulation of excess water. When prolactin is administered to these hypophysectiomized teleosts, they are again able to survive in fresh water. Prolactin effects osmoregulation in fishes through inhibition of sodium excretion by the gill, by changes in branchial water permeability, and by decreases in sodium excretion by the kidneys (3, 239). In rats, prolactin blocks the diuretic and natriuretic response to isotonic and hypotonic saline expansion, but not to whole blood expansion (240). A possible explanation of these results is that saline expansion increases back-diffusion through dilated intercellular spaces in the proximal tubule while blood does not, and prolactin may prevent the dilatation of the intercellular spaces (240).

Buckman and Peake (241) presented evidence for a role for prolactin in osmoregulation in man. Hypotonic saline and water decreased plasma prolactin concentrations 10 percent to 15 percent, while hypertonic saline markedly increased prolactin levels. In contrast, Adler et al. (242) could not confirm these results. They found that administration of a water load caused a very small increase in prolactin. There was no change after hypotonic or hypertonic saline. They argue that the design of the experiments by Buckman and Peake may have accounted for their findings—that is, the hypertonic saline may have caused pain which in turn stimulated release of prolactin. Berl et al. (243) stimulated endogenous prolactin secretion by administration of thyrotropin-releasing hormone, and found no change in renal function; hypotonic and hypertonic infusions failed to charge serum prolactin levels, and these investigators concluded that prolactin is probably not important for salt water metabolism in man.

Administration of bromoergocryptine, a drug which inhibits prolactin secretion, increases urinary sodium and potassium excretion in rats (244), and in man bromoergocryptine inhibits the rise of plasma aldosterone which normally occurs after furosemia-induced sodium diuresis (245). In the rat, sodium depletion was found to increase both plasma prolactin levels and aldosterone production (246). However, Gomez-Sanchez (247) could not find any increase in prolactin levels after sodium depletion in the rat. Furthermore, prolactin levels are increased following thyrotropin-releasing hormone injections in man, without any change in plasma aldosterone, and prolactin levels are elevated in a variety of conditions such as pituitary tumors and galactorrhea without pituitary tumors, and in these situations aldosterone excretion and plasma levels are normal.

Although there is a variety of experimental evidence suggesting that prolactin can influence salt and water metabolism in mammals, the clinical evidence does not support any significant physiological role for prolactin in water and electrolyte metabolism in man. Prolactin levels may be low or high in a variety of conditions with no obvious change in the blood electrolytes, aldosterone secretion, or salt and water excretion. Nevertheless, prolactin may play some minor role or synergize with other hormones in altering electrolyte balance, but future studies are needed to clarify the role of prolactin in salt and water homeostasis in man.

CATECHOLAMINES

The importance of the catecholamines for electrolyte homeostasis appears to be primarily in their role as neurotransmitters, both to stimulate secretion of hormones with more direct effects on electrolytes, and to control circulatory pressure and flow.

Renal nerve stimulation (45, 47, 52) infusion of catecholamines into the intact kidney (44–47) or application of catecholamines to kidney slices (48, 49) all stimulate renin release, an action which is blocked by beta-adrenergic inhibitors (50, 51). The physiological significance of this reponse to the catecholamines is uncertain, but this is one rationale for treating hypertension with beta-adrenergic blocking agents (51).

Stressful situations which cause sympathetic nervous system discharge are associated with inhibition of ADH release and a resultant diuresis. Although infusion of large amounts of epinephrine can stimulate ADH secretion (248), it appears unlikely that this is physiologically significant. In the kidney, the catecholamines may inhibit the response of the renal tubules to ADH (249), a phenomenon which can be demonstrated in the isolated toad bladder where the action of the catecholamines can be shown to block both sodium and water permeability and the sodium transport effects of ADH (250–251). Both in the kidney (252) and in the amphibian bladder (250, 251) it can be shown that it is the alpha-adrenergic effects of the catecholamines which inhibit the increase in cAMP which occurs in response to ADH. On the other hand it has been proposed that the beta-adrenergic effects of catecholamines enhance the response to ADH (250). Recently, specific cell receptors for stimulation of cAMP production by the β-agonist isoproterenol have been identified in the distal convoluted tubule and cortical collecting tubule of the rabbit (253).

Although it is difficult to separate a direct effect of the catecholamines on renal tubular sodium transport from effects mediated by hemodynamic changes, studies of the isolated perfused kidney (254) or using micropuncture techniques (255) have recently provided support for clearance studies (256) which indicated a direct tubular effect of both catecholamines and renal sympathetic nerves. In these studies it was shown that renal nerve stimulation or infusion of catecholamines increases tubular sodium reabsorption without changes in renal blood flow or glomerular filtration rate.

Thus there is considerable evidence for direct and indirect renal effects of the catecholamines, but their role in body fluid and electrolyte homeostasis remains unclear. Furthermore, their actions to increase blood pressure, to cause renal vasoconstriction, or to cause redistribution of blood within the vascular space can all be expected to have complex indirect effects on control of electrolyte metabolism in the intact organism.

GROWTH HORMONE

Growth hormone has an anabolic effect on all tissues. It has no specific direct effect on electrolytes but indirectly results in retention of sodium, potassium, and water which is appropriate for the tissue growth and may have direct and indirect effects on divalent ion metabolism (see Chap. 8).

ENDOCRINE ABNORMALITIES COMMONLY ASSOCIATED WITH ELECTROLYTE DISTURBANCE

ADRENOCORTICAL INSUFFICIENCY

The clinical manifestations of adrenocortical hormone insufficiency are determined by the degree of insufficiency, whether the insufficiency is chronic or acute, and whether secretion of some or all corticosteroids is insufficient. The degree of insufficiency depends upon the ability of the adrenal cortex to secrete its hormones, and more importantly upon the needs of the organism. A patient with partial loss of adrenocortical function might function reasonably well if unstressed and given ready access to salt, but this same person would be in danger if subjected to trauma, surgical stress, or sodium restriction. Except for enzymatic disorders leading to specific corticosteroid insufficiencies, which will be considered subsequently, the states of adrenocortical insufficiency can best be considered by classifying them into primary and secondary types. Primary adrenocortical insufficiency is due to failure of the gland to secrete adequate amounts of hormone, even with maximal stimulation.

Secondary adrenocortical insufficiency occurs because of insufficient stimulation of the adrenal gland by the trophic hormones ACTH and angiotensin. Rarely, insufficiency of ACTH secretion may occur with preservation of secretion of other anterior pituitary trophic hormones, but most commonly there is insufficient secretion of all trophic hormones in pituitary insufficiency. Destruction of the anterior pituitary gland may result from surgical or irradiation ablation, from nonsecretory pituitory tumors, from infarction, from metastatic tumors, or from a variety of infil-trative, infectious, or granulomatous diseases. Supracellar tumors, trauma, infection, hydrocephalus, or infiltrative diseases may lead to loss of hypothalamic releasing or inhibiting factors and secondarily cause adenohypophyseal dysfunction. Thus the systemic manifestations of anterior pituitary disease are protean and depend upon the degree of abnormality of secretion of each of the pituitary trophic hormones. Total loss of pituitary trophic hormones, as may occur after surgical hypophysectomy, is rapidly fatal if hormonal replacement is withheld and is characterized by nausea, vomiting, prostration, vascular collapse, and hyperthermia. Incomplete hypopituitarism is much more common, and the systemic manifestations may be much more subtle with gonadal failure secondary to gonadotrophic insufficiency being most prominent. Hypothyroidism due to loss of thyrotrophic hormone is very common, and secondary adrenocortical failure due to ACTH insufficiency is next most common. As with primary adrenocortical insufficiency, secondary insufficiency is rarely complete, and the manifestations, which are similar, depend in large part on the demands of stresses put upon the patient. Since the primary effect of ACTH is control of cortisol synthesis and secretion, glucocorticoid insufficiency characterizes ACTH insufficiency, and patients with anterior hypopituitarism may not have disturbances of mineral metabolism or require mineralocorticoid hormone replacement. With profound or long-standing hypopituitarism, however, adrenal cortical atrophy may become so severe that the zona glomerulosa becomes unresponsive to stimulation by angiotensin or by increases of plasma potassium concentration, and the patient may develop renal sodium wasting and potassium retention, hypotension, and hyperkalemia.

Secondary hypoaldosteronism can result from inadequate stimulation of the adrenal cortex by angiotension. Since angiotensin II generation is dependent upon adequacy of renin substrate, renin, and converting enzyme, then theoretically deficiencies of any of these could lead to low angiotensin generation and secondary hypoaldosteronism. The only clinically important state of angiotensin insufficiency identified to date is hyporeninism. This condition occurs most commonly in older individuals with mild to moderate degrees of renal failure, is characterized by varying degrees of hyperkalemia, and appears to be due to an inability of the diseased kidney to secrete renin normally in response to the usual stimuli (see section on aldosterone above). Diabetes mellitus may also be associated with abnormally low renin secretion, and a number of patients with hyporeninemic hypoaldosteronism have been diabetic (see section on diabetes below). It has only recently become recognized that renal prostaglandins are involved with renal renin secretion, and it has been shown that inhibition of prostaglandin synthesis by nonsteroidal anti-inflammatory agents such as indomethacin may lower renin secretion sufficiently to cause hypoaldosteronism and hyperkalemia in some patients with renal disease (257).

Primary adrenocortical insufficiency is due to loss of substance of the adrenal cortex due to surgery, infection, hemorrhage, autoimmune processes, or replacement by amyloid or malignant tumor. The consequence is loss of both cortisol and aldosterone. In mild states of insufficiency, and without stress on the individual, the condition may be chronic and fairly well tolerated if adequate dietary sodium chloride is available. Impaired distal renal tubular transport, in the face of inadequate mineralocorticoid stimulation, may result in urinary sodium wasting and retention of potassium and hydrogen ion, the net result of which is ECF volume contraction, hyperkalemia, and metabolic acidosis. Decreased renal perfusion results from glucocorticoid insufficiency and from the contracted ECF volume, and mild renal insufficiency may be seen. With further adrenal insufficiency the blood pressure falls, cardiac size is diminished, cardiac output falls, and complete circulatory collapse is imminent and may be precipitated by even mild stress. Anorexia and diarrhea are manifestations of the steroid deficiency and hasten the development of ECF contraction and vascular collapse.

Deficiencies in adrenocorticoid hormone secretion also occur with inborn defects in adrenal steroidogenic enzymes. In such cases, there is usually insufficient function of a single enzyme resulting in an accumulation of the precursor molecules and the metabolites of these precursors (Fig. 23-3). If there is an impairment of cortisol synthesis, the hypothalamo-pituitary negative feedback system is disturbed, resulting in increased ACTH secretion, stimulation of steroiddogenesis, and further accumulation of the steroid precursors. The blood level of cortisol may finally reach an adequate level for basal function, but there may be little or no reserve and the individual may be in danger of adrenal insufficiency in times of stress. The price the individual pays for this minimally adequate cortisol level, however, is increased ACTH secretion and increased synthesis of all steroid compounds proximal to the defective enzymatic step. These precursor steroids, many of which are not normally secreted by the adrenal cortex, spill over into the circulation where they produce physiological responses (258, 259).

Two of these disorders, those due to deficiencies of the C_{21}-hydroxylase or the C_{11}-hydroxylase enzymes, are usually referred to as "adrenogenital syndrome" because overproduction of the 17-ketosteroid hormones results in virilization of female children or isosexual precosity in males (258–262). The most common of these is C_{21}-hydroxylase deficiency, an inherited disorder transmitted in an autosomal recessive manner with variable penetrance resulting in different degrees of C_{21}-hydroxylase enzyme activity. This disorder usually presents itself in two different ways. Approximately half of the affected individuals show a sodium-wasting tendency with very low aldosterone secretion even when the patient is sodium depleted. The aldosterone deficiency also results in potassium and hydrogen ion retention and the serum electrolytes of these patients are characterized by hyponatremia, hyperkalemia, and metabolic acidosis. The urinary sodium concentration and the 24-h sodium excretion are excessive, and the patients frequently compensate for this by voluntarily ingesting large quantities of salt. The remainder of the patients with C_{21}-hydroxylase deficiency appear to synthesize sufficiently adequate amounts of aldosterone to maintain electrolyte balance. Various explanations have been proposed to explain the two manifestations of C_{21}-

hydroxylase deficiency. One commonly held theory proposes that there are two isoenzymes of C_{21}-hydroxylase, one for the cortisol synthetic pathway in the zona fasciculata and one for the aldosterone pathway in the zona glomerulosa (260, 263). In the salt-wasting form of the disease, both isoenzymes are deficient; if only the isoenzyme of the cortisol pathway is deficient, aldosterone may be synthesized and electrolyte balance maintained. Another theory proposes that the salt-losing form represents a more profound enzyme deficiency resulting in loss of both glucocorticoid and mineralocorticoid secretion (258). In fact, cortisol secretion is much lower in the salt-losing compared with the non-salt-losing type. In both types, treatment consists of glucocorticoid hormone replacement, but in the salt-wasting form of this disorder mineralocorticoid hormone replacement is necessary as well.

A defect in 11β-hydroxylation results in the hypertensive form of congenital adrenal hyperplasia (261, 262, 264). The predominant precursors which accumulate in this enzymatic deficiency are deoxycorticosterone (DOC) and 11-deoxycortisol. As in the C_{21}-hydroxylation defect there is overproduction of adrenal androgens, resulting in virilization. Most of the patients with this form of adrenal hyperplasia have hypertension, presumably because of the sodium which is retained by the kidney in response to the mineralocorticoid effect of the DOC. The sodium retention and resultant ECF volume expansion suppress renal renin secretion. Renin responsiveness to sodium depletion is intact, but aldosterone secretion fails to increase during a low-salt diet, presumably because the 11β-hydroxylase defect prevents conversion of DOC to aldosterone. However, when ACTH secretion is suppressed and DOC production falls, the secretion of aldosterone can be shown to increase in response to a low-sodium diet, indicating that the defect in 11-hydroxylation of DOC in zona glomerulosa is not complete. Two peculiar but unexplained clinical findings in 11β-hydroxylase deficiency are the failure of some affected persons to become hypertensive and the rarity of mineralocorticoid-induced serum electrolyte abnormalities such as hypokalemic alkalosis which one might expect to be caused by the excessive DOC production (261). Treatment consists of glucocorticoid hormone replacement.

Two further forms of congenital adrenal hyperplasia are associated with underproduction of adrenal sex steroids and with electrolyte abnormalities. Deficiency of 3β-hydroxysteroid dehydrogenase (3β-HSD) results in decreased synthesis of cortisol, aldosterone, and sex steroids (258, 259, 265). Salt wasting is severe, and many infants with this defect do not survive.

Another rare but fascinating picture occurs with 17-hydroxylase deficiency in adrenals and gonads resulting in male pseudohermaphroditism and sexual infantilism in the female (266, 267). Since 17-hydroxylation is not involved in the mineralocorticoid synthetic pathway, the synthesis of aldosterone precursors is increased in response to the excessive ACTH which is caused by cortisol deficiency. Secretion of aldosterone itself is decreased. This can be explained by the mineralocorticoid effect of DOC which is formed in excess and causes sodium retention, hypertension, hypokalemia, and suppression of renin secretion. The blood pressure and electrolyte abnormalities respond to glucocorticoid hormone replacement, but correction of the sexual defects requires sex hormone replacement.

Even rarer are 18-hydroxylase deficiency and 18-dehydrogenase deficiency (268–271). Only aldosterone synthesis is impaired, and cortisol and sex steroid secretion are normal. Children with these deficiencies have shown profound salt wasting with dehydration, hyponatremia, and hyperkalemia. Treatment with mineralocorticoid hormones is necessary, but there is a peculiar tendency of salt wasting to ameliorate with age.

ADRENOCORTICOID HORMONE EXCESS

The steroid hormones of the adrenal cortex fall into three broad categories based upon their tissue effects: the glucocorticoids, the mineralocorticoids, and the weak sex hormones. The clinical manifestations of an excess quantity of any cortical hormone depend upon its relative potency to bring about changes in intermediary metabolism, mineral metabolism, anabolism or catabolism, virilization or feminization. Most of the cortical hormones have some effect on both intermediary metabolism and mineral metabolism, although the potency of the effects varies widely among the individual compounds (Table 23-1).

The clinical picture brought about by an excess of hormones whose principal action is glucocorticoid is commonly known as Cushing's syndrome (the term *Cushing's disease* should be reserved for instances of Cushing's syndrome brought on by excessive pituitary secretion of the adrenocorticotrophic hormone, ACTH). This disease state may be brought about (1) by excessive secretion of ACTH by the pituitary resulting in bilateral hyperplasia of the adrenal cortex, (2) by excessive steroid production by a benign adrenal cortical adenoma, (3) by excessive steroid production by an adrenal cortical carcinoma, (4) by the adrenal cortical response to an ACTH-like hormone produced by a remote neoplasm (the ectopic ACTH syndrome), or (5) by the administration of exogenous natural or synthetic steroid hormones or adrenocorticotrophic substances. Although the glucocorticoid hormones have only slight mineralocorticoid activity, they may be present in sufficiently large amounts in Cushing's syndrome to produce abnormalities in electrolyte metabolism. Potassium and hydrogen ions are lost in the urine due to the mineralocorticoid effect on the distal portions of the renal tubule, and a state of hypokalemic alkalosis may result. The catabolic actions of the glucocorticoid hormones cause loss of cellular potassium and greatly contribute to the generalized depletion of total body potassium. The presence of hypokalemic alkalosis in Cushing's syndrome is considered an ominous sign, for it indicates the presence of an enormous amount of glucocorticoid hormone, and the most likely causes are either adrenal cortical carcinoma or ectopic ACTH production by a nonendocrine tumor (272). A feature of adrenal cortical carcinoma which may contribute to the likelihood of development of electrolyte disturbance is altered steroid synthesis. Inadequate 11β-hydroxylation is common in tumors and may result in excessive secretion of deoxycorticosterone which has much greater mineralocorticoid activity than does cortisol (273, 274).

Electrolyte disturbances may also be brought about indirectly by the effects of glucocorticoid hormones on the cardiovascular system and the kidney. Hypertension is common in Cushing's syndrome, and this may ultimately lead to heart failure, edema formation, and renal failure. Furthermore, the glucocorticoid hormones cause demineralization of bone and hypercalciuria which may lead to nephrocalcinosis and the formation of renal calculi. Hypokalemic alkalosis, if present, would exacerbate this situation. These renal lesions cause interstitial nephritis, urinary tract infection, loss of urinary concentrating ability, and may ultimately lead to renal failure.

In contrast to the clinical picture of glucocorticoid excess, which is frequently associated with nonglucocorticoid manifestations such as electrolyte disturbances, virilization, and feminization, states of mineralocorticoid excess are usually characterized by the singular effects of these hormones on blood pressure and electrolyte metabolism (see also Chap. 14). Primary aldosteronism, as originally described, is caused by excessive aldosterone secretion from a solitary adrenal adenoma arising from the zona glomerulosa and associated with suppression and atrophy of the remaining normal zona glomerulosa (275). The high plasma levels of aldosterone act on the renal tubule to cause sodium retention and secretion of potassium and hydrogen. Similar effects of aldosterone on cation transport occur in other tissues such as colon (64, 65, 69) and salivary (67, 68) and sweat glands (66), but it is the renal action which appears most important in production of the hypokalemic alkalosis that is characteristic of primary aldosteronism. In addition to the low serum potassium concentration and the high bicarbonate concentration, an elevation of the serum sodium concentration into the high-normal range is usually seen. The urinary electrolyte pattern of the patient with primary aldosteronism is usually normal, reflecting the dietary intake. Urinary potassium conservation, which one would expect in the hypokalemic patient, is not seen, however, and administration of an excessive amount of sodium either in the diet or by intravenous administration causes a characteristic kaliuresis (276). On the other hand, restriction of dietary sodium, particularly when associated with adequate potassium intake, can prevent urinary potassium wasting and hypokalemia. Although the patient with primary aldosteronism has a greater than normal total body sodium content, there is characteristically no edema or other sign of fluid overload unless some other fluid-retaining state such as heart failure supervenes. This is because of the ability of the kidney to escape from the sodium-retaining effects of aldosterone and to regain a new state of sodium balance in which excretion is equal to intake, even though the total body content of salt and water is modestly increased (95). Probably as a result of the increased total body sodium in primary aldosteronism, there is a striking natriuretic response to a salt load. Patients with this disease who are given intravenous saline develop a natriuresis which is greater than that seen in salt-loaded subjects with essential hypertension, and both excrete the salt load more rapidly than do normotensive subjects (277, 278). Two other hallmarks of primary aldosteronism which are the results of the aldosterone-induced sodium retention are hypertension and decreased renin secretion. These are discussed more fully in Chap. 14. Because primary aldosteronism due to an adrenal adenoma can produce hypertension in the absence of hypokalemia, and because this disease is surgically curable, it is important to evaluate plasma renin activity and aldosterone in all hypertensives who are not responsive to the most basic antihypertensive regimen.

In recent years it has become recognized that many patients with the hallmarks of primary aldosteronism, such as hypertension, hypokalemia, low plasma renin activity and high plasma and urinary aldosterone do not have an aldosterone-producing adenoma but instead have bilateral adrenal cortical hyperplasia, frequently with micronodular or macronodular appearance. The distinction between aldosteronism due to a solitary nodule and that due to bilateral cortical hyperplasia is important, because although their clinical manifestations are identical, the patients with hyperplasia do not respond favorably to subtotal or even total adrenalectomy and frequently remain hypertensive postoperatively (279–281).

A large fraction of the population of hyperten-sive patients can be shown to have low plasma renin activity but normal aldosterone levels. Like patients with primary aldosteronism, these patients show an exaggerated natriuretic response to an intravenous saline load (277, 278). Usually, the serum electrolyte concentrations are normal, and to date no satisfactory explanation can be given to account for the suppressed plasma renin activity, or to explain the fact that the aldosterone secretion rate may be normal even though the patient appears to be volume-expanded and the plasma renin activity is suppressed. There is evidence to suggest that aldosterone secretion may be maintained by ACTH in this clinical state (282).

Secondary aldosteronism is a state of increased secretion of aldosterone which occurs in response to the demands of the body to expand the ECF volume. Such disease states are characterized by edema, and typical examples are congestive heart failure, cirrhosis, and the nephrotic syndrome. Secondary aldosteronism is also a normal physiological response to dehydration and hemorrhage. In the usual developmental sequence, water and electrolytes are lost from the intravascular space, and the resultant decrease in renal perfusion stimulates renin secretion which in turn stimulates aldosterone secretion. If the renal tubules are capable of a normal response to the increased blood levels of aldosterone, the concentration of sodium in the urine becomes very small. Urinary potassium and hydrogen ion losses do not become excessive, however, because in these hypovolemic states the reabsorption rate of glomerular filtrate in the proximal tubule is high and very little sodium is actually delivered to the aldosterone-sensitive distal tubular sodium reabsorbing sites. Consequently, the hypokalemic alkalosis so typical of primary aldosteronism does not develop in secondary aldosteronism. Two further characteristics of secondary aldosteronism are failure of the kidney to escape from the salt-retaining effects of the aldosterone, and normal suppression of aldosterone secretion if the renal perfusion should be sufficiently restored to normal that renin secretion rate returns to normal.

Entirely different clinical pictures are seen in patients with states of excessive aldosterone secretion which result from adrenocortical stimulation by renin from tumors of the kidney or from juxtaglomerular hyperplasia. There are now several reported occurrences of hemangiopericytoma, or juxtaglomerular tumor (283, 284). These tumors are usually benign and may be localized by renal arteriography or by catheterization of the renal veins for determination of plasma renin activity. The clinical picture caused by these tumors consists of hyperreninemia, secondary hyperaldosteronism, hypertension, and hypokalemia. A similar clinical picture can result from excessive renin secretion by Wilms's tumor (285) and clear-cell carcinoma of the kidney (286).

Recognition of juxtaglomerular cell hyperplasia dates from 1962 when Bartter described a 5-year-old retarded boy and a 25-year-old immature man, both of whom had hypokalemia, metabolic alkalosis, normotension, increased plasma renin concentration, increased urinary aldosterone excretion, and hyperplasia of the juxtaglomerular apparatus on renal biopsy (287). Patients with the syndrome exhibit two other important features: the blood pressure response to angiotensin II administered intravenously is subnormal (287–289), and there is an abnormality in renal tubular reabsorption of sodium (290, 291). A greater than normal fraction of filtered sodium is delivered to sites in the distal nephron where potassium is secreted, and a greater than normal fraction of sodium delivered to the distal nephron is excreted into the urine.

The pathogenesis of Bartter's syndrome is not clearly understood, and there is a question as to the homogeneity of the disease process among the reported cases. Bartter originally suggested that the insensitivity to the pressor action of angiotensin II which characterizes the syndrome led to renal hypoperfusion and secondary hyperreninemia and hyperaldosteronism. Others have suggested that renal tubular sodium wasting is the basic defect (290, 291). Both the proximal tubule and the thick ascending limb of Henle's loop have been implicated as a site of defective sodium reabsorption (292, 293). Studies by Tomko et al. (293) in a middle-aged patient with Bartter's syndrome suggested a proximal tubular defect because of increased sodium clearance and free

water clearance. Although normal sodium balance has been demonstrated in some cases, decreased sodium reabsorption in the proximal tubule or loop of Henle may still exist with supranormal reabsorption of sodium in the distal nephron to offset the proximal defect. If this set of events were to occur, however, there should be no volume depletion with secondary hyperreninemia and hyperaldosteronism.

Recent studies have implicated renal prostaglandins as playing a role in the pathogenesis of the syndrome (294, 295). As mentioned previously, prostaglandins may stimulate the release of renin from the kidney and may inhibit tubular reabsorption of sodium. Prostaglandin production in vascular tissue may exert vasodepressor effects and can attenuate the vascular response to vasopressor agents. The clinical features of Bartter's syndrome have been observed in a patient with hyperplasia of renomedullary interstitial cells and presumably with overproduction of prostaglandins (296). Furthermore, several workers have reported excess excretion of urinary prostaglandins in the syndrome, while inhibition of prostaglandin synthesis has been shown to lower the elevated urinary excretion of prostaglandin and return the serum potassium to normal. In three patients with Bartter's syndrome treated with indomethacin, the hyperreninemia and hyperaldosteronism were partially or completely corrected, urinary sodium excretion diminished to less than intake, and potassium balance became positive (295). More recent studies, however, indicate that with prolonged indomethacin treatment, patients with Bartter's syndrome show a return of hyperreninemia and hypokalemia (297).

Pseudo-Bartter's syndrome presents a clinical picture similar to Bartter's syndrome and occurs in patients who are mentally disturbed and who produce the syndrome by surreptitious vomiting, chronic use of diuretics or of laxatives (298, 299). The patients with surreptitious vomiting have some discrete clinical findings that make the diagnosis suspect. They may develop parotid enlargement, and renin levels are quite high, while aldosterone levels as a result of low serum potassium are lower than expected in view of the high renin. Urine is alkaline and chloride excretion is extremely low. It may be difficult to confirm a diagnosis in these patients since they are extremely clever in avoiding detection of vomiting. Those patients who surreptitiously take diuretics may be diagnosed by measurement of diuretics in the urine. This syndrome of pseudo-Bartter's is probably more common than true Bartter's syndrome and is best treated with psychiatric therapy.

Excessive secretion of other adrenal steroid hormones with mineralocorticoid activity may occur because of enzymatic defects in steroid synthesis which are found in adrenal cortical tumors or in congenital adrenal hyperplasia. These are described above under Adrenocortical Insufficiency and Cushing's Syndrome.

Electrolyte disturbances brought about by administration of exogenous mineralocorticoid hormones are extremely rare. Perhaps this is because primary adrenocortical insufficiency, which is virtually the only indication for administration of mineralocorticoid hormones, is a rare disorder. It appears likely that hyporeninemic hypoaldosteronism will be recognized with increasing frequency because of the greater availability of renin and aldosterone assays and because of increased awareness of the problem, and this will lead to more frequent use of mineralocorticoid hormones for replacement therapy. More frequent use, of course, will lead to more frequent incidence of complications. The complications of mineralocorticoid hormone administration such as sodium retention and hypokalemic alkalosis are the same as those of excess endogenous mineralocorticoid hormone secretion and are functions of dose and the sensitivity of the patient to the hormone. An individual with normal heart, kidneys, and peripheral circulation who is given a mineralocorticoid hormone in a dose that exceeds his needs will develop renal escape from the salt-retaining effects of the hormone but will continue to waste potassium and hydrogen ions in the urine. The potassium and hydrogen ion loss may be extreme if dietary sodium intake is high, and the subject will develop hypokalemia and metabolic alkalosis. A patient with overt or incipient heart failure, with hepatic cirrhosis, or with severe hypoalbuminemia may not be able to escape from the renal sodium-retaining effect of the administered

mineralocorticoid hormone and may continue to retain sodium and water to the point of anasarca and pulmonary edema.

Extracts of the licorice plant, *Glycyrrhiza glabra*, contain a substance, glycyrrhizinic acid, which has properties like mineralocorticoid hormones (300–302). The crude extract is best known for its use in flavoring of candies, and it has also found use in the flavoring of pharmaceuticals. The observation that licorice extract was beneficial for gastric ulcer lead to its administration in the treatment of this disease, and it was soon recognized that individuals treated with this substance developed hypokalemia and hypertension just as if they had been given deoxycorticosterone (this observation was made before the isolation and synthesis of aldosterone). It was subsequently found that both the mineralocorticoid activity and the ulcer-healing property could be attributed to glycyrrhizinic acid, the glucuronide derivative of glycyrrhetinic acid. A succinate derivative of glycyrrehtinic acid, carbenoxolone, is currently used in some parts of the world to treat gastric ulcer, and like the parent compound it too has mineralocorticoid properties and causes hypertension and hypokalemic alkalosis. It is interesting to note that both the ulcer-healing properties and the mineralocorticoid actions of these compounds are blocked by the aldosterone antagonist spironolactone.

THYROID DISORDERS

Patients with hyperthyroidism are in a hypermetabolic state and exhibit circulatory disorders which can best be described as hyperdynamic. A large number of the clinical manifestations are due to increased activity of the sympathetic nervous system, although the findings such as fine tremor, tachycardia, sweating, and staring eyes may be absent or less prominent in older patients, those with so-called apathetic thyrotoxicosis. In most hyperthyroid patients, heat generation from thyroid thermogenesis (see above) is increased, and dissipation of this heat may lead to increased evaporative water loss from the skin and lungs, and thus to dehydration. Dehydration, hypernatremia, and vascular collapse are major manifestations of thyroid storm.

Renal blood flow and GFR may be high in patients with hyperthyroidism (118, 119), and though these changes are not directly associated with diuresis, there is an inability of the kidney to elaborate a maximally concentrated urine even after administration of ADH (126, 127). The mechanism by which thyroid hormone impairs renal concentrating ability is unknown, but it does not appear to be a direct interference with the action of ADH on the renal tubule, for it can be shown in vitro that the effects of ADH and thyroxin on epithelia are actually additive (303). Hypothalamic and posterior pituitary control of ADH secretion are probably intact in hyperthyroidism as evidenced by a normal increase in free water reabsorption after intravenous administration of hypertonic saline (127). It appears most likely that the increase in total renal blood flow includes an increase in medullary blood flow which in turn causes a reduction of the medullary interstitial solute concentration gradient, thus preventing maximal concentration of the urine even in the presence of ADH (128).

High-output cardiac failure commonly occurs in long-standing untreated hyperthyroidism. The consequences of renal sodium retention and accumulation of edema fluid are the same as in heart failure of any etiology, but the heart itself is particularly resistant to the actions of digitalis in thyrotoxicosis.

Hypercalcemia may be seen in hyperthyroidism (127, 305) and provides another mechanism for an indirect effect of thyroid hormone on renal function and electrolyte and water balance. Early in the course of the disease, or with mild elevations of serum calcium concentration, there may be polyuria and failure to concentrate the urine maximally due to inhibition of the effect of ADH on the renal tubule. The presence of hypercalcemia in the thyrotoxic patient does not explain the renal resistance to the urine-concentrating effect of vasopressin described above, however, for vasopressin resistance can be demonstrated in eucalcemic patients (127).

Hypothyroidism is associated with proportionate reductions in GFR and renal blood flow (117–119), and with weight gain, edema, and an increase in total body exchangeable sodium (305, 306). Upon administration of thyroid hormone, there is a diuresis of water and sodium. Despite these indicators of a volume-expanded state, however, the blood volume is decreased, and there is evidence that both proximal and distal tubules are unable to reabsorb sodium normally (132). The serum sodium concentration is usually normal, and the GFR reduced so that the filtered load of sodium delivered to the tubules is reduced; nevertheless, fractional reabsorption is lower than normal and does not increase in response to mineralocorticoid hormone administration (132).

Hypothyroidism is also associated with an inability to dilute the urine maximally and to excrete a water load (121, 122). This phenomenon appears to be due to the decreased glomerular filtration, which in turn results in decreased delivery of filtrate to the diluting segment of the renal tubule. Despite this inability to excrete water maximally and the decrease in fractional tubular reabsorption of sodium, hyponatremia is rare in hypothyroidism, and when it occurs it may be due to excessive secretion of ADH (123, 125).

The inability to excrete a water load in hypothyroidism clinically resembles that seen in primary or secondary adrenocortical insufficiency (120). In adrenal insufficiency, however, the administration of glucocorticoid hormones restores renal water excretion to normal. As described in the section on glucocorticoid hormones, adrenal insufficiency not only reduces GFR but it also lowers the osmotic threshold for ADH secretion. In hypothyroidism there is no evidence for an abnormality in control of ADH secretion except for the rare example of the syndrome of inappropriate ADH secretion. In states of combined diabetes insipidus and hypothyroidism the effect of the hypothyroidism to reduce free water excretion may actually be beneficial, and administration of thyroid hormone may initiate a massive diuresis (307).

Hypothyroidism is associated with structural changes demonstrable on renal biopsy and consisting of glomerular basement-membrane thickening, increased mesangial matrix, thickened capillary walls, and cellular inclusions (308–309).

These changes, which are reversible upon treatment of the hypothyroid state, may explain the common occurrence of proteinuria in myxedema (309) and perhaps the rare occurrence of the nephrotic syndrome as well.

DIABETES MELLITUS (see also Chap. 24)

The most common disturbance of the serum electrolytes which is observed in insulin deficiency is hyponatremia. As detailed above, this abnormality develops primarily as a result of the osmotic activity of high concentrations of glucose in the extracellular fluid and may also result from the hyperlipidemia which commonly occurs in diabetes or from water retention secondary to chlorpropamide treatment.

With the development of diabetic ketoacidosis, other abnormalities occur which are due primarily to the generation of organic acids. Since glucose cannot gain entry into the cells because of insulin lack, adipose cells begin to hydrolyze triglycerides and release fatty acids into the circulation which are metabolized in the liver to acetoacetic acid and β-hydroxybutyric acid. Plasma buffering of these acids leads to reduction of the bicarbonate concentration (lower plasma or serum CO_2 content) as bicarbonate is consumed to form carbonic acid which is excreted as expired CO_2 by the lungs. Cells participate in the process of buffering the keto acids by taking up hydrogen ions into the cytoplasm in exchange for potassium, which is the cation in greatest abundance in the cytoplasm. The increased extracellular potassium concentration that results from this shift of potassium from ICF to ECF compartments leads to renal potassium excretion by two principal mechanisms: increased glomerular filtration of potassium, and stimulation of secretion of aldosterone which acts on the renal tubule to cause potassium secretion.

Presence of the acetoacetate and β-hydroxybutyrate bases in the extracellular fluid after the hydrogen ion has been dissipated results in another abnormality of the serum electrolytes, the "anion gap." Ordinarily, the difference between the sum of the concentrations of the cations sodium and potassium and the sum of the concentrations of the anions chloride and bicarbonate is equal only to some 10 to 15 meq/L, and this can be accounted for by anionic plasma proteins and small amounts of phosphate. When anions such as those of the keto acids accumulate in the ECF they result in lowering of the measured anions (chiefly by HCO_3 consumption). Since the keto acids are not determined in the standard serum electrolyte examination, there appears to be a "gap" between the sums of the cations and anions. The expression "increased undetermined anion," though more lengthy, is more meaningful than "anion gap." This useful clinical concept has wide applicability (310, 311).

The dehydration of ketoacidosis, which may be profound, plays an important part in the electrolyte disturbances by increasing the extracellular concentration of glucose and potassium and by stimulating renin secretion. The increased aldosterone secretion which is stimulated by renin exacerbates the potassium wasting.

Thus the serum electrolytes of the diabetic in ketoacidosis will show low sodium and bicarbonate concentrations and a normal to high potassium concentration. The total body content of potassium is reduced, as is the content of sodium and water.

Some diabetics may develop profound hyperglycemia and dehydration with little or no acidosis (312–314). This condition, referred to as hyperosmolar coma, occurs most often in individuals who are past middle age, who have mild or previously subclinical diabetes mellitus, have some other chronic disease, and have some impairment of renal function. The hyperglycemia appears to develop over a period of several days, and the osmotic effect of the extracellular glucose results in a shift of water from the intracellular to the extracellular compartments. The high blood glucose also causes an osmotic diuresis which leads to profound dehydration and urinary loss of sodium and potassium. In contrast to the ketosis and metabolic acidosis which occur with insulin deficiency in younger diabetics, individuals with hyperosmolar coma have little or no production of acetoacetate and β-hydroxybutyrate. The reasons for the relative absence of ketoacidosis in most cases of hyperosmolar coma are unclear. In some large series, it has been observed that the plasma levels of free fatty acids, the substrate for hepatic production of keto acids, are lower in hyperosmolar coma than in diabetic ketoacidosis (313, 314). This may be because of secretion of small amounts of insulin which, although unable to maintain normal glucose utilization, are able to inhibit lipolysis (313–315). Another explanation may be a reduced rate of ketone body production by the liver, despite adequate substrate availability (316). Whatever the reason, the lack of ketoacidosis in this clinical state is characteristic and probably allows the more prolonged course, thus permitting an even greater degree of dehydration than in ketotic diabetic coma. As a result of the combined and sometime opposing factors affecting fluid and electrolyte distribution and excretion, the serum electrolyte concentrations may take almost any pattern but most often show high-normal sodium and potassium concentrations, normal chloride concentration, and mildly reduced bicarbonate concentration. The blood urea nitrogen and creatinine concentrations are usually elevated, with a disproportionate urea nitrogen elevation reflecting the dehydration and reduced renal perfusion. Urinary sodium wasting continues despite volume contraction because of the osmotic effect of the filtered glucose, and potassium wasting occurs as a result of both the osmotic diuresis and the secondary aldosteronism induced by the dehydration.

Finally, an extremely serious complication of uncontrolled ketotic or nonketotic diabetes is the development of lactic acidosis. In any situation in which tissue hypoxia occurs, anaerobic glycolysis results in the production of excessive amounts of lactic and pyruvic acids. This situation frequently follows the dehydration of diabetic hyperosmolar coma or ketoacidosis and may be exacerbated or precipitated by administration of biguanide oral hypoglycemic agents. Lactic acidosis is also seen in other examples of reduced tissue perfusion such as surgical or septic shock. In any case, the excess extracellular fluid concentrations of lactic and pyruvic acids lead to consumption of bicarbonate buffers and lowering of serum bicarbonate concentration. The lactate and pyruvate anions themselves increase the concentration of undetermined anions and increase the "anion gap" as discussed above. Therapy is directed at correction of the vascular insufficiency, hypoxia, acidosis, and dehydration, but despite vigorous administration of insulin, bicarbonate, saline fluids, and oxygen, the mortality from lactic acidosis is extremely high.

REFERENCES

1. Bentley, P. J.: *Endocrines and Osmoregulation. A Comparative Account of the Regulation of Water and Salt in Vertebrates,* Springer-Verlag OHG, Berlin, 1971.

2. Maetz, J.: Salt and water metabolism, in E. J. W. Barrington and C. B. Jorgensen (eds.), *Perspectives in Endocrinology,* Academic Press, Inc., New York, 1968, pp. 47–162.

3. Keynes, R. D.: From frog skin to sheep rumen: A survey of transport of salts and water across multicellular structures, *Quart. Rev. Biophysics,* **2:**177–281, 1969.

4. Lev, A. A., and W. McD. Armstrong: Ionic activities in cells, *Curr. Top. Membr. Transp.,* **6:**59, 1975.

5. Armstrong, W. McD.: The cell membrane and biological transport, in E. E. Selkurt (ed.), *Physiology,* 4th ed., Little, Brown and Company, Boston, 1976, pp. 1–38.

6. Hoffman, J. F.: Ionic transport across the plasma membrane, in G. Weissman and R. Claiborne (eds.), *Cell Membranes. Biochemistry, Cell Biology and Pathology,* H. P. Publishing Company, New York, 1975, p. 95.

7. Bittar, E. E.: Regulation of ion transport by hormones, in E. E. Bittar (ed.), *Membranes and Ion Transport,* Interscience Publishers, New York, 1971, vol. 3, p. 297.

8. Herrera, F. C.: Frog skin and toad bladder, in E. E. Bittar (ed.), *Membranes and Ion Transport,* Interscience Publishers, New York, 1971, vol. 3, p. 1.

9. Giebisch, G. (ed.): *Electrophysiology of Epithelial Cells,* F. K. Schattauer Verlag, Stuttgart, 1971.

10. Ullrich, K. J.: Permeability characteristics of the mammalian nephron, in J. Orloff and R. W. Ber-

liner (eds.), *Handbook of Physiology*, sec. 8, *Renal Physiology*, American Physiological Society, Washington, D.C., 1973, p. 377.

11. Erlij, D.: Solute transport across isolated epithelia, *Kidney Int.*, **9**:76, 1976.

12. Diamond, J. M.: The epithelial junction: Bridge, gate and fence, *Physiologist*, **20** (1):10, 1977.

13. Douglas, W. W.: Stimulus-secretion coupling: The concept and clues from chromaffin and other cells, *Br. J. Pharmacol.*, **34**:451, 1968.

14. Matthews, E. K.: Calcium and hormone release, in A. W. Cuthbert (ed.), *Calcium and Cellular Function*, Macmillan & Co., Ltd., London, 1970, p. 163.

15. Rasmussen, H., and N. Nagata: Hormones, cell calcium and cyclic AMP, in A. W. Cuthbert (ed.), *Calcium and Cellular Function*, Macmillan & Co., Ltd., London, 1970, p. 198.

16. Thorn, N. A.: Role of calcium in secretory processes, in N. A. Thorn and O. H. Petersen (eds.), *Secretory Mechanisms of Exocrine Glands, Proceedings of the Alfred Benzon Symposium VII*, Munksgaard, Copenhagen, 1974, p. 305.

17. Feldman, D., J. W. Funder, and I. S. Edelman: Subcellular mechanisms in the action of adrenal steroids, *Am. J. Med.*, **53**:545, 1972.

18. Funder, J. W., D. Feldman, and I. S. Edelman: The roles of plasma binding and receptor specificity in the mineralocorticoid action of aldosterone, *Endocrinology*, **92**:994, 1973.

19. Funder, J. W., D. Feldman, and I. S. Edelman: Glucocorticoid receptors in the rat kidney: The binding of tritiated-dexamethasone, *Endocrinology*, **96**:1005, 1973.

20. Fuller, P. J., and J. W. Funder: Mineralocorticoid and glucocorticoid receptors in human kidney, *Kidney Int.*, **10**:154, 1976.

21. Baxter, J. D., M. Schambelan, D. T. Matulich, B. J. Spindler, A. A. Taylor, and F. C. Bartter: Aldosterone receptors and the evaluation of plasma mineralocorticoid activity in normal and hypertensive states, *J. Clin. Invest.*, **58**:579, 1976.

22. Moses, A. M., J. L. Gabrilove, and L. J. Soffer: Simplified water loading test in hypoadrenocorticism and hypothyroidism, *J. Clin. Endocrinol. Metab.*, **18**:1413, 1958.

23. Aubry, R. H., H. R. Nankin, A. M. Moses, and D. H. P. Streeten: Measurement of the osmotic threshold for vasopressin release in human subjects, and its modification by cortisol, *J. Clin. Endocrinol. Metab.*, **25**:1481, 1965.

24. Hierholzer, K., and M. Wiederholt: Some aspects of distal tubular solute and water transport, *Kidney Int.*, **9**:198, 1976.

25. Stolte, H., J. P. Brecht, M. Wiederholt, and K. Hierholzer: Einfluss von Adrenalektomie und Glucocorticoiden auf die Wasserpermeabilität Corticaler Nephronabschnitte der Rattenniere, *Pfluegers Arch.*, **299**:99, 1968.

26. Ackerman, G. L., and C. L. Miller: Role of hypovolemia in the impaired water diuresis of adrenal insufficiency, *J. Clin. Endocrinol. Metab.*, **30**:252, 1970.

27. Oparil, S., and E. Haber: The renin-angiotensin system, *N. Engl. J. Med.*, **291**:389, 446, 1974.

28. Laragh, J. H., and J. E. Sealey: The renin-angiotensin-aldosterone hormonal system and regulation of sodium, potassium and blood pressure homeostasis, in J. Orloff and R. W. Berliner (eds.), *Handbook of Physiology*, sec. 8, *Renal Physiology*, American Physiological Society, Washington, D.C., 1973, p. 831.

29. Erdös, E. G.: Angiotensin I converting enzyme, *Circ. Res.*, **36**:247, 1975.

30. Soffer, R. L.: Angiotensin-converting enzyme and the regulation of vasoactive peptides, *Annu. Rev. Biochem.*, **45**:73, 1976.

31. Oparil, S., C. A. Sanders, and E. Haber: In-vivo and in-vitro conversion of angiotensin I to angiotensin II in dog blood, *Circ. Res.*, **26**:591, 1970.

32. Aiken, J. W., and J. R. Vane: The renin-angiotensin system: Inhibition of converting enzyme in isolated tissues, *Nature*, **228**:30, 1970.

33. Blair-West, J. R., J. P. Coghlan, D. A. Denton, J. W. Funder, B. A. Scoggins, and R. D. Wright: The effect of the heptapeptide (2-8) and hexapeptide (3-8) fragments of angiotensin II on aldosterone secretion, *J. Clin. Endocrinol. Metab.*, **32**:575, 1971.

34. Goodfriend, T. L., and M. J. Peach: Angiotensin III: (Des-aspartic acid[1])-angiotensin II. Evidence and speculation for its role as an important agonist in the renin-angiotensin system., *Circ. Res.*, **36** (suppl.):I38, 1975.

35. Lohmeier, T. E., J. O. Davis, and R. H. Freeman: Des-asp[1]-angiotensin II: Possible role in mediat-

ing responses of the renin-angiotensin system, *Proc. Soc. Exp. Biol. Med.*, **149**:515, 1975.

36. Thurau, K., and J. Mason, The intrarenal function of the juxtaglomerular apparatus, in K. Thurau (ed.), *Kidney and Urinary Tract Physiology*, MTP International Review of Science, Physiology Series One, University Park Press, Baltimore, 1974, vol. 6, p. 357.

37. Davis, J. O., and R. H. Freeman: Mechanisms regulating renin release, *Physiol. Rev.*, **56**:1, 1976.

38. Dluhy, R. G., R. H. Underwood, and G. H. Williams: Influence of dietary potassium on plasma renin activity in normal man, *J. Appl. Physiol.*, **28**:299, 1970.

39. Brunner, H. R., L. Baer, J. E. Sealey, G. G. Ledingham, and J. H. Laragh: Influence of potassium administration and of potassium deprivation on plasma renin in normal and hypertensive subjects, *J. Clin. Invest.*, **49**:2128, 1970.

40. Vander, Arthur J.: Direct effects of potassium on renin secretion and renal function, *Am. J. Physiol.*, **219**:455, 1970.

41. Shade, R. E., J. O. Davis, J. A. Johnson, and R. T. Witty: Effects of renal arterial infusion of sodium and potassium on renin secretion in the dog, *Circ. Res.*, **31**:719, 1972.

41. Nash, F. D., H. H. Rostorfer, M. D. Bailie, R. L. Wathen, and E. G. Schneider: Renin release: Relation to renal sodium load and dissociation from hemodynamic changes, *Circ. Res.*, **22**:473, 1968.

43. Wright, F. S., and J. P. Briggs: Feedback regulation of glomerular filtration rate, *Am. J. Physiol.*, **233**:F1, 1977.

44. Wathen, R. L., W. S. Kingsbury, D. A. Stouder, E. G. Schneider, and H. H. Rostorfer: Effects of infusion of catecholamines and angiotensin II on renin release in anesthetized dogs, *Am. J. Physiol.*, **209**:1012, 1965.

45. Vander, A. J.: Effects of catacholamines and the renal nerves on renin secretion in anesthetized dogs, *Am. J. Physiol.*, **209**:659, 1965.

46. Gordon, R. D., O. Küchel, G. W. Liddle, and D. P. Island: Role of the sympathetic nervous system in regulating renin and aldosterone production in man, *J. Clin. Invest.*, **46**:599, 1967.

47. Johnson, J. A., J. O. Davis, and R. T. Witty: Effects of catecholamines and renal nerve stimulation on renin release in the nonfiltering kidney, *Circ. Res.*, **29**:646, 1971.

48. Aoi, W., M. B. Wade, D. R. Rosner, and M. H. Weinberger: Renin release by rat kidney slices in vitro: Effects of cations and catecholamines, *Am. J. Physiol.*, **227**:630, 1974.

49. Weinberger, M. H., W. Aoi, and D. P. Henry: Direct effect of β-adrenergic stimulation on renin release by the rat kidney slice in vitro, *Circ. Res.*, **37**:318, 1975.

50. Michelakis, A. M., and R. G. McAllister: The effect of chronic adrenergic receptor blockade on plasma renin activity in man, *J. Clin. Endocrinol. Metab.*, **34**:386, 1972.

51. Bühler, F. R., J. H. Laragh, E. D. Vaughn, Jr., H. R. Brunner, H. Gavras, and L. Baer: The antihypertensive action of propranolol. Specific antirenin responses in high and normal renin forms of essential, renal, renovascular and malignant hypertension, *Am. J. Cardiol.*, **32**:511, 1973.

52. Aoi, W., D. P. Henry, and M. H. Weinberger: Evidence for a physiological role of renal sympathetic nerves in adrenergic stimulation of renin release in the rat, *Circ. Res.*, **38**:123, 1976.

53. Williams, G. H., J. P. Cain, R. G. Dluhy, and R. H. Underwood: Studies of the control of plasma aldosterone concentration in normal man. I. Response to posture, acute and chronic volume depletion, and sodium loading., *J. Clin. Invest.*, **51**:1731, 1972.

54. Weinberger, M. H., D. C. Kem, C. Gomez-Sanchez, N. J. Kramer, B. T. Martin, and C. A. Nugent: The effect of dexamethasone on the control of plasma aldosterone concentration in normal recumbent man, *J. Lab. Clin. Med.*, **85**:957, 1975.

55. Blair-West, J. R., J. P. Coughlan, D. A. Denton, J. R. Goding, M. Wintour, and R. D. Wright: The control of aldosterone secretion, *Rec. Prog. Horm. Res.*, **19**:311, 1963.

56. Davis, J. O., J. Urquhart, and J. T. Higgins, Jr.: The effects of alterations of plasma sodium and potassium concentration on aldosterone secretion, *J. Clin. Invest.*, **42**:597, 1963.

57. Bartter, F. C., and W. B. Schwartz: The syndrome of inappropriate secretion of antidiuretic hormone, *Am. J. Med.*, **42**:790, 1967.

58. Fichman, M. P., and J. E. Bethune: The role of adrenocorticoids in the inappropriate antidiuretic

hormone syndrome, *Ann. Int. Med.*, **68**:806, 1968.

59. Nolph, K. D., and R. W. Schrier: Sodium, potassium and water metabolism in the syndrome of inappropriate antidiuretic hormone secretion, *Am. J. Med.*, **49**:534, 1970.

60. Cannon, P. J., R. P. Ames, and J. H. Laragh: Relation between potassium balance and aldosterone secretion in normal subjects and in patients with hypertensive or renal tubular disease, *J. Clin. Invest.*, **45**:865, 1966.

61. Himathongkam, T., R. G. Dluhy, and G. H. Williams: Potassium-aldosterone-renin interrelationships, *J. Clin. Endocrinol. Metab.*, **41**:153, 1975.

62. Cooke, C. R., J. S. Horvath, M. A. Moore, T. Bledsoe, and W. G. Walker: Modulation of plasma aldosterone concentration by plasma potassium in anephric man in the absence of a change in potassium balance, *J. Clin. Invest.*, **52**:3028, 1973.

63. Sharp, G. W. G., and A. Leaf,: Effects of aldosterone and its mechanism of action on sodium transport, in J. Orloff and R. W. Berliner (eds.), *Handbook of Physiology*, sec. 8, *Renal Physiology*, American Physiological Society, Washington, D.C., 1973, p. 815.

64. Levitan, R., and F. J. Ingelfinger: Effect of d-aldosterone on salt and water absorption from the intact human colon, *J. Clin Invest.*, **44**:801, 1965.

65. Richards, P.: Mineralocorticoids and rectal potential difference, *Lancet*, **2**:798, 1973.

66. McConahay, T. P., S. Robinson, and J. L. Newton: d-Aldosterone and sweat electrolytes, *J. Appl. Physiol.*, **19**:575, 1964.

67. Wotman, S., F. J. Goodwin, I. D. Mandel, and J. H. Laragh: Changes in salivary electrolytes following treatment of primary aldosteronism, *Arch. Int. Med.*, **124**:477, 1969.

68. Gruber, W. D., H. Knauf, and E. Frömter: The action of aldosterone on Na^+ and K^+ transport in the rat submaxillary main duct, *Pfluegers Arch.*, **344**:33, 1973.

69. Edmonds, C. J., and R. C. Godfrey: Measurement of electrical potential of the human rectum and pelvic colon in normal and aldosterone-treated patients, *Gut*, **11**:330, 1970.

70. Beevers, D. G., J. J. Morton, M. Tree, and J. Young: Rectal potential difference in the diagnosis of aldosterone excess, *Gut*, **16**:36, 1975.

71. Crabbé, J.: Stimulation of active sodium transport by the isolated toad bladder with aldosterone in vitro, *J. Clin. Invest.*, **40**:2103, 1961.

72. Sharp, G. W. G., and A. Leaf: Biological action of aldosterone in vitro, *Nature*, **202**:1185, 1964.

73. Crabbé, J., and P. DeWeer: Action of aldosterone and vasopressin on the active transport of sodium by the isolated toad bladder, *J. Physiol.*, **180**:560, 1965.

74. Sharp, G. W. G., C. H. Coggins, N. S. Lichstenstein, and A. Leaf: Evidence for a mucosal effect of aldosterone on sodium transport in the toad bladder, *J. Clin. Invest.*, **45**:1640, 1966.

75. Fimognari, G. M., G. A. Porter, and I. S. Edelman: The role of the tricarboxylic acid cycle in the action of aldosterone on sodium transport, *Biochim. Biophys. Acta*, **135**:89, 1967.

76. Herman, T. S., G. M. Fimognari, and I. S. Edelman: Studies on renal aldosterone-binding proteins, *J. Biol. Chem.*, **243**:3849, 1968.

77. Edelman, I. S., and G. M. Fimognori: On the biochemical mechanism of action of aldosterone, *Rec. Prog. Horm. Res.*, **24**:1, 1968.

78. Sharp, G. W. G.: Transport across the epithelial membrane with particular reference to the toad bladder, in E. J. Harris (ed.), *Transport and Accumulation in Biological Systems*, Butterworth & Co. (Publishers), Ltd., London, 1972, p. 147.

79. Higgins, J. T., Jr., L. Cesaro, B. Gebler, and E. Frömter: Electrical properties of amphibian urinary bladder epithelia. I. Inverse relationship between potential difference and resistance in tightly mounted preparations, *Pfluegers Arch.*, **358**:41, 1975.

80. Higgins, J. T., Jr., B. Gebler, and E. Frömter: Electrical properties of amphibian urinary bladder epithelia. II. The cell potential profile in necturus maculosus, *Pfluegers Arch.*, **371**:87, 1977.

81. Wright, F. S.: Increasing magnitude of electrical potential along the renal distal tubule, *Am. J. Physiol.*, **220**:624, 1971.

82. Malnic, G., and G. Giebisch: Some electrical properties of distal tubular epithelium in the rat, *Am. J. Physiol.*, **223**:797, 1972.

83. Malnic, G., M. DeMello Aires, and G. Giebish: Potassium transport across renal distal tubules during acid-base disturbances, *Am. J. Physiol.*, **221**:1192, 1971.

84. Gennari, F. J., M. B. Goldstein, and W. B. Schwartz: The nature of the renal adaptation to chronic hypocapnia, *J. Clin. Invest.*, **51**:1722, 1972.

85. Gennari, F. J., and J. J. Cohen: The role of the kidney in potassium homeostasis: Lessons from acid-base disturbances, *Kidney Int.*, **8**:1, 1975.

86. Alexander, E. A., and N. G. Levinsky: An extra-renal mechanism of potassium adaptation, *J. Clin. Invest.*, **47**:740, 1968.

87. Adler, S.: An extrarenal action of aldosterone on mammalian skeletal muscle, *Am. J. Physiol.*, **218**:616, 1970.

88. Schambelan, M., J. R. Stockigt, and E. G. Biglieri: Isolated hypoaldosteronism in adults: A renin-deficiency syndrome, *N. Engl. J. Med.*, **287**:573, 1972.

89. Weidmann, P., R. Reinhart, M. H. Maxwell, P. Rowe, J. W. Coburn, and S. G. Massry: Syndrome of hyporeninemic hypoaldosteronism and hyperkalemia in renal disease, *J. Clin. Endocrinol. Metab.*, **36**:965, 1973.

90. Weidmann, P., M. H. Maxwell, P. Rowe, R. Winer, and S. G. Massry: Role of the renin-angiotensin-aldosterone system in the regulation of plasma potassium in chronic renal disease, *Nephron*, **15**:35, 1975.

91. Goldfarb, S., M. Cox, I. Singer, and M. Goldberg: Acute hyperkalemia induced by hyperglycemia: Hormonal mechanisms, *Ann. Int. Med.*, **84**:426, 1976.

92. Relman, A. S., and W. B. Schwartz: The effect of DOCA on electrolyte balance in normal man and its relation to sodium chloride intake, *Yale J. Biol. Med.*, **24**:540, 1952.

93. Davis, J. O., and D. S. Howell: Comparative effect of ACTH, cortisone and DCA on renal function, electrolyte excretion and water exchange in normal dogs, *Endocrinology*, **52**:245, 1953.

94. August, J. T., D. H. Nelson, and G. W. Thorn: Response of normal subjects to large amounts of aldosterone, *J. Clin. Invest.*, **37**:1549, 1958.

95. Rovner, D. R., J. W. Conn, R. J. Knopf, E. L. Cohen, and M. T. Y. Hsueh: Nature of renal escape from the sodium retaining effect of aldosterone in primary aldosteronism and in normal subjects, *J. Clin. Endocrinol. Metab.*, **25**:53, 1965.

96. Davis, J. O., J. E. Holman, C. C. J. Carpenter, J. Urquhart, and J. T. Higgins, Jr.: An extra-adrenal factor essential for chronic renal sodium retention in presence of increased sodium-retaining hormone, *Circ. Res.*, **14**:17, 1964.

97. Higgins, J. T., Jr.: Escape from sodium-retaining effects of deoxycorticosterone in hypotensive and hypertensive dogs, *Proc. Soc. Exp. Biol. Med.*, **134**:768, 1970.

98. Levinsky, N. G., and R. C. Lalone: The mechanism of sodium diuresis after saline infusion in the dog, *J. Clin. Invest.*, **42**:1261, 1963.

99. DeWardener, H. E., I. H. Mills, W. F. Clapham, and C. J. Hayter: Studies on the efferent mechanism of the sodium diuresis which follows the administration of intravenous saline in the dog, *Clin. Sci.*, **21**:249, 1961.

100. Levinsky, N. G.: A critical appraisal of some of the evidence for natriuretic hormone, *Proc. V Int. Cong. Nephrol.*, Mexico City, 1972, p. 162.

101. Klahr, S., and H. J. Rodriguez: Natriuretic hormone, *Nephron*, **15**:387, 1975.

102. Dirks, J. H., J. Cirksena, and R. W. Berliner: The effect of saline infusion on sodium reabsorption by the proximal tubule of the dog, *J. Clin. Invest.*, **44**:1160, 1965.

103. Watson, J. F.: Effect of saline loading on sodium reabsorption in the dog proximal tubule, *Am. J. Physiol.*, **210**:781, 1966.

104. Robson, A. M., P. L. Srivastava, and N S. Bricker: The influence of saline loading on renal glucose reabsorption in the rat, *J. Clin. Invest.*, **47**:329, 1968.

105. Baines, A. D.: Effect of extracellular fluid volume expansion on maximum glucose reabsorption rate and glomerular tubular balance in single rat nephrons, *J. Clin. Invest.*, **50**:2414, 1971.

106. Schneider, E. G., J. W. Strandhoy, L. R. Willis, and F. G. Knox: Relationship between proximal sodium reabsorption and excretion of calcium, magnesium and phosphorus, *Kidney Int.*, **4**:369, 1973.

107. Higgins, J. T., Jr., and A. E. Meinders: Quantitative relationship of renal glucose and sodium reabsorption during ECF expansion, *Am. J. Physiol.*, **229**:66, 1975.

108. Landau, R. L., D. M. Bergenstal, K. Lugibihl, and M. E. Kascht: The metabolic effects of pro-

gesterone in man, *J. Clin. Endocrinol. Metab.*, **15:**1194, 1955.

109. Landau, R. L., and K. Lugibihl: Inhibition of sodium-retaining influence of aldosterone by progesterone, *J. Clin. Endocrinol. Metab.*, **18:**1237, 1958.

110. Kagawa, C. M.: Blocking urinary electrolyte effects of desoxycorticosterone with progesterone in rats, *Proc. Soc. Exp. Biol. Med.*, **99:**705, 1958.

111. Kagawa, C. M., F. M. Sturtevant, and C. G. Van Arman: Pharmacology of a new steroid that blocks salt activity of aldosterone and desoxycorticosterone, *J. Pharmacol. Exp. Ther.*, **126:**123, 1959.

112. Kagawa, C. M.: Mineralocorticoid-blocking properties of a progesterone-like derivative (SC-11835), *Endocrinology*, **74:**724, 1964.

113. Helmer, O. M., and W. E. Judson: Influence of high renin substrate levels on renin-angiotensin system in pregnancy, *Am. J. Obstet. Gynecol.*, **99:**9, 1967.

114. Laragh, J. H., J. E. Sealey, J. G. G. Ledingham, and M. A. Newton: Oral contraceptives: Renin, aldosterone and high blood pressure, *J. Am. Med. Assoc.*, **201:**918, 1967.

115. Weinberger, M. H., R. D. Collins, A. J. Dowdy, G. W. Nokes, and J. A. Leutscher: Hypertension induced by oral contraceptives containing estrogen and gestagen: Effects on plasma renin activity and aldosterone excretion, *Ann. Int. Med.*, **71:**891, 1969.

116. Gibson, J. G., Jr., and A. W. Harris: Clinical studies of blood volume. Hyperthyroidism and myxedema, *J. Clin. Invest.*, **18:**59, 1939.

117. Corcoran, A. C., and I. H. Page: Specific renal functions in hyperthyroidism and myxedema. Effects of treatment, *J. Clin. Endocrinol. Metab.*, **7:**801, 1947.

118. Hlad, C. J., Jr., and N. S. Bricker: Renal function and I[131] clearance in hyperthyroidism and myxedema, *J. Clin. Endocrinol. Metab.*, **14:**1539, 1954.

119. Ford, R. V., J. C. Owens, G. W. Curd, Jr., J. H. Moyer, and C. L. Spurr: Kidney function in various thyroid states, *J. Clin. Endocrinol. Metab.*, **21:**548, 1961.

120. Crispell, K. R., W. Parson, and P. Sprinkle: A cortisone-resistant abnormality in the diuretic re-

sponse to ingested water in primary myxedema, *J. Clin. Endocrinol. Metab.*, **14:**640, 1954.

121. Bleifer, K. H., J. L. Belsky, L. Saxon, and S. Papper: The diuretic response to administered water in patients with primary myxedema, *J. Clin. Endocrinol. Metab.*, **20:**409, 1960.

122. Papper, S., and R. G. Lancestremere: Certain aspects of renal function in myxedema, *J. Chronic Dis.*, **14:**495, 1961.

123. Goldberg, M., and M. Reivich: Studies on the mechanism of hyponatremia and impaired water excretion in myxedema, *Ann. Intern. Med.*, **56:**120, 1962.

124. Emmanouel, D. S., M. D. Lindheimer, and A. I. Katz: Mechanism of impaired water excretion in the hypothyroid rat, *J. Clin. Invest.*, **54:**926, 1974.

125. Pettinger, W. A., L. Talner, and T. F. Ferris: Inappropriate secretion of antidiuretic hormone due to myxedema, *N. Engl. J. Med.*, **272:**362, 1965.

126. Weston, R. E., H. B. Horowitz, J. Grossman, J. B. Hanenson, and L. Leiter: Decreased antidiuretic response to beta-hypophamine in hyperthyroidism, *J. Clin. Endocrinol. Metab.*, **16:**322, 1956.

127. Wijdeveld, P. G. A. B., and A. P. Jansen: Renal concentrating and water-excreting capacity in hyperthyroidism, *Clin. Chim. Acta*, **5:**618, 1960.

128. Cutler, R. E., H. Glatte, and J. T. Dowling: Effect of hyperthyroidism on the renal concentrating mechanism in humans, *J. Clin. Endocrinol. Metab.*, **27:**453, 1967.

129. Bradley, S. E., G. P. Bradley, and F. Stéphan: Role of structural inbalance in the pathogenesis of renal dysfunction in the hypothyroid rat, *Trans. Assoc. Am. Physicians*, **85:**344, 1972.

130. Eiler, J. J., T. L. Althausen, and M. Stockholm: Effect of thyroxin on maximum rate of transfer of glucose and Diodrast by renal tubules, *Am. J. Physiol.*, **140:**699, 1944.

131. Holmes, E. W., Jr., and V. A. DiScala: Studies on the exaggerated natriuretic response to a saline infusion in the hypothyroid rat, *J. Clin. Invest.*, **49:**1224, 1970.

132. Vaamonde, C. A., M. J. Sebastianelli, L. S. Vaamonde, E. L. Pellegrini, R. S. Watts, E. L. Klinger, Jr. and S. Papper: Impaired renal tubular reabsorption of sodium in hypothyroid man, *J. Lab. Clin. Med.*, **85:**451, 1975.

133. Ismail-Beigi, F., and I. S. Edelman: Mechanism

of thyroid calorigenesis: Role of active sodium transport, *Proc. Natl. Acad. Sci. U.S.A.*, **67**:1071, 1970.

134. Ismail-Beigi, F., and I. S. Edelman: Effects of thyroid status on electrolyte distribution in rat tissues, *Am. J. Physiol.*, **225**:1172, 1973.

135. Edelman, I. S., and F. Ismail-Beigi: Thyroid thermogenesis and active sodium transport, *Recent Prog. Horm. Res.*, **30**:235, 1974.

136. Edelman, I. S.: Thyroid thermogenesis, *N. Engl. J. Med.*, **290**:1303, 1974.

137. Cole, C. H., and R. W. Waddell: Alteration in intracellular sodium concentration and ouabain-sensitive ATPase in erythrocytes from hyperthyroid patients, *J. Clin. Endocrinol. Metab.*, **42**:1056, 1976.

138. Anderson, W. A. D.: Hyperparathyroidism and renal disease, *Arch. Pathol.*, **27**:753, 1939.

139. Epstein, F. H., D. Beck, F. A. Carone, H. Levitan, and A. Manitius: Changes in renal concentrating ability produced by parathyroid extract, *J. Clin. Invest.*, **38**:1214, 1959.

140. Carone, F. A., F. H. Epstein, D. Beck, and H. Levitan: The effects upon the kidneys of transient hypercalcemia induced by parathyroid extract, *Am. J. Pathol.*, **36**:77, 1960.

141. Bell, N. H., F. delGreco, and J. A. Colwell: Primary hyperparathyroidism and salt-wasting nephropathy, *J. Chronic Dis.*, **28**:601, 1975.

142. Chase, L. R., and G. D. Aurbach: Parathyroid function and the renal excretion of 3′ 5′-adenylic acid, *Proc. Natl. Acad. Sci. U.S.A.*, **58**:518, 1967.

143. Chase, L. R., and G. D. Aurbach: Renal adenyl cyclase: Anatomically separate sites for parathyroid hormone and vasopressin, *Science*, **159**:545, 1968.

144. Morel, F., D. Chabardes, and M. Imbert: Target sites of antidiuretic hormone (ADH) and parathyroid hormone (PTH) along the segments of the nephron, *Adv. Nephrol.*, **5**:283, 1975.

145. Knox, F. G., E. G. Schneider, L. R. Willis, J. W. Strandhoy, C. E. Ott, J.-L. Cuche, R. S. Goldsmith, and C. D. Arnaud: Proximal tubule reabsorption after hyperoncotic albumin infusion. Role of parathyroid hormone and dissociation from plasma volume, *J. Clin. Invest.*, **53**:501, 1974.

146. Schneider, E. G.: Effect of parathyroid hormone

secretion in sodium reabsorption by the proximal tubule, *Am. J. Physiol.*, **229**:1170, 1975.

147. Muldowney, F. P., D. V. Carroll, J. F. Donohue, and R. Freaney: Correction of renal bicarbonate wastage by parathyroidectomy: Implications in acid-base homeostasis, *Q. J. Med.*, **40**:487, 1971.

148. Ardaillou, R., P. Vuagnat, G. Milhaud, and G. Richet: Effets de la thyrocalcitonine sur l'excrétion rénale des phosphates, du calcium et des ions H^+ chez l'homme, *Nephron*, **4**:298, 1967.

149. Cochran, M., M. Peacock, G. Sachs, and B. E. C. Nordin: Renal effects of calcitonin, *Br. Med. J.*, **1**:135, 1970.

150. Ardaillou, R., G. Milhaud, F. Rousselet, P. Vuagnat, and G. Richet: Effet de la thyrocalcitonine sur l'excrétion rénale du sodium et du chlore dhez l'homme normal, *C. R. Acad. Sci. (Paris)*, **264**:3037, 1967.

151. Haddad, J. G., Jr., S. J. Birge, and L. V. Avioli: Effects of prolonged thyrocalcitonin administration on Paget's disease of bone, *N. Engl. J. Med.*, **283**:549, 1970.

152. Rasmussen, H., C. Anast, and C. Arnaud: Thyrocalcitonin, EGTA and urinary electrolyte excretion, *J. Clin. Invest.*, **46**:746, 1967.

153. Cramer, C. F., C. O. Parkes, and D. H. Copp: The effect of chicken and hog calcitonin on some parameters of Ca, P, and Mg metabolism in dogs, *Can. J. Physiol. Pharmacol.*, **47**:181, 1969.

154. Clark, J. D., and A. D. Kenny: Hog thyrocalcitonin in the dog: Urinary calcium, phosphorus, magnesium and sodium responses, *Endocrinology*, **84**:1199, 1969.

155. Pak, C. Y. C., B. Ruskin, and A. Casper: Renal effects of porcine thyrocalcitonin in the dog, *Endocrinology*, **87**:262, 1970.

156. Loreau, N., C. Lepreux, and R. Ardaillou: Calcitonin-sensitive adenylate cyclase in rat renal tubular membranes, *Biochem. J.*, **150**:305, 1975.

157. Chabardes, D., M. Imbert-Teboul, M. Montégut, A. Clique, and F. Morel: Distribution of calcitonin-sensitive adenylate cyclase activity along the rabbit kidney tubule, *Proc. Natl. Acad. Sci. U.S.A.*, **73**:3608, 1976.

158. Andre, R., and J. Crabbé: Stimulation by insulin of active sodium transport by toad skin. Influence of aldosterone and vasopressin, *Arch. Int. Physiol. Biochim.*, **74**:538, 1966.

159. Christlieb, A. R.: Diabetes and hypertensive vascular disease: Mechanisms and treatment, *Am. J. Cardiol.*, **32**:592, 1973.

160. Katz, M. A.: Hyperglycemia-induced hyponatremia—calculation of expected serum sodium depression, *N. Engl. J. Med.*, **289**:843, 1973.

161. Jenkins, P. G., and C. Larmore: Hyperglycemia-induced hyponatremia, *N. Engl. J. Med.*, **290**:573, 1974.

162. Waugh, W. H.: Utility of expressing serum sodium per unit of water in assessing hyponatremia, *Metabolism*, **18**:706, 1969.

163. Steffes, M. W., and E. F. Freier: A simple and precise method of determining true sodium, potassium and chloride concentrations in hyperlipemia, *J. Lab. Clin. Med.*, **88**:683, 1976.

164. Meinders, A. E., J. L. Touber, and L. A. deVries: Chlorpropamide treatment in diabetes insipidus, *Lancet*, **2**:544, 1967.

165. Michelis, M. F., and H. V. Murdaugh: Selective hypoaldosteronism: An editorial revisited after 15 years, *Am. J. Med.*, **59**:1, 1975.

166. Perez, G. O., L. Lespier, J. Jacobi, J. R. Oster, F. H. Katz, C. A. Vaamonde, and L. M. Fishman: Hyporeninemia and hypoaldosteronism in diabetes mellitus, *Arch. Int. Med.*, **137**:852, 1977.

167. Weeks, J. R.: Prostaglandins. Introduction, *Fed. Proc.*, **33**:37, 1974.

168. Bergstrom, S., and B. Samuelsson (eds.): *Prostaglandins*, Interscience Publishers, Inc., New York, 1967.

169. Larsson, C., and E. Anggard: Regional differences in the formation and metabolism of prostaglandins in the rabbit kidney, *Eur. J. Pharmacol.*, **21**:30, 1973.

170. Morrison, A. R., K. Nishikawa, and P. Needleman: Unmasking of thromboxane A_2 synthesis by ureteral obstruction in the rabbit kidney, *Clin. Res.*, **25**:442A, 1977.

171. Lonigro, A. J., N. A. Terragno, K. U. Malik, and J. C. McGiff: Differential inhibition by prostaglandins of the renal actions of pressor stimuli, *Prostaglandins*, **3**:595, 1973.

172. Frolich, J. C., B. J. Sweetman, K. Carr, and J. A. Oates: Assessment of the levels of PGA_2 in human plasma by gas chromatography–mass spectrometry, *Prostaglandins*, **10**:185, 1975.

173. Frolich, J. C., B. J. Sweetman, K. Carr, J. W. Hollifield, and J. A. Oates: Prostaglandin production in renal medulla. Paper presented at 48th meeting of American Oil Chemists Society, Philadelphia, October 1974.

174. Crowshaw, K.: Incorporation of (1-^{14} C) arachidonic acid into the lipids of rabbit renal slices and conversion to prostaglandins E_2 and F_2, *Prostaglandins*, **3**:607, 1973.

175. Crowshaw, K., and J. C. McGiff: Prostaglandins in the kidney: A correlative study of their biochemistry and renal function, in M. P. Sambhi (ed.), *Excerpta Med. Int. Workshop Conf. Mechanisms Hypertension*, 1973, p. 254.

176. Carr, A. A.: Hemodynamic and renal effects of prostaglandin, PGA_1, in subjects with essential hypertension, *Am. J. Med. Sci.*, **259**:21, 1970.

177. Lee, J. B., J. C. McGiff, H. Kannegiesser, Y. Y. Aykent, J. G. Mudd, and T. F. Frawley: Prostaglandin A_1: Antihypertensive and renal effects. Studies in ·patients with essential hypertension, *Ann. Intern. Med.*, **74**:703, 1971.

178. Martinez-Maldonado, M., M. N. Tsaparas, G. Eknoyan, and W. N. Suki: Renal actions of prostaglandins: Comparison with acetylcholine and volume expansion, *Am. J. Physiol.*, **222**:1147, 1972.

179. Gross, J. B., and F. C. Bartter: Effects of prostaglandins E_1, A_1 and F_2 on renal handling of salt and water, *Am. J. Physiol.*, **225**:218, 1973.

180. Johnston, H. H., J. P. Herzog, and D. P. Lauler: Effect of prostaglandin E_1 on renal hemodynamics, sodium and water excretion, *Am. J. Physiol.*, **213**:939, 1967.

181. McGiff, J. C., K. Crowshaw, and D. H. Itskovitz: Prostaglandins and renal function, *Fed. Proc.*, **33**:39, 1974.

182. McGiff, J. C., K. Crowshaw, N. A. Terragno, and A. J. Lonigro: Release of a prostaglandin-like substance into renal venous blood in response to angiotensin II, *Circ. Res.*, **27**(suppl. 1):I121, 1970.

183. Itskovitz, H. D., and J. McGiff: Hormonal regulation of the renal circulation, *Circ. Res.*, **34**(suppl. 1):I65, 1974.

184. Aiken, J. W., and J. R. Vane: Intrarenal prostaglandin release attenuates the renal vasoconstrictor activity of angiotensin, *J. Pharmacol. Exp. Ther.*, **184**:678, 1973.

185. Tannenbaum, J., J. A. Splawinski, J. A. Oates, and A. S. Nies: Enhanced renal prostaglandin production in the dog. I. Effect on renal function, *Circ. Res.*, **36**:197, 1975.

186. McGiff, J. C., K. Crowshaw, N. A. Terrango, A. J. Lonigro, J. C. Strand, M. A. Williamson, J. B. Lee, and K. K. Ng: Prostaglandin-like substances appearing in canine renal venous blood during renal ischemia. Their partial characterization by pharmacologic and chromatographic procedures, *Circ. Res.*, **27**:765, 1970.

187. McGiff, J. C., H. D. Itskovitz, and N. A. Terragno: The actions of bradykinin and eledoisin in the canine isolated kidney: Relationships to prostaglandins, *Clin. Sci. Mol. Med.*, **49**:125, 1975.

188. Bailie, M. D., J. A. Barbour, and J. B. Hook: Effects of indomethacin on furosemide-induced changes in renal blood flow, *Proc. Soc. Exp. Biol. Med.*, **148**:1173–1176, 1975.

189. Williamson, H. E., W. A. Bourland, and G. R. Marchand: Inhibition of ethacrynic acid induced increase in renal blood flow by indomethacin, *Prostaglandins*, **8**:297, 1974.

190. Cadnapaphornchai, P., G. A. Aisenbrey, A. L. McCool, K. M. McDonald, and R. W. Schrier: Intrarenal humoral substances and hyperemic responses to ureteral occlusion (abstract), in *Proc. 7th Annu. Meeting Am. Soc. Nephrol.*, Washington, D.C., 1974, p. 15.

191. Herbaczynska-Cedro, K., and J. R. Vane: Contribution of intrarenal generation of prostaglandin to autoregulation of renal blood flow in the dog, *Circ. Res.*, **33**:428, 1973.

192. Venuto, R. C., T. O'Dorisio, T. F. Ferris, and J. H. Stein: Prostaglandins and renal function. II. The effect of prostaglandin inhibition on autoregulation of blood flow in the intact kidney of the dog, *Prostaglandins*, **9**:817–828, 1975.

193. Anderson, R. J., M. S. Taher, R. E. Cronin, K. M. McDonald, and R. W. Schrier: Effect of beta-adrenergic blockade and inhibitors of angiotensin II and prostaglandins on renal autoregulation, *Am. J. Physiol.*, **229**:731–736, 1975.

194. Owen, T., I. Ehrhart, J. Weidner, F. Haddy, and J. Scott: Effects of indomethacin (I) on blood flow, reactive hyperemia (RH) and autoregulation (AR) in the dog kidney, *Fed. Proc.*, **33**:348, 1974.

195. Vander, A. J.: Direct effects of prostaglandin on renal function and renin release in anesthetized dog, *Am. J. Physiol.*, **214**:218, 1968.

196. Strandhoy, J. W., C. E. Ott, E. G. Schneider, L. R. Willis, N. P. Beck, B. B. Davis, and F. G. Knox: Effects of prostaglandin E_1 and E_2 on renal sodium reabsorption and Starling forces, *Am. J. Physiol.*, **226**:1015, 1974.

197. Kirschenbaum, M. A., and J. H. Stein: The effect of inhibition of prostaglandin synthesis on urinary sodium excretion in the conscious dog, *J. Clin. Invest.*, **57**:517–521, 1976.

198. Lipson, L. C., and G. W. Sharp: Effect of prostaglandin E_1 on sodium transport and osmotic water flow in the toad bladder, *Am. J. Physiol.*, **220**:1046, 1971.

199. Barry, E., and W. Hall: Stimulation of sodium movement across frog skin by prostaglandin E_1, *J. Physiol. (London)*, **200**:83P, 1969.

200. Zusman, R. M., B. V. Caldwell, P. J. Mulrow, and L. Speroff: The role of prostaglandin A in the control of sodium homeostasis and blood pressure, *Prostaglandins*, **3**:679, 1973.

201. Larsson, C., and E. Anggard: Regional differences in the formation and metabolism of prostaglandins in the rabbit kidney, *Eur. J. Pharmacol.*, **21**:30, 1973.

202. Grantham, J. J., and J. Orloff: Effect of prostaglandin E_1 on the permeability response of the isolated collecting tubule to vasopressin, adenosine 3',5'-monophosphate and theophylline, *J. Clin. Invest.*, **47**:1154, 1968.

203. Orloff, J., J. S. Handler, and S. Berkstrom: Effect of prostaglandin (PGE₁) on the permeability response of toad bladder to vasopressin, theophylline and adenosine 3',5'-monophosphate, *Nature*, **205**:397, 1965.

204. Ozer, A., and G. W. Sharp: Effect of prostaglandins and their inhibitors on osmotic water flow in the toad bladder, *Am. J. Physiol.*, **222**:674, 1972.

205. Wong, P. Y. D., J. R. Bedwani, and A. W. Cuthbert: Hormone action and the levels of cyclic AMP and prostaglandins in the toad bladder, *Nature (New Biol.)*, **238**:27, 1972.

206. Albert, W. C., and J. S. Handler: Effect of PGE₁, indomethacin and polyphloretin phosphate on toad bladder response to ADH, *Am. J. Physiol.*, **226**:1382, 1974.

207. Flores, J., P. A. Witkum, B. Beckman, and G. W.

Sharp: Stimulation of osmotic water flow in toad bladder by prostaglandin E_1. Evidence for different compartments of cyclic AMP, *J. Clin. Invest.*, **56**:256–262, 1975.

208. Beck, N. P., T. Kaneko, U. Zor, J. Field, and B. B. Davis: Effects of vasopressin and prostaglandin E_1 on the adenyl cyclase-cyclic 3′,5′-adenosine monophosphate system of the renal medulla of the rat, *J. Clin. Invest.*, **50**:2461, 1971.

209. Anderson, R. J., T. Berl, K. D. McDonald, and R. W. Schrier: Evidence for an in vivo antagonism between vasopressin and prostaglandin in the mammalian kidney, *J. Clin. Invest.*, **56**:420–426, 1975.

210. Berl, T., W. Czaczkes, W. and C. R. Kleeman: Effect of prostaglandin synthesis inhibition on the renal action of vasopressin: Studies in man and the rat, *Proc. 8th Ann. Meeting Am. Soc. Nephrol.*, Washington, D. C., 1975, p. 72.

211. Carlson, L. A., L. Ekelund, and L. Oro: Circulatory and respiratory effects of different doses of prostaglandin E_1 in man, *Acta Physiol. Scand.*, **75**:161, 1969.

212. Tan, S. Y., and P. J. Mulrow: Inhibition of the renin-aldosterone response to furosemide by indomethacin, *J. Clin. Endocrinol. Metab.*, **45**:174–176, 1977.

213. Data, J. L., W. J. Crump, M. G. Frazer, J. C. Frolich, and A. S. Nies: Prostaglandins: A role in baroreceptor control of renin release, *Proc. 58th Annu. Meeting Endocrine Soc.*, San Francisco, p. 228.

214. Franco, R., S. Y. Tan, and P. J. Mulrow: Renin release in an in vitro superfusion system of rat kidney slices: Effect of prostaglandins, *Clin. Res.*, **25**:594A, 1977.

215. Jaffe, B. M., C. W. Parker, G. R. Marshall, and P. Needleman: Renal concentration of prostaglandin E in acute and chronic renal ischemia, *Biochem. Biophys. Res. Commun.*, **49**:799, 1972.

216. Pugsley, D. J., L. J. Beilin, and R. Peto: Renal prostaglandin synthesis in the Goldblatt hypertensive rat, *Circ. Res.*, **36** (suppl):I81, 1975.

217. Sirois, P., and D. J. Gagnon: Release of renomedullary prostaglandins in normal and hypertensive rats, *Experientia*, **30**:1418, 1974.

218. Dunn, M. J.: Renal prostaglandin synthesis in the spontaneously hypertensive rat, *J. Clin. Invest.*, **58**:862, 1976.

219. Armstrong, J. M., G. J. Blackwell, R. J. Flower, J. C. McGiff, K. M. Mullane, and J. R. Vane: Genetic hypertension in rats is accompanied by a defect in renal prostaglandin catabolism, *Nature*, **260**:582, 1976.

220. Romero, J. C., and C. G. Strong: The effect of indomethacin blockade of prostaglandin synthesis on blood pressure of normal rabbits and rabbits with renovascular hypertension, *Circ. Res.*, **40**:35, 1977.

221. Hornych, A., J. Bedrossian, and J. Bariety: Prostaglandins and hypertension in chronic renal diseases, *Clin. Nephrol.*, **4**:144, 1975.

222. Patak, R. V., B. K. Mookerjee, C. J. Bentzel, P. E. Hysert, M. Babej, and J. B. Lee: Antagonism of the effects of furosemide by indomethacin in normal and hypertensive man, *Prostaglandins*, **10**:649, 1975.

223. Moncada, S., E. A. Higgs, and J. R. Vane: Human arterial and venous tissues generate prostacyclin (prostaglandin X), a potent inhibitor of platelet aggregation, *Lancet*, **1**:18, 1977.

224. Rioux, F., and D. Regoli: In vitro production of prostaglandins by isolated aorta strips of normotensive and hypertensive rats, *Can. J. Physiol. Pharmacol.*, **53**:673, 1975.

225. Greenburg, S.: Evidence for enhanced venous smooth muscle turnover of prostaglandin-like substance in portal veins from spontaneously hypertensive rats, *Prostaglandins*, **11**:163, 1976.

226. Muirhead, E. E., G. Germain, B. E. Leach, J. A. Pitcock, P. Stephenson, B. Brooks, W. L. Brosius, E. G. Daniels, and J. W. Hinman: Production of renomedullary prostaglandins by renomedullary interstitial cells grown in tissue culture, *Circ. Res.*, **31**(suppl. 2):II161, 1972.

227. Muirhead, E. E.: Role of the renal medulla in hypertension, in G. H. Stollerman (ed.), *Advances in Internal Medicine*, Year Book Medical Publishers, Inc., Chicago, 1974, vol. 19, p. 81.

228. Scicli, A. G., O. A. Carretero, A. Hampton, P. Cortes, and N. P. Oza: Site of kininogenase secretion in the dog nephron, *Am. J. Physiol.*, **230**:533–536, 1976.

229. Margolius, H. S., D. Horwitz, R. Geller, R. W. Alexander, J. R. Gill, Jr., J. J. Pisano, and H. R.

Keiser: Urinary kallikrein excretion in normal man. Relationships to sodium intake and sodium-retaining steroids, *Circ. Res.*, **35**:812–819, 1974.

230. Margolius, H. S., D. Horwitz, J. J. Pisano, and H. R. Keiser: Urinary kallikrein excretion in hypertensive man. Relationships to sodium intake and sodium-retaining steroids, *Circ. Res.*, **35**:820–825, 1974.

231. Hong, S. -C., and L. Levine: Stimulation of prostaglandin synthesis by bradykinin and thrombin and their mechanisms of action on MC5-5 fibroblasts, *J. Biol. Chem.*, **251**:5814–5816, 1976.

232. Gimbrone, M. A., Jr., and R. W. Alexander: Angiotensin II stimulation of prostaglandin production in a cultured human vascular endothelium, *Science*, **189**:219–220, 1975.

233. Alexander, R. W., and M. A. Gimbrone: Stimulation of prostaglandin E synthesis in cultured human umbilical vein smooth muscle cells, *Proc. Nat. Acad. Sci. U.S.A.*, **73**:1617–1620, 1976.

234. Hagemann, M. H., A. H. Stephenson, and A. J. Lonigro: Effect of blockade of prostaglandin synthesis on the renal vasodilator response to bradykinin, *Clin. Res.*, **23**:505A, 1975.

235. Lockett, M. F., and C. N. Roberts: Hormonal factors affecting sodium excretion in the rat, *J. Physiol.*, **167**:581, 1963.

236. Lockett, M. F., and B. Nail: A comparative study of the renal actions of growth and lactogenic hormones in rats, *J. Physiol.*, **180**:147, 1965.

237. Lockett, M. F.: A comparison of the direct renal action of pituitary growth and lactogenic hormones, *J. Physiol.*, **181**:192, 1965.

238. Horrobin, D. F., I. J. Lloyd, A. Lipton, P. G. Burstyn, N. Durkin, and K. L. Muirui: Actions of prolactin on human renal function, *Lancet*, **2**:352, 1971.

239. Ensor, D. M., and J. N. Ball: Prolactin and osmoregulation in fishes, *Fed. Proc.*, **31**:1615, 1972.

240. Lucci, M. S., H. H. Bengele, and S. Solomon: Suppressive action of prolactin on renal response to volume expansion, *Am. J. Physiol.*, **229**:81–85, 1975.

241. Buckman, M. T., G. T. Peake, and G. Robertson: Hyperprolactinemia influences renal function in man, *Metabolism*, **25**:509–516, 1976.

242. Adler, R. A., G. L. Noel, L. Wartofsky, and L. G. Frantz: Failure of oral water loading and intra-venous hypotonic saline to suppress prolactin in man, *J. Clin. Endocrinol. Metab.*, **41**:383–389, 1975.

243. Berl, T., N. Brautbar, M. Ben-David, W. Czaczkes, and C. Kleeman: Osmotic control of prolactin release and its effect on renal water excretion in man, *Kidney Int.*, **10**:158–163, 1976.

244. Richardson, B. P.: Evidence for a physiological role of prolactin in osmoregulation in the rat after its inhibition by 2-bromo alpha ergokryptine, *Br. J. Pharmacol.*, **47**:623P, 1973.

245. Edwards, C. R. W., P. A. Miall, J. P. Hanker, M. O. Thorner, E. A. Al-Dujaili, and G. M. Besser: Inhibition of the plasma-aldosterone response to furosemide by bromocriptine, *Lancet*, **2**:903–905, 1975.

246. Relkin, R., and M. Adachi: Effects of sodium deprivation on pituitary and plasma prolactin, growth hormone and thyrotropin levels in the rat, *Neuroendocrinology*, **11**:240, 1973.

247. Gomez-Sanchez, C., O. B. Holland, J. R. Higgins, D. C. Kem, and N. M. Kaplan: Circadian rhythms of serum renin activity and serum corticosterone, prolactin and aldosterone concentrations in the male rat on normal and low-sodium diets, *Endocrinology*, **99**:567, 1976.

248. O'Connor, W. J., and E. B. Verney: The effect of increased activity of the sympathetic system in the inhibition of water diuresis by emotional stress, *Q. J. Exp. Physiol.*, **33**:77, 1945.

249. Fisher, D. A.: Norepinephrine inhibition of vasopressin antidiuresis, *J. Clin. Invest.*, **47**:540, 1968.

250. Handler, J. S., R. Bensinger, and J. Orloff: Effect of adrenergic agents on toad bladder response to ADH, 3′-5′-AMP and theophyllin, *Am. J. Physiol.*, **215**:1024, 1968.

251. Omachi, R. S., D. E. Robbie, J. S. Handler, and J. Orloff: Effects of ADH and other agents on cyclic AMP accumulation in toad bladder epithelium, *Am. J. Physiol.*, **226**:1152, 1974.

252. Beck, N. P., S. W. Reed, H. V. Murdaugh, and B. B. Davis: Effects of catecholamines and their interaction with other hormones on cyclic 3′-5′-adenosine monophosphate of the kidney, *J. Clin. Invest.*, **51**:939, 1972.

253. Morel, F., D. Chabardès, and M. Imbert: Functional segmentation of the rabbit distal tubule by

microdetermination of hormone-dependent adenylate cyclase activity, *Kidney Int.*, **9**:264, 1976.

254. Besarab, A., P. Silva, L. Landsberg, and F. H. Epstein: Effect of catecholamines on tubular function in the isolated perfused rat kidney, *Am. J. Physiol.*, **233**:F39, 1977.

255. Bello-Reuss, E., D. L. Trevino, and C. W. Gottschalk: Effect of renal sympathetic nerve stimulation on proximal water and sodium reabsorption, *J. Clin. Invest.*, **57**:1104, 1976.

256. Slick, G. L., A. J. Aguilera, E. J. Zambroski, G. F. DiBona, and G. J. Kaloyanides: Renal neuroadrenergic transmission, *Am. J. Physiol.*, **229**:60, 1975.

257. Tan, S. Y., R. Shapiro, and P. J. Mulrow: Renal prostaglandins exert major influence on the renin-aldosterone axis and on K^+ homeostasis, *Clin. Res.*, **25**:598A, 1977.

258. New, M. I., and L. S. Levine: Congenital adrenal hyperplasia, *Adv. Hum. Genet.*, **4**:251, 1973.

259. Bongiovanni, A. M., and A. W. Root: The adrenogenital syndrome, *N. Engl. J. Med.*, **268**:1283, 1342, 1391, 1963.

260. Bongiovanni, A. M.: Adrenogenital syndrome: Uncomplicated and hypertensive forms, *Pediatrics*, **21**:661, 1958.

261. Gandy, H. M., E. H. Keutmann, and A. J. Izzo: Characterization of urinary steroids in adrenal hyperplasia: Isolation of metabolitis of cortisol, compound S, and desoxycorticosterone from a normotensive patient with adrenogenital syndrome, *J. Clin. Invest.*, **39**:364, 1960.

262. New, M. T., and M. P. Seaman: Secretion rates of cortisol and aldosterone precursors in various forms of congenital adrenal hyperplasia, *J. Clin. Endocrinol. Metab.*, **30**:361, 1970.

263. Bryan, G. T., B. Kliman, and F. C. Bartter: Impaired aldosterone production in "salt-losing" congenital adrenal hyperplasia, *J., Clin. Invest.*, **44**:957, 1965.

264. Green, O. C., C. J. Migeon, and L. Wilkins: Urinary steroids in the hypertensive form of congenital adrenal hyperplasia, *J. Clin. Endocrinol. Metab.*, **20**:929, 1960.

265. Bongiovanni, A. M.: Unusual steroid pattern in congenital adrenal hyperplasia: Deficiency of 3β-hydroxydehydrogenase, *J. Clin. Endocrinol. Metab.*, **21**:860, 1961.

266. Biglieri, E. G., M. A. Herron, and N. Burst: 17-Hydroxylation deficiency in man, *J. Clin. Invest.*, **45**:1946, 1966.

267. Goldsmith, O., D. H. Solomon, and R. Horton: Hypogonadism and mineralocorticoid excess. The 17-hydroxylase deficiency syndrome, *N. Engl. J. Med.*, **277**:673, 1967.

268. Ulick, S., E. Gautier, K. K. Vetter, J. R. Markello, S. Yaffe, and C. U. Lowe: An aldosterone biosynthetic defect in a salt-losing disorder, *J. Clin. Endocrinol. Metab.*, **24**:669, 1964.

269. Visser, H. K., and W. S. Cost: A new hereditary defect in the biosynthesis of aldosterone: Urinary C_{21}-corticosteroid pattern in three related patients with a salt-losing syndrome suggesting an 18-oxidation defect, *Acta Endocrinol. (Kbh.)*, **47**:589, 1964.

270. Rappaport, R., F. Dray, J. C. Legrand, and P. Royer: Hypoaldostéronisme congénital familial par defaut de la 18-OH-déhydrogénase, *Pediatr. Res.*, **2**:456, 1968.

271. David, R., S. Golan, and W. Drucker: Familial aldosterone deficiency: Enzyme defect, diagnosis and clinical course, *Pediatrics*, **41**:403, 1968.

272. Bagshawe, K. D.: Hypokalemia, carcinoma and Cushing's syndrome, *Lancet*, **2**:284, 1960.

273. Lipsett, M. B., and H. Wilson: Adrenocortical cancer: Steroid biosynthesis and metabolism evaluated by urinary metabolites, *J. Clin. Endocrinol. Metab.*, **22**:906, 1962.

274. Crane, M. G., and J. J. Harris: Desoxycorticosterone secretion rates in hyperadrenocorticism, *J. Clin. Endocrinol. Metab.*, **26**:1135, 1966.

275. Conn, J. W.: Primary aldosteronism: New clinical syndrome, *J. Lab. Clin. Med.*, **45**:3, 1955.

276. Espiner, E. A., J. R. Tucci, P. I. Jagger, and D. P. Lauler: Effect of saline infusions on aldosterone secretion and electrolyte excretion in normal subjects and patients with primary aldosteronism, *N. Engl. J. Med.*, **277**:1, 1967.

277. Krakoff, L. R., F. J. Goodwin, L. Baer, M. Torres, and J. H. Laragh: The role of renin in the exaggerated natriuresis of hypertension, *Circulation*, **42**:335, 1970.

278. Luft, F. C., C. E. Grim, L. R. Willis, J. T. Higgins, Jr., and M. H. Weinberger: Natriuretic response to saline infusion in normotensive and hypertensive man. The role of renin suppression in

exaggerated natriuresis, *Circulation*, **55**:779, 1977.

279. Biglieri, E. G., M. Schambelan, P. E. Slaton, and J. R. Stockigt: The intercurrent hypertension of primary aldosteronism, *Circ. Res.*, **27** (suppl. I):I195, 1970.

280. Biglieri, E. G., J. R. Stockigt, and M. Schambelan: Adrenal mineralocorticoids causing hypertension, *Am. J. Med.*, **52**:623, 1972.

281. Baer, L., S. C. Sommers, L. R. Krakoff, M. A. Newton, and J. H. Laragh: Pseudoprimary aldosteronism: An entity distinct from true primary aldosteronism, *Circ. Res.*, **27** (suppl. I):I203, 1970.

282. Grim, C. E., J. Winnacker, T. Peters, and G. Gilbert: Low renin, "normal" aldosterone and hypertension: Circadian rhythm of renin, aldosterone, cortisol and growth hormone, *J. Clin. Endocrinol. Metab.*, **39**:247, 1974.

283. Robertson, P. W., A. Klidjian, L. K. Harding, G. Walters, M. R. Lee, and A. H. T. Robb-Smith: Hypertension due to a renin-secreting renal tumor, *Am. J. Med.*, **43**:963, 1967.

284. Kihara, I., S. Kitamura, T. Hoshino, H. Seida, and T. Watanabe: A hitherto unreported vascular tumor of the kidney. A proposal of "juxtaglomerular cell tumor," *Acta Pathol. Jap.*, **18**:197, 1968.

285. Mitchell, J. D., T. J. Baxter, J. R. Blair-West, and D. A. McCardie: Renin levels in nephroblastoma (Wilm's tumor). Report of a renin-secreting tumor, *Arch. Dis. Child.*, **45**:376, 1970.

286. Hollifield, J. W., D. L. Page, C. Smith, A. M. Michelakis, E. Staab, and R. Rhamy: Renin-secreting clear cell carcinoma of the kidney, *Arch. Int. Med.*, **135**:859, 1975.

287. Bartter, F. C., P. Pronove, J. R. Gill, and R. C. MacCardle: Hyperplasia of the juxtaglomerular complex with hyperaldosteronism and hypokalemic alkalosis, a new syndrome, *Am. J. Med.*, **33**:811, 1962.

288. Catanzaro, F., J. Bourgoignie, P. Serirat, and H. M. Perry, Jr.: Angiotensin-infusion test: Correlation with renin activity in peripheral venous blood, *Arch. Int. Med.*, **122**:10, 1968.

289. Brackett, N. C., Jr., M. Koppel, R. E. Randall, Jr., and W. P. Nixon: Hyperplasia of the juxtaglomerula complex with secondary aldosteronism without hypertension (Bartter's syndrome), *Am. J. Med.*, **44**:803, 1968.

290. Cannon, P. J., J. M. Leeming, S. C. Sommers, R. W. Winters, and J. H. Laragh: Juxtaglomerular cell hyperplasia and secondary hyperaldosteronism (Bartter's syndrome): A reevaluation of the pathophysiology, *Medicine (Baltimore)*, **47**:107, 1968.

291. White, M. G.: Bartter's syndrome. A manifestation of renal tubular defects, *Arch. Int. Med.*, **129**:41, 1972.

292. Chaimovitz, C., J. Levi, O. S. Better, L. Oslander, and A. Benderli: Studies on the site of renal salt loss in a patient with Bartter's syndrome, *Pediatr. Res.*, **7**:89, 1973.

293. Tomko, D. K., B. P. Y. Yeh, and W. F. Falls: Bartter's syndrome. Study of a fifty-two year old man with evidence for a defect in proximal tubular sodium reabsorption and comments on therapy, *Am. J. Med.*, **61**:111–118, 1976.

294. Fichman, M. P., N. Telfer, P. Zia, P. Speckart, M. Golub, and R. Rude: Role of prostaglandins in the pathogenesis of Bartter's syndrome, *Am. J. Med.*, **60**:785–787, 1976.

295. Gill, J. R., J. C. Frolich, R. E. Bowden, A. A. Taylor, H. R. Keiser, H. W. Feyberth, J. A. Oates, and F. C. Bartter: Bartter's syndrome. A disorder characterized by high urinary prostaglandins and a dependence of hyperreninemia on prostaglandin synthesis, *Am. J. Med.*, **61**:43–51, 1976.

296. Verberckmoes, R., B. vanDamme, J. Clement, A. Amery, and P. Michielsen: Bartter's syndrome with hyperplasia of renomedullary cells: Successful treatment with indomethacin, *Kidney Int.*, **9**:302–307, 1976.

297. Bartter, F. C.: Personal communication.

298. Wolff, H. P., P. Vecsei, K. Kruck, S. Roscher, J. J. Brown, G. O. Dusterdieck, A. F. Lever, and J. I. S. Robertson: Psychiatric disturbance leading to potassium depletion, sodium depletion, raised plasma renin concentration and secondary aldosteronism, *Lancet*, **1**:257, 1968.

299. Ben-Ishay, D., M. Levy, and D. Birnbaum: Self-induced secondary hyperaldosteronism simulating Bartter's syndrome, *Isr. J. Med. Sci.*, **8**:1835, 1972.

300. Molhuysen, J. A., J. Gerbrandy, L. A. de Vries, J. C. de Jong, J. B. Lenstra, K. P. Turner, and

J. G. G. Borst: A liquorice extract with deoxycortone-like action, *Lancet,* **2:**381, 1950.

301. Conn, J. W., D. R. Rovner, and E. L. Cohen: Licorice-induced pseudoaldosteronism, hypertension, hypokalemia, aldosteronopenia, and suppressed plasma renin activity, *JAMA,* **205:**492, 1968.

302. Salassa, R. M., V. R. Mattox, and J. W. Rosevear: Inhibition of the "mineralocorticoid" activity of licorice by spironolactone, *J. Clin. Endocrinol. Metab.,* **22:**1156, 1962.

303. Marusic, E., and J. Torretti: Synergistic action of vasopressin and thyroxine on water transfer on the isolated toad bladder, *Nature,* **202:**1118, 1964.

304. Baxter, J. D., and P. K. Bondy: Hypercalcemia of thyrotoxicosis, *Ann. Intern. Med.,* **65:**429, 1966.

305. Aikawa, J. K.: The nature of myxedema: Alterations in serum electrolyte concentrations and radiosodium space and in exchangeable sodium and potassium contents, *Ann. Intern. Med.,* **44:**30–39, 1956.

306. Munro, D. S., H. Renschler, and G. M. Wilson: Exchangeable potassium and sodium in hyperthyroidism and hypothyroidism, *Metabolism,* **7:**124, 1958.

307. Hare, K., D. M. Phillips, J. Bradshaw, G. Chambers, and R. S. Hare: The diuretic action of thyroid in diabetes insipidus, *Am. J. Physiol.,* **141:**187, 1944.

308. DiScala, V. A., M. Salomon, E. Grishman, and S. Churg: Renal structure in myxedema, *Arch. Pathol.,* **84:**474, 1967.

309. Salomon, M. I., V. DiScala, E. Grishman, J. Brener, and J. Churg: Renal lesions in hypothyroidism: A study based on kidney biopsies, *Metabolism,* **16:**846, 1967.

310. Emmett, M., and R. G. Narins: Clinical use of the anion gap, *Medicine,* **56:**38, 1977.

311. Oh, M. S., and H. J. Carroll: The anion gap, *N. Engl. J. Med.,* **297:**814, 1977.

312. McCurdy, D. K.: Hyperosmolar hyperglycemic nonketotic diabetic coma, *Med. Clin. N. Am.,* **54:**683, 1970.

313. Gerich, J. E., M. M. Martin, and L. Recant: Clinical and metabolic characteristics of hyperosmolar nonketotic coma, *Diabetes,* **20:**228, 1971.

314. Arieff, A. I., and H. J. Carroll: Hyperosmolar nonketotic coma with hyperglycemia: Clinical features, pathophysiology, renal function, acid-base balance, plasma-cerebrospinal fluid equilibria and the effects of therapy in 37 cases, *Medicine (Baltimore),* **51:**73, 1972.

315. Henry, D. P., and R. Bressler: Serum insulin levels in nonketotic, hyperosmotic diabetes mellitus, *Am. J. Med. Sci.,* **256:**150, 1968.

316. Foster, D. W.: Insulin deficiency and hyperosmolar coma, *Adv. Inter. Med.,* **19:**159, 1974.

24

Diabetic acidosis and coma

CHARLES R. KLEEMAN
ROBERT G. NARINS

The severely uncontrolled diabetic is a patient in great danger. When this is appreciated and treatment based on sound pathophysiologic principles is promptly and systematically administered, the response will be overwhelmingly gratifying to both physician and patient. As mentioned by Hockaday and Alberti (1), the essence of optimum management is to lower the 5 to 15 percent mortality still reported from major centers. Some have considered this percentage an irreducible minimum, but we must only accept this opinion temporarily while we work to understand and remove the factors responsible for this mortality.

INSULIN DEFICIENCY

The fundamental cause of diabetic ketoacidosis, nonketotic hyperosmolar or hyperglycemic coma, and combined diabetic ketoacidosis and lactic acidosis is a relative or absolute deficiency of insulin. While "normal" amounts of insulin (radioimmunoreactive) have frequently been detected in the circulation of these patients, these concentrations are obviously inadequate for the degree of hyperglycemia and/or the metabolic state of the patient. The major causes of insulin deficiency are the following:

1. The patient fails to take insulin or fails to take an adequate amount. This usually is due to the patient's lack of understanding of his disease and its treatment, probably because the physician has not properly instructed him. Occasionally a patient will develop some disorder which causes rather marked anorexia. Because of this and the fear of insulin reactions, he will stop taking insulin entirely. This, of course, will make little difference in mild to moderate diabetes; however, in severe or moderately severe diabetes the failure to take insulin for a day or two, particularly in association with lack of food intake, may lead to the rapid development of acidosis.
2. Infections, to which the diabetic patient is susceptible, may be obvious at the time of examination or may require special studies for detection, such as blood and urine cultures. The intelligent patient with diabetes will often give himself additional amounts of insulin during an obvious infectious process.
3. Surgical emergency, severe trauma, myocar-

dial infarction, and severe emotional stress represent other frequent precipitating causes. Severe emotional stress is a particularly common cause of uncontrolled diabetes in the juvenile patient.

4. The abrupt onset of a failure of insulin formation or secretion in the juvenile diabetic patient leads to severe ketoacidosis or coma as the initial indication of diabetes mellitus.

5. Acute hemorrhagic pancreatitis in the absence of true diabetes mellitus is a rare cause. Mild abnormalities in carbohydrate metabolism are often seen in this disorder, but occasionally pancreatitis may precipitate a frank, severe diabetic acidosis.

6. Chronic, severe overinsulinization with repeated hypoglycemic reactions may lead to deglycogenation of the liver and severe ketosis, disproportionate to the extent of glycosuria and hyperglycemia.

7. An associated endocrine disorder develops which significantly antagonizes the metabolic effects of insulin, e.g., acromegaly, Cushing's syndrome, thyrotoxicosis, or pheochromocytoma.

8. In patients with latent or subclinical diabetes, acute deficiency may be produced by massive overeating, particularly of carbohydrate, or by parenteral alimentation exceeding the borderline insulin secretory capacity of the pancreas.

The magnitude of the role of glucagon in uncontrolled diabetes mellitus and diabetic acidosis remains controversial. The concentration of glucagon in the plasma is markedly raised in diabetic ketoacidosis (2). It also increases rapidly soon after *deprivation of insulin* in diabetic patients (3, 4). However, it is quite clear that there must be a deficiency of insulin for glucagon to contribute to a significant sustained rise in plasma glucose, fatty acids, and ketones (5) and that pharmacologically induced glucagonemia to three to six times that of the basal levels does not impair glucose tolerance in normal subjects or cause deterioration of diabetic control as long as insulin is available (5).

Insulin lack causes alterations of intermediary metabolism which in turn result in life-threatening disorders of water, electrolyte, and acid-base homeostasis. The altered carbohydrate, fat, and protein metabolism effects predictable changes in acid production and in the distribution and excretion of body water and electrolytes.

HYPERGLYCEMIA, HYPEROSMOLALITY, AND INTERNAL SHIFTS OF FLUID

The lack of insulin immediately leads to an impaired glucose utilization by almost all tissues (brain excluded) and an excessive hepatic production of glucose from noncarbohydrate sources (gluconeogenesis). Both processes, underutilization and excessive production, cause a progressive increase in the glucose concentration of blood and extracellular fluids. In the absence of insulin, the cells are relatively impermeable to glucose, and therefore the increasing hyperglycemia creates a progressive rise in the effective osmotic pressure of the extracellular fluids. The calculation of the osmotic contribution of glucose is presented in Fig. 24-1. As the osmolality of the extracellular fluid (ECF) increases, there is a continuous diffusion of water from the cells to the extracellular compartment as osmotic equilibrium is maintained. This process leads to progressive intracellular dehydration which would be

---

Millimole (mmol) ≡ Molecular weight (MW) in milligrams
MW glucose = 180
∴ 1 mmol = 180 mg

Since each mmol of glucose accounts for 1 mosm, every 180 mg/dL rise of blood glucose causes a 10 mosm/L rise.

If blood glucose is 180 mg/dL, then each 100 mL has 180 mg (or 1 mmol), and each liter has 1800 mg (or 10 mmol).

Divide blood glucose (mg/dL) by 18 to get its osmotic contribution.

Figure 24-1. The method of calculating the osmotic contribution of glucose to the blood.

accompanied by an expansion of the ECFs were it not for the continued loss of water and solutes (sodium, potassium, chloride) from the extracellular space to the exterior as the uncontrolled diabetic state proceeds. This will be discussed more fully in a subsequent section.

In brief, the increasing concentration of glucose in the blood (ECF) causes a shift of water out of the cells; this in turn dilutes the remaining extracellular solutes, the most important of which are the sodium salts. This process is illustrated in Fig. 24-2.

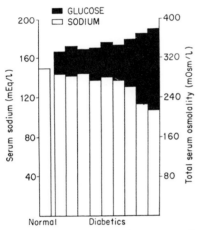

Figure 24-2. The relationship between the concentrations of glucose and sodium and the total serum osmolality in diabetic acidosis. (*After J. P. Peters,* Metabolism, *1:223, 1952.*)

It is apparent from Fig. 24-2 that although the osmolality of the total body fluid progressively increases during uncontrolled hyperglycemia (a reflection of the increased glucose concentration and of the overall loss of water in excess of the major solutes or electrolytes), the sodium and chloride concentration in the ECF is usually normal or low in the untreated patient. While the chloride level may be further reduced by vomiting, the hyponatremia is a reflection not of salt loss in excess of water but of a dilution of the residual extracellular sodium by water from the cells. This phenomenon is the major cause of the hyponatremia and hypochloremia present in diabetic ketoacidosis. It is obvious that any loss by way of the kidney or gastrointestinal (GI) tract of

these ions from the extracellular space would contribute to the *magnitude* of the hyponatremia and hypochloremia for any given degree of osmotically induced movement of water from the cells. A further contribution to the lowering of the serum sodium may be its movement into the cells as they become progressively depleted of potassium (see Chap. 4). Rarely, severe hyperlipemia as is seen in acute xanthoma diabeticorum may contribute to a spurious, or fictitious, hyponatremia (see Chaps. 3 and 12). Under these circumstances, all the solutes dissolved in the aqueous phase of the blood or plasma are reduced.[1]

If, despite the hyperglycemia, serum sodium is normal or even elevated, this indicates an even more profound degree of water loss from the body in excess of sodium than is seen in the average case of severe ketoacidosis and is most characteristic of the nonketotic hyperosmolar diabetic coma (see below). The combination of hypernatremia and profound hyperglycemia is seen most often in the older patient with uncontrolled diabetes in whom progressive glycosuria and polyuria continue for many days to weeks with minimal, if any, ketonemia and acidosis. Thus, the patient is usually not seen in the hospital until high degrees of water loss have occurred (see below).

Glucose, sodium and its attendant anions, and urea make up the major solutes of the plasma. From their values the total osmolality of the body fluids can be calculated:

$$P_{osm} = 2([Na^+]) + \frac{BUN\ mg/dl}{2.8} + \frac{blood\ glucose\ mg/dl}{18} \quad (24\text{-}1)$$

The serum osmolality may also be determined directly by measuring the freezing point of the plasma by means of an osmometer. A calculated osmolality that greatly exceeds the measured osmolality would suggest the possibility of severe hyperlipemia which, of course, can always be de-

---

[1] When a unit volume of plasma or serum contains an abnormally large proportion of lipid, the water phase is proportionately reduced.

tected by the lactescence of the plasma. The authors have found that the direct measurement of the serum osmolality is of great value in calculating the total deficit of body water in the patient with diabetic acidosis. The normal osmolality of the body fluids is about 285 mosm/L. If the osmolality of a patient with diabetic acidosis is 314 mosm/L, this represents a 10 percent increment in solute concentration, or approximately a 10 percent *decrement* in total body water. If the calculated normal total body water is 40 L, a 10 percent loss would be 4 L. This calculation assumes that no solute has been lost from the body fluids; this is obviously not true in diabetic acidosis. However, the authors have observed that the positive water balance during the first 48 h of treatment correlates quite well with the deficit calculated from serum osmolality. This empirical observation suggests that the increment in solute concentration contributed to the body fluids from the elevated blood sugar level approximates the decrement that would occur from the electrolyte loss.

GLYCOSURIA AND RENAL LOSSES OF WATER AND ELECTROLYTES

As the blood sugar rises, the filtered load of glucose progressively increases and exceeds the threshold for its renal tubular resorption; glucose then appears in the urine in increasing amounts. This carbohydrate, like any other nonresorbed solute (osmotic diuretic), prevents the resorption of water and sodium salts, leading to a progressive increase in urine flow. Figure 24-3 illustrates the effect of glycosuria during diabetic acidosis on the rate of urinary flow and electrolyte loss. This osmotic diuresis is the *major* cause of sodium, chloride, and water losses in severe diabetic acidosis. Glycosuria may exceed 50 g/h, or 277 mosm/h (Fig. 24-3). The concentration of sodium and chloride in the urine during this glucose diuresis is usually between 50 and 100 meq/L but may be as low as 10 to 25 meq/L if the stimulus for sodium conservation is marked and the simultaneous rate of glomerular filtration is below normal. This is characterisitic of the concentration of these electrolytes in the urine dur-

ing any severe osmotic diuresis (see Chaps. 3 and 13). The *hypotonic* nature of the urine with respect to sodium and chloride should be emphasized. The loss of body fluid as a consequence of osmotic diuresis can be visualized as a combination of isotonic saline and free water, i.e., 1 L of urine during osmotic diuresis diagrammatically represented as:

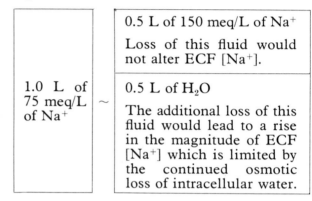

| 1.0 L of 75 meq/L of Na^+ | ~ | 0.5 L of 150 meq/L of Na^+ Loss of this fluid would not alter ECF $[Na^+]$. |
| | | 0.5 L of H_2O The additional loss of this fluid would lead to a rise in the magnitude of ECF $[Na^+]$ which is limited by the continued osmotic loss of intracellular water. |

As dehydration increases, the glomerular filtration and renal blood flow progressively decrease, and the patient may be oliguric or even anuric in spite of the marked hyperglycemia. In the treatment of the severely dehydrated oliguric patient, fluid replacement will reexpand the extracellular volume, causing renal hemodynamics to improve

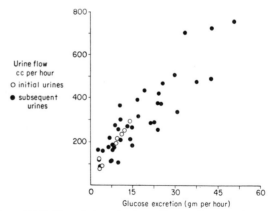

Figure 24-3. The relation of urinary flow to the excretion rate of glucose during diabetic acidosis. Initial urines are those obtained at the beginning of therapy, subsequent are those obtained during therapy. (*From D. W. Seldin and R. Tarail,* J. Clin. Invest., *29:552, 1950.*)

and urinary volume to increase progressively, and glycosuria may actually increase in spite of a falling blood sugar level. Stated differently, as the glomerular filtration rate (GFR) increases, the filtered load of glucose, a function of $P_g \times$ GFR, will increase despite a decrease in the concentration of glucose in the ECF or blood. A corollary to the above is that the presence of chronic or acute renal disease such as acute tubular necrosis, diabetic glomerulosclerosis, glomerulonephritis and/or nephrosclerosis will reduce the GFR per nephron and thus decrease the filtered load of glucose or ketones for any given increase in blood level, and hyperglycemia and ketonemia may exist with little or no sugar or ketones in the urine (an abnormally high renal threshold for these substances).

POTASSIUM LOSS

Little mention has been made of the effect of the glycosuria and the osmotic diuresis on the renal loss of potassium. Although osmotic diuresis does slightly increase the renal excretion of potassium, this effect is much less than its effect on the excretion of sodium and chloride. The major causes for the loss of potassium in diabetic acidosis are as follows (6):

1. Lean-tissue breakdown, with the liberation of approximately 3 meq of potassium per gram of nitrogen lost. This is due to the starvationlike state created by the intermediary metabolic defect associated with insulin deficiency and the marked hypersecretion of adrenal glucocorticoids which accompanies severe uncontrolled diabetes mellitus (7, 8).
2. The progressive depletion of tissue stores of glycogen. Normally, 1 meq of potassium is "deposited" in the cells with every 3 g of glycogen. As the latter is utilized and not repleted, the "freed" potassium is excreted. Severe diabetic acidosis in the adult may cause a 200- to 300-g deficit of glycogen with its accompanying 70 to 100 meq of potassium.
3. The loss of intracellular water (cellular dehydration) is a strong stimulus for the loss or net flux of potassium from body cells (9) and its

continued high rate of excretion in the urine as part of the "dehydration reaction" (see Chap. 13). Because the sustained hyperglycemia in uncontrolled diabetes causes the continued withdrawal of cellular water, this stimulus for potassium loss persists until the cellular deficit of water is corrected.

4. The deficiency of insulin may well prevent cells from maintaining the highest or optimal intracellular/extracellular concentration ratio for potassium (10, 11, 12). Therefore, K^+ may more readily diffuse out of cells along its electrochemical gradient into the ECF and then into the urine. This action of insulin is not dependent on or secondary to its effect on glucose transport.
5. The increased secretion of aldosterone (13) caused by the profound depletion of sodium and extracellular volume enhances the renal loss of potassium for any given metabolic state and rate of sodium excretion.
6. Severe anorexia and vomiting, which would prevent the ingestion of potassium-containing foods necessary for the correction of the developing deficit of potassium. Sustained vomiting would cause the loss of almost 10 to 20 meq of potassium per liter of vomitus.

Therefore, in summary, the combination of ongoing cellular losses of K^+ and continued renal potassium wasting results in the severe defects observed. Despite the marked deficit of potassium produced by these derangements, the serum potassium level is usually normal or elevated when the patient with untreated diabetic acidosis enters the hospital. The factors which tend to elevate the initial level of potassium in the serum are (1) metabolic acidosis per se (Chap. 3), (2) defects in the intermediary metabolic processes, e.g., inadequate tissue oxygenation, impaired generation of ATP for the $Na^+-K^+-ATPase$, which are essential for the maintenance of the concentration gradient for potassium between the cell and extracellular fluid, (3) the deficiency of insulin (see No. 4 above), (4) functional renal impairment due to loss of intravascular volume, hypotension, and marked intrarenal vasoconstriction which would lower the renal clearance of potassium for any given metabolic setting. In this latter context, an

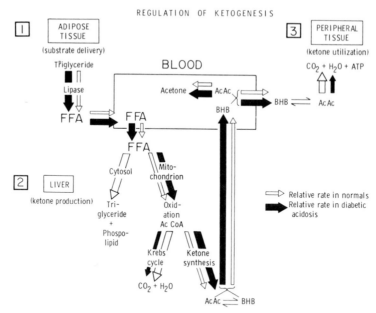

Figure 24-4. Scheme of the three elements of net ketone production. See text for details. Abbreviations: FFA: free fatty acids; AcCoA: acetyl-coenzyme A; AcAc: acetoacetic acid; βHB: beta-hydroxybutyric acid; ATP: adenosine triphosphate.

unusually high serum potassium should also bring to mind the syndrome of hyporeninemic hypoaldosteronism in the diabetic patient (12) (see Chaps. 14 and 23). The presence of a low serum potassium level prior to therapy therefore indicates an especially profound degree of potassium depletion.

LEAN TISSUE AND NITROGEN LOSS

The patient with uncontrolled diabetes with moderate acidosis often has a progressive loss of appetite, so his caloric intake decreases. This lack of calories, together with the loss of the normal nitrogen-sparing effect of carbohydrates when there is a relative or absolute deficiency of insulin, leads to progressive tissue breakdown and negative nitrogen balance. The increased endogenous production of urea secondary to this tissue breakdown causes an increase in the blood urea nitrogen out of proportion to the degree of renal impairment or to the increase in serum creati-

nine. It also causes a marked increase in the renal excretion of urea, which contributes a further osmotic effect in addition to that of the glycosuria. The destruction of tissue protein is associated with the liberation of intracellular potassium, phosphorus, and magnesium which are lost from the body through the urine in increasing amounts as diabetic acidosis proceeds, and which, of course, must be returned to the individual during treatment and the recovery phase when lost protoplasm is being repleted.

KETOGENESIS

The generation and maintenance of net keto acid production involves the interaction of three basic elements (Fig. 24-4): (1) adipose tissue, (2) the liver, and (3) extrahepatic tissue. Free fatty acids (FFA), derived from adipose tissue, serve as substrate for hepatic ketogenesis, and the ketones are finally metabolized by such extrahepatic tissues as muscle and brain. In the uncontrolled diabetic state, alterations of each of the above elements result in massive overproduction of ketone acids and life-threatening ketoacidosis.

The conversion of triglycerides to FFA by adipose tissue is largely controlled by a hormone-sensitive lipase (14). Certain hormones (e.g., epinephrine and glucocorticoids) enhance cAMP formation; this, in turn, activates the lipase, resulting in enhanced lipolysis and FFA mobilization. In contrast to the other hormones, insulin impairs lipase activity by inhibiting adenylate cyclase, thereby reducing cAMP. Reduced insulin activity, therefore, unleashes lipase and allows large amounts of FFAs to gain access to the circulation.

The liver's ability to rapidly metabolize FFA limits its plasma concentration, preventing a significant fall in pH due to FFA, per se. The entry of FFA into hepatocytes is largely governed by their plasma concentration. Upon entry into the liver cell, rapid conversion to the metabolically active coenzyme A (CoA) derivative occurs in the cytosol. A small fraction of the active fatty acid forms triglyceride and phospholipid while the remainder is transported into the mitochondrion where it is oxidized. Transport of fatty acids through the inner mitochondrial membrane requires that they first be converted to their carnitine derivatives by an enzyme located on the membrane's outer surface. At the inner surface, CoA replaces carnitine and the activated fatty acid may now be oxidized to the 2-carbon, acetyl-CoA (15). It has recently been shown that glucagon stimulates the entry of FFA into the mitochondrion by enhancing the formation of the carnitine derivative. The hyperglucagonemia which accompanies ketoacidosis may, therefore, enhance the ketogenic potential of the liver by facilitating the availability of FFA to the biosynthetic site of ketones (16).

Further metabolism of acetyl-CoA is effected by enzymes of the Krebs cycle to carbon dioxide and water, or by other intramitochondrial enzymatic pathways to ketone acids. In uncontrolled diabetes mellitus, there is much evidence to suggest that cycle activity is diminished, thereby forcing acteyl-CoA to form ketones (17). Acetoacetic acid is the first ketone formed from acetyl-CoA

and will slowly and nonenzymatically decarboxylate to form acetone (Fig. 24-4). The conversion of the strong acetoacetic acid to the nonacid, acetone, represents one form of metabolic buffering, since this reaction prevents the acetoacetic acid's hydrogen ion from expressing its physicochemical activity. Since acetone is nonmetabolizable and since it is excreted far less efficiently than the others ketones, it may remain in the blood for many hours following the normalization of ketogenesis by insulin (18). In this setting, acetone may cause a positive nitroprusside test, creating the confusing picture of the treated diabetic whose blood sugar and bicarbonate have normalized but whose serum ketones remain positive (19). The normal bicarbonate and absence of an elevated anion gap indicate that acetoacetic *acid* is not present and that the positive nitroprusside reaction most likely reflects acetone.

The third ketone body is β-hydroxybutyric acid which is the reduction product of acetoacetic acid (Fig. 24-4). These two ketones, β-hydroxybutyric and acetoacetic acid, are interconvertible, and their relative concentrations depend upon the availability of reduced pyridine nucleotide ($NADH_2$). The latter, in turn, is largely regulated by the availability of oxygen to the tissues. It follows, therefore, that with tissue hypoxia, as in shock, pneumonia, etc., when $NADH_2$ is abundant, the β-hydroxybutyric acid/acetoacetic acid ratio will elevate. Since β-hydroxybutyric acid, at any concentration, is nonreactive to nitroprusside, ketosis will be obscured when tissue hypoxia obtains. Thus, hypotensive, acidotic diabetics whose semiquantitative nitroprusside tests (tablets, powder, or dipsticks) reveal zero to moderate ketosis may actually be "hiding" massive amounts of ketones as the unmeasurable β-hydroxybutyric acid. With fluid and insulin therapy, total ketone production will fall, but increased tissue perfusion and oxygenation will drive the β-hydroxybutyric acid to the measurable acetoacetic acid form, giving the false impression of worsening or non-improving ketosis.

Since the renal excretion of β-hydroxybutyric acid and acetoacetic acid is extremely efficient, it is common to see ketonuria in the absence of ketonemia in patients with only mild ketosis. The only time the reverse occurs, i.e., ketonemia without ketonuria, is when severe acute or chronic renal failure is present.

The liver, unlike peripheral tissue, is unable to metabolize the ketone acids it synthesizes. The β-hydroxybutyric acid and acetoacetic acid are taken up from the circulation by such tissues as muscle and kidney and oxidized to carbon dioxide and water. Although not well studied in humans, there is substantial data from animal studies to indicate that the peripheral catabolism of ketones is depressed in uncontrolled diabetes (20). Recent studies in humans are compatible with this observation (21).

In summary, the absence of insulin initiates a series of reactions which result in severe overproduction of keto acids. Increased fat mobilization and glucagon release provide substrate and stimulate the controlling hepatic biosynthetic reactions of ketogenesis. A decreased peripheral utilization may further increase the circulating level of keto acids. Thus, the diabetic state is associated with the stimulation of all three of the basic elements involved in ketogenesis.

ACID-BASE CHANGES

UNCOMPLICATED DKA

The normal response to ketone acid overproduction is reflected by biochemical changes in plasma and functional alterations in lungs and kidney. Changes in all three areas are directed toward prevention of life-threatening acidosis.

As β-hydroxybutyric acid and acetoacetic acid gain access to the extracellular space, blood buffers are progressively titrated in an effort to limit the acidifying process. Bicarbonate, the most easily measured of the blood buffers, is consumed, and its anionic charge is replaced by the negatively charged β-hydroxybutyrate and acetoacetate. The acidosis is manifested by the fall in bicarbonate and reciprocal rise in the anion gap (AG) (19). The latter represents those anions, other than chloride and bicarbonate, which offset sodium's positive charge: $AG = Na^+ - (Cl^- + HCO_3^-) = 10$ to 12 meq/L (normal). In pure diabetic ketoacidosis, the increment in the anion gap above normal equals the amount of circulating keto acid and consequently also equal the meq/L decrement in serum bicarbonate. With therapy, the ketones are converted to bicarbonate by muscle, a process which at once normalizes the serum bicarbonate and anion gap.

Respiration is stimulated by the acidemia and the consequent decrease in P_{CO_2} and carbonic acid acts to bring arterial pH back toward normal. This labored, deep ventilation was first described in 1874 by Kussmaul in his report of an obese, 35-year-old diabetic. She was described as "... breathing loud, rapid and the respiratory movements strikingly large. Powerful costal abdominal inspirations alternating with powerful expirations" (22). It takes approximately 12 to 24 h for a given degree of acidosis to elicit a maximal respiratory response (23). The expected fall in P_{CO_2} that is appropriate for a given degree of systemic acidosis is defined by the following formula which relates the observed total CO_2 to the expected arterial P_{CO_2}. P_{CO_2} (mmHg) $= 1.5$ (total CO_2) $+ 8 \pm 2$ (24). A ketoacidotic patient with a total CO_2 of 10 meq/L ought to have a P_{CO_2} of 23 (±2) mmHg. If the observed P_{CO_2} were less than 21 or greater than 25 mmHg, a superimposed respiratory disorder would be diagnosed (see Chap. 6).

The renal response to diabetic ketoacidosis is similar to that seen in other metabolic acidoses. The tubules reabsorb all filtered bicarbonate, thereby conserving alkali and acidifying the urine. The major urinary buffers, phosphate and ammonia, are titrated, effecting the excretion of large amounts of acid. Under the stimulus of systemic acidosis, renal synthesis and excretion of ammonia increases markedly and the combined excretion of titratable acid plus ammonium accounts for the seven- to tenfold increase in acid excretion during severe ketoacidosis (25). There is some evidence, however, indicating that ketones may suppress renal ammonia synthesis, thereby limiting the maximal increase that could otherwise occur in severe ketoacidosis (26).

It is important to recognize that it usually takes from many hours to several days for ketoacidosis to develop when insulin is removed (25). The abrupt sudden onset of acidosis should immediately suggest the possibility of lactic acidosis (see below), the presence of a toxin, and/or renal failure.

COMPLICATED (MIXED) ACID-BASE DISORDERS

A number of pathophysiologic changes occur in uncontrolled diabetes which may further complicate acid-base metabolism. When a metabolic alkalosis or respiratory acidosis or alkalosis is superimposed upon ketoacidosis, a "mixed" acid-base disorder is said to exist (see Chap. 6). The most common mixed disturbances seen in diabetes are as follows.

Mixed ketoacidosis and metabolic alkalosis

It is quite common for the vomiting which frequently complicates ketoacidosis to superimpose a metabolic alkalosis on the preexisting ketoacidosis. A similar picture may also develop from overzealous therapy with alkali. Table 24-1 outlines the serum electrolytes and acid-base parameters found in this mixed disorder.

Vomiting or alkali therapy, while replenishing circulating bicarbonate, either exerts no effect or may increase ketone anions (27). Consequently, the pH, P_{CO_2}, and bicarbonate may normalize, while the anion gap remains elevated. This highlights the importance of the anion gap in diagnosing acid-base disorders (Chap. 6, ref. 19). Less severe alkaloses will only partially correct the bicarbonate, in which case the increment in the anion gap will exceed the decrement in bicarbonate.

With therapy, the ketones are metabolized to alkali and the final serum bicarbonate concentra-

Table 24-1

	NORMAL	DKA	VOMITING OR NaHCO₃ THERAPY PLUS DKA
Na, meq/L	140	140	145
K	4	5	4
Cl	105	105	95
CO₂	25	10	25
AG	10	25	25
pH	7.40	7.23	7.40
P_{CO_2}, mmHg	40	22	40

Table 24-2

	NORMAL	DKA	RESPIRATORY ALKALOSIS PLUS DKA
Na, meq/L	140	140	139
K	4	5	4
Cl	105	105	106
CO₂	25	10	8
AG	10	25	25
pH	7.40	7.23	7.44
P_{CO_2}, mmHg	40	22	12

tion will equal the sum of this regenerated bicarbonate plus the additional amount due to vomiting or therapy. Thus, reversal of ketoacidosis unmasks the metabolic alkalosis.

Mixed ketoacidosis and respiratory alkalosis

Diabetics have an increased susceptibility to infection, especially pneumonia and gram-negative sepsis, and these infections will often precipitate an episode of ketoacidosis. Since pneumonia and endotoxemia cause hyperventilation (28), it is not uncommon to see respiratory alkalosis superimposed upon diabetic ketoacidosis. These processes have offsetting effects on pH but additive effects on bicarbonate concentration. It is common, therefore, to find a normal pH with a strikingly low serum bicarbonate. An example is shown in Table 24-2. In this example, the severe hyperventilation decreased the serum carbonic acid concentration so markedly that the pH moved toward the frankly alkalemic range. The further depression of total CO_2, in the face of normalization of pH, emphasizes the fact that the serum total CO_2, by itself, does not give enough information to appropriately evaluate acid-base disorders (see Chap. 6).

It is very common to see a similar mixed acid-base disorder develop in the recovery phase of any severe metabolic acidosis, including ketoacidosis. Bicarbonate, P_{CO_2}, and pH all begin to increase as acetoacetate and β-hydroxybutyrate are metabolized to bicarbonate. During this stage, respiratory compensation recovers more slowly than serum bicarbonate, resulting in a sustained lowering of P_{CO_2} while bicarbonate approaches normal. By consequence, the pH rapidly normalizes or may even move into the frankly alkaline range. By 12 to 24 h, respiration normalizes and acid-base balance returns. Therapy with $NaHCO_3$ during the acidemic phase will tend to worsen this "alkaline overshoot" by further elevating the serum bicarbonate concentration at a time when the P_{CO_2} is inappropriately low. If careful attention has been paid to reexpansion of the ECF volume with saline and the needed potassium replacement, it is unlikely that the kidney will retain this additional bicarbonate. In the face of normovolemia, normokalemia, and hypocapnia, the kidney tends to excrete bicarbonate (see Chap 6.)

CLINICAL EVALUATION OF KETOSIS

A number of semiquantitative tests based on the nitroprusside reaction (Ketostix, Acetest tablets or powder) are used for the detection of ketosis. The chemical reaction is strongest with acetoacetic acid, weak with acetone, and nonreactive with β-hydroxybutyric acid. The serum acetoacetic acid concentration is high enough in the great majority of patients with diabetic ketoacidosis to give a positive nitroprusside reaction. In the presence of tissue hypoxia, however, the severity or even the very presence of ketonemia may go unrecognized because the bulk of ketones reside in the β-hydroxybutyric acid form, which is nitroprusside-negative. Since the β-hydroxybutyric acid/acetoacetic acid ratio is subject to much variability, it is not surprising that a poor correlation exists between the serum nitroprusside test and the exact quantitative assessment of total ketones (29).

As previously noted, substantial levels of acetone may remain in the serum following clearing of acetoacetic acid and β-hyroxybutyric acid. The positive nitroprusside reaction in this setting does not reflect ongoing ketosis which would, of course, signal the need for more insulin, but rather indicates the natural evolution of resolving ketosis (18).

Thus, a positive test for acetoacetic acid is very helpful in diagnosing ketoacidosis, but a trace positive or negative test does not rule it out. It follows that a negative test in an acidotic diabetic may reflect either a mixed keto-lactic acidosis or a pure lactic acidosis. In this setting, therapy with insulin should be begun and specific tests for β-hydroxybutyric acid and lactic acid carried out.

During therapy of ketoacidosis, changes occur in the βHB/AcAc ratio and serum acetone which impose important restrictions on the interpretation of the degree of positivity of the serum Acetest. Because of these uncertainties, the authors no longer rely on the Acetest, in serial plasma dilution, to dictate insulin needs.

A confusing picture is sometimes presented by patients with "euglycemic diabetic ketoacidosis" (30). This group also presents with severe ketoacidosis, but with a normal to slightly elevated blood sugar. It almost always occurs in known diabetics who are insulin dependent and who have taken their insulin dose on the day of admission. The pathophysiology of this syndrome is still to be worked out. Therapy is similar to hyperglycemic ketoacidosis, but glucose-containing solutions are used from the outset.

It is important to remember that there are other causes of ketosis which must be distinguished from diabetic ketoacidosis and which may simulate the picture of "euglycemic diabetic ketoacidosis" (see Table 24-3).

Table 24-3

DISORDER	DEGREE OF KETOSIS	BLOOD SUGAR	CLUE TO DIAGNOSIS
Starvation	+1 − +2	Low−Normal	History; serum $HCO_3 \geq 17$ meq/L
High-fat diet	+1 − +2	Normal	Diet history
Drugs/toxins			
Paraldehyde (31)	+1 − +2	Normal	History; paraldehyde odor on breath
Isopropyl alcohol (32)	+1 − +4	Normal−Low	Ketosis due to acetone; normal HCO_3 and anion gap
Alcoholic ketosis (33)	+2 − +4	Low−Normal	Recent binge, vomiting
von Gierke's disease (34)	+2 − +4	Low	Hypoglycemia, hepatomegaly

The severe ketoacidosis sets off a chain of aggravating physiologic changes.

1. There is a marked peripheral vasodilatation, in spite of hypotension, causing the cherry-red skin and mucous membranes which are so characteristic of the patient in severe diabetic acidosis. This peripheral vasodilation leads to an increased cutaneous insensible water loss which further aggravates the fluid deficit.
2. Loss of appetite and excessive nausea and vomiting follow the ketoacidosis, so that thirst cannot be satisfied.
3. Further sodium chloride, potassium, and water losses occur through the vomitus.

It is felt by most that the diffuse and/or localized abdominal pain seen in association with many cases of diabetic acidosis is secondary to the ketoacidosis per se. This abdominal pain has often been misdiagnosed as an acute surgical emergency. An important point that differentiates this from other acute surgical abdominal conditions is that the loss of appetite followed by nausea and vomiting in diabetic acidosis *always* precedes the abdominal pain. This sequence is in contrast to that seen in most surgical emergencies. The characteristic polymorphonuclear leukocytosis, which may be secondary to the dehydration, acidosis, and adrenal cortical stimulation, further confuses the picture and may actually reach leukemoid proportions of 40,000 to 50,000 white blood cells per cubic millimeter of blood. Diabetic acidosis and coma may be precipitated by a fulminant, acute, hemorrhagic pancreatitis. In this situation the abdominal pain will be persistent and severe. The hypotension will be very resistant to water, electrolytes, and even blood replacement, and the patient will fail to improve during therapy in contrast to the improvement of the patient in the usual diabetic coma. These are all clues to the possible presence of acute pancreatitis.

With respect to the diagnosis of acute pancreatitis associated with diabetic ketosis, plasma amylase levels may be greatly elevated without pancreatic inflammation or any disorder of exocrine function of the pancreas. In fact, Warshaw and associates (35) have recently demonstrated that the elevated serum amylase observed in at least 50 percent of their patients with diabetic ketoacidosis was, in six out of seven cases, of salivary and not pancreatic origin when isoenzyme analysis of the plasma was carried out by polyserylamide-gel electrophoresis. Finn and Cope (36) documented that during recovery the decrease of the amylasemia parallels the fall in blood sugar level, suggesting a relationship between the abnormal carbohydrate metabolism and the elevated serum amylase level. Recently, the value of the amylase clearance/creatinine clearance ratio in the diagnosis of true acute pancreatitits in diabetes and in other states with impaired renal function has been documented (37).

Source	Osmolality	Sodium concentration
Skin and Lungs	0 (Distilled Water)	0
Renal	ISO or Hypertonic	25 - 100 mEq/L
Vomitus	Isotonic	50 - 80 mEq/L

Figure 24-5. The qualitative characteristics of the fluids lost during diabetic acidosis with respect to their total osmolality and sodium concentration.

QUANTITATIVE WATER AND ELECTROLYTE LOSSES

Figures 24-5 and 24-6 summarize the characteristics of the water and electrolyte losses in uncontrolled diabetic acidosis (8, 38–41). It is readily apparent that all avenues of sodium and chloride loss are hypotonic to the normal body fluids, i.e., the water losses are in excess of the simultaneous sodium losses. Thus, the water loss in diabetic acidosis represents the most serious form of hypertonic dehydration and leads to extreme intracellular depletion of fluids. The water losses through the skin, lungs, and gastrointestinal tract

		Range
Water	= 75 - 100 cc/kg	
Na^+	= 8 mEq/kg	(5 - 10)
Cl^-	= 5 mEq/kg	(3 - 10)
K^+	= 6 mEq/kg	(3 - 11)
Nit.	= 0.5 gm/kg	

Figure 24-6. Average losses of water, nitrogen, and electrolytes in severe diabetic acidosis. Derived from balance studies during recovery phase. The values represent those available in the literature (see Refs. 8, 39–42) and from the authors' series.

are aggravated by the usual inability of the patient to replace water because of anorexia, vomiting, or coma. The extreme depletion of body fluids from all spaces leads to a relentless contraction of the vascular volume, to hypotension and often shock. As in all states associated with a depletion of the vascular volume and increased blood viscosity, there is a progressive reduction in renal blood flow and GFR (42) which further impairs renal compensatory mechanisms, thus leading to a more rapidly developing and severe acidosis. To emphasize the adverse role of hypovolemia per se, Porte and associates (43) showed that the administration of appropriate salt solutions, *without insulin,* greatly inhibited the development of ketoacidosis following withdrawal of insulin from insulin-dependent diabetic subjects. Further, it has been shown that hemorrhagic or hypovolemic hypotension and shock can seriously impair the output of insulin from the pancreas, and that this is due to norepinephrine or alpha-adrenergic inhibition of insulin secretion (43, 44).

The sustained renal ischemia even in the absence of acute organic renal failure may cause transient albuminuria and appearance of granular casts in the urine which may be erroneously attributed to an associated acute or chronic renal disease. However, if the severe renal ischemia is sustained, actual acute tubular necrosis may be superimposed upon the prerenal azotemia and will greatly complicate the diagnostic and therapeutic problems (see Chap. 15).

Figure 24-6 presents average values for water, electrolyte, and nitrogen losses which are incurred during severe diabetic acidosis (8, 38–41). These values should be remembered, for they give the physician an empirical starting point in estimating the total deficit that developed prior to the patient's hospitalization. It will be noted that magnesium and phosphate, although lost in large quantities during severe uncontrolled diabetes mellitus, have not been included.

To date, no carefully controlled randomized studies have appeared in the adult or pediatric literature on the use of parenteral inorganic phosphorus as a component of the early (first 24 to 36 h) treatment of diabetic acidosis and coma, and its effect on morbidity and mortality. Franks and associates (45) in the late 1940s treated 10 patients with diabetic ketoacidosis with 1.3 to 2.6 g of elemental phosphorus given rapidly during the early hours of parenteral fluid therapy, and they compared this group with patients receiving saline only and with another 11 receiving glucose and saline. He concluded, "The administration of sodium phosphate was accompanied with (a) a tendency toward improved utilization of carbohydrate (b) a rise in plasma chloride and in carbondioxide combining power (c) an apparent retention of fluid in the vascular system (d) a rapid clearing of the mental state and (e) a statistically significant decrease in fatality rate. The results of this study suggest that the therapeutic regimen in diabetic coma should include the parenteral administration of sodium phosphate 4 to 8 hours after the first dose of insulin." Before Franks' study (45), Guest and Rapoport (46) had carried out extensive experiments in animals and humans showing the marked derangement in inorganic and organic phosphate metabolism in the red blood cells during diabetic ketoacidosis. Today it is clear that acute phosphate depletion and severe hypophosphatemia, as seen before and during the treatment of these patients, may produce clinically significant abnormalities in the central and peripheral nervous system, skeletal muscles, oxygen transport by the red cells, and phagocytic and migratory capacity of the white cells (47, 48, 49). Despite this, we still cannot clearly recommend the addition of phosphorus to our early parenteral therapy of diabetic acidosis and coma.

Many of our comments regarding phosphorus also apply to magnesium—the hypomagnesemia and total body depletion in uncontrolled diabetes (41), the physiologic abnormalities accompanying its acute depletion, and the absence of controlled studies of its effect when included in our early parenteral fluid therapy. If hyperphosphatemia and hypermagnesemia are avoided, we see no reason why these ions should not be added to our solutions and we hope that conclusive information on this point will be forthcoming.

TREATMENT

The fundamental physiologic principles which have been presented govern therapy in all cases;

however, each case must be individualized. There is no substitute for careful clinical and laboratory observation of each patient. Only through rigorous observation can one properly evaluate the patient's needs and response to therapy. This type of observation is far more important than the slight to moderate differences in the approach to therapy that can be seen from institution to institution or from one "authority" to another. In fact, given the meticulous hour-to-hour care necessary and a few basic principles, the major morbidity and mortality are primarily related to the patient's associated disorders and even the patient's socioeconomic status.

GENERAL POINTS TO BE FOLLOWED AND REMEMBERED

1. The patient must be examined by the physician frequently and completely for clinical changes; the observation and care of the patient in diabetic acidosis *cannot* be left to the nursing staff.
2. Diabetic acidosis is never associated with fever unless some complication is present. "Prophylactic" antibiotics should not be used, but antibiotic therapy should be initiated if the patient is febrile and a careful effort, with appropriate cultures, has been made to determine the cause of the fever.
3. Young adults appear much less dehydrated than they actually are. A history of the patient's weight just prior to the onset of his acute illness is extremely important. If the patient can be weighed on admission, weight loss is a good approximation of the magnitude of fluid loss. Allow for a tissue loss (protein and fat) of 1 lb/day for each day that the patient has not eaten prior to admission, or ½ lb/day if food intake has been curtailed but not stopped altogether.
4. All deep reflexes should be checked very carefully on the initial physical examination. This and the electrocardiogram are the best methods for following a rapidly decreasing serum potassium. In spite of the marked potassium depletion, the serum potassium level on admission is usually normal or elevated, and the

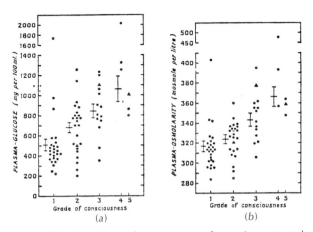

Figure 24-7. (a) Relation between state of consciousness and plasma glucose in 70 episodes of diabetic ketoacidosis. (b) Relation between state of consciousness and calculated plasma osmolarity in 70 episodes of diabetic ketoacidosis. (*From Fulop.*)

electrocardiogram may show peaking of the T waves, suggestive of potassium intoxication (see above).
5. The patient with severe diabetic ketoacidosis is frequently stuporous and relatively unresponsive, and at times in frank coma. It is clear that the level of consciousness is best correlated with the magnitude of hyperglycemia and hyperosmolality of the body fluids noted at the time of the patient's admission (Fig. 24-7) (50). This depression of the sensorium is usually readily responsive to the corrective therapy. However, at times after the initial clearing, the patient may once again become stuporous or semicomatose despite biochemical improvement in the metabolic parameters in the serum, or a patient mentally clear on admission may follow this same untoward course. As noted earlier, Posner and Plum (51) in selected cases have correlated this worsening state with the development of severe cerebrospinal fluid acidosis as the blood pH returns toward normal (Fig. 24-8). Sporadic cases have been described (52, 53) where the patient after initial clearing of the sensorium suddenly lapsed into deep coma with falling blood pressure, tachycardia, often with fever, and shortly expired despite progressive improvement in the abnormal blood chemistry values. Post-

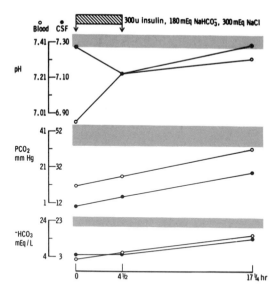

Figure 24-8. Data in Case 1. The ordinates for pH, P_{CO_2}, and bicarbonate concentration in blood (open circles) and cerebrospinal fluid (black circles), respectively, have different values at the same point. When arterial–cerebrospinal fluid difference is normal, the circles superimpose. The shaded areas represent the normal range for both blood and cerebrospinal fluid. In this patient, the cerebrospinal fluid pH was normal on admission when the blood was profoundly acidotic, and the cerebrospinal fluid itself became acid as the serum pH was corrected. The cerebrospinal fluid pH fell at 4½ h because the cerebrospinal fluid P_{CO_2} rose in parallel with the blood P_{CO_2} but the cerebrospinal fluid bicarbonate did not change.

mortem examination has consistently demonstrated severe cerebral edema (52–56). Fulop (56) has suggested that prior to therapy the prolonged hyperglycemia has caused a significant rise in the glucose concentration in the interstitial and intracellular space of the brain despite the blood-brain barrier. As the blood sugar level falls rapidly during effective therapy, there is a reversal of the gradient of glucose concentration between the blood and the brain, the osmotic pressure of the blood falls below that of the brain, and the water moves into the interstitial and intracellular space of the brain, causing severe cerebral edema. However, increased content of glucose in the brain makes up only a small part of the increase in brain osmol content during sustained hyperglycemia. The content of glucose has never been reported to exceed 25 percent of plasma glucose levels. When the glucose concentration in the plasma is *rapidly* reduced with insulin to normal or near normal values in animals with experimental diabetic coma, brain content of glucose falls at the same rate as does the glucose in the plasma with no evidence of retention in the brain (57, 58). Despite this, total brain osmolality falls at a significantly slower rate than does that of the plasma, causing an osmotic gradient between brain and plasma and the rapid development of brain edema. A substantial portion of the increase in total osmol content of the brain consists of measured solutes such as Na^+ (11%), Cl^- (8%), K^+ (26%), but the largest part consists of undetermined or ideogenic osmols (45%). This osmolar generation is the direct result of the insulin therapy, for comparably rapid lowering of plasma glucose with peritoneal dialysis does not cause an increase in brain solute content and does not cause cerebral edema (57, 58). In the majority of the reported cases of brain edema complicating treatment of ketoacidosis, blood glucose was rapidly reduced to levels close to 100 mg/dL. It may be possible to prevent the effects of insulin leading to brain edema by avoiding overly rapid reduction of blood glucose to normal during the total therapy of diabetic coma. Attempts to treat the cerebral edema with mannitol, glucocorticoids, etc. have not been successful.

6. A decision as to catheterization of the bladder may be made on the following bases:

a. If the individual is lucid and can void spontaneously and if rectal or vaginal examination discloses no evidence of prostatic enlargement or cystocele, catheterization is not necessary, and the patient should be allowed to void spontaneously.

b. If a large residual urine is suspected in a conscious patient, the patient should void and be immediately catheterized *one time only* to check the residual urine and obtain a urine culture. The catheter should then be removed.

c. If the individual is stuporous or if urine specimens cannot be obtained, an indwelling catheter with a sterile sealed drainage system may be inserted but must be removed as soon as the patient becomes lucid enough to void spontaneously. *The physician should make every effort to avoid catheterizing the patient in diabetic acidosis or coma* because of the danger of causing a urinary tract infection or a serious exacerbation of an already existing one.

7. With respect to the question of admitting the patient with mild ketoacidosis to the hospital, it is always better to err on the side of being overly cautious and to hospitalize. At times the physician may know his patient so well and be so convinced of the patient's intelligence and reliability that he may choose to treat mild ketosis and mild dehydration on an ambulatory basis. The patient under the doctor's direction initiates hourly oral feedings with juices, water, salted broth, dietetic carbonated drinks, and hourly subcutaneous injections of 5 to 10 units of regular insulin. Urines are checked hourly for sugar and ketones and this treatment continued until ketonuria is cleared and there has been a significant decrease in the degree of glycosuria. The patient can then be placed on a schedule of one dose of regular insulin before each meal for a day or two prior to reinstituting usual insulin regimen. Failure of the patient to respond promptly to the above "ambulatory approach" should lead to the necessary hospitalization.

INSULIN ADMINISTRATION

Randomized studies (59, 60) have shown that the speed of recovery from ketoacidosis does not correlate with the total dose of insulin used, when cumulative doses ranging from 125 to 800 units were studied. Nevertheless, physicians continue to treat with large doses, justifying their use in the deep-rooted notion that acidosis and ketosis induce an acute state of insulin resistance (61, 62). Hundreds of units of insulin have been and are still being used in an effort to overcome this presumed resistance, and dosage is often based on complicated formulas that add to the mystique which surrounds therapy of ketoacidosis.

In recent years, many studies have appeared which clearly demonstrate that ketoacidosis may be safely, simply, and effectively treated with cumulative doses of regular insulin well under 100 units (63–69). Continuous infusion of 4 to 8 units/h or hourly intramuscular or subcutaneous injections of 5 to 10 units have been shown to lower blood sugar smoothly, improve ketosis, and repair acidosis at rates indistinguishable from those achieved with conventional, higher-dose regimens (67, 68). Table 24-4 is taken from the prospective study of Kitabchi et al. (67) which compared conventional, intermittent high-dose insulin therapy with low-dose intramuscular (IM) therapy. No significant difference in the time required to reverse the hyperglycemia, ketosis, or acidosis was observed between the two groups. Six of the 24 high-dose and none of the low-dose subjects became hypoglycemic during therapy. Hypokalemia occurred in 7 subjects from the high-dose group whereas it developed in only 1 of the low-dose subjects. These data underscore

Table 24-4. Comparison of results with high-dose and low-dose therapy

	HIGH DOSE	LOW DOSE	p
Number of patients	24	24	
Glucose ≤ 250 mg/dL	4.5 ± 0.8*	6.7 ± 0.8*	NS†
HCO_3 > 15 meq/L	11.6 ± 1.6*	11.1 ± 1.2*	NS
pH > 7.3	6.9 ± 1.3*	8.3 ± 0.9*	NS
Acetone < 1:2	10.3 ± 1.2*	12.0 ± 1.8*	NS
Alertness	11.1 ± 2.6*	7.5 ± 1.5*	NS
Insulin given (U) to achieve glucose of			
250 mg/dL	263.4 ± 45.3	46 ± 5	<0.001
Total fluid (mL) 1st 6 h	4233.4 ± 284	4006 ± 200	NS
Number of patients with hypoglycemia	6	0	

* Hours ± SEM of therapy until value achieved.

† NS = not significant.

the effectiveness of low-dose therapy and suggest that it may achieve normoglycemia and normokalemia more smoothly than does high-dose therapy.

These dosage schedules achieve serum insulin levels of 20 to 200 μU/mL (68, 70). These concentrations have previously been shown to be optimal for glucose transport in normal subjects (71). The ability of these same levels to reverse effectively and rapidly the hyperglycemia and ketosis in uncontrolled diabetics tends to negate the idea that ketosis and/or acidemia induce biologically significant degrees of insulin resistance in the great majority of ketoacidotic patients. Similar conclusions were reached by Hockaday and Alberti (1) who found no difference in insulin sensitivity in patients whose initial pH ranged from 6.90 to 7.25.

Low-dose insulin schedules which have proven effective are outlined below.

Intramuscular and subcutaneous therapy

In normotensive patients, regular insulin therapy is initiated with 0.2 unit/kg given by deep IM injection. Doses of 5 to 10 units are given intramuscularly each hour thereafter until the blood sugar reaches 250 mg/dL and the ketoacidosis clears. At this time further insulin is given every 2 h subcutaneously. Subsequent subcutaneous (SC) doses are based on blood sugar or on the glucose content of double voided urine specimens. It is important to underscore the need for repeated tests of the blood sugar and frequent doses of SC regular insulin. There is a tendency for many physicians to relax their therapy and vigilance once acute ketoacidosis has been reversed. Ketoacidosis and hyperglycemia are quick to return unless the patient's ongoing need for insulin is met. If the patient is hypotensive initially, insulin should be given intravenously since absorption from hypoperfused muscle may be erratic. Once the blood pressure has stabilized, IM or SC therapy may be used. Following its initial rapid decline, consequent to rehydration, the blood sugar will continue to fall by 75 to 100 mg/dL per h (68, 69). This value may be used to anticipate when the blood sugar will reach 250 mg/dL and therapy with glucose-containing solutions begun. Blood should be collected for serum enzyme studies prior to initiating IM therapy since these injections will traumatize muscle and increase serum enzyme levels.

Continuous intravenous therapy

The binding of insulin to the glass and plastic used for its infusion potentially decreases the dose delivered to the patient. This will not significantly affect delivery, however, if sufficiently high concentrations of regular insulin are used and the tubing is rinsed with the solution. If 100 units of regular insulin are added to 1 L of normal saline, and if the tubing is "washed out" with the first 50 mL, the remaining fluid will accurately deliver the desired dose (72). This high concentration and the washout procedure apparently saturate the insulin-binding sites. One milliliter per minute of this solution will deliver 6 units of insulin per hour, a dose sufficient for most patients. Fluid is best delivered with an infusion pump, but in its absence a pediatric infusion set may be safely and conveniently employed. As noted with IM therapy, when the blood sugar reaches 250 mg/dL, and if the ketosis has cleared, one should switch to SC therapy.

The simplicity of low-dose IM, SC, or intravenous (IV) therapy coupled with its ability to effect smooth reversal of the biochemical abnormalities and to minimize hypoglycemia and hypokalemia make the low-dose regimen more attractive to the authors. Regardless of which therapy and dose of insulin the physician selects, and they may be equally effective (68, 69, 70), it is absolutely critical to follow serum electrolytes and biochemical parameters. One must be prepared to increase or decrease insulin therapy depending upon the patient's response. The patient who is truly resistant to insulin may require many hundreds of units before a response is obtained. If the blood sugar has remained unchanged or increased 1 to 2 h after initiating therapy, as outlined above, the patient should be given 100 units of regular insulin intravenously. The dose may be doubled every 1 to 2 h (100, 200, 400, etc.) if no response is obtained. This degree of resistance is rarely met.

ALKALI THERAPY

The accession of strong ketone acids to extracellular space causes progressive loss of bicarbonate, fall in systemic pH, and compensatory decrease in P_{CO_2}, as was previously noted. With therapy, β-hydroxybutyrate and acetoacetate are metabolized to bicarbonate, thereby reversing the ketoacidosis. If the patient retains every millimol of ketone produced, its eventual oxidative conversion to alkali will return the serum bicarbonate to exactly normal. To the extent that sodium β-hydroxybutyrate and sodium acetoacetate are lost in the urine, a true bicarbonate deficit would exist which could only be replenished by renal synthesis or by exogenous replacement.

Many have argued that since insulin therapy reverses the biochemical abnormalities, including the bicarbonate deficit, alkali therapy is not only unnecessary but may in fact be detrimental. Others have felt that patients with severe degrees of acidosis, i.e., pH less than 7.15 and bicarbonate equal to or less than 8 meq/L, were at substantial risk from their low pH and therefore have advocated early therapy with alkali.

The perceived need for alkali is based on the following observations:

1. Insensitivity of peripheral tissues to insulin occurs in acidosis (61, 62). It might, therefore, be expected that alkali therapy would allow insulin to exert its full effects more rapidly. As noted above, the physiological importance of this acid inhibition has recently been seriously questioned (64, 65).
2. Profound hemodynamic effects of acidosis may lead to life-threatening pulmonary edema, hypotension, and shock (73). Acidosis directly impairs myocardial contractility but simultaneously causes the release of epinephrine. The positive inotropic effect of the latter largely offsets the inhibitory effect of low pH (74). However, when the pH falls below 7.15, the catechol effect is inhibited, thereby unmasking the negative inotropic effects of acidosis. These low pHs cause venous constriction and arteriolar dilatation leading to a decrease in venous capacitance and peripheral vascular resistance. The fall in capacitance forces more

blood into the pulmonary and arterial circuits while arteriolar dilatation leads to hypotension. Thus, greater demands are placed on a compromised myocardium, potentially leading to pulmonary edema, hypotension, and shock.
3. Acidosis induces widespread metabolic defects which may disrupt cellular function (75). Defects in glycolysis and lactate consumption are two such examples (76, 77).

The undesirable effects of alkali therapy have received much attention of late and are briefly outlined below:

1. In their oft-quoted paper, Posner and Plum (51) describe two ketoacidotic diabetics whose mental status worsened during sodium bicarbonate therapy (Fig. 24-8). Their cerebrospinal fluid (CSF) pH fell by 0.15 and 0.12 units respectively, when their state of consciousness worsened. It has been argued that the increase in ECF pH, consequent to alkali therapy, acts on peripheral chemoreceptors to diminish alveolar ventilation, thereby raising the P_{CO_2}. Since carbon dioxide, but not bicarbonate, rapidly enters the CSF, the brain is primarily exposed to the acidifying effects of P_{CO_2}. Thus, in the early phase of alkali therapy, when ECF pH is rising, a paradoxical fall in cerebrospinal fluid (CSF) pH occurs which alters cerebral function. In time, bicarbonate will also enter the CSF and cause its pH to return toward control levels.

Thus, on the basis of these two patients, the widespread belief has developed that CSF acidosis and stupor are significant and common complications of alkali therapy. Subsequent studies, however, have shown that CSF pH falls during conventional therapy of ketoacidosis regardless of whether or not bicarbonate is used (78, 79). In fact, the decline in CSF pH in diabetics treated with bicarbonate (-0.12 ± 0.02) was not significantly different from those treated without alkali (0.07 ± 0.05) (78, 79). It is of interest that the fall in CSF pH that routinely occurred in diabetics who did not suffer any central nervous system (CNS) dysfunction closely approximated that of Posner's and Plum's two patients. These observations cast doubt on the importance of the fall in CSF pH. In the opinion of the authors, the occurrence of worsening of the state of consciousness with alkali therapy is so rare that it should not strongly influence the decision to use bicarbonate.

2. Hemoglobin's affinity for oxygen is greatly influenced by acid-base changes. Low pH decreases affinity (Bohr effect) and thereby enables hemoglobin to "unload" more oxygen at the tissue level (80). When the red blood cell (RBC) glycolytic intermediate, 2,3-diphosphoglycerate (2,3-DPG), is abundant, hemoglobin's affinity for oxygen also falls, whereas affinity rises when a dearth of 2,3-DPG exists (81). Acidosis, by impairing RBC glycolysis, causes the 2,3-DPG content to fall (46, 49, 82). Thus, acidosis exerts positive and negative effects on hemoglobin-oxygen binding, and these effects need not occur simultaneously.

Although the Bohr effect is induced rapidly, the RBC 2,3-DPG content falls only slowly (Table 24-5). The predominance of the Bohr effect in early acidosis tends to increase tissue oxygenation, but the fall in 2,3-DPG, which occurs in time, counters the Bohr effect and thereby returns hemoglobin-oxygen affinity to baseline (84).

Rapid normalization of pH during alkali treatment reverses the Bohr effect more rapidly than RBC 2,3-DPG can be replenished.

During this transient state of imbalance, when 2,3-DPG is low and the Bohr effect is absent, oxygen will be more tightly bound to hemoglobin, and tissue oxygen delivery might suffer. This observation has been used as a caveat to enjoin physicians from the injudicious use of bicarbonate.

The authors are presently unaware of any evidence which, when critically reviewed, proves that alkali therapy in any way impairs tissue oxygenation in patients. In fact, Munk et al. (84) demonstrated that hemoglobin's affinity for oxygen increased during therapy of juvenile ketoacidosis, regardless of whether or not bicarbonate was given. It is the opinion of the authors that the imperfections in our understanding of how acid-base changes influence tissue oxygenation are presently far too great to justify withholding alkali in diabetics.

3. The "alkaline overshoot" which tends to occur with therapy may be exacerbated by $NaHCO_3$ therapy. This has been discussed above.

One must bear in mind that arterial pH is exquisitely sensitive to small changes in serum bicarbonate in patients with severe diabetic ketoacidosis. The bicarbonate/carbonic acid ratio defines the pH. When low absolute levels of bicarbonate prevail, an additional, even small, change effects large changes in the ratio, and thereby in the pH. This point helps to put matters

Table 24-5. Effects of acid-base changes on hemoglobin-oxygen affinity

STAGE OF ACIDOSIS	2,3-DPG*	BOHR EFFECT	NET CHANGE IN HEMO-GLOBIN-OXYGEN AFFINITY	POTENTIAL EFFECT ON TISSUE OXYGENATION
Initial acute acidosis	Remains normal	Present	Fall (<basal)	Increased
Steady-state acidosis	Low	Present	Return to basal	Return to basal
Initial response to alkali	Remains low	Absent	Rise	Decreased

* 2,3-Diphosphoglycerate.

Table 24-6. Effects of small changes in serum HCO_3 and P_{CO_2} on pH in severe diabetic ketoacidosis

	NORMAL	SEVERE DKA	FURTHER MINIMAL FALL IN HCO_3	ACUTE MINIMAL RISE IN P_{CO_2}	COMBINED CHANGES IN HCO_3 AND P_{CO_2}	MINIMAL RISE IN HCO_3
HCO_3, meq/L	24	5.0	2.5	5.0	2.5	8.0
P_{CO_2}, mmHg	40	16.0	16.0	30.0	30.0	16.0
pH	7.40	7.12	6.83	6.84	6.54	7.32

into perspective. As shown in Table 24-6, a further 2.5 meq/L fall in serum bicarbonate in a typical patient with severe ketoacidosis would be expected to lower the pH from 7.12 to 6.83. Hypotension with lactic acidosis, unchecked ketoacidosis, or even the dilutional acidosis caused by rapid saline infusions could cause this small decline in bicarbonate and precipitate sudden, severe worsening of acidosis. In the same patient, a small, sudden elevation of P_{CO_2} is shown to result in a similar catastrophic fall in pH. It should be obvious that such patients are in precarious balance. This sensitivity to bicarbonate may also be used to the patient's advantage. A small *increase* in bicarbonate from 5.0 to 8.0 meq/L will elevate the pH from the dangerously low value of 7.12 to the far safer figure of 7.32 (Table 24-6). In the authors' opinion, the benefits derived from small doses of bicarbonate far outweigh any theoretical or as yet poorly defined side effect.

Sodium bicarbonate is clearly the alkali of choice for parenteral therapy. Other sources of base, such as sodium lactate, must first be metabolized to bicarbonate before becoming effective. As was pointed out by Schwartz and Waters (85), one cannot always rely on this metabolic conversion to occur, thus these indirect forms of alkali are less dependable.

When the initial pH is ≤ 7.15 and the serum bicarbonate ≤ 8 meq/L, therapy should be begun with 44 to 88 meq of sodium bicarbonate in adults and 0.5 to 1.0 meq/kg in children. Hypotensive patients and those whose bicarbonate concentration is < 5 meq/L should be given larger doses based on their deficits (see Chap. 6).

WATER AND SODIUM REPLACEMENT

It is clear that the net overall loss of salt (NaCl) and water in diabetic ketoacidosis and coma is quite hypotonic to the normal extracellular fluid and can be approximated by one-half normal (0.45%) saline over even a more dilute solution in hyperosmolar ketotic or nonketotic coma. This being the case, the final total "mix" of the solutions used in therapy must approach this hypotonic deficit. Failure to use hypotonic fluid in the overall replacement therapy of these patients may lead to hyperosmolality, manifested by hypernatremia and hyperchloremia. This may mean that more salt than necessary has been given during the process of total correction of the water deficit. The hypernatremia will delay the rehydration of the cells, and the renal excretion of any excess salt will contribute to a continued osmotic diuresis even after glycosuria has been corrected. That we have stressed the hypotonic nature of the fluid losses should not be taken to mean that it is best to initiate the intravenous therapy with hypotonic solution. The latter, in the form of 0.45% saline, can certainly be used even from the beginning in the patient who has no hypotension or signs of shock. However, it must be remembered that isotonic saline will support the blood and interstitial fluid volume far better than one-half normal saline despite the fact that it will delay or lead to a slower correction of the *intracellular* water deficit. When the more hypotonic solution is given and the blood sugar is falling in response to effective insulin therapy, the major part of the administered water will move intracellularly, correcting the intracellular dehydration, but, at times, at the expense of the optimum reexpansion of the plasma and interstitial volume. As rapid rehydration of the cells, especially those of the brain, may not be most physiologically sound, and as we have stressed the serious adverse effects of continuing hypovolemia, it seems most rational to administer isotonic saline as the initial replacement solution. The rate and amount will depend on the observed state of the circulation. The greater the degree of hypotension, the faster and larger will be this replacement. In general, a rate of 500 to 1000 mL/h is satisfactory, and when the blood pressure and pulse have stabilized, one can switch to the 0.45% normal saline with or without 5% dextrose depending upon whether the blood sugar has fallen below 300 mg/dL.

All replacement fluids should be administered intravenously in the treatment of the diabetic "comas" until the patient is also able to take fluids by mouth. The inadequacy of subcutaneous administration of fluid, particularly hypotonic salt or solutions of carbohydrate, cannot be too strongly emphasized. Fluids administered subcutaneously may not improve the circulation, and further clinical deterioration may occur as plasma electrolytes move into the subcutaneous site of a hypodermoclysis in response to osmotic demands of the hypotonic fluids administered. No absolute arbitrary statement can be made with regard to the use of alkali solutions (sodium bicarbonate or sodium lactate) in the treatment of diabetic acidosis (see above). However, it is the authors' opinion that in the overwhelming number of cases, bicarbonate and/or lactate solutions are unnecessary and, at times, even deleterious to the smooth and rapid acid-base and metabolic recovery of the patient. Alkali administration need be initiated only if the original acidosis is profound, i.e., when plasma bicarbonate is less than 8 meq/L (pH less than 7.15) or when replacement with saline solution and insulin does not bring about a distinct increase in the plasma bicarbonate and pH by the sixth hour of therapy. It has been suggested (61, 62), but not definitely shown in studies of human beings (63, 64), that acidosis per se interferes with the action of insulin. If alkali is used, it can be given in varying amounts as an isotonic mixture of hypertonic (880 meq/L) sodium bicarbonate and one-half normal saline.

BLOOD, PLASMA, AND VOLUME EXPANDERS

Volume expanders such as blood, plasma, and isooncotic albumin have a definite place in the treatment of diabetic acidosis. It is imperative that severe hypotension and shock be corrected as rapidly as possible. If after the first hour of electrolyte and water replacement a sustained hypotension is not ameliorated, blood or plasma should be immediately administered. Shock secondary to fluid and electrolyte loss is more rapidly corrected when the blood or plasma accompanies the electrolyte and water replacement (86). It should be stressed that adrenergic substances such as norepinephrine or dopamine are not effective in correcting oligemic shock, and severe acidosis must be corrected to allow the circulatory system to respond to the patient's own endogenously produced catecholamines. Secondary hypotension or shock developing 4 to 8 h after initiating therapy usually indicates (1) rapid development of hypokalemia, (2) myocardial infarction, (3) overwhelming sepsis, or (4) gastrointestinal or internal hemorrhage.

GLUCOSE (AND FRUCTOSE) ADMINISTRATION

Glucose solutions with or without electrolytes should be initiated when the blood sugar has fallen to approximately 250 mg/dL. There is little point in administering glucose when the blood sugar level is still markedly elevated, for this will only potentiate the hyperglycemia and cellular dehydration and enhance glycosuria and renal salt and water loss. However, carbohydrate replacement is an integral part of the overall treatment of diabetic acidosis. The total body stores of carbohydrate are markedly diminished in spite of the hyperglycemia. In the average adult case of severe diabetic acidosis, approximately 50 g of carbohydrate is available in the extracellular fluid, whereas the total body depletion of glycogen stores may range from 200 to 400 g. It is not unusual during therapy to see the blood sugar decrease to hypoglycemic levels *without* an appreciable clearing of the plasma ketonemia. This is simply because when insulin is administered, the amount of glucose available in the extracellular fluids is rapidly utilized for glycogenesis but is inadequate to reverse the process of excessive ketogenesis.

It is appropriate at this point to discuss the present role, if any, of fructose in the treatment of diabetic acidosis (87, 88). This hexose, unlike glucose, does not require insulin for transcellular transport and can be used as a glucose substitute by all tissues, with the exception of the CNS. Once inside the cell, fructose enters an intermediary metabolic point that bypasses some of the early steps of the Emden-Myerhoff pathway required for glucose breakdown and utilization. Therefore, fructose can be utilized in a surprisingly normal manner in the insulin-requiring patient with uncontrolled diabetes. However, despite the theoretical benefits, fructose has five drawbacks to its use in the treatment of diabetic acidosis:

1. Fructose cannot be utilized by the central nervous system and therefore cannot correct the clinical manifestations of a hypoglycemic reaction. If fructose is used early in the treatment, it should be replaced by glucose solutions when the blood sugar has decreased significantly.
2. If fructose is infused at a rate much greater than 1 g/kg body weight per hour its metabolism causes a very rapid production of lactic and pyruvic acids (89). When these are liberated into the extracellular fluids, they may actually potentiate the acidosis in spite of clearing of all the plasma ketones. The authors have observed this phenomenon when treating mild diabetic acidosis with fructose solutions alone. This acidosis may also occur in nondiabetic subjects receiving fructose at the above rate (89).
3. Fructose is considerably more expensive than glucose as a replacement solution.
4. The two- to three-carbon fragments derived from fructose metabolism in the liver can be rapidly channeled into new glucose molecules which, in the absence of insulin, can be liberated into the circulation and contribute to the maintaining of hyperglycemia.
5. Fructose may be falsely measured as glucose in many of the presently utilized automated techniques for plasma sugar determination. In view of these qualifications, there seems no practical or beneficial reason for the use of fructose solutions as replacement therapy.

POTASSIUM REPLACEMENT

Potassium salts should be added to therapy when the blood sugar begins to decrease or when the electrocardiogram, blood pressure, or peripheral deep reflexes suggest a significant decrease in serum potassium. This occasionally may occur as early as 2 h after initiation of therapy if the patient shows a very prompt response, or rarely may be noted on the first electrocardiogram or blood specimen if potassium depletion is profound (90). Under these circumstances one must be prepared to administer potassium early, particularly if a secondary fall in blood pressure occurs. This emphasizes the importance of having an initial control electrocardiogram prior to, or shortly after, starting treatment in diabetic acidosis. In the authors' experience, potassium is usually begun 6 h after the initiation of therapy. Potassium is usually administered at a rate of 20 to 40 meq/h intravenously, if urinary flow is adequate. Otherwise, it may be given at somewhat less than 20 meq/h along with careful electrocardiographic monitoring. It is important to remember that potassium depletion itself can produce shock and that a patient in severe diabetic acidosis with anuria may still be profoundly potassium-depleted. Under these circumstances, this ion should still be administered to correct any marked electrocardiographic abnormalities or secondary hypotension if they should occur. Certainly, however, when in doubt, one should err on the low side in potassium replacement in the anuric or oliguric patient.

Potassium chloride is the salt that is usually administered in the treatment of diabetic acidosis. At times, as much as 200 to 300 meq is given during the first 24 h of therapy. Since the chloride ion is distributed primarily in the extracellular space while potassium moves to an intracellular site in exchange for hydrogen ion (see Chap. 3), potassium can actually potentiate a mild acidosis of a hyperchloremic type even after the ketonemia has been completely corrected. Potassium phosphate or potassium acetate salts do not produce this mild acidosis. The acetate ion is metabolized, and the phosphate ion moves into the intracellular site with potassium to replace the intracellular deficit of phosphate.

ORAL REPLACEMENTS

If a patient is conscious and lucid, has not been nauseated or been vomiting, and shows no evidence of gastric dilatation, he may be carefully started on liquid or soft small feedings and potassium-containing fluids such as dilute orange juice by mouth early in the course of therapy; otherwise, it is probably better to wait 12 to 24 h before introducing any form of oral replacement. The authors have not found that gastric aspiration is necessary in every patient with diabetic acidosis or coma. If the patient has shown clinical evidence of gastric dilatation, such as (1) profound vomiting, (2) left upper quadrant tympany with or without an obvious succussion splash, or (3) an emesis that has a coffee-grounds appearance or is oily in consistency, but is benzidine- or guaiac-negative, a Levin tube is inserted, the stomach is aspirated as completely as possible, and the tube may be left in place for 12 to 24 h.

MISCELLANEOUS MEASURES

A diabetic coma flow sheet should be put on the wall by the patient's bedside, and the recorded information should be as complete as possible. Fractional urine specimens are checked at hourly intervals for volume, specific gravity, qualitative sugar, and acetone. One must remember that the urinary acetone may still be 4 plus when the plasma has decreased virtually to zero by qualitative testing. In following the patient's course, the authors rely much more heavily on blood sugar, electrolytes and plasma acetone determinations than on measurements in the urine. The most important reason for collecting urine in diabetic acidosis is to measure its volume, or hourly output. This enables one to evaluate the magnitude of the continued urinary loss of fluid during corrective therapy. It is not unusual for a patient who has a deficit of 6 or 7 L to receive this volume in the first 12 h of therapy. During this time, the patient may excrete 5 of these 7 L because of the sustained glycosuria. If this is not known, a false impression of the net magnitude of the replacement will be obtained.

Specific gravity or, preferably, osmolality measurements on the urine samples are of physiologic interest and may be of some clinical value. Isosthenuria in the dehydrated, acidotic patient with sugar in the urine may indicate the presence of acute or chronic tubular injury. Secondly, if the patient has been receiving hypotonic replacement, the excretion of an obviously hypotonic urine (less than 200 mosm/L or specific gravity of less than 1.008) after continuous therapy indicates that hydration is complete. At this point, the patient with relatively normal kidneys responds to the hypotonic fluid with a characteristic water diuresis. Although large amounts of glucose in the urine may elevate the specific gravity, at this phase of therapy quantitative glucose output is usually quite low.

During recovery from diabetic coma or acidosis, the blood sugar, plasma ketones, and electrolytes should be measured every 2 h, and creatinine, urea, magnesium, and phosphorus at least every 4 h.

PATHOPHSIOLOGY AND CLINICAL ASPECTS OF HYPEROSMOLAR, HYPERGLYCEMIC, NONKETOACIDOTIC DIABETIC COMA

Warburg, in 1925, reported that diabetic coma (hyperglycemia and coma) could occur without acetonuria (91). Because the majority of these patients suffered from renal disease, he concluded that this biochemical syndrome was due to the reduced kidney function. It is of interest that some of these patients had neither hyperventilation (Kussmaul type) nor acetone on their breath. Since 1955, an increasing number of patients with marked alteration in their sensorium (stupor to coma) and extreme hyperglycemia, 800 mg/dL or more, but without ketoacidosis have been described (53, 54, 93–99). However, it must be emphasized that at least 50 percent of these patients have acidosis, albeit not ketoacidosis (52, 53).

CLINICAL ASPECTS

Although the majority of these patients are elderly, with either no previous diagnosis of diabetes or with very mild maturity-onset diabetes, hyperosmolar, hyperglycemic, nonketotic diabetic coma has been described on occasion even in young patients and children with insulin-dependent diabetes who previously had episodes of frank ketosis (95, 96) or in whom the diabetes was first discovered during the hyperosmolar coma (96). A precipitating factor can usually be documented as accompanying or preceding the hyperosmolar state: pancreatitis (97), pancreatic carcinoma (94), severe burns (98), corticosteroid therapy (99), peritoneal dialysis (100), hemodialysis (101), treatment with antimetabolites (102), administration of Dilantin (103), vascular disease, and infection (102). Hyperglycemia has also been reported in hypothermia (104). A common finding has been increased carbohydrate intake or total parenteral alimentation before the development of hyperglycemic coma in these patients; this may play an important role in the development of this syndrome (52, 53, 98, 103).

Frequently, polyuria, polydipsia, and loss of weight precede the gradual development of impairment of consciousness (lethargy to deep coma, depression, irritability, and hallucination), but these symptoms may be overshadowed by those of the associated illness. Furthermore, the syndrome may occur without excessive glycosuria and polyuria in burn patients with very large insensible (pulmonary and skin) water loss (105) and in patients with severe chronic renal failure during peritoneal dialysis (100). As the process progresses, the clinical syndrome will fall into two categories, hypovolemic and neurologic, both due to the intense hypertonic dehydration. In contrast to the usual diabetic coma with ketosis, fever may be found in a great percentage of these patients and was seen in all six children de-

scribed by Rubin et al. (96). This fever may be due to the associated complications (see above) and/or the effect on the CNS of the hypertonic dehydration per se. It is of interest that *hypothermia* is common in patients with sustained hypoglycemia.

Seizures and focal neurologic signs may be interpreted as cerebrovascular accidents, but the frequent reversibility of the neurologic symptoms, signs, and electroencephalographic abnormalities, with control of the metabolic imbalance (106), points to a direct relationship between the hyperosmolality and the neurologic findings (Table 24-7). At times, intracerebral and subarachnoid bleeding may occur, with or without a generalized hemorrhagic tendency (98). The bleeding is due to noninflammatory rupture of the capillaries secondary to the severe cellular dehydration (107).

Abdominal pain when present may be due either to an intra-abdominal complication or the uncontrolled metabolic state, as discussed in the previous section on diabetic acidosis.

It is significant that both acetone on the breath and Kussmaul's respiration are absent. Air hunger is reported as an unusual presenting symptom, but it probably occurs in patients with coexistent lactic acidosis or uremic acidosis (108).

LABORATORY FINDINGS

Marked hyperosmolality due to the water depletion, hyperglycemia, and, frequently, hypernatremia, associated with little or no ketoacidosis, are the common laboratory features. The extreme hyperglycemia is an obligatory finding, frequently reaching 1000 mg/dL, or more; a case in France

Table 24-7. Neurological symptoms and signs in hyperglycemic, hyperosmolar coma

TYPE	TOPOGRAPHICAL ORIGIN	CHARACTERISTICS
Alterations or loss of consciousness; hallucinations and other psychic disturbances	Cerebral cortex	Rarely absent; deep coma the rule
Focal dysfunction (aphasia, hemiparesis, unilateral hyperreflexia, and unilateral Babinski reflex)	Cerebral cortex	May be seen independently of seizures; may be prolonged (1 week)
Seizures	Cortex and/or thalamus	Focal as a rule; common
Hyperthermia	Hypothalamus	Very frequent

Source: From Maccario (106).

with a blood sugar level of 4800 mg/dL has been reported (109). Serum or plasma osmolality may be above 400 mosm/kg plasma water. If an osmometer is not available, the osmolality of the plasma can be estimated using a simple equation [Eq. (24-1)] (under Movements of Water and Solutes). Hypernatremia (greater than 145 meq/L) and hyperchloremia (greater than 107 meq/L) may or may not be present. Hypernatremia is obviously indicative of a greater degree of water depletion, for, as explained earlier, hyperglycemia per se causes hyponatremia due to osmotic withdrawal of water from the cells and dilution of the residual sodium in the extracellular fluid. A rise of 100 mg/dL in the measured plasma glucose is associated with a decrease in plasma sodium of approximately 1.6 meq/L. As the concentration of glucose increases in the extracellular fluid, it exerts an osmotic effect which draws water out of cells. The continuous osmotic equilibrium dampens the measured rise in plasma glucose so that a measured increase of 100 mg/dL actually reflects the addition of slightly more glucose to the plasma (about 102 mg/dL). As with ketoacidosis, despite the presence of normokalemia or occasionally hyperkalemia, potassium depletion of a serious degree is usually present. Elevated blood urea nitrogen level is indicative of organic and/or functional reduction of GFR, excessive back-diffusion of urea across the renal tubules due to the late oliguria, which leads to a greater decrease in urea than in creatinine clearance, and enhanced lean-tissue breakdown. Because of the back-diffusion of urea and the lean-tissue breakdown, blood urea nitrogen is frequently increased proportionately more than the serum creatinine, their ratio greatly exceeding the normal one of 10:1. While impaired renal blood flow secondary to the dehydration, hemoconcentration, and hypovolemia is a major cause of the reduced GFR, many of these patients have demonstrated underlying organic renal disease prior to the development of hyperosmolar nonketotic diabetic (HNKD) coma. This point has been stressed by Arieff and Carroll (52), and the renal disease may well contribute to the magnitude of the hyperglycemia. The hypovolemia also causes enough reduction in organ perfusion to cause tissue hypoxia with resulting lactic acidosis. However, plasma bicarbonate in the majority of cases is above 18 meq/L with blood pH near normal. Characteristically, the urine will show 4+ glycosuria with minimal, if any, ketonuria. The hematocrit, hemoglobin, and the polymorphonuclear leukocyte count are usually increased, the number of leukocytes at times approaching 50,000 per cubic millimeter. While hemoconcentration is readily explained by the degree of dehydration per se, other mechanisms must be involved in the polymorphonuclear leukocytosis. Plasma insulin levels in these patients

Table 24-8. Laboratory differential of a diabetic patient in coma

	KETOACIDOSIS	HYPEROSMOLAR	LACTIC ACIDOSIS	HYPOGLYCEMIC
Plasma				
Glycemia	$\uparrow\uparrow$	$\uparrow\uparrow\uparrow\uparrow$	$\uparrow$ or N	
Ketonemia	$+++$	—— *	—— *	——
pH	$\downarrow$	N	$\downarrow$	N
Bicarbonate	$\downarrow$	N	$\downarrow$	N
Lactic acid	N	N	$\uparrow$	N
[Na⁺]	$\downarrow$	$\uparrow$N or $\downarrow$	$\downarrow$ or N	N
[K⁺]	$\uparrow$ or N	$\uparrow$N or $\downarrow$	$\uparrow$ or N	N
Osmolality	$\uparrow$	$\uparrow\uparrow\uparrow$	N	N
Blood urea nitrogen	$\uparrow$	$\uparrow\uparrow$	$\uparrow$	N
Urine				
Glycosuria	$++++$	$++++$	$++++$ or ——	——
Ketonuria	$++++$	——	——	—— or $++$

—— = negative.

* At times, β-hydroxybutyric acid may be elevated in the plasma but is not detected by the Ketostix or Acetest methods (see earlier discussion).

are certainly low (5 to 30 μU/mL) for the degree of hyperglycemia but greater than the levels found in most patients with ketoacidosis (52, 53).

Table 24-8 summarizes the laboratory findings that may be of value in the differential diagnosis of comatose states associated with uncontrolled diabetes.

PATHOGENESIS (FIG. 24-9)

Hyperosmolality

The cause of the hyperosmolar state is identical to that described earlier in the chapter in the section on diabetic ketoacidosis, although the degree of water depletion or hypertonic dehydration is considerably greater (see Table 24-9). Due to the earlier depression of the sensorium in this older-age group of patients, they fail to "keep up" with their renal and extrarenal water losses by oral ingestion of water.

However, in many patients with this syndrome, the intense thirst often leads them to the excessive use of beverages containing carbohydrates (juices), and the blood sugar level rises further; in other cases, extreme hyperglycemia is caused by parenteral administration of hypertonic glucose solutions.

The presence of detectable insulin (52, 53, 109, 111) in the plasma of these patients suggests that prior to the development of the severe sustained hyperglycemia, the insulin levels may well have been significantly higher. Seltzer and Harris (112) have shown that in the patient with adult-onset diabetes, a continuous 7-day infusion of glucose, with sustained hyperglycemia, at first caused an increase in plasma insulin which later fell below the preinfusion concentration. In contrast, the normal controls maintained their increased levels of insulin throughout the infusion despite comparable degrees of hyperglycemia. This demonstrable "low insulin reserve" of the patient with

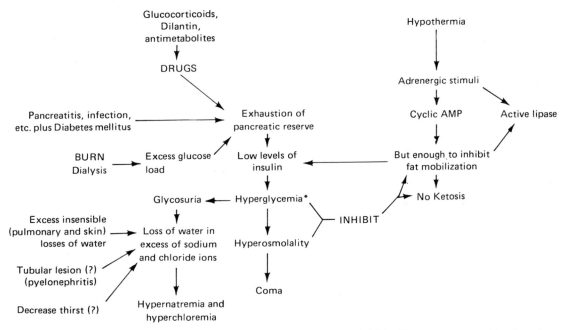

*Underlying renal disease with reduced GFR will cause a more rapid and greater rise in blood sugar by decreasing the renal "run-off" or glycosuria for any given increase in plasma glucose.

Figure 24-9. Physiopathology of hyperglycemic, hyperosmolar coma.

Table 24-9. Deficits of water and electrolytes in patients with nonketotic coma

	H_2O, L	Na^+, meq	K^+, meq
Mean	9.1	407	137
Range	4.8–12.6	152–664	42–242

	H_2O, mL/kg BODY WEIGHT	NA^+, meq/kg BODY WEIGHT	K^+, meq/kg BODY WEIGHT
Mean	119	5.3	1.8
Range	60–165	1.9–8.5	0.5–3.1

From Arieff (53).

adult-onset diabetes simply contributes to further hyperglycemia. Further, Mandell and Fellers (113) found, in infants and young children (2 to 36 months), that hypertonic (hypernatremic) dehydration associated with acute gastroenteritis caused hyperglycemia up to 685 mg/dL with apparent inappropriately low insulin response. The blood sugar levels returned to normal after correction of the dehydration. Antimetabolites (102) and Dilantin (103) may predispose to this syndrome by inhibiting insulin synthesis or secretion, glucocorticoids by increasing gluconeogenesis and decreasing peripheral utilization of glucose. Administration of large amounts of carbohydrate may also play a role in the severe hyperglycemia associated with islet-cell damage in burned patients (98). Hyperglycemia during hypothermia is associated with a decreased secretion of insulin. The latter may be due to an increased activity of the adrenergic nervous system, since in this condition adrenergic blocking agents allow insulin levels to rise and to be corrected (113a). The hyperosmolar and hyperglycemic state associated with peritoneal dialysis with hypertonic glucose solutions is discussed in detail in Chap. 12.

Nonketotic state

The absence of significant ketonemia and ketonuria in diabetic patients with concomitant marked hyperglycemia (> 800 mg/dL) must be due to either enhanced utilization or limited production of keto acids. The data available to date suggest the latter as the correct explanation (52, 53, 114).

There is little doubt that any effective level of circulating insulin will contribute significantly to the absence of ketosis. Zierler and Rabinowitz

(115) have shown that in the human forearm the amount of insulin necessary to promote glucose transport is ten times greater than that which inhibits fat mobilization. Since fat mobilization is required for ketone body production, it is possible to have a concentration of insulin which would allow dissociation of ketosis and hyperglycemia. The greater frequency of this syndrome in maturity-onset rather than growth-onset diabetes would be predicted since insulin levels are normal or elevated in the adult diabetic patient (116). Also, Seltzer and Harris (112) did not observe ketosis in spite of hyperglycemia and very low serum levels of insulin in diabetic patients during 7 days' continuous infusion of glucose. Mirsky et al. (117) demonstrated a direct relationship between blood glucose and glucose utilization and an inverse relationship between blood glucose and blood ketone levels, showing that hyperglycemia per se is antiketogenic (Fig. 24-10). Therefore, it is probable that the marked and prolonged hyperglycemia observed in the nonketotic hyperglycemic state can cause sufficient glucose utilization in the face of insulin insufficiency to prevent the development of ketosis. Finally, Gerich and associates (118) found that severe water deprivation in fasted rats, while leading to impaired glucose tolerance and hyperglycemia, actually inhibited both FFA mobilization from fat stores and ketone body production. They postulated a role of the hyperosmolar dehydration in the pathogenesis of HNKD coma.

COMA

The similarity between the neurologic disturbance in hyperglycemic and other hyperosmolar states suggests a common etiologic mechanism, and this has been discussed earlier in this chapter. Luse and Harris (119) have described the pathologic changes that may be seen by electron microscopy in association with severe hyperosmolar dehydration. These consist of massive shrinking of the oligodendroglial cytoplasm, decrease in oligodendroglial processes about the vessels, vacuolation of the endothelial cells, and increased density of the nerves.

THERAPY

In the authors' experience, these patients may need as little as 50 to as much as 500 units regular insulin the first 24 h (Fig. 24-11) administered by the method proposed earlier in this chapter. With respect to electrolyte and water replacement, the same principles also discussed earlier

apply to these patients with the exception that their average water requirements are twice those of the patient with nonhyperosmolar diabetic ketoacidosis (Fig. 24-6). If the patient is conscious and not vomiting, water may be administered by mouth; or, if he is unconscious, water may also be given per rectum. Ten or more liters may be necessary and must be pushed until a good state of hydration is achieved. Until this point is reached (12 to 24 h), the frequently observed early oliguria may persist.

While the mortality rate is high, early recognition and correct management may considerably reduce the mortality, since the metabolic alteration is potentially reversible.

After recovering from the acute episode, many of these patients return to a state of clinically mild diabetes mellitus, often controlled by diet alone. This indicates that after recovery these pa-

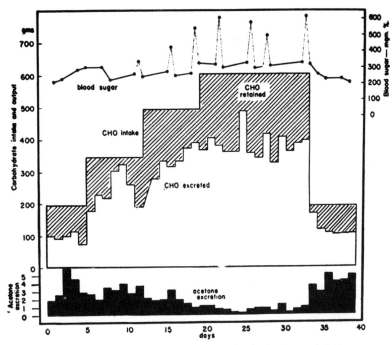

Figure 24-10. Effect of exogenous insulin deprivation and the influence of a high carbohydrate intake in an adult diabetic. The dashed lines off the blood sugar curve refer to the highest blood sugars observed during the day. Insulin administration was stopped at zero days.

tients have enough residual insulin secretory reserve to support their usual requirements (105, 120).

LACTIC ACIDOSIS

Stable diabetics usually have a normal plasma lactate (less than 1.5 meq/L), whereas 9 to 15 percent of acutely ill, acidotic diabetics have levels in excess of 5 meq/L (121, 53, 122, 123). This lactic acidosis, whether occurring alone or in combination with ketoacidosis, adds significantly to the morbidity and mortality of diabetes mellitus. An increased understanding of the biochem-

istry and physiology of lactic acid metabolism has emerged over the past several years. In the discussion that follows, these biochemical and physiologic principles will be used as a framework for the understanding of lactic acidosis in the diabetic.

PATHOPHYSIOLOGY

To understand the pathogenesis of lactic acidosis, one must first realize that cellular metabolism of lactic acid is inextricably linked with the metabolism of glucose, pyridine nucleotides, adenosine triphosphate (ATP) and pyruvic acid

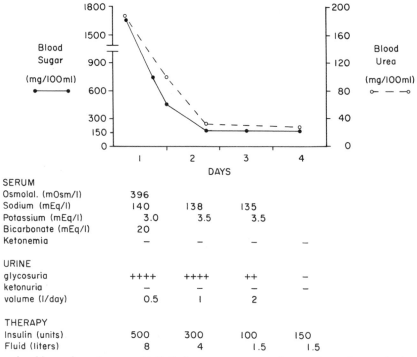

SERUM				
Osmolal. (mOsm/l)	396			
Sodium (mEq/l)	140	138	135	
Potassium (mEq/l)	3.0	3.5	3.5	
Bicarbonate (mEq/l)	20			
Ketonemia	−	−	−	−
URINE				
glycosuria	++++	++++	++	−
ketonuria	−	−	−	−
volume (l/day)	0.5	1	2	
THERAPY				
Insulin (units)	500	300	100	150
Fluid (liters)	8	4	1.5	1.5

Figure 24-11. An example of hyperglycemic coma. M. D. F., female, 52 years old, not previously known to be diabetic, mentioned polyuria and polydipsia for 15 days before admission and intake of about 5 to 6 L daily of sugar-containing soft drinks. She had been unconscious for 1 day. On admission she was comatose and extremely dehydrated, and her breathing was not acidotic. Blood pressure was 90/50 mmHg. Further physical examination was noncontributory. As can be seen in the figure, the patient had on admission severe hypoglycemia and high blood urea levels without acidosis or ketosis. She was treated with hypotonic saline (NaCl 0.45%) plus 800 units of regular insulin within the first 48 h. After recovery, the patient was discharged on a low-caloric diet and chlorpropamide (0.5 g daily).

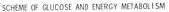

SCHEME OF GLUCOSE AND ENERGY METABOLISM

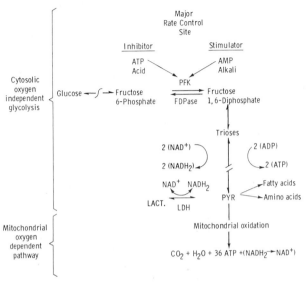

Figure 24-12. Scheme of anaerobic and aerobic glucose metabolism. Abbreviations: ATP = adenosine triphosphate; AMP = adenosine monophosphate; Lact = lactic acid; LDH = lactate dehydrogenase; NAD$^+$ = nicotine adenine dinucleotide, oxidized form; NADH$_2$ = nicotine adenine dinucleotide, reduced form; PYR = pyruvic acid; FDPase = fructose diphosphatase.

(Fig. 24-12). It appears that the cellular content of ATP plays a central role in this system, and that factors which alter its level may cause major acid-base changes.

Energy released during intermediary metabolism is captured and stored as ATP which, in turn, serves as the energy source for many vital cellular functions. The ability of ATP to inhibit several of the key enzymes of energy metabolism allows a negative-feedback loop to develop which stabilizes cellular energy reserves. In this system, a fall in ATP stimulates metabolic reactions which synthesize more of this high-energy phosphate. The phosphofructokinase (PFK) reaction (Fig. 24-12) is a major rate-limiting step in anaerobic glycolysis, and its activity increases when cellular ATP stores fall. The resulting increase in glycolysis generates 2 mmol each of ATP, pyruvic acid, and reduced pyridine nucleotide (NADH$_2$) for every mmol of glucose catabolized. In the presence of oxygen and mitochondria, py-

ruvic acid may be completely combusted to CO_2 and water, and in the process generate an additional 36 mmol of ATP. Mitochondria will also oxidize the NADH$_2$, thereby ensuring a steady supply of oxidized pyridine (NAD$^+$) thereby enabling glycolysis to continue unimpaired. Thus, the ATP yield and the efficiency of cellular energy metabolism is greatest in the presence of oxygen, which allows for the use of oxidative mitochondrial reactions.

As the supply of oxygen to tissues becomes limited, ATP production and NADH$_2$ oxidation switch from the highly efficient but oxygen-requiring mitochondrial processes to the inefficient but oxygen-independent cytosolic reactions. In order to maintain adequate rates of ATP production, anaerobic glycolysis must now increase markedly thereby greatly increasing the synthesis of pyruvic acid and NADH$_2$. The cytosolic enzyme lactate dehydrogenase (LDH), by catalyzing the conversion of pyruvic to lactic acid, also oxidizes $NADH_2$, thereby providing enough NAD^+ to allow glycolysis to continue unabated. Thus, lactic acidosis is the price which cells must pay in order to stabilize energy stores during hypoxia.

When the tissues are resupplied with oxygen, the LDH reaction regenerates pyruvic acid and $NADH_2$ from lactate and NAD^+. Aerobic mitochondrial reactions now oxidize pyruvate and $NADH_2$ and thereby replenish depleted tissue stores of ATP.

Extrahepatic tissues normally produce more pyruvic and lactic acid than can be catabolized by reactions other than LDH. By consequence, large amounts of these acids reach the circulation daily. Estimates made in man suggest that 1500 to 1900 mmol of lactate is turned over on a daily basis (124, 125). Net lactate production, however, is minimal since the liver takes up the vast bulk of lactate and metabolizes it to CO_2, water, and glucose. The bicarbonate consumed by lactic acid in the periphery is regenerated by the liver as it metabolizes the lactate. This balance between peripheral production and hepatic consumption not only plays a major role in glucose homeostasis, but also has vital implications for acid-base balance. If the liver were required to regenerate 1500 mmol/day of bicarbonate, severe acute or chronic liver disease ought to be associated with overwhelming lactic acidosis. That this fails to occur (126, 127) suggests that either lactate production decreases in liver failure or that other tissues are capable of assuming the liver's metabolic role.

The presence of hyperlacticemia always indicates an imbalance between lactate production and utilization. Serum lactate elevation may be caused by an increased rate of production which overwhelms consumption by the liver and other tissues or to a failure of utilization in the face of normal production. Combinations of excess production and decreased utilization, of course, may also be etiologic.

The etiology and prognosis of hyperlacticemia has been related to prevailing serum lactate/pyruvate (L/P) ratios. As originally proposed by Huckabee (128), elevations of serum lactate associated with increased serum L/P ratios reflected tissue hypoxia and augured a poor prognosis. This conclusion was based upon the following data and assumptions.

The diffusion of pyruvate and lactate into the ECF results in an L/P ratio of 4 to 10/1, under normal circumstances (129). Increments in pyruvate production, unassociated with tissue hypoxia, will result in proportionate elevations of serum lactate and pyruvate and a stable L/P ratio. Glucose and pyruvate infusions (129), and acute alkaloses (129) provide such examples. When hypoxia is present, the associated increase in $NADH_2$ increases the fraction of pyruvate converted to lactate (Fig. 24-12), thereby increasing the L/P ratio. Hypoxic lactic acidosis is generally far more ominous than the variety associated with normal tissue oxygen utilization. The significance of the L/P ratio has been lessened, however, by recent observations indicating that an increased ratio may occur in a variety of situations in which tissue oxygenation is normal. Inspection of Eq. (24-2) shows that hydrogen ions are

$$Pyr^- + NADH_2$$
$$+ H^+ \overset{LDH}{\rightleftharpoons} Lact^- + NAD^+ \qquad (24\text{-}2)$$

reactants in the LDH reaction. Thus, in severe acidosis, the plethora of hydrogen ions will, by mass action, shift the reaction to the right, thereby increasing the L/P ratio. Several aerobic metabolic reactions, like the oxidation of fat and alcohol, generate abundant amounts of $NADH_2$. The increase in the steady-state level of $NADH_2$ induces a similar increase in the L/P ratio, despite normal tissue oxygenation.

In general, the cause of lactic acidosis is usually apparent and little additional clinical benefit accrues from the measurement of pyruvate and calculation of the L/P ratio. Patients with idiopathic lactic acidosis, as originally described by Huckabee (130), whose acidosis cannot be attributed to any recognized cause, must be extremely rare. Fulop has recently questioned whether lactic acidosis is ever idiopathic (131).

MAJOR CAUSES OF LACTIC ACIDOSIS IN DIABETICS

Patients with diabetes mellitus are not immune to any of the causes of lactic acidosis which are detailed in Chap. 6. There is no convincing evidence, however, to suggest that any metabolic defect exists in diabetes which sensitizes patients to this disease. The tolerance of diabetics to lactate infusions or to the lactic acidosis of exercise is no different from that of normal controls (132). There are, however, three conditions, frequently found in diabetes, which may cause lactic acidosis. These complicating events are fructose therapy (also see earlier discussion), shock, and phenformin ingestion.

Fructose

Unlike glucose, which must pass through the rate-limiting PFK reaction, fructose enters the glycolytic pathway at the triose level (Fig. 24-12). By entering the metabolic scheme at a point beyond the major rate-limiting step, fructose is more freely converted to pyruvate and lactate. Moreover, the rapid phosphorylation of fructose in the liver decreases hepatic ATP levels, resulting in enhanced glycolysis and lactic acid production (133). When given rapidly (0.5 g/kg/h), fructose can cause the plasma lactate concentration to increase by 3 to 5 meq/L. In normal subjects, this will have only minor effects on acid-base balance since serum bicarbonate will fall to only 20 to 22 meq/L. Patients in profound ketoacidosis, however, are far more sensitive to a 3 to 5 meq/L fall in bicarbonate. As illustrated in Table 24-6, a typical patient with severe ketoacidosis may have an initial serum bicarbonate of 5 meq/L. A 3 meq/L fall, consequent to fructose therapy, would lower this patient's pH to less than 7.0. Because of its acidifying potential and for the reasons already stated (see earlier discussion), the authors do not recommend the use of fructose in the therapy of diabetic ketoacidosis.

Hypotension and shock

The acidemia and profound fluid and electrolyte losses that attend diabetic ketoacidosis commonly cause hypotension and shock. The tissue hypoxia that results will compromise pyruvate oxidation and cause lactic acidosis. In addition to stimulating lactic acid production, the hypoxia will shift acetoacetic acid to β-hydroxybutyric acid, thereby making the diagnosis of ketoacidosis difficult. The superimposition of lactic acidosis on an es-

tablished ketoacidosis can acutely lower pH to catastrophic levels.

Phenformin therapy

Many cases of lactic acidosis have been reported in diabetics taking oral hypoglycemic biguanides (134). Phenformin is the class of biguanide most extensively marketed in the United States and most frequently implicated in lactic acidosis. Absolute proof linking phenformin to this disorder is still wanting; however, available data are so incriminating that a cause-and-effect relationship is difficult to avoid. A brief review of this evidence follows.

1. Cohen and Woods (122) have shown that in 34 patients with phenformin-associated lactic acidosis, in whom the duration of phenformin therapy was noted, 24 (71 percent) developed their acidosis within 2 months of initiating therapy.
2. A number of reports have shown that an overdose of phenformin can cause severe lactic acidosis in nondiabetics (135–138).
3. Blood levels of phenformin have been extremely elevated in all acidotic patients in whom they were measured (122, 139).
4. Phenformin appears to diminish lactate tolerance in humans. Infusions of sodium lactate or the generation of endogenous lactate with alcohol or exercise results in higher peak serum lactate levels and a slower decline when examined following the ingestion of phenformin (140).
5. The mechanism by which phenformin lowers blood sugar remains controversial. The inhibition of oxidative metabolism, the inhibition of gluconeogenesis, and the inhibition of GI absorption of glucose are three current postulates for which there are extensive experimental support (141, 142, 143). These metabolic derangements could stimulate lactic acid production by muscle and impair its utilization by liver and thereby result in elevated serum lactate levels.
6. Finally, the large number of cases being reported in diabetics becomes persuasive especially when no other cause of lactic acidosis,

other than phenformin ingestion, is apparent (144).

The authors believe that the weight of available evidence strongly suggests that phenformin promotes lactic acidosis in diabetics. The incidence of phenformin-associated lactic acidosis is difficult to assess. In a prospective analysis of 204 patients taking the drug, 3 developed lactic acidosis (145). If this figure is substantiated, phenformin could account for more than 1000 deaths annually (146).

Phenformin is catabolized and excreted by the liver and kidney (147). Its excretion, which depends upon glomerular filtration and tubular secretion, decreases early in the course of renal failure (148). It has been argued that an intercurrent illness, e.g., myocardial infarction or dehydration, decreases phenformin catabolism and excretion, resulting in increasing plasma concentrations. In a manner analogous to the lactic acidosis associated with phenformin overdose, the elevated plasma levels, perhaps in combination with compromised tissue perfusion, leads to lactic acidosis. Much more work remains, however, before final clarification of the mechanism of lactic acidosis takes place.

CLINICAL AND LABORATORY FINDINGS

The clinical presentation is similar to diabetic ketoacidosis. Progressive dyspnea, abdominal pain, nausea and vomiting with diminishing state of consciousness characterize the clinical picture. Signs of dehydration and extracellular fluid volume contraction are found in 50 to 65 percent of patients (134). Hypothermia, with rectal temperatures less than 36.5°C, were found in approximately half of the patients reviewed by Dembo et al. (134). Laboratory data are consistent with a severe, high anion gap metabolic acidosis in which arterial pH is commonly below 7.10. The plasma lactate is generally well in excess of 10 meq/L and the L/P ratio will often exceed 50. The altered redox state will also elevate the β-hydroxybutyric acid/acetoacetic acid ratio (see above), making the diagnosis of any associated ketosis difficult. Thus, short of doing a specific test for β-hydroxy-

butyric acid, there is no way for the clinician to be absolutely certain that he is not dealing with a mixed keto-lactic acidosis. Blood sugar is usually normal but occasionally may reach frankly hypoglycemic levels. The white blood cell count is frequently elevated along with the blood urea nitrogen and creatinine, as expected in dehydrated, acidotic patients.

DIAGNOSIS AND THERAPY

The diagnosis of pure lactic acidosis or mixed keto-lactic acidosis ultimately depends upon demonstration of increased plasma levels of lactic acid. Since an acidosis is defined as a *process* which generates acid, without regard to the prevailing pH of blood or to the amount of acid accumulated, any elevation of lactate, in the strictest sense, represents lactic acidosis. The *significance* of lactic acid accumulation, however, is related to the plasma concentration as well as to the prevailing level of plasma bicarbonate. It should be apparent, for example, that the significance of a 2.5 meq/L increase in plasma lactate will be vastly different when superimposed upon a normal serum bicarbonate concentration from when it develops in a ketoacidotic patient whose serum bicarbonate had been 5.0 meq/L (Table 24-6).

The presence of lactic acidosis may be suspected in severely acidotic diabetics whose serum ketones are negative or only weakly positive. Life-threatening ketosis may still be the major metabolic abnormality, but some degree of lactic acidosis is usually also present.

The prognosis for phenformin-associated lactic acidosis is poor, with an expected mortality of 42 to 66 percent (134, 139, 144). This far exceeds the mortality in ketoacidosis and probably relates to the older age of the patients taking phenformin. The more severe acidemia and the absence of therapeutic agents that can dramatically reverse lactic acid production the way that insulin reverses ketoacid production in ketoacidosis also play important roles. The three main principles which underlie therapy of this disorder are (1) attempt to decrease net lactic acid production, (2) provide enough alkali to prevent the adverse hemodynamic effects of acidemia, (3) prevent volume overload which attends $NaHCO_3$ therapy by use of diuretics or dialysis.

Since many of these patients are dehydrated and hypotensive when initially seen, a component of hypoxic lactic acidosis may be present in addition to that induced by phenformin. The judicious use of oxygen and volume expansion with bicarbonate-containing solutions (see below) can be lifesaving at this stage.

We recommend early use of parenteral insulin to treat this disorder. As previously discussed, profound lactic acidosis can completely mask an associated ketosis, and since a significant number of these patients are also ketotic (133, 139, 144), the use of insulin is critical to their management. If plasma β-hydroxybutyric acid levels are normal or if the patient's elevated anion gap is totally explained by the plasma lactate, insulin therapy may be discontinued. There is some evidence, however, to suggest that insulin therapy may also decrease lactic acid production. Lactic acid is not only produced from glucose, but certain amino acids may also serve as precursors. Insulin can decrease the release of these amino acids from muscle and thereby decrease lactic acid production (149). Moreover, insulin may also stimulate the activity of pyruvate dehydrogenase, thereby stimulating pyruvate and lactate oxidation. The evidence supporting a therapeutic role for insulin in decreasing net lactic acid production is presently only suggestive. The mortality of phenformin-associated lactic acidosis is so high that the potential benefits from insulin therapy should be considered in all patients regardless of whether ketosis is present or not. Since patients are usually not hyperglycemic, enough glucose must be given with the insulin to prevent hypoglycemia. The dosage of parenteral insulin is the same as recommended for ketoacidosis (see earlier discussion).

Sodium bicarbonate should be infused at rates sufficient to maintain arterial pH greater than or equal to 7.15. After initial loading doses, a sustaining infusion of 146 meq/L $NaHCO_3$ (four 50-mL ampuls of $NaHCO_3$ added to 1000 mL 5% dextrose in water) is used to maintain the desired pH. Rates of infusion must be individualized, and the physician must be prepared to quickly alter this rate depending upon the arterial pH and bicarbonate. It is not unusual for patients to require more than 100 meq of $NaHCO_3$ per hour. As lactic acid production declines and hourly bicarbonate requirements diminish, it is important to discontinue bicarbonate therapy even though the patient's serum level has risen to only 10 to 15 meq/L. At this stage, as the presumed effects of phenformin are disappearing, the patient begins to metabolize serum lactate to bicarbonate. The two factors which determine what the final serum bicarbonate concentration will be are the amount of administered $NaHCO_3$ that is retained and the amount of bicarbonate resynthesized from lactate. During the induction of acidosis, each 1 meq of titrated bicarbonate is replaced by 1 meq of lactate. If only trivial amounts of lactate are lost in the urine, catabolism of the retained amount should normalize the serum bicarbonate. Thus, a metabolic alkalosis often develops due to additive effects of the administered and retained $NaHCO_3$ and to the bicarbonate resynthesized from lactate. This alkalosis may be minimized if exogenous $NaHCO_3$ is discontinued early and the patient is allowed to increase his serum bicarbonate by metabolizing his lactate. Continued hyperventilation will add a respiratory component to the alkalosis. Acetazolamide (250 to 500 mg oral or intravenous) may be helpful in restoring plasma volume and serum bicarbonate.

Volume overload and congestive heart failure frequently result from the very large loads of $NaHCO_3$ required to treat this disorder. This complication can be avoided by the judicious use of potent diuretics or dialysis in patients with impaired renal function.

Furosemide or ethacrynic acid should be used only after the physician is certain that initial volume depletion has been repaired. At this point, diuretics should be given in amounts sufficient to cause sodium and water losses equivalent to the quantity being given by vein. The NaCl diuresis will ensure that sufficient "space" remains available for the needed alkali. One should anticipate using intravenous doses of 40 to 100 mg of diuretic every 1 to 2 h. The sodium chloride losses of 50 to 100 meq/L and potassium losses of 20 to 30 meq/L and urine volumes of 0.5 to 1.5 L/h may be achieved. The sodium lost in the urine may be replaced as the bicarbonate salt, while urinary potassium losses may be replaced hourly as KCl. Careful hemodynamic measurements must be followed along with hourly serum and urinary electrolytes.

Those patients whose renal function does not permit the use of diuretics must be treated with dialysis. Dialysis should not be used until it becomes apparent that volume overload will develop without it. Fluid may be removed and alkali given via the dialysis bath, while additional $NaHCO_3$ may be given by vein, in replacement of the fluid removed by dialysis. The standard dialysis bath uses lactate as its source of alkali, and, therefore, is an inappropriate choice for therapy of this disorder. The pharmacy can make 2-L dialysis fluid containing 135 meq/L of Na, 30 meq/L of K, 95 meq/L of Cl, 40 meq/L of HCO_3, and 1.5 to 4.5% glucose. Calcium cannot be added since it precipitates with bicarbonate.

There are presently no data defining the dialyzability of phenformin. If it turns out that the drug can be removed by dialysis, earlier use of this therapeutic modality may become indicated.

REFERENCES

1. Hockaday, T. D. R., and K. G. M. Alberti: Diabetic coma, *Clin. Endocrinol. Metabol.*, **1**(3):751, 1972.
2. Muller, W. A., G. R. Faloona, and R. H. Unger: Hyperglucagonemia in diabetic ketoacidosis, *Am. J. Med.*, **54**:52, 1973.
3. Gerich, J. E., E. Tsalikian, M. Lorenzi, J. H. Karam, and D. M. Bier: Plasma glucagon and alanine responses to acute insulin deficiency in man, *J. Clin. Endocrinol. Metab.*, **40**:526, 1975.
4. Alberti, K. G. M. M., N. J. Christensen, J. Iversen, and H. Orskov: Role of glucagon and other hormones in development of diabetic ketoacidosis, *Lancet*, **2**:1307, 1975.
5. Felig, P., J. Wahren, R. Sherwin, and R. Hendler: Insulin, glucagon, and somatostatin in normal physiology and diabetes mellitus, *Diabetes*, **25**:1091, 1976.

6. Butler, A. M., N. B. Talbot, C. H. Burnett, J. R. Stanbury, and E. A. McLachlan: Metabolic studies in diabetic coma, *Trans. Assoc. Am. Physicians*, **60**:102, 1947.
7. Jacobs, H. S., and J. D. N. Nabarro: Plasma II-hydroxycorticosteroid and growth hormone levels in acute medical illnesses, *Br. Med. J.*, **2**:595, 1969.
8. Butler, A. M.: Parenteral fluid therapy in diabetic coma, *Acta Paediatr. Scand.*, **38**:59, 1949.
9. Makoff, D. L., J. A. DaSilva, B. J. Rosenbaum, et al.: Hypertonic expansion, acid-base and electrolyte changes, *Am. J. Physiol.*, **218**:1201, 1970.
10. Zierler, K. L.: Effect of insulin on potassium efflux from rat muscle in the presence and absence of glucose, *Am. J. Physiol*, **198**:1066, 1960.
11. Hiatt, N., T. Yamakawa, and M. B. Davidson: Necessity for insulin in the transfer of excess infused K^+ to intracellular fluid, *Metabolism*, **23**:43, 1973.
12. Goldfarb, S., M. Cox, I. Singer, and M. Goldberg: Acute hyperkalemia induced by hyperglycemia. Hormonal mechanisms, *Ann. Intern. Med.*, **84**:426, 1976.
13. Christlieb, A. R., J.-P. Assal, N. Katsilambros, G. H. Williams, G. P. Kozak, and T. Suzuki: Plasma renin activity and blood volume in uncontrolled diabetes. Ketoacidosis, a state of secondary aldosteronism, *Diabetes*, **24**:190, 1975.
14. Sneyd, J. G. T., J. D. Corbin, and C. R. Park: The role of cyclic AMP in the action of insulin, in N. Back, L. Martini, and R. Paoletti (eds.), *Pharmacology of Hormonal Polypeptides and Proteins*, Plenum Press, New York, 1968, p. 367.
15. Kopec, B., and I. B. Fritz: Comparison of properties of carnitine palmityltransferase II, and preparation of antibodies to carnitine palmotyltransferases. *J. Biol. Chem.*, **248**:4069, 1973.
16. McGarry, J. D., and D. W. Foster: Ketogenesis and its regulation, *Am. J. Med.*, **61**:9, 1976.
17. Krebs, H. A.: Rate control of the tricarboxylic acid cycle, *Adv. Enzyme Regul.*, **8**:335, 1970.
18. Sulway, M. J., and J. M. Malins: Acetone in diabetic ketoacidosis, *Lancet*, **2**:736, 1970.
19. Emmett, M., and R. G. Narins: Clinical use of the anion gap, *Medicine (Baltimore)*, **56**:38, 1977.
20. Balasse, E. D., and R. J. Havel: Turnover rate and oxidation of ketone bodies in normal and diabetic dogs, *Diabetologia*, **6**:36, 1970.

21. Wildenhoff, K. E.: Blood ketone body disappearance rate in diabetics and normals after rapid infusion of DL-3-hydroxybutyrate, studies before and after diabetic treatment, *Acta Med. Scand.*, **200**:79, 1976.

22. Major, R. H.: *Classic Description of Disease*, Charles C Thomas, Publisher, Springfield, Ill., 1959, p. 247.

23. Pierce, N. F., D. S. Fedson, R. C. Brigham, R. C. Mitra, R. B. Sack, and A. Mondal: The ventilatory response to acute base deficit in humans, *Ann. Intern. Med.*, **72**:633, 1970.

24. Albert, M. S., R. B. Dell, and R. W. Winters: Quantitative displacement of acid-base equilibrium in metabolic acidosis, *Ann. Intern. Med.*, **66**:312, 1967.

25. Atchley, D. W., R. F. Loeb, D. W. Richards, Jr., E. M. Benedict, and M. E. Driscoll: On diabetic acidosis, *J. Clin. Invest.*, **12**:297, 1933.

26. Lemieux, G., P. Vinay, P. Robitaille, G. E. Plante, Y. Lussier, and P. Martin: The effect of ketone bodies on renal ammoniagenesis, *J. Clin. Invest.*, **50**:1781, 1971.

27. Lipsky, S. R., B. J. Alper, M. E. Rubini, W. F. Van Eck, and M. E. Gordon: The effects of alkalosis upon ketone body production and carbohydrate metabolism in man, *J. Clin. Invest.*, **33**:1269, 1954.

28. Simmons, D. H., J. Nicoloff, and L. B. Guze: Hyperventilation and respiratory alkalosis as signs of gram negative bacteremia, *JAMA*, **197**:2196, 1960.

29. Alberti, K. G. M. M., and T. D. R. Hockaday: Rapid blood ketone body estimation in the diagnosis of diabetic ketoacidosis, *Br. Med. J.*, **2**:565, 1972.

30. Munro, J. F., I. W. Campbell, A. C. McCuish, and L. J. P. Duncan: Euglycemic diabetic ketoacidosis, *Br. Med. J.*, **2**:578, 1973.

31. Hadden, J. W., and R. T. Metzner: Pseudoketosis and hyperacetaldehydemia in paraldehyde acidosis, *Am. J. Med.*, **47**:642, 1969.

32. Ashkar, F. S., and R. Miller: Hospital ketosis in the alcoholic diabetic, a syndrome due to isopropyl alcohol intoxication, *South Med. J.*, **64**:1409, 1971.

33. Fulop, M., and H. D. Hoberman: Alcoholic ketosis, *Diabetes*, **24**:785, 1975.

34. Howell, R. F., D. M. Ashton, and J. B. Wyngaarden: Glucose-6-phosphatase deficiency glycogen storage disease. Studies on the interrelationships of carbohydrate lipid and purine abnormalities, *Pediatrics*, **29**:553, 1962.

35. Warshaw, A. L., E. R. Feller, and K. Lee: On the cause of raised serum amylase for diabetic ketoacidosis, *Lancet*, **1**:929, 1977.

36. Finn, R., and S. Cope: The plasma amylase in diabetic coma, *Diabetes*, **12**:2, 141, 1963.

37. Warshaw, A. L., and A. F. Fuller: Specificity of increased renal clearance of amylase in diagnosis of acute pancreatitis, *N. Engl. J. Med.*, **292**:325, 1975.

38. Butler, A. M.: Diabetic coma, *N. Engl. J. Med.*, **243**(17):648, 1950.

39. Atchley, D. W., R. F. Loeb, D. W. Richards, Jr., E. M. Benedict, and M. E. Driscoll: A detailed study of electrolyte balances following the withdrawal and reestablishment of insulin therapy, *J. Clin. Invest.*, **12**:297, 1933.

40. Franks, M., R. F. Berris, N. O. Kaplan, and G. B. Meyers: Metabolic studies in diabetic acidosis. II. Effect of administration of sodium phosphate, *Arch. Intern. Med.*, **81**:42, 1948.

41. Nabarro, J. D. N., A. G. Spencer, and J. M. Stowers: Metabolic studies in severe diabetic ketosis, *Q. J. Med.*, **21**:225, 1952.

42. Ruebi, F. C.: Glomerular filtration rate, renal blood flow and blood viscosity during and after diabetic coma, *Circ. Res.*, **1**:410, 1953.

43. Porte, D.: Sympathetic regulation of insulin secretion, its relation to diabetes mellitus, *Arch. Intern. Med.*, **123**:252, 1969.

44. Cerchio, G. M., P. A. Persico, and H. Jeffey: Inhibition of insulin release during hypovolemic shock, *Metabolism*, **22**:1449, 1973.

45. Franks, M., R. F. Berris, N. O. Kaplan, and G. B. Meyers: Metabolic studies in diabetic acidosis. II. Effect of administration of sodium phosphate, *Arch. Intern. Med.*, **81**:42, 1948.

46. Guest, G. M., and S. Rapaport: Organic acid soluble phosphorus compounds of the blood, *Physiol. Rev.*, **21**:41, 1941.

47. Lee, D. B. N., and C. R. Kleeman: Phosphorus depletion in man, in G. Banks (ed.), McGaw Medical Monographs, November 1976.

48. Klock, J. C., H. E. Williams, and W. C. Mentzer:

Hemolytic anemia and somatic cell dysfunction in severe hypophosphatemia, *Arch. Intern. Med.,* **134:**360, 1974.

49. Craddock. P. R., Y. Yaivata, L. Van Senten, et al.: Acquired phagocyte dysfunction. A complication of the hypophosphatemia of parenteral hyperalimentation, *N. Engl. J. Med.,* **290:**1403, 1974.

50. Fulop, M., H. Tannenbaum, and N. Dreyer: Ketotic hyperosmolar coma, *Lancet,* **2:**635, 1973.

51. Posner, J. B., and F. Plum: Spinal-fluid pH and neurologic symptoms in systemic acidosis, *N. Engl. J. Med.,* **277:**605, 1967.

52. Arieff, A. I., and H. J. Carroll: Nonketotic hyperosmolar coma with hyperglycemia: Clinical features, pathophysiology, renal function, acid-base balance, plasma-cerebrospinal fluid equilibria and the effects of therapy in 37 cases, *Medicine (Baltimore),* **51:**73, 1972.

53. Arieff, A. I.: Kidney, water, and electrolyte metabolism in diabetis mellitus, in B. M. Brenner and F. C. Rector (eds.), *The Kidney,* W. B. Saunders Company, Philadelphia, 1976, vol. II, p. 1257.

54. Fitzgerald, M. G., D. J. O'Sullivan, and J. M. Malins: Fatal diabetic ketosis, *Br. Med. J.,* **1:**247, 1961.

55. Young, E., and R. F. Bradley: Cerebral edema with irreversible coma in severe diabetic ketoacidosis, *N. Engl. J. Med.,* **276:**12, 1967.

56. Fulop, M.: Cerebral edema in severe diabetic ketoacidosis, *N. Engl. J. Med.,* **276:**1445, 1967.

57. Arieff, A. I., and C. R. Kleeman: Studies on the mechanisms of cerebral edema in diabetic comas. I. Effect of hyperglycemia and rapid lowering of plasma glucose in normal rabbits, *J. Clin. Invest.,* **52:**571, 1973.

58. Arieff, A. I., and C. R. Kleeman: Cerebral edema in diabetic comas. II. Effects of hyperosmolality, hyperglycemia and insulin in diabetic rabbits, *J. Clin. Endocrinol. Metab.,* **38:**1057, 1974.

59. Smith, K., and H. E. Martin: Response of diabetic coma to various insulin dosages, *Diabetes,* **3:**287, 1954.

60. Shaw, C. E., Jr., G. E. Hurwitz, M. Schmukler, S. H. Brager, and S. P. Bessman: A clinical and laboratory study of insulin dosage in diabetic acidosis: Comparison with small and large doses, *Diabetes,* **2:**23, 1962.

61. Walker, B. B., D. N. Phear, F. I. R. Martin, and C. W. Baird: Inhibition of insulin by acidosis, *Lancet,* **2:**964, 1963.

62. Mackler, B., H. Lichenstein, and G. M. Guest: Effects of ammonium chloride acidosis on the action of insulin in dogs, *Am. J. Physiol.,* **166:**191, 1951.

63. Genuth, S. M.: Constant intravenous insulin infusion in diabetic ketoacidosis, *JAMA,* **223:**1348, 1973.

64. Moseley, J.: Diabetic crises in children treated with small doses of intramuscular insulin, *Br. Med. J.,* **1:**59, 1975.

65. Hannan, T. J., and G. M. Stathers: Constant low-dose insulin infusion in severe diabetes mellitus, *Med. J. Aust.,* **1:**11, 1976.

66. Campbell, L. V., L. Lazarus, J. H. Casey, and E. W. Kraegen: Routine use of low-dose intravenous insulin infusion in severe hyperglycemia, *Med. J. Aust.,* **2:**519, 1976.

67. Kitabchi, A. E., V. Ayyagari, S. M. O. Guerra, and Medical House Staff: The efficacy of low-dose vs. conventional therapy of insulin for treatment of diabetic ketoacidosis, *Ann. Intern. Med.,* **84:**633, 1976.

68. Alberti, K. G. M. M., T. D. R. Hockaday, and R. C. Turner: Small doses of intramuscular insulin in the treatment of diabetic coma, *Lancet,* **2:**515, 1973.

69. Stenvert, L. S., M. D. Drop, J. M. Bertrand, M. D. Duvald-Arnould, A. E. Gober, J. H. Hersheh, M. D. McEnergy, and H. C. Knowles: Low dose intravenous insulin infusion vs. subcutaneous insulin injections: A controlled comparative study of diabetic ketoacidosis, *Pediatrics,* **59:**733–738, 1977.

70. Kaufman, I. A., M. A. Keller, and W. L. Nyhan: Diabetic ketosis and acidosis: The continuous infusion of low doses of insulin, *J. Pediatr.,* **87:**846, 1975.

71. Cristensen, N. J., and H. Orskov: The relationship between endogenous serum insulin concentration and glucose uptake in the forearm muscles of nondiabetics, *J. Clin. Invest.,* **47:**1262, 1968.

72. Peterson, L., J. Caldwell, and J. Hoffman: Insulin absorbance to polyvinylchloride surfaces with implications for constant-infusion therapy, *Diabetes,* **25:**72, 1976.

73. Wildenthal, K.: The effects of acid-base disturbances on cardiovascular and pulmonary function, *Kidney Int.*, **1**:375, 1972.

74. Wildenthal, K., D. S. Mierzwiak, R. W. Myers, in human blood, *J. Appl. Physiol.*, **12**:485, 1958. on left ventricular performance, *Am. J. Physiol.*, **214**:1352, 1968.

75. Relman, A. S.: Metabolic consequences of acid-base disorders, *Kidney Int.*, **1**:347, 1972.

76. Halperin, M. L., H. P. Connors, A. S. Relman, and M. L. Karnovsky: Factors that control the effect of pH on glycolysis in leukocytes, *J. Biol. Chem.*, **244**:384, 1969.

77. Hems, R., B. D. Ross, M. N. Berry, and H. A. Krebs: Gluconeogenesis in the perfused rat liver, *Biochem. J.*, **101**:284, 1966.

79. Ohman, J. L., Jr., E. B. Marliss, T. T. Aoki, C. S. Munichoodappa, V. V. Kahnna, and G. P. Kozak: The cerebrospinal fluid in diabetic ketoacidosis, *N. Engl. J. Med.*, **284**:382, 1971.

79. Assal, J., T. T. Aoki, F. M. Manzano, and G. P. Kozak: Metabolic effects of sodium bicarbonate in management of diabetic ketoacidisos, *Diabetes*, **23**:405, 1974.

80. Severinghaus, J. W.: Oxyhemoglobin dissociation curve correction for temperature and pH variation in human blood, *J. Appl. Physiol.*, **12**:485, 1958.

81. Chanutin, A., and R. R. Churnish: Effect of organic and inorganic phosphates on oxygen equilibrium of human erythrocytes, *Arch. Biochem. Biophys.*, **121**:96, 1967.

82. Kanter, Y., J. R. Gerson, and A. N. Bessman: 2, 3 Diphosphoglycerate, nucleotide phosphate, organic and inorganic phosphate levels during the early phases of diabetic ketoacidosis, *Diabetes*, **26**:429–433, 1977.

83. Bellingham, A. J., J. C. Detter, and C. Lenfant: Regulatory mechanisms of hemoglobin-oxygen affinity in acidosis and alkalosis, *J. Clin. Invest.*, **50**:700, 1971.

84. Munk, P., M. H. Freedman, H. Levison, and R. M. Ehrlich: Effect of bicarbonate on oxygen transport in juvenile diabetic ketoacidosis, *J. Pediatr.*, **84**:510, 1974.

85. Schwartz, W. B., and W. C. Waters: Lactate vs. bicarbonate, *Am. J. Med.*, **32**:831, 1962.

86. Winkler, A. W., T. S. Danowski, and J. R. Elkinton: Role of colloid and of saline in treatment of shock, *J. Clin. Invest.*, **25**:220, 1946.

87. Miller, M., W. R. Drucker, J. E. Owens, J. W. Craig, and H. Woodward, Jr.: Metabolism of intravenous fructose and glucose in normal and diabetic subjects, *J. Clin. Invest.*, **31**:115, 1952.

88. Darragh, J. H., R. A. Womersley, and W. H. Meroney: Fructose in the treatment of diabetic ketosis, *J. Clin. Invest.*, **32**:1214, 1953.

89. Bergstrom, J., E. Hultman, and A. E. Roch-Norland: Lactic acid accumulation in connection with fructose infusion, *Acta Med. Scand.*, **184**:359, 1968.

90. Abramson, E., and R. Arky: Diabetic acidosis with initial hypokalemia, *JAMA*, **195**:115, 1966.

91. Warburg, E: Diabetic coma with uremia, *Acta Med. Scand.*, **61**:301, 1925.

92. Sament, S., and M. B. Schwartz: Severe diabetic stupor without ketosis, *S. Afr. Med. J.*, **31**:893, 1957.

93. Danowski, T. S., and J. D. N. Nabarro: Hyperosmolar and other types of nonketoacidotic coma in diabetes, *Diabetes*, **14**:162, 1965.

94. Jackson, W. P. U., and R. Forman: Hyperosmolar nonketotic diabetic coma, *Diabetes*, **15**:714, 1966.

95. Kolodny, H. D., and L. Sherman: Hyperglycemic nonketotic coma in insulin-dependent diabetes mellitus, *JAMA*, **203**:119, 1968.

96. Rubin, H. M., R. Kramer, and A. Drash: Hyperosmolality complicating diabetes mellitus in childhood, *J. Pediatr.*, **74**:117, 1969.

97. Halmos, P. B., J. K. Nelson, and R. C. Lowry: Hyperosmolar non-ketoacidotic coma in diabetes, *Lancet*, **1**:675, 1966.

98. Rosenberg, S. A., D. K. Brief, J. M. Kinney, M. G. Herrera, R. E. Wilson, and F. D. Moore: The syndrome of dehydration, coma and severe hyperglycemia without ketosis in patients convalescing from burns, *N. Engl. J. Med.*, **272**:931, 1965.

99. Pyorala, K., O. Suhonen, and P. Pentikainen: Steroid therapy and hyperosmolar non-ketotic coma, *Lancet*, **1**:596, 1968.

100. Boyer, J., G. N. Gill, and F. H. Epstein: Hyperglycemia and hyperosmolality complicating peritoneal dialysis, *Ann. Intern. Med.*, **67**:368, 1967.

101. Potter, D. J.: Death as a result of hyperglycemia without ketosis—a complication of hemodialysis, *Ann. Intern. Med.*, **64**:399, 1966.

102. Spenney, J. G., C. A. Eure, and R. A. Kreisberg:

Hyperglycemic, hyperosmolar, nonketoacidotic diabetes, *Diabetes,* **18:**107, 1969.

103. Goldberg, E. M., and S. S. Sanbar; Hyperglycemic, nonketotic coma following administration of Dilantin (diphenylhydantoin), *Diabetes,* **18:**101, 1969.

104. Wyne, V.: Electrolyte disturbances associated with failure to metabolize glucose during hypothermia, *Lancet,* **2:**575, 1954.

105. Oakes, D. D., P. H. Schreibman, R. S. Hoffman, and R. A. Arky: Hyperglycemic, nonketotic coma in the patient with burns: Factors in pathogenesis, *Metabolism,* **18:**103, 1969.

106. Maccario, M.: Neurological dysfunction associated with nonketotic hyperglycemia, *Arch. Neurol.,* **19:**525, 1968.

107. Finberg, L., C. Luttrell, and H. Redd: Pathogenesis of lesions in the nervous system in hypernatremic states, *Pediatrics,* **23:**46, 1959.

108. Daughaday, W. H., R. J. Lipicky, and D. C. Rasinski: Lactic acidosis as a cause of nonketotic acidosis in diabetic patients, *N. Engl. J. Med.,* **267:**1010, 1962.

109. Larcan, A., C. Huriet, P. Vert, and G. Thibant: Non-acidiketosic metabolic comas in diabetics, *Diabetes,* **11:**99, 1963.

110. Henry, D. P., and R. Bressler: Serum insulin levels in non-ketotic hyperosmotic diabetes mellitus, *Am. J. Med. Sci.,* **256:**150, 1968.

111. Johnson, R. D., J. W. Conn, C. J. Dykman, S. Pek, and J. I. Starr: Mechanisms and management of hyperosmolar coma without ketoacidosis in the diabetic, *Diabetes,* **18:**111, 1969.

112. Seltzer, H. S., and V. L. Harris: Exhaustion of insulogenic reserve in maturity-onset diabetic patients during prolonged and continuous hyperglycemic stress, *Diabetes,* **13:**6, 1964.

113. Mandell, F., and F. X. Fellers: Hyperglycemia in hypernatremic dehydration, *Clin. Ped.,* **13:**367, 1974.

113a. Baum, D., and D. Porte, Jr.: Adrenergic regulation of the inhibition of insulin release in hypothermia, *Diabetes,* **17**(suppl. 1):298, 1968.

114. Chaikoff, I. L., and S. Soskin: Utilization of acetoacetic acid by normal and diabetic dogs before and after evisceration, *Am. J. Physiol.,* **87:**58, 1928.

115. Zierler, K., and D. Rabinowitz: Roles of insulin and growth hormone, based on studies of forearm metabolism in man, *Medicine (Baltimore),* **42:**385, 1963.

116. Yalow, R. S., S. M. Glick, J. Roth, and S. A. Berson: Plasma insulin and growth hormone levels in obesity and diabetes, *Ann. N.Y. Acad. Sci.,* **131:**357, 1965.

117. Mirsky, I. A., A. N. Franzblau, N. Nelson, and W. E. Nelson: The role of excessive carbohydrate intake in the etiology of diabetic coma, *J. Clin. Endocrinol. Metab.,* **1:**307, 1941.

118. Gerich, J., J. C. Penhos, R. A. Gutman, and L. Recant: Effect of dehydration and hyperosmolarity on glucose, free fatty acid and ketone body metabolism in the rat, *Diabetes,* **22:**264, 1973.

119. Luse, S. A., and B. Harris: Brain ultrastructure in hydration and dehydration, *Arch. Neurol.,* **4:**131, 1961.

120. Liberman, B., B. L. Wajchenberg, and P. R. Maroko: Hyperosmolar nonketotic diabetic coma, *Rev. Bra. Pesqui. Med. Biol.,* **1:**133, 1968.

121. Watkins, P. J., J. S. Smith, M. G. Fitzgerald, and J. M. Malins: Lactic acidosis in diabetes, *Br. Med. J.,* **1:**744, 1969.

122. Cohen, R. D., and H. F. Woods: *Clinical and Biochemical Aspects of Lactic Acidosis,* Blackwell Scientific Publications, Ltd., Oxford, 1976.

123. Fulop, M., H. D. Hoberman, J. H. Rascoff, N. A. Bonheim, N. P. Dreyer, and H. Tannenbaum: Lactic acidosis in diabetic patients, Arch. *Intern. Med.,* **136:**987, 1976.

124. Kreisberg, R. A., L. F. Pennington, and B. R. Boshell: Lactate turnover and gluconeogenesis in obesity, effect of phenformin, *Diabetes,* **19:**64, 1970.

125. Searle, G. L., and R. R. Cavalieri: Determination of lactate kinetics in the human analysis of data from single injection vs. continuous infusion methods, *Proc. Soc. Exp. Biol. Med.,* **139:**1002, 1972.

126. Prytz, H., and A. C. Thomsen: Acid-base status in liver cirrhosis. Disturbances in stable, terminal, and porta-caval shunted patients, *Scand. J. Gastroenterol.,* **11:**249, 1976.

127. Record, C. O., K. G. M. M. Alberti, and D. H. Williamson: Metabolic studies in experimental liver disease resulting from d(+) galactosamine administration, *Biochem. J.,* **130:**37, 1972.

128. Huckabee, W. E.: Relationships of pyruvate and lactate during anaerobic metabolism: I. Effects of

infusion of pyruvate or glucose and of hyperventilation, *J. Clin. Invest.*, **37**:244, 1958.

129. Tranquada, R. E., W. J. Grant, and C. R. Peterson: Lactic acidosis, *Arch. Intern. Med.*, **117**:192, 1966.

130. Huckabee, W. E.: Abnormal resting blood lactate. II. Lactic acidosis, *Am. J. Med.*, **30**:840, 1961.

131. Fulop, M., and H. D. Hoberman: Is lactic acidosis spontaneous? *N. Y. State J. Med.*, Jan. 24, 1977.

132. Anderson, J., W. D. Thomas, and R. W. S. Tomlinson: Pyruvate and lactate excretion in diabetes mellitus after sodium lactate, *Br. Med. J.*, **2**:1114, 1966.

133. Woods, H. F., and K. G. M. M. Alberti: Dangers of intravenous fructose, *Lancet*, **2**:1354, 1972.

134. Dembo, A. J., E. B. Marliss, and M. L. Halperin: Insulin therapy in phenformin-associated lactic acidosis. A case report, biochemical considerations, and review of the literature, *Diabetes*, **24**:28, 1975.

135. Strauss, F. G., and M. A. Sullivan: Phenformin intoxication resulting in lactic acidosis, *Johns Hopkins Med. J.*, **128**:278, 1970.

136. Bingle, J. P., G. W. Storey, and J. M. Winter: Fatal self-poisoning with phenformin, *Br. Med. J.*, **3**:752, 1970.

137. Cohen, R. D., J. D. Ward, A. J. S. Brain, C. R. Murray, T. M. Savege, and R. A. Iles: The relation between phenformin therapy and lactic acidosis, *Diabetologia*, **9**:43, 1973.

138. Davidson, M. B., W. R. Bozarth, D. R. Challoner, and C. J. Goodner: Phenformin hypoglycaemia and lactic acidosis, *N. Engl. J. Med.*, **275**:886, 1966.

139. Assan, R., C. Heuclin, F. Lemaire, and J. F. Attali: Phenformin-induced lactic acidosis in diabetic patients, *Diabetes*, **24**:791, 1975.

140. Hermann, L. S.: Biguanide and lactate metabolism. A review, *Dan. Med. Bull.*, **20**:65, 1973.

141. Steiner, D. F., and R. H. Williams: Respiratory inhibition and hypoglycemia by biguanides and decamethylenediguanide, *Biochim. Biophys. Acta,* **30**:329, 1958.

142. Schafer, G.: Site specific uncoupling and inhibition of energy transfer by biguanides, *Biochim. Biophys. Acta*, **93**:279, 1964.

143. Caspary, W. F., and W. Crentzfeldt: Inhibition of intestinal amino acid transport by blood sugar lowering biguanides, *Diabetologia*, **9**:6, 1973.

144. Fulop, M., and H. D. Hoberman: Phenformin-associated metabolic acidosis, *Diabetes,* **25**:292, 1976.

145. Williams, R. H., and J. P. Palmer: Farewell to phenformin for treating diabetes mellitus, *Ann. Intern. Med.*, **83**:567, 1975.

146. Narins, R. G.: Acid-base metabolism, in H. Gonick (ed.), *Current Nephrology*, Pinecliff Medical Publishing Co., Los Angeles, 1977, vol. I.

147. Wick, A. N., C. J. Steward, and G. S. Serif: Tissue distribution of C^{14}-labelled betaphenethylbiguanide, *Diabetes*, **9**:163, 1960.

148. Bosanac, P., S. B. Yablon, D. Alkalay, A. S. Relman, and R. G. Narins: Phenformin (DBI) tolerance and its renal tubular secretion in man (abstract), *Am. Soc. Nephrol.*, **9**:9, 1976.

149. Cahill, G. F., Jr., T. T. Aoki, and E. B. Marliss: Insulin and muscle protein, in D. F. Steiner and N. Freinkel (eds.), *Handbook of Physiology*, sec. 7, vol. 1, *Endocrine Pancreas*, American Physiological Society, Washington, D.C., 1977, pp. 563–577.

25

Fluid and electrolyte metabolism during pregnancy

THOMAS F. FERRIS

PHYSIOLOGIC CHANGES DURING PREGNANCY

Pregnancy is associated with many changes in normal physiology. Frequently the mechanism of the altered physiology is not clear, and although one can postulate a teleologic role in some instances, most of the changes do not yield to such speculative endeavors. However, the changes occurring with pregnancy provide insight into normal control mechanisms.

ARTERIAL PRESSURE AND BLOOD VOLUME

Arterial blood pressure falls during pregnancy, and, although cardiac output increases 30 to 40 percent, it is accompanied by a dramatic fall in total systemic resistance (1). Although it was originally suggested that the fall in resistance was due to the uteroplacental blood flow acting as an arteriovenous shunt, the decrease in resistance in fact occurs in the first trimester, prior to any great development of the uterine vasculature. Also, in the third trimester, when uterine blood flow is highest, arterial blood pressure increases slightly.

The range of normal blood pressure in non-pregnant women is inapplicable to a consideration of blood pressure in pregnancy. In pregnancy, mean arterial pressure is lowest, 72 ± 9 mmHg, at about the 22d week of gestation and rises to 82 ± 8 mmHg by the 40th week (2). Thus, a blood pressure of 120/80 (mean arterial pressure 93 mmHg) is elevated in pregnancy. The arterial pressure in the second trimester has prognostic significance, since it has been found that there is an increase in stillbirths, frequency of interuterine fetal growth retardation, and toxemia when mean arterial pressure is 90 mmHg or more (3).

The cause of the decrease in peripheral resistance is not known, but recent findings of elevated plasma prostaglandin E (PGE) in human pregnancy are of interest (4) (Fig. 25-1). Prostaglandins of the E series are potent vasodilators and antagonize the vasoconstrictor effect of both angiotensin and norepinephrine (5). High levels of PGE have been found in uterine vein blood of pregnant rabbits (6), dogs (7), and monkeys (8). The concentration of PGE measured by immunoassay in the uterine vein of pregnant rabbits is 172 ± 48 ng/mL compared to 0.75 ± 0.3 ng/mL in renal vein (6). Whether all the increased peripheral PGE is synthesized in the uterus and pla-

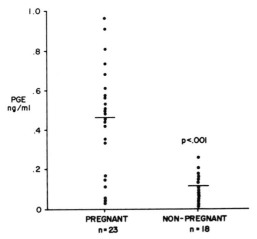

Figure 25-1. Prostaglandin E measured by immunoassay in peripheral vein of pregnant women and nonpregnant controls. (*From Bay et al.*)

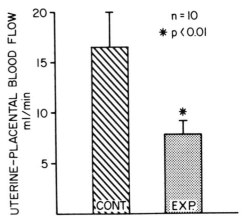

Figure 25-2. The effect of prostaglandin inhibition on uterine-placental blood flow in pregnant rabbits. (*From Venuto et al.*)

centa is unclear. Experiments by Golub et al. (9) have demonstrated in humans that approximately 66 percent of PGE injected into the right ventricle is immediately inactivated during passage through the lung circulation. However, the extraordinary increase in uteroplacental PGE secretion in pregnancy might produce the high PGE levels in the arterial circulation. It is also possible that pregnancy increases synthesis of PGE in all blood vessels and smooth muscles. Smooth-muscle relaxation occurs in the genitourinary, gastrointestinal, and respiratory tracts during pregnancy (10).

Venuto et al. (11) have demonstrated the importance of prostaglandin synthesis in regulating uteroplacental blood flow.

Indomethacin or meclofenamate, potent inhibitors of prostaglandin synthetase, bring about a striking reduction in uterine blood flow in the pregnant rabbit (Fig. 25-2). The reduction in uteroplacental flow is accompanied by a fall in uterine vein PGE concentration.

Accompanying the reduction in blood pressure there is increase in both renin and aldosterone secretion beginning in the first trimester (12) (Fig. 25-3). Plasma renin activity increases to approximately 15 times nonpregnant levels (13) as the result of a threefold increase in renin substrate and an eightfold increase in plasma renin con-

centration. Plasma angiotensin II is similarly elevated, 78 ± 24 pg/mL, compared to a range of 5 to 35 pg/mL in nonpregnant women (12). It appears that the elevated plasma angiotensin is important in maintaining arterial pressure, since angiotensin blockade with Saralasin causes significant hypotension in pregnant animals (14).

The increased secretion of renin and aldosterone during pregnancy has been postulated to be necessary to overcome the natriuretic effect of the

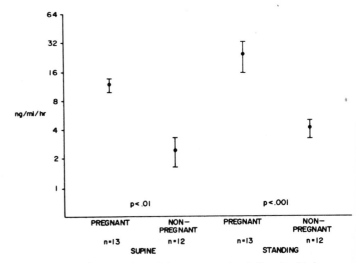

Figure 25-3. Plasma renin activity on unrestricted diets in third trimester pregnant women and nonpregnant controls. (*From Bay et al.*)

increase in glomerular filtration rate (GFR) and the elevated progesterone secretion in pregnancy. However, there is no evidence that pregnancy is a salt-losing state. Bay et al. (4) have demonstrated that sodium balance in pregnant women is maintained on a 10-meq sodium intake over a 7-day period (Fig. 25-4), but that on a 300-meq sodium intake, elevated plasma renin and aldosterone persist (Fig. 25-5). Thus, pregnant women conserve sodium normally but are unable to suppress plasma renin or aldosterone on a high-sodium diet to the values of nonpregnant women. This suggests that a mechanism other than sodium balance maintains the elevated renin secretion of pregnancy. Vasodilatation is known to increase renin secretion as seen during administration of diazoxide, hydralazine, and nitroprusside. It is of note that these drugs also cause sodium retention and concomitant increases in cardiac output, renal blood flow, and GFR. Thus, vasodilatation, possibly due to increased PGE synthesis, could explain both the reduction in systemic resistance and the salt retention with extracellular fluid (ECF) expansion in pregnancy.

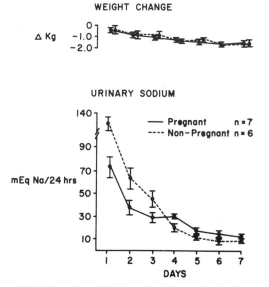

Figure 25-4. The effect of 7 days of a 10-meq Na intake in third trimester pregnant women and nonpregnant controls. Note the similar weight loss and the ability of the pregnant women to conserve Na normally. (*From Bay et al.*)

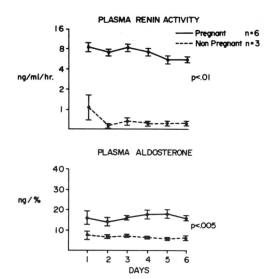

Figure 25-5. The effect of 6 days of a 300-meq Na intake on plasma renin activity and aldosterone in pregnant and nonpregnant women. Note that plasma renin activity and plasma aldosterone remained elevated in the pregnant women despite similar urinary Na excretion in both groups, approximately 300 meq daily. (*From Bay et al.*)

Urinary kallikrein has also been found elevated in pregnancy (15). Like renin, it increases in the first trimester and remains elevated throughout gestation. Since urinary kallikrein is increased both by angiotensin and PGE infusions, the increased excretion might be due to increased plasma concentration of both in pregnancy.

Although vasodilatation could increase renin secretion, it would not necessarily explain the resistance to angiotensin which occurs as early as the 14th week of pregnancy (16). This resistance is not due simply to the elevated plasma renin since infusions of albumin or saline decrease plasma renin in pregnant women without increasing sensitivity to angiotensin (17). The studies by Brunner et al. (18) demonstrating the importance of angiotensin receptor affinity in determining sensitivity to angiotensin may have relevance. Pregnancy is similar to conditions on a low-sodium diet where receptor affinity is diminished. Increased PGE synthesis could account for the decrease in angiotensin sensitivity. There are interesting similarities between pregnancy and Bartter's syndrome, a clinical condition associated with insensitivity to angiotensin and increased urinary PGE excretion (19, 20). With treatment of Bartter's syndrome with indomethacin, urinary PGE excretion and plasma renin activity fall as angiotensin sensitivity returns towards normal. Thus, the decrease in angiotensin sensitivity in Bartter's syndrome is thought to be due to increased PGE synthesis. Similarly, in pregnancy, where PGE synthesis is increased, the rise in renin secretion may occur to compensate for the resistance to angiotensin sensitivity which develops. Thus, both renin and PGE may act in concert to maintain arterial blood pressure during pregnancy.

The increase in plasma volume and ECF volume which occurs in pregnancy is not dependent upon increased mineralocorticoid secretion since Addisonian women have had normal pregnancies without need for increasing the dose of mineralocorticoid during the pregnancy (21). This also argues against a natriuretic effect of elevated progesterone secretion's causing the increased aldosterone secretion with pregnancy. Estrogen secretion increases in pregnancy, and pharmacologic doses of estrogen can cause salt retention (22). Although renal tubular receptors for estrogen have been described (23) it seems unlikely that estrogen has a mineralocorticoid effect during pregnancy since this would suppress renin and aldosterone secretion. Estrogen might, however, cause sodium retention by vasodilating the vascular bed with an increase in renal sodium absorption. The salt retention with estrogen would then be independent of increased mineralocorticoid secretion but caused by increase in vascular capacity.

Blood volume increases approximately 50 percent in pregnancy with expansion of both plasma volume and red cell mass (24). Since the increase in plasma volume is greater than that of red cell mass, a "physiologic anemia" occurs in pregnancy. This may reduce blood viscosity and be another factor in reducing vascular resistance.

GLOMERULAR FILTRATION RATE

GFR increases as early as the second month of gestation, along with an increase in renal blood flow. The increased GFR is reflected in the low mean blood urea nitrogen (BUN), 8.7 ± 1.8 mg/dL, and serum creatinine, 0.46 ± 0.6 mg/dL, seen in normal pregnancy (29). Whether the increase in glomerular filtration is due entirely to the increase in renal plasma flow is not known. Studies have indicated approximately a 50 percent increase in both. Bucht found the insulin clearance in 23 women increased from 122 ± 24 to 170 ± 23 mL/min from the 8th to the 32d week of pregnancy (26). Filtration fraction remains constant until late in pregnancy, when a disproportionate increase in filtration over renal plasma flow occurs (27). The increasing filtration fraction could indicate an increase in efferent arteriolar resistance, since blood pressure and angiotensin sensitivity increase slightly in the third trimester (2, 16). Also, serum protein concentration falls approximately 1 g/dL in late pregnancy, which would reduce plasma oncotic pressure by approximately 7 mmHg (28). If glomerular hydrostatic pressure, proximal tubule pressure, and the ultrafiltration coefficient of the glomerulus remain constant, a fall in oncotic pressure would increase glomerular filtration and filtration fraction.

RENAL BLOOD FLOW

The 30 to 50 percent increase in renal blood flow during pregnancy is in part due to the increase in cardiac output. However, blood flow does not simply increase to all organs; no increase in cerebral or hepatic blood flow has been detected. Thus, a disproportionate decrease in renal vascular resistance must occur during pregnancy. It is tempting to speculate that an increase in renal PGE synthesis diminishes renal vascular resistance. Infusions of PGE are known to reduce renal vascular resistance in humans.

Early studies which reported a decline in renal blood flow in the last trimester were done on pregnant women lying supine. This position reduces venous return because of the gravid uterus compressing the inferior vena cava and will give spurious values for cardiac output as well as GFR and renal blood flow. When measurements of cardiac output and renal blood flow are made with the pregnant woman lying on her side, no decrease is found in the third trimester.

Growth hormone produces renal vasodilatation, increased renal blood flow, and ECF volume expansion, but growth hormone levels are low during pregnancy. Human somatomammotrophin, which is immunologically and chemically similar to human growth hormone, increases in pregnancy and is measurable as early as the 6th week of gestation (30). However, whether somatomammotrophin and growth hormone have similar effects on the kidney is not known, and increases in somatomammotrophin with hydatidiform mole and choriocarcinoma have not been reported to cause vascular dilation and increased renal blood flow.

RENAL TUBULAR FUNCTION

Glomerular-tubular balance

The increase in GFR during pregnancy necessitates an equal increase in sodium reabsorption by the nephron if extraordinary losses of sodium are to be prevented. With a sodium concentration of 140 meq/L in glomerular filtrate and a GFR of 100 mL/min the daily filtered sodium is 20,160 meq. Increasing GFR to 150 mL/min increases sodium filtration to 30,240 meq/day. The increase in GFR during pregnancy necessitates an equal increase in sodium reabsorption by the nephron if extraordinary losses of sodium are to be prevented. The renal tubules must thus reabsorb some 10,000 meq more sodium in pregnancy to prevent sodium wasting.

Glucosuria

Up to 40 percent of pregnant women have glucosuria, which is due in part to the inability of the proximal tubules to increase glucose reabsorption in parallel with filtration. Christensen found the renal threshold for glucose in pregnancy to be 155 ± 17 mg/dL compared to 196 ± 6 mg/dL in nonpregnant women (31). Since he found the tubular maximum for glucose transport (Tm_g) essentially the same in pregnant and control women, he felt the reduced threshold during pregnancy was due to the increased filtration. Welsh and Sims measured inulin clearance and Tm_g in 29 pregnant women, 16 without and 13 with glucosuria (32). GFR was the same in both groups, but

maximum reabsorption of glucose was significantly lower in pregnant women with glucosuria (310 ± 18 mg/min) or in nonpregnant women (366 ± 16 mg/min). There is normally an increase in Tm_g with increase in GFR, and Tm_g may appear normal in pregnant women with glucosuria if not considered in relation to the high GFR accompanying pregnancy. Figure 25-6 demonstrates that pregnancy displaces the slope of the regression line of Tm_g on inulin clearance to the right, but pregnant women with glucosuria have an even greater decrease in Tm_g when related to GFR. Since the glucosuric women were not studied again after pregnancy, it is not known whether Tm_g fell during pregnancy or whether glucosuria developed with the increase in filtered load in women who had initially lower Tm_g. Some investigators (33) feel the frequency of glucosuria during pregnancy is so high that it is misleading in detecting latent diabetes. However, glucosuria in pregnancy cannot be completely discounted, for some reports have indicated latent or asymptomatic diabetes in 20 percent of pregnant women with glucosuria (34). These women

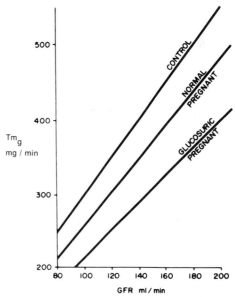

Figure 25-6. Regression lines of maximum tubular glucose absorption (Tm_g) on GFR in nonpregnant control women, pregnant women without glucosuria, and pregnant women with glucosuria. (*After Welsh and Sims.*)

are usually patients with a strong family history of diabetes and a history of having delivered large babies.

Aminoaciduria

In addition to glucosuria, aminoaciduria develops during pregnancy. Wallraff et al. (35) and Christensen et al. (36) found that excretion of many amino acids was increased with corresponding reductions in plasma amino acid levels. In the case of histidine, at least, the percentage of filtered amino acid reabsorbed is decreased. An increase in urinary histidine serves as the basis for one test for detection of pregnancy. Cortisone administration causes a pattern of aminoaciduria similar to that in pregnancy (37), and the aminoaciduria of pregnancy has been interpreted as indicating increased cortisol effect on the renal tubules. Whether or not cortisone similarly reduces Tm_g is unknown.

The aminoaciduria and tendency to glucosuria in pregnancy may be due to increased delivery of filtrate out of the proximal tubule. There is limited capacity for glucose and amino acid absorption in the distal tubule. Thus, the normal capacity to conserve sodium in pregnancy points to increased reabsorption of sodium distal to the proximal tubule, an effect possibly mediated by the high plasma aldosterone of pregnancy.

GLUCOSE HOMEOSTASIS DURING PREGNANCY

Pregnancy is associated with a profound change in fuel metabolism caused both by the fetal demand for glucose and amino acids and by the development during pregnancy of resistance to insulin. The rate of glucose utilization is increased from 2 to 3 mg/kg per min in nonpregnant women to approximately 6 mg/kg per min in pregnancy (39). The metabolic demands of the fetus are thought to be met entirely by glucose, and glycogen stores in liver and muscle in the fetus are greater than those in adults.

In pregnancy circulating levels of glucose and amino acids are reduced, whereas free fatty acids and ketones are increased. The metabolic state is similar to starvation, with a tendency towards fasting hypoglycemia (38). During fasting, blood glucose levels are approximately 15 to 20 percent lower in pregnant women, and there is an exaggeration of the ketonemia which occurs with starvation. Thus, the pregnant woman has an increased tendency to ketosis during dehydration or vomiting, and severe caloric restriction poses a greater risk of hypoglycemia. In spite of the hypoglycemic potential of pregnancy, diabetes is apt to develop in genetically predisposed women with reversion of carbohydrate metabolism to normal postpartum. Insulin secretion is increased in pregnancy in response to both ingestion of glucose and amino acids (40). Fasting insulin concentration, however, is reduced probably because of the hypoglycemia (41). Thus, insulin resistance and potential hypoglycemia coexist in pregnancy.

The cause of the insulin antagonism which develops during pregnancy is unknown but, at least in part, is related to increased secretion of chorionic somatomammotrophin, estrogen, progesterone, and cortisol. Chorionic somatomammotrophin is a polypeptide which is secreted throughout pregnancy with a tenfold or more increase in concentration in the last half of pregnancy (30). Chemically and immunologically it is similar to growth hormone and, like growth hormone, it causes an impairment in glucose tolerance when infused in nonpregnant subjects. The placenta secretes estrogen and progesterone during pregnancy, and both are known to act as insulin antagonists (42, 43). In addition to these steroids, plasma cortisol increases during pregnancy (44), which would contribute to the diabetogenic state of pregnancy. However, in spite of all these factors' causing insulin antagonism, diabetes presenting during pregnancy is uncommon.

ADRENAL HORMONES

Plasma cortisol rises progressively during pregnancy. Originally the increase was thought to be due to the increase in transcortin concentration, which rises from 33 mg of protein per liter to approximately 70 mg of protein per liter of plasma, but free cortisol is also elevated (44). The increase in transcortin is also induced by estrogen administration to nonpregnant women. In spite of the elevated plasma cortisol, urinary excretion of 17-hydroxycorticosteroids decreases during pregnancy. The cause is an actual decrease in cortisol secretion rate during gestation. Cortisol production was found to be 15.5 mg per 24 h in 13 pregnant women compared to 18 mg per 24 h in nonpregnant controls (45). A similar change in cortisol secretion occurs in patients receiving estrogen. Thus, the half-life of cortisol is prolonged; this may reflect impairment of the liver's ability to metabolize cortisol in pregnancy.

Following adrenocorticotropic hormone (ACTH), a greater rise in plasma cortisol occurs in the pregnant woman, but the pituitary is less responsive as measured by the metyrapone test (46). It has been suggested that the elevated plasma cortisol is a response to diminished intracellular binding of cortisol in the hypothalamus and pituitary because of competitive binding by progesterone (47).

Aldosterone secretion increases markedly in pregnancy, the rise occurring as early as the 15th week. In the last trimester the aldosterone secretion rate is approximately 10 times that in nonpregnant women (48). Although the elevated secretion rate of progesterone would antagonize the renal tubular effect of aldosterone, varying dietary sodium alters aldosterone secretion without parallel change in progesterone secretion. In pregnant women studied in our laboratory, mean midday plasma aldosterone in the third trimester on an unrestricted diet was 29 ± 8 ng/dL compared to 7.8 ± 1 ng/dL in nonpregnant women. Aldosterone excretion, which was under 18 μg per 24 h in nonpregnant women was 66 ± 10 μg per 24 h in pregnant women in the third trimester (4).

A feature of pregnancy is the failure to develop hypokalemia in spite of elevated aldosterone secretion and normal sodium intake. This has been thought to be due to progesterone antagonizing the effect of aldosterone at the renal tubule, but there is evidence that responsiveness to aldosterone is diminished in pregnancy independent of a change in progesterone secretion (49).

CALCIUM AND PHOSPHORUS METABOLISM

The pregnant woman requires 1.5 to 2 g of calcium intake daily during the last half of pregnancy to maintain calcium balance. The fetus contains approximately 25 to 30 g of calcium, and most of this is retained during the second half of pregnancy. Significant increases in calcium turnover have been found in pregnant women in advance of the fetal skeletal mineralization (50). The use of calcium supplements throughout pregnancy assures an adequate intake of calcium, but on a normal calcium diet osteomalacia is unusual during pregnancy. Total serum calcium concentration falls during pregnancy, the lowest values being in the eighth month of gestation. This decrease in calcium is due to the hypoalbuminemia which develops in pregnancy; ionized calcium is unchanged (51). Despite the fetal demands for calcium, urinary excretion of calcium is increased, possibly because of the increase in glomerular filtration which occurs. However, plasma phosphate concentration remains unchanged throughout pregnancy so that the increase in glomerular filtration does not affect phosphate clearance.

Except for the last 4 to 6 weeks of pregnancy, parathyroid hormone (PTH) is within the normal range. However, it rises to markedly elevated values at term (52). The reason for the elevated PTH in late pregnancy is not clear. There does not seem to be a correlation between serum calcium and parathormone concentration, and no differences have been found between maternal and cord blood PTH levels. Serum alkaline phosphatase is elevated during pregnancy and reaches a peak of two to four times normal at term. The source of the alkaline phosphatase is the placenta (53). It decreases rapidly after delivery, reaching normal levels about 20 days postpartum. Whether placental alkaline phosphatase is involved in the increased calcium turnover of pregnancy is not known.

PLASMA SODIUM CONCENTRATION

Plasma osmolality decreases approximately 10 mosm/kg H_2O in pregnancy; this is reflected in a decrease in sodium concentration of 5 meq/L at term. The water retained in excess of sodium occurs primarily in the last trimester and may be caused by elevated antidiuretic hormone (ADH) secretion. Weir et al. (54), using a radioimmunoassay technique, have found plasma arginine vasopressin concentration to be between 4 and 8 pg/mL in nonpregnant women but was 9.7 ± 0.9 pg/mL in pregnancy. Although the difference between the two groups was not significant, the fact that plasma ADH tended to be higher when serum tonicity was lower would indicate an increase in secretion relative to tonicity in pregnancy. The cause of this increased ADH secretion is not clear. An increase in effective blood volume could induce an increase in ADH secretion, but this stimulus should be present from early pregnancy if the stimulus is similar to that increasing renin secretion.

In 1938 Chesley demonstrated that approximately 66 percent of pregnant women failed to concentrate the urine to 1.022 sp gr or greater following a Fishberg concentration test (55). Also, in patients with diabetes insipidus worsening of the polyuria and antagonism to injected pitressin has been reported (56). Because of the increase in GFR during pregnancy, distal delivery of filtrate may be increased with resultant increase in urinary volume. Elevated PGE synthesis in pregnancy could also be a factor. Prostaglandins of the E series are known to antagonize the hydroosmotic effect of ADH at the collecting tubule, and conceivably the increased requirement of pitressin during pregnancy may be a reflection of increased renal PGE synthesis. However, in spite of possible antagonism to ADH, serum tonicity falls in late pregnancy.

Since there is evidence that angiotensin increases both thirst and ADH secretion, the decreased tonicity could be a reflection of elevated renin secretion (57). However, hyponatremia develops only in the last 6 weeks of pregnancy, and plasma angiotensin is increased throughout pregnancy.

One cause of hyponatremia in late pregnancy could be increased secretion of oxytocin. Oxytocin has an antidiuretic effect, and when infused to induce labor at a rate of 45 μU or more per minute the effect is equal to maximal doses of vasopressin (58). Thus, with the induction of labor with oxytocin care must be taken to restrict water. Severe hyponatremia has occurred when such precautions have not been observed. In some circumstances the diagnosis of eclampsia has been made, but subsequent determination of serum sodium has indicated that hyponatremia was the cause of the convulsion.

ARTERIAL pH DURING PREGNANCY

Arterial P_{CO_2} in normal pregnancy is approximately 30 mmHg compared to normal values of 40 mmHg (59). The hyperventilation causes an increase in renal bicarbonate excretion, so plasma bicarbonate in normal pregnancy is 16 to 20 meq/L. The reduction in plasma bicarbonate and mild respiratory alkalosis has little significance except in situations where a metabolic acidosis, e.g., ketoacidosis or lactic acidosis, supervenes, in which case total buffering capacity is reduced.

The increased ventilation throughout pregnancy is due to increased tidal volume without increase in respiratory rate. However, P_{O_2} does not increase and may actually decrease, because of the decrease in pulmonary diffusing capacity in late pregnancy. There is a great deal of evidence to suggest that the increased ventilation in pregnancy is due to increase in progesterone secretion which lowers the threshold of the respiratory center to carbon dioxide. Reductions in arterial P_{CO_2} similar to those in pregnancy have been induced in nonpregnant subjects by administering progesterone (60). Estrogens have an effect upon respiration similar to progesterone and may also contribute to the hyperventilation.

EDEMA

Dependent edema of the feet and ankles occurs in up to 80 percent of women during pregnancy. It appears usually late in the day and clears overnight. The cause is high venous and capillary pressure in the legs due to increased venous capacitance and pressure of the gravid uterus upon the inferior vena cava, as well as the reduction in plasma oncotic pressure. Generalized edema of the face and hands is more often a sign of early toxemia, but it may occur in up to 20 percent of normotensive women during pregnancy. Since the incidence of edema is so high during pregnancy, there has been difficulty in demonstrating a positive correlation between edema and the development of toxemia in some studies. The problem could be resolved by correlating arterial blood pressure with the sodium retention. With toxemia, the salt retention which occurs accompanies a rise in arterial blood pressure. The dependent edema of normal pregnancy is not associated with change in arterial blood pressure. Postural edema can be treated by moderate salt restriction and bed rest.

There is controversy concerning the use of diuretics during pregnancy. Finnerty (61) reported that the prophylactic use of a thiazide in women at high risk of developing toxemia decreased the incidence of the disease, but this has not been confirmed by others (62). Gant (63) has reported that diuretic therapy reduces the metabolic clearance rate of dehydroepiandrosterone (DHEA) which is dependent upon placental conversion of DHEA to estrone and estrodiol. Although these findings have been interpreted to indicate reduced placental perfusion, there is controversy over whether DHEA clearance can be used as a measure of uterine blood flow (64). The reduced clearance may reflect a change in placental function induced by diuretics. However, in Finnerty's patients no increase in fetal loss or other complications occurred with the use of the diuretics throughout pregnancy, and there are several large published series and innumerable pregnant women who have been treated with diuretics throughout pregnancy without untoward effects (65, 66). Thus, the routine use of diuretics, like the use of any drug, is not justified in pregnancy, but there is no clinical evidence that they do harm.

RENAL DISEASES IN PREGNANCY

The effect of pregnancy on various renal diseases is covered in a recent review of the subject (67). There are certain renal diseases, however, which have particular pertinence in a discussion of pregnancy.

Acute renal failure (see also Chap. 15)

In women developing acute renal failure early in pregnancy, infection of the uterus is the most common cause. *Clostridium welchii* and *Streptococcus pyogenes* are the usual offending organisms following a septic abortion. The characteristic feature of clostridial uterine infection is septicemia with intravascular hemolysis, hemoglobinemia, and renal failure. Infection is the most common cause of death in this group of women, mortality rates being approximately 30 percent. Emptying the uterus of infected and necrotic tissue is essential, and hysterectomy is occasionally necessary when uterine perforation or extensive myometrial necrosis is suspected (68). Irreversible renal failure in this group of patients is unusual, and with adequate therapy for renal failure, recovery of function can be expected.

The development of acute renal failure in late pregnancy is usually associated with toxemia of pregnancy and a related obstetric complication. In one series (69), 62 percent of women developing acute renal failure in late pregnancy had toxemia and 25 percent had preceding eclampsia. The great danger of acute renal failure in late pregnancy is the high incidence (approximately 25 percent) of cortical necrosis. This is a rare complication in nonpregnant patients, and its occurrence in pregnancy is related to the increased incidence of intravascular coagulation during pregnancy. The basic pathologic change in cortical necrosis is intimal hyalinization of the arcuate arteries, which represents organization of thrombi, and further thrombus formation in interlobar arteries, afferent arterioles, and glomeruli. These women frequently develop renal failure with evidence of a consumptive coagulopathy, hemolysis, helmet or burr cells on peripheral smear, fibrin split products in the serum, and reduced clotting factors and fibrinogen in the blood. Pregnancy is associated with several changes and complications that may predispose to intravascular coagulation: (1) an increase in clotting factors (70); (2) the increased risk of gram-negative infection during pregnancy which may activate a Shwartzmanlike reaction with intravascular clotting; (3) preeclampsia, in which hypertension and arteriolar constriction may cause endothelial cell injury which acts as a nidus for platelet thrombi; (4) the frequency of abruptio placentae in preeclampsia with the release of thromboplastic material from the placenta into the circulation (71); (5) hemorrhage and shock from an obstetric complication. Jaundice, hepatic necrosis, myocarditis, and convulsions are frequently seen with acute renal failure in late pregnancy and are probably systemic manifestations of the generalized consumptive phenomenon (72, 73).

The diagnosis of cortical necrosis should be considered when oliguria exceeds 14 to 21 days. A renal biopsy is helpful in establishing the diagnosis; intracortical calcification may be found on x-ray as early as 1 week after development of the disease but cannot be depended on to confirm the presence of the disease (74, 75). Although cortical necrosis has been thought to have a uniformly fatal outcome, there have been several documented cases of oliguria lasting up to 60 days with recovery of some renal function (76, 77). There is evidence that the juxtamedullary nephrons may be spared in cortical necrosis, and hypertrophy and hyperfunction of these nephrons may occur with time. Similarly, the process may be patchy, and some areas of kidney may ultimately recover if sufficient time elapses. Slow increase in the GFR has been documented in these patients for up to 3 years after the acute insult (78). Many patients have received renal transplants following bilateral cortical necrosis.

Postpartum renal failure

In 1968 Wagoner, Holley, and Johnson in the United States (79) and Robson et al. (80) in Great Britain described the syndrome of postpartum renal failure. The disease consists of the rapid development of renal failure 2 to 10 weeks postpartum with findings at autopsy of malignant nephrosclerosis. Three of four patients reported by Robson had hypertension during pregnancy, but the three patients of Wagoner had normotensive pregnancies. Peripheral smears were not available in Wagoner's cases, but in the British series there was evidence of microangiopathic hemolytic anemia with reticulocytosis and fragmented red blood cells on peripheral smear. The disease has been termed "postpartum hemolytic-uremic syndrome." The pathologic changes in the kidneys are fibrin deposits in glomeruli and afferent arterioles as well as marked intimal hyperplasia, attributed to organization of fibrin deposits in the arcuate and interlobular arteries. The cause of the disease is unknown; an unusual sensitivity to oxytocin has been postulated, but the intravascular coagulation to which pregnant women are predisposed is probably more important. In this regard it is of note that of the 37 adults with hemolytic-uremic syndrome reported in the literature between 1966 and 1973, only 3 were men (81); 22 of the 34 women were either within 10 weeks of delivery (13 patients) or were taking oral contraceptives (9 patients). In children, the hemolytic-uremic syndrome is self-limited and recovery rate is approximately 70 percent (82), however 73 percent of adults either die or may require chronic hemodialysis (83, 84). There is evidence that heparin therapy may be beneficial, and it merits a trial in any patient in whom the diagnosis is documented by renal biopsy. The cause of the hemolytic-uremic syndrome during pregnancy and in the postpartum period is unclear. However, the similarity of the hemolytic-uremic syndrome to the generalized Shwartzman reaction is striking (71). In the nonpregnant rabbit, the Shwartzman reaction results in fibrin deposits in the lungs, liver, and spleen after the first injection of endotoxin, with deposits in the glomeruli following the second injection 24 h later. In the pregnant rabbit, however, fibrin deposits occur in the lungs, liver, spleen, and kidneys after the first injection of endotoxin. In 1947 Beeson (85) demonstrated that blockade of the reticuloendothelial system with Thorotrast resulted in fibrin deposits in the kidney following the first injection of endotoxin. It has been postulated that pregnancy causes a similar reticuloendothelial system blockade so that any stimulus causing activation of clotting might be more apt to result in fibrin deposition in the kidney (86). During pregnancy it is possible that thromboplastic material is constantly released from the placenta into the circulation. Thromboplastin and fibrin are known to be taken up by reticuloendothelial cells and would predispose the pregnant woman to a generalized Shwartzman reaction similar to that in animals with reticuloendothelial system blockade. Since vasoconstriction can activate localized intravascular coagulation, the coexistence of preeclampsia in many of these patients would be an added risk factor for development of the disease. Why the disease occurs postpartum is perplexing but may be related to the release of thromboplastic material from the involuting uterus or to an aberration in the return of the clotting factors to nonpregnant levels.

Pregnancy following renal transplantation

Although most patients on long-term hemodialysis for chronic renal failure are amenorrheal; resumption of menses follows transplantation if renal function becomes normal. Contraceptive measures are essential in these women if pregnancy is to be avoided. In women desirous of becoming pregnant it is probably wise to wait 1 year following a related donor homograft and 2 years after a cadaveric transplant to be reasonably certain of stable renal function. The chance of a successful pregnancy following transplantation is excellent; 16 of 18 reported pregnancies have resulted in live births (87, 88).

Cesarean section was required in two of five pregnancies in one series, but all six deliveries in another were vaginal. Because of the placement of the transplanted kidney in the pelvis, compression of the kidney by the fetal head may occur before and during labor. The use of simultaneous intravenous pyelography and pelvimetry at term has been recommended to determine the feasibility of vaginal delivery. Uniform reduction in creatinine clearance after the 32d week of gestation was found in one series and attributed to compression of the kidney by the fetus, but this reduction was not seen by others. (If clearances are obtained in the supine position, a reduction in GFR occurs in all pregnant women after the 32d week of gestation because of interference by the uterus with venous return from the vena cava.) Compression of the renal vessels during delivery, if it occurs, is transient and not of sufficient magnitude to necessitate cesarean section.

In three of the eight pregnancies reported by Penn there was evidence of preeclampsia with the development of hypertension, proteinuria, and reduced GFR. At 12 weeks one woman developed preeclampsia, which necessitated a therapeutic abortion. The other two delivered living infants, although one died postpartum because of prematurity. Hypertension and proteinuria disappeared following delivery, and renal function returned to the prepartum level. Although it was suggested that fetal cells might have entered the maternal circulation, inducing development of graft-directed antibodies and causing the reduction in renal function, it seems more likely that the transient reduction in renal function was due to preeclampsia in these women. Impairment of renal function during late gestation in transplanted kidneys does not return to prepartum levels following delivery in some instances.

Two children born to parents with renal transplants have had congenital defects. One had pulmonary valvular stenosis; the other child, whose father was on immunosuppression therapy following a renal homograft, had multiple defects: a large myelomeningocele, bilateral dislocated hips, and talipes equinovarus (89). The incidence of congenital defects in children of renal transplant parents is low and has been estimated to be about 5.3 percent.

The combination of steroid and immunosuppression therapy in the mother may be the cause of problems in the neonatal period. In one series of six live infants, one died of prematurity, one had pneumonitis with the respiratory distress syndrome but subsequently recovered, and two had evidence of adrenocortical insufficiency with lymphopenia, hyponatremia, and hyperkalemia. The clinical syndrome was felt to be analogous to congenital thymic aplasia; chest x-rays failed to reveal a thymic shadow in the infants.

TOXEMIA OF PREGNANCY

Toxemia occurs usually in late pregnancy and is characterized by hypertension, edema, and, usually, proteinuria, which disappear postpartum. Historically, convulsions have been the hallmark of toxemia, and the entity has been subdivided into eclampsia (from the Greek word *eclampsis*, "a sudden flash") and preeclampsia, based upon whether a convulsion has or has not occurred. Since the causes of the hypertension and of the proteinuria in toxemia are different, it is to be expected that hypertension would be more prominent in some patients and proteinuria in others. The disease has a bimodal frequency with peak incidence in young primiparous and in older multiparous women. When toxemia occurs in the absence of proteinuria, particularly in multiparous women, it may be an early manifestation of essential hypertension diathesis occurring during pregnancy.

MECHANISM OF HYPERTENSION

The cause of the increase in peripheral resistance in toxemia is unknown, but there are several factors which must be examined. One phenomenon common to all forms of hypertension is increased sensitivity to vasopressor substances; hypersensitivity to angiotensin and norepinephrine has been demonstrated in toxemia (90). The increased sensitivity to angiotensin precedes the hypertension and occurs as early as the 14th week in women who subsequently develop toxemia (16) (Fig. 25-7). The increased sensitivity of arterioles to vasopressor substances could be due to either increased reactivity of vascular smooth muscle or structural thickening of the vessel wall. An increase in wall/lumen ratio from swelling will lead to an augmented response to pressor stimuli. Increased contents of sodium, water, potassium, chloride, and calcium in the arteries of hypertensive animals and humans have been demonstrated (91), and swelling of the renal arterioles has been described in renal biopsies from toxemic women (29). Such swelling affords a mechanical advantage in contraction, and an increase in intracellular sodium may also alter the resting electric potential. Intracellular calcium is known to be important in activating contractile proteins, and there is now evidence that sodium entry into the arterial wall increases the movement of calcium across muscle surface membranes. In view of the small volume of these arteriolar muscle cells, the amount of calcium that

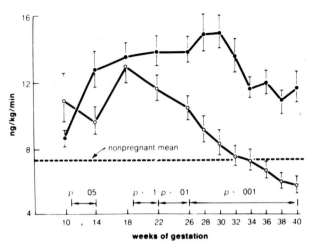

Figure 25-7. Angiotensin sensitivity measured as nanograms of angiotensin per kilogram per minute needed to raise diastolic blood pressure 20 mmHg in pregnant women. Note the decrease in sensitivity to angiotensin as early as the 10th week of gestation. In women who developed toxemia (open circles) a progressive increase in sensitivity occurred beginning at the 18th week. With the development of overt toxemia, after 32 weeks, sensitivity had increased to levels greater than in nonpregnant women. (*From Gant et al.*)

enters in this way might be sufficient to raise intracellular calcium to a level that could augment contraction. Thus, sodium and water entry into the arteriolar cells would affect peripheral resistance not only by reduction in lumen size but also by altering intracellular calcium concentration, causing greater activation of contractile proteins.

There are several other aspects to the salt retention occurring in toxemia which would increase blood pressure. The development of edema occurs during an increase in renal resistance and with reduction in renal blood flow and GFR so that the normal increase of sodium excretion in response to hypertension is prevented. The salt retention occurs also in the face of an increase in systemic resistance, so exquisite sensitivity to volume expansion is present.

There is a large amount of clinical evidence indicating that reduction in uterine blood flow is associated with toxemia. The higher incidence of disease in primiparous women may be related to the less developed uterine vasculature. Anatomic studies in women have demonstrated the caliber of the uterine arteries in multiparous women to be greater than in the primigravid state (92). Uteroplacental ischemia was postulated as a cause of toxemia by Young as early as 1914 (93), and Page and Ogden in 1939 (94) induced acute hypertension in pregnant dogs by clamping the aorta below the level of the renal arteries. Attempts to produce chronic hypertension during pregnancy in experimental animals by reduction in uterine blood flow have usually been unsuccessful due to abortion, premature delivery, or because of the development of collateral circulation around the clamp. However, balloons inserted in the uterine horns of pregnant cats and dogs cause a rise in blood pressure (95), and uteroplacental ischemia induced by placing Z-sutures through the placenta and uterus (96) or by constriction of the aorta induce hypertension. Cavanaugh et al. (97) reported hypertension and proteinuria in pregnant baboons in the third trimester of pregnancy after applying clamps to the uterine artery (64).

Gant et al. (98) have demonstrated a reduction in the clearance of dehydroepiandrosterone sulfate in pregnant women prior to the development of clinically evident toxemia. As mentioned previously, dehydroepiandrosterone sulfate clearance, dependent on conversion to estrogens by the placenta, may not be a valid measure of uteroplacental blood flow.

UTERINE RENIN

The presence of a substance with reninlike characteristics in the placenta, but not the uterus, of pregnant cats was first reported by Stakemann in 1960 (99). Gross et al. (100) reported finding a reninlike material in rabbit uterus and placenta, and his studies were extended by Ferris et al. (101, 102), who demonstrated that uterine renin persisted for up to 72 h after nephrectomy and was not altered by changes in sodium intake. Symonds et al. (103) demonstrated that cell cultures of human chorion and uterine muscle synthesized renin. The highest concentration is in blood vessels of the myometrium (104). Whether uterine renin is identical with renal renin or represents an isoenzyme is not clear. Molecular weights determined by gel filtration are the same,

and the enzymes are identical with respect to mobility on disk electrophoresis, but small K_m differences have been reported (105). In vitro perfusion of the isolated rabbit uterus with Tyrode solution causes renin to be released into the perfusate (106), and reduction in uterine perfusion by either ligation of the uterine arteries or hemorrhagic hypotension increases uterine secretion in the nephrectomized pregnant rabbit (107). Human amniotic fluid contains a high concentration of prorenin, a larger molocule, which may escape into the circulation and explain the discrepancy between plasma renin and angiotensin in some pregnant women (108).

The role uterine renin plays in normal pregnancy is not clear. The high plasma renin concentration of pregnancy does not seem to be of uterine origin since in the pregnant rabbit a high salt intake depresses plasma and renal renin with no change in uterine renin concentration. In normotensive pregnant women no difference between uterine arterial and venous concentrations of renin has been detected at cesarean section (109).

Experiments in pregnant animals indicate that uterine renin may be of importance in regulating uterine blood flow. Angiotensin increases uterine blood flow in the pregnant rabbit (107) and dog (7) with diminution in uterine vascular resistance. Although angiotensin has a variable vasoconstrictor effect upon vascular beds, the vasodilatation in the uterine circulation is unique. The effect of angiotensin seems specific, since the rise in uterine blood flow occurs with a nonpressor dose of angiotensin with no increase occurring with a pressor dose of norepinephrine. The uterine vasodilatation with angiotensin might be caused by increased synthesis of PGE. Experiments in pregnant dogs, monkeys, and rabbits have demonstrated that angiotensin increases uterine PGE secretion. The increase in uterine PGE synthesis could act locally to dilate the uterine vasculature. Thus, uterine renin may act primarily as a tissue enzyme regulating uterine flow by increasing uterine angiotensin and PGE synthesis.

Toxemia is associated with variable plasma renin (110, 111) and angiotensin concentration (12), usually lower than in normotensive pregnancies. Since there is increased sensitivity to angiotensin in toxemia, the concentration of plasma renin and angiotensin does not measure its physiological effect. If insensitivity to angiotensin in pregnancy is dependent upon PGE synthesis, a reduction in synthesis could alter sensitivity. Thus, a reduction in uteroplacental blood flow could induce hypertension by either reduction in uterine PGE synthesis or increase in uterine renin secretion. The combination of a small but inappropriate release of uterine renin in a setting of increased angiotensin sensitivity could induce hypertension. A great deal more work is obviously necessary in this area to determine if a change in PGE synthesis occurs with or precedes the development of hypertension to explain the gradual increase in sensitivity to angiotensin which develops in women with toxemia (Fig. 25-6).

The findings by Gant et al. (112) that women who ultimately develop toxemia demonstrate a rise in blood pressure when lying supine probably reflects increased sensitivity to angiotensin. Lying supine increases plasma renin concentration because of compression of the inferior vena cava by the gravid uterus with reduction in cardiac output and renal blood flow. The rise in blood pressure in response to this maneuver is physiologically similar to an infusion of angiotensin.

RENAL FUNCTION IN TOXEMIA

There is a reduction in GFR with the development of toxemia, but since GFR is increased in pregnancy, such a reduction can occur with the GFR remaining in the normal nonpregnant range. Bucht (113) found the inulin clearance in toxemia was about 62 percent of that in normal pregnant women. Renal blood flow fell similarly to 62 to 84 percent of values found in pregnant controls, but the studies were hampered by determinations of para-aminohippuric acid clearance at low urine flow rates.

Urate production in pregnancy is normal, but urate clearance increases so mean plasma urate in pregnant women is 3.57 ± 0.7 mg/dL. The in-

creased clearance may reflect both increased filtered urate as well as increased renal plasma flow increasing delivery of urate to tubular secretory sites. With the development of toxemia plasma urate rises to approximately 5 mg/dL in mild toxemia and to over 7.5 mg/dL in severe toxemia (114). Plasma urate is a better criterion than BUN, blood pressure, or proteinuria in assessing the severity of toxemia. The cause of the decrease in urate clearance with toxemia is not completely clear. Handler (115) suggested that increased plasma lactate from an ischemic uterus inhibited urate secretion. He was unable, however, to find a significant elevation in blood lactate in patients with mild toxemia in whom a reduction in urate clearance was present, and this has been confirmed by others (116). In women with eclampsia, elevation in blood lactate secondary to the convulsion might account, in part, for the diminished urate clearance. Both convulsions and hypertension elevate blood lactate, and this would decrease urate clearance.

Volume depletion diminishes urate clearance, and urinary sodium excretion has a linear correlation with urate clearance in pregnancy (117). Increasing filtration fraction with angiotensin and norepinephrine diminishes urate clearance (118) which might be mediated either by an increase in peritubular capillary oncotic pressure increasing urate reabsorption or to diminished delivery of urate to the secretory site. Whether a rise in filtration fraction occurs in toxemia is unclear.

RENAL PATHOLOGY

Significant changes in the glomeruli in toxemia were first described in 1918 by Lohlein (119), and subsequently Fahr (120) called attention to the swelling of capillary wall. In 1933 Baird and Dunn (121) noted uneven thickening of the capillary basement membrane and were struck by the bulky endothelial cells in which the cytoplasm appeared foamy. The first electron microscopic study of the glomerulus in toxemia (122) demonstrated the striking swelling of endothelial cells of the glomerular capillaries with deposits of a fibrinlike material within and under the endothelial cells. This report was confirmed by Spargo (123) who called the lesion "glomerular capillary endotheliosis." Vassalli (124) demonstrated by immunofluorescent staining that the deposits in the glomeruli were fibrinogen or one of its derivatives. There was no evidence of soluble antigen-antibody complexes in the glomeruli, and by immunofluorescence the occasional presence of IgG or IgM in the glomeruli is thought to represent nonspecific trapping.

Pregnant ewes develop a disease which is quite similar to toxemia, with convulsions, proteinuria, and reduction in GFR in response to stress (73). The changes in the glomeruli by both light and electron microscopy are indistinguishable from human toxemia. However, hypertension does not occur, and it is of note that plasma renin does not increase in ovine pregnancy and the ovine uterus and amniotic fluid do not contain renin.

Although the glomeruli appear bloodless, capillary thrombosis is rare unless associated with acute renal failure or cortical necrosis. There is little proliferation of either endothelial or epithelial cells, and the afferent arterioles and arcuate arteries are not thickened when compared to those of control subjects. Complete resolution of these glomerular changes has been reported by some to occur as early as 4 weeks postpartum (123), whereas others have noted their persistence for as long as 2 years in some instances (124). The absence of immunologic damage to the glomerulus in toxemia points to direct endothelial cell injury with local activation of intravascular coagulation. Similar glomerular lesions have been produced in rabbits by thromboplastin infusions (125). Some authors have found the glomerular changes in only a small percentage of multiparous women presenting with toxemia. McCartney (126) studied 152 multiparous women with chronic hypertension and superimposed toxemia and found that only 14 percent had the characteristic lesion of the glomerulus. In contrast, in 62 primigravidas with toxemia the characteristic lesion was found in 44 (71 percent); 16 (26 percent) of these primiparous women with toxemia also had chronic renal disease. Pollak and Nettles (29) found characteristic features of toxemia in 72 percent of their cases. Since the glomerular pa-

thology best correlates with the proteinuria, the characteristic pathologic findings would not be present in all toxemic women. The spectrum of proteinuria in toxemia can range from nephrotic levels, 10 to 30 g per 24 h, to as low as 500 mg per 24 h. In multiparous women hypertension is most prominent and proteinuria mild or absent.

LIVER PATHOLOGY

Two types of lesions occur in the liver during toxemia: (1) localized hemorrhages in the periportal areas which later become replaced by fibrin and (2) various grades of ischemic lesions ranging from very small areas of damage to large infarcts. These lesions are usually never seen if the toxemia is clinically mild but are found in two-thirds of patients with eclampsia. Rarely, large subcapsular hematomas develop over the liver and rupture into the peritoneal cavity with fatal results. The cause of these large subcapsular hematomas is unclear. Some originate deep in the liver (127), but most seem to arise from the capsule itself. Of 51 cases with subcapsular hematoma, 35 had toxemia, 14 had eclampsia. Recent reports indicate that fibrin deposits demonstrated by immunofluorescence are present in the hepatic vasculature in toxemia (128).

CENTRAL NERVOUS SYSTEM

The most common cause of death in eclampsia is cerebral hemorrhage, and evidence of hemorrhage is found in about 60 percent of patients who die within 2 days of the onset of the convulsions. The hemorrhages are both small petechial hemorrhages, which microscopically show thrombosis of precapillaries with infarction, and large hematomas. These thrombi are always in close proximity to areas of hemorrhage. This would suggest that the changes in the brain are primarily due to intense cerebral vasoconstriction with secondary thrombosis of small vessels (129). Multiple areas of ischemic softening are scattered throughout the brain but are not hemorrhagic. Frequently a single large hemorrhage into the white matter, the basal ganglia, or pons can occur, producing a subarachnoid hemorrhage. The coma which often occurs in eclampsia is due in many patients to cerebral hemorrhage.

In patients with eclampsia who develop cerebral hemorrhage the blood pressure rise frequently appears insufficient to cause the rupture of the arteries. It is possible that fibrin deposits in cerebral capillaries results in ischemic changes.

An unusual cause of headache and convulsions in the postpartum period is central vein thrombosis. Thrombosis most commonly develops in a vein over the parietal cortex. The convulsions may be indistinguishable from those of eclampsia. The cause of postpartum cerebral venous thrombosis is unclear, but it may be related to the postpartum hypercoagulable state, which may also account for postpartum phlebothrombosis and renal failure (130, 131).

MISCELLANEOUS PATHOLOGIC CHANGES

The adrenal cortex in patients with severe toxemia appears ischemic and can have widespread hemorrhages. Although usually these lesions are not sufficient to cause adrenal insufficiency, such findings in the adrenal cortex must alert the clinician to the possibility of postpartum adrenal insufficiency following severe toxemia.

Several reviews of placental pathology have been published (132, 133), but no uniformity of opinion exists concerning whether there is a specific lesion of the placenta in toxemia.

CLINICAL FEATURES OF TOXEMIA

A useful classification of toxemia would be a modification of that adopted by the American Committee of Maternal Welfare.

I. Acute toxemia of pregnancy (onset after the 24th week)
  A. Preeclampsia
  B. Eclampsia (when a convulsion has occurred)

II. Chronic hypertensive vascular disease or renal disease with pregnancy.
  A. Without superimposed acute toxemia.
    1. Hypertension or renal disease known to antedate pregnancy.
    2. Hypertension or renal disease discovered in pregnancy.
  B. With superimposed acute toxemia.

The clinical onset of toxemia is insidious and may not be accompanied by symptoms. The usual sequence is edema and hypertension followed by proteinuria, although occasionally proteinuria precedes hypertension. Headaches, visual disturbances, epigastric pain and apprehension are frequent symptoms. Toxemia usually begins after the 32d week of pregnancy but may begin earlier, particularly in women with preexisting renal disease or hypertension. It can occur during the first trimester with a hydatidiform mole. The disease can occur postpartum with hypertension and convulsions usually 24 to 48 h after delivery, although it has been reported as long as 7 days postpartum. The physical examination frequently demonstrates generalized puffy edema, particularly of the face and hands. Diastolic hypertension is prominent with systolic pressures below 160 mmHg in most cases. Systolic blood pressure over 200 mmHg with toxemia usually points to the presence of underlying essential hypertension. Funduscopic examination will reveal segmental arteriolar narrowing with a wet, glistening fundus indicative of retinal edema. Hemorrhages and exudates are rare but may occur following convulsions. Unilateral or bilateral retinal detachments can occur in toxemia and are associated with sudden blindness. Detachment is caused by intraocular edema, and usually spontaneous reattachment of the retina follows diuresis and control of the hypertension. Careful examination of the heart and lungs must be made to determine if congestive heart failure is present. The degree of central nervous excitability is assessed by careful determination of the spinal reflexes.

The incidence of toxemia of pregnancy varies widely, ranging from 2 percent of all deliveries in the Far East to 29.9 percent in Puerto Rico. In the United States the incidence is approximately 7 percent, but in Aberdeen, Scotland, MacGillivray et al. (2) found a 24.2 percent incidence of hypertension in primigravidas and 8 percent in multiparous patients. The incidence will depend upon the criteria used for the diagnosis. Pressures in excess of 125/75 mmHg prior to 32 weeks' gestation are associated with significant increases in fetal risk, as are pressures over 125/85 mmHg at term (134). MacGillivray accepts a 14 mmHg rise in diastolic blood pressure during pregnancy as evidence of toxemia. Certainly an elevation of 20 mmHg or more in systolic blood pressure and 10 mmHg or more in diastolic pressure during pregnancy should be considered abnormal regardless of the absolute values obtained. Although there is a fall in blood pressure during the second trimester, the rise from the second trimester to term should not exceed 15 mmHg in either diastolic or systolic pressure.

Toxemia is frequent in women with twin pregnancies, diabetes, hydramnios, and hydatidiform mole. There seems to be no increased incidence of preeclampsia in blacks. Approximately one-third of women who have toxemia will develop the disease in a subsequent pregnancy, and in women who develop toxemia with subsequent pregnancies, 50 percent develop fixed essential hypertension. The disease is more common in the lower socioeconomic classes in which obesity and short stature seem more common.

Edema with toxemia

Chesley (135) analyzed 10,591 cases of toxemia and found that 72 percent gained less than 30 pounds during the pregnancy, while 88 percent of women who gained more than 30 pounds had normotensive pregnancies. Thus, excessive weight gain during pregnancy does not necessarily predispose to toxemia. The association of obesity with toxemia is probably similar to that of obesity with essential hypertension. It does not cause the hypertension, but in the hypertensive patient, weight gain increases arterial pressure.

Although edema in pregnancy is usually not pathologic, edema can be a manifestation of toxemia. When generalized edema develops in pregnancy, blood pressure usually rises, and increased sensitivity to angiotensin can be demonstrated (16). The cause of the increased sodium retention in toxemia, as in other clinical conditions associated with edema, is not clear. Since plasma renin and angiotensin are frequently lower in toxemia, an increase in aldosterone secretion would not occur. One factor increasing sodium absorption is the reduced GFR occurring in toxemia. Since the renal tubular cells must reabsorb extraordinary amounts of sodium during pregnancy because of increase in filtration, any reduction in glomerular filtration might cause greater fractional reabsorption of sodium.

Clinical evidence of vasoconstriction in toxemia is found in the retina where arteriolar vasoconstriction is prominent and in the hemoconcentration which frequently is present. In toxemic patients, plasma volume is reduced because of venous vasoconstriction, which increases capillary pressure. Reduction in plasma volume with hemoconcentration is seen in other states in which circulating vasoconstriction plays a role, e.g., pheochromocytoma and renal artery stenosis.

The extent to which the hypertension of toxemia represents volume expansion or vasoconstriction varies with each patient. Both mechanisms are important, as evidenced by toxemic patients with striking edema and other patients with equal hypertension in whom edema is minimal. Studies on the prophylactic use of thiazides in preventing toxemia have been conflicting (61, 62), but use of a diuretic throughout pregnancy examines only the question whether high salt intake causes toxemia and not whether sodium worsens toxemia.

Similarly, the hemoconcentration of toxemia has been interpreted to indicate that plasma expanders are necessary in toxemia (136). Since the cause of the hemoconcentration is not extracellular volume depletion, but vasoconstriction, expansion of vascular volume does not correct the pathophysiologic state. The use of a vasodilator will relieve vasoconstriction, and reconstitution of plasma volume will occur as mobilization of fluid sequestered in the interstitium enters the vascular space. The use of plasma expanders to correct hemoconcentration is contraindicated in the presence of hypertension. However, the initial use of diuretics as antihypertensive agents when hemoconcentration is present could be questioned. The immediate need is for relief of vasoconstriction.

Patients with toxemia being treated with a low salt intake and diuretics can develop hypovolemia which will reduce renal blood flow and worsen the azotemia (137). This can occur in any patient being treated with diuretics and only indicates that care must be taken to prevent volume depletion with diuretics after blood pressure control has been achieved.

LABORATORY FEATURES

Hematologic findings

Pregnancy is associated with an increase in clotting factors and mild activation of the clotting mechanism (70). Normotensive pregnant women who have had renal biopsies demonstrate on immunofluorescent staining slight deposits of fibrin in glomeruli (124). Although circulating levels of fibrinogen and other clotting factors in toxemia are similar to those of normal pregnant women, the platelet count is frequently depressed, and toxemia consistently is associated with increased amount of cryofibrinogen in the blood (138, 139). The presence of cryofibrinogen in toxemia indicates that a fibrin monomer is present, and since fibrinolysis is depressed in pregnancy, circulating fibrin deposited in the glomerulus might not be lysed (140). Evidence of platelet damage in toxemia is the demonstration that platelet adhesiveness is increased compared to that of normal pregnancy (71). The increase in acid phosphatase found in some toxemic patients is thought to represent acid phosphatase liberated from platelets during intravascular destruction.

Patients with severe toxemia may develop a hemolytic-uremic syndrome which may be transitory or prolonged (139). Marked fragmentation of red blood cells is seen on smear and may be associated with the development of renal cortical necrosis. The cause of the intravascular coagulation may be release of trophoblastic material from the placenta. Since the maternal blood channel of the placenta, the intervillous space, becomes a source of fibrin deposits with placental senescence, the premature or disproportionate senescence of the placenta in toxemia may be pertinent.

Toxemia is associated with thrombocytopenia (70), and the diagnosis is frequently confused with idiopathic or thrombotic thrombocytopenic purpura (141). The presence of hypertension or a significant rise in arterial pressure during the pregnancy accompanying the thrombocytopenia should alert the physician to the presence of toxemia.

There are other diseases with multiple system involvement occurring during or immediately after pregnancy that might have as a common cause intravascular clotting. Acute fatty liver of pregnancy (72), postpartum myocardiopathy (142), tetracycline hepatotoxicity in pregnancy (143), acute cortical necrosis (144), recurrent thrombotic thrombocytopenic purpura with pregnancy (141), and postpartum necrosis of the anterior pituitary (145) are also frequently associated with toxemia of pregnancy and could be manifestations of small-vessel thrombosis occurring either during or immediately after pregnancy. A review of the 41 published cases of acute fatty liver of pregnancy revealed that 22 patients had either toxemia clinically or characteristic renal changes at postpartum examination in association with pathologic changes in brain, pancreas, and kidneys. Kunelis (143) was the first to point out the multisystem nature of this disease and that virtually all patients dying of acute fatty liver of pregnancy had elevation of BUN but only minimal elevation of serum glutamic oxaloacetic transaminase (SGOT) and serum glutamic pyruvic transaminase (SGPT). This is quite unlike viral hepatitis, which results in acute hepatic failure and death.

Urinary findings

Of 35 patients with preeclampsia, Pollak and Nettles found 24 had abnormalities of the urinary sediment (29). The abnormalities were minor; only 5 patients had more than 10 red blood cells per high power field. Of the 35 cases, 6 had casts, both erythrocyte and epithelial, but there were no casts in the urine of 21 patients with characteristic changes of toxemia on renal biopsy. Thus, most patients with toxemia have negative urine sediment, although a few will have microscopic hematuria and red blood cell casts. Significant hematuria with casts points to a preceding or acute glomerulonephritis. The amount of proteinuria is variable. It can range from under 1 g to more than 300 g.

Figure 25-8 depicts a postulated series of events which could explain the pathophysiology of toxemia.

TREATMENT

The first aim of treatment should be prevention of toxemia. Proper prenatal care with attention to adequate but not excessive weight gain, vitamin supplementation, and monitoring of blood pressure reduces the incidence of toxemia. Poor blacks in the southern United States have a high incidence of toxemia (146), but there is no correlation between toxemia and nutrition in India (147) or in Australia (148). The World Health Organization Expert Committee has stated, "There seems to be no scientific basis for believing that deficiency or excess of any essential nutrient predisposes to preeclampsia and eclampsia." (149)

The poor, however, in many countries suffer a higher incidence of toxemia. In the United States the relationship between income and maternal death might be partly explained on the basis of availability of medical care, but in Jerusalem where this is not as great a factor, the toxemia rate in illiterate women is twice that of matched control subjects (150). Since the poor are more apt to have children at early and late ages, this may be one factor explaining the increased incidence.

The most important feature in the prevention and treatment of toxemia is the recognition by obstetricians that a rise in blood pressure greater than 15 mmHg (systolic) or 10 mmHg (diastolic) during pregnancy is significant and that the development of proteinuria is always an indication for hospitalization. Hospitalization will allow the course of the hypertension, proteinuria, and renal function to be followed closely.

Initial therapy is bed rest in a room that is darkened to prevent photic stimuli. Blood pres-

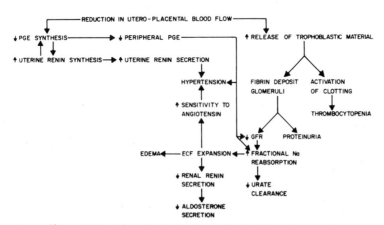

Figure 25-8. A hypothesis for the pathophysiology in toxemia. Diminished uteroplacental blood flow leads to a possible decrease in uterine synthesis of PGE but an increase in renin synthesis. In addition, fibrin deposits in glomeruli caused a reduction in GFR and sodium retention.

sure, pulse, respirations, and urine volume are carefully monitored. In the conscious patient there is no need for an indwelling catheter, but in patients having convulsions or in a comatose state, an indwelling catheter is warranted to carefully evaluate urine output. In the patient with mild toxemia, i.e., blood pressure no higher than 140/90 mmHg, therapy consists of bed rest, sedation with phenobarbital or diazepam (Valium), salt restriction to 500 to 1000 mg daily, and, if edema is present, 50 mg hydrochlorothiazide or 40 mg furosemide orally. These measures usually suffice in controlling the hypertension. Baseline BUN and plasma creatinine and uric acid concentration are determined, and 24-h urine collection for volume and total protein excretion is obtained. Daily weights are a guide to the extent of the diuresis. The level of serum uric acid before institution of diuretic therapy is an excellent guide to the severity of the toxemia. If the uric acid is greater than 4.5 mg/dL and the patient has not been on diuretics or had a recent convulsion, this degree of hyperuricemia is virtually diagnostic of toxemia. Levels of uric acid above 5.5 mg/dL are indicative of severe toxemia. Extremely high levels can be seen in eclamptic patients following a convulsion, in which intense muscular effort has caused elevation of plasma lactate which further decreases uric acid clearance (115). Essential hypertension occurring in pregnancy does not cause significant change in the serum urate concentration. A serum uric acid below 4 mg per 100 mL with hypertension in pregnancy is most consistent with essential hypertension.

If therapy results in a reduction in pressure to below 120/80 mmHg, proteinuria is less than 150 mg per 24 h, renal function is normal, and there is no evidence of central nervous system (CNS) hyperexcitability, the patient can be followed as an outpatient. The serum urate concentration correlates better with minimal disease than BUN or creatinine levels. Patients with preeclampsia have normal tubular function, so concentrated urine with high specific gravity, greater than 1.020, is frequent.

When the patient has severe hypertension, i.e., blood pressure greater than 140/90 mmHg, more potent antihypertensive therapy should be initiated. Although magnesium sulfate has a mild antihypertensive effect, it primarily diminishes CNS excitability and acts as an anticonvulsant. The advantage of magnesium as an anticonvulsant and antihypertensive in toxemia resides in its long-established use by obstetricians and their confidence in using the drug. More potent antihypertensive drugs are far more effective, however, in lowering blood pressure.

Hydralazine (Apresoline), 25 to 50 mg every 6 h orally, is effective when used in conjunction with a diuretic (151). To prevent the reflex tachycardia which may occur with hydralazine, propranolol, 40 mg every 6 h, may be added. In one patient with chronic hypertension taking 160 to 240 mg propranolol daily throughout pregnancy, growth retardation of the fetus and postnatal hypoglycemia and bradycardia has been reported (152).

In severe toxemia in which diastolic blood pressure is greater than 110 mmHg, parenteral antihypertensive therapy is indicated. If the diastolic pressure is below 120 mmHg, 500 mg methyldopa and 40 to 80 mg furosemide are given intravenously and repeated every 6 h. Since methyldopa is a CNS depressant, it may be of benefit in a patient with hyperexcitability and usually does not cause undue somnolence. Since parenteral methyldopa requires 6 to 8 h for maximum effect, immediate control of blood pressure can be accomplished with parenteral hydralazine, 25 mg given intramuscularly, or 25 to 50 mg in 500 mL glucose and water intravenously.

When the diastolic blood pressure is 120 mmHg or greater, 300 mg diazoxide intravenously can be given rapidly with 40 to 80 mg furosemide. Finnerty (153) has treated 61 severe toxemics, 2 with eclampsia, with diazoxide and furosemide, resulting in an average diuresis of 16 lb prior to delivery. There were no maternal deaths and only four fetal deaths, with an incidence of prematurity of 37 percent. Fetal mortality was as low in Finnerty's series as the 11 percent reported in a series in which hypertension was not treated (154). Michael has also reported excellent results with diazoxide in 53 severe toxemics with control of blood pressure in all and without evidence of fetal distress (155). The only side effect of diazoxide was the cessation of labor in about 50 percent of the patients, probably as a result of the generalized smooth-muscle relaxant effect of the drug. The use of diazoxide in pregnant ewes lowered arterial pressure but did not decrease uterine blood flow or have an adverse effect upon fetal hemodynamics (156). Administration of oxytocic agents immediately restarted labor.

After reduction of the blood pressure has been accomplished and the patient's clinical state stabilized, delivery of the fetus is indicated in severe toxemia. In rare instances where fetal survival is questionable the pregnancy can be continued, but constant hospitalization is required. The patient should be maintained on 500 to 1000 mg sodium per day and diuretics given until edema disappears, at which time they should be discontinued. Oral antihypertensive drugs should be used if needed. Measurements of fetal development are helpful, utilizing urinary estriol and pregnanediol determinations as well as lecithin/sphingomyelin ratios in amniotic fluid (157). When toxemia is associated with low urinary estriol excretion one can presume that intrauterine growth has ceased and delivery is indicated. If elevation of the BUN persists in spite of blood pressure control, delivery is indicated since fetal growth or maturation is not likely in the presence of azotemia. Eclampsia is always an indication for delivery once the blood pressure and convulsions have been controlled. Eclampsia indicates severe disease, and convulsions increase maternal and fetal mortality.

In the preeclamptic patient either phenobarbital or diazepam can be used for sedation and an anticonvulsant. Although phenobarbital crosses the placenta, its margin of safety is high in infants.

EFFECT OF TREATMENT ON UTERINE BLOOD FLOW

There are few studies of the uterine circulation in toxemia. Assali (158), using the nitrous oxide technique, demonstrated increased uterine vascular resistance with decreased flow. Utilizing electromagnetic flow probes in pregnant dogs and ewes the uterus has been reported to increase flow with increasing perfusion pressure (159). However, in pregnant rabbits, using radioactive microspheres to measure uterine blood flow, Venuto et al. have demonstrated that uterine blood flow is constant over a range of blood pressure from 75 to 112 mmHg (11) (Fig. 25-9). Relief of vasoconstriction should increase perfusion of the uterus, par-

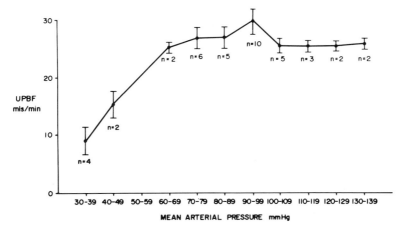

Figure 25-9. The effect of varying perfusion pressure on uteroplacental blood flow in the pregnant rabbit. Arterial pressure was raised by carotid ligation and lowered by antihypertensive drugs. n = number of observations at each arterial pressure level. Note the constancy of uterine blood flow with mean arterial pressures ranging from 60 to 69 mmHg. (*From Venuto et al.*)

ticularly if cardiac output increases. Both hydralazine and diazoxide increase cardiac output, and methyldopa reduces blood pressure with little or no change in cardiac output. Although dehydroisoandrosterone clearance has been found to be reduced with antihypertensive therapy with either diuretics (63) or hydralazine (160) there is no evidence for increased fetal mortality in treated toxemic patients. Since the major cause of maternal mortality in toxemia is cerebral vascular hemorrhage, one must at all costs prevent such a maternal catastrophe, and the evidence is conclusive that antihypertensive agents prevent cerebral vascular accidents in hypertensive diseases (161).

THE REMOTE CONSEQUENCES OF TOXEMIA

In follow-up of toxemic women, subsequent hypertension is more common, but whether toxemia caused the hypertension is still open to question (162). Many feel that toxemia, like hypertension induced by contraceptive drugs (163), differentiates those women who will ultimately develop essential hypertension. The effect of toxemia on the induction of hypertension is difficult to evaluate since many women with underlying renal disease and hypertension are included in every series of toxemic patients. Similarly, the influence of obesity and race, known to be factors in the development of essential hypertension, has been ignored in many studies on the long-term follow-up of women with toxemia of pregnancy. Bechgaard et al. (164) found the incidence of hypertension in 372 women 15 years after toxemia to be 25 percent plus an unknown proportion of the 8 percent who had died in the 15-year period. Epstein found that 15 years after toxemia 37 percent of patients in the Yale series were hypertensive compared with 7 percent of the control group (165). Harbert et al. (166) give an incidence of hypertension after eclampsia of 15 percent, whereas Fritzsch et al. (167), in a follow-up of 19 eclamptic patients, found that 4 were hypertensive, 1 had chronic glomerulonephritis, and 7 had chronic interstitial nephritis.

The two most careful studies of this problem have been done by Epstein (165) and Chesley

(168). Epstein restricted his study to white women with hypertension, proteinuria, and edema. However, half the patients were multiparous. When examined 15 years after the episode of toxemia the incidence of hypertension (blood pressure greater than 150/90 mmHg) was three times greater than control women of the same age and weight who had normotensive pregnancies. No evidence of residual renal disease or urinary tract infection was found in the toxemic group. Since the incidence of hypertension was similar in siblings of both groups Epstein concluded that toxemia predisposed women to the development of hypertension.

In contrast, Chesley restricted his study to 270 primiparous women surviving eclampsia over a 20-year period at the Margaret Hague Maternity Hospital. By eliminating preeclamptic and multiparous patients, he felt he was excluding essential hypertension during pregnancy. Since approximately 40 percent of hypertensive women have decreased blood pressure during pregnancy, often to the normal range, the development of hypertension late in pregnancy can be misleading. In Chesley's follow-up the remote mortality over 20 years was the same as in unselected women. The frequency distribution curve of diastolic blood pressure was identical in women having had primiparous eclampsia and in several epidemiologic studies of unselected women. However, in both black and white women having eclampsia with multiparous pregnancies the remote mortality was 2.6 to 3.8 times greater than expected. Thus, eclampsia was associated with a higher incidence of subsequent hypertension only in multiparous women.

It is of interest that diabetes was 5 times as common on follow-up examination in primiparous women developing eclampsia and 10 times the expected rate in multiparous eclamptic women. The increased incidence of toxemia may be related to the fact that prediabetic women have large babies. This could not be documented because of the absence of birth weights in many of Chesley's patients but may be an important factor in the development of toxemia.

Some have argued that Chesley's figures are pertinent only to eclamptic women and that preeclamptic patients are frequently hypertensive for longer periods and would have a greater incidence of subsequent hypertension. This argument presumes that duration, rather than severity, of toxemia causes subsequent hypertension and that eclampsia occurs suddenly. The evidence would indicate, however, that eclampsia is most often the result of a prolonged and neglected preeclamptic state. Although eclamptic patients are rapidly delivered, most have little or no prenatal care, and the length of time they have been hypertensive is usually unknown. In Chesley's series, when blood pressure was recorded prior to the episode of eclampsia, in nearly half of the patients preeclampsia had been present for at least 3 weeks and in about 12 percent it had been present for more than 6 weeks before convulsions occurred.

Of Chesley's 207 primiparous white eclamptic patients, 148 had later pregnancies, and 69 suffered recurrent toxemia. Thus, 25 percent of these cases had at least two toxemic pregnancies, and yet the prevalence of hypertension was not increased over a control population. The recurrence of toxemia was only 25 percent in women who developed toxemia with the first pregnancy. Singh et al. (169) reported a higher incidence of later hypertension only in women having preeclampsia in more than one pregnancy.

Bryans et al. (170) followed 168 white women and 167 black women for 1 to 44 years after eclampsia and compared their mean blood pressure with blood pressures found in several epidemiologic studies. Diastolic pressure of primiparous black women was no higher than that of control subjects, and the prevalence of hypertension in the white women with eclampsia was not increased. Multiparous eclamptic women, however, had a higher prevalence of later hypertension, and blood pressure was higher in relatives of multiparous eclamptic women.

REFERENCES

1. Lees, M. M., S. H. Taylor, F. B. Scott, and M. G. Kerr: A study of cardiac output at rest throughout pregnancy, *J. Obstet. Gynaecol. Br. Commonw.*, **74:**319, 1967.
2. MacGillivray, I., G. A. Rose, and B. Rowe: Blood pressure survey in pregnancy, *Clin. Sci.*, **37:**395, 1969.
3. Page, E. W., and R. Christianson: The impact of mean arterial pressure in the middle trimester on the outcome of pregnancy, *Am. J. Obstet. Gynecol.*, **125:**740, 1976.
4. Bay, W. H., R. Greenspan, and T. F. Ferris: Factors controlling plasma renin and aldosterone in pregnancy, *Circ. Res.* In press.
5. Horton, E. W.: Prostaglandins at adrenergic nerve endings, *Br. Med. Bull.*, **29:**148, 1973.
6. Venuto, R., T. O'Dorisio, J. H. Stein, and T. F. Ferris: The effect of prostaglandin inhibition on uterine blood flow, *J. Clin. Invest.*, **55:**193, 1975.
7. Terragno, N. A., D. A. Terragno, D. Pacholczyk, and J. C. McGiff: Prostaglandins and the regulation of uterine blood flow in pregnancy, *Nature*, **249:**57, 1974.
8. Speroff, L., R. V. Haning, E. J. Ewaschuk, S. L. Alberino, and F. X. Kieliszek: Uterine artery blood flow studies in pregnant monkeys, in M. D. Lindheimer, A. I. Katz, and F. R. Zuspan (eds.), *Hypertension in Pregnancy*, John Wiley & Sons, Inc., New York, 1976, p. 315.
9. Golub, M., P. Zia, M. Matsuma, and R. Horton: Metabolism of PGA and E in man, *J. Clin. Invest.*, **56:**1404, 1975.
10. Burrow, G. N., and T. F. Ferris (eds.), Toxemia and hypertension, in *Medical Complications During Pregnancy*, W. B. Saunders Company, 1975, pp. 53–104.
11. Venuto, R., J. W. Cox, J. H. Stein, and T. F. Ferris: Regulation of uterine blood flow in the pregnant rabbit, *J. Clin. Invest.*, **57:**700, 1976.
12. Weir, R. J., J. J. Brown, R. Fraser, A. F. Lever, et al.: Plasma renin, renin substrate, angiotensin II and aldosterone in hypertensive disease of pregnancy, *Lancet* **1:**291, 1973.
13. Vallotton, M. B., C. Godard, and R. Gaillard: Assessment of the renin-angiotensin system, aldosterone, and cortisol in mother and fetus at term, in M. D. Lindheimer, A. I. Katz, and F. R. Zuspan (eds.), *Hypertension in Pregnancy*, John Wiley & Sons, Inc., New York, 1976, p. 281.
14. Ferris, T. F., R. C. Venuto, and W. H. Bay: Studies of the uterine circulation in the pregnant rabbit, in M. D. Lindheimer, A. I. Katz, and F. R. Zuspan (eds.), *Hypertension in Pregnancy*, John Wiley & Sons, Inc., New York, 1976, p. 351.

15. Elebute, O. A. and I. H. Mills: Urinary kallikrein in normal and hypertensive pregnancies, in M. D. Lindheimer, A. I. Katz, and F. R. Zuspan (eds.), *Hypertension in Pregnancy,* John Wiley & Sons, Inc., New York, 1976, p. 329.

16. Gant, N. F., G. L. Daley, S. Chand, P. J. Whalley, and P. C. MacDonald: A study of angiotensin II pressor response throughout primigravid pregnancy, *J. Clin. Invest.,* **52:**2682, 1973.

17. Cunningham, F. G., K. Cox, and N. F. Gant: Further observations on the nature of pressor responsitivity to AII in human pregnancy, *Obstet. Gynecol.,* **46:**581, 1975.

18. Brunner, J., P. Change, R. Wallach, J. E. Sealey, and J. H. Laragh: Angiotensin II vascular receptors: Their avidity in relationship to sodium balance, the autonomic venous system and hypertension, *J. Clin. Invest.,* **51:**58, 1972.

19. Gill, J. R., J. C. Frolich, R. E. Bowden, A. A. Taylor, H. R. Keiser, H. W. Seyberth, J. A. Oates, and F. C. Bartter: Bartter's syndrome: A disorder characterized by high urinary prostaglandins and a dependence of hyperreninemia on prostaglandin synthesis, *Am. J. Med.,* **61:**43, 1976.

20. Fichman, M. P., N. Telfer, P. Zia, P. Speckart, M. Golub, and R. Rude: Role of prostaglandins in the pathogenesis of Bartter's syndrome, *Am. J. Med.,* **60:**785, 1976.

21. Normington, E. A. M., and D. Davies: Hypertension and oedema complicating pregnancy in Addison's disease, *Br. Med. J.,* **1:**148, 1972.

22. Johnson, J. A., J. O. Davis, J. S. Baumber, and E. G. Schneider: Effect of estrogen and progesterone on electrolyte balances in normal dogs, *Am. J. Physiol.,* **219:**1691, 1970.

23. DeVries, J. R., J. H. Lukens, and D. D. Fanestil: Estradiol renal receptor molecules and estradiol dependent antinatriuresis, *Kidney Int.,* **2:**95, 1972.

24. Prichard, J. A.: Studies of red cell mass in pregnancy, *Anesthesiology,* **26:**393, 1965.

25. Brenner, B. M., J. L. Troy, T. M. Daugherty, W. M. Deen, and C. R. Robertson: Dynamics of glomerular ultrafiltration in the rat: Plasma flow dependence of GFR, *Am. J. Physiol.,* **223:**1184, 1972.

26. Bucht, J.: Studies on renal function in man: With special reference to glomerular filtration and renal plasma flow in pregnancy, *Scand. J. Clin. Lab. Invest.,* **3** (suppl. 3): 1, 1951.

27. Sims, E. A. H., and K. E. Krantz: Serial studies of renal function during pregnancy and the puerperium in normal women, *J. Clin. Invest.,* **37:**1764, 1958.

28. Robertson, E. G.: Increased erythrocyte fragility in association with osmotic changes in pregnancy serum, *J. Reprod. Fertil.,* **16:**323, 1968.

29. Pollak, V. C., and J. B. Nettles: The kidney in toxemia of pregnancy: A clinical and pathological study based on renal biopsies, *Medicine (Baltimore),* **39:**469, 1960.

30. Grumbach, M. M., S. L. Kaplan, J. J. Sciarra, and I. M. Burr: Chorionic growth hormone prolactin (CGP): Secretion, disposition, biologic activity in man, and postulated function as the "growth hormone" of the second half of pregnancy, *Ann. N.Y. Acad. Sci.,* **148:**501, 1968.

31. Christensen, P. J.: Tubular reabsorption of glucose during pregnancy, *Scand. J. Clin. Lab. Invest.,* **10:**364, 1958.

32. Welsh, G. W., and E. A. H. Sims: The mechanisms of renal glucosuria in pregnancy, *Diabetes,* **9:**363, 1960.

33. Fine, J.: Glycosuria of pregnancy, *Br. Med. J.,* **1:**205, 1967.

34. Wright, A. D., H. G. Dixon, and G. F. Joplin: Diabetes and latent diabetes in pregnancy, *Br. Med. Bull.,* **24:**25, 1968.

35. Wallraff, E. B., E. C. Brodie, and A. L. Borden: Urinary excretion of amino acids in pregnancy, *J. Clin. Invest.,* **29:**1542, 1950.

36. Christensen, P. J., J. W. Date, F. Schonheyder, and K. Volqvartz: Amino acids in blood plasma and urine during pregnancy, *Scand. J. Clin. Lab. Invest.,* **9:**52, 1957.

37. Zinneman, H. H., U. S. Seal, and R. P. Doe: Urinary amino acids in pregnancy following progesterone and estrogen, *J. Clin. Endocrinol. Metab.,* **27:**397, 1967.

38. Felig, P.: Diabetes mellitus, in G. N. Burrow and T. F. Ferris (eds.), *Medical Complications During Pregnancy,* W. B. Saunders Company, Philadelphia, 1975, p. 170.

39. Page, E. W.: Human fetal nutrition and growth, *Am. J. Obstet. Gynecol.,* **104:**378, 1969.

40. Tyson, J. E., A. C. Barnes, T. J. Merimee, and V. A. McKusick: Isolated growth hormone deficiency: studies in pregnancy, *J. Clin. Endocrinol. Metab.,* **31:**147, 1970.

41. Felig, P., and V. Lynch: Starvation in human pregnancy: Hypoglycemia, hypoinsulinemia, and hyperketonemia, *Science*, **170**:990, 1970.

42. Spellacy, W. N., W. C. Buhi, and S. A. Birk: The effect of estrogens on carbohydrate metabolism: Glucose, insulin and growth hormone studies on one hundred and seventy-one women ingesting Premarin, mestranol, and ethinyl estradiol for six months, *Am. J. Obstet. Gynecol.*, **114**:378, 1972.

43. Kalkhoff, R. K., B. L. Richardson, and P. Beck: Relative effects of pregnancy, human placental lactogen and prenisone on carbohydrate tolerance in normal and subclinical diabetic subjects, *Diabetes*, **18**:153, 1969.

44. Kopelman, J. J., and M. Levitz: Plasma cortisol levels and cortisol binding in normal and preeclamptic pregnancies, *Am. J. Obstet. Gynecol.*, **108**:925, 1970.

45. Migeon, C. J., F. M. Kenny, and F. H. Taylor: Cortisol production rate. VIII. Pregnancy. *J. Clin. Endocrinol. Metab.*, **28**:661, 1968.

46. Beck, P., C. J. Eaton, I. S. Young, and H. S. Kupperman: Metyrapone response in pregnancy, *Am. J. Obstet. Gynecol.*, **100**:327, 1968.

47. Baxter, J. D., and P. H. Forsham: Tissue effects of glucocorticoids, *Am. J. Med.*, **53**:573, 1972.

48. Watanabe, M., C. I. Meeker, M. J. Gray, E. A. H. Sims, and S. Solomon: Secretion rate of aldosterone in normal pregnancy, *J. Clin. Invest.*, **42**:1619, 1963.

49. Watanabe, M., C. I. Meeker, M. J. Gray, E. A. H. Sims, and S. Solomon: Aldosterone secretion rates in abnormal pregnancy, *J. Clin. Endocrinol. Metab.*, **25**:166, 1965.

50. Heany, R. P., and T. G. Skillman: Calcium metabolism in normal human pregnancy, *J. Clin. Endocrinol. Metab.*, **33**:661, 1971.

51. Burrow, G. N.: Adrenal, pituitary and parathyroid disorders, in G. N. Burrow and T. F. Ferris (eds.), *Medical Complications During Pregnancy*, W. B. Saunders Company, Philadelphia, 1975, p. 242.

52. Cushard, W. B., Jr., M. A. Creditor, J. M. Canterbury, and E. Reiss: Physiologic hyperparathyroidism in pregnancy, *J. Clin. Endocrinol. Metab.*, **34**:767, 1972.

53. Boyer, S. H.: Alkaline phosphatase in human sera and placentae. Starch gel electrophoresis reveals many phosphatase components including a polymorphism in placentae, *Science*, **134**:1002, 1961.

54. Weir, R. J., A. Doig, R. Fraser, J. J. Morton, J. Parboosingh, J. I. S. Robertson, and A. Wilson: Studies of the renin-angiotensin system, cortisol, DOC, and ADH in normal and hypertensive pregnancy, in M. D. Lindheimer, A. I. Katz, and F. R. Zuspan (eds.), *Hypertension in Pregnancy*, John Wiley & Sons, Inc., New York, 1976, p. 251.

55. Chesley, L. C.: Renal function tests in the differentiation of Bright's disease from so-called specific toxemia of pregnancy, *Surg. Gynecol. Obstet.*, **67**:481, 1938.

56. Warren, J. C., and R. S. Jernstrom: Diabetes insipidus and pregnancy, *Am. J. Obstet. Gynecol.*, **81**:1036, 1961.

57. Fitzsimmons, J. T.: The physiological basis of thirst, *Kidney Int.*, **10**:3, 1976.

58. Abdaul-Karim, R., and N. S. Assali: Renal function in human pregnancy. V. Effects of oxytocin on renal hemodynamics and water and electrolyte excretion, *J. Lab. Clin. Med.*, **57**:522, 1961.

59. Blechner, J. N., J. R. Cotter, V. G. Stenger, C. M. Hinkley, and H. Prystowsky: Oxygen, carbon dioxide and hydrogen ion concentrations in arterial blood during pregnancy, *Am. J. Obstet. Gynecol.*, **100**:1, 1968.

60. Lyons, H. A., and R. Antonio: The sensitivity of the respiratory center in pregnancy and after the administration of progesterone, *Trans. Assoc. Am. Physicians*, **72**:173, 1959.

61. Finnerty, F. A., Jr., and F. J. Bepko: Lowering the perinatal mortality and prematurity rate. *JAMA*, **195**:429, 1966.

62. Krauss, G. W., J. R. Marchese, and S. S. C. Yen: Prophylactic use of hydrochlorathiazide in pregnancy, *JAMA*, **198**:1150, 1966.

63. Gant, N. F., J. D. Madden, P. K. Siiteri, and P. C. MacDonald: The metabolic clearance rate of DHEA III. The effect of thiazide diuretics in normal and future preeclamptic pregnancy, *Am. J. Obstet. Gynecol.*, **123**:159, 1975.

64. Clewell, W., and G. Meschia: Relationship of metabolic clearance rate of DHEA to placental blood flow: A mathematical model, *Am. J. Obstet. Gynecol.*, **125**:507, 1976.

65. Landesman, R., O. Aguero, K. Wilson, B. LaRussa, W. Campbell, and O. Penaloza: The prophylactic use of chlorothalidone in pregnancy, *J. Obstet. Gynaecol. Br. Commonw.*, **1004,** 1965.

66. Redman, C. W. G., L. T. Berlin, J. Bonnar, and M. K. Qunsted: Fetal outcome in trial of antihypertensive treatment in pregnancy, *Lancet,* **11:**753, 1976.

67. Ferris, T. F.: Renal disease, in G. N. Burrow and T. F. Ferris (eds.), *Medical Complications During Pregnancy,* W. B. Saunders Company, Philadelphia, 1975, p. 1.

68. Bornstein, D. L., A. N. Weinberg, M. N. Swartz, and L. J. Kunz: Anaerobic infections: Review of current experience, *Medicine (Baltimore),* **46:**207, 1967.

69. Smith, K., J. C. M. Browne, R. Shackman, and O. M. Wrong: Acute renal failure of obstetric origin, *Lancet,* **2:**351, 1965.

70. Bonnar, J., C. W. G. Redman, and K. W. Denson: The role of coagulation and fibrinolysis in preeclampsia, in M. D. Lindheimer, A. I. Katz, and F. R. Zuspan (eds.), *Hypertension in Pregnancy,* John Wiley & Sons, Inc., New York, 1976, p. 85.

71. McKay, D. G.: Clinical significance of the pathology of toxemia of pregnancy, *Circulation,* **30** (suppl. 2): 66, 1964.

72. Hatfield, A. K., J. H. Stein, J. N. Greenberger, R. W. Abernathy, and T. F. Ferris: Idiopathic acute fatty liver of pregnancy, *Am. J. Dig. Dis.,* **17:**167, 1972.

73. Ferris, T. F., P. B. Herdson, M. S. Dunnill, and M. R. Lee: Toxemia of pregnancy in sheep: A clinical physiological and pathological study, *J. Clin. Invest.,* **48:**1643, 1969.

74. Rieselbach, R. E., S. Klahr, and M. S. Bricker: Diffuse bilateral cortical necrosis: A longitudinal study of the functional characteristics of residual nephrons, *Am. J. Med.,* **42:**457, 1967.

75. Riff, R. M.: Renocortical necrosis: Partial recovery after 49 days of oliguria, *Arch. Intern. Med.,* **119:**518, 1967.

76. Kleinknecht, D., J. P. Grunfeld, P. C. Gomez, J. F. Moreau, and R. Garcia-Torres: Diagnostic procedures and long term prognosis in bilateral renal cortical necrosis, *Kidney Int.,* **4:**390, 1973.

77. Walls, J. Jr., W. J. Schorr, and D. N. S. Kerr: Prolonged oliguria with survival in acute bilateral cortical necrosis, *Br. Med. J.,* **4:**220, 1968.

78. Effersoe, P., F. Raaschou, and A. C. Thomsen: Bilateral renal cortical necrosis: A patient followup over 8 years, *Am. J. Med.,* **33:**455, 1962.

79. Wagoner, R. D., K. E. Holley, and W. F. Johnson: Accelerated nephrosclerosis and postpartum acute renal failure in normotensive patients, *Ann. Intern. Med.,* **69:**237, 1968.

80. Robson, J. S., A. M. Martin, and V. A. Buckley: Irreversible postpartum renal failure: A new syndrome, *Q. J. Med.,* **37:**423, 1968.

81. Finkelstein, F. O., M. Kashgarian, and J. P. Hayslett: Clinical spectrum of postpartum renal failure, *Am. J. Med.,* **57:**649, 1974.

82. Tune, B. M., T. F. Leavitt, and T. J. Gribble: The hemolytic uremic syndrome in California: A review of 28 cases, *J. Pediatrics,* **82:**304, 1973.

83. Erickson, C. C., M. D. Lagios, P. Schoenfield, and R. Cohen: Effect of bilateral nephrectomy in postpartum nephrosclerosis, *Arch. Intern. Med.,* **128:**448, 1971.

84. Luke, R. G., R. R. Siegel, W. Talbert, and N. Holland: Heparin treatment for postpartum renal failure with microangiopathic hemolytic anemia, *Lancet,* **2:**750, 1970.

85. Beeson, P. B.: Effect of reticulo-endothelial blockade on immunity to the Shwartzman phenomenon, *Proc. Soc. Exp. Biol. Med.,* **64:**46, 1947.

86. McKay, D. G.: A partial synthesis of the generalized Shwartzmann reaction, *Fed. Proc.,* **22:**1373, 1963.

87. Merkatz, I. R., G. H. Schwartz, and D. S. David: Resumption of female reproductive function following renal transplantation, *JAMA,* **216:**1749, 1971.

88. Penn, I., E. Makowski, W. Droegemueller, C. G. Halgrimson, and T. E. Starzl: Parenthood in renal homograft recipients, *JAMA,* **216:**1755, 1971.

89. Tallent, M. B., R. L. Simmons, and J. S. Najerian: Birth defects in child of male recipient of kidney transplant, *JAMA,* **211:**1854, 1970.

90. Talledo, O., L. Chesley, and F. Zuspan: Renin-angiotensin system in normal and toxemic pregnancies, *Am. J. Obstet. Gynecol.,* **100:**218, 1968.

91. Tobian, L., and J. T. Binion: Tissue cations and water in arterial hypertension, *Circulation,* **5:**754, 1952.

92. Beker, J. C.: Aetiology of eclampsia, *J. Obstet. Gynecol. Br. Commonw.,* **55:**756, 1948.

93. Young, J.: The aetiology of eclampsia and albuminuria and their relation to accidental hemorrhage, *J. Obstet. Gynaecol. Br. Emp.,* **26:**1, 1914.

94. Page, E. W., and E. Ogden: The physiology of hypertension in eclampsia, *Am. J. Obstet. Gynecol.*, **38**:230, 1939.

95. VanBouwdijk Bastiaanse, M. A., and J. D. Mastbloom: Kidney and pregnancy, ischemia of the gravid uterus in dogs, *Acta Gynaecologic (Basel)*, **127**:1, 1949.

96. Berger, M., and D. Cavanaugh: Toxemia of pregnancy, the hypertensive effect of acute experimental placental ischemia, *Am. J. Obstet. Gynecol.*, **87**:293, 1963.

97. Cavanaugh, D., P. S. Rao, and K. Tung: Toxemia of pregnancy: The development of an experimental model in the primate, *Obstet. Gynecol.*, **39**:637, 1972.

98. Gant, N. J., H. T. Hutchinson, P. K. Siiteri, and P. C. MacDonald: Study of the metabolic clearance rate of dehydroisoandrosterone sulfate in pregnancy, *Am. J. Obstet. Gynecol.*, **111**:555, 1971.

99. Stakemann, G.: A renin-like pressor substance found in the placenta of the cat, *Acta Pathol. Microbiol. Scand.*, **50**:350, 1960.

100. Gross, F., G. Schaechtelin, M. Ziegler, and M. Berger: A renin-like substance in the placenta and uterus of the rabbit, *Lancet*, **1**:914, 1964.

101. Ferris, T. F., P. Gorden, and P. J. Mulrow: Rabbit uterus as a possible site of renin synthesis, *Am. J. Physiol.*, **212**:703, 1967.

102. Ferris, T. F., P. Gorden, and P. J. Mulrow: Rabbit uterus as a source of renin, *Am. J. Physiol.*, **212**:698, 1967.

103. Symonds, E. M., M. A. Stanley, and S. L. Skinner: Production of renin by in vitro cultures of human chorion and uterine muscle, *Nature*, **217**:1152, 1968.

104. Eskildsen, P. C.: Location of renin in rabbit uterus by help of microdissection, *Acta Path. Microbiol. Scand.*, **80**:241, 1972.

105. Anderson, R. C., P. N. Herbert, and P. J. Mulrow: A comparison of properties of renin obtained from the kidney and uterus of the rabbit, *Am. J. Physiol.*, **215**:774, 1968.

106. Ryan, J. W., and T. F. Ferris: Release of a renin-like enzyme from the pregnant uterus of the rabbit, *Biochem. J.*, **105**:160, 1967.

107. Ferris, T. F., J. H. Stein, and J. Kauffman: Uter-ine blood flow and uterine renin secretion, *J. Clin. Invest.*, **51**:2828, 1972.

108. Day, R. P., J. A. Luetscher, and C. M. Gonzales: Occurrence of big renin in human plasma, amniotic fluid and kidney extracts, *J. Clin. Endocrinol. Metab.*, **40**:1078, 1975.

109. Oparil, S., J. Low, E. N. Ehrlich, and M. D. Lindheimer: The renin-angiotensin system in mother and fetus at cesarean section: A preliminary communication, in M. D. Lindheimer, A. I. Katz, and F. R. Zuspan (eds.), *Hypertension in Pregnancy*, John Wiley & Sons, Inc., New York, 1976, p. 287.

110. Brown, J. J., D. L. Davies, P. B. Doak, A. F. Lever, J. I. S. Robertson, and P. Trust: Plasma renin concentration in hypertensive disease of pregnancy, *Lancet*, **2**:1219, 1965.

111. Tapia, H. R., C. E. Johnson, and C. E. Strong: Renin-angiotensin system in normal and in hypertensive disease of pregnancy, *Lancet*, **2**:847, 1972.

112. Gant, N. J., S. Chand, R. J. Worley, P. T. Whalley, V. D. Crosby, and P. C. MacDonald: A clinical test useful for predicting the development of acute hypertension in pregnancy, *Am. J. Obstet. Gynecol.*, **120**:1, 1974.

113. Bucht, J., and L. Werko: Glomerular filtration rate and renal blood flow in hypertensive toxemia of pregnancy, *J. Obstet. Gynaecol. Br. Emp.*, **60**:157, 1953.

114. Boyle, J. A., S. Campell, A. M. Duncan, W. R. Greig, and W. W. Buchanan: Serum uric acid levels in normal pregnancy with observations on the renal excretion of urate in pregnancy, *J. Clin. Pathol.*, **19**:501, 1966.

115. Handler, J. S.: The role of lactic acid in the reduced excretion of uric acid in toxemia of pregnancy, *J. Clin. Invest.*, **39**:526, 1960.

116. Fadel, H. E., G. Northrop, and H. R. Misenhimer: Hyperuricema in pre-eclampsia: A reappraisal, *Am. J. Obstet. Gynecol.*, **125**:640, 1976.

117. Torres, C., L. J. Schewitz, and V. E. Pollak: The effect of small amounts of ADH on sodium and urate excretion in pregnancy, *Am. J. Obstet. Gynecol.*, **94**:654, 1966.

118. Ferris, T. F., and P. Gorden: The effect of angiotension and norepinephrine upon urate clearance in man, *Am. J. Med.*, **44**:359, 1968.

119. Lohlein, M.: Zur Pathogenese der Nierenkrankh-

erten Nephritis and Nephrose mit besonderer Besichtigung der nephropathia Gravidarum, *Dtsch. Med. Wochenschr.*, **44**:1187, 1918.

120. Fahr, T.: Uber Marenveranderungen bei Eklampsie, *Zentralbl. Gynaekol.*, **44**:991, 1920.

121. Baird, D., and J. S. Dunn: Renal lesions in eclampsia and nephritis of pregnancy, *J. Pathol. Bacteriol.*, **37**:291, 1933.

122. Farquhar, M.: The nephrotic syndrome, in *Proc. 10th Annu. Conf.*, National Kidney Disease Foundation, New York, 1959, p. 2.

123. Spargo, B., C. P. McCartney, and R. Winemiller: Glomerular capillary endotheliosis in toxemia of pregnancy, *Arch. Pathol.*, **68**:593, 1959.

124. Vassalli, P., R. H. Morris, and R. T. McCluskey: The pathogenic role of fibrin deposition in the glomerular lesions of toxemia of pregnancy, *J. Exp. Med.*, **118**:467, 1963.

125. Mauter, W., J. Chung, E. Grishman, and S. Dachs: Pre-eclamptic nephropathy: An electron microscopic study, *Lab. Invest.*, **11**:518, 1962.

126. McCartney, C. P.: Renal morphology and function among patients with pre-eclampsia and gravida with essential hypertension, *Clin. Obstet. Gynecol.*, **11**:506, 1968.

127. Slattery, L. R., R. M. Abrams, E. R. Berebaum, S. B. Labor, and B. Avon: Spontaneous hematoma of the liver during pregnancy, *Obstet. Gynecol.*, **32**:664, 1968.

128. Arias, F., and R. Mancilla-Jimenez: Hepatic fibrinogen deposits in pre-eclampsia, *N. Engl. J. Med.*, **295**:578, 1976.

129. Sheehan, J. L., and J. B. Lynch: *Pathology of Toxemia of Pregnancy*, The Williams and Wilkins Company, Baltimore, 1973.

130. Burstein, R., N. Alkjaersig, and A. Fletcher: Tromboembolism during pregnancy and the postpartum state, *J. Lab. Clin. Med.*, **73**:838, 1971.

131. Hyde, E., D. Joyce, V. Gurevich, P. T. Flute, and S. Barvera: Intravascular coagulation during pregnancy and the puerperium, *J. Obstet. Gynecol. Br. Commonw.*, **80**:1059, 1973.

132. Anderson, W. R., and D. G. McKay: Electron microscopic study of the trophoblast in normal and toxemic placentas, *Am. J. Obstet. Gynecol.*, **95**:1134, 1966.

133. Benirschke, K., and S. G. Driscoll: *The Pathology of the Human Placenta*, Springer-Verlag, Berlin, 1967.

134. Friedman, E. A., and R. K. Neff: Pregnancy outcome as related to hypertension, edema and proteinuria, in M. D. Lindheimer, A. I. Katz, and F. R. Zuspan (eds.), *Hypertension in Pregnancy*, John Wiley & Sons, Inc., New York, 1976, p. 13.

135. Chesley, L. C.: Weight changes and water balance in normal and toxic pregnancy, *Am. J. Obstet. Gynecol.*, **48**:565, 1944.

136. Cloeren, S. E., and T. H. Lippert: Effect of plasma expanders in toxemia of pregnancy, *N. Engl. J. Med.*, **287**:1356, 1972.

137. Palomaki, J. F., and M. D. Lindheimer: Sodium depletion simulating deterioration in a toxemic pregnancy, *N. Engl. J. Med.*, **282**:88, 1970.

138. McKay, D. G., and A. E. Covey: Cryofibrinogenemia in toxemia of pregnancy, *Obstet. Gynecol.*, **23**:508, 1964.

139. Brain, M. C., K. B. Kuah, and H. G. Dixon: Heparin treatment of hemolysis and thrombocytopenia in pre-eclampsia, *J. Obstet. Gynaecol. Br. Commonw.*, **74**:702, 1967.

140. Henderson, A. H., D. J. Pugsley, and D. P. Thomas: Fibrin degradation products in pre-eclamptic toxemia and eclampsia, *Br. Med. J.*, **3**:545, 1970.

141. Piver, M. S., S. A. Lisker, N. Rowan, L. L. Weber, J. I. Brody, and L. H. Beizer: Thrombotic thrombocytopenic purpura during pregnancy, *Am. J. Obstet. Gynecol.*, **100**:302, 1968.

142. Burch, G. E., T. D. Giles, and C. U. Tsui: Postpartal cardiomyopathy, *Cardiovasc. Clin.*, **4**:270, 1972.

143. Kunelis, C. T., J. L. Peters, and H. A. Edmondson: Fatty liver of pregnancy and its relationship to tetracycline therapy, *Am. J. Med.*, **38**:359, 1965.

144. Kleinknecht, D., J. P. Grunfeld, P. C. Gomez, J. F. Moreau, and R. Garcia-Torres: Diagnostic procedures and long term prognosis in bilateral renal cortical necrosis, *Kidney Int.*, **4**:390, 1973.

145. Sheehan, H. L.: Neurological complications of pregnancy, *Proc. R. Soc. Med.*, **32**:584, 1939.

146. Clemendor, A., S. Sall, and E. Herbilas: Achalasia and nutritional deficiency during pregnancy, *Obstet. Gynecol.*, **33**:106, 1969.

147. Chaudhuri, S. K.: Relationship of protein-caloric malnutrition with toxemia of pregnancy, *Am. J. Obstet. Gynecol.*, **107**:33, 1970.

148. Hankin, M. E., and E. M. Symonds: Body weight, diet and preeclamptic toxemia of pregnancy, *Aust.*

N.Z. J. Obstet. Gynaecol., **4:**156, 1962.

149. World Health Organization: Expert Committee on Pregnancy and Lactation, WHO Techn. Rep. Ser., vol. 302, 1965.

150. Davies, A. M., J. W. Czaczkes, E. Sadovsky, R. Prywes, P. Weiskoph, and V. V. Sterk: Toxemia of pregnancy in Jerusalem, *Isr. J. Med. Sci.,* **6:**253, 1970.

151. Johnson, G. T., and R. B. Thompson: A clinical trial of I. V. apresoline in management of toxemia of late pregnancy, *J. Obstet. Gynecol. Br. Commonw.,* **65:**360, 1958.

152. Gladstone, G. G., A. Hordof, and W. M. Gersony: Propranolol administration during pregnancy: Effects on fetus, *J. Pediatr.,* **86:**962, 1975.

153. Finnerty, F. A., Jr.: Hypertensive emergencies, in J. N. Laragh (ed.), *Hypertension Manual,* Yorke Medical Books, New York, 1974.

154. Zuspan, F. P., and M. C. Ward: Improved fetal salvage in eclampsia, *Obstet. Gynecol.,* **26:**893, 1965.

155. Michael, C. A.: Intravenous diazoxide in the treatment of severe toxemia of eclampsia, *Aust. N.Z. J. Obstet. Gynaecol.,* **13:**143, 1973.

156. Nuwazhid, B., C. R. Brinkman, B. Katchen, S. Symchowicz, H. Martinek, and N. S. Assali: Maternal and fetal hemodynamic effects of diazoxide, *Obstet. Gynecol.,* **46:**197, 1975.

157. Tyson, J. E.: Obstetrical management of the pregnant diabetic, *Med. Clin. North Am.,* **55:**961, 1971.

158. Assali, N. S., R. A. Douglas, Jr., W. W. Baird, D. B. Nicholson, and R. Suyemoto: Uteroplacental blood flow in toxemic pregnancy, *Am. J. Obstet. Gynecol.,* **66:**248, 1953.

159. Assali, N. S., L. W. Holm, and N. Segal: Regional blood flow and vascular resistance of the fetus in uterine action of vasoactive drugs, *Am. J. Obstet. Gynecol.,* **83:**809, 1962.

160. Gant, N. F., J. D. Madden, P. K. Siiteri: The metabolic clearance of DHEA IV effects of induced hypertension, hypotension and natriuresis in normal and hypertensive pregnancies, *Am. J. Obstet. Gynecol.,* **124:**143, 1976.

161. Freis, E. D.: The treatment of hypertension, *Am. J. Med.,* **52:**664, 1972.

162. Sloan, W. C., C. V. Florey, R. M. Acheson, and D. M. Kessner: Epidemiologic methods in the study of blood pressure in relatives of toxemic primiparae, *Am. J. Epidemiol.,* **91:**553, 1970.

163. Woods, J. W., W. A. Algary, and F. M. Stier: Induction of hypertension with oral contraceptives (abstract), *Circulation,* **45-46** (suppl. 2): 82, 1972.

164. Bechgaard, P., C. Andreassen, and E. Heitel: Ultimate prognosis of hypertension following toxemia, in N. F. Morris and J. C. M. Browne (eds.), *Nontoxemic Hypertension in Pregnancy,* Little, Brown and Company, Boston, 1958.

165. Epstein, F. H.: Late vascular effect of toxemia of pregnancy, *N. Engl. J. Med.,* **271:**391, 1938.

166. Harbert, G. M., H. A. Claiborne, H. S. McGaughey, L. A. Wilson, and W. N. Thornton: Convulsive toxemia, *Am. J. Obstet. Gynecol.,* **100:**336, 1967.

167. Fritzsch, W., M. Birnbaum, W. Flach, and E. P. Issel: Spatschaden nach Eklampsia, *Zentralbl. Gynaekol.,* **92:**1009, 1970.

168. Chesley, L. C., J. E. Annitto, and R. A. Cosgrove: Long term followup study of eclamptic women, *Am. J. Obstet. Gynecol.,* **101:**886, 1968.

169. Singh, M. M., I. MacGillivray, and R. G. Mahaffy: A study of the long term effects of preeclampsia on blood pressure and renal function, *J. Obstet. Gynaecol. Br. Commonw.,* **81:**903, 1974.

170. Bryans, C. I., Jr., W. L. Southerland, and R. B. Zuspan: Eclampsia: A long term followup study, *Obstet. Gynecol.,* **21:**701, 1963.

26

Fluid and electrolyte disorders and the central nervous system

ALLEN I. ARIEFF / R. WILLIAM SCHMIDT

INTRODUCTION

Cerebral dysfunction is among the most prominent clinical manifestations of many patients who have disorders of fluid, electrolyte, and acid-base metabolism. The spectrum of such disorders which may result in cerebral dysfunction includes either increases and/or decreases in plasma (or blood) concentration of sodium (Na^+), glucose, phosphate, hydrogen (H^+) ion, carbon dioxide (CO_2), bicarbonate, oxygen, calcium (Ca^{2+}), and ketones. In addition, certain states such as uremia, hyponatremia, and dialysis dementia (1–3) have their primary effects on the central nervous system (CNS).

There is an exhaustive neurochemical literature which deals with changes in brain water, electrolytes, and acid-base components. However, much of this literature is appreciated only by neurochemists and those in closely related disciplines. Very little of this literature is known to clinicians; thus much information which is potentially of therapeutic and diagnostic importance has not been assimilated into clinical medicine.

In this chapter, we will review the relationship between systemic abnormalities of water, electrolytes, and acid-base metabolism and the brain from two vantage points: (1) effects of systemic abnormalities on the CNS, (2) effects of CNS lesions on renal function, water, and electrolytes.

EFFECTS OF SYSTEMIC DISEASE STATES ON BRAIN WATER AND ELECTROLYTES

IONIC CONSTITUENTS AND ACID-BASE BALANCE OF NORMAL BRAIN AND CEREBROSPINAL FLUID (CSF)

Osmotically active solute

The principal osmotically active constituents of brain, unlike those of extracellular fluid, consist of both organic and inorganic solutes. The major inorganic constituents of the brain, and their approximate concentrations (mmol/kg wet weight) in the cerebral cortex of mammalian species (rat, cat, dog, human) are Na^+ (50 to 60 mmol/kg), K^+ (85 to 100 mmol/kg), Cl^- (35 to 45 mmol/kg), Ca^{2+} (1 to 2.8 mmol/kg), Mg^{2+} (5 to 6 mmol/kg), and bicarbonate (10 to 12 mmol/kg) (4–6).

It is obvious that the sum of inorganic brain cations far exceeds that of inorganic anions. The total brain cation concentration is about 170 mmol/kg wet weight, while anions, including Cl^-, bicarbonate, sulfates, phosphates, and organic acid anions (such as lactate, glutamine, glutamate, and N-acetylaspartate) are at most about 85 mmol/kg wet weight (5). The remaining brain intracellular anions are probably polyionic lipids and proteins. Since most brain Cl^- is extracellular, the bulk of intracellular anions are doubtless organic and macromolecular (5). In addition, there are also minute quantities in the brain of certain trace metals, such as copper, manganese, zinc, iron, tin, aluminum, and rubidium (1, 5, 7, 8).

The actual osmotic activity of any of the aforementioned constituents is not entirely clear. Most Ca^{2+} and Mg^{2+} is probably bound and not osmotically active (4). The principal intracellular osmotically active cation is K^+, and a substantial portion of intracellular Na^+ is also probably osmotically active (4, 7). The role of organic phosphates in brain osmoregulation also has not been well studied (9). The osmotic activity in brain of amino acids and other organic acids is uncertain, although these substances appear to play a major role in osmotic adaptation in the cells of many invertebrates (10, 11) and amphibians (12). Those organic intracellular metabolites which are probably osmotically active include glutamate, aspartate, lactate, pyruvate, and alanine (13).

There is a substantial amount of evidence, both in man (14–16) and experimental animals (17–19), that there may be changes in plasma osmolality where the apparent net loss or gain of cellular water and solute does not account for the expected change in tissue osmolality (assuming that intracellular and extracellular osmolality are in dynamic equilibrium) (20–22). In these instances there may be apparent inactivation of intracellular solute (14, 16) or a gain in solute which is not due to commonly measured substances (18, 19, 23). This undetermined solute has been called "idiogenic osmols" (17–19). Furthermore, there is a substantial body of evidence which suggests that the brain undergoes osmotic adaptation to hyperosmolar states in a manner which is distinctly different from that of other tissues. For example, in birds and mammals, mus-

cle and nucleated red blood cells may adapt to hyperosmolar states by loss of water and gain in cation (17, 18, 24), while brain adapts primarily by de novo generation of solute by as yet unexplained mechanisms (17, 19, 25). However, these mechanisms apparently are not activated immediately, and as a result, overly rapid induction of hyperosmolality (increase of plasma osmolality by at least 35 mosm/kg) may be lethal (26, 27). Furthermore, the adaptive mechanisms may in themselves provoke functional derangements in the brain. Patients or experimental animals that are chronically hyperosmolar are generally symptomatic and may be comatose (23), while patients or laboratory animals with chronic hyponatremia who do not have brain edema frequently have alterations of sensorium (23).

Acid-base status of brain and CSF

There have been a substantial number of studies dealing with the acid-base status of brain and cerebrospinal fluid (CSF). Those dealing with the CSF are generally far less controversial because of the ready applicability of commonly used techniques for direct measurement of gases in CSF (28, 29). The steady-state relationships between acid-base components in arterial blood versus cisternal CSF in man are shown in Fig. 26-1. In general, bicarbonate concentration is similar in blood and CSF (about 24 mmol/L). The arterial pH (about 7.40) is higher than that in CSF (about 7.32) because P_{CO_2} in CSF (about 48 mmHg) is higher than that in blood (about 40 mmHg).

The CSF protein concentration (about 40 mg/dL) is minute compared to that in plasma (about 7 g/dL). However, despite this apparent inferior buffering capacity, the pH of CSF remains remarkably constant despite substantial changes in arterial pH. In those conditions characterized by acute alterations in systemic P_{CO_2} (respiratory alkalosis and acidosis) there are acute alterations in pH and P_{CO_2} of CSF which are directionally similar to those in arterial blood (29, 30). However, the changes in CSF pH are initially less than those in arterial blood, and within 1 h, compensatory mechanisms have been initiated (31). In acute respiratory alkalosis, there is an increase

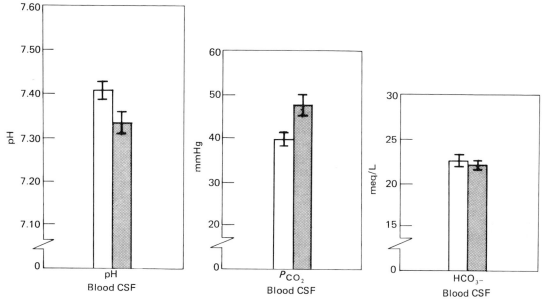

Figure 26-1. The relationship between acid-base balance in arterial blood versus cisternal CSF in human subjects. (*Data summarized from Katzman and Pappius*)

in the CSF concentrations of both lactate and other, as yet unidentified, organic acids (6, 32, 33), which results in a decrease of CSF pH towards normal (34). This compensation is nearly complete after 4 to 6 h (Fig. 26-2). With an arterial pH of about 7.65, the simultaneously determined intracellular pH (pH_i) of brain will rise from 7.05 to 7.23 after 1 h with an arterial P_{CO_2} of 15 mmHg, but after 2 h, it has returned to normal values (Fig. 26-2).

In acute respiratory acidosis (arterial P_{CO_2} above 80 mmHg), there is initially a significant decline in pH of CSF. Within 1 to 2 h, bicarbonate concentration of CSF begins to rise (6, 31, 35), but compensation is only minimal after 4 to 6 h (6, 35). By contrast, although pH_i of brain falls from 7.05 to 6.88 after 1 h of hypercapnia, it returns to normal after 3 h of sustained hypercapnia (6).

In acute metabolic disturbances of acid-base balance, effects on pH in CSF are only minimal. When arterial pH was lowered from 7.40 to 7.18 by infusion of HCl, there was no significant alteration in pH of CSF (35). Similarly, when $NaHCO_3$ was infused to increase arterial pH from

7.40 to 7.53, the pH of CSF was unaltered (35). It appears that neither bicarbonate nor hydrogen ion can readily cross the blood-CSF barrier, but this barrier is readily permeable to CO_2.

CSF electrolytes

CSF is different from plasma in several important respects. Since CSF is essentially protein-free and has no cells, the "unmeasured anion," i.e., the difference between measured cations and measured anions, is close to zero. In general, the CSF $[Na^+ + K^+]$ is similar to $[Cl^- + HCO_3]$. There is considerable variation among mammalian species, but in general the CSF $[Na^+]$ is similar to that of plasma. However, when Na^+ is expressed as mmol/kg water, its concentration is higher in plasma than in CSF (36). Because of the osmotic equilibrium between plasma and CSF, changes in CSF $[Na^+]$ generally parallel those of plasma.

In contrast to Na^+, the CSF $[K^+]$ is relatively constant, being essentially independent of the plasma $[K^+]$. In human subjects, the $[K^+]$ in CSF

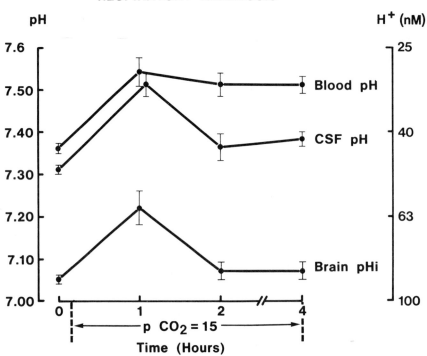

RESPIRATORY ALKALOSIS

Figure 26-2. Changes in pH of CSF and blood, and in brain intracellular pH (pH_i) during 4 h of hypocapnia. With arterial pH maintained at approximately 7.52, brain pH_i increases from 7.05 to 7.23 after 1 h, and pH of CSF similarly rises. After 2 or 4 h, however, brain pH_i is normal. pH of CSF approaches normal values, but after 4 h, it is still significantly greater (p less than 0.01). (*From Arieff, Kerian, Massry, and DeLima.*)

remained at about 3.0 meq/L despite variations of plasma K^+ between 3.4 and 5.8 meq/L (37). In experimental animals, CSF K^+ did not change despite marked variation in plasma K^+ induced by either K^+ loading or K^+ depletion (38). However, in some patients with severe hypokalemia (plasma K^+ below 2 meq/L), CSF $[K^+]$ as low as 2.4 to 2.6 meq/L has been described (36). In studies published since 1954, the CSF K^+ in 56 normal human subjects ($\pm$ SD) has been found to be 2.89 $\pm$ 0.26 meq/L (36). In the goat, rabbit, dog, and cat, $[K^+]$ in cisternal CSF has a range of only 2.52 to 2.98 meq/L (36). There are at least two mechanisms which serve to maintain CSF K^+ in this narrow range. There is a carrier-mediated trans-

port of K^+ across the choroid plexus from blood into the CSF. There is also exchange of CSF K^+ with brain K^+. Although the evidence is not conclusive, both of these mechanisms probably require active transport processes.

In virtually all mammalian species, the CSF $[Ca^{2+}]$ is between 2 and 3 meq/L. Calcium is secreted by the choroid plexus into the CSF. Since protein concentration in CSF is minimal, virtually all Ca^{2+} in CSF is ionized and not protein-bound. It has long been suggested that the CSF $[Ca^{2+}]$ was similar to ionized Ca^{2+} in plasma. However, using modern methodology to measure Ca^{2+}, the ionized $[Ca^{2+}]$ in plasma is still found to be consistently greater than that in CSF (39).

However, there is also a potential difference between CSF and plasma of about +5 mV (40). When this electrochemical gradient is taken into account, there is electrochemical equilibrium for Ca^{2+} between CSF and plasma in normal human subjects. However, it is still most unlikely that plasma ionized Ca^{2+} and CSF Ca^{2+} are in equilibrium. When plasma Ca^{2+} is altered by Ca^{2+} infusion, parathyroidectomy, parathyroid hormone administration, ethylenediaminetetraacetic acid (EDTA), uremia, or vitamin D intoxication, there is little if any change in the Ca^{2+} in CSF (36, 41, 42). Therefore, the bulk of evidence suggests that Ca^{2+} in CSF is maintained by active secretory processes at the choroid plexus and is not directly related to plasma ionized Ca^{2+} levels.

The Mg^{2+} level in CSF of human subjects is slightly higher than that of plasma. In studies of 1033 patients, Mg^{2+} in CSF was 2.41 meq/L while that in plasma was 1.82 meq/L (36). The consistency of CSF Mg^{2+} at a higher level than plasma suggests that there must be active secretion of Mg^{2+} into CSF, probably at the choroid plexus. Intravenous infusion of $MgSO_4$ to elevate plasma Mg^{2+} levels results in a small rise of CSF Mg^{2+} at very high plasma levels. Elevations in plasma Mg^{2+} of 270 to 700 percent result in a rise of CSF Mg^{2+} of only 20 to 25 percent (36, 43). In animals with renal failure, a 30 percent rise in plasma Mg^{2+} did not affect CSF Mg^{2+} (42). However, a Mg^{2+}-deficient diet did result in a small decrement of CSF Mg^{2+} (44) in rabbits. In patients with hypomagnesemia (serum Mg^{2+} below 2.14 meq/L), CSF Mg^{2+} is somewhat less than normal (45).

CHARACTERISTICS OF THE BLOOD-BRAIN BARRIER

Brain extracellular space

In general, extracellular space (ECS) is thought of as that fluid compartment which is outside of cells. However in practice, the ECS is defined as that fluid compartment which is available for the distribution of a particular marker. The ECS is determined as the ratio of distribution of the marker in the tissue to its distribution in a reference fluid which is considered to represent extracellular fluid (46). If plasma is used as the extracellular fluid, it must be corrected for the Donnan effect (see Chap. 1). This concept is especially difficult when applied to the brain. There is essentially a dual circulation of fluids about the brain (both blood and CSF). The vast bulk of evidence suggests that the CSF is identical with, and a continuation of, the extracellular fluid of the brain (46–48). The measurement of ECS assumes that the marker has equilibrated between tissue and extracellular fluid. There is a tendency for any substance entering the brain via the blood to be siphoned off into the CSF, so that equilibration may not be reached. There is a similar tendency for any substance administered via the CSF to be siphoned off via the bloodstream. Collectively, these tendencies are known as the "sink action" of the CSF (49). In addition, several extracellular markers, such as thiocyanate and sulfate, are actively removed from the CSF by active transport systems at the choroid plexus (47). To attain the equilibrium conditions between CSF and brain necessary to determine ECS, the same concentration of extracellular marker must be present in both plasma water and CSF. This can be attained by simultaneous administration of the extracellular marker in these two compartments (47). Several different in vivo techniques have been employed (6, 50, 51).

A number of different markers have been used to determine the brain ECS. These include endogenous Cl^- (usually corrected for intracellular Cl^-, which is about 7 percent of total Cl^-), $^{36}Cl^-$, thiocyanate, Na^+, $^{23}Na^+$, sulfate, inulin, sucrose, and bromide (46, 47). In addition, brain ECS has also been estimated by electron microscopy, tissue diffusion profiles, and measurement of cortical electric impedance (47). Early studies employing either electron microscopy or extracellular markers given only via the bloodstream revealed an ECS of less than 5 percent, but these findings have been shown to be due to fixation artifact or the sink action of the CSF (46, 47, 49). When brain ECS is appropriately determined in mammalian cerebral cortex by any of the aforementioned techniques, i.e., either by simultaneous blood and CSF administration of chemical extracellular markers, by measurement of cortical electric impedance, or by evaluation of cerebral cortex diffusion profiles, the range is from 15 to 25 percent, with a mean value of about 20 percent (47). Segments of the ECS appear to be in free communication only with the bloodstream and other parts only with the CSF (51).

Anatomy of the blood-brain barrier

When a nonmetabolizable, nontoxic substance is administered via the bloodstream such that steady-state conditions are maintained for several hours, it will achieve a similar volume of distribution throughout most cell systems. Examples of such substances, include inulin, sulfate, salicylic acid, antipyrine, and urea. However, for a given time interval (up to 4 h), none of the aforementioned will achieve a concentration in brain which is as high as its concentration in other tissues such as liver or muscle (52). This selective behavior of the brain, whereby passage of certain substances out of the blood is restricted, has been called the blood-brain barrier. Some of the earlier experiments whereby the existence of such a barrier was demonstrated utilized vital dyes. Ehrlich in 1882 (53) showed that many dyes when injected intravenously stained most tissues in the body except the brain. Lewandowsky in 1900 found that Prussian blue reagent did not pass from blood to brain (54) and Goldman in 1909 reported similar findings with trypan blue (55).

Several factors have been shown to influence the rate of passage of a substance from blood to brain. These include the K_a, configuration, molecular size, charge, and lipid solubility. Lipid-soluble substances penetrate the blood-brain barrier much more rapidly than non-lipid-soluble ones. For example, one of the reasons that thiopental and amobarbital act more rapidly than phenobarbital is because of their greater lipid solubility. For weak acids and bases, the partition parameter determines their entry in the brain—weak acids tend to be excluded and weak bases concentrated (56).

The anatomical delineation of the blood-brain barrier is complex and has been described in great detail elsewhere (52, 57). It will be only briefly reviewed here. The principal components of the blood-brain barrier are the brain capillaries, the astrocytic processes (end-feet processes), the thick brain capillary basement membrane, and the thick cell wall (Fig. 26-3). In contrast to capillaries elsewhere in the body, the brain capillary basement membranes function as an epithelial sheet. Brain capillaries are made of a single layer of endothelial cells, with a dense cytoplasm containing few vesicles. In contrast to other capillaries, brain endothelial cells are connected by tight junctions that act to form a continuous cell layer. A basement membrane surrounds the cells, and this is in turn covered by the glial cells, whose astrocytic processes cover about 85 percent of the capillary surface (52, 57). The intracerebral arterioles and venules are also covered by continuous endothelial cell layers with tight junctions. Both the astrocytic end-feet processes which surround the capillaries and the thick neuronal cell walls probably constitute the bulk of the blood-brain barrier. The thick lipid cell wall would tend to exclude those small molecules which pass out of cerebral capillaries but are not lipid-soluble.

EFFECTS OF ACUTE RESPIRATORY DISTURBANCES ON BRAIN WATER, ELECTROLYTES, AND ACID-BASE STATUS

The clinical manifestations of the water and electrolyte abnormalities accompanying acute respiratory disorders have been well described in Chap. 6 and elsewhere (58). It is well known that respiratory alkalosis, acidosis, and hypoxia all can have profound effects on the central nervous system.

Respiratory acidosis

Respiratory acidosis is frequently associated with depression of sensorium as manifested by lethargy, stupor, or obtundation (59). Coma may supervene with substantial degrees of CO_2 retention (arterial P_{CO_2} above 60 mmHg). The quantification of symptoms which are referable to CO_2 retention is complicated by the fact that "pure" hypercapnia is rare without concomitant hypoxia.

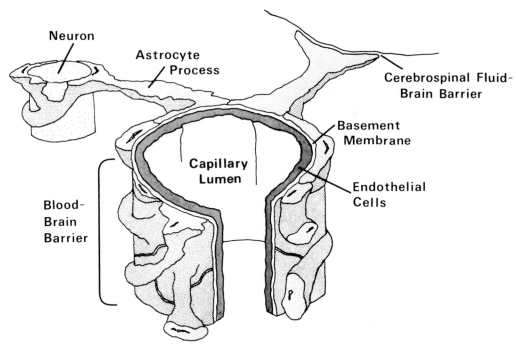

Figure 26-3. Diagrammatic rendition of the blood-brain barrier. The principal components are the astrocytic foot processes, endothelial cells with tight junctions, and a thick capillary basement membrane. The CSF-brain barrier consists primarily of choroid plexus and ependyma. (*Original drawing by Bob Surface of Medical Research Graphics, San Francisco, Calif.*)

Patients with chronic obstructive pulmonary disease or bronchial asthma virtually always have hypoxia with hypercapnia. Nonetheless, by examining separately the effects on the CNS of hypoxia and hypercapnia, it should be possible to ascertain some of the effects of each.

With the induction of acute hypercapnia (P_{CO_2} = 80 to 90 mmHg) without hypoxia (arterial P_{O_2} above 70 mmHg), there are similar decrements in pH of both arterial blood and CSF (29, 60). There is thus no barrier to the penetration of CO_2 into the CSF (29). However, largely because of an increase in cerebral blood flow, the P_{CO_2} in CSF will rise relatively less than arterial P_{CO_2}, resulting in a smaller decline of pH in CSF (61). Within 1 h after the P_{CO_2} is elevated, there is a gradual rise in the bicarbonate concentration in CSF, such that pH of CSF begins to rise towards normal values. These changes precede any alterations in arterial bicarbonate concentration. After 3 h with arterial P_{CO_2} maintained at 80 to 90 mmHg, the CSF bicarbonate has risen (in the dog) from 20 to 25 meq/L. However, after 6 h of hypercapnia, the pH of CSF is still significantly below normal values (29, 62). After 1 day of hypercapnia, pH in CSF is normal, while CSF bicarbonate is 35 meq/L, significantly above normal. However, arterial pH is still acidotic, demonstrating the lag between systemic compensation by the kidneys versus CSF compensation via transport across the choroid plexus (62). The renal compensatory mechanisms for respiratory acidosis are discussed in Chap. 6. The increased bicarbonate concentration in CSF is secreted by the choroid plexus. Although it is not entirely clear whether hypercapnia or CSF acidemia is the stimulus for increased secretion of bicarbonate, it is clear that bicarbonate is formed at the choroid plexus and

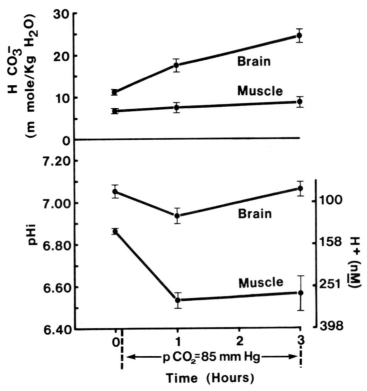

Figure 26-4. Changes in brain (cerebral cortex) and skeletal muscle during 3 h of respiratory acidosis (arterial pH = 7.07). Intracellular pH (pH$_i$) of both brain and muscle fall significantly within 1 h. Within 3 h, brain pH$_i$ is normal, but that of muscle remains significantly acidotic. Return of brain pH$_i$ to normal values is largely accomplished by a rise in calculated brain bicarbonate concentration (from 11.3 to 24.4 mmol/kg H$_2$O), but during this time interval, muscle bicarbonate concentration does not change. (*From Arieff, Kerian, Massry, and DeLima.*)

transported against a concentration gradient into the CSF. The process is carbonic anhydrase–dependent and can be largely blocked by the action of acetazolamide (29).

The compensatory mechanisms of brain in animals with acute respiratory acidosis are more rapid than those in blood or CSF. With acute hypercapnia (P_{CO_2} = 80 to 90 mmHg) in the dog, arterial pH falls from 7.36 to 7.07 in 1 h, while the simultaneously measured intracellular pH (pH$_i$) in brain (cerebral cortex) is 6.90 versus a normal value of 7.06 (Fig. 26-4). However, after only 30 to 60 min of hypercapnia, the calculated cerebral cortex bicarbonate concentration has increased to 57 percent above the normal value (6, 63). After 3 h of hypercapnia, with no change whatsoever in arterial pH, brain pH$_i$ has returned to normal values (Fig. 26-4). The brain bicarbonate is now 24.4 meq/kg H$_2$O (normal value = 11.3 meq/kg H$_2$O). Within 3 h, with both arterial and CSF P_{CO_2} maintained at about 85 mmHg, brain was able to normalize its pH$_i$ by generation of bicarbonate (6, 63).

The means by which the brain restores its pH$_i$ to normal during respiratory acidosis are complex. There is substantial generation of bicarbonate by brain, most of which takes place within the first 30 min (63). The mechanisms by which the brain generates bicarbonate are unclear, although they are probably not secondary to the action of carbonic anhydrase, as acetazolamide does not block brain bicarbonate generation (64). There are, however, several other means by which the brain might generate bicarbonate. Numerous reactions in the brain produce CO_2, particularly those that involve decarboxylation. There could be direct hydroxylation of gaseous CO_2 to bicarbonate, as occurs in some elasmobranch fish (65). Other CO_2-producing reactions in brain include metabolism of glucose via the Krebs (tricarboxylic acid) cycle, and conversion of glutamic acid to γ-aminobutyric acid (66) in which CO_2 in brain may possibly be carbonic acid or bicarbonate (67). Furthermore, most of these reactions are intimately linked to glucose metabolism, since glutamic acid is produced via the Krebs cycle, and pyruvate, a product of the metabolism of glucose via the Embden-Meyerhof pathway (glycolysis), is a precursor of most amino acids found in brain. Several steps in the metabolism of glucose are pH-dependent, and it is quite possible that intracellular acidosis might shift equilibriums to favor certain CO_2-producing reactions (66).

There also appears to be a fixed amount of nonbicarbonate buffer in brain, which is equivalent to about 33 mmol of buffer per kilogram of brain tissue (68). After the initial 2 to 3 h of hypercapnia, there is a marked upward shift in the brain CO_2 dissociation curve (62), so that brain buffering capacity increases with increasing P_{CO_2}. There is also probably increased conversion of glutamic acid to α-ketoglutamic acid, with liberation of NH_3 (69). The metabolism of glutamic acid could remove a potential source of H^+ ion, while increased production of NH_3 could buffer additional H^+ ion by conversion to NH_4 (69).

Thus, buffering by the brain in respiratory acidosis results from many complex, interacting factors.

While cerebral compensation of acute hypercapnia is apparently complete within 4 h, the same is not true of other tissues. In skeletal muscle, for instance, after 1 h of respiratory acidosis, the pH_i has declined from 6.85 to 6.53. After 3 h of hypercapnia, however, muscle pH_i and bicar-

bonate concentration are unaltered (Fig. 26-4) while brain pH_i is normal.

Respiratory alkalosis

Respiratory alkalosis in man is frequently observed with several systemic disease states which include bronchial asthma, hepatic cirrhosis, salicylate intoxication, hypoxia, sepsis, and certain lesions of the brain. In the aforementioned conditions, the related symptoms are usually those of the underlying disorder rather than the alkalosis, per se. Modest acute respiratory alkalosis may be accompanied by only mild symptoms (paresthesias, dizziness). However, more severe alkalosis (pH 7.52 to 7.65) in patients with respiratory insufficiency and hypoxia can result in a symptom complex of hypotension, seizures, asterixis, myoclonus, and coma, with a mortality exceeding 75 percent (70).

The arterial P_{CO_2} is the primary regulator of cerebral blood flow (71), but there is also an effect of brain extracellular pH (72). Hypocapnia is a potent cerebral vasoconstrictor. This effect is utilized clinically during anesthesia, when hyperventilation (to induce hypocapnia) can effectively decrease intracranial volume and relieve cerebral swelling (73). By contrast, both hypercapnia and hypoxia are potent cerebral vasodilators (72).

With acute hypocapnia in experimental animals, there is an initial rise in the brain pH_i (6, 68, 74). Almost immediately, there is a decline in brain bicarbonate concentration (68) with a rise in brain concentration of lactate (6, 68, 75, 76). Within 2 h, with arterial P_{CO_2} maintained below 20 mmHg, brain pH_i has returned to control values (Fig. 26-5). The return of brain pH_i to normal occurs concomitant with the fall of brain bicarbonate, which in turn is almost stoichiometic with the increase in lactate (Fig. 26-5) (6, 68, 75). There is also a rise of lactate and fall in bicarbonate in CSF, but the CSF lactate is not high enough to account for the observed decline in CSF bicarbonate (6, 77, 78).

In addition to the rise in brain lactate, there is also a change in the brain CO_2 dissociation curve (62, 74), such that brain buffering capacity is de-

Cerebral Cortex

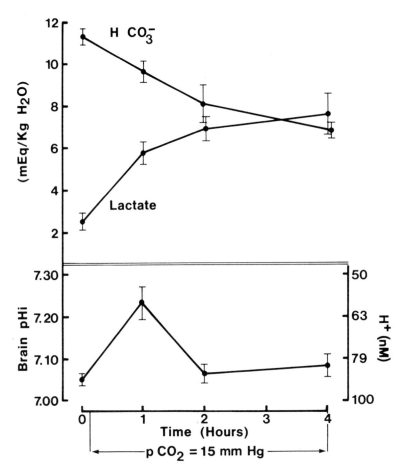

Figure 26-5. Changes in brain lactate, bicarbonate, and intracellular pH (pH$_i$) during 4 h of respiratory alkalosis. With onset of hypocapnia, brain pH$_i$ initially rises, but after approximately 1 h, it begins to fall towards normal. Accompanying decrease in brain pH$_i$, there is a sustained rise in brain lactate with a corresponding fall in brain bicarbonate. After 4 h with arterial pH maintained at approximately 7.52, rise in brain lactate (from 2.5 to 7.6 mmol/kg H$_2$O) is similar to fall in brain bicarbonate (from 11.3 to 6.9 mmol/kg H$_2$O), and brain pH$_i$ is normal. (*From Arieff, Kerian, Massry, and DeLima.*)

creased. There is no associated change in brain concentration of adenosine triphosphate (ATP), adenosine diphosphate (ADP), phosphocreatine, or creatine (75). The decrease in brain buffering capacity did not relate with the finding that there were no alterations in brain concentration of glutamic acid, glutamine, or NH$_3$ (60). Thus, although brain buffering capacity is decreased during hypocapnia, the biochemical mechanisms are not known.

In patients with acute respiratory alkalosis, there is a significant decline in cerebral blood flow which correlates well with marked slowing of the EEG (79). There is also an increase in jugular venous K$^+$ and a decline in [Na$^+$].

Thus, within 2 h of the onset of respiratory alkalosis, the brain, after an initial rise in pH_i, has restored its pH_i to normal (Fig. 26-5). This is accomplished primarily by cerebral vasoconstriction leading to a reduction in cerebral blood flow and increased anaerobic metabolism (72, 79). Although high-energy phosphate compounds are not affected, there is an increase in brain lactate, leading to a fall in brain bicarbonate (6, 68, 75). The aforementioned sequence appears to represent the brain's primary response to acute respiratory alkalosis.

EFFECTS OF METABOLIC ACID-BASE DISTURBANCES ON BRAIN

In contrast to the investigation of respiratory abnormalities, relatively little investigation has been carried out on the effects of metabolic disorders of acid-base metabolism on the central nervous system.

Metabolic acidosis

Metablic acidosis has been induced in laboratory by animals means of HCl or NH_4Cl infusion (80, 81). In some animals, with arterial pH of 7.06 and plasma bicarbonate of 6 meq/L, the brain pH_i fell by 0.29 pH units, with no change in the brain extracellular space (81). In other studies, however, metabolic acidosis in rats (NH_4Cl injection, arterial pH = 7.31) had no effect on brain pH_i or bicarbonate concentration (80).

In rabbits with lactic acidosis (arterial pH = 7.09), brain pH_i was not directly measured, but there was a significant increase in brain lactate concentration (from 3.9 to 18.1 mmol/kg), so that brain pH_i probably fell (82). In rats with diabetic ketoacidosis (plasma ketones = 9.5 mmol/L), there was no change in brain pH_i (83). Thus, it appears that metabolic acidosis has a small and inconsistent effect upon brain pH_i.

Metabolic alkalosis

Metabolic alkalosis has been produced in hypocapnic rats and dogs by infusing $NaHCO_3$ (80, 81,

84). In rats with arterial pH of 7.80 (P_{CO_2} = 16 mmHg, bicarbonate = 25 meq/L), there were increases in brain lactate and pyruvate concentrations, with an increase in lactate/pyruvate ratio from 16 to 24 (84). There was no significant change in brain pH_i (7.12) when compared to normal values (7.09). In normocapnic dogs or rats, when arterial pH was raised to 7.52 to 7.71 by $NaHCO_3$ infusion (plasma bicarbonate = 34 meq/L), there was also no significant change in brain pH_i. In brain of the alkalotic rats, there was also no change in brain ATP, ADP, AMP, or phosphocreatine (71). Therefore, in experimental animals, metabolic alkalosis (arterial pH of 7.52 to 7.80) has essentially no effect on brain intracellular pH, there is only a minimal rise in brain lactate concentration, and there is no change in brain bicarbonate (80, 81, 84).

RENAL FAILURE

Acute renal failure

The central nervous system manifestations of uremia include a continuum of signs and symptoms of dysfunction (2). Early symptoms may include loss of recent memory and impaired ability to concentrate, with depression, delusions, and slurring of speech. As renal failure progresses, these may include abnormalities of gait, action tremor, multifocal myoclonus, asterixis, and gradually increasing depression of sensorium, with inability to perform routine mental tasks. With more advanced renal failure, there may be seizures and, eventually, coma. These clinical characteristics will often fluctuate from day to day in any given patient, so that intervals of lucidity may be intermixed with delusions, depression, and stupor. The neurologic manifestations of uremia are generally similar whatever the underlying renal disease—glomerulonephritis, pyelonephritis, diabetes—with the possible exception of patients whose renal failure is due to primary hyperparathyroidism (85, 86).

Electroencephalograms (EEGs) have been studied in a large number of patients with chronic renal failure, as well as in some patients with acute renal failure (87–92). In general, patients with renal failure demonstrate a generalized slowing of background frequencies, loss of normal alpha rhythm, a shift in the percent EEG power from higher (above 9 Hz) to lower (less than 7 Hz) frequencies and an increase in the burst index. These findings are somewhat non-specific, but there may also be a myoclonic response to photic stimulation at different frequencies, which may be more specific for uremia (88). Similar findings are present in experimental animals with renal failure (42). The EEG tends to worsen both during and for several hours after hemodialysis (92–94). There is an initial period of stabilization (up to 6 months) when the EEG may deteriorate, but it then tends to approach

normal values in patients who continue to be treated with chronic dialysis (95).

The cause of the EEG abnormalities observed in uremic patients is unclear. Hagstram (88) noted a correlation of worsened EEG findings with hyperphosphatemia. However, hyperphosphatemia leads to hypocalcemia (96), which stimulates parathyroid hormone (PTH) secretion. Thus, it may be that a significant common denominator of the EEG abnormalities present in uremia is an effect of PTH on brain (42, 86, 90). In experimental animals with acute renal failure, many of the EEG abnormalities can be shown to be related to a direct effect of PTH on brain, leading to an elevated brain content of Ca^{2+} (42). Preliminary studies in patients with acute renal failure suggest a similar pathogenesis (90). Figure

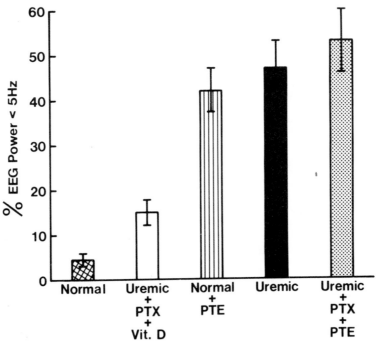

Figure 26-6. Percent EEG power for frequency classes below 5 Hz in five experimental groups of animals. The area (or power) occupied by frequency classes below 5 Hz is similar in normal animals and in uremic parathyroidectomized animals. The EEG power for frequencies below 5 Hz is significantly increased in uremic animals with intact parathyroid glands and in both uremic parathyroidectomized and normal animals receiving parathyroid extract (PTE). (*From Guisado, Arieff, and Massry.*)

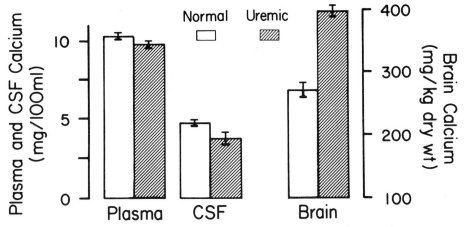

Figure 26-7. The brain Ca²⁺ content in brain of normal dogs and of those with 3½ days of acute renal failure (serum creatinine = 11 mg/dL). Despite a significant rise in brain Ca²⁺, there is essentially no change in Ca²⁺ concentration of plasma and CSF. (*From Arieff and Massry.*)

26-6 shows the percent EEG power less than 5 Hz in animals with renal failure, either with or without an excess of PTH in plasma. Figure 26-7 shows brain Ca²⁺ content in normal versus uremic dogs. It can be seen that the EEG is abnormal only in those animals with high plasma levels of PTH and elevated brain Ca²⁺ content.

In patients with acute renal failure, the EEG is abnormal within 48 h of the onset of renal failure (90) and is generally not affected by dialysis (87, 90, 92) over a period of up to 3 weeks. During this interval, patients with acute renal failure have been shown to have elevated levels of PTH in plasma (97). Several months after return of renal function, plasma PTH levels are normal. Although there are a multitude of factors which contribute to uremic encephalopathy (2, 88), many investigators have shown no correlation between encephalopathy and any of the commonly measured indicators of renal failure (blood urea nitrogen, creatinine, bicarbonate, pH, potassium) (87–92). Thus, PTH may be a major "uremic toxin."

There are many studies of brain composition in both patients and experimental animals with renal failure. In experimental animals with acute renal failure, all investigators have found that there is no evidence of cerebral edema, as evidenced by normal brain water content (6, 98–100). The permeability of brain is altered in the uremic state. Fishman and Raskin (98) have shown that there is increased permeability to ¹⁴C-labeled sucrose, with a more rapid entry of this carbohydrate into cerebral tissues. There was inhibition of the entry of ¹⁴C-labeled penicillin into brain (101), but no effect on entry of sulfate (98, 100). In addition, there was delayed equilibration of ²⁴Na⁺ but accelerated entry into brain of ⁴²K⁺ (101), suggesting alterations in the "sodium pump" in uremia. The delayed entry into brain of penicillin may reflect accumulation in brain of other organic acids which inhibit or saturate a common transport system. The permeability of brain to another weak organic acid, ¹⁴C-labeled dimethadione, was unaltered by uremia (6).

Alterations of cerebral metabolism which might be related to the aforementioned changes in permeability have also been studied in animals with renal failure. In brain of rats with acute renal failure, van den Nort and coworkers (102) found that creatine phosphate, ATP, and glucose were increased, but there were corresponding de-

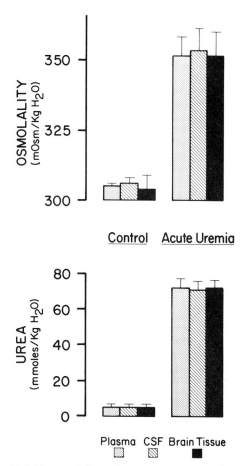

Figure 26-8. The osmolality and urea concentration in brain, CSF, and plasma of normal dogs, and dogs with acute renal failure for 3½ days (serum creatinine = 11 mg/dL). It can be seen that there is no significant difference in urea concentration or osmolality between the 3 compartments (for urea, 1 mmol/L = 2.8 mg/dL of BUN). (*From Arieff, Massry, Barrientos, and Kleeman.*)

have noted a diminution of brain $Na^+ -K^+-$ATPase in more severely uremic animals, while Mg^{2+}-dependent ATPase was normal. It is possible, although unproved, that the diminished brain Na^+-K^+-ATPase activity may be somehow related to observed alterations in equilibration of Na^+ and K^+ in uremic brain (101), as well as to the diminished brain content of Na^+ observed in dogs with acute renal failure (100).

Other studies of uremic brain have revealed decreased cerebral oxygen consumption (2, 104). There may also be impaired removal of organic acids from the brain via the choroid plexus due to saturation of transport mechanisms (2). The accumulation of organic acids in brain could interfere with neurotransmission.

In animals with either acute or chronic renal failure, urea concentration and osmolality are similar in brain, CSF, and plasma (Fig. 26-8) (100, 105). The content of H_2O, K^+, and Mg^{2+} is normal (41, 98–100), but Na^+ content is decreased (100). The functional significance of the

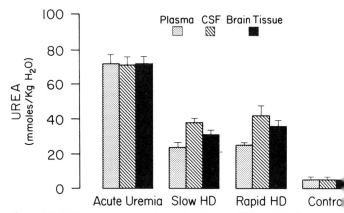

Figure 26-9. The urea concentration in plasma, CSF, and brain (cerebral cortex) of uremic animals treated with either rapid or slow hemodialysis (HD) and normal animals. Urea concentration is similar in all three compartments in both normal and uremic animals. After either slow or rapid HD, the urea gradient between brain and plasma is 6 to 8 mmol/kg H_2O and the difference is not significant (p greater .05). There is, however, a significant difference between urea concentration in plasma and that in CSF after either rapid or slow HD (p less than 0.01). Brackets are mean ±SE. (*After Arieff, Massry, Barrientos, and Kleeman.*)

creases in creatine, AMP, ADP, and lactate. Total brain adenine nucleotide content and Na^+-K^+-dependent ATPase (Na^+-K^+-ATPase) were normal. The uremic brain had an impaired ability to utilize ATP and was thus unable to produce ADP, AMP, and lactate from ATP at normal rates. There was a corresponding decrease in the brain's metabolic rate, along with elevated glucose and low lactate levels. Other workers (103) low brain Na^+ is not known, but preliminary studies suggest that it is also decreased in patients with acute renal failure (90). The solute content of brain in animals with acute renal failure is such that essentially all of the increase in brain osmolality is due to an increase of brain urea concentration (Figs. 26-9, 26-10). However, in animals with chronic renal failure, about half of the increase in brain osmolality is due to the presence of undetermined solute (idiogenic osmols) in brain (Fig. 26-10). The idiogenic osmols are accompanied by decrements in brain content of Na^+ and K^+ (105).

In animals who have acute renal failure and metabolic acidosis, the pH_i of brain, and skeletal muscle as well, is normal (6, 106) (Fig. 26-11). In patients with renal failure, pH_i has been reported to be normal in both skeletal muscle (107)

and leukocytes (108), as well as in the "whole body" (109). The pH of CSF has also been shown to be normal in both patients and laboratory animals with renal failure (94, 100, 110, 111). Thus, despite the presence of extracellular metabolic acidosis, intracellular buffering capacity is able to maintain a normal pH_i in brain, muscle, white blood cells, and most other tissues as well, in both man and laboratory animals.

Chronic renal failure

There have been very few studies of the brain in either patients or laboratory animals with chronic renal failure. With chronic renal failure, the EEG findings are similar to those observed in patients with acute renal failure (see above). In general, for the initial 3 to 6 months of dialytic therapy,

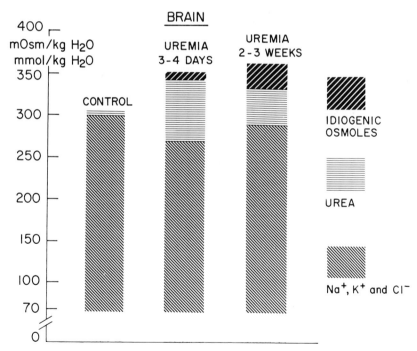

Figure 26-10. Effects on brain solute of acute (3 to 4 days) or chronic (2 to 3 weeks) renal failure in dogs. In animals with acute renal failure, plasma creatinine is 10.8 ± 0.8 mg/dL; in those with chronic renal failure, GFR is less than 10 mL/min. In dogs with acute renal failure, essentially all the increase in brain osmolality is due to an increase in urea concentration. With chronic renal failure, about half the increase in brain solute is due to idiogenic osmols. (*From Arieff, Guisado, and Lazarowitz.*)

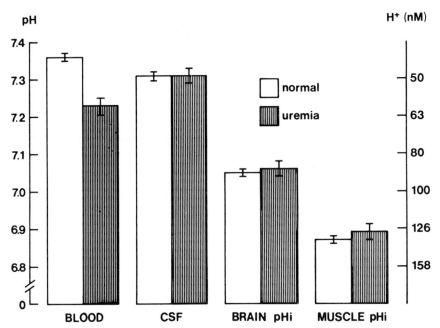

Figure 26-11. The pH of arterial blood and cerebrospinal fluid (CSF), and the intracellular pH (pH$_i$) in brain (cerebral cortex) and skeletal muscle. In animals with uremia (serum creatinine, 11.8 ± 0.4 mg/dL), there was a significant fall in arterial pH. However, there was no change in pH of CSF or of the pH$_i$ in brain or muscle. (*From Arieff, Guisado, Massry and Lazarowitz.*)

the EEG either does not change or may in fact worsen. After this time, there is generally gradual improvement in the EEG; among patients maintained on chronic dialysis for over 1 year, the EEG may actually appear to be normal (2, 91, 92, 95).

Pathologically, studies of brain in over 400 patients dying with chronic renal failure have been reported (112–114). Subdural hemorrhages are very common in dialyzed subjects, being reported in about 1 to 3 percent of cases (112, 114). In addition, intracerebral hemorrhages are present in about 6 percent of dialyzed patients who expire and are usually associated with hypertension (114). Histologically, the changes in brain are probably nonspecific. By biochemical and histologic criteria (113), cerebral edema is not a part of chronic renal failure. Generalized but variable neuronal degeneration is often present but is in-

consistent as to location (113, 115). Among patients dying of uremia per se, there is some necrosis of the granular layer of cerebral cortex (113). Small intracerebral hemorrhages and necrotic foci are seen in about 10 percent of uremic patients (113, 114). Focal glial proliferation is found in only 2 percent of uremic patients, and no consistent evidence of (toxic) encephalitis is observed. In general, then, the cerebral changes associated with uremia are nonspecific and are probably related more to the underlying disease state.

There are few available studies of brain water and electrolytes in animals with chronic renal failure. These suggest that brain H_2O, Na^+, K^+, and Cl^- are similar to normal values (105, 116) and that brain Ca^{2+} is modestly elevated (86). Brain and plasma urea levels are similar (105), and a substantial amount of solute in brain of animals with chronic renal failure is not due to commonly measured solutes such as Na^+, K^+, Cl^-, Ca^{2+}, Mg^{2+}, lactate, and glucose. This undetermined solute has been designated as "idiogenic osmols" and may be related to accumulation of organic acids in the brain (6, 105).

Dialysis disequilibrium syndrome. In patients with chronic renal failure who are treated with maintenance dialysis, there are numerous systemic abnormalities. Most prominent among the manifestations of chronic renal failure are renal osteodystrophy, anemia, cardiovascular disorders, and malnutrition, all of which have been discussed elsewhere (117). There are also several central nervous system disorders which may occur in chronic dialysis patients. These disorders seem to occur as a consequence of the dialytic therapy and include dialysis disequilibrium syndrome and dialysis encephalopathy.

Dialysis disequilibrium syndrome (DDS) is a symptom complex which characteristically occurs late in the course of, or several hours after, hemodialysis. From a purely mechanical and technical standpoint, it is quite possible to correct most of the abnormal blood chemistry values found in uremic patients to acceptable levels in much less time than is commonly done. The efficiency of hemodialysis can be increased by increasing blood and/or dialysate flow rates. However, when this is done and blood urea nitrogen (BUN) is rapidly lowered, patients often manifest a symptom complex which may include headache, nausea, emesis, blurring of vision, muscular twitching, disorientation, hypertension, tremors, and seizures. This syndrome has been called DDS. Although DDS has been reported in all age groups, it is more common among younger patients, particularly the pediatric age group (118). Despite many studies on the composition of both CSF and plasma in patients with DDS, there is as yet no single laboratory value or constellation of values which has been found to be consistently abnormal. The syndrome is most often associated with rapid hemodialysis of patients with acute renal failure, but it has also been reported following maintenance hemodialysis of patients with chronic renal failure (119).

In its mildest form, DDS may be manifested by no more than restlessness and severe headache, which may occur during or soon after hemodialysis (120). This is commonly followed by nausea and vomiting, often accompanied by blood pressure elevation. These symptoms may be accompanied by disorientation and tremors, which may progress to seizures, with or without cardiac arrhythmias (121). Seizures have usually been of the grand mal type (89, 122). Focal seizures have been observed, but these are often due to preexisting focal neurologic disease (89). Most patients will recover from these symptoms, but recovery may take several days, at which time dialysis may again be necessary. In some patients, seizures may lead to coma, and death may ensue (122–124).

The EEG findings in patients with uremia consist of increased slow wave activity, increased spike wave activity, and bursts of delta wave activity, with loss of normal alpha rhythm (89, 92, 94). During and immediately after hemodialysis, the EEG findings may deteriorate. There is almost complete loss of alpha wave activity, with a further increase in theta and delta wave activity (93, 94, 124). These EEG changes may occur with or without DDS.

The CSF pressure has consistently been found to be normal in uremia, both in man (94, 124) and in experimental animals (99, 100, 126). Following hemodialysis of uremic man or experimental animals, the CSF pressure generally rises, whether dialysis is slow or rapid, regardless of the presence or absence of DDS (94, 99, 100, 124, 127). There is some evidence that intraocular pressure may also increase during dialysis (128). The presence of elevated CSF pressure is felt by many to indicate cerebral edema. However, an increase in CSF pressure may be secondary to increased CSF volume, increased cerebral blood flow, or increased brain water content (cerebral edema) (129), all of which will increase intracerebral volume. In the experimental animal, it has been consistently observed that CSF pressure will increase during hemodialysis, whether or not cerebral edema is present (99, 100). The most likely explanation for this phenomenon is that during hemodialysis there is a more rapid removal of urea from both brain and plasma than from CSF. The rate of removal of urea from brain closely parallels its rate of removal from plasma (100). This relationship is demonstrated in Fig. 26-9, which shows the urea concentration in brain (cerebral cortex), plasma, and cisternal CSF in uremic animals and in animals treated with either rapid or slow hemodialysis. Regardless of the rate with which urea was cleared from plasma in these studies, the urea gradient between plasma and brain was only about 6 mmol/kg H_2O. However, the urea concentration of CSF was 14 to 19 mmol/kg H_2O higher than that of plasma. The delayed clearance of urea from CSF probably accounts for virtually the entire osmotic gradient which is observed between CSF and plasma after hemodialysis. This osmotic gradient presumably leads to a net movement of water into the CSF, resulting in a rise in CSF pressure which is independent of the presence of brain edema.

In general, patients who are to be treated with dialysis will initially have a lower than normal arterial pH and plasma [HCO_3^-]. Most standard dialysate solutions contain HCO_3^- precursor (acetate or lactate) at a concentration of about 32 meq/L. Thus, hemodialysis can be expected to increase arterial pH and [HCO_3^-] by the addition of HCO_3^- to the extracellular fluid. Under such circumstances, one would expect that as normalization of the arterial pH occurs, arterial P_{CO_2}, which is low in patients with chronic uremia because of the presence of acidemia, would tend to rise. A rise in arterial P_{CO_2} would also be associated with a rise in the P_{CO_2} of CSF. However, it has been demonstrated that during, after, and between hemodialyses, arterial P_{CO_2} does not change appreciably (94, 130). Thus, one also would not expect the P_{CO_2} of CSF to change. However, several studies in dialysis patients have demonstrated that during hemodialysis there may be a substantial rise in the P_{CO_2} of lumbar CSF with a concomitant fall in its pH (111). Studies on the cisternal CSF of uremic dogs treated with rapid hemodialysis have revealed that in all such animals who developed DDS, pH of CSF fell (100). The fall in CSF pH was the result of both a rise in P_{CO_2} and a fall in [HCO_3^-]. It appears that in both man and experimental animals with DDS, there is a fall in CSF pH and a rise in CSF P_{CO_2} without a concomitant rise in P_{CO_2} of blood. Part of the reason that such findings have not been observed in all patients treated with rapid hemodialysis may be the fact that lumbar, rather than cisternal, CSF has been examined (94). Under circumstances where there are abrupt changes in systemic acid-base parameters, lumbar CSF may not accurately reflect changes in cisternal CSF (131). In addition, there are many methodological errors possible in measurement of CSF acid-base values (29).

There have been only limited studies of brain pathology in patients with DDS. In most patients thus far who have been examined postmortem, brain swelling has been observed (122, 132, 133). In addition, tentorial herniation has often been present (122, 132). Of particular note is the fact that many patients who died with seizure disorders during or after hemodialysis were considered to have DDS. Autopsy of these patients has often revealed the unsuspected presence of preexisting CNS disease such as subdural hematoma or intracerebral hemorrhage (114, 122, 132–137). At this time, there have been no neuropathologic studies of the CNS in patients dying with DDS.

In addition to DDS, there are other clinical situations associated with renal failure and hemodialysis which may result in syndromes similar to DDS. These conditions include (1) hypoglycemia, (2) hyponatremia, (3) subdural hematoma, (4) uremia per se, (5) nonketotic hyperosmolar coma with hyperglycemia, (6) depletion syndrome, (7) cerebral embolus secondary to shunt declotting, (8) excessive ultrafiltration leading to seizures, (9) acute cerebrovascular accident, (10) dialysis dementia, (11) dialysis proportioning system malfunction. All of the aforementioned clinical conditions may present with symptoms which are similar to DDS (1, 2, 89, 100, 133–144). Because of these factors, DDS remains a diagnosis of exclusion, with uncertain etiology.

Based upon the consistent finding of elevated CSF pressure and the presence of brain edema in patients dying with DDS, it has been felt that cerebral edema is a primary factor in the pathogenesis of DDS. The cause of the cerebral edema is uncertain, and many theories have been proposed to explain its occurrence.

During hemodialysis, both osmolality and urea

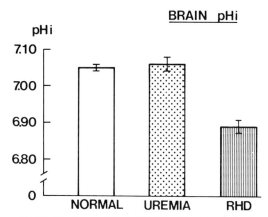

Figure 26-12. The intracellular pH (pH$_i$) of brain (cerebral cortex) in normal dogs, uremic dogs, and uremic dogs treated with rapid hemodialysis (RHD). Following rapid hemodialysis, there is a significant decline in the pH$_i$ of brain. (*From Arieff, Guisado, Massry and Lazarowitz.*)

concentration of CSF fall at a slower rate than that of plasma (93, 94, 125, 145, 146). On the basis of this observation, it has been suggested that after hemodialysis, there might be retention of urea in brain, resulting in brain osmolality higher than that of plasma. The increased brain osmolality could result in a net movement of water into brain, leading to cerebral edema (93, 147). This so called "reverse urea" effect has been the most frequently advanced theory for the pathogenesis of DDS. However, experimental evidence has not supported the aforementioned concept. Actual analysis of brain tissue in uremic animals treated with rapid hemodialysis has revealed no significant difference between urea concentration of plasma and brain (99, 100, 127). Thus, it appears unlikely that the "reverse urea" effect is important in the pathogenesis of DDS.

In addition to the delayed clearance of urea from the CSF, there is also evidence of a paradoxical acidosis in CSF. Cowie and coworkers found that in some patients treated with rapid hemodialysis, there is a fall in pH of the CSF despite a rise in arterial pH (111). A similar fall in pH of CSF occurs after rapid hemodialysis of experimental animals with acute renal failure (6, 100). It has been suggested that a fall in the pH of CSF may contribute to depression of senso-

rium (28). It has also been suggested that intracellular acidosis of brain cells, by altering intracellular binding of cations (Na$^+$ and K$^+$), may raise brain intracellular osmolality. Such an increase of osmolality could lead to brain edema (148). Recent studies in uremic animals have shown that following rapid hemodialysis, where the plasma urea is lowered by about 48 mmol/L in less than 2 h, there is a significant decrement in the intracellular pH of cerebral cortex (Fig. 26-12), from 7.05 to 6.88 (6). This fall in cerebral cortex intracellular pH is accompanied by a significant rise in cerebral cortex water content (Fig. 26-13). Thus, it is possible that rapid hemodialysis may in some manner lead to an increase in brain H$^+$ ion content, with a subsequent rise in intracellular osmolality. That a rise in intracellular osmolality can lead to tissue swelling has been well demonstrated in the red blood cell (149). Such a sequence may underlie the pathophysiology of DDS.

The solute which contributes to the observed rise of brain intracellular osmolality has not been precisely identified. Changes in brain content of measured solutes—Na$^+$, K$^+$ Cl$^-$, Ca^{2+}, Mg^{2+}, lactate, glucose—did not account for the observed changes in brain osmolality (100). The decrement in bicarbonate concentration of both CSF and brain suggests the de novo appearance of organic acids. These organic acids could be produced by breakdown of proteins or polypeptides,

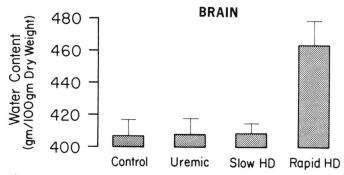

Figure 26-13. The brain (cerebral cortex) water content in normal dogs, uremic dogs, and dogs treated with either slow or rapid hemodialysis (HD). Rapid HD results in a significant increment of brain water content (cerebral edema). (*After Arieff, Massry, Barrientos, and Kleeman.*)

or by metabolic interconversion, such as glutamine to glutamic acid (148). Such metabolic processes could increase brain osmolality by several different mechanisms, such as (1) generation of NH_3 (148, 150), (2) displacement of bound intracellular Na^+ and K^+ by H^+ ions donated by organic acids, or by NH_4^+ ions, and (3) increased osmotic activity of organic acid anions formed by breakdown of larger protein molecules (150). The unidentified solute is commonly referred to as "idiogenic osmols" (17–19).

The treatment of DDS is conjectural at best. Several investigators have "treated" this syndrome by addition of osmotically active solute (glucose, urea, fructose, NaCl, mannitol) to the dialysate. The purpose of such maneuvers has been to minimize rapid alterations in plasma osmolality during dialysis (119, 124, 151, 152). However, for the most part, such manipulations have been carried out on stable chronic dialysis patients. Additionally, these patients were usually dialyzed slowly, with only minimal change in plasma urea and osmolality during dialysis. It is difficult to evaluate a treatment for DDS when it is used in patients who generally do not develop the syndrome. Additional studies are needed in patients with acute renal failure, or in those with chronic renal failure undergoing their initial few hemodialyses. Evaluation of the efficacy of prevention of DDS by addition of solute to the dialysate must await these additional investigations.

In both man and experimental animals, the occurrence of DDS can be largely prevented by use of "slow" dialysis, i.e., low blood flow rates (less than 200 mL/min) with a short duration of hemodialysis (less than 4 h) at frequent intervals (every 1 to 2 days) (89, 100, 127, 147, 153). Thus, until additional therapy becomes available, DDS can probably be best prevented in those individuals who are most likely to develop DDS by employing short, frequent dialyses at low blood flow rates.

Dialysis encephalopathy. A progressive, generally fatal neurological syndrome has been described in patients being treated with chronic hemodialysis (1, 143). Most patients have been treated with hemodialysis for at least 3 years before the onset of symptoms (115). The earliest sign of the syndrome is stuttering speech progressing to dysarthria, dyspraxia, and dysphagia. Early personality changes consisted of impaired memory, loss of ability to concentrate, personality changes, and psychosis manifested by depression and paranoia. Within 6 months of the onset of symptoms, most patients are unable to communicate verbally. Neurological signs gradually develop; they consist of bizarre involuntary limb movements, facial grimacing, myoclonic jerks, asterixis, motor apraxia, facial weakness, and generalized tremulousness.

The EEG shows a characteristic pattern which has been described by several different investigators at medical centers in the United States[1] (1, 115, 143, 154). There are bursts of diffuse slow wave (4 to 7 Hz) activity with spike waves and loss of normal alpha activity. Initially, the EEG findings are paroxysmal, often with relatively normal interludes. As the syndrome progresses, there are fewer and fewer normal interludes. Dialysis encephalopathy may first be suspected when a patient on chronic hemodialysis develops a worsening of the EEG. However, it should be stressed that any of the EEG changes reported in patients with dialysis dementia may also be present in patients with severe or poorly treated uremia. The EEG changes alone are not specific enough to enable one to make the diagnosis of dialysis dementia.

Pathological studies on brain of patients dying with dialysis encephalopathy have not revealed any consistent abnormalities. Some investigators have reported that the brains have been histologically normal[2] (1, 115, 143, 155); others have found evidence of various histological abnormalities. These abnormalities include cortical gliosis (1, 155) and atrophy (154). In patients in whom there was more extensive neuropathologic study of the brain, there was cytoplasmic and nuclear shrinkage, and in neurons there was increased lipofuscin pigment, loss of Nissl substance, and nuclear hyperchromicity (115). There was also astrocytic proliferation and evidence of neuronal

---

[1] A. I. Arieff, V. C. Lazarowitz: Unpublished data, 1975–1977.

[2] J. Wolinsky, A. I. Arieff: Unpublished data, 1977, and S. Price: Unpublished data, 1977.

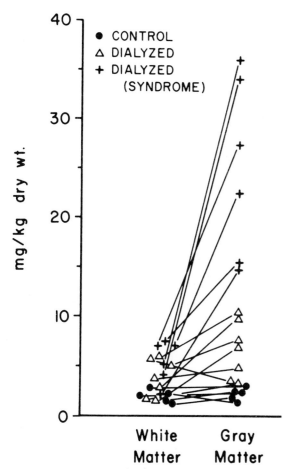

Figure 26-14. Aluminum levels in brain gray and white matter of control subjects and uremic patients with and without encephalopathy syndrome. (*From Alfrey, LeGendre, and Kaehny.*)

dropout (115). Other histological changes were also observed, but these were inconsistent (115). The aforementioned changes were then compared to histological changes in brain of both chronic dialysis patients without dialysis encephalopathy and patients with chronic renal failure not treated with dialysis (115). In patients treated with hemodialysis but without dialysis encephalopathy, histological changes were similar to those of patients with dialysis encephalopathy. In patients with chronic renal failure not treated with dialysis, the aforementioned changes were either minimal or absent. Thus, at this time, his-

tological changes in brain of patients with dialysis encephalopathy must be regarded as nonspecific and inconsistent. Perhaps in the future, more advanced neurolopathologic techniques will reveal some hitherto undetected lesion. The previously described changes, although nonspecific, actually most resemble the changes found in several "slow virus" infections of the CNS such as Jakob-Creutzfeldt disease or kuru[3] (156). Patients with these diseases often have symptoms similar to those of patients with dialysis encephalopathy. Despite the similar clinical presentations of patients with either dialysis dementia or Alzheimer's disease (presenile dementia), gross and histologic changes characteristic of Alzheimer's disease (157) have not been observed in patients with dialysis encephalopathy. The differences in histologic findings and their nonspecificity suggest that dialysis encephalopathy is in fact a multifactorial disease process, with several different disease processes converging to a common clinical presentation. A similar clinical picture may be observed in patients with several different types of dementia (157), such as Pick's disease, kuru, Jakob-Creutzfeldt disease, and Huntington's chorea.

Although histological examination of cerebral tissue has not been rewarding in patients with dialysis encephalopathy, there have been some promising biochemical findings.

It has been reported (1, 8) that in brain (cerebral cortex) of patients with dialysis encephalopathy, there is increased content of tin (Sn^{2+}) and aluminum (Al^{3+}). Subsequent investigation revealed that Sn^{2+} was also elevated in brain of patients with chronic renal failure but without dialysis encephalopathy. However, Al^{3+} has been demonstrated to be significantly higher in cerebral cortex of patients with dialysis encephalopathy (Fig. 26-14) than in chronic hemodialysis patients without encephalopathy, or in undialyzed patients with chronic renal failure (8, 158). However, we[4] have recently had the opportunity to study three patients with chronic renal failure

[3] J. R. Barringer: Personnel communication, 1977.

[4] A. I. Arieff, D. Armstrong, and V. C. Lazarowitz: Unpublished data, 1976–1977.

(creatinine clearance less than 20 mL/min) who had been taking $Al(OH)_3$ for at least 5 years before death. The Al^{3+} content in cerebral cortex (6 to 15 mg/kg dry weight) of these patients was only slightly less than reported in patients with dialysis encephalopathy. Thus, a high Al^{3+} content in cerebral cortex may also be related to the duration of $Al(OH)_3$ therapy in patients with renal insufficiency.

Apparently, some Al^{3+} is absorbed following oral administration of aluminum-containing antacids such as $Al(OH)_3$ or $Al_2(CO_3)_3$ (159, 160). The retention of Al^{3+} is greater in patients with renal failure than in normal subjects (160), but it is minimal in any case. In normal subjects ingesting 2.2 g of Al^{3+} over 3 days, plasma Al^{3+} increased only from 6.5 to 14.2 $\mu g/L$, or an increased whole body Al^{2+} of about 0.13 mg (for a 70-kg human), which represents only 0.006 percent of the ingested dose. However, over a period of years in patients with no renal function, this amount may be significant. It is also possible that an increase in body Al^{3+} stores may be the result of Al^{3+} contamination from other sources, such as Al^{3+} in water, aluminum pipes, or Al^{3+} leaked from anodes (158). Granted that Al^{3+} content is high in brain of patients with dialysis encephalopathy, this in no way shows that the Al^{3+} contributes to the encephalopathy. Aluminum content is also elevated in brain of patients with other types of dementia, such as Alzheimer's disease and senile dementia (161) and may in fact represent a nonspecific finding common to dementia (162). Studies which purport to show toxic effects of Al^{3+} salts are for the most part unconvincing. A toxic and fatal syndrome has been claimed to follow oral administration of Al^{3+} salts (163) in rats. However, normal rats given high amounts of $Al(OH)_3$ orally apparently died of aspiration pneumonia (163). When this was avoided by giving rats oral $Al(OH)_3$ by nasogastric tube, no toxic effects were observed (164). Syndromes induced in animals by giving $Al(OH)_3$ either intraperitoneally or subcutaneously, by "painting" Al^{3+} salts on the exposed brain, or by subarachnoid injection of Al^{3+} salts are obviously not analagous to any clinical situation and thus do not require further comment (163, 165, 166).

In addition to Al^{3+}, calcium (Ca^{2+}) has also been shown to be elevated in brain of patients with dialysis encephalopathy (1, 154). Other trace metals may be increased in cerebral tissues (167) of patients with dementia. For example, increased levels of Mg^{2+} have been demonstrated in brain of patients with Sturge-Weber syndrome (168) or striatonigral degeneration (169). Thus, at the present time, the etiology of dialysis encephalopathy must be regarded as unknown, and the possible role of aluminum-containing antacids is unclear.

There is no known satisfactory treatment for patients with dialysis encephalopathy. None of those reported in the literature thus far have survived, usually dying within 18 months of the time of diagnosis. There have been 3 additional cases[5] observed at Stanford University Medical Center and University of California, San Francisco School of Medicine, and 7 cases[6] at the University of British Columbia Medical Center, Vancouver, B. C., Canada in 3 years (1975–1977). All 10 died within 1½ years of the onset of symptoms of dialysis encephalopathy. The syndrome is not helped by increased frequency of dialysis or even by renal transplantation (1, 115). Definitive therapy must await a better understanding of the pathogenesis of this disorder.

DIABETIC COMAS (See also Chap. 24)

Coma, as a complication of diabetes mellitus, has been described for over 100 years (170). When used in reference to diabetic patients, the term is usually a misnomer. In fact, most of these patients do have some depression of sensorium, which usually takes the form of impaired response to verbal or painful stimuli, but some patients are alert and responsive and are therefore not comatose. In the strict sense, one should not diagnose diabetic "coma" unless there is at least some depression of sensorium, usually to a state of obtundation (171, 172). Obtundation can be defined as a state of dull indifference, where increased stimulation is required to evoke a response (172). If one excludes stroke, there are at least four syndromes of metabolic derangements

---

[5] A. I. Arieff: Unpublished data, 1975–1977.

[6] J. Price: Unpublished data, 1975–1977.

associated with diabetes which can be classified as diabetic comas. These are (1) diabetic ketoacidosis; (2) nonketotic hyperosmolar coma with hyperglycemia (nonketotic coma); (3) hypoglycemia; and (4) lactic acidosis. There is an abundance of clinical descriptions of these entities (173–178). Although there has been much fruitful investigative work on the biochemical derangements which characterize these clinical entities, the actual cause of coma is not known in any of them.

Diabetic ketoacidosis

Diabetic ketoacidosis is a metabolic abnormality which is characterized by hyperglycemia (blood glucose above 250 mg/dL) and metabolic acidosis (arterial pH below 7.25 and/or plasma bicarbonate less than 16 meq/L) due to hyperketonemia [plasma acetoacetate + β-hydroxybutyrate above 7 mmol/L (plasma acetest greater than 2+ at a 1:1 dilution)], with depression of sensorium to at least a state of obtundation. The disorder is most common among juvenile or growth-onset diabetic patients.

The pathogenesis of diabetic ketoacidosis has been adequately reviewed elsewhere (175, 178–182). Despite over 100 years of clinical and experimental investigation, the pathogenesis of coma in this disorder has not been elucidated. There are several important theories which will be briefly reviewed.

Ketonemia. There have been many suggestions that hyperketonemia per se may be important in the genesis of coma in patients with diabetic ketoacidosis. The only experimental studies which relate to this problem were performed prior to 1940, and they have yet to be confirmed. It has been reported that in rabbits, infusion of either acetoacetic acid or sodium acetoacetate resulted in coma (183). Under similar circumstances, infusion of either β-hydroxybutyric acid or sodium β-hydroxybutyrate did not result in coma, although some of these animals had unexplained deaths (183). Infusion of HCl to achieve a similar plasma bicarbonate as was obtained with β-hydroxybutyric acid infusion did not result in coma (183). These studies suggest that acetoacetate may somehow affect cerebral function in a way

such that coma results. Studies by Kety and coworkers (184) in patients with ketoacidosis are somewhat supportive of this concept in that they demonstrate a continuing fall in cerebral utilization of oxygen with increasing plasma ketone levels. Furthermore, the brain can probably metabolize β-hydroxybutyrate to γ-hydroxybutyrate, a substance which is an anesthetic agent (185). Thus, hyperketonemia may impair cerebral oxygen utilization and also have an anesthetic effect, both of which may contribute to depression of sensorium.

Metabolic acidosis. Metabolic acidosis is probably not an important cause of coma in ketoacidotic subjects. Acidosis per se is usually not associated with coma in patients with a variety of systemic diseases such as uremia, cholera (28, 186, 187), and hypercapnia (188, 189). Furthermore, infusion or ingestion of acid (HCl or NH_4Cl) to induce acute metabolic acidemia does not cause coma in laboratory animals (183, 190) or man (28, 191).

There has been some evidence suggesting that depression of sensorium correlates not with arterial pH but rather with the pH of CSF (28). However, subsequent investigation has failed to confirm these earlier impressions. There was no apparent relationship between depression of sensorium and pH of CSF in patients with nonketotic coma (171), in subjects with cholera who were treated with $NaHCO_3$ (186), or in patients with ketoacidosis who received intravenous $NaHCO_3$ (192, 193). In the latter two groups of patients, despite the fact that pH of CSF fell after administration of intravenous $NaHCO_3$, there was actually an improvement in sensorium. It is thus most likely that intracellular pH of brain, rather than pH of CSF, actually correlates with depression of sensorium. Since there is a generally poor correlation between pH of CSF versus brain intracellular pH (6, 29, 194–196), especially in metabolic disorders, it may be that in the earlier studies (28), conditions were such that brain intracellular pH and pH in CSF had undergone similar changes.

In rats with diabetic ketoacidosis, brain intracellular pH is probably normal, (83), as is lactate concentration (83, 197). The CSF pH is also usually normal in patients with ketoacidosis (193,

198). Thus, it is unlikely that brain intracellular pH is depressed in keotacidotic subjects. However in patients with severe acidemia (pH less than 7.00), there is probably a decrement in brain intracellular pH. Such cerebral intracellular acidosis can impair the conversion of glucose 6-phosphate to pyruvate by inhibition of phosphofructokinase in brain (199). Subsequent inhibition of the Krebs cycle could then lead to coma.

Cerebral hypoxia. Hypoxia is a well-known cause of coma (172). Patients with ketoacidosis have several abnormalities which might theoretically predispose to hypoxia, such as hyperviscosity of the blood (200) and decreased cerebral oxygen consumption (184). If hypoxia were severe, there could be a fall in brain intracellular pH due to increased brain lactate, as well as a decrease in brain high-energy phosphate compounds. Neither sequence is likely to occur. In animals with ketoacidosis, brain intracellular pH is probably normal (83), as is brain lactate (197). Total brain adenine nucleotides are also normal (83, 197). If the action of Na^+–K^+–ATPase in brain were impaired, there should be increases in brain Na^+ and decreases in K^+. Preliminary studies in animals do not support this hypothesis. Thus, at the present time, there is no data to support an important role for cerebral hypoxia in the pathogenesis of coma associated with ketoacidosis.

Hyperosmolality. It has been conclusively shown that hyperosmolality per se can induce coma in laboratory animals (202, 203). However, it is unlikely that extracellular hyperosmolality is often a cause of coma in ketoacidotic patients. Many patients with high plasma osmolality are alert, while those with lower levels of extracellular osmolality may be comatose (204). In both patients and laboratory animals, it appears that plasma osmolality must exceed 350 mosm/kg before there is depression of sensorium (171, 202, 203). In 438 ketoacidotic patients with coma, the mean plasma osmolality was only 322 mosm/kg (205). Overall, however, there is a significant correlation between depression of sensorium and extracellular osmolality (Fig. 26-15). Thus, hyperosmolality probably contributes to depression of sensorium at levels in excess of 340 mosm/kg (198) but is not a primary factor.

Other factors. Intravascular deposition of fibrin

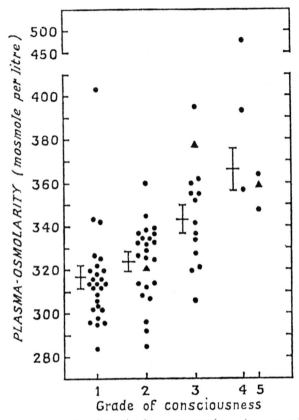

Figure 26-15. The relationship between state of consciousness and plasma osmolality (calculated) in 70 patients with diabetic ketoacidosis. Increasing numbers on abscissa denote increasing depression of sensorium. (*From Fulop, Tannenbaum, and Dreyer.*)

has recently been demonstrated in brains of patients dying with ketoacidotic coma. The fibrin deposition was associated with ischemic tissue damage (206). Studies of the coagulation system in these patients demonstrated thrombocytopenia with advanced elevated plasma fibrinogen levels. The hypothesis has been put forth that cerebral intravascular coagulation, by occluding small vessels and producing local ischemia, may play a major role in production of coma in ketoacidotic patients. The presence of such cerebral intravascular fibrin deposition, even if confirmed by others (207), is probably not a major or consistent abnormality. In all probability, coma in diabetic ketoacidosis is caused by a number of factors acting in combination. There is hyperviscosity of the blood and impaired cerebral oxygen utilization. There is probably some direct effect on brain of acetoacetate, and perhaps β-hydroxybutyrate as well, which tends to produce coma. During diabetic ketoacidosis, about one-half of the brain's source of energy may come from ketones, so their metabolites probably accumulate in the brain. It also may be that certain metabolites of glucose (fructose 6-phosphate, glucose 6-phosphate, citrate, acetyl-CoA) which accumulate in the brain of ketoacidotic animals manifest central nervous system toxicity. Hyperosmolality is present to varying degrees in all patients with diabetic ketoacidosis and may play some role in depression of sensorium. Disseminated intravascular coagulation appears to be present in some patients with diabetic ketoacidosis. Such a coagulopathy could result in localized areas of cerebral hypoperfusion, which may accelerate depression of sensorium. Finally, many patients with diabetic ketoacidosis have severe associated medical conditions such as sepsis, myocardial infarction, and pneumonia. These diseases may in themselves lead to depression of sensorium. The multiplicity of factors undoubtedly accounts for the fact that no single variable, such as arterial pH, plasma ketone levels, pH of CSF, plasma osmolality, or blood glucose concentration can consistently be correlated with depression of sensorium.

Nonketotic coma (See also Chap. 24)

Nonketotic hyperosmolar coma with hyperglycemia (nonketotic coma) is characterized by hyperglycemia (plasma glucose above 600 mg/dL) and hyperosmolality (plasma osmolality above 350 mosm/kg) without significant ketonemia (plasma acetest less than 2+ at a 1:1 dilution), and with depression of sensorium to at least a stupor (173). The pathogenesis of nonketotic coma has been extensively studied, and in all probability it represents a heterogenous entity. There is interplay between free fatty acid mobilization and metabolism, insulin secretion, growth hormone, dehydration, and hyperosmolality. These various pathogenic features have been discussed elsewhere (173, 175, 205).

Neurologic manifestations are prominent in patients with nonketotic coma. About 36 percent of patients are initially diagnosed as having an acute stroke (173), with about 27 percent having either hemiparesis or Babinski sign. About 10 to 15 percent of patients with nonketotic coma present with seizures (138, 173, 208, 209). The seizures are usually of a focal nature, although grand mal seizures and myoclonus are frequent (138, 208), as are other focal neurologic findings. The seizures are usually resistent to conventional anticonvulsant therapy (208, 209).

Focal neurologic changes have included aphasia, homonymous hemianopsia, hemisensory defects, hemiparesis, hyperreflexia, and both simple and complex visual hallucinations. In general, most of the aforementioned changes are reversible following correction of the metabolic abnormalities. Evidence of brainstem dysfunction in the form of tonic eye deviation and nystagmus has also been reported, suggesting at least occasional involvement of the vestibular system. A variety of autonomic nervous system changes, such as hyperpnea and hypertension, may also be observed. This variety of neurologic changes in patients with nonketotic coma cannot be explained by a single structural lesion, but rather appears to represent a widespread functional disturbance which affects all levels of the nervous system (138, 208).

The multiplicity of neurological involvement often suggests the presence of acute cerebral parenchymal damage, but cerebral angiography and neuropathologic examinations usually fail to disclose structural abnormalities correlating with the clinical observations. Furthermore, in surviving patients, the prompt resolution of the neurologic deficit without persistent sequelae suggests that acute vascular accidents or other structural lesions are an unlikely explanation for the clinical findings. The mean age of patients presenting with nonketotic coma is about 62 years (173), and most of them have some sort of preceding vascular abnormality, such as old infarcts, cerebral arteriosclerosis, or lacunar states (209). It is possible that localized areas of vascular insufficiency may render certain neuronal groups more sensitive to the metabolic changes of nonketotic coma, resulting in transient functional neurologic changes. A similar phenomenon has been observed in experimental animals who are allowed to recover from hemiparesis induced by unilateral cerebral artery ligation (210). When acute hyperosmolality is induced in these animals, there is the reappearance of neurologic deficits which correspond functionally to the anatomic areas of the brain previously subjected to the acute vascular insult.

The mechanisms by which hyperosmolality may induce neuronal discharges leading to seizure activity are not well known. In the clinical situation, seizure activity is very rare in ketoacidotic patients (204) but is present in about 15 percent of those patients with nonketotic coma (138, 209). Thus, hyperketonemia may in some manner suppress the effects of hyperosmolality on the CNS. In both ketoacidosis and nonketotic coma, there is probably some suppression of Krebs cycle activity in the brain. In ketoacidosis (in the rat), there is accumulation of citrate in the brain (83). Additionally, hyperosmolality per se can inhibit

Krebs cycle activity (27). With Krebs cycle inhibition, the energy supply of brain may be met, at least in part, by metabolism of ketones, lactate, glutamate, and perhaps other amino acids as well (211, 212). In particular, γ-aminobutyric acid (GABA) is found in high concentrations only in nervous tissue (213, 214). GABA has been shown to be a cortical depressant, raising the seizure threshold (215). In the brain, GABA can be metabolized to succinate via the GABA shunt, which is an alternative to the Krebs cycle for the conversion of α-ketoglutarate to succinate (216). The GABA shunt can provide up to 40 percent of the brain's energy requirement under certain circumstances (216). Thus, in patients with nonketotic coma, it may be that increased metabolism of GABA lowers the seizure threshold (217). Conversely, in ketoacidotic animals, brain tissue levels of GABA are normal (218), which may in part account for the absence of seizures.

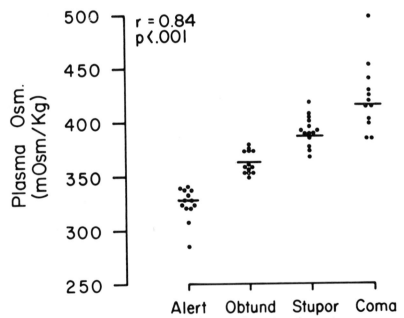

Figure 26-16. The relationship between depression of sensorium and plasma osmolality (osm) in 53 patients with blood glucose greater than 600 mg/dL but without ketoacidosis. In calculating the correlation coefficient (r), alertness was counted as 1, obtundation (obtund) as 2, stupor as 3, and coma as 4. For each group, plasma osmolality is significantly different from that of the adjacent group(s) (p less than 0.01). (*From Arieff and Carroll.*)

Clinically, depression of sensorium in patients with either ketoacidosis or nonketotic coma has been found to correlate with extracellular hyperosmolality (Figs. 26-15, 26-16), but not with hyperglycemia, or pH of either blood or CSF (171, 192, 193, 198). The mechanisms by which hyperosmolality can induce coma are unclear. There is a general impression that hyperglycemia, as is the case with other acute hyperosmolar states (105), should cause cerebral dehydration. However, evidence in both patients and laboratory animals with hyperglycemia suggest that this is not the case. Patients who die with nonketotic coma have not been reported to show evidence of cerebral dehydration. In fact, of 14 patients with nonketotic coma where there was postmortem examination of the brain, none had evidence of cerebral dehydration (105, 173, 219, 220–222) and several had cerebral edema (219, 223, 224).

In laboratory animals, rapid elevation of plasma glucose by infusion of 2.87 *M* glucose (1 mL/min) causes cerebral dehydration and death in 60 to 90 min (225). However, when plasma glucose in rabbits is elevated to about 1100 mg/dL in 1 h, the sequence of events in brain is different (17). After

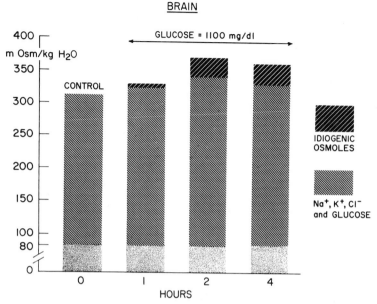

Figure 26-18. Comparison of effects on brain solute composition of 1 to 4 h of hyperglycemia. After 1 h of glucose infusion, virtually all the increase in brain solute is due to increase in concentration of glucose and electrolytes. After 2 or 4 h of hyperglycemia, about half the increase in brain solute is due to presence of undetermined solute. (*From Arieff, Guisado and Lazarowitz.*)

1 to 2 h of hyperglycemia, there is an initial decrease in brain-water content (Fig. 26-17). However, when plasma glucose is then maintained at about 1100 mg/dL for 4 to 6 h, brain water content returns to normal values. By comparison, under similar circumstances, skeletal muscle water content falls significantly after 2 h and remains depressed (Fig. 26-18). The secondary increase of brain water to normal values is accompanied by an increase in brain osmol content such that brain and plasma osmolality are similar. This increase in brain osmol content is only partially accounted for by changes in brain content of measured solute—glucose, lactate, sorbitol, myoinositol, urea, Na^+, K^+, or Cl^-—the remainder consisting of idiogenic osmols (Fig. 26-18). The generation of idiogenic osmols during hyperglycemia thus enables the brain to achieve osmotic equilibrium with plasma despite less loss of water and/or gain in solute than would be expected if the brain were a more perfect osmometer. Such a mechanism is probably homeostatic,

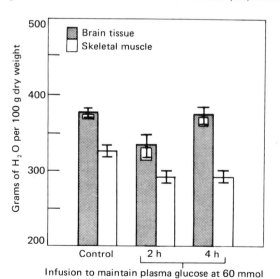

Figure 26-17. Brain and muscle water content. After 2 h of hyperglycemia, there is a loss of about 10 percent in both brain and muscle water content. After 4 h of hyperglycemia, the brain water content is the same as in controls, but muscle water content remains low. (*From Guisado and Arieff.*)

permitting the brain to maintain its intracellular volume and inorganic solute concentration within the normal range at a time when plasma osmolality is markedly elevated. In animals with experimental nonketotic coma, generation of idiogenic osmols by brain appears to be a response to hyperglycemia rather than to hyperosmolality per se. When plasma osmolality is elevated to similar levels (about 350 mosm/kg) over a 4- to 6-h period by infusion of either mannitol or glycerol (226, 227), essentially all of the increase in brain osmolality is due to loss of water by brain, with a subsequent increase in brain $[Na^+]$, $[K^+]$, and $[Cl^-]$ (Fig. 26-19). The identity of the idiogenic osmols in brain has not been established at this time.

There have been several possible explanations advanced to explain the adaptive processes of the brain to hyperglycemia. It has been suggested by some that the brain might synthesize fructose, sorbitol, or myoinositol in quantities such that brain intracellular osmolality would be increased by similar levels as that of plasma (228, 229). Others have suggested that glucose might enter

brain cells to achieve intracellular concentrations of sufficient magnitude to equalize plasma and brain osmolalities (223). However, all of these theories have been effectively invalidated by experimental evidence. During hyperglycemic states in laboratory animals, brain glucose concentration has been only about 20 to 30 percent of plasma glucose (17, 218, 227–230). The theories concerning possible generation of fructose, myoinositol, or sorbitol by brain were based upon findings of increased levels of sorbitol in CSF during hyperglycemia states (228). However, during hyperglycemic states in laboratory animals, brain concentration of sorbitol has never been present in osmotically significant amounts (17, 227, 229, 231). Also, it may be that the elevated levels of fructose and sorbitol observed in the CSF of hyperglycemic animals are produced not by the brain, but by spinal nerve roots (232). Similarly, myoinositol levels in brain have not been shown to increase substantially during hyperglycemia (17, 229).

Although the identity of the idiogenic osmols in brain is not yet known, they may represent changes in the intracellular binding of cations (Na^+ and K^+). At least 20 percent of brain K^+ is normally nonexchangeable (4) and thus is probably osmotically inactive. Similarly about 20 percent of brain Na^+ is also not exchangeable (4). Various types of osmotic stress can alter the brain intracellular binding of Na^+ and K^+ in vitro (7). Also hyperosmolality induced by intravenous infusion of NaCl decreases the amount of bound Na^+ and K^+ in brain (105) in vivo. Although the effects on brain have not yet been directly evaluated, an intracellular acidosis will increase cellular osmolality in other cells, such as red blood cells (149), by displacement of bound K^+ ion with H^+ ion. Such a phenomenon may well occur in cerebral cortex as well (6).

Thus, the adaptation of brain to hyperglycemic states depends on the interaction of several factors which may occur within the brain, including dehydration, some gain in measured solute, and generation of idiogenic osmols. The net effect upon brain volume will be based on the rapidity, duration, and degree of the hyperglycemia, as well as on various characteristics of individual patients.

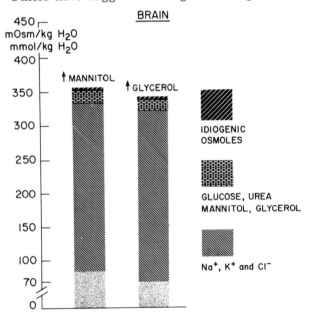

Figure 26-19. Effects on brain solute of hyperosmolality induced by infusions of either mannitol or glycerol for 6 h. Essentially all the increase in brain osmolality is due to increases in measured solute, with virtually no generation of idiogenic osmols. (*From Arieff, Guisado, and Lazarowitz.*)

Hypoglycemia

The neurologic manifestations of hypoglycemia are well known and may include tremulousness, cold sweating, headache, and confusion. In addition, a multitude of neurologic signs and symptoms, such as delirium, hypothermia, brainstem dysfunction, strokelike illness, and focal or generalized seizures may occur (172, 211). Such neurological manifestations may progress to coma and death (172).

Although it is commonly felt that hyperinsulinemia is virtually synonymous with hypoglycemia, there are other causes as well. Hypoglycemia is commonly induced by a wide variety of drugs (233), including alcohol (234), non-insulin-secreting tumors (235), and starvation (236).

The symptoms of hypoglycemia are diverse. In addition to the aforementioned neurologic abnormalities, there is a wide spectrum of more subtle changes. Some patients with hypoglycemia are asymptomatic (236), while others may manifest moderate hysteria and hypochondriasis (237), and still others may display irrational and maniacal behavior (238). In general, symptoms depend somewhat on the rapidity with which plasma glucose is lowered rather than the absolute level of plasma glucose (211). Women may be asymptomatic with plasma glucose levels of 35 mg/dL after 72 h of fasting (236), while rapidly lowering plasma glucose to such a level would generally provoke seizures (211).

The symptoms of hypoglycemia, as well as autopsy findings, suggest the presence of increased intracranial pressure, and it is possible that cerebral edema may underlie many of the symptoms of hypoglycemic coma. In both patients and experimental animals dying with hypoxia, the gross and microscopic findings in the brain are similar to those seen with hypoglycemia. It has thus been postulated that the pathophysiologic events underlying the symptomatology and coma in these two conditions may be similar (172, 211, 239). It has also been suggested that with either hypoglycemia or hypoxia, a decrease in cerebral oxygenation, might disrupt cell membrane bound Na^+–K^+–ATPase, with a net movement of Na^+ into brain (239). This increment in brain Na^+ would raise brain osmolality which in turn could cause a movement of water into brain, and hence cerebral edema would ensue.

Other studies have shown that hypoglycemia does not cause a significant fall in brain ATP or phosphocreatine (240, 241), leading to the postulate that hypoglycemic coma may result from a lack of certain specific energy-supplying substrates, such as glucose and its metabolites. Such metabolites might include alanine, GABA, ketones, lactate, and glutamate, which can probably serve as energy sources for the brain under hypoglycemic conditions (211, 242). Recently, it has been suggested that the neurologic manifestations of hypoglycemia might have at least two components.

Seizures observed soon after the onset of hypoglycemia are probably related to increased transport of Na^+ and K^+ into brain cells. The resultant increase in cerebral osmolality probably leads to some degree of cerebral swelling. The increase in cerebral volume and K^+ content correlates temporarily with the occurrence of grand mal seizures in experimental animals (243). Between the times animals are having grand mal seizures, they are alert and responsive to stimuli. Biochemically, although there is hypoglycemia (plasma glucose less than 40 mg/dL), brain glucose concentration is normal (about 2 mmol/kg intracellular H_2O). Thus, seizures observed early (within 2 h) in the course of hypoglycemia occur when both brain glucose (243) and high-energy phosphate compounds (241) are normal.

Late (after 3 h) in the course of hypoglycemia, coma ensues. The coma is associated with a significant decrement in brain glucose (241, 243) and in other energy-supplying substrates, such as glutamate and lactate (243). However, even in comatose animals, brain ATP and phosphocreatine are normal (241).

The EEG alterations associated with hypoglycemia have been extensively described (176). In general, with increasing hypoglycemia there is a slowing of the dominent alpha rhythm (8 to 12 Hz) to 6 to 7 Hz. The alpha rhythm persists but is no longer the dominant frequency. These changes occur at plasma glucose levels of 50 to 70 mg/dL. Theta waves (4 to 7 Hz) appear with plasma glucose below 50 mg/dL, and if plasma glucose continues to fall, there will be asynchronous irregular waves, with eventual flattening of the EEG. The plasma glucose levels where such changes occur will vary markedly among individual patients. With correction of the hypoglycemia, the EEG will change towards normal in the reverse order (244). If irreversible brain damage has occurred, the EEG will not revert to normal.

HYPONATREMIA (See also Chap. 12)

Hyponatremia is probably the most common electrolyte abnormality seen in a general hospital population. It is seen in association with many different systemic disease states. Hyponatremia is always the result of dilution and may occur in the presence or absence of depletion of total body Na^+. The etiologies of hyponatremia are diverse and include iatrogenic causes, such as diuretic administration (245), excessive parenteral fluids (246), and a wide variety of pharmacologic agents (247). Self-induced hyponatremia has been reported in both adults and infants ingesting excessive quantities of water (248–251) and in habitual beer-drinking adults (252, 253). Other causes of hyponatremia are related to the inability to appropriately excrete free water, most commonly in hospitalized patients who are given water, usually intravenously, in excess of their ability to excrete it. Iatrogenic overhydration may occur in patients who have normal renal diluting capacity, such as those who receive massive amounts of intravenous dextrose in water, or distilled water during bladder irrigation for prostate surgery (254). However, because individuals with normal kidney function are able to excrete at least 10 mL/min free water (255), acute hyponatremia occurs more frequently in patients who are water-loaded in the presence of conditions which may impair free water excretion. Such conditions include congestive heart failure, syndrome of inappropriate ADH secretion, renal failure, liver disease, or use of any of a long list of drugs (247). Voluntary water intoxication is rare but has been reported in polydipsic patients who are frequently psychotic (248).

The mortality in patients with acute hyponatremia (serum Na^+ less than 120 meq/L per 12 h) is substantial (over 50 percent), but mortality is much less in patients whose hyponatremia has developed over a period of days to weeks (Fig. 26-20).

Symptoms of acute hyponatremia patients

The symptoms of hyponatremia are dependent on the etiology, magnitude, and acuteness of the condition. In general, symptoms of sustained hyponatremia which are due to a combination of Na^+ depletion and water ingestion (256) differ markedly from those which accompany acute water intoxication. The symptoms of water intoxication are related to both the extent of the fall in serum Na^+ and to the rapidity with which serum Na^+ is lowered.

Neurological manifestations of acute water intoxication usually are not observed until plasma Na^+ has fallen below 125 meq/L (257, 258) and they include nausea, emesis, muscular twitching, grand mal seizures, and coma. Acute (less than 24 h) water intoxication (plasma Na^+ less than 125 meq/L) has a mortality above 50 percent (Fig. 26-20) (246, 248, 251, 252, 254, 257, 259) with a substantial morbidity (usually brain damage). However, when plasma Na^+ is slowly (several days to several weeks) lowered to 125 meq/L or less by salt depletion and water ingestion, patients usually are less symptomatic (254, 256, 258, 260).

In experimental animals with acute water intoxication, coma and seizures may be seen when serum Na^+ is acutely lowered to levels of about 120 meq/L over a period of 2 h (254). When serum Na^+ is reduced to 122 meq/L over 2 to 3 days, however, most animals are asymptomatic (254). More profound hyponatremia (serum Na^+ = 110 meq/L or lower) usually results in varying degrees of lethargy, coma, and seizures (254, 261). Thus, in both patients and experimental animals, the neurological manifestations seem to correlate grossly both with the degree of hyponatremia and with the rapidity of the fall in serum Na^+.

Symptoms of chronic hyponatremia

Patients with chronic hyponatremia usually have less fulminant symptoms and a far lower morbidity and mortality (Fig. 26-20). In a classic exper-

MORTALITY IN 74 ADULT PATIENTS WITH HYPONATREMIA

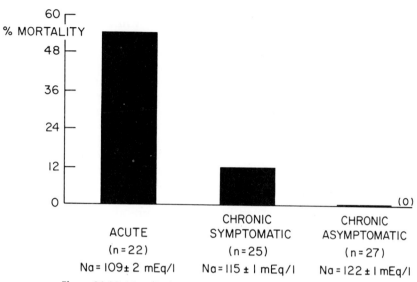

Figure 26-20. Mortality in patients with hyponatremia. A mortality rate of 55 percent in adults with acute hyponatremia is contrasted with a 12 percent mortality rate in symptomatic adults with chronic hyponatremia. No deaths were seen in adults with chronic asymptomatic hyponatremia. (*Data and figure from Covey and Arieff.*)

iment, individuals were maintained for 11 days on a salt-free diet, with frequent exposure to a high ambient temperature to cause excessive perspiration, combined with a high water intake (262). Their mean serum Na^+ concentrations fell from 147 to 131 meq/L. These subjects all experienced constant thirst, impaired sensation of taste, and anorexia, and several experienced muscle cramps. All had a feeling of general exhaustion, with dyspnea on exertion and dulling of sensorium. Other studies have shown that in individuals with a greater depression of serum Na^+ (120 to 130 meq/L), symptoms of nausea, emesis and abdominal cramps may occur (256, 263). With even more severe hyponatremia (below 115 mmol/L), subjects may manifest weakness, lethargy, restlessness, confusion, delirium and impaired mentation (187). In addition, muscular twitching is often present, and convulsions may occur (252, 254, 257, 264, 265). Many other neurological abnormalities have been reported in patients with chronic hyponatremia, including focal weakness,

hemiparesis, ataxia, and Babinski sign (252, 256).

By contrast, symptoms of acute water intoxication appear to differ substantially from those which can be attributed to Na^+ depletion per se, although the differences may actually be due to the rapidity with which plasma Na^+ is lowered. Neurological manifestations of acute water intoxication usually are not observed until plasma Na^+ has fallen below 125 meq/L (257, 258, 260). They may include nausea, emesis, and muscular twitching, as well as seizures and coma.

Chronic hyponatremia is common in patients with any of several edematous states such as congestive heart failure, renal insufficiency, or liver failure, in all of which both total body water and Na^+ are increased (266). Chronic hypernatremia is also frequently seen in patients with the syndrome of inappropriate secretion of antidiuretic hormone (SIADH), which may be caused by tumor (most characteristically oat-cell carcinoma of the lung), central nervous system disease, acute intermittent porphyria, or lung disease. Among hospitalized patients, an inappropriate ADH-like syndrome is commonly seen with the administration of various drugs, including oral hypoglycemics, tricyclic antidepressant agents, anticancer agents, diuretics, clofibrate, and analgesics (247). Chronic hyponatremia may also be seen in patients with salt-losing states, such as salt-losing renal disease, excessive sweating, Addison's disease, and gastrointestinal loss (267), and has also been reported in patients ingesting massive quantities of beer (252). Finally, evidence has been presented recently suggesting a lowered cerebral threshold for ADH release in certain chronically ill patients. These patients apparently have "reset osmostats," which are manifested as sustained hyponatremia in the face of intact ability to excrete free water (268).

Chronic hyponatremia in children is less frequent, although acute water intoxication with seizures and altered sensorium has been reported. Inappropriate ADH syndromes are seen in children (269) as well as adults. In addition, in a recent study of small-for-gestational-age infants, Day and coworkers (270) found hyponatremia, which was frequently asymptomatic, in 28 percent of the infants. These infants appeared to have an unexplained high renal loss of sodium and in addition were given inadequate electrolyte replacement in their feedings.

Patients with chronic hyponatremia often have neurological symptoms which may include seizures (254), depression of mental status (apathy to frank coma), hemiparesis (252, 257), Babinski signs, rigidity, and asterixis (271). The psychiatric literature includes several cases of patients with occult hyponatremia who were admitted for evaluation of abrupt changes in personality while other patients with chronic hyponatremia may display no symptoms at all (254, 267, 270). The central nervous system symptoms are for the most part reversible with recognition and prompt correction of the hypotonicity (271), although cases of irreversible neurological damage probably resulting from hyponatremia have been reported (246, 254).

In unselected hyponatremic patients, the degree of hyponatremia does not always correlate with the severity of symptoms (254). One patient with a serum Na^+ of 115 meq/L may be asymptomatic, while another whose Na^+ is 120 meq/L may present in frank coma. The mental status of 65 consecutive hospitalized hyponatremic patients whose plasma Na^+ was 128 meq/L or less is plotted against plasma Na^+ in Fig. 26-21. There is in general a good correlation, albeit considerable overlap. Similar findings have been reported by others (256), where some patients with serum Na^+ of 108 to 132 mmol/L had severe neurological manifestations and others with Na^+ of 117 to 133 mmol/L were asymptomatic. In general, however, when plasma Na^+ is below 120 mmol/L, most patients have some depression of sensorium and many have seizures (Fig. 26-21).

Hyponatremia: electroencephalographic changes

EEG abnormalities in hyponatremia are common but also nonspecific (246). The most common changes are a loss of normal alpha wave activity with irregular discharges of high amplitude, slow (4 to 7 Hz) wave activity (272). These changes are more obvious over the posterior than the anterior portion of the head, and they tend to be more severe with lower levels of serum Na^+. The EEG findings usually returned to normal after correction of the hyponatremia (252, 271, 272).

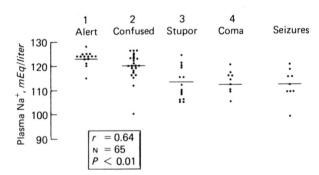

Figure 26-21. The relationship between plasma Na^+ concentration and depression of sensorium in 65 patients with plasma Na^+ of 128 meq/L or less. It can be seen that although there is a highly significant overall correlation, substantial overlap among groups of patients is present. All patients who had seizures had plasma Na^+ of less than 121 meq/L. (*From Arieff, Llach, and Massry.*)

Hyponatremia: pathology

Very few pathological studies of the brain in patients who have died of hyponatremia have been reported. In one of the first published cases, a patient who had absorbed 9000 mL of tap water was studied 1 h after death (259). Although not actually measured, the calculated serum Na^+ was less than 120 meq/L. Examination of the cranial contents revealed obliteration of the subarachnoid space. The cerebral gyri were flattened, sulci were largely obliterated, there was uniform enlargement of the brain in all directions, and the ventricles were reduced in size. Microscopically, there was increased vacuolization and swelling of supportive (glial) structures, with cellular swelling apparently confined to white matter. An ad-

ditional postmortem examination in a patient who died of acute water intoxication revealed gross brain edema with both uncal and tonsillar herniation (251). In one other patient who died 3 weeks after an episode of acute water intoxication, no cerebral edema was present (246).

Several investigators have studied the effects of acute water intoxication on brain in experimental animals. In general, all have found that there is considerably less swelling in brain than in other tissues (liver, muscle) studied (261, 273, 274). Edema is present in both gray and white matter of brain (261, 275), although more so in white matter (276). The blood-brain barrier is judged to be generally intact in water-intoxicated animals (no penetration into brain of parenterally administered trypan blue) (275).

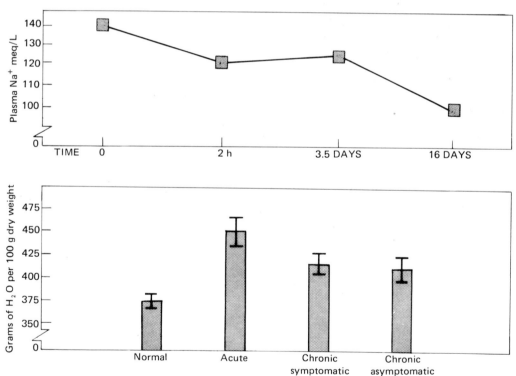

Figure 26-22. Brain water in normal rabbits, and three groups of hyponatremic animals. In animals in which plasma Na^+ is lowered to 119 meq/L in 2 h, brain water is 17 percent above normal values. When plasma Na^+ is lowered more gradually over either 3½ or 16 days, brain water is increased only 7 percent. There is no difference in brain water when symptomatic and asymptomatic chronically hyponatremic animals are compared. Brackets indicate ± SE. (*From Covey and Arieff.*)

Microscopically, cellular swelling appears to be confined to astrocytes, with sparing of neuronal elements (275, 278). Phase microscopy of brain in water-intoxicated rats (278) revealed mild perivascular glial swelling with severe swelling of astrocytes. Electron microscopy showed no damage to cytoplasmic organelles, intact mitochondria, and normal tight junctions. There was no evidence of damage to neurons or oligodendrocytes, and the extracellular space was enlarged.

Hyponatremia: effects of brain water and electrolytes

Brain water and electrolyte content in hyponatremic animals has been evaluated by a number of different laboratories. Interpretation of the results reported by different authors is made difficult by the variety of animal species used and the different degrees of hyponatremia achieved. In general, however, the increase in brain water content seems to be greatest in animals with acute hyponatremia (1 to 4 h) (Fig. 26-22). During chronic hyponatremia, however, the increase in brain water content is lower than that predicted by the extent of the hyponatremia and also lower than that seen in other tissues (261, 273).

Thus, it appears that the actual increase in brain water content in response to hyponatremia is somehow limited by various mechanisms (Fig. 26-22). Brain electrolyte content (mmol/kg dry weight) is somewhat decreased in animals made hyponatremic over a period of 1 to 2 h (Fig. 26-23). When hyponatremia is induced over longer periods of time, there is a significant fall in brain content of Na^+, K^+, and Cl^- (Fig. 26-23). In general, the fall in brain content of Na^+ and K^+ in animals with chronic hyponatremia is proportional to the fall in serum Na^+ level (Fig. 26-23), although there is also a decrease in brain amino acid content (279). The principal mechanism which limits the extent of brain swelling in response to prolonged hyponatremia would appear to be the observed decrement in brain electrolyte content, chiefly Na^+ and K^+. This is further substantiated by the decline in brain osmolality observed in hyponatremic animals (254). Brain osmolality is significantly higher than that of serum in animals made acutely hyponatre-

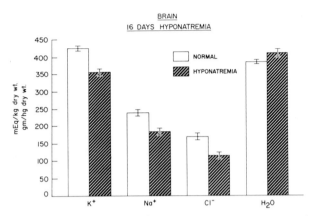

Figure 26-23. Brain content of Na^+, K^+, Cl^- and water in normal animals and in rabbits with hyponatremia ($\downarrow$Na) of 16 days' duration (plasma Na^+ = 99 meq/L). It can be seen that in the $\downarrow$Na animals, brain water content is 7 percent above normal and brain content of Na^+, K^+, and Cl^- is 17 to 37 percent below normal values. The loss of electrolytes by brain prevented a larger gain in brain water. Shaded bars represent $\downarrow$Na animals and brackets are mean ± SE. (*From Arieff, Llach, and Massry.*)

mic (2 h). When similar degrees of hyponatremia are induced over a period of several days, brain osmolality progressively falls, eventually reaching levels similar to plasma (254).

Thus, the fall in brain osmolality limits the extent of water gain by brain by reducing the osmotic gradient induced by the acute fall in serum Na^+.

The change in brain composition which is of greatest order of magnitude in animals with acute hyponatremia is an increase in brain water content, whereas in chronic hyponatremia, there is a lesser gain in brain water, but a significant fall in both Na^+ and K^+ content (Fig. 26-24). Several observers have suggested that the encephalopathy associated with hyponatremia may be related to the decrease in brain K^+ which is seen in experimental animals (258, 274). There is some evidence which suggests that the degree of encephalopathy in acutely hyponatremic rats does not correlate either with the serum Na^+ level or the brain content of Na^+ or K^+ (261). In acutely water-intoxicated rats, the effects of hyponatremia on brain function appeared to be related to brain edema per se, which occurred before the brain was able to undergo compensatory changes to adapt to the fall in serum Na$^+$. In animals with chronic hyponatremia, however, significant decrements in brain content of both Na$^+$ and K$^+$ were present (Fig. 26-23).

Recently, transport systems for both the release and reuptake of neurotransmitter amino acids have been shown to exist in synaptosomes of brain and spinal cord (280). A Na$^+$ gradient is assumed to be one of the major sources of energy for transport of such metabolites against a concentration gradient (281). In brain and spinal cord synaptosomes, the neurotransmitter amino acid

transport systems are almost totally Na$^+$-dependent (280, 282), and amino acid uptake in brain slices is largely inhibited by the absence of Na$^+$ (283).

Hyponatremia, then, may affect brain function by any of several mechanisms. Initially, the symptoms of acute hyponatremia are probably due to brain swelling, with a secondary increase of intracranial pressure. With more prolonged hyponatremia (more than 3 to 4 h), the brain becomes depleted of both Na$^+$ and K$^+$, thereby limiting the increase in brain cell volume. The loss of brain Na$^+$ may result in both an inhibition of brain energy metabolism and interference with neurotransmitter amino acid release at the synaptic level. These changes may directly affect brain function and may in part be responsible for the encephalopathy of hyponatremia.

Acute water intoxication: therapy (See also Chap. 12)

Despite a substantial amount of literature pertaining to both patients and experimental animals with acute symptomatic hyponatremia, there is surprisingly little available information as to the appropriate therapeutic approach. There is general agreement that if hyponatremia is due to a specific underlying medical illness (cirrhosis, congestive heart failure, Addison's disease), therapy should be directed primarily at this process. However, in the patient with acute symptomatic hyponatremia, there is apparently no unanimity of opinion as to appropriate therapy. Most internal medicine textbooks (284, 285) agree that acute symptomatic hyponatremia is a medical emergency and suggest the use of hypertonic (500 to 860 mM) NaCl. However, these same sources caution against treating hyponatremia "too rapidly" because of the possible dangers of congestive heart failure or cerebral hemorrhage. There are few actual recommendations as to how much hypertonic NaCl to infuse over how rapid a period of time, and even less supporting data.

The paucity of such recommendations reflects the fact that it is not known how fast one can safely raise plasma Na$^+$ in patients with acute hyponatremia or how long it takes for acute hypo-

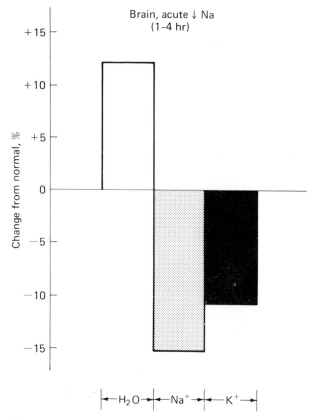

Figure 26-24. Changes in brain content of water, Na$^+$, and K$^+$ in animals with acute (1 to 4 h) hyponatremia. With a fall in plasma osmolality, an osmotic gradient favors the net movement of water into brain, with brain water increasing to 13 percent above control values. There is also a loss by brain of Na$^+$ and K$^+$ (by 11 to 16 percent), with a resultant fall in brain osmolality, so that the increase in brain water is lessened. (*From Arieff and Guisado.*)

natremia to cause permanent brain damage. Studies directed at the aforementioned problems, in either patients or experimental animals, have yet to be undertaken. It is known that in patients, acute water intoxication with plasma Na^+ below 125 mmol/L can cause irreversible brain damage within 12 h (246, 251, 254, 259), but the time span whereby recovery of cerebral function is possible is not known. It is known that in patients, rapid infusion or ingestion of large quantities of hypertonic NaCl can cause congestive heart failure and subdural and intracerebral hemorrhage, with a prohibitive morbidity and mortality (286–289), while hyponatremia, per se, appears to decrease cardiac output (127). However, either the infusion of 862 mM NaCl at a rate of about 70 mmol/h, or establishment of a negative free water balance of about 600 mL/h will usually elevate plasma Na^+ by 2 to 3 mmol/L per h (254, 290). These forms of therapy are continued until the patient undergoes definite symptomatic improvement, or until plasma Na^+ has been increased above 130 mmol/L. Both procedures appear to be relatively safe, and until more definitive data is available, therapy of acute symptomatic water intoxication should probably be based on similar maneuvers.

HYPERNATREMIA (See also Chap. 12)

A number of central nervous system lesions have been reported to cause hypernatremia; these have been reviewed elsewhere (23, 291–293). In addition to lesions in the central nervous system, there are a number of medical conditions which are commonly associated with hypernatremia, the preponderance of which are quite different in children and in adults.

In infants, gastroenteritis with diarrhea is the most common cause (291, 294, 295) while in elderly individuals, hypernatremia is often associated with infirmity and inability to freely obtain water, leading to gradual desiccation (292). Small children may also become hypernatremic after accidental administration of a high solute load, particularly accidental substitution of NaCl for sugar in preparation of formula (296, 297) or improper dilution of concentrated formulas (298).

Other causes of hypernatremia include nasogastric hyperalimentation, nonketotic hyperosmolar coma, acute renal failure, renal tubular damage, dialysis, dehydration secondary to elevated ambient temperature, pituitary or renal diabetes insipidus, sea water ingestion, and hyperadrenocorticoid states. These have been discussed elsewhere (3, 291, 292). More recently hypernatremia has been reported in association with renal transplantation (299). Generally, diabetes insipidus is associated with hypernatremia only under circumstances where the patient is unable to freely obtain water or when the lesion responsible for the diabetes insipidus results in a decrease of thirst. There may also be a whole new class of hypernatremic patients who have not been previously diagnosed. Excessive administration of hypertonic solutions of $NaHCO_3$ to critically ill patients suffering cardiac arrest was associated with a dangerously elevated plasma osmolality (377 ± 7 mosm/kg) in 12 patients, none of whom survived (287). Similarly, administration of large quantities of $NaHCO_3$ to newborn infants has been associated with hypernatremia and intracranial hemorrhage, with a mortality of 71 percent (288). Severe hypernatremia has also been observed in patients inadvertently receiving intravenous hypertonic NaCl for therapeutic abortion (289), and may also occur in patients with lactic acidosis who receive large quantities of intravenous $NaHCO_3$ (174).

Neurological symptoms are among the more prominent manifestations of hypernatremia in patients at both extremes of age, and they frequently alert the physician to the possible existence of a hypernatremic state. In children the majority of cases of hypernatremia are associated with readily reversible underlying systemic illnesses, and it appears that neurological damage is the primary cause of mortality and morbidity (300–304). In adults, by contrast, hypernatremia is frequently associated with a grave underlying systemic disorder. It is thus less easy to attribute mortality and morbidity to the hypernatremia per se, although neurological manifestations are nearly always present (3, 305). In addition to the variations in the neurological manifestations of hypernatremia which may be seen with age, the eventual mortality and morbidity also seem to vary with the rapidity with which the hypernatremic state is attained.

Symptoms of hypernatremia

In children, the mortality of acute hypernatremia (plasma Na^+ above 160 meq/L for less than 24 h) exceeds 40 percent, and it is above 10 percent when the hypernatremia develops over a period of several days (Fig. 26-25). Most children who present with chronic (more than 48 h) hypernatremia have had gastroenteritis with diarrhea (302, 303). It appears that these children became gradually dehydrated over a number of days (302). A second large group of children have had infections which have resulted in fever with tachypnea (294, 301). Other causes of hypernatremia in the pediatric age group are far less common (23). Hypernatremic children often manifest a characteristic clinical picture which has been described elsewhere (294, 306). About 67 percent of such patients have symptoms referable to the central nervous system. Most have marked irritability and they often emit a high-pitched cry. Depression of sensorium is characteristically present, and this varies from moderate lethargy to frank coma. Normal muscle tone is the rule, but many patients have varying degrees of increased muscle tone, and some develop frank seizure activity (294, 302) Meningeal signs are not usually present on admission. The most frequent abnormality found on lumbar puncture is an elevated CSF protein concentration, without pleocytosis (307). Although most of these patients are not diabetic, many are hyperglycemic and may also have hyperkalemia, metabolic acidosis, and hypocalcemia (302, 307, 308). Seizures are not commonly observed in patients with chronic hypernatremia, but after therapy is begun, up to 40 percent may exhibit seizure activity (300). A similar sequence is observed in hypernatremic rabbits whose serum Na^+ is rapidly lowered to normal with intravenous 140 mM (2.5%) glucose in water (309).

Both morbidity and mortality of children with chronic hypernatremia are substantial. The mortality in different series is between 10 percent and 71 percent (Fig. 26-25), and morbidity is very high. Among 100 patients studied by Macaulay and Watson (304), 8 sustained brain damage: 1 had tetraplegia and 7 were either retarded, hyperkinetic, or clumsy. Among 32 hypernatremic patients who were successfully treated and then followed for up to 8 years, 1 was monoplegic, 2 had seizure disorders, and 8 had abnormal EEG findings (300).

In infants with acute hypernatremia, the most commonly observed symptoms are emesis, fever, and labored respiration. Spasticity may be observed, grand mal seizures occur in almost all patients, and coma is frequent (303). Neurologic abnormalities, such as hemiparesis and Babinski sign, are common. Both morbidity and mortality are imposing. In the Binghamton, New York, salt-poisoning episode, 14 infants in a hospital nursery were accidentally given formula containing 739 to 1170 meq of NaCl per liter (297). Of the 14, 11 had symptoms which included muscular twitching or frank convulsions, vomiting, and respiratory distress. The mean serum Na^+ in the 14 patients was 199 meq/L. These acutely hypernatremic infants displayed signs of avid thirst until they were quite ill. Fever was common in older infants, although not in neonates. Mortality rate was formidable (43 percent) (Fig. 26-25), although 1 infant with a peak serum Na^+ of 274 meq/L survived with treatment. Among 7 other

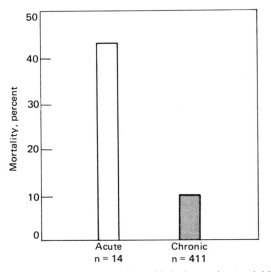

Figure 26-25. Comparison of the published mortality in children who became hypernatremic (serum Na^+ above 100 meq/L) over a few hours, and that of children who became hypernatremic over several days. (*From Covey and Arieff.*)

children with dehydration and hypernatremia, all survived, but 6 of the 7 had severe brain damage (310).

Acute hypernatremia is less common than chronic hypernatremia in adults and is generally a result of acute solute loading when it does occur. It has been reported with the accidental introduction of hypertonic NaCl into maternal circulation during therapeutic abortion (289) and with the use of NaCl as an emetic (291). Particularly fulminant symptoms have occurred with malfunction of either hemodialysis or peritoneal dialysis proportioning systems (140, 144). Hot climate has caused an acute rise in serum Na^+ over a few hours (311). Acute hypernatremia can occur in patients with heatstroke (312), in those who drown in sea water (which has a Na^+ content of 450 to 500 meq/L), and has also been described in at least one retarded adult who ingested massive quantities of table salt (313). Acute hypernatremia is probably not uncommon among patients who are resuscitated following cardiac arrest after having been given large amounts of intravenous $NaHCO_3$ (287).

Hypernatremia in adults usually occurs as a chronic process where the symptoms are obscured by those of other concomitant diseases which are often of a catastrophic nature (292, 305, 314). Because of these associated medical conditions, the presenting symptoms are usually not attributable to hypernatremia per se. The sensation of thirst, often intense, may not be verbalized because affected patients frequently have depression of sensorium. The physical signs commonly associated with dehydration, such as altered skin turgor and sunken eye sockets, may not be apparent because of the usual effects of aging (187). Lethargy, stupor, or coma may be present to varying degrees. Muscle irritability and convulsions have been reported (307, 315) but are unusual, and it may be difficult to separate effects of hyperosmolality from the effects of therapy.

SYMPTOMS OF HYPEROSMOLALITY: ANIMALS

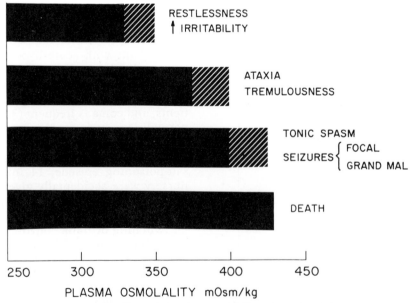

Figure 26-26. Effects of acute hyperosmolality on symptomatology in experimental animals. Crosshatched areas represent the range of plasma osmolality for each group of manifestations. (*From Arieff, Guisado, and Lazarowitz.*)

Symptoms similar to those observed in patients have been produced in experimental animals with acute hypernatremia. In rabbits infused with 1000 mM NaCl, severe central nervous system symptoms began to appear when plasma osmolality had reached 350 mosm/kg. Initially the animals became alternately restless and lethargic, and they then went on to develop nystagmus and ataxia, muscular twitching and trembling. Stupor ensued. Many died of respiratory failure, usually at a plasma osmolality of about 430 mosm/kg (26, 27) (Fig. 26-26). A similar picture has been observed in kittens made hypernatremic by intraperitoneal injection of hypertonic NaCl (18) and in animals with hyperosmolar states achieved by infusion of similar osmotic loads of sucrose or mannitol (27).

Hypernatremia: electroencephalographic changes

In experimental animals, hyperosmolality results in a progressive slowing of background EEG frequencies, but no spikes or paroxysmal discharges are seen even in the presence of paroxysmal jerking of the body (26, 27). These changes suggest alterations at different levels of the nervous system, and probably of spinal cord or peripheral nerve trunks as well since the paroxysmal jerks and tonic contractures do not disappear after spinal cord or sciatic nerve section (26).

Other EEG abnormalities are observed at the time symptoms of hyperosmolality become manifest. There is a generalized reduction in voltage, disappearance of fast activity, and the appearance of bursts of 4 to 5 per second spindlelike activity. There is gradual progression to 1 to 3 per second high-voltage waves, with cessation of EEG activity at the time of respiratory arrest (27). The EEG changes appear to be reversible with correction of plasma osmolality to normal (27).

Electroencephalograms obtained in patients with hypernatremia have generally been normal. However, the EEGs of 10 of 52 hypernatremic children studied by Bruck (302) showed a decrease in amplitude similar to that observed in experimental animals, with generalized slowing of the background rhythm. All but 2 had returned to normal with 2 to 40 days after treatment. The

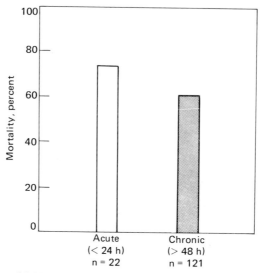

Figure 26-27. Comparison of published mortality of acute and chronic hypernatremia for adults. When one considers that adults with hypernatremia resulting from such grave conditions as stroke with dehydration, lactic acidosis, resuscitation from cardiac arrest, and hyperglycemic nonketotic coma comprise the bulk of published cases, it is not surprising that eventual mortality is formidable. (*From Covey and Arieff.*)

2 persistently abnormal EEGs showed typical seizure discharges.

Hypernatremia: mortality

The mortality of chronic hypernatremia in children ranges from 7 percent to 29 percent and is summarized in Fig. 26-25.

Mortality in children with acute hypernatremia averages 43 percent, and about two-thirds of survivors have neurological sequelae (3) (Fig. 26-25). Because of associated medical conditions which in themselves carry grave prognoses, it is much more difficult to assess the mortality and morbidity of chronic hypernatremia in adults. Figure 26-27 summarizes the experience in the literature for adults with sustained (over 48 h) hypernatremia (serum Na$^+$ above 160 meq/L). When one recalls that included in this table are such serious underlying conditions as resuscitation from cardiac arrest (289), nonketotic hyperosmolar coma (314) and acute stroke with dehydration (292), it is not surprising that it is associated with a 60 percent mortality. However, from the experience in children, who generally are without chronic underlying disease, it is highly probable that hypernatremia per se adds considerably to the mortality and morbidity of the underlying condition.

Hypernatremia: anatomic changes in the brain

In acute hypernatremia, as fluid from the intracellular space moves into the extracellular compartment to establish osmotic equilibrium, the cells initially lose volume (105). In the brain, this loss of volume may put mechanical traction on delicate cerebral vessels to produce vascular damage (18).

Autopsies performed on children who died from acute salt poisoning have provided much of our information about the anatomical lesions produced in humans by acute hypernatremia (303). In these children, there is evidence of widespread cerebral vascular damage. Capillaries and veins are markedly congested, with subcortical parenchymous hemorrhage and subarachnoid bleeding. Venous thromboses, sometimes leading to infarction, and occlusion of major venous sinuses have been observed. Although cerebral edema has been noted in some patients, it is more likely the result of overly rapid rehydration therapy rather than the hypernatremia per se.

The anatomical brain damage produced by acute hyperosmolality has also been studied in experimental animals. Shrunken, grossly dehydrated brains, engorged vessels, and petechial hemorrhages were observed in rabbits made hyperosmolar (mean plasma osmolality of 396 mosm/kg) by the infusion of 1000 mM NaCl, with a 76 percent mortality. Similar findings were observed in kittens made hypernatremic by intraperitoneal injection of hypertonic saline and sodium bicarbonate. At necropsy 85 percent of the animals had subdural hemorrhage with xanthrochromia of the CSF, and 7 percent had subdural hematoma (18).

Similar findings of hemorrhage and congested cerebral vessels have been observed in children dying of chronic hypernatremia (304). In chronically hypernatremic animals, dehydration and

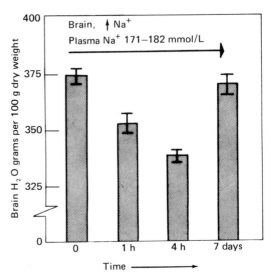

Figure 26-28. Effects of sustained hypernatremia (↑Na) on brain water content in rabbits. With plasma Na⁺ maintained at 171 to 182 mM for 1 to 4 h, there is a significant loss of brain water. However, when plasma Na⁺ is maintained above 171 mM for 1 week, brain water content returns to normal values. (*From Arieff, Guisado, an Lazarowitz.*)

vascular congestion are present (279), although hemorrhagic changes are usually not seen (105).

Effects of hypernatremia on brain water and electrolytes

The effects of acute and chronic hypernatremia on brain water and electrolytes in experimental animals is summarized in Figs. 26-28 and 26-29, which show results obtained by several different investigators working with different animal species. In animals with acute hypernatremia (mean serum Na⁺ of 178 meq/L) of less than 3 h duration there is an abrupt decrease in brain water (Fig. 26-28) and a rise in intracellular Na⁺ and Cl⁻ concentration (Fig. 26-29). Potassium content increases minimally (105). Acutely, the increase in measured intracellular osmolality of the brain can be essentially all accounted for by the observed increases in measured brain electrolyte (Na⁺, K⁺, Cl⁻) concentration (Fig. 26-29).

After several days of sustained hypernatremia, however, brain water content is almost normal (105). In rabbits who have been hypernatremic

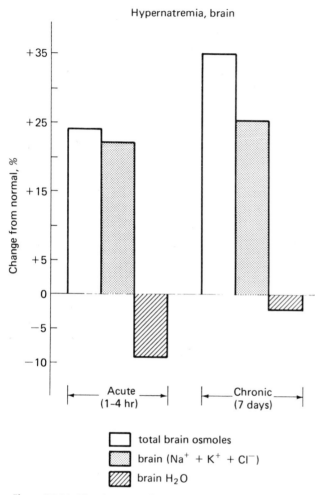

Hypernatremia, brain

total brain osmoles

brain (Na$^+$ + K$^+$ + Cl$^-$)

brain H$_2$O

Figure 26-29. The changes in brain osmol content (mosm/kg dry weight), brain content of Na$^+$ + K$^+$ + Cl$^-$ (mmol/kg dry weight), and brain water content (g H$_2$O per 100 g dry weight) in animals with experimental hypernatremia. Brain osmolality has been estimated by assuming osmolality of plasma and brain to be equal in a steady state. In animals with acute hypernatremia (1 to 4 h), brain osmolality increases due both to a loss in water and gain in solute. Brain water content is 9 percent below control values. Brain osmol content is increased by 24 percent above normal values, with virtually all of the increase accounted for by increases in Na$^+$, K$^+$ and Cl$^-$. In chronically hypernatremic animals, brain osmolality is also elevated, but most of the increase is due to a gain in brain solute. Brain water content is similar to normal values. Brain osmol content is 35 percent above control levels, but most of the increase is not accounted for by changes in brain content of Na$^+$, K$^+$, Cl$^-$, but is due to undetermined solute (idiogenic osmols). (*From Arieff and Guisado.*)

(mean serum Na$^+$ of 173 meq/L) for seven days, brain water content is normal, in spite of the fact that in these same animals there is still a marked loss of intracellular water in muscle tissue (105). Total brain Na$^+$ and Cl$^-$ remain elevated, but the increase in measured electrolytes (Na$^+$, K$^+$, Cl$^-$) is not sufficient to account for all of the measured increase in brain osmolality (Fig. 26-29). In other words, there is the appearance of unmeasured solute which accounts for about 60 percent of the increase in brain intracellular osmolality in chronically (1 week) hypernatremic animals. The solute ("idiogenic osmols") begins to appear after several hours of hypernatremia and is as yet uncharacterized. In several different laboratories (105, 279, 316) a rise in intracellular amino acids (glutamine, alanine, aspartate, glutamate) has been observed in the brains of chronically hypernatremic animals and appears to contribute at least in part to the rise in brain osmolality (Fig. 26-30). Similar findings have been reported in

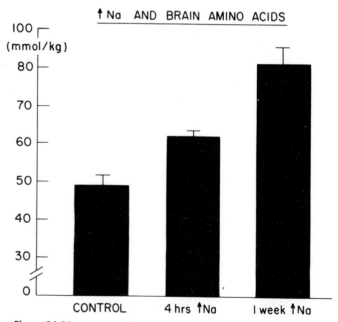

Figure 26-30. Amino acid levels in brain of rabbits who had hypernatremia (↑Na) for either 4 h or 1 week. There is a significant increase in brain amino acid concentration after 4 h of hypernatremia. After 1 week of hypernatremia, with an increase in brain osmolality of 80 mosm/kg H$_2$O, brain amino acids have increased by 33 mosm/kg. (*From Arieff, Guisado, and Lazarowitz.*)

hypernatremic brain studied in vitro (317). Other possible mechanisms might include the disassociation of intracellular protein-salt complexes, the action of hydrolytic enzymes in lysozymes activated by hyperosmolality, or some changes in intracellular metabolism leading to accumulation in brain of other small-molecular-weight substances (150, 307). Thus, it appears that the brain may have adaptive mechanisms not found in other body tissues (318) which serve to defend cellular volume. By the generation of idiogenic osmols the brain is able to achieve osmotic equilibrium with plasma by internal adaptive mechanisms which serve to minimize the loss of brain water.

In a teleologic sense, it would appear advantageous to maintain a normal cerebral cellular volume in the face of changes in plasma osmolality. Abrupt shrinkage of the brain could lead to tearing of cerebral vessels and meninges, with subsequent subdural hemorrhage, as has been described in patients and animals with acute hypernatremia (307). Thus, from a clinical standpoint, the ability of the brain to generate idiogenic osmols to maintain cellular volume intact is beneficial to survival. In this sense, it is of interest that the brains of some vertebrates who live parts of their lives in both saltwater and freshwater environments appear to have the ability to adapt to the changing osmotic environment by altering intracellular amino acid content (12).

Hypernatremia: therapy

Hypernatremia is associated with a significant mortality, in both infants and elderly individuals (Figs. 26-25 and 26-27). The problem is of considerable magnitude in both age groups. In studies from several different medical centers, the reported incidence of severe hypernatremia exceeds one patient per hospital per month in elderly individuals (23), with a slightly higher incidence in children (3, 23). Despite the magnitude of the problem, there is little hard data available on the quantitative aspects of therapy of severe hypernatremia. It has been shown in patients and experimental animals that hyperosmolality per se is potentially lethal (Figs. 26-25, 26-26, and 26-27). However, overly rapid treatment of hypernatremia

by infusion of hypotonic solutions can cause seizures and cerebral edema, which may also be lethal (144, 287, 289, 309, 320).

Most investigators agree that patients with hypernatremic dehydration should be treated with fluid which provides free water in excess of electrolytes. In both children and adults, fluid therapy is usually calculated so as to be administered over a period of about 48 h (291, 294). Despite such recommendations, little data in humans or animals is available as to the ideal rate of fluid administration. Fatal cases of cerebral edema, as well as permanent brain damage, have occurred when hypernatremia was completely corrected within 24 h (144, 300, 302), while seizures with cerebral edema occur in more than 50 percent of hypernatremic rabbits when plasma Na^+ is reduced from 185 to 142 mmol/L in 4 h (309). The aforementioned studies highlight the dangers of overly rapid correction of hypernatremia. However, they also point out the fact that there is really no data which has demonstrated how fast one can safely lower plasma Na^+ in hypernatremic states. Currently accepted therapeutic regimens for treating hypernatremia in adults or children have recently been reviewed (3, 291, 294).

NEUROLOGIC FACTORS IN SALT AND WATER BALANCE

INTEGRATION OF COMPLEX PERIPHERAL AFFERENTS

The mechanisms which allow precise regulation of extracellular fluid volume and its electrolyte composition have long been regarded as the domain of the renal physiologist and clinical nephrologist. Knowledge of the regulation of excretory fluid composition has formed a primary base for the understanding of how salt and water balance are normally regulated. Less well understood are the CNS mechanisms which monitor the complex of peripheral afferent signals involving volume, pressure, and osmolality, integrate them with the input of central afferents such as osmolality, memory, and psychosocial factors, and then effect directed behavioral patterns to allow acquisition of appropriate amounts of salt and water. We do not wholly understand why craving for salt occurs or what constitutes thirst. We do, however, understand that the perception or misperception of these complex sensations can affect behavioral patterns of eating and drinking such that renal regulation of salt and water balance can then act.

EFFECTING OF DIRECTED OR PERCEPTION-BASED BEHAVIORAL PATTERNS

Water perception (See also Chap. 12)

Primary drinking. Thirst is a complex, subjective sensation. It is derived from the combined input of pharyngeal and hypothalamic osmoreceptors and intravascular volume receptors of the heart, lung, and major blood vessels. Because of difficulty in characterizing thirst, it is usual to describe thirst in terms of the patterns of stimuli which result in water drinking. Both primary and secondary forms of water drinking have been recognized and characterized (Table 26-1). Primary water drinking results from decreases in total body water or from shifts in body water from intracellular to extracellular sites. A rise in extracellular fluid osmolality, either as the result of the

Table 26-1. Mechanisms of thirst

I. CAUSES OF PRIMARY WATER DRINKING
A. Cellular dehydration
1. Water deprivation
2. Extracellular hyperosmolality
3. Potassium depletion
B. Extracellular fluid volume depletion
1. Shock
2. Hemorrhage
3. Diarrhea (e.g., cholera)
4. Extracellular fluid sequestration (e.g., ascites, congestive heart failure, nephrotic syndrome)

II. CAUSES OF SECONDARY WATER DRINKING
A. Circadian rhythms
B. Oropharyngeal osmoreceptors
C. Stress, anticipation
D. Hyperthermia
E. Circulating catecholamines
F. Angiotensin II

loss of water from the body (dehydration) or as the result of an increased amount of solute added to extracellular fluid (hyperosmolality) causes a shift in balance of intracellular and extracellular water and results in cellular dehydration. Osmoreceptors, localized at least in part in the paraventricular nuclei of the diencephalon, appear capable of responding to cellular dehydration and effecting both the sensation of thirst and the action of drinking. Injection of very small amounts of hypertonic NaCl into the third ventricle of the brain will also effect an immediate and vigorous drinking response (293, 322). Similarly, injection of hypertonic NaCl into the carotid artery, a stimulus previously used to test the capacity of the brain to release vasopressin, causes an immediate sensation of thirst and will induce water drinking (293, 323, 324).

Primary water drinking may also occur as a result of a decrease in extracellular fluid volume without any apparent change in extracellular or intracellular osmolality. Thus, under conditions of acute hemorrhage, severe diarrhea, or isotonic dehydration, thirst will occur and drinking results. Because vascular stretch receptors localized in the aortic arch, carotid sinus, left atrium, and pulmonary veins appear to be primarily responsible for the monitoring of "effective" extracellular fluid volume (324, 325), it is also typical to see thirst and primary water drinking in patients who have cardiogenic shock, nephrotic syndrome, or severe ascites, conditions in which total extracellular volume is markedly increased, yet effective intravascular volume is diminished (324, 325).

Secondary drinking. In contrast to primary water drinking, where the action occurs in response to a loss of water, secondary water drinking is regarded as a form of anticipatory behavior. In secondary water drinking, no direct and immediate need for water exists, and the drinking is rather in anticipation of future water needs. Perception of such needs, by its very nature, is complex and interdependent upon activity patterns, dietary patterns, social behavior, and mood. The mechanisms involved are largely unknown but appear to involve circadian rhythms, oropharyngeal stimuli, visual stimuli, and learned behavioral patterns (293). They appear to intertwine

considerably with stimuli producing feeding behavior, and are largely geared to produce an excessive water intake, relying upon the kidney to
subsequently correct the excess. Such drinking
behavior can be readily observed in patients who
have ingested a hypertonic glucose solution or a
dry meal—long before any change in plasma volume or osmolality can be perceived. Extremes of
secondary water drinking may also be seen in patients who manifest psychogenic water drinking
or in "normal" subjects accumulating the increased fluid intake common to social gatherings.
The neural control mechanisms by which secondary drinking is controlled have not yet been
fully elucidated. Spontaneous drinking may be
partially controlled by neural elements in the
zona incerta, which is a rostral extension of the
midbrain reticular system and is located just dorsal to the lateral hypothalamus. Small lesions restricted to the zona incerta in rats have been
shown to reduce total daily intake of water by 20
to 50 percent. However, these rats did drink both
in the absence of food and following periods of
water deprivation, and their water intake in response to osmotic stress was also normal
(326–328). Thus, the only consistent change in
drinking patterns observed after the zona incerta
lesions was a reduction in the amount of water
consumed in excess of needs (326).

Early experiments investigating the neural control of water intake have suggested the presence
of an osmosensitive region in the diencephalon.
Damage to the lateral preoptic area in the dog
abolished spontaneous drinking in response to
hypertonic NaCl infusion without affecting increased water intake in response to dehydration.
Permanent alteration of thirst mechanisms can be
produced by symmetrical lesions which either involve the most lateral part of the lateral hypothalamus or invade the internal capsule and optic
tracts, the subthalamus, and the base of the brain,
but do not involve the fornix or the anterior hypothalamus. When animals in whom such lesions
have been induced are allowed to recover, they do
not increase their water intake in response to
either water deprivation, intravenous injection of
hypertonic NaCl, or hyperthermia. Additionally,
they do not reduce their water intake when over-

hydrated, and they fail to drink after intravenous
administration of hyperoncotic colloid. Lesions of
the lateral hypothalamus may also affect thirst
mechanisms by interruption of fiber tracts that
pass through the hypothalamus. Bilateral lesions
which are anterior or posterior to the hypothalamus may produce the same syndromes as do lateral hypothalamic lesions (329). Histologic studies of lateral hypothalamic lesions suggest that
the medial forebrain bundle may be as important
as the lateral hypothalamus proper in the control
of food and water intake. The medial forebrain
bundle is a major projection system that traverses
the entire lateral hypothalamic area and carries
fibers from the septal and hippocampal areas to
the limbic midbrain area, periaqueductal gray
matter, and the reticular formation of the tegmentum. Cholinergic stimulation of these areas
(septum, hippocampal amygdala, limbic midbrain
tegmentum) can also induce drinking (329).

Whether water perception is based upon primary or secondary stimuli, other factors may affect that perception. Catecholamines, renin, angiotensin, and prostaglandins have all been noted
to affect drinking behavior under experimental
conditions. Both atropine and isoproterenol can
stimulate water drinking. Thirst may be a prominent symptom in patients with hyperreninemic
hypertension, and it may be relieved by nephrectomy (330). A role for the kidney in extracellular
regulation of thirst has also been proposed, since
maneuvers such as vena cava ligation are less effective as a stimulus for drinking in the nephrectomized than in the intact animal (329). Further
support for this postulate relates to the observation that parenteral administration of extracts
from renal cortex can increase drinking in nephrectomized rats (331). This renal dipsogenic extract is similar to renin (329).

**Hormonal effects: renin-angiotensin and renal
"dipsogenic extract."** Renin secretion and plasma
angiotensin levels are increased in most forms of
primary water drinking, and it is probable that angiotensin II is important in causing thirst. Intravascular infusion of renin or angiotensin II can
elicit drinking (332). Certain areas of the brain
such as the subfornical organ (333) and the organum vasculosum of the lamina terminalis in

the third ventricle (334, 335) are extremely sensitive to angiotensin. Stimulation of these areas will result in drinking. Ablation of angiotensin activity or blockage of angiotensin effect with saralasin (a competitive inhibitor of angiotensin II) will inhibit the dipsogenic effect of angiotensin (335, 336). A renal "dipsogenic extract" (337), renin, is capable of stimulating drinking, and this effect can be blocked by saralasin, suggesting that the effect is mediated by angiotensin. Intravenous infusion of catecholamines can stimulate renin release into the circulation. The renin leads to increased production of angiotensin II, which may be in part responsible for the thirst associated with increased adrenergic activity.

Of considerable recent interest with respect to the normal role of renin and of angiotensin in dipsogenic behavior is the discovery that intracranial injection of renin evokes a drinking response in experimental animals (338) and that a separate renin-angiotensin system exists within the brain (339, 340). The physiologic role of this system is unknown at present, but an important regulatory role seems possible. A close interaction between angiotensin II and dopamine in the stimulation of drinking has been described (335, 341). Blockage of dopamine-mediated drinking by haloperidol also blocks the dipsogenic effects of angiotensin II. The dipsogenic effects of angiotensin can be enhanced by increasing brain dopamine levels by blocking dopamine β-hydroxylase with ALA-31 (341) providing further evidence of angiotensin-catecholamine interaction in brain. An apparently separate central cholinergic dipsogenic system also exists. Acetylcholine can stimulate drinking by an effect which is blocked by atropine and appears to be largely separate from the angiotensin-catecholamine dipsogenic effect (335, 341).

To further complicate the system, recent evidence also implicates the prostaglandins in the regulation of thirst. Prostaglandin E_1, when injected intracranially, may cause thirst (342). This observation may correlate with recent studies of Berl et al. (343), who reported that in severe hypokalemia, polydipsia appears to be independent of the effects of hypokalemia upon urine-concentrating ability (343). Moreover, it has also been demonstrated that hypokalmeia causes a marked increase in circulating prostaglandin E_1 levels (344). The observations will require confirmation, but they suggest a potentially important role for prostaglandins in the regulation of thirst.

Clinical disorders of thirst. Disorders which involve thirst as an appropriate symptom should be clearly differentiated from actual disorders of the thirst mechanism (Table 26-2). The severe polydipsia of diabetes insipidus is dramatic but entirely appropriate because loss of the perception of thirst would result in the patient developing severe consequences of uncontrolled polyuria, such as hyperosmolality and hypotension. In our experience, the patient with combined loss of thirst perception and vasopressin secretion is extremely difficult to control. The thirst associated with diabetes mellitus, with severe vomiting (e.g., in pyloric stenosis), with severe diarrhea (e.g., in cholera), with nephrogenic diabetes insipidus, or with cardiogenic shock are all examples of appropriate thirst. In all of these situations the thirst mechanism has been activated by either a redistribution of body water or by a reduction of body

Table 26-2. Clinical states of increased thirst

I. NORMAL THIRST MECHANISMS
A. Extracellular fluid volume depletion: isotonic dehydration, hemorrhage, cardiogenic shock, severe vomiting, diarrhea, diuretic therapy, diabetes insipidus, nephrogenic diabetes insipidus, diabetes mellitus
B. Intracellular fluid volume depletion: diabetes mellitus, hypernatremic dehydration, other hyperosmolar states, ? hypokalemia
C. Hyperpyrexic states

II. ABNORMAL THIRST MECHANISMS—HYPERDIPSIA
A. Hyperreninemic states—malignant hypertension
B. Oropharyngeal osmoreceptor blockade—nerve sectioning, abnormal salivary gland function (e.g., Sjogren's syndrome)
C. Psychogenic water drinking
D. Pharmacologic blockage—atropine, antihistamines

III. ABNORMAL THIRST MECHANISMS—HYPODIPSIA
A. Hypothalamic destruction—trauma, encephalitis, eosinophilic granuloma, histiocytosis, hydrocephalus, subarachnoid hemorrhage, cerebrovascular occlusions
B. Bilateral nephrectomy
C. Adrenergic blockage—propranolol, haloperidol
D. Angiotension blockage—saralasin

water and represents a normal action of the thirst mechanism in response to its normal stimuli.

Pathologic thirst can be defined as thirst which persists despite the existence of normal hydration or overhydration and is seen in a variety of clinical states. Pathologic thirst has been demonstrated in hyperreninemic states as well as in hypercalcemic and severe hypokalemic states. Metastatic tumor, cerebral inflammatory diseases, and cerebral trauma may also produce pathologic thirst—presumably because of stimulation of the activity of cerebral dipsogenic centers. Psychogenic water drinking is a dramatic example of pathologic polydipsia. In the typical patient, both water intake and urine volumes are large (above 6 L/day) but signs and symptoms of water intoxication are rare. The ingestion of such large volumes of water may result in temporary impairment of renal concentrating capacity, the latter brought about as the result of having to excrete large volumes of "free water" in order to maintain external water balance.

Pathologic hypodipsia has been observed in many clinical states which involve damage to the supraopticohypophyseal system or to the thirst centers themselves. Management of the patient with both diabetes insipidus and hypodipsia is extremely difficult and often unsuccessful. Patients presenting with primary hypodipsia alone are unusual but have been reported in association with slow-growing intracranial tumors such as craniopharyngiomas, gliomas, ectopic pinealomas, and with Hand-Schüller-Christian disease. Such patients usually present with a history of weakness, stupor, and weight loss, and often appear to be grossly dehydrated. In contrast to the patient with hypodipsia and diabetes insipidus who may have a similar clinical picture, the patient with isolated hypodipsia has a reduced urine output with an appropriately high urine osmolality. Caution must be exercised in making a diagnosis of primary hypodipsia. Because of the complexity of perception of thirst and the initiation of a drinking response, any cerebral trauma or pharmacologic depressant of cerebral function may mimic this disorder.

It is probable that many patients with so called "essential" hypernatremia (345) in fact have lesions of the supraopticohypophyseal system. Many patients with essential (cerebral) hypernatremia have been known to have osmoreceptor dysfunction secondary to cerebral damage (346) or trauma (347). In these patients, ADH elaboration is at least partially intact, the renin-aldosterone axis is normal, and the patients can produce a concentrated or dilute urine in response to appropriate stimuli (345–348).

Neurologic control of water conservation (see also Chap. 12). Equally important in considering the mechanisms of water perception to thirst, which might be regarded as a mechanism to cause water repletion, is the complex hypothalamic-renal mechanism responsible for water conservation. In the brain, clusters of specialized neurons primarily localized in the paraventricular and supraoptic nuclei of the anterior hypothalamus (349) are responsible for the synthesis of the decapeptide, vasopressin. A vasopressin analogue, vasotocin, exists in all living nonmammalian vertebrates including elasmobranchs and cyclostomes (350). In mammals the hormone is synthesized and packaged into specialized neurosecretory granules in which it appears to be associated with a specialized protein, neurophysin (351). The neurosecretory granules, once formed, move by axoplasmic streaming down the extended axons and are stored in bulbous terminations. The largest (and most easily damaged) tract is the supraopticohypophyseal tract which terminates in pars nervosa of the pituitary (Fig. 26-31). A second pathway of importance terminates in the zona externa of the median eminence of the hypothalamus and, because of its location, secretes into the hypophyseal portal venous system (352, 353). The importance of this location may be twofold: (1) there is some evidence to suggest that vasopressin or neurophysin may be important in modification of the rate of delivery or activity of anterior pituitary release factors such as corticotrophin (354–356), and (2) the location is important in the partial preservation of antidiuretic activity in patients developing a lesion of the supraopticohypophyseal tract (350). Lesions occurring below the median eminence result in retrograde degeneration of injured neurons, but the neurons terminating in the median eminence

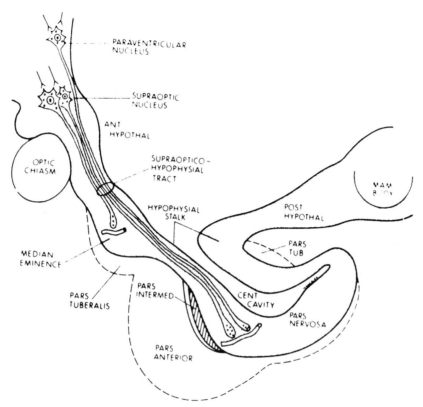

Figure 26-31. Schematic diagram of the neurosecretory tracts of the hypothalamus and pituitary (pars nervosa). (*From Hays.*)

persist and subsequently provide a partial vasopressin secretory capability. A third tract of axons appears to terminate on the surface of the third ventricle of the brain near the median eminence and organum vasculosum of the lamina terminates (357). These axons appear to secrete into the CSF (358). The importance and role of this tract is unclear, although it may have important effects on memory consolidation (359). The specialized ends of the axons terminate on the basement membrane of capillaries (Fig. 26-32). The stored neurosecretory granules are released as the result of depolarizing impulses which originate in the hypothalamic nuclei and are propagated down the axonal tracts to the neurosecretory terminals. The process of release is strongly Ca^{2+}-dependent and involves the extrusion of both vasopressin and neurophysin into the systemic circulation.

The fact that both an actapeptide and a protein carrier are released simultaneously (360) suggests that the process is one of exocytosis. The following steps appear necessary for the release of vasopressin (ADH): (1) propagation of impulses from the hypothalamic nuclei down the neurohypophyseal stalk to the axonal terminations in the pars nervosa of the pituitary body, (2) depolarization of the axonal end processes, (3) influx of Ca^{2+} in the axonal cytosol, (4) fusion of the granulocytic vesicle membrane with the axonal cell membrane, (5) extrusion of the neurophysin-vasopressin material and their dissociation, and (6) endocytosis of the vesicle membrane during or following cell repolarization.

Sachs and coworkers (361) have performed a series of experiments which have done much to enable us to understand the mechanisms which

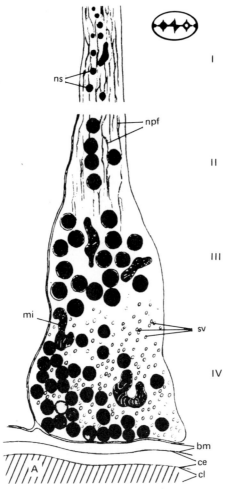

Figure 26-32. Diagram of the different regions (I-IV) of a neurosecretory axon demonstrating neurosecretory granules (ns) and empty synaptic vesicles (sv). Note the close anatomic relationship of the axon to the basement membrane (bm), capillary endothelium (ce), and capillary lumen (cl). Mitochondria (mi) and neuroprotofibrils (npf) are also noted. (*From H. M. Gershenfeld, et al., Endocrinology, 66:741, 1960.*)

determine how much ADH will be released in response to a given stimulus. These (362) and similar studies suggest that the vasopressin pool which is available for release is heterogenous. There is a ready release pool which comprises perhaps 10 to 20 percent of resting glandular vasopressin content. Once this pool is released,

the neurohypophysis may continue to release vasopressin from other storage sites, but only at a much reduced rate. Recovery and repletion of the ready release pool is a slow process.

Regulation of vasopressin release. A large number of physiologic and pharmacologic stimuli are capable of causing vasopressin release (Table 26-3). In terms of normal physiologic regulation of vasopressin release, however, such a list can be generally simplified into osmotic and volume stimuli. The concept that secretion of vasopressin is regulated under normal conditions by the osmolality of body water originated from the studies of Verney and associates (362). They showed that the release of an antidiuretic substance was controlled by intracranial osmoreceptors sensitive to changes in blood concentration of Na^+ and certain other solutes (362). Until very recently, largely due to an inability to measure accurately physiologic quantities of vasopressin in blood, little has been added to these original

Table 26-3. Factors stimulating or inhibiting vasopressin secretion

I. STIMULI

A. Primary factors
  1. Loss in osmoreceptor cell intracellular water due to systemic hyperosmolality
  2. Decreases in "effective" intravascular volume as perceived by
    a. Carotid sinus and aortic arch baroreceptors
    b. Left atrial and pulmonary venous capacitance
  3. Pain, severe emotional stress
B. Secondary factors
  1. Increased hypothalamic temperature
  2. Pharmacologic agents such as acetylcholine, carbachol, isoproterenol, nicotine, morphine, barbiturates, epinephrine, Mecholyl, prostaglandin E

II. INHIBITORS

A. Primary factors
  1. Osmoreceptive cell distention due to systemic hyposmolality
  2. Increased "effective" intravascular volume
    a. Increased peripheral vascular resistence
    b. Extracellular fluid volume expansion
B. Secondary factors
  1. Hypothermia
  2. Pharmacologic agents such as alcohol, diphenylhydantoin, atropine, norepinephrine

studies. Immunoassays capable of measuring arginine vasopressin directly in the low concentrations present in body fluids have now been reported (363–365), leading to increased understanding of osmoreceptor function. Robertson and colleagues (363) have clarified several important points relative to the relationship between changes in plasma osmolality and plasma arginine vasopressin levels. In normal subjects plasma vasopressin levels rise progressively and rapidly as plasma osmolality (P_{osm}) rises above 280 mosm/kg. An approximation of plasma vasopressin (366) levels can be made using the formula of Robertson et al.: PAVP = 0.38 ($P_{osm} = 280$) with PAVP expressed in pg/mL (366). Under normal circumstances an increase in plasma vasopressin levels to the range of 5 to 6 pg/mL is sufficient in normal hydropenic subjects to raise urinary osmolality to maximum levels. For urine osmolality (U_{osm}), the relationship $U_{osm} = 250$ (PAVP − 0.25) has been described and has a high degree of correlation over a wide range of urinary osmotic loads (363). Of importance is the recognition that the osmoreceptive mechanism is an extremely sensitive regulator of vasopressin secretion. A 1 percent change in plasma osmolality (about 3 mosm/kg) is sufficient to evoke detectable changes in plasma vasopressin levels and marked changes in U_{osm} (approximately 100 mosm/kg). The entire range of urine osmolalities achievable in man can be attained by change in PAVP from 0.5 to 5.0 pg/mL. This requires only a change in P_{osm} from 250 mosm/kg to 293 mosm/kg.

The relationship between plasma osmolality and vasopressin secretion is subject to modification by a variety of factors. Most important clinically is the observation that not all osmotically active substances are equally effective in evoking a response. In Table 26-3 the various stimuli and inhibitors of ADH secretion are summarized. Certain solutes, typically Na^+ salts and mannitol, appear potent in evoking a response from the osmoreceptive centers. Under normal conditions, Na^+ and its associated anions contribute over 95 percent of the osmotically active materials in plasma. Changes in the concentrations of these ions account for almost all the normal variations in plasma osmolality and osmoregulatory re-

sponses. Some normal plasma solutes such as urea and glucose do not exert much osmoregulatory effect. Hypertonic NaCl or mannitol injected or infused into the carotid artery evokes a rapid release of vasopressin (362), whereas hypertonic glucose may actually have the reverse effect (366). The explanation for such differences may be related to differences in the permeability of osmoreceptive cells to such solutes—passive permeability being low to Na^+ but high to urea. As a result, changes in plasma osmolality due to changes in plasma Na^+ could result in much greater changes in intracellular volume than could be expected for glucose or urea. The clinical importance of this observation is that it suggests that the polyuria of diabetes mellitus may be due not only to an osmotic diuresis but also to a fall in plasma vasopressin levels or a relative insensitivity of the osmoreceptive centers to other stimuli.

Blood pressure and/or blood volume appear to be major factors altering the normal relationship between plasma osmolality and vasopressin secretion. Reducing blood volume by 7 to 15 percent in humans alters the set point for vasopressin release to osmotic stimuli and may, by direct stimuli from baroreceptors in the aortic arch, left atrium, and pulmonary veins, result in a release of vasopressin even though plasma osmolality is unaltered. The mechanism appears rather insensitive, however, and is unlikely to serve much function in normal day-to-day variation of water excretion. Extracellular fluid volume expansion will also impede vasopressin secretion in response to osmotic stimuli (367). Beyond a certain level (about 10 percent volume depletion in man) (366, 368), marked alteration in the osmoreceptor sensitivity occurs. If the threshold for secretion is reduced to the level of the existing plasma osmolality, vasopressin release may occur without any change in osmolality. This undoubtedly accounts for the sudden increase in plasma vasopressin levels seen in hypovolemic states. Clinically such a distinction of priorities becomes important in understanding the logic of hemodilution and water retention in such states as congestive heart failure, nephrotic syndrome, ascites, or the hepatorenal syndrome.

A variety of pharmacologic agents will modify circulating plasma vasopressin levels, either by accentuating or by inhibiting secretion (Tables 26-3, 26-4). Several cholinergic (i.e., acetylcholine, bethanechol) and β-adrenergic agents (i.e., isoproterenol) are capable of stimulating ADH release while other agents, most importantly ethanol, norepinephrine, and diphenylhydantoin, cause an inhibition of release. Under normal circumstances vasopressin release varies in response to changes in plasma osmolality. In addition, however, a whole spectrum of relationships may exist which are the result of many other factors, such as changes in extracellular volume, anxiety, changes in body temperature, pharmacologic agents, and corticosteroid and thyroid hormone levels.

PATHOLOGIC SYNDROMES RESULTANT FROM A FAILURE OF WATER PERCEPTION (See also Chap. 12)

Diabetes insipidus

Diabetes insipidus is a clinical syndrome which develops as a result of failure of the hypothalamic neurosecretory cells to produce or release vasopressin in sufficient quantities to permit normal water homeostasis. In contrast to other syndromes which mimic diabetes insipidus, such as nephrogenic diabetes insipidus, vasopressin secretion is insufficient to maintain normal water conservation. Only under conditions of marked plasma hypoosmolality and profound water diuresis are plasma vasopressin levels in patients with diabetes insipidus comparable to levels in normal subjects.

The clinical syndrome of central diabetes insipidus has been well characterized experimentally. For a complete and persistent state of diabetes insipidus to be produced in experimental animals, the lesion must encompass not only the neurohypophysis and pituitary stalk but also the supraoptic nuclei, so that the axons which terminate in the median eminence are also destroyed. If the lesion fails to involve the median eminence and/or supraoptic nuclei, then the experimental animal will characteristically experience an initial complete loss of neurohypophyseal function. This will be followed sometime thereafter by partial recovery and the persistence of a very mild form of diabetes insipidus. The outstanding characteristic of the syndrome is the abrupt onset of polyuria (10 to 20 L/day) with the simultaneous onset of polydipsia (unless the patient is comatose or has simultaneously sustained damage to the thirst centers). The urine is invariably hypotonic (specific gravity usually less than 1.005 and urinary osmolality below 200 mosm/kg) and remains hypotonic despite severe systemic hyperosmolality. Only with severe dehydration, when

Table 26-4. Clinical conditions of increased vasopressin activity

I. APPROPRIATE CAUSES OF INCREASED SECRETION

A. Hyperosmolality—dehydration, hypernatremia, nephrogenic diabetes insipidus

B. Functional hypovolemia—"effective" intravascular volume depletion, shock, hemorrhage, constrictive pericarditis, pulmonary embolism, dehydration, congestive heart failure, cirrhosis with ascites, nephrotic syndrome, hepatorenal syndrome, chronic obstructive pulmonary disease, nephrogenic diabetes insipidus, postobstructive diuresis, Addison's disease

C. Fear, severe emotional stimuli

D. Iatrogenic causes—diuretics, restricted salt or water intake

II. INAPPROPRIATE CAUSES OF INCREASED VASOPRESSIN SECRETION

A. Tumors—bronchogenic carcinoma (oat-cell type), adenocarcinoma of pancreas, adenocarcinoma of duodenum, Hodgkin's disease, lymphosarcoma, lymphoma thymoma, ? primary neural tumors

B. Pulmonary infections (may in part involve I.B. above)—tuberculosis, pneumococcal pneumonia, pulmonary aspergillosis, pulmonary abscesses, viral pneumonitis

C. Neurologic injury—brain tumors, subdural hematomas, concussions, skull fractures, viral encephalitides, tuberculous and other infectious meningitides, cerebral vascular thrombosis, paroxysmal seizure disorders, Guillain-Barré syndrome, diffuse cerebral atrophy.

D. Iatrogenic causes—electroconvulsive therapy, vasopressin therapy, morphine meperidine, barbiturates, anesthetics, nicotine, ? cyclophosphamide, ? clofibrate, ? vincristine, carbechol

III. MISCELLANEOUS OR UNKNOWN CAUSES

Myxedema, systemic lupus erythematosis, acute intermittent porphyria, intermittent or continuous positive pressure ventilation (may be caused by I.B. above)

vascular collapse occurs and GFR declines dramatically, does urine osmolality approach plasma levels.

Pathophysiology. Both in humans and in experimental animals, the syndrome is characterized by a triphasic pattern of evolution following injury (369–372). Immediately following the inciting event, polyuria and polydipsia develop. Within hours, however, there is a second phase, which is characterized by increasing tonicity of the urine with falling urine volume. In many respects it appears that this is a normalization of function, but it is not. Water-loading tests performed during this phase paradoxically demonstrate an inability to dilute the urine and excrete the water load. In fact the water retention may be very abnormal and produce profound systemic hypoosmolality and symptoms of water intoxication. This phase is a period of increased ADH release into the circulation, which probably represents release of vasopressin from damaged and degenerating neurons. The phase may last for days before it subsides and is replaced by the third and most persistent phase—that phase characterized by continuous polyuria and polydipsia.

There may be a "fourth phase" to the syndrome; this often develops in patients who have only partial damage to the hypothalamic centers. In these patients gradual, but not complete, recovery of vasopressin secretory capacity may occur, often months after the original injury. The patient will then be left with partial diabetes insipidus. In some cases the ADH deficiency will be extremely mild and demonstrable only under very rigid conditions. Most patients who develop diabetes insipidus as the result of either trauma or surgery will recover some neurohypophysal function.

Etiology. Trauma is one of the most common causes of diabetes insipidus (350). Trauma may take the form of basal skull fractures or other forms of head trauma without evident fractures. Cryohypophysectomy, pituitary stalk sections, and yttrium implants have produced diabetes insipidus, as has Sheehan's syndrome.

About half of all cases of central diabetes insipidus are idiopathic. They may be congenital and/or familial in presentation (although such cases are rare) and have been variably described to be transmitted as an autosomal dominant trait with incomplete sex-dependent penetrance or as a sex-linked recessive. These cases appear at any age and are not associated with defects in anterior pituitary function. Subjects with this disorder have a marked decrease in the number of paraventricular and supraoptic neurons with increased gliosis in these areas, suggesting neuronal degeneration rather than a defect in synthesis or release of ADH (64). This contrasts with the hereditary form of diabetes insipidus observed in Brattleboro rats where the defect appears to be in the synthesis and release of vasopressin and neurophysin (352, 373). Much less common causes (Table 26-5) are (1) suprasellar and intrasellar tumors of primary or metastatic origin, especially breast carcinoma, (2) encephalitis and meningitis, (3) histiocytosis such as eosinophilic granuloma or Schüller-Christian syndrome, (4) sarcoidosis, (5) tuberculosis, and (6) vascular lesions such as aneurysms and atheroembolic disease.

Table 26-5 Etiology of the SIADH syndrome

I. NEUROHYPOPHYSEAL VASOPRESSIN PRODUCTION
A. Brain tumor
B. Encephalitis
C. Meningitis
D. Subdural hematoma
E. Subarachnoid hemorrhage
F. Brain abscess
G. Concussions, convulsions
H. Guillain-Barré syndrome
I. Acute intermittent porphyria
J. Electroconvulsive therapy

II. ECTOPIC VASOPRESSIN PRODUCTION
A. Bronchogenic carcinomas
B. Hodgkin's disease
C. Lymphoma, thymoma
D. Pancreatic adenocarcinoma
E. Other adenocarcinomas
F. Tuberculosis

III. OCCULT VASOPRESSIN RELEASE
A. Pneumococcal pneumonia
B. Chronic obstructive pulmonary disease (COPD)
C. Aspirgillosis, lung abscess
D. Viral pneumonia

Of the usual causes of diabetes insipidus, tumors deserve comment because of several specific and unusual features. Anterior pituitary adenomas rarely, if ever, produce diabetes insipidus, despite their capacity to displace the posterior pituitary lobe entirely. To produce diabetes insipidus, tumors must displace the posterior lobe and also must involve the median eminence and/or neurohypophysal nuclei. Examples of tumors which may do this are the craniopharyngiomas, pinealomas, and suprasellar cysts (374). Metastatic tumors may also produce diabetes insipidus; the most common of such metastatic tumors is carcinoma of the breast. Such tumors invariably produce diabetes insipidus before they spread sufficiently to involve the adenohypophysis (375).

Clinical features. Occurrence of diabetes insipidus is equally distributed between the sexes, and the primary abnormality is the excretion of large volumes of hypotonic urine. The onset is so characteristically abrupt that if the patient described a slowly developing polyuria, other causes should be considered more likely. The degree of polyuria varies with the level of residual vasopressin secretion. Since normally 10 to 15 percent of glomerular filtrate reaches the collecting duct, this in effect sets the limits on urine volume, and normally one can anticipate maximum urine volumes of 15 to 20 L/day. Nocturia rather than polyuria is the usual patient complaint, and often the correct diagnosis is confused with other causes of nocturia such as congestive heart failure. Continuous thirst is a hallmark of the disease, and for unknown reasons, patients with diabetes insipidus have a marked preference for ice-cold water (376). The perception of thirst is an important and appropriate defense mechanism. Patients unable to perceive thirst and effect a drinking response (e.g., unconscious, postneurosurgical patients) are in grave danger of rapid, severe hypertonic dehydration. If the patient truly has diabetes insipidus, water deprivation, even as a diagnostic test, is dangerous and should be undertaken only under careful supervision and monitoring. The large water turnover eventually produces a severe functional hydronephrosis and hydroureter. Bladder capacity may be increased markedly. Such hydrodynamic changes are functional and not, of themselves, harmful.

Diagnosis. Until very recently, the inability to measure plasma vasopressin levels accurately has hampered the clinician in the effort to differentiate diabetes insipidus from other causes of polyuria. As a result, a profusion of tests involving dehydration, nicotine stimulation, cigarette smoking, and hypertonic NaCl infusion have been developed. Such tests generally seek to correlate urinary osmolality or specific gravity with stimuli known to evoke vasopressin release. The recent development of accurate immunoassays for arginine vasopressin and their commercial availability should simplify and increase the precision of diagnosis (363).

The absence of severe polyuria does not rule out the diagnosis of central diabetes insipidus. In patients with severe dehydration, shock, or congestive heart failure, both renal blood flow and single-nephron GFR may be severely reduced. Under such circumstances both fractional proximal tubular reabsorption and fractional distal tubular reabsorption of water may be increased—even in the absence of vasopressin. Urine volumes then may be very much reduced (approximately 3000 mL/day) and urine osmolality increased to the levels of plasma or even slightly greater.

The "reset osmostat." Resetting of the osmoresponsiveness of supraoptic and paraventicular nuclei cells, a "reset osmostat," has been proposed to account for some cases of sustained hypernatremia (348). Such patients have often been found to have normal renal concentrating and diluting capability, but they modulate vasopressin release at an increase plasma osmolality (345). Such a hypothesis is attractive, particularly since it has been demonstrated in laboratory models that osmoreceptor modulation of vasopressin release can continue at a different threshold of sensitivity when intravascular volume depletion has been produced. It appears to be more probable that such individuals actually have a partial diabetes insipidus; the sustained hypernatremia probably reflects a compromise state between the heightened stimuli needed for vasopressin release, and suppression of stimuli for thirst in order to reduce urine volumes to tolerable levels. Careful study of the vasopressin secretory capacity in response to standardized osmotic stimuli in such patients has not been performed to date. Until such studies are obtained, the "reset osmostat" phenomenon remains speculative as a clinical entity, at least with respect to hypernatremic states (366).

Treatment. The mainstay in therapy for cases of central diabetes insipidus is the administration of replacement amounts of vasopressin. The material is available both in an aqueous form for immediate intravenous infusion and in a more slowly absorbable form that can be injected intramuscularly for sustained, slow action. Both methods are effective, but the best long-term control is with the use of the latter form. This material, supplied as vasopressin tannate (5 units/mL) in peanut oil, can be administered once a day with good results.

Once the diagnosis of diabetes insipidus has been established and therapy initiated, the physician often assumes that the condition is stable and requirements for exogenous vasopressin will be persistent. This is often not the case. With time, the patient with severe diabetes insipidus may recover, sometimes to the point where the abnormality is undetectable. Periodic reevaluation is essential to prevent water overload in these patients. Moreover, partial recovery of vasopressin secretory capacity may permit use of other agents, such as oral chlorpropamide or nasal sprays of synthetic vasopressin analogues, both of which can potentiate endogenous vasopressin activity and may thus allow stoppage of intramuscular injections.

Several oral agents have been employed in the control of polyuria. With the exception of the sulfonyl ureas such as chlorpropamide, these agents are either ineffective and/or dangerous in patients with diabetes insipidus. Thiazide diuretics have been used with modest success in nephrogenic diabetes insipidus. They act by causing a NaCl diuresis, extracellular fluid volume contraction, and, as a result, a decrease in distal tubular delivery of fluid to be excreted. While this therapy can be used in central diabetes insipidus, it does leave the patient mildly dehydrated in order to achieve a reduction in urine volume. Acetaminophen, clofibrate, and indomethacin all have been reported to have an antidiuretic effect in patients with diabetes insipidus. None of these agents, however, have been satisfactorily demonstrated to augment control of diabetes insipidus. Their use should be discouraged since most potent agents are generally available.

Sulfonylurea compounds such as chlorpropamide and tolbutamide were accidentally discovered to have antidiuretic effects (377). Subsequently it has been demonstrated that these agents, particularly chlorpropamide, can be effective in control of the patient with partial diabetes insipidus (378, 379). The sulfonylureas act upon the distal tubule and collecting duct epithelium to increase water reabsorption, but they require the presence of small amounts of vasopressin to be effective (380, 381). The antidiuretic activity of tolbutamide is weak. Chlorpropamide has been found to have a much greater effect and may be given orally. As an initial approximation, the dosage is about 250 to 500 mg once or twice daily in adults (378). In some patients, particularly those with mild forms of diabetes insipidus, low dosage with chlorpropamide can achieve satisfactory control and provide a simple and acceptable mode of therapy.

Syndromes of excessive and inappropriate secretion of vasopressin (SIADH)

Dilutional hyponatremia is a common abnormality in hospitalized patients. The many factors which can lead to hyponatremia are discussed in Chap. 18, but when carefully studied, the majority of patients with dilutional hyponatremia will have plasma vasopressin levels which are "inappropriate" with respect to the concurrent plasma osmolality. This recognition has lead to considerable confusion about the significance of such vasopressin levels, resulting in frequent misdiagnosis of SIADH.

The appropriateness of any level of vasopressin secretion requires recognition of the fact that vasopressin secretion is the consequence of several concurrent stimuli to the hypothalamus and is not the exclusive consequence of changes in extracellular osmolality (382). Tables 26-4 and 26-5 provide a basis for separating appropriate causes of dilutional hyponatremia from truly inappropriate causes of dilutional hyponatremia. Inappropriate ADH secretion can perhaps be best defined as those clinical situations in which vasopressin secretion is persistent despite the absence of all known normal osmotic and nonosmotic stimuli for secretion.

Several factors may alter the relationships between osmolality and vasopressin release. These factors can be divided into two categories: (1) alterations in effective intravascular volume and (2) alterations in cerebral cortical and thalamic input to the hypothalamic nuclei as the result of fear and/or pain.

Baroreceptor mechanisms are known to exist in the carotid sinus, aortic arch, cardiac atria, and pumonary vasculature. Sensory fibers from these receptors appear to enter the central nervous system by way of the vagus nerve and cervical sympathetic nerves. Destruction of these nerves will markedly reduce the vasopressin secretory response to volume depletion. Such experimental observations give strong support to the hypothesis that functional hypovolemia may evoke an increase in vasopressin secretion and account for some cases of dilutional hyponatremia. Several clinical states are associated with functional hypovolemia and with avid retention of salt and water by the kidney. Dehydration and hemorrhage are two obvious examples as both are associated with a decrease in total body Na^+ and total body water. Vasopressin release in response to such changes may result in dilutional hyponatremia, which is inappropriate to the maintenance of a constant osmolality but is appropriate toward restoration of intravascular volume.

Decreases in intravascular volume (hemorrhage, cardiogenic shock, peripheral edema, ascites) may decrease hydrostatic pressure in the capillaries surrounding the proximal renal tubules, thereby increasing reabsorption of salt and water in that segment. The resulting decrease in distal delivery of NaCl to the loop of Henle may then impede formation of a hypotonic tubular fluid and, as a result of a decreased capacity to form free water, impede free water excretion even in the absence of vasopressin (383). Thus, many of the patients reported to have SIADH may actually have a "reset osmostat" syndrome and may only reflect our current inability to completely define "appropriate." Only about 20 percent of patients with SIADH have actually totally lost osmoregulatory effect on vasopressin (366).

Clinical states of inappropriate dilutional hyponatremia. In recent years considerable attention has been drawn to the clinical syndrome of SIADH (384). These patients appear to be clinically normovolemic with normal renal and adrenal function, and they present with severe hyponatremia and hypoosmolality. Despite the hypoosmolality, these patients excrete a less than maximally dilute urine which contains normal amounts of Na^+. The syndrome has been recognized in association with a variety of pathologic conditions as listed in Table 26-5. Two groups of causes of this syndrome can be recognized. In the first group there is excessive production of vasopressin from the neurohypophysis as the result of either central nervous system injury or stimulation. In the second group there is also excessive production of vasopressin (or of polypeptides which have vasopressinlike activity), but the source is probably not the neurohypophysis. Most of the cases in this latter group are the result of polypeptide secretion from tumors (385–388), but it has been found in the lung tissue of patients with tuberculosis (389). The actual synthesis of vasopressin from amino acid precursors has been demonstrated in such tumors (388). In a third group, most notably patients with pneumococcal pneumonia, the source of the vasopressin is unclear.

In all groups of patients with SIADH the characteristics are similar. The patient has marked hypoosmolality which is associated with an inappropriately high (i.e., less than maximally dilute urine osmolality). Actual urine osmolality will range widely, sometimes even being higher than plasma osmolality. After demonstration of a less than maximally dilute urine in the presence of plasma hypoosmolality, the diagnosis of SIADH is made primarily by exclusion. The combination of a urine osmolality above 50 mosm/kg with a high–normal urinary Na^+ concentration in a patient with systemic hypoosmolality, no known defect in free water generation, and no known defect in "effective" intravascular volume establishes the diagnosis of SIADH.

Therapy of inappropriate vasopressin secre-

Table 26-6 Conditions mimicking SIADH

I. DEFECTS IN FREE WATER GENERATION

A. Chronic renal failure
B. Decreased distal delivery—multiple causes including shock, hepatorenal syndrome, severe congestive heart failure
C. Use of diuretics affecting the thick ascending limb, loop of Henle, furosemide, ethacrynic acid
D. Chronic, severe hypokalemia
E. Bartter's syndrome, myxedema

II. ENHANCED DISTAL WATER REABSORPTION

A. Chlorpropamide, tolbutamide
B. Phosphodiesterase inhibition—theophylline, aminophylline therapy
C. ? Glucocorticoid deficiency

tion. Depending upon the etiology and severity of SIADH, several avenues of therapy are open. In those patients who have SIADH without clinical manifestations of hyponatremia, severe water restriction alone may be sufficient therapy. After a period of several days, increased water intake can be permitted with careful monitoring. In those cases in which vasopressin is produced by tumors, the syndrome may recur rapidly if water restriction is removed. These individuals require additional forms of therapy as described below.

Patients with severe dilutional hyponatremia (serum Na^+ below 120 meq/L) have an extremely high mortality rate (23). Many such individuals will demonstrate clinical signs of acute water intoxication, and more urgent therapy is required. The administration of "loop" diuretics, such as furosemide, coupled with the administration of hypertonic NaCl has been described as an extremely effective form of therapy (290). It is important to recognize that the administration of small amounts of hypertonic NaCl alone may suppress proximal Na^+ reabsorption, as well as increase delivery of fluid to the loop of Henle and enhance free water generation, both of which may worsen the problem. The relatively large volumes of hypertonic NaCl which would be required could cause additional extracellular fluid volume expansion in a patient who is already expanded. Moreover the rapid renal excretion of NaCl in these patients limits the effectiveness of such therapy (390). For this reason, it seems appropriate to couple a diuretic such as furosemide with

hypertonic NaCl infusion to impede free water generation and produce a diuresis which is hypotonic to the infusate. Rapid reversal of the hyponatremia is possible using this therapy, but caution is necessary because of the rapid changes in osmolality and the risks of overtreatment.

Both lithium (391) and demeclocycline (392) have been recently described as therapeutic agents in patients with chronic SIADH. Declomycin appears to be preferable both because of lack of significant CNS depressant effects and its dose-dependent and predictable effects upon the collecting duct (except in patients with cirrhosis).

NEUROLOGIC FACTORS AFFECTING Na^+ BALANCE

Regulation of Na^+ intake

The importance of thirst in control of water balance is well recognized, but less well known is the possible role of salt perception in the regulation of external salt balance. There is important evidence which suggests that salt intake is regulated and is an important factor in the regulation of Na^+ balance, both normally and in pathophysiologic states such as Addison's disease.

Patients with Addison's disease often demonstrate a marked preference for salty foods. A dramatic salt-craving tendency—patients literally eating handfuls of crystalline salt—is not uncommon (393). The heightened salt intake is important in external homeostasis for such patients. When salt intake is restricted to normal amounts, patients with Addison's disease have been known to develop adrenal crisis and die (394).

Little is known about the mechanisms involved in such perception of increased salt need, but certain factors seem important. Rats subjected to adrenalectomy will develop an enhanced preference for NaCl solutions instead of tap water and can thus maintain themselves in the absence of adrenal steroids. Section of the facial nerve in such animals destroys their capacity to distinguish saline from tap water, and they quickly die (395). The gustatory perception of saltiness is known to relate to the taste buds in the anterior two-thirds of the tongue (in humans). These taste buds are innervated by small sensory fibers which travel through the chorda tympani of the facial nerve. Destruction of the chorda tympani in humans will remove the ability to perceive saltiness in foods. The localization of salt perception to discrete nuclei in the thalamus does not appear to occur in humans. Cortical projections of such perception are diffuse, and the interaction between taste, volume perception, and salt craving is virtually unknown.

Neurologic factors in Na^+ excretion

There is no compelling evidence that renal nerves are required for regulation of Na^+ excretion in humans. Studies of human renal allograft function (396) have revealed that in transplanted kidneys, external salt balance can be maintained. Experimental pharmacologic or surgical denervation of the kidney has been reported to cause natriuresis, but increased Na^+ excretion can probably be ascribed to increases in GFR (397). However, neurologic factors do play a role in regulation of renal Na^+ reabsorption. Cervical spinal cord section in dogs abolishes the natriuretic response to whole blood infusion (398). Chronic cardiac denervation results in a marked blunting in the natriuretic response to intravenous NaCl infusion (399). Increases in total peripheral vascular resistence probably can also modify the response to NaCl infusion. Both patients with essential hypertension and subjects receiving norepinephrine infusions have an accentuated response to volume expansion when compared to normal subjects. Adrenergic blockage reduces or abolishes this effect, but interruption of parasympathetic fibers in the thorax does not significantly alter the natriuretic response to volume expansion.

The role of the brain in Na^+ excretion

Claude Bernard (400) observed in rats that puncture of the floor of the fourth ventricle just anterior to the facial colliculus results in diuresis. Lesions in the posterior hypothalamus of rats produce a severe salt-wasting syndrome (400), but similar lesions in the anterior hypothalamus do not. Homer Smith (401) was probably the first to suggest that the brain elaborates a hormone which is responsible for regulation of Na^+ excretion. A multitude of studies have subsequently attempted to demonstrate the existence of such a substance and to localize its site of production. At best such experiments have yielded equivocal data (402).

Additionally, Anderson and coworkers (403) have demonstrated that infusion of hypertonic NaCl into the third ventricle of the brain of a goat results in a marked natriuresis, a decrement in free water clearance, and an increase in blood pressure. Although these observations suggest the existence of a substance other than vasopressin which might be a natriuretic hormone (404, 405), there has been no clear confirmation. Although it has been 20 years since Smith postulated the existence of the material (401), the issue is far from resolved at the present time.

Cerebral salt-wasting syndrome

There have been several reports in the literature which suggest that intracranial injuries, such as subdural hematomas and brainstem infarcts, may be associated with "salt-losing states" (258). However, intracranial lesions have also been associated with hyponatremia due to SIADH. It is possible that many of the reports of "cerebral salt wasting" are unrecognized cases of SIADH. At the present time there is little evidence to support the existence of a primary cerebral salt-losing syndrome in humans.

ACUTE RENAL FAILURE AND THE BRAIN

Acute renal failure has been described in association with several neuropathologic states. Grand mal seizures have been reported to produce acute tubular necrosis (406–409) and bilateral cortical necrosis with juxtamedullary nephron sparing (407). Severe frontal lobe hemorrhages have also been reported to be associated with acute tubular necrosis (406). It seems improbable that such cases can all be ascribed to renal vasoconstriction, although such a possibility cannot be excluded. Some cases may be the result of a severe, if transient, reduction in blood pressure either during the seizure or in the postictal state. In addition, it is also possible that myoglobinuria is a complicating factor in some cases of acute renal failure associated with seizures (410). Similar observations have been reported in patients who have undergone electroconvulsive therapy (406, 408, 409).

However, there have been a large number of reported cases of acute renal failure associated with intracranial lesions where there is no other obvious cause for the renal failure. Sitprija and Tangchai (407) reviewed 16 patients who had renal failure associated with intracranial lesion, 12 of whom did not survive. Of these 16 patients, 10 were young (22 to 47 years) and had no reason to have renal failure other than the intracranial lesion (407).

Reduction in renal blood flow and renal cortical ischemia can be induced by electrical stimulation of cerebral cortex (408, 409). Acute tubular necrosis can actually be induced in cats by electrical stimulation of the anterior signoid gyrus (408).

It appears likely that in both humans and experimental animals, cerebral lesions can cause acute tubular necrosis (406). The mechanisms are unclear at this time but are probably related to renal vasoconstriction. In humans, most lesions which cause renal failure are located in the posterior and orbital regions of the frontal lobe (406).

REFERENCES

1. Alfrey, A. C., J. M. Mishell, J. Burks, S. R. Contiguglia, H. Rudolph, E. Lewin, and J. H. Holmes: Syndrome of dyspraxia and multifocal seizures associated with chronic hemodialysis, *Trans. Am. Soc. Artif. Intern. Organs*, **18**:257, 1972.
2. Raskin, N. H., and R. A. Fishman: Neurologic disorders in renal failure, *N. Engl. J. Med.*, **294**:143, 204, 1976.
3. Covey, C. M., and A. I. Arieff: Disorders of sodium and water metabolism and their effects on the central nervous system, in B. M. Brenner and J. H. Stein (eds.), *Contemporary Issues in Nephrology*, vol. 1, Churchill Livingstone, New York, 1978, pp. 212–241.
4. Katzman, R., and H. M. Pappius: Brain ions, in *Brain Electrolytes and Fluid Metabolism*, The Williams & Wilkins Company, Baltimore, 1973, pp. 111–134.
5. Tower, D. B.: Inorganic constituents, in A. Lajtha (ed.), *Handbook of Neurochemistry* **I**, *Chemical Architecture of the Nervous System*, Plenum Press, New York, 1969, pp. 1–24.
6. Arieff, A. I., A. Kerian, S. G. Massry, and J. DeLima: Intracellular pH of brain: Alterations in acute respiratory acidosis and alkalosis, *Am. J. Physiol.*, **230**:804, 1976.
7. Hanig, R. C., and M. H. Aprison: Determination of calcium, copper, iron, magnesium, manganese, potassium, zinc and chloride in several brain areas, *Anal. Biochem.*, **21**:169, 1967.
8. Alfrey, A. C., G. R. LeGendre, and W. D. Kaehny: The dialysis encephalopathy syndrome: Possible aluminum intoxication, *N. Engl. J. Med.*, **294**:184, 1976.
9. Bessman, S. P.: Osmotic implications of changes in metabolic intermediates in the brain, *Proc. Am. Soc. Neurochem.*, **7**:103, 1976.
10. Florkin, M., and E. Schoffeniels: Isosmotic intracellular regulation, in *Molecular Approaches to Ecology*, Academic Press, New York, 1969, pp. 89–111.
11. Forster, R. P., and L. Goldstein: Intracellular osmoregulatory role of amino acids and urea in marine elasmobranchs, *Am. J. Physiol.*, **230**:925, 1976.
12. Baxter, C. F., and C. L. Ortiz: Amino acids and the maintenance of osmotic equilibrium in brain tissue, *Life Sci.*, **5**:2321, 1966.
13. Rapoport, S. I.: Permeability and osmotic properties of the blood brain barrier: Osmotic edema, in *Blood Brain Barrier in Physiology and Medicine*, Raven Books, Abelard-Schuman, Limited, New York, 1976, pp. 118–119.
14. Carroll, H. J., R. Gotterer, and B. Altshuler: Exchangeable sodium, body potassium, and body water in previously edematous cardiac patients; Evidence for osmotic inactivation of cation, *Circulation*, **32**:185, 1965.
15. Welt, L. G., J. Orloff, D. M. Kydd, and J. E. Olt-

man: An example of cellular hyperosmolarity, *J. Clin. Invest.*, **29:**935, 1950.

16. Elkinton, J. R., A. W. Winkler, and T. S. Danowski: Inactive cell base and the measurement of changes in cell water, *Yale J. Biol. Med.*, **17:**383, 1944.

17. Arieff, A. I., and C. R. Kleeman: Studies on mechanisms of cerebral edema in diabetic comas: Effects of hyperglycemia and rapid lowering of plasma glucose in normal rabbits, *J. Clin. Invest.*, **52:**571, 1973.

18. Finberg, L., C. Luttrell, and H. Redd: Pathogenesis of lesions in the nervous system in hypernatremic states: Experimental studies of gross anatomic changes and alterations of chemical composition of the tissues, *Pediatrics*, **23:**46, 1959.

19. McDowell, M. E., A. V. Wolf, and A. Steer: Osmotic volumes of distribution: Idiogenic changes in osmotic pressure associated with administration of hypertonic solutions, *Am. J. Physiol.*, **180:**545, 1955.

20. Appelboom, J. W. T., W. A. Brodsky, W. S. Tuttle, and I. Diamond: The freezing point depression of mammalian tissues after sudden heating in boiling distilled water, *J. Gen. Physiol.*, **41:**1153, 1958.

21. Arieff, A. I., C. R. Kleeman, A. Keushkerian, and H. Bagdoyan: Brain tissue osmolality: Method of determination and variations in hyper- and hypoosmolar states, *J. Lab. Clin. Med.*, **79:**334, 1972.

22. Maffly, R. H., and A. Leaf: The potential of water in mammalian tissues, *J. Gen. Physiol.*, **42:**1257, 1959.

23. Arieff, A. I., and R. Guisado: Effects on the central nervous system of hypernatremic and hyponatremic states, *Kidney Int.*, **10:**104, 1976.

24. Kregenow, F. M.: The response of duck erythrocytes to hypertonic media, *J. Gen. Physiol.*, **58:**396, 1971.

25. Baxter, C. F., J. H. Thurston, A. I. Arieff, and S. P. Bessman: Organic molecules involved in the osmotic regulation of nervous tissue, *Proc. Am. Soc. Neurochem.*, **7:**14, 1976.

26. Dodge, P. R., J. F. Sotos, I. Gomstorp, D. Deviro, M. Levy, and T. Rabe: Neurophysiologic disturbances in hypertonic dehydration, *Trans. Am. Neurol. Assoc.*, **87:**33, 1962.

27. Sotos, J. F., P. R. Dodge, P. Meara, and N. B. Talbot: Studies in experimental hypertonicity. 1. Pathogenesis of the clinical syndrome, biochemical abnormalities and cause of death, *Pediatrics*, **26:**925, 1960.

28. Posner, J. B., and F. Plum: Spinal fluid pH and neurologic symptoms in systemic acidosis, *N. Engl. J. Med.*, **277:**605, 1967.

29. Katzman, R., and H. M. Pappius: Acid-base balance in the cerebrospinal fluid, in *Brain Electrolytes and Fluid Metabolism*, The Williams & Wilkins Company, Baltimore, 1973, pp. 224–245.

30. Davson, H.: The cerebrospinal fluid, in *A Textbook of General Physiology*, 4th ed., The Williams & Wilkins Company, Baltimore, 1970, pp. 714–750.

31. Lee, J. E., J. B. Posner, and F. Plum: Buffering capacity of cerebrospinal fluid in acute respiratory acidosis in dogs, *Am. J. Physiol.*, **217:**1035, 1969.

32. Plum, F., and J. B. Posner: Blood and cerebrospinal fluid lactate during hyperventilation, *Am. J. Physiol.*, **212:**864, 1967.

33. Wichser, J., and H. Kazemi: CSF bicarbonate regulation in respiratory acidosis and alkalosis, *J. Appl. Physiol.*, **38:**504, 1975.

34. Hornbein, T. F., and E. G. Pavlin: Distribution of H^+ and HCO_3^- between CSF and blood during respiratory alkalosis in dogs, *Am. J. Physiol.*, **228:**1149, 1975.

35. Pavlin, E. G., and T. F. Hornbein: Distribution of H^+ and HCO_3^- between CSF and blood during respiratory acidosis in dogs, *Am. J. Physiol.*, **228:**1145, 1975.

36. Katzman, R., and H. M. Pappius: Cerebrospinal fluid ions, in *Brain Electrolytes and Fluid Metabolism*, The Williams & Wilkins Company, Baltimore, 1973, pp. 75–110.

37. Bradbury, M. W. B., J. Stubbs, I. E. Hughes, and P. Parker: The distribution of potassium, sodium, chloride and urea between lumbar cerebrospinal fluid and blood serum in human subjects, *Clin. Sci.*, **25:**97, 1963.

38. Bradbury, M. W. B., and C. R. Kleeman: Stability of the potassium content of cerebrospinal fluid and brain, *Am. J. Physiol.*, **213:**519, 1967.

39. Ames, A., M. Sakanoue, and S. Endo: Na, K, Ca, Mg, and Cl concentrations in choroid plexus fluid

and cisternal fluid compared with plasma ultra-filtrate, *J. Neurophysiol.*, **27**:672, 1964.

40. Held, D., V. Fencl, and J. R. Papenheimer: Electrical potential of cerebrospinal fluid, *J. Neurophysiol.*, **27**:942, 1964.

41. Arieff, A. I., and S. G. Massry: Calcium metabolism of brain in acute renal failure: Effects of uremia, hemodialysis and parathyroid hormone, *J. Clin. Invest.*, **53**:387, 1974.

42. Guisado, R., A. I. Arieff, and S. G. Massry: Changes in the electroencephalogram in acute uremia: Effects of parathyroid hormone and brain electrolytes, *J. Clin. Invest.*, **55**:738, 1975.

43. Oppelt, W. W., I. MacIntyre, and D. P. Rall: Magnesium exchange between blood and cerebrospinal fluid, *Am. J. Physiol.*, **205**:959, 1963.

44. Bradbury, M. W. B., C. R. Kleeman, H. Bagdoyan, and A. Berberian: The calcium and magnesium content of skeletal muscle, brain, and cerebrospinal fluid as determined by atomic absorption flame photometry, *J. Lab. Clin. Med.*, **71**:884, 1968.

45. Woodbury, J., K. Lyons, R. Carretta, A. Hahn, and J. F. Sullivan: Cerebrospinal fluid and serum levels of magnesium zinc, and calcium in man, *Neurology (Minneap.)*, **18**:700, 1968.

46. Davson, H.: The extracellular space of brain and cord, in *Physiology of the Cerebrospinal Fluid*, J & A Churchill Ltd., London, 1967, p. 107.

47. Katzman, R., and H. M. Pappius: Fluid compartments, in *Brain Electrolytes and Fluid Metabolism*, The Williams & Wilkins Company, Baltimore, 1973, pp. 33–48.

48. Brightman, M. W., R. R. Shivers, and L. Prescott: Morphology of the walls around fluid compartments in nervous tissue, in H. F. Cserr, J. D. Fenstermacher, and V. Fencl (eds.), *Fluid Environment of the Brain*, Academic Press, Inc., New York, 1975, pp. 3–29.

49. Oldendorf, W. H., and H. Davson: Brain extracellular space and the sink action of the CSF, *Arch Neurol.*, **17**:196, 1967.

50. Bourke, R. S., E. S. Greenberg, and D. B. Tower: Variation of cerebral cortex fluid spaces in vivo as a function of species brain size, *Am. J. Physiol.*, **208**:682, 1965.

51. Levin, E., A. I. Arieff, and C. R. Kleeman: Evidence of different compartments in the brain for

extracellular markers, *Am. J. Physiol.*, **221**:1319, 1971.

52. Crone, C.: General properties of the blood brain barrier with special emphasis on glucose, in H. F. Cserr, J. D. Fenstermacher, and V. Fencl (eds.), *Fluid Environment of the Brain*, Academic Press, Inc., New York, 1975, pp. 33–46.

53. Erlich, P.: *Das Sauerstoff-Bedurfnis des Organismus, Eine Farbenanalytische Studie*, pp. 69–72, Berline, 1885. (Cited in Bakay, *Cerebral Edema*, Charles C Thomas, Springfield, Ill., 1965.)

54. Lewandowsky, M.: Aur Lehre Von Der Cerebros-spinalflüssigkeit: *Z. Klin. Med.*, **40**:480, 1900.

55. Goldman, E. E.: Die Aussere und Innere Sekretion des Gesunden und Gesunden und Kranken Organismus im Lichte der "Vitalen Farbung," *Beitr. Z. Klin. Chir.*, **64**:192, 1909.

56. Rapoport, S. I.: Regulation of drug entry into the nervous system, in *Blood Brain Barrier in Physiology and Medicine*, Raven Books, Abelard-Schuman, Limited, New York, 1976, pp. 153–176.

57. Rapoport, S. I.: Sites and functions of the blood-brain barrier, in *Blood Brain Barrier in Physiology and Medicine*, Raven Books, Abelard-Schuman, Limited, New York, 1976, pp. 43–86.

58. Berger, A. J., R. A. Mitchell, and J. W. Severinghaus: Regulation of respiration, parts 1, 2 and 3, *N. Engl. J. Med.*, **297**:92–97, 138–143, 194–201, 1977.

59. Refsum, H. E.: Relationship between state of consciousness and arterial hypoxemia and hypercapnia in patients with pulmonary insufficiency breathing air, *Clin. Sci.*, **25**:361, 1963.

60. Pavlin, E. G., and T. F. Hornbein: Distribution of H^+ and HCO_3^- between CSF and blood during metabolic acidosis in dogs, *Am. J. Physiol.*, **228**:1134, 1975.

61. Fencl, V., J. R. Vale, and J. A. Broch: Respiration and cerebral blood flow in metabolic alkalosis and acidosis in humans, *J. Appl. Physiol.*, **27**:67, 1969.

62. Kazemi, H., D. C. Shannon, and E. Carvallo-Gil: Brain CO_2 buffering capacity in respiratory acidosis and alkalosis, *J. Appl. Physiol.*, **22**:241, 1967.

63. Ponten, U.: Consecutive acid-base changes in blood, brain tissue and cerebrospinal fluid during

respiratory acidosis and baseosis, *Acta Neurol. Scand.*, **42**:455, 1966.

64. Kjallquist M., M. Nardini, and B. K. Siesjo: The effect of acetazolamide upon tissue concentrations of bicarbonate, lactate, and pyruvate in the rat brain, *Acta Physiol. Scand.*, **77**:241, 1969.

65. Maren, T. H.: Bicarbonate formation in cerebrospinal fluid: Role in sodium transport and pH regulation, *Am. J. Physiol.*, **222**:885, 1972.

66. Roberts, E., and K. Kuriyama: Biochemical-physiological correlations in studies of the gamma-aminobutyric acid system, *Brain Res.*, **8**:1, 1968.

67. Pollay, M.: Transport mechanisms in the choroid plexus, *Fed. Proc.*, **33**:2064, 1974.

68. Pontén, U.: Acid-base changes in rat brain tissue during acute respiratory acidosis and baseosis, *Acta Physiol. Scand.*, **68**:152, 1966.

69. Kazemi, H., N. S. Shore, V. E. Shih, and D. C. Shannon: Brain organic buffers in respiratory acidosis and alkalosis, *J. Appl. Physiol.*, **34**:478, 1973.

70. Kilburn, K. H.: Shock, seizures, and coma with alkalosis during mechanical ventilation, *Ann. Intern. Med.*, **65**:977, 1966.

71. Severinghaus, J. W., and N. Lassen: Step hypocapnia to separate arterial from tissue pCO_2 in the regulation of cerebral blood flow, *Circ. Res.*, **20**:272, 1967.

72. Betz, E.: Cerebral blood flow: Its measurement and regulation, *Physiol. Rev.*, **52**:595, 1972.

73. Shenkin, H. A., and W. F. Bouzarth: Clinical methods of reducing intracranial pressure, *N. Engl. J. Med.*, **282**:1465, 1970.

74. Roos, A.: Intracellular pH and buffering power of rat brain, *Am. J. Physiol.*, **221**:176, 1971.

75. Granholm, L., and B. K. Siesjo: The effects of hypercapnia and hypocapnia upon the cerebrospinal fluid lactate and pyruvate concentrations and upon the lactate, pyruvate, ATP, ADP, phosphocreatine and creatine concentrations of cat brain tissue, *Acta Physiol. Scand.*, **75**:257, 1969.

76. Leusen, I., and G. Demeester: Lactate and pyruvate in the brain of rats during hyperventilation, *Arch. Int. Physiol. Biochim.*, **74**:25, 1966.

77. Van Vaerenbergh, P. J. J., G. Demeester, and I. Leusen: Lactate in cerebrospinal fluid during hyperventilation, *Arch. Int. Physiol. Biochim.*, **73**:738, 1965.

78. Nara, Y., A. S. Geha, and A. E. Baue: Blood and cerebral lactate metabolism during sustained hyperventilation in anesthetized intact dogs, *Surgery*, **69**:940, 1971.

79. Gotoh, F., J. S. Meyer, and Y. Takagi: Cerebral effects of hyperventilation in man, *Arch. Neurol.*, **12**:410, 1965.

80. Siesjo, B. K., and U. Ponten: Acid-base changes in the brain in nonrespiratory acidosis and alkalosis, *Exp. Brain Res.*, **2**:176, 1966.

81. Kibler, R. F., R. P. O'Neill, and E. D. Robin: Intracellular acid-base relations of dog brain with reference to the brain extracellular volume, *J. Clin. Invest.*, **43**:431, 1964.

82. Arieff, A. I., A. Kerian, and R. Guisado: Spontaneous lactic acidosis: Effects on central nervous system and intracellular pH, *Kidney Int.*, **8**:405, 1975.

83. Ruderman, N. B., P. S. Ross, M. Berger, and M. N. Goodman: Regulation of glucose and ketone-body metabolism in brain of anesthetized rats, *Biochem J.*, **138**:1, 1974.

84. Granholm, L., and B. K. Siesjo: The effect of combined respiratory and nonrespiratory alkalosis on energy metabolites and acid-base parameters in the rat brain, *Acta Physiol. Scand.*, **81**:307, 1971.

85. Mallette, L. E., J. P. Bilezikian, D. A. Heath, and G. D. Aurbach: Primary hyperparathyroidism: Clinical and biochemical features, *Medicine*, **53**:127, 1974.

86. Cogan, M., C. Covey, A. Arieff, A. Wisniewski, and O. Clark: Effects of hyperparathyroidism on the central nervous system, *Am. J. Med.*, (in press).

87. Locke, S. J. P. Merrill, and H. R. Tyler: Neurologic complications of acute uremia, *Arch. Intern. Med.*, **108**:75, 1961.

88. Hagstam, K. E.: EEG frequency content related to chemical blood parameters in chronic uremia, *Scand. J. Urol. Nephrol.*, **7** (suppl. 1): 1, 1971.

89. Tyler, H. R.: Neurologic disorders in renal failure, *Am. J. Med.*, **44**:734, 1968.

90. Cooper, J. D., V. C. Lazarowitz, and A. I. Arieff: Neurodiagnostic abnormalities in patients with acute renal failure, *J. Clin. Invest.*, **61**:1448, 1978.

91. Jacob, J. D. P. Gloor, O. H. Elwan, J. B. Dossetor, and V. R. Pateras: Electroencephalographic changes in chronic renal failure, *Neurology*, **15**:419, 1965.

92. Kiley, J., and O. Hines: Electroencephalographic evaluation of uremia, *Arch. Intern. Med.,* **116:**67, 1965.

93. Kennedy, A. C., A. I. Linton, S. Renfrew, R. G. Luke, and A. Dinwoodie: The pathogenesis and prevention of cerebral dysfunction during dialysis, *Lancet,* **1:**790, 1964.

94. Hampers, C. L., P. B. Doak, M. N. Callaghan, H. R. Tyler, and J. P. Merrill: The electroencephalogram and spinal fluid during hemodialysis, *Arch. Intern. Med.,* **118:**340, 1966.

95. Kiley, J. E., M. W. Woodruff, and K. L. Pratt: Evaluation of encephalopathy by EEG frequency analysis in chronic dialysis patients, *Clin. Nephrol.,* **5:**245, 1976.

96. Slatopolsky, E., S. Caglar, J. P. Pennell, D. B. Taggart, J. M. Canterbury, E. Reiss, and N. S. Bricker: On the pathogenesis of hyperparathyroidism in chronic experimental renal insufficiency in the dog, *J. Clin. Invest.,* **50:**492, 1971.

97. Massry, S. G., A. I. Arieff, J. W. Coburn, G. Palmieri, and C. R. Kleeman: Devalent ion metabolism in patients with acute renal failure; studies on the mechanism of hypocalcemia, *Kidney Int.,* **5:**437, 1974.

98. Fishman, R. A., and N. H. Raskin: Experimental uremic encephalopathy, *Arch. Neurol.,* **17:**10, 1967.

99. Pappius, H. M., J. H. Oh, and J. B. Dossetor: The effects of rapid hemodialysis on brain tissues and cerebrospinal fluid of dogs, *Can. J. Physiol. Pharmacol.,* **45:**129, 1967.

100. Arieff, A. I., S. G. Massry, A. Barrientos, and C. Kleeman: Brain water and electrolyte metabolism in uremia: Effects of slow and rapid hemodialysis, *Kidney Int.,* **4:**177, 1973.

101. Fishman, R. A.: Permeability changes in experimental uremic encephalopathy, *Arch. Intern. Med.,* **126:**835, 1970.

102. van den Noort, S., R. E. Eckel, K. Brine, and J. T. Hrdlicka: Brain metabolism in uremic and adenosine-infused rats, *J. Clin. Invest.,* **47:**2133, 1968.

103. Minkoff, L., G. Gaertner, M. Darab, C. Mercier, and M. L. Levin: Inhibition of brain sodium-potassium ATPase in uremic rats, *J. Lab Clin. Med.,* **80:**71, 1972.

104. Scheinberg, D.: Effects of uremia on cerebral blood flow and metabolism, *Neurology,* **4:**101, 1954.

105. Arieff, A. I., R. Guisado, and V. C. Lazarowitz: The pathophysiology of hyperosmolar states, in T. E. Andreoli, J. J. Grantham, and F. C. Rector, Jr. (eds.), *Disturbances in Body Fluid Osmolality,* The American Physiological Society, Bethesda, Maryland, 1977, pp. 227–250.

106. Arieff, A. I., R. Guisado, S. G. Massry, and V. C. Lazarowitz: Central nervous system pH in uremia and the effects of hemodialysis, *J. Clin. Invest.,* **58:**306, 1976.

107. Maschio, G., G. Bazzato, E. Bertaglia, D. Sardini, and G. Mioni: Intracellular pH and electrolyte content of skeletal muscle in patients with chronic renal acidosis, *Nephron,* **7:**481, 1970.

108. Levin, G. E., and D. N. Baron: Leucocyte intracellular pH in patients with the metabolic acidosis of renal failure, *Clin. Sci.,* **52:**325, 1977.

109. Tizianello, A., G. De Ferrari, G. Gurreri, and N. Acquarone: Effects of metabolic alkalosis, metabolic acidosis and uraemia on whole-body intracellular pH in man, *Clin. Sci.,* **52:**125, 1977.

110. Pauli H. G., C. Vorburger, and F. Reubi: Chronic derangements of cerebrospinal fluid acid-base components in man, *J. Appl. Physiol.,* **17:**993, 1962.

111. Cowie, J., A. T. Lambie, and J. S. Robson: The influence of extracorporeal dialysis on the acid-base composition of blood and cerebrospinal fluid, *Clin. Sci.,* **23:**397, 1962.

112. Leonard, A., and F. L. Shapiro: Subdural hematoma in regularly hemodialyzed patients, *Ann. Intern. Med.,* **82:**650, 1975.

113. Olsen, S.: The brain in uremia, *Acta Psychiat. Scand.,* **36** (suppl. 156): 1, 1961.

114. Rotter, W., and P. Roettger: Comparative pathologic-anatomic study of cases of chronic global renal insufficiency with and without hemodialysis, *Clin. Nephrol.,* **1:**257, 1974.

115. Burks, J. S., A. C. Alfrey, J. Huddlestone, M. D. Norenberg, and E. Lewin: A fatal encephalopathy in chronic haemodialysis patients, *Lancet* **1:**764, 1976.

116. Cooper, J. D., R. Guisado, and A. I. Arieff: Peripheral neuropathy and acute renal failure: Studies in patients and animals, *Clin. Res.,* **24:**396A, 1976.

117. Gotch, F. A., and K. K. Kreuger: Adequacy of dialysis, *Kidney Int.*, **7** (suppl. 2):S1, 1975.

118. Grushkin, C. M., B. Korsch, and R. N. Fine: Hemodialysis in small children, *JAMA*, **221**:869, 1972.

119. Porte, F. K., W. J. Johnson, and D. W. Klass: Prevention of dialysis disequilibrium syndrome by use of high sodium concentration in the dialysate, *Kidney Int.*, **3**:327, 1973.

120. Fukushige, M., O. Tado, S. Matsuki, M. Mizoguchi, H. Tanaka, and H. Nihira: Hemodialysis with Kiil-type artificial kidney: Clinical study on disequilibrium syndrome, *Acta. Urol. Jap.*, **17**:89, 1971.

121. Mawdsley, C.: Neurological complications of hemodialysis, *Proc. R. Soc. Med.*, **65**:871, 1972.

122. deC Peterson, H., and A. G. Swanson: Acute encephalopathy occurring during hemodialysis, *Arch. Intern. Med.*, **113**:877, 1964.

123. Kretchmar, L. H., W. M. Green, C. W. Waterhouse, and W. L. Parry: Repeated hemodialysis in chronic uremia, *JAMA*, **184**:1030, 1963.

124. Kennedy, A. C.: Dialysis disequilibrium syndrome, *Electroencephalogr. Clin. Neurophysiol.*, **29**:206, 1970.

125. Funder, J., and J. O. Wieth: Changes in cerebrospinal fluid composition following hemodialysis, *Scand. J. Clin. Lab. Invest.*, **19**:301, 1967.

126. Gilliland, K. G., and R. M. Hegstrom: The effect of hemodialysis on cerebrospinal fluid pressure in uremic dogs, *Trans. Am. Soc. Artif. Intern. Organs*, **9**:44, 1963.

127. Wakim, K. G.: Predominance of hyponatremia over hypo-osmolality in simulation of the dialysis disequilibrium syndrome, *Mayo Clin. Proc.*, **44**:433, 1969.

128. Sitprija, V., and J. H. Holmes: Preliminary observations on the change in intracranial pressure and intraoccular pressure during hemodialysis, *Trans. Am. Soc. Artif. Intern. Organs*, **8**:300, 1962.

129. Rosomoff, H. L., and F. T. Zugibe: Distribution of intracranial contents in experimental edema, *Arch. Neurol.*, **9**:26, 1963.

130. Rosenbaum, B. J., J. W. Coburn, J. H. Shinaberger, and S. G. Massry: Acid-base status during the interdialytic period in patients maintained with chronic hemodialysis, *Ann. Intern. Med.*, **71**:1105, 1969.

131. Plum, F., and R. W. Price: Acid-base balance of cisternal and lumbar cerebrospinal fluid in hospital patients, *N. Engl. J. Med.*, **289**:1346, 1973.

132. Chazan, B. I., S. B. Rees, M. C. Balodimos, D. Younger, and D. B. Ferguson: Dialysis in diabetics, *JAMA*, **209**:2026, 1969.

133. Arieff, A. I., and S. G. Massry: Dialysis disequilibrium syndrome, in S. G. Massry and A. L. Sellers (eds.), *Clinical Aspects of Uremia and Dialysis*, Charles C Thomas, Publisher, Springfield, Ill., 1976, pp. 34–52.

134. Siddiqui, J. Y., A. E. Fitz, R. L. Lawton, and W. M. Kirkendall: Causes of death in patients receiving long-term hemodialysis, *JAMA*, **212**:1350, 1970.

135. Talalla, A., H. Halbrook, B. H. Barbour, and T. Kurze: Subdural hematoma associated with long-term hemodialysis for chronic renal disease, *JAMA*, **212**:1847, 1970.

136. Weber, D. L., T. Reagan, and M. Leeds: Intracerebral hemorrhage during hemodialysis, *New York State J. Med.*, **72**:1853, 1972.

137. Leonard, C. D., C. Weil, and B. H. Scribner: Subdural hematomas in patients undergoing hemodialysis, *Lancet*, **2**:239, 1969.

138. Maccario, M.: Neurological dysfunction associated with non-ketotic hyperglycemia, *Arch. Neurol.*, **19**:525, 1968.

139. Rigg, G. A., and B. A. Bercu: Hypoglycemia: A complication of hemodialysis, *N. Engl. J. Med.*, **277**:1139, 1967.

140. Bluemle, L. W.: Current status of chronic hemodialysis, *Am. J. Med.*, **44**:749, 1968.

141. Gaan, D., N. P. Mallick, R. A. L. Brewis, and Y. K. Seedat: Cerebral damage from declotting Scribner shunts, *Lancet*, **2**:77, 1969.

142. Potter, D. J.: Death as a result of hyperglycemia without ketosis: A complication of hemodialysis, *Ann. Intern. Med.*, **64**:399, 1966.

143. Mahurkar, S. D., S. K. Dhar, R. Salta, L. Meyers, E. C. Smith, and G. Dunea: Dialysis dementia, *Lancet*, **1**:1412, 1973.

144. Smith, R. J., M. R. Block, A. I. Arieff, M. J. Blumenkrantz, and J. W. Cobrun: Hypernatremic hyperosmolar coma complicating chronic peritoneal dialysis, *Proc. Clin Dialy. & Trans. Forum*, **4**:96, 1974.

145. Kato, T., K. Sawanishi, J. Kawamura, H. Uey-

ama, Y. Miyake, A. Yamashita, and T. Okabe: Biochemical studies of hemodialysis, especially on dialysis disequilibrium, *Acta Urol. Jap.,* **14:**641, 1969.

146. Rosen, S. M., K. O'Connor, and S. Shaldon: Haemodialysis disequilibrium, *Br. Med. J.,* **2:**672, 1964.

147. Maher, J. F., and G. E. Schreiner: Hazards and complications of dialysis, *N. Engl. J. Med.,* **273:**370, 1965.

148. Bito, L. Z., and R. E. Myers: On the physiological response of the cerebral cortex to acute stress (reversible asphyxia), *J. Physiol. (London),* **221:**349, 1972.

149. Davson, H.: Ionic equilibria, bioelectric potentials, and active transport, in *A Textbook of General Physiology,* The Williams & Wilkins Company, Baltimore, 1970, p. 550.

150. Fishman, R. A.: Cell volume, pumps, and neurologic function: Brain's adaptation to osmotic stress, in F. Plum (ed.), *Brain Dysfunction in Metabolic Disorders,* Raven Books, Abelard-Schuman, Limited, New York, 1974, pp. 159–171.

151. Gutman, R. A., R. O. Hickman, G. E. Chatrian, and B. H. Scribner: Failure of high dialysis-fluid glucose to prevent the disequilibrium syndrome, *Lancet,* **1:**295, 1967.

152. Rodrigo, F., J. Shideman, R. McHuch, T. Buselmeier, and C. Kjellstrand: Osmolality changes during hemodialysis, *Ann. Intern. Med.,* **86:**554, 1977.

153. Kerr, D. N. S., R. W. Elliott, J. W. Osselton, D. Barwick, and R. Ashcroft: Fast and slow haemodialysis compared in patients on regular dialysis, *Proc. Eur. Dial. Transplant Assoc.,* **3:**282, 1966.

154. Ball, J. H., D. E. Butkus, and D. S. Madison: Effect of subtotal parathyroidectomy on dialysis dementia, *Nephron,* **18:**151, 1977.

155. Barratt, L. J., and J. R. Lawrence: Dialysis-associated dementia, *Aust. N.Z. J. Med.,* **5:**62, 1975.

156. Gibbs, C. J., and D. C. Gajdusek: Isolation and characterization of the subacute spongiform encephalopathies in man: Kuru and Creutzfeldt-Jacob disease, *J. Clin. Pathol.,* **25:**84, 1970.

157. McHugh, P. R.: Dementia, in P. B. Beeson and W. McDermott (eds.), *Cecil-Loeb Textbook of Medicine,* 13th ed., W. B. Saunders Company, Philadelphia, 1971, pp. 102–107.

158. Flendrig, J. A., H. Kruis, and H. A. Das: Aluminum and dialysis dementia, *Lancet,* **1:**1235, 1976.

159. Kaehny, W. D., A. P. Hegg, and A. C. Alfrey: Gastrointestinal absorption of aluminum from aluminum-containing antacids, *N. Engl. J. Med.,* **296:**1389, 1977.

160. Berlyne, G. M., J. Ben-Ari, D. Pest, J. Weinberger, M. Stern, G. R. Gilmore, and R. Levine: Hyperaluminaemia from aluminum resins in renal failure, *Lancet,* **2:**494, 1970.

161. Crapper, D. R., S. S. Krishnan, and S. Quittkat: Aluminum, neurofibrillary degeneration and Alzheimer's disease, *Brain,* **99:**67, 1976.

162. Dialysis dementia: Aluminum again? (editorial), *Lancet,* **1:**349, 1976.

163. Berlyne, G. M., J. B. Ari, E. Knopf, R. Yagil, G. Weinberger, and G. M. Danovitch: Aluminum toxicity in rats, *Lancet,* **1:**564, 1972.

164. Arieff, A. I., D. Armstrong, J. D. Cooper, and V. C. Lazarowitz: Brain aluminum, renal failure and dementia, *Kidney Int.,* **12:**477, 1977.

165. Kopeloff, L. M., S. E. Barrera, and N. Kopeloff: Recurrent convulsive seizures in animals produced by immunologic and chemical means, *Am. J. Psychiatry,* **98:**881, 1942.

166. Klatzo, I., H. Wisniewski, and E. Streicher: Experimental production of neurofibrillary degeneration, I. Light microscopic observations, *J. Neuropathol. Exp. Neurol.,* **24:**187, 1965.

167. Lyle, W. H.: Dialysis dementia, *Lancet,* **2:**271, 1973.

168. Duckett, S., G. Lyon, and P. Galle: Mise en evidence de magnesium dans les calcifications cerebrales de la maladie de Sturge-Weber, *C.R. Acad. Sci. (D)* (Paris), **282:**113, 1976.

169. Duckett, S., R. Escourolles, F. Gray, et al.: Striatonigral degeneration: Electron-probe study, *Acta Neuropathol. (Berl.),* **32:**269, 1975.

170. Ketones and coma (editorial), *N. Engl. J. Med.,* **284:**328, 1971.

171. Arieff, A. I., and H. J. Carroll: Cerebral edema and depression of sensorium in nonketotic hyperosmolar coma, *Diabetes,* **23:**525, 1974.

172. Plum, F., and J. B. Posner: Metabolic brain diseases causing coma, in *Diagnosis of Stupor and Coma,* F. A. Davis Company, Philadelphia, 1966, pp. 132–136.

173. Arieff, A. I., and H. J. Carroll: Nonketotic hyper-

osmolar coma with hyperglycemia: Clinical features, pathophysiology, renal function, acid-base balance, plasma-cerebrospinal fluid equilibria and the effects of therapy in 37 cases, *Medicine (Baltimore)*, **51**:73, 1972.

174. Waters, W. C. III, J. D. Hall, and W. B. Schwartz: Spontaneous lactic acidosis, *Am. J. Med.*, **35**:781, 1963.

175. Gerich, J. E., M. M. Martin, and L. Recant: Clinical and metabolic characteristics of hyperosmolar nonketotic coma, *Diabetes*, **20**:228, 1971.

176. Marks, V., and F. C. Rose: Electroencephalopathy, in *Hypoglycemia*, Blackwell Scientific Publications Ltd., Oxford, 1965, pp. 304–316.

177. Asfeldt, V. H.: Ketoacidosis diabetica. A prognostic and therapeutic study of 119 consecutive cases, *Dan. Med. Bull.*, **12**:103, 1965.

178. Martin, H. E., K. Smith, and M. L. Wilson: The fluid and electrolyte therapy of severe diabetic acidosis and ketosis. A study of twenty-nine episodes (twenty-six patients), *Am. J. Med.*, **24**:376, 1958.

179. McGarry, J. D., and D. W. Foster: Regulation of ketogenesis and clinical aspects of the ketotic state, *Metabolism*, **21**:471, 1972.

180. Wieland, O.: Diabetic acidosis: Biochemical aspects, in B. S. Liebel and G. A. Wrenshall (eds.), *On the Nature and Treatment of Diabetes*, Excerpta Medica Foundation, New York, 1965, pp. 533–544.

181. McGarry, J. D., and D. W. Foster: Ketogenesis and its regulation, *Am. J. Med.*, **61**:9, 1976.

182. Felig, P.: Diabetic ketoacidosis, *N. Engl. J. Med.*, **290**:1360, 1974.

183. Schneider, R., and H. Droller: Relative importance of ketosis and acidosis in production of diabetic coma, *Q. J. Exp. Physiol.*, **28**:323, 1938.

184. Kety, S. S., B. D. Polis, C. S. Nadler, and C. F. Schmidt: The blood flow and oxygen consumption of the human brain in diabetic acidosis and coma, *J. Clin. Invest.*, **27**:500, 1948.

185. Guisado, R., and A. I. Arieff: Neurological manifestations of diabetic comas: Correlation with biochemical alterations in the brain, *Metabolism*, **24**:665, 1975.

186. Pierce, N. F., D. S. Fedson, K. L. Brigham, S. Permutt, and A. Mondal: Relation of ventilation during base deficit to acid-base values in blood and spinal fluid, *J. Appl. Physiol.*, **30**:677, 1971.

187. Weiner, M. W., and F. H. Epstein: Signs and symptoms of electrolyte disorders, in M. H. Maxwell and C. R. Kleeman (eds.), *Clinical Disorders of Fluid and Electrolyte Metabolism*, McGraw-Hill Book Company, New York, 1972, pp. 629–661.

188. Dufano, M., and S. Ishikawa: Hypercapnia: Mental changes and extrapulmonary complications, *Ann. Intern. Med.*, **63**:829, 1965.

189. Huang, Y. H., and G. J. Mogenson: Differential effects of incertal and hypothalamic lesions on food and water intake, *Exp. Neurol.*, **43**:276, 1974.

190. Pitts, R. F., and R. S. Alexander: The nature of the renal tubular mechanism for acidifying the urine, *Am. J. Physiol.*, **144**:239, 1945.

191. Pitts, R. F., W. D. Lotspeich, W. A. Schiess, J. L. Ayer, and P. Miner: The renal regulation of acid-base metabolism in man. I. The nature of the mechanism for acidifying the urine, *J. Clin. Invest.*, **27**:48, 1948.

192. Assal, J. P., T. T. Aoki, F. M. Manzano, and G. P. Kozak: Metabolic effects of sodium bicarbonate in management of diabetic ketoacidosis, *Diabetes*, **23**:405, 1974.

193. Ohman, J. L., E. B. Marliss, T. T. Aoki, C. S. Munichoodappa, V. V. Khanna, and G. P. Kozak: The cerebrospinal fluid in diabetic ketoacidosis, *N. Engl. J. Med.*, **284**:283, 1971.

194. Siesjo, B. K.: The regulation of cerebrospinal fluid pH, *Kidney Int.*, **1**:360, 1972.

195. Siesjo, B. K., and A. Kjallquist: A new theory for the regulation of the extracellular pH in the brain, *Scand. J. Clin. Lab. Invest.*, **24**:1, 1969.

196. Kjallquist, A., M. Nardini, and B. K. Siesjo: The regulation of extra- and intracellular acid-base parameters in the rat brain during hyper- and hypocapnia, *Acta Physiol. Scand.*, **76**:485, 1969.

197. Blackshear, P. J., and K. G. M. M. Alberti: Experimental diabetic ketoacidosis, *Biochem. J.*, **138**:107, 1974.

198. Fulop, M., H. Tannenbaum, and N. Dreyer: Ketotic hyperosmolar coma, *Lancet*, **2**:635, 1973.

199. Folbergrova, J., V. MacMillan, and B. K. Siejo: The effect of hypercapnic acidosis upon some glycolytic and Krebs cycle-associated intermedi-

ates in the rat brain, *J. Neurochem.,* **19:**2507, 1972.

200. Reubi, F. C.: Glomerular filtration rate, renal blood flow and blood viscosity during and after diabetic coma, *Circ. Res.,* **1:**410, 1953.

201. Arieff, A. I., J. Garty, and A. Kerian: Diabetic ketoacidosis: Complications of therapy in an experimental model, *Clin. Res.,* **24:**153A, 1976.

202. Dodge, P. R., J. D. Crawford, and J. H. Probst: Studies in experimental water intoxication, *Arch. Neurol.,* **3:**513, 1960.

203. Sotos, J. F., P. R. Dodge, and N. B. Talbot: Studies in experimental hypertonity. II. Hypertonicity of body fluids as a cause of acidosis, *Pediatrics,* **30:**180, 1962.

204. Nabaroo, J. D. N.: Hyperosmolar non-ketotic coma, in B. S. Leibel and G. A. Wrenshall (eds.), *On the Nature and Treatment of Diabetes,* Excerpta Medica Foundation, New York, 1965, pp. 551–562.

205. Foster, D. W.: Insulin deficiency and hyperosmolar coma, *Adv. Intern. Med.,* **19:**159, 1974.

206. Timperley, W. R., F. E. Preston, and J. D. Ward: Cerebral intravascular coagulation in diabetic acidosis, *Lancet,* **1:**952, 1974.

207. Anderson, J. M., G. A. Machin, I. McKinlay, and D. Thistlethwaite: Diabetic ketoacidosis and intracerebral thrombosis, *Lancet,* **1:**1341, 1974.

208. Maccario, M., C. P. Messis, and E. F. Vastola: Focal seizures as a manifestation of hyperglycemia without ketoacidosis, *Neurology,* **15:**195, 1965.

209. Daniels, J. C., S. Chokroverty, and K. D. Barron: Anacidotic hyperglycemia and focal seizures, *Arch. Intern. Med.,* **124:**701, 1969.

210. Posner, J. B., A. G. Swanson, and F. Plum: Acid-base balance in cerebrospinal fluid, *Arch. Neurol.,* **12:**479, 1965.

211. Marks, V., and C. Rose: Cerebral metabolism and hypoglycemia, in *Hypoglycemia,* Blackwell Scientific Publications Ltd., Oxford, 1965, pp. 52–61.

212. Stone, W. E., J. K. Tews, K. E. Whisler, and D. J. Brown: Incorporation of carbon from glucose into cerebral amino acids, proteins and lipids, and alterations during recovery from hypoglycemia, *J. Neurochem.,* **19:**321, 1972.

213. Himwich, W. A., and H. C. Agrawal: Amino acids: Free amino acid pool of central nervous system, in A. Lajtha (ed.), *Handbook of Neurochemistry,* vol. 1, *Chemical Architecture of the Central Nervous System,* Plenum Press, Plenum Publishing Corporation, New York, 1969, pp. 33–38.

214. Roberts, E., M. Rothstein, and C. F. Baxter: Some metabolic studies of gamma-aminobutyric acid, *Proc. Soc. Exp. Biol. Med.,* **97:**796, 1958.

215. Hayashi, T.: Inhibition and excitation due to GABA in the central nervous system, *Nature,* **182:**1076, 1958.

216. Baxter, C. D.: The nature of gamma-aminobutyric acid, in A. Lajtha (ed.), *Handbook of Neurochemistry,* vol. 3, *Metabolic Reactions in the Nervous System,* Plenum Press, Plenum Publishing Corporation, New York, 1970, pp. 289–353.

217. Curtis, D. R., and J. C. Watkins: The pharmacology of amino acids related to gamma-aminobutyric acid, *Pharmacol. Rev.,* **17:**347, 1965.

218. Flock, E. V., G. M. Tyce, and C. A. Owen, Jr.: Glucose metabolism in brains of diabetic rats, *Endocrinology,* **85:**428, 1969.

219. Rubin, H. M., R. Kramer, and A. Drash: Hyperosmolality complicating diabetes mellitus in childhood, *J. Pediatr.,* **74:**177, 1969.

220. DiBenedetto, R. J., J. A. Crocco, and J. L. Soscia: Hyperglycemic non-ketotic coma, *Arch. Intern. Med.,* **116:**74, 1965.

221. Halmos, P. B., J. K. Nelson, and R. C. Lowry: Hyperosmolar non-ketoacidotic coma in diabetes, *Lancet,* **1:**675, 1966.

222. Jackson, W. P. U., and R. Forman: Hyperosmolar non-ketotic diabetic coma, *Diabetes,* **15:**714, 1966.

223. Fernandez, J. P., J. T. McGinn, and R. S. Hoffman: Cerebral edema from blood-brain glucose differences complicating peritoneal dialysis second membrane syndrome, *N.Y. State J. Med.,* **68:**677, 1968.

224. Hayes, T. M., and C. J. Woods: Unexpected death during treatment of uncomplicated diabetic ketoacidosis, *Br. Med. J.,* **4:**32, 1968.

225. Van Harreveld, A., N. K. Hooper, and J. T. Cusick: Brain electrolytes and cortical impedance, *Am. J. Physiol.,* **201:**139, 1961.

226. Guisado, R., A. I. Arieff, and S. G. Massry: Ef-

fects of glycerol infusion on brain water and electrolytes, *Am. J. Physiol.*, **227**:865, 1974.

227. Arieff, A. I., and C. R. Kleeman: Cerebral edema in diabetic comas. II. Effects of hyperosmolality, hyperglycemia and insulin in diabetic rabbits, *J. Clin. Endocrinol. Metab.*, **38**:1057, 1974.

228. Clements, R. S. Jr., L. D. Prockop, and A. I. Winegrad: Acute cerebral edema during treatment of hyperglycaemia, *Lancet*, **2**:384, 1968.

229. Prockop, L. D.: Hyperglycemia, polyol accumulation, and increased intracranial pressure, *Arch. Neurol.*, **25**:126, 1971.

230. Thurston, J. H., R. E. Hauhart, E. M. Jones, and J. L. Ater: Effects of alloxan diabetes, anti-insulin serum diabetes, and non-diabetic dehydration on brain carbohydrate and energy metabolism in young mice, *J. Biol. Chem.*, **250**:1751, 1975.

231. Stewart, M. A., W. R. Sherman, M. M. Kurien, G. I. Moonsammy, and M. Wisgerhof: Polyol accumulations in nervous tissue of rats with experimental diabetes and galactosaemia, *J. Neurochem.*, **14**:1057, 1967.

232. Gabbay, K. H.: The sorbitol pathway and the complications of diabetes, *N. Engl. J. Med.*, **288**:831, 1973.

233. Seltzer, H. S.: Drug-induced hypoglycemia, *Diabetes*, **21**:955, 1972.

234. Freinkel, N., R. A. Arky, D. L. Singer, A. K. Cohen, S. J. Bleicher, J. B. Anderson, C. K. Silbert, and A. E. Foster: Alcohol hypoglycemia, *Diabetes*, **14**:350, 1965.

235. Chowdhury, F., and S. J. Bleicher: Studies of tumor hypoglycemia, *Metabolism*, **22**:663, 1973.

236. Merimee, T. J., and J. E. Tyson: Stabilization of plasma glycose during fasting, *N. Engl. J. Med.*, **291**:1275, 1974.

237. Anthony, D., S. Dippe, F. D. Hofeldt, J. W. Davis, and P. H. Forsham: Personality disorder and reactive hypoglycemia: A quantitative study, *Diabetes*, **22**:664, 1973.

238. Silverstein, M. N., K. G. Wakim, and R. C. Bahn: Hypoglycemia associated with neoplasia, *Am. J. Med.*, **36**:415, 1964.

239. Duffy, T. E., S. R. Nelson, and O. H. Lowry: Cerebral carbohydrate metabolism during acute hypoxia and recovery, *J. Neurochem.*, **19**:959, 1972.

240. Tarr M., D. Brada, and F. E. Samson, Jr.: Cerebral high energy phosphates during insulin hypoglycemia, *Am. J. Physiol.*, **203**:690, 1962.

241. Ferrendelli, J. A., and M. M. Chang: Brain metabolism during hypoglycemia, *Arch. Neurol.*, **28**:173, 1973.

242. Nemoto E. M., J. T. Hoff, and J. W. Severinghaus: Cerebral lactate metabolism in insulin-induced hypoglycemic dogs, *Physiologist*, **14**:202, 1971.

243. Arieff, A. I., T. Doerner, H. Zelig, and S. G. Massry: Mechanisms of seizures and coma in hypoglycemia: Evidence for a direct effect of insulin on electrolyte transport in brain, *J. Clin. Invest.*, **54**:654, 1974.

244. Cadilhas J., M. Ribstein, and R. Jean: EEG et troubles metaboliques, *Rev. Neurol.*, **100**:270, 1959.

245. Fichman, M. P., H. Vorherr, C. R. Kleeman, and N. Telfer: Diuretic-induced hyponatremia, *Ann. Intern. Med.*, **75**:853, 1971.

246. Lipsmeyer, E., and G. L. Ackerman: Irreversible brain damage after water intoxication, *JAMA*, **196**:286, 1966.

247. Miller, M., and A. Moses: Drug-induced states of impaired water excretion, *Kidney Int.*, **10**:96, 1976.

248. Wright, R.: Overdosing on water, *Newsweek*, March 14, 1977, p. 46.

249. Crumpacker, R. W., and R. L. Kriel: Voluntary water intoxication in normal infants, *Neurology*, **23**:1251, 1973.

250. Mendelson, W. B., and P. C. Deza: Polydipsia, hyponatremia, and seizures in psychotic patients, *J. Nerv. Ment. Dis.*, **162**(2):140, 1976.

251. Raskind, M.: Psychosis, polydipsia, and water intoxication: Report of a fatal case, *Arch. Gen. Psychiatry*, **30**:112, 1974.

252. Demanet, J. C., M. Bennyns, and C. Stevens-Rocmans: Coma due to water intoxication in beer drinkers, *Lancet*, **2**:1115, 1971.

253. Hilden, T., and T. L. Svendsen: Electrolyte disturbances in beer drinkers, *Lancet*, **2**:245, 1975.

254. Arieff, A. I., F. Llach, and S. G. Massry: Neurological manifestations and morbidity of hyponatremia: Correlation with brain water and electrolytes, *Medicine (Baltimore)*, **55**:121, 1976.

255. Bartter, F. C.: Hyper- and hypo-osmolality syndromes, *Am. J. Cardiol.*, **12**:650, 1963.

256. Stormont, J. M., and C. Waterhouse: The genesis of hyponatremia associated with marked overhydration and water intoxication, *Circulation,* **24**:191, 1961.

257. Swanson, A. G., and O. A. Iseri: Acute encephalopathy due to water intoxication, *N. Engl. J. Med.,* **258**:831, 1958.

258. Katzman, R., and H. M. Pappius: Hyponatremia and water intoxication, in *Brain Electrolytes and Fluid Metabolism,* The Williams & Wilkins Company, Baltimore, 1973, p. 291.

259. Helwig, F. C., C. B. Schultz, and D. E. Curry: Water intoxication: Report of a fatal case with clinical, pathological and experimental studies, *JAMA,* **104**:1569, 1935.

260. Wynn, V.: Water intoxication and serum hypotonicity, *Metabolism,* **5**:490, 1956.

261. Rymer, M. M., and R. A. Fishman: Protective adaption of brain to water intoxication, *Arch. Neurol.,* **28**:49, 1973.

262. McCance, R. A.: Experimental sodium chloride deficiency in man, *Proc. R. Soc. London Biol.,* **119**:245, 1936.

263. Weissman, P. N., L. Shenkman, and R. I. Gregerman: Chlorpropamide hyponatremia, *N. Engl. J. Med.,* **284**:65, 1971.

264. Scott, J. C., J. S. Welch, and I. B. Berman: Water intoxication and sodium depletion in surgical patients, *Obstet. Gynecol.,* **26**:168, 1965.

265. Saphir, W.: Chronic hypochloremia simulating psychoneurosis, *JAMA,* **129**:510, 1945.

266. Edelman, I. S., J. Leibman, M. P. O'Meara, and L. W. Birkenfeld: Interrelations between serum sodium concentration, serum osmolarity and total exchangeable sodium, total exchangeable potassium and total body water, *J. Clin. Invest.,* **37**:1236, 1958.

267. Fuisz, R. E.: Hyponatremia, *Medicine (Baltimore),* **42**:149, 1963.

268. DeFronzo, R., M. Goldberg, and Z. S. Agus: Normal diluting capacity in hyponatremic patients, *Ann. Intern. Med.,* **84**:538, 1976.

269. Varavithya, W., and S. Hellerstein: Acute symptomatic hyponatremia, *J. Pediatr.,* **71**:269, 1967.

270. Day, G., I. Radde, J. W. Balfe, and G. W. Chance: Electrolyte abnormalities in very low birthweight infants, *Pediatr. Res.,* **10**:522, 1976.

271. DeTroyer, A., and J. C. Demanet: Clinical, biological and pathogenic features of the syndrome of inappropriate secretion of antidiuretic hormone, *Q. J. Med.,* **45**:521, 1976.

272. Pampiglione, G.: The effect of metabolic disorders on brain activity, *J. R. Coll. Physicians Lond.,* **7**:347, 1973.

273. Holliday, M. A., M. N. Kalayci, and J. Harrah: Factors that limit brain volume changes in response to acute and sustained hyper- and hyponatremia, *J. Clin. Invest.,* **47**:1916, 1968.

274. Dila, C. J., and H. M. Pappius: Cerebral water and electrolytes: An experimental model of inappropriate secretion of antidiuretic hormone, *Arch. Neurol.,* **26**:85, 1972.

275. Wasterlain, C. G., and J. B. Posner: Cerebral edema in water intoxication I. Clinical and chemical observations, *Arch. Neurol.,* **19**:71, 1968.

276. Herschkowitz, N., B. B. McGillivray, and T. N. Cumings: Biochemical and electrophysiological studies in experimental cerebral edema, *Brain,* **88**:557, 1965.

277. Luse, S. A., and B. Harris: Brain ultrastructure in hydration and dehydration, *Arch. Neurol.,* **4**:139, 1961.

278. Wasterlain, C. G., and R. M. Torack: Cerebral edema in water intoxication. II. An ultrastructural study, *Arch. Neurol.,* **19**:79, 1968.

279. Thurston, J. H., R. E. Hauhart, E. M. Jones, and J. L. Ater: Effects of salt and water loading on carbohydrate and energy metabolism and levels of selected amino acids in the brain of young mice, *J. Neurochem.,* **24**:953, 1975.

280. Bennett, J. P., W. J. Logan, and S. H. Snyder: Aminoacids as central nervous transmitters: The influence of ions, aminoacid analogues, and ontogency on transport systems for L-Glutamic and L-Aspartic acids and glycine into central nervous synaptosomes of the rat, *J. Neurochem.,* **21**:1533, 1973.

281. Schultz, S. G., and P. F. Currant: Coupled transport of sodium and organic solute, *Physiol. Rev.,* **50**:637, 1970.

282. Lajtha, A., and H. Sershen: Inhibition of aminoacid uptake by the absence of sodium in slices of brain, *J. Neurochem.,* **24**:667, 1975.

283. Lahiri, S., and A. Lajtha: Cerebral aminoacid transport in vitro. I. Some requirements and

properties of uptake, *J. Neurochem.*, **11**:77, 1964.

284. Schwartz, W. B.: Disorders of fluid, electrolyte and acid-base balance: Hyponatremia, in P. B. Beeson and W. McDermott (eds.), *Textbook of Medicine*, W. B. Saunders Company, Philadelphia, 1975, pp. 1581–1584.

285. Welt, L. G.: Disorders of fluids and electrolytes: Comments on correction of hypo- and hypernatremia, in M. M. Wintrobe, G. W. Thorn, R. D. Adams, E. Braunwald, K. J. Isselbacher, and R. G. Petersdorf (eds.), *Harrison's Principles of Internal Medicine*, McGraw-Hill Book Company, New York, 1974, pp. 1348–1349.

286. Luttrell, C. N., and L. Finberg: Hemorrhagic encephalopathy induced by hypernatremia. I. Clinical, laboratory and pathological observations, *AMA Arch. Neurol. Psychiat.*, **81**:424, 1959.

287. Mattar, J. A., M. H. Weil, H. Shubin, and L. Stein: Cardiac arrest in the critically ill, *Am. J. Med.*, **56**:162, 1974.

288. Simmons, M. A., E. W. Adcock, H. Bard, and F. C. Battaglia: Hypernatremia and intracranial hemorrhage in neonates, *N. Engl. J. Med.*, **291**:6, 1974.

289. DeVillota, E. D., J. M. Cavanilles, L. Stein, H. Shubin, and M. H. Weil: Hyperosmolar crisis following infusion of hypertonic sodium chloride for purposes of therapeutic abortion, *Am. J. Med.*, **55**:116, 1973.

290. Hantman, D., B. Rossier, R. Zohlman, and R. Schrier: Rapid correction of hyponatremia in the syndrome of inappropriate secretion of antidiuretic hormone: An alternative treatment to hypertonic saline, *Ann. Intern. Med.*, **78**:870, 1973.

291. Ross, E. J., and S. B. M. Christie: Hypernatremia, *Medicine (Baltimore)*, **48**:441, 1969.

292. Zierler, K. L.: Hyperosmolarity in adults: A critical review, *J. Chronic Dis.*, **7**:1, 1958.

293. Park, R., R. Guisado, and A. I. Arieff: Nutrient deficiencies in man: Water, in *CRC Handbook of Nutrition and Food*, CRC Press, West Palm Beach, Fla., in press.

294. Finberg, L.: Hypernatremic (hypertonic) dehydration in infants, *N. Engl. J. Med.*, **289**:196, 1973.

295. Rapoport, S.: Hyperosmolarity and hyperelectrolytemia in pathological conditions of childhood, *Am. J. Dis. Child.*, **74**:682, 1947.

296. Elton, N. W., W. J. Elton, and J. P. Nazareno: Pathology of acute salt poisoning in infants, *Am. J. Clin. Pathol.*, **39**:252, 1963.

297. Finberg, L., J. Kiley, and C. N. Luttrell: Mass accidental salt poisoning in infancy: A study of a hospital disaster, *JAMA*, **184**:187, 1963.

298. Colle, E., E. Ayoub, and R. Raile: Hypertonic dehydration (hypernatremia): The role of feedings high in solutes, *Pediatrics*, **22**:5, 1958.

299. Popovtzer, M. M., W. F. Pinggera, J. H. Holmes, C. G. Halgrimson, and T. E. Starzl: Hypernatremia, *Arch. Intern. Med.*, **127**:1129, 1971.

300. Morris-Jones, P. H., I. B. Houston, and R. C. Evans: Prognosis of the neurological complications of acute hypernatremia, *Lancet*, **2**:1385, 1967.

301. Banister, A., S. Siddiqi, and G. W. Hatcher: Treatment of hypernatremic dehydration in infancy, *Arch. Dis. Child.*, **50**:179, 1975.

302. Bruck, E., G. Abal, and T. Aceto: Pathogenesis and pathophysiology of hypertonic dehydration with diarrhea, *Am. J. Dis. Child.*, **115**:122, 1968.

303. Finberg, L.: Pathogenesis of lesions in the nervous system in hypernatremic states. I. Clinical observations of infants, *Pediatrics*, **23**:40, 1959.

304. Macaulay, D., and M. Watson: Hypernatremia as a cause of brain damage, *Arch. Dis. Child.*, **42**:485, 1967.

305. Knowles, H. C.: Hypernatremia, *Metabolism*, **5**:508, 1956.

306. Skinner, A. L., and F. C. Moll: Hypernatremia accompanying infant diarrhea, *Am. J. Dis. Child.*, **92**:562, 1956.

307. Katzman, R., and H. M. Pappius: Hypernatremia and hyperosmolarity, in *Brain Electrolytes and Fluid Metabolism*, The Williams & Wilkins Company, Baltimore, 1973, pp. 278–290.

308. Stevenson, R. E., and F. P. Bowyer: Hyperglycemia with hyperosmolar dehydration in non diabetic infants, *J. Pediatr.*, **77**:818, 1970.

309. Hogan, G. R., P. R. Dodge, S. R. Gill, S. Master, and J. F. Sotos: Pathogenesis of seizures occurring during restoration of plasma tonicity to normal in animals previously chronically hypernatremic, *Pediatrics*, **43**:54, 1969.

310. Finberg, L., and H. E. Harrison: Hypernatremia in infants: An evaluation of the clinical and biochemical findings accompanying this state, *Pediatrics*, **16**:1, 1955.

311. Toor, M., E. Wertheimer, S. Massry, and J. B.

Rosenfeld: Development and correction of hyper-natremia during a two hour hike at 42°C at Sodom, *Harefuah*, **57**:244, 1959.

312. Levine, J. A.: Heatstroke in the aged, *Am. J. Med.*, **47**:251, 1969.

313. Johnston, J. G., and W. O. Robertson: Fatal ingestion of table salt by an adult, *West. J. Med.*, **126**:141, 1977.

314. Nellis, G. F.: The hyperosmolar non-ketoacidotic diabetic syndrome: A clinical study, Drukkerij Van Denderen B. V., Groningen, Amsterdam, 1975, pp. 203–211.

315. Sparacio, R. R., B. Anziska, and H. S. Schutta: Hypernatremia and chorea: A report of two cases, *Neurology*, **26**:46, 1976.

316. Lockwood, A. H.: Acute and chronic hyperosmolality: Effects on cerebral amino acids and energy metabolism, *Arch. Neurol.*, **32**:62, 1975.

317. Fishman, R. A., and P. H. Chan: Changes in ammonia and amino acid metabolism induced by hyperosmolality in vivo and in vitro, *Trans. Am. Neurol. Assoc.*, **101**:1, 1976.

318. Kregenow, F. M.: The response of duck erythrocytes to hypertonic media, *J. Gen. Physiol.*, **58**:396, 1971.

319. Shank, R. P., and C. F. Baxter: Metabolism of glucose, amino acids, and some related metabolites in the brain of toads (Bufo boreas) adapted to fresh water or hyperosmotic environments, *J. Neurochem.*, **21**:301, 1973.

320. Cameron, J. M., and A. D. Dayan: Association of brain damage with therapeutic abortion induced by amniotic-fluid replacement: Report of two cases, *Br. Med. J.*, **1**:1010, 1966.

321. Andersson, B.: Polydipsia caused by intrahypothalamic injections of hypertonic NaCl solutions, *Experimentia*, **8**:157, 1952.

322. Thornborough, J. R., S. S. Passo, and A. B. Rothballer: Receptors in cerebral circulation affecting sodium excretion in the cat, *Am. J. Physiol.*, **225**:138, 1973.

323. Hickey, R. C., and K. Hare: The renal excretion of chloride and water in diabetes insipidus, *J. Clin. Invest.*, **23**:768, 1944.

324. Gauer, O. H., and J. P. Henry: Circulatory basis of fluid volume control, *Physiol. Rev.*, **43**:423, 1963.

325. Henry, J. P., P. D. Gupta, J. P. Meehan, R. Sinclair, and L. Share: The role of afferents from the low pressure system in the release of anti-diuretic hormone during non-hypotensive hemmorrhage, *Can. J. Physiol. Pharmacol.*, **46**:287, 1968.

326. Bass, D., C. Kleeman, M. Quinn, A. Henschel, and A. Hegnauer: Mechanisms of acclimatization to heat in man, *Medicine (Baltimore)*, **34**:323, 1955.

327. Berliner, R.: Outline of renal physiology, in M. Strauss and L. Welt (eds.), *Diseases of the Kidney*, Little, Brown and Company, Boston, 1971, pp. 31–86.

328. Zuker, I. H., and G. Kaley: Natriuresis induced by intracarotid infusion of hypertonic sodium chloride, *Am. J. Physiol.*, **230**:427, 1976.

329. Fitzsimmons, J. T.: Thirst, *Physiol. Rev.*, **52**:468, 1972.

330. Rogers, P. W., and N. A. Kurtzman: Renal failure: Uncontrollable thirst and hyper reninemia: Cessation of thirst with bilateral nephrectomy, *JAMA*, **225**:1236, 1973.

331. Fitzsimmons, J. T.: The role of a renal thirst factor in drinking induced by extracellular stimuli, *J. Physiol. (London)*, **201**:349, 1969.

332. Fitzsimmons, J. T., and B. J. Simons: The effect on drinking in the rat of intravenous infusion of angiotensin given alone or in combination, *J. Physiol. (London)*, **203**:45, 1969.

333. Simpson, J. B., A. N. Epstein, and J. S. Camardo: Dose-response analysis of angiotensin-induced drinking at subfornical organ (SFO) and third ventricle, *Physiologist*, **18**:391, 1975.

334. Hoffman, W. E., and M. I. Phillips: Blockage of blood pressure and drinking responses to angiotensin by anterior third ventricle obstruction, *Fed. Proc.*, **34**:374, 1975.

335. Fitzsimmons, J. T.: Physiological basis of thirst, *Kidney Int.*, **10**:3, 1976.

336. Simpson, J. B., A. N. Epstein, and J. S. Camardo: Ablation or competitive blockade of some subfornical organ (SFO) prevents thirst of intravenous angiotensin, *Fed. Proc.*, **24**:374, 1975.

337. Stevenson, J. A.: Neural control of food and water intake, in W. Haymaker, E. Anderson, and W. H. Nauta (eds.), *The Hypothalamus*, Charles C Thomas, Publisher, Springfield, Ill., 1969, pp. 524–621.

338. Fitzsimmons, J. T.: The effect on drinking of peptide precursors and of shorter chain peptide

fragments of angiotensin II injected into the rat's diencephalon, *J. Physiol. (London)*, **214**:295, 1971.

339. Ganten, D., J. Marquez, P. Granter, K. Hayduk, K. Karsunky, R. Boucher, and J. Genest: Renin in dog brain, *Am. J. Physiol.*, **221**:1733, 1971.

340. Fischer-Farrero, C., V. Nahmod, D. Goldstein, and S. Finkielman: Angiotensin and renin in rat and dog brain, *J. Exp. Med.*, **133**:353, 1971.

341. Fitzsimmons, J. T., and P. E. Setler: The relative importance of central nervous catecholaminergic and cholinergic mechanisms in drinking in response to angiotensin and other thirst stimuli, *J. Physiol. (London)*, **250**:613, 1975.

342. Ramwell, P. W., and J. E. Shaw: Biological significance of the prostaglandins, *Recent Prog. Horm. Res.*, **26**:139, 1970.

343. Berl, T., R. J. Anderson, G. Aisenbrey, S. Linas, and R. Schrier: On the mechanism of polyuria in potassium depletion: The role of polydipsia, *Clin. Res.*, **25**(2):136A, 1977.

344. Leksell, L.: Influence of prostaglandin E_1 on cerebral mechanisms involved in the control of fluid balance, *Acta Physiol. Scand.*, **98**:85, 1976.

345. DeRubertis, F. R., M. F. Michelis, and B. B. Davis: "Essential" hypernatremia, *Arch. Intern. Med.*, **134**:889, 1974.

346. Travis, L. B., W. F. Dodge, J. D. Waggener, and C. Kashemsant: Defective thirst mechanisms secondary to a hypothalamic lesion, *J. Pediatr.*, **70**:915, 1967.

347. Golonka, J. E., and J. A. Richardson: Postconcussive hypoerosmolality and deficient thirst, *Am. J. Med.*, **48**:261, 1970.

348. Sridhar, C. B., G. D. Calvert, and H. K. Ibbertson: Syndrome of hypernatremia, hypodipsia, and partial diabetes insipidus: A new interpretation, *J. Clin. Endocrinol. Metab.*, **38**:890, 1974.

349. Kleeman, C. R., and R. Cutler: The neurohypophysis, *Annu. Rev. Physiol.*, **25**:385, 1963.

350. Hays, R. M.: Vasopressin, *N. Engl. J. Med.*, **295**:659, 1976.

351. Archer R., J. Chauvet, and G. Olivry: Sur l'existence d'une hormone unique neurohypophysaire: Relation entre l'oxytocin, la vasopressine et la protein de Van Dyke extradites de la neurohypophyse du boenf, *Biochem. Biophys. Acta.*, **22**:428, 1956.

352. Zimmerman, E. A., and A. G. Robinson: Hypothalamic nuclei secreting vasopressin and neurophysin, *Kidney Int.*, **10**:12, 1976.

353. Zimmerman, E. A., P. W. Carmel, M. K. Husain, M. Ferin, M. Tannenbaum, A. G. Frantz, and A. G. Robinson: Vasopressin and neurophysin: High concentrations in monkey hypophyseal portal blood, *Science*, **182**:925, 1973.

354. Watkins, W. B., P. Schwabedal, and R. Bock: Immunological chemical demonstration of a CRF associated neurophysin in the external zone of the rat median eminence, *Cell Tissue Res.*, **152**:411, 1974.

355. Hedge, G. A., M. B. Yates, R. Marcus, and F. E. Yates: Site of action of vasopressin causing corticotrophin release, *Endocrinology*, **79**:328, 1966.

356. Yates, F. E., S. M. Russell, M. F. Dallman, G. A. Hedge, S. M. McCann, and A. P. S. Dhariwal: Potentiation by vasopressin of corticotrophin release induced by corticotrophin releasing factor, *Endocrinology*, **88**:3, 1971.

357. Scott, D. E., G. P. Kozlowski, and M. N. Sheridan: Scanning electroenmicroscopy in the ultra structural analysis of the mammalian cerebral ventricular system, *Int. Rev. Cytol.*, **37**:349, 1974.

358. Vorherr, H., W. B. Bradbury, M. Hoghoughi, and C. R. Kleeman: Antidiuretic hormone in cerebrospinal fluid during endogenous and exogenous changes in its blood level, *Endocrinology*, **73**:246, 1968.

359. Van Wimersma Greidanus, T. J. B., B. Bohus, and D. De Weid: The role of vasopressin in memory process, *Prog. Brain Res.*, **42**:135, 1975.

360. Douglas, W. W.: How do neurones secrete peptides? Exocytosis and its consequences including "synaptic vesicle" formation in the hypothalamoneurohypophyseal system, *Prog. Brain Res.*, **39**:21, 1973.

361. Sachs, H. L., L. Share, J. Osinchak, and A. Carpie: Capacity of the neurohypophysis to release vasopressin, *Endocrinology*, **81**:775, 1967.

362. Verney, E. B.: The antidiuretic hormone and the factors which determine its release, *Proc. R. Soc. London Biol.*, **135**:25, 1947.

363. Robertson, G. L., E. A. Mahr, S. Athar, and T. Sinha: Development and clinical application of a new method for the radioimmunoassay of arginine vasopressin in human plasma, *J. Clin. Invest.*, **52**:2340, 1973.

364. Beardswell, C. G.: Radioimmunoassay of arginine vasopressin in human plasma, *J. Clin. Endocrinol. Metab.*, **33**:254, 1971.

365. Shimamoto, K., T. Murase, and T. Yamaji: A heterologous radioimmunoassay for arginine vasopressin, *J. Lab. Clin. Med.*, **87**:338, 1976.

366. Robertson, G. L., R. L. Shelton, and S. Athar: The osmoregulation of vasopressin, *Kidney Int.*, **10**:25, 1976.

367. Dunn, F. L., T. J. Brennan, A. E. Nelson, and G. L. Robertson: The role of blood osmolality and volume in regulating vasopressin secretion in the rat, *J. Clin. Invest.*, **52**:3212, 1973.

368. Goetz, K. L., G. C. Bond, and W. E. Smith: Effect of moderate hemorrhage in humans on plasma ADH and renin, *Proc. Soc. Exp. Biol. Med.*, **147**:277, 1974.

369. Hollingshead, W.: The interphase of diabetes insipidus, *Mayo Clin. Proc.*, **39**:92, 1964.

370. Gastineau, C., A. Frethem, H. Svien, G. Magid, and T. Kearns, Hyponatremia from section of pituitary stalk for diabetic retinopathy, *Mayo Clin. Proc.*, **42**:400, 1967.

371. Hollingshead, W. H.: The interphase of diabetes insipidus, *Mayo Clin. Proc.*, **39**:92, 1964.

372. Randall, R. V., E. C. Clark, H. W. J. Dodge, and L. G. Love: Polyuria after operation for tumors in the region of the hypophysis and hypothalamus, *J. Clin. Endocrinol.*, **20**:1614, 1966.

373. Berl, T., R. J. Anderson, K. M. McDonald, and R. W. Schrier: Clinical disorders of water metabolism, *Kidney Int.*, **10**:117, 1976.

374. Puschett, J. B., and M. Goldberg: Endocrinopathy associated with pineal tumor, *Ann. Intern. Med.*, **69**:203, 1969.

375. Duchen, G. W.: Metastatic carcinoma in the pituitary gland and hypothalamus, *J. Path. Bacteriol.*, **91**:347, 1966.

376. Thomas, W. C.: Diabetes insipidus, *J. Clin. Endocrinol. Metab.*, **17**:565, 1957.

377. Arduino, F., F. P. J. Ferraz, and J. Rodrigues: Antidiuretic action of chlorpropamide in idiopathic diabetes insipidus, *J. Clin. Endocrinol. Metab.*, **26**:1325, 1966.

378. Vallet, H. L., M. Prasad, and R. B. Goldbloom: Chlorpropamide treatment of diabetes insipidus in children, *Pediatrics*, **45**:246, 1970.

379. Wales, J. K., and T. R. Fraser: The clinical use of chlorpropamide in diabetes insipidus, *Acta Endocrinol. (Kbh)*, **68**:725, 1971.

380. Ingelfinger, J., and R. M. Hays: Evidence that chlorpropamide and vasopressin share a common site of action, *J. Clin. Endocrinol. Metab.*, **29**:738, 1969.

381. Miller, M., and A. M. Moses: Potentiation of vasopressin action by chlorpropamide in vivo, *Endocrinology*, **86**:1024, 1970.

382. Rydin, H., and E. B. Verney: The inhibition of water diuresis by emotional stress and muscular exercise, *J. Exp. Physiol.*, **27**:343, 1938.

383. Moses, A. M., M. Miller, and D. Streeten: Quantitative influence of blood volume expansion on the osmotic threshold for vasopressin release, *J. Clin. Endocrinol. Metab.*, **27**:655, 1967.

384. Schwartz, W. B., W. Bennett, S. Curelop, and F. C. Bartter: Syndrome of renal sodium loss and hyponatremia probably resulting from inappropriate secretion of antidiuretic hormone, *Am. J. Med.*, **23**:529, 1957.

385. Utiger, R. D.: Inappropriate antidiuresis and carcinoma of the lung: Vasopressin in tumor extracts by immunoassay, *J. Clin. Endocrinol. Metab.*, **26**:970, 1966.

386. Marks, L. J., B. Berde, L. A. Klein, J. Roth, S. R. Goonan, D. Blumen, and D. C. Nabseth: Inappropriate vasopressin secretion and carcinoma of the pancreas, *Am. J. Med.*, **45**:967, 1968.

387. Voherr, H., S. Massry, R. Utiger, and C. R. Kleeman: Antidiuretic principle in malignant tumor extracts from patients with inappropriate ADH syndrome, *J. Clin. Endocrin. Metab.*, **28**:162, 1968.

388. George, J. M., C. C. Capen, and A. S. Phillips: Biosynthesis of vasopressin in vitro and ultrastructure of a bronchogenic carcinoma, *J. Clin. Invest.*, **51**:141, 1972.

389. Voherr, H., S. Massry, R. Fallet, L. Kaplan, and C. R. Kleeman: Antidiuretic principle in tuberculous lung tissue of a patient with pulmonary tuberculosis and hyponatremia, *Ann. Intern. Med.*, **72**:383, 1970.

390. Bartter, F. C., and W. B. Schwartz: The syndrome of inappropriate secretion of antidiuretic hormone, *Am. J. Med.*, **42**:790, 1967.

391. White, M. G., and C. D. Fetner: Treatment of the syndrome of inappropriate secretion of antidi-

uretic hormone with lithium carbonate, *N. Engl. J. Med.*, **292:**915, 1975.

392. De Trover, A., and J. C. Demanet: Correction of antidiuresis by demeclocycline, *N. Engl. J. Med.*, **292:**915, 1975.

393. Wilkins, L., and C. P. Richter: Great craving for salt by children with cortico adrenal insufficiency, *JAMA*, **114:**866, 1940.

394. Richter, C. P.: Total self regulatory functions in animals and human beings, *Harvey Lectures*, **38:**63, 1943.

395. Richter, C. P.: Salt taste thresholds of normal and adrenalectomized rats, *Endocrinology*, **24:**367, 1939.

396. Bricker, N. S., W. Guild, J. Reardan, and J. Merrill: Observations on the functional capacity of the denervated homotransplanted kidney with parallel studies on the identical twin donor, *J. Clin. Invest.*, **35:**1364, 1956.

397. Kamm, D. E., and N. G. Levinsky: The mechanism of denervation natriuresis, *J. Clin. Invest.*, **44:**93, 1965.

398. Pierce, J. W., and H. Sonnenberg: Effects of spinal section and renal denervation on the renal response to blood volume expansion, *Can. J. Physiol. Pharmacol.*, **43:**211, 1965.

399. Gilmore, J. P., and W. M. Daggett: Response of chronic cardiac denervated dog to acute volume expansion, *Am. J. Physiol.*, **210:**509, 1966.

400. Cort, J. H.: *Electrolytes, Fluid Dynamics and the Nervous System*, Academic Press, Inc., New York, 1965.

401. Smith, H. W.: Salt and water volume receptors: An exercise in physiologic apologetics, *Am. J. Med.*, **23:**623, 1957.

402. Schrier, R. W., and H. E. De Wardner: Tubular reabsorption of sodium ion: Influence of factors other than aldosterone and glomerular filtration rate, *N. Engl. J. Med.*, **285:**1231, 1971.

403. Andersson, B., M. F. Dallman, and K. Olsson: Evidence for a hypothalamic control of renal sodium excretion, *Acta Physiol. Scand.*, **75:**496, 1969.

404. Cort, J. H.: Saluretic activity of blood during carotid occlusion, *Am. J. Physiol.*, **215:**921, 1968.

405. Cort, J. H., and B. Lichardus: The natriuretic activity of jugular vein blood during carotid occlusion, *Physiol. Bohemoslov.*, **12:**497, 1963.

406. Steinmetz, P. R., and J. E. Kiley: Renal tubular necrosis following lesions of the brain, *Am. J. Med.*, **29:**268, 1960.

407. Sitprija, V., and R. Tangcha: Renal failure in intracranial lesions: Evidence of function of juxtamedullary nephrons, *Am. J. Med.*, **54:**241, 1973.

408. Clute, K. F., and G. W. Fitzgerald: Anuria following electroshock therapy, *Can. Med. Assoc. J.*, **59:**426, 1948.

409. Goodman, L.: Lower nephron nephrosis following electroconvulsive therapy: Report of two fatalities, *J. Nerv. Ment. Dis.*, **112:**130, 1950.

410. Grossman, R. A., R. W. Hamilton, B. W. Morse, A. A. Penn, and M. Goldberg: Non traumatic rhabdomyolysis and acute renal failure, *N. Engl. J. Med.*, **291:**807, 1974.

27

The effects of acute and prolonged fasting and refeeding on water, electrolyte, and acid-base metabolism

ERNST J. DRENICK

INTRODUCTION

Throughout history, people have fasted voluntarily for a variety of reasons. Ritual fasts, intended to "cleanse," have been popular in many lands and cultures. Even today, fasting is practiced by religious and various faddist groups, occasionally with disastrous results. Fasts have been used as a form of political protest by prominent persons. While generally considered painful and cruel, fasting is actually not too difficult to tolerate, as long as water is available, because hunger subsides within a few days. Only rarely have prolonged voluntary fasts been fatal, as happened, for instance, with Terence MacSwiney, an Irish patriot, who fasted for 74 days. Capitalizing upon the popular concept of the cruel tortures resulting from fasting, a number of "professional" fasters exhibited themselves in county fairs around the turn of the century. The earlier scientific observations were carried out in such "hunger artists," and, among them, the classic and most detailed description of such an individual, who fasted 31 days, led to the publication of a 400-page volume by Benedict in 1915 (1).

The privations suffered by survivors from ships or aircraft during World War II prompted investigations into water and minimum food requirements. Short fasts under variable conditions, with and without water or salt, in cold or hot environments, with and without exercise, were carefully studied in the succeeding years. Fasting was suggested as a suitable treatment for obesity by Folin and Denis (2) in 1915, and numerous writers have made similar recommendations since then. Fasting was thought to be beneficial in the therapy of epilepsy, and careful studies of fasts in lean epileptic children were published by Gamble et al. in 1923 (3). More recently, in Russia, prolonged fasts were considered beneficial in the treatment of mental illnesses.

The bulk of information regarding prolonged fasting was gathered in obese subjects when it became apparent that fasts of several months could be tolerated without serious difficulties (4). Many physiologic changes were observed, and studies in lean volunteers have shown that the effects of fasting are quite similar in obese and normal-weight subjects.

To be familiar with the physiology of fasting is useful because obese subjects are now commonly treated by fasting and because unintentional privation of food is encountered not too rarely in elderly disabled patients.

Acute fasting of 48 to 72 h, results primarily in water and electrolyte loss. With prolonged fasts, the consequences of tissue catabolism and the ketoacidosis become more prominent, and, eventually, clinically significant depletion phenomena will appear. The two phases are not clearly separable and can be discussed more logically as one continuing process. Unless specifically stated, the data presented relate to fasting in the presence of an ample water intake.

This chapter is concerned primarily with mineral and water metabolism in fasting. Observations of alterations in serum levels and changes in excretion have provided most of the data. In fasting, the kidneys are the main avenue for disposal of various solutes, because fecal elimination in many subjects ceases altogether. Sweat glands are not an important organ in this regard, because, during fasting, sweat production is reduced and mineral content of sweat decreases. While respiration aids in the control of the acidosis and in the disposal of water, the expired air is not a vehicle for the excretion of significant amounts of acetone.

ENERGY SOURCES AND REQUIREMENTS

To explain the mineral and fluid balances in fasting, it is necessary first to know the quantity and kind of body tissues consumed. To do this accurately, nitrogen excretion has to be measured to permit calculation of protein loss. Total calorie consumption is determined by calorimetry. Total calories minus protein calories reveals the number of fat calories plus carbohydrate calories consumed. The measurement of the respiratory quotients permits the further breakdown into the fat and carbohydrate calories. In long fasts, the contribution of glycogen is insignificant.

Most of the more reliable energy balance data during fasting were obtained within the confines of metabolic balance wards. Reasonable daily energy expenditures during fasting have been found to amount to about 1800 calories for lean subjects (1) and 2500 calories for the obese (130 to 150 kg) (5). The data below apply to subjects in these weight categories, but they are approximations, limited in accuracy by the diversity of weight and physical activity levels.

Figure 27-1 demonstrates the daily energy expenditures for lean and obese subjects and the proportional contribution of calories by glycogen, fat, and protein.

Energy requirements decrease by 25 to 30 percent in the course of 3 to 4 weeks of fasting. This is brought about by a decrease in voluntary activity, a fall in basal metabolism, and, with the diminishing weight burden, a lowered calorie cost of physical effort. Not only the total amount of endogenous fuel consumed but also its relative composition changes during the first month's

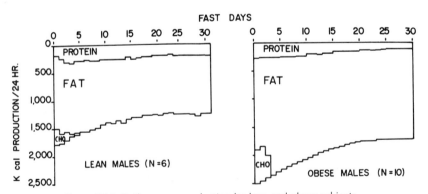

Figure 27-1. Daily energy production by lean and obese subjects during a 1-month fast. The contribution of calories from carbohydrate ceases after a few days while fat and protein calories diminish with the length of the fast.

fasting. Glycogen stores supply a significant portion of the calorie requirements during only the first 3 days. Protein catabolism rises initially and then decreases slowly over a period of 3 to 4 weeks to remain virtually constant subsequently at a level of about 22 to 25 g/day.

If small amounts of protein are then fed, the negative nitrogen balance can be eliminated over a period of 3 weeks. As little as 55 g/day has been found sufficient to produce this effect (5), stimulating the introduction of "modified fasting" as a treatment modality (6, 7).

Fat consumption reaches a peak of about 150 g in the lean and 250 g in the obese during the first week and then declines gradually. After 3 to 4 weeks of fasting, fat utilization in the obese subject seems to stabilize.

TOTAL BODY WATER BALANCE

In theory, the determination of body water loss in fasting could be carried out in a number of ways which are less cumbersome than via the indirect approach of nitrogen balances and calorimetry; it should be possible to analyze body compartments before and after weight loss, utilizing isotope or dye dilution, body radiation counting chambers, or densitometry. However, these methods have proved very unreliable, particularly when applied in short fasting periods. With deuterium and tritium dilutions, for example, the calculated body water losses were found to be greater than total weight loss in a number of instances (8, 9).

Although balance studies also have their uncertainties and inaccuracies, these studies have provided the most reliable data regarding body water loss. Figure 27-2 illustrates daily total weight loss during 1 month's fasting for groups of lean and obese subjects. If the combined weights of anhydrous endogenous nutrients consumed are subtracted from total weight loss, the difference represents weight of lost body water with its solutes contained in it. For a group of lean subjects, this total body water loss amounted to 7.1 L and for an obese group to 11.8 L in the course of a 1-month fast.

In lean subjects the rate of body water loss is highest in the first 5 days; it diminishes rapidly, and after 10 days a fairly stable average loss is maintained, though fluctuations from one day to the next can be substantial. The general pattern

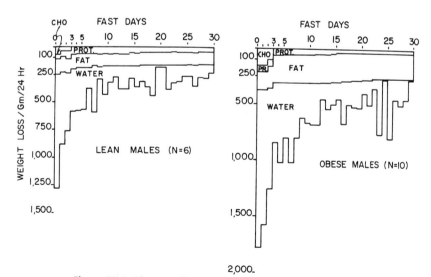

Figure 27-2. The contribution to daily and total weight loss by water loss and consumption of anhydrous endogenous nutrients during fasting.

of water loss in the obese is similar but quantitatively larger.

EXTRACELLULAR FLUID

By far the greatest part, probably two-thirds, of the early water loss elicited by fasting originates in the extracellular compartment, including the vascular space and the lumen of the gastrointestinal tract. Accordingly, the preexisting size of this compartment will, in large measure, determine the magnitude of the early weight loss. In most healthy lean individuals, extracellular fluid (ECF) volume is a fairly constant fraction of body weight, and acute weight loss with fasting is proportional to initial body weight. In obese patients, ECF contributes a much less constant fraction to body weight; body size, however, is not the only factor for obese patients. Water retention, in the absence of congestive heart failure, is a common phenomenon in the obese, and the early weight losses seem influenced by the degree of prior water retention. While very severely overweight subjects usually retain more water, this is not always the case.

The loss of volume from the vascular compartment in lean subjects seems to be limited to the first 10 days of fasting but may reach approximately 20 percent of the original plasma volume. In absolute figures, this represents a fall of the plasma volume from 2800 mL initially to 2300 mL. In obese subjects the fall in plasma volume ceases after 2 weeks of fasting. In three different studies, the mean decrement in plasma volumes was found to range from 400 to 660 mL. Basal plasma volumes in the obese tend to be greater than in lean subjects, so that although of the same magnitude as in normal-weight subjects, the proportional decrease is considerably less in the obese than in the lean (12 to 20 percent).

Various methods, some direct, some derived from electrolyte loss, have been employed to determine compartmental fluid changes. All have great handicaps, and as a result the published values vary greatly. Sodium loss as an indirect measure of extracellular water loss in acute fasting cannot be used with too much confidence, because in acidosis sodium may be mobilized from bone or even lean tissue and lead to erroneously high estimates of ECF loss. In the later phase of fasting, when sodium excretion is largely blocked, extracellular water may be cleared while the sodium originally contained in it is simultaneously shifted into cells or into bone.

Chloride is considered a better indicator of changes in the ECF compartment, and indeed, sodium loss is considerably greater than chloride loss. With chloride excretion as the basis of calculation, lean males were found to lose an average of 1.6 L in the first 2 days and a total of 1.9 L of ECF within 5 days of fasting (range 1.2 to 2.7 L) (10). Using sodium loss as a measure, a fall of 2.5 L in ECF in 6 days of fasting was calculated by Gamble (11). A 1.0-L fall in 5 days was found by another writer for 12 males in whom thiocyanate space was measured (12). In yet another study of lean subjects fasting 10 days, a 3.3-L fall in ECF was found on the basis of direct fluid balance measurements (13).

ECF loss within the first 15 days of fasting in nonedematous obese patients amounted to 4.7 L if calculated on the basis of sodium excretion and 3.6 L when based on chloride excretion. In edematous obese subjects, as much as 8.3 L was lost from the ECF compartment within 15 days and before sodium excretion ceased. Subsequently, despite virtually complete sodium conservation, the remaining edema continued to recede gradually.

While the magnitude of ECF loss in the latter stages of prolonged fasting is small or nil in nonedematous subjects, estimates would suggest that in edematous obese patients any weight loss in excess of 450 g/day represents ECF loss. On a theoretical basis, there is actually some evidence for the belief that in lean subjects ECF, relative to the diminishing size of the remaining body mass, may slowly increase. Total body tissue mass continues to decrease while total body sodium is maintained at a constant level. Therefore, in order to preserve stable electrolyte concentrations in plasma and interstitial fluid, the fluid compartment may have to expand. Careful balance measurements by Benedict seem to support this hypothesis. In his study, a slightly positive water balance relative to the size of the residual tissues was shown after the eighth day of fasting. Whether this relative increase in body water content involves the intracellular as well as the interstitial fluid compartment is uncertain.

INTRACELLULAR WATER

Intracellular water is liberated from many tissues as a result of consumption of glycogen and body protein stores.

Glycogen is present primarily in liver and muscle. The liver contains about 200 g, laid down with three times this amount of water. With fasting, nearly 60 percent of this glycogen store is expended in the first 2 to 3 days (14), releasing about 400 mL of water. Muscle glycogen content decreases to one-half normal within 2 days. Assuming that 1 kg of wet muscle contains 15 g of glycogen and that the average muscle mass of a 70-kg human amounts to 35 kg, then another 600 to 700 mL of glycogen-bound water is made available to the body pool during the first 2 to 3 days of fasting.

The oxidation of protoplasmic protein releases bound intracellular water incidental to its oxida-

tion in a ratio of 3 g of water for each 1 g of protein. The daily consumption of protein in lean subjects during the first few days of fasting follows a constant pattern. The same amount of nitrogen is excreted on the first fast day as on the last day of food intake. Protein catabolism as measured by nitrogen excretion increases slightly on day 2 and reaches a peak of about 12 g, equal to 75 g of protein, on the third or fourth day. Subsequently, protein sparing becomes increasingly effective, and after 4 weeks of fasting nitrogen excretion declines to a stable minimum of about 7 g/day. Figure 27-3 illustrates the cumulative nitrogen losses for obese subjects with corresponding intracellular water release. Protein catabolism and, therefore, cell water losses are lower in females, explaining, at least in part, the fact that females lose weight less rapidly than males.

In all fasting subjects, protein catabolism tends to rise and diminish in the same pattern, but protein sparing in the obese improves to a greater extent throughout the first month, and, overall, less protein is catabolized in the obese than in lean subjects. After the first month nitrogen excretion continues at a constant rate from day to day, even if fasting periods are extended to 4

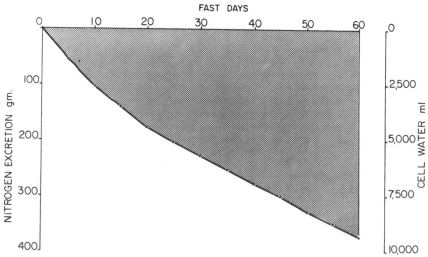

Figure 27-3. Total cumulative nitrogen losses during 2 months of fasting. Cell water loss is derived from nitrogen loss by multiplication with a factor of 26. Loss rates diminish progressively during the first month but are stable thereafter.

months. Daily nitrogen losses for obese males average 3 to 4 g after the first 30 fast days, and the rate of release of cellular water is maintained at a constant rate. Extremely obese subjects excrete more nitrogen, but the correlation with degree of overweight is not linear. A subject weighing twice as much as another loses only about 30 percent more nitrogen during the first month of fasting. The differences in protein catabolism, then, are not a major factor in determining the rate of weight loss or the extent of water loss in different subjects.

In addition to bound intracellular fluid, a certain volume of water is produced daily during fasting from the oxidation of endogenous food components. For practical purposes, these nutrients are triglyceride and protein. The oxidation of 1 g of protein generates 0.41 g of water. The measurement of excreted nitrogen permits precise determination of oxidative water derived from protein catabolism. The differences between lean and obese subjects are relatively insignificant in this regard. Within the first month of fasting the oxidation of an average 1200 g of dry protein adds about 500 mL to the available pool of body water.

The amount of sugar oxidized is insignificant. The oxidation of glycogen from muscle and liver stores involves approximately 350 g, producing 175 mL of water in the first 2 days.

Oxidation of fat remains important in generating newly formed water, as a progressively larger proportion of the energy requirements during fasting is met by triglyceride. Oxidation of 1 g produces 1.07 g of water. An average lean male who consumes 3600 g of his endogenous fat within 31 days of fasting will produce almost 4000 mL of exodative water. During a 24-h period in a lean fasting subject, this source adds approximately 150 mL of water to the body pool. This quantity falls to about 120 mL after 2 weeks and remains stable for the remainder of the month.

In an obese subject the quantity of fat consumed is even higher, because total energy expenditure and the proportion of fat in the fuel mixture are greater. A 2250-cal daily energy expenditure, provided by oxidation of fat, represents a consumption of 280 g of triglyceride and production of roughly 300 mL of oxidative water per day. This source of water may supply 20 percent of total daily excretory volume. A puzzling manifestation among fasting patients is the disappearance of thirst despite a marked contraction of ECF and cellular water content (see Chap. 12). In fact, fasting subjects consume only minute amounts of water spontaneously. Many find the taste of water offensive. However, because of the endogenous sources of water described above, a minimum of 800 mL water intake per day suffices to provide an adequate volume for the excretion of solutes by the kidneys.

Clinically, the decrease in body water and cellular fluid content is accompanied by dryness of skin and mucous membranes. To the patients, the loss of cellular and interstitial water becomes apparent by the looseness of rings on fingers or looseness of dentures. The contraction of plasma contributes to the development of orthostatic hypotension, one of the more important complications of fasting. Volume depletion also elicits the increased secretion of aldosterone (see below). The hematocrit rises in the early phase of fasting and increases of 2 to 3 vol percent are common. Similarly, the concentration of plasma protein has been noted to rise transiently. Other sequels of the contraction of plasma volume include decreased renal perfusion, resulting in a decrement of glomerular filtration of as much as 50 percent. Diminution of hepatic perfusion results in abnormal sulfobromophthalein (BSP) retention, in cholestasis, and occasionally in raised serum bilirubin levels.

URINARY VOLUME AND OSMOLALITY

Urine output in acute fasting reflects the mobilization of body water from various compartments. In lean as well as obese subjects drinking a constant quantity of water per day, urine volume is maximal in the first 2 days and diminishes gradually thereafter. If ad libitum water intake is permitted, urine volume may fall to very low levels (less than 400 mL) in the later phases of fasting, because intake is spontaneously reduced. If an intake of about 2 L/day is enforced, output equals intake within the first 2 to 3 days and diminishes somewhat within 20 days (Fig. 27-4).

Urine osmolality and specific gravity are maxi-

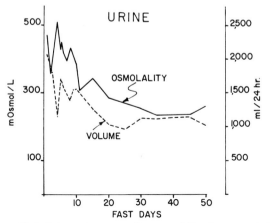

Figure 27-4. Urine volume as well as osmolality decreases during the first month of fasting. Water intake ad lib.

mal in the initial days of fasting and fall gradually with continued fasting, which may be partially due to impaired renal concentrating ability.

MINERAL LOSSES

SODIUM

If fasting is then begun abruptly after a normal food intake, the general pattern of sodium loss in the urine appears to be very similar in virtually all lean and obese subjects. Excretion is highest on the first day and then diminishes rapidly. The individual differences in magnitude of sodium loss very likely are the result of differences in body stores of sodium and water. The size of these stores depends on the level of dietary salt intake and, in the obese, on their variable degree of "inappropriate" salt and water retention before the fast. Figure 27-5A demonstrates acute daily sodium losses in groups of lean and obese subjects without overt edema during the first 15 days of fasting. Cumulative losses within 15 days in these two groups averaged 350 and 600 meq respectively. Figure 27-5B demonstrates daily sodium excretion over a 60-day period of fasting in a group of obese subjects, and separately is shown the excretion curve for a very obese man who was frankly edematous but not in congestive failure. Cumulative losses in 2 months in these obese

subjects averaged 930 meq and reached 1300 meq in the obese edematous subject.

The major portion of the sodium excreted in the first 6 days of fasting probably originates in the ECF compartment. Cumulative sodium excretion in the urine corresponds reasonably well to the isosmotic contraction of the ECF compartment. Additionally, there is some evidence that bone sodium is mobilized during the acute early phase of fasting before sodium excretion ceases.

If low-sodium diets are fed in the prefast period, sizable quantities of sodium are lost then, and subsequently the sodium diuresis coincident

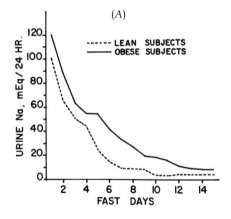

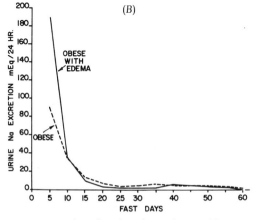

Figure 27-5. (A) Daily sodium loss during the initial fast period for groups of lean and obese subjects decreases rapidly. (B) Massive sodium loss occurs in obese subjects but optimum sodium conservation occurs after 15 to 20 days in edematous and nonedematous subjects.

with fasting is much reduced (12). The pattern of fasting sodium excretion in these circumstances assumes a different character (16). Sodium loss is small on the first day, begins to rise on the second day, peaks on day 4 or 5, and abates up to day 10, after which renal conservation becomes increasingly competent.

The cause and pattern of salt loss occurring despite a prior salt-restriction period have been ascribed to the effect of the developing metabolic acidosis (see below), for if a sodium diuresis is induced in subjects prior to fasting, first by a period of low intake and then by a period of metabolic acidosis due to ammonium chloride loading, then the sodium loss during the fast period proper is further reduced (17). However, even after a prefast adaptation to low sodium intake plus an ammonium chloride–induced metabolic acidosis, a definite though small increase in sodium loss still occurs (Fig. 27-6). Thus, a minor cause of sodium loss, accounting for, perhaps up to 10 percent of the total, has yet to be clarified. It may be that keto acid excretion rises so abruptly that some sodium is needed to maintain ionic balance in the urine. The further reduction in sodium excretion to almost total conservation is facilitated by the marked rise in ammonium production which peaks after 10 to 15 days and provides an ample supply of cations.

In lean and obese subjects, sodium excretion virtually ceases after fasting 10 to 15 days. In the

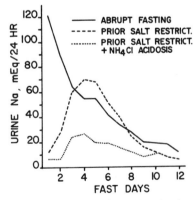

Figure 27-6. Sodium loss during the natriuretic phase of fasting depends on the dietary regimen prior to fasting. The highest losses follow normal salt intake, the lowest if salt was restricted and a period of acid loading preceded the fast.

edematous fasting subject, salt excretion also ceases even though the edema may still persist. However, with continued fasting, edema slowly recedes while serum sodium concentration remains stable. Although sodium excretion stops, protoplasmic protein, containing about 30 meq of sodium per kg, continues to be catabolized. If the ECF compartment and lean tissue mass continue to shrink, the sodium concentration in plasma and interstitial fluid should rise unless sodium can be concentrated in sites where storage in an osmotically inactive form is possible. Total muscle sodium may increase two- to threefold after 2 months of fasting. Whether bone and collagen also participate as storage sites for the gradually developing retention of sodium is not known.

The mechanisms responsible for renal sodium conservation in fasting have been studied (18), but only partial answers and some conflicting data have been forthcoming. Decreased plasma volume during fasting should stimulate renin and aldosterone secretion; nevertheless, these changes have not been consistently found (19). In addition to decreased glomerular filtration, increased proximal sodium resorption undoubtedly contributes to sodium retention (see Chap. 3). Potassium depletion results in sequestration of sodium in the intracellular compartment, so that administration of potassium chloride in a fasting subject may increase sodium secretion (Fig. 27-7) (see Chap. 4).

Recently, the reduction in plasma insulin levels and the rise in glucagon concentrations has been found to play a role in the genesis of the initial natriuresis of fasting (20). Glucagon has been shown to rise in early fasting in proportion to sodium excretion, and exogenous glucagon effected an increase in urinary sodium loss.

Because of the ample sodium stores and the limited period of sodium loss in total fasting, clinical depletion symptoms are unusual. On rare occasions fluctuating losses leading to depletion phenomena have been recorded (21). Serum sodium levels tend to remain unchanged throughout fasting. Supplementation with sodium during fasting is not beneficial except, possibly, in those subjects who lose weight at an unusually rapid rate. In such subjects, dizziness or fainting, the sequelae of the contraction of the plasma compartment, can sometimes be avoided or amelio-

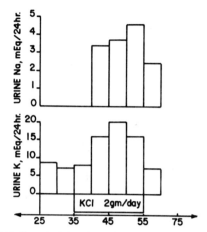

Figure 27-7. The administration of a potassium supplement after 35 days of fasting effects a significant sodium loss in a subject who, at that point, had no detectable urinary sodium.

rated by the administration of sodium and the resulting repletion of fluid.

POTASSIUM

During fasting, particularly during the initial phases, large quantities of potassium are lost in the urine (22). The source of potassium, in the absence of any intake, is primarily lean tissue. The concentration of potassium in various body tissues differs. Ratios of 2 meq of potassium to 1 g of lean tissue nitrogen are considered to prevail for whole body lean tissue. In muscle, the ratio is closer to 3 meq of potassium to 1 g of muscle nitrogen. If 1 kg of lean tissue is catabolized in fasting, about 60 meq of potassium may be released. In the first month's fasting, lean tissue catabolism may furnish as much as 300 meq of potassium to the body pool. Therefore, actual depletion of the remaining tissues would occur only if the rate of excretion exceeded the rate of release of potassium from catabolized tissue.

In addition to release from protoplasmic sources, potassium is released from glycogen stores. Assuming a glycogen consumption of about 400 g in the first 2 to 3 days and a ratio of 3 g of glycogen to 1 meq of potassium, then about 130 meq of this cation will be released and made

available from glycogen stores in liver and muscle.

The renal mechanisms of potassium loss are described in detail in Chap. 4

The magnitude of daily urinary potassium loss varies. In lean subjects, it has been found to average from 33 to 41 meq/day over a 10-day fast period. In a group of obese subjects, during the first 10 days' fast, urine loss averaged 41 meq. However, over prolonged periods, for instance after 1 month's fasting, the potassium loss in lean subjects remains about 15 meq/day, whereas obese patients at this stage lose less than one-half that amount. This difference may represent more efficient protein sparing in the obese fasting subject who is able to utilize the ample adipose tissue stores.

Total losses in the urine for the first month of fasting vary from 480 to 820 meq in different subjects, demonstrating the great range in renal capability to conserve potassium. Figure 27-8 illustrates potassium balances for two groups of obese fasting subjects, one with and one without potassium supplementation. In the absence of a potassium intake, renal conservation improves over the initial 15 to 20 days of fasting to such a degree

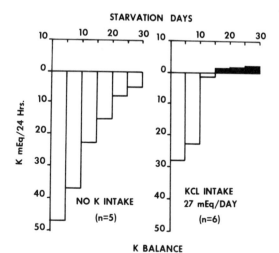

Figure 27-8. Potassium balances reveal that depletion takes place during the first 15 days despite progressive conservation if potassium is withheld and repletion after 15 days if potassium chloride supplements are given.

that, in many subjects, after this period the amount of potassium released from catabolized tissue equals excretion rates. Even more effective potassium conservation in some subjects would permit, in theory, a partial repletion of the re-maining lean tissue even though no potassium was ingested. On the other hand, in patients with continued high excretion rates, tissue depletion is reflected in a gradually falling serum potassium level. This is the exception rather than the rule,

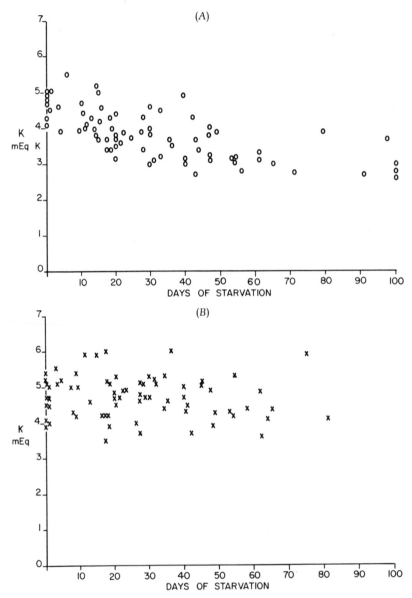

Figure 27-9. (A) and (B). Random serum potassium levels in fasting subjects decrease gradually. With a potassium supplement, levels remain unchanged.

and only rarely are the serum levels of less than 3 meq/L seen after 2 or more months of fasting (Fig. 27-9*A* and *B*). If 2 g potassium chloride per day is administered, repletion takes place after an initial negative balance period lasting about 15 days.

Various maneuvers can be employed to modify potassium excretion during fasting in an attempt to minimize depletion. The intake, prior to fasting, of a diet low in potassium or the consumption of a low-calorie, low-potassium diet tends to induce renal potassium conservation. If a fast is started subsequently, potassium loss is smaller. Figure 27-10 demonstrates that the potassium excretion/nitrogen loss ratio can be markedly lowered. Group 1 represents this potassium/nitrogen ratio in subjects commencing a fast abruptly; in group 2, a low-calorie diet preceded the fast; in group 3, a potassium supplement was given with fasting started abruptly; and in group 4, a low-calorie diet preceded the potassium-supplemented fast. The first group lost proportionately the largest quantity of potassium, and the last group experienced no deficit at all.

Attempts have been made to determine the degree of potassium depletion by measuring total body potassium content. ^{40}K and ^{42}K isotopes

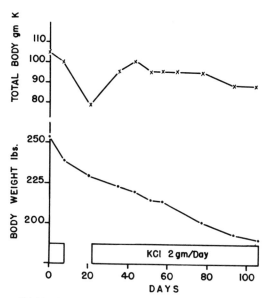

Figure 27-11. Discontinuation of potassium supplementation in the early fast period permits an acute fall in total body potassium and repletion with reinstitution of the supplement. The slow decrease after day 40 signifies loss of lean tissue.

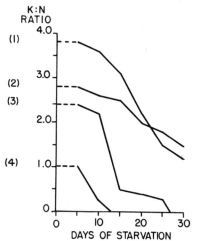

Figure 27-10. Urinary potassium (milliequivalents) to nitrogen (grams) in fasting ratios reveal that most potassium is lost if fasting is started abruptly (1). Less potassium is excreted if a low-calorie diet precedes the fast (2) or if a potassium supplement is given (3), and no deficit occurs if a low-calorie diet is fed before and a supplement given during fasting (4).

have been utilized. The accuracy of this technique is doubtful, though some results appear to conform to balance data. Figure 27-11 illustrates the acute decrease in body potassium when a supplement was temporarily stopped in the early phase of fasting and there was subsequent repletion with potassium chloride. The slow decrease in the later phases represents the catabolism of protoplasmic matrix and the release and excretion of the potassium contained in it.

Despite the lack of overt evidence of potassium depletion, as demonstrated by hypokalemia, certain clinical events are probably ascribable to tissue potassium deficit. It has been postulated that potassium depletion of renal tissue may account for the inability of the kidney to maintain an appropriately low urine pH during fasting though a metabolic acidosis persists. The fasting kidney loses the capacity to depress the urine pH after ammonium chloride loading. After supplementation with potassium, this impairment is reversed (23). Furthermore, potassium depletion was thought to account for the inability of the kidney to effect appropriate concentration of the urine, and this defect, too, is thought to be preventable by potassium supplementation (24). Postural hypotension has been ascribed to possible potassium depletion of smooth muscle cells in arteriolar walls, leading to impairment of vascular tone. However, potassium supplementation does not avert the development of this symptom. Electrocardiographic changes commonly associated with acute potassium depletion do not appear in fasting.

MAGNESIUM AND CALCIUM

Detailed data on magnesium loss in fasting are available only for obese subjects. The origin of the excreted magnesium is probably lean tissue protoplasm and bone. The proportionate contribution from either of these two sources is not known but seems to be variable. The rate of loss is relatively high in the first 5 to 10 days; subsequently, a slower excretion continues throughout fasting.

Magnesium losses in fasting obese subjects are shown in Fig. 27-12. Gross losses are substantial,

and even after correction for lean tissue catabolism, the additional loss of magnesium among fasting subjects ranged from 150 to 450 meq in a 2-month period. Average loss amounted to almost 400 meq. Assuming 2200 meq as the normal total body magnesium content in an average 70-kg male, the net loss after fasting ranged from 10 to 20 percent (average: 17 percent) of body stores. The large differences in magnesium loss among various subjects are unexplained. There is only a vague correlation with initial body weight.

Plasma levels during fasts up to 60 days show no consistent trend. In one group of 18 fasting subjects, approximately equal numbers showed no change, slight increases, and moderate declines. Red blood cell magnesium content similarly failed to reveal any consistent trends; however, presumably, during a 40- to 50-day fast, the majority of the red cell population remained alive from the prefast period, and magnesium content throughout the life span of a red cell is thought to be stable.

In those subjects who, during fasting, continue to form stools, significant quantities of magnesium are eliminated via this route. These losses

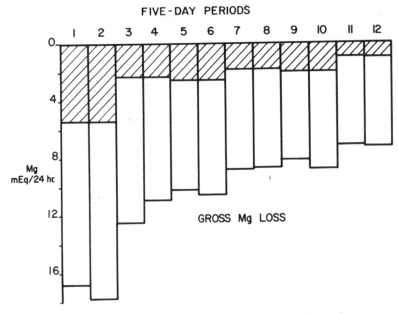

Figure 27-12. Daily magnesium loss declines gradually during the first month of fasting. The shaded areas represent fecal magnesium.

are in excess of fecal nitrogen loss and demonstrate that the intestine can function as an excretory organ for magnesium.

The greater portion of magnesium leaves the body through the kidneys. Fasting subjects excrete four to five times as much magnesium as do patients consuming magnesium-free but equicaloric diets. With fasting, a consistent pattern of urinary magnesium excretion is noted in all subjects. It is similar to that of calcium but unlike that of sodium and potassium (Fig. 27-13). Magnesium excretion rises throughout the first 7 days of fasting to an average peak of 13 meq/day, and then excretion recedes to a stable minimum of about 7 to 10 meq.

Of this daily loss, 2 to 4 meq can be accounted for as magnesium released from catabolized lean tissue. The remaining 5 to 7 meq represents magnesium derived from either depleted lean tissue stores or from bone deposits, or both. No information is available proving that bone stores are depleted in prolonged fasting. Muscle specimens have been examined in six subjects who fasted 2 months without magnesium supplementation. In these, significant muscle tissue depletion occurred. Instead of a normal magnesium content of about 80 meq/kg of dry fat-free tissue, the concentration in the fasting subjects ranged from 51 to 69 meq/kg (average: 63 meq magnesium per kilogram of dry muscle tissue). This degree of depletion of muscle would suggest that only one-half of the deficit originated in lean tissue. The rest may have been contributed by bone stores.

One cause of magnesium loss is the metabolic

acidosis produced by fasting. The pattern of rising and diminishing magnesium loss parallels the increase and decrease of the acidosis. It seems likely, therefore, that magnesium is utilized to neutralize part of the excess acid radicals in the urine. No definite symptoms have been ascribed to magnesium depletion during fasting. Tetanic carpal spasm is an infrequent complication of fasting. Though magnesium depletion has been linked with this symptom, there is inadequate evidence that these manifestations are causally connected.

Calcium losses in fasting are only slightly larger than those of magnesium, though body calcium stores are at least fifty times greater. Figure 27-14 demonstrates absolute quantities of calcium excretion compared to magnesium excretion in a group of fasting obese male subjects. Total losses during a 50-day period ranged from 550 to 900 meq. The pattern of excretion from day to day is also similar to that of magnesium. It is possible that calcium carbonate released from bones helps to buffer the acids formed endogenously during fasting.

The source of the large amounts of calcium lost in prolonged fasting undoubtedly is bone, though actual analyses of bone calcium content after fasting are not available. Despite the large calcium deficit in fasting, no decrease in serum calcium levels occurs, and no ill effects arise. Supplementation with calcium salts during fasting reduces the negativity of the calcium balance (25), but there is no evidence that any benefits derive from such a maneuver.

ACID-BASE CHANGES

During fasting, phosphate and sulfate make up the acid residue of catabolized lean tissue protoplasm. With the breakdown of each 100 g of (wet) lean tissue, 11 meq of acid excess—that is, acid originating in this same quantity of tissue but not balanced by base—enters the ECF and requires disposition (26). In the urine, these acid radicals and keto acids have to be balanced by an equivalent quantity of NH_4 plus titratable acidity and some fixed base (see Chap. 24).

All these processes alter acid-base balance in

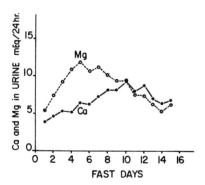

Figure 27-13. Magnesium and calcium excretion pattern during the first 15 days of fasting in obese subjects.

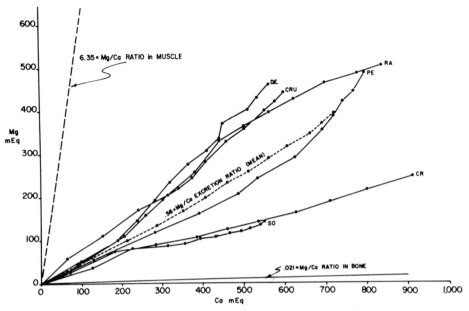

Figure 27-14. Magnesium losses are compared with calcium losses in six subjects. The points along the curves denote 5-day periods. Widely differing excretion rates of both minerals produce dissimilar degrees of depletion.

the serum, although only to a relatively minor degree and only transiently. Blood pH falls to a low of 7.30 to 7.36 between the sixth and eleventh days of fasting and then rises slowly. The same pattern appears in serum bicarbonate, which decreases in amounts equivalent to the increase in organic acids. Average lows of 16.7 meq/L are found on the tenth day. A gradual improvement to 20 to 24 meq/L follows over the next 20 days. Hyperventilation occurs in response to the metabolic acidosis, resulting in a drop in P_{CO_2} to 31 to 36 mmHg. The respiratory compensation subsides within 20 to 25 days. Virtually normal acid-base balance is then maintained for the entire fast period (Fig. 27-15).

The development of a metabolic acidosis is reflected in the urine by a fall in pH beginning on the second day and reaching a minimum in the range of 4.8 to 5.23 between the fourth and sixth day. Subsequently, despite the continuing ketosis and acidosis in blood, the urine pH gradually rises, returning to baseline levels between the tenth and fifteenth day of fasting (Fig. 27-16).

Urine titratable acidity reaches its peak at about double the baseline levels around the end of the first week of fasting. Maximum values range from 40 to 70 meq per 24 h. This pattern parallels the

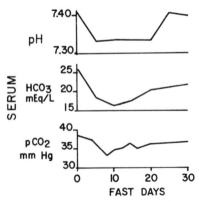

Figure 27-15. Mean changes in serum pH, bicarbonate concentration, and P_{CO_2} in a group of fasting obese subjects reveal a mild acidosis and almost complete restoration to original levels within 25 days.

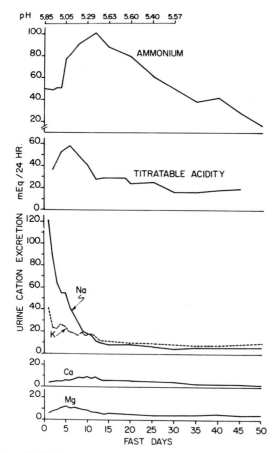

Figure 27-16. Mean urine cation excretion for a group of fasting obese men reflects the increasing metabolic acidosis during the first 2 weeks and subsequent amelioration.

increase in phosphate excretion which makes up the predominant portion of titratable acidity buffer. The secondary decrease in phosphate excretion coincides with the rising urine pH.

Urinary ammonium rises continuously throughout the first 10 days of fasting. Fivefold increases above baseline values, up to a maximum of 150 meq daily, reveal that the majority of hydrogen ion excess is excreted in this mode. The peak of ammonium excretion coincides with the low point of blood pH. This may be expected because acidosis, specifically renal tissue acidosis, favors accelerated deamination of glutamine, increased gluconeogenesis, and enhanced ammonia diffusion into the urine. Ammonia, being strongly

alkaline, may contribute to the paradoxical rise in urine pH after the sixth day of fasting.

The sequence of changes in urinary anion excretion is shown in Fig. 27-17. The pattern of gradual decreases involves all acid radicals except keto acids. The most drastic decrease is manifested in chloride excretion, which falls to about 5 meq/day within 2 weeks of fasting, paralleling the pattern of diminishing sodium loss.

Sulfate excretion peaks on the fifth to seventh day at about 50 meq/day and then decreases to an average of 20 to 30 meq/day. Though quantitatively variable from one subject to the next, the loss of sulfate after the first 15 fast days is directly proportional to nitrogen loss, and the respective

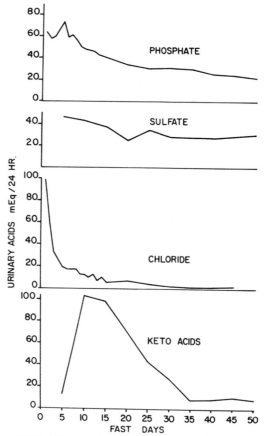

Figure 27-17. Urinary anion excretion in prolonged fasting reveals a decline of acid radicals while keto acid excretion rises to peak after 15 to 20 days of fasting.

amounts resemble the proportions of nitrogen to sulfur present in muscle tissue. The relative excess of sulfate over nitrogen in the initial fasting period may be a reflection of catabolism of tissue which contains sulfur in higher concentrations than lean tissue on the whole.

Phosphate loss in urine is extensive but without ill effects, presumably because of the ample stores in bone. Up to 80 meq/day is lost; but, again, this excretion rate is rapidly reduced, and after 15 to 20 days the average daily output ranges from 20 to 30 meq.

Urinary carbonic acid does not contribute significantly to the excreted acid load in fasting because urine pH is too low.

No changes of any significance occur in serum levels of chloride and phosphate during fasting.

KETOSIS

If a subject with expendable fat stores continues to fast for more than 2 to 3 days, his energy requirements are met increasingly by catabolism of fat, while glycogen stores become progressively depleted. Ketosis develops as glucose oxidation falls below the critical 3 percent of total energy turnover, the minimum required for complete combustion of fat to its final end products, carbon dioxide and water.

In essence, the metabolic fuel mixture providing energy during fasting in normal or in obese subjects consists of an endogenous ketogenic diet in which fat may contribute up to 90 percent of the calories. Only chronically emaciated patients whose adipose stores are reduced to less than 10 percent of normal seem to be unable to furnish enough triglyceride to produce a ketosis with fasting. The ketones in serum and ECF contribute to the mild metabolic acidosis. The most prevalent keto acid is β-hydroxybutyrate (80%), but considerable amounts of acetoacetate and some acetone are also present.

The concentration of ketones in the serum is a function of the rate of production versus the combined rate of utilization in tissue and excretion via kidneys and lungs. Increased lipolysis is manifested by an increase of serum free fatty acids (FFA), reaching twice normal levels within 48 h of fasting. Increasing fatty acid oxidation and decreasing fatty acid synthesis supply the substrate for a markedly increased formation of acetoacetate by the liver. β-hydroxybutyric acid is derived from acetoacetate by reduction, while decarboxylation of acetoacetate produces acetone. The actual stimulus to ketone production may be the fall in insulin secretion that accompanies the reduction in blood glucose levels (27).

The concentration of ketones in the serum of fasting subjects varies markedly, and no obvious reasons for these differences are known. The rates of increase of acetoacetate in lean and obese groups differ slightly, with the more rapid rise noted in the lean subjects. However, within 18 h of fasting, the levels for both groups tend to be the same.

On day 1 of fasting, the concentrations of acetoacetate and β-hydroxybutyrate are approximately equal. Subsequently, butyrate rises progressively and at a more rapid rate than acetoacetate, so that by day 8 the ratio in the serum is about 4:1.

Total ketone levels also rise more rapidly in lean than in obese subjects and more rapidly in lean females than in lean males. The differences diminish progressively, and after 4 to 5 days ketone levels are similar in the two sexes and all weight categories.

Figure 27-18 demonstrates random serum ketone levels in a group of obese subjects fasting up to 50 days. Peaks are reached after 30 to 40 days. After a slight subsequent decline, ketone concentrations tend to remain reasonably stable.

Urinary excretion of acetoacetate and butyrate also begins to increase within 12 h after the last meal, and progressively increasing quantities of ketone bodies are lost. In a lean subject, a peak excretion of 7 g/day was found after 20 days' fasting. Subsequently, there was a moderate fall in output to about 5 g/day, and this excretion rate continued throughout 1 month of fasting. In obese subjects, the urinary acetoacetate ranged from 14 to 20 mol/day during peak excretion, that is, after 10 to 15 days of fasting. Average β-hydroxybutyrate excretion at the 15-day interval peaked at 110 mol per 24 h (Fig. 27-19). Renal

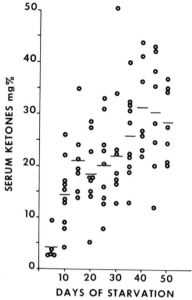

Figure 27-18. Random and mean serum ketone levels rise during the first 30 to 40 days of fasting.

clearance rates have been calculated at 8 to 10 mL/min. This large quantity of organic acids represents a major portion of acid radicals requiring neutralization in the urine.

The development and persistence of ketoacidosis is of clinical significance in prolonged fasting, primarily because keto acids and uric acid compete for renal tubular transport sites. Therefore, as keto acids accumulate in the serum, urate clearance and excretion are partially blocked. The persistent hyperuricemia may lead to the development of acute gouty arthritis and renal urate calculi. These events arose in fasting subjects who did not have a history of gout and had normal serum uric acid levels before fasting. The use of allopurinol prevents the development of hyperuricemia. Probenecid is somewhat less effective in curbing the initial rise in serum urate, but actual gouty attacks are prevented. Figure 27-19 demonstrates absolute rises above baseline levels of uric acid in groups of fasting subjects with and without treatment to control hyperuricemia.

There have been no other proved physiologic disturbances ascribable to the ketosis, though some have felt that it may be responsible for the surprising lack of hunger in prolonged fasting. Recently, it has been shown that during fasting keto acids largely replace glucose as the primary fuel for the central nervous system, supplying 75 percent of the needed calories (28). The gradual decrease in plasma ketone levels after 40 to 50 days of fasting may be a reflection of more efficient utilization, possibly by muscle. A reduction in energy requirements with a concomitant decrease in lipolysis may also contribute to the decrease in the severity of the ketosis.

REFEEDING

During refeeding following a period of fasting, most acid-base abnormalities are promptly re-

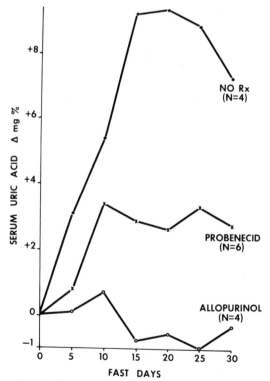

Figure 27-19. Serum urate concentrations increase during fasting. With uricosuric agents the increase is held to less than half, and a slight decrease follows with allopurinol.

versed. If hyperuricemia has prevailed during fasting, the disappearance of the ketosis improves urate excretion, and larger quantities of uric acid are excreted while serum levels rapidly diminish. Positive balances are observed for all minerals which have been excreted during fasting. If glucose and water are given orally after 3 days of fasting and before sodium excretion has become minimal, a marked diminution of renal sodium excretion follows. This is associated with a reduction of water excretion (3, 29). A similar effect has been noted following refeeding with protein but not with fat (30). Intravenous glucose infusions effect a lowering of sodium excretion within 2 h and simultaneously raise renal concentrating capability. Refeeding with glucose, after prolonged fasting, induces rapid disappearance of the ketosis and a lessened excretion of calcium, magnesium, and phosphorus without any significant changes in urinary sodium (31).

During realimentation following prolonged fasting, phenomena involving abnormal water and salt retention tend to develop. These events are variable depending on the type and quantities of food ingested and the salt content. Also, the length of the preceding fast and the degree of obesity at the time of refeeding seem related to the severity of "refeeding edema."

Some degree of increase in body water content is expected and represents simply restoration of normal hydration of tissues. ECF and plasma water are repleted. Glycogen is deposited with bound water. In addition, protein is resynthesized if as little as 30 g of protein is eaten daily. This occurs even when the entire diet does not exceed a total of 300 cal and despite a continuing negative calorie balance. However, the period of a positive nitrogen balance is only transient unless food intake is increased to approximately 1000 cal. At any rate, 3 g of water is bound in newly formed protoplasm with every gram of protein resynthesized. The repletion of glycogen plus bound water represents a weight gain of approximately 1.5 kg. About 0.2 kg is retained as intestinal water.

The magnitude of disproportionate body water increment with refeeding in obese subjects may range from 5 to 11 L. These amounts are accumulated over a refeeding period of from 20 to 26 days, but the period of excessive water retention is self-limited.

All body compartments and tissues share in the accumulation and expansion of water stores. The interstitial water increases most drastically, and, beyond restoration of normal hydration, marked pitting edema may occur. Serum sodium and osmolality decrease slightly. The gain in body water is associated with a drastically positive sodium balance. The severity of water and salt retention can be curbed to a significant degree if small amounts of sodium are ingested during the fasting period. The clinical observation of "dilution anemia" coincides with, and is a manifestation of, the period of maximal water retention. Restoration of a more normal blood pressure and disappearance of the orthostatic hypotension occur with this phase.

At the end of this water retention period and despite a constant diet and salt intake a spontaneous diuresis occurs, resulting in an abrupt weight loss over a period of up to 2 weeks. In addition to the mechanisms involved in water and salt retention after short fasts, hormonal effects elicited by prolonged fasting have been invoked as causes. Persistently increased rates of aldosterone secretion may contribute to salt and water retention. Levels of antidiuretic hormone (ADH) in plasma are normal in this phase and responses to either water or salt loading are physiological. The mechanism effecting the downward adjustment in body water following the water retention period has not been elucidated.

CLINICAL PROBLEMS IN FASTING AND ITS PRACTICAL MANAGEMENT

In morbidly obese subjects who may have been hospitalized for a variety of illnesses, a rapid and extensive weight loss is often desirable. Among such conditions are maturity-onset diabetes, hypertension, gout, cardiac ischemia, or cerebral ischemic disease. Various surgical procedures may have to be postponed to make surgery feasible or easier, or to render a repair more likely to be permanent. Herniorrhaphies, surgery on varicose veins, cholecystectomies, and orthopedic surgery of spine or weight-bearing joints belong in this category.

Prolonged fasting induces a rapid, continuous reduction in weight; but problems can occur that are peculiar to fasting and are not seen with moderately restricted diets.

While the initial fasting diuresis is desirable in patients with the Pickwickian syndrome and in obese subjects with marked peripheral edema, the rapid shift of electrolytes can bring about distressing side effects. Fatal cardiac irregularities occurred in 2 out of a group of 12 subjects who were treated with diuretics (32). Diuretics and digitalis should not be used while a fast is instituted. The extensive fluid loss brings about a marked fall in plasma and ECF volume and a reduction of cellular water. Postural hypotension may develop gradually or precipitously and may become so serious as to require refeeding. Postural hypotension can be a distinct hazard to those patients who have ischemic disease of the brain or heart. To minimize the danger, the rate of fluid loss can be slowed by the administration of 1.0 g of sodium bicarbonate daily. Hot showers and hot tub baths should be avoided, particularly in the morning hours, when the postural hypotension is apt to be most marked. A common complaint of intermittent muscle spasms may be related to the rapid compartmental shift or loss of sodium. If obesity is complicated by hypertension, no blood pressure–lowering medication should be administered during fasting or during semistarvation regimens, because the hypotensive effects of the reducing regimen and of drug treatment may be additive and unpredictably drastic. Fasting, in itself, is usually accompanied by a gradual and progressive fall in blood pressure, which occurs long before normal weight is restored.

Another sequel of the fall in plasma volume is a functional impairment of glomerular filtration and hepatic perfusion. Transient increases in serum creatinine of up to 2 mg/dL can occur. Marked rises in BSP retention of up to 40 percent have been noted (33). Some patients notice transient blurring of vision. The rehydration that follows refeeding promptly reverses these abnormalities.

Body potassium depletion may contribute to some of the ill effects, for instance, postural hypotension (see Chap. 4). One of the routine measures during fasting includes the administration of 20 mL of a 10% sugar-free KCl solution per day. Significant depletion can thus be avoided.

Hyperuricemia invariably develops in prolonged fasting. If suitable measures are taken, hyperuricemia can be avoided. Allopurinol, 200 mg t.i.d., seems to be preferable, though probenecid, 2 g daily, is generally satisfactory. Ideally, medication should be started several days before the fast. Without these measures, serum urate levels may increase to greater than 20 mg/dL, and several instances of secondary gout have been encountered (34). These episodes occurred anytime after 1 month of fasting in subjects who initially had normal urate levels and no history of gout. A second complication, also preventable by medication and an ample intake of water, is the development of renal urate stones. The formation of these calculi is aided by the acid pH of the urine, the low urine volume, and the persistent hyperuricemia.

The rise in serum keto acids is the primary cause for a metabolic acidosis. No evidence of any clinically significant symptoms resulting from the mild metabolic acidosis has been observed. No treatment is necessary.

In the absence of exogenous carbohydrate, blood sugar levels decline gradually and may fall to levels as low as 40 mg/dL. The fall is slow and does not elicit symptoms of hypoglycemia. The blood sugar levels of obese diabetic subjects tend to fall to normal or slightly subnormal levels with fasting. One case of acute porphyria has been reported, possibly precipitated by the lack of carbohydrate intake in a susceptible subject (35).

The maximum practical fasting periods should not exceed 2 months. On occasion a patient may insist on continuing a fasting regimen beyond 2 months. With careful monitoring this is feasible; but in general after about 60 days, nausea, hypotension, lassitude, and weakness usually become troublesome. An ample intake of water must be strongly encouraged, and a minimum of 2 L/day is suggested. The voluntary intake of water is often minute, and urine volume may become precariously low.

Because of the physiologic changes caused by fasting, possible contraindications to fasting include gout or hyperuricemia with family history of gout, myocardial infarction or cerebrovascular accidents of recent origin, or chronic renal disease. These are important when the physiologic changes brought about by fasting are considered. Routine test procedures and the medications to minimize potential hazards related to disordered fluid or electrolyte balance should include the following:

Allopurinol	600 mg/day
10% KCl solution (sugarless)	20 mL/day
Sodium bicarbonate (prn)	1.0 g/day
Blood pressure—recumbent and upright	daily
Urine acetone (ketone reagent strip)	daily
Serum creatinine	weekly
Serum uric acid	weekly
Complete blood count	weekly

More complete descriptions of routine management have been published (36).

With refeeding, a marked weight gain is generally observed. This is the result of expansion of intracellular and extracellular fluid space, possibly mediated by high aldosterone levels. The fluid retention may become severe enough to cause manifest edema if salt intake with refeeding is unrestricted. The "refeeding edema" seems self-limited. A spontaneous diuresis occurs after 10 days to 3 weeks.

In general the problems associated with fasting are predictable and easily recognizable. Most can be prevented, and the treatment is simple. If results are unsatisfactory, refeeding invariably relieves fast-induced disorders of fluid and electrolyte metabolism.

REFERENCES

1. Benedict, F. G.: *A Study of Prolonged Fasting*, Carnegie Institution, Washington, 1915.
2. Folin, O., and W. Denis: On starvation and obesity, with special references to acidosis, *J. Biol. Chem.*, **21**:183, 1915.
3. Gamble, J. L., G. S. Ross, and F. F. Tisdall: The metabolism of fixed base during fasting, *J. Biol. Chem.*, **57**:633, 1923.
4. Drenick, E. J., E. Swendseid, W. H. Blahd, and G. Tuttle: Prolonged starvation as treatment for severe obesity, *JAMA*, **187**:100, 1964.
5. Apfelbaum, M., P. Boudon, D. Lacatis, et al.: Effects metaboliques de la diete protidique chez 41 sujects obeses, *Presse. Med.*, **78**:1917, 1970.
6. Blackburn, G. L., J. P. Flatt, G. H. A. Clowes, T. E. O'Donnell, and T. E. Hensle: Protein-sparing therapy during periods of starvation with sepsis or trauma, *Ann. Surg.*, **177**:588, 1973.
7. Genuth, S. M., J. H. Castro, and V. Vertes: Weight reduction in obesity by outpatient semi-starvation, *JAMA*, **230**:978, 1974.
8. Gilder, H., N. Cornell, W. R. Grafe, J. R. MacFarlane, J. W. Asaph, W. T. Stubenbord, G. M. Watkins, J. R. Rees, and B. Thorbjarnarson: Components of weight loss in obese patients subjected to prolonged starvation, *J. Appl. Physiol.*, **23**:304, 1967.
9. Smith, R., and E. J. Drenick: Changes in body water and sodium during prolonged starvation for extreme obesity, *Clin. Sci.*, **31**:437, 1966.
10. Winkler, A. W., T. S. Danowski, J. R. Elkinton, and J. P. Peters: Electrolyte and fluid studies during water deprivation and starvation in human subjects, and the effect of ingestion of fish, or carbohydrate, and of salt solutions, *J. Clin. Invest.*, **23**:807, 1944.
11. Gamble, J. L.: Physiological information gained from studies on the life raft ration, *Harvey Lectures*, **42**:247, 1946–1947.
12. Taylor, H. L., A. Henschel, O. Mickelsen, and A. Keys: Some effects of acute starvation with hard work on body weight, body fluids and metabolism, *J. Appl. Physiol.*, **6**:613, 1953–1954.
13. Consolazio, C. F., L. O. Matoush, H. L. Johnson, R. A. Nelson, and H. J. Krzywicki: Metabolic aspects of acute starvation in normal humans (10 days), *Am. J. Clin. Nutr.*, **20**:672, 1967.
14. Hultman, E.: Muscle glycogen in man determined in needle biopsy specimens: Method and normal values, *Scand. J. Clin. Lab. Invest.*, **19**:209, 1967.

15. Strauss, M. B., E. Lamdin, W. P. Smith, and D. J. Bleifer: Surfeit and deficit of sodium, *Arch. Intern. Med.*, **102**:527, 1958.

16. Stinebaugh, B. J., and F. X. Schloeder: Studies on the natriuresis of fasting. I. Effect of prefast intake, *Metabolism*, **15**:828, 1966.

17. Schloeder, F. S., and B. J. Stinebaugh: Studies on the natriuresis of fasting. II. Relationship to acidosis, *Metabolism*, **15**:838, 1966.

18. Bloom, W. L., and W. Mitchell, Jr.: Salt excretion of fasting patients, *Arch. Intern. Med.*, **106**:321, 1960.

19. Kjellberg, J., M. Piscator, and J. Castenfors: Urinary proteins and plasma renin activity during total starvation, *Acta Med. Scand.*, **190**:519, 1971.

20. Saudek, C. D., P. R. Boulter, and R. A. Arky: The natriuretic effect of glucagon and its role in starvation, *J. Clin. Endocrinol. Metab.*, **36**:761, 1973.

21. Runcie, J.: Urinary sodium and potassium excretion in fasting obese subjects, *Br. Med. J.*, **3**:22, 1971.

22. Drenick, E. J., W. G. Blahd, F. R. Singer, and M. Lederer: Body potassium content in obese subjects and potassium depletion during prolonged fasting, *Am. J. Clin. Nutr.*, **18**:278, 1966.

23. Schloeder, F. X., and B. J. Stinebaugh: Defect of urinary acidification during fasting, *Metabolism*, **15**:17, 1966.

24. Rubini, M. E.: Water excretion in potassium-deficient man, *J. Clin. Invest.*, **40**:2215, 1961.

25. Bolinger, R. E., B. P. Lukert, R. W. Brown, L. Guevara, and R. Steinberg: Metabolic balance of obese subjects during fasting, *Arch. Intern. Med.*, **118**:3, 1966.

26. Gonick, H. C., G. Goldberg, and D. Mulcare: Reexamination of the acid-ash content of several diets, *Am. J. Clin. Nutr.*, **21**:898, 1968.

27. Foster, D. W.: Studies in the ketosis of fasting, *J. Clin. Invest.*, **46**:1283, 1967.

28. Owen, O. E., A. P. Morgan, H. G. Kemp, J. M. Sullivan, M. G. Herrera, and G. F. Cahill, Jr.: Brain metabolism during fasting, *J. Clin. Invest.*, **46**:1589, 1967.

29. Bloom, W. L.: Carbohydrates and water balance, *Am. J. Clin. Nutr.*, **20**:157, 1967.

30. Katz, A. I., D. R. Hollingsworth, and F. H. Epstein: Influence of carbohydrate and protein on sodium excretion during fasting and refeeding, *J. Lab. Clin. Med.*, **72**:93, 1968.

31. Brickman, A. S., E. J. Drenick, I. F. Hunt, and J. W. Coburn: Studies of water (H_2O) and electrolyte (E) retention (R) following carbohydrate administration (CH) to fasting (F) obese subjects (abstract), *Clin. Res.*, **17**:167, 1969.

32. Spencer, I. O. B., and M. B. Durh: Death during therapeutic starvation for obesity, *Lancet*, **1**:1288, 1968.

33. Verdy, M.: BSP retention during total fasting, *Metabolism*, **15**:769, 1966.

34. Drenick, E. J., J. L. Fisler, and H. F. Dennin: The effect of allopurinol on the hyperuricemia of fasting, *Clin. Pharmacol. Ther.*, **12**:68, 1971.

35. Knudsen, K. B., M. Sparberg, and F. Lecocg: Porphyria precipitated by fasting, *N. Engl. J. Med.*, **277**:350, 1967.

36. Drenick, E. J.: Prolonged fasting, in W. L. Asher (ed.), *Treating the Obese*, Medcom Press, New York, 1974, p. 95.

28

Intestinal bypass operation: Physiological changes, complications and treatment

ERNST J. DRENICK

INTRODUCTION

Surgical procedures intended for permanent relief of morbid obesity have been performed with increasing frequency over the last 20 years. By 1976, between 12,000 and 20,000 such operations had been carried out in the United States. The bypass operations were designed to produce a state of "controlled malabsorption" by excluding dietary calories from all but about 10 percent of the absorptive area of the small bowel. The procedure was welcome to compulsive eaters, because it was expected that the operation would produce a progressive weight loss even if excessive calorie intake continued. Physicians charged with the treatment of morbidly obese patients have been willing to consider the surgical approach because conservative treatment has been largely unsuccessful in such patients.

Morbid, refractory obesity carries its own morbidity and mortality. A surgical procedure may therefore be justifiable if it assures a predictable weight loss to normal or near normal levels; however, if the risks, the mortality, the incidence of complications, and the economic costs of surgical treatment were to exceed those of untreated obes-

ity, the wisdom of the surgical approach would remain in question, at least from the point of view of the physician. Definitive studies to establish whether the surgical or the conservative approach results in less harm to the individual have not been carried out. Risk benefit ratios are very difficult to assess in these circumstances because the patients' perspective differs greatly from that of the physician. In many instances, the quality of life for a morbidly obese individual can be so miserable that surgical candidates are perfectly willing to accept all risks, postoperative complications, and setbacks as the price for a satisfactory weight loss.

Both acute and chronic complications of this operation are common. Although the operation has been performed for 20 years, new complications still turn up, and others may be encountered in years to come. Although a number of the complications have appeared rather forbidding in the past, more recent investigations have clarified their pathogenesis, and more or less effective countermeasures can now be employed. Considering the ever-increasing population of bypass patients, physicians must become familiar with the pathogenesis and treatment of the various complications, which, in a number of instances, have been life threatening or actually fatal. In this chapter the emphasis will be on those physiologic and pathophysiologic changes which involve electrolyte disorders. Numerous other complications not involving such problems will not be discussed in detail.

THE OPERATION

The earliest report of a bypass procedure was published by Payne et al. (1) in 1963. In this operation, a 15-in segment of proximal jejunum was anastomosed to the transverse colon. Although it results in an extensive weight loss, this type of bypass has been largely abandoned, because in many patients it was followed by unmanageable diarrhea and severe fluid and electrolyte disorders. The mortality rate was high. Yet, one

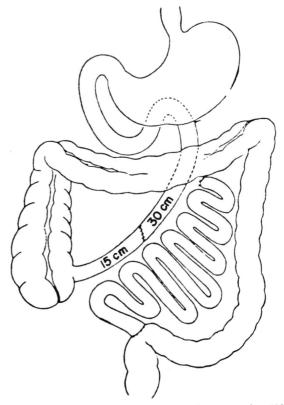

Figure 28-2. End-to-end jejunoileal bypass, Scott procedure (12).

should be aware that in a number of institutions this particular bypass procedure is still being performed, and all of the complications discussed below are frequently encountered in severe degree with this type of bypass.

Two operations are commonly used at present. The first, shown in Fig. 28-1 as developed by Payne, DeWind et al., is the end-to-side bypass in which the proximal 14 in of jejunum are anastomosed to the ileum at a point 4 in proximal to the ileocecal valve (1). The second operation, devised by Scott et al. and Salmon et al. (2, 3) employs an end-to-end anastomosis of variable lengths of proximal jejunum and distal ileum, with the bypassed small bowel segment anastomosed to drain into the colon (Fig. 28-2). Various sites along the course of the large bowel have been selected for this later anastomosis, including the cecum, the transverse colon, and the sigmoid.

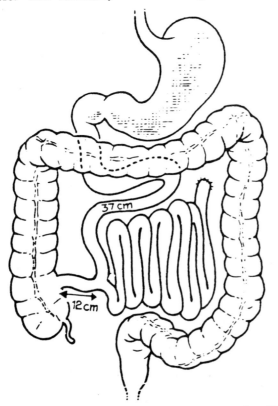

Figure 28-1. End-to-side jejunoileal bypass, Payne procedure (45).

WEIGHT LOSS

The rate of weight loss and the extent of the eventual weight reduction are determined by a number of factors which are highly variable, and for this reason no precise prediction can be offered to any one individual as to how successful the operation will be. Most observers agree that the shorter the functioning segment, the greater the eventual weight loss (4). However, this is not an absolute determinant; rather it appears that the ratio of the total length of small bowel present before operation versus the length of functioning small bowel after operation may be the critical factor (5). Those patients with a lesser total length of bowel and presumably more efficient absorptive capability per unit surface area before surgery tend to lose less weight than those who have a very long bowel at the time of surgery, given the same segment length of functioning small bowel after the operation. If more than 25 in is left in continuity, weight loss is very slow

and sometimes negligible, regardless of the respective lengths of the jejunal or ileal segment (5). A second determinant of weight loss is the initial weight excess of the patient. Since it requires a greater quantity of calories to sustain a very large subject in caloric equilibrium a finite calorie deficit will produce a greater weight loss in a very heavy individual than in a moderately obese subject.

The pattern of weight loss is characterized by an initial steep decline over the first 6 months, followed by a progressive weight reduction proceeding for 1 to 1½ years at a reasonably linear rate. Weight usually stabilizes at a plateau level which is from 15 to 25 percent above ideal weight. In a not insignificant number of bypass patients a secondary weight gain may eventually occur, regardless of the type of operative procedure, although the gain appears to be more common and greater following end-to-side jejunoileostomy. In Fig. 28-3, mean weight losses as percent decrease from baseline are shown at var-

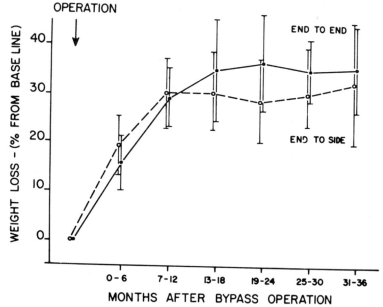

Figure 28-3. Percent weight loss following two types of bypass procedures in weight-matched groups. The data are expressed as mean ±1 SD. The percent loss is significantly different between the two procedure types at the 0- to 6-month, 13- to 18-month, and 19- to 24-month time periods (15, 23, 49–52).

ious intervals after bypass. These data have been collected from several different institutions, but the means shown have no predictive value for the individual patient. Figure 28-4 demonstrates a slightly better weight loss for the end-to-end bypass procedure. Unknown variables, such as absorptive adaptation or food intake exceeding the malabsorptive losses, may minimize the initial weight loss or eventually facilitate a secondary weight gain. On the other end of the spectrum, isolated patients may lose weight rapidly and to excess, primarily due to bypass-induced complications, and may reach the point of emaciation. Because of the extreme differences in response to the operation, some authors found that the only variables showing significant correlation with rate of weight loss were initial weight and length of intestine left in continuity (6).

FACTORS CONTRIBUTING TO WEIGHT LOSS

Among several mechanisms producing weight loss after bypass, the earliest is the stress cata-

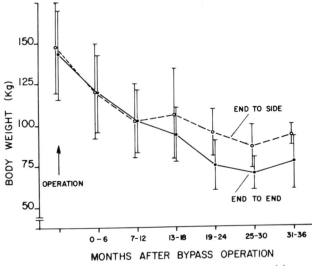

Figure 28-4. Body weight losses (kg) after two types of bypass procedures in weight-matched groups. The data are expressed as mean ±1 SD. The absolute weight is significantly different between the two groups at the 19- to 24-month time periods (1, 3, 12, 14, 46, 47).

bolic phase immediately after surgery. This response can be prevented by parenteral nutrition, but since the response is complex and because it is probably unnecessary to furnish the customary preoperative quantities of energy-supplying nutrients to a grossly obese patient, parenteral nutrition is rarely employed.

In the early postoperative stage, after eating is resumed, the great majority of patients tend to eat much less than before the operation. This is partly the result of counselling by the physician, who generally advises smaller portions and a low-fat diet. But more importantly, the patient empirically limits his intake in order to avoid digestive distress. The patient spontaneously adopts a greatly reduced total daily food intake (7–10). In one group of bypass patients, calorie consumption decreased from a mean of 4900 to 3100 kcal during the first 6 months but later stabilized at 3500 kcal/day (11).

The most obvious mechanism of weight loss is malabsorption, as discussed below. Failure to lose weight in the anticipated manner has been explained in several ways. Over time, a number of adaptive processes occur which tend to enhance absorptive capability. Gastric emptying time increases from a mean of 95 min before operation to 152 min 6 months after bypass. This diminishes the tendency to overload the shortened small bowel, thereby avoiding reactive hyperperistalsis and increased diarrhea (12). A second factor favoring increased absorptive capacity is nutrient reflux into the excluded ileal segment. Since readily absorbable nutrients can enter the bypassed segment, regardless of the site of anastomosis, the absorptive surface of the functioning segment is enlarged to a variable extent. Reflux can be observed in virtually all patients and lasts for 1 to 5 h as demonstrated by addition of contrast medium to a meal (12). The distance of reflux into the excluded ileum varies from a few centimeters to more than 60 cm. During reoperation a normal diameter of ileum and normal mucosal thickness is seen in the bypassed ileum proximal to the ileosigmoidostomy, suggesting normal function. Higher up in the defunctionalized loops, intestinal atrophy and narrowing of the luminal diameter indicates that reflux does not reach this area (13).

Improved absorption can also be inferred from the anatomical findings on reoperation 1 year or longer after bypass. In one series, the length of the functioning bowel segment had increased between 25 to 83 percent over the original measurements (13). The diameter of this segment also had increased 1 to 2 cm. However the histological appearance of villi did not seem to be altered, and enzyme content of the epithelial cells remained constant. Evidence in support of adaptive improvement in absorption was obtained by examining vitamin B_{12} excretion with Schilling tests. After an initial fall in plasma levels, test results reverted to normal 18 months to 2 years after bypass.

Finally, a few patients manage to outeat the malabsorption by ingesting small quantities of highly nutritious foods at frequent intervals. With careful planning, the patient can consume large amounts of carbohydrates and other nutrients without eliciting increased diarrhea with greater caloric waste. Although such instances are unusual, some patients have achieved food consumption far in excess of preoperative intake, and failure to lose weight was the disappointing end result.

BODY COMPOSITION

The aim of the bypass operation is to produce fat loss without a decrease in lean tissue mass. Body composition has been examined by several observers (14, 15). Figure 28-5 demonstrates changes in various body compartments over an extended period after the operation. Although the proportionate reduction in fat content is obviously the major change, lean tissue appears to be reduced as well, with the greatest decrement occurring in the initial 6 months after the operation.

Total body water decreases to a lesser extent, implying that body hydration is relatively greater. Perturbations of body water content in either direction are common after the bypass operation.

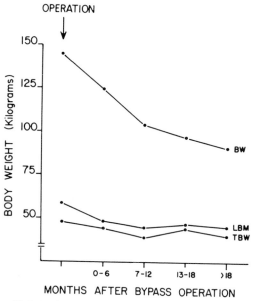

Figure 28-5. Body composition changes after end-to-end bypass operation (14). BW = body weight, LBM = lean body mass, TBW = total body water.

Excess fluid loss and sequestration in extracellular space or intestinal lumen can occur alternately in the same patient at different time periods. Diarrhea-induced dehydration or nutritional edema may greatly alter total body water content.

MALABSORPTION OF NUTRIENTS

The stools produced following bypass are characteristic of ileal resection and ileal disease. Depending on the kinds of food and the overall quantities consumed, watery steatorrhea alternates with semisolid, mushy feces. On ad lib diets, the mean quantities of fecal fat show a gradual increase (Fig. 28-6) suggesting that greater voluntary intake follows improved appetite and health. The variability in fecal fat is considerable from subject to subject and from day to day depending on intake and severity of diarrhea. Daily fecal fat excretion has been observed to vary from

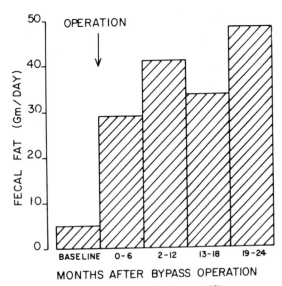

Figure 28-6. Fecal fat before and after bypass (48).

14 to 150 g. Nitrogen excretion also tends to rise with time, both in absolute amounts and as a percentage of ingested protein. This signifies that the finite absorptive capability produces progressively greater wasting of protein as intake is increased. Up to 90 percent of ingested triglyceride and over 30 percent of protein are excreted. The precise quantities of carbohydrates wasted are not known, since after bacterial degradation measurements in feces are uncertain.

The energy content of feces, as estimated by Crisp (8), was 504 kcal/day 4 months after the operation and gradually increased to 593 kcal/day after 24 months. The loss rose in concert with increased food consumption.

DIARRHEA

Although controlled malabsorption is the exclusive aim of intestinal bypass operations, the procedure actually results in a complex of physiologic and pathologic alterations affecting the intestinal tract and distant organs. It produces, first, a short-bowel syndrome, and, second, bacterial overgrowth in the excluded loops of small bowel. Both contribute to the development of the majority of serious complications related to fluid, acid-base, and electrolyte disorders.

In the initial stage after the operation, fluid losses occur due to diarrhea. This may start only after several days and becomes more acute with resumption of oral feedings. Intravenous fluids can compensate for fecal losses. Until adaptation to the short bowel has occurred, diarrhea continues and may produce as much as 6 L of fecal fluid a day. The severity of the diarrhea is highly unpredictable, and unfortunately, in contrast to the progressive improvement of patients who have had a large segment of small bowel resected, in bypass patients the diarrhea may fail to diminish.

At least two mechanisms for this diarrhea have been postulated in addition to the rapid transit effect of a short bowel. First, bile acids, no longer adequately reabsorbed in the remaining ileum, reach the colon in excessive quantities. High concentrations of bile acids are known to induce fluid secretion into the colon, favoring watery diarrhea. Secondary bile acids, the products of bacterial degradation, are present in large quantities in bypass patients and are thought to be particularly irritating to the mucosa. Second, enteric bacteria, acting upon fatty acids in the lower bowel, produce hydroxy-fatty acids. These acids, equivalent to castor oil, impair absorption and stimulate secretion of water into the colon. Mild intercurrent illnesses, unrelated to the bypass, may cause disproportionately severe diarrhea.

Accurate data for fecal weight are unavailable for large groups of bypass patients. Difficulties in collection and day to day variability make meaningful data difficult to obtain. In a small group of patients, daily excretion varied from normal quantities to 2400 g/day 2 years after the operation. The mean daily output after stabilization was 1060 g per 24 h.

The frequency of bowel movements varies widely from "constipation" to as many as 30 bowel movements per day. Danowski (16) reported that 50 percent of the patients had fewer than 6 bowel movements per day 5 to 7 months after bypass; the remainder had between 6 and 20 per day. Distressing diarrhea persisted at 1 year after the operation in at least 25 percent of the patients (3). Intolerance of certain foods, eating

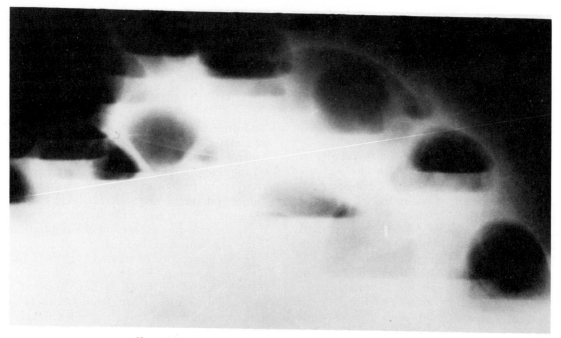

Figure 28-7. Gas-fluid levels in distended loops of bypassed small bowel and colon denoting bypass enteropathy.

large quantities, and drinking iced liquids accentuated the severity of the diarrhea.

Refluxing of large quantities of enteric fluid into the excluded small-bowel loops occurs commonly. Stagnation in the bypassed segment and in the colon is frequently seen (Fig. 28-7). Evacuation at irregular intervals contributes to the erratic exacerbations of diarrhea.

ELECTROLYTE LOSSES

Severe electrolyte losses are common in diarrheal diseases and are consequently frequent in bypass patients. Up to 40 percent of the patients develop signs of depletion during the first year; the incidence decreases to 5 percent subsequently. The losses can be extensive, rapid, recurrent, and difficult to treat. Of bypass patients, 10 to 15 percent, including those with intractable, chronic diarrhea, will at some time require rehospitalization for treatment of acute electrolyte depletion.

Table 28-1 lists the quantities of various elec-

trolytes present in feces as percent of the amounts ingested. It should be pointed out, however, that measurements of fecal excretion for all nutrients and electrolytes as well as for fluid are of a precarious nature, and truly reliable data are very difficult to obtain. First of all, in the diarrheal stage micturition is frequently involuntarily accompanied by defecation, with unknown loss of sample fractions. The patient's cooperation is not easily obtained, because the collection procedure is onerous and difficult. An additional obstacle to obtaining precise collecting data is the fact that the excluded loops of small bowel and a distended colon act as reservoirs which are evacu-

Table 28-1. Stool electrolytes following jejunoileal bypass, percent of intake, means, N = 7

	UP TO 6 MONTHS	7–12 MONTHS	> 12 MONTHS
K	22.1	35.1	31.3
Na	13.3	23.6	45.4
Ca	60.8	104.6	95.4
Mg	44.1	60.7	83.5

ated at variable intervals and to a variable degree; thus, 24-h or 3-day collections provide only approximate measurements. Furthermore, the severity of the diarrhea is totally unpredictable, and with exacerbations, electrolyte losses may rise sharply.

POTASSIUM

Potassium depletion is the most frequently reported electrolyte derangement. In one series of patients, hypokalemia (less than 3.5 meq/L) was recorded in 19 percent of males and 27 percent of females (17) despite potassium supplementation. Without such, most patients became transiently hypokalemic at one time or another during the first 6 months after the operation. In a second series (16) hypokalemia of less than 3.0 meq/L occurred in 18 percent of patients.

Potassium depletion can be explained on the basis of fecal losses if intake, as is often the case, remains restricted. The quantities usually lost in feces are about threefold greater than in normals, both in absolute amounts and as a percentage of intake. Daily losses in a period when diarrhea was only moderate ranged as high as 44 meq. During severe exacerbations, losses could not be determined accurately and may have been considerably greater. At present, no data are available regarding aldosterone levels or secretion rates in bypass patients, but it is possible that aldosterone may increase in response to volume depletion, enhancing potassium secretion by the colonic mucosa. Furthermore, unknown quantities of potassium are secreted into the functioning and, perhaps, into the bypassed small bowel. Since transit time is shortened and a "diarrheal state" prevails, secreted potassium may escape reabsorption. Severe hypokalemia with levels below 2.7 meq/L has been reported rarely (16). This degree of depletion was associated with marked muscle weakness. Additional symptoms ascribed to potassium depletion in these patients were numbness, tingling, cramping, and nausea. Among 300 patients, 16 percent required rehospitalization for intravenous administration of potassium (17). Two

cardiac deaths, attributable to hypokalemia, have been reported (18, 19). However, severe hypokalemia was not encountered beyond 2 years after the bypass operation.

SODIUM AND CHLORIDE

Sodium losses in feces as a fraction of intake are of a magnitude similar to losses of potassium and greatly exceed normal fecal sodium content, which usually remains below 5 meq per 24 h. In contrast to potassium, sodium absorption in the colon and ileum may be relatively efficient. Aldosterone levels rise with hypovolemia and this hormone may be involved in the regulation of sodium absorption at these sites (19).

Hyponatremia or excessive hypernatremia have not been noted in the spectrum of bypass-induced electrolyte abnormalities. Danowski noted a mean increase in serum sodium from 141 to 143 meq/L accompanying increases in serum chloride to 107 meq/L in one-third of the patients. Several instances of a rather mild hyperchloremic acidosis, responsive to bicarbonate supplements, have been cited by DeWind (17). The cause of the development of hyperchloremia is unclear. Serum phosphorus and bicarbonate concentrations remained unchanged when measured for up to 7 months after the operation.

CALCIUM AND MAGNESIUM

Calcium losses in feces following bypass are substantial and result from a combination of various mechanisms, including steatorrhea, rapid transit, short bowel, and low vitamin D levels (20). While normal obese subjects retained 21 percent of ingested calcium, some bypass patients absorbed only 8 percent (21). Careful determinations in patients with severe diarrhea have shown that fecal calcium can be equal to ingested calcium at 6 months and 1 year after bypass (Table 28-1). In addition, one must consider continuing urinary calcium losses, which, although diminished in bypass patients, range from 25 to greater than 100 mg per 24 h. Thus, many patients are in negative calcium balance. Whether this is a chronic or intermittent process is unknown. A longer ileal segment (36 cm or more), left in continuity, favors better calcium absorption and lower fecal losses.

Magnesium is absorbed throughout the small bowel, and absorption decreases in proportion to reduction in bowel length. If no magnesium is ingested or absorbed, as happens in fasting, net secretion causes moderate but slow losses from body stores. These losses are accentuated in the presence of steatorrhea or watery diarrhea. The losses after bypass are substantial when diarrhea is severe and approach fractional calcium losses in magnitude. In absolute quantities, up to 30 meq of magnesium may be lost in 24 h.

Manifest hypocalcemia (less than 8.5 mg/dL) was observed in 20 percent of females and 24 percent of male bypass patients in one large series (17). It is noteworthy that serum calcium may fall to extremely low levels very quickly. Some of the most severe instances of hypocalcemia, with serum concentrations of 3 to 4 mg/dL, developed within 2 to 3 weeks after surgery.

Clinical manifestations of hypocalcemia and hypomagnesemia are relatively infrequent despite the high incidence of subnormal serum concentrations. Muscle cramping, paresthesias, and anxiety have been regarded as symptoms of calcium depletion (17). Tetany is rare but has been mentioned several times as a consequence of hypocalcemia and/or hypomagnesemia (3, 22). The administration of these cations by vein promptly abolished the tetany. One death has been ascribed to calcium depletion (23); however, this event was not clearly substantiated by low serum calcium levels or other clinical evidence. Ample oral supplements, given prophylactically, have been generally adequate to prevent critical depletion.

It is of interest that the severe magnesium depletion in bypass patients produced a failure both of parathyroid hormone (PTH) release in response to hypocalcemia and of target organ responsiveness to this hormone. Serum calcium levels increased only after intravenous (IV) administration of magnesium, which effected an acute release of PTH and secondary rise in serum calcium (24).

The potential long-range effects of impaired calcium, magnesium, and vitamin D absorption have not been studied extensively or over extended time periods after the operation. However, even after relatively short intervals, three of six bypass patients had abnormal bone biopsies, with abnormalities ranging from slight increases in osteoclasts and mild osteomalacia to overt osteitis fibrosa (20).

Although it was shown in one series that by 18 months to 2 years adaptation improved mineral and vitamin D absorption (20), subnormal serum levels persisted unless supplements were furnished.

PROTEIN DEPLETION

Protein depletion is a not unexpected sequel of bypass surgery. Various causes contribute to this undesirable effect. The planned malabsorption is but one mechanism and is probably not the critical factor. In one group of otherwise healthy bypass patients, nitrogen excretion was 2.5 g/day and did not exceed 7 g (25). Reduced food intake plus malabsorption results in significantly lowered serum albumin levels in about 50 percent of bypass patients (20). Levels generally reach a nadir at about 6 to 12 months after the operation, and more nearly normal levels are restored thereafter by improved absorption and greater intake. In the absence of additional complications albumin concentrations usually remain above 3.0 mg/dL thereafter.

During the hypoproteinemic phase, a number of related manifestations, such as hair loss, a mild to moderate anemia, and muscular weakness are common. In some patients, the skin has remained atrophic. A mild degree of edema may persist indefinitely, presumably the result of hypoproteinemia and increased vascular permeability. An increased susceptibility to infections as a result of impaired immune responses has been ascribed to protein malnutrition.

Rapid and acute protein depletion may occur as

the result of complications of the bypass operation and will be discussed below.

Treatment with protein supplements is helpful, but not universally effective, because oral administration of greater quantities can exacerbate the diarrhea and produce greater losses. The lowered serum albumin levels contribute to the observed decreases in concentration of protein-bound serum electrolytes.

BYPASS ENTEROPATHY

Beyond the consequences produced by the short bowel and the bile and fatty acid diarrhea, bypass patients are prone to develop a syndrome which has been termed bypass enteropathy. This is a chronic inflammatory process involving the excluded loops of small bowel, equivalent to a blind-loop syndrome. The colonic flora invading the bypassed loops causes a nonspecific inflammation of the mucosa which in turn produces enteric and distant organ disease. Most frequently, when surgical exploration has been undertaken, the bacterial population in the excluded loops paralleled the fecal spectrum in number and type of organisms.

The incidence of this syndrome is very high, but the symptoms and signs may be mild and ascribed to malabsorption. Depending on the selection of criteria, as many as 80 percent of bypass patients may have this symptom complex in some degree. Its presence is suggested by a variable set of complaints which include intermittent, distressing abdominal bloating with increasing or pernicious diarrhea, anorexia, nausea and vomiting, fever, rectal burning and pain, and precipitous weight loss. Exacerbations of the enteropathy cause the most severe fluid and electrolyte derangements after bypass and necessitate most readmissions to the hospital for treatment of acute electrolyte depletion states.

The drugs commonly used to control diarrhea—notably opiates such as codeine or diphenoxylate hydrochloride—are useless or harmful in bypass enteropathy. While inhibiting peristalsis of the functioning bowel, these drugs also inhibit peristalsis in the excluded bowel segment, increasing the stasis and stagnation of luminal contents. Thus the inflammatory process is accentuated and its ill effects enhanced.

Extreme lowering of serum calcium and magnesium levels in bypass patients appears to coincide with exacerbations of the bypass enteropathy. A number of systemic complications of bypass have also been related to this syndrome; among these are arthritis, skin lesions, vasculitis (26), possibly the hepatic changes, and nonspecific visceral granulomatous disease (27). Pneumatosis intestinalis (28) and pseudoobstruction of the colon with massive chronic distention have been observed in association with bypass enteritis. However, it is not known if pseudoobstruction is in fact a part of the syndrome or an entity of different origin. Although distressing, this complication in itself does not seem to cause acute or severe electrolyte depletion. Increasing hepatic steatosis with marked dysfunction has been noted with the syndrome. Under these circumstances, protein synthesis can be impaired, adding to the severity of hypoproteinemia and its consequences.

The most extensive protein depletion states have been observed in association with bypass enteropathy. Serum albumin has been observed to fall from 4.7 to 2.1 mg/dL within 18 days after the operation. The rapid development of marked hypoproteinemia has its origin in active, exudative protein in addition to the usual anorexia, and the catabolic effect of fever and stress and malabsorption. Exudative fecal protein loss may reach 17 g/day (26). The cumulative effect of these losses over an extended period is an undesirable and excessive weight loss with severe protein calorie malnutrition (Fig. 28-8).

Treatment of enteropathy is generally successful if begun early. Nutritional support, intravenous correction of electrolyte depletion, and suppression of blind-loop overgrowth are essential. If the patient fails to respond, dismantling of the bypass is indicated, because hepatic deterioration may ensue with graver prospects and greater surgical risk. Metronidazole or broad-spectrum antibiotics have proved valuable in re-

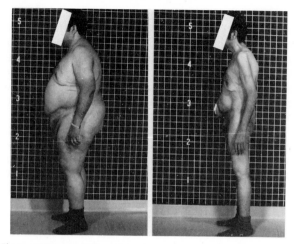

Figure 28-8. Emaciation due to bypass enteropathy with exudative enteric protein loss.

ducing the anaerobic organisms, the most likely offenders. Both the enteric and the systemic manifestations improve if enteropathy is managed in this fashion.

URINARY CHANGES

Alterations in quantity and quality of urine and of urinary constituents are to be expected in bypass patients. The prominent causes for the observed changes are the persistent diarrhea and the damaging effect of bile acids and hydroxy-fatty acids upon the colonic mucosa, resulting in secretion of fluid into the gut and in diversion of fluid from the kidneys. Urine volumes in our patients decreased by 16 to 20 percent, from a mean of 2000 mL to 1650 mL/day (Fig. 28-9). Patients who developed renal stones were noted to have even lower mean volumes, under 1000 mL per day (16). Specific gravity remained unaltered, presumably due to fecal loss of minerals. Creatinine excretion decreased, as may be expected in patients whose lean body mass diminishes. In addition, creatinine clearance had fallen from a mean of 178 to 108 mL/min 1 year after bypass. Diminished renal function or pathologic urinary constituents do not appear unless hyperoxaluria damages the urinary tract.

HYPEROXALURIA, STONE FORMATION, AND OXALATE NEPHROPATHY

Normally, only a small amount of oxalic acid, about 20 to 40 mg/day, is excreted in the urine. The origin of urinary oxalate is primarily dietary. A fraction of ingested oxalate is absorbed by passive diffusion through the wall of the large bowel. Most is normally eliminated in the feces as the insoluble calcium oxalate salt; however, in patients with steatorrhea of any cause, the large quantities of unabsorbed fatty acids present in the lower bowel are thought to compete with oxalic acid for available calcium ions to form insoluble calcium soaps. The surplus oxalic acid radicals have to bind to cations other than calcium, and in these more soluble forms, oxalic acid is absorbable in the colon. It has been demonstrated that bypass patients absorbed almost four times as much of ingested ^{14}C-labeled oxalate as did normals. Absorbed oxalate is transported through the bloodstream to the kidneys, where insoluble calcium oxalate may form.

Hyperoxaluria of a variable degree appears in all bypass patients, and abundant crystal formation is commonly observable in their urine. Crystaluria occurs at acid or alkaline urine pH; in some patients, stone formation in the renal pelvis or deposition of calcium oxalate crystals within the parenchyma of the kidney may occur. In one large series of 543 patients (29), the incidence of

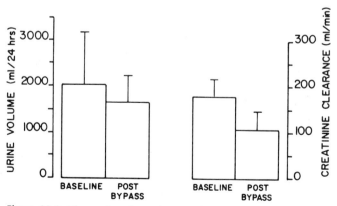

Figure 28-9. Change in urine volume and creatinine clearance after bypass operations (N = 7).

stone passage was 17 percent. In other series the incidence varied from 4.3 to as high as 30 percent (30, 31). Nephrolithiasis tended to develop between 6 to 12 months after the operation in over half the stone formers, with decreasing frequency up to the fourth postoperative year. About 60 percent of stone passages were single episodes, but over 10 percent of sufferers had multiple attacks, with some patients passing several stones per month. The majority of stones are small in size, but jagged. The chemical makeup is almost always pure calcium oxalate.

Spontaneous passage of stones is the rule, but in some patients the rate of stone growth is rapid; within a few months the stones may become too large to pass through the ureters (Fig. 28-10) and nephrolithotomy may become necessary.

Possible cofactors leading from crystal to stone formation have been proposed. Urine volume falls after the bypass. Specific gravity of urine has not been uniformly higher in stone formers. Oxalate and calcium excretion in stone formers and non-stone-formers has been of the same magnitude, that is, about 120 mg of oxalate and 160 mg of calcium per 24 h. Some patients were noted to have passed stones repeatedly with marginally elevated urine oxalate excretion, while others with urine oxalate levels four- to sixfold greater than normal failed to develop nephrolithiasis. Thus undefined individual differences in the capacity to inhibit crystal formation and aggregation remain a significant factor.

A number of measures have been employed to lessen oxaluria and the likelihood of stone formation. A diet low in oxalate is the primary form of treatment. Such a regimen has lowered 24-h

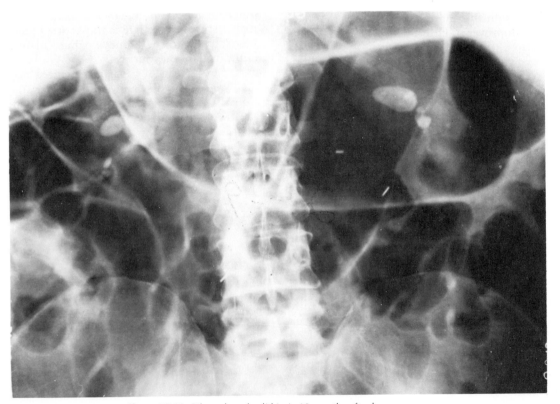

Figure 28-10. Bilateral nephrolithiasis 18 months after bypass operation. Note bowel distention due to enteropathy.

urinary oxalate in bypass patients from 140 to 24 mg. A significant quantity of urinary oxalate may be derived from ascorbic acid (32) if it is consumed and absorbed in large amounts. About one-half of ingested ascorbate is converted to oxalic acid. It appears reasonable, therefore, to limit vitamin supplements to a tolerable amount. Endogenous oxalate production may contribute to the total body pool and the excretory load; for this reason measures to limit absorption of metabolic precursors have been recommended. Taurine administration has been suggested as a possible means to reduce absorption of glycine, an oxalate precursor (33). However, clinically, no consistent benefits have been observed. It is now held that very little of the oxalate appearing in the urine is derived via endogenous metabolic pathways.

The amount of fat ingested and the resulting steatorrhea was found to be unrelated to urinary oxalate excretion by Dobbins (34), while Earnest (35) and Anderson (36) found that urinary oxalate decreased with institution of a low-fat diet and with diminishing steatorrhea. It is generally recommended, despite conflicting evidence regarding utility, that fat intake should be low. Substitution of medium-chain triglyceride substituting for dietary fat may reduce oxaluria by about 30 percent (37).

A rational means to reduce oxalate absorption in the colon may be oral administration of calcium in large quantities (3). Abundant calcium would permit formation of calcium soaps, while surplus calcium still remained available for binding to oxalic acid with precipitation of insoluble calcium oxalate. Another avenue to accomplish reduced colonic oxalate absorption is the ingestion of cholestyramine, which is thought to absorb soluble oxalate salts (38). Unfortunately, many bypass patients find cholestyramine unpalatable and distressing in the presence of disturbed gastrointestinal function.

As might be expected from observations in primary hyperoxaluria, bypass patients with hyperoxaluria are prone to develop impairment of renal function as well. Renal failure due to interstitial nephritis with parenchymal oxalate deposition was described in a bypass patient by Cryer et al. (39). Renal tubular dysfunction (40) may be an early phenomenon. Irreversible end-stage renal failure may ensue, requiring hemodialysis (41) or renal transplants. Reconstitution of normal bowel continuity is necessary to prevent progression of the process, but it neither reverses existing damage to renal parenchyma nor improves function.

The incidence of renal oxalosis following bypass is unknown, but it may occur in the absence of stone formation. In one small series, 2 out of 32 patients had developed histological evidence of oxalate nephropathy with markedly impaired renal function.

In the routine care of bypass patients it is essential that a sensitive renal function test be included as part of the follow-up examinations. A progressive fall in creatinine clearance may be the signal of significant renal damage requiring a biopsy for documentation of oxalate-induced nephropathy. The severity of the process may dictate dismantling of the bypass.

In addition to the undesirable sequelae of the bypass operation discussed above, a host of other complications have been observed (9). These range from the immediate and late complications of any abdominal surgery to the development of gallbladder stones, anorectal gastrointestinal hemorrhagic disease, manifestations of renal failure, and many others.

CLINICAL PROBLEMS PECULIAR TO POSTBYPASS PATIENTS AND THE PRACTICAL MANAGEMENT

Several problems which require appropriate intervention arise after intestinal bypass operations. In some respects, the treatment in this situation has to differ from the therapy usually employed for relief of the particular anomaly; this is true, for instance, for the treatment of diarrhea or renal stone formation.

Those problems which occur frequently or repeatedly in the same patient will be mentioned.

DIARRHEA

Considering the various contributory causes described in the text of this chapter, several therapeutic measures are indicated.

A. Dietary measures
1. Small, multiple meals
2. Low fat content, substitution of medium-chain triglycerides for saturated fats
3. Low sugar content
4. No liquids for 30 min after solid food
5. Liquids in small quantities
6. No iced liquids
7. No concentrated sugar-containing drinks
B. Medications
1. Calcium carbonate, preferably in liquid form, containing 6 to 12 g elemental calcium per 24 h
2. Methylcellulose (bulk-forming agent to absorb luminal liquid)
3. Cholestyramine can be tried if bile acids are a factor in causing the diarrhea, 4 g q.i.d.
4. Antibiotics (if enteropathy is evident) against anaerobic organisms
   a. Metronidazole, 250 mg, 2 tablets q.i.d. until improved, repeat when necessary
   b. Clindamycin
5. Antibiotics against aerobic organisms
   a. Ampicillin

ELECTROLYTE DEPLETION (Ca, Mg, K)

A. Mild cases
1. Oral supplements—administer during the time of day when diarrhea is least likely to occur
2. Suggested dosage
   a. Calcium—4 to 12 g/day (as carbonate, gluconate, or lactate)
   b. Magnesium—50 meq/day (as magnesium oxide)
   c. Potassium—40 to 60 meq/day (as potassium chloride)
   d. Vitamin D—recommended daily dose × 3
B. Severe or symptomatic depletion
1. Calcium gluconate—IV
2. Magnesium sulfate—IV and IM
3. Potassium chloride—IV
4. Vitamin D—recommended daily dose × 3

DEHYDRATION

A. Mild cases
1. Oral liquids—small quantities, frequent intervals, at room temperature
B. Severe cases
1. IV fluids (with electrolytes as needed) to compensate for total fluid output plus insensible loss

HYPERCHLOREMIC ACIDOSIS (USUALLY MILD)

A. Oral sodium bicarbonate

PROTEIN DEPLETION

A. Mild cases
1. Oral protein supplements in liquid suspension 90 to 120 g
2. Oral amino acid mixtures
B. Severe cases
1. IV hyperalimentation—plus oral protein supplements if tolerated (45)
2. IV essential amino acids (43)
3. Avoid diuretics if edema is present
4. Metronidazole, if bypass enteropathy with exudative protein loss is suspected as a factor in protein depletion
C. Intractable depletion
1. Feeding jejunostomy of proximal excluded jejunum for infusion of nutrients, fluid and electrolytes (44)

HYPEROXALURIA AND STONE FORMATION

A. Proceed as follows:
1. Maintain hydration and low urine specific gravity by drinking large quantities, but in small amounts at frequent intervals to avoid exacerbation of diarrhea
2. Low fat diet
3. Low oxalate diet
   a. Avoid vitamin concentrates (ascorbic acid is a source for oxalate)
4. Calcium carbonate 6 to 12 g/day

5. Aluminum hydroxide antacids containing 3.5 g elemental aluminum/day
6. Cholestyramine 4 g t.i.d.
7. Don't restrict calcium intake
8. Don't use thiazide diuretics

REFERENCES

1. Payne, J. H., L. T. DeWind, and R. R. Commons: Metabolic observations in patients with jejunocolic shunts, *Am. J. Surg.*, **106:**273–289, 1963.
2. Scott, H. W., Jr., R. Dean, H. J. Shull, et al.: New considerations in use of jejunoileal bypass in patients with morbid obesity, *Ann. Surg.*, **177:**723–735, 1973.
3. Salmon, P. A.: The results of small intestine bypass operations for the treatment of obesity, *Surg. Gynecol. Obstet.*, **132:**965–979, 1971.
4. Weismann, R. E.: Surgical palliation of massive and severe obesity, *Am. J. Surg.*, **125:**437–446, 1973.
5. Bray, G. A., R. E. Barry, and J. R. Benfield, et al.: Intestinal bypass operation as a treatment for obesity, *Ann. Intern. Med.*, **85:**97–109, 1976.
6. Juhl, E., F. Quaade, and H. Baden: Weight loss in relation to the length of small intestine left in continuity after jejunoileal shunt operation for obesity, *Scand. J. Gastroenterol.*, **9:**219–221, 1974.
7. Mulcare, D. B., H. F. Dennin, and E. J. Drenick: Effect of diet on malabsorption after small bowel bypass, *J. Am. Diet. Assoc.*, **57:**331–334, 1970.
8. Crisp, A. H., R. S. Kalucy, T. R. E. Pilkington, et al.: Some psychosocial consequences of ileojejunal bypass surgery, *Am. J. Clin. Nutr.*, **30:**109–120, 1977.
9. Iber, F. L., and M. Cooper: Jejunoileal bypass for the treatment of massive obesity. Prevalence, morbidity, and short- and long-term consequences, *Am. J. Clin. Nutr.*, **30:**4–15, 1977.
10. Bray, G. A., R. E. Barry, J. R. Benfield, et al.: Intestinal bypass surgery for obesity decreases food intake and taste preferences, *Am. J. Clin. Nutr.*, **29:**779–783, 1976.
11. Barry, R. E., J. Barisch, G. A. Bray, et al.: Intestinal adaptation after jejunoileal bypass in man, *Am. J. Clin. Nutr.*, **30:**32–42, 1977.
12. Quaade, F., E. Juhl, and K. Feldt-Rasmussen: Blind-loop reflux in relation to weight loss in obese patients treated with jejunoileal anastomosis, *Scand. J. Gastroenterol.*, **6:**537–541, 1971.
13. Sherman, C. D. Jr., W. W. Faloon, and M. S. Flood: Revision operations after bowel bypass for obesity, *Am. J. Clin. Nutr.*, **30:**98–102, 1977.
14. Scott, H. W. Jr., A. B. Brill, and R. R. Price: Body composition in morbidly obese patients before and after jejunoileal bypass, *Ann. Surg.*, **182**(4):395–404, 1975.
15. Morgan, A. P., and F. D. Moore: Jejunoileostomy for extreme obesity: Rationale, metabolic observations, and results in a single case, *Ann. Surg.*, **166:**75–82, 1965.
16. Danowski, T. S., D. W. Clare, S. Nolan, et al.: Prospective study of jejunoileal bypass in obesity. 1. Clinical manifestations in first 5 to 7 months, *Obesity and Bariatric Med.*, **4**(3):108–114, 1975.
17. DeWind, L. T., and J. H. Payne: Intestinal bypass surgery for morbid obesity, *JAMA*, **236:**2298–2301, 1976.
18. Starkloff, G. B., J. F. Donovan, K. R. Ramach, et al.: Metabolic intestinal surgery: Its complications and management, *Arch. Surg.*, **110:**652-657, 1975.
19. Fikri, E., and R. R. Cassella: Jejunoileal bypass for massive obesity: Results and complications in fifty-two patients, *Ann. Surg.*, **179:**460–464, 1974.
20. Teitelbaum, S. L., J. D. Halverson, M. Bates, et al.: Metabolic intestinal surgery: Its complica-D after jejunal-ileal bypass for obesity: Evidence of an adaptive response, *Ann. Intern. Med.*, **86:**289–293, 1977.
21. Danö, P., and C. Christiansen: Calcium absorption and bone mineral contents following intestinal shunt operation in obesity: A comparison of three types of operation, *Scand. J. Gastroenterol.*, **9:**775–779, 1974.
22. Bendezu, R., R. G. Wieland, S. G. Green, et al.: Certain metabolic consequences of jejunoileal bypass, *Am. J. Clin. Nutr.*, **29:**366–370, 1976.
23. DeMuth, W. E., and H. S. Rottenstein: Death associated with hypocalcemia after small-bowel

short circuiting, *N. Engl. J. Med.*, **270**:1239–1240, 1964.

24. Rude, R. K., S. B. Oldham, and F. R. Singer: Functional hypoparathyroidism and parathyroid hormone end-organ resistance in human magnesium deficiency, *Clin. Endocrinol.*, **5**:209–224, 1976.

25. Scott, H. W. Jr., D. H. Law, IV, H. H. Sandstead, et al.: Jejunoileal shunt in surgical treatment of morbid obesity, *Ann. Surg.*, **171**(5):770–782, 1970.

26. Drenick, E. J., M. E. Ament, S. M. Finegold, et al.: Bypass enteropathy: An inflammatory process in the excluded segment with systemic complications, *Am. J. Clin. Nutr.*, **30**:76–89, 1977.

27. Passaro, E., Jr., E. J. Drenick, and S. E. Wilson: Bypass enteritis: A new complication of jejunoileal bypass for obesity, *Am. J. Surg.*, **131**:169–174, 1976.

28. Drenick, E. J., M. E. Ament, S. M. Finegold, et al.: Bypass enteropathy: Intestinal and systemic manifestations following small-bowel bypass, *JAMA*, **236**:269–272, 1967.

29. Gregory, J. G., E. B. Starkloff, E. Miyai, et al.: Urologic complications of ileal bypass operation for morbid obesity, *J. Urol.*, **113**:521, 1975.

30. Wise L., and T. Stein: Biliary and urinary calculi: Pathogenesis following small bowel bypass for obesity, *Arch. Surg.*, **110**:1043–1047, 1975.

31. Dickstein, S. S., and B. Frame: Urinary tract calculi after intestinal shunt operations for the treatment of obesity, *Surg. Gynecol. Obstet.*, **136**:257–260, 1973.

32. Atkins, G. L., B. M. Dean, W. J. Griffin, et al.: Quantitative aspects of ascorbic acid metabolism in man, *J. Biol. Chem.*, **239**(9):2975–2980, 1964.

33. Admirand, W. H., D. Earnest, and H. Williams: Hyperoxaluria and bowel disease (abstract), *Clin. Res.*, 562, 1973.

34. Dobbins, J. W., and H. J. Binder: Importance of the colon in enteric hyperoxaluria, *N. Engl. J. Med.*, **296**:298–301, 1977.

35. Earnest, D. L.: Perspectives on incidence, etiology, and treatment of enteric hyperoxaluria, *Am. J. Clin. Nutr.*, **30**:72–75, 1977.

36. Andersson, H., and R. Jagenburg: Fat-reduced diet in the treatment of hyperoxaluria in patients with ileopathy, *Gut*, **15**:360–366, 1974.

37. Earnest, D. L., H. E. Williams, and W. H. Admirand: A physiochemical basis for treatment of enteric hyperoxaluria (abstract), *Clin. Res.*, **23**:439A, 1975.

38. Smith, L. H., H. Fromm, and A. F. Hofmann: Acquired hyperoxaluria, nephrolithiasis, and intestinal disease: Description of a syndrome, *N. Engl. J. Med.*, **286**:1371–1375, 1972.

39. Cryer, P. E., A. J. Garber, D. Hoffsten, et al.: Renal failure after small intestinal bypass for obesity, *Arch. Intern. Med.*, **135**:1610–1612, 1975.

40. Vainder, M., and J. Kelly: Renal tubular dysfunction secondary to jejunoileal bypass, *JAMA*, **235**(12):1257–1258, 1976.

41. Barbour, B. H., D. Mitchell, B. Joseph, et al.: Maintenance hemodialysis after jejunalileal anastomosis therapy for obesity (abstract), *Proc. Am. Soc. Nephrol. Ann. Meeting*, November 21–23, 1976, p. 27.

42. Ames, F. C., E. M. Copeland, D. C. Leeb, et al.: Liver dysfunction following small-bowel bypass for obesity nonoperative treatment of fatty metamorphosis with parenteral hyperalimentation, *JAMA*, **235**(12):1249–1252, 1976.

43. Heimburger, S. L., E. Steiger, P. LoGerfo, et al.: Reversal of severe fatty hepatic infiltration after intestinal bypass for morbid obesity by calorie-free amino acid infusion, *Am. J. Surg.*, **129**(3):229–235, 1975.

44. Pace, W. G., J. W. Large, and N. R. Thomford: A modification of the jejunoileal bypass, *Am. J. Surg.*, **128**:631–632, 1974.

45. Scott, H. W., Jr.: Intestinal bypass operations in treatment of massive obesity, *Hosp Practice*, pp. 104–112, November 1972.

46. Schwartz, H., and H. E. Jensen: Jejuno-ileostomy in the treatment of obesity, *Acta. Chir. Scand.*, **139**:551–556, 1973.

47. Brill, A. B., H. H. Sandstead, and R. Price, et al.: Changes in body composition after jejunoileal bypass in morbidly obese patients, *Am. J. Surg.*, **123**:49–56, 1972.

48. Faloon, W. W., A. Rubulis, J. Knipp, et al.: Fecal fat, bile acid, and sterol excretion and biliary lipid changes in jejunoileostomy patients, *Am. J. Clin. Nutr.*, **30**:21–31, 1977.

29

Clinical physiology of heat exposure

JAMES P. KNOCHEL

PHYSIOLOGY OF HEAT STRESS

THERMOREGULATION

The ability to maintain a relatively constant temperature is critical to body homeostasis. This homeostatic process involves several regulatory mechanisms which balance loss and gain of body heat. In response to a rise of body temperature above normal, whether the heat is derived from the environment (exogenous) or the body itself (endogenous), certain physiologic adaptations occur which allow the individual to deal efficiently with the excess heat load. The capacities of these physiologic mechanisms to buffer the effect of high ambient temperatures are very great, but, like all physical systems, they have limitations. Failure to dissipate a heat load efficiently may adversely affect normal physiological processes, aggravate preexisting diseases, and cause certain well-defined disease states.

Three factors determine the thermal balance of the body: metabolic heat production, heat exchange between the organism and its surroundings, and heat loss by the evaporation of sweat.

Heat production by basal metabolism occurs continuously at a rate ranging between 60 and 70 large calories per hour in the average adult.[1] Heat production increases markedly with exercise, and for brief periods may exceed 1000 kcal/h during intense physical work (1). By definition, one large calorie will increase the temperature of one kilogram of water one degree Celsius. Because of physical differences, the sudden addition of 70 kcal to a 70-kg person is theoretically sufficient to elevate body temperature approximately 0.8°C. This would occur if there were no means to dissipate the added heat.

Heat is exchanged between the body and its surroundings by three physical mechanisms. The first, radiation, is exchange of heat between the body and an object by electromagnetic waves. The second, convection, entails exchange of heat between skin and adjacent streaming currents of air or liquids. The third, conduction, the least important in quantitative terms, is transfer of heat down a gradient between the skin and another object with which the skin is in contact.

Heat exchange becomes limited or even re-

[1] In this discussion, a large calorie, or kcal, will be referred to simply as a calorie.

versed if the ambient air temperature equals or exceeds that of the body surface and if air movement stops. If the requirement to cool the body exceeds the capacity for heat exchange by radiation, convection, and conduction, sweating must occur to permit heat loss by vaporization of water. Each 1.7 mL of sweat vaporized will relieve the body of 1 kcal of heat load. Maximum rates of sweat vaporization are related to dryness as well as air movement. In a hot climate, the limit of the body's ability to dissipate a heat load is a function of its capacity to sweat and of the environment's capacity to support vaporization of sweat. The maximum sweat rate in an untrained, unacclimatized person may approach 1.5 L/h (2). While complete vaporization of this quantity of sweat could theoretically relieve an 882-kcal heat load (1500 ÷ 1.7 = 882), such physical efficiency is never attained, since 20 percent or more of sweat may be lost by dripping (3), and such sweat rates cannot be sustained. Under environmental conditions which prevent loss of heat by direct physical means, the upper limits of heat dissipation are approached at caloric expenditures of 650 kcal/h (4). Sustained work in excess of this rate may cause hyperpyrexia.

When the environmental temperature equals or exceeds that of the body surface and the air is saturated with moisture, a progressive rise of body temperature is inevitable. Even under basal conditions, the predicted rise of body temperature would be 1.1°C (2°F) per hour (Fig. 29-1). More important, the temperature rise under a moderate work-load expenditure of only 300 kcal/h will exceed 5°C (9.0°F per hour) (2). This physical fact supports the clinical observation that once sweating ceases in an individual subjected to heat stress, frank hyperpyrexia may appear with dramatic rapidity.

Heat acclimatization

Acclimatization to heat is a physiologic process by which an individual becomes able to tolerate heat stress safely and comfortably. During this process, profound adaptations take place that involve the cardiovascular, endocrine, and exocrine systems. A critical factor in the human ability to

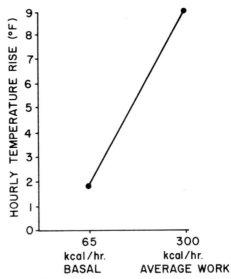

Figure 29-1. Relationship between the rate of body temperature rise compared to heat production in an environment that favors neither heat loss nor heat gain from the body.

tolerate physical work in the heat is the status of physical training. An unacclimatized person who is in excellent physical condition, however, can withstand a given heat stress much more easily than one who is not. In many respects, physical conditioning per se produces changes similar to those of heat acclimatization. Quite obviously, when defining acclimatization, one must qualify the term to answer the question, Acclimatization to what? The level of adaptation which permits one to tolerate sedentary activity in an uncomfortably hot climate does not ensure survival under conditions of hard, prolonged physical work.

Physiologic responses to work in the heat

A person working steadily in the heat may become febrile. Besides basal heat production of approximately 70 kcal, the subject may also derive up to 150 kcal/h by irradiation from the sun (2). To this load is added the heat produced by work. Heat produced under various conditions is shown in Table 29-1.

The capacity to dissipate heat may be so limited that work of even moderate intensity will cause fever. Two excellent examples illustrate the

Table 29-1. Energy expenditure during different types of physical activity

Work	kcal/h
Shoveling	570
Hand sawing	450
Walking (4 mph)	340
Pushing wheelbarrow	300
Carrying bricks	216
Light assembly work	108
Typing	84
Competitive sports*	
Football	102
Wrestling	114
Hockey	173
5-mile run	360
Basketball	344
Swimming (20 min)	220

* Calories expended per event in addition to basal requirement.
Source: From Passmore and Durnin (1); and Buskirk (47).

intensity of heat produced by exercise. First, muscle temperature may reach 41.1°C (106°F) or more during intense work (5). Second, the heat of metabolism independent of muscular contraction may be enormous. In one study (6) of unacclimatized young men before and after exercising 1 h in the heat [48.9°C (77°F) wet-bulb temperature], at work loads of 50 percent of maximal O_2 utilization, hepatic venous temperature was noted to rise as high at 41.6°C (107°F), while the simultaneous rectal temperature was only 40.0°C (104°F). These studies have two important implications. First, not only are the biochemical processes in muscle cells during contraction a major source of heat, but hepatic metabolism, e.g., gluconeogenesis and glycogenolysis, is also a major source of heat. Second, core (rectal) temperature, conventionally used as an index of heat load, may substantially underestimate temperatures elsewhere in the body during hard work.

The cardiovascular response to hard work in the heat. During hard work in a hot environment, there may occur a serious deficit in effective arterial volume. The ability to tolerate this stress depends on the integrity and critical responsiveness of the cardiovascular system. Muscular work, independent of environmental heat, results in

massive shunting of blood to skeletal muscle, so-called exercise hyperemia.

Muscle blood flow varies in almost direct proportion to the degree of work and ranges from 1 mL per 100 g/min at rest to more than 20 to 40 times this value during intense exercise (7). A 70-kg male has about 30 kg of skeletal muscle. If he runs while carrying a heavy load and utilizes approximately two-thirds of muscle mass, the shunt to his muscle vasculature could be as high as 4 L/min.

Besides blood shunted to skeletal muscle, a substantial loss of plasma volume into muscle cells may also occur during hard work. The major fuel for muscular contraction during intense exercise is muscle glycogen. As glycogen or other substrates are broken down, many smaller intermediary products are formed. Since the cell membrane is relatively less permeable to the intermediary products of glycolysis than to water, powerful osmotic forces are generated within muscle cells. At least during the early period of exercise, glycolysis induces movement of water from plasma in quantities averaging 10 percent or more of the inflowing arterial volume (8). Finally, the effective volume of body fluids is also diminished by losses of sweat.

Heat generated by muscular contraction is conducted to blood flowing through the dilated muscle vascular bed. The heated blood is returned to the heart and in turn to hypothalamic centers. Hypothalamic responses induce dilatation of skin vessels and secretion of sweat by the sweat glands. This important response is the Benzinger reflex (9). In classic experiments, Benzinger showed that a rise in intracranial temperature increases peripheral blood flow and sudomotor activity. Peripheral blood flow rises by approximately 15 mL/min for every 0.01°C increase in temperature. Hellon and Lind (10) showed that simple exposure to heat induced a rise of forearm (cutaneous) blood flow from 4 mL/dL arm volume per minute to 12 mL/min. Neither core nor skin temperature but the temperature of blood reaching the anterior hypothalamus controls this response.

As blood and body temperature rise during work, the rise of blood flow to muscle and skin could produce potentially serious hypotension were it not for intense splanchnic vasoconstriction (11, 12). Examining the response of resting normal subjects to hyperthermia induced by water-perfused suits, Rowell and his associates (13) showed that elevation of the skin temperature to 40.5°C was associated with a rise of arterial blood temperature up to 39.4°C, up to a 125 percent increase in cardiac output, a 15 to 60 percent reduction of hepatic blood flow, and a net rise of splanchnic vascular resistance of as much as 120 percent. However, diminished splanchnic blood flow is inadequate to compensate for the combined loss of plasma water into muscle, increased vascular capacitance resulting from dilatation of vessels in skeletal muscle and skin, and loss of extracellular fluid volume as sweat. The net effect is a sharp diminution of effective arterial volume.

The central circulatory response to the fall of effective arterial volume is decreased venous return, an increased heart rate, and a decreased stroke volume. If heart rate and venous return are adequate, cardiac output may remain the same or rise; but if sufficient hyperthermia occurs, cardiac output as well as stroke volume will fall sharply.

Gold (14) studied volunteers exposed to dry heat for 2 h at 54.5°C (130°F) or 1 h at 71.1°C (160°F). Although hazardous, the study was of practical importance, since during hot weather similar temperatures may occur in closed, parked automobiles, enclosed attics, and boiler rooms. Exposure to such extreme heat initially elicited signs of a hyperkinetic circulation, but as heat storage rose, mean venous pressure increased from 40 to nearly 200 mmH$_2$O. Cardiac output was estimated in one subject. It initially rose, but as deterioration appeared, it fell. Each subject was removed from the heat chamber when collapse was imminent (this was based on abnormal sensations of lightheadedness and a facial color change from pinkish red to almost ashen gray). At this point, some of the subjects began to cease sweating. Gold suggested that the primary event in the circulatory collapse of heat pyrexia was high output cardiac failure and that sweating ceases because of the rising venous pressure.

Rowell and his coworkers studied hemodynamic responses of 10 unacclimatized, untrained men to 50 percent to 80 percent maximal exercise in temperatures of 26.5°C (78°F) and 43.3°C (110°F) (13). At the higher temperature, exercise was associated with diminished cardiac output, stroke volume, and central blood volume. The average heart rate rose from 174 beats per minute at 25.6°C (78°F) to 195 beats per minute at 43.3°C (110°F). Of great importance, the greater heat strain while working at 43.3°C was not associated with a higher oxygen utilization. Williams and his associates (15) demonstrated that, as an individual performs work at a level approaching his maximum oxygen utilization under conditions of high environmental temperature, requirements for augmented cardiac output to maintain skin and muscle blood flow are met only by additional cardioacceleration. Under these conditions, stroke volume and, eventually, cardiac output fall.

Cutaneous blood flow probably decreases drastically as exhaustion appears during exercise in heat (16). Since delivery of heated blood to the body surface is impaired, the ability to dissipate heat from the skin is jeopardized. In conjunction with diminished sweat production that eventually occurs during protracted heat loads (17, 18), mounting hyperpyrexia would be anticipated if similar work were continued. Whether or not the decreased cutaneous blood flow is related to the piloerection and chilly sensations sometimes noted as a prodrome to acute heatstroke is unknown.

From the foregoing evidence, it seems clear that the keystone of human ability to tolerate hard work in a hot environment is the capacity to increase and to sustain cardiovascular performance.

Endocrine response to heat stress. Either simple exposure to heat or performance of physical work in the heat may be accompanied by profound changes of endocrine function. However, endocrine function cannot be assessed only by concentrative changes of plasma hormones. During simple exposure to intense heat, plasma volume contracts; consequently, the concentration of any substance bound to plasma proteins will rise modestly. Similarly, hard work in the heat, by profound diminution of renal blood flow, glomerular filtration rate (GFR), and splanchnic blood flow, could alter distribution, decrease excretion, or affect metabolism of the hormone in question. Furthermore, the altered state of the circulation and metabolism brought about by either acclimatization to heat or physical training could conceivably alter many factors controlling its disposition. Therefore, demonstration that the concentration of a substance rises during hard work in the heat does not necessarily indicate that it was released from its site of production or storage.

These hypothetical considerations are exemplified in a report by Mitra et al. (19) concerning their observations on growth hormone secretion in response to acute versus chronic heat stress in cattle. They showed that, whereas acute exposure led to an abrupt increase of growth hormone concentration in plasma, chronic heat exposure was associated with a diminished rate of secretion, decreased plasma concentration, decreased fractional turnover rate, and increased volume of distribution. Such studies need to be done in humans in order to characterize the endocrine response to performance of work in a hot environment. The following data are presented with the foregoing reservations in mind.

Either hard work or acute heat exposure activates the renin-angiotensin system and increases production of aldosterone (20, 21, 22, 23, 24). The rise of plasma renin activity is less pronounced under a given degree of heat stress in an acclimatized individual. In studies conducted in young soldiers in basic military training in hot weather (23) plasma renin activity was elevated to values more than 10 times normal in samples collected before arising in the morning, even when sodium intake exceeded 300 meq/day. Similarly, in relation to sodium intake, both excretion and secretion of aldosterone were considerably greater than normal. Although this response of aldosterone production is probably of critical importance for eventual acclimatization, its role in the immediate response to work in the heat is perhaps less important, as there is evidence that the onset of biologic activity of aldosterone is delayed up to 2 h (25). Observations on young men before and after 1 h in a sauna (46 to 51°C, water content 46 g/kg of bathing air) showed that plasma renin activity,

angiotensin II, and aldosterone rose significantly (26). Although no measurements were obtained, it was speculated that acute volume depletion was the likely stimulus for these changes. Observations from the same laboratory on the effects of running exercises on plasma renin activity, angiotensin II, and aldosterone showed even more pronounced changes (27).

In a recent study (28), it was found that plasma aldosterone at rest was slightly lower after heat acclimatization. As mentioned earlier, this could well be compatible with an increased metabolic clearance rate even in the presence of increased production of the hormone.

Either physical work or heat is a potent stimulus for growth hormone release (29, 30). Growth hormone causes retention of salt and water (31). Its action could conceivably be equally important to that of renin, angiotensin, and aldosterone in acclimatization.

Hale and his associates (32) detected no change of plasma adrenocorticotropic hormone concentration in normal subjects exposed to a temperature of 49°C (120°F) for 45 min. While some have found that plasma cortisol concentration rises briefly during exposure to intense heat or during hard physical work (33), this has not been observed by others (28). Excretion of 17-hydroxycorticosteroids or 17-ketosteroids into the urine does not change after acclimatization or training (59).

Kotchen and his associates (22) examined norepinephrine, epinephrine, and renin in response to graded exercise. By their method of analysis, neither norepinephrine nor renin activity rose in trained subjects until they exercised at 70 percent or more of the maximum work capacity. Plasma epinephrine concentration rose only with maximal exercise. The effect of heat per se on plasma catecholamine concentration in man apparently has not been reported. Fiorica and his associates (34) observed no change in plasma catecholamine concentration during acute heat exposure in dogs. Hasselman and his coworkers (35) found that men working in temperatures of 37 to 40°C (98.6 to 104.0°F) excreted smaller quantities of catecholamines in their urine than when working at 22 to 30°C (71.6 to 86°F). The meaning of this report is obscured by the fact that performance of work in a hot climate is associated with a pronounced fall of GFR and renal blood flow (36) that could account for diminished catecholamine excretion independent of the rate of release.

Renal functional response to heat stress. The renal response to hard work in the heat has been well characterized. Neither GFR nor renal plasma flow change appreciably during moderate work. In contrast, Radigan (34) showed that exposure to a temperature of 51°C (123.8°F) at rest produced an average 39 percent fall in renal plasma flow and a 21 percent fall in GFR. Both fell further during work in the heat. These changes are associated with oliguria and diminished sodium excretion (36, 37). Individuals living in hot climates are often unable to concentrate urine to normal maximal values (38). This is ordinarily not severe enough to cause polyuria, although frank polyuria unresponsive to posterior pituitary extract was described in some British soldiers stationed in the Libyan desert during World War II (39). Since frank polyuria is so unusual in people living in hot climates, one must seriously question whether any true relationship exists. Nevertheless, mild or moderate polyuria could favor development of dehydration.

The prevailing urine pH is lower in persons living in hot climates (40, 41, 42, 43). There could be a relationship between low urine pH and the higher incidence of uric acid stones in residents of hot regions (41).

Serum creatinine concentration, when measured conventionally as creatinine chromogen, may actually fall after an individual has acutely produced large quantities of sweat (23, 44, 45, 46). For example, a normal individual may display a decline of serum creatinine from 1.2 to 0.8 meq/dL after several days in the heat. This can be explained by the fact that certain noncreatinine chromogens measured as creatinine are readily excreted in sweat but not in urine (45). If creatinine clearance is calculated using data obtained by measuring creatinine chromogens, as is done conventionally by current automated techniques, one could mistakenly assume that GFR had risen. This result would be spurious; however, it should be recognized that *after* a normal subject be-

comes physically conditioned in the heat, resting GFR, measured by inulin clearance, does rise by approximately 20 percent (23).

Effect of heat stress on blood composition

Simple exposure to a high ambient temperature induces hyperventilation, a fall in blood P_{CO_2}, and acute respiratory alkalosis. At least at the outset, serum $[K^+]$ may fall as much as 1.0 meq/L, probably as a result of the alkalosis (47). If exposure is sufficient to increase body temperature to about 39°C, serum K may rise rather than fall (48). Hyperkalemia thus induced occurs despite increasingly intense respiratory alkalosis. Dehydration is not entirely responsible for the hyperkalemia. Potassium release from cells could also occur as a consequence of increased metabolism caused by heating, and at least part of the hyperkalemia could occur by means of decreased K excretion by the kidney.

Hypernatremia and hyperchloremia may also occur during heat exposure. The major factor responsible appears to be elaboration of sweat, a hypotonic fluid, without adequate water replacement.

After acclimatization, serum K tends to become somewhat lower, Na and Cl higher.

A low normal serum K also occurs in highly trained marathon runners (49). These changes, seen in heat-acclimatized and in physically trained humans, are of interest since they occur despite expansion of body water spaces (23). The same biochemical and volume changes occur in patients with primary aldosteronism; however, in contrast to the case with primary aldosteronism, heat-acclimatized or trained humans do not display hypertension or metabolic alkalosis. The low normal serum K in the trained or acclimatized person occurs without K deficiency (23). Relevant observations on these parameters are discussed below.

Serum phosphorus concentration declines continuously during exposure to heat, as temperature continues to rise (48). Hypophosphatemia also occurs as a result of respiratory alkalosis independently of fever (50). Since it occurs in the face of a declining urine phosphorus excretion, it must reflect increased cellular uptake of phosphorus. Magnesium concentration in plasma rises very slightly during exposure to heat (51).

PHYSIOLOGIC FEATURES OF A HEAT-ACCLIMATIZED AND PHYSICALLY CONDITIONED HUMAN

The following is a classic description of heat acclimatization from William Bean's (52) observation of soldiers training in the California desert during World War II:

When fit, adequately trained men are exposed to high temperature and high relative humidity, they are incapable of work for long periods. Compared with their performance in a temperate environment, the pulse is higher, internal and skin temperatures are higher, and the blood pressure, especially in the erect position, is unstable. The face and upper part of the body are flushed, the eyes and nasal mucosa may be injected, causing lacrimation and sniffles; hands and feet exhibit edema; the rate of sweating increases considerably. There is a sense of overwhelming oppression which rapidly takes the spirit out of men. Trifling work is fatiguing and more burdensome work rapidly leads to exhaustion. A throbbing headache may develop and reach cruel intensity. Dizziness occurs and is accentuated by the standing position. Dyspnea may be a problem. Thirst, which rapidly becomes intense if water is withheld, proves a guide to needed water replacement since the loss is never voluntarily replaced during work. Nausea, vomiting and loss of appetite are commonplace. Lack of coordination reduces efficiency. Eyes become glazed and stare vacantly. Apathy may be interrupted by outbursts of irritability. Judgment and morale decline. Occasionally, hysteria or hyperventilation with tetany may add to their bizarre signs and symptoms. The walking man may collapse and the standing man may faint. Unwillingness to continue work and the onset of physical disability may rapidly disorganize a well disciplined and efficient unit. Such a severe and alarming illness has commonly produced almost complete ineffectiveness. Contrast with this picture that of the same man after four or five days of work in the heat. He now performs his work with only slightly higher pulse and temperature than in a comfortable environment. He is cheerful, alert and vigorous. No longer does he exhibit the flushed, sometimes edematous skin and engorged mucous membranes of earlier exposures. He can stand without fear of syncope even after four

hours of continuous work. Water is drunk eagerly although thirst is still not an adequate incentive for complete fluid replacement. Sweating continues at a rapid rate somewhat greater than on the first exposure. Thus, the essential gains of cardiovascular-thermal acclimatization have been made, though improvement may continue at a slow rate for days or weeks.

Cardiovascular adaptations and training

Three critical cardiovascular adaptations occur under conditions of heat stress that permit an individual to perform work comfortably in a hot environment (53, 54). These are an increased maximal cardiac output, a decreased peak heart rate, and an increased stroke volume (11, 55). These adaptations facilitate efficient delivery of heated blood from muscle and viscera to the body surface, where heat can be dissipated. A classic feature of the heat-acclimatized state is a smaller increment in rectal temperature with a given quantity of exercise. This results not only from the enhanced capacity of the cardiovascular system to propel blood and facilitate heat dissipation but also from the increased metabolic efficiency acquired by physical training. A large body of evidence has accumulated during the past few years showing that not only are mechanisms of oxygen delivery to muscle increased by training, but there also occurs a marked increase in myoglobin content (56) and the density of mitochondria per unit of muscle mass (57). Since energy utilization is nearly 20 times more efficient by oxidative (mitochondrial) than by anaerobic metabolism, these adaptations would not only explain the increased potential for oxygen utilization with training but also provide a solid chemical-structural explanation for the mechanism underlying enhanced metabolic efficiency. Thus, heat production during a given quantity of work will be less in a trained man, and heat strain will be proportionately less.

Sweat volume and composition

A major feature of the heat-acclimatized state is a drastic alteration in the composition and volume of thermal sweat. The first recognition that

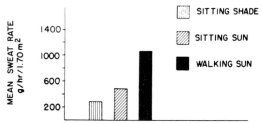

Figure 29-2. Heat load versus rate of sweat production.

sweat [Na⁺] diminishes as an individual becomes acclimatized is credited to Dill and his associates (58). Their observations have been amply confirmed; the fall in sweat [Na⁺] and rise in the volume of sweat produced in response to a given work load are physiologic hallmarks of the heat-acclimatized state.

The relationships between heat stress and the volume of sweat produced before and after acclimatization have been extensively studied. Typical findings from such studies are shown in Figs. 29-2, 29-3, 29-4, and 29-5. The volume of sweat rises in proportion to the heat load (Fig. 29-2) and the volume of sweat produced at any body temperature is higher after acclimatization (Figs. 29-3, 29-4). Of great importance, hydration will simultaneously enhance sweat production and ameliorate the rise of body temperature over a given series of heat loads induced by walking (Fig. 29-5).

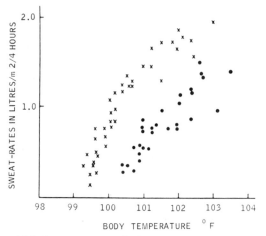

Figure 29-3. Sweat rate versus body temperature before and after acclimatization. [*From Wyndham et al.*]

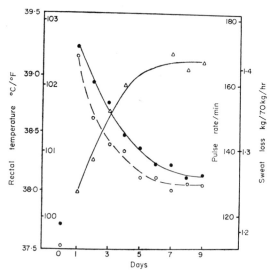

Figure 29-4. Daily (serial) sweat rate, temperature and sweat Na. [*From Leitheid and Lind, as adapted from Lind and Bass.*]

It seems to be the common experience of those performing work in a hot climate that sweat production during initial exposure to heat may be much more voluminous than that after acclimatization has occurred. This disparity between physiologic observations made by climatologists and subjective impressions of people working in hot climates may have some basis in fact. Many physiologic studies of heat acclimatization that demonstrate increased sweat production during the acclimatizing process have been conducted under artificial conditions in the laboratory and usually have not been of more than several weeks' duration. In contrast, Adam and his associates (59) studied the effects of standardized heat exposure on British troops during a period of 6 months. During the first 2 weeks, they noted that sweat production increased in response to a given heat exposure, but during the following 5-month period, there was a progressive decline of sweat output in response to the same stimulus. The same conclusion has recently been reached by Dasler and his associates (60). These investigators examined sweat production under conditions of work in the heat and attributed the eventual decline of sweat production to increased physio-

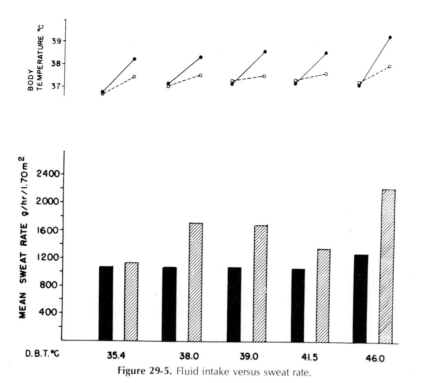

Figure 29-5. Fluid intake versus sweat rate.

logic efficiency brought about by the heat-acclimatized state. The bulk of evidence would suggest that diminished sweat production in response to a given work load after prolonged acclimatization to heat is probably the result of enhanced metabolic efficiency induced by physical training and is a reflection of less endogenous heat production under conditions of work.

The role of aldosterone in sodium conservation

Considerable evidence indicates that aldosterone excretion in the urine is higher during acclimatization and probably remains higher in subjects living in tropical environments than in those in temperate environments (20). There is also evidence that increased production of aldosterone may be essential for acclimatization. Robinson and his coworkers (61) have shown that a large intake of NaCl may suppress the normal decline of sweat [Na+] in response to heat exposure. These studies were conducted under conditions

of minimal heat stress and thus may not be applicable to natural heat acclimatization in which intense physical work is a component. Other studies (62) have shown that aldosterone secretion and excretion remain inordinately high in relation to Na intake not only in individuals training in the heat but also under the same conditions of training during cool weather. The latter observations indicate an important effect of physical activity independent of heat stress.

Diminished [Na+] of thermal sweat is due to the action of aldosterone (Fig. 29-6), as proved experimentally by Ladell (63) and others (64, 65, 66). These authors have shown that, after administration of desoxycorticosterone or aldosterone or in individuals naturally acclimatized to heat, administration of spironolactone leads to a prompt rise of sweat [Na+].

Sweat gland responsiveness to exogenous aldosterone is somewhat sluggish in comparison to the response of the kidney. The renal response occurs within hours, whereas the decline in sweat

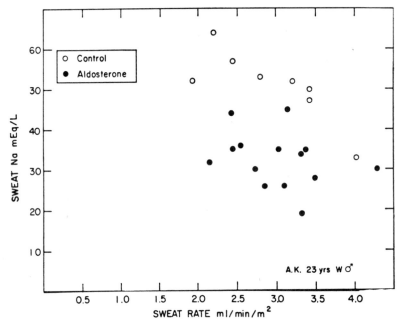

Figure 29-6. Sweat rate versus sweat Na. [*From Grand et al.*]

[Na+] requires 1 or 2 days to appear and does not reach its lowest value for 5 or more days (65).

Acclimatization to heat is associated with increments of blood volume (67, 68), plasma volume, extracellular fluid (ECF) volume, and total body water (55, 69).

The volumes of plasma, ECF, and total body water rise in correlation with the increased cardiac output in response to work during the process of acclimatization to heat (55). In our own studies (23) on individuals training in a moderately warm climate, there was a mean rise of ECF volume of 9.6 percent and an increase of total body water of 6.7 percent. Yoshimura (70) described higher values for blood and plasma volume in subjects studied during hot as compared to those studied in cool weather. Desai and his associates (71) showed markedly higher values for total exchangeable sodium (^{24}Na) and sodium space in subjects residing in a warm, humid climate than in those living in a temperate climate.

People who are acclimatized to work in the heat display venous distention at rest. It is most evident over the forearm and dorsum of the hand but may be present in the jugular veins as well. This reflects a normally increased blood volume; venous pressure is normal.

Conn and his associates have made major contributions (64, 72, 73) to our understanding of the physiologic state of acclimatization to heat and have shown that this state is quite analogous to that produced by prolonged administration of aldosterone to normal man. Thus, given an individual consuming a normal quantity of sodium chloride, administration of aldosterone or desoxycorticosterone leads to sodium retention by the kidneys, a modest weight gain, and decreased concentration of sodium in sweat. After several days, a new steady state is achieved characterized by sodium excretion into the urine equal to intake. However, extracellular volume remains modestly expanded. This so-called "escape," i.e., reappearance of sodium in the urine despite continued administration of aldosterone, does not occur in the sweat glands. Continued excretion of sodium into the urine in the presence of unrelenting sodium conservation by sweat glands closely resembles some but certainly not all of the characteristic findings in normal humans following acclimatization to heat. The foregoing evidence strongly supports the notion that retention of salt and water sufficient to allow for physiologic expansion of body fluid compartments is necessary for heat acclimatization. Aldosterone very likely plays a key role in this process. The possibility exists that other hormones, e.g., growth hormone, may also play a role.

Exogenous administration of the mineralocorticoid desoxycorticosterone does not induce acclimatization as determined by usual measurements of response to heat stress (74). However, Braun and his associates (38) suggested that aldosterone administration does exert a favorable effect on certain hemodynamic and thermal responses to exercise in the heat. Evidence obtained from other experimental studies (75, 76) suggests that aldosterone exerts an inotropic effect on the heart, but this is not a property of desoxycorticosterone.

ENVIRONMENTAL HEAT ILLNESS

In 1929, Wakefield and Hall (77) reviewed the history of disease resulting from excessive environmental heat. A characteristic of severe illness such as heatstroke has been its propensity to occur in catastrophic numbers. In Peking, in July of 1743, 11,000 persons are said to have perished from the effects of an intense, prolonged heat wave. In 1873, Gihon described a condition known as adynamia, observed in sailors who became ill while working in ship boiler rooms and in those subjected to sweatbox punishment. The temperature in those rooms often reached 71°C (170°F). Woodruff (78) described the death of 123 of 186 British soldiers imprisoned for one night in the infamous Black Hole of Calcutta.

Heatstroke is sometimes called siriasis (78) based on a biblical reference that it occurred coincidentally with the appearance of the dog star, Sirius, that could be seen in the twilight and followed the sun throughout the summer.

A complete classification of heat illness has been prepared by the Climatic Physiology Committee of the Medical Research Council of Great Britain (79). Those conditions germane to this textbook include heat cramps, heat syncope, heat edema, heat exhaustion, and heatstroke.

HEAT SYNCOPE

A person in good health who squats for 1 min and suddenly stands upright often feels a bit faint and may show tachycardia and hypotension. If the same person does the same maneuver after exposure to a high ambient temperature or working in the heat for several hours, these symptoms may be more pronounced; indeed, the person may faint. When syncope occurs in a person who has been briefly exposed to a high environmental temperature, and no other cause is apparent, the diagnosis of heat syncope may be made.

The pathogenesis of this disorder is apparently vasodilatation, postural pooling of blood, diminished venous return to the heart, reduction of cardiac output, and cerebral ischemia. As soon as sufficient salt and water have been retained as a result of acclimatization, syncope no longer occurs.

In some individuals who become potassium-deficient by sweating (see below) or by other means, syncope may be due to autonomic insufficiency. Biglieri has shown (80) that hypokalemia may lower blood pressure, impair vascular responsiveness to catecholamines, and blunt cardioacceleration otherwise produced by hypotension. Correction of hypokalemia rapidly reverses these abnormalities.

Heat syncope will occur more commonly in persons with cardiovascular disease and especially in anyone who has a deficit of salt and water.

Usually, treatment for heat syncope is unnecessary. Indeed, the patient commonly awakens before the audience regains their wits. He or she should be allowed to rest in the shade or a cooler environment.

HEAT EDEMA

Slight edema of the ankles and dependent parts is extremely common in persons who are unacclimatized. It occurs within a day or two after entering a hot climate, is invariably mild and noticed more by women, and vanishes during acclimatization.

The cause of heat edema appears to be salt and water retention resulting from interaction of several factors. These could include salt supplementation, oliguria secondary to heat-induced vasodilatation, increased aldosterone production, and perhaps increased growth hormone production.

The only effect of heat edema is its unpleasing appearance. Treatment is not required. Indeed, it is unwise to offer such a patient a diuretic, since it could not only interfere with acclimatization but also induce K loss.

HEAT CRAMPS

This is an acute disorder of skeletal muscle characterized by brief, intermittent, often excruciating cramps in muscles that have been subjected to intensive work. They often occur in men whose physical condition is superior and who are well acclimatized. The classical description of this disorder was published by Talbott (81).

As a descriptive term, heat cramp is a misnomer. Exposure to heat per se does not elicit muscle cramps. Tetany during exposure to high environmental temperature appears to result from hyperventilation and acute respiratory alkalosis, and it is clearly distinguishable from muscle cramps (82). It is believed that muscle cramps result from an acute deficiency of Na after adequate replacement of the water loss incurred by sweating. Thus, such patients are hyponatremic.

Role of hyponatremia and its pathogenesis

Three factors are characteristic of individuals predisposed to heat cramps. First, due to their acclimatized state, they are able to produce sweat in large quantities in response to hard muscular work. Second, they consume adequate amounts of water to replace the sweat losses. Third, they fail to replace Na losses. Acclimatization is associated with diminished sweat [Na$^+$]; nevertheless, [Na$^+$] in sweat still rises sharply as the rate of sweat production rises. This is explained by the fact that the [Na$^+$] of sweat at its site of formation in the secretory coil of the gland is equal to that

in plasma water (40). At low sweat rates, there is time for Na to be reabsorbed as the precursor fluid passes along the duct. However, at high flow rates, there is insufficient contact time for Na reabsorption to occur, and [Na$^+$] in the final sweat is much higher (Fig. 29-7).

The highly conditioned and acclimatized person is able to produce large volumes of sweat and thus is paradoxically endangered by the capacity to lose larger quantities of Na than an unacclimatized person. Moreover, maintenance of hydration will facilitate a higher sweat rate than would occur under conditions of dehydration (Fig. 29-5). The maximum sweat rate for unacclimatized individuals is 1.5 L/h, while for acclimatized individuals it is 2.5 L/h. The [Na$^+$] in sweat produced is 100 meq/L for the former group and 70 meq/L for the latter group. Therefore, the maximum Na loss is 150 meq/h for unacclimatized individuals and 175 meq/h for acclimatized individuals.

The mechanism responsible for heat cramps is not known. Thus, whether heat cramps represent *cramps* (with the implication that they occur in response to electrical phenomena—i.e., in conjunction with action potentials) or contractures (implying electrical silence) (84) has not been examined. Although the putative cause of cramps is hyponatremia, one should remain skeptical, since comparable hyponatremia occurs under a variety

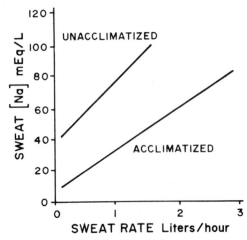

Figure 29-7. Relationship of sweat (Na$^+$) to sweat rate in the acclimatized and unacclimatized human.

of other circumstances in which cramps seldom, if ever, occur. For example, in acute water intoxication, muscular cramps are unusual. However, one cannot dispute the fact that Na (perhaps also Cl) is somehow implicated in heat cramps, since administration of salt leads to rapid relief. Accordingly, it seems pertinent to speculate on the possible mechanism whereby hyponatremia might induce skeletal muscle cramps.

Hypothetical mechanism

Contraction of skeletal muscle occurs by interaction of the contractile proteins actin and myosin. In the resting state, their interaction is inhibited by troponin. Contraction is facilitated by liberation of calcium ions from their site of storage. Calcium ions thus freed into the sarcoplasm react with troponin, nullify its influence, and permit actin and myosin to interact. Active transport of calcium back into the sarcoplasmic reticulum reverses the process and reestablishes the relaxed state. Presumably, the ionic species exchanging for calcium is sodium. Sodium enters the muscle cell from ECF when the cell surface increases its permeability to sodium during excitation.

A $Na^+ - Ca^{2+} - ATPase$ has been isolated from skeletal muscle microsomes (85). Possibly its role is to reduce the concentration of free calcium ions by entrapping them. It is conceivable that hyponatremia might decrease the number of sodium ions entering the cell and so interfere with activation of this adenosine triphosphatase. Sequestration of calcium ions in the sarcoplasmic reticulum might also be prevented. In turn, interaction of myosin and actin would persist and relaxation could not occur.

Since cramps tend to follow intensive muscular work, they might also result from deficient supplies of energy substrates to provide fuel for active transport processes. However, heat cramps are promptly relieved by replacement of sodium deficits, but not by ingestion of glucose (81).

Clinical features

Heat cramps tend to occur toward the end of the working day, while, walking home or having ar-

rived, on relaxing, or on taking a cool shower. Muscle cramps *during* exercise, such as those experienced by football players, may thus be quite different. The paroxysms of painful cramping tend to last no more than a few minutes and ordinarily disappear spontaneously. Rarely, heat cramps involve muscles of the anterior abdominal wall, simulating an acute surgical abdomen. Although one might expect that muscle necrosis and myoglobinuria could follow severe episodes of muscle cramps, to my knowledge these have not been reported, nor has the possibility been examined. Similarly, the possibility that creatine phosphokinase activity or other enzyme values may rise in this condition has not been examined. However, in detailed observations on laborers in the steel mills of Youngstown, Ohio, Talbott and his associates (86) described marked creatinuria in those with muscle cramps, hyponatremia, dehydration, and slight to moderate fever. In those patients, the rate of creatine excretion was marked (up to 75 mg/h) and would be compatible with muscle injury. Most individuals who sustain heat cramps soon discover that ingestion of salt during work is effective prophylaxis. In the event of severe, repeated, unrelenting cramps, oral or intravenous salt solutions rapidly relieve all symptoms.

According to the currently accepted definition of heat cramps, if any systemic symptoms or findings coexist with simple muscular cramps, the disorder should be identified as heat exhaustion.

HEAT EXHAUSTION

This is the most common clinical disorder resulting from work in a high temperature. Although most cases occur during heat waves, heavy sweating incident to intense muscular work, even in temperate climates, may lead to profound losses of body water or sodium chloride and may culminate in every symptom and finding of classical heat exhaustion.

Although pure forms rarely occur, one may divide heat exhaustion into that associated with predominant dehydration and that associated with predominant salt depletion.

Heat exhaustion due to predominant water depletion

An individual working in a hot environment does not voluntarily replace the volume of water lost by sweating, but usually maintains a negative water balance that averages 1 percent or 2 percent of his total body weight (87). This dehydration may impair maximum physical performance. Moroff and Bass (88) have shown that water administration in excess of need improves physical performance under conditions of heat stress. Classically, heat exhaustion due to predominant water loss occurs when the supply of water is limited. It is common in soldiers or laborers in the desert who ingest salt without adequate water, and in infants or enfeebled adults who are unable to express their desire for water. The latter type of patient may become seriously water-depleted while retaining normal stores of sodium; as a result, hypernatremia and hypertonic dehydration occur (see also Chap. 12). Intracellular water is depressed. Oliguria is the rule, and the urine contains very little sodium. Symptoms include intense thirst, fatigue, weakness, discomfort, anxiety, and impaired judgment. Marked central nervous system dysfunction eventually becomes prominent manifested by hyperventilation, paresthesias, tetany, agitation, hysteria, muscular incoordination, and in some patients, psychosis. Terminally, these patients demonstrate delirium, hyperthermia, and coma. This form of heat exhaustion is treacherous, if unrecognized or untreated, it may terminate in heat stroke. Physical examination shows dehydration. Body temperature is almost invariably elevated.

Should circulatory failure or a convulsion supervene, the rise of body temperature accelerates and heat stroke rapidly supervenes.

Heat exhaustion due to predominant salt depletion

The classic clinical description of this disorder was published by McCance (89, 90). It occurs when large volumes of thermal sweat are replaced by adequate water but inadequate salt. It differs from heat cramps in two major respects, namely, it is accompanied by systemic symptoms and tends to occur in unacclimatized persons. Marked dehydration or weight loss do not occur, and the volume of urine and sweat remains normal. In contrast to subjects with heat exhaustion due to water depletion, these patients tend not to complain of intense thirst. Interstitial fluid volume contracts, and the intracellular space expands. Plasma volume, due to the oncotic pressure of serum proteins, tends to be better maintained than interstitial volume.

Symptoms consist of profound weakness, fatigue, severe frontal headache, giddiness, anorexia, nausea, vomiting, diarrhea, and skeletal muscle cramps. As in heat cramps, painful contractions tend to occur in those muscles fatigued by work and are apt to be precipitated by large quantities of water. Such patients may appear haggard, with pallid, clammy, inelastic skin. Hypotension and tachycardia are prominent. In contrast to heat exhaustion due to water depletion, body temperature usually remains normal or subnormal, but if dehydration supervenes as a result of vomiting, body temperature may rise. Sodium chloride deficiency in these individuals may exceed 1000 mmol.

Heat exhaustion is usually associated with deficits of both salt and water. Accordingly, symptoms may be manifold. In view of the common occurrence of fever, headache, malaise, fatigue, myalgias, and sometimes even vomiting and diarrhea, it is not surprising that such patients are sometimes given the diagnosis of "summer flu." Administration of acetylsalicylic acid to such persons who are performing muscular work may paradoxically increase body temperature (91). Treatment for heat exhaustion should be individualized. In most cases, the patient will need no more than lightly salted liquids and rest. In more severe cases, especially those with a rapid pulse and orthostasis, it is advisable to measure serum $[Na^+]$ and examine the urine.

Treatment

In the presence of hypernatremia and a scanty, concentrated urine, the predominant water deficiency may be severe. A simple method to approximate the water deficit is based upon the assumption that total body water (TBW) has been reduced in inverse proportion to the elevation of serum [Na$^+$]. For example, a patient whose normal weight was 70 kg presents with a serum [Na$^+$] of 165 meq/L. The patient's normal TBW may be estimated as 60 percent of body weight, or 42 L. The product of normal serum [Na$^+$] and normal TBW divided by his observed sodium is 35.6. This figure is the prevailing volume of TBW. Therefore, 42−35.6 or 6.4 L represents the patient's water deficit (see also Chap. 12).

The rate of administration should be carefully controlled. Excessively rapid correction of hypernatremia may cause convulsive seizures. It is prudent to administer no more than one-half of the total deficit during the first 2 to 4 h. Water should be given orally if at all possible. If the intravenous route is necessary, the solution of choice is 5% dextrose. Care should be taken to avoid severe hyperglycemia and hypokalemia. When serum Na has fallen to 150 meq/L, hypotonic saline (0.45%) may be substituted. As the point of correction is approached, symptomatic improvement should be evident. The volume and Na content of the urine will increase; its specific gravity will decline. In some patients who have had severe dehydration and hypernatremia, several days may elapse before cerebral function returns to its original state.

Those whose deficit is predominantly salt are generally easier to treat. If administration of salted liquids by mouth is not possible, normal saline or in severe cases, hypertonic saline (3%) may be given intravenously. The required quantity of Na is easily calculated by multiplying the difference between 140 and the observed serum [Na$^+$] by the volume of TBW in liters. Usually, one should not administer more than one-half this quantity as hypertonic saline. The remainder may be given as normal saline over a period of 6 h.

HEATSTROKE

Heatstroke is a catastrophic disorder characterized by hyperpyrexia [a rectal temperature of more than 40.6°C (105°F)], delirium, coma, and anhidrosis. The older terms *heat apoplexy* and *sunstroke* are now considered archaic.

Although heatstroke is the least common of the disorders associated with heat stress, it is the most important since it may occur in epidemic form, carries up to 80 percent mortality, and imposes severe persistent disability in many survivors.

Predisposing factors in normal humans

A variety of factors may increase susceptibility to heatstroke (Table 29-2). Important among these are deficits of salt and water and any acute febrile state which adds to the environmental heat load. Febrile reactions to immunizations are especially important. In young, healthy individuals, lack of acclimatization is perhaps the most common predisposing factor.

As noted by Dreosti in 1935 (92), there are apparently normal individuals who are unable to tolerate heat. In such persons, normal acclimatization does not occur. When forced to work in the heat or when exposed to a sufficiently high temperature at rest, such a person risks serious illness. Even with modest work, rectal temperature rises (93). The cause of the heat intolerance is

Table 29-2. Heatstroke: Predisposing factors

I. PREDISPOSING FACTORS IN NORMAL HUMANS
A. Salt and water depletion
B. Infection
C. Fever with immunization
D. Lack of acclimatization
E. Heat intolerance
F. Obesity

II. DISEASES PREDISPOSING TO HEAT ILLNESS
A. Cardiovascular disease
B. Diabetes mellitus
C. Malnutrition
D. Acute or chronic alcoholism
E. Impaired sweat production
1. Prickly heat (miliaria)
2. Sweat gland injury after heatstroke or barbiturate poisoning
3. Scleroderma
4. Healed thermal burns
5. Ectodermal dysplasia
6. Sweat gland ductal obstruction in diabetes mellitus
7. Congestive heart failure
F. Potassium deficiency

unknown. A recent study (94) suggests that during heat stress, afflicted individuals may not be capable of translocating interstitial fluid into the vascular compartment as efficiently as normal people. Measures to detect such individuals have successfully decreased the incidence of heat injury among laborers in the gold mines of South Africa (95). Unfortunately, similar measures have not been considered in this country to detect individuals at risk among football players, distance runners, or military recruits.

Another common impediment to heat tolerance is obesity. Every farmer is aware that his 1000-lb hog may not survive an August heat wave. Every physician is aware that his patients with morbid obesity have great difficulty in times of intense heat. Even children with moderate obesity may experience severe heat strain during exercise. Haynes and his associates (96) showed that rectal temperatures rose significantly more in obese boys after standardized exercise. In another study (97), the same investigators showed that overweight prepuberal girls could not perform as well in the heat as obese boys.

Diseases predisposing to heatstroke

Some of the illnesses that increase the risk of heatstroke are also shown in Table 29-2. The keystone of defense against environmental heat is cardiovascular integrity. Thus, any cardiovascular disease may impair heat tolerance (98). To illustrate this point, Burch and his associates (99, 100) examined the effects of high temperature [32.2°C (90°F)] and humidity (75 percent) on 23 patients with congestive heart failure. Heart failure became more overt, cardiac output failed to rise normally, some developed angina pectoris with electrocardiographic changes, and some demonstrated a rise of venous pressure. Daily and Harrison (101) showed that, in rats, saline expansion, which was well tolerated at a normal temperature, led to fatal pulmonary edema during hyperthermia.

Virtually any chronic disabling disease increases the risk of heatstroke. Especially notable are diabetes mellitus, malnutrition, and acute or chronic alcohol abuse. The short-term effects of ethanol on heat balance are well known. In cold climates, patients with ethanol-induced coma are commonly hypothermic from heat loss via the skin due to cutaneous vasodilatation. Similar vasodilatation under conditions of high environmental temperature may permit a gain of body heat by identical means and may lead to serious hyperpyrexia.

A brief period of moderate or heavy consumption of alcohol may permit loss of acclimatization. Those who perform hard physical work commonly experience discomfort, lightheadedness, and weakness when work is resumed after an evening or weekend of drinking. In my own experience, the incidence of heatstroke in drinking laborers is greater on Monday than on other days of the week.

Impairment of sweat production has been associated with a higher incidence of heatstroke. One of the most common causes is miliaria (prickly heat). Sweat-gland injury or necrosis may follow acute heatstroke (101) and may account for persistent heat intolerance noted by some persons who survive. Barbiturate poisoning may also cause sweat-gland necrosis (102), which might explain the occasional occurrence of heatstroke in patients intoxicated with barbiturates. Sweat-gland entrapment may occur with advanced scleroderma (103) or in patients who have survived extensive burns (77). Obstructive periductal lymphocytic infiltration of sweat glands has been described in an elderly diabetic patient with fatal heatstroke (104). Sweat glands may be absent in patients with ectodermal dysplasia (105). Malfunction of sweat glands with inability to conserve sodium and resulting salt and water deficiency in patients with cystic fibrosis (106) increases their susceptibility to heatstroke. Impaired sweat production at the time of thermal stress occurs in patients with congestive heart failure (107) and in those receiving certain drugs, including those used in the treatment of parkinsonism, such as benztropine mesylate (Cogentin) (108), atropine (109) and other anticholinergics, phenothiazines and antihistamines (110). A variety of other drugs rarely cause idiosyncratic hyperpyrexia. These include lysergic acid diethylamide (LSD) (111), methyldopa (112), and propylthiouracil. Body temperature of 42.2°C (108°F) has been observed in severe salicylate poisoning (113). In that case, violent muscular activity probably contributed to the fever. Ingestion of normal doses of acetylsalicylic acid may paradoxically cause fever during exercise (95). A list of drugs commonly implicated in heatstroke is shown in Table 29-3.

The potential importance of potassium deficiency in the pathogenesis of heatstroke has been suggested (62, 114) because of the common finding of hypokalemia and other evidence suggestive of depletion of this ion in individuals who produce large volumes of sweat in response to hard work in hot climates.

Evidence for potassium deficiency in heatstroke and its occurrence during acclimatization to heat

Of 121 patients with acute heatstroke whose serum $[K^+]$ was measured at admission, a value of less than 3.5 meq/L was observed in 46 percent (62, 79, 115, 116, 117, 118, 119, 120). Although

Table 29-3. Drugs increasing risk of environmental heat injury

CLASS OF DRUG	EXAMPLE	POSSIBLE MECHANISM
Diuretics	Benzodiathiazinines, furosemide; ethacrynic acid, acetazolamide	Salt depletion and dehydration
Anticholinergics	Atropine, belladonna	Suppression of sweating
Antiparkinsonians	Procyclydine, HCl, benzotropine mesylate	Suppression of sweating
Phenothiazines	Chlorpromazine, promethazine	Suppression of sweating and possibly disturbed hypothalamic temperature regulation
Tricyclics	Tranylcypromine	Increased motor activity and increased heat production
Antihistamines	Diphenhydramine	Supresion of sweating
Butyrophenones	Haloperidol	Possible disturbed hypothalamic temperature regulation and failure to recognize thirst
Sympatho-mimetic amines	Dextroamphetamine, phenmetrazine	Increased psychomotor activity

exposure to heat may be accompanied by hyperventilation, respiratory alkalosis, and hypokalemia, the development of significant fever as a result of heat exposure (48) or performance of hard physical work in the heat is almost invariably accompanied by hyperkalemia due to release of K from muscle (121) and liver (122). When K-deficient men become febrile during heat exposure, hyperkalemia does not occur (48). Severe lactic acidosis (arterial blood pH 6.9 and lactate 11.2 mmol/L) has been identified in patients with stress-induced heatstroke (123). Since acute acidosis should induce a shift of K from cells to plasma (47), an abnormally low serum $[K^+]$ in the presence of acute lactic acidosis suggests potassium deficiency.

During World War II, Ladell (39) observed that a number of British troops in the Libyan desert became intensely polyuric after prolonged exposure to hot climates. In some, urine volumes exceeded 8 L/day and did not diminish after injection of posterior pituitary extract. Edholm observed daily urine volumes exceeding 10 L/day under similar circumstances (124). Although potassium measurements were not made in these soldiers, their polyuria could conceivably have been the result of hypokalemic nephropathy.

Sobel and his associates (125) reported vacuolar changes in renal tubular epithelium, hypokalemia, and polyuria in a number of United States Air Force trainees who sustained acute heatstroke. These findings are also compatible with kaliopenic nephropathy. Polyuria could substantially augment the usual water deficits that exist under such conditions and could increase susceptibility to water-deficiency heat exhaustion and heatstroke.

The mechanism responsible for such extreme polyuria is not clear. Elaboration of urine volumes of the magnitude reported by Ladell (39) and Edholm (124) is distinctly unusual in potassium-deficient patients and suggests that intake of solute and water were disproportionately high. The fact that such observations have been made only on military subjects might be compatible with the latter notion, since large intakes of sodium chloride are customarily encouraged under such conditions. I have observed that total solute output into the urine in soldiers in basic military training who ingest 350 mmol of sodium chloride and a diet containing 146 g of protein may attain values as high as 1500 mosm (126). If such a large quantity of osmotically active particles were excreted in individuals elaborating 8 L of urine daily, urine solute concentration would be 188 mosm/kg of water. If such conditions prevail, a disturbance of thirst must also be invoked as an additional mechanism to explain the marked polyuria observed in those subjects. Hyperreninemia occurs under these conditions (126). It has been implicated as a cause of thirst (127).

Several investigators have estimated potassium balance during acclimatization to heat. Bass and his coworkers (53) examined young men exposed 12 h/day at a temperature of 48.9°C (120°F), relative humidity 28 percent, and who estimated an average daily potassium loss of 15 meq in excess of intake. When they were exposed to heat, their work consisted only of walking for four 30-min periods daily.

Gordon (128) exposed two volunteer subjects to 31.1°C (88°F), 40 percent relative humidity for 6 h/day, 5 days/week for 3 weeks, while they ingested 25 meq of potassium daily. On each day of the study, the subjects vigorously exercised on a bicycle for 30 min, alternating with 30-min rest periods; potassium deficits in these two subjects were 161 and 192 meq.

Streeten and his associates (129) measured potassium balance in four subjects exposed to a temperature ranging from 32.2 to 37.8°C (90 to 100°F) and humidity of 60 to 70 percent for 7 h for 15 to 23 days. Work was not undertaken, and all subjects wore rubber suits to insure collection of all sweat. Potassium intake was more than 100 meq each day. Exclusive of fecal potassium losses, cumulative values for potassium balance during the period of heat exposure in these four subjects were −24, −169, −180, and −411 meq. Potassium excretion in both sweat and urine rose substantially following saline infusions. In all subjects, urinary excretion of aldosterone, estimated by a bioassay procedure, was also substantially higher during the period of heat exposure.

Frank hypokalemia was not observed in any of the aforementioned studies (18, 117, 129).

The level of physical activity in the studies discussed (18, 129) was not so intense as that undertaken by young athletes or military recruits who are at high risk of developing heatstroke. These individuals have been shown to secrete up to 12 L or more of sweat per day, and since [K$^+$] in sweat may range up to 9 meq/L (130), K losses in sweat exceeding 100 meq/day could readily occur. Since dietary intake of K does not ordinarily exceed 100 meq, additional losses of K in urine and feces could generate a severe deficit in a relatively short period of time.

The possibility that serious K depletion might occur under such conditions was examined by measuring serial values for exchangeable ^{42}K in healthy, unacclimatized young soldiers undergoing basic military training in the hot summer and in the cooler winter months (23). As indicated in Fig. 29-8, those training in the hot weather sustained a mean K deficit of 517 meq by the eleventh day of their training. In comparison, those studied in cooler weather showed the expected steady rise of total body K coincident with the increase of lean body mass. All subjects had been maintained on a constant diet containing 106 meq K throughout the periods of observation. Despite large losses of K in sweat at the time they were maximally deficient, K excretion into the urine was inappropriately high and ranged from 41 to 79 meq/day. Simultaneously, the [Na$^+$]/[K$^+$] ratio

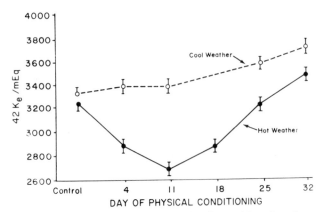

Figure 29-8. Comparison of average total exchangeable radioactive potassium in six military recruits training in hot weather with average values for nine training in cool weather. The interval between the control study and training day 4 was seven days.

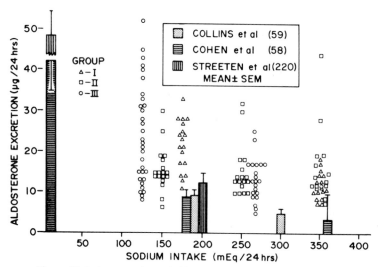

Figure 29-9. A comparison of aldosterone excretion and intake of sodium. Group I represents subjects undergoing basic military training in hot weather; group II represents those training in cooler climates. The bars represent values reported by other investigators using identical analytical methods for normal subjects nor performing strenuous physical work. [*From Knochel et al. (132)*]

in their sweat was very low, reflecting activity of aldosterone on sweat glands. Finally, excretion and secretion of aldosterone (Figs. 29-9, 29-10) and, in many instances, plasma renin activity appeared to be high with respect to Na intake (131, 132, 133, 134, 135). Based on these studies, it was concluded that intense physical work in the heat stimulates higher production of renin and aldosterone than would occur in nonexercising subjects on similar Na intakes. Aldosterone overproduction under these conditions might have induced mineralocorticoid escape. Thus, aldosterone, in the presence of conditions permitting excretion of large amounts of Na into the urine, could facilitate continued excretion of K by the kidney despite serious K depletion. Consequently, the kidney played a role in the genesis of K depletion in those subjects. Although it has not been proved, it would seem highly possible that excessive Na intake could well enhance K losses by the kidney. Although excretion and secretion of aldosterone appeared excessively high in terms of Na intake in all of our subjects during physical conditioning, this relationship appeared to be less

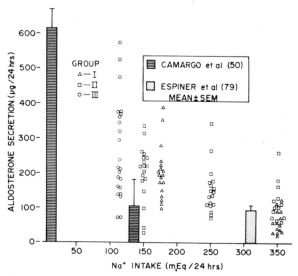

Figure 29-10. A comparison of aldosterone secretion and intake of sodium. Group I represents subjects undergoing basic military training in hot weather; group II and group III represent those training in cooler climates. The bars represent values reported by other investigators using identical analytic methods for normal subjects not performing strenuous physical work. [*From Knochel et al. (132)*]

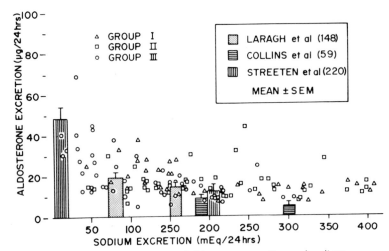

Figure 29-11. A comparison of aldosterone excretion and sodium excretion. Group I represents subjects undergoing basic military training in hot weather; group II and group III represent those training in cooler climates. The bars represent values reported by other investigators using identical analytic methods for normal subjects not performing strenuous physical work.

impressive when excretion and secretion of aldosterone were considered in terms of Na excretion into the urine (Figs. 29-11, 29-12). Despite large intakes of Na, large quantities of aldosterone were excreted in urine, establishing a situation analogous to one of a much lower Na intake. This suggests that excretion and secretion of aldosterone were more or less physiologic (131, 133, 134, 135, 136), although they are sufficient in quantity to stimulate tubular secretion of K despite simulta-

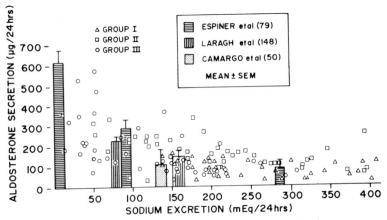

Figure 29-12. A comparison of aldosterone secretion and sodium excretion. Group I represents subjects undergoing basic military training in hot weather, group II and group III represent those training in cooler climates. The bars represent values reported by other investigators using analytic methods for normal subjects not performing strenuous physical work.

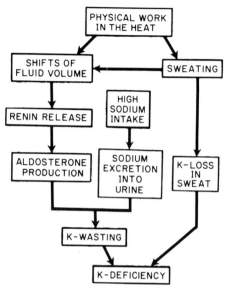

Figure 29-13. Hypothetical mechanism to explain K deficiency during work in the heat.

neous K deficiency. The series of events interacting to produce K deficiency under these conditions is shown in Fig. 29-13.

Comparison of exchangeable ^{42}K with simultaneous aldosterone secretory rates in those subjects studied in hot weather who became K-deficient suggested that the two were related (Fig. 29-14). It has been observed repeatedly that K deficiency is associated with suppression of aldosterone production (137). Although our observations were limited in number, the possibility exists that the transient fall of aldosterone secretion was the result of K deficiency. Indeed, this pattern of aldosterone secretion was not observed in men undergoing conditioning in cooler climates who did not become K-deficient.

There are several other possible harmful consequences of potassium deficiency in people undergoing intensive training in the heat that appear worthy of consideration. Biglieri and his associates (80) have shown that postural hypotension, syncope, and failure of cardioacceleration on assumption of the erect posture may occur with potassium deficiency. Postural hypotension and syncope are commonly observed in young men during physical conditioning in hot climates. The exact mechanism responsible for postural hypo-

tension with potassium deficiency is unknown. However, it has been well established that potassium deficiency is associated with marked hyporesponsiveness to the vasoconstrictive action of catecholamines (80, 138).

Potassium deficiency may impair release of growth hormone (139). Observations that growth hormone release occurs with work as well as with heat exposure (30) and its possible role in stimulating retention of salt and water (31) suggest importance in heat acclimatization. The possible interference with its normal release during thermal stress by potassium could have important implications.

Potassium deficiency could seriously jeopardize energy transformations necessary for performance of hard work as well as the ability to become physically conditioned. Thus, potassium deficiency suppresses insulin release in response to a hyperglycemic stimulus (139), glucose intolerance occurs (14), and the ability to synthesize glycogen in skeletal muscle is impaired (136,

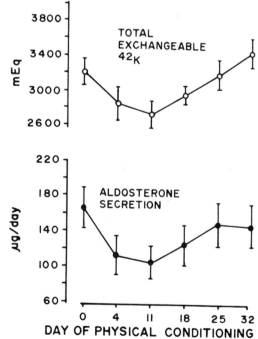

Figure 29-14. A comparison of serial values (mean ± SEM) for total exchangeable potassium and aldosterone secretion in six subjects undergoing intensive physical conditioning in hot weather.

140). The ability to increase muscle glycogen content is a requirement for physical conditioning and is a major factor facilitating endurance for hard physical work (141). The possibility that potassium deficiency may interfere with glycogen synthesis and prevent a biochemical adaptation facilitating the conditioned state has been confirmed experimentally in this laboratory (142).

Potassium deficiency per se may be associated with elevated activity of lactic acid dehydrogenase (LAD) serum glutamic oxaloacetic transaminase (SGOT), and creatine phosphokinase (CPK) in humans (143, 144) and dogs (145). This can occur independently of muscular exercise. Studies from our laboratory (146) showed that dogs with advanced potassium deficiency demonstrated subnormal muscle membrane potential followed by release of CPK. This suggested loss of integrity of the muscle cell membrane as a result of potassium deficiency.

In a situation possibly analogous to that produced by advanced potassium deficiency, namely, depolarization of the skeletal muscle membrane by metabolic inhibitors, Zierler (147) has demonstrated enhanced permeability of the membrane to muscle aldolase.

Rhabdomyolysis occurs very commonly in young men with stress-induced heat injury. It may occur in apparently normal individuals who, before adequate physical conditioning has been attained, undertake severe, prolonged muscular work. For example, it has been observed repeatedly during the first few days of military training and is often the result of repetitious, violent calisthenics such as "squat jumps." Clearly, such individuals are not potassium deficient. However, rhabdomyolysis has also been observed in a number of patients with potassium deficiency of diverse causes, (148, 149) especially when it occurs in conjunction with retention of sodium.

Potassium is a potent vasodilator. It is released from contracting skeletal muscle fibers, and its rising concentration in interstitial fluid is thought to dilate arterioles, mediating the normal rise of muscle blood flow during exercise (150). In potassium-deficient dogs studied during exercise, it has been shown that potassium ions are not released from skeletal muscle, muscle blood flow

does not rise normally, and necrosis follows, possibly the result of ischemia (145). Those studies (145) suggested that potassium deficiency might contribute to the high incidence of rhabdomyolysis observed in young people under conditions of prolonged physical exertion.

Additional studies from this laboratory show that potassium-deficient dogs demonstrate a sharp fall of cardiac output and develop acute pulmonary edema with exercise (151).

If the foregoing observations can be extrapolated to potassium-deficient humans performing sustained hard work, they could not only explain the occurrence of muscle necrosis by means of ischemia but also suggest that potassium deficiency could impair cardiovascular performance sufficiently to prevent adequate heat dissipation. In support of this, it has been well demonstrated in certain experimental animals that potassium deficiency, in conjunction with sodium loading, may readily induce myocardial necrosis (152) and impair cardiac performance (153). As a consequence, potassium deficiency could conceivably play a major role in the pathogenesis of rhabdomyolysis as well as hyperpyrexia. This hypothesis is illustrated in Fig. 29-15.

Clearly, there is no reason to implicate potassium deficiency in any more than a small fraction

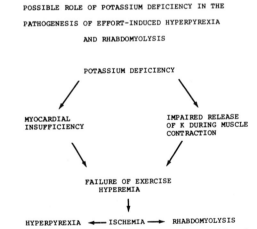

Figure 29-15. A hypothesis characterizing the possible role of potassium deficiency in the pathogenesis of exertional hyperpyrexia and rhabdomyolysis.

of the cases of heatstroke. In most instances, there is no evidence that potassium deficiency preceded the illness. In others, heatstroke occurs within the first 3 days of heat exposure. In those patients, it does not seem possible that significant potassium deficiency could have occurred. Thus, it seems that potassium deficiency could play a contributory role in the pathogenesis of heatstroke when it appears in subjects who have produced voluminous quantities of sweat for one week or more. In those instances, it may contribute heavily to the associated morbidity.

Clinical spectrum of heatstroke

Classical heatstroke. Clinical descriptions of classical heatstroke are based on observations made by several authors on clusters of cases during heat waves. Typical of the latter were reports by Ferris and associates (118), Austin and Berry (116), and more recently by Levine (117). In the report by Ferris et al. (118), all cases occurred within 8 consecutive days when ambient temperatures ranged between 38.9 and 41.1°C (102 and 106°F). Of his 44 cases, only 3 were less than the age of 40 years. Two of those 3 were alcoholics and the other had an acute respiratory infection superimposed on postpartum anemia and malnutrition. In 100 selected cases reported by Austin and Berry (116), most patients were more than 60 years of age; 84 percent had cardiovascular disease and 30 percent had previous histories of admissions to the hospital for alcoholism.

Levine (117) reported on 25 patients with fatal hyperpyrexia whose average age was 78.4 years; 72 percent had arteriosclerotic heart disease and 12 percent had hypertension or hypertensive heart disease.

The foregoing reports are typical of circumstances preceding that form of heatstroke observed during sustained waves of high environmental temperature. Thus, after several days of temperatures often exceeding 37.9°C (100°F) or when environmental temperature is perhaps lower but accompanied by high relative humidity, that portion of the population who are aged, chronically ill, or enfeebled will be at high risk (154). A point to be strongly emphasized in the pathogenesis of heatstroke in this group of patients concerns the nature of the heat stress. Not only are the temperature and humidity high, but both are usually sustained through the day and night for several days. Thus, active perspiration is continuous but eventually fails, body temperature rises sharply, and classical heatstroke rapidly supervenes. One should be especially alert for such cases in the event of an electrical power shortage. In larger cities, many persons live in poorly ventilated apartments that can be cooled only by air conditioning. Many who live under such conditions never subject themselves to sufficient heat to become acclimatized. During "brownouts" they are at extreme risk of developing heat injury.

Prodromal symptoms in these patients may be absent, with the first manifestation being sudden collapse. They are commonly found wandering about in a state of stupor. Other patients develop weakness, dizziness, nausea, and fainting spells for a period of 2 or 3 days before their collapse. Some complain of frontal headache, weakness, and a feeling of excessive body heat. Muscle cramps may occur but are unusual since sodium deficiency is not characteristic. Of those survivors who are able to recall their prodromal period, about half state that sweating ceased before the onset of their collapse. In some, this has been associated with a sensation of coldness and the appearance of gooseflesh. It is to be noted that convulsive seizures are generally *not* observed in acute heatstroke but are commonly observed as the patient is being cooled therapeutically.

Some patients who develop this form of heatstroke undergo a prodrome characteristic of predominant water-depletion heat exhaustion. This is especially prominent among persons in nursing homes or other chronic invalid care facilities where attendant care is marginal and there is no provision of adequate water to restore extensive losses of sweat.

The typical physical findings of heatstroke, nearly hyperpyrexia, coma, and hot, dry skin are based on observations made on patients like the foregoing. Specifically, the notation in the reports of Austin and Berry (116) and Ferris and his associates (118) that sweating was totally absent in 100 percent of their patients and in 84 percent of the patients reported by Levine (117) has established the clinical finding of a hot, dry skin as a virtual prerequisite for the diagnosis of heatstroke. Moreover, anhidrosis in such patients has led to the notion that fatigue of the sweating mechanism occupies the key position among factors thought to play a role in the pathogenesis of classical heatstroke.

Based on clinical observations that patients with heatstroke commonly displayed a hot, dry skin, Thaysen and Schwartz (17) and later Schwartz and Itoh (155) showed that, during prolonged exposure to the heat, the rate of sweat secretion could not be sustained for more than 6 h despite a rising body temperature. Furthermore, the sweat volume response to methacholine became blunted and, finally, the local response to methacholine in patients with heatstroke was only 1 to 2 percent of that observed in normal subjects. They concluded that their findings indicated "fatigue" of the sweat glands and suggested that this phenomenon played a role in the pathogenesis of heatstroke. This view has been challenged by Gilat and his associates (156), who noted that even when so-called "fatigue" had occurred, the rate was substantially higher than values observed at rest. They argued that, since the sweat rate had not fallen substantially, sweat-gland fatigue cannot be considered important in the pathogenesis of heat stroke. The same authors have also leveled criticism at the suggestion made by Ladell (157) that hyperthermia per se is the cause of sweat-gland fatigue. Gilat and his coworkers (156) studied the change of rectal temperature in eight highly trained, heat-acclimatized Israeli soldiers during a march of 31.5 km while carrying a standard load of 35 kg. Five of the eight had rectal temperatures ranging from 41.5 to 42.4°C (106.7 to 108.3°F) on completion of the march. They were allowed rest stops and water. Dehydration averaged only 0.9 L. Active sweating had persisted in all. Three were euphoric and restless. At the time of the hyperthermia, all were considered to demonstrate early, albeit transient, symptoms of heatstroke. Consideration of these data and the observations on 38 cases of exertion-induced heatstroke in which sweating was observed despite hyperpyrexia indicates clearly that sweat-gland failure is not always the critical factor in all patients with heatstroke. These findings were in agreement with those made in 1925 by Kuo and his associates (158), who published detailed observations on four normal subjects exposed to intense heat stress imposed by a dry-bulb temperature of 72°C (162°F) and wet-bulb temperature of 40.8°C (118°F). They observed that the major effects of heat exposure, including stupor, that appeared when rectal temperatures had risen to values ranging from 39.5°C (103.1°F) to 40.8°C (105.4°F), occurred before sweating diminished. They postulated that sweat-gland exhaustion could not explain the sudden diminution of sweating, since profuse, generalized sweating reappeared promptly if the subjects were removed from the heat chamber to a cool environment. Sweat-gland fatigue and failure must exist in some patients, especially elderly ones with classical heatstroke who have dry, hot skin without evidence of sweating. The rapid reappearance of sweating after it had subsided in the normal subjects observed in short-term studies by Kuo (158) may in fact have little relationship to sweat-gland failure that occurs after sweating has been protracted in patients who have incurred heatstroke. Those subjects forming the basis of Gilat's observations (156) were healthy young men performing virtually superhuman feats for which adequate heat-dissipating means were not available. In this latter group, the total duration of physical activity required to produce hyperthermia is usually measured in minutes or hours, whereas elderly patients with classical anhidrotic heatstroke have usually been sweating at least for a day or more and therefore would be more likely to have incurred failure of the sweat mechanism.

Exertion-induced heatstroke. Descriptions of classical heatstroke as described in invalids or in the elderly population stand in sharp contrast to observations made on patients who incurred heatstroke in association with physical exertion (159, 160, 161, 162, 163). Analysis of the literature and personal observations both generate the impression that the majority of cases occur in association with events that increase endogenous heat production and have clearly established that sweating persists in more than 50 percent of the total number of cases. Thus, it is clear that fatal heatstroke can occur in perfectly healthy, highly acclimatized and physically conditioned individuals when the physical means to dissipate heat is exceeded by endogenous heat production. In the United States, the majority of such cases appear to occur in marathon runners (160, 162), football players (123, 159), and military recruits (62, 161, 163). In both groups, sustained, often extraordinary physical exertion commonly precedes heatstroke. In the case of football players, many are young, highly competitive, inexperienced, and overenthusiastic, and consequently they do not pace themselves. In contrast, serious heat illness is virtually unknown among professional football players. In military recruits, the mandate to achieve a superior physical condition and the fear of being sent through a second course of recruit training would appear to substitute for the competitive zeal seen in the athlete. Although prophylactic measures to forestall or prevent heatstroke have been widely publicized, (164, 165, 166) one occasionally observes certain practices in physical conditioning programs that undoubtedly favor the propensity to incur heatstroke (126). Flagrant among these is the false notion that water deprivation accelerates physical conditioning—during football practice sessions, water has been provided as a tepid, salted solution containing dissolved oatmeal in order to discourage its consumption. Another example is the provision of only salted water in canteens for soldiers in basic training. Overzealous administration of salt supplements is also very common. Without question, salt supplements are mandatory during the first week or so of conditioning in hot climates. However, provision of water is much more important. Ingestion of excessive sodium and insufficient water is a potentially lethal practice and undoubtedly accounts for cases of severe water-depletion heat exhaustion that culminate in frank heatstroke. Another potentially disastrous practice is based on the notion that strenuous exercise, such as long-distance running, in hot climates while clothed in impervious plastic sweat clothing, will safely accelerate weight loss in overweight athletes (123).

The following description is considered quite typical of exertional heatstroke in a football player.

Patient 1. A 20-year-old football player was brought to the emergency room after collapsing during practice. Several hours before, he became extremely irritable and, for no apparent reason, provoked arguments and made threats to several of his close friends. Thereafter, he babbled incoherently and ran wildly about the field before collapsing. Football practice had been underway for 10 days. The temperatures had not been higher than 32.2°C (90°F), but the peak daily humidity exceeded 50 percent. Physical examination showed a heavily built man who was totally unresponsive with hot, flushed, moist skin. His pupils were equal in size, widely dilated, and did not respond to light. Eye grounds were normal. Rectal temperature was greater than 42.2°C (108°F), pulse rate was 160 beats per minute, blood pressure was 80/0 mmHg, and respirations were deep at a rate of 30 per minute. While he was on the examining table, cooling was effected by placing the patient in a wake of a large fan and by rubbing him with ice for 90 min until his rectal temperature reached 38.9°C (102°F). On cooling, his blood pressure rose to 100/60 mmHg. The patient became tremulous and had a series of grand mal seizures. These were followed by a rise of rectal temperature to 41.7°C (107°F). Sweating did not appear. One hour later, he became frankly cyanotic, and although only 800 mL of fluid had been administered intravenously, he showed signs compatible with frank pulmonary edema. Reinstitution of cooling measures and intermittent positive pressure respiration produced improvement.

Laboratory findings showed a white blood cell count of 18,000 per cubic millimeter with 82 percent polymorphonuclear cells and a platelet count of 46,000 per cubic millimeter. Serum potassium was 2.7 meq/L and total carbon dioxide was 8.9 mmol/L. Arterial blood pH was 7.19 and arterial carbon dioxide pressure (Pa_{CO_2}) was 28 mmHg. On the second day, the urine was scanty in volume, dark, and showed a positive test for heme pigment. Serum glutamic oxaloacetic transaminase activity was 2640 units (normal range, 2 to 12 units). Serum creatine phosphokinase activity exceeded 100,000 IU/L.

During the next 18 h, although the patient's temperature was kept below 38.9°C (102°F), he remained in coma. Babinski reflexes and ankle clonus were present bilaterally. Widespread petechial hemorrhages were evident. His electrocardiogram showed ST-T changes compatible with posterior myocardial ischemia. On the following day, 34 h after admission, scleral icterus was observed. Total urine output since admission had been only 400 mL. Due to a rapidly rising serum urea nitrogen concentration, hemodialysis was performed, effecting a weight loss of 1.4 kg and diminution of serum urea nitrogen concentration from 175 to 90 mg/dL. At its completion, the patient had another convulsive seizure and died. During the seizure, serum potassium concentration had risen from 4.2 to 8.0 meq/L.

This case illustrates several important points:

1. Frank heatstroke occurs in otherwise healthy young people even though sweating has not ceased.
2. In heavily built individuals who achieve higher levels of muscular work, hyperthermia is often severe. This may be correlated with widespread hemorrhagic necrosis involving skeletal muscle, myocardium, liver, kidney, and brain.
3. The onset of hyperthermia may be preceded by psychotic behavior (119).
4. Thrombocytopenia is the rule and is probably the result of disseminated intravascular coagulation.
5. In severe cases, shock and acute pulmonary edema have been observed before fluid replacement, and these presumably indicate either acute left ventricular failure or a disturbance of pulmonary vascular permeability. The possibility that lactic acidosis impaired left ventricular function in this patient should be considered (167, 168).
6. Evidence of rhabdomyolysis exists in virtually all cases.
7. Death commonly occurs as a result of acute hyperkalemia either following a convulsive seizure or as a result of extensive rhabdomyolysis with acute renal failure.
8. Hypokalemia at the time of admission is common and, in those individuals who have been sweating profusely for a week or more, may represent serious potassium depletion.

Such cases of fulminating heatstroke classically occur among those subjected to sustained, intense physical activity in hot climates. In these patients, metabolic heat production either supersedes their capability of heat dissipation despite favorable environmental conditions or cannot be dissipated because of clothing that prevents vaporization of sweat. A good example of the latter is the football player whose leather-lined gear may cover 30 percent or more of body surface; Mathews demonstrated (169) that, under such conditions, strain due to heat stress may be increased markedly.

The persistence of sweating in some of these cases is of critical importance since it may obscure the diagnosis. Thus, when such an individual collapses, the skin may feel hot and moist. As sweat vaporizes, the skin may become cooler, thereby making recognition difficult. In some, rectal temperature recorded at a depth of 19 cm or more will disclose frank hyperpyrexia. However, there are other patients who present with an identical history to that just described who remain in coma and demonstrate a moist skin and a rectal temperature of 39 to 50°C (102 to 104°F). Except for the lack of frank hyperpyrexia, these patients show all classical findings and complications of exertional heatstroke. In such cases, it is assumed that body temperature was probably higher initially but lowered itself spontaneously as exertion ceased and sweat was vaporized.

Many such cases of effort-induced heatstroke have been observed in military recruits (62, 170, 171, 125, 161, 163, 172) as well as in highly trained soldiers whose requirements for performance exceed human tolerance (156, 173). Similarly higher incidence is being recognized among marathon runners who perform under adverse climatic conditions (160, 162) and football players during preseason conditioning in the late summer (12, 83).

Severe, fulminating, exertional heatstroke with rhabdomyolysis has also been noted in cases of amphetamine poisoning (171). Extreme hyperpyrexia [rectal temperature 43.3°C (110°F)] in conjunction with profound muscular rigidity has occurred in a patient who ingested 10 mg of dextroamphetamine and 10 mg of the monoamine oxidase inhibitor tranylcypromine (175). Hyperpyrexia with extreme hyperactivity has also been reported after ingestion of LSD (111). Hyperpyrexia is a common manifestation of massive amphetamine overdosage (176, 177). That it is at least partially the result of physical hyperactivity and the associated endogenous heat production by skeletal muscle is suggested by the occurrence of hyperkalemia following administration of amphetamines to experimental animals (178) and prevention of hyperthermia by curare (179). For similar reasons, exertion-induced heatstroke has been observed in extremely agitated psychotic patients (120) and, perhaps of equal importance, in patients experiencing alcoholic withdrawal. The following case reports are further illustrative.

Patient 2. A 21-year-old man was admitted to the Psychiatry Service on August 7, 1969, because of hyperactivity, poor judgment, insomnia, agitation, and confusion. He was treated with large doses of chlorpromazine hydrochloride, benztropine mesylate, and fluphenazine hydrochloride. He remained confused and hyperactive. On the afternoon of August 13, he complained of dryness of his mouth. The next morning he was hot, showed dry skin, and could not be aroused. His rectal temperature exceeded 42.2°C (108°F). His blood pressure was 60/40 mmHg, pulse was 140 beats per minute and regular, temperature was 41.7°C (107°F), and respirations were 36 per minute. The right pupil was fixed and measured 10 mm. He was totally unresponsive to deep pain and showed generalized flaccidity. Arterial blood gas measurement showed Pa_{O_2} of 89 mmHg, Pa_{CO_2} was 27.5 mmHg, pH was 7.4, and oxygen saturation was 96%. Laboratory values showed serum sodium 136 meq/L, serum potassium 4.2 meq/L, serum chloride 103 meq/L, total carbon dioxide 19 mmol/L, total bilirubin 1.5 mg/dL, and platelet count 10,000 per cub millimeter. His prothrombin time was 24 s with a control of 13 s. His partial thromboplastin time was 49 with a control of 35. Fibrinogen concentration was 287 mg/dL. The urine showed findings compatible with the presence of myoglobin.

The patient's temperature was lowered to 38.9°C (102°F) by rubbing with ice bags. Despite cooling, his blood pressure did not respond and it was necessary to use vasopressors to maintain blood pressure. Heparin therapy was instituted. Repeat serum electrolyte determinations showed a sodium concentration of 135 meq/L, potassium 2.7 meq/L, chloride 95 meq/L, and total carbon dioxide 14 mmol/L. During the next 3 days, the patient had convulsive seizures and showed evidence of progressive renal insufficiency. He died on the third day following the onset of heatstroke.

This patient's heatstroke was considered to have resulted from physical exertion incident to psychotic agitation. His overwhelming endogenous heat load produced by continuous physical activity could not be dissipated, probably due to the action of drugs known to impair sweating.

The next case illustrates another common problem; heatstroke in the patient experiencing alcoholic withdrawal.

Patient 3. A 45-year-old painter was admitted for treatment of a vertebral fracture sustained in a fall. He had been a known alcoholic for many years and had been treated previously for delirium tremens.

Initial physical examination showed localized tenderness over the spine and impaired motion of the lower extremities due to pain. A slight tremor of the outstretched hands was evident. Initial laboratory results were within normal limits. During the first and second hospital days the patient displayed anorexia and vomited several times after meals. On his third hospital day, he became irrational and disoriented, requiring restraint and sedation. Physical examination showed a constant tremor, severe agitation, and extreme generalized sweating. He was treated with paraldehyde and chlorpromazine. Laboratory findings at this time showed the following values: serum potassium 2.8 meq/L; serum sodium, 137 meq/L; serum chloride, 95 meq/L, and total carbon dioxide, 32 mmol/L. Because of persistent drenching sweats, the patient was given 2 to 3 L of intravenous fluids per day. On the evening of the fourth day, he passed a small quantity of benzidine-positive urine. The pigment appeared to be myoglobin by electrophoresis. His serum was clear. Blood drawn that evening showed a serum CPK activity of 1750 IU/mL and SGOT level of 2420 units.

On the fourth hospital day, the patient had a convulsive seizure. His rectal temperature immediately thereafter was 41.7°C (107°F), and he was still sweating. Although cooling was accomplished rapidly, the patient remained unresponsive, flaccid, and anuric. Extensive muscular edema appeared. He died on the fifth hospital day.

This case illustrates again that heatstroke can occur in hospitalized patients whose disease, treatment, or both impair mechanisms by which heat can be dissipated. The patient had classical delirium tremens accompanied by persistent overactivity producing an overwhelming endogenous heat load. Undoubtedly, this was abetted by dehydration and salt depletion due to inadequate fluid replacement, vomiting, and profuse diaphoresis. Although the patient displayed no evidence or findings suggestive of alcoholic myopathy at the time of admission, such a condition might have predisposed to acute muscular injury following prolonged agitation and convulsive seizures. Potassium deficiency might also be implicated in this patient's rhabdomyolysis.

Pathology of heatstroke

Tissue damage by heat. The effect of fever per se on function and structure of tissue has not been extensively studied. Burger and Fuhrman showed (180, 181) that animal tissues incubated in vitro at 42°C (107.6°F) and intact animals whose body temperature was maintained at 43°C (109.4°F) for 1 h showed pronounced metabolic disturbances. These included increased ammonia production by the cerebral cortex and diminished oxygen utilization by the liver. It is well known that fever per se may induce sulfobromophthalein sodium retention (182, 183, 184).

Gupta and his associates (185) examined the effect of artificially induced fever in normal human subjects and showed that serum glutamic pyruvic transaminase (SGPT) activity was abnormally elevated 24 and 48 h after the peak of fever. Spurr (186) showed that increasing the temperatures of dogs to 41.5°C (106.7°F) for 1 h/day for 4 days elicited pronounced elevations of SGPT, SGOT, and isocitric dehydrogenase activity in hepatic venous plasma.

Muscular exercise may also produce increased activity of SGPT, SGOT, LAD, CPK, all of which exist in high concentration in skeletal muscle. Since intense exercise may produce fever, the possibility exists that the increased enzyme activity that follows exercise could be partially the result of thermal injury to skeletal muscle. It is quite clear that the elevation of body temperature following a given work load is appreciably less after training. Similarly, in both experimental animals and humans, the rise in activity of these enzymes is higher after a given quantity of exercise in the unconditioned state than after training (187, 188, 189).

Based on the change in pattern of LAD isozyme activity after marathon running, Rose and his associates (190) suggested that the source of the enzymes was not the myocardium bur rather skeletal muscle, liver, or both. However, at least two groups of investigators have shown that levels of LAD isozymes of myocardial origin rise after exercise in untrained rats and could be correlated with evidence of histologic damage in the heart (188, 191). These events did not occur after training. Although they are of obvious importance, neither the CPK nor the LAD isozyme response to heavy exertion in unconditioned man has been characterized.

Further evidence that the enzyme rise after exercise may reflect skeletal muscle damage as well as hepatic damage has also been reported by Garbus et al. (188, 170), who showed that rhabdomyolysis occurred after exercise in untrained rats but not in trained rats.

The demonstrations by these investigators that temperatures within the range attainable by physiologic processes may produce chemical and trophic disturbances could have important implications. Thus, observations by Gilat and his associates (156) that rectal temperature in normal, physically conditioned men performing strenuous exercise may rise up to 42°C (107.6°F) and the observations by Rowell and his associates (6) that temperature of hepatic venous blood is higher than core temperature during exercise leads to the notion that thermal cellular injury could possibly be induced by extreme exercise in normal subjects.

Clinical pathology of heatstroke. The classic description of the pathologic findings in fatal cases of heatstroke was published by Malamud et al. (172).

Myocardial damage is common. Characteristically, subendocardial hemorrhages occur beneath the left interventricular septum. Fragmentation and rupture of muscle fibers are also common. We have observed extensive transmural myocardial infarction in a young man with stress-induced heatstroke (62). Careful dissection of all coronary vessels at the time of autopsy disclosed no evidence whatever of occlusive disease.

A recent report described a fatal case of heatstroke in a young football player who showed hemorrhagic infarction of an anterior papillary muscle (159).

Kew and his coworkers reported their observations on 26 patients with exertional heatstroke (192). Seventeen of the 26 showed abnormalities of myocardial LAD isoenzymes and electrocardiographic disturbances. In two fatal cases, findings were confined to myofibrillar degeneration and interstitial edema.

The possible mechanism whereby frank myocardial infarction or patchy myocardial necrosis occurs in the absence of coronary artery occlusion is unclear. Hyperthermic rats develop pulmonary edema with saline loads (68). That hypotension with low coronary flow could conceivably be responsible for myocardial damage is supported by experimental studies in which large doses of isoproterenol hydrochloride have been used to induce myocardial necrosis. It is perhaps also noteworthy that induction of myocardial necrosis by vasopressor agents occurs experimentally much more readily in the presence of potassium deficiency (193).

Evidence of kidney damage is very common in patients with acute heatstroke. Mild proteinuria and modest abnormalities of the urinary sediment are found in virtually all of these patients. In those with heat illness induced by physical exertion, acute renal insufficiency occurs in approximately 25 percent of cases. Four reports (43, 170, 173, 194) have emphasized that severe, often fatal, heat illness with acute oliguric renal failure may occur in association with physical effort in hot climates and not necessarily be attended by hyperpyrexia. In contrast, in patients who develop classical heatstroke as a result of simple exposure to high temperature, acute renal insufficiency occurs only in 5 percent (62). In patients whose heatstroke is induced by physical effort, a large array of conditions exist that could conceivably contribute to the pathogenesis of acute renal failure. Thus, they may be partially dehydrated, excrete an acid urine, and they are often markedly hyperuricemic despite the excretion of larger quantities of uric acid than normal in their urine (43, 194). Uric acid nephropathy has been observed in such patients. Second, potassium deficiency may exist and has been regarded by some authors as capable of depressing glomerular filtration rate and renal plasma flow as well as inducing tubular damage (195). Third, the nephrotoxic effects of myoglobin in a concentrated, acid

urine and its association with acute tubular necrosis is well known. Finally, the possibility of glomerular injury consequent to disseminated intravascular coagulation in acute heatstroke has been well described (130). A hypothetical scheme to explain the mechanism of heat stress nephropathy is shown in Fig. 29-16.

In 15 marine recruits with exertional heatstroke, O'Donnell administered 12.5 g of mannitol upon arrival at the dispensary. This was followed by infusions of crystalloid containing 12.5 g of mannitol per liter. None of these patients developed acute renal failure (161).

Patients whose heatstroke is complicated by acute tubular necrosis may recover fully with careful management (170). However, a recent report by Kew and his associates (130) has described subtle, progressive impairment of renal function in four patients who recovered from heatstroke but whose renal biopsy specimens demonstrated interstitial nephritis. The cause of this finding was not apparent. Consideration might be given to the possibility that these effects are the outcome of tubular or interstitial damage due to urate nephropathy (194).

Damage to the central nervous system in heatstroke is a universal finding in fatal cases. Changes in the brain generally consist of edema,

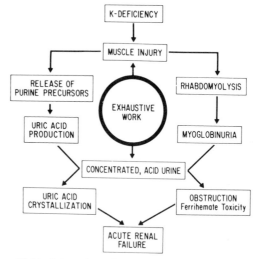

Figure 29-16. A hypothetical scheme to explain the role of exhaustive muscular work and K deficiency in the pathogenesis of "heat-stress nephropathy."

patchy congestion, and diffuse petechial hemorrhages. The hypothalamus is not ordinarily damaged. Striking changes occur in the cerebellum which show marked deterioration or disappearance of Purkinje cells. In all instances, parenchymal changes of the central nervous system occur in direct relationship to the severity and duration of hyperthermia. The predominance of alterations in cerebellar structure correspond to the clinical picture of central nervous system damage in patients who survive severe heatstroke. These patients' findings often resemble cerebellar ataxia with marked dysarthria and dysmetria (196).

Evidence of liver damage is very common (197), and jaundice occurs commonly in patients surviving more than 2 days. In approximately 5 percent of cases, jaundice may become intense. Histologic findings include perisinusoidal edema and patchy necrosis which may be predominantly centrolobular. Ordinarily, patients who survive show no residual impairment of liver function.

Pancreatitis has also been observed (62). In the latter instance, it was sufficiently severe to cause common bile duct obstruction.

Evidence of skeletal muscle damage or rhabdomyolysis, displayed by elevation of CPK activity in serum and myglobinuria, occurs in a large percentage of patients whose heat injury is induced by intensive physical exertion. Although release of myoglobin from muscle may be accompanied by extreme hyperkalemia and consequently may pose a serious hazard to life, those who survive may completely recover their skeletal muscle function (170). To my knowledge significant rhabdomyolysis has been observed almost exclusively in patients whose heatstroke followed physical exertion or occurred in assocation with other hyperkinetic states such as amphetamine intoxication, psychotic agitation, delirium tremens, or severe convulsions. It is unusual in classical heatstroke.

Electron microscopic studies have disclosed pathologic alterations of the subcellular components of sweat glands (198). This might explain the occasional observation that patients who have survived severe heatstroke display a residual impairment in their ability to sweat and demonstrate a persistent susceptibility to the effects of environmental heat.

Coagulation disorders in fatal heatstroke are common. Petechial hemorrhages and ecchymoses are often striking. These changes have been characteristically attributed to increased capillary permeability, impaired production of clotting factors by the liver, and thrombocytopenia (199). In 1962, Shibolet (115) pointed out that hypofibrinogenemia and severe fibrinolysis occur in heatstroke. Since that time, characteristic features of disseminated intravascular coagulation have been confirmed by several authors (144, 161, 200, 201). It is now well recognized that this process occurs very commonly in severe cases of heatstroke and has been held responsible for the widespread tissue damage observed in this condition (202). Experimental evidence published by Bedrak et al. (203) shows that people merely exposed to heat demonstrate enchanced blood fibrinolytic activity without depression of plasma fibrinogen concentration. The same authors showed that activation of the fibrinolytic state by heat exposure is less marked following acclimatization (204). Studying dogs, Bedrak (205) showed that fibrinolytic activity and depression of plasma fibrinogen concentration resulted from muscular exercise in the heat and, as in humans, was ameliorated by acclimatization. Moxley and his associates (206) confirmed these findings in humans and showed that trained subjects show slightly higher values for euglobulin activity that was not considered biologically important. In contrast, Schrier and his associates (207) described increased plasma fibrinogen concentrations in military recruits during the early days of their training.

Virtually all patients with frank heatstroke show evidence of disseminated intravascular coagulation (DIC). Usually, thrombocytopenia is evident by the end of the first 24 h. In most cases, recovery is complete by the end of the fifth to seventh day. More severe cases show severe thrombocytopenia which is most severe by the end of the second to third day, is associated with hypofibrinogenemia and elevated concentrations of split fibrin products in both blood and urine. These findings may persist in severe cases. Commonly, hemorrhage associated with DIC is a major cause of death in those patients with extremely severe heatstroke who survive the initial hyperthermia. It appears to be especially prominent in cases of heatstroke that occur after physical exertion.

Kew and his coworkers (208) examined SGOT, SGPT, LAD, and CPK activities in the serum of 53 patients with heatstroke and found substantial elevations in all. Their data suggest that SGOT of less than 1000 units (normal, 10 to 35 units) indicates a favorable outcome, whereas higher values were commonly associated with severe complications and death. Furthermore, nine patients with comparable hyperpyrexia who showed either normal or only slightly elevated values for LAD and SGOT were subsequently shown to have an infection responsible for their fever and not to be victims of heatstroke.

Hypocalcemia, sometimes of profound degree (i.e., concentrations less than 4 mg/dL in serum), has been observed in patients with heatstroke. It is associated with extensive injury to skeletal muscle. It has been observed early in the course of the disease even before frank azotemia has appeared, as illustrated by patient 2 of this series. It is not due to hypoalbuminemia. Profound hypocalcemia has been observed in a patient with malignant hyperpyrexia accompanied by extensive rhabdomyolysis (209) and in patients with acute renal failure due to idiopathic rhabdomyolysis (2).

Meroney et al. (210) observed that patients with posttraumatic acute renal failure demonstrated disproportionate elevations of serum phosphorus in the presence of extensive devitalization of skeletal muscle. The degree of hyperphosphatemia was inversely related to the severity of hypocalcemia. Infusion of Ca induced only evanescent elevation of $[Ca^{2+}]$. They exploited these observations by studying dogs that were nephrectomized and subjected to skeletal muscle trauma. They showed that injected isotopic calcium (^{45}Ca) became sequestered in devitalized muscle 10 times more rapidly than in either normal animals or those subjected to nephrectomy alone. Their observations, subsequently confirmed by others (211), would seem to provide an explanation for the hypocalcemia that is so commonly observed in such patients.

More recently it has been shown that hypercalcemia may also occur in patients with rhabdomyolysis (2, 211) (see also Chap. 19). In contrast to hypocalcemia, hypercalcemia usually appears during the second week. It may be accompanied by conjunctival injection and pruritus, which are thought to reflect the action of excessive parathormone (118, 212). In some of these patients, plasma parathormone concentration has been elevated despite hypercalcemia (2, 211), thereby suggesting transient hyperparathyroidism. It is worth emphasizing that hypercalcemia in some of these instances has definitely preceded the diuretic phase of acute renal failure (213) resulting from myoglobinuria independently of heatstroke (42, 214). Moreover, hypercalcemia in patients with heatstroke has been reported only in those with acute oliguric renal failure in association with antecedent severe muscle or soft-tissue injury. Although it is highly speculative, it seems possible that such profound hypocalcemia early in the course of acute renal failure in conjunction with extensive tissue destruction and calcium deposition may provide a powerful stimulus to parathyroid hyperplasia and overproduction of parathormone. Thus, if the intensity of hypocalcemia were sufficient to result in a transient autonomous hyperparathyroid state somewhat analogous to that of chronic uremia, the transient appearance of frank hyperparathyroidism could be readily explained. Obviously, serial estimations of parathormone, serum calcium, and associated indices of increased parathyroid activity throughout the course of this illness are necessary to substantiate the notion that early profound hypocalcemia is the responsible factor for the subsequent appearance of hypercalcemia.

Hypophosphatemia may occur transiently in patients with heatstroke. It has been observed early in the course and generally resolves spontaneously. Levels in serum less than 0.9 mg/dL have been observed. One possible factor underlying hypophosphatemia in acute heatstroke might be acute respiratory alkalosis. In one of our own cases, when serum phosphorus was 0.9 mg/dL, arterial pH was 7.45 and P_{CO_2} was 24 mmHg. In this patient, total muscle phosphorus content was normal. In normal subjects, serum phosphorus does not fall to this level unless much more severe respiratory alkalosis is induced (215). This suggests that other mechanisms responsible for hypophosphatemia may be involved in patients with acute heatstroke.

Acid-base disturbances are common in patients with acute heatstroke. Normal humans, when exposed to a high environmental temperature, characteristically hyperventilate and may develop tetany. As a result of hyperventilation and respiratory alkalosis, they may develop hypokalemia and hypophosphatemia. Patients with mild or moderate heatstroke reflect this characteristic and accordingly display mild to moderate respiratory alkalosis. The respiratory alkalosis observed in mild heatstroke stands in sharp contrast to the relatively severe respiratory alkalosis that may be observed in heat exhaustion (216). The reason for the less intense respiratory alkalosis in heatstroke may be related to the greater suppression of consciousness in the latter condition. In contrast, patients with exertional heatstroke usually have metabolic acidosis which is identifiable when appropriate measurements are conducted early. Whole blood lactate concentration usually ranges from 8 to 12 mmol/L (123). However, in patients with agitation, convulsions, hyperthermia and cardiovascular collapse, values exceeding 20 mmol/L have been observed. In all these cases, hyperventilation is sufficiently intense to depress arterial P_{CO_2}. It is never sufficient to elevate blood pH to normal. In patients with extremely severe classical (nonexertional) heatstroke, lactic acidosis may also be observed.

Severe lactic acidosis can usually be explained by circulatory shock with diminished perfusion of muscle as well as enhanced lactate production from skeletal muscle due to pronounced muscular activity. Lactate production by the liver also increases during severe exertion consequent to gluconeogenesis and glycolysis. Rowell et al. (6) observed that it attained rather astronomical proportions during heat stress. If laboratory measurement of lactate is unavailable, it may be suspected if the anion gap in serum electrolytes exceeds 20 meq/L ([Na + K] − [Cl + HCO$_3$]).

Treatment of heatstroke

General measures. The therapeutic cornerstone for successful treatment of heatstroke is elimination of hyperthermia. Delay in cooling probably represents the single most important factor leading to death or residual serious disability in those who survive. Reasons underlying delays in cooling are two in number. The first is failure to recognize heatstroke and to appreciate the seriousness of hyperpyrexia. It is to be emphasized over and over that heatstroke is an extreme medical emergency. As a precaution, physicians should properly instruct ambulance attendants, paramedics, football coaches, trainers, or nurses in hospital emergency rooms in the diagnosis of this disorder. During heat waves, it is wise for ambulances to carry ice so that treatment may be initiated on the spot. In our own experience, patients who have collapsed and who have been identified as suffering from heatstroke by firemen, have been actively treated enroute to the hospital and have even regained consciousness before arrival at the emergency room. Survival is the rule in such cases. The second cause of delay in treatment is lack of proper cooling facilities at the hospital. In those geographic areas, industries, or football training camps where heatstroke may potentially occur, one should anticipate its occurrence and be ready with an effective plan of action.

Two recent publications illustrate the benefits of early recognition, anticipated provision of facilities, and aggressive treatment. O'Donnell (161) treated 15 consecutive marine recruits from Parris Island, South Carolina. All survived without morbidity. Beller and Boyd (163) treated 13 consecutive cases of exertional heatstroke in army recruits. All survived without morbidity. Although statistics are not available, I would estimate mortality in such cases in hospitals where preparations have not been made would be approximately 50 percent.

Once the diagnosis of heatstroke is made, an intravenous line should be established as quickly as possible to permit access to the circulation. If the patient is comatose, and if properly trained personnel are available, the patient should undergo tracheal intubation. This is done since many of these patients vomit and will first display convulsive seizures during cooling with the associated risk of aspiration. Rectal temperature should be recorded preferably using a thermistor. This should be inserted into the rectum to a depth of 20 cm. Because of their length, standard thermometers measure anal temperature, not core temperature. Having accomplished these initial maneuvers, the patient should thereupon be immersed in a tub of ice water and briskly massaged to stimulate exchange of heat. This procedure may induce severe pain in the hands of the attendants and requires that several individuals be available in order to alternate efforts. Cooling may also be effected by rubbing the body surface briskly with plastic bags containing ice while the body is wet down with water. This is effective provided it can be carried out in the wake of a large fan in an air-conditioned room. By either means body temperature may be lowered to 38°C (102.2°F) within as little as 60 min or less. When the core temperature reaches 40°C (102°F), cooling measures should be stopped since body temperature will ordinarily continue to fall. Convulsions, if they should occur at this time, may prevent a further fall of body temperature. Indeed a convulsion may be followed by a recurrence of hyperthermia. Intravenous chlorpromazine, 50 mg given at the initiation of treatment, is very useful to prevent tremors and convulsions that appear during the cooling period. It may be repeated every 4 h if necessary (217, 218, 219).

A good number of these patients will display profound hypotension at the time of admission. While this may result from impairment of myocardial performance (220), it is more often the result of translocation of blood volume to the dilated superficial vessels in the skin. Thus, it is not necessarily the result of total body volume deficit. Cooling ordinarily restores blood pressure to normal by means of cutaneous vasoconstriction. Therefore, large volumes of intravenous fluids for the purpose of elevating blood pressure should not be utilized in the early treatment period since once cooling is induced, return of blood to the central circulation may cause acute pulmonary edema. If cooling does not restore the blood pressure, 250 to 500 cc of normal saline should be rapidly infused. If this is not effective, a vasopressor such as Aramine should be used. Norepinephrine should be avoided since it induces intense peripheral vasoconstriction and may prolong the hyperthermic period. Dextran

should be avoided since it may impair platelet function and thereby promote hemorrhage (221).

Once the patient has been cooled it may be anticipated that hyperthermia will recur within 3 or 4 h. This is especially true in those patients who are unable to sweat. Cooling measures must be reinstituted accordingly. Recovery of ability to sweat may require several weeks.

The most important laboratory measurements at the time of admission consist of arterial blood gases, pH, serum electrolyte concentrations, and a complete blood count including platelets. Baseline values for prothrombin time, partial thromboplastin time, fibrinogen and fibrin split products should be obtained if available. When possible, blood lactate concentration should be determined since lactic acidosis occurs commonly in patients whose heatstroke is induced by muscular exercise. As in other circumstances, lactic acidosis may become much worse once hypotension is corrected due to a washout of lactate and hydrogen ions from skeletal muscle. If arterial pH is low in this type of patient and there is no evidence of impaired gas exchange by the lungs, one can safely assume that the low pH is the result of acute lactic acidosis. Under the latter circumstance, arterial P_{CO_2} would usually be in the vicinity of 28 mmHg. Pulmonary edema has been observed in patients with exertion-induced heatstroke even when fluids have not been administered. This could well be the result of acute lactic acidosis and should warrant consideration of bicarbonate therapy.

Treatment of complications. *Disseminated Intravascular Coagulation.* This has been documented in a large number of patients with acute heatstroke. This is especially likely in that form induced by muscular exertion. Thrombocytopenia, decreased fibrinogen concentration, and elevated fibrin split products in serum occur in the bulk of patients with heatstroke. Purpura is very common on the second or third day. At the present time there appears to be no clear-cut indication for heparin therapy in such patients, but it may be considered if there is evidence of gross hemorrhage. Bleeding has also been ascribed to fibrinolysis. Treatment with E-aminocaproic acid has been recommended for fibrinolysis. However, most authorities would agree that its use is extremely hazardous and probably provides no long-term benefit. Indeed, recent evidence suggests that it may cause rhabdomyolysis (222). Some of the bleeding diathesis in patients with heatstroke is also due to decreased production of clotting factors in the liver due to acute liver injury. Peripheral eosinophilia, possibly due to purpura, may appear during the recovery period. Mild hemolysis is also common.

Rhabdomyolysis. Elevated CPK activity in serum is present in nearly all cases of exertional heatstroke but occurs less often in classical heatstroke. This usually indicates rhabdomyolysis. There are three imminent dangers of rhabdomyolysis. These are (1) hyperkalemia with its attendant dangers of cardiotoxicity, (2) myoglobinuria and its attendant danger of acute renal failure, and (3) shock as a result of sequestration of fluid into injured muscle cells.

Loss of circulatory volume into injured muscle cells may be so severe that up to 12 L of normal saline may be required on the first day of treatment in order to maintain blood pressure. Such large volumes of fluid unavoidably lead to edema of the involved skeletal muscle. This complication may have the dire consequence of vascular compression if it should involve the extremities. It tends to occur on the third or fourth day and may be responsible for a second episode of acute muscle necrosis, heralded by a second rise of CPK activity and sometimes myoglobinuria. If this "second-wave phenomenon" appears imminent, one must observe the patient's extremities carefully. Should there appear evidence of vascular compression such as loss of arterial pulsations, blanching, coldness, or neuropathy, one should strongly consider fasciotomy.

Acute Renal Failure. (See also Chap. 15.) This occurs in about 5 percent of patients with classical heatstroke and in about 30 percent of patients with exertional heatstroke. Mannitol has been advocated as an effective agent to prevent acute renal failure. Accordingly, it has been reported that the early use of mannitol may prevent this complication in patients with acute heatstroke (162). Acute renal failure is commonly directly related to the severity of muscle necrosis and hyperuricemia. Its recognition requires careful monitoring of urine output, body weight, and fluid administration. The common occurrence of acute renal failure in such patients demands early examination of the urine for specific gravity or osmolality, myoglobin, measurement of the urine/plasma concentration ratio for urea nitrogen and the urine [Na$^+$] as aids in identification of acute renal failure. If the urine is concentrated, contains little Na (e.g., less than 20 meq/L) and the urine/plasma concentration ratio for urea nitrogen is above 10:1, one can be reasonably certain that acute tubular necrosis does not exist. However, if the urine is isotonic to plasma, the urine/plasma urea nitrogen concentration ratio is less than 5:1 and the urine [Na$^+$] is high, acute tubular necrosis is likely. (Previous administration of diuretics will obscure the meaning of urine [Na$^+$].) If there is evidence of acute renal failure, the patient may be given 100 mg or more of furosemide intravenously in conjunction with 25 g of 20 percent mannitol. If diuresis follows, it should be sustained by fluids and furosemide as needed.

Hypokalemia and Hyperkalemia. Hypokalemia occurs in about one-half of the cases. It does not ordinarily require treatment in classical heatstroke since it is usually related to acute respiratory alkalosis. In patients with exertion-induced heatstroke, it often represents frank K depletion. Even in these patients, hypokalemia is usually transient since release of K$^+$ from injured tissues frequently corrects the hypokalemia and often leads to hyperkalemia. The latter is especially apt to occur in the presence of oliguria and often requires use of agents to lower serum [K$^+$] or reverse its electrocardiographic effects. Aggressive hemodialysis is often necessary.

Hypernatremia. This is commonly observed. Its treatment is detailed in the section on heat exhaustion.

Hypocalcemia. Although calcium levels even less than 4 mg/dL have been observed and levels between 4 and 5 mg/dL are common in acute heatstroke, tetany is highly unusual. Calcium administration should be avoided if possible since it will cause deposition of calcium carbonate and calcium phosphate in skeletal muscle.

Hyperuricemia. In some patients, especially

those with exercise-induced heatstroke, hyperuricemia may be profound (223). I have observed three patients whose serum uric acid concentration at the time of admission ranged between 35 and 48 mg/dL in the presence of a normal blood urea nitrogen. When such extreme hyperuricemia is observed, consideration might be given to the use of allopurinol. However, under usual circumstances hyperuricemia is much less intense. In these situations it will usually resolve spontaneously.

Nonketotic, Hyperosmolar Coma. Hyperglycemia, with levels of glucose in the vicinity of 1000 mg/dL, has been observed in some patients with heatstroke who have survived 7 days or more. This appears to be more common in children. In all cases widespread skeletal muscle injury has been evident. In most instances, hyperglycemia can be ascribed to excessive administration of glucose in conjunction with renal insufficiency.

Electrocardiographic Abnormalities. Alterations of the electrocardiogram consisting of inverted T waves, depressed S-T segments, conduction defects, and arrhythmias are common (192). These do not necessarily indicate structural damage to the heart. However, on rare occasions frank myocardial infarction has occurred in the absence of coronary artery occlusion (62, 159). Due to common association of hypokalemia, one should be extremely judicious concerning the use of digitalis.

Central Nervous System Dysfunction. Patients with heatstroke are commonly obtunded for several days following recovery from hyperthermia. Although a broad range of functional disorders occurs, recovery may be complete (173). Abnormalities of cerebellar function are especially common in patients with sustained severe heatstroke. While these abnormalities may be transient, some patients will show persistent defects including disorders of ocular movement and ataxia. In the early stages of heatstroke and usually in the presence of hyperthermia, the pupils may be widely dilated, irregular, and sometimes unresponsive to light. In contrast to other situations, this does not indicate cerebral death since all the abnormalities may disappear within several hours following ap-

propriate cooling. Nuchal rigidity has been observed in acute heatstroke. Although this is not ordinarily associated with pleocytosis, one of our cases demonstrated blood in the subarachnoid space at autopsy. The spinal fluid usually shows no more than a modest elevation of protein concentration in patients with frank heatstroke.

Differential diagnosis of heatstroke

Under ordinary circumstances, little difficulty should be experienced in identifying classical heatstroke. One should not rely on the presence of dry skin to confirm the diagnosis, since a perspiring patient with hyperpyrexia is an equal candidate for thermal tissue injury.

Hypothalamic damage resulting from heatstroke is uncommon. In contrast, hyperthermia may occur in patients with hypothalamic lesions. Chesanow (224) has pointed out that "hypothalamic hyperthermia" should be suspected by (1) a uniformly high temperature without the peaks and troughs seen in sepsis; (2) anhidrosis, which may be unilateral; (3) resistance to antipyretic drugs; and (4) the presence of disorders reflecting damage to adjacent structures, such as diabetes insipidus.

Tornblom (225) reviewed several case reports of fatal idiopathic hyperthermia that occurred on the first to sixth day after removal of insulinomas. The cause of hyperthermia in these patients is unknown.

Confusion may arise in certain patients with meningitis accompanied by an unusually high fever since patients with heatstroke sometimes demonstrate nuchal rigidity. In classical heatstroke, spinal fluid may be blood-tinged at times and show an elevated protein concentration. Pleocytosis is not a feature.

Malignant hyperpyrexia is an uncommon abnormality characterized by the occurrence of extreme hyperpyrexia (up to 44.5°C, or 112°F) during or following general anesthesia (226). Susceptible individuals may demonstrate persistently elevated CPK activity in serum. Since it carries 70 percent mortality, its prevention or recognition in susceptible persons is of vital importance.

Although the height of fever in acute meningococcemia, typhus, Rocky Mountain spotted fever, or falciparum malaria does not ordinarily reach the levels seen in heatstroke, delirium and appearance of hemorrhagic skin manifestations certainly warrant their consideration in the differential diagnosis. Midbrain hemorrhage may occur in certain alcoholic patients and may be accompanied by hyperthermia. In some, hyperthermia would seem to be the result of the accompanying agitation and related metabolic heat production rather than a primary disturbance in thermal regulation. As evidenced by patient 3, frank heatstroke can occur as a complication of delirium tremens.

Prognosis

The physician who anticipates the occurrence of heatstroke and who has a well-conceived plan for its treatment, competent help, and adequate facilities will save the lives of the majority of such patients. Under these conditions, the outcome should be successful in as many as 95 percent of cases. In contrast, sporadic cases, which are often unanticipated and, as a consequence, temporarily neglected, carry a much higher mortality. In military recruits or young football players in whom heatstroke is associated with physical exertion, heatstroke tends to be severe and associated with many complications. However, even in severe cases, if cooling procedures are performed in aggressive fashion and when otherwise fatal complications are anticipated, most patients will survive.

REFERENCES

1. Passmore, R., and J. V. G. A. Durnin: Human energy expenditure, *Physiol. Rev.*, **35**:801, 1955.
2. Leonard, A., and R. J. Nelms, Jr.: Hypercalcemia in diuretic phase of acute renal failure, *Ann. Intern. Med.*, **73**:137, 1970.
3. Consalazio, C. F., R. E. Johnson, and L. J. Pecora: *Physiological Measurements of Metabolic Function in Man*, McGraw-Hill Book Company, New York, 1963.
4. Adolph, E. F., and D. B. Dill: Observations on water metabolism in the desert, *Am. J. Physiol.*, **123**:369, 1938.
5. Assmussen, E., and O. Boje: Body temperature and capacity for work, *Acta Physiol. Scand.*, **10**:475, 1945.
6. Rowell, L. B., et al.: Splanchnic blood flow and metabolism in heat-stressed man, *J. Appl. Physiol.*, **24**:475, 1968.
7. Barcroft, H.: Circulation in skeletal muscle, in *Handbook of Physiology: A Critical Comprehensive Presentation of Physiologic Knowledge and Concepts*, Williams & Wilkins Co., Baltimore, 1963, pp. 1353–1386.
8. Schlein, E. M., D. Jensen, and J. P. Knochel: The effect of plasma water loss on assessment of muscle metabolism during exercise, *J. Appl. Physiol.*, **34**:568, 1973.
9. Benzinger, T. H.: On physical heat regulation and the sense of temperature in man, *Proc. Natl. Acad. Sci. USA*, **46**:645, 1959.
10. Hellon, R. F., and A. R. Lind: The influence of age on peripheral vasodilatation in a hot environment, *J. Physiol.*, **141**:262, 1958.
11. Rowell, L. B., et al.: Hepatic clearance of indocyanine green in man under thermal and exercise stress, *J. Appl. Physiol.*, **20**:384, 1965.
12. Rowell, L. B., et al.: Redistribution of blood flow during sustained high skin temperature in resting man, *J. Appl. Physiol.*, **28**:415, 1970.
13. Rowell, L. B., et al.: Reductions in cardiac output, central blood volume and stroke volume with thermal stress in normal men during exercise, *J. Clin. Invest.*, **45**:1801, 1966.
14. Gold, J.: Development of heat pyrexia, *JAMA*, **173**:1175, 1960.
15. Williams, C. G., et al.: Circulatory and metabolic reactions to work in the heat, *J. Appl. Physiol.*, **17**:625, 1962.
16. Barger, A. C., et al.: Venous pressure and cutaneous reactive hyperemia in exhaustive exercise and certain other circulatory stresses, *J. Appl. Physiol.*, **2**:81, 1949.
17. Thaysen, J. H., and I. L. Schwartz: Fatigue of sweat glands, *J. Clin. Invest.*, **34**:1719, 1955.
18. Schwartz, I. L., and J. H. Thaysen: Excretion of sodium and potassium in human sweat, *J. Clin. Invest.*, **35**:144, 1956.

19. Mitra, R., G. I. Christison, and H. D. Johnson: Dynamics of growth hormone secretion in chronically heat-stressed cattle (abstract), *Fed. Proc.*, **30**:209, 1971.

20. Collins, K. J., and J. S. Weiner: Endocrinologic aspects of exposure to high environmental temperatures, *Physiol. Rev.*, **48**:785, 1968.

21. Bozovic, L., J. Castenfors, and M. Piscator: Effect of prolonged, heavy exercise on urinary protein excretion and plasma renin activity, *Acta Physiol. Scand.*, **70**:143, 1967.

22. Kotchen, T. A., et al.: Renin, norepinephrine and epinephrine responses to gradual graded exercise, *J. Appl. Physiol.*, **31**:178, 1971.

23. Knochel, J. P., L. N. Dotin, and R. J. Hamburger: Pathophysiology of intense physical conditioning in a hot climate: I. Mechanisms of potassium depletion, *J. Clin. Invest.*, **51**:242, 1972.

24. Finberg, J. P. M., Miriam Katz, H. Gazit, and G. M. Berlyne: Plasma renin activity after acute heat exposure in nonacclimatized and naturally acclimatized man, *J. Appl. Physiol.*, **36**:519, 1974.

25. Barger, A. C., R. D. Berlin, and J. F. Tulenko: Infusion of aldosterone, 9-α-fluorohydrocortisone and antidiuretic hormone into the renal artery of normal and adrenalectomized, unanesthetized dogs: Effect on electrolyte and water excretion, *Endocrinology*, **62**:804, 1958.

26. Kosunen, K. J., A. J. Pakarinen, K. Kuoppasalmi, and H. Adlercreutz: Plasma renin activity, angiotensin II, and aldosterone during intense heat stress, **41**:323, 1976.

27. Kosunen, K. J., and A. J. Pakarinen: Plasma renin, angiotensin II, and plasma and urinary aldosterone in running exercise, *J. Appl. Physiol.*, **41**:26, 1976.

28. Bonner, R. M., M. H. Harrison, C. J. Hall, and R. J. Edwards: Acclimatization on intravascular responses to acute heat stress in man, *J. Appl. Physiol.*, **41**:708, 1976.

29. Schalch, D. S.: The influence of physical stress and exercise on growth hormone and insulin secretion in man, *J. Lab. Clin. Med.*, **69**:256, 1967.

30. Okada, Y., T. Matsuoka, and Y. Kumahara: Human growth hormone secretion during exposure to hot air in normal adult male subjects, *J. Clin. Endocrinol.*, **34**:759, 1972.

31. Biglieri, E. G., C. D. Watlington, and P. H. Forsham: Sodium retention with HGH and its subfractions, *J. Clin. Endocrinol. Metab.*, **21**:361, 1961.

32. Hale, H. B., et al.: Blood adrenocorticotrophic hormone and plasma corticosteroids in men exposed to adverse environmental conditions, *J. Clin. Invest.*, **136**:1642, 1957.

33. Collins, K. J., et al.: The plasma glucocorticoid response to environmental heat stress, *J. Physiol.*, **194**:33, 1968.

34. Fiorica, V., et al.: Sympathico-adrenomedullary activity in dogs during acute heat exposure, *J. Appl. Physiol.*, **22**:16, 1967.

35. Hasselman, M., G. Schaaf, and B. Metz: Influence respective du travail de la temperature ambiante et de la privation de sommeil sur l'excretion urinaire de catecholamines chez l'hormone normal, *C. R. Soc. Biol. (Paris)*, **154**:197, 1960.

36. Radigan, L. R., and S. Robinson: Effects of environmental heat stress and exercise on renal blood flow and filtration rate, *J. Appl. Physiol.*, **2**:185, 1949.

37. Castenfors, J.: Renal function during exercise, *Acta Physiol. Scand.*, **70** (suppl. 293):1, 1967.

38. Katz, A. I., S. Massry, J. Agmon, and M. Toor: Concentration and dilution of urine in permanent inhabitants of hot regions, *Isr. J. Med. Sci.*, **1**:968, 1965.

39. Ladell, W. S. S., J. C. Waterlow, and M. F. Hudson: Desert climate: Physiological and clinical observations, *Lancet*, **2**:491, 1944.

40. Kanter, G. S.: Heat and excretion in man, *J. Appl. Physiol.*, **7**:533, 1955.

41. Frank, M. A., A. Atsmon, A. DeVries, and L. N. Posener: A study of urine volume and some urinary constituents with a view to the etiology of urolithiasis in a hot climate, *New Istanbul Contrib. Clin. Sci.*, **6**:20, 1963.

42. Grossman, H. H., and H. Lange: Hypercalcemia in acute renal failure, *Ann. Intern. Med.*, **69**:1332, 1968.

43. Schrier, R. W., et al.: Nephropathy associated with heat stress and exercise, *Ann. Intern. Med.*, **67**:356, 1967.

44. Conn, R. B., Jr.: Fluorimetric determination of creatine, *Clin. Chem.*, **6**:537, 1960.

45. Bass, D. E., and I. T. Dobalian: Ratio between

true and apparent creatinine in sweat, *J. Appl. Physiol.*, **55**:555, 1953.

46. Knochel, J. P., and W. W. Carter: The role of muscle cell injury in the pathogenesis of acute renal failure after exercise, *Kidney Int.*, **10**:S-58, 1976.

47. Burnell, J. M., et al.: The effect in humans of extracellular pH change on the relationship between serum potassium concentration and extracellular potassium, *J. Clin. Invest.*, **35**:935, 1956.

48. Coburn, J. W., R. C. Reba, and F. N. Craig: Effect of potassium depletion on response to acute heat exposure in unacclimatized man, *Am. J. Physiol.*, **211**:117, 1966.

49. Rose, K. D.: Warning for million: Intense exercise can deplete potassium, *Physician and Sportsmedicine*, **3**:67, 1975.

50. Totel, G. L.: Physiological responses to heat of resting man with impaired sweating capacity, *J. Appl. Physiol.*, **37**:346, 1974.

51. Beller, G. A., J. T. Maher, L. H. Hartley, D. E. Bass, and W. E. C. Wackers: Changes in serum and sweat magnesium levels during work in the heat, *Aviat. Space Environ. Med.*, **46**(5):709, 1975.

52. Bean, W. B. quoted in W. A. Sodeman (ed.), *Pathologic Physiology*, W. B. Saunders Company, Philadelphia, 1956, p. 234.

53. Bass, E. E., et al.: Mechanisms of acclimatization to heat in man, *Medicine (Baltimore)*, **34**:323, 1955.

54. Saltin, B., et al.: *Response to Exercise After Bed Rest and After Training*, American Heart Association Monograph 23, American Heart Association, Inc., New York, 1968.

55. Wyndham, C. H., et al.: Changes in central circulation and body fluid space during acclimatization to heat, *J. Appl. Physiol.*, **25**:586, 1968.

56. Pattengale, P. K., and J. O. Holloszy: Augmentation of skeletal muscle myoglobin by a program of treadmill running, *Am. J. Physiol.*, **213**:783, 1967.

57. Gollnick, P. D., and D. W. King: Effect of exercise and training on mitochondria of rat skeletal muscle, *Am. J. Physiol.*, **216**:1502, 1969.

58. Dill, D. B., F. G. Hall, and H. T. Edwards: Changes in composition of sweat during acclimatization to heat, *Am. J. Physiol.*, **123**:412, 1938.

59. Adam, J. M., et al.: Physiological responses to hot environments of young european men in the tropics: II and III. Further studies on the effects of exposure to varying levels of environmental stress, *Med. Res. Counc. Spec. Rep. Ser. (Lond.)*, **55**:381, 1955.

60. Dasler, A. R., and E. Hardenbergh: Decreased sweat rate in heat acclimatization (abstract), *Fed. Proc.*, **30**:209, 1971.

61. Robinson, S., R. K. Kincaid, and R. E. Rhamy: Effect of salt deficiency on the salt concentration in sweat, *J. Appl. Physiol.*, **3**:55, 1950.

62. Knochel, J. P., W. R. Beisel, E. G. Herndon, E. S. Gerard, and E. G. Barry: The renal cardiovascular, hematologic and serum electrolyte abnormalities of heat stroke, *Am. J. Med.*, **30**:299, 1961.

63. Ladell, W. S. S., and R. J. Shepard: Aldosterone inhibition and acclimatization to heat (abstract), *J. Physiol.*, **160**:19, 1962.

64. Conn, J. W.: Aldosteronism in man: Some climatological aspects, *JAMA*, **183**:775, 1963.

65. Collins, K. J.: The action of exogenous aldosterone on the secretion and composition of drug-induced sweat, *Clin. Sci.*, **30**:207, 1966.

66. Furman, K. I., and G. Beer: Dynamic changes in sweat electrolyte composition induced by heat stress as an indication of acclimatization and aldosterone activity, *Clin. Sci.*, **24**:7, 1963.

67. Barcroft, J. C., et al.: On the relation of external temperature to blood volume, *Philos. Trans. R. Soc. Lond.*, **211**:445, 1922.

68. Bazett, H. C.: The effect of heat on the blood volume and circulation, *JAMA*, **111**:1841, 1938.

69. Bass, D. E., and A. Henschel: Responses of body fluid compartments to heat and cold, *Physiol. Rev.*, **36**:128, 1956.

70. Yoshimura, H.: Seasonal changes in human body fluid, *Jap. J. Physiol.*, **8**:165, 1958.

71. Desai, N. D., et al.: Total body exchangeable sodium and radio sodium space in Indians from warm and humid climate, *Indian J. Med. Sci.*, **21**:300, 1967.

72. Streeten, D. H. P., et al.: Secondary aldosteronism: Metabolic and adrenocortical responses of normal men to high environmental temperatures, *Metabolism*, **9**:1071, 1960.

73. Conn, J. W.: The mechanism of acclimatization to heat, *Adv. Intern. Med.*, **3**:373, 1949.

74. Robinson, S., R. K. Kincaid, and R. K. Phamy:

Effects of desoxycorticosterone acetate on acclimatization of men to heat, *J. Appl. Physiol.*, **2**:399, 1950.

75. Lichten, P. R., et al.: Inotropic effect of aldosterone on the myocardium of normal dogs (abstract), *Fed. Proc.*, **22**:358, 1964.

76. Tanz, R. D.: Studies on the inotropic action of aldosterone on isolated cardiac tissue preparations, including the effects of pH, ouabain and SC-8109, *J. Pharmacol. Exp. Ther.*, **135**:71, 1962.

77. Wakefield, E. G., and W. W. Hall: Heat injuries: A preparatory study for experimental heat stroke, *JAMA*, **89**:92, 1929.

78. Woodruff, P.: *The Men Who Ruled India*, vol. 1, *The Founders of Modern India*, Jonathan Cape, Ltd., London, 1954.

79. Weiner, J. S., and G. O. Horne: A classification of heat illness, *Br. Med. J.*, **1**:1533, 1958.

80. Biglieri, E. G., and M. B. McIlroy: Abnormalities of renal function and circulatory reflexes in primary aldosteronism, *Circulation*, **33**:78, 1966.

81. Talbott, J. H.: Heat cramps, *Medicine*, **14**:232, 1935.

82. Iampietro, P. R.: Heat-induced tetany, *Fed. Proc.*, **22**:884, 1963.

83. Bulmer, M. G., and G. D. Forwell: The concentration of sodium in thermal sweat, *J. Physiol.*, **132**:115, 1956.

84. Layzer, R. B., and L. P. Rowland: Cramps, *N. Engl. J. Med.*, **385**:31, 1971.

85. Rubin, B. B., and A. M. Katz: Sodium and potassium effects on skeletal muscle microsomal adenosine triphosphatase and calcium uptake, *Science*, **158**:1189, 1967.

86. Talbott, J. H., et al.: The ill effects of heat upon workmen, *J. Indust. Hyg. Toxicol.*, **19**:258, 1937.

87. Adolph, E. F.: *Physiology of Man in the Desert*, Interscience Publishers, Inc., New York, 1947.

88. Moroff, S. V., and D. E. Bass: Effects of overhydration on man's physiological responses to work in the heat, *J. Appl. Physiol.*, **20**:267, 1965.

89. McCance, R. A.: Medical problems in mineral metabolism: III. Experimental sodium chloride deficiency in man, *Proc. R. Soc. London Biol.*, **119**:245, 1936.

90. McCance, R. A.: Medical problems in mineral metabolism: III. Experimental human salt deficiency, *Lancet*, **1**:823, 1936.

91. Woodbury, D. M.: Analgesic-antipyretics, anti-inflammatory agents, and inhibitors of uric acid synthesis salicylates and cogeners, phenacetin & congeners, indomethacin, calchicine, alloysurinal, in L. S. Goodman and A. Gilmon (eds.), *The Pharmacological Basis of Therapeutics*, 4th ed., p. 314, 1970.

92. Dreosti, G. L.: Problems arising out of temperature and humidity in deep mining in the Witwatersrand, *J. S. African Chem. Min. Met.*, **36**:102, 1935.

93. Wyndham, C. H.: The problems of heat intolerance in man, in J. O. Hardy, A. P. Gagge, and J. A. Stolwijk (eds.), *Physiological and Behavioural Temperature Regulation*, Charles C Thomas, Publisher, Springfield, Ill., 1970, pp. 324–341.

94. Senay, L. C., and R. Kok: Body fluid responses of heat-tolerant and intolerant men to work in a hot wet environment, *J. Appl. Physiol.*, **40**:55, 1976.

95. Wyndham, C. H.: The physiology of exercise under heat stress, *Ann. Rev. Physiol.*, **35**:193, 1973.

96. Haymes, E. M., R. J. McCormick, and E. R. Buskirk: Heat tolerance of exercising lean and obese prepubertal boys, *J. Appl. Physiol.*, **39**:457, 1975.

97. Haymes, E. M., E. R. Buskirk, J. L. Hudgson, H. M. Lundegren, and W. C. Nicholas: Heat tolerance of exercising lean and heavy prepubertal girls, *J. Appl. Physiol.*, **36**:566, 1974.

98. Adolph, E. S., and W. B. Fulton: The effects of exposure to high temperatures upon the circulation in man, *Am. J. Physiol.*, **67**:573, 1923.

99. Burch, G. E., and A. Hyman: Influence of a hot and humid environment upon cardiac output and work in normal man and in patients with chronic congestive heart failure at rest, *Am. Heart J.*, **53**:665, 1957.

100. Ansari, A., and G. E. Burch: Influence of hot environments on the cardiovascular system, *Arch. Intern. Med.*, **123**:371, 1969.

101. Daily, W. M., and T. R. Harrison: A study of the mechanism and treatment of experimental heat pyrexia, *Am. J. Med. Sci.*, **215**:42, 1948.

102. Leavel, U. W.: Sweat gland neurosis in barbiturate poisoning, *Arch. Dermatol.*, **100**:218, 1969.

103. Buchwald, I., and P. J. Davis: Scleroderma with fatal heat stroke, *JAMA*, **201**:270, 1967.

104. Bleisch, V.: Clincopathologic conference: A 65-

year-old woman with heat stroke, *Am. J. Med.*, **43**:113, 1967.

105. MacQuaide, D. H. G.: Congenital absence of sweat glands, *Lancet*, **2**:531, 1944.

106. Di Sant'Agnese, P. A., et al.: Sweat electrolyte disturbances associated with childhood pancreatic disease, *Am. J. Med.*, **15**:777, 1953.

107. Burch, G. E.: Influence of environmental temperature and relative humidity on the rate of water loss through the skin in congestive heart failure in a subtropical climate, *Am. J. Med. Sci.*, **211**:181, 1946.

108. Litman, R. E.: Heat stroke in parkinsonism, *Arch. Intern. Med.*, **89**:562, 1952.

109. Chapman, J., and W. B. Bean: Iatrogenic heat stroke, *JAMA*, **161**:1375, 1956.

110. Gottschalk, P. B., and J. E. Thomas: Heat stroke, *Mayo Clin. Proc.*, **41**:470, 1966.

111. Friedman, S. A., and S. E. Hirsch: Extreme hyperthermia after LSD ingestion, *JAMA*, **217**:1549, 1971.

112. Parker, W. A.: Methldopa hyperpyrexia (editorial), *JAMA*, **228**:1097, 1974.

113. Schreiner, G. E.: The role of hemodialysis (artificial kidney) in acute poisoning, *Arch. Intern. Med.*, **102**:896, 1958.

114. Knochel, J. P., and R. M. Vertel: Salt loading as a possible factor in the production of potassium depletion, rhabdomyolysis and heat injury, *Lancet*, **1**:659–661, 1967.

115. Shibolet, S., S. Fisher, and T. Gilat: Fibrinolysis and hemorrhages in fatal heat stroke, *N. Engl. J. Med.*, **266**:169, 1962.

116. Austin, M. G., and J. W. Berry: Observations on 100 cases of heat stroke, *JAMA*, **161**:1525, 1956.

117. Levine, J. A.: Heat stroke in the aged, *Am. J. Med.*, **47**:251, 1969.

118. Ferris, E. B., Jr., et al.: Heat stroke: Clinical and chemical observations on 44 cases, *J. Clin. Invest.*, **17**:249, 1938.

119. Baxter, C. R., and P. E. Teschan: Atypical heat stroke, with hypernatremia, acute renal failure, and fulminating potassium intoxication, *Arch. Intern. Med.*, **101**:1040, 1958.

120. Bale, P. M., A. F. Calvert, and E. Hirst: Skeletal muscle necrosis in heat stroke, *Am. J. Clin. Pathol.*, **50**:440, 1968.

121. Kilburn, K. H.: Muscular origin of elevated plasma potassium during muscular exercise, *J. Appl. Physiol.*, **21**:675, 1966.

122. Spurr, G. G., and G. Barlow: Tissue electrolytes in hyperthermic dogs, *J. Appl. Physiol.*, **28**:13, 1970.

123. Ruppert, R. D., et al.: The mechanism of metabolic acidosis in heat stroke (abstract), *Clin. Res.*, **12**:356, 1964.

124. Edholm, O. G.: Comments on symposium on heat acclimatization, *Fed. Proc.*, **23**:907, 1963.

125. Sobel S., et al.: Renal mechanisms in heat stroke (abstract), *Clin. Res.*, **11**:252, 1963.

126. Knochel, J. P.: Dog days and siriasis, How to kill a football player (editorial), *JAMA*, **233**:513, 1975.

127. Rogers, P. W., and N. A. Kurtzman: Renal failure, uncontrollable thirst, and hyperreninemia, *JAMA*, **225**:1236, 1973.

128. Gordon, R. S., and H. L. Andrews: Potassium depletion under heat stress, *Fed. Proc.*, **25**:1372, 1966.

129. Streeten, D. H. P., et al.: Secondary aldosteronism: Metabolic and adrenocortical responses of normal men to high environmental temperatures, *Metabolism*, **9**:1071, 1960.

130. Kew, M. C., C. Abrahams, and H. C. Seftel: Chronic interstitial nephritis as a consequence of heat stroke, *Q. J. Med.*, **39**:189, 1970.

131. Collins, R. E., et al.: Abnormally sustained aldosterone secretion during salt loading in patients with various forms of benign hypertension; relation of plasma renin activity, *J. Clin. Invest.*, **49**:1415, 1970.

132. Cohen, E. L., J. W. Conn, and D. R. Rovner: Postural augmentation of plasma renin activity and aldosterone excretion in normal people, *J. Clin. Invest.*, **46**:481, 1967.

133. Streeten, D. H. P., et al.: Studies on the renin-aldosterone system in patients with hypertension and in normal subjects, *Am. J. Med.*, **46**:844, 1969.

134. Espiner, E. A., et al.: Effect of saline infusions on aldosterone secretion and electrolyte excretion in normal subjects and patients with primary aldosteronism, *N. Engl. J. Med.*, **277**:1, 1967.

135. Camargo, C. A., et al.: Decreased plasma clearance and hepatic extraction of aldosterone in pa-

tients with heart failure, *J. Clin. Invest.*, **44**:356, 1965.

136. Laragh, J. H., J. E. Sealey, and S. C. Sommers: Patterns of adrenal secretion and urinary excretion of aldosterone and plasma renin activity in normal and hypertensive subjects, *Circ. Res.*, **18**(suppl. 1):1, 1966.

137. Cannon, P. J., R. P. Ames, and J. H. Laragh: Relation between potassium balance and aldosterone secretion in normal subjects and in patients with hypertensive or renal tubular disease, *J. Clin. Invest.*, **45**:865, 1966.

138. Fukuchi, S., et al.: The relationship between vascular reactivity and extracellular potassium, *Tohoku J. Exp. Med.*, **85**:181, 1965.

139. Conn. J. W.: Hypertension, the potassium ion and impaired carbohydrate tolerance, *N. Engl. J. Med.*, **273**:1135, 1965.

140. Bergstrom, J., and E. Hultman: The effect of thiazides, chlorthalidone and furosemide on muscle electrolytes and muscle glycogen in normal subjects, *Acta Med. Scand.*, **180**:363, 1966.

141. Karlsson, J., and B. Saltin: Diet, muscle glycogen and endurance performance, *J. Appl. Physiol.*, **31**:203, 1971.

142. Blachley, J., J. Long, and J. P. Knochel: The effect of potassium (K) deficiency on resting muscle glycogen (G) content and its response to exercise, *Clin. Res.*, **21**:39, 1974.

143. Graig, F. A., and F. M. Jacobius: Elevated serum enzyme levels associated with hypokalemia (abstract), *Ann. Intern. Med.*, **66**:1059, 1967.

144. Weber, M. B., and J. A. Blakely: The hemorrhagic diathesis of heat stroke, *Lancet*, **1**:1190, 1969.

145. Knochel, J. P., and E. M. Schlein: On the mechanism of rhabdomyolysis in potassium depletion, *J. Clin. Invest.*, **51**:1750, 1972.

146. Bilbrey, G. L., N. W. Carter, and J. P. Knochel: Skeletal muscle resting membrane potential in potassium deficiency, *J. Clin. Invest.*, **52**:3011, 1973.

147. Zierler, K. L.: Increased muscle permeability to aldolase produced by depolarization and by metabolic inhibitors, *Am. J. Physiol.*, **193**:534, 1958.

148. Gross, E. G., J. D. Dexter, and R. G. Roth: Hypokalemic myopathy with myoglobinuria associated with licorice ingestion, *N. Engl. J. Med.*, **274**:602, 1966.

149. Achor, R. W. P., and L. A. Smith: Nutritional deficiency syndrome with diarrhea resulting in hypopotassemia, muscle degeneration and renal insufficiency: Report of a case with recovery, *Mayo Clin. Proc.*, **32**:297, 1955.

150. Kjellmer, I.: Potassium ion as a vasodilator during muscular exercise, *Acta Physiol. Scand.*, **63**:460, 1965.

151. Knochel, J. P., F. D. Foley, Jr., and H. L. Walker: Effect of potassium (K) depletion on cardiac output and lactate response to exercise in the dog, *Mineral and Electrolyte Metabolism*, in press.

152. Darrow, D. C., and H. C. Miller: Production of cardiac lesions by repeated injections of desoxycorticosterone acetate, *J. Clin. Invest.*, **21**:601, 1942.

153. Gale, H. H.: Contractile mechanics of papillary muscles from rats with experimentally induced cardiac necrosis (abstract), *Physiologist*, **14**:145, 1971.

154. Ellis, F. P., F. Nelson, and L. Pincus: Mortality during heat waves in New York City July 1972 and August and September 1973, *Environ. Res.*, **10**:1, 1975.

155. Schwartz, I. L., and S. Itoh: Fatigue of the sweat glands in heat stroke (abstract), *J Clin. Invest.*, **35**:733, 1956.

156. Gilat, T., S. Shibolet, and E. Sohar: Mechanism of heat stroke, *J. Trop. Med. Hyg.*, **66**:204, 1963.

157. Ladell, W. S.: Disorders due to heat, *Trans. R. Soc. Trop. Med. Hyg.*, **51**:189, 1957.

158. Kuo, K. W., et al.: Sweating with heat stroke, *J. Oriental Med.*, **22**:98, 1925.

159. Barcenas, C., H. P. Hoeffer, and J. T. Lie: CPC obesity, football, dog days and siriasis: A deadly combination, **92**:237, 1976.

160. Green, L. H., S. I. Cohen, and G. Kurland: Fatal myocardial infarction in marathon racing, *Ann. Intern. Med.*, **84**:704, 1976.

161. O'Donnell, T. F., Jr.: Acute heat stroke: Epidemiologic, biochemical, renal and coagulation studies, *JAMA*, **234**:824, 1975.

162. CPC: Extreme physical effort in summer heat followed by collapse, stupor, purpura, jaundice and azotemia, *Am. J. Med.*, **18**:659, 1955.

163. Beller, F. A., and A. E. Boyd: Heat stroke: A report of 13 consecutive cases without mortality de-

spite severe hyperpyrexia and neurologic dysfunction, *Milit. Med.*, **140**(7):464, 1975.

164. Buskirk, E. R., and D. E. Bass: Climate and exercise, in W. R. Johnson and E. R. Burkirk (eds.), *Science and Medicine of Exercise and Sport*, 2d ed., Harper & Row, Publishers, Incorporated, New York, 1974.

165. Murphy, R. J., and W. F. Ashe: Prevention of heat illness in football players, *JAMA*, **194**:650, 1965.

166. Spickard, A.: Heat stroke in college football and suggestions for prevention, *South. Med. J.*, **61**:791, 1968.

167. Wildenthal, K., et al.: Effects of lactic acidosis on left ventricular performance, *Am. J. Physiol.*, **214**:1352, 1968.

168. Altland, P. D., and B. Highman: Effects of exercise on serum enzyme values and tissues of rats, *Proc. Soc. Exp. Biol. Med.*, **125**:999, 1967.

169. Mathews, D. K., E. L. Fox, and D. Tanzi: Physiological responses during exercise and recovery in a football uniform, *J. Appl. Physiol.*, **26**:611, 1969.

170. Vertel, R. M., and J. P. Knochel: Acute renal failure due to heat injury: An analysis of ten cases associated with a high incidence of myoglobinuria, *Am. J. Med.*, **43**:435, 1967.

171. Kendrick, W. C., A. R. Hull, and J. P. Knochel: Rhabdomyolysis and shock following intravenous amphetamine administration. In press.

172. Malamud, N., W. Haymaker, and R. P. Custer: Heat stroke: A clinocopathologic study of 125 fatal cases, *Milit. Surg.*, **99**:397, 1946.

173. Shibolet, S., R. Coll, and T. Gilat, et al.: Heat stroke: Its clinical picture and mechanism in 36 cases, *Q. J. Med.*, **36**:525, 1967.

174. Fox, E. L., et al.: Effects of football equipment on thermal balance and energy cost during exercise, *Res. Q. Am. Assoc. Health Phys. Educ.*, **37**:332, 1966.

175. Krisko, I., E. Lewis, and J. E. Johnson, III: Severe hyperpyrexia due to tranylcypromine-amphetamine toxicity, *Ann. Intern. Med.*, **70**:559, 1969.

176. Ginsberg, M. D., M. Hertzman, and W. W. Schmidt-Nowara: Amphetamine intoxication with coagulopathy, hyperthermia and reversible renal failure, *Ann. Intern. Med.*, **73**:81, 1970.

177. Zalis, E. G., and L. F. Parmlay, Jr.: Fatal amphetamine poisoning, *Arch. Intern. Med.*, **112**:822, 1963.

178. Moore, K. E.: Effects of D-amphetamine on plasma and tissue electrolyte concentrations of aggregated and of hyperthyroid mice, *Proc. Soc. Exp. Biol. Med.*, **122**:292, 1966.

179. Zalis, E. G., G. Kaplan, and G. D. Lundberg: Acute lethality of the amphetamines in dogs and its antagonism by curare, *Proc. Soc. Exp. Biol. Med.*, **118**:557, 1965.

180. Burger, F. J., and F. A. Fuhrman: Evidence of injury of tissues after hyperthermia, *Am. J. Physiol.*, **206**:1062, 1964.

181. Burger, F. J., and F. A. Fuhrman: Evidence of injury by heat in mammalian tissues, *Am. J. Physiol.*, **206**:1057, 1964.

182. Machella, T. E.: The relationship of bromsulphalein retention to the fever of natural *P. falciparum* malaria, *Am. J. Med. Sci.*, **213**:81, 1947.

183. Hicks, M. H., et al.: The effect of spontaneous and artificially induced fever on liver function, *J. Clin. Invest.*, **27**:580, 1948.

184. Mendeloff, A. I., et al.: Studies in bromsulfalein: Factors alerting its disappearance from the blood after a single intravenous injection, *Gastroenterology*, **13**:222, 1949.

185. Gupta, N. N., R. M. L. Mehrotra, and N. L. J. Agarwal: Evaluation of functional and morphological status of liver during pyrexia, *J. Assoc. Physicians, India*, **11**:747, 1963.

186. Spurr, G. B.: Serum enzymes following repetitive hyperthermia, *Proc. Soc. Exp. Biol. Med.*, **139**:698, 1972.

187. Fowler, W. M., Jr., et al.: Changes in serum enzyme levels after exercise in trained and untrained subjects, *J. Appl. Physiol.*, **17**:943, 1962.

188. Garbus, J., B. Highman, and P. D. Altland: Serum enzymes and lactic dehydrogenase isoenzymes after exercise and training in rats, *Am. J. Physiol.*, **207**:467, 1964.

189. Fowler, W. M., Jr., et al.: The effect of exercise on serum enzymes, *Arch. Phys. Med. Rehabil.*, **49**:554, 1968.

190. Rose, L. I., J. E. Bousser, and K. H. Cooper: Serum enzymes after marathon running, *J. Appl. Physiol.*, **29**:355, 1970.

191. Papadopoulos, N. M., A. A. Leon, and C. M.

Bloor: Effects of exercise on plasma and tissue levels of lactate dehydrogenase and isoenzymes in rats, *Proc. Soc. Exp. Biol. Med.*, **125**:999, 1967.

192. Kew, M. C., B. K. Tucker, I. Bersohn, and H. C. Seftel: The heart in heatstroke, *Am. Heart J.*, **77**:324, 1969.

193. Selye, H., and E. Bajusz: Conditioning by corticoids for the production of cardiac lesions with noradrenaline, *Acta Endocrinol.*, **30**:183, 1959.

194. Knochel, J. P., L. N. Dotin, and R. J. Hamburger: Heat stress, exercise and muscle injury: Effects of urate metabolism and renal function, *Ann. Intern. Med.*, **81**:321, 1974.

195. Schwartz, W. B., and A. S. Relman: Effects of electrolyte disorders on renal function, *N. Engl. J. Med.*, **276**:383, 1967.

196. Mehta, A. C., and R. N. Baker: Persistent neurological deficits in heat stroke, *Neurology*, **20**:336, 1970.

197. Herman, R. H., and B. H. Sullivan, Jr.: Heat stroke and jaundice, *Am. J. Med.*, **27**:154, 1959.

198. Baba, N., and R. D. Ruppert: Alteration of eccrine sweat gland in fatal heat stroke, *Arch. Pathol.*, **85**:669, 1968.

199. Wright, D. O., and J. T. Cuttino: Purpuric manifestations of heat stroke: Studies of prothrombin and platelets in 12 cases, *Arch. Intern. Med.*, **77**:27, 1946.

200. Perchick, J. S., A. Winkelstein, and R. K. Shadduck: Disseminated intravascular coagulation in heat stroke, *JAMA*, **231**:480, 1975.

201. Knochel, J. P.: Disseminated intravascular coagulation in heat stroke response to heparin therapy (editorial), *JAMA*, **231**:496, 1975.

202. Sohal, R. S., et al.: Heat stroke: An electron microscopic study of endothelial cell damage and disseminated intravascular coagulation, *Arch. Intern. Med.*, **122**:43, 1968.

203. Bedrak, E., G. Beer, and K. I. Fuhrman: Fibrinolytic activity and heat stress, *Israel J. Exp. Med.*, **11**:1, 1963.

204. Bedrak, E., G. Beer, and K. I. Fuhrman: Fibrinolytic activity and muscular exercise in heat, *J. Appl. Physiol.*, **19**:469, 1964.

205. Bedrak, E.: Effect of muscular exercise in a hot environment on canine fibrinolysis in blood in inactive and exercising men, *J. Appl. Physiol.*, **20**:1307, 1965.

206. Moxley, R. T., P. Brakman, and T. Astrup: Resting levels of fibrinolysis in blood in inactive and exercising men, *J. Appl. Physiol.*, **28**:549, 1970.

207. Schrier, R. W., et al.: Renal metabolic and circulatory responses to heat and exercise, *Ann. Intern. Med.*, **73**:213, 1970.

208. Kew, M., I. Bersohn, and H. Seftel: The diagnostic and prognostic significance of the serum enzyme changes in heat stroke, *Trans. R. Soc. Trop. Med. Hyg.*, **65**:325, 1971.

209. Denborough, M. A., et al.: Biochemical changes in malignant hyperpyrexia, *Lancet*, **1**:1137, 1970.

210. Meroney, W. H., et al.: The acute calcification of traumatized muscle, with particular reference to acute post-traumatic renal insufficiency, *J. Clin. Invest.*, **36**:825, 1956.

211. Fortner, R. W., et al.: Acute renal insufficiency in heat stress injury (abstract), *Am. Soc. Nephrol.*, **5**:23, 1971.

212. Massry, S. G., et al.: Intractable pruritus as a manifestation of hyperparathyroidism in uremia, *N. Engl. J. Med.*, **279**:697, 1968.

213. Leonard, C. D., and E. R. Eichner: Acute renal failure and transient hypercalcemia in idiopathic rhabdomyolysis, *JAMA*, **211**:1539, 1970.

214. Butikofer, E., and J. Molleyres: Akute Ischamische Muskelnekrosen, Reversible Muskelverkalkungen und Sekondare Hyperkalcamie bei Akuter Anurie, *Schweiz Med. Woschenschr.*, **98**:961, 1968.

215. Mostellar, M. E., and E. P. Tuttle, Jr.: The effects of alkalosis on plasma concentration and urinary excretion of inorganic phosphate in man, *J. Clin. Invest.*, **43**:138, 1964.

216. Boyd, A. E., and G. A. Beller: Heat exhaustion and respiratory alkalosis, *Ann. Intern. Med.*, **83**:835, 1975.

217. Jesati, R. M.: Management of severe hyperthermia with chlorpromazine and refrigeration, *N. Engl. J. Med.*, **254**:426, 1956.

218. Ho-Ch'ang, Y., et al.: Chlorpromazine and heat reducing measures in treatment of heat stroke, *China Med. J.*, **77**:174, 1958.

219. Hoagland, R. J., and R. H. Bishop: A physiologic treatment of heat stroke, *Am. J. Med. Sci.*, **241**:415, 1961.

220. O'Donnell, T. F., Jr., and G. H. A. Clowes, Jr.:

The circulatory abnormalities of heat stroke, *N. Engl. J. Med.*, **287**:734, 1972.

221. Langdell, R. D., et al.: Dextran and prolonged bleeding time, *JAMA*, **166**:346, 1958.

222. Rizza, R. A., S. Sclonick, and C. L. Conley: Myoglobinuria following aminocaproic acid administration, *JAMA*, **236**:1845, 1976.

223. Nolph, K. D., M. E. Whitcomb, and R. W. Schrier: Mechanisms for inefficient peritoneal dialysis in acute renal failure associated with heat stress and exercise, *Ann. Intern. Med.*, **71**:317, 1969.

224. Chesanow, R. L.: A 65 year old woman with heat stroke, *Am. J. Med.*, **41**:415, 1961.

225. Tornblom, N.: Hyperinsulinism with fatal postoperative hyperthermia, *Acta. Med. Scand.*, **170**:757, 1961.

226. Kalow, E., et al.: Metabolic error of muscle metabolism after recovery from malignant hyperthermia, *Lancet*, **2**:895, 1970.

30

Fluid, electrolyte, and acid-base abnormalities in pediatrics

LAURENCE FINBERG

INTRODUCTION

Children differ from adults anatomically, physiologically, and biochemically, to say nothing of psychologically and socially. Here we are not concerned with the last two; but differences in chemical anatomy, in water physiology, and in developmental biochemistry justify a special chapter on pediatrics in a volume about water and electrolytes otherwise focused on adult disorders.

Because disorders of water homeostasis place the infant and child in a particularly vulnerable role, pediatricians have been strong contributors to the modern clinical science of electrolyte physiology, a field of career endeavor, at one time at least, appropriate for a pediatrician-scientist. The most noteworthy of the pediatric contributors to this field were J. L. Gamble and D. C. Darrow, whose seminal studies were published between 1920 and 1960. They, in effect, translated the work of the physical chemists Arrhenius, Van't Hoff, Gibbs, Henderson, and Van Slyke into biologic terms and thence moved to clinical application. Third and fourth generations of their students are now adapting physiology to molecular biology without, as yet, improving very much upon the clinical insights of earlier decades.

The younger the children, the greater are the differences between children and adults. Not only are there differences qualitatively and quantitatively, but the ongoing process of developmental maturation in and of itself provides a difference of clinical concern. Several important points along the age continuum may be identified because each poses specific clinical problems or vulnerabilities.

First chronologically is the prematurely born infant, a fetus untimely brought to extrauterine circumstance and ill equipped for it. He or she comes with an excess of body water even by term-infant standards and a very large visceral organ mass compared to muscle and other tissue. The pulmonary system is vulnerable to disorder, and the renal system is immature in function. In fact, all homeostatic systems are underdeveloped. Nutrition, at least temporarily, will be less available. The therapeutic devices available to support ventilation and temperature regulation strain water and acid-base homeostasis. Second is the neonatal period for term-born infants. Less fragile than the immaturely born, the newborn period, nonetheless, represents a time of very rapid change and adjustment as well as rapid growth with compositional change. Third is the period of infancy following the neonatal, lasting from about 1 month to about 16 months of age (longer, up to 30 months, for the undernourished), a time of continued dependency for thirst needs and high vulnerability to nutritional failure and gastrointestinal fluid-losing disease. Next is middle childhood to about the onset of puberty, a period of developmental movement toward adult features. Finally, there is adolescence—the final but turbulent transition to adult form and function.

In the subsequent sections of this chapter we shall consider in turn the relevant comparative inorganic chemical anatomy of these periods; next, the metabolic peculiarities imposed by growth, changing composition, and the relationship of surface to size; then, the changing influence on the various regulators of homeostasis. Finally, we shall consider the specific disease entities important in pediatrics—important because of prevalence and risk or because of exclusive occurrence during infancy or childhood.

BODY COMPOSITION (See also Chaps. 1 and 12)

FLUID PARTITION

In approaching clinical problems of fluid balance, one should know the chemical anatomy of the various compartments of the body which contain water and which are separated from one another by boundaries and compositional differences. For the adult, Fig. 30-1 and Table 30-1 from Edelman and Leibman (1) summarize water distribution in a 70-kg adult male. The fundamental division is into two parts, water and solute within cells (ICF) and water and solute outside of cells (ECF). The portions of extracellular water not available for quick transfer, e.g., that in bone and dense connective tissue, are of lesser magnitude in children and are, in any event, not considered in short-term problems. The transcellular water, principally the fluid of gastrointestinal lumen, is also considered outside the body though in a steady-state relationship to the extracellular fluid.

EXTRACELLULAR FLUID

Infants and children differ in water distribution from the adult as shown in Fig. 30-2 from Friis-Hansen (2). Table 30-2 (3) from the same author gives data for the postnatal periods. These differences have major importance when plans for therapy of disordered composition are to be made. The progressive drop in the total body water (TBW) fraction of body weight with age occurs,

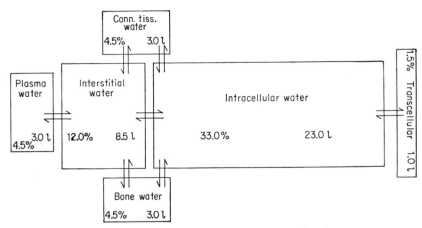

Figure 30-1. Body water compartments in a normal 70-kg man shown as a percentage of body weight in liters. (*After Edelman and Leibman*)

Table 30-1. Body water distribution in a healthy young adult male*

COMPARTMENT	PERCENT OF BODY WEIGHT	PERCENT OF TOTAL BODY WATER	LITERS
Plasma	4.5	7.5	3
Interstitial lymph	12	20	8.5
Dense connective tissue and cartilage	4.5	7.5	3
Inaccessible bone water	4.5	7.5	3
Transcellular	1.5	2.5	1
Total extracellular	27	45	19
"Functional" extracellular†	21	35	14.5
Total body water	60	100	42
Total intracellular	33	55	23

* All figures rounded to nearest 0.5.
† Minus bone water and transcellular water.
Source: After Edelman and Leibman.

after the first weeks, largely because of addition of fat to total body mass. Increased skeletal mass plays a like role after puberty.

The relatively small skeletal and muscle mass of the newborn and small infant whose organs, e.g., liver, skin, brain, and kidney, are proportionately large, means that cell constituents of the ICF at early ages are slightly different from those of older infants. Malnourished patients have a more infantile pattern of cell distribution than nourished infants.

A surprising amount of fat appears in the healthy infant, reaching by about 6 months of age more than 20 percent of weight. It remains high and then falls as a fraction of body mass during childhood (4). An alternate way of expressing the TBW for purposes of calculation is to think of it as a relatively constant 70 percent of the lean body mass (LBM). For individual clinical problems, this is useful because one may make a rough estimate of the fat content of an individual, by inspection knowing the average data for the appropriately nourished at each age. Clearly, the marasmic infant, for example, has negligible fat content. For clinical purposes, from about 3 months to 9 years the ECF may be estimated to be 25 percent of the LBM and the total water as 70 percent of the LBM.

INTRACELLULAR FLUID

The intracellular fluid contains potassium and magnesium as principal cations, and phosphate, proteinate, sulfate, and bicarbonate as principal anions (see Chap. 1). This composition differs strikingly from the solute of the ECF, which has sodium, chloride, and bicarbonate predominating, much as was the situation in the primeval sea. Inasmuch as the muscle cell is dominant by mass (60 percent of cell mass) and also representative of all but highly specialized cells, that tissue

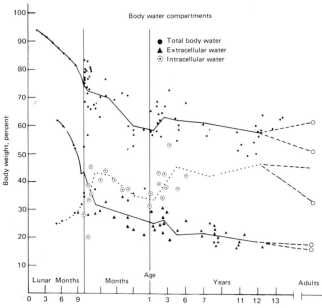

Figure 30-2. TBW, ECW, and ICW as percentages of body weight in infants and children, compared to corresponding values for the fetus and adults.

Table 30-2. Distribution of body water between extracellular and intracellular fluid as a percent of body weight

AGE	TOTAL WATER	EXTRA-CELLULAR WATER	INTRA-CELLULAR WATER	EXTRACELLULAR WATER/INTRACELLULAR WATER
0–1 day	79	43.9	35.1	1.25
1–10 days	74	39.7	34.3	1.16
1–3 months	72.3	32.2	40.1	0.80
3–6 months	70.1	30.1	40	0.75
6–12 months	60.4	27.4	33	0.83
1–2 years	58.7	25.6	33.1	0.77
2–3 years	63.5	26.7	36.8	0.73
3–5 years	62.2	21.4	40.8	0.52
5–10 years	61.5	22	39.5	0.56
10–16 years	58	18.7	39.3	0.48

Source: After Friis-Hansen, using the volume of distribution of deuterium oxide for total body water and of thiosulfate for extracellular water. Intracellular water is obtained by subtracting the average of extracellular water from total body water.

will be used as the prototype. Muscle cells contain no chloride (in the millimolar concentration range) and very little sodium (about 5 to 8 meq/L of cell water). In the discussion which follows, the ICF is treated as an actual solution with virtually all of the water molecules free to move and those ions not chemically bound to protein similarly participating in the ionic equilibriums which characterize such solutions. This concept has been challenged in varying degrees, as has the concept that sodium ions are extruded from the cell by an active transport system (5, 6). Others have disputed the doubters (7). While the precise mechanism of these phenomena remains controversial, the physiologist and clinician may continue to regard the system as permitting rapid free movement of water everywhere and the cellular compartment as excluding Na^+ and Cl^- ions, at least insofar as studies of dehydration and rehydration are concerned. Because whether correct in mechanism or not, the cell fluid and the extracellular fluid interact in physiologic experiments and clinical situations in accord with these assumptions and dynamics.

The exclusion of Na^+ and Cl^- from cell water (relatively) gives these ions a very particular physiologic role, i.e., the quantity of NaCl present in the effective fluid system determines the division of water between the ICF and the ECF. The concentration of these ions, of course, will be determined by the volume of water as well as by the content of solute; hyponatremia thus may occur with either an expanded or a contracted ECF, with radically different significance. On the other hand, because of renal overflow and the toxicity of added cell solute, a hypernatremic state almost always means a reduction in cell water volume, though the ECF may vary from high to low.

The special anatomy of the capillaries and the interior membranes of the brain cause this organ to behave with respect to water shifts as though it were a single cell (see also Chap. 26) (8, 9). The anatomic difference consists of tight junctions between adjacent endothelial cells. This functional "blood-brain" barrier means that water moves with customary rapidity along concentration gradients, but solutes, even crystalloids, move slowly. Glucose (in physiologic, not pathologic, concentration) and perhaps some of its metabolites move as elsewhere in the body owing to facilitated diffusion, but sodium and other ions take hours to equilibrate (9). Thus, osmolal gradients cause the brain as a whole to swell or shrink (10). If a hypernatremic disequilibrium is introduced in muscle tissue, water will leave cells and expand the tissue ECF, leaving tissue volume unchanged but redistributed. In the central nervous system (CNS), the critical boundary is not the cell membrane but the capillary endothelium, so the entire organ will shrink. Conversely the reverse gradient will cause water to flow into the brain, and the organ will swell (see Chap. 26).

ECF-PLASMA

The extracellular compartment has one very physiologically important subcompartment, the blood plasma. Plasma contains 6 to 7 g of protein/dL (1.5 to 2 mosm/kg) which essentially remains intravascular. Since protein carries an electric charge, a Gibbs-Donnan equilibrium occurs, causing slight differences in ionic composition between plasma and interstitial fluid. The plasma volume is maintained, despite hydrostatic pressure from the cardiac pump, by the small osmotic gradient in accordance with Starling's law.

In clinical problems, the two main divisions, ICF and ECF, and a subcompartment of the ECF, the plasma, are of prime physiologic importance. Subtractions or additions to any of them may be expressed as mass (weight) and thus as a proportion of body weight. Each of the three significant "spaces" has a unique chemical anatomy, and the mechanisms that maintain or fail to maintain the integrity of each is understood sufficiently to make rational restoration when disturbances occur.

METABOLIC TURNOVER

CALORIES AND WATER

In contradistinction to considerations of composition that relate to mass, water turnover relates to expenditure of energy that is not a function of mass alone. Water expenditure is directly linked to heat (caloric) expenditure. Most of the energy output of homeothermic animals is dissipated as heat and carries water directly with it by insensible water loss from skin and lungs, and indirectly by leaving waste products of metabolism for excretion in the urine. The infant with small mass and large surface has a much higher heat and water loss per kilogram than do older children and adults (11). Table 30-3 summarizes the differences, indicating clearly the special vulnerability of the infant to disturbances in water balance whether from increased loss, impaired intake, or both. The high heat production of the infant is due in part to the relatively high proportion of weight taken by body organs which do not slow their rates of heat production during periods of stress.

INSENSIBLE WATER LOSS (IWL)

The three fixed continuing losses for homeothermic infants are (1) insensible water loss (skin and lungs), (2) the urine, and (3) a small amount in the normal stool. All of these are dependent on caloric expenditure, which will be expressed as kcal or Calories. Each may vary from changes in the environment or from a disorder. To start, one may look at the basal state: resting, no food intake, 37°C temperature, and a neutral 20°C, 40 percent humidity environment. Under these conditions, the insensible loss has been variously measured between 42 and 48 mL per 100 kcal expended with very close agreement over many

Table 30-3. Basal water requirements in relation to age, weight, and surface area

AGE	WEIGHT, kg	SURFACE AREA, m²	cal/kg	BASAL METABOLISM, cal/24 h	BASAL WATER REQUIREMENT, mL/24 h
Newborn	3.2	0.2	45–50	150	125
1 week	3.3	0.2	60	200	200
3 months	5	0.25	54	270	270
6 months	8	0.35	50	400	400
12 months	10	0.45	50	500	500
3 years	15	0.60	47	700	700
5 years	20	0.80	45	900	900
8 years	30	1.05	37	1100	1100
13 years	60	1.70	27	1600	1600

years and with varied methodologies. A loss of 45 mL per 100 kcal will be used here—about 30 mL through the skin and 15 mL through the lung. Abnormal water loss through skin (sweat) or lung (hyperventilation) will dissipate 1 kcal for every 1.85 mL of water or 0.54 kcal/mL. Sweating, an active process, involves loss of electrolyte; IWL does not.

URINE

Urine losses from metabolism are more variable owing to the capacity of the kidney to concentrate and dilute the solute of the urine. Because of renal disease, many patients have a fixed urine solute concentration of 300 mosm/kg; others during illness probably have a similar limitation from extrarenal factors; and, finally, infants have a lower concentration ceiling (700 mosm/kg compared to 1500 mosm/kg) for about a year. These considerations make it clinically prudent to assume the urine produced to have a concentration of 300 mosm/kg as being well within clinical margins of safety and to accept an excess of administered water to achieve this. At this concentration, obligatory urine losses will be about 50 to 55 mL per 100 kcal expended. Thus, if a small amount is assumed for stool, the net needs at basal condition per 100 kcal will be 45 mL for IWL, 50 for urine, and 5 for stool, or 100 mL per 100 kcal equivalent to 1 mL/kcal expended!

NONBASAL CONDITIONS

As caloric expenditure goes up, water losses will increase at the same rate. Offsetting these losses in part is a product of metabolism, the water of oxidation, amounting to 12 mL per 100 kcal. A rise in body temperature increases heat and water losses about 13 percent per degree Celsius (12). Muscle activity also increases heat and water loss, as does dietary intake and hyperventilation. At the bedside, detailed calculation of all these factors cannot be done, nor does it prove necessary since many empiric observations have determined reasonable guidelines. Uncommonly a pa-

tient will be at basal condition defined as no elevation of temperature, intrinsic or ambient, no movement, and a normal breathing rate. For most infants, when there is no sustained hyperthermia, hyperventilation, or excessive activity, but there are fluctuating small changes in all of these functions, an allotment of water requirements (or heat expenditure) may be taken as 1½ times basal. When one of the three is extreme (e.g., sustained high-grade fever), about twice basal will be lost, and in the very unusual event of all three variables being simultaneously extreme (e.g., maintained fever, convulsions, hyperventilation), three times basal will be needed. This empiric range has proved clinically useful under many and varied circumstances.

ELECTROLYTE TURNOVER

In children the obligatory electrolyte losses are small and are governed by the same general principles as for adults. Sodium and chloride are well conserved by the intact organism. Potassium losses ensue whenever there is urine output. The range of permissible sodium and chloride for safe intake by the healthy infant is from 0.1 to 10 meq per 100 kcal expended. A generally safe allotment for parenteral fluids where some sodium salt is convenient to protect against hemolysis is 2 to 3 meq per 100 kcal. The potassium range of safety is much narrower, but again 2 to 3 meq per 100 kcal is a reasonable allowance. When treating infants with very large electrolyte deficits, the daily requirements are essentially negligible (especially sodium and chloride) and may be disregarded.

The most important summary statement for this section on turnover is to remind the therapist that water turnover needs relate not directly to mass, but to energy expenditure, and unlike the replacement of losses from mass, turnover needs may not be expressed accurately as a percentage of weight across various age levels. Surface area may be used, as a usual function and a useful index of energy expenditure, but the newborn, the obese, and the edematous patients are exceptions and should be so regarded.

REGULATING SYSTEMS AFFECTING HOMEOSTASIS

In addition to the special consideration of age, appropriate chemical anatomy, and the special vulnerability owing to high turnover rates of water, immature homeostatic regulator mechanisms need consideration. These contribute to vulnerability in the infant and child, and some are age-related in a developmental sense. We shall consider here only those that presently seem of greatest clinical relevance in hydration disorders: diet regulation and gastrointestinal function, renal excretion of solute and water, the hydrogen ion buffer capacities, and calcium and phosphorus regulation. In this chapter only the irregular functioning occurring in childhood either because of the diseases to which children are subjected or the immature state of the regulator distinguishing the child will be discussed.

FACTORS AFFECTING WATER AND SOLUTE INTAKE

The biologic mechanisms for thirst and for urine concentration are present in earliest infancy though limited by the totally dependent state of the infant with respect to intake and by renal immaturity with regard to maximal urine concentration. Although thirst may be demonstrated, the ability of the infant to signal this sensation is restricted to responsiveness to proffered liquid, neither language nor locomotion being possible. Thirst will also be indiscriminate in that hypernatremic infants have been observed to drink heavily salted solutions when offered.

The very young infant grows very rapidly, requiring, therefore, a high caloric intake per unit mass; 10 to 12 percent of calories, optimally, will be from protein. Before going further, an analysis of customary diets offered to infants is in order. The usual mainstay of the diet for infants involves a mammalian milk. Human milk provides high-quality protein (8 percent of calories, but of high biologic value), low solute (Na, Cl, K), and a Ca/P of 2:1 (by weight) and an energy density of 0.67 kcal/mL. Cow milk also has high-quality protein at 18 to 22 percent of calories (more urea for excretion), relatively high mineral content

(Na, Cl, K), including high Ca and P in a ratio of 1.25. Caloric density is also 0.67 kcal/mL. In the United States, infants during the early months, when milk represents virtually the whole diet, consume prepared formulas from cow milk; these are made to simulate human milk in protein and mineral contents. In practice, the solute content falls between the two natural milks, and the excess solute must be excreted by the kidney. In addition, there are vegetable protein mixtures marketed whose protein content must be higher (to be adequate) because of its biologic inferiority.

All this is clinically important because milk diets, though entirely liquid, have about the same nutritional characteristics (protein, carbohydrate, fat, minerals, and water) as the mixed diets of children and adults. Refeeding such a diet immediately after illness to an infant, particularly one still in a catabolic state, poses the same kind of solute stress that a full diet has for the older person, but the per-kilogram load of renal excretory solute is much higher for the infant because his Calorie-per-kilogram expenditure is also much higher.

To recapitulate, infants have a high energy expenditure, a high water turnover, and a rapid rate of growth. Liquid diets other than human milk provide an excess of solute for urinary excretion. The dependent, uncommunicative state of the infant reduces choice of intake. The high turnover rate produces vulnerability to mild interference with intake and in turn leads to pathophysiologic disturbance after a brief insult.

RENAL REGULATION OF SOLUTE AND WATER

The underlying physiology has been reviewed in Chaps. 7, 12, and 13. First consider states of excess solute presented for excretion. A high-protein end-product expenditure, whether from intake or from tissue breakdown of the rapidly metabolizing infant, presents a high urea load for renal excretion. Rapid insensible water loss (without electrolyte) will lead the kidney to be influenced by simultaneous stimuli of increased sodium concentration and slight hypovolemia. The response will not lessen the hypernatremia because the sodium concentration in urine will usually not exceed that of the plasma water. The hypernatremia may be corrected naturally only through an intact and responsive thirst mechanism; the kidney's evolutionary development does not produce the expected teleologic result. On the other hand, the renal capacity for sodium conservation is extraordinary when situations of sodium deprivation obtain.

Next, states with loss of ECF water also occur. There are a number of situations where antidiuretic hormone (ADH) activity reduces urine output while a catabolic state, usually an infection, causes release of water from cells. This results in endogenous cell water entering the ECF while not being promptly excreted. Acute severe infections and CNS injury are two such occurrences; suppurative meningitis has both triggering elements present. No hazard comes to the patient unless an exogenous water load is superimposed, with the kidney responding to ADH, continuing to produce a concentrated low volume of output; then water intoxication may supervene. Because the amount of water given to children for daily turnover needs has been understood to be large (per kilogram) such overloads have occurred frequently in infants cared for by the unwary during clinical management of either severe infections, especially those of the CNS, or during maintenance following CNS trauma.

In summary, again owing to the high normal water turnover, the homeostatic limits for water excretion are brought quickly into focus when infants become sick. Unlike adult patients, where days elapse before problems occasioned by water retention become obvious, only hours elapse for infants. On the other hand, too much awareness by clinicians of these water-retentive states has sometimes led to ill-advised restraint in fluid administration. They may then fail to replace the deficit of water and salt while focusing their attention on the limited ability to excrete water. Such an error is even more grievous than overloading with water, though either may have serious consequences. Deficit replacement requiring water and solute is a priority secondary to plasma volume restoration in dehydrated states.

ACID-BASE HOMEOSTASIS (See also Chap. 6)

Newborn and prematurely born infants have less homeostatic buffering capacity than do older children. They may be said to have normally a mild physiologic metabolic acidosis. Although pH norms run only slightly lower (7.30 to 7.38), CO_2 contents in serum are usually 20 to 22 meq/L rather than the 25 to 27 meq/L seen after puberty. How much this is due to deficient carbonic anhydrase (newborn only), to high metabolic acid production because of rapid turnover, or to renal immaturity in excreting nonvolatile acids is not often clear. The situation creates then an obvious though mild additional physiologic vulnerability in maintaining pH. The hazard is offset during active growth by skeletal retention. In addition, at all times, infants present a more rapid adaptive clinical response to what would appear to be an extreme circumstance in the adult. Thus, dehydrated infants with CO_2 contents below 6 meq/L may appear surprisingly well and, in fact, may recover well, without specific alkali therapy, once volume replacement and good renal output are achieved.

CALCIUM-PHOSPHORUS HOMEOSTASIS (See also Chaps. 8 and 19)

Ionized calcium levels in ECF are quite constant in children as they are in adults. Newborn infants, on the other hand, have less secure calcium homeostasis, and when stressed either by nonspecific illness or by a phosphate dietary load, they often become hypocalcemic. How much is due to transient immaturity of parathyroid function and how much to vitamin D metabolism and other factors remains unclear. Renal excretion of phosphate during infancy is such that levels of phosphorus in serum of 6.5 to 7.5 mg/dL are usual for 3 to 4 months and levels of 5.5 to 7.0 are common during the first year. All during childhood the mean normal level remains over 4.5 mg/dL. Only with puberty does the phosphorus value in serum fall to the adult range. These differences suggest that clinical attention be paid to calcium and phosphate levels, especially in neonates, whenever disturbances in hydration occur. Hypocalcemia is the most common abnormality of clinical significance.

COMMON PHYSIOLOGIC DISTURBANCES AND THEIR CORRECTION

Regardless of fundamental etiology, there are certain disturbances of physiology that require a diagnostic approach to pathophysiology (as distinct from etiology—thus, "isotonic dehydration" not "*Salmonella typhimurium* enteritis"). The clinical elements and laboratory data that define the disturbance also point the way to rational restorative management. Whatever the disturbance in hydration, a systematic plan of diagnostic analysis will be helpful. Such a process should take up each element of the disturbance that will be useful in formulating a therapeutic plan. We recommend the following appraisals in order: (1) volume, (2) osmolal status, (3) H^+ ion disturbance, (4) cell ion losses (primarily K^+), (5) ionized Ca changes. The respective measurements that should be sought are (1) weight and weight change; (2) serum $[Na^+]$; (3) pH, HCO_3^-, PCO_2; (4) $[K^+]$ and $[HCO_3^-]$ (not always useful); and (5) Ca or Ca^{2+} levels. Clinical history and examination findings are usually sufficient for first approximations, especially for the first two appraisals. These two factors should be given therapeutic priority over the others unless there is concomitant or previous injury to kidney or lungs. In most clinical circumstances, correction of volume and osmolal disturbances will usually lead to correction of the other three disturbances when renal and pulmonary function return, if addition of K to intake is also remembered. The five points of analysis are stressed in the discussion of specific hydration disorders that follows.

ISOTONIC CONSTRICTION OF BODY FLUIDS (ISOTONIC DEHYDRATION)

Clinical analysis

Most of the problems of infancy that lead to dehydration come from gastrointestinal disease in which increased water and salt losses and reduced intake in varying proportion result in loss of body fluids, both water and salts. At least two-thirds of the time, under present circumstances in the developed areas, Na salts and water are lost in physiologic proportion so that $[Na^+]$ in the serum (and ECF) is in the normal range (142 ± 6 meq/L). As indicated above, the problem may be usefully analyzed for five considerations: volume, osmolality, H^+ ion, ICF losses, and Ca homeostasis. Each point of the analysis should start from the specific historical pathogenesis, take into account physical findings, and eventually be confirmed with quantitative analyses. Laboratory analyses are not required to begin therapy and particularly not for the most urgent steps, though an accurate weight must be determined. As already stated, the first two points of analysis are usually much more important than the last three.

Consideration of *volume* should begin with the history and with careful observation for signs of early circulatory impairment or changes in the skin elasticity, in order to estimate the fluid deficit. Hypovolemia produces most of the signs. The details of this evaluation are discussed at length in Chap. 11 and elsewhere (13). The earliest objective evidence of isotonic constriction of body fluids is detectable when about 5 percent of body weight has been lost over a 24-h period. Tachycardia and dry skin and membranes present at that time. When 10 percent has been lost, marked circulatory impairment evidenced by coolness and mottling of extremities and loss of skin turgor becomes manifest. Loss of skin elasticity in infants and sunken eyeballs at any age add to the clinical evidence. When 15 percent weight loss occurs in this time, a moribund or near-moribund state is present. Thus, a rough but clinically satisfactory estimate into mild, moderately severe, and severe may be made with reasonable confidence corresponding to losses of 5, 10, and 15 percent of body weight over a 1- or 2-day period. This amount restated as 50, 100, or 150 mL/kg constitutes the deficit which should usually be essentially replaced by 24 to 30 h of therapy.

Next for consideration in the volume review is the estimation of the obligatory losses mandated by energy expenditure for an ensuing time period, arbitrarily usually taken to be 24 h. If there is low-grade, intermittent high-grade, or absence of fever, and if there is mild activity and only slight hyperpnea—all common circumstances—the maintenance water allowance should be about 1½ times the basal need (see Table 30-3).

Finally, consideration must be given to ongoing abnormal losses occasioned by the disease process. Most infantile diarrhea will abate on cessation of intake; some will continue. Diabetes insipidus will surely continue, tube drainage of the stomach may be watched, etc. All such abnormal losses may be measured at appropriate intervals as they occur; this should be done whenever such losses are sizable.

Combining the estimate of the deficit and the estimated obligatory losses gives a tentative volume of water to be administered for the first 24 h. Additions for observed ongoing abnormal losses will be made as necessary. Rate of administration will be considered after analysis is complete.

The status of body *osmolality* is a shorthand way of estimating the sodium salt losses by clinically estimating shifts in the proportions of fluid in the main body fluid compartments. Since a shift to or from the ECF may produce disturbance quite independent of volume change, one looks for evidence by history, by physical examination, and by chemical analyses for either hyper- or hyponatremic states. More details of this analysis are discussed later in this chapter when hypernatremia is discussed and in Chap. 12. Still greater detail may be found elsewhere (9). The optimal early management depends upon recognizing both volume changes and water shifts, if any. A judgment that the usual isotonic constriction is occurring implies that the deficit portion of the therapy should be replaced by a fluid resembling ECF, i.e., one containing Na^+ in a concentration of about 150 meq/L, since experience shows that most (more than two-thirds) of the loss comes from this compartment during isotonic constriction. The ongoing water losses will require no accompanying electrolyte if the deficit has been judged greater than 5 percent of weight because the implied losses of salt are so much greater than the small amount required for daily physiologic losses. At this point in the analysis,

then, both water volume and sodium replacement have been given a first approximation as a rough but clinically reasonable estimate.

Next, consideration of the H^+ *ion* disturbance or *acid-base* disorder should occur. Most dehydrating illnesses of infants result in a metabolic acidosis or acidemia because of organic acid accumulation from ketosis and coexistent oliguria secondary to hypovolemia and consequent low renal perfusion. Low peripheral perfusion may add lactic acid. Unless the problem is very severe or there is a coexistent renal or underlying metabolic problem, restoration of volume to the depleted compartments (especially the plasma) and provision of water for urine formation, thereby permitting excretion of nonvolatile acid, will suffice without need for specifically calculated alkali administration. For patients who have either no H^+ disturbance or those who are acidotic, it is advisable to give a physiologic amount of base anion (HCO_3^-, lactate or acetate) so as not to obligate renal work in excretion of excess chloride. Thus, ordinarily about one-fifth to one-third of the anions should be as base; the remainder as Cl^-. Only rarely must specific base replacement be calculated or more than a physiologic proportion of basic anion be given. When necessary, this calculation may be done by using 30 percent of the body weight as a distribution space for quick changes and 50 percent of body weight for more chronic (greater than 4 hours) changes. These volumes are based on experimental data and do not correspond to a physiologic compartment. When such calculations are employed, it should be recognized that a number of dynamic equilibriums are involved and laboratory work-up is highly advisable.

Replacement of ICF ions in practice means K^+ replacement. At present no evidence for early administration of Mg or PO_4 has appeared. K^+ losses are almost always present when the abnormal body fluid losses are either from the gastrointestinal tract or in the urine. Both acidosis and alkalosis enhance K^+ losses in the urine as well. Thus, optimal treatment calls for replacement of K^+ so that water will return to cells and the clinical results of K^+ depletion, intestinal ileus, and hypotonus of muscle, remit. Parenteral K^+ should await established urine flow. Amounts of 3 meq/kg per day in concentrations up to 40 meq/L are appropriate. Very special circumstances may call for even higher concentrations, and it is the rate per minute per kilogram that is the limiting factor. Too much may flood the ECF, producing cardiac arrhythmias, including standstill. About 0.02 meq/kg per min or 1 meq/kg per h is an approximate upper limit of tolerance by intravenous administration. Most patients do well on the lower concentrations, which are safer, and indeed the best clinical rule is to give K^+ orally whenever possible.

Calcium homeostasis depends upon the mineral skeleton–ECF steady state and the systems which regulate it. Dehydration may cause phosphate and sulfate retention via hypovolemia and oliguria. Increased concentration of these anions tends to depress ionized calcium levels in ECF. On the other hand, a lowered pH has a reverse effect. In the newborn, whose control of ionized calcium is labile, and in the hypernatremic states (see below), special concern should be given to the effects of the dehydration and those of prospective therapy. For most other patients, physiologic mechanisms will suffice without special therapeutic concern.

Having now estimated volume, ECF cation (sodium), ECF anion (chloride and base), and ICF cation (potassium) needs, the next step in planning is to determine how to mix the water and salts, the route to administer them, in what order, and at what rate. For purposes of timing, there may exist an emergency insofar as plasma volume restoration is concerned; next will follow the need for the ECF expansion to support plasma volume; and finally the cells must be rehydrated for optimal function. All of these things may occur pari passu, but the order of emphasis should be as given above. This suggests three phases for the first 24 h of therapy, when a realistic goal should be substantially complete restoration of all body compartments after isotonic constriction has occurred. These phases may conveniently and rationally be labeled *emergency, repletion,* and *early recovery.*

As an example, assume an estimated deficit of 10 percent of mass, or 100 mL/kg. Assume also an age where 1½ times basal indicates another 100 mL/kg of water will be expended in the next 24 h, and, finally, assume that continued abnormal losses will be covered by direct observations. The deficit fluid should contain about 150 meq/L of sodium. The maintenance water needs no electrolyte. Acidosis has been presumed but not judged urgent, so physiologic amounts only of anion (20 to 25 percent) will be of base, the rest of chloride. Finally, a potassium deficit greater than or equal to 3 meq/kg will be assumed because of the type of illness.

Phases of therapy

An *emergency* phase exists if plasma volume is reduced to the point of objective evidence of circulatory impairment, no matter how minor. This phase should be rapid (about 20 to 40 min) and end when circulation is well restored and preferably (though not invariably) urine production is established. A solution containing protein will be highly effective here, particularly one with about 5% albumin. Single-donor plasma, modified plasma, whole blood, or 4% albumin solutions are examples. Empirically we know that 20 mL/kg of body weight may be administered to a dehydrated patient intravenously over 20 min with impunity. When this is done, it is best followed, in infants, by another rapid infusion of 20 mL/kg of 10% glucose in water. This adds momentarily to plasma volume, supplies calories to starving tissues, reversing ketosis, and provides water for immediate renal excretion.

If protein solutions are not available, glucose and electrolyte solutions may be substituted (see also Chap. 10). We prefer 10% glucose in this phase, others use 5% glucose, and yet others use salts alone (e.g., Ringer lactate). Conclusive evidence for superiority of one of these regimens does not exist. For any of them to have the same effect upon plasma volume as a 5% albumin solution, about four times as much would be needed. In practice, half this much, 40 mL/kg, suffices over 30 to 40 min. The possible advantages in 10% glucose are the same as those indicated above when it is used as a second step. When used as a first step, electrolyte should be added; a recommended amount is sodium 75 to 80 meq/L, chloride 55 to 60 meq/L, and HCO_3^- or some other base (lactate, acetate) 20 meq/L. When no glucose is used, the salt concentration should be approximately isotonic. The volume of water given (40 mL/kg) is subtracted from the estimated day's total of 200 mL/kg, leaving 160 mL/kg for the remaining hours. An emergency or "IV push" phase of treatment is very important for these patients. Attempts at gradual restoration of body fluids frequently fail because of the downward spiral of physiologic functions dependent on circulation. Small infants (under 4 kg) or malnourished infants should preferably receive a solution containing albumin.

The *repletion* phase should last for 5 to 8 h. The emphasis will be on expansion of ECF now that plasma volume and circulation are restored. A marker will be urine production. The clinician may use either oral or parenteral administration here. For simplicity, a parenteral route will be described here, one necessitated when vomiting or anorexia preclude oral intake, but one less flexible than a regimen that includes the intestinal tract. The rate of administration should be such that when this phase is completed (6 to 8 h from start of therapy) one-half of the 24-h allotment of fluid has been given, 100 mL/kg in the example. There should be glucose in the fluid, 5% in concentration, and sodium, 70 to 75 meq/L, chloride, 50 to 55 meq/L and HCO_3 (lactate, acetate), 20 meq/L. Potassium as acetate or chloride may be added at 20 to 25 meq/L as soon as urine formation is assured; the anion proportions should be sustained.

The *early recovery* phase should continue with the same fluid (potassium now required unless anuria has been demonstrated), but at a slower rate to deliver the second half of the 24-h allotment over 16 to 18 h. The emphasis is on cell hydration, and often the oral route may be used for this part of the therapy.

To recapitulate: First analyze and diagnose the five physiologic components of the disturbance. Estimate the impact on volume including deficit, obligatory requirements, and ongoing pathologic losses. Next assess whether or not evidence exists for shifts of fluid within body compartments. At this point either a tentative diagnosis of isotonic constriction is made or another postulate is entertained (the others are discussed below). Clinical evidence of H^+ disturbance are sought, an approximation of K deficit is made, and brief consideration of a Ca problem is given. Following analysis, therapy is planned from the appraisal and implemented in three phases: The emergency period lasts 30 to 60 min and emphasizes restoration of circulation (plasma volume). The repletion period lasts 6 to 8 h and restores the ECF while bringing the intake to half the original volume estimated for 24 h. The final 16 h of the first 24 h emphasizes cell water restoration and gives the second half of the day's estimate plus any additional observed pathologic losses.

HYPERNATREMIC DEHYDRATION

When a hypernatremic state develops, the pathogenesis will have been different from isotonic constriction in that water losses will have been proportionally greater than salt losses. The clinical details may be so obscured that precise early diagnosis of this disturbance may be accomplished only about half the time. Frequently evidence of CNS involvement will be manifest and circulatory signs less evident for each degree of volume depletion (9). This combination strongly suggests a hypernatremic state. CNS involvement in hypernatremic dehydration may be brought about in several ways. Two are of special importance. Hemorrhage may occur when the osmolal gradient develops rapidly (9). This probably represents capillary rupture resulting from a rapidly shrunken brain within a closed cranial bony "box." Evidence for this pathogenesis has been presented from the pathology observed and from the fact that the phenomenon may be prevented in experimental animals by maintaining CSF volume through an infusion directly into the CSF (9). The mechanism for these volume changes was discussed earlier and comes from the tight junctions between endothelial cells in the CNS that produce the blood-brain barrier which slows solute flux while permitting normal water flow.

Hemorrhage occurs regularly in severe salt poisoning and in about one-third of patients with the disturbance secondary to enteritis. Indirect evidence from morbidity studies suggest about 8 percent of survivors may have had hemorrhage. Sites most involved include the cerebellum and areas near the sagittal sinus, but involvement of all portions of the CNS has been observed. Thrombosis often follows hemorrhage and may extend the damage.

A second and more puzzling phenomenon is the development of "idiogenic osmols," the presence of which is associated with nervous system symptoms (see Chap. 26). These osmols are not restricted to the CNS but appear to occur there in a higher concentration than in muscle, perhaps owing to the more complete exclusion of sodium from the nonchloride space within the brain (see Chap. 26). Briefly, when a hyperosmolal state is induced, measurement and calculations of the colligative properties of tissue indicate that osmols appear in cell water from material not previously contributing to the osmotic activity, hence the word "idiogenic" (9). This solute adds to the attractiveness of cells for water during rehydration if rehydration is rapid. In the case of the CNS, such swelling may be both symptomatic and deleterious.

Subclinical depression of ECF calcium occurs about 30 to 40 percent of the time in hypernatremic states, though rarely does clinical tetany occur. The mechanism for this remains obscure and appears somehow related to body potassium deficits (16).

Each of the phenomena described above may be responsible for some of the CNS symptoms seen regularly during hypernatremic dehydration (see also Chaps. 11 and 26). The range of symptoms is from mild disturbance in consciousness, most commonly seen as marked lethargy when undisturbed coupled with hyperirritability when stimulated by touch, light, or sound, to coma and convulsions. This status may progress to muscle twitchings and generalized convulsions. Muscle hypertonicity is commonplace, and nuchal rigidity may be confused with that caused by meningitis.

As already noted, tetany is rare, and hemorrhage, though of great importance because of potential danger to life and because of its sequelae,

occurs in no more than 30 to 35 percent of even the fatal outcomes. The idiogenic osmols, however, have been found to be a regular concomitant, and if not causal of the symptoms, they are at least a biologic marker of interest.

Yet another interesting feature of hypernatremic states is the frequent occurrence of hyperglycemia independent of food intake (14, 15). On occasion, levels of over 1000 mg/dL have been encountered. A few studied patients have been insulinopenic (15); this implies that the glucose will not enter cells well and, therefore, the glucose molecules will join the sodium salts as extracellular obligates and worsen the osmolal disturbance, desiccating cells further.

Because circulation is often preserved, there may be no need for an emergency phase. If the volume depletion exceeds 10 percent of mass, there may be circulatory deficit as well. In these patients, the emergency phase should be managed with a 5% albumin solution if at all possible, 20 mL/kg (10, 13). After this, and for the many patients for whom the emergency phase may be omitted, the principle of therapy is very gradual replacement of water over time so that the brain does not swell. Swelling will occur if low [Na^+] solutions are delivered rapidly owing to the blood-brain capillary boundaries referred to earlier (8, 9). Such swelling may be avoided by using higher (greater than 60 meq/L) [Na^+], but this tends at best to make the patient edematous and at worst (because of possible continued water losses) to make him more hypernatremic. The recommended regimen (Na, 20 to 30 meq/L) which gradually replaces estimated deficit over a 48-h (or slightly longer) period has worked well.

These patients usually have volume deficits when CNS symptoms appear amounting to about 10 percent of mass. The sodium content of the patient is relatively high, but there may be an absolute deficit; the case is similar for chloride ion, which often is even less deficient. Acidosis and acidemia are common but not obligatory except in severe salt poisoning. Potassium losses are often extreme, and their replacement is a key to restoring water to cells.

In planning therapy, then, volume administration for deficit should be distributed over at least

48 h; and the rate, after a brief emergency phase of 20 min when necessary, should be constant over the whole period. The 48-h volume should be the sum of the deficit plus 2 days' IWL requirements plus any observed abnormal losses. Fluid [Na^+] should be 20 to 30 meq/L, K (maximal to prevent an osmotic gradient from causing brain swelling), 40 meq/L, and the anions in accordance with the acid-base status. Ten milliliters of 10% calcium gluconate per 500 mL of fluid is safe and on rare occasions will abort symptomatic hypocalcemia (9,10). Insulin should not be given for the transitory hyperglycemia. Doing so is the physiologic equivalent of giving water rapidly. The brain will then swell. Thus, administration of glucose is also safe, though perhaps lower concentration (2½ to 3%) might be preferable to those usually recommended.

HYPONATREMIC DEHYDRATION (See also Chaps. 3 and 13)

Hyponatremic states tend to occur when a body fluid is being lost and replacement for it, oral or parenteral, consists of water with little or no electrolyte. In United States practice, this occurs in about 10 percent of hospitalized infants with dehydration. The ECF becomes strikingly depleted, and accordingly circulation suffers. Analysis of the disturbance must take the pathogenesis into account, and estimates are made as in the preceding examples. If, however, the sodium depletion is extreme and renal function has been compromised, the emergency phase may require the administration of a hypertonic sodium solution in order to restore body water distribution by taking water out of swollen cells. To do this, the sodium deficit must be calculated from its osmotic distribution, the TBW (70 percent of the lean body mass).[1] Replacement may be given with either M or $M/2$ (1000 or 500 meq/L) balanced sodium salts (Cl plus base as anions) intravenously. A customary and cautious approach is to give half the calculated deficit, wait 1 or 2 h, obtain labor-

[1] E.g., a 5-kg undernourished infant with [Na^+] of 110 meq/L in serum would have a deficit of Na 3.5 × 30 or 105 meq (5 × 0.70 = 3.5; 140 − 110 = 30).

atory confirmation, and then, if results are as expected, give the second half. Isotonic saline will usually be ineffective because urine losses of sodium may be paradoxically large. Potassium deficits may be considerable and should be corrected as in isonatremic constriction problems. Once ECF volume has been restored, these patients are best managed in the same manner as patients with isonatremic body fluid constriction disturbances with early replacement of deficit.

SPECIFIC ETIOLOGIC PROBLEMS OF INFANTS AND CHILDREN

INFECTIOUS INFANTILE ENTERITIS (DIARRHEA)

Diarrheal disease in malnourished infants remains a major killer in undeveloped countries and a significant source of morbidity in developed ones. Regardless of the specific agent (bacteria, virus, or toxin) the immediate problem is fluid and nutritional restoration, and success depends upon prompt and accurate therapy. Vomiting, which cuts off oral intake, heralds the period of rapid dehydration and usually leads to hospitalization. In the United States, two-thirds of those hospitalized have isotonic constriction of body fluid, about 25 percent (with occasional "epidemic" of 75 to 90 percent) are hypernatremic (Na^+ greater than 150 meq/L of serum), and about 10 percent are hyponatremic. With severe marasmus or kwashiorkor, hyponatremia is very common and seems to represent in part an adaptive state.

Patients with enteritis are usually acidotic because (1) stool water is slightly more alkaline than ECF, i.e., there is loss of base, (2) starvation leads to ketosis, (3) enteric organisms produce metabolic acid which is absorbed, (4) reduced tissue perfusion leads to lactic acid production, and (5) most importantly, oliguria limits excretion of nonvolatile acid. Thus, the acidemia once present develops rapidly and is usually coupled with azotemia. Potassium losses are high because stool water is usually high in this ion.

Table 30-4 contains data on stool water from 80 United States infants with nonspecific diarrhea

Table 30-4. Infants with diarrhea: Electrolyte concentrations in stool water (15)

ION	RANGE	1ST QUARTILE	MEDIAN meq/l	3D QUARTILE	MEAN	CV*
Na	5.3–150	37.4	60.5	88.2	65.2	56.2
Cl	3.9–129	19.8	46.8	71.4	50.6	64.0
K	11.5–117	31.8	41.3	52.5	45.0	45.8
Na$^+$, K	35–202	88	110	131	110	25.8

* Coefficient of variation = $\dfrac{\text{standard deviation}}{\text{mean}} \times 100$

showing the wide range of electrolyte concentration (17). No association with type of etiology is found with particular concentrations of Na$^+$ and K$^+$. An exception (not in Table 30-4) is Asiatic cholera, where the stool water resembles an ultrafiltrate of the plasma and the consequent disturbance reflects the high sodium losses. K$^+$ losses in United States infants range from 3 to 15 meq/kg, and Na$^+$ losses from 3 to 10 meq/kg (10, 13). Management of these patients requires support of nutritional disturbance beyond water and mineral losses; this necessitates clinical skill in refeeding. Amino acid solutions may be useful, and oral disaccharides may have to be avoided.

Most clinicians begin oral intake either during the early recovery period (or even immediately after the emergency phase) or following that phase with a solution containing carbohydrate plus electrolytes such as sodium and potassium salts (10). Recently some have advocated a single solution for all parts of the world. Others, including this author, prefer to use a concentrated sodium solution (Na$^+$, 90 to 120 meq/L) for victims of cholera and a more dilute solution (Na$^+$, 50 meq/L) for temperate zone infants of developed countries. Using the higher concentration in the noncholera areas will invite a significant incidence of hypernatremia.

The chronic protein-calorie malnourished states known as marasmus (primarily calorie deprivation) and kwashiorkor (protein or protein plus calorie deprivation) frequently have associated electrolyte changes, most often reduced solute concentration in cells and adaptive hyponatremia.

For such patients with chronic hyponatremia, a rapid rise in [Na$^+$] in serum of 10 to 15 meq/L (e.g., from 130 to 145) will result in the same disturbance that occurs in a well-nourished infant when sodium increases from 140 to 155. There is much greater difficulty in assessing these patients, however, and quite possibly different parts of the world have special problems because of differing dietary habits and the inadequacy of many diets.

HIGH-SOLUTE DIETS

In some parts of the world (Great Britain, Spain) the introduction of inexpensive dry milk as an infant food has led to high-solute ingestion by infants. Most of the problem has been traceable to improper dilution by families through misunderstanding the importance of water and the risk of high solute. In the United States, the offering of protein supplements or improper dilution of powdered and evaporated feeds may produce the same problem, though, in practice, less commonly. Skim milk preparations, sometimes boiled, have produced a problem in the United States. The best management may require peritoneal dialysis in addition to the regimen for hypernatremic dehydration (9, 10).

Dialysis should be reserved for those infants judged to have a clear excess of sodium. When the technique is carried out, a 7½ to 8% glucose solution containing no electrolyte is advised. Lower concentrations of glucose will result in uptake of water to the ECF from the peritoneal space, making withdrawal difficult or inefficient. The high glucose levels produced in the patient produce a temporary offset to the electrolyte being removed, thereby achieving the desired slow rate (as glucose enters cells and is metabolized) of correction of the osmolal disturbance. Intravenous therapy should accompany dialysis to supply water and potassium needs.

PYLORIC STENOSIS

Hypertrophic pyloric stenosis leads to vomiting secondary to high gastrointestinal obstruction. The resultant disturbance is one of the few in which there is a metabolic alkalosis. Therapy should include use of only neutral salts of Na^+ and K^+; i.e., no base. On rare occasion NH_4Cl may be indicated to speed appropriate restoration of a physiologic pH. Two meq/kg of the acidic salt may be given together with NaCl and KCl. Potassium losses are large from renal excretion of K^+ in alkalosis.

RENAL TUBULAR ACIDOSIS (See also Chap. 18)

There are both congenital and acquired forms, and there are both distal and proximal tubular varieties. In all of these, excess bicarbonate is excreted in the urine for the metabolic status of the patient's plasma; i.e., there is bicarbonate wastage with resultant acidosis. Physiologic fluids may be restored by long-term, regular administration of bicarbonate. The dosage ranges from 1 to 5 meq/kg per day depending on the type of disturbance. The acquired forms are usually reversible in a few months or even sooner.

CONGENITAL K^+ LOSERS

A number of young children have chronic renal K^+ wastage. Some of this group have entities classified as Bartter's syndrome (18, 19). Some have pseudohyperaldosteronism or Liddle's syndrome (20), and some defy classification. All have low K^+ levels in tissue and in ECF; all have a chronic metabolic alkalosis. In all of them therapy is partially unsatisfactory. They tend to be dwarfed presumably because of inability to sustain cell mass. Large oral K^+ loads are either excreted in the urine or become intolerable to the bowel. Therapy with K^+ and K^+-retaining diuretics (e.g., triamterene) have some benefit. Trials with prostaglandin inhibitors have been recently suggested (21).

CONGENITAL CHLORIDE LOSERS

Over 30 years ago Gamble (22) and Darrow (23) each described a patient whose stools contained excess chloride ion. Since then at least another 15 to 20 such patients have been recognized. Since they have increased bicarbonate generation and subsequent K^+ loss, they also are alkalotic and potassium-deficient. The same electrolyte defect may also occur in cystic fibrosis of the pancreas (24). Management consists of supplying daily KC1, 3 to 5 meq/kg per day.

NEPHROGENIC DIABETES INSIPIDUS

A rare X-linked defect in water excretion makes such patients' renal tubules unresponsive to ADH. Like patients with ADH deficiency, these patients obligatorily excrete enormous amounts of urine each day. They quickly become hypernatremic unless water is provided, and management during infancy is very difficult during every minor illness. Natriuretic diuretics provide some help by reducing free water clearance, but the relief is only partial. High daily water intake must be sustained.

ABSENCE OF THIRST

Another rare group of patients are those with congenital absence of thirst. They will also become hypernatremic, and they may be trained to drink fixed quantities of water each day. Occasionally head injury or surgery causes an acquired form of this defect, sometimes complicated by simultaneous diabetes insipidus. Achieving the appropriate therapeutic regimen will be difficult but possible with meticulous attention to weight change and use of small doses of Pitressin in oil for those with diabetes insipidus.

CYSTIC FIBROSIS OF THE PANCREAS

Patients with cystic fibrosis have unusually high (60 to 120 meq/L) concentrations of NaCl in their sweat. Thus, when subjected to environmental heat stress, salt replacement is essential to avoid serious extracellular fluid depletion. Replacement with ordinary solutions or oral water results in a hyponatremic state of the symptomatic variety, i.e., ECF depletion. The ordinary infant formulas, made low in salt for normals, will provide inadequate NaCl for these patients during periods of sustained heat stress. The salt intake has to be doubled over that of the formula during infancy.

SURGERY IN CHILDREN AND PARENTERAL NUTRITION

Trauma, including burns and major surgery, interferes with intake and leads to ADH production independent of osmolality. Head injuries and neurosurgery may be followed by particularly complex fluid problems because either diabetes insipidus or increased ADH output may occur, or both, sequentially. When transient diabetes insipidus occurs, we prefer to use Pitressin in oil for a 24- to 48-h effect and then to be very cautious to avoid water volume overload.

Total or partial parenteral nutrition may be necessary for children with alimentary tract abnormalities or disease. The general principles are like those for adults (Chap. 10), but it is necessary to remember the higher caloric and water requirements per kilogram in the younger ages. All the minerals and accessory foodstuffs should be given proportional to calories administered and not proportional to mass in adult terms.

SPECIAL PROBLEMS OF THE PREMATURELY BORN INFANT

The tiny prematurely born infant frequently has ventilatory failure because of hyaline membrane disease or another pulmonary problem. The use of assisted ventilation increases water loss owing to rapid rate and from low humidity. Artificial heating devices, frequently with radiant heat, also increase water losses from the skin. On the other hand, the basal metabolic rate is relatively slow, and it is physiologic to lose water in the first days of life. Attempts to humidify O_2 administration with supersaturation mist may produce the opposite problem, water intoxication.

With all of these variables, the neonatologist must consider, almost hourly, the patient's water and electrolyte status, as well as the acid-base status disturbed by disordered oxygenation and faulty CO_2 expiration. No simple rules may be promulgated, so varied are the problems. However, all of the principles are the same, and with care they may be rationally applied to good effect (25, 26, 27).

Earlier reference was made to the fragile acid-base homeostasis of the infant. This may be so exaggerated for the prematurely born infant in the early weeks that diets, even those modified to simulate human milk, may carry more acidic radicals (PO_4, SO_4) than the immature kidney will excrete. A "late metabolic acidosis" then may supervene (28). Either prevention or small doses of sodium bicarbonate (2 to 4 meq/kg per day) will manage the problem. Finally, water and sodium homeostasis may also go easily awry on types of intakes perfectly acceptable in older infants, leading to hyponatremic states (29, 30). Again, monitoring and adjustment of sodium intake easily corrects such disturbances.

REFERENCES

1. Edelman, I. S., and J. Leibman: Anatomy of body water and electrolytes, *Am. J. Med.*, **27**:256, 1959.
2. Friis-Hansen, B. J.: Body water compartments in children, *Pediatrics*, **28**:169, 1961.
3. Friis-Hansen, B. J.: Changes in body water during growth, *Acta Paediatr. Scand.*, **110** (suppl.), 1958.
4. Fomon, S. J.: Body composition of the male reference infant during the first year of life, *Pediatrics*, **40**:863, 1967.
5. Ling, G. N., and C. L. Walton: What retains water in lung cells? *Science*, **191**:293, 1976.
6. Ling, G. N.: *A Physical Theory of the Living State*, Blaisdell Publishing Company, New York, 1962.
7. Palmer, L. G., and J. Guloti: Potassium accu-

mulation in muscle: A test of the binding hypothesis, *Science*, **194**:521, 1976.

8. Reese, T. S., and M. J. Karnoresky: Fine structural localization of a blood-brain barrier to exogenous perocidase, *J. Cell Biol.*, **34**:207, 1967.

9. Finberg, L.: Hypernatremic dehydration, *Advances in Pediatrics*, **16**:325, 1969.

10. Finberg, L.: Diarrheal dehydration, in R. W. Winters (ed.), *The Body Fluids in Pediatrics*, Little, Brown and Company, Boston, 1973, p. 349.

11. Darrow, D. C.: The significance of body size, *Am. J. Dis. Child.*, **98**:416, 1959.

12. DuBois, E. F.: The basal metabolism in fever, *JAMA*, **77**:352, 1921.

13. Finberg, L.: The management of the critically ill child with dehydration secondary to diarrhea, *Pediatrics*, **45**:1029, 1970.

14. Stevenson, R. E., and F. P. Bowyer: Hyperglycemia with hyperosmolal dehydration in nondiabetic infants, *J. Pediatr.*, **77**:818, 1970.

15. Mandell, F., and F. X. Fellers: Hyperglycemia in hypernatremic dehydration, *Clin. Ped.*, **13**:367, 1974.

16. Finberg, L.: Experimental studies of the mechanisms producing hypocalcemia in hypernatremic states, *J. Clin. Invest.*, **36**:434, 1957.

17. Finberg, L., C. S. Cheung, and E. Fleishman: The significance of the concentrations of electrolytes in stool water, *Am. J. Dis. Child.*, **100**:809, 1960.

18. Bartter, F. C., P. Pronove, J. R. Gill, and R. C. McCardle: Hyperplasia of the juxtaglomerular complex with hyperaldosteronism and hypokalemic alkalosis, *Am. J. Med.*, **33**:811, 1962.

19. Sann, L., M. David, P. Richard, D. Floret, J. Sassard, C. A. Bizollon, and R. Francois: Effect of sodium restriction and angiotensin II infusion in Bartter's syndrome, *Pediatr. Res.*, **10**:971, 1976.

20. Liddle, G. W., T. Bledsoe, and W. S. Coppage: A familial renal disorder simulating primary aldosterone secretion, in E. C. Boulieu and P. Robel (eds.), *Aldosterone*, Blackwell Scientific Publications, Ltd., Oxford, 1963, p. 353.

21. Bartter's syndrome (editorial), *Lancet*, **2**:721, 1976.

22. Gamble, J. L., K. R. Fahey, A. B. Appleton, and E. MacLachlan: Congenital alkalosis with diarrhea, *J. Pediatr.*, **26**:509, 1945.

23. Darrow, D. C.: Congenital alkalosis with diarrhea, *J. Pediatr.*, **26**:519, 1945.

24. Hochman, H. I., R. Feins, R. Rubin, and J. Gould: Chloride losing diarrhea and metabolic alkalosis in an infant with cystic fibrosis, *Arch. Dis. Child.*, **51**:390, 1976.

25. Driscoll, J. M., Jr., and W. C. Heird: Maintenance fluid therapy during the neonatal period, in R. W. Winters (ed.), *The Body Fluids in Pediatrics*, Little, Brown and Company, Boston, 1976, p. 265.

26. Sinclair, J. C.: Pathophysiology of hyaline membrane disease, in R. W. Winters (ed.), *The Body Fluids in Pediatrics*, Little, Brown and Company, Boston, 1976, p. 279.

27. Mellins, R. B.: Cardiorespiratory disorders in children, in R. W. Winters (ed.), *The Body Fluids in Pediatrics*, Little, Brown and Company, Boston, 1976, p. 457.

28. Kildeberg, P.: Late metabolic acidosis of premature infants, in R. W. Winters (ed.), *The Body Fluids in Pediatrics*, Little, Brown and Company, Boston, 1976, p. 338.

29. Day, G. M., I. C. Radde, J. W. Balfe, and G. W. Chance: Electrolyte abnormalities in very low birthweight infants, *Pediatr. Res.*, **10**:522, 1976.

30. Ray, R. N., G. W. Chance, I. C. Radde, et al.: Late hyponatremia in very low birthweight infants (<1.3 kilograms), *Pediatr. Res.*, **10**:526, 1976.

Index